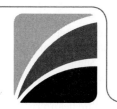

Women's Health Care
in Advanced Practice Nursing

Ivy M. Alexander, PhD, APRN, ANP-BC, FAANP, FAAN, is clinical professor of nursing and director of Advanced Practice Programs at the University of Connecticut (UConn) School of Nursing. She maintains a clinical practice at UConn Health Internal Medicine in downtown Storrs. Her clinical, scholarly, and research interests are in midlife women's health care. She has worked extensively with menopause and osteoporosis management and has published and presented widely regarding these subject areas, including two books, which have been translated into Spanish, Greek, and Italian. She has been principal investigator on studies evaluating women's relationships with their primary care providers; Black women's perceptions of menopause, midlife health risks, and self-management techniques used to manage menopause symptoms and reduce health risks; and osteoporosis risks and management. She has consulted for national and international companies such as Athena Medical Products, Medscape, Wyeth-Ayerst, Duramed Pharmaceuticals, Pfizer, Eli Lilly, Roche, Venus Medical Communications, Amgen, and Datamonitor.

Versie Johnson-Mallard, PhD, ARNP, WHNP-BC, FAANP, FAAN, Robert Wood Johnson Nurse Faculty Scholar alumna, is a National Certification Corporation board–certified women's health nurse practitioner, faculty, and chair of Family, Community and Health System Science at the University of Florida College of Nursing. Scientific discovery and funding were with the Robert Wood Johnson Foundation, Department of Health and Human Services Office on Women's Health, National Institute of Nursing Research (NINR), and National Cancer Institute (NCI) under the National Institutes of Health (NIH). Sexual and reproductive health clinical inquiry was the impetus to advance scientific knowledge about innovative educational interventions designed to promote reproductive health and cancer prevention among young adults.

Dr. Johnson-Mallard's teaching, clinical practice, research, and publications are in the area of women's health, sexual and reproductive health promotion, human papillomavirus (HPV)/cancer screening/prevention/vaccination, and behavior change in response to culturally appropriate educational interventions. Dr. Johnson-Mallard provides consultation to partners who share interest in the development of education material, clinical guidelines, and policy around reproductive health and cancer prevention.

Elizabeth A. Kostas-Polston, PhD, APRN, WHNP-BC, FAANP, FAAN, is a Robert Wood Johnson Foundation Nurse Faculty Scholar alumna and board-certified women's health nurse practitioner who holds a dual appointment as assistant professor in the Daniel K. Inouye Graduate School of Nursing at the Uniformed Services University of the Health Sciences, and Saint Louis University School of Medicine, Department of Otolaryngology, Head and Neck Surgery. She received her bachelor of science in nursing from Arizona State University, a master of science in nursing with specialization in women's health (obstetrics, gynecology, and primary care of women) from the University of Florida, and a doctor of philosophy from Loyola University Chicago. As a nurse scientist and Robert Wood Johnson Foundation Nurse Faculty Scholar, her scholarship is focused on ensuring the effective translation of knowledge for new approaches to health promotion, disease prevention, and the diagnosis, treatment, and management of HPV-related cancers. In support of her training, she was selected as a fellow and completed postdoctoral studies in genetics, genomics, and molecular biology at the National Institutes of Health/National Institute of Nursing Research. The primary aim of Dr. Kostas-Polston's clinical practice is to improve the health of women and their families. Toward this end, she works with others interested in the development of health promotion and disease-prevention strategies, evidence-based clinical guidelines, and health policy focused on sexual and reproductive and HPV-related cancer prevention.

Catherine Ingram Fogel, PhD, RNC, FAAN, is a research professor emeritus at the University of North Carolina at Chapel Hill School of Nursing. She is the author of several texts on women's health, including the award-winning *Women's Health Care* and the first edition of *Women's Health Care in Advanced Practice Nursing*, and has authored numerous research and clinical articles on women's health. For more than 35 years, she has had both a sustained research program and clinical practice with incarcerated women. Her research has increased nursing's awareness and understanding of the health problems of incarcerated women and their complicated lives. Fogel was the principal investigator on one National Institutes of Health (NIH)-funded grant focusing on prevention of sexually transmitted infections and HIV in women prisoners; another NIH-funded grant exploring the experiences of parenting from prison; a Centers for Disease Control and Prevention (CDC)-funded grant to deliver a sexually transmitted infection (STI) risk reduction intervention to HIV-infected women living in the Southeast, and an additional CDC-funded grant to adapt a proven HIV risk-reduction intervention to incarcerated women. Dr. Fogel was also a coinvestigator on a federally funded grant to determine if a comprehensive intervention, supporting seek–test–and–treat, can result in significant reduction in the potential for HIV-infected prisoners to retransmit their virus after release.

Fogel is a member of the American Nurses Association and Sigma Theta Tau and a fellow of the American Academy of Nursing. She was certified as a women's health care nurse practitioner in 1982. She received a North Carolina Community Service Award for her work with women prisoners and the 1993 Association of Women's Health, Obstetric and Neonatal Nurses (AWHONN) National Excellence in Clinical Practice Award.

Nancy Fugate Woods, PhD, RN, FAAN, is professor in the Department of Family and Child Nursing at the University of Washington. Since the late 1970s, she has led a sustained program of research in the field of women's health. Her collaborative research has resulted in an improved understanding of women's transition to menopause, including physical and emotional factors; has advanced nursing care for midlife women; and has provided women with a better understanding of their health. In 1989, Dr. Woods helped establish the Center for Women's Health Research at the University of Washington.

Dr. Woods has served as president of the American Academy of Nursing, the North American Menopause Society, and the Society for Menstrual Cycle Research. She helped set research agendas as a member of the National Institutes of Health (NIH) Women's Health Task Force and Office of Women's Health Research Advisory Council. Her honors include election to the Institute of Medicine of the National Academies and to the American Academy of Nursing. She received the American Nurses Foundation Distinguished Contribution to Nursing Research Award and, in 2003, received the Pathfinder Award from the Friends of the National Institute for Nursing Research. She earned a BS in nursing from the University of Wisconsin, Eau Claire, in 1968; an MN from the University of Washington in 1969; and a PhD in epidemiology from the University of North Carolina, Chapel Hill, in 1978.

Women's Health Care in Advanced Practice Nursing

Second Edition

Ivy M. Alexander, PhD, APRN, ANP-BC, FAANP, FAAN

Versie Johnson-Mallard, PhD, ARNP, WHNP-BC, FAANP, FAAN

Elizabeth A. Kostas-Polston, PhD, APRN, WHNP-BC, FAANP, FAAN

Catherine Ingram Fogel, PhD, RNC, FAAN

Nancy Fugate Woods, PhD, RN, FAAN

EDITORS

SPRINGER PUBLISHING COMPANY

NEW YORK

Springer Publishing Company, LLC
11 West 42nd Street
New York, NY 10036
www.springerpub.com

Acquisitions Editor: Elizabeth Nieginski
Composition: Newgen KnowledgeWorks

ISBN: 978-0-8261-2748-8
e-book ISBN: 978-0-8261-9431-2
Test Bank ISBN: 978-0-8261-2755-6
PowerPoint ISBN: 978-0-8261-2749-5
Case Studies and Resources ISBN: 978-0-8261-9445-9

Qualified instructors may request supplements by emailing textbook@springerpub.com

16 17 18 19 20/ 5 4 3 2 1

The author and the publisher of this Work have made every effort to use sources believed to be reliable to provide information that is accurate and compatible with the standards generally accepted at the time of publication. Because medical science is continually advancing, our knowledge base continues to expand. Therefore, as new information becomes available, changes in procedures become necessary. We recommend that the reader always consult current research and specific institutional policies before performing any clinical procedure. The author and publisher shall not be liable for any special, consequential, or exemplary damages resulting, in whole or in part, from the readers' use of, or reliance on, the information contained in this book. The publisher has no responsibility for the persistence or accuracy of URLs for external or third-party Internet websites referred to in this publication and does not guarantee that any content on such websites is, or will remain, accurate or appropriate.

Library of Congress Cataloging-in-Publication Data
Names: Alexander, Ivy M., editor. | Johnson-Mallard, Versie, editor. | Kostas-Polston, Elizabeth A., editor. |
  Fogel, Catherine Ingram, 1941-editor. | Woods, Nancy Fugate, editor.
Title: Women's health care in advanced practice nursing / Ivy M. Alexander, Versie Johnson-Mallard,
  Elizabeth A. Kostas-Polston, Catherine Ingram Fogel, Nancy Fugate Woods, editors.
Description: Second edition. | New York, NY: Springer Publishing Company, LLC, [2017] | Includes bibliographical
  references and index.
Identifiers: LCCN 2016020144| ISBN 9780826127488 | ISBN 9780826194312 (eBook) | ISBN 9780826127556 (test bank) |
  ISBN 9780826127495 (powerpoints) | ISBN 9780826194459 (case studies and resources)
Subjects: | MESH: Women's Health Services | Nursing Care | Women's Health | Nurse Practitioners | Health Promotion
Classification: LCC RT42 | NLM WA 309.1 | DDC 613/.04244—dc23
LC record available at https://lccn.loc.gov/2016020144

Printed in the United States of America by Bradford & Bigelow.

The editors dedicate this book to the nurse practitioners who provide excellent, individualized care to women.

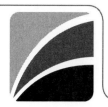

Contents

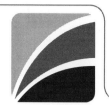

Contributors

Ivy M. Alexander, PhD, APRN, ANP-BC, FAANP, FAAN
Clinical Professor and Director of Advanced Practice Programs
University of Connecticut School of Nursing
Adult Nurse Practitioner
UConn Health
Storrs, Connecticut

Angela Frederick Amar, PhD, RN, FAAN
Assistant Dean for BSN Education
Associate Professor
Nell Hodgson Woodruff School of Nursing
Emory University
Atlanta, Georgia

Deborah Antai-Otong, MS, APRN, PMHCNS-BC, FAAN
Department of Veterans Administration
VISN 17 Continuous Readiness Officer
Behavioral Health Consultant
Arlington, Texas

Candi Bachour, PharmD
Resident
University of Tennessee Health Science Center
Memphis, Tennessee

Rachel Oldani Bender, MSN, WHNP-BC
Women's Health Care Nurse Practitioner
Women's Health Care Specialists
St. Peter's, Missouri

Adrienne Berarducci, PhD, ARNP, BC, FAANP
Associate Professor
University of South Florida
Tampa, Florida

Richard S. Bercik, MD
Assistant Professor
Department of Obstetrics, Gynecology, and Reproductive Science
Department of Urology
Yale School of Medicine
New Haven, Connecticut

Judith Berg, PhD, RN, WHNP-BC, FAAN, FAANP
Clinical Professor
College of Nursing
University of Arizona
Tucson, Arizona

Tara F. Bertulfo, DNP, RN, ARNP
Clinical Assistant Professor
Georgia Baptist College of Nursing
Mercer University
Atlanta, Georgia

Candace Brown, MSN, PharmD
Professor of Clinical Pharmacy and Psychiatry
University of Tennessee Health Science Center
Memphis, Tennessee

Janice Camp, RN, MSN, MSPH, CIH, COHNS
Principal Lecturer Emeritus
Department of Environmental and Occupational Health Sciences
University of Washington
Seattle, Washington

Susan Caverly, PhD, ARNP, BC
Director of Psychiatric Services and the Integrated Cognitive
    Therapies Program
Therapeutic Health Services
Clinical Professor
Psychosocial & Community Health Department
School of Nursing
University of Washington
Seattle, Washington

JiWon Choi, PhD, RN
Assistant Adjunct Professor
Department of Social & Behavioral Sciences
Institute for Health & Aging
University of California, San Francisco
San Francisco, California

Barbara B. Cochrane, PhD, RN, FAAN
Professor in Family and Child Nursing
The de Tornyay Endowed Professor for Healthy Aging
Director, de Tornyay Center for Healthy Aging
University of Washington School of Nursing
Seattle, Washington

Cheryl L. Cooke, PhD, DNP, ARNP, PMHNP-BC
Associate Professor
University of Washington Bothell
Bothell, Washington

Caroline Dorsen, PhD, FNP-BC
Assistant Professor
New York University College of Nursing
Affiliated Investigator
Center for Drug Use and HIV Research (CDUHR)
New York, New York

Deborah G. Feigel, PA-C
Lakeview Health Systems
(Formerly Multidisciplinary Breast Clinic and Department of
    General Surgery)
Mayo Clinic Florida
Jacksonville, Florida

Lisa L. Ferguson, DNP, WHNP-BC
Adjunct Faculty
Department of Family, Community, and Health System Science
College of Nursing
University of Florida
Gainesville, Florida

Robert Gildersleeve, MD
Assistant Clinical Professor
Department of OB/GYN
University of Connecticut School of Medicine
Farmington, Connecticut
Clinical Preceptor
Yale University School of Nursing
New Haven, Connecticut

Meredith Goff, RN, CNM, MS
Midwife; Director of Prenatal Services
Outer Cape Health Services
Wellfleet, Massachusetts

Catherine Ingram Fogel, PhD, RNC, FAAN
Research Professor Emeritus
School of Nursing
University of North Carolina at Chapel Hill
Chapel Hill, North Carolina

Tracie Harrison, PhD, RN, FAAN
Associate Professor
School of Nursing
University of Texas at Austin
Austin, Texas

Leslie J. Heron, RN, BSN, MN, APRN, FNP-BC, NC-BC
Nurse Practitioner
Seattle Cancer Care Alliance, Survivorship Clinic
Fred Hutchinson Cancer Research Center, Survivorship Program
Seattle, Washington

Gail M. Houck, PhD, RN, PMHNP
Professor
Department of Family and Child Nursing
University of Washington
Seattle, Washington

Heather Hutchins-Wiese, PhD, RD
Assistant Professor
Dietetics and Human Nutrition
School of Health Sciences
Eastern Michigan University
Ypsilanti, Michigan

Seja Jackson, MS, APRN, AAHIVS
HIV Specialist
Burgdorf Health Center
St. Francis Hospital and Medical Center
Hartford, Connecticut

Annette Jakubisin Konicki, PhD, APRN, ANP-BC, FNP-BC
Associate Clinical Professor
University of Connecticut School of Nursing
Storrs, Connecticut

Naomi Jay, PhD, NP, RN
Nurse Practitioner
USCF ANCRE Center
Mount Zion Hospital
San Francisco, California

Versie Johnson-Mallard, PhD, ARNP, WHNP-BC, FAANP, FAAN
Chair, Department of Family, Community, and Health
    System Science
Robert Wood Johnson Nurse Faculty Scholar Alumna
University of Florida, College of Nursing
Gainesville, Florida

Heather C. Katz, DNP, RN, MSN, WHNP-BC
Chief, Quality Management Division
USA MEDDAC
Fort Knox, Kentucky

Lilyan Kay, MS, MPH, CNM (Ret), FNP-BC
Georgetown University School of Nursing and Health Sciences
Family Nurse Practitioner Program
Washington, DC

Kathleen Kelleher, APNC, CBCN, DMH
Nurse Practitioner
Breast Surgery
Chilton Medical Center
Drew University Health Services
Pompton Plains, New Jersey

**Elizabeth A. Kostas-Polston, PhD, APRN, WHNP-BC,
    FAANP, FAAN**
Assistant Professor; Daniel K. Inouye Graduate School of Nursing
Uniformed Services University of the Health Sciences
Robert Wood Johnson Nurse Faculty Scholar Alumna;
    Women's Health Nurse Practitioner
Bethesda, Maryland

Cara J. Krulewitch, PhD, CNM, FACNM
Adjunct Associate Professor
School of Medicine
Uniformed Services University of the Health Sciences
Bethesda, Maryland

Elizabeth Kusturiss, MSN, CRNP
Nurse Practitioner in Sexual Medicine
Center for Pelvic Medicine
Academic Urology
Rosemont, Pennsylvania

Devangi Ladani, MS, APRN, AGPCNP-BC
Nurse Practitioner
University of Connecticut
Storrs, Connecticut

Carol A. Landis, PhD, RN, FAAN
Assistant Professor
New York University College of Nursing
Affiliated Investigator
Center for Drug Use and HIV Research (CDUHR)
New York, New York

Danielle LaRosa, MS, APRN, FNP-BC
Nurse Practitioner
Optum
Rocky Hill, Connecticut

Jenna LoGiudice, PhD, CNM, RN
Assistant Professor
Egan School of Nursing and Health Studies
Fairfield University
Fairfield, Connecticut

Allison McCarson, DNP, MSN, CNM
United States Government
American College of Nurse Midwives
Colorado Springs, Colorado

Regina A. McClure, AACN, RN
Capt., U.S. Air Force NC
Walter Reed National Military Medical Center
Bethesda, Maryland

Emily Miesse, BSE, CLC, FNP-C
Advanced Practice Nurse Practitioner
Shoreline Medical Associates
Madison, Connecticut

Ellen Sullivan Mitchell, PhD
Associate Professor Emeritus
Family and Child Nursing
University of Washington, School of Nursing
Seattle, Washington

Selina A. Mohammed, PhD, MPH, RN
Associate Professor
School of Nursing and Health Studies
University of Washington Bothell
Bothell, Washington

Tina M. Chasse Mulinski, MSN, APRN
Nurse Practitioner
The Cardiology Group
St. Vincent's Multispeciality Group
Hamden, Connecticut

Kristi Rae Norcross, DNP, CNM
Certified Nurse Midwife
Lt Col, U.S. Air Force
San Antonio Military Medical Center
San Antonio, Texas

Karin V. Nyström, MSN, APRN, FAHA
Stroke Coordinator
Yale New Haven Stroke Center
Yale New Haven Hospital
New Haven, Connecticut

Ellen F. Olshansky, PhD, RN, WHNP-BC, FAAN
Professor and Chair
Department of Nursing
School of Social Work
University of Southern California
Los Angeles, California

Debbie Postlethwaite, RNP, MPH
Assistant Director
Biostatistical Consulting Unit
Division of Research, Kaiser Permanente
Oakland, California

Richard M. Prior, DNP, FNP-BC, FAANP
Chief Nursing Officer
Ireland Army Community Hospital
Fort Knox, Kentucky

**Theresa G. Rashdan, DNP, CPNP-PC, FNP-C,
CPNP-AC, CNS, RN**
Assistant Professor
University of South Florida
Tampa, FL
Advanced Registered Nurse Practitioner
BayCare
Plant City/Lutz, Florida

Heather Dawn Reynolds, CNM, MSN, FACNM
Associate Professor
Yale University School of Nursing
Orange, Connecticut

Cherrilyn F. Richmond, MS, APRN, FNP, WHNP-BC
Women's Health Nurse Practitioner
Clinical Researcher, Yale School of Nursing Preceptor
Yale Urogynecology and Reconstructive Pelvic Surgery
Department of OB/GYN
Yale University School of Medicine
New Haven, Connecticut

Diane C. Seibert, PhD, ARNP, FAANP, FAAN
Professor
Interim Associate Dean for Academic Affairs
Daniel K. Inouye Graduate School of Nursing
Uniformed Services University
Bethesda, Maryland

Barbara J. Silko, ARNP, PhD
Nurse Practitioner, Gynecology Oncology
University of Washington Medical Center and Seattle Cancer
   Care Alliance
Seattle, Washington

Katherine Simmonds, MS, MPH, WHNP-BC
Assistant Professor and Coordinator
Women's Health NP Specialty
MGH Institute of Health Professions
Charlestown, Massachusetts

Anna G. Small, MSN, JD, CNM
Corporate Director of Compliance
Shriners Hospitals for Children
Tampa, Florida

Susan Kellogg Spadt, PhD, CRNP, IF, CST
Director of Female Sexual Medicine
Academic Urology Center for Pelvic Medicine
Rosemont, Pennsylvania
Professor OB/GYN
Drexel University College of Medicine
Philadelphia, Pennsylvania

Lisa Stern, RN, MSN, MA
Vice President of Medical Services
Planned Parenthood Northern California
Volunteer Clinical Faculty
University of California San Francisco
San Francisco, California

Marianne T. Stone-Godena, CNM, MSN
Assistant Professor Maternal-Newborn Nursing
Rhode Island College
Providence, Rhode Island

Diana Taylor, PhD, RN, FAAN
Professor Emerita, Family Health Care Nursing Department
Faculty, Advancing New Standards in Reproductive Health
   (ANSIRH)
Bixby Center for Global Reproductive Health
University of California, San Francisco
San Francisco, California

Kathryn Tierney, MSN, APRN-BC, FNP
Family Nurse Practitioner
Middlesex Hospital MultiSpecialty Group
Middletown, Connecticut

Lauren Vo, MS, AGPCNP-BC, APRN
Nurse Practitioner
University of Connecticut
Storrs, Connecticut

Deborah Ward, RN, PhD, FAAN
Health Sciences Clinical Professor
Betty Irene Moore School of Nursing
University of California–Davis Health System
Sacramento, California

Candy Wilson, PhD, APRN, WHNP-BC
Nurse Scientist
U.S. Air Force Acupuncture and Integrative Medicine Center
Malcolm Grow Medical Clinics and Surgery Center (MGMCSC)
Joint Base Andrews, Maryland

Catherine G. Winkler, PhD, MPH, RN
Adjunct Faculty
Fairfield University
Fairfield, California

Catherine Takacs Witkop, MD, MPH, Col, USAF, MC
Associate Professor, PMB and OB/GYN
Program Director, General Preventive Medicine Residency
Uniformed Services University of the Health Sciences
Bethesda, Maryland

Matthew Witkovic, MS
Family Nurse Practitioner
University of Connecticut
Storrs, Connecticut

Nancy Fugate Woods, PhD, RN, FAAN
Professor, Biobehavioral Nursing, and Dean Emeritus
University of Washington School of Nursing
Seattle, Washington

Heather M. Young, PhD, RN, FAAN
Dignity Heath Dean's Chair in Nursing Leadership
Dean and Professor
Betty Irene Moore School of Nursing
Associate Vice Chancellor for Nursing
University of California, Davis
Davis, California

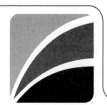

If you picked up *Women's Health Care in Advanced Practice Nursing, Second Edition,* to advance your "learning curve," I congratulate you. After reading it, I am certain you will agree with me that this text represents a must-read for advanced practice nurses and other providers who deliver health care to women—at any age and at any stage. The importance of this new edition of *Women's Health Care in Advanced Practice Nursing* cannot be overstated. It is edited by long-standing noted icons in our field of nursing (Catherine Ingram Fogel and Nancy Fugate Woods), along with new members of the editorial team: Ivy M. Alexander, Versie Johnson-Mallard, and Elizabeth A. Kostas-Polston, each of whom brings unique clinically informed scholarship to the team. As an adult nurse practitioner clinician scholar, Ivy M. Alexander has focused on midlife women's health and health care, especially menopause and osteoporosis. In her scholarly emphases, Versie Johnson-Mallard, a women's health nurse practitioner, sheds new light on women's sexual and reproductive health, including HPV/cancer screening and prevention and behavioral change in response to culturally appropriate educational interventions. In the laboratory as well as the clinic, Elizabeth A. Kostas-Polston, a women's health nurse practitioner, addresses health-promotion and disease-prevention strategies focused on sexual and reproductive health and HPV-related cancer prevention. This next generation of leaders in women's health and health care has identified contributors who are scholars in many areas important to women's health; all are not only knowledgeable, but passionate about women's health knowledge discovery and its application to transformative health care.

For almost any advancement, I believe that three aspects help move the needle toward positive change: seeing possibilities, framing, and timing. This book is visionary, leading, and timely. Regarding the importance of seeing possibilities, the foundational editors were way ahead of the curve in mainstream health care by focusing on women and their health. Fogel and Woods conceived of the first version of this book in the early 1980s, when women's health was narrowly defined for health care (it was mostly about the reproductive phase, and biomedicine dominated), and the study of women's health lacked popularity and certainly was not comprehensive. Regarding the impact of framing for the book, the editors departed from the typical biomedical approach and articulated a framework that speaks directly to us in nursing, focusing on what I call *health ecology* (women within their environments or what some refer to as the *context of their lives*). In this new edition of the book, you will be immersed in this frame in Part I. Regarding the influence of timing, with their early grasp on what would come to be a widespread emphasis on women and their health, the editors focus their own discovery and practice scholarship over time, becoming notable experts who are able to interprofessionally network and link with other prominent experts. Thus, the authors of this book represent the "best in class" for conveying contemporary and futuristic perspectives.

Several of the contributing authors to this book have participated, as I do, in the Women's Health Expert Panel (WHEP) of the American Academy of Nursing. These are peer-nominated and elected nurse scholars from academia and health care practice who focus on applying knowledge to shape policy and clinical practice. They and the other chosen contributors are the *thought leaders* who are most informed about women's health and whose analytic thinking is the most informative. Collectively, as members of the WHEP, we have published and spoken publicly on what is crucial to the health of women and critiqued exposés written by those in other disciplines to call attention to missing links within the national women's health research and clinical services policy agendas. Linking to the transformations spurred by the Patient Protection and Affordable Care Act (ACA), attention has swung toward a national prevention strategy as articulated especially by the National Prevention Council, U.S. Preventive Services Task Force, and the Institute of Medicine. Part II of this book brings to you the most well-versed current perspectives for the application of preventive care (and health-promotion care) for women across the life span. We all know that, generally, women often seek health care for bothersome symptoms associated with chronic physical or emotional conditions, reproductive (pregnancy) or sexual health–related conditions, and the consequences of violence. In Part III, you can update your knowledge on the most prominent women's health issues that engage health care providers.

I am sure you can sense by my comments in this Foreword that I feel fortunate to be able to urge you to read this most *forward-looking* book. In today's health care delivery world, and as epitomized in this book, I am inspired to see that for knowledge to be applied to women's health, a health ecology frame is becoming increasingly valued. Regional politics aside, everywhere I look, be it in acute or community settings, advanced practice registered nurses (APRNs) are being sought after, I believe, because they bring the value added of a holistic approach. No group is better positioned to model the elements brought forward by this book than women's health APRNs. So whether you are a passionate advocate for, thinking about becoming, on the path to becoming, or actually are an APRN in women's health, this book should be your provocative and affirming handbook—an accelerant for helping ensure that you are an influential women's health provider, scholar, leader, policy maker, and spokesperson.

Joan L. Shaver, PhD, RN, FAAN
Professor and Dean
University of Arizona College of Nursing
Tucson, Arizona

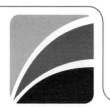

Preface

Women's health has been defined from a variety of perspectives. Women themselves describe articulately what it means to be healthy. Often their descriptions allude to experiencing the absence of illness or symptoms but more often to being able to perform their roles in life, having the capacity to respond to stress and strain, and experiencing high-level wellness.

This text originated in the 1970s as Catherine Ingram Fogel and Nancy Fugate Woods recognized the need for resources for nurses and nursing students who were interested in the emerging area of women's health. The grandmother of this text was first conceived and birthed in 1981, revised and updated in 1995 and again in 2008, and has paralleled the history of the original editors and contributors, as we moved from our young adult years in the midst of the Women's Health Movement of the 1970s and 1980s to our more mature years as we prepared this edition of *Women's Health in Advanced Practice Nursing* and forged a new collaborative with editors of a younger generation.

Over the past four decades, nursing scholars have studied women's health through the lenses of feminist theory, nursing theory, and now through critical, postcolonial, and womanist theory. In a relatively short period of history, and propelled by a fusion of the U.S. feminist movement of the late 20th century and the popular health movement, scholars redefined *women's health* as more than women's reproductive health to include a holistic view of what it means to be a healthy woman. Indeed, women's health as a discipline has been transformed from gynecology to "Gyn Ecology," an understanding of women's health in the context of everyday life. An ecological perspective implies that the multiple environments in which women live their lives, including the influence of the society, culture, institutions, community, and families, need to be considered. During this period, women's health scholars engaged women in redefining their own health as inclusive of well-being and not simply a compendium of women's diseases. Clinicians and researchers alike redefined being healthy as the processes of attaining, regaining, and retaining health, consistent with the nursing theories of the time. Moreover, a life-span view became imperative as scholars came to appreciate that women's health at one part of the life span influenced their chances for health later in life.

Thinking about women's health from this new perspective implied putting women at the center of clinical services as well as research, focusing on women's health in the context of their lives. New frameworks for understanding women's health shaped by feminism and feminist theory now guide research and clinical scholarship. Scholars of revisionist views of feminist theory challenged investigators to consider the intersectionality of women's identities and the consequences for health. One's gender is only one component of who one is: gender, race/ethnicity, social class, sexual orientation and gender identity, and disability/ableness all intersect in influencing one's chances for health. In addition, frameworks prompted by globalization reinforce the need to use many different lenses in viewing the health of women around the world. The efforts of the 1980s and 1990s to integrate women's health literature across disciplines enlarged the perspectives with which communities of nurse scholars and clinicians have come to view women and their health.

Over the past four decades, we have seen dramatic changes in the nature of nursing practice, including that of advanced practice nurses. A rarity in the 1970s, advanced practice nurses are now an essential part of the health care workforce, providing an ever-increasing proportion of primary care for women. As educational programs transition, the push for educating all advanced practice nurses about women's unique health care problems and appropriate models of care has escalated.

Part I, Women's Lives, Women's Health, views women's health as inextricably linked to the context in which women live their lives, making it impossible to understand women's health without appreciating the challenges and opportunities they face in everyday living. Understanding women's lived experiences has become key to understanding their well-being and chances for health. In this section of the text, we consider women and their health as viewed from a population perspective, using national data to paint a picture of morbidity, mortality, health, and well-being, as well as the use of health care. Women have long been attracted to work in health care, and both their distribution and the challenges associated with being a health care provider and practicing in one of the many health professions is explored. The emergence of a clinical scholarship of women's health, in contrast to gynecology and obstetrics, gave rise to a need to transform women's health research as well as models of care and health policy. Women-sensitive models of care have emerged over the past two decades; some of these have been influential in shaping the delivery of services in a variety of health care settings. Recognition of the diversity of U.S. society prompted consideration of health care for special populations of women, and appreciation of women's rights to health care warrants our attention to the legal aspects of women's health care, especially as the legal aspects of women's health care continue to be contested. Feminist frameworks for women's health offer an updated view of the many lenses through which we can understand women's health as we care for women.

Part II, Health Promotion and Prevention for Women, draws attention to the work of health promotion and prevention, reflected both in women's own self-care as well as professional services. Viewed through the lenses introduced in Part I, women's health is a multidimensional experience, most of which is managed by women themselves, with occasional encounters with health professionals. What women do to stay healthy has been studied by numerous disciplines with a wide range of activities. Women often assume the role as agents of health for their families and demonstrate a high level of interest in health-related information. Indeed, they frequently justify paying attention to their own health in relation to their need to care for their families. They manage their own and family members' illnesses, often simultaneously providing illness-related care to their children, partners, and parents. The everyday activities that create health are often the purview of women's work; these include meal planning and preparation, family activities, sleep and rest patterns, and the like. Women are active in obtaining information about their health and often express a desire to work with a health professional who respects their knowledge about their own health and how to promote it. At the same time, women seek health-promotion advice from professionals to help sort out valid information and recommendations about keeping healthy. Women experience their health as embodied: We are and simultaneously live in our bodies. From the early days of the feminist movement of the 20th century, when women used plastic speculums to view their vaginas and cervices, demystification of women's bodies became part of women's health care. As women, we continue to be attentive to some of the unique aspects of our bodies, such as the menstrual cycle and menopause. In Part II, we trace experiences of health and health promotion in young, midlife, and older women as a foundation for understanding well-woman's health. The emergence of the emphasis on the well women in wellness visits prompts us to consider the questions: What is a healthy woman? What is a mentally healthy woman? How does one attain and maintain optimal health? Health practices span nutrition, exercise/activity, and sleep, each of which demonstrably shapes our health. In an era of personalized health care, we examine the influence of the contemporary "omics" sciences as a foundation for understanding emerging approaches to diagnosis and delivery of health care. Women's multiple roles in society commonly include employment, in addition to their family roles, and the majority of family caregivers are women: We examine both of these contexts for women's health and the implications for health care. Women's sexual health, including special considerations for women who are lesbians, transgender, bisexual, and questioning, warrants special attention of health care providers, as does the management of fertility. As women anticipate having children, both preconception health promotion and prenatal care are essential.

Part III, Managing Symptoms and Women's Health Considerations, includes an array of problems that account for a growing portion of advanced nursing practice. Women may find that health professionals do not take their complaints seriously, promoting their frustration and dissatisfaction with health care. Part III includes information about topics that touch women's lives and about which many seek information and validation from health professionals. Although women's uniquely experienced reproductive health problems are important, so also are health problems that are not unique to women but may be experienced uniquely, such as heart disease. A variety of reproductive-related health problems, as well as general problems such as chronic illnesses, are the focus of many health care visits.

In Part III, we address an array of health problems that are unique to women (such as women's reproductive health problems), are more prevalent in women (such as breast cancer), and are diagnosed and managed in different ways for women (such as thyroid disorders, diabetes, and heart disease). Among these considerations are those that are linked most directly to reproductive health care, including breast health, care for transgender and gender reassignment, sexual health problems and dysfunctions, vulvar and vaginal health problems, perimenstrual and pelvic symptoms and syndromes, urological and pelvic floor health problems, sexually transmitted infections, women's experiences of HIV/AIDS, human papillomavirus, gynecologic cancers, menopause, osteoporosis, unintended pregnancy, infertility, high-risk childbearing, and intrapartum and postpartum care. In this section, we also recognize that many women's health problems are not only those related to reproductive system function, but also those that include mental health challenges, substance abuse, violence against women, cardiovascular diseases, endocrine-related problems, chronic illness, and disability.

Several exciting online resources are available for each chapter. Case studies provide real-world application of the materials. Resources are available for literature, websites, and smartphone applications to access further information. Test bank review questions reflect the most salient points of the content. Additionally, PowerPoint presentations for each chapter can be used as instructional aids or for review of content. This ancillary material is available to qualified instructors by emailing Springer Publishing Company at textbook@springerpub.com.

Ivy M. Alexander
Versie Johnson-Mallard
Elizabeth A. Kostas-Polston
Catherine Ingram Fogel
Nancy Fugate Woods

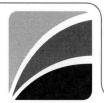

Acknowledgments

The editors gratefully acknowledge the outstanding work of the many contributing authors whose excellence in research and patient care has added so much to this book. We also acknowledge the assistance of Springer Publishing Company staff, especially Elizabeth Nieginski, Rachel Landes, Lindsay Claire, and Joanne Jay.

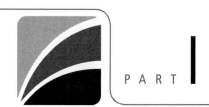

PART I

Women's Lives, Women's Health

CHAPTER 1

Women and Their Health

Versie Johnson-Mallard • Nancy Fugate Woods

Women's health can be viewed from a multiplicity of perspectives. Women, themselves, are articulate in their descriptions of what it means to be healthy. Often their descriptions not only allude to the absence of illness or symptoms, but also include the ability to perform their life roles, the capacity to respond to stress and strain, and the experience of high-level wellness, and this pattern is consistent among both young and older women (Perry & Woods, 1995; Woods et al., 1988). Women's health is inextricably linked to the context in which women live their lives, making it impossible to understand women's health without an appreciation of the context in which they live their lives. Understanding women's lived experiences in the family unit, community, and work has become key to understanding their chances for health and well-being.

The 20th century witnessed a remarkable change in our understanding of women's health and saw extraordinary improvements in the health and well-being of women in the United States resulting from an increase in access to care, research, policy, and innovative approaches to health care. Our understanding of women's health and unique challenges—informed by research that extends from genomic molecular events to behavioral, psychological, societal, and economic phenomena—continues as one of the most exciting challenges of scientific inquiry and political inquiry. Despite the progress, the health of women in the United States remains subject to wide disparities. These disparities among women overall are readily apparent for specific populations of women based on socioeconomic status, education, and race/ethnicity. Recent trends in women's demographics—including educational attainment, employment status, health insurance, family composition, reproduction, and access to health care—suggest an increasingly complex social context (Pew Research Center, 2013). An understanding of women's health issues, if it is to be truly comprehensive, must consider such factors and trends.

The first section of this chapter describes selected sociodemographic characteristics of women in the United States. Some of the most notable of these characteristics at the beginning of the 21st century are the changing educational status of women and racial/ethnic populations. The second section presents selected measures of health status.

These include mortality, morbidity, and health care access and utilization. Next, we discuss the complicated interplay between and steadily changing scientific knowledge regarding the areas of biology and environment. We conclude with an exploration of the future directions for women's health, including global health trends.

■ SOCIAL CONTEXT FOR WOMEN'S HEALTH

In 2013, the U.S. population of women was estimated at 161 million, with women outnumbering men at 4.0 million to 2.0 million at the age of 85 years and older. Who are these women and how healthy are they? To understand the health of women in the U.S. social context, we present the most recently available data on selected social characteristics of women, with a focus on the changing population demographics. Differences in the life circumstances of women are influenced through a number of pathways, many of which are not yet understood. Considering the health of women within their broad sociostructural environment is important in light of race/ethnicity and socioeconomic status, all of which have an impact on women's health. Gender differences in some aspects of health status are presented when the differences are remarkable. Notably, data regarding women's health are limited and often are not available by important demographic characteristics. Race/ethnic variation is discussed when the data sources are available. We recognize the limitations of reporting demographics such as race and ethnicity, because definitions vary over time, and data are inconsistently available for small but growing populations. Furthermore, reporting can obscure the diversity within and among subgroups of women. For example, the Asian/Pacific Islanders category includes more than 25 heterogeneous groups, and no distinction is made in terms of their immigration status. The category "Black" includes African Americans whose families have lived in the United States for generations as well as more recent immigrants such as refugees from war-torn countries such as Somalia. In addition, Hispanic origin is separated by the Census Bureau as an ethnicity not a race. In 2012, about 9 million Americans chose two or more racial categories when asked about their race (U.S. Census Bureau, 2012). Also, because detailed racial/ethnic information is frequently unavailable, and because socioeconomic status and cultures of ethnic and racial groups may vary dramatically with important health consequences, racial labeling may mask notable health differences and thus should be considered with caution. Finally, given the strong association between socioeconomic status as measured by family income, poverty threshold, or level of education and the health of women, differences are also noted when data permit.

Growth

America is becoming a more racially diverse country. The social demographics of multiracial Americans in the United States are growing at a rate three times as fast as the population as a whole (Pew Research Center, 2015). As of June 2015, youth in America born between 1982 and 2000, termed *millennials*, number 83.1 million—one quarter of the nation's population. Racial/ethnic diversity among millennials is noteworthy: 44.2% were from a minority race or ethnic group in 2015. Those younger than 5 years were even more diverse, now the majority minority in this age cohort at 50.2% (U.S. Census Bureau, 2011).

In 2015, the total female population was racially and ethnically diverse and was composed of White (71.3%); Black (12.5%); Hispanic (11.5%); Asian/Pacific Islander (3.9%); and American Indian, Eskimo, and Aleutian (1%) (U.S. Census Bureau, 2015). Population growth rates are higher among the Hispanic population than among White non-Hispanic or Black subgroups. Moreover, the growth of the Hispanic population is likely to continue, as Hispanic women compose a large proportion of the population of reproductive age and have the highest fertility rates. In fact, by the year 2050, population projections indicate that Hispanic, Black, American Indian, and Asian adolescents will constitute 56% of the total adolescent population (U.S. Census Bureau, 2011).

Immigration

The United States is largely a nation of immigrants, and the immigrant population is increasing. Since 2012, foreign women (51.4%) outnumber foreign men. Indeed, in 2013, approximately 14% of the population was foreign born compared with 10% in 1999 (Pew Research Center, 2015). Among the immigrant population, 47% were born in Latin American and Caribbean countries, with 28% from Asia, 12% from Europe, and 7% from other areas of the world. The continuing influx of immigrants contributes to growing racial/ethnic diversity in the U.S. population.

Immigrants and refugees of the 21st century are not as well educated as the professionals of the 1950s and 1960s, because many immigrants now come from poverty-stricken countries, such as Ethiopia, or are survivors of war-ravaged nations, such as Bosnia, Kosovo, and Somalia. Notably, descendants of these immigrants and refugees represent the largest segment of U.S. population growth, a trend that is predicted to continue. Second-generation U.S.-born children of immigrants are likely to hold a college degree;

11.6% of immigrants hold master's, professional, or doctorate degrees (Burnside, Brown, Burger, Hamilton, Moses, & Bettencourt, 2012; statistical portrait of the foreign born). Their share in poverty is lower, and they are as well off as the overall adult population (Pew Research Center, 2015).

Regardless of the country of origin, most immigrants confront challenges such as linguistic differences and changes in financial status on arriving in the United States. The process of immigration can affect health status and behaviors adversely through disruption of social networks; new exposure to racial and class-based discrimination; differential adverse environmental exposures; and adjustment to new language, culture, and values. For example, rates of obesity, smoking, alcohol, and illicit drug use tend to increase among Mexicans who immigrate to the United States. In contrast, foreign-born Mexican immigrant women are reported to have better birth outcomes than U.S.-born Mexican women, which may result from such protective factors as strong family support and cultural ties (Center for American Progress, 2014).

Linguistic Differences

The United States is not known for being multilinguistic, leading to marked linguistic challenges for some, but not all, immigrant populations. For example, among foreign-born Blacks, most of whom are from island nations such as the Dominican Republic, Haiti, Jamaica, and Trinidad, English proficiency is common. In contrast, more traditional Hispanic immigrants often have limited English proficiency. Similarly, Asian/Pacific Islander women, who emigrate from more than 20 countries, may speak one of more than 1,000 different languages. When immigrant women enter health care organizations, their level of English proficiency combined with the provider's potential lack of linguistically and culturally competent health care skills can lead to the underutilization of health care services and unintended adverse health outcomes. Linguistic differences may play a role in family dynamics and social, educational, and employment opportunities for immigrants.

Educational Attainment

Educational attainment is one of the most important influences on economic well-being among women and has a profound impact on women's health. Graduating from high school and college significantly improves women's health and well-being by increasing economic security and providing the literacy skills necessary to navigate the health care system. Conversely, lacking a high school diploma may cause women to have lower earnings, greater difficulty in obtaining health care, as well as be more likely to engage in substance abuse and suffer from other adverse health consequences. Although the U.S. overall trends reflect a more educated population, significant differences in educational attainment persist with regard to gender and race/ethnicity. Persons with less than a high school education have death rates at least double those with education beyond high school. Nonetheless, the educational attainment of women indicates a dramatic improvement for a group that has historically been less educated, and these differences have been decreasing in recent years.

Women's progress in educational attainment is striking in comparison with that in 1969 to 1970, when men earned the majority of every type of postsecondary degree: During 2010 to 2014, women earned more than half of all associate, bachelor's, master's, and doctoral or professional degrees (Ryan & Bauman, 2016). The proportion of doctoral or first professional degrees earned by women rose from 9.6% in 1969 to 1970 to 51.4% in 2010 to 2014. Women now comprise almost 69% of all college students in graduate and undergraduate programs (Ryan & Bauman, 2016).

Despite the narrowing in educational attainment between women and men, persisting differences among racial/ethnic groups may contribute to restricted employment opportunities and decreased financial solvency for less-educated women. Racial/ethnic disparities in education are evident. Although nearly 35% of all women 25 to 29 years of age had earned a college degree in 2009 to 2014, less than 16% of Hispanic Native Hawaiian or Pacific Islander (10.4%), non-Hispanic American Indian/Alaska Native (14%), and Hispanic women (15.5%) had a college degree. Non-Hispanic Black (approximately 22%), non-Hispanic Asian (62.7%), and non-Hispanic White women (41%) were most likely to have a bachelor's degree. In 2012, 91% of women 25 to 29 years of age had earned a high school or general equivalency diploma (Women's Health USA, 2013).

Employment

The proportion of women to men in the workforce has changed from previous generations. In 2014, approximately 60% of women 16 years and older were in the labor force compared with 70.5% of men, reflecting a dramatic change in women's labor force participation from 43% in 1970. Women with children younger than 18 years of age are in the labor force—nearly 71% in 2013 compared with 47% in 1975. Labor force participation is related to women's roles, with nearly 60% of married mothers with children younger than 2 years to 80% of unmarried women or separated mothers with children 6 to 17 years of age (Women's Health USA, 2013).

The highest percentage of women in the labor work force by age is 40 to 44 years. Estimates from the U.S. Department of Labor, Bureau of Labor Statistics, are that 72% are age 25 to 54 years, 56.5% are 55 to 64 years, and 11% are 65 years and older (Ryan & Bauman, 2016). The labor force participation rates of women have been increasing across age groups, except among young and older women. Women accounted for 51% of the employed in occupations such as lawyers (33%) and registered nurses at 91%. (See Chapter 2 for further discussion of women's work in health care.) Regardless of gender, the Asian labor force is projected to increase most rapidly, and the Hispanic labor force is projected to be larger than the Black labor force because of faster population growth. Changes in labor force participation also varied by age and occupation.

Employment can have beneficial or negative effects on the well-being of women. Previous research reports show inconsistent findings on how employment affects women's health. Although some studies report an association between employment and good health as measured by self-esteem, perceived health, and physical functioning (Hoyt & Murphy, 2016; Pugliesi, 1995), others report that excessive strain is associated with poor health (Amick et al., 1998; Mcdonald, Jackson, Vickers, & Wilkes, 2016). The increase in the percentages of women with children and two-parent families who are employed outside the home highlights the importance of child care issues and support systems for women faced with multiple responsibilities.

The United States is one of the few industrialized countries that does not provide paid maternity leave and health benefits guaranteed by law. Although the 1993 Family and Medical Leave Act (FMLA) guarantees unpaid leave to workers in businesses with 50 or more employees, the FMLA disproportionately excludes low-wage workers who often work in smaller businesses (Commission on Family and Medical Leave, 1996). For example, in 1996, nearly half of U.S. working women were not eligible for FMLA protection. Furthermore, among workers eligible for family or medical leave, 64% reported that, although they needed leave, they could not take it because they needed the income. In 1996, the United States dramatically altered its welfare program with the passage of the Personal Responsibility and Work Opportunity Reconciliation Act (PRWORA), which ended federal administration of welfare and replaced it with block grants to the states. This cash assistance program, known as Temporary Aid to Needy Families (TANF), imposes lifetime limits on benefits, more stringent work requirements, and a host of behavioral mandates. The PRWORA ended entitlement to child care for families that receive welfare and established the Child Care Development Fund block grant; however, the law did not require states to make child care available. Notably, sanctions penalize women for deviation from prescribed behaviors (i.e., mandated immunization, paternity identification, and family planning services) by cutting some or all of their benefits (Chavkin, 1999). Although no federal program is in place to follow women after they stop receiving TANF, state-specific studies have reported on women's subsequent employment and income (Heymann & Earle, 1999; Parrott, 1998; Regenstein, Meyer, & Hicks, 1998). Overall, most women report that they did not receive paid sick leave, paid vacation, or health benefits. The working conditions faced by mothers who had been on welfare previously are worse in part because of their significant lower levels of education, which increases the likelihood of their having to work in poorer conditions, including part-time positions that lack benefits (U.S. Department of Health and Human Services, 1998). Essentially, women who leave TANF to work often need to work under conditions that prevent them from fulfilling their parental responsibilities.

Veteran Status

Women account for an increasing proportion of veterans of the U.S. Armed Forces: 2.5 million or 10.3% of all living veterans. Projections are that, by 2030, women will account for 15% of all veterans, reflecting a similar proportion of active duty military personal. Nearly half of women veterans are from the Gulf War era and more recent conflicts, including Operation Enduring Freedom (OEF), Operation Iraqi Freedom (OIF), and Operation New Dawn (OND). Continuous changes in the military roles of women as well as their multiple deployments and blurring of combat and non-combat operations suggest that the needs of these women may differ greatly from those of women veterans from previous eras. Women veterans are younger than their male counterparts, with 21% younger than 35 years compared with 7% of male veterans, and women account for a much smaller proportion of veterans older than 65 years (45% for men, 16% women). The poverty rate is higher than for male veterans: 10% of women veterans live below the poverty level versus 16% of male veterans. Military sexual trauma (MST), sexual assault, and/or severe and threatening sexual harassment occurring during military service have been identified in 15% of women and 7% of men. MST, along with deployment to war zones and combat exposure, increases the risk of posttraumatic stress disorder, depression, and substance abuse. Efforts to provide gender-sensitive care for women veterans are discussed in Chapter 3.

Economic Status

Earnings of employed women rise with increasing education, but a gender gap persists, with women full-time workers earning 19% to 25% less than men at every level of education. For example, women with a high school diploma earn an average weekly income of $554 compared with men, who earn $720. Women are more likely than men to be among the working poor, those in the workforce but living below the poverty level. Being among the working poor is most common among women aged 16 to 19 and 20 to 24 years (15.7% and 18.3%, respectively) and among Black (14.5%) and Hispanic (13.8%) women (Women's Health USA, 2013). Between 1979 and 2013, women's earnings have increased 20% in more than 2 decades. Specifically, in 1979, women's earnings were 62% and 82% of those in 2013, represented as a proportion of men's earnings (Ryan & Bauman, 2016), making it more likely that women who are employed will also be overrepresented among the poor. In families in which both women and men are employed, working wives contribute 37% of their families' incomes. Only 18% of wives earn more than their husbands. Despite increases in income for women and overall declines in poverty, nearly 15% of U.S. women live in poverty compared with 11% of adult men (U.S. Census Bureau, 2012).

Nearly 25% of Hispanic, non-Hispanic Black, and non-Hispanic American Indian/Alaska Native women live in poverty (Table 1.1). Poverty is most prevalent among non-Hispanic American Indian/Alaska Native women (27.7% overall live in poverty), with 34.2% of those age 18 to 44 years, 22.3% of those age 45 to 64 years, and 12.9% of those 65 years and older. Non-Hispanic Black women have comparable rates of poverty (overall 25.7%), with 29.2% of those 18 to 44 years of age, 22.5% of those age 45 to 64 years, and 20.5% of those 65 years and older. Rates for Hispanics are similar to those for non-Hispanic Black women. Non-Hispanic White women are least likely to live in poverty (10.6%), similar to rates (11.9%) of non-Hispanic Asian women.

TABLE 1.1	Persons Below Poverty Level, by Selected Characteristics in the United States, 2012 (%)	
RACE/ ETHNICITY	ALL PERSONS	FEMALE HOUSEHOLDER, NO SPOUSE PRESENT
White	12.7	44.2
Black	27.2	53.3
Asian	11.7	33.0
Hispanic or Latino	25.6	54.7
White, non-Hispanic	9.7	36.5

Adapted from National Center for Health Statistics (2014a).

Poverty status is related to age: Regardless of race/ethnicity, women 45 to 64 and 65 years of age and older are less likely to experience poverty than those aged 18 to 44. Poverty status is also related to educational attainment: Although nearly one third of women aged 25 years without a high school diploma live in poverty, only 16% of those with a high school diploma, 11.5% with some college education, and 4.9% with a bachelor degree or higher lived in poverty. Poverty also varies with household composition. Married-couple families were least likely to be poor (6.2%), but households headed by a single adult female, were twice as likely to be poor compared with those headed by a single adult male (31% vs. 16% respectively) (DeNavas-Walk & Proctor, 2014).

Before the most recent recession, the median household income was not statistically different at $51,759 and $51,939 for women and men, respectively (DeNavas-Walk & Proctor, 2014). However, in 2013, household earnings were 8% lower than the 2007 median before the recession and 8.7% lower than the median household income peak in 1999 ($56,895). During 2013, women working full-time earned 78% of men's earnings: Mean earnings were $39,157 for women and $50,033 for men. It is noteworthy that the female-to-male earnings ratio has not changed since 2007. For the third consecutive year, the number of people in poverty was not statistically different from the previous year's estimate, but 45.3 million people lived in poverty (U.S. Census Bureau, 2013).

Household Composition

Dramatic changes in family formation and marriage patterns have occurred since the mid-1960s, with increasing proportions of women and men postponing marriage, and there has also been a significant increase in the percentage of people who never marry. In 2014, half of adults aged 18 years and older did not live with a spouse (Figure 1.1). About 13% of women older than 18 years were heads of their households, 15% lived alone, 14% lived with relatives, and 8% lived with nonrelatives (DeNavas-Walk & Proctor, 2014). Young women who were 18 to 24 years old were most likely to live with relatives (59%) and nonrelatives

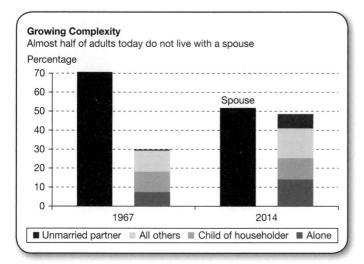

FIGURE 1.1
Living arrangements of adults age 18 years and older.
Source: Current Population Survey. Annual Social and Economic Supplement, 1967–2014.

(17%), but more than 60% of women 35 to 64 years were living with a spouse. Being a head of household with no spouse present was most common for women 25 to 44 years old. Women 65 years and older were likely to be living alone or with a spouse. In 2012, non-Hispanic Black women were most likely to be single heads of households with family members present (27.5%), and non-Hispanic Asian and White women were least likely to be single heads of households (7.6% and 9.4%).

Same-sex couples account for about 1% of households, with female couples accounting for about 53% of these households in 2011. Nearly one quarter of female same-sex couples have children compared with 11% of same-sex male couple. Households with same-sex couples have higher levels of educational attainment than opposite-sex couples, with 52% of male same-sex householders and 46% of female same-sex householders having a college degree, compared with 36% of opposite-sex couple householders (Women's Health USA, 2013).

Caregivers

In addition to contributing solely or significantly to their family's income through employment, many women are the main caregivers of children and aging parents for their families. Given that women disproportionately carry the responsibility for family caregiving, they may struggle to meet the demands of both work and family care. Caregiving for women is discussed in detail in Chapter 18.

Reproductive Trends

FERTILITY

The general fertility rate for the United States relates the number of births to the number of women of childbearing age. In 2008, the overall fertility rate was 68.6 per 1,000 women of

childbearing age, and in 2013, it was 62.9 in 2014 (Hamilton, Martin, Osternam, & Curtin, 2015). The 2013 birthrates increased slightly (1%) in 2014 among non-Hispanic Black, non-Hispanic White, and Hispanic women. Births among Asian women increased by 6% in 2014. In contrast, among American Indian women, birthrates decreased by 2%.

BIRTHRATES FOR TEENAGERS

The drop in U.S. birthrates for teenagers was first noted after 2007, dropping 7% annually. The annual number in 2014 was 24.2 births per 1,000 women aged 15 to 19 years, a historic low. Birthrates among teenagers fell from 11% for women 15 to 17 years and for women 18 to 19 years declined 8%.

SINGLE-PARENT CHILDBEARING

After rising 13-fold from 1940 through 1990, the rate of increase of nonmarital childbearing slowed during the 1990s. The birthrate among unmarried women increased between 2000 and 2005 from 44.1 births per 1,000 unmarried women aged 15 to 44 years to 47.2 and then declined to 45.2% in 2012 (Monte & Ellis, 2014). Several key factors contributed to the number of nonmarital births through 2012, including increased birthrates and steep increases in the number of unmarried women of childbearing age. Also, the number of women of childbearing age (defined as between 15 and 44 years) increased substantially from the mid-1960s through the early 1990s—reflecting the impact of the baby boom. Furthermore, increasing proportions of women and men delayed marriage beginning in the 1960s, a trend that is not abating.

■ HEALTH STATUS INDICATORS

Health status indicators, one of the simplest ways to understand health status across populations, include using data on mortality, morbidity, and access to and utilization of health services. The following health status indicators are selected primarily based on whether they had a marked impact on women's quality of life, functioning, or well-being; affected a large proportion of women or a subgroup of women; or reflected an important emerging health issue. When data are available and differences for key health conditions are notable, we provide prevalence or incidence estimates based on race/ethnicity and gender. Moreover, given the strong relationship between health and income, which is especially important for women who represent the majority of the poor in the United States, we report health measures by socioeconomic differences.

Life Expectancy

Life expectancy is a key indicator of health status worldwide, and mortality rate is the measure of the number of deaths per unit of the population. The life expectancy of U.S. women has nearly doubled since the turn of the 20th century, from 48 years in 1900 to a record high of 81 years in 2015 (Women's Health USA, 2013). Indeed, a baby girl born in 2011 in the United States has a life expectancy of 81.1 years, 4.8 years longer than her male counterpart who is expected to live an average of 76.3 years. Overall, women are expected to outlive men by an average of 5 to 6 years, and this varies by race/ethnicity. Hispanic women have the longest life expectancy: They are expected to live 83.7 years compared with 78.9 years for Hispanic men. In contrast, non-Hispanic Black women have a life expectancy of 77.8 years compared with 71.6 for Black men (Women's Health USA, 2013). However, by age 65 years, these differences narrow and life expectancy becomes more similar for White and Black women. Life expectancy data are not available for Asian, Native Hawaiian, and other Pacific Islander and American Indian/Alaska Native populations. Although life expectancy has increased since 1970 for both women and men, women's life expectancy increased less than that for men (8.6% vs. 13.7% for men). There is a worrisome increase in women's mortality rates in more than 40% of U.S. counties but this occurred for males in only 3.4% of counties (Women's Health USA, 2013).

Although the United States has the highest health care expenditures as a percentage of gross domestic products than other developed countries, the life expectancy for women is lower in the United States than in several other developed countries (Table 1.2).

Causes of Death

In 1900, the leading causes of mortality among U.S. women included infectious diseases, pregnancy, and childbirth. In the 20th century, significant progress was made toward increasing the years of life for most Americans, and regardless of race/ethnicity or gender, Americans live longer than ever before. Presently, the chronic conditions of heart disease, cancer, respiratory disease, and stroke account for more than half of U.S. women's deaths and are the leading causes of mortality for women (Table 1.3).

TABLE 1.2	Women's Life Expectancy at Birth for Selected Countries, 2013	
COUNTRY	LIFE EXPECTANCY (YEARS)	RANK
Japan	87	1
Spain	86	2
France	85	3
Switzerland	85	3
Australia	85	3
Israel	84	4
Sweden	84	4
Greece	84	4
Ireland	83	5
Denmark	82	6
Costa Rica	81	7
United States	81	7
Panama	81	7
Thailand	79	9
El Salvador	77	11
Fiji	73	15
India	68	19
Haiti	64	23
Afghanistan	62	25
Congo	60	27
Somalia	56	31
Chad	53	34
Sierra Leone	46	36

Source: National Center for Health Statistics (2014a).

TABLE 1.3	Selected Causes of Death for Women, 2010
CAUSE OF DEATH	AGE-ADJUSTED DEATH RATE FOR WOMEN PER 100,000 POPULATON
All causes	634.9
Diseases of the heart	143.3
Ischemic heart disease	84.9
Cerebrovascular diseases	38.3
Malignant neoplasms	146.7
Trachea, bronchus, lung	38.1
Colon, rectum, and anus	13.3
Breast	22.1
Chronic lower respiratory diseases	38
Influenza and pneumonia	13.1
Chronic liver diseases and cirrhosis	6.2
Diabetes mellitus	17.6
Alzheimer's disease	27.3
HIV	1.4
Unintentional injuries	25.6
Motor vehicle-related injuries	6.5
Suicide	5.0
Homicide	2.3
Poison	7.5

Source: National Center for Health Statistics (2014a, Table 20, p. 86).

Although women have a longer life expectancy than men, they do not necessarily live those extra years in good physical and mental health. In 2011, Mississippi, followed by West Virginia, had the highest death rate; Hawaii had the lowest (Figure 1.2). As a nation we are doing well; however, data supports that a few states remain burdened with health status indicators of high mortality rates for men and women, calling for unique and targeted systems interventions.

HIV is claiming an increasing number of young women's lives and is comparable to death rates from homicide. Unintentional injuries and suicides also account for a relatively large number of women's deaths.

Leading causes of death vary by age, with unintentional injury leading the cause of death for women 18 to 44 years of age and the third leading cause for 45- to 65-year-olds. Suicide and homicide are the fourth and fifth causes for

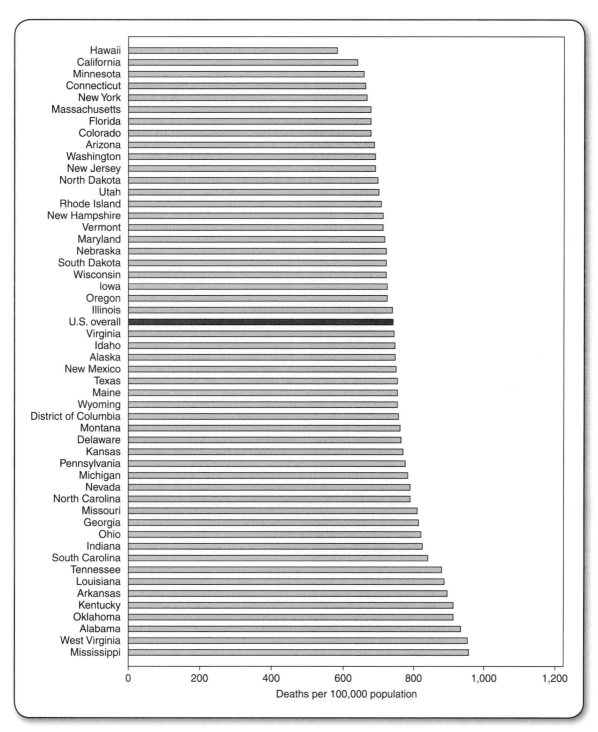

FIGURE 1.2

Comparison of state death rates. Rates per 100,000 population were calculated based on postcensal population as of July 1, 2011, U.S. residents only.

Source: National Vital Statistics System (2012).

18- to 44-year-olds, and HIV and pregnancy complications account for the ninth and tenth leading causes for 18- to 44-year-olds. Liver disease is in the top 10 for all women younger than 65 years of age. Alzheimer's disease and flu/pneumonia are leading causes of death for women 65 years and older (Table 1.4).

Compared with previous years, the 2010 reported causes of death decreased for women with diseases of the heart, cerebrovascular system, malignant neoplasms, influenza, and pneumonia (Centers for Disease Control and Prevention [CDC]/National Center for Health Statistics [NCHS], 2012). In addition, there are differences in the

leading causes of death for women of different racial/ethnic groups. Although the heart disease mortality rate is two thirds higher for Black women than White women, Hispanic, American Indian, and Asian women had lower rates than did White women. Cancer was the second most common cause of death of women in the United States.

Table 1.5 provides estimates of years of life lost before age 75 years according to selected causes of death for women. In addition, there are differences in the years of life lost for the leading causes of death for women of different racial/ethnic groups. In particular, Black women have the greatest number of life years lost for every cause of death

TABLE 1.4	Ten Leading Causes of Death Among Women Aged 18 Years and Older, by Age, 2010			
RANK	TOTAL (%)	18–44 YEARS (%)	45–64 YEARS (%)	65 YEARS AND OLDER (%)
1	Heart disease (23.8)	Unintentional injury (24.0)	Cancer (38.3)	Heart disease (25.9)
2	Cancer (22.4)	Cancer (19.5)	Heart disease (16.2)	Cancer (19.4)
3	Stroke (6.3)	Heart disease (9.8)	Unintentional injury (5.7)	Stroke (7.0)
4	Chronic lower respiratory disease (6.0)	Suicide (7.1)	Chronic lower respiratory disease (4.8)	Chronic lower respiratory disease (6.4)
5	Alzheimer's disease (4.8)	Homicide (3.9)	Stroke (3.7)	Alzheimer's disease (5.9)
6	Unintentional injury (3.5)	Stroke (2.6)	Diabetes (3.4)	Diabetes (2.6)
7	Diabetes (2.8)	Diabetes (2.3)	Liver disease (2.9)	Flu & pneumonia (2.4)
8	Flu and pneumonia (2.2)	Liver disease (2.2)	Suicide (1.9)	Kidney disease (2.2)
9	Kidney disease (2.1)	HIV (2.0)	Septicemia (1.7)	Unintentional injury (2.1)
10	Septicemia (1.5)	Pregnancy complications (1.6)	Kidney disease (1.6)	Septicemia (1.5)

Adapted from Women's Health USA (2013).
Source: Centers for Disease Control and Prevention, National Center for Health Statistics (2012), National Vital Statistics System (2012).

TABLE 1.5	Age-Adjusted Years Lost Before 75 Years for Selected Cause of Death, by Race/Ethnicity in the United States, 2010				
ALL FEMALES	AGE-ADJUSTED YEARS LOST	BLACK	WHITE	HISPANIC	AMERICAN INDIAN	ASIAN
All causes	4,994.0	9,832.5	6,342.8	4,795.1	6,771.3	3,061.2
Diseases of heart	593.6	1,691.1	900.9	598.1	820.9	400.1
Cerebrovascular diseases	149.1	358.1	142.7	150.4	129.7	148.3
Malignant neoplasms	1,301.0	1,796.7	1,375.8	951.2	929.5	874.7
Influenza and pneumonia	60.7	109.8	66.7	57.5	99.3	38.4
Alzheimer's disease	12.6	10.0	12.4	8.4	8.8	3.2
Suicide	163.7	196.4	430.0	193.6	437.9	199.7
Homicide	94.9	821.2	138.7	238.0	256.4	68.8

than all other racial/ethnic groups of women except for suicide and Alzheimer's disease. Years of life lost were greatest for malignant neoplasms and heart disease for women. These estimates reflect the younger age at which women die from cancer and heart disease, as well as the large proportion of the population for whom cerebrovascular disease is a leading cause of death (Table 1.6). There has been a decrease in suicide rates in the case of women, the highest rates being in American Indian women younger than 75 years of age. In contrast, homicide rates have increased for Asians, American Indians, and Hispanics, and the greatest increase is noted among Black women (Health, U.S., 2013).

Morbidity

Morbidity is a generic measure that assesses the quantity of health in a given population and is easy to interpret and compare across populations and time. The incidence of specific outcomes such as injuries, chronic conditions, mental illness, and activity limitations are summary measures of morbidity, which are presented in this section.

INJURIES

In 2012, 37.4 million medically attended episodes of injury and poisoning were reported among the U.S. civilian noninstitutionalized population (CDC, 2012). The age-adjusted injury and poisoning episode rate for women was 79% lower than the rate for men. Falls was the only category of external causes for which the rate for women exceeded that for men (47.2 vs. 37.6 per 1,000 persons, respectively). The higher rate of falls among women is likely because of the higher number of women who are older than 45 years and especially 65 years and older, for whom the rate of falls for women was twice that for men. Poisoning death rates have become the leading mechanism, with most caused by drugs, specifically prescription pain medications. Women have a greater prevalence of chronic pain and are more vulnerable to prescription pain medication dependency (Women's Health USA, 2013).

VIOLENCE AGAINST WOMEN

Violence is a term that encompasses a broad range of maltreatment against women and men. Violence and abuse against women refer to the combination of the following five major components of such maltreatment: physical violence, sexual violence, threats of physical and/or sexual violence, stalking, and psychological/emotional abuse (U.S. Census Bureau, 2015; Women's Health USA, 2013). Physical violence, sexual violence, threats of physical and/or sexual violence, and psychological aggression by a current

TABLE 1.6	Age-Adjusted Cancer Incidence Rates for Selected Cancer Sites in Women: Number of New Cases per 100,000 population, 2010					
ALL FEMALES	**AGE-ADJUSTED YEARS LOST**	**BLACK**	**WHITE**	**HISPANIC**	**AMERICAN INDIAN**	**ASIAN**
Cancer, all sites	415.6	396.2	367.6	303	314	435.4
Lung/bronchus	47.3	51.4	36.4	28.4	24.2	51.2
Colon/rectum	34.2	45.3	41.0	33.3	30.6	34.7
Breast	126.6	121.2	90.5	97.8	85.5	135
Cervix uteri	7.1	8.3	8.3	6.3	10.3	6.1
Corpus and uterus, not otherwise specified	27.4	24.4	27.5	22.1	20.3	28.3
Ovary	13.2	8.9	11.9	9.4	11.7	13.2
Oral cavity and pharynx	6.2	5.2	a	5.1	4.0	6.6
Stomach	4.7	8.3	13.0	8.7	9.2	3.6
Pancreas	10.7	14.9	12.0	10.2	10.1	10.8
Urinary bladder	9.3	6.9	a	4.6	4.4	10.2
Non-Hodgkins lymphoma	17.8	12.4	12.5	11.7	15.5	18.1
Leukemia	10.7	8.6	7.7	5.6	8.6	11

[a]Data not available.
Adapted from National Center for Health Statistics (2014a; see Table 42, p. 155).

or former spouse or dating partner compose the narrower category of intimate partner violence (IPV). Available data suggest that violence against women is a significant public health problem in the United States. Approximately 36% of women 18 years and older reported having experienced rape, physical violence, and/or stalking by an intimate partner, whereas nearly half reported having experienced psychological aggression (Women's Health USA, 2013).

IPV prevalence varies with sexual orientation, with bisexual women (57%) being more likely than lesbian (40%) or heterosexual women (32%) to report lifetime experiences of physical IVP, including slapping, pushing, or shoving and severe acts such as being choked, beaten, or burned. Bisexual women are also more likely to report experiencing severe physical violence, including being choked or beaten (49%) than lesbian (29%) or heterosexual women (24%). Both bisexual and lesbian women reported higher rates of psychological aggression, including name-calling, humiliation, or coercion by an intimate partner (76%, 63%, and 48%, respectively; Women's Health USA, 2013) (see Chapters 20 and 21).

Although these data indicate the high prevalence of the problem, reporting of violence against women remains inconsistent. Although some experts believe that studies overestimate the extent of violence against women, others believe that there is underestimation. To date, few national studies report on women who are immigrants, homeless, disabled, or in the military or other institutionalized situations, which may be populations at significantly greater risk of violence against women.

EMERGING INFECTIONS

Infectious diseases continue to affect all people, regardless of gender, age, ethnic background, lifestyle, and socioeconomic status. They cause suffering and death and impose an enormous financial burden in the United States. Many infectious diseases have been conquered by modern interventions such as vaccines and antibiotics. New diseases are constantly emerging, including Zika, Ebola, severe acute respiratory syndrome, Lyme disease, and hantavirus pulmonary syndrome; others reemerge in drug-resistant forms, including malaria, tuberculosis, and bacterial pneumonias. Among women, populations of particular concern include pregnant women, immigrants, and refugees. For example, if a pregnant woman acquires an infection, it can increase the infant's risk of preterm delivery, low birth weight, long-term disability, or death. Although many of these adverse birth outcomes could be prevented by prenatal care, access to and utilization of prenatal care are disparate by race/ethnicity and socioeconomic status. For example, infants born to American Indian and Black women have the highest neonatal death rates because of infectious diseases than any other group (CDC, Infant mortality in populations, 2013).

ZIKA VIRUS

The Zika virus has a potential impact on sexual and reproductive health of women in the United States. Brazil and Colombia were first to report instances of Zika in the United States. Zika was first isolated in Uganda. Zika, named from a forest in Uganda, is a single-stranded RNA virus. The Zika virus is common in areas of Africa, Asia, and Pacific Islands (CDC, 2016). Dissemination of accurate and current information is critical to prevent panic and myths.

A single-stranded RNA virus, Zika, was first isolated in 1947 from a monkey in the Zika forest (CDC, 2016). The Zika virus has been isolated in sperm, urine, and blood (CDC, 2016). It is spread primarily by mosquito bite, and transmitted by pregnant women to fetus, through blood and sexual contact. The illness is usually mild with symptoms lasting for several days to a week (CDC, 2016). Common symptoms are fever, rash, joint pain, and conjunctivitis. There is no specific antiviral; treatment is symptom management (e.g., rest, fluids, analgesics, and antipyretics; Foy et al., 2011). Health care providers are encouraged to report suspected cases to their state or local health departments to facilitate diagnosis and mitigate the risk of local transmission.

Birth defects such as microcephaly, seizure, intellectual difficulty, and developmental delays have resulted in the babies of women affected during pregnancy. Close monitoring for growth and development is the current management of such infants. Prevention is the primary way of combating the spread of the virus by avoidance of mosquito bites, postponement of travel to areas with Zika, and avoidance of exposure to the virus before, during, and after conception.

HUMAN PAPILLOMAVIRUS

Human papillomavirus (HPV) is the most common sexually transmitted infection (STI) among young adults in the United States (WHO, n.d.). It is estimated that roughly 14 million people will be newly infected in 2016. HPV currently infects about 27% of women in the United States between the ages of 14 and 59 years (CDC, 2015). STIs tend to disproportionately affect women and minorities and are more prevalent in the southern United States.

Generally, when people talk about HPV, the focus is on women, but it does not mean HPV cannot affect men. More than half of men who are sexually active in the United States will have HPV at some time in their life. About 1% of sexually active men in the United States have genital warts at any one time. Four hundred men who get HPV-related cancer of the penis, 1,500 men who get HPV-related cancer of the anus, 5,600 men who get cancers of the oropharynx (back of the throat), have been exposed to a high-risk strain of HPV. The human papillomavirus can remain dormant for months or years before showing signs and symptoms. Low-risk strains of HPV can cause genital warts in both men and women. Genital warts are the first symptom seen in low-risk HPV strains. However, high-risk HPV rarely causes initial symptoms. Genital warts appear as small bumps in the genital area or around the anus. They can be small or large, raised or flat, and even shaped like cauliflower. Pregnant women with genital warts should be counseled concerning the low risk for warts on the larynx (recurrent respiratory papillomatosis) in their infants or children.

In most HPV infections (90%), the virus is self-limiting, without any clinical symptoms, and resolves on its own.

However, when the virus is persistent, lasting longer than 6 to 8 months, or when it is joined by other HPV genotypes there is a greater likelihood of developing cervical cancer precursor cells or an invasive epithelial lesion. HPV is a major etiological factor in the development of benign cervical papillomas as well as cervical cancer. Ten percent of HPV cases become persistent and cause more severe health problems ranging from genital warts to cervical cancer. Ninety percent of all cervical cancer cases are caused by a high-risk type of HPV (see Chapter 32).

HUMAN IMMUNODEFICIENCY VIRUS

In 2011, 23% of all people living with HIV in the United States were women, and they accounted for about 21% of estimated new cases. Although HIV and AIDS disproportionately affect men who have sex with men, a substantial proportion of HIV/AIDS diagnoses occur among women; in particular approximately two of three new diagnoses involve non-Hispanic Black women (40/100,000). White women (2/100,000 women) have the lowest rates of HIV diagnosis, with Hispanic (7.9/100,000), non-Hispanic American Indian/Alaska Native (5.5/100,000), and non-Hispanic women of multiple races (7.5/100,000) having higher rates. Among Black women, HIV affects 40 per 100,000 women (Women's Health USA, 2013).

The CDC estimated that between 120,000 and 160,000 adult and adolescent females were living with HIV infection, including those with AIDS (CDC, 2015). Between 1992 and 2015, the number of persons living with AIDS increased in all groups as a result of the 1993 expanded AIDS case definition and, more recently, improved survival among those who have benefited from the new combination drug therapies. During that period, a growing proportion of women was living with AIDS, reflecting the ongoing trend in populations affected by the epidemic. In 1992, women accounted for 14% of persons living with AIDS. By 1998, the proportion had grown to 20%. Thus, in just over a decade, the proportion of all AIDS cases reported among adult and adolescent women more than tripled, from 7% in 1985 to 23% in 1999. The epidemic has increased most dramatically among Black and Hispanic women (Misra, 1999). Notably, the AIDS epidemic is far from over. Cases of HIV infection reported among 13- to 24-year-olds, of whom nearly 50% are female, are increasing for this age group who had reported recent high-risk behavior.

CHRONIC CONDITIONS

Chronic conditions are often debilitating and contribute significantly to key causes of death among women. There is a complex and long-term interplay between chronic conditions and health across a woman's life span. Although women live longer than men, women also experience greater morbidity at younger ages and utilize health services at higher rates than men. As women progress from childbearing ages through menopause and to postmenopause years, the prevalence of chronic conditions increases, with an associated shift to conditions linked to environmental factors.

Overall, the pattern and magnitude of chronic conditions vary markedly by gender. Women were more likely to report arthritis, cataracts, orthopedic impairment, goiter or thyroid disease, diabetes, hypertension, varicose veins, chronic bronchitis, asthma, and chronic sinusitis; men were more likely to report visual impairment, hearing impairment, and heart disease.

The burden of chronic diseases occurs disproportionately among poor women. Chronic conditions are reported more frequently by low-income and less-educated women (CDC, 2015; Misra, 1999). Based on National Health Interview Survey (NHIS) data, low income was correlated with the occurrence of diabetes, asthma, hypertension, and thyroid disease (National Center for Health Statistics, 2014b). Additionally, the differences in chronic conditions by racial/ethnic populations can differ dramatically. For example, American Indians/Alaska Natives were three times more likely to have had diabetes and end-stage renal disease than Asians/Pacific Islanders and six times more likely to have had these conditions than Whites. Blacks were twice as likely as Asians/Pacific Islanders to have diabetes and end-stage renal disease and four times more likely to have these conditions than Whites (Golden et al., 2015).

In 2014, the age-adjusted incidence of diagnosed type 2 diabetes was 6.5 per 1,000 for women. The reproductive age of 18 to 44 years complicated by type 2 diabetes can be an additional superimposed chronic medical concern for primary care providers. The average age at diagnosis for Whites was 55.4 years, and for Blacks it was 49 and 55.4 years in 2011. Overall, from 1997 to 2011, little to no change in median age at diagnosis has been noted in all race/ethnic groups (Figure 1.3).

Pain conditions are also common in women, especially low back pain and migraine or severe headache. Arthritis is the most common cause of disability among U.S. adults. Although osteoarthritis is the most common, types of arthritis that primarily affect women are lupus, fibromyalgia, and rheumatoid arthritis. Arthritis is more common among women than among men (25% vs. 19%), and increases with age, with 34% of women 45 to 64 years and 55.7% of those older than 65 years having been diagnosed with arthritis. In addition, arthritis prevalence differs by race/ethnicity. More than 25% of non-Hispanic White, non-Hispanic Black, non-Hispanic American Indian/Alaska Native, and non-Hispanic women of multiple races report having been diagnosed with arthritis compared with 19.6% of Hispanic women and 12.9% of non-Hispanic Asian women. Arthritis prevalence is associated with obesity, with 33% of obese women and 19% of neither overweight nor obese women reporting (Women's Health USA, 2013).

Vision loss and hearing loss are both sources of disability for women. Trouble seeing affects approximately 10% of women, whereas hearing difficulty or deafness affects approximately 1.5% (National Center for Health Statistics, 2014b). Although cancer was considered a fatal disease in the early part of the 20th century, it has become a chronic disease for many because survival rates have increased. The leading cause of death among women between 35 and 84 years of age, lung and bronchial cancer now is the leading cause of cancer deaths in women, followed by breast cancer

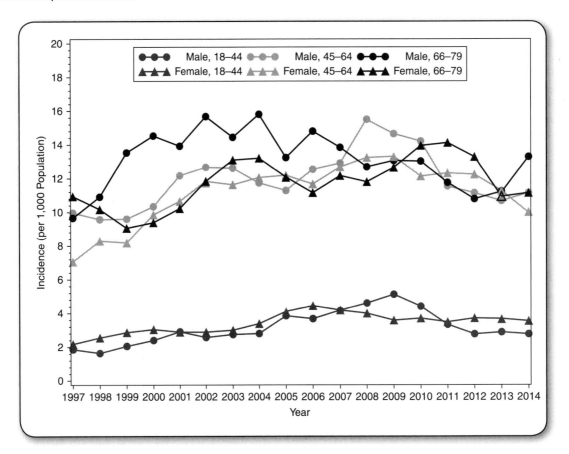

FIGURE 1.3

Age-adjusted incidence of diabetes per 1,000 by age and sex, 1997 to 2014.

Sources: Centers for Disease Control and Prevention (CDC), National Center for Health Statistics, Division of Health Interview Statistics, data from the National Health Interview Survey. Data computed by personnel in CDC's Division of Diabetes Translation, National Center for Chronic Disease Prevention and Health Promotion.

(responsible for 26% and 15% of cancer deaths, respectively). As seen in Table 1.6, colorectal, pancreatic, and ovarian cancers were also major causes of cancer among women. Because survival rates for different types of cancer differ, the most common types of cancer are not always the most common cause of cancer deaths. Lung and bronchial cancer occurs in only 52.4 per 100,000 women compared with breast cancer, which occurs in 118.7 per 100,000 women, but death rates are higher for lung and bronchial cancer because of the lower survival rates (Women's Health USA, 2013). Breast cancer, which is the second most common form of malignancy in U.S. women, has racial disparities. Although 12% to 29% more White women than Black women are diagnosed with breast cancer, Black women are 28% more likely than White women to die from the disease. Also, the 5-year breast cancer survival rate is 69% among Black women compared with 85% for White women.

Heart disease and stroke are the first and third causes of death for women in the United States. Although much attention has focused on the diagnosis and treatment of women with heart disease, an important understanding is the disability associated with these two diseases. Both heart disease and stroke are associated with increasing age, but like other diseases, these vary with socioeconomic status and race/ethnicity. Although similar proportions of

non-Hispanic Black and White women experience heart disease, a higher proportion of non-Hispanic American Indian/Alaska Native and non-Hispanic multiracial women experience heart disease. Stroke incidence increases with age: Rates are 6.1% for women 65 to 74 years of age but 10.9% for those 75 years and older. Also, stroke is more prevalent among those living in poverty, and the proportion of women with stroke decreases from 4.5% for those with incomes less than 100% of the poverty level to 1.8% of those with incomes more than 400% of the poverty level (Women's Health USA, 2013).

Chronic obstructive pulmonary disease (COPD) also is an important source of chronic illness and disability for women, as well as the fourth leading cause of death among U.S. women aged 18 years and older. Approximately 6% of women report having COPD and its prevalence increases with age (11% of women 65–74 years and 10.4% of women 75 and older). COPD varies with race/ethnicity and poverty level. It is most common among non-Hispanic American Indian/Alaska Natives (8.6%) and non-Hispanic women of multiple races (9.9%), followed by non-Hispanic White women (7%), non-Hispanic Black women (6%), Hispanic women (4.9%), and non-Hispanic Asian Women (2.6%). Women living with incomes less than 100% of the poverty level are twice as likely to report COPD as those with an income of 400% of poverty level (10% vs. 4.6%; Women's Health USA, 2013).

Hypertension is common among women, with 27.5% of women having been diagnosed with high blood pressure. Approximately 12% of women have uncontrolled hypertension. Hypertension increases with age, and approximately 75% of women 65 years and older have hypertension. Racial/ethnic variation is evident: More than 40% of non-Hispanic Black women have hypertension compared with 25% of non-Hispanic Whites (Women's Health USA, 2013).

Osteoporosis is more prevalent among women than men and increases with age. Approximately 9% of women have been diagnosed with osteoporosis. One in four women 65 years and older reports having been diagnosed. Non-Hispanic White and Mexican American women 65 years and older were more likely to have been diagnosed with osteoporosis than non-Hispanic Black women (29% and 27% vs. 12.9%). Risk of bone fractures among older women is associated with osteoporosis and may lead to disability and death (Women's Health USA, 2013).

Although overweight and obesity are not diseases, they are associated with increased risk of numerous diseases, including hypertension, type 2 diabetes, cardiovascular and liver diseases, arthritis, some types of cancer, and reproductive health risks. There is little racial/ethnic variation in being underweight, but approximately 37% of non-Hispanic White women were of normal weight (body mass index [BMI], 18.5–24.9) compared with 16.7% of non-Hispanic Black women and 20.5% of Mexican American women. Obesity has increased significantly among non-Hispanic Black and Mexican American women (58% and 45%, respectively). Obesity increases with age (from 26% of women 18–24 years of age and 40% of women 45 years and older) and is more common among women living in households with incomes below the poverty level 45% compared with 29% of those with incomes 300% of the poverty level (Women's Health USA, 2013).

REPRODUCTIVE AND GYNECOLOGIC CONDITIONS

Both reproductive and gynecologic conditions affect a considerable proportion of women. Dysmenorrhea and vulvodynia cause discomfort that interferes with some women's normal activities, but other conditions, such as endometriosis, uterine fibroids, and ovarian cysts, affect fertility and reproductive functioning. Endometriosis and uterine fibroids affected 5.6% and 6.1% of women 15 to 44 years of age, respectively, in 2010. The prevalence of both increases with age, and they are most common among women 35 to 44 years of age (10% and 13%, respectively, for endometriosis and fibroids). Racial/ethnic differences are noteworthy, with 12.3% of non-Hispanic Black women, 5.6% of White women, and 4.2% of Hispanic women experiencing uterine fibroids. Non-Hispanic White women are most likely to experience endometriosis (6.9%) compared with 3.4% of Black and 3.9% of Hispanic women. These two conditions are most often responsible for hysterectomy. Infertility is estimated to affect 14% of all U.S. women 15 to 44 years of age. Infertility increases from 7.3% of women

15 to 24 years of age to 19.6% of those 40 to 44 years of age (Women's Health USA, 2013). In addition to age, endometriosis, obesity, and polycystic ovary syndrome are associated with infertility.

MENTAL ILLNESS

Mental illnesses affect women and men differently. Scientists are only beginning to understand the contribution of various biological and psychosocial factors to mental health and mental illness in both women and men. Research on women's health—which has grown substantially in the last 30 years—helps to clarify the risk and protective factors for mental disorders in women and to improve women's mental health treatment outcomes.

Depressive disorders include major depression, dysthymic disorder (a less severe but more chronic form of depression), and bipolar disorder (manic-depressive illness). In the United States, nearly 10 million women (8.5%) and 5.5 million men (4.9%) were affected by a major depressive episode between 2007 and 2010. Notably, major depression is the leading cause of disease burden among females aged 12 years and older in the United States (CDC, 2014). Figure 1.4 illustrates the differences between men and women reporting symptoms of depression. For all age groups, a higher percentage of women reported higher scores.

Although depression is not the only mental illness that affects women more often than men, it is significant because of its common occurrence, recurrence, and effects on functioning. The prevalence of major depressive episode varies with race/ethnicity. Non-Hispanic White and non-Hispanic multiracial women were most likely to report a major depressive episode during the past year (9.6% and 10.9% respectively). Non-Hispanic Asian women were the least likely to report a major depressive episode in the past year (4.6%). Age influences the prevalence of depressive episodes, with 9% to 11% of women below retirement age versus 2.7% of women aged 65 years and older reporting a major depressive episode (Women's Health USA, 2013). The important influences of income, education, and marital status, as well as age and race/ethnicity, need to be considered in studies of depression.

The main risk factor for developing Alzheimer's disease—a dementing brain disorder that leads to the loss of mental and physical functioning and eventually to death—is increased age. Although the number of new cases of Alzheimer's disease is similar in older adult women and men, the number of existing cases is twice as high among women as among men, with women older than 65 years constituting 3.2 million diagnosed cases. Alzheimer's disease death rates have increased between 2000 and 2010 by about 40%, from 141.2 to 196.9 deaths per 100,000 people. The greater prevalence and mortality among women appear to be related to their longevity rather than to an increased sex-specific disease risk (Women's Health USA, 2013).

Caregivers of people with Alzheimer's disease are usually wives and daughters, with women constituting 70% of the 15.4 million Americans who provide unpaid care for a person with Alzheimer's or another dementia (Women's

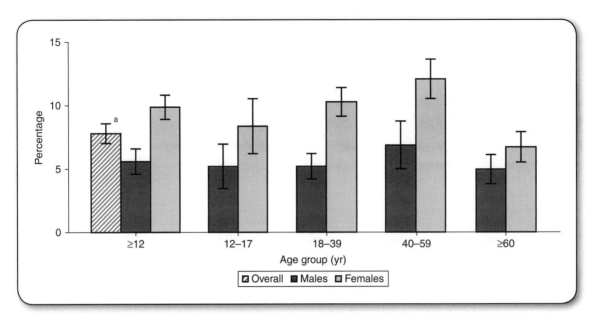

FIGURE 1.4

Depression among persons 12 years or older in the United States, 2007–2010. Current depression was determined based on responses to the Patient Health Questionnaire, which asks about symptoms of depression during the preceding 2 weeks. Depression was defined by a score of greater than or equal to 10 of a possible total score of 27.

[a]95% confidence interval.

Source: Centers for Disease Control (2012), United States, National Health and Nutrition Examination Survey, 2007–2010.

Health USA, 2013). The chronic stress often associated with caregiving for someone with dementia can contribute to mental health problems for the caregiver (see Chapter 18). Because women in general are at greater risk of depression than men, and as caregivers are much more likely to suffer from depression than the average person, women caregivers of people with Alzheimer's disease may be particularly vulnerable to depression.

Mental issues such as schizophrenia, depression, bipolar disorders, Alzheimer's disease, and obsessive-compulsive disorders affect nearly one in five Americans each year. Nearly 70% of adults with a diagnosed mental disorder do not receive treatment. Among all areas of health care, the mental health field is beset by disparities in the availability of and access to services occurring by means of financial barriers and stigmatization (Reeves et al., 2011).

The first Surgeon General's report on mental health underscored the close relationship between mental and physical health (U.S. Department of Health and Human Services, 1999). Comorbid conditions are common among those diagnosed with mental illness, and it is not unusual for women to experience both depression and substance abuse. About 6% of women diagnosed with major depressive disorder were three times as likely to report substance-use disorder as those who did not, but men were more likely than women to experience a substance-use disorder (11.9% vs. 6%; Women's Health USA, 2013). In addition, women with mental health problems also experience chronic illnesses such as diabetes or hypertension, and some health problems are exacerbated by psychotherapeutic medications.

WOMEN'S PERCEPTION OF THEIR HEALTH AND LIMITATIONS IN FUNCTIONING

Many women who experience chronic illness, whether mental or physical, also experience limitation of activity related to their conditions. About 17% of women report limitations related to chronic illness: Nearly 10% report fair or poor health, by their own assessment and self-assessed health status, severe psychological distress, and 3.7% report serious psychological distress (National Center for Health Statistics, 2014a).

ACTIVITY LIMITATIONS

Women's quality of life is affected by their ability to carry out daily activities at work, at home, and in the community. Adverse health affects all aspects of women's lives, particularly their ability to engage in daily activities. Activity limitation caused by a physical, mental, or emotional health problem is a broad measure of health functioning for women. Women were nearly twice as likely as men to report activity limitation in 2011 to 2012 (17% compared with 9%). Activity limitation caused by chronic conditions was substantially higher among women with lower family incomes (Women's Health USA, 2013).

Health Care Access and Utilization

Women in the United States obtain health care services through a variety of sources. Numerous factors, including affordability and availability of services and information about how and why it is important to access and utilize such services, affect their access to these services. Given the consolidation of the health care system, the shift to managed care, and decreased public funding of health care and health-related programs, the changes in health care delivery have serious implications for women's health care utilization. Although women commonly enter the health care delivery system for pregnancy prevention or pregnancy-related services, these reproductive health services are typically provided separately from other aspects of women's health care. Health services organizations for women include private- and public-sector groups. For women, the fragmentation of care, lack of coordination of services, and discontinuities in the health care delivery system contribute to higher costs to individual women and both deficiencies and excesses in care.

Access to health care is important for preventive care and for prompt treatment of illness and injuries. Indicators of health care access and utilization include use of preventive services, outpatient care, and inpatient care, and access to these varies by health insurance status, poverty status, and race/ethnicity. Women's access to health care services is seriously compromised by inadequate health insurance, and women without health insurance generally cannot obtain appropriate health care. Despite the *Healthy People 2020* objective that all people in the United States have health insurance coverage, in 2011, nearly 16% of U.S. women were uninsured (Women's Health USA, 2013). Although little is known about how women obtain basic health care in the United States, national survey data report that women are more likely than men to have a usual source of care, have more outpatient visits, have more hospital stays (even excluding maternity stays), use home health services, and use nursing homes.

PUBLICLY FUNDED HEALTH PROGRAMS

The two major publicly funded health programs are Medicare and Medicaid. Medicare is funded by the federal government and reimburses the elderly and disabled for their health care. Medicaid is funded jointly by federal and state governments to provide health care for the poor. Although Medicaid eligibility and benefits vary by state, Medicare and Medicaid health care utilization and costs often vary dramatically by state. Women are more likely to

qualify for Medicaid given their disproportionate share of poverty. More than two thirds of 18- to 64-year-old women are covered by publicly funded insurance, accounting for more than two thirds of Medicaid and 13% of Medicare recipients, and 20% have dual coverage. Approximately 9.4% of women in this age group rely on other sources, (e.g., the military; Women's Health USA, 2013).

The Patient Protection and Affordable Care Act promises to have dramatic effects on women's access to health care as well as to a variety of preventive services. See Chapter 3 for a more detailed discussion of this coverage for women.

PRIVATELY FUNDED HEALTH CARE

Approximately 67% of U.S. women younger than 65 years had some form of private health insurance, most of which is obtained through the workplace. As the health insurance marketplace continues to rapidly change as new types of managed care products emerge, the share of an employee's total compensation for health insurance and the use of traditional fee-for-service medical care continues to decline markedly. Approximately 13% of women had public insurance and 19.5% were uninsured. Health insurance coverage varies by race/ethnicity, with non-Hispanic Whites having coverage (75.4%), non-Hispanic Black (55%), but less than 50% of non-Hispanic American Indian/Alaska Natives and Hispanics (46.6% and 45.3%, respectively) having coverage. Public coverage is most common among non-Hispanic Black and non-Hispanic American Indian/Alaska Natives (37% vs. 30%; Women's Health USA, 2013). Although women and men report similar levels of enrollment for private insurance, enrollment varies significantly by race/ethnicity and poverty status (Table 1.7).

HEALTH CARE PAYMENT AND EXPENDITURES

Major sources of payment for health care in the United States include the government and employers. The United States continues to spend more on health care than any other industrialized country, and health spending is increasing rapidly (National Center for Health Statistics, 2005). The expenditures for prescription drugs increased more rapidly than any other type of health expenditure. The United States continues to spend a larger proportion of its

TABLE 1.7	Men's and Women's Health Insurance Status, 2012		
CHARACTERISTICS	**% OF POPULATION WITH PRIVATE HEALTH INSURANCE**	**% OF POPULATION WITH MEDICAID**	**% OF POPULATION WITH NO HEALTH INSURANCE**
Female	61.9	19.3	15.6
Male	61.8	16.3	18.8

Source: National Center for Health Statistics (2014a; Tables 122, p. 350; 124, p. 356; 125, p. 359).

gross national product on health care than any other major industrialized country. Much of U.S. health care spending is directed to care for chronic diseases and conditions that reflect the aging population.

PREVENTION SERVICES

The use of prevention services has substantial positive effects on the long-term health status of women. The use of several different types of preventive services has been increasing; however, disparities in their use according to income and by race/ethnicity persist among all persons.

The importance of promoting wellness and preventing illness among women involves screening for conditions such as breast, cervical, and colorectal cancer. Regular mammographic screening for women aged 50 years and older is effective in reducing deaths from breast cancer. In 2013, approximately 65% of women aged 65 years and older had had a mammogram within the previous 2 years. Among those 40 years and older, the proportion of women receiving mammograms was 64% or greater for all racial/ethnic groups except multiracial women. The proportion of women receiving mammograms was higher among those with greater levels of education (53% for those who had not completed high school) and much lower (36%) for women who were uninsured than for those with private insurance (74%) or Medicaid (64%). The percentage of women 18 to 44 years of age and 45 to 64 years was relatively high (80% and 77%, respectively), but the proportion older than 65 years dropped to 47%, consistent with changing guidelines about screening. Women who reported having Pap tests within the previous 3 years differed by race/ethnicity. The reported prevalence was as follows: non-Hispanic Black women, 78%; non-Hispanic White women, 73%; Hispanic women, 74%; American Indian/Alaskan Native women, 73%; and Asian women, 68%.

Finally, colorectal cancer is the third leading cause of cancer-related deaths among women after lung and breast cancer. Early detection and treatment can substantially reduce the risks associated with colorectal cancer for people aged 50 years and older. Other preventive strategies relevant to women include the HPV vaccine to prevent cervical cancer, anal cancer, and genital warts. In 2011, only approximately 30% of young women 18 to 26 years of age had at least one dose. The lowest rates are among Hispanics (21.6%) and non-Hispanic Asians (21.4%), and the highest rates are among non-Hispanic Whites and Blacks (33.6% and 29.7%, respectively; Women's Health USA, 2013). In 2011, only 65% of women 65 years of age and older received pneumococcal vaccines. For women older than 65 years, non-Hispanic Whites and non-Hispanic multirace women had the highest rates (68.6% and 78.8%, respectively). For other groups of women, rates were 45% to 50% (Women's Health USA, 2013). The preventive care provisions of the Patient Protection and Affordable Care Act should improve access to these preventive services by expanding health insurance access and requiring new plans to cover U.S. Preventive Services Task Force (USPSTF)-recommended preventive services and well-woman visits without co-payments required (Women's Health USA, 2013).

OUTPATIENT CARE

Important changes in the delivery of health care in the United States are driven in large part by the need to contain rising costs. One significant change has been a decline in the use of inpatient services and an increase in outpatient services such as outpatient surgery and hospice care. From 2009 to 2011, nearly 87% of women had a usual source of care, a place where they could go when sick, such as an office for health professionals or health center, but not an emergency department. More than 90% of women who have private or public insurance coverage had a usual source of care compared with only 56% who were uninsured. In addition to varying health insurance coverage, having access to a usual source of care varies with race/ethnicity. Nearly 89% of non-Hispanic White women, 85% of non-Hispanic Black women, 85% of American Indian/Alaska Natives, 85.7% of Asians, 85% of Native Hawaiian/Pacific Islanders, and 82% of multirace women but only 78.6% of Hispanics reported a usual source of care (Women's Health USA, 2013). Having a usual source of care is more commonly experienced by older women who are most likely to have health insurance: Nearly 97% of those older than 65 years had a usual source of care compared with nearly 79% of women 18 to 34 years of age (Women's Health USA, 2013).

Although women frequently enter the health care delivery system with reproductive health concerns, they seldom have the opportunity to benefit from primary care that is comprehensive and coordinated. Regardless of the type of provider or reason for accessing care, women's health care delivery in the United States remains fragmented. An estimated 80% of women report that they have a usual source of care, which is predominately in physician offices. Among physician providers, family practitioners, general internists, and OB/GYNs provide the majority of basic health care to women; however, women may rely on multiple providers (Women's Health USA, 2013). For example, 33% of women aged 18 years and older reported seeing an OB/GYN and an additional primary care provider for their regular care. Women who used two or more physicians for regular care were more likely to be younger, have private insurance, and have higher income than women who used only one physician. Also, these women were more likely to have more annual visits and to receive more clinical preventive services. Among women who relied on only one physician, 39% reported using a family practitioner or an internist, 16% used an OB/GYN, 3% used a specialist, and 10% had no regular physician. Finally, despite estimates that more than 100,000 advanced practice nurses deliver primary health care, less than 2% of women report using nonphysician providers as a regular source of care.

Women made the majority of their health care visits to physicians' offices, with the number increasing as women aged. A similar pattern with age was found for hospital inpatient visits and emergency departments, with the latter especially pronounced for women 75 years and older (Table 1.8; National Center for Health Statistics, 2014a).

In 2007, an estimated 1,459,000 women received home health care, with 31% of patients younger than 65 years.

TABLE 1.8	Women's Visits to Offices, Outpatient Settings, and Departments, 2010: Per 100 Persons			
AGE	ALL SETTINGS	PHYSICIAN OFFICES	HOSPITAL OUTPATIENT	DEPARTMENTS
Younger than 18 years	322	252	33	37
18–44 years	415	323	35	57
45–54 years	450	372	37	40
55–64 years	546	469	46	31

Of the remainder of women patients, 18% were 65 to 74 years, 29% 75 to 84 years, and 22% older than 85 years. In addition, 1,045,100 women received hospice care during that same year in the United States. *Hospice care* is defined as a program of palliative and supportive care services that provides physical, psychological, social, and spiritual care for dying persons, their families, and loved ones. Of the patients enrolled in hospice care, 17% were younger than 65 years, with the remainder accounting for hospice care divided among those 65 to 74 years (15%), 75 to 84 years (29%), and 85 years and older (38%). There is a striking increase in the use of each service as women age. The most common admission diagnoses for home health care include malignant neoplasms; diabetes; diseases of the nervous system and sense organs, circulatory, respiratory, and musculoskeletal systems; decubitus ulcers; and fractures. Primary admission diagnoses for hospice care include malignant neoplasms and diseases of the heart and respiratory system.

The proportion of women living in nursing homes is also noteworthy. More than 1,061,000 women resided in nursing homes during 2007, with only 6.4 per 100,000 younger than 65 years of age. Of women 65 to 74 years of age, 98 per 100,000 resided in nursing homes, and of those 75 to 84 years about 423 per 100,000 resided in nursing homes, increasing after age 85 years to 1,651 per 100,000 (National Center for Health Statistics, 2014a). Differences in marital status between older women and men are reflected in both their living arrangements, such as in a nursing home, and in their relationship to their informal caregivers. Women tend to care for their spouses or partners, and, as they age, they find themselves living alone (about 30%). Although most men were cared for by a spouse, lived with family members, and had a primary caregiver with whom they lived, women were more likely to live alone or with nonfamily members. Notably, the primary caregiver of most women was a relative other than a spouse—most often a child or child-in-law.

As more people live to the oldest ages and because the incidence of many debilitating illnesses such as diabetes, dementia, and osteoporosis increases with age, the number of elderly nursing home residents will continue to grow and issues surrounding long-term care will become increasingly important. The majority of nursing home residents were White, widowed, and functionally dependent women. The leading admission diagnoses for elderly nursing home residents (both men and women) were diseases of the circulatory system, followed by mental disorders.

INPATIENT CARE

Hospitalization is dependent not only on a woman's medical condition, but also on her ability to access and use ambulatory health care. Delaying or not receiving timely and appropriate care for chronic conditions and other health problems may lead to the development of more serious health conditions that require hospitalization. Utilization of inpatient services has declined, as has the number of beds in community hospitals. The National Hospital Discharge Survey is the principal source of national data on the characteristics of patients discharged from nonfederal short-stay hospitals.

Hospital costs are the highest of any type of health care service. For example, in 2010, mean health care expenses of women older than 18 years who had an expense were greatest for hospital inpatient services at $15,792 per person, compared with home health services at $5,066, hospital outpatient services at $2,529, and office-based services at $1,645. Prescription medications cost women an average of $1,617 per person and emergency room services, $1,461 on average. Dental services cost an average of $677 per woman (Women's Health USA, 2013). The average cost of total health care services per woman was $6,066 in 2010. Women paid approximately 14.4% of these expenses out of pocket. When they are hospitalized, women have shorter average lengths of stay than men (4.5 vs. 5.5 days in 2010), but the pattern of diagnoses and procedures varied between women and men in large part because of hospitalizations for pregnancy-related causes (including deliveries and diagnoses associated with pregnancy). For women younger than 18 years of age, pneumonia, asthma, injuries, and fractures account for the major reasons for hospitalization. For women 18 to 44 years, HIV infection, childbirth, alcohol and drug problems, serious mental illness, diseases of the heart, intervertebral disc disorders, injuries, and fractures constitute major reasons for hospitalization. For women 45 to 64 years, major reasons for hospitalization are cancer, diabetes, alcohol and drug problems, diseases of the heart, stroke, pneumonia, injuries, and fractures. For those 65 to 74 years old, major causes of hospitalization are cancer, diabetes, serious mental illness, disease of the heart, stroke, pneumonia, osteoarthritis, injuries, and hip fracture. For those 75 years and older, primary causes of hospitalization include cancer, diabetes, serious mental illness, diseases of the heart, stroke, pneumonia, osteoarthritis, injuries, and hip fracture.

ORAL CARE

Dental health care is essential for oral health and for the prevention and treatment of tooth decay and infection. In 2011, women were more likely than men to have a dental visit (65% vs. 58%). Dental visits were more common among women with household incomes 400% of poverty (82%) compared with women with incomes less than 100% of poverty (42.6%). Cost represents a significant barrier for women in accessing dental care. Only 20% of adults have dental insurance. In 2011, 16% of women did not obtain needed care because they could not afford it. The rate for women not getting needed care was greater for women with public insurance (23%) and for those who were uninsured (36%; Women's Health USA, 2013).

Health Behaviors

All people engage in behaviors that are either helpful or harmful to themselves and others, with consequences to their health and well-being that will have both immediate and long-term effects. Many of these patterns of behavior are associated with morbidity and mortality. Exercising, not smoking, not using drugs, drinking alcohol in moderation, and good nutrition can improve or maintain women's general health and well-being and can also reduce the risk of selected morbidities and the consequences of such morbidities.

PHYSICAL ACTIVITY

The 1996 Surgeon General's report on physical activity and health reported that three quarters of U.S. adults exercise during their leisure time (U.S. Department of Health and Human Services, 1996). Despite the implementation of the Title IX, Education Amendments of 1972, which provides for equal opportunity for women in school sporting activities, one third of women report no leisure-time physical activity. Women's multiple roles in the workplace and at home compete with leisure-time physical activity. The 2008 Physical Activity Guidelines for Americans recommend that adults should engage in at least 2.5 hours of moderate-intensity or 1.25 hours of vigorous-intensity aerobic activity (e.g., jogging) per week or a combination of both plus muscle-strengthening activities on at least 2 days per week (see Chapter 14). In 2011, 16.6% of women met the recommendations for both adequate aerobic and muscle-strengthening activity versus 24% of men. Women were a lot less likely to meet muscle-strengthening activity recommendations compared with aerobic activity (19.8% vs. 43.9%). Physical activity varied with education and race/ethnicity. Women with a college degree were more than twice as likely to meet aerobic activity guidelines as women without a high school diploma (59.3% vs. 25.9%) and muscle-strengthening guidelines (30.4% vs. 7.6%). White women and non-Hispanic women of multiple races were more likely to report adequate aerobic activity and muscle-strengthening activity than women of other race/ethnic groups; 23% of non-Hispanic women of White and multiple races reported adequate levels of muscle-strengthening activity versus 15% or less among other groups of women (Women's Health USA, 2013). Some unintended adverse health consequences can result from physical activity. For example, exercise undertaken incorrectly can lead to musculoskeletal injuries and metabolic abnormalities. Also, excessive exercise among girls during puberty can result in the female athlete triad: disordered eating, amenorrhea, and osteoporosis (see Chapter 14).

NUTRITION

Given the established relationship between nutrition and health, the majority of health promotion behavior changes are nutrition related. The nutritional status of adult women is the culmination of nutrient intake, metabolism, and utilization over their life span. Although the link between nutrition and good health is established (see Chapter 13), women's eating patterns are affected by numerous societal factors that reflect the cultural and socioeconomic landscape of the 21st century. These factors include increased employment outside the home, consumption of convenience foods, meals eaten away from home, single woman–headed households, and tobacco use. For many reasons such as professional fulfillment, economic necessity, and TANF, women of all age groups are employed and thus burdened by the multiple responsibilities of employment, child care, and home management, which leaves minimal time and energy to prepare well-balanced, home-cooked meals for themselves and their families. Because nutrition is a modifiable factor for numerous chronic diseases, the *Healthy People 2020* nutritional initiative includes objectives that concern weight gain, obesity, dietary intake, and nutrients (folate, calcium, and iron), which directly impact women's health. In 2007 to 2010, 43% of women reported that they had consumed fast food. On average, those who did consumed about 25% of their total daily calories from these items. Fast food consumption declined with age, such that 59% of women aged 18 to 24 years consumed fast food compared with 22.9% of women 65 years and older. More than half of non-Hispanic Black women consumed fast food (55.5%), followed by 47.8% of Mexican American women and 41.4% of non-Hispanic White women. Consumption of sugar-sweetened beverages varied with household income, with 60% of women with incomes less than 200% of poverty compared with 36.3% of women with incomes of 400% of poverty. Sugar-drink consumption ranged from 43% among non-Hispanic White women to 66.1% of non-Hispanic Black women (Women's Health USA, 2013).

Federal programs of the U.S. Department of Agriculture provide help to low-income families in obtaining food. The Supplemental Nutrition Assistance Program (SNAP), formerly the Federal Food Stamp Program, provides benefits for purchasing foods to individuals and families with incomes usually below 130% of poverty. In 2011, SNAP served a record high of 44.1 million people per month, about one in seven Americans. Among households that relied on SNAP, 5.1 million (24.5%) were female-headed households with children. They accounted for 52% of all SNAP households with children. In addition, the Special

Supplemental Nutrition Program for Women, Infants, and Children (WIC) also serves low-income women and families by providing supplementary nutritious foods, nutrition education, breastfeeding support, and referrals to health and social services. In 2012, WIC served nearly 2.1 million pregnant women and mothers, accounting for 23.5% of WIC participation. In addition, more than 75% of the 8.9 million individuals receiving WIC benefits were infants and children.

Food security, having access at all times to enough food for an active, healthy life, is becoming a more prevalent issue in the United States. Households with low food security have multiple food access issues, but little if any reduced food intake. Those with very low food security have reduced food intake and disrupted eating patterns. In 2011, nearly 18 million households experienced food insecurity for one or more members at some point in the year. Very low food security increased from 5.4% to 5.7% in 2011, returning to levels seen in 2008 and 2009 during the recession. Food security varies with household composition. Women and men living alone had similar rates of food insecurity (15%), but female-headed households with children and no spouse were more likely than male-headed households with no spouse to experience food insecurity (36.8% vs. 24.9%). Also female-headed households were more likely than male-headed households to experience very low food security (11.5% vs. 75%; Women's Health USA, 2013).

SUBSTANCE ABUSE

Substance abuse may have a profound impact on the current and future health of women. Women who use illicit substances are more likely to have poor nutrition and serious morbidity and to die from drug overdose, suicide, and violence. Furthermore, studies report an increased risk of mental disorders, including major depression, anxiety disorders, and posttraumatic stress disorder (Kessler et al., 1997). Rates of substance use and choice of substance vary by gender, age, race/ethnicity, educational attainment, and poverty status.

Federal law defines illicit drugs as marijuana, cocaine, heroin, hallucinogens, stimulants, inhalants, and nonmedical use of prescription-type psychotherapeutic drugs, such as pain medications, and sedatives. The number of poisoning deaths, most of which are drug related, has increased, including those tracked to use of prescription pain medications, and have surpassed motor vehicle accidents as the leading cause of fatal injury in the United States. From 2009 to 2011, 6.7% of women (vs. 11% of men) aged 18 years and older used an illicit drug within the previous month. Most commonly used were marijuana (4.9% for women) and psychotherapeutic drugs (nonmedical use; 2.3%). Less than 1% of women used cocaine, heroin, hallucinogens, or inhalants. Among women, 17% of those 18 to 25 years of age reported using an illicit drug during the previous month compared with less than 5% of women 50 years and older. Non-Hispanic Asian women and Hispanic women were less likely than women of other racial/ethnic groups to report using illicit

drugs in the previous month. Illicit drug use was more common among non-Hispanic women of multiple races (9%) and non-Hispanic White women (97.5%) than among non-Hispanic Black women (6.7%; Women's Health USA, 2013).

Although women are more likely than men to be lifetime abstainers, women appear to suffer more severe consequences than men do after shorter duration of less alcohol intake. From 2009 to 2011, 21% of women reported consuming four or more drinks on a single occasion over the course of about 2 hours (binge drinking) and 7.3% reported heavy drinking (consuming on average more than one drink per day). Drinking patterns are related to both household income and age and race/ethnicity. At incomes of 200% of poverty level, women and men were equally likely to drink heavily (8.2%), and binge drinking tended to increase with income. Nearly 38% of women aged 18 to 25 years reported binge drinking in the previous month compared with 6.2% of those 65 years and older. Heavy drinking was also more common among young women (11.4%) and decreased to less than 7% of women aged 35 years and older. Binge drinking ranged from 9% among non-Hispanic Asian women to about 25% of non-Hispanic White and native Hawaiian/other Pacific Islander women (Women's Health USA, 2013).

Cigarette smoking is the major preventable cause of mortality among adult women and leads to an increased risk of cancer, heart disease, stroke, reproductive health problems, and pulmonary conditions. Once women start smoking, they continue to smoke for a number of reasons, including nicotine addiction, stress management, struggles against depression, and weight management. Women are less likely to report smoking than men, with approximately one in four women reportedly smoking. From 2009 to 2011, the prevalence of smoking among women was highest among American Indian women (33.9%) and lowest among non-Hispanic Asian women (6.9%; Table 1.9). Notably, the prevalence of smoking was lower among women with more education (11.8% of those with a college degree vs. 32% of those without high school education. Smoking cessation is an important way to reduce the risk of poor health. From 2009 to 2011, 8% to 9% of those who had ever smoked daily and who had smoked in the previous 3 years did not smoke in the previous year. The proportions of adults who quit smoking vary with education attainment, being greatest among women with college degrees (12.2%). The Patient Protection and Affordable Care Act provides tobacco-cessation treatment and counseling without cost sharing (Women's Health USA, 2013).

Overall, the profile of health-promoting behaviors for women shows that activity levels decrease with age and that only about 20% of young adult women engage in regular physical activity that meets guidelines for aerobic and muscle-strengthening activity. Fat and carbohydrate intake remains relatively stable at 50% and 33%, respectively, across the life span, but total number of kilocalories taken in decreases with age. The proportion of women at a healthy weight (not overweight or obese) increases as women age.

TABLE 1.9	Percentage of Women Who Currently Smoke Cigarettes, by Age and Race, 2012		
AGE (YEARS)	ALL WOMEN	WHITE	BLACK OR AFRICAN AMERICAN
18–24	14.5	16.9	7.4
25–34	19.4	20.7	17.3
35–44	16.1	17.6	11.2
45–64	18.9	19.4	20.4
65 and older	7.5	7.5	9.1

Source: National Center for Health Statistics (2013).

Changing Women's Health

BIOLOGICAL AND ENVIRONMENTAL FACTORS

The last decade of the 20th century was a time of significant advances in women's health. Prompted by the feminist movement of the 1960s and 1970s, increasing attention to women's health brought changes in health services, such as freestanding birth centers, development of academic coursework in women's health for professionals and the general public, and advances in research about women's health. Each of these changes portends enhanced possibilities for women's health during the 21st century. The consequences of advanced understanding of women's health through research may be the most dramatic in the decades ahead.

THE HUMAN GENOME

Research focused on the human genome has revealed new understandings about sex differences that may have profound implications for women's health. Not only have new insights about sex differences in the genetic bases for phenotypic differences between men and women revolutionized this field, but also some genetic discoveries have been made that may drive health consequences for women. An Institute of Medicine (2001) report provides significant evidence that sex does matter. Being male or female is linked to differences in health and illness, and these differences are influenced by genetic, physiological, environmental, and experiential factors. Although in many instances sex differences can be traced to the effects of reproductive hormones, hormones are no longer a universal explanation for these differences. Research on understanding the human genome has provided a basis for learning about the molecular and cellular mechanisms that underlie sex-specific differences in phenotype. Many of these new understandings warrant further investigation. Sexual genotype (XX in females and XY in males) has effects far beyond elaboration of reproductive hormones. Genes on sex chromosomes can be expressed differently in females and males. Single or double copies of the genes, meiotic effects, X-chromosome inactivation, and genetic imprinting are a few of the phenomena involved. X-chromosome inactivation is the random silencing of one or the other X-chromosome that takes place during early embryonic development. X-chromosome inactivation, which occurs about the time of implantation, is a unique biochemical process in that it occurs only in females. Females inherit a paternally imprinted X-chromosome, unlike males, who inherit only a maternally imprinted X-chromosome. A subset of genes on the X-chromosome may escape inactivation. As a result, females can get double doses of certain genes. The Y-chromosome has a host of actively transcribed genes that are expressed throughout the male body but are absent from the female body.

Although the new biological discoveries are important to the understanding of women's health, it remains important to recall that these sex differences are not the same as gender differences. Sex differences refer to differences that are biologically driven, whereas gender refers to differences that are socially influenced: self-representation as male or female and social responses to one's phenotype. There are many differences between males and females in basic cellular biochemistries that can affect health, and many do not arise only because of hormonal differences between the sexes. Research is in progress on the functions and effects of X-chromosome– and Y-chromosome–linked genes in somatic as well as germ cells. Mechanisms of influence of genetic sex differences in biological organization (cell, organ, organ system, and organism), effects of genes versus the effects of hormones, and sex differences across the life span remain to be fully understood.

ENVIRONMENTS FOR WOMEN'S HEALTH

The effects of women's environmental exposures on their health have gained scientific attention (Haynes et al., 2000). As a basis for its work, the Federal Interagency Working Group on Women's Health and the Environment of the Department of Health and Human Services defined environment to include the home, school, indoor and outdoor workplaces, public and private facilities and outdoor spaces, and health care services and recreational settings. Women's health can be affected by the products women use in these settings as well as by contact with physical, chemical, and biological toxicants in air, water, soil, food, and other organisms. In addition, lifestyle, substances ingested, and economic circumstances can influence health. There are multiple mechanisms by which environmental exposures can influence health. For example, environmental chemicals may increase or decrease signaling molecules by mimicking or blocking effector molecule signals that disrupt signal pathways.

How populations differ in their susceptibility and how susceptibility changes over time may be explained in part by focusing on the intersection of genetic and environmental influences—for example, understanding how environmental agents with estrogenic-like activity interact with genes. Study of endocrine disruptors and their potentially adverse health effects could contribute significantly to improving women's health through curtailment of environmental exposures. In addition, studies of genetic susceptibility to environmental exposures—for example, the *NATZ* gene, which determines slow acetylation among smokers and its effect on breast cancer—may help reduce risk if these biological indicators become readily available to women.

Finally, as we have come to appreciate the disparities in health experienced by many populations of women, we are beginning to understand the utility of the concept of gender disparities. Health disparities exist when there are differences in the incidence, prevalence, mortality, and burden of disease and other adverse health outcomes when compared with the general population. Sociocultural environments form the context for women's lives and have profound effects on their health and that of future generations. The critical intersection of gender, race/ethnicity, class, and age shapes the environments that influence women's chances for health. Consequently, it is difficult to attribute gender disparities in health to biology, environments, physiology, or human experience. The intersection of gender with other characteristics often determines women's

- Exposures to toxins
- Social relations such as those linked to low social and economic status
- Racism
- Sexism
- Heterosexism
- Stress
- Tobacco/alcohol/other substance use

Sociocultural as well as physical and chemical environments thus form the context for women's lives and have profound effects on their health and that of future generations. It is therefore critical to consider women's health from an integrative perspective and to move beyond research describing the nature of women's health problems to that which engages women in the study of solutions to their health problems. Likewise, it is critical to consider both the individual experience of health as well as the community's health. A multilevel approach to health is important in order to institute the kinds of programs that are likely to be successful in improving women's chances for good health.

GLOBALIZATION

A final important factor influencing women's health in the 21st century is globalization. As economic forces move women into a global economy, some would point out that the world continues to be an unsafe place for girls and women. Meleis (2005) asserted that the gender divide compromises the safety of women. Women are at risk for violence, rape, trafficking, and abuse. Their mortality and injury rates reflect the limited definition of the nature and type of work they do. Conditions expose them to infections such as HIV/AIDS, pregnancy and birthing cycles, and unsafe abortions owing to the inadequacy and inaccessibility of health services. Meleis urges several urgent actions to enhance safe womanhood, not just safe motherhood. Among these are addressing health risks associated with women's work, marriage, violence, reproductive rules, and access to resources. The education of young girls sets their horizons by determining their options for work. How work is defined limits consideration of the nature, burden of double and triple shifts, and hazards of work that are not currently considered in the economic and labor statistics or health studies. Marriage defines many women and obligates them to provide services and resources to husbands and families, as well as shoulder the burdens of multiple roles. Battering and abuse of girls and women, trafficking, and access to income through sex work all put women at great health risk, including for HIV/AIDS. Wars and terrorism increase women's chances of rape and burden. Pregnancy, birth, and motherhood also escalate the risk of poor health for women. Finally, health care services that are fragmented, inaccessible, and focused on disease rather than prevention and health promotion become a source of overload for women. The invisibility of women's health care issues on national and international agendas intensifies the risk for women.

Meleis proposes that a fundamental change is necessary in the conceptual framework for women's health. She recommends using a human rights framework that is guided by a focus on women's life situations and experiences as a starting point for considering health. Stigma, exploitation, and oppression are key concepts in understanding women's health. Second, she urges redefinition of women's work from employment to a multidimensional framework that includes the amount of energy, activity, and space occupied; the amount and quality of time; the resources for their work; and the results, values, and meaning of their work. Third, she recommends development of policies that acknowledge women's perspectives, experiences, and life context, as well as give women a platform and advocacy to have their voices heard in the policy arena. Finally, Meleis recommends that societies consider women the center of the family and the community, expecting them to be the agents for continuity of values, gatekeepers, integrators, and guardians of social capital. This implies placing women's health at the forefront of foreign policy and international consciousness in war and peace. (This discussion is continued in Chapter 3.)

■ THE FUTURE DIRECTIONS OF WOMEN'S HEALTH

Notable advances have been achieved in the scope and depth of women's health and health care research in the last century. However, major challenges continue to emerge; these challenges are influenced by socioeconomic and environmental trends; genetic, hormonal, and biological determinants; globalization; and other social issues. Future and emerging issues for women's health in the 21st century need to address the effects of demographic and sociocultural change on women's health and also focus on the impact of such changes on the health care system and the ability of women to access appropriate high-quality care. The need to broaden research topics and to take into account populations that have been inadequately studied to date is essential. In general, although health care providers are committed to doing everything possible to promote women's health, the range of clinical and public health interventions is often limited, access to health care is inequitable, and the research evidence specific to women remains incomplete. Therefore, when considering future directions in research, one should ask whether study results will advance the ability to improve women's health and whether health care providers are being educated adequately to promote women's health!

■ REFERENCES

Amick, B. C., Kawachi, I., Coakley, E. H., Lerner, D., Levine, S., & Colditz, G. A. (1998). Relationship of job strain and iso-strain to health status in a cohort of women in the United States. *Scandinavian Journal of Work Environment and Health, 24*(1), 54–61.

Burnside, W. R., Brown, J. H., Burger, O., Hamilton, M. J., Moses, M., & Bettencourt, L. (2012). Human macroecology: Linking pattern and process in big-picture human ecology. *Biological Reviews, 87*(1), 194–208.

Center for American Progress. (2014). *The facts on immigration today.* Center for American Progress Immigration Team. Washington, DC. Retrieved from www.americanprogress.org

Centers for Disease Control and Prevention (CDC). (2012). National Health and Nutrition Examination Survey, 2007–2010. *Morbidity and Mortality Weekly Report, 60*(51), 1747. Retrieved from http://www.cdc.gov/mmwr/preview/mmwrhtml/mm6051a7.htm?s_cid=mm6051a7_w#x2013

Centers for Disease Control and Prevention (CDC). (2013). National Center for Health Statistics, Division of Health Interview Statistics, data from the National Health Interview Survey. *NCHS Data Brief 178*(178), 1–8.

Centers for Disease Control and Prevention (CDC). (2014). Depression in the U.S. household population, 2009–2012. *National Center for Health Statistics, Division of Health Interview Statistics,* NCH Data Brief No. 172.

Centers for Disease Control and Prevention. (2016). *Zika and sexual transmission.* Retrieved from http://www.cdc.gov/zika/transmission/sexual-transmission.html

Centers for Disease Control and Prevention CDC/National Center for Health Statistics (NCHS). (2012). Final data for 2010. *National Vital Statistics, 61*(4). Hyattsville, MD. Retrieved from http://www.cdc.gov/nchs/data/nvsr/nvsr61/nvsr61_04.pdf

Chavkin, W. (1999). What's a mother to do? Welfare, work, and family. *American Journal of Public Health, 89*(4), 477–479.

Commission on Family and Medical Leave. (1996). *A workable balance: Report to Congress on family and medical leave.* Washington, DC: U.S. Department of Labor.

DeNavas-Walk, C., & Proctor, B. D. (2014). *Income and poverty in the United States: 2014 current population reports.* U.S. Census Bureau, 60–252.

Foy, B. D., Kobylinski, K. C., Foy, J. L. C., Blitvich, B. J., Travassos da Rosa, A., Haddow, A. D., . . . Tesh, R. B. (2011). Probable non–vector-borne transmission of zika virus, Colorado, USA. *Emerging Infectious Diseases, 17*(5), 880–882. Retrieved from http://doi.org/10.3201/eid1705.101939

Golden, C., Driscoll, A. K., Simon, A. E., Judson, D. H., Miller, E. A., & Parker, J. D. (2015). Linkage of NCHS population health surveys to administrative records from Social Social Security Administration and Center for D=Medicare & Medicaid Services. *Vital Health Statistics, 1*(58), 2–53. Hyattsville, MD: National Center for Health Statistics.

Hamilton, B. E., Martin, J. A., Osternam, M. J. K., & Curtin, S. C. (2015). *Birth: Preliminary data tor 2014.* National Vital Statistics (NVVs, reports, 64 No. 6.). Hyattsville, MD: National Center for Health Statistics.

Haynes, S., Lynch, B. S., Biegel, R., Malliou, E., Rudick, J., & Sassaman, A. P. (2000). Women's health and the environment: Innovations in science and policy. *Journal of Women's Health and Gender-Based Medicine, 3,* 245–272.

Heymann, S. J., & Earle, A. (1999). The impact of welfare reform on parents' ability to care for their children's health. *American Journal of Public Health, 89,* 502–505.

Hoyt, C. L., & Murphy, S. E. (2016). Managing to clear the air: Stereotype threat, women, and leadership.

Institute of Medicine, Committee on Understanding the Biology of Sex and Gender Differences. (2001). *Exploring the biological contributions to human. Does sex matter?* Washington, DC: National Academy of Sciences.

Kant, A. K, Schatzkin, A., Harris, T. B., Ziegler, R., & Block, G. (1993). Dietary diversity and subsequent mortality in the First National Health and Nutrition Examination Survey epidemiologic follow-up study. *American Journal of Clinical Nutrition, 57*(3), 434–440.

Kessler, R. C., Crum, R. M., Warner, L. A., Nelson, C. B., Schulenberg, J., & Anthony, J. C. (1997). Lifetime co-occurrence of *DSM-III-R* alcohol abuse and dependence with other psychiatric disorders in the National Comorbidity Survey. *Archives of General Psychiatry, 54*(4), 313–321.

Mcdonald, G., Jackson, D., Vickers, M. H., & Wilkes, L. (2016). Surviving workplace adversity: A qualitative study of nurses and midwives and their strategies to increase personal resilience. *Journal of Nursing Management, 24*(1), 123–131.

Meleis, A. (2005). Safe womanhood is not safe motherhood: Policy implications. *Health Care for Women International, 26,* 464–471.

Misra, D. (1999). Women's experience of chronic diseases. In H. A. Grason, J. E. Hutchins, & G. B. Silver (Eds.), *Charting a course for the future of women's and perinatal health. Vol. 2: Review of key issues* (pp. 137–146). Baltimore, MD: Women's and Children's Health Policy Center, Johns Hopkins School of Public Health.

Monte, L. M., & Ellis, R. (2014). *Fertility of women in the United States: 2012: Population characteristics. Current Population Reports* (pp. 520–575). Washington, DC: U.S. Census Bureau.

National Center for Health Statistics. (2005). *Health, United States, 2005 with chartbook on trends in the health of Americans.* Hyattsville, MD: Author.

National Center for Health Statistics. (2014a). *Health, United States, 2013 with Special Feature on Prescription Drugs.* Hyattsville, MD: Author.

National Center for Health Statistics. (2014b). Summary health statistics hearing trouble, vision, and teeth trouble among adults age 18 and over: United States, 2014. *National Health Interview Survey, A-6a,* 1–9.

National Vital Statistics System. (2012). *Mortality public use data files, 2011.* Retrieved from www.cdc.gov/nchs/data_access/vitalstatsonline.htm

Parrott, S. (1998). *Welfare recipients who find jobs: What do we know about their employment and earnings?* Washington, DC: Center on Budget and Policy Priorities.

Perry J., & Woods, N. F. (1995). Older women and their images of health: A replication study. *ANS Advances in Nursing Science, 18*(1), 51–61.

Pew Research Center. (2013). *Social and demographic trends: 10 findings about women in the workplace.* Retrieved from http://www.pewsocialtrends.org/2013/12/11/10-findings-about-women-in-the-workplace

Pew Research Center. (2015). U.S. immigrant population projected to rise, even as share falls among Hispanics, Asians. Retrieved from http://www.pewresearch.org/fact-tank/2015/03/09/u-s-immigrant-population-projected-to-rise-even-as-share-falls-among-hispanics-asians

Pugliesi, K. (1995). Work and well-being: Gender differences in the psychological consequences of employment. *Journal of Health and Social Behavior, 36*(1), 57–71.

Reeves, W. C., Strine, T. W., Pratt, L. A., Thompson, W., Ahluwalia, I., Dhingra, S. S., … Safran, M. A.; Centers for Disease Control and Prevention (CDC). (2011). Mental illness surveillance among adults in the United States. *Morbidity and Mortality Weekly Report, 60*(3), 1–32.

Regenstein, M., Meyer, J. A., & Hicks, J. D. (1998). *Job prospects for welfare recipients: Employers speak out.* Washington, DC: Urban Institute.

Ryan, C., & Bauman, K. (2016). Educational attainment in the United States: 2015. *Population Characteristics Current Population Reports,* 20–578.

Trussell, J. (2011). Contraceptive failure in the United States. *Contraception, 83,* 397–404.

U.S. Census Bureau. (NewsRoom 2011). *2010 census shows American's diversity.* Retrieved from https://www.census.gov/newsroom/releases/archives/2010_census/cb11-cn125.html

U.S. Census Bureau. (2012). *Population: Section 1 U.S. Census Bureau, Statistical Abstract of the United States 2012.* Retrieved from http://www2.census.gov/library/publications/2011/compendia/statab/131ed/tables/pop.pdf

U.S. Census Bureau. (2015). *Monthly population estimates for the United States: April 1, 2010 to December 1, 2016.* Retrieved from http://www.census.gov/newsroom/press-releases/2016/cb16-110.html

U.S. Department of Health and Human Services. (1996). *Physical activity and health: A report of the Surgeon General.* Washington, DC: U.S. Government Printing Office.

U.S. Department of Health and Human Services. (1998). *Characteristics and financial circumstances of TANF recipients, July–September 1997.* Washington, DC: Author.

U.S. Department of Health and Human Services. (1999). *Mental health: A report of the Surgeon General—Executive summary.* Rockville, MD: U.S. Department of Human Services, Substance Abuse and Mental Health Services Administration, Center for Mental Health Services, National Institutes of Health, National Institute of Mental Health.

Women's Health USA. (2013). Retrieved from http://mchb.hrsa.gov/whusa13/dl/pdf/hsu.pdf

Woods, N. F., Laffrey, S., Duffy, M., Lentz, M. J., Mitchell, E. S., Taylor, D., & Cowan, K. A. (1988). Being healthy: Women's images. *ANS Advances in Nursing Science, 11*(1), 36–46.

World Health Organization. (n.d.). *Sexual and reproductive health.* Retrieved from http://www.who.int/reproductivehealth/topics/sexual_health/sh_definitions/en

World Health Organization (WHO), Department of Reproductive Health and Research, Johns Hopkins Bloomberg School of Public Health/Center for Communication Programs (CCP). (2011). *Knowledge for health project. Family planning: A global handbook for providers* (2011 update). Baltimore, MD; Geneva, Switzerland: CCP and WHO.

CHAPTER 2

Women as Health Care Providers

Diana Taylor

■ HEALTH CARE WORKFORCE IN THE UNITED STATES

The delivery of health services is one of the largest industries in the United States, with about 19 million jobs (Centers for Disease Control and Prevention [CDC], 2014; The Center for Health Workforce Studies, 2014) either in the health sector or in health occupations employment outside of the health sector, accounting for more than 13% of the total U.S. workforce. Between 2002 and 2012, employment in the country's health sector grew by more than 22%, whereas employment in other sectors remained stable. About two thirds of all health care jobs are in hospitals (38%) and offices of health care practitioners, and one quarter are in nursing homes (16%) or other ambulatory or personal care facilities (Bureau of Labor Statistics [BLS], 2013b). Of the total workforce in 2012, RNs (18%) were the single largest health occupation, followed by nursing assistants (10%), personal care aides (8%), and home health aides (6%) (BLS, 2013b). Embedded within these statistics is the fact that the current health care workforce does not reflect the nation's diversity. In the United States, women are overrepresented in the health workforce compared with the total population. Although people of color represent more than 25% of the total U.S. population, only 10% are health professionals.

Rapid changes in economic, demographic, and health care system factors are driving reform in the U.S. health workforce. There are imbalances among geographic and functional health workforce shortages, health care reform, and development of health care workers to meet the population and health service needs. These health workforce imbalances intersect with continuing systems of oppression and inequities across gender, race, and economic status. Given these changes and inequities, the future health care workforce will be increasingly female, young, racially/ethnically diverse, and not U.S. born, at or below the poverty level, and at a low level of educational attainment.

In this chapter, we provide an overview of the current U.S. health care workforce; trends for the future; and critical drivers, disparities, and challenges to ensure an adequate supply and distribution of well-prepared health workers to meet the nation's health care needs. Since women dominate the current and future health care workforce, we focus on how gender, and other elements that intersect with gender, shapes, strengthens, and empowers women as the primary health care workforce to meet current and future population and health service needs.

■ U.S. HEALTH OCCUPATIONS AND PROVIDERS

Definitions of *health care providers* (people and places) are rooted in history; their evolution is shaped by social, economic, and political forces. With the rapid and massive changes in the U.S. health care system, system redesign is occurring along with a redefinition of health care workers' roles. These changes are influenced by multiple determinants: the form of government, definitions of health, social values, costs, society's expectations for the health care system, and the political power of various players. Embedded within these structures and determinants of the U.S. health care system are significant disparities in the health workforce by health occupation, gender, race, and culture.

The term health care provider refers to people who provide care to patients and the settings or systems in which health services are provided. More than 545,000 establishments make up the health services industry with four general segments:

- Hospitals (public and private)
- Nursing and personal care facilities (excluding residential, mental retardation, mental health, substance-abuse, and other residential care facilities)
- Home health care
- Ambulatory care settings (excluding home health care, but including medical and diagnostic laboratories, offices and clinics of doctors of medicine, offices and clinics of dentists, offices and clinics of other health practitioners [chiropractors, optometrists, podiatrists, occupational/physical therapists, psychologists, speech/hearing therapists, nutritionists, and alternative medicine practitioners], outpatient care centers [kidney dialysis centers, drug treatment clinics, mental health centers, and rehabilitation centers], medical and diagnostic laboratories, and other ambulatory health services [ambulance and helicopter transport services, blood and organ banks, pacemaker monitoring services, and nonhospital surgical centers]; BLS, 2013; U.S. Department of Labor, 2015a)

Among the U.S. working-age population, health occupations are defined and found among the Bureau of Labor Statistics (BLS) Occupational Employment Statistics' categories/groupings (BLS, 2015a) created by the 2010 Standard Occupational Classification (SOC) system (U.S. Department of Labor, 2010b) and represent the U.S. health workforce.[1] The SOC is used by federal statistical agencies to classify workers into occupational categories for the purpose of data collection and analysis, with cross-references with the U.S. BLS (fastest growing occupations), the BLS Occupational Employment Statistics (employment and wage estimates), and the U.S. Census Bureau's American Community Survey (ACS; current demographic data).[2] In addition to the U.S. BLS, the National Center for Health Workforce Analysis (NCHWA), a unit of the Health Resources and Services Administration (HRSA) of the U.S. Department of Health and Human Services (USDHHS), uses these labor and census data to further estimate the supply and demand for health workers in the United States as well as to develop tools and resources to inform decision making on health care workforce investments in order to produce a health care workforce of sufficient size and skill to meet the nation's health care needs (HRSA, 2014).[3]

Using the SOC[4] system (U.S. Census Bureau, 2012), the largest category of health workers is the health care practitioners and technical occupations, with health diagnosing and treating practitioners (e.g., health professionals such as RNs/advanced practice registered nurses [APRNs], physicians, pharmacists, dentists, physician assistants, speech/language pathologists, chiropractors, occupational/physical/respiratory therapists, dietitians/nutritionists, optometrists) and health technologists and technicians (e.g., health practitioner support technologists and technicians, licensed practical and licensed vocational nurses [LPN/LVNs], dental hygienists, diagnostic-related technologists/technicians, emergency medical technicians/paramedics, medical/clinical laboratory technicians, medical record/health information technicians, and dispensing opticians) accounting for more than half of the health care workforce (HRSA, 2014). Other occupations within the SOC categories of health care support occupations (nursing, psychiatric, and home health aides; medical, dental, and physical therapy assistants) and personal care and service occupations (personal care aides) account for one third of health care workers. Another 15% to 20% of the health care workforce is in the SOC categories of office and administrative support occupations (i.e., medical secretaries), community/social service occupations (i.e., counselors and social workers), life/social science occupations (i.e., psychologists), and management occupations.[5]

The NCHWA regularly publishes a summary of data on the size and characteristics of U.S. health occupations based on the U.S. government's SOC system. The most recent summary in the *U.S. Health Workforce Chartbook*, published in November 2013, is based on U.S. Census Bureau data from the ACS Public Use Microdata Sample (PUMS) 2008–2010 (HRSA, 2013a). The U.S. Health Workforce Chartbook estimates the total number of individuals in the occupation or occupational grouping, the percentage of females, the percentage of health workers older than age 55,

and the highest and lowest number of workers per 100,000 in the working-age population across the 50 states. A more recent NCHWA report summarized the gender and racial/ethnic diversity of U.S. health occupations for 2010 to 2012 (HRSA, 2015d).

In the most recent *U.S. Health Workforce Chartbook* (HRSA, 2013a), health occupation titles were grouped (differently from the 2010 SOC categories) into four categories for ease of reporting: Part I comprises clinicians (physicians, physician assistants, RNs including APRNs, LPNs, pharmacists, and oral health professions, including dentists, dental hygienists, and dental assistants); Part II presents additional clinician categories (chiropractors, veterinarians, and vision health professionals, including optometrists and dispensing opticians) and occupations concerned with health care administration duties (medical/health service managers and medical secretaries); Part III reports on health-related technologists and technicians as well as aides and assistants; and Part IV describes behavioral (psychologists, counselors, and social workers) and allied health (physical therapists and assistant/aides, dietitians/nutritionists, occupational therapists, respiratory therapists, speech-language pathologists, and massage therapists) occupations.

In 2010, 14 million individuals were classified as health workers, representing approximately 10% of the U.S. workforce (HRSA, 2013a). The largest health occupations or groupings in 2008 to 2010 were RNs (approximately 2,825,000); nursing, psychiatric, and home health aides (2,329,000); personal care aides (1,023,000); physicians (861,000); medical assistants and other health care support occupations (845,000); and LPN/LVNs (690,000). More than half of the 35 occupations or occupational groupings (HRSA, 2013a) are greater than 70% female, with dental hygienists, dental assistants, medical secretaries, and speech-language pathologists being more than 95% female. There are significant variations in age across occupations, from dentists and psychologists (more than 30% being older than 55 years) to emergency medical technicians and paramedics, dental assistants, and physical therapist assistants and aides (fewer than 8% being older than 55 years).

▪ SOCIOCULTURAL FRAMEWORK: WOMEN AS PAID HEALTH CARE PROVIDERS

One of the most striking developments of the post–World War II period has been the increase in women working outside the home. Worldwide, women now make up 47% of the total U.S. paid labor force, and 58% of women are now in the labor force (BLS, 2013b). Despite these advances, women remain concentrated in particular sectors of the economy, such as service jobs (U.S. Department of Labor, 2010a). Despite equal opportunity laws, women have not achieved parity with men's earnings, and many continue to be crowded into female "employment ghettos" such as factories and hospitals.

In 2014, the U.S. civilian workforce included more than 140 million full- and part-time employed workers; 53% were men, and 47% were women. Nearly 40% of working women were employed in traditionally female occupations such as social work, nursing, and teaching. Less than 10% of men are employed in these occupations. In spite of advances in educational preparation (the number of women with college degrees tripled from 1970 to 2012), women face a pay gap in nearly every occupation. In 2013, among full-time, year-round workers, women were paid 78% of what men were paid; the pay gap is worse for women of color and increases with age (American Association of University Women [AAUW], 2015; Department for Professional Employees [DPE], 2015; Institute for Women's Policy Research [IWPR], 2014; U.S. Department of Labor, 2015b; see Table 2.1).

Across the world, women provide the majority of paid (and unpaid) health care. In the United States, women are overrepresented in the health workforce compared with the total population. Although men represent a larger proportion of the overall U.S. working-age population, women represent the majority of workers in 27 of 32 health occupations, accounting for more than 80% of workers in nearly half (15 of 32) of these occupations (HRSA, 2014). Although women are making significant advances in the traditionally male occupations of medicine, dentistry, pharmacy, and some highly technical occupations, they continue to far outnumber men in the traditionally female occupations: nurse, occupational and physical therapist, dietitian/nutritionist, dental assistant/dental hygienist, nursing assistant, and health aide/technician. In general, the majority of the pay gap between men and women in health occupations widens in the highest

TABLE 2.1	Women Workers in Selected Health Occupations, United States, 1995 & 2014						
		WOMEN (% OF TOTAL)			AVERAGE EARNINGS $/WEEK FOR FULL-TIME WORKERS		
HEALTH OCCUPATION	TOTAL WORKERS IN 1,000s	1995	2014 (BLS, 2014a)	MEDIAN AGE (YRS)	ALL	WOMEN	MEN
Total employed ≥ age 16 years	146,305	46.1	46.9	42.3	791	719	871
Dental hygienists	175	99.4	97.1	41	975	951	–
Dental assistants	273	98.5	96.6	37	535	535	–
Medical assistants	508	–	92.8	34	546	539	–
Dieticians and nutritionists	123	93.2[a]	92.4	47	919	875	–
Occupational therapists	111	90.5	92.4	41	1,146	1,139	–
Nurse practitioners	128	–	91.5	45	1,619	1,682	–
Registered nurses	2,888	93.1	90	45	1,090	1,076	1,190
Licensed practical nurses	641	95.4	89	43	539	539	539
Aides: nursing, psychiatric, home health	1,980	89.4[b]	88.5	41	539	539	539
Physician assistants	84	53.2	74.5	40	1,619	–	–
Clinical laboratory technicians	294	71.7	74	45	824	818	878
Physical therapists	193	70.2	69.8	40	1,387	1,307	1,478
Pharmacists	214	36.2	56.3	41	1,995	1,902	2,176
Physicians	1,014	24.4	36.7	47	1,661	1,246	2,102
Dentists	192	13.4	29.1	52	1,908	–	–

[a]Dieticians only. Nutritionists not included in 1995 data.
[b]Nursing aides, orderlies, and attendants included in 1995 data.
Source: Figures for the total number of workers and for the percentage of those workers that were women in 2014 are from Bureau of Labor Statistics (2014a). Figures for the percentage of the total number of workers that were women in 1995 are from Bureau of Labor Statistics (1995). Figures for the average earnings per week for full-time workers are from U.S. Department of Labor (2015a, 2015b).

paying ones such as medicine and dentistry. For example, women physicians and surgeons earn 71% of what their male counterparts earn, even after controlling for age, race, hours, and education (Goldin, 2014). Except for dental hygienists who have no gender pay inequity, male dentists make 26% more, male nurses make 11% more, and male pharmacists make 9% more than their female counterparts (Goldin, 2014).

In addition to gender, the health care workforce is more racially diverse than the U.S. population and has increased in racial/ethnic diversity over the past decade. In 2014, the racial distribution in the United States was 62% non-Hispanic Whites; 12% Black/African American; 17% Hispanic; 5.2% Asian/Pacific Islander; and less than 1% American Indian/Alaskan Native. By 2060, these proportions will shift quite dramatically, as there will no longer be any clear racial/ethnic majority because the minority population is projected to rise to 56% of the total in 2060, compared with 38% in 2014. Less than 45% will be non-Hispanic White; 13%, Black/African American; 29%, Hispanic origin; almost 10%, Asian/Pacific Islander; and less than 1%, American Indian, Eskimo, and Aleut (U.S. Census Bureau, 2015a). Around the time the 2020 Census is conducted, more than half of the nation's children are expected to be part of a minority race/ethnic group. This proportion is expected to continue to grow so that by 2060, just 36% of all children (people younger than 18 years) will be single-race non-Hispanic White, compared with 52% today. By 2060, the nation's foreign-born population would reach nearly 19% of the total population, increased from 13% in 2014 (U.S. Census Bureau, 2015b).

The trends in racial/ethnic diversity vary considerably by occupation, although minorities tend to be more highly represented among the lower skilled occupations. The share of African American non-Hispanics saw the largest gain in share of the health workforce (16.9% in 2004 to 18.2% in 2013), which is a larger increase compared with the U.S. population trends (14.0% in 2004 to 14.8% in 2013). Hispanics gained representation in the health care workforce (8.5% in 2004 to 10.9% in 2013), though at a slightly slower rate compared with the U.S. population (14.2% in 2004 to 17.1% in 2014) (Snyder, Stover, Skillman, & Frogner, 2015; see Table 2.2).

The statistics presented in Table 2.1 illustrate the demographic characteristics of women workers in selected paid health care occupations.[6] In 2012, 74% of pharmacists, 72% of physicians, 79% of RNs, and 81% of dentists were White (non-Hispanic) compared with 78% White (non-Hispanic) in the U.S. working-age population (HRSA, 2015d). Overall, Whites and Asians are more represented among the occupations found within the health diagnosing and treating practitioners subcategory—occupations that often require many years of education or training—than in the U.S. working-age population altogether. Conversely, Hispanics, Black/African American, American Indians/Alaska Natives, Pacific Islanders, and individuals reporting multiple or other race are, in general, far less underrepresented in

this subcategory. However, Asians are underrepresented in two occupations—APRNs (4%) and speech-language pathologists (2%).

Among the health technologists and technicians subcategory, Blacks have the largest representation (25%) among LPNs, nearly twice their representation in the overall U.S. workforce. However, Hispanics are underrepresented in all occupations in this subcategory. Similar to the health technical occupations, there is varying racial/ethnic representation among all the health care support occupations—occupations that generally require fewer years of education or training. For example, Blacks have their highest proportion among nursing, psychiatric, and home health aides (38%), whereas Hispanics have their highest representation among dental assistants (23%), both of which are greater proportion than in the overall national workforce. In addition, American Indians/Alaska Natives and Pacific Islanders have the largest proportion of workers (1.2% and 0.6%, respectively) among personal care aides (personal care and service occupation). Conversely, Whites have their lowest representation among nursing, psychiatric, and home health aides (54%; HRSA, 2014).

In general, Tables 2.1 and 2.2 do not present surprising information. Many authors have compared the proportion of women in the health occupations and explored the gender and racial hierarchies in the health labor force (Brown, 1982; Butter, 1985; HRSA, 2014; Levinson & Lurie, 2004; Marieskind, 1980; Olson, 2011). The statistics are followed and updated annually by the federal government and published in various government reports available to the public (e.g., reports from the U.S. Census Bureau, Department of Labor, BLS, and Bureau of Health Professions). More recently, the federal government has focused on the diversity of American health care workers through the establishment of a Women's Bureau of the Department of Labor and NCHWA at HRSA's Bureau of Health Workforce. There is a rising awareness of the need to collect and analyze data regarding the national, regional, and state differences of personnel working in the U.S. health care delivery system, including gender, class, and race/ethnic factors.

The occupations listed in Tables 2.1 and 2.2 are not all of those on which information is available, but they provide a good representation and clear picture of the continued gender and racial/ethnic disparity in paid health care roles. In Table 2.1, the occupations are listed in order of proportion of women in selected health occupations for 2014 (U.S. Department of Labor, 2014a, 2015a, 2015b, 2015c) and compared with 1995 data. Notably, the large numbers of nursing aides and medical assistants, of which approximately 90% or more are women, account for the majority of women in all health care occupations. Clearly, women, particularly women of color, are clustered in jobs and occupations that are lower in pay, lower in status, and less autonomous than the jobs of most men in the health care field (BLS, 2013b; Butter, Carpenter, Kay, & Simmons, 1987; Doyal, 1995; Fisher, 1995; HRSA, 2014; Olson,

TABLE 2.2	Racial and Ethnic Diversity of Workers in Selected Health Occupations, United States, 2010–2012 (Percentage)							
HEALTH OCCUPATION	WHITE (NON-HISPANIC)	HISPANIC OR LATINO	BLACK/ AFRICAN AMERICAN (NON-HISPANIC)	ASIAN (NON-HISPANIC)	AMERICAN INDIAN AND ALASKA NATIVE	NATIVE HAWAIIAN AND OTHER PACIFIC ISLANDER	MULTIPLE/ OTHER RACE (NON-HISPANIC)	NON-HISPANIC OR LATINO
Working age population ≥ 16 years	77.6	15.5	13.6	6.0	0.7	0.2	2.0	84.5
Dental hygienists	91.6	5.7	2.9	3.6	0.4	—[a]	1.5	94.3
Dental assistants	81.1	22.5	8.8	6.9	1.0	–	2.2	77.5
Dentists	80.5	6.1	3.3	14.5	–	–	1.5	93.9
Physicians	72.2	6.0	5.3	20.0	0.2	0.03	2.2	94.0
Medical assistants	72.6	19.0	18.4	5.3	0.8	0.4	2.4	81.0
Dieticians and nutritionists	76.0	9.1	15.4	6.6	0.6	–	1.2	90.9
Occupational therapists	87.2	4.3	5.0	6.3	–	–	1.2	95.7
Advanced practice registered nurses[b]	89.5	4.4	5.2	4.0	–	–	1.1	95.6
Registered nurses	78.6	5.4	10.7	8.8	0.4	0.1	1.4	94.6
Licensed practical nurses	68.2	8.2	25.0	4.1	0.7	0.1	1.8	91.8
Aides: nursing, psychiatric, home health aides	54.0	13.4	37.5	5.1	1.0	0.2	2.3	86.6
Physicians assistants	81.6	10.8	8.0	7.2	0.3	–	2.9	89.2
Clinical lab technicians and technologists	68.5	9.2	14.9	13.3	0.7	0.2	2.4	98.2
Physical therapists	82.8	4.2	4.2	11.4	0.2	–	1.2	95.8
Pharmacists	73.7	4.0	5.9	18.0	0.2	–	1.8	96.0

[a] Absent numbers indicate estimates with relative standard errors ≥ 20% or there is no data present in the 2010–2014 American Community Survey, Public Use Microdata Sample (ACS PUMS) for this subgroup.
[b] Includes nurse anesthetists, midwives and nurse practitioners.
Source: Health Resources and Services Administration (2015d).

2011). There are significant variations in age across occupations, from dentists and psychologists, with more than 30% older than 55 years, to emergency medical technicians and paramedics, dental assistants, and physical therapist assistants/aides, with fewer than 8% older than 55 years (HRSA, 2013a). Among the health professions occupations, one quarter of U.S. physicians and 20% of pharmacists are older than 55 years. Detailed information on demographics (including age and race/ethnicity data), workforce settings, and geographic distribution of the U.S. health workforce, as well as more information about the data and methods, can also be found in the *U.S. Health Workforce Chartbook* and the *Technical Documentation for the Chartbook* at http://bhpr.hrsa.gov/healthworkforce/index.html

The health care industry has seen constant job growth over the past two decades, even during the most recent recession, when health care added 428,000 jobs and the rest of the economy lost 7.5 million jobs (Frogner, Spetz, Parente, & Oberlin, 2015; Wood, 2011). Health care employment is expected to rise, in large part because of the growing elderly population that typically requires more health care services, as well as the implementation of the Patient Protection and Affordable Care Act (ACA) of 2010 (Cuckler et al., 2013). Recent projections from the HRSA expect the majority of the increase in primary care demand will be caused by demographics and the remaining 20% will be caused by changes in demand under the ACA (HRSA, 2013a).

Workforce supply and capacity are also cyclical. The total number of individuals working in a profession is affected both by capacity (those trained and authorized to provide services in question) and by actual supply (qualified individuals who want to work). As provider shortages become apparent, educational programs expand, producing more graduates, and legal scopes of practice may grant broader practice authority to some professions in underserved areas. At the same time, practice models shift to integrate new workers into care delivery, effectively expanding capacity. Efforts to increase capacity may coincide with economic trends producing higher-than-anticipated numbers of individuals wanting to work. Evidence of the cyclical nature of workforce supply is the recent undersupply followed by oversupply of nurses and pharmacists (Buerhaus, Auerbach, & Staiger, 2009; Zavsdski, 2014).

Health care occupations in the 21st century will have more women in them and will be more ethnically diverse than they are today in terms of the number and proportion of women occupying jobs in the health workforce. Trends in supply and demand as well as other implications of gender and ethnic diversity among the health workforce will be explored further. First, we highlight some historical factors.

Historical Perspectives

In prehistoric eras, both men and women shared the activities of healing—herbs and roots were gathered and dispensed to those who were ailing. However, records suggest that gender divisions began even during these early times. Women tended to fulfill the caregiver and midwifery role, and men tended to be medicine givers (Dock & Stewart, 1938). Religion and medicine were united very early with medicine men and later physicians became priests, whereas nuns provided nursing care. Although knowledge of women as midwives, doctors, and healers in antiquity is fragmented, clearly these women existed as evidenced by writings from the 5th century BCE: Metrodora (woman doctor and midwife) and Hygieia (daughter of Asclepius and practiced preventive healing) (Parker, 1997). Although the majority of physicians have been men, since the 19th century, nurses in the United States and Europe have been almost exclusively women[7] (Choy, 2003; D'Antonio, 2010).

During the 19th century, few women received a formal education, and few were formally employed outside the home. Women in the 1800s were struggling to define a role for themselves in society through the women's suffrage movement of the 1840s as well as through the early women's health organizations of the time (Ehrenreich & English, 1973). Among other reasons, science was used to justify limiting women to inferior positions in society. Hamilton (1885, in Ehrenreich & English, 1973) wrote

that "the best education for girls, then, is that which best prepares them for the legitimate duties of womanhood" (p. 319; e.g., wife, mother, homemaker). He further asserted that attainment of high intellectual culture exacts too great a price and results in a "ruined or physically damaged constitution" (p. 321). Hamilton based his theory about education for women on a set of assumptions about physical and intellectual differences among the sexes. With respect to women, he described how "brain work" competes with the "vital forces of the body," and that such a diversion of "nerve power" to the mental labor involved in education could only lead to "greatly impaired or permanently ruined health, a life of sterility, general unhappiness, and uselessness" (p. 320). Furthermore, poor women, slaves, and domestic workers were ordered to provide caregiving services in homes.

Beginning in the mid-1800s, Florence Nightingale and other nursing reformers reframed these statements to argue that the role of trained nurse allowed women to harness their innately feminine caring traits and contribute meaningfully to society (Reverby, 1987a). Women who sought education as physicians also appealed to social beliefs about women's attributes, balancing what historian Regina Morantz-Sanchez has called "sympathy and science" (Morantz-Sanchez, 1985). During this critical period of transition in U.S. medical history, urbanization, immigration, and the growth of hospitals led to a gradual replacement of family members as caregivers to reliance on professional nurses and physicians (Rosenberg, 1995).

The landmark Flexner Report, promulgated in 1910, set forth new and more "scientific" standards for medical education (e.g., increasing the number of years of education required of medical school applicants). The report consolidated and formalized ideals that had already been circulating among medical elites. It resulted in the closure of many schools that had previously educated women and Black physicians. Although many medical schools, such as Johns Hopkins, accepted women, they did so in very small numbers, meaning that the numbers of women physicians actually decreased during the early 20th century (Ludmerer, 1988). As standards of entry were tightened and the American Medical Association (AMA) and state medical organizations gained more power over the medical profession, it became more difficult for women, Jewish people, and people of color to access medical education (Starr, 1982). The number of women in the medical profession continued to decrease through the 1950s. Social changes during the 1960s changed the trajectory of women in medicine. The feminist movement, affirmative action programs, and women's own determination led women to seek higher education, particularly in the traditionally male medical careers. With expansion and rapid change in the health care system, new careers (not the traditional professions of nursing, medicine, pharmacy, or dentistry) are emerging in allied health occupations that now compose 60% of all health-related jobs.

Beginning in the early 1990s, health care workforce policy planning and development under private–public partnerships were formed to assist health professionals, workforce policy makers, and educational institutions in responding to the challenges of the changing health care system. Between

1991 and 2008, the Pew Health Professions Commission chronicled several major health system trends, including cost-containment, consumer involvement, access to care, workforce regulation, shifts in demographics and disease burdens, and critical challenges for the U.S. health care workforce. The Pew Commission's fourth and final report titled *Recreating Health Professional Practice for a New Century* offered recommendations that affect the scope and training of all health care professional groups, as well as 21 competencies for all health care workers for the 21st century (Commission & O'Neil, 1998) and linked population needs with health care workforce capacity and competencies and not merely titles.

With better health care workforce data and private–public partnerships, the Institute of Medicine (IOM) has led a number of reports that challenge the Flexnerian paradigm in which the focus has been on degrees and specialized training rather than on aligning population needs with health care worker training and entry into practice. The IOM 2010 report titled *The Future of Nursing: Leading Change, Advancing Health* thoroughly examined how nurses' roles, responsibilities, and education should change to meet the needs of an aging, increasingly diverse population and to respond to a complex, evolving health care system (IOM, 2011b). The report calls on the nation's leaders and stakeholders to act on recommendations in key areas to strengthen and empower the 3 million (largely women) nurses: advancing educational transformation, leveraging nursing leadership, removing barriers to practice and care, promoting nursing diversity, and fostering interprofessional collaboration. This report was followed by the 2011 workshop report, *Allied Health Workforce and Services* (IOM, 2011b), which called for a better model for the location and financing of allied health care education and for the reintegration of allied health into the care delivery system. Although governments have always played a role in promoting health care workforce training and regulation, state-based strategies are emerging, and they implement new practice models that more quickly meet the needs of populations and practitioners.

As we move into the next decade of the paid health workforce history, we provide an overview of the major health care professions groups—those with the most women (nurses) and those with the fewest women (physicians, dentists, and pharmacists), followed by a summary of the allied health workforce. Using nomenclature from BLS (2015a) 2010 SOC system (U.S. Department of Labor, 2015d), we describe these four frontline health care professionals as health diagnosing treating practitioners and describe the allied health workers as health technologists and technicians and health care support occupations.

Health Diagnosing and Treating Practitioners

Three health care occupations—medicine, dentistry, and pharmacy—are identified as traditionally male in Table 2.1, which also identifies them as the highest paid health occupations (Cain et al., 2014; *The New England Journal of Medicine* [NEJM], 2014). There is a considerable literature on women in medicine, less on women in dentistry

and pharmacy. Women are changing the practice of these formerly male professions. With an undersupply of physicians in primary care, women physicians are helping to transform the practice of medicine by their dominance in primary care fields. However, shortages are looming for both dentistry and pharmacy. More than half of the practicing pharmacists are women, compared with 32% in 1990, the pharmacy work environment is changing (more part-time workers). In subsequent sections, we will focus on women in medicine as representative of the challenges facing women in these male-identified occupations as well as highlight some unique aspects of women in dental and pharmacy occupations.

■ DISCUSSION

First, we describe the largest women-dominated health professional group—RNs and midwives. RNs, including APRNs, among whom 90% are women, account for the largest group of health diagnosing and treating practitioners (approx. 2.8 million RNs and APRNs; HRSA, 2015d).

Nursing's Roles in Providing Health Care: RNs and APRNs

Florence Nightingale is traditionally associated with the advent of modern trained nursing and midwifery. Nightingale asserted that "every woman is a nurse" (Nightingale, 1992). The development of nursing in the United States began during the mid-1800s and was strongly influenced by the public health and hospital-based programs established in England by Nightingale. The 19th century saw the organization of hospitals as centers for care for the sick as well as the organization of medical education and profession of nursing. In the late 1850s, Elizabeth Blackwell, a friend of Florence Nightingale and the first American woman to become a physician, was instrumental in promoting Nightingale's methods for nursing education (e.g., practical experiential training in the hospital setting). Nursing became a respectable occupation for women by the end of the 19th century because of the pioneering and collaborative efforts of Nightingale and Blackwell—along with other pioneers such as Dorothea Dix (who established nursing care in asylums for the mentally ill), Isabel Hampton Robb (who established the first school of nursing based on Nightingale's model), Lillian Wald and Mary Brewster (who established public health nursing in the United States), Mary Breckinridge (nurse-midwifery leader), and Lavinia Dock and Adelaide Nutting (who published texts on the science and theory of nursing practice) (Jamieson & Sewall, 1944).

Nurses make up the single largest health profession in the United States (HRSA, 2013b). There were 2.8 million RNs (including APRNs) and 690,000 LPNs working in the field of nursing or seeking nursing employment in 2008 to 2010 (U.S. Department of Labor, 2012). They perform a variety of patient care duties and are critical to the delivery of health care services across a wide array of settings, including ambulatory care clinics, hospitals, nursing homes, public health facilities, hospice programs, and home health agencies.

Distinctions are made among different types of nurses according to their education, role, and the level of autonomy in practice. LPNs typically receive training for a year beyond high school and, after passing the national NCLEX-PN® exam, become licensed to work in patient care. LPNs provide a variety of direct care services, including administration of medication, taking of medical histories, recording of symptoms and vital signs, and other tasks as delegated by RNs, physicians, and other health care providers. RNs usually have a bachelor's degree in nursing, a 2-year associate's degree in nursing, or a diploma from an approved nursing program. They must also pass a national exam, the NCLEX-RN®, before they are licensed to practice. The scope of RN responsibilities is more complex and analytical than that of LPNs. RNs provide a wide array of direct care services such as administration of treatments, care coordination, disease prevention, patient education, and health promotion for individuals, families, and communities. RNs may choose to obtain advanced clinical education and training to become APRN defined by four titles—certified nurse-midwife (CNM), certified registered nurse anesthetist (CRNA), clinical nurse specialist (CNS), and nurse practitioner (NP). APRNs usually have a master's degree, although some complete doctoral-level training, and often focus in a clinical specialty area.

About 445,000 RNs (16%) and 166,000 LPNs (24%) lived in rural areas. The per-capita distribution of RNs varied substantially across states (HRSA, 2013b), with fewer RNs per 100,000 population working in the West and Southwest states (i.e., California, Idaho, Nevada, New Mexico, Oklahoma, Texas, Utah, Wyoming) and more RNs per 100,000 population working in the Northeast and Midwest states (i.e., Delaware, Iowa, Maine, Massachusetts, Montana, Nebraska, North/South Dakota, Pennsylvania). The nursing workforce grew substantially in the past decade, with the number of RNs growing by more than 500,000 (24%) and LPNs by more than 90,000 (16%) and outpaced growth in the U.S. population.

The average RN is a White, married, middle-aged mother working full time in a hospital. Over the past decade, RNs and LPNs are becoming more diverse. The proportion of non-White RNs increased from 20% to 25%, a 25% increase, and the proportion of men in the RN workforce increased to almost 10%, a 12.5% increase. Owing to growth in new entrants, the absolute number of RNs younger than 30 has increased. However, with one third of the nursing workforce older than 50 years of age, the overall age of RNs has increased during the past decade (HRSA, 2013b). Currently, more than half of the RN workforce (55%) holds a bachelor's or higher degree.

The annual median wage for a RN was $66,640 in 2014. The highest paid 10% of RNs made more than $98,880, whereas the bottom 10% earned less than $45,880. The states with the highest RN employment levels also have the highest average wages, ranging from California ($98,400), New York ($77,110), Texas ($68,590), Pennsylvania ($66,570), and Florida ($62,570). The top-paying states for RNs are concentrated in the West and Northeast regions,

with annual wages ranging from $83,000 (Oregon), $86,000 (Alaska and Massachusetts), and $88,000 (Alaska) to $98,000 (California).

Although annual earnings of RNs are above average for all workers (approximately $34,750; U.S. Department of Labor, 2015c), they are markedly lower than physician, dentist, and pharmacist earnings (Table 2.1) and below those for physical therapists and dental hygienists (HRSA, 2013a). However, because of slow recovery from the 2008 to 2009 recession, average annual staff RN wages and benefits in private hospitals have declined, with an average annual decrease in real wages (inflation-adjusted) of 0.8% (HRSA, 2015d; McMenamin, 2014). In 1988, more than two thirds of nurses worked in hospital settings; about 7% worked in nursing homes, community or public health settings, or ambulatory sites; and the remaining 11% worked in nursing education, student health, occupational, and private-duty nursing (O'Neil, 1993). Although hospitals remain the major employer of nurses, results from the 2012 National Sample Survey of Registered Nurses (NSSRN) indicate a trend away from the hospital as the setting for the principal nursing position (HRSA, 2013a). In 2013, more than half of RNs worked in hospitals, which included surgical centers (58%), with about one third (30%) employed in home health care (6.3%), nursing care facilities (7%), community/public health settings, or ambulatory settings such as health practitioner offices (7%) and outpatient care centers (6%) (HRSA, 2013a).

One of the important changes in health professions over the past 50 years has been the development of advanced practice nursing (HRSA, 2012a), and the more autonomous APRN roles of CNM, CNS, CRNA, and NP. APRNs are prepared by education and certification to assess, diagnose, and manage patient problems, order tests, and prescribe medications. As with RNs, boards of nursing (BONs) in each state license and regulate the practice of APRNs (National Council of State Boards of Nursing [NCSBN], 2012). The majority of APRNs are employed in physician/other practitioner offices and outpatient care centers with less than one third of NPs (26%), CNMs (29%), and CRNAs (30%) employed by hospitals (HRSA, 2013a).

Depending on the data source, APRNs represent approximately 9% of the national RN population. Although the number of employed APRNs have been estimated more than 250,000, according to the U.S. government (HRSA, 2013a) in 2012, there were 158,000 employed NPs (110,000), CNMs (12,400), and CRNAs (35,600) (U.S. Department of Labor, 2014a). However, the number of licensed NPs in the United States was estimated at 154,000 by the HRSA-conducted 2012 National Sample Survey of Nurse Practitioners (NSSNP) to provide accurate national estimates of the NP workforce (HRSA, 2012a). As CNSs are not recognized by statute in all states, neither the BLS nor the HRSA provides regular reports; NSSRN estimated that there were nearly 60,000 CNSs in 2010 (HRSA, 2010).

According to multiple data sources (American Association of Nurse Anesthetists [AANA], 2009; HRSA, 2012b; Sipe, Fullerton, & Schuiling, 2009) dated 2008 to 2012, demographic characteristics among the three groups of nurses in advanced practice are similar for mean age

(48 years) and race (90% non-Hispanic White), but differ on gender. The CNM and NP groups are predominately women (99% and 93%, respectively), whereas the CRNA group is nearly half men (45%). APRNs are less diverse than the RN population, with 4.4% Hispanic and 5% Black/African American APRNs.

Within the NP workforce, nearly half were working in primary care practices or facilities. However, about three quarters of NPs report having been certified in a primary care specialty such as internal medicine (13%), pediatrics (3%), psychiatry/mental health (6%), women's health (9%), and palliative care/pain management (2%) (Auerbach et al., 2012; HRSA, 2012b). As of 2012, more than half worked in ambulatory care settings, including private physician or NP practices and private or federal community health clinics.

CNMs and NPs who are employed full-time have similar average salaries in the $95,000 range (BLS, 2014b, 2014c, 2014d); CRNAs employed full-time earn significantly more on average ($154,000). In many states, APRNs care for a high number of Medicaid, uninsured, and minority patients in both the inner city and rural communities (Skillman, Kaplan, Fordyce, McMenamin, & Doescher, 2012; Yoon, Grumbach, & Bindman, 2004). The geographic distribution of APRNs varies by state regulations limiting their practice to the full scope of their ability and training. States with the highest number of APRNs include New York, California, Texas, Florida, and Massachusetts; CRNAs are most prevalent in Pennsylvania, Florida, Minnesota, Texas, and California (HRSA, 2013a).

The recent economic recession has resulted in a temporary RN surplus because of deferred retirements and enrollment/graduation surges in nursing programs (McMenamin, 2013). Although there will always be a need for traditional hospital nurses, a large number of new nurses will be needed in home health care (to perform complex procedures in patients' homes), long-term care (for older, sicker patients and rehabilitation for stroke, head injury, or Alzheimer's disease patients), and ambulatory care (for patients having same-day surgery, rehabilitation, chemotherapy [IOM, 2011b], chronic disease management, primary care, and preventive services). The BLS (2013b) projects that 700,000 additional RN jobs will become available between 2010 and 2020, with the largest share in hospitals but also in high growth areas such as home health (55% growth), community care facilities for the elderly (50% growth), outpatient clinics (45% growth), and health practitioner offices (45% growth). Although new and less-experienced RN graduates are frustrated by lack of jobs now, the demand for RNs in the future looks bright. Having a full and growing pipeline of new nurses today will be prepared to address the "tsunami of RN retirements" that is predicted in the next decade (McMenamin, 2014).

Employment of CRNAs, CNMs, and NPs is expected to grow 31% from 2012 to 2022, much faster than the average for all occupations. Growth will occur because of an increase in the demand for health care services. Several factors, including ACA legislation and the resulting newly insured, an increased emphasis on preventive care, and the large, aging baby-boom population will contribute to this demand. APRNs, combining nursing and medical knowledge and skills, can perform many of the same services as physicians and will be needed to provide primary care services (U.S. Department of Labor, 2014a).

Medicine

As of 2014, there are more than 1 million licensed physicians and surgeons in the United States, and 37% of them were women (BLS, 2014a). As indicated in Table 2.1, the proportion of physicians who are women increased from 24% in 1995. During the past three decades, the proportion of physicians who are female has risen from 8% to nearly one in three (HRSA, 2008). Recent trends suggest that within the next two decades, women will constitute nearly half the physician workforce. The increase in the number of new physicians who are female means that male physicians tend to be older, on average, than female physicians. The AMA (2006) reports that in 2004, approximately 36% of active male physicians were younger than 45 years compared with approximately 61% of active female physicians.

There are few data about the proportion of minority women physicians, but ethnic diversity in medicine has been slow to improve. In 1989 and 2010, 3% of all physicians were Black (Hart-Brothers, 1994). Approximately one in four Americans is either Black or Hispanic, yet together these two minority groups constitute only 11% of the physician workforce (see Table 2.2). In contrast, Asian physicians were overrepresented (20%) compared with 6% of Asians in the total workforce in 2014. In 2014, the number of Black physicians doubled to 6%, equal to Latino(a)s (U.S. Department of Labor, 2014b). However, in the past decade, the number of Black women physicians has increased more rapidly than the number of male physicians in the United States. These women have made it into a traditionally male work world, and, although they are at the top of the health care occupations hierarchy, they face problems similar to those faced by women in other occupations and in society as a whole.

The proportion of physicians who are women varies substantially by medical specialty, with women more likely to choose primary care specialties over surgical or other subspecialties. Among those specialties with more than 10,000 physicians, the two specialties with the highest proportion of female physicians are general pediatrics (52%) and obstetrics and gynecology (41%). The two specialties with the smallest proportion of female physicians are orthopedic surgery (4%) and urology (5%) (HRSA, 2008). Novielli, Hojat, Park, Connella, and Veloski (2001) report that differences between male and female physicians in choice of medical career path stem not from experience, but rather from personal preference. The authors find that women starting medical school are more likely than men to express a desire to practice in a nonsurgical specialty. Furthermore, during medical school, women are more likely than men to be dissuaded from entering a surgical specialty. Of those new enrollees in medical school who expressed an initial preference for a surgical specialty, the proportion that eventually entered a nonsurgical residency program was higher for women than men. Similarly, of those new enrollees in medical school who expressed an initial interest in a nonsurgical specialty, the proportion that eventually entered a nonsurgical residency program was higher for women than for men.

The work settings of physicians are primarily in private offices (40%) and hospitals, with hospital percentages varying from 25% to 42% depending on the source (HRSA, 2013a). Between the passage of the ACA in 2010 and 2015, 16 million people in the United States gained access to health care. More people with health coverage, combined with an aging population living longer, make for a predicted shortage of up to 124,000 physicians by 2025 (BLS, 2015b; Cooper, 2013; DHHS, 2015).

In spite of projected shortages, physician supply will likely increase but will be muted by other factors that will probably reduce growth. New technologies will allow physicians to treat more patients in the same amount of time, and the increased use of physician assistants and NPs may be used to reduce costs at hospitals and outpatient care facilities (BLS, 2015b). In addition, the increasing proportion of physicians who are women and are older, and who typically work fewer hours per year compared with their younger male colleagues, suggests that total hours of physician services provided is increasing less rapidly than the number of licensed physicians (HRSA, 2008).

As described in the history of the development of nursing, the history of women in medicine is clearly linked with women's social and political history. It is not surprising that women faced resistance in seeking entrance into the medical profession. In the 19th century, when women were organizing and fighting for their political (right to vote) and social (right to work outside the home and own property) rights and some women were fighting to establish nursing as a respectable career for women, others were arguing that women ought to be physicians "by virtue of their natural gifts as healers and nurturers" (Morantz-Sanchez, 1985). Although the feminist movement of the 19th century helped women gain access to medical education and careers, at the same time the feminist movement also incited a strong resistance to women in medicine (Shryock, 1967).

The early relative success in the 1850s in opening medicine to women was minimized or reversed in the late 19th and early 20th centuries. During this time, the Flexner Report was contracted by the Carnegie Corporation and published in 1910. The wealth of the industrial revolution had allowed the development of organized philanthropy, and medical reform was a high priority for these new foundations. In the name of standardizing (in accordance with the Johns Hopkins medical education model) and ensuring the quality of medical education, the majority of smaller, less well-endowed and well-supported medical schools that trained women and minority physicians were effectively closed. Although this process eliminated ineffective and dangerous small schools and led to the current model of undergraduate study followed by medical school then 3 to 8 years of residency, depending on the specialty, it also eliminated those that were effective and successful but unable to finance the newly required facilities. Without access to training opportunities, the number of women

physicians decreased markedly. Not until the 20th-century women's movement, which gained momentum in the 1960s, did women begin to increase significantly in numbers and proportion of medical school applicants, admissions, and graduates (Walsch, 1977).

Making it into the world of medicine, however, does not mean making it within the world of medicine—if making it means status and monetary success. The average physician earned $187,000 in 2012, with full-time women physicians still making only 59% of their male colleague's wages (BLS, 2015b). This abysmal gap could be related to the lower paying specialties typically chosen by women, or it could stem from a lack of opportunity in higher paying, leadership positions. Ross (2001) notes that payment for services rendered does not discriminate by physician gender, and he proposes that income differences between men and women likely reflect a voluntary trade-off between earnings and lifestyle beyond those factors controlled for (Ness & Ukoli, 2001). Additional factors that might explain the difference in average earnings of male and female physicians are that, compared with their male colleagues, female physicians might see fewer patient per hour and be less likely to participate in night and weekend call activities.

Physician wages vary greatly among the specialties, with the highest paying specialties of surgery and oncology paying nearly three times internal medicine and pediatrics. The most extreme difference is $83 per hour (Leigh, Tancredi, Jerant, & Kravitz, 2010). Primary care physicians' total compensation is less than that of specialists, and their income is increasing at a slower rate. The gap in income, combined with various other factors such as high medical school debt and professional prestige, influences the decisions of recent medical school graduates.

In 2006 to 2008, women graduating from U.S. medical schools were substantially underrepresented among residents in the high-paying specialties of neurosurgery, orthopedics, urology, otolaryngology, general surgery, and radiology. Conversely, 47% of women had specialized in internal medicine and 75% in pediatrics, the lower paying specialties (Jagsi, Griffith, DeCastro, & Ubel, 2014). Whether these specialty choices reflect women's preferences for practice type and environment (possibly shaped by the genders who dominate them) or reflect a subtle pressure to choose "appropriate" specialties, gender segregation within medical specialties continues, with a higher proportion of women being at the bottom of the medical hierarchy. In a 1998 survey of women physicians (Frank, Harvey, & Elon, 2000), although most were satisfied with their medical career and choice of specialty, many would not become physicians if starting their careers again because of work stress, harassment, and poor control over their work environment (MomMD, 2004; Reed, Jernstedt, & McCormick, 2009).

The discrimination that women physicians have faced in medicine has been well documented (Friedman, 1994; Lorber, 1984; Morantz-Sanchez, 1985; Walsch, 1977). The problems of combining a family with a demanding medical career have been explored with the not-surprising finding that women physicians feel the most strain in their personal lives, some strain in their family role, and minimal strain in their professional role (Bickel, 2000; Ducker, 1986; Frank et al., 2000). Women physicians, like women in general, sacrifice their own health and well-being for the sake of others. Women physicians struggle to combine a family life and a career (More & Greer, 2000; Woodward, Cohen, & Ferrier, 1990). A female surgery resident who is married starts out "with a strike against her" because her attention is assumed to be divided between her career and her marriage/family responsibilities (Burnley & Burkett, 1986). The struggles that men physicians face in combining a family and a career are not documented in the literature on physicians; therefore comparisons are not currently possible. However, there is an indication among young physicians, both men and women, to reduce the traditionally long and rigorous training and practice schedules and to find ways to maintain a more healthy balance among their professional, family, and medical leadership responsibilities (Friedman, 1994; MomMD, 2016). There is also indication that the disparities in earnings between men and women physicians have begun to shrink. Although physician earnings are one of the highest of any occupation, women physicians earn about two thirds of men physicians' mean annual income (U.S. Department of Labor, 2015a). With the growth of managed care, the ACA, and an increase of salaried physicians (for both men and women), gender differences in earnings are declining.

The increase in the number of women in medicine may be related to a decline in men's applications to medical schools, as well as older men physicians leaving the practice. Medicine has been seen as a less attractive career choice for well-educated men (who have the greatest career options) because of constraints on professional fees and salaries, the expansion of managed care arrangements, and increasing government regulation of health care services (Ginzberg & Minogiannis, 2004). Women may be in a more advantageous position because their values tend to be more congruent with the shape of the new health care system. Many prefer salaried employment, many are attracted to primary care specialties, and many prefer the flexibility that medicine offers them to extend or contract their hours of work.

An unfortunate outcome of the increased number of women in medicine has been an increase in distancing behavior among women physicians and other women health care workers, especially nurses. Surveys in the past decade support the view that women physicians are no more collaborative in their relationships than men physicians (Fagin, 1994). Articles written by women physicians indicate that the problem may be worse when both professionals are women, because women physicians must demonstrate their differences from women nurses, thereby increasing their status while lowering nurses' status (National League for Nursing, 1990; Ulrich, 2010). Lorber (1987) and Wilson (1987) sum up the issues by stating that women physicians face a choice—either they can align themselves with men physicians and perpetuate physician dominance of the health care system or they can align themselves with other women and work toward change of the health care system. More recent evidence suggests that lack of physician understanding about and respect for other health care worker's knowledge and scope of practice may be more important than gender differences between physicians and other health workers (Ulrich, 2010).

Twenty years ago, both men and women patients preferred women physicians (up to three times more often), especially in the areas of obstetrics and gynecology, family practice, internal medicine, and psychiatry (Ahmad, Gupta, Rawlins, & Stewart, 2002; Fenton, Robinowitz, & Leaf, 1987). This gender preference has lessened with time. In a 1999 study of more than 8,000 women, only just more than half preferred a female gynecologist, and 42% had no gender preference (Schmittdiel, Selby, Grumbach, & Quesenberry, 1999). In certain specialties, physician preference is more linked to reason for the treatment and physician characteristics as male or female, independent of the actual gender (Dusch, O'Sullivan, & Ascher, 2014). In surgery, a 2014 study showed that 78% of patients had no preference for the orthopedic surgeon's gender, and any preference, if shown, was not statistically significant (Abghari et al., 2014).

Whether the increasing proportion of women physicians will result in women influencing the practice of medicine or whether the established medical profession will influence women physicians—or a combination of the two—the status of women physicians will continue to be linked with the status of women in society.

PHARMACY

Pharmacists represent the third largest health professional group in the United States, with about 214,000 active pharmacists in 2014 (U.S. Department of Labor, 2015b). Most pharmacists are employed and practice in hospitals and medical centers (23%) or retail stores with pharmacies (43%; U.S. Department of Labor, 2015b). Smaller numbers of pharmacists are employed by pharmaceutical manufacturers, managed care and health insurance plans, consulting groups, long-term care facilities, home health care, and universities.

The entry to work is typically 6 years of education to obtain a doctor of pharmacy degree. The graduate must then pass national- and state-level licensure exams. The pharmacist has the option of 1 to 2 years in residency for advanced clinical or academic work (U.S. Department of Labor, 2015b), thus preparing pharmacists to take on more complex clinical roles such as counseling patients, advising other health professionals on drug use issues, and participating in disease management programs.

Pharmacists practicing today provide a much broader range of services than they did in the past. A 2014 national survey of working pharmacists showed the most common services offered are medication therapy management (60%) and immunizations (53%). These services greatly increased in the past decade from 13% of respondents offering medication therapy management and 15% administering immunizations. In the same survey, half of pharmacists working in large chain stores reported offering health screenings. This compares with less than 10% in 2004 (American Association of Colleges of Pharmacy [AACP], 2014a).

There has been an unprecedented demand for pharmacists and for pharmaceutical care services. Although the overall supply of pharmacists has increased in the past decade and will continue to grow 14% until 2022, slightly above the average for all professions, growth will not meet demand. Some of the factors identified as contributing to the shortage include advances in new drug development and dispensing technology, changes in the organization of pharmaceutical distribution through pharmacy benefit management programs and growth of chain pharmacy stores, rapid expansion in the number of medications dispensed, increased numbers of pharmacy technicians, and greater range of opportunities for clinical pharmacists (Knapp, 1999; DHHS, 2000).

Pharmacists are some of the highest paid health professionals. The 2012 median annual pay was $117,000. The highest annual wage was $132,160, made by pharmacists working in California, which employs the most pharmacists in the United States (BLS, 2015d). The wage gap of women pharmacists is better compared with other professions; they earn 87% of their male colleagues, rather than 82% (see Table 2.1).

As with many professions, pharmacy has seen changes in workforce demographics over the past three decades, particularly for gender. In 1970, women pharmacists accounted for 13% of the pharmacy workforce, progressing to nearly 54% in 2012 and 56% in 2014 (see Table 2.1). The racial/ethnic diversity of licensed pharmacists in the United States is improving, but like other high-paying health professions, it does not represent the diversity of the U.S. population. In 2010, the majority of pharmacists were White (72%) and Asian (17%), with much smaller representation of Black (6%), and Hispanic/Latino(a) (4%). Pharmacists are aging. In 2000, 78% of pharmacists were younger than 40 years. In 2014, 72% were older than 41 years, with fully 37% older than 56 years (AACP, 2014b; HRSA, 2013a). This compares with the total U.S. 2014 workforce, which is 42% older than 40 years (U.S. Department of Labor, 2015b).

Of the three highest paid health professionals—physicians, dentists, and pharmacists—the growth of women in pharmacy has been most impressive. What aspect of education, training, policy, reimbursement, or work environment has supported this growth? Goldin and Katz in a 2012 National Bureau of Economic Research working paper suggest it is the move away from self-employed pharmacists and interchangeability of pharmacists in their workflow, allowing for job sharing and part-time work (Goldin & Katz, 2012). How can the other professions learn from this change?

DENTISTRY

As cosmetic dental services increase in demand and the aging baby-boom generation needs dental work, the employment of dentists is projected to grow 18% from 2014 to 2024 (BLS, 2015c). Oral health care is provided by dentists and dental hygienists, with support from dental assistants, which includes 152,000 dental hygienists and 284,000 dental assistants (HRSA, 2013a). Dental care focuses on oral health and oral function provided by general dentists, dental specialists, and dental hygienists. Most dentists practice as generalists, in sharp contrast with medicine, where the number of specialist physicians far exceeds generalists.

Once focused on treatment, today the focus is on preventive aspects of oral health care. Similar to all other health professionals, technological advances, market evolution, health insurance, and demographic changes have substantially altered the types and quality of dental services.

Studies continue to link oral health to overall health. Medications such as painkillers and diuretics can reduce saliva flow that washes away bacteria in the mouth, diabetes can lower the body's resistance to infections, and oral cancer risk increases with age. Functional dental services have increased in demand as baby boomers age. Consumers are living longer and keeping their teeth longer, reflecting an increasing demand for implants, bridges, and cosmetic services. The U.S. public is increasingly interested in the prevention of dental disease, good occlusion, pain-free joint and jaw function, good lip function for speech, and skeletal harmony in their faces for an attractive appearance. There is also a need for holistic dental providers with the capacity to consider overall health status. Concurrently, there has been a deterioration in oral health according to two government studies that found over one third of the U.S. population has no access to community water fluoridation and more than 108 million children and adults lack dental care (IOM, 2011a).

Dental services are commonly provided in private clinic settings and most commonly by solo-practice dentists or groups with two or three dentists. In 2014, approximately one of four dentists reported being self-employed. There is no consensus on the optimal number and ratio of health professionals to meet the population's health care needs. However, in the 1990s, growth in dental services fell below overall population growth (Brown & Lazar, 1999). According to 2012 data, more than 30% of dentists were older than 55 years in contrast to the 8% of dental assistants who are older than 55 years (HRSA, 2013a). Even as the employment of dentists is expected to grow faster than any other profession, it will not meet the population needs (BLS, 2015c). The demand for dentists will grow by 10%, but the supply will only grow by 6% (HRSA, 2015c).

The median annual wage for dentists was $149,310 in May 2012. The lowest 10% earned less than $73,840, and the top 10% earned $187,200 or more. Earnings vary according to the number of years in practice, location, hours worked, and specialty. Data are not available for gender differences in wages for male and female dentists (see Table 2.1; U.S. Department of Labor, 2015b).

The rate of growth in the number of women in dentistry has been substantial, with almost a 50% increase in women dentists over the past 20 years. In 1980, women represented 14% of new graduates in dentistry; by 1996, the proportion had increased to 36%. Although women represented only 2% of practicing dentists in 1980, they represented almost 22% in 2005 and 25% in 2012 (American Dental Association [ADA], 1999; BLS, 2013a; HRSA, 2015d; U.S. Department of Labor, 2006). Compared with the number of women in medicine and pharmacy, the number of women in dentistry lags, with only one of four dentists being women, compared with a 1:2 ratio for pharmacy and a 1:3 ratio for medicine. Although earnings are high for dentists, the traditional solo practice model may be a deterrent for women entering the profession who want to balance work and family and prefer group or part-time practice.

Similar to the other health professions, dentists and dental hygienists/assistants do not represent the race/ethnicity of the U.S. population (see Table 2.2). The majority of dentists are non-Hispanic White (81%), with 3.3% African American and 14.5% Asian (HRSA, 2015d). Approximately 6% of dentists and dental hygienists are Latino(a) compared with 23% of dental assistants. Yet dental care is seen as the greatest unmet need by low-income and minority communities. Although dental care has historically been segregated from other health care services, innovative workforce models are being tested across the country to address the needs of the elderly, disabled, and low-income populations in the context of their existing community and public health systems (Mertz, 2014).

ALLIED HEALTH CARE SUPPORT OCCUPATIONS AND PERSONAL CARE/SERVICE OCCUPATIONS

Although there is no single definition of the allied health workforce or list of allied health occupations, the 2013 *U.S. Health Workforce Chartbook* (HRSA, 2013a) lists these occupations by categories of dietitians/nutritionists; allied health therapists and their assistants (physical therapy, occupational therapy, respiratory therapy, speech-language pathology, massage therapy); technologists and technicians (health diagnosing/treating practitioner support, medical/clinical laboratory, diagnostic related, medical records/health information, and paramedic/emergency medical technicians); and aides and assistants (medical, nursing, psychiatric, home health aides, personal care aides). According to this 2013 report, these allied health care workers[8] make up more than half of the nation's health care workforce. Although there is no unified definition, allied health care workers are generally considered to be a large cluster (more than 200 occupational titles) of health care–related professions and personnel whose functions include assisting, facilitating, or complementing the work of health professionals and other specialists in the health care system, and who choose to be identified as allied health personnel. All definitions exclude dentists and physicians, and most exclude registered nurses, pharmacists, physician assistants, clinical psychologists, counselors, and social workers. The federal government has defined an *allied health care professional* as a professional who has a certificate, associate degree, bachelor's degree, master's degree, doctoral degree, or postbaccalaureate training in science relating to health care and who shares in the responsibility for the delivery of health care and related services (U.S. Government Publishing Office [GPO], 2015). Health care workforce experts do not recommend regularizing the allied health definition nor do they draw rigid distinctions among the terms *profession*, *occupation*, or *field* that prevent the continued evolution of the health care workforce (IOM, 2011b).

Although estimates vary widely, data from 2010 suggest that 60% of the total health care workforce (approximately 7 million workers) is employed as allied health workers. Health care support occupations—medical, nursing, psychiatric, home health assistants and personal care aides—account for the largest group of allied health workers with more than 4 million workers (approximately 60% of the allied health workforce); half of this group are nursing/psychiatric/home health aides (2.3 million workers). Technologists/technicians represent about 20% of the allied health workforce (1.5 million), and another 15% are allied health therapists and nutritionists/dietitians (800,000) (HRSA, 2013a).

The allied health workforce lacks diversity by gender but is more ethnically diverse than the health diagnosing and treating practitioners. Women make up a large proportion of the workforce in most of these occupations (80%–85%). The largest proportion of female allied health workers is within the therapists, health care support, health technologists/technicians, and personal care service categories. A recent report of the NCHWA (HRSA, 2015d) highlights the proportion of women in selected allied health occupations: dental hygienists/assistants and speech-language therapists (96% women), nutritionists and occupational therapists (90% women), health records technologists/technicians and nursing, medical and home health aides (87% women), clinical laboratory/diagnostic technologists/technicians (72% women), physical therapists/assistants (70% women), and respiratory therapists (66% women). Men outnumber women in only one occupational category—emergency medical technicians and paramedics (HRSA, 2015d).

Racial/ethnic diversity is increased in the health care support and personal care occupations that require fewer years of education or training. Ethnic minority women are overrepresented in the lowest paying allied health occupations such as nursing assistants and personal care aides. Black/African Americans (14% of U.S. working population) are overrepresented in the areas of nursing/psychiatric/home health assistant (37.5%), personal care aide (28%), and medical assistant (18%) fields, but are equitably represented in the respiratory therapist (13.5%), medical/clinical laboratory technician (15%), and health information technician (18%) fields. Although Hispanics (16% of U.S. working population) are underrepresented in almost all of the allied health worker categories, they have the highest representation among dental assistants (23%). Conversely, non-Hispanic Whites have their lowest representation among nursing/psychiatric/home health assistants (54%) and personal care aides (59%).

The majority of technical allied health jobs are in hospitals: 80% of respiratory therapists, 60% of clinical laboratory technologists, and more than half of radiology technicians. Dieticians, emergency medical technicians, and occupational and physical therapists are often employed by private contractors or state and local governments (public health departments). The majority of the lowest paid allied health workers are in nursing and personal care facilities and home health care. Two thirds of the 845,000 medical assistants are employed in clinics or doctors' offices, and more than half of the 2.4 million nursing, psychiatric, and home health aides work in nursing care or long-term care facilities (HRSA, 2013a). The service and support occupations attract many workers with little or no specialized education or training. In general, education and technical training is directly linked with earnings and wages for all health care workers, including allied health workers (see Table 2.1). Although a high school diploma and on-the-job training are the minimum qualifications for entry into most of the lowest paid occupational categories, some college education or technical training is necessary for the technical and higher paid allied health occupations.

The median annual earnings for the lowest paid groups of personal care, nursing, and home health aides ($20,000 to $24,000) was less than the average annual wage for all workers ($35,000) (U.S. Department of Labor, 2014a). Medical record and health information technicians are projected to be the fastest growing occupations because of rapid growth in the number of medical tests, treatments, and procedures that will likely be increasingly scrutinized by third-party payers, regulators, courts, and consumers. Although technical jobs often have higher wages, these occupations are often unstable for long-term employment. These technology-driven jobs (e.g., radiation imaging) have limited scopes of practice, and new technology will reduce the need for workers. Overall within the allied health occupations, there is less of a gender–wage gap, with women allied health workers earning 80% to 90% of men's salaries (U.S. Department of Labor, 2015b). Although some authors have suggested that this disparity could reflect men's higher levels of responsibility rather than unequal pay for the same work, others point to the fact that, in the occupations with the most women (e.g., dental assistants and dietitians), they earn less than similar categories of workers that have more men (AAUW, 2015; Morrison & Gallagher Robins, 2015; Muller, 1994).

It has been widely believed that these jobs—because they tend to be thought of as women's jobs—are neither physically hazardous nor particularly stressful. In a recent report, low-wage women workers are more likely to have inflexible and unpredictable work schedules, have impossible childcare choices, and be vulnerable to discrimination and harassment (Gallagher Robins & Frohlich, 2014). Dietary workers report that they often prepare healthier foods professionally than they consume at home. Another myth is that women are working part time to supplement a husband's salary. In a 1993 study (Himmelstein, Lewontin, & Woolhandler, 1996), many poor and minority women, especially single African American mothers, were concentrated in the allied and auxiliary health occupations that did not provide worker benefits or health insurance. In 2010, more than 38% of low-wage workers lacked health insurance from any source, increased from 16% in 1979 (Schmitt, 2012). Although the ACA has significantly improved women's access to affordable health insurance, workers in these jobs may still face barriers to health insurance coverage and services they need, including reproductive health care services. Even with affordable health insurance, the ACA leaves an important share of low-wage workers, especially low-wage Latino(a), African American, and Asian workers, as well as many immigrant workers, without coverage (Di Julio, Firth, & Brodie, 2015). Compared with other occupational sectors, there are more occupational injuries and illness in hospitals and nursing homes, and these affect the lower paid workers more frequently (BLS, 2013a; Colligan,

Smith, & Hurrell, 1977; Occupational Safety and Health Administration [OSHA], 2013; U.S. Department of Labor, 2005).

Allied health positions—in particular, medical assistants and home health aides—are expected to grow rapidly in the next 10 years, by approximately 45% (Taché & Chapman, 2006; U.S. Department of Labor, 2012). In one of the higher paying allied health occupations, the demand for dental hygienists is increasing in response to the increasing need for dental care and the greater substitution of hygienists for services previously performed by dentists.

■ HEALTH CARE WORKFORCE DRIVERS AND DISPARITIES: INTERSECTIONS OF GENDER, RACE/ETHNICITY, ECONOMIC STATUS, AND POPULATION NEEDS

The health care system is undergoing major change, which has direct implications for the health care workforce. We are moving from acute care treatment to ambulatory care focused on the prevention of chronic disease. With innovations in technology and communications, the professional hierarchy will flatten to utilize a diverse health care team focused on consumers and cost-effectiveness. Legislative and demographic drivers include ACA implementation population growth that is increasingly diverse combined with an aging population.

Other trends include the growing problems in financing care for the uninsured and vulnerable populations (e.g., the working and nonworking poor, people with AIDS, the homeless, the chronically mentally ill, and frail elderly people needing long-term care) and the changing patterns of disease created by changing demographics and social trends (e.g., the aging population, the drug epidemic, environmental diseases, or deaths from violence). An aging population will require more home health care services and new technologies; health networks will become larger and more complex, requiring more managerial and support workers. When the ACA is fully implemented, an estimated 32 million people will be insured, and many will be seeking a source for primary care (Goodell, Dower, & O'Neil, 2011; O'Neil, 2003). The maldistribution of primary care providers appears to be a more significant problem than overall shortage.

A shift from hospital care to less expensive ambulatory and home care is occurring, partially because of a focus on (and funding for) disease prevention and health promotion, as well as cost-containment and self-care practices by many Americans. According to a recent study of health workforce demand, 3 to 4 million new health care jobs (20%–26% increase over current levels) will be created over the next decade (Frogner et al., 2015). The ambulatory care sector will see the largest gain in jobs, mostly because there will be growth in home health care and its workers have the lowest level of education. The fastest growing health occupations, such as medical assistants and pharmacy technicians, require no more than a high school diploma, with the ACA driving almost half of the jobs growth for medical secretaries, assistants, and pharmacy aides/technicians

(Spetz, Frogner, Lucia, & Jacobs, 2014). It is unfortunate that a high rate of poverty exists in these areas of anticipated job growth; for example, one in five workers in home health services is at or below the federal poverty level and has a higher rate of work disability (Frogner & Spetz, 2013, 2015; Frogner et al., 2015). Given these trends and projections, the health care workforce will be increasingly female, younger, racially/ethnically diverse, and non-U.S. born, with low income and low education.

Challenges Facing the Health Care Workforce

These trends point to the challenges of a mismatch across growing populations, a lack of workforce capacity, workforce shortages, and the need to develop health care workers. Challenges of the future concern people shortages, unmet training needs, maldistribution of services and providers, and imbalances across gender and racial diversity. Challenges will also include shifting from a mind-set of who is available to what is needed; overcoming convictions about who can and should do what; redesigning training so that incumbent health care workers are equipped with the skills needed to improved equity, quality, and safety; and investing in short- and long-term strategies to cultivate the necessary human capital to overcome shortages and develop a diverse health workforce that represents U.S. society, that is fairly compensated, and that does not discriminate. A major challenge in diversifying the health care workforce is to address gender (Hess et al., 2015; Newman, 2014) and racial inequities (Snyder et al., 2015) and the complex and intersecting historical, cultural, structural, and interpersonal patterns of discrimination (Aspen Institute; Byrd & Clayton, 2003; Collins, 1998; Davis, 2011; Jones, 2000; Redwood, 2015; Schulz & Mullings, 2006).

Gender and Racial Determinants and Inequities

According to a 2003 systematic review, differences in population characteristics, such as race/ethnicity, class, culture, and gender, are at the root of many of the present health and health system problems in the United States. Contrary to articulating gender, race, and class as distinct social categories, intersectionality (a theory posited by U.S. Black feminists, who challenged the notion of a universal gendered experience) postulates that these systems of oppression are mutually constituted and work together to produce inequality (Davis, 1981; Collins, 1990; Schulz & Mullings, 2006). Only until recently has there been a focus on the critical intersection among and between gender, race/ethnicity, economic inequality, sexual orientation, "abledness," sexual violence, genetic determinants, and a competent and productive health care workforce. Women and men as workers are shaped simultaneously by race-, class-, and gender-based systems of hierarchy as well as by ability/disability, sexual orientation, and age. Moreover, ecosocial theory integrates the body, mind, and society in understanding the health impact of social conditions and structural inequities, as well

as the ways that gender, race, and culture become interwoven in life (Hammarström et al., 2014).

Although this chapter focuses primarily on disparities associated with gender and race, much of the impact of these inequities also apply across other population dimensions. Marked differences in the intersecting social determinants, such as poverty, low socioeconomic status (SES), and lack of access to care, exist along racial/ethnic lines and have been shown to contribute to poor health outcomes on (DHHS, n.d.; MacDorman & Mathews, 2011; Sondik, Huang, Klein, & Satcher, 2010) historically linked to exclusion or discrimination.

Although the status for women in the workforce has improved over the past several decades, many women still struggle for equality in many occupations, and wage gaps persist. Despite high levels of education (women are earning postsecondary degrees at a faster rate than men are), and strong representation in professional and technical occupations, women still face persistent wage and earnings gap. Although a number of factors may influence the differences in earnings between men and women in the aggregate (such as higher numbers of women in lower paying occupations), the wage gap continues even within individual occupations. Women are also more likely than men to leave and then reenter the workforce if they have children, which may affect accrued seniority or promotions; yet even this is insufficient to explain the entire persistent gap (DPE, 2015).

In addition, the United States has been undergoing racial change throughout its history but never before at the pace and in the manner occurring now. Discrimination and racism continue to be a part of the fabric and tradition of American society and have adversely affected minority populations, the health care system in general, and the health care workforce. *Discrimination*, as defined in the *American Heritage Dictionary*, is

> Making a difference in treatment or favor on a class or categorical basis while disregarding individual merit; acting on the basis of prejudice; and the denial of equal opportunity (i.e. for education, employment, promotions, loans, housing, and health care).

Discrimination of this nature is not always easy to identify; however, its consequences are quite concrete. Prejudice and bias, on the other hand, involves thoughts, attitudes, insensitivity, and ignorance, not actual behaviors or demonstrable denials of opportunity. Prejudice frequently leads to discrimination. A prominent and particularly negative form of prejudice in America is racism. Too often racism is manifested in the attitudes of health care providers toward patients and their coworkers of different racial/ethnic groups as well as the structural- and system-level factors that maintain inequities and discriminatory patterns. Racism has an adverse impact on the health care environment and on those receiving health care services.

According to global labor standards, *workplace discrimination* is defined as:

> Practices that place individuals in a subordinate or disadvantaged position in the workplace or labor

market because of characteristics (race, religion, sex, political opinion, national extraction, social origin, or other attribute) that bear no relation to the person's competencies or the inherent requirements of the job. (International Labour Organization [ILO], 2015, p. 1)

In the health care arena, health care providers may be victims as well as perpetrators of gender and racial discrimination. Selective mistreatment undermines the work experiences of individuals who are identified with groups that are the targets of discriminatory behaviors. Although discrimination occurs on multiple levels—job, housing, and education inequities—it is complicated for women and racial minorities. Poverty, racism, and gender inequalities intersect to create "structural violence" whereby unequal opportunity and marginalization persist for many in the health workforce (Rhodes et al., 2012).

GENDER DISCRIMINATION

Gender discrimination, has been defined as any distinction, exclusion, or restriction made on the basis of socially constructed gender roles and norms that prevents a person from enjoying full human rights (World Health Organization [WHO], 2001). Gender discrimination can take many forms such as wage discrimination, occupational gender segregation, sexual harassment, or conduct that creates an intimidating, hostile, or humiliating school or work environment. Gender discrimination can be less overt such as the exclusion of informal or home health workers from protective labor legislation (i.e., overtime payment requirements).

How gender discrimination has affected women in health care has been explored by a number of scholars (Ashley, 1976; Cleland, 1971; Darbyshire, 1987; Doyal, 1995; Hochschild, 1983; Levitt, 1977; Marini, 1989; Reverby, 1987a, 1987b; Tijdens, de Vries, & Steinmetz, 2013; Weaver & Garrett, 1983). Most historians attribute the discrepancy in compensation between men and women in the health occupations to gender discrimination and to lack of social value on caring work (Reverby, 1987b). Ashley describes the discriminatory attitudes toward women that institutionalized their servitude in hospitals and points out the far-reaching effects of sexism on the quality and delivery of health care in U.S. hospitals. Roberts (1983) explored oppression and oppressed group behavior in nursing, discussing how oppression has fostered the horizontal violence of nurse against nurse. Hochschild (1983) linked the work of "caring" with occupational activities and economics. In a study of women service workers, she described how women are expected to sell their "emotional labor"—to pretend to have positive feelings they are not experiencing and to deny their negative responses in order to make others feel they are being cared for in a safe environment (Hochschild, 1983). This often results in "emotional dissonance"—core stress in which the task of managing an estrangement between self and feeling and between self and behavior. Although women in jobs with the greatest responsibility reported the most stress, it was those with the least say over their working lives who suffered the worst effects. Hochschild also reported that this experience leads to burnout and a loss

of self as feelings and emotions became dulled as a defense against an intolerable situation. Subsequent studies have found that women workers with the least autonomy, job status, or control in their work suffered from physical and emotional disorders resulting in significant economic impact (Doyal, 1995; Hochschild, 1983).

Marini (1989) first described wage gaps in segregated occupations: The more an occupation is female-identified, the lower the wages for that occupation. A more recent study (Tijdens et al., 2013) found that "female" tasks and skills are devalued in the labor market, supporting the links among occupational segregation/composition, gender–wage gap, and discrimination. Moreover, even when women choose the same jobs as men, the wage gap persists. For example, male surgeons earn almost 40% more per week than their female counterparts. In real terms, this means that a female surgeon earns $756 less per week than her male colleague, which adds up to nearly $40,000 over the course of 1 year (Baxter, 2015).

More recent research suggests that there has been a lack of concerted attention to gender discrimination within the health care workforce because of the lack of clarity and consensus about what it is and how it manifests itself in the health workforce (Newman, 2014). Newman reviewed the literature on definitions, types, and effects of gender discrimination. Gender inequalities and discrimination contribute to clogged health worker educational pipelines, recruitment bottlenecks, workplace absenteeism, attrition, and worker maldistribution. Other negative effects of gender discrimination include lower productivity because of stress and low morale, which further limits the pool of motivated frontline health care workers to cope with current and future health challenges. Research on nurses found that they experienced moral distress associated with perceived poor ethical climate, such as the dissonance between a lack of respect for colleagues or patients and the nurse's perceived lack of decision making power (Lamiani, Borghi, & Argentero, 2015).

RACIAL/ETHNIC DISCRIMINATION

Racial/ethnic disparities and discrimination in health care occur in the context of broader historic and contemporary social, structural, and economic inequality, with evidence of persistent racial/ethnic discrimination in many sectors of American life. African Americans, Hispanics, American Indians/Pacific Islanders, and some Asian American subgroups are disproportionately represented in the lower socioeconomic ranks, in lower quality schools, and in poorer paying jobs (Nelson, 2002). These disparities can be traced to many factors, including historic patterns of legalized segregation, structural racism, and discrimination. It is unfortunate that discrimination remains, as evidenced by how much of American social and economic life remains ordered by race/ethnicity, with people of color disadvantaged relative to Whites.

Reviews of hundreds of studies conducted in different parts of the country indicate significant differences in health care received by persons of different racial/ethnic backgrounds. Differential treatment and access to care in most studies could not be explained by such factors as socioeconomic status (SES), insurance coverage, stage or severity of disease, comorbidities, type and availability of health care services, and patient preferences (Mayberry, Mili, & Ofili, 2000). Despite efforts to address diversity of the health care workforce over the past 30 years, entrenched structural inequities exist in health care professional education and within health care institutions (Schroeder & DiAngelo, 2010). Although institutions focus on promoting cultural competence within the health professional workforce, issues of power, White privilege, and racism/antiracism are not systematically addressed. More and more evidence suggests that if institutionalized racism is addressed by health care systems (including education programs), other levels of racism, such as internalized and personally mediated racism, will resolve themselves (Jones, 2000).

Most of the health care workforce data on racial discrimination comes from health professions literature on physicians and nurses. The representation of many minorities (e.g., African Americans, Hispanics, and Native Americans) within health professions is far below their representation in the general population. Physician surveys conducted in the 1990s established that racial/ethnic discrimination was common in the health care workplace. A 1995 national study among academic physicians found that nearly half of nonracial majority physicians had experienced racial/ethnic discrimination in the workplace. Another national study, conducted in 1993 and 1994 among female physicians, found that approximately 60% of nonracial majority respondents reported racial/ethnic discrimination at work (Palepu et al., 1998). Furthermore, physicians from nonmajority backgrounds are generally less satisfied with their careers and less likely to be promoted than their majority colleagues with similar academic productivity. The proportion of physicians who reported that they had experienced racial/ethnic discrimination "sometimes, often, or very often" during their medical career was substantial among nonmajority physicians (71% of Black, 45% of Asian, 63% of "other" race, and 27% of Hispanic/Latino[a], compared with 7% of White physicians, all $p < .05$). Similarly, the proportion of nonmajority physicians who reported that they experienced discrimination in their current work setting was substantial (59% of Black, 39% of Asian, 35% of "other" race, 24% of Hispanic/Latino[a], and 21% of White physicians) (Nunez-Smith et al., 2009).

In a 2002 report, the IOM found "strong but circumstantial evidence for the role of bias, stereotyping, and prejudice" (p. 178) in perpetuating racial health disparities (Nelson, 2002). Although explicit race bias is rare among health professionals, an unconscious preference for Whites compared with Blacks is commonly revealed on tests of implicit bias (Chapman, Kaatz, & Carnes, 2013). Implicit racial bias has been implicated in the failure to achieve greater inclusion of Black students in medical education; the percentage of Black men among all medical school graduates has declined over the past 20 years (Ansell & McDonald, 2015). Although nurses are a historically oppressed group, the profession as a whole, like physicians, has not adequately addressed their complicity in the relative silence on race and the role they have in perpetuating racial health care disparities (Hall & Fields, 2013).

Hall and Fields point out that the majority of nurses are White and that racism perpetuated by Whites is more prevalent than that of any other people of color. Allen (2006) writes of nursing education as a factory perpetuating racial inequities and White privilege.

Institutional racism at the level of health care systems and health professions training has been described as a critically important factor in maintaining discriminatory practices. The institutional climate for discrimination in education and health care systems is influenced by several elements of the institutional context, including the degree of structural diversity; the historical legacy of inclusion or exclusion of students, clinicians, and faculty of color; the psychological climate (i.e., perceptions of the degree of racial tension and discrimination on campus or institution); and the behavioral dimension (i.e., the quality and quantity of interactions across diverse groups and diversity-related education; Grumbach, Coffman, Rosenoff, & Munoz, 2001; Gurin, Dey, Hurtado, & Gurin, 2002; Hurtado, Milem, Clayton-Pedersen, & Allen, 1999; Smedley, Butler, & Bristow, 2004). More recent evidence shows that the long-standing inequities within medicine, nursing, and health care institutions continue because of the lack of acknowledgment of "Whiteness" as a source of structural advantage within the health professions, education, and health care institutions (Schroeder & DiAngelo, 2010).

In a 2004 IOM report (Smedley et al., 2004), a review of the evidence indicated that reducing discrimination and bias among the health care workforce and service is associated with improved access to care for racial/ethnic minority patients, greater patient choice and satisfaction, better patient–provider communication, and better educational experiences for health professionals, students, and practitioners. Efforts to increase the proportions of people of color in health care professions have met with limited success and have been hampered by gross inequalities in educational opportunity for students of different racial/ethnic groups. The costs associated with health professions training pose a significant barrier for many students of color. Tuition and other educational costs have climbed steadily along with increasing student debt, whereas sources of grant aid have decreased.

Racial discrimination in the job market continues to persist (Emmons & Noeth, 2015). Higher education has not leveled the playing field in terms of occupational success or wage gaps. White and Asian college graduates do much better than their counterparts without college, whereas college-graduate Hispanics and Blacks do much worse proportionately. The Black unemployment rate has consistently been twice as high as the rate for Whites even among college graduates. Blacks and Latino(a)s at all educational levels, including those with college and advanced degrees, earn less than their White counterparts; this means lower lifetime earnings, less ability to save, and less likelihood to receive help from family for education costs.

Encouraging, however, are the emerging advocacy efforts, as well as sustainable antiracist action, within the health professions. Recently, health professional leaders have called on their communities to advocate against the implicit bias among professionals that is adversely affecting the health of all minorities and Black patients in particular. Mary Bassett, New York City health commissioner, suggests that health care professionals should be accountable for battling the racism that contributes to poor health (Bassett, 2015). Nursing professors, Joanne Hall and Becky Fields, have called on White nurses to talk to other White nurses about how marginalizing racial disparities are perpetuated in nursing practices, the development of knowledge, and education (Hall & Fields, 2013). In response to the killings of unarmed Black men, a national student-led campaign (White Coats 4 Black Lives) was initiated to call attention to biases among health professionals, in learning environments, and in administrative decision making that leads to disparities in the medical community and, ultimately, the health of people (White Coats 4 Black Lives, 2015). Mandated action within educational institutions to make real and sustained change includes faculty and staff workshops (e.g., undoing racism workshops in school of nursing), top leadership commitment,[9] institutionally certified mission statements, and institutional maintenance and support for the antiracist efforts (Schroeder & DiAngelo, 2010).

■ FUTURE DIRECTIONS

Strengthening the Health Care Workforce for a Preferred Future

Strengthening the nation's health and human services infrastructure involves addressing the critical shortage of primary care physicians, nurses, behavioral health providers, long-term care workers, and community health workers (CHWs) in the United States. With growing national diversity, disparities, inequities, and discrimination within the health care workforce must be addressed as well. National and global policy reforms have been initiated that focus on fiscal, legislative, and workforce policies to ensure the balance, mix, and distribution of health care workers necessary for a well-functioning, cost-efficient health system in the 21st century (Derksen & Whelan, 2009).

A growing body of literature indicates that many health care workforce problems, especially in public systems, have been focusing on the "hardware" issues (i.e., infrastructure, technology, economics) but not on the "software" issues of health care systems (i.e., human and social aspects). In attempts to reform health systems, the "economic reductionism and technocratic structuralism" fail to take into account the everyday organizational reality of what goes on inside health care delivery systems. Health care workers are not simply robots nor are they angels who have only the best interest of the patients at heart, but they are thinking, reflexive people who internalize and perpetuate the social norms of the societies in which they live and work (Govender & Penn-Kekana, 2008).

Until recently, little has been done to change health professions or health care worker enactment of these norms and biases or to include such workers as change agents

in education or health care delivery. Furthermore, little attention has focused on the dynamic between health care workers and the health care delivery system. In the current market-driven system, health care workers are treated as problems (liabilities and expenses) rather than as part of a solution (critical and participatory resources). The usual business approach of focusing on supply and demand fails to capture one of the fundamental problems that health care workers and professionals face today—the environment of care. Underpinning these health care workforce changes are the shifts in the larger work environment that limit economic mobility and livable wages: Stable jobs are being replaced with quasi-formal employment, freelancing, and mixed-earning strategies (e.g., a home health aide who drives for Uber or contracts through TaskRabbit.com), which lack basic benefits such as health insurance, dental and vision care, paid vacation, paid sick leave, or paid paternal leave (Carlton & Rockfeller Foundation, 2015).

WHAT IS BEING DONE AND WHAT MORE SHOULD BE DONE

Developing and maintaining a health care workforce that meets the needs of the population and the health service system require multiple approaches. These include policy reforms and private–public partnerships that create good jobs for all workers while addressing diversity and discrimination, working in teams, and empowering women.

Private–Public Investments and Policy Reforms • The federal government is stepping up its investment in the health care workforce and creating policy levers for sustainable change. The 2010 ACA (2015) includes critical funding for new as well as existing efforts to diversify the nation's health care workforce through academic programs, mentoring, and employment opportunities. Increasing and modernizing the health care workforce is a major goal of the ACA. The health reform law contains dozens of provisions related to health care workforce issues, including strengthening of primary care through payment reform, academic and financial assistance programs, and examination of the changing role of frontline health care workers such as NPs, who are increasingly providing primary care to medically underserved communities.

The president's 2015 budget initiative proposed major new investments to build the health care workforce and improve the delivery of health care services, particularly primary care services across the nation. Key components of the budget included a new HRSA grant program geared toward modernizing graduate medical education, major expansion of the National Health Service Corps (incentivizing health professionals to serve in primary care and medically underserved communities), and extension of enhanced Medicaid primary care payments through calendar year 2015 (DHHS, 2014). Established in 1982, HRSA is the primary federal agency of the DHHS responsible for improving access to health care by strengthening the health care workforce, building healthy communities, and achieving health equity. As health insurance coverage expansions that began in 2014 continue nationwide, HRSA's health care workforce programs seek to provide targeted support for health professions and for parts of the country where shortages of health professionals exist. Reorganization of HRSA's health workforce efforts occurred in 2014 under the Bureau of Health Workforce (HRSA, 2015a) with a focus on the following programs: scholarship, loan, and loan-repayment programs for health care professionals (addresses primary care professionals in underserved communities), health professions training grants (support diversity, interprofessional practice and training in geriatrics for primary care professionals), graduate medical education, health workforce analysis (improves research for health care workforce policy decisions), and health care workforce shortage designation and analysis. To this end, the budget provides a total of $1.8 billion for HRSA workforce programs (about 2.3% of DHHS budget in 2015 and twice that 5 years ago), a total that includes $1.2 billion in mandatory funding, to expand the nation's health care workforce capacity and to target health workforce resources to where they are needed most.

The 2015 HRSA budget included $530 million in mandatory funding for a new program, Targeted Support for Graduate Medical Education. This new competitive grant program funded teaching hospitals, children's hospitals, and community-based consortia of teaching hospitals and/or other health care entities to expand residency training, with a focus on ambulatory and preventive care, in order to advance the ACA's goals of higher value health care that reduces long-term costs. The 2015 HRSA Budget (HRSA, 2015b) also provided for two new workforce initiatives, including $10 million to support a new Clinical Training in Interprofessional Practice program to increase the capacity of community-based primary health care teams to deliver quality care. In addition, the budget provided $4 million to fund new Rural Physician Training Grants to help rural-focused training programs recruit and graduate students who are most likely to practice medicine in underserved rural communities. In addition, HRSA continues funding for health care professions programs—nursing, oral health, primary care, geriatric, behavioral health, and public health care workforce development and training.

Partnerships between the federal government and private philanthropy have expanded health care workforce development, especially HRSA partnerships with the Robert Wood Johnson Foundation (RWJF; interprofessional education/practice, diversity, nursing workforce; RWJF, 2015), the John A. Hartford Foundation (geriatric workforce), and the Josiah Macy Jr. Foundation (primary care workforce). As the largest philanthropy dedicated to the health and health care in the United States, RWJF has been the leader of a number of important initiatives to strengthen the health care workforce and support the preparation of a diverse and well-trained leadership and workforce to meet the nation's current and future health care needs (Ladden & Maher, 2014). For example, leadership programs prepare health care professionals for success in a complex and changing health environment and enable them to lead systemic change (www.rwjf.org). Specific RWJF workforce initiatives aim to identify and develop innovations and policies to develop the dental, medical, nursing, and public health workforce in order to make health systems work better. For example, The Primary Care Team: Learning from Effective Ambulatory Practices (PCT-LEAP; RWJF, 2012) initiative is identifying changes in policy, workforce, culture, education, and training related to primary care that can improve the way practices function. The program studies 30 high-functioning primary care practices to learn what they do to maximize the contributions of health care professionals and other staff. Policies that affect nursing, primary care, interprofessional collaboration in education and in providing care, public health, and oral health will be specifically addressed. In addition, the RWJF has advanced women in the workforce through a decade of investment to strengthen the nursing workforce. Many of the RWJF's nursing programs support recommendations from the IOM's report, *The Future of Nursing: Leading Change, Advancing Health* (2010), which provides a blueprint for transforming the nursing profession to improve health care and meet the needs of diverse populations. These recommendations are being implemented through The Future of Nursing: Campaign for Action, a collaboration between RWJF and AARP (www.champion-nursing.org).

Improving Health Workforce Diversity • In a 2009 report, HRSA, along with the Office of Public Health and Science, concluded that health education pipeline program interventions can exert a meaningful, positive effect on student outcomes and that enrichment programs and academic support programs are promising interventions to improve academic performance and increase interest and enrollment in health profession programs (U.S. Department of Health and Human Services, Health Resources and Services Administration, Bureau of Health Professions, Office of Public Health and Science, Office of Minority Health, 2009). In a follow-up review, an HRSA-funded workforce studies center has summarized the effectiveness of pipeline programs that seek to recruit and retain minorities into the health workforce (Snyder et al., 2015). In their analysis of recent published and gray literature (2009–2014), minimal evidence was found to demonstrate the long-term success of programs on the change in the representation of racial/ethnic minorities in the health professions. Some efforts have been found to be effective at increasing the interest, application, and enrollment of racial/ethnic minorities into health profession schools, such as medicine or dentistry, yet there is still a missing link in the pipeline among entry, persistence, graduation, and pursuit of a career. Professional schools have implemented a variety of programs to support racial/ethnic minorities, including mentoring programs, professional development, academic and social supports, and financial supports, yet evidence regarding the longer term effectiveness of such programs in retaining and graduating students or facilitating a professional career is lacking (Read, Vessey, Amar, & Cullinan, 2013; Schroeder & DiAngelo, 2010).

In their review, Snyder et al. (2015) recommend (a) expanding pipeline or pathway efforts to diversify the behavioral health workforce and the allied health occupations; (b) tailoring programs to specific populations and contexts; and (c) specifying contextual factors that have an impact on the retention of racial/ethnic minorities once they are in the education program as well as the profession. Even if minorities successfully graduate and obtain jobs as nurses, doctors, and allied health professionals will they stay?

As part of a national campaign to recruit and prepare a more diverse and culturally competent nursing workforce, 41 state action coalitions are working on diversity initiatives and are weaving them into their education, leadership, and practice work. Outcomes from these initiatives are showing modest, but steady, positive results. Between 2010 and 2014, the percentage of minority students in baccalaureate nursing programs increased 3.3% (from 26.8% to 30.1%), the percentage of minority students in master's nursing programs increased 5.8% (from 26.1% to 31.9%), and the percentage of minority students in doctoral nursing programs increased 6.5% (from 23.2% to 29.7%). Examples from Connecticut and Vermont demonstrate innovations in both diversity and team-based practice (Campaign for Action, 2014, 2015).

The health care industry can take lessons from other business sectors that value a diverse, productive, and healthy workforce. In the decades since Congress passed the Civil Rights Act of 1964, corporations have experimented with dozens of diversity measures such as diversity training, diversity performance evaluations for mangers, affinity networks, mentoring programs, diversity councils, and diversity managers. A large-scale study of 829 companies found that companies that give diversity councils or diversity managers responsibility for getting more women and minorities into good jobs typically demonstrate significant increases in the diversity of managers (Dobbin, Kalev, & Kelly, 2007). So do companies that create formal mentoring programs. Much less effective are diversity training sessions, diversity performance evaluations for managers, and affinity groups for women and minorities. In the average workplace, networking programs lead to slight increases for White women and decreases for Black men. Although these groups give people a place to share their experiences, they often bring together people on the lowest rungs of the corporate ladder. They may not put people in touch with what they need to know or whom they need to know in order to move up (Campaign for Action, 2014). Mentoring programs, by contrast, appear to help women and minorities. They show positive effects for Black women, Latino(a)s, and Asians. Moreover, in industries with many highly educated workers who are eligible for management jobs, they also help White women and Black men. Mentor programs put aspiring managers in contact with people who can help them move up, both by offering advice and by finding them jobs (Dobbin et al., 2007).

Tackling racism and discrimination—both personally and in the workplace—is daunting and often viewed as divisive. It has been suggested that White professionals acknowledge and address White racial domination to advance critical thinking, institutional reform, and public advocacy to address racial (and gender) inequities and discrimination (Bassett, 2015; Read et al., 2013; Schroeder & DiAngelo, 2010). Equally important is development of an "appropriate Whiteness" by those in the dominant culture to avoid continued marginalization by implicit or explicit

takeover of the antiracist movement by the very people it is meant to affect (Gillborn, 2013; Higginbotham, 1984).

Although more research is needed to examine the effects of racial inequality, alone and in combination with other forms of social inequality (e.g., class, gender, sexual identity), it is also critical for White professionals to lead discussions among themselves and with their students about the history of power, bias, and racism in the United States and within the health care workforce. As so eloquently stated by Martin Luther King more than 50 years ago, "In the end, we will remember not the words of our enemies, but the silence of our friends; and there comes a time when silence is betrayal" (King, 1965). White professionals must themselves grapple with processes that lead to worsening conditions faced by many people of color, specifically impoverishment, segregation, incarceration, environmental threats, and related health consequences. Talking about discrimination is an important first step; using counter-stereotypical exemplars and strategies to override biases must be part of the conversation (Stone & Ajayi, 2013; Vedantam, 2013).

Renewed efforts are needed to reform health care institutions—to hire, promote, train, and retain staff of diverse backgrounds to fully represent the diversity of the populations served. Engaging the assets and knowledge from communities of color and heeding their beliefs and perspectives, as well as hiring staff from within these communities, will help identify and promote effective policies (Bassett, 2015). Hall and Fields (2013) advocate for "positive profiling" to address and prevent racial health disparities and inequities. They suggest nurses can use evidence to remove barriers to care and implement strategies to avoid the potential for implicit racism that results in delays in care, reduced referrals, or suboptimal treatment.

In terms of broader advocacy, health professionals can and should not sit on the sidelines. Rather, by virtue of their ethical codes of practice, health care professionals have an obligation to participate in health justice groups and nonviolent demonstrations. Some may write editorials or lead forums and teach-ins; engage their politicians to demand change in law, policy, and practice; and work within and across the health professions to advocate for equality. As health care professionals, we must break the silences in whatever way we can. According to Loretta Ross (2012)—reproductive justice feminist—we all have a role to play in seeking and building a movement against oppression in which every human being is included, and equality is a milestone in the process. There are historical and recent examples of feminist thinking, racial politics, and the role of racial majorities and minorities in contesting racism and sexism and in demanding civil rights, voting rights, equal employment, and educational opportunities (Higginbotham, 1984; Roberts & Jesudason, 2014).

Institutional and Workplace Policies That Make a Difference for All Women • Women and racial/ethnic minorities are also changing the work environment and culture and creating a more humane work life. With more women in the workforce, industries outside of health care are recognizing the value of women's talent as well as temperament. Some research findings suggest that women take a more long-term, contextual view toward solving complex problems and often conduct business with fewer trappings of rank or hierarchy (Devillard, Graven, Lawson, Paradise, & Sancier-Sultan, 2012; Drucker, 1992; Fisher, 1999; Rosin, 2012). Women workers, managers, and professionals have demonstrated skills related to attention to detail, sensitive listening, and empathetic responses, as well as an ability to motivate, organize, and direct others. Many believe that, in the field of international development, women's grassroots organizations will be the most significant economic catalysts and forces for social justice in the 21st century (Fisher, 1999). As traditional corporations are decentralizing and building staff networks based on teams of equals, they have found that women are often skilled at constructing and maintaining these networks. Women also gravitate to companies that offer flexible work arrangements in order to balance work and family, and this in turn influences the number of such options available in the market.

The health care industry can take lessons from other business sectors that value a diverse, productive, and healthy workforce. Several studies have suggested that organizations that develop women perform better than those that do not. Since 2007 (Devillard et al., 2012), the consulting firm McKinsey has released research reports, titled *Women Matter*, about gender diversity and corporate performance. The first report, *Women Matter 1* (Desvaux, Devillard, & Baumgarten, 2007), demonstrated a correlation between a company's performance and the proportion of women serving on its executive board. In McKinsey's *Women Matter 2010* report (Devillard et al., 2102), companies showed that gender diversity was best supported within an ecosystem consisting of management commitment (executive champion with established targets for gender diversity), women's development programs (skills development and networks to master corporate codes and raise ambitions/profiles), and a set of enablers (human resource policies/processes, family/personal support mechanisms, indicators to track improvements).

Some successful hospitals have focused on improving the work environment, finding that shared governance and shared leadership creates a more satisfying work environment (Cheung & Aiken, 2006; Peterson, 2001). Other important attributes of health care services with effective administrative structures and quality patient care include participatory management, enhanced communication, adequate staffing, and investment in the development of nurses and staff. These organizations are involving staff—because they are closest to patients—in defining and developing the practice of care. Recognizing the link between cost and quality, some health care organizations are involving nurses in the financial management of their units. Many pioneering primary care practices are implementing innovative staffing models that make better use of their frontline staff, delegating more tasks to qualified prebaccalaureate health care workers (Blash, 2014).

Some policy makers suggest that the health system is a core institution and argue that it should be seen as a space in which to begin to challenge gender norms that have a negative impact on the nature of health care workers and patients (Govender & Penn-Kekana, 2008). Interventions recommended to redress gender biases and discrimination in the health care system call for action on multiple levels, such as integrating gender into health care institutions and integrating gender into health care worker training. A first step in eliminating gender bias in the workplace is to understand it. For example, in one large company, they found that in the promotion process, women were judged by their performance, whereas men were judged on their potential. This same gender bias existed in recruitment: Recruiters were much more critical of female than male candidates (Devillard et al., 2012). Based on this research, companies have established training courses to change gender perceptions and biases. In order to reward and retain highly trained staff, many health care systems are offering career development as part of their practice change model, providing career ladders with promotions both within and beyond the job category, wage increases, quality bonuses, educational reimbursement, and other nonsalary incentives. Career development for frontline workers may provide a broader benefit, enabling local health care organizations to serve as "economic engines" for the communities they serve, providing not only culturally competent health care to patients, but also economic opportunity and upward mobility to the health care workers who often originate from those same communities. Gender consciousness and gender sensitivity (Govender & Penn-Kekana, 2008) should be part of the basic and continuing training of all health care workers. Learning awareness of the gender dynamics that exist has an impact on how and when men and women seek care and how they talk about their symptoms in interactions with health care workers.

Policies that make it easier for women to have children and stay employed can make a difference. One study suggests that a lack of "family-friendly" policies, such as paid leave and a right to work part time, have contributed to nearly 30% of the decline in female labor force participation (Blau & Kahn, 2013; Goldfarb, 2014). Because working less than full time has been found to be a risky career move—shown by a number of studies that fewer part-time workers advance in their careers—companies are institutionalizing flexible working options (Devillard et al., 2012). Newer research suggests that the gender gap in pay would be considerably reduced and might vanish altogether if companies did not have an incentive to disproportionately reward individuals who labored long hours and worked particular hours. Goldin (2014) recommends that a solution for reducing the gender pay gap is workplace flexibility in terms of hours and location. For example, female pharmacists make 91% of what men make, partly because of technology that allows them to work remotely with flexible hours.

Anticipating women's career needs and planning for them can encourage women to return to work after maternity leave or take on the challenge of a promotion. Identifying women of high potential with the aim of getting them further along in their career paths before they have children has been instituted by some companies because more senior women tend to be more likely to return to work. Institutional strategies for recruiting women and minorities into health care careers means starting early—educating young women and boys about opportunities in high school and offering summer internships. Women's empowerment strategies from low-resource countries and low-wage workers in the United States can also inform the U.S. health care system (Gallagher Robins & Frohlich, 2014; IOM, Cuff, Patel, & Perex, 2015).

Many people within health care have already recognized that the new health care system will require health workers with different skills, attitudes, and values (O'Neil, 1993, 2003). As the boundaries of health care professions change, there is a growing demand for the skills of collaboration, effective communication, and teamwork. With less of a focus on competition and cheaper alternatives to professionals (e.g., NPs can provide equal or better care than primary care doctors; certified nursing assistants [CNAs] and CHWs substituting for RNs), there will be a move away from "task shifting" to team-based development with the "team at the table" and development of the whole team. In the health care workforce, the changing needs of patients suggest that medical care will be only one part of a person's health care needs. Rather than using medicine, a vertical "captain of the ship" model, as the standard for all health care, the foundational model is turning to focus on team-based care built on population health needs and provider competencies. With women as the dominant workforce in health care delivery, promoting and rewarding the skills and abilities of women will only improve health care delivery. Including women's experiences and concerns as a source of organizational vision can put the "care" back into health care. The attributes that are most valuable in today's workplace—social intelligence, open communication, the ability to sit still and focus—are, at a minimum, not predominantly male.

Focusing on gender diversity and nondiscrimination of women in the health care workforce does not mean the end of men. In fact, it seems that men have been lagging behind women in recent years and not adapting to a postindustrial work world that needs both high-tech and high-touch skills. Workplaces that avoid "women-only" solutions find that men will take advantage of programs such as onsite childcare, career planning, and flextime options. Critical will be the focus on human potential across the workplace regardless of gender, race, class, and other social determinants or inequities.

Women health care workers bring to the curing and caring arts compassion, patience, a precision touch, people skills, an interest in healing as a team, a tendency to seek holistic therapies, and a view of the patient as a whole person with social and psychological needs. In addition to the need for national and institutional policy change to reduce discrimination and empower women and people of color in the health care workforce, the challenge to women health care providers will be to work together across their multiple diversities and structural intersections. Just as women physicians must work with other women health care workers, nurses will be moving from a direct care role to a new role of organizing and coordinating teams of caregivers. Tensions currently exist about how to delegate, how to manage the workload and be accountable for outcomes, and how to provide for the growth and development of

multiple caregivers and other support staff. Nurses and women physicians must consider delegation, along with shared governance, as another form of empowerment. Delegation must be learned, practiced, evaluated, and improved. The work environment must be created in which delegation is supported and valued and positive outcomes are rewarded. A critical element of the redesign will be the evaluation of the effectiveness of health care provider roles. As we are making monumental changes in how we care for patients, we must also evaluate whether we are improving patient care or making it worse.

■ WOMEN AS UNPAID HEALTH CARE PROVIDERS

Clearly, health care is women's work, with the majority of health care providers being women. Turning the phrase around presents another truth—women's work is health care. Much of the work that women do in their unpaid, private lives is health care for themselves and their families. The "caring tricycle" of women is often a lifetime of responsibility that begins with the care of children, continues into middle age with the care of an aging parent, and culminates in old age with the responsibility for a frail partner (Doyal, 1995; Hochschild, 1983). Almost always a labor of love, it can also be a crushing burden for women who must balance work and other family responsibilities with the constant caregiving of vulnerable, dependent humans (see Chapter 4).

The arguments used to gain women's access into the paid fields of health care were based on women's natural talents and interests in caring for their families. Chodorow (1996) argued that women's greater interest in and ability to care for family members is a socially constructed gender difference, not a biologically determined difference. The ancient, socially proscribed roles of food gathering, cultivation, and preparation and of keeping the home environment clean and safe, as well as the biological role of bearing and caring for children, had singularly prepared women to care for the health and welfare of society.

Today, women still do the majority of domestic work—housework, shopping, cooking, and caregiving—regardless of whether they are employed outside of the home (Bianchi & Milkie, 2010; Brody, 1994; Hook, 2010). Although men's participation in some routine housework, notably cooking, has risen in recent years, women have the domestic management role, with the overall responsibility for running the household. They are usually more responsible for planning and organization, maintaining harmony, managing relationships, and performing the emotion work necessary for family life (Craig & Powell, 2015; Mattingly & Sayer, 2006). Women's subjective experience is that they have to run the household and family without domestic help (Crabb, 2015). The facts that more women are in the labor force and that the two-income family is fast becoming a necessity rather than a luxury have not altered women's socially proscribed roles and their primary responsibility for the care of children.

One way of evaluating the socially recognized importance of women as health care providers for the family is an exploration of the marketing aimed at women as the health care decision maker for the family (e.g., the "ask Doctor Mom" commercial for cough medicine). Women provide health care and also decide from whom and where they will seek help for themselves and their families. To guide women consumers toward healthy choices in providing family health care, women are also targeted by food product advertisements that promote healthy children, heart health, low fat, low sugar, and smart buying as healthy buying, including all types of food products from soup to peanut butter. The importance of a clean house, clean clothes, and healthy exercise—not to mention a beautiful body, preferably looking like a fashion model—is primarily advertised using women models and targeted to women who are responsible for the health and welfare of their families (Graham, 1985; Kurtzleben, 2012).

Beyond the standard of daily health care provided by women in families is the role of health care provider for the ill and infirm in the family (Finch, 1983; National Alliance for Caregiving [NAC], 2009; Robinson, 1997). Nearly 66 million adults serve as unpaid family caregivers in the United States, constituting the largest source of long-term care in the nation (Spillman & Black, 2005). With two of every three caregivers a female (CDC, 2004; Spillman & Black, 2005), family caregiving is still largely women's work. Although the proportion of male caregivers has slowly risen over the past 20 years, it still lags far behind. In 2011, the "average" U.S. caregiver is a 49-year-old woman who works outside the home and spends nearly 20 hours per week providing unpaid care to her mother for nearly 5 years. Almost two thirds of family caregivers are female (65%) and more than eight in 10 are caring for a relative or friend aged 50 years or older (Feinberg, Reinhard, Houser, & Choula, 2011).

Systematic reviews of family caregiving studies over the past 30 years reveal that family care can have negative effects on the caregivers' own financial situation, retirement security, physical and emotional health, social networks, careers, and ability to keep their loved one at home. The impact is particularly severe for caregivers of individuals who have complex chronic health conditions and both functional and cognitive impairments (Feinberg et al., 2011). In the 2011 update of a study of the contributions and costs of family caregiving, it was estimated that the value of unpaid contributions of family caregiving was estimated at $450 billion in 2009, which vastly exceeds the value of paid home care. For women, the total individual amount of lost wages because of leaving the labor force early and/or reducing their hours of work as a result of caregiving responsibilities equaled $142,693, with additional lost social security benefits ($131,351) and lost pension benefits (conservatively estimated at $50,000) for a total of $324,044 in 2011 (MetLife, 2011). As men are more likely to pay for family caregiving, their lost wages were about 60% of women caregivers, and the total economic impact on working male caregivers was estimated at $283,716.

Although elderly spouses provide care to each other when one of them becomes ill or disabled, because of the discrepancy in life expectancy between men and women, most caregiving spouses are women. Daughters outnumber sons by about four to one as primary caregivers to disabled parents and are the largest group of helpers for the disabled elderly (Brody, 1994; Feinberg et al., 2011; Robinson, 1997). More recent research on gender disparities in family caregiving show that women are more likely to commit to particularly arduous caregiving, including hands-on care that involves bathing and using the toilet. Men, on the whole, are less apt to get their hands dirty—and they feel less guilt about hiring help than women do.

Elaine Brody (1981) was the first to define the role of "women in the middle" as those women having primary responsibility for dependent children as well as assuming care for their elderly parents and in-laws as the advances of medical science and public health have resulted in an extended life span. U.S. demographics are not encouraging for this group of women in the middle. The population is expected to become much older, with nearly one in five U.S. residents aged 65 years and older in 2030 (U.S. Census Bureau projections, 2000; Vincent & Velkoff, 2010). Only 4% of the total U.S. population was aged 65 years or older in 1900. In 1990, 12% of the population was 65 years or older, which was projected to be 14% in 2010 and is projected to be 21% by the year 2050 (Day, 1992; Vincent & Velkoff, 2010). The number of the oldest old (i.e., people older than 85 years) has also increased dramatically to almost 6 million in 2010 and is expected to increase to 9 million in 2030 and 19 million in 2050 (U.S. Census Bureau, 2000; Vincent & Velkoff, 2010).

Not all people older than 65 years are infirm; in fact, most are in good health. However, the increasing disability and episodic health needs of this age group rely primarily on daughters or daughters-in-law for assistance. The aging of the population has combined with a decrease in the birthrate (4 per family in 1900 to 1.2 per family in 1997). This means that there will be an increase in the number of needy elderly in the population corresponding to a decrease in the number of women (or men) available to provide health care assistance. Almost no data are available on the numbers of women providing care to children with serious ongoing health conditions, and most of this care is rendered without appearing on the ledgers of the nations' economy (Stein, Bauman, & Jessop, 1994). Advanced technology has improved the life span of many disabled children, allowing them to live at home but requiring significant caretaking. These caretakers, the women in the middle, will likely attend to the needs of their aging and young dependent family members to the detriment of their own health needs (Bull, 2001; Hoffmann & Mitchell, 1998).

It is not only the increase in the numbers of elderly in the population that has placed additional burdens on women as family health care providers. The changes resulting from the implementation of Medicare reimbursement policies—which effectively limits the amount of time any particular patient stays in the hospital—have resulted in patients being discharged sooner and sicker than in the past. The majority of these patients are discharged home with the assumption that home care is cheaper than hospital care and just as safe, if not beneficial, after a certain stabilized point in recovery

(Bull, Bowers, Kirschling, & Neufeld, 1990; Landers, 2010; Naylor & Sochalski, 2010; Picot, 1995; Robinson, 1997; Toles, Abbott, Hirschman, & Naylor, 2012). Much of this at-home care—from assistance with daily living activities to complex cancer pain and treatment management to managing the ever-changing demands of the Alzheimer's patient or the ventilator-assisted child—is provided by women, either an unpaid family member or a home health aide (Brody, 1994; Landers, 2010; Talley & Crews, 2007; Toles et al., 2012). An increasing body of evidence demonstrating the importance and the effectiveness of coordinated transitions between hospital and home, the Transitional Care Model (TCM) uses a transitional care nurse to deliver and coordinate the care of high-risk older adults within and across all health care settings and caregivers (Naylor & Sochalski, 2010). Research on the TCM shows that patient satisfaction is increased among patients receiving TCM and that TCM lessens the burden among family members by reducing the demands of caregiving and improving family functioning.

Beyond the family health care needs that women attend to, women are volunteer community activists in promoting health care. Whether it is campaigning for safe living environments in the inner city, combating toxic waste hazards, working for clean water and proper sanitation in developing countries, or advocating for reproductive justice and economic equity, women are leaders in identifying the problems and organizing the solutions (Doyal, 1995; *Ms. Magazine*, 2015; National Partnership for Women & Families, 2015; Pizurki, Mejia, Butter, & Ewart, 1987; SisterSong, 2015). WHO has recognized the importance of women as health care providers in its emphasis on "Women, Health and Development" in the efforts for "Health for All by the Year 2000" through the mechanisms of primary, preventive health care (Pizurki et al., 1987). To improve accountability in the implementation of global and national goals, the WHO Commission on Social Determinants of Health (Sen, Ostlin, & George, 2007) has called for engagement of community-based activists and leaders through WHO Gender, Equity and Rights Teams focused on gender equality, women's empowerment, and health equity (WHO, 2015).

At national, local, and state levels, women are organizing and advocating for new models of delivering health care that links the intersections of gender, race, and health with economic and social justice (All Above All, 2015; National Latina Institute for Reproductive Health [NLIRH], 2015; National Partnership for Women & Families, 2015; National Women's Law Center [NWLC], 2015; Taylor & Dower, 1997). On a national level, the National Partnership for Women and Families (2015) was an early organization to advocate for the intersection of workplace fairness, family-friendly workplace policies, health care access, and reproductive rights. Organizations are building coalitions and training women to mobilize to change the structural inequities inherent in work and health care systems as well as politics (CoreAlign, 2015; SisterSong, 2015).

But who cares for the caregivers? Little is known about the costs to the system when family caregivers are deterred from entering the labor force, quit their jobs or work part-time, or are less efficient in their jobs because of caregiving responsibilities. As women's wages are generally lower than men's, women are more likely than men to leave paid employment to become unpaid family caregivers. Although there is evidence that more employers are providing incentives to women workers in the form of child and elder care services, the tension remains among changing values—new values about women's roles as paid workers and traditional values of women remaining the primary caregivers and health care providers for the family.

■ SUMMARY

Health care has been and will continue in the near future to be women's work, and this work cannot be separated from women's lives. Although the increasing numbers of women doctors, dentists, and pharmacists receive a lot of attention and praise for "making it in a man's world," the majority of paid and unpaid health care providers are women, with unskilled, minority women at the bottom of the employment ladder. Federal and institutional policies will continue to support diversity in the health care workforce, with an emphasis on collaboration and team-based care advanced by new technologies. The challenge to health care systems lies in their ability to empower the workforce and create equitable solutions for all health care workers. The challenge for women health care providers will be to participate in the evolving definitions of what their contributions should produce versus the historical traditions of professional authority. Women's talents for caregiving, working in teams, and long-term problem solving provide the basis for real solutions to the current health care dilemmas, including workplace solutions to institutional gender bias and racial discrimination at all levels of the health care workforce.

■ ACKNOWLEDGMENT

I would like to acknowledge the colleagues who made significant contributions to this chapter. They all made this a much improved and richer chapter. First, to Dr. Carol Leppa as the lead author in the first edition of *History of Women's Health Nurses*; to Lisa Stern, NP, MS, a PhD candidate in the history of health sciences, for her update of the women's health professional history; to Dr. Monica McLemore and Dr. Candace Burton for their contribution to the section on intersectionality of discrimination of health care providers (both individuals and institutions); and to Kim Hildebrandt-Cardozo, CNM, MS, for her critical review of the history and current status of women as health care providers.

■ NOTES

1. These occupational categories have limitations. Before 2010, for example, registered nursing made no distinction between NPs, nurse midwives, and RNs. The nursing aides, orderlies,

and attendants occupational category also includes multiple job titles, levels of training, and certifications and were separated into separate job categories in 2010. Some job titles in a health setting may not necessarily reflect similar Occupational Employment Statistics (OES) occupational classifications, which may cause some problems in reporting. For example, confusion may result from the differences in defining a home health aide as any individual providing services in the home or as one who completes home health aide certification requirements (http:// bhpr.hrsa.gov/index.html).

2. For more detailed information on the data sources, definitions, methods, and SOC categories, see *Sex, Race, and Ethnic Diversity of U.S. Health Occupations (2010–2012) Technical Documentation* at http://bhpr.hrsa.gov/healthworkforce/index.html

3. The National Center for Health Workforce Analysis (NCHWA; http://bhpr.hrsa.gov/healthworkforce/index.html), which is the data and statistics unit of the DHHS/HRSA, provides data resources for county, state, national, and global workforce estimation and analysis. In addition, the NCHWA develops the national infrastructure for workforce data management, supports state governments and organizations to improve workforce data, and supports state/regional health workforce research centers through a grant program.

4. Variation in definitions reflects the changes in standards and measurement. The BLS estimates occupational employment statistics every 2 years using the classifications developed by the SOC system. However, the SOC is revised every 10 years; 2010 was the last revision.

5. More detailed information on the work settings can be found on the U.S. Census Bureau website: www.census.gov/eos/www/ naics. (U.S. Department of Health and Human Services, Health Resources and Services Administration, National Center for Health Workforce Analysis (2014).

6. For the national perspective, the primary source of national data on the racial and ethnic mix of the health care workforce is the American Community Survey (ACS), which is an annual nationally representative household survey conducted by the U.S. Census Bureau. Data on the diversity of the pipeline of workers are available through the Integrated Postsecondary Education Data System (IPEDS) for those in occupations requiring at least a postsecondary award; however, data are not available for those with less than a postsecondary award.

7. There are non Euro-American examples, such as in the Philippines, which had long traditions of male nurses (Choy, 2003; D'Antonio, 2010).

8. Despite the linguistic confusion associated with the term *allied health worker*, it continues to be used by federal and state agencies to refer to supporting staff—therapists, technicians, clerks, aides, assistants, and a few other workers not classified as dentists, doctors, or nurses.

9. Nancy Woods used her power position as dean of the School of Nursing to end the silence surrounding institutional racism at the University of Washington School of Nursing with a public apology. Her action paved the way for continuing antiracist work in the school and the university (Schroeder & DiAngelo, p. 254).

■ REFERENCES

Abghari, M. S., Takemoto, R., Sadiq, A., Karia, R., Phillips, D., & Egol, K. A. (2014). Patient perceptions and preferences when choosing an orthopaedic surgeon. *The Iowa Orthopaedic Journal, 34*, 204–208.

Affordable Care Act (ACA). (2015). *Affordable Care Act*. Retrieved from http://www.hhs.gov/healthcare/rights

Ahmad, F., Gupta, H., Rawlins, J., & Stewart, D. E. (2002). Preferences for gender of family physician among Canadian European-descent and South-Asian immigrant women. *Family Practice, 19*(2), 146–153.

All Above All. (2015). *All above all for abortion coverage*. Retrieved from http://allaboveall.org

Allen, D. G. (2006). Whiteness and difference in nursing. *Nursing Philosophy: An International Journal for Healthcare Professionals, 7*(2), 65–78.

American Association of Colleges of Pharmacy (AACP). (2014a). *2014 National pharmacist workforce survey*. Retrieved from http://www .aacp.org/resources/research/pharmacyworkforcecenter/Documents/ FinalReportOfTheNationalPharmacistWorkforceStudy2014.pdf

American Association of Colleges of Pharmacy (AACP). (2014b). *2014 National pharmacist workforce survey results: Demographic information of licensed pharmacists as percentages, 2000–2014*. Retrieved from http://www.aacp.org/resources/research/pharmacyworkforce center/Documents/PWC-demographics.pdf

American Association of Nurse Anesthetists (AANA). (2009). *Certified registered nurse anesthetists fact sheet*. Retrieved from http://www .aana.com/ceandeducation/becomeacrna/Pages/Nurse-Anesthetists-at -a-Glance.aspx

American Association of University Women (AAUW). (2015). *The simple truth gender pay gap*. Retrieved from http://www.aauw.org/ files/2015/02/The-Simple-Truth_Spring-2015.pdf

American Dental Association (ADA). (1999). *ADA dental workforce model: 1997–2020*. Chicago, IL: Author.

Ansell, D. A., & McDonald, E. K. (2015). Bias, Black lives, and academic medicine. *The New England Journal of Medicine, 372*(12), 1087–1089.

Ashley, J. A. (1976). *Hospitals, paternalism, and the role of the nurse*. New York, NY: Columbia University, Teachers College.

Aspen Institute. (2011). *Glossary for understanding the dismantling structural racism/promoting racial equity analysis*. Retrieved from http://www.aspeninstitute.org/sites/default/files/content/docs/rcc/ RCC-Structural-Racism-Glossary.pdf

Auerbach, D. I., Pearson, M. L., Taylor, D., Battistelli, M., Sussell, J., Hunter, L. E.,...Schneider, E. C. (2012). *Nurse practitioners and sexual and reproductive health services: An analysis of supply and demand*. Retrieved from http://www.rand.org/pubs/technical_reports/ TR1224.html

Bassett, M. T. (2015). #BlackLivesMatter—A challenge to the medical and public health communities. *The New England Journal of Medicine, 372*(12), 1085–1087.

Baxter, E. (2015). *How the gender wage gap differs by occupation*. Washington, DC: Center for American Progress. Retrieved from https:// www.americanprogress.org/issues/women/news/2015/04/14/110959/ how-the-gender-wage-gap-differs-by-occupation

Bianchi, S. M., & Milkie, M. A. (2010). Work and family research in the first decade of the 21st century. *Journal of Marriage and Family, 72*(3), 705–725.

Bickel, J. (2000). Women in academic medicine. *Journal of the American Medical Women's Association, 55*(1), 10–12, 19. Retrieved from http://www.ncbi.nlm.nih.gov/pubmed/10680399

Blash, L. (2014). *Innovative workforce models highlight the value of pre-baccalaureate health care workers*. Retrieved from http://www .brookings.edu/blogs/the-avenue/posts/2014/09/08-health-care -workforce-models-blash

Blau, F. D., & Kahn, L. M. (2013). *Female labor supply: Why is the U.S. falling behind?* Retrieved from http://ftp.iza.org/dp7140.pdf

Brody, E. M. (1981). "Women in the middle" and family help to older people. *The Gerontologist, 21*(5), 471–480.

Brody, E. M. (1994). Women as unpaid caregivers: The price they pay. In E. Friedman (Ed.), *An unfinished revolution: Women and health care in America* (pp. 67–86). New York, NY: United Hospital Fund.

Brown, C. (1982). Women workers in the health service industry. In E. Fee (Ed.), *Women and health: The politics of sex in medicine* (pp. 105–116). New York, NY: Baywood.

Brown, L. J., & Lazar, V. (1999). Trends in the dental health work force. *Journal of the American Dental Association (1939), 130*(12), 1743–1749.

Buerhaus, P. I., Auerbach, D. I., & Staiger, D. O. (2009). The recent surge in nurse employment: Causes and implications. *Health Affairs (Project Hope), 28*(4), w657–w668.

Bull, M. J. (2001). Interventions for women as family caregivers. *Annual Review of Nursing Research*, 19, 125–142.

Bull, M. J., Bowers, J. E., Kirschling, J. M., & Neufeld, A. (1990). *Factors influencing family caregiver burden and health. Western Journal of Nursing Research*, 12(6), 758–776.

Bureau of Labor Statistics. (1995). *Current population survey, health occupations by gender*. Retrieved from http://www.bls.gov/cps/aa1995/aat11.txt

Bureau of Labor Statistics. (2012). *Employed persons by detailed occupation and age, 2012 annual averages*. Retrieved from www.bls.gov/cps/occupation_age.xls

Bureau of Labor Statistics (BLS). (2013a). *Caring for our caregivers: Facts about hospital worker safety*. Retrieved from http://docplayer.net/130691-Caring-for-our-caregivers.html

Bureau of Labor Statistics (BLS). (2013b). *Industry-occupation matrix data, by occupation*. Retrieved from http://www.bls.gov/emp/ep_table_108.htm

Bureau of Labor Statistics (BLS). (2014a). *Labor force statistics from the current population survey*. Retrieved from http://www.bls.gov/cps/cpsaat11.htm

Bureau of Labor Statistics (BLS). (2014b). *Occupational employment and wages, May 2014; 29–1151 nurse anesthetists*. Retrieved from http://www.bls.gov/oes/current/oes291151.htm

Bureau of Labor Statistics (BLS). (2014c). *Occupational employment and wages, May 2014; 29–1161 nurse midwives*. Retrieved from http://www.bls.gov/oes/current/oes291161.htm

Bureau of Labor Statistics (BLS). (2014d). *Occupational employment and wages, May 2014; 29–1171 nurse practitioners*. Retrieved from http://www.bls.gov/oes/current/oes291171.htm

Bureau of Labor Statistics (BLS). (2015a). *Occupational employment statistics: May 2014 occupation profiles*. Retrieved from http://www.bls.gov/oes/current/oes_stru.htm

Bureau of Labor Statistics (BLS). (2015b). *Occupational outlook handbook, physicians and surgeons*. Retrieved from http://www.bls.gov/ooh/healthcare/physicians-and-surgeons.htm

Bureau of Labor Statistics (BLS). (2015c). *Occupational outlook handbook: Dentists*. Retrieved from http://www.bls.gov/ooh/healthcare/dentists.htm

Bureau of Labor Statistics (BLS). (2015d). *Occupational outlook handbook: Pharmacists*. Retrieved from http://www.bls.gov/ooh/healthcare/pharmacists.htm#tab-1

Burnley, C. S., & Burkett, G. L. (1986). Specialization: Are women in surgery different? *Journal of the American Medical Women's Association (1972)*, 41(5), 144–7, 151.

Butter, I. H. (1985). *Sex and status: Hierarchies in the health workforce* (Vol. 1). Washington, DC: American Public Health Association.

Butter, I. H., Carpenter, E. S., Kay, B. J., & Simmons, R. S. (1987). Gender hierarchies in the health labor force. *International Journal of Health Services: Planning, Administration, Evaluation*, 17(1), 133–149.

Byrd, W. M., & Clayton, L. A. (2003). Racial and ethnic disparities in healthcare: A background and history. *Unequal treatment: Confronting racial and ethnic disparities in health care* (pp. 455–527). Washington, DC: Institute of Medicine of the National Academies.

Cain, J., Campbell, T., Congdon, H. B., Hancock, K., Kaun, M., Lockman, P. R., & Evans, R. L. (2014). Pharmacy student debt and return on investment of a pharmacy education. *American Journal of Pharmaceutical Education*, 78(1), 5. Retrieved from http://www.ncbi.nlm.nih.gov/pmc/articles/PMC3930253

Campaign for Action. (2014). *Innovative pilot program aims to improve diversity in the nursing workforce in Connecticut*. Retrieved from http://campaignforaction.org/community-post/innovative-pilot-program-aims-improve-diversity-nursing-workforce-connecticut

Campaign for Action. (2015). *Encouraging diversity in the nursing workforce from LNA to nursing faculty*. Retrieved from http://campaignforaction.org/community-post/encouraging-diversity-nursing-workforce-ina-nursing-faculty

Carlton, A., & Rockfeller Foundation. (2015). *Good jobs should matter to both employers and employees*. Retrieved from https://www.rockefellerfoundation.org/blog/good-jobs-should-matter-to-both-employers-and-employees

Center for Health Workforce Studies. (2014). *The health care workforce in New York: Trends in the supply and demand for health workers.* Retrieved from http://chws.albany.edu/archive/uploads/2014/08/nytracking2014.pdf

Centers for Disease Control and Prevention (CDC). (2004). *Current home health care patients*. Retrieved from http://www.cdc.gov/nchs/data/nhhcsd/curhomecare00.pdf

Centers for Disease Control and Prevention (CDC). (2014). *Healthcare workers*. Retrieved from http://www.cdc.gov/niosh/topics/healthcare

Chapman, E. N., Kaatz, A., & Carnes, M. (2013). Physicians and implicit bias: How doctors may unwittingly perpetuate health care disparities. *Journal of General Internal Medicine*, 28(11), 1504–1510.

Cheung, R., & Aiken, L. H. (2006). Hospital initiatives to support a better-educated workforce. *The Journal of Nursing Administration*, 36(7–8), 357–362.

Chodorow, N. J. (1996). Theoretical gender and clinical gender: Epistemological reflections on the psychology of women. *Journal of the American Psychoanalytic Association*, 44(Suppl.), 215–238.

Choy, C. C. (2003). *Empire of care: Nursing and migration in Filipino American history*. Durham, NC: Duke University Press.

Cleland, V. (1971). Sex discrimination: Nursing's most pervasive problem. *The American Journal of Nursing*, 71(8), 1542–1547.

Colligan, M. J., Smith, M. J., & Hurrell, J. J. (1977). Occupational incidence rates of mental health disorders. *Journal of Human Stress*, 3(3), 34–39.

Collins, P. H. (1990). Black feminist thought in the matrix of domination. In P. H. Collins (Ed.), *Black feminist thought: Knowledge, consciousness, and the politics of empowerment* (pp. 221–238). Boston, MA: Unwin Hyman.

Collins, P. H. (1998). It's all in the family: Intersections of gender, race, and nation. *Hypatia*, 13(3), 62–82.

Cooper, B. (2015). The Women of #BlackLivesMatter. *Ms. Magazine*, winter. Retrieved from http://www.msmagazine.com/Winter2015/index.asp

Cooper, R. A. (2013). Unraveling the physician supply dilemma. *Journal of American Medical Association*, 310(18), 1931–1932.

CoreAlign. (2015). *CoreAlign*. Retrieved from www.corealign.org

Crabb, A. (2015). *The wide drought*. Sydney, Australia: Random House.

Craig, L., & Powell, A. (2015). *Gender divisions of domestic work: Housework shares when adult children live with mom and dad*. San Diego, CA: Population Association of America Annual Meeting.

Cuckler, G. A., Sisko, A. M., Keehan, S. P., Smith, S. D., Madison, A. J., Poisal, J. A., … Stone, D. A. (2013). National health expenditure projections, 2012–22: Slow growth until coverage expands and economy improves. *Health Affairs (Project Hope)*, 32(10), 1820–1831.

D'Antonio, P. (2010). *American nursing: A history of knowledge, authority, and the meaning of work*. Baltimore, MD: Johns Hopkins University Press.

Darbyshire, P. (1987). Nurses and doctors. The burden of history. *Nursing Times*, 83(4), 32–34.

Davis, A. Y. (1981). *Women, race and class*. New York, NY: Random House.

Davis, A. Y. (2011). *Women, race, & class*. New York, NY: Vintage.

Day, J. C. (1992). *Population projections of the United States, by age, sex, race, and Hispanic origin: 1992 to 2050*. Washington, DC: U.S. Department of Commerce, Economics and Statistics Administration, Bureau of the Census.

Department for Professional Employees (DPE). (2015). *Professionals in the workplace: women in the professional workforce*. Retrieved from http://dpeaflcio.org/wp-content/uploads/Women-in-the-Professional-Workforce-2015.pdf

Derksen, D. J., & Whelan, E.-M. (2009). *Closing the health care workforce gap: Reforming federal health care workforce policies to meet the needs of the 21st century*. Washington, DC: Center for American Progress Action Fund.

Desvaux, G., Devillard, S., & Baumgarten, P. (2007). *Women matter: Gender diversity, a corporate performance driver*. Retrieved from http://www.mckinsey.com/client_service/organization/latest_thinking/women_matter

Devillard, S., Graven, W., Lawson, E., Paradise, R., & Sancier-Sultan, S. (2012). *Women matter 2012: Making the breakthrough* (pp. 1–26). New York, NY: McKinsey and Company.

Di Julio, B., Firth, J., & Brodie, M. (2015). *California's previously uninsured after the ACA's second open enrollment period*. Retrieved from

http://kff.org/health-reform/report/californias-previously-uninsured
-after-the-acas-second-open-enrollment-period

Discrimination. (2015). In *American Heritage Dictionary: The Free Dictionary*. (2015). Retrieved from http://www.thefreedictionary.com/discrimination

Dobbin, F., Kalev, A., & Kelly, E. (2007). Diversity management in corporate America. *Contexts-American Sociological Association, 6*(4), 21–27.

Dock, L., & Stewart, I. (1938). *A short history of nursing schools*. New York, NY: GP Putnam's sons.

Doyal, L. (1995). What makes women sick: Gender and the political economy of health. *British Medical Journal, 311*, 577.

Drucker, P. F. (1992). *Managing for the future*. New York, NY: Truman Talley Books/Plume.

Ducker, D. G. (1986). Role conflict in women physicians: A longitudinal study. *Journal of the American Medical Women's Association (1972), 41*(1), 14–16.

Dusch, M. N., O'Sullivan, P. S., & Ascher, N. L. (2014). Patient perceptions of female surgeons: How surgeon demeanor and type of surgery affect patient preference. *The Journal of Surgical Research, 187*(1), 59–64.

Ehrenreich, B., & English, D. (1973). Witches, midwives, and nurses: A history of women healers. New York, NY: The Feminist Press.

Emmons, W. R., & Noeth, B. J. (2015). Why didn't higher education protect Hispanic and Black wealth? *In the Balance, 12*, 1–3.

Fagin, C. (1994). Women and nursing, today and tomorrow. *An unfinished revolution: Women and health care in America*. New York, NY: United Hospital Fund of New York.

Feinberg, L., Reinhard, S. C., Houser, A., & Choula, R. (2011). Valuing the invaluable: 2011 update: The growing contributions and costs of family caregiving. Washington, DC: AARP Public Policy Institute.

Fenton, W. S., Robinowitz, C. B., & Leaf, P. J. (1987). Male and female psychiatrists and their patients. *The American Journal of Psychiatry, 144*(3), 358–361.

Finch, J. (1983). *Labour of love: Women working and caring*. Boston, MA: Routledge and Kegan Paul.

Fisher, H. (1999). *The first sex*. New York, NY: Random House.

Fisher, S. (1995). *Nursing wounds: Nurse practitioners, doctors, women patients, and the negotiation of meaning*. New Brunswick, NJ: Rutgers University Press.

Flexnor, A. (1910). *Carnegie Bulletin: Medical education in the U.S. and Canada*. Bulletin No. 4. New York, NY: The Carnegie Foundation for Advancement of Teaching.

Frank, E., Harvey, L., & Elon, L. (2000). Family responsibilities and domestic activities of U.S. women physicians. *Archives of Family Medicine, 9*(2), 134–140.

Friedman, E. (1994). *An unfinished revolution: Women and health care in America*. New York, NY: United Hospital Fund.

Frogner, B., & Spetz, J. (2013). *Affordable Care Act of 2010: Creating job opportunities for racially and ethnically diverse populations*. Washington, DC: Joint Center for Political and Economic Studies.

Frogner, B., & Spetz, J. (2015). *Entry and exit of workers in long-term care*. Retrieved from http://healthworkforce.ucsf.edu/sites/health workforce.ucsf.edu/files/Report-Entry_and_Exit_of_Workers_in_Long-Term_Care.pdf

Frogner, B. K., Spetz, J., Parente, S. T., & Oberlin, S. (2015). The demand for health care workers post-ACA. *International Journal of Health Economics and Management, 15*(1), 139–151.

Gallagher Robins, K., & Frohlich, L. (2014). *Underpaid, overloaded, and overrepresented: Findings from NWLC's new report on women in low-wage jobs*. Retrieved from http://www.nwlc.org/our-blog/underpaid-overloaded-and-overrepresented-findings-nwlcs-new-report-women-low-wage-jobs

Gillborn, D. (2013). Understanding White privilege: Creating pathways to authentic relationships across race. *British Journal of Educational Studies, 61*(4), 507–509.

Ginzberg, E., & Minogiannis, P. (2004). *U.S. healthcare and the future supply of physicians*. New Brunswick, NJ: Transaction.

Goldfarb, Z. (2014). *Women are disappearing from the workforce: Here's how to fix that*. Retrieved from http://www.washingtonpost.com/news/wonkblog/wp/2014/08/12/women-are-disappearing-from-the-workforce-heres-how-to-fix-that

Goldin, C. (2014). A grand gender convergence: Its last chapter. *The American Economic Review, 104*(4), 1091–1119.

Goldin, C., & Katz, L. F. (2012). *The most egalitarian of all professions: Pharmacy and the evolution of a family-friendly occupation*. Retrieved from www.nber.org/papers/w18410

Goodell, S., Dower, C., & O'Neil, E. (2011). Primary care workforce in the United States. *The Synthesis Project, 22*(4), 2–4.

Govender, V., & Penn-Kekana, L. (2008). Gender biases and discrimination: A review of health care interpersonal interactions. *Global Public Health, 3*(Suppl. 1), 90–103.

Graham, H. (1985). Providers, negotiators and mediators: Women as the hidden carers. *Women, Health and Healing* (pp. 25–52). New York, NY: Tavistock.

Grumbach, K., Coffman, J., Rosenoff, E., & Munoz, C. (2001). *Trends in underrepresented minority participation in health professions schools* (pp. 185–207). Washington, DC: National Academy of Sciences.

Gurin, P., Dey, E., Hurtado, S., & Gurin, G. (2002). Diversity and higher education: Theory and impact on educational outcomes. *Harvard Educational Review, 72*(3), 330–367.

Hall, J. M., & Fields, B. (2013). Continuing the conversation in nursing on race and racism. *Nursing Outlook, 61*(3), 164–173.

Hammarström, A., Johansson, K., Annandale, E., Ahlgren, C., Aléx, L., Christianson, M., . . . Verdonk, P. (2014). Central gender theoretical concepts in health research: The state of the art. *Journal of Epidemiology and Community Health, 68*(2), 185–190.

Hart-Brothers, E. (1994). Contributions of women of color to the health care of America. In E. Friedman (Ed.), *An unfinished revolution: Women and healthcare in America* (pp. 205–222). New York, NY: United Hospital Fund of New York.

Health Resources and Services Administration (HRSA). (2008). *The physician workforce: projections and research into current issues affecting supply and demand*. Retrieved from http://bhpr.hrsa.gov/healthworkforce/supplydemand/medicine/physiciansupplyissues.pdf

Health Resources and Services Administration (HRSA). (2010). *The registered nurse population: Findings from the 2008 national sample survey of registered nurses*. Retrieved from http://bhpr.hrsa.gov/healthworkforce/rnsurveys/rnsurveyfinal.pdf

Health Resources and Services Administration (HRSA). (2012a). *Highlights from the 2012 national sample survey of nurse practitioners*. Retrieved from http://bhpr.hrsa.gov/healthworkforce/supply demand/nursing/nursepractitionersurvey/npsurveyhighlights.pdf

Health Resources and Services Administration (HRSA). (2012b). *National sample survey of nurse practitioners*. Retrieved from http://bhpr.hrsa.gov/healthworkforce/supplydemand/nursing/nursepractitionersurvey/index.html

Health Resources and Services Administration (HRSA). (2013a). *The U.S. health workforce chartbook*. Retrieved from http://bhpr.hrsa.gov/healthworkforce/supplydemand/usworkforce/chartbook/index.html

Health Resources and Services Administration (HRSA). (2013b). *The U.S. nursing workforce: Trends in supply and education*. Retrieved from http://bhpr.hrsa.gov/healthworkforce/supplydemand/nursing/nursing workforce/nursingworkforcefullreport.pdf

Health Resources and Services Administration (HRSA). (2015a). *Bureau of Health Workforce*. Retrieved from http://www.hrsa.gov/about/organization/bureaus/bhw/index.html

Health Resources and Services Administration (HRSA). (2015b). *HHS FY2015 budget in brief*. Retrieved from http://www.hhs.gov/about/budget/fy2015/budget-in-brief/hrsa/index.html

Health Resources and Services Administration (HRSA). (2015c). *National and state-level projections of dentists and dental hygienists in the U.S., 2012–2025*. Retrieved from http://bhpr.hrsa.gov/healthworkforce/supplydemand/dentistry/nationalstatelevelprojectionsdentists.pdf

Health Resources and Services Administration (HRSA). (2015d). *Sex, race, and ethnic diversity of U.S. health occupations (2010–2012)*. Retrieved from http://bhpr.hrsa.gov/healthworkforce/supplydemand/usworkforce/diversityushealthoccupations.pdf

Hess, C., Milli, J., Hayes, J., Hegewisch, A., Mayayeva, Y., Roman, S., . . . Augeri, J. (2015). *The status of women in the States: 2015*. Retrieved from http://statusofwomendata.org/app/uploads/2015/02/Status-of-Women-in-the-States-2015-Full-National-Report.pdf

Higginbotham, E. B. (1984). *Righteous discontent: The women's movement in the black Baptist church, 1880–1920* (pp. 258–304). Cambridge, MA: Harvard University Press.

Himmelstein, D. U., Lewontin, J. P., & Woolhandler, S. (1996). Medical care employment in the United States, 1968 to 1993: The importance of health sector jobs for African Americans and women. *American Journal of Public Health, 86*(4), 525–528.

Hochschild, A. R. (1983). *The managed heart: Commercialization of human feeling.* Berkeley, CA: University of California Press.

Hoffmann, R. L., & Mitchell, A. M. (1998). Caregiver burden: Historical development. *Nursing Forum, 33*(4), 5–11.

Hook, J. L. (2010). Gender inequality in the welfare state: Sex segregation in housework, 1965–2003. *American Journal of Sociology, 115*(5), 1480–1523.

Hurtado, S., Milem, J., Clayton-Pedersen, A., & Allen, W. (1999). *Enacting diverse learning environments: Improving the climate for racial/ethnic diversity in higher education.* ASHE-ERIC Higher Education Report, Vol. 26, No. 8, ERIC.

Institute for Women's Policy Research (IWPR). (2014). *The gender wage gap by occupation 2014 and by race and ethnicity.* #C431. Retrieved from http://www.iwpr.org/publications/pubs/the-gender-wage-gap-2014

Institute of Medicine (IOM). (2010). *The future of nursing: Leading change, advancing health.* Committee on the Robert Wood Johnson Foundation Initiative on the Future of Nursing. Washington, DC: National Academies Press, Institute of Medicine.

Institute of Medicine (IOM). (2011a). *Advancing oral health in America.* Retrieved from https://iom.nationalacademies.org/~/media/Files/Report%20Files/2011/Advancing-Oral-Health-in-America/Advancing%20Oral%20Health%202011%20Report%20Brief.pdf

Institute of Medicing (IOM). (2011b). *Allied health workforce and services: Workshop summary.* Board on Health Services. Washington, DC: National Academies Press, Institute of Medicine.

Institute of Medicine (IOM); Cuff, P., Patel, D., & Perex, M. (2015). *Empowering women and strengthening health systems and services through investing in nursing and midwifery enterprise: Lessons from lower-income countries: Workshop summary.* Washington, DC: National Academies Press.

International Labour Organization (ILO). (2012). Q&As on business, discrimination and equality. Retrieved from http://www.ilo.org/empent/areas/business-helpdesk/faqs/WCMS_DOC_ENT_HLP_BDE_FAQ_EN/lang--en/index.htm

Jagsi, R., Griffith, K. A., DeCastro, R. A., & Ubel, P. (2014). Sex, role models, and specialty choices among graduates of U.S. medical schools in 2006–2008. *Journal of the American College of Surgeons, 218*(3), 345–352.

Jamieson, E. M., & Sewall, M. F. (1944). *Trends in nursing history.* Philadelphia, PA: W. B. Saunders.

Jones, C. P. (2000). Levels of racism: Theoretical framework and gardener's tale. *American Journal of Public Health, 90*(8), 1212–1215. Retrieved from http://www.cahealthadvocates.org/_pdf/news/2007/Levels-Of-Racism.pdf

King, M. L., Jr. (1957). *Loving your enemies' sermon.* In Clayborne Carson (Ed.), A Knock at Midnight: Inspiration from the Great Sermons of Martin Luther King, Jr. (p. 37). New York, NY: IPM/Warner Books.

Knapp, K. K. (1999). Charting the demand for pharmacists in the managed care era. *American Journal of Health-System Pharmacy: Official Journal of the American Society of Health-System Pharmacists, 56*(13), 1309–1314.

Kurtzleben, D. (2012). Vive la difference: Gender divides remain in housework, child care. *U.S. News & World Report.* Retrieved from http://www.usnews.com/news/articles/2012/06/22/vive-la-difference-gender-divides-remain-in-housework-child-care

Ladden, M., & Maher, N. (2014). A transformative program, ahead of its time. *Nursing Outlook, 62*(6), 482–490.

Lamiani, G., Borghi, L., & Argentero, P. (2015). When healthcare professionals cannot do the right thing: A systematic review of moral distress and its correlates. *Journal of Health Psychology.* doi: 10.1177/1359105315595120. Retrieved from http://hpq.sagepub.com/content/early/2015/07/29/1359105315595120.full.pdf+html

Landers, S. H. (2010). Why health care is going home. *New England Journal of Medicine, 363*(18), 1690–1691.

Leigh, J. P., Tancredi, D., Jerant, A., & Kravitz, R. L. (2010). Physician wages across specialties: Informing the physician reimbursement debate. *Archives of Internal Medicine, 170*(19), 1728–1734.

Levinson, W., & Lurie, N. (2004). When most doctors are women: What lies ahead? *Annals of Internal Medicine, 141*(6), 471–474.

Levitt, J. (1977). Men and women as providers of health care. *Social Science & Medicine, 11*(6–7), 395–398.

Lorber, J. (1984). *Women physicians: Careers, status, and power* (Vol. 281). London, UK: Routledge and Kegan & Paul.

Lorber, J. (1987). A welcome to a crowded field: Where will the new women physicians fit in? *Journal of the American Medical Women's Association (1972), 42*(5), 149–152.

Ludmerer, K. M. (1988). *Learning to heal: The development of American medical education.* New York, NY: Basic Books.

MacDorman, M., & Mathews, T. (2011). CDC health disparities and inequalities report—United States, 2011. *Morbidity and Mortality Weekly Report Surveillance Summaries, 60*(Suppl.), 1–109.

Marieskind, H. I. (1980). *Women in the health system: Patient providers, and programs.* St. Louis, MO: C. V. Mosby.

Marini, M. M. (1989). Sex differences in earnings in the United States. *Annual Review of Sociology, (15),* 343–380.

Mattingly, M. J., & Sayer, L. C. (2006). Under pressure: Gender differences in the relationship between free time and feeling rushed. *Journal of Marriage and Family, 68*(1), 205–221.

Mayberry, R. M., Mili, F., & Ofili, E. (2000). Racial and ethnic differences in access to medical care. *Medical Care Research and Review, 57*(Suppl. 1), 108–145.

McMenamin, P. (2013). *Economic prospects for RNs: 2013 and beyond.* Retrieved from http://nursingworld.org/MainMenuCategories/ANAMarketplace/ANAPeriodicals/AmericanNurseToday/Archive/2013-ANT/ANT-Mar13/Issues-up-close-Mar13.pdf

McMenamin, P. (2014). New BLS data on staff nurse compensation and inflation-adjusted wages. *Nursing Economic$, 32*(6), 320–322.

Mertz, E. (2014). *Putting oral health back in the picture.* Retrieved from http://futurehealth.ucsf.edu/Public/Publications-and-Resources/Content.aspx?topic=HT_July_2014_Putting_Oral_Health

MetLife. (2011). *The MetLife study of caregiving costs to working caregivers: Double jeopardy for baby boomers caring for their parents.* Retrieved from https://www.metlife.com/assets/cao/mmi/publications/studies/2011/Caregiving-Costs-to-Working-Caregivers.pdf

MomMD. (2004). *Challenges facing women in medicine.* Retrieved from http://www.mommd.com/challenges.shtml

MomMD. (2016). *Physicians giving up medicine.* Retrieved from http://www.mommd.com/givingup.shtml

Morantz-Sanchez, R. (1985). Sympathy and science. *Women physicians in American medicine.* Chapel Hill, NC: University of North Carolina Press.

More, E. S., & Greer, M. (2000). American women physicians in 2000: A history in progress. *Journal of the American Women's Medical Association, 55*(1), 6–9. Retrieved from http://escholarship.umassmed.edu/lib_articles/49

Morrison, A., & Gallageher Robins, K. (2015). *The women in the low-wage workforce may not be who you think.* Retrieved from http://www.nwlc.org/resource/chart-book-women-low-wage-workforce-may-not-be-who-you-think

Muller, C. (1994). Women in allied health professions. In E. Friedman (Ed.), *An unfinished revolution: Women and health care in America* (pp. 177–203). New York, NY: United Hospital Fund.

National Alliance for Caregiving (NAC). (2009). *Caregiving in the U.S.* Retrieved from http://www.caregiving.org/data/04execsumm.pdf

National Council of State Boards of Nursing (NCSBN). (2012). *A health care consumer's guide to advanced practice registered nursing.* Retrieved from https://www.ncsbn.org/APRN_Brochure_June2012.pdf

National Latina Institute for Reproductive Health (NLIRH). (2015). *Who we are.* Retrieved from http://www.latinainstitute.org/en/mission-vision-values-0

National League for Nursing. (1990). *Nurses of America media project.* New York, NY: NLN.

National Partnership for Women & Families. (2015). Retrieved from http://www.nationalpartnership.org

National Women's Law Center (NWLC). (2015). Retrieved from http://www.nwlc.org

Naylor, M. D., & Sochalski, J. A. (2010). Scaling up: Bringing the transitional care model into the mainstream. *Issue Brief (Commonwealth Fund), 103,* 1–12.

NEJM Career Center. (2014). Compensation in the physician specialties: Mostly stable. *New England Journal of Medicine (NEJM).*

Retrieved from http://www.nejmcareercenter.org/article/compensation-in-the-physician-specialties-mostly-stable

Nelson, A. (2002). Unequal treatment: Confronting racial and ethnic disparities in health care. *Journal of the National Medical Association, 94*(8), 666–668.

Ness, R., & Ukoli, F. (2001). Salary equity among male and female internists. *Annals of Internal Medicine, 134*(9, Pt. 1), 798–799.

Newman, C. (2014). Time to address gender discrimination and inequality in the health workforce. *Human Resources for Health, 12*, 25.

Nightingale, F. (1992). *Notes on nursing: What it is, and what it is not.* Philadelphia, PA: Lippincott Williams & Wilkins.

Novielli, K., Hojat, M., Park, P., Connella, J., & Veloski, J. (2001). Career choice: Glass ceiling or glass slipper. *Academic Medicine, 76*(10), S58–S61.

Nunez-Smith, M., Pilgrim, N., Wynia, M., Desai, M. M., Jones, B. A., Bright, C.,…Bradley, E. H. (2009). Race/ethnicity and workplace discrimination: Results of a national survey of physicians. *Journal of General Internal Medicine, 24*(11), 1198–1204.

Occupational Safety and Health Administration (OSHA). (2013). *Worker safety in hospitals, caring for caregivers.* Retrieved from https://www.osha.gov/dsg/hospitals

O'Neil, E. H. (1993). *Health professions education for the future: Schools in service to the nation.* San Francisco, CA: Pew Health Professions Commission.

O'Neil, E. H. (2003). *Emerging workforce issues. Proceedings of the California Health Care Foundation Leadership Program.* Sacramento, CA: CHCF.

Olson, S. (2011). *Allied health workforce and services: Workshop summary.* Washington, DC: National Academies Press.

Palepu, A., Carr, P. L., Friedman, R. H., Amos, H., Ash, A. S., & Moskowitz, M. A. (1998). Minority faculty and academic rank in medicine. *Journal of the American Medical Association, 280*, 767–771.

Parker, H. (1997). Women doctors in Greece, Rome, and the Byzantine empire. In L. R. Furst (Ed.), *Women Healers and Physicians: Climbing a Long Hill,* (pp. 131–150). Lexington, KY: University of Kentucky.

Peterson, C. A. (2001). Nursing shortage: Not a simple problem—No easy answers. *Online Journal of Issues in Nursing, 6*(1), 1.

Pew Health Professions Commision & O'Neil, E. H. (1998). *Recreating health professional practice for a new century: The fourth report of the Pew Health Professions Commission.* Pew Health Professions Commission, Center for the Health Professions, University of California, San Francisco.

Picot, S. J. (1995). Rewards, costs, and coping of African American caregivers. *Nursing Research, 44*(3), 147–152.

Pizurki, H., Mejia, A., Butter, I., & Ewart, L. (1987). *Women as providers of health care.* Geneva, Switzerland: WHO.

Read, C. Y., Vessey, J. A., Amar, A. F., & Cullinan, D. M. (2013). The challenges of inclusivity in baccalaureate nursing programs. *Journal of Nursing Education, 52*(4), 185–190.

Redwood, Y. (2015). *Advancing health equity in turbulent times.* Retrieved from http://www.gih.org/files/FileDownloads/Advancing_Health_Equity_CHF_August_2015.pdf

Reed, V. A., Jernstedt, G. C., & McCormick, T. R. (2009). A longitudinal study of determinants of career satisfaction in medical students. *Medical Education Online, 9*, 11. Retrieved from http://www.med-ed-online.org/res00089.htm

Reverby, S. (1987a). A caring dilemma: Womanhood and nursing in historical perspective. *Nursing Research, 36*(1), 5–11.

Reverby, S. (1987b). *Ordered to care: The dilemma of American nursing, 1850–1945.* New York, NY: Cambridge University Press.

Rhodes, T., Wagner, K., Strathdee, S. A., Shannon, K., Davidson, P., & Bourgois, P. (2012). Structural violence and structural vulnerability within the risk environment: Theoretical and methodological perspectives for a social epidemiology of HIV risk among injection drug users and sex workers. *Rethinking social epidemiology* (pp. 205–230). New York, NY: Springer.

Roberts, D., & Jesudason, S. (2014). Movement intersectionality: The case of race, gender, disability, and genetic technologies. *Du Bois Review, 10*(2), 313–328. Retrieved from http://journals.cambridge.org/action/displayAbstract?fromPage=online&aid=9142652&fileId=S1742058X13000210

Roberts, S. J. (1983). Oppressed group behavior: Implications for nursing. *Advances in Nursing Science, 5*(4), 21–30.

Robert Wood Johnson Foundation (RWJF). (2012). *Robert Wood Johnson Foundation announces new program to help primary care practices use their workforce more effectively.* Robert Wood Johnson Foundation. Retrieved from http://www.rwjf.org/en/library/articles-and-news/2012/03/robert-wood-johnson-foundation-announces-new-program-to-help-pri.html

Robert Wood Johnson Foundation (RWJF). (2015). Health policy workforce briefs. *Health policy workforce.* Retrieved from http://www.rwjf.org/en/library/features/health-policy/workforce.html

Robinson, K. M. (1997). Family caregiving: Who provides the care, and at what cost? *Nursing Economic$, 15*(5), 243–247.

Rosenberg, C. E. (1995). *The care of strangers: The rise of America's hospital system.* Baltimore, MD: Johns Hopkins University Press.

Rosin, H. (2012). *The end of men: And the rise of women.* London, UK: Penguin.

Ross, G. S. (2001). Salary equity among male and female internists. *Annals of Internal Medicine, 134*(9, Pt. 1), 798–799.

Ross, L. (2012). A feminist vision: No justice—no equity. *Equality…how much further?* Retrieved from http://www.ontheissuesmagazine.com/2010summer/2010summer_Ross.php

Schmitt, J. (2012). *Health-insurance coverage for low-wage workers, 1979–2010 and beyond.* Washington, DC: Center for Economic and Policy Research. Retrieved from http://www.cepr.net/documents/publications/health-low-wage-2012–02.pdf

Schmittdiel, J., Selby, J. V., Grumbach, K., & Quesenberry, C. P. (1999). Women's provider preferences for basic gynecology care in a large health maintenance organization. *Journal of Women's Health & Gender-Based Medicine, 8*(6), 825–833.

Schroeder, C., & DiAngelo, R. (2010). Addressing whiteness in nursing education: The sociopolitical climate project at the University of Washington School of Nursing. *Advances in Nursing Science, 33*(3), 244–255.

Schulz, A. J., & Mullings, L. (2006). *Gender, race, class, and health: Intersectional approaches.* San Francisco, CA: Jossey-Bass.

Sen, G., Ostlin, P., & George, A. (2007). *Unequal unfair ineffective and inefficient. Gender inequity in health: Why it exists and how we can change it.* Final report to the WHO Commission on Social Determinants of Health. Geneva, Switzerland: WHO.

Shryock, R. H. (1967). Medicine in America: Historical essays. *American Journal of the Medical Sciences, 253*(5), 154.

Sipe, T. A., Fullerton, J. T., & Schuiling, K. D. (2009). Demographic profiles of certified nurse-midwives, certified registered nurse anesthetists, and nurse practitioners: Reflections on implications for uniform education and regulation. *Journal of Professional Nursing: Official Journal of the American Association of Colleges of Nursing, 25*(3), 178–185.

SisterSong. (2015). *Sister Song: Women of Color Reproductive Justice Collective.* Retrieved from http://www.sistersong.net

Skillman, S., Kaplan, L., Fordyce, M., McMenamin, P., & Doescher, M. (2012). *Understanding advanced practice registered nurse distribution in urban and rural areas of the United States using National Provider Identifier Data.* Seattle, WA: University of Washington.

Smedley, B. D., Butler, A. S., & Bristow, L. R. (2004). *In the nation's compelling interest: Ensuring diversity in the health care workforce.* Washington, DC: National Academies Press.

Snyder, C. R., Stover, B., Skillman, S. M., & Frogner, B. K. (2015). *Facilitating racial and ethnic diversity in the health workforce.* Retrieved from http://depts.washington.edu/uwrhrc/uploads/FINALREPORT_Facilitating%20Diversity%20in%20the%20Health%20Workforce_7.8.2015.pdf

Sondik, E. J., Huang, D. T., Klein, R. J., & Satcher, D. (2010). Progress toward the *Healthy People 2010* goals and objectives. *Annual Review of Public Health, 31*, 271–281.

Spetz, J., Frogner, B., Lucia, L., & Jacobs, K. (2014). *The impact of the Affordable Care Act on new jobs.* Retrieved from http://www.bigideasforjobs.org/wp-content/uploads/2012/03/Spetz_Lee_Final.pdf

Spillman, B. C., & Black, K. J. (2005). *Staying the course: Trends in family caregiving.* Washington, DC: AARP Public Policy Institute.

Starr, P. (1982). *The social transformation of American medicine.* New York, NY: Basic Books.

Stein, R., Bauman, L., & Jessop, D. (1994). Women as formal and informal caregivers of children. *An unfinished revolution: Women and health care in America* (pp. 103–120). New York, NY: United Hospital Fund.

Stone, T. E., & Ajayi, C. (2013). "There comes a time when silence is betrayal": Racism and nursing. *Nursing & Health Sciences, 15*(4), 407–409.

Taché, S., & Chapman, S. (2006). The expanding roles and occupational characteristics of medical assistants: Overview of an emerging field in allied health. *Journal of Allied Health, 35*(4), 233–237.

Talley, R. C., & Crews, J. E. (2007). Framing the public health of caregiving. *American Journal of Public Health, 97*(2), 224–228.

Taylor, D., & Dower, K. (1997). Toward a women-centered health care system: Women's experiences, women's voices, women's needs. *Health Care for Women International, 18*(4), 407–422.

Tijdens, K., de Vries, D. H., & Steinmetz, S. (2013). Health workforce remuneration: Comparing wage levels, ranking, and dispersion of 16 occupational groups in 20 countries. *Human Resources for Health, 11*, 11.

Toles, M. P., Abbott, K. M., Hirschman, K. B., & Naylor, M. D. (2012). Transitions in care among older adults receiving long-term services and supports. *Journal of Gerontological Nursing, 38*(11), 40–47.

Ulrich, B. (2010). Gender diversity and nurse–physician relationships. *AMA Journal of Ethics, 12*(1), 41–45. Retrieved from http://journalofethics.ama-assn.org/2010/01/msoc1–1001.html

U.S. Census Bureau. (2000). *Statistical abstract of the United States: 2000* (120th ed.). Washington, DC: Author.

U.S. Census Bureau. (2012). *America community survey.* Retrieved from https://www.census.gov/programs-surveys/acs/data.html

U.S. Census Bureau. (2015a). *New Census Bureau report analyzes U.S. population projections.* Retrieved from https://www.census.gov/newsroom/press-releases/2015/cb15-tps16.html

U.S. Census Bureau. (2015b). *Projections of the size and composition of the U.S. Population: 2014 to 2060.* Retrieved from https://www.census.gov/content/dam/Census/library/publications/2015/demo/p25–1143.pdf

U.S. Department of Health and Human Services. (n.d.). *A nation free of disparities in health and health care: HHS action plan to reduce racial and ethnic health disparities.* Retrieved from http://minorityhealth.hhs.gov/npa/files/plans/hhs/hhs_plan_complete.pdf

U.S. Department of Health and Human Services (DHHS). (2000). *The pharmacist workforce: A study of the supply and demand for pharmacists.* Retrieved from http://bhpr.hrsa.gov/healthworkforce/supplydemand/pharmacy/pharmacistsupplydemand.pdf

U.S. Department of Health and Human Services (DHHS). (2014). *A 21st century health care workforce for the nation.* Retrieved from http://aspe.hhs.gov/sites/default/files/pdf/76796/rpt_healthcareworkforce.pdf

U.S. Department of Health and Human Services (DHHS). (2015). *The Affordable Care Act is working.* Retrieved from http://www.hhs.gov/healthcare/facts-and-features/fact-sheets/aca-is-working/index.html

U.S. Department of Health and Human Services, Health Resources and Services Administration, Bureau of Health Professions, Office of Public Health and Science, Office of Minority Health. (2009). *Pipeline programs to improve racial and ethnic diversity in the health professions: An inventory of federal programs, assessment of evaluation approaches, and critical review of the research literature.* Retrieved from http://bhpr.hrsa.gov/healthworkforce/supplydemand/usworkforce/pipelinediversityprograms.pdf

U.S. Department of Health and Human Services, Health Resources and Services Administration, National Center for Health Workforce Analysis. (2014). *Sex, race, and ethnic diversity of U.S. Health occupations (2010–2012),* Rockville, MD: Author.

U.S. Department of Labor. (2005). *Occupational employment projections to 2014: Fastest growing occupations, 2004–2014, Table 2, November 2005 Monthly Labor Review.* Retrieved from http://www.bls.gov/opub/mlr/2005/11/art5full.pdf

U.S. Department of Labor. (2006). *Occupational employment statistics.* Retrieved from http://www.bls.gov/oes/home.htm

U.S. Department of Labor. (2010a). *Quick stats on women workers.* Retrieved from www.dol.gov/wb/factsheets/QS-womenwork2010.htm

U.S. Department of Labor. (2010b). *Standard occupational classification.* Retrieved from http://www.bls.gov/soc

U.S. Department of Labor. (2012). *Occupational outlook handbook.* Retrieved from http://www.bls.gov/ooh/a-z-index.htm

U.S. Department of Labor. (2014a). *Occupational outlook handbook, nurse anesthetists, nurse midwives, and nurse practitioners.* Retrieved from http://www.bls.gov/ooh/healthcare/nurse-anesthetists-nurse-midwives-and-nurse-practitioners.htm

U.S. Department of Labor. (2014b). *Women in the labor force: A databook* (Report 1049). Retrieved from http://www.bls.gov/opub/reports/cps/women-in-the-labor-force-a-databook-2014.pdf

U.S. Department of Labor. (2015a). *Labor force statistics from the current population survey.* Retrieved from http://www.bls.gov/cps/cpsaat39.htm

U.S. Department of Labor. (2015b). *Labor force statistics from the current population survey.* Retrieved from http://www.bls.gov/cps/tables.htm

U.S. Department of Labor. (2015c). *May 2014 national occupational employment and wage estimates United States.* Retrieved from http://www.bls.gov/oes/current/oes_nat.htm

U.S. Department of Labor. (2015d). *Standard occupational classification.* Retrieved from http://www.bls.gov/soc

U.S. Government Publishing Office (GPO). (2015). 42 U.S.C. 295P—DEFINITIONS. Retrieved from http://www.gpo.gov/fdsys/granule/USCODE-2010-title42/USCODE-2010-title42-chap6A-subchapV-partF-sec295p

Vedantam, S. (2013). *How to fight racial bias when it is silent and subtle.* Retrieved from http://www.npr.org/sections/codeswitch/2013/07/19/203306999/How-To-Fight-Racial-Bias-When-Its-Silent-And-Subtle

Vincent, G. K., & Velkoff, V. A. (2010). *The next four decades: The older population in the United States: 2010 to 2050.* U.S. Department of Commerce, Economics and Statistics Administration, U.S. Census Bureau. Washington, DC: U.S. Department of Commerce.

Walsch, M. R. (1977). *"Doctors wanted: No women need apply": Sexual barriers in the medical profession 1835–1975.* New Haven, CT: Yale University Press. Retrieved from http://www.americanscientist.org/bookshelf/pub/doctors-wanted-no-women-need-apply-and-the-hidden-malpractice

Weaver, J. L., & Garrett, S. D. (1983). Sexism and racism in the American health care industry: A comparative analysis. In E. Fee (Ed.), *The Politics of Sex in Medicine* (pp. 79–104). New York, NY: Baywood.

White Coats 4 Black Lives. (2015). Retrieved from http://www.whitecoats4blacklives.org

Wilson, M. P. (1987). Making a difference—Women, medicine, and the twenty-first century. *Yale Journal of Biology and Medicine, 60*(3), 273–288.

Wood, C. A. (2011). Employment in health care: A crutch for the ailing economy during the 2007–09 recession. *Monthly Labor Review, 134*(4), 13–18.

Woodward, C. A., Cohen, M. L., & Ferrier, B. M. (1990). Career interruptions and hours practiced: Comparison between young men and women physicians. *Canadian Journal of Public Health (Revue Canadienne De Santé Publique), 81*(1), 16–20.

World Health Organization (WHO). (2001). Transforming health systems: Gender and rights in reproductive health: A training manual for health managers. Retrieved from http://www.who.int/reproductivehealth/publications/gender_rights/RHR_01_29/en

World Health Organization (WHO). (2015). *WHO at the UN Commission on the Status of Women (CSW).* Retrieved from http://www.who.int/life-course/news/who-at-csw/en

Yoon, J., Grumbach, K., & Bindman, A. B. (2004). Access to Spanish-speaking physicians in California: Supply, insurance, or both. *Journal of the American Board of Family Practice/American Board of Family Practice, 17*(3), 165–172.

Zavadski, K. (2014). *The pharmacy school bubble is about to burst; one of America's most reliable professions is producing too many graduates and not enough jobs.* Retrieved from https://newrepublic.com/article/119634/pharmacy-school-crisis-why-good-jobs-are-drying

CHAPTER 3

Women and Health Care

Nancy Fugate Woods • Ellen F. Olshansky • Deborah Ward

What have we accomplished in our efforts to improve women's health care during the 20th century? Women have pushed for a redefinition of women's health that transcends the boundaries of reproductive health care and incorporates a life-span view that accommodates their health from the perinatal period to the end of life. Women have helped reconfigure the delivery of women's health care by challenging existing systems to replace fragmentation with integration and coordination of health care services. Women have demanded services unique for women such as birthing centers and menopause clinics.

What would women like to claim as 21st-century achievements in women's health care? Here are a few claims for the early part of the 21st century. Among a long list of aspirations for enhancing women's health care, we would like to claim the following.

■ The greater conceptual clarity of sex, gender, and related concepts has prompted health professionals to demonstrate growing recognition of the importance of gender awareness as essential to avoiding bias in the delivery of services, as well as educating future health professionals and conducting research.
■ Health care professionals are prepared to provide comprehensive women's health care using gender-sensitive models that span women's lives.
■ Researchers design studies in collaboration with women, analyze changes in women's health data and compare them to men and male and female vertebrate animals, seek new methodologies and methods to optimize the inclusion of heterogeneous populations of women, and translate their findings directly to clinical and public health practice and for women, themselves.
■ The analysis of problems women face in obtaining appropriate, gender-sensitive health care has prompted policy changes to promote access to comprehensive, coordinated, integrated women's health care that is associated with higher levels of satisfaction, higher rates of use of preventive services, and reduced morbidity and mortality.
■ Global research efforts have underscored the importance of gender inequality as experienced in many countries and its relationship to patterns of morbidity

and mortality and provided evidence to propel changes to promote women's health and enhance the care women receive while ensuring equity.
■ Around the world women's contributions to health and health care in their countries are valued, compensated, counted, and accounted for in the gross domestic product, and countries are accountable to women in providing gender-appropriate and equitable care.

In this chapter we:

1. Examine concepts of sex and gender as a basis for considering gender-sensitive health care
2. Review sexism and gender bias as they have existed in U.S. health care, education of health professionals, and research
3. Explore advances in the education of health care professionals to provide women's health care
4. Analyze changes in women's health research to guide care (translation)
5. Propose a gender-sensitive approach to health care for women, including integration for sexual and reproductive health (SRH) in primary care and life-span approaches
6. Analyze policy challenges within our existing health care "systems" in the United States, including progress and promise of health care reform and the Patient Protection and Affordable Care Act (ACA)
7. Consider a global view of women and health care

■ SEX, GENDER, AND HEALTH CARE FOR WOMEN

The definition and differentiation of *sex* and *gender* have been important contributions to the study of women's health and health care. Since the second wave of feminism in 1960s and 1970s in the United States, we have seen acknowledgment of the importance of understanding sex and gender, as both are related to health. During most of the 20th century, *sex* was used to guide research about men and women irrespective of the focus of the work being either biological or sociocultural. Contemporary theory and research about sex and gender have revised the thinking of many health professionals about what it means to be female (sex) and what being a woman means within the context of our society (gender).

In documents about women's health care and research, sex has been viewed as biologically determined, based on chromosomal patterns and the effects of sex hormones on reproductive organ development. Scientists formulating the National Institutes of Health (NIH) Agenda for Women's Health (USPHS, 1992) distinguished between the biological definitions of *male* and *female* based on chromosomal sex and introduced the consideration of gender. Scientific interest in chromosomal and biological elements of sex has been fueled by genomics research (Institute of Medicine [IOM], 2001).

Definitions of *sex* have emanated from biomedicine and more recent developments in gender-specific medicine, whereas social scientists have defined *gender* as a social category that includes changing definitions of appropriate roles, division of labor, economic power, and political influence. When seen as static differences, both sex and gender have been viewed through dualistic lenses through which *sex* became defined as male or female based on the reproductive organs and functions and *gender* was viewed as a person's representation of self as male or female, rooted in biology and shaped by one's environment, experience, and socialization. The limitations of these definitions may preclude a view of the interplay of sex and gender that allows for the influence of the body and of culture and history, as they simultaneously influence health and behavior. In addition, scholars have emphasized the importance of analyzing gender in relation to other power structures such as class, race/ethnicity, and sexuality (Hammarström et al., 2014).

Concepts of sex and gender continue to be revised as the binaries of male and female are being reexamined to accommodate the human experience of both sex and gender. A recent analysis of sex, gender, intersectionality, embodiment, gender equality, and gender equity examined their importance to health research (Hammarström et al., 2014). Hammarström et al. propose that sex, in interaction with gender, offers the potential for the analysis of sex as a continuum with various options that include not only X- and Y-chromosomes, hormonal levels, and internal and external genitalia, but also opens up the possibility to view sex and gender as integration of body–mind–context. These considerations can be viewed not only at the level of the individual, but also at the level of social structures in which gender relations are integrated, including labor markets and the health care system.

Hammarström et al. (2014) include the concepts of intersectionality and embodiment to further expand our thinking about sex and gender. Intersectionality is grounded in assumptions of heterogeneity within groups of women and men, prompting recognition that individuals are defined by multiple intersecting dimensions. Women simultaneously have a gender, class, ethnicity, ability/disability, sexual orientation, and age. The addition of these dimensions to gender further guides consideration of equality and equity, denoting populations whose risk for discrimination and bias is unique (Hammarström et al., 2014). Embodiment focuses on how one's body interacts with environments. Body–mind is viewed holistically, in contrast to the split between body and mind, in which the lived body functions as mind–body–world. Social embodiment prompts consideration of social processes and gender relations as they relate to health. Moreover, ecosocial theory integrates the body, mind, and society in understanding the health impact of social conditions, how sex and gender become interwoven in life.

Gender equality and gender equity aid analysis of the distribution of opportunities, resources, and responsibilities between women and men. Equality concerns equal rights, or the absence of gendered discrimination, and gender equity concerns the needs of the genders. Notions of sameness–difference reflect concerns about equality, whereas fairness reflects concerns about equity, concepts important to understanding policy. Do policies advocate equality, the absence of discrimination, and gender equity as meeting the needs of both women and men?

Krieger's tutorial "Genders, Sexes, and Health: What Are the Connections—and Why Does It Matter?" pointed out that gender relations can influence the expression and the interpretation of biological traits and that sex-linked biological characteristics can contribute to or amplify gender differentials in health. Krieger also includes a definition of *sexism* as inequitable gender relationships and references it to institutional and interpersonal practices by which dominant gender groups accrue privilege by subordinating other gender groups and justify these practices via ideologies of innate superiority, difference, or deviance (Krieger, 2003). Based on clear definitions of sex and gender, she provides instructive case examples of the differential roles of gender relations and sex-linked biology on health outcomes. As an example, gender relations can be a determinant of men versus women using physical violence against intimate partners (gender relations affect exposure to intimate partner violence) at the same time that sex-linked biology affects exposure (sex as a determinant of muscle strength and stamina and body size). Thus the health outcome of a lethal assault is related to the greater physical strength and size of men and the gender-related skills and training in inflicting and warding off attack.

Current thinking in health care admonishes health professionals to uncouple sex and gender in an effort to establish "gender equal" health care. Bachmann and Mussman (2015) consider the marginalization of the transgender community and advocate for a redefinition of what constitutes "normal" male and female. They point out research that indicates sexual preference is not binary, with bisexuality being reported as a sexual option, and that neither sexual preferences nor gender identity are binaries. These concepts are discussed further in Chapters 20 and 25.

Sex and gender have different and multifaceted influences on health and health care, and both have played a role in shaping federal policy. In 1985, the Task Force Report on Women's Health set in motion a series of events that included the development of the Office of Research on Women's Health (ORWH) at the NIH in 1990, development of the first NIH Research Agenda on Women's Health in 1991, and establishment of the Centers of Excellence (CoEs) for Women's Health Care in 1996. Although this body of work clearly focused on both sex and gender, the U.S. Public Health Services (USPHS) Task Force Report offered an early definition of women's health as focusing on health problems specific to women, more common or more serious in women, having distinct causes or manifestations in women, having different treatment or outcomes in women, and having high morbidity and/or mortality in women (USPHS, 1985). The Task Force also recommended that both biomedical and behavioral research should be expanded to ensure emphasis on these areas. Consequences of the Task Force's efforts included three objectives for the ORWH: ensuring that issues pertaining to women were adequately addressed (diseases, disorders, and conditions unique to, more prevalent among, or far more serious in women for which there are different risk factors or interventions for women than for men); ensuring appropriate participation in clinical research, especially clinical trials; and fostering increased involvement of women in biomedical research, emphasizing their decision-making roles in clinical medicine and research. The inclusion of women in NIH-funded health research was required, and this inclusion criterion has since been extended to minorities (underrepresented ethnic groups). In the early reports that emanated from USPHS and NIH, sex and gender were sometimes used interchangeably, but in documents dating from the 2001 IOM Report *Exploring the Biological Contributions to Human Health: Does Sex Matter?* clear distinction was made more frequently between sex and gender (IOM, 2001).

■ SEX AND GENDER DIFFERENCES, GENDER BIAS, AND HEALTH CARE

The social and health sciences literature provides evidence of the complex influences of sex and gender in delivering personal health services, educating health professionals, and researching women's health. Investigators have found evidence of sex and gender differences and bias in diagnosis, treatment, prescription of medications, and hospitalization. This body of work contributed important understanding about practices that need to be corrected in the interest of gender equality and gender equity. As noted in Chapter 1, women and men experience many common types of health problems, but there are health problems that are unique to women or are much more prevalent among women than men. Thus one would anticipate sex differences in the incidence and prevalence of health problems. Gender differences also would arise from the ways in which women and men are socialized. Sex and gender bias occurs in situations in which differences are attributed to women and men that result in one sex or gender receiving care that is unequal or inequitable. Some examples of the complexity of sex and gender differences and bias in health care are explored in the following sections.

Mental Health and Mental Illness

Classic studies (Aslin, 1977; Broverman, Broverman, Clarkson, Rosenkrantz, & Vogel, 1970) demonstrated that women judged to behave in gender-appropriate ways were also judged to be psychologically less healthy than men and that the gender of a therapist can influence expectations about women's mental health (see Chapter 12 for further discussion). Assumptions about one sex (female) as inherently less healthy introduced bias into the judgments of actual health.

Gender has been associated with mental health and illness because of sex and gender differences in the presentation and prevalence of various types of mental illnesses and the assumptions about gender underlying ways in which women and men are diagnosed with mental illness. The American Psychiatric Association (APA, 2013) notes that the prevalence of psychiatric disorders varies between men and women. Women demonstrate higher rates than men of many psychiatric disorders: mood, anxiety, eating, sleep, personality, somatoform, dissociative, obsessive-compulsive spectrum, and impulse control, as well as late-onset schizophrenia with prominent mood symptoms and dementia of the Alzheimer's type (APA, 2013). Of note is the greater prevalence of depression among women. A variety of explanations have been proposed to account for these differences. Some propose that gender role socialization encourages girls and women to express symptoms and discourages these behaviors in boys and men. Others attribute gender differences in mental health to the tendency of women to internalize and men to externalize symptoms/disorders. Still others implicate the more stressful nature of girls' and women's lives, including adverse early experiences of abuse, as well as gender stereotypes about women's and men's mental health.

A recent study of gendered mental disorders examined masculine and feminine stereotypes about mental disorders and their relationship to stigma. Boysen, Ebersole, Canser, and Coston (2014) found that people held gendered stereotypes about mental disorders, with a masculine stereotype consisting of externalizing disorders such as antisocial personality and substance use and a feminine stereotype of internalizing disorders such as anxiety and mood. The masculine disorders and symptoms elicited more stigma than feminine disorders. Whether men and women fall into gender-neutral diagnostic categories as a result of gender-neutral evaluations or are guided into gender-biased diagnoses as a result of gender-biased evaluations by health professionals is an important question that continues to be studied.

The intricate interweaving of socially constructed definitions of gender and their relation to diagnostic taxonomies is also illustrated by the continuing controversies surrounding various diagnoses in revisions of the *Diagnostic and Statistical Manual of Mental Disorders* (DSM), the standardized diagnostic manual that forms the basis for diagnosis and treatment, not to mention billing and data collection. Recent investigations of premenstrual dysphoric disorder (PMDD) illustrate the controversies over a menstruation-related mood disorder and their potential consequences on women's health (Zachar & Kendler 2014). Proposals to include PMDD as a diagnosis in the *DSM* (3rd rev. ed.; *DSM-III-R*; and 4th ed.; *DSM-IV*; APA, 1994) prompted an intense debate, but PMDD was recently included in the *Diagnostic and Statistical Manual of Mental Disorders* (5th ed.; *DSM-5*; APA, 2013) without significant objection.

Concerns about stigmatizing a normal part of women's menstrual cycles had justified not including PMDD in the *DSM-III-R*. Instead of including it in the manual, the APA included a section labeled "late luteal phase dysphoric disorder" (LLPDD) in an appendix. *DSM-IV* retained the diagnosis in the appendix, but changed the label from LLPDD to PMDD. In 2013, the APA included PMDD as a diagnosis.

A number of factors encouraging the inclusion of PMDD in the *DSM-5* include potential economic effects, social–political consequences, ethical concerns, conservative attitudes, and peer pressure. A recent interview study of mental health clinicians involved in the consideration of PMDD inclusion in the *DSM-IV* revealed several elements of their decision processes that guided their thinking. Reasons given for including PMDD in the main *DSM-IV* included agreement on PMDD symptoms and their time course, recognition of benefits of treatment, and the use of a biomedical model for understanding psychiatric disorders. Those who favored deleting PMDD from *DSM-IV* raised issues such as the likelihood of false-positive diagnosis of PMDD, questionable diagnostic validity of the psychological symptoms, and the belief that premenstrual syndrome (PMS) and PMDD were embedded in cultural assumptions about gender roles. Feminist values and negative social consequences were additional reasons for deleting PMDD from *DSM-IV*. Reference was made to the earlier diagnosis of hysteria and the likelihood of PMDD being used against women or masking the real reasons for women's anger and distress. Another issue was the conviction that the diagnosis of PMDD was being advocated by pharmaceutical manufacturers who stood to profit from sales of medications.

Reasons given for retaining PMDD in the *DSM-IV* appendix included philosophical ideas regarding the nature of disorders: PMDD was seen as an exacerbation of an existing condition, but not a mood disorder because of the inclusion of many somatic symptoms, such as bloating. Some expressed opinions that higher standards of evidence should be available to support the inclusion of PMDD in the *DSM*, weighed with the risk of having a diagnosis that could be used against women. Peer pressure may have been a factor for some of the participants in the *DSM-IV* decision process (Zachar & Kendler, 2014).

Of interest is the fact that the *DSM-5* revision attracted controversies over several decisions but not over PMDD. Several reasons were offered for the lack of debate, including generational changes among feminists who objected to *DSM-IV* decisions and availability of additional research on the validity and treatment of PMDD. At the same time, there were concerns about sexism influencing these decisions, as reflected in a failure to recognize that women's distress was related to cultural roles and powerlessness (Zachar & Kendler, 2014).

In the same time frame that Zachar and Kendler (2014) published their investigation, Browne (2015) asked if premenstrual dysphoric disorder was really a disorder. She asserted that PMDD was a socially constructed disorder that pathologizes understandable anger and distress that women experience. Moreover, she notes that PMDD is culture-bound, not a universal syndrome, for example, it is not commonly reported in Asia. Browne argues that PMDD symptoms are caused not by a mental disorder but instead by one's environment and that such distress should be recognized without being defined as a pathology. Browne recommends a feminist solution: changing attitudes toward women's suffering instead of pathologizing women's anger and distress.

These two sets of analyses of PMDD as a diagnosis illustrate the underlying processes by which a contested diagnosis gains acceptance despite consideration of evidence that it is socially constructed. Moreover, these analyses raise important questions about motivations that drive professional decisions to identify new diagnoses. Are health professionals induced to create new diagnoses in the interest of helping women who experience distress? In advancing the position of all women in society? In the interest of gender equality? Gender equity? To what extent was gender disparity or gender bias involved in these deliberations?

Medical Diagnosis and Treatment

The history of women's medical diagnosis is similarly rife with now-discredited categories such as hysteria (Leavitt, 1984). Indeed, there is evidence that links the gender of patients to the type of diagnosis health professionals assign to them. Whether these differences are attributable to health professionals' gender stereotypes or bias or to gender differences in the presentation of symptoms and associated prevalence of disease is challenging to interpret.

Heart disease is the leading cause of death for U.S. women, yet diagnosing and treating cardiac events in women remain fraught with challenges. One challenge in the diagnosis of cardiac events is the differences in symptoms women and men report. Instead of the classic chest pain reported by men, women often report different types of symptoms. In one study of women and men in a myocardial infarction (MI) registry, women were more likely to complain of pain in the left shoulder/arm/hand, throat/jaw, upper abdomen and between the shoulder blades; vomiting and nausea; dyspnea; fear of death; and dizziness than men. Moreover, women were more likely to report more than four symptoms. There were no significant differences in the reporting of chest pain, feelings of pressure or tightness, diaphoresis, pain in the right shoulder/arm/hand, and syncope. Although women and men did not differ in reports of the chief acute MI symptoms (chest pain, feelings of tightness or pressure, and diaphoresis), women were more likely to report additional symptoms (Kirchberger, Heier, Kuch, Wende, & Meisinger, 2011). The consequence of gender differences in symptom reporting is that women may be less likely to be allocated the highest priority in getting emergency care by first responders providing ambulance service (Coventry, Bremner, Jacobs, & Finn, 2013).

Recent research findings illustrate the complexity of gender effects in the presentation of symptoms as well as the management and health outcomes in patients with ST-segment elevation myocardial infarction (STEMI). Leurent et al. (2014) examined whether female gender was associated with higher in-hospital mortality using data from 5,000 patients from a registry of STEMI in France. Several hypotheses have been suggested to account for increased female mortality from MI that include more serious comorbidity, longer times to revascularization, and use of less optimal reperfusion strategies. There remains a question of whether female gender is a risk factor for in-hospital death from STEMI. Significant differences between women's and men's experiences before reaching the hospital were noted, including a smaller proportion of women using the emergency medical ambulance service and fewer having significant ST-segment elevation on electrocardiography before hospital admission, and less direct access to the cardiac catheterization lab in case of angioplasty. The average time of ischemia was longer for female than male patients, with delayed treatment at all stages, including pain onset to calling for help, call to hospital door time, and door to balloon or thrombo-aspiration time. Lower rates of some reperfusion techniques in women were apparent. In-hospital morbidity and mortality rates were higher in women, and hospital stay was longer. The mortality for women was twice than that for men and affected primarily women younger than 69 years. Evidence of excess mortality in the hospital for women remained even after adjustments for characteristics of the patients and time to revascularization and the revascularization technique used.

These results present several dilemmas for interpretation: Were the deaths attributable to differences in time to seeking care? Did women call for help later than men after experiencing chest pain? If so, why did women call later? Did they not associate their symptoms with MI? Were women diagnosed less accurately in the absence of ST-segment elevation? Did women receive different treatment? Why did they have less access to the cardiac catheterization lab? Did those who did not survive die from a different disease process (e.g., rupture of the coronary artery plaque that immediately occluded their arteries vs. a more gradual development of plaque that gradually reduced coronary artery blood flow)? How much of the excess mortality was attributable to sex differences in the disease process versus gender difference in the response to chest pain or other symptoms? And to gender bias in treatment?

Pharmacotherapy

Sex and gender differences as well as sexism influence the prescription of medications. During the late 20th century, physicians recommended over-the-counter medications to young women (and minority group patients) more than they did to men (Pradel, Hartzema, Mutran, & Hanson-Divers, 1999). Three quarters of all psychotropic medications were prescribed for women (Fankhauser, 1997). Women are subsequently at higher risk than men for adverse drug reactions; women on antidepressants (two thirds of all antidepressant prescriptions are for women) experienced more—and more severe—side effects than did men. Complications from pharmaceutical use of all kinds disproportionately affect women; office visits for medication-related morbidity are greatest for women aged 65 to 74 years (Aparasu, 1999).

Because women appear to experience more medication-related adverse reactions, and if they are the targets of over-the-counter drug advertising and physician recommendations for over-the-counter drugs, it could be speculated that clinicians' expectations and market forces might be powerful determinants of the care women receive. Might men physicians (and other prescribers) embrace certain expectations about women's behavior and adjustment and tend to determine that women are more in need of psychotropic drugs, for example, than their equally troubled but more reticent men patients? Do women request medication more than men and, if so, why? It is not known what the U.S. population of women has as a baseline standard of demand and need for care, apart from the products and services eagerly sold to them. As Ruiz and Verbrugge (1997) stated:

> We know little about how men and women voluntarily adopt some risk behaviours and risk exposures, their different perceptions of symptoms and expression of complaints, how their milieux of social support affect health and health behaviour, and their behavioral strategies for treating and adjusting to health problems. (p. 106)

The conditions that lead women more than men to use medicaments of all kinds await full explication. The historic development of women as herbalists clearly arose from their role as family nurse and healer (Ehrenreich & English, 1973). An argument can be made that faith in pharmaceutical therapy is a logical association with what has been called women's culture—a culture of connection and mutual aid rather than the individualism associated with male culture. Under this theoretical construct, women would be more likely to use drugs of all kinds—from diet pills to megavitamins—whereas men are more apt to be socialized to ignore or endure symptoms such as low energy, despondency, or overeating.

Women's physiology is increasingly thought to play a role in treatment. Sex differences in the pharmacokinetics of antidepressants may be influenced by female sex hormones and oral contraceptives. In a recent review of sex differences in response to antidepressant pharmacotherapy, Damoiseaux, Proost, Jiawan, and Melgert (2014) explored evidence for differences in pharmacokinetic properties, including absorption, distribution, metabolism, and excretion of medications, in women and men. Recent research indicates that sex hormones may influence all pharmacokinetic processes. Women experience variation in hormone levels throughout their life span, potentially influencing their response to antidepressants as well as occurrence of adverse events. Depression symptoms have been associated with deficiencies in norepinephrine, dopamine, and/or serotonin, and the presentation of symptoms in women includes a greater tendency to experience negative emotions. Because women and men appear to react differently to antidepressant therapy, these differences may be because of pharmacokinetic differences that may be attributable to sex hormone effects, and thus differences may occur in relation to the menstrual cycle, with use of oral contraceptives, and at other times of hormonal shifts such as the menopausal transition. Because estrogen modulates the neurotransmitters (norepinephrine, serotonin, and dopamine) related to depression, sex differences in the effects of psychotropic drugs affecting these neurotransmitters are not surprising. There are several sex differences in pharmacokinetic processes that include absorption and bioavailability, distribution, metabolism, and excretion. One possible example is the effect of progesterone on prolonging the gut transit time of drugs, providing greater opportunity for absorption of medications. Another is the influence of the cytochrome P450 enzymes. Women have higher CYP3A4 activity and the CYP enzymes play a major role in the metabolism of antidepressants. CYP enzymes are modulated by estradiol. Physiological variation during the menstrual cycle has multiple potential effects on pharmacokinetics, with multiple possible consequences for psychotherapeutic drugs prescribed for depression. For example, increasing the metabolism of antidepressant substrates may result in a lower plasma concentration and possibly lower efficacy, requiring an increase in the dose of the medication. This is of consequence in pregnant women given that clinical trials frequently exclude pregnant women. The sex differences in response to antidepressants discussed here alert clinicians to the possibility that sex-linked biology (e.g., hormonal influences) plays an important role in modulating the effects of these medications and requires careful consideration of appropriate dose of them.

Surgery

Famous studies by Wennberg and others demonstrated a national pattern of extreme variability in physician practice patterns (Wennberg & Cooper, 1999). This variability is influenced by factors such as the practice patterns of regional peers, style and location of medical school training, and penetration by specialty practice. Patient gender has also been found to influence rates and types of surgery.

Gynecology was one of the first specialty areas to fall under the scrutiny of women's health care analysts. As of 1980, the hysterectomy had become the most frequently performed major operation for women of reproductive years. At that time, the American College of Obstetricians and Gynecologists estimated that 15% of hysterectomies were performed to remove cancer, 30% to remove noncancerous fibroids, 35% for pelvic relaxation or prolapse, and 20% for sterilization (Scully, 1980). A hysterectomy should not be performed as an elective procedure or when more conservative treatment will suffice, and yet it was estimated that one third of hysterectomies and half of cesarean sections performed in the United States were unnecessary (Seaman, 1972). More recent evidence continues to demonstrate that nonclinical factors (physician characteristics such as background, training, experience, and practice style) play a statistically significant role in this surgical decision (Geller, Burns, & Brailer, 1996).

Cardiology and cardiovascular surgery exemplify another specialty practice arena studied for its utilization by gender. Although the risk of developing coronary artery disease has increased for women and decreased for men since 1950, women were less likely than men to be referred promptly for cardiac surgical consultation (Schwartz et al., 1997). In a survey of 720 physicians responding to a computerized survey instrument, women and Black patients were significantly less likely to be referred for cardiac catheterization than men and White patients (Schulman et al., 1999). Black women were least likely of all groups to be referred. The authors concluded that, after careful controls were applied, race and patient gender independently influenced the management of chest pain. The lower rates of referral for cardiac catheterization found in this study illustrate the importance of intersectionality of gender and race that creates unique levels of risk for women.

■ WOMEN'S HEALTH SCHOLARSHIP AND RESEARCH

Women's health scholarship, including theory and research, began to flourish in the 1970s in the wake of the resurgence of a women's health movement that focused on demystifying women's health and enhancing women's access to appropriate health care. One important element of this scholarship was a broad vision of women's health that transcended the limits of reproductive health and emphasized an integrated, holistic view inclusive of women's bodies, as well as their minds and emotions, in place of a fragmented view of women's health (reproductive/nonreproductive, body/mind) and focused more broadly on health and well-being, not only diseases of women (Mc Bride & Mc Bride, 1991). Nursing was quick to embrace the new view of women's health. Indeed, Mc Bride and Mc Bride (1993) encouraged us to think about women's health as Gyne-Ecology, viewing women's health in the context of their lives, not merely gynecology. Academic programs such as the Women's Health and Healing Program at the University of California, San Francisco, School of Nursing and the development of a Women's Health Program at the University of Illinois, Chicago (Dan, 1994; Ruzek, Olesen, & Clarke, 1997), led to the development of the Society for Menstrual Cycle Research and other academic programs focusing on women. In 1989, just 3 years after the National Institute of Nursing Research was established, it funded the first Center for Women's Health Research at the University of Washington.

Transitions in Women's Health Scholarship

The transition in thinking about women's health has been dramatic, given that early efforts to redefine women's health began to emerge in the 1960s and 1970s, an era punctuated by the Title X Family Planning Program, the landmark U.S. Supreme Court decision *Roe v. Wade* (U.S. Reports, 1973) protecting women's rights to choose whether or not to continue a pregnancy, and establishment of women's self-help clinics such as the Los Angeles Women's Feminist Women's Health Center and the Boston Women's Health Book Collective (Boston Women's Health Book Collective, 1974; Ruzek, 1978; Weissman, 1998).

Transitions in scholarly works about women's health have been apparent: Scholars have incorporated new frameworks for studying women and employed new methodologies and methods. Novel conceptualization of women's health put women at the center of inquiry, integrated feminist theory, incorporated theoretical models of health and illness specific to women, and emphasized the importance of context in studying health from a holistic perspective, incorporating consideration of person–environment relationships and social determinants of health. Integrating biological, psychosocial, and cultural dimensions of health and emphasizing life transitions as the focus of nursing scholarship represent significant transitions (Andrist & MacPherson, 2001; Taylor & Woods, 2001). Noteworthy was the attention given to the social context of women's lives that drew scholar's attention to the consideration of racism, sexism, classism, and heterosexism (Taylor, Olesen, Ruzek, & Clarke, 1977; Taylor & Woods, 1996).

Methodological considerations led to the development of science that would serve emancipatory ends: Scholars no longer relied solely on empiricist methodology, and the integration of interpretive, naturalistic methodologies as well as critical methodology marked a body of emergent scholarship in nursing in the 1980s. This work emphasized the development of knowledge for and with women instead of about women: New knowledge was seen as a tool of empowerment and liberation (Andrist & MacPherson, 2001). Changing methodologies prompted investigators to engage in reflexivity, considering the impact of their relationships with the women who participated in their studies, cocreating new knowledge. Investigators were encouraged to think of themselves as situated knowers whose positions influenced what they were able to see and know.

In 2000, a review of nursing research related to women's health revealed contributions in a variety of areas, including parenting, employment, caregiving, disparities in health experienced by lesbians, menstrual cycle, menopause, stress, fatigue, sleep, violence against women, and women's decision making related to their health (Taylor & Woods, 2001). These topics reflected everyday concerns of women, many of them neglected before the 1980s.

Over the past three decades there have been important transitions in the scholarship of women's health. Among these are a transition from topics that were sex or gender ignorant or that assumed male as the norm to research topics grounded in the understanding of the relationship of women's lives to their health. Central among society's assumptions regarding women is the inherent otherness of women; in this context, normal, positive physiological functions were seen as pathologic. For example, many menstrual cycle studies conducted before the 1980s were designed to detect the problems women experience because they menstruate (e.g., a hypothesized propensity for illness, violent crimes, or accidents). The new scholarship emphasized understanding menstruation as normative, seeking to learn from women about their lived experiences.

Federal Support for Women's Health Research

In 1985, the USPHS Task Force on Women's Health Issues published a two-volume report in which members recommended expanding biomedical and behavioral research that would include the study of conditions uniquely relevant to women across the life span, more prevalent among women than among men, or in which risk factors were different for women versus men, as well as treatment approaches that differed for women versus men (USPHS, 1985). In 1986, the NIH Advisory Committee on Women's Health recommended that investigators include women in research, especially in clinical trials; justify exclusion of women from research when appropriate; and evaluate gender differences in their findings. Because of a slow response to these recommendations, the Congressional Caucus for Women's Issues drafted the Women's Health Equity Act of 1990, which set in motion a series of events that included a Government Accounting Office study of expenditures of NIH funds on women's health research and the eventual establishment of the ORWH at the NIH in 1990. The ORWH was directed to ensure women's health issues were adequately addressed, especially those unique to women, including those for which risk factors differed from those for men, and approaches to care differed. The inclusion of women in clinical trials and the engagement of women as investigators in biomedical research were also part of the original mission (USPHS, 1992). In 1991, the landmark Women's Health Initiative Study was initiated, and Dr. Bernadine Healey, the first woman NIH director, was appointed.

In 1991, the ORWH convened a Task Force on Opportunities for Research on Women's Health that developed research recommendations focusing on women's health (USPHS, 1992). This volume included a life-span view of women's health, and panelists considered science as it intersected with topics such as reproductive biology, early developmental biology, aging processes, cardiovascular function and disease, malignancy, and immune function and infectious disease. A significant contribution of this agenda was the panelists' ability to transcend the boundaries of the disease-focused institutes of NIH and focus on both reproductive and nonreproductive health issues important to women. This agenda has since been updated for the 21st century (USPHS, 1999) and again in 2010 (USPHS, 2010).

The 1999 Agenda for Research on Women's Health, including seven volumes, reflected important efforts at promoting a new level of intellectual vigor in addressing women's health (see ORWH at http://orwh.od.nih.gov and USPHS, 1999). The 1999 agenda grew from an inclusive process in which women's health advocates as well as scientists participated in regional and national meetings and heard public testimony. Explicit consideration of various groups of women representing America's ethnic groups and those living with disabilities enriched the agenda-setting process. The final reports reflected the deliberations and recommendations from these hearings and assessed the current status of research on women's health. Gaps in knowledge, sex and gender differences that may influence women's health and factors that affect health of women from various populations were topics of discussion. Enhancing prevention, diagnosis, and treatment was an explicit focus of discussion, as was the development of strategies to improve the health status of women regardless of race/ethnicity, age, or other characteristics. In addition, career issues for women scientists were addressed in the report.

Research topics spanned a wide range of health issues. Among these were disorders and consequences of alcohol, tobacco, and other drug use; behavioral and social science aspects of women's health; bone and musculoskeletal disorders; cancer; cardiovascular diseases; digestive diseases; immunity and autoimmune diseases; infectious diseases and emerging infections; mental disorders; neuroscience; oral health; pharmacological issues; reproductive health; and urologic and kidney conditions. Chapters also address the use of sex and gender to define and characterize differences between men and women. A special consideration was research design for studies of women, addressing special populations of women, racial/ethnic and cultural diversity, and multidisciplinary perspectives. Although promising, the 1999 agenda gave little emphasis to the health consequences of poverty in women, the power differential between men and women that influences health, and the gendered allocation of work in U.S. society. Moreover, the global perspective needed to examine the consequences of economic development and social policy on women's health was missing (Woods, 2000).

One special initiative of the ORWH has been the development and funding of the Specialized Centers of Research (SCORs). This innovative interdisciplinary research program focuses on sex differences and major medical conditions affecting women. SCORs support research integrating basic, clinical, and translational research approaches to incorporating a sex and gender focus. Eleven SCOR awards are co-funded by ORWH and the National Institute on Aging, National Institute of Arthritis and Musculoskeletal and Skin Diseases, Eunice Kennedy Shriver National Institute of Child Health and Human Development, National Institute of Diabetes and Digestive and Kidney Diseases, National Institute on Drug Abuse, National Institute of Mental Health, and U.S. Food and Drug Administration (FDA). Some of the topics addressed by the SCORs include addiction and health, substance abuse relapse, fetal antecedents to sex differences in depression, irritable bowel syndrome and interstitial cystitis, pelvic floor disorders, molecular and epidemiological factors and urinary tract infections, gender-sensitive treatment for tobacco dependence, neurovisceral sciences and pain, sex differences in musculoskeletal disorders, intrauterine environment and polycystic ovary syndrome, vascular dysfunction, and cognitive decline (NIH, 2002).

The Building Interdisciplinary Research Careers in Women's Health (BIRCWH) is a mentored career development program that aims to increase the number of women's health and sex differences investigators. This program contributes to the development of future scientists in women's health and sex differences and is already revealing best practices in interdisciplinary mentoring for research careers (Domino, Bodurtha, Nagel, & Building Interdisciplinary Research Careers in Women's Health Directors, 2011; Guise, Regensteiner, & Building Interdisciplinary Research Careers in Women's Health Directors, 2012).

A 2001 IOM report *Exploring the Biological Contributions to Human Health: Does Sex Matter?* alerted scientists to the fact that biological sex differences were important, but often ignored in research, especially research using animals or cells/tissues. Nearly a decade later, Zucker and Beery (2010) reaffirmed the finding that consideration of sex difference in cellular and animal studies is not yet the norm. A recently issued NIH notice focuses on the consideration of sex as a biological variable in NIH-funded research, stipulating that sex as a biological variable will be factored into research designs, analyses, and reporting in vertebrate animal and human studies, to be effective in 2016 (USPHS, 2015).

The year 2010 was a watershed year for women's health research, marked by the publication of the ORWH report "Moving into the Future with New Dimensions and Strategies: A Vision for 2020 for Women's Health" (USPHS, 2010) and the IOM Report *Women's Health Research: Progress, Pitfalls, and Promise* (IOM, 2010). The updated ORWH research agenda included six new goals to address contemporary issues:

1. Increase sex differences research in basic sciences studies
2. Incorporate findings of sex and gender differences in the design and applications of new technologies, medical devices, and therapeutic drugs
3. Actualize personalized prevention, diagnostics, and therapeutics for girls and women
4. Create strategic alliances and partnerships to maximize the domestic and global impact of women's health research
5. Develop and implement new communication and social networking technologies to increase the understanding and appreciation of women's health and wellness research
6. Employ innovative strategies to build a well-trained, diverse, and vigorous women's health research workforce

In the same year, the IOM of the National Academy of Sciences (IOM, 2010) published the report *Women's Health Research: Progress, Pitfalls, and Promise*. The IOM committee was charged with "examining what research on women's health has revealed; how that research has been communicated to providers, women, the public, and others; and identify gaps in those areas" (p. 2). The committee was directed to identify examples of successful dissemination of findings, paying particular attention to how the communication influenced women's use of care and preventive services, and to make recommendations where appropriate.

The IOM committee focused on health conditions that were specific to women, more common or more serious in women, had distinct causes or manifestations in women, had different outcomes or treatments for women, or had high morbidity and/or mortality in women. Seven recommendations from the IOM committee included:

1. U.S. government agencies and other relevant organizations sustain/strengthen focus on women's health, including research spectrum of genetic, behavioral, and social determinants of health and change over lifetimes.

2. The NIH, the Agency for Healthcare Research and Quality, and the Centers for Disease Control and Prevention develop targeted initiatives to increase research on populations of women with highest risks and burdens of disease.

3. Research on women emphasizes promotion of wellness and quality of life; conditions that have high morbidity and affect quality of life; development of better measures or metrics to compare health condition effects, interventions, and treatments; end points to include quality of life outcomes (functional status or functionality, mobility, and pain) in addition to mortality.

4. Cross-institute initiatives in the NIH support research on common determinants and risk factors that underlie multiple diseases and on interventions to decrease the occurrence or progression of diseases in women—urge NIH ORWH and Office of Behavioral and Social Sciences Research collaboration.

5. Government and other funding agencies ensure adequate research participation by women, analysis of data by sex, and reporting of sex-stratified analyses.

6. Research emphasis should be on how to translate research findings into practice and public health policies rapidly and at practitioner and overall public health systems levels.

7. U.S. Department of Health and Human Services (DHHS) appoint a task force to develop evidence-based strategies to communicate and market to women health messages based on research results.

Both the ORWH and the IOM reports emphasized understanding the determinants of health, especially sex and gender differences, as well as life-span considerations. Compared with the ORWH report, the IOM report emphasized the importance of social and environmental determinants of health. The IOM committee commented on scientific progress in the understanding conditions affecting women, study of vulnerable groups of women, and use of appropriate research methods. Both reports emphasized the importance of accelerating the translation of research findings into practice and policy implications and communicating with women about their health.

The IOM committee (IOM, 2010) judged research on the following set of conditions to have made major progress: breast cancer, cervical cancer, and cardiovascular disease. Conditions that had some progress included depression, osteoporosis, and HIV/AIDS. Conditions judged to have little scientific progress included unintended pregnancy, maternal morbidity/mortality, autoimmune diseases, alcohol and drug addiction, lung cancer, gynecologic cancers other than cervical cancer, nonmalignant gynecologic disorders, and Alzheimer's disease.

Shaver, Olshansky, and Woods for the American Academy of Nursing Women's Health Expert Panel (2013) offered comments relative to both the 2010 ORWH Research Agenda and the IOM Report on Women's Health Research. Their recommendations included:

1. Expanding the development and testing of gender-sensitive interventions—this requires giving voice to women's experiences and perspectives, incorporating complexities and diversities of women's experiences, integrating reflexivity in research, and promoting empowerment and emancipation. Gender-sensitive interventions affirm gender equity by considering needs and preferences of genders and do not privilege the experiences of either gender. Gender-tailored or gender-specific interventions are designed for one gender based on differences and preferences (Im & Meleis, 2001). Women-specific interventions are grounded in the reality of women's lives, unique responsibilities, and biology as exemplified by the SUCCESS program for smoking cessation for pregnant women (Albrecht, Kelly-Thomas, Osbonre, & Ogbagaber, 2011; Li & Froelicher, 2010).

2. Attending to the intersectionality of gender with other health determinants—essential to the translation of research findings to services. Women simultaneously are Black, Hispanic, poor, heterosexual, and living with disabilities (Hankivsky et al., 2007; Kazanjian & Hankivsky, 2008).

3. Rebalancing emphasis on behavioral, integrative, and pharmacological therapeutics—requires emphasis on nonpharmacologic therapies such as lifestyle modification. The integration of biological aspects of appetite regulation and metabolism, as well as behavioral, social, psychological, physical environments of everyday living (such as oppressive social and built environments, in understanding obesity) exemplifies this rebalancing.

4. Increasing the study of underemphasized conditions disproportionately affecting women (e.g., functional or stress-related disorders). Examples include studies of osteoporosis and incontinence as they develop over the course of the life span.

5. Enhancing scientific attention to unintended pregnancies and sexually transmitted infections (STIs)—requires attention to the dynamics that promote unintended pregnancy as well as combined, multimodal interventions aimed at prevention, such as providing education about and access to contraceptives, slowing rates of sexual initiation, and enhancing condom use (Jemmott & Jemmott, 1992; Jemmott, Jemmott, Hutchinson, Cederbaum, & O'Leary, 2008; Jemmott, Jemmott, & O'Leary, 2007). Supporting women in coercive relationships to choose contraception and avoid unprotected sex is an important component (Teitelman, Tennille, Bohinski, Jemmott, & Jemmott, 2011).

6. Expanding investigations of prevention and treatment consequences of violence against women—includes study of life-span consequences of violence for girls and women as well as outcomes of military sexual trauma (MST) for women in the military (Yano et al., 2011). The interrelationship of STIs, violence, and unintended pregnancy is an important consideration.

7. Increasing studies of effective technologies and their use to support women as they age and in their caregiving roles—includes adapting communication technologies to detect health problems and provide real-time feedback of health information.

8. Accelerating testing of the models for translating research findings directly to the public—can include using communication technologies to convey health information to women and requiring investigators to develop communication and dissemination plans for their studies (Shaver et al., 2013).

Helpful research on women's health will not come about from pouring old wine in new bottles. Many have advocated for a reformulation of science, clear views of women's experiences through lenses ground by women. This could include qualitative methods of analysis that are reaching new levels of rigor and reproducibility. It could include the interpretation of biological uniqueness as a sign of health rather than deviance or illness. And reformulated science could include designing research *for* rather than *on* women, with liberating rather than oppressive results (Woods, 1992).

Simply adding a cohort of women to a study designed to illuminate issues grounded in thinking about men or increasing the proportion of women researchers in a male-dominated field will not solve the problem of advancing a more complete understanding of women's health. What is necessary is a reexamination of the nature of science that will foster a better understanding of the health of the many populations of women and serve emancipatory ends (Woods, 1992, p. 1).

Research Policy and Funding

As women's health research agendas for the nation have changed, so have policies to support new visions for women's health research. The NIH Revitalization Act of 1993 mandated that the NIH establish guidelines for including women and minorities in clinical research (NIH, 1994). Starting in 1995, all NIH-sponsored research had to comply with those guidelines, which mandated that women and minorities be included in the research; that cost could not preclude such inclusion; and that outreach, recruitment, and retention efforts would be supported (NIH Tracking/Inclusion Committee, 2002). The FDA also instituted a 1993 policy change regarding women: To gain FDA approval of pharmaceuticals, drug companies were required to include women in clinical trials, study gender differences in phase 3 (safety and efficacy) trials, and study gonadal hormone interactions with new drugs (Herz, 1997).

The peer-review process exerts at least an indirect influence on women's health research. The Center for Scientific Review of the NIH, which sets guidelines and policy for research review, now explicitly includes gender, ethnicity, and geographic distribution among its principles for reviewer selection (Center for Scientific Review, 2002).

Of note, the research efforts of the largest single group of health care professionals—nurses—were not organizationally included in the NIH until 1986, when the National Center for Nursing Research was established. One of the smallest of the institutes, the nursing center received some $144 million in the 2016 budget, compared with much larger budgets for institutes focusing on prevalent diseases in the United States (www.nih.gov).

Funding for training new investigators in women's health has been established by NIH's ORWH via the BIRCWH program, as well as for programs for nascent scientists among high school girls and women already established in biomedical careers but who encounter barriers that limit their advancement. In addition, the ORWH has funded SCORs described earlier. The picture for funding health care research relevant to women has improved, but careful observers should bear in mind the continued disproportion and not forget the abysmal baseline from which it started and that limits funding in an era of incremental budget increases.

Women are not the only group who may be coerced and/or mistreated in research studies, but they deserve special attention from prospective researchers in regard to issues of power and information. Sechrest (1975) was an early reporter on the coercion and power that can be applied to foster women's participation in research projects. She noted that early research on oral contraceptives took advantage of relatively uniformed and low-resource Puerto Rican women who had few options for avoiding pregnancy. Financial incentives or provision of free medical care for women and their children may also be irresistible elements in recruiting. Continuing examination of ethics related to women's health research is warranted.

■ SEX, GENDER, AND EDUCATION OF HEALTH PROFESSIONALS

Analyses of professional education materials, as well as influential advertising directed toward health professionals, demonstrate a history of continuing sex and gender bias. Early work revealed inaccurate information in medical texts concerning subjects such as the strength of women's sexual drives, the roles of the vagina and clitoris in orgasm, and the incidence and prevalence of female sexual dysfunction (Scully & Bart, 1973). One text portrayed women as inherently sick and asserted that the feminine core consisted of masochism, passivity, and narcissism. At the same time, the text advised physicians to counsel their women patients to simulate orgasms if they were not orgasmic with their husbands.

Naomi Wolf, in her 1997 book *Promiscuities* on sexual coming-of-age, provided the lecture we never had on the clitoris. Identified and well-described in 1559 by the Venetian scientist Renaldus Columbus, the clitoris was described by midwives, anatomists, and physicians through the 18th century (Wolf, 1997). But when sexual purity and ill health for women were popularized, and as the home and family were separated into their own private spheres in the 19th century, information on this sexual organ, along with cognizance of female sexual desire, was suppressed. Wolf argues that Freud was hardly the first authority to examine and misunderstand the clitoris, and she reminds readers that generations of social critics suggested that close attention to female anatomy and physiology could improve intimate relationships. The authors of *A New View of a Woman's Body* (Federation of Feminist Women's Health Centers, 1991) examined the basic research on the anatomy and physiology of the clitoris and have clarified the role of the clitoris as a vital sexual organ whose existence was omitted from medical texts. Illustrations of women's genitals in professional textbooks through the 1980s frequently excluded the clitoris.

Textbooks and advertisements aimed at gynecologists have reinforced the status and intellectual asymmetry between patients and doctors (Fisher, 1986). "By controlling women and their reproductive capacities," wrote Fisher, "medical domination functioned to sustain male domination" (p. 160). A newer generation of critic suggests that both texts and advertisements have moved away from portraying women as inferior and victim and instead are portraying women as invincible to illness and especially age, so long as they make the right choices about their behavior and the medical goods and services they purchase (Kaufert & Lock, 1997). "Health is the new virtue for women as they age.... [I]f she allows her body to deteriorate, then she becomes unworthy, undeserving of support" (Kaufert & Lock, 1997, p. 86). Being characterized as invincible is not much of an improvement over being characterized as a victim, when both stereotypes prevent development of health care providers and systems that respond to women's complex and various needs.

Progress in Health Professional Education

Some improvements in care for women have been brought about by national initiatives, such as the establishment of women's health offices in various federal agencies (USPHS, NIH, and FDA) and women's health services at the Veterans Administration (VA). Nonetheless, evidence suggests that the progress in enhancing health professionals' education in women's health and health care has been slow and incremental.

Efforts to change the capacity of the health care workforce to deliver comprehensive women's health care have attempted to reduce fragmentation in service delivery by assembling teams and creating structures such as Women's Health Centers to deliver care. In 1996, the USPHS funded the creation of CoEs in Women's Health at multiple sites in the United States. These had important missions that involved creating new models of care for women, educating health professionals in these models, supporting interdisciplinary clinical research, and mentoring. These are described in more detail in our discussion, Gender-Sensitive Health Care.

Essential to improving the capacity for delivering comprehensive women's health care is the education of health professionals in ways that expose students to:

- Curricula that include current knowledge about women's health based on research on sex and gender differences, among other topics
- Practitioner role models who exhibit sensitivity to and awareness of women's health issues
- Models of service delivery that are gender sensitive and comprehensive
- Organizations that reflect positive values about women and their contributions to the health professions as well as to the larger society
- Faculty with expertise in comprehensive women's health and health care and commitment to advancing

comprehensive care for women (Writing Group for the 1996 American Academy of Nursing Expert Panel on Women's Health Issues, 1997)

Slow integration of gender-specific information in professional curricula can be attributed to faculty's lack of awareness of scientific evidence, lesser value placed on this information, bloated curricula that already exceed reasonable amounts of content, and resistance to curricular change by those who struggle to maintain areas of knowledge they value more highly.

A recommended strategy for fostering health professions education about women's health and health care includes promoting faculty development in women's health; comprehensive health care for women through continuing professional education (including nursing, medicine, pharmacy, etc.) offers the opportunity to integrate updated scientific information, as exemplified in the DHHS Office on Women's Health (OWH) professional education materials. Another option is assessment of specific competencies of faculty and credentialing through specialty board examination in practice disciplines (e.g., nursing and medicine), which afford opportunity to evaluate what providers know. Certification by examination in areas of expertise, such as the North America Menopause Society Menopause Practitioner Examination is one example of a postgraduate certification of expertise (see www.menopause.org). Other strategies include use of interdisciplinary and interprofessional team teaching, introduction of standardized patients demonstrating complex women's health issues, and incorporation of comprehensive and current scientific resources through online libraries accessible across educational institutions and practice settings in which students are placed. Finally, creating and maintaining an audit of exemplary clinical practicum sites (e.g., the CoEs in Women's Health Care) provide a rich resource for educational programs.

Wood, Blehar, and Mauery (2011) urged efforts to "improve women's health and basic sex differences educational curricula for trainees and continuing education for practitioners for all members of today's new interdisciplinary health care teams" (p. 102) and specified the inclusion of nurses, nurse practitioners, physician assistants, dentists, health psychologists, dietitians, and physical therapists as well as physicians (p. 102). Because research is ultimately connected to the preparation of health professionals and in turn to the quality of care provided, the use of tax dollars to prioritize opportunities for research on sex differences and women's health, as well as cross-disciplinary research ensuring communication of findings to current and future health professionals, merits high priority.

The DHHS, Health Resources and Services Administration (HRSA), OWH report on Women's Health Curricula (2013) summarized the deliberations of expert panels on interprofessional education focusing on women's health curricula. Among the expert panel recommendations are those related to:

- Conceptual approaches to women's health content and key content areas for collaboration
- Assessment of institutional readiness for integrating women's health education

- Creation of collaborative opportunities in women's health
- Teaching of recommendations for interprofessional education in women's health

A proposed conceptual framework for Interprofessional Women's Health education is organized by three theoretical perspectives and five major content areas. The three theoretical perspectives include those related to the social determinants of health, life-span approach, and cultural considerations. Social determinants of health were identified as central in understanding health inequities, access to care, and environmental and social contexts shaping well-being. The Commission on the Social Determinants of Health (2008) from the World Health Organization (WHO) provided an elaboration of individual (race/ethnicity, socioeconomic status, and gender) and contextual (immediate surroundings, environmental conditions, workplace dangers, and larger cultural patterns, including gender norms) characteristics. Among these are gender inequality, access to care, and experiences related to poverty. Life-span approaches encourage consideration of a woman's current context, role, and life demands, as well as an appreciation for the cumulative experiences affecting her health from the pregnancy experiences of one's mother through one's old age. (Osteoporosis is not a disease of old age but one of cumulative bone health across the life course.) Cultural considerations, as defined in this report, include points of intersection of gender, race/ethnicity, nativity, sexual identity, and sexual orientation, among other characteristics. Intersectionality is a theoretical approach foundational to understanding the diversity of women's health experiences.

The five key content areas proposed for interprofessional curricula include role of the health professional, biological considerations, selected conditions, behavioral health, and wellness and prevention. Table 3.1 includes common content areas across the health professions identified by the HRSA panel.

This report also includes strategies for promoting collaboration across health professions and several teaching recommendations for interprofessional education in women's health.

The implementation of curricular recommendations, such as those in the DHHS/HRSA report on Women's Health Curricula (2013), focuses the challenges for faculty. Essential to this transformative effort will be faculty development efforts that infuse both theoretical perspectives of women's health and research findings about women's health and health care.

Susan Wood (Wood et al., 2011, p. 103) leaves us with some challenging questions:

- As access to health care coverage becomes more prevalent for women, "will health professionals have the capacity and skills to provide quality care?"
- With expanded comparative effectiveness research (and pragmatic trials as well as other innovative research approaches), "will knowledge about sex and gender differences with clinical relevance be translated into practice?"

TABLE 3.1	Common Content Areas in Women's Health Across the Health Professions
AREA	**SAMPLE TOPICS**
Role of the health professional	Ethics Knowledge of other health professions Gender in provider–patient communication Patient-centered decision making Interprofessional education
Biological considerations	Age Sex Genetics Hormonal influences Pharmacokinetics and pharmacodynamics
Selected conditions	Autoimmune disorders Cardiovascular disease Endocrine disorders Endometriosis Infectious disease, especially HIV Pregnancy and breastfeeding, especially medications taken during pregnancy and periodontal health in pregnancy Metabolic disorders Musculskeletal health Neurological conditions
Behavioral and mental health	Anxiety/stress Depression/bipolar disorders Domestic/intimate partner violence Eating behaviors/disorders Sexual behavior Substance abuse Traumatic experiences
Wellness and prevention	Access to care Environmental health Exercise physiology Hormonal transitions Nutrition Oral health Reproductive choice, family planning, and obstetrics Preventive health screening and immunizations Work–family balance

Adapted from U.S. Department of Health and Human Services, Health Resources and Services Administration, Office of Women's Health (2013, p. 14).

- How will new knowledge about women's health be mainstreamed throughout health professional curricula and continuing professional education?

Wood challenges us to think about the necessity of transforming curricula to promote comprehensive women's health care. The DHHS/HRSA report on Women's Health Curricula provides a starting point for future ventures in women's health professional education.

In addition to HRSA, the Office for Research on Women's Health at the NIH has funded Career Development awards, the BIRCWH that were created to promote fellowship training for medical residents and postdoctoral trainees in other disciplines. These programs have enlarged the capacity for preparing investigators for team science and were discussed earlier in this chapter (Domino et al., 2011; Guise et al., 2012).

HEALTH CARE FOR WOMEN: NEW MODELS

A notable shift in health care over the past few decades has been from a monopolistically physician-centered and traditionally authoritarian manner of delivering personal health services to a pluralistic array of clinicians, healers, and approaches to cure and care. Moving over time from word of mouth to the telephone book, and more recently the Internet, services as diverse as acupuncture and music therapy are entering the everyday consumer vocabulary. At the end of the 20th century, mainstream clinical groups were surprised and even shocked to learn that more visits are paid to alternative than to mainstream clinicians (Eisenberg et al., 1998). At the end of the 20th century, women used alternative therapies more than men (49% vs. 38%); higher income persons and those with college education were more likely to use alternative therapies, but the national use of at least one alternative treatment was 42%, a significant increase from 34% in 1990 (Eisenberg et al., 1999). An expansion in women's use of complementary and alternative health care resources was noted, especially in the wake of the findings from the Women's Health Initiative Study. Newton, Buist, Keenan, Anderson, and LaCroix (2002) surveyed women in the Group Health plan, learning that 76.1% used any of the therapies, 43.1% used stress management, 37.0% used over-the-counter alternative remedies, 31.6% used chiropractic, 29.5% used massage therapy, 22.9% used dietary soy, 10.4% used acupuncture, 9.4% used naturopathic or homeopathic therapies, and 4.6% used herbalists. Among women who used these therapies, 89% to 100% found them to be somewhat or very helpful (Newton et al., 2002).

The lure of 12-plus billion dollars in consumer buying power alone has been enough to bring window-dressing and even some fundamental change to health care service delivery. Although the evolution of some models of women's personal health care delivery has been the result of humanistic movements within some of the professions, women themselves have had a profound influence on the structure of personal health services. In some instances, such as the increasing use of midwives, traditional modes of health care, often culturally linked, have come into wider use (Paine, Dower, & O'Neil, 1999). In other instances, women have created new kinds of services, such as self-help clinics, caregiver support teams, and resource groups on the Internet. In some cases, professionals appropriated women's efforts, creating modified forms of personal health services that remain firmly under the control of professionals (e.g., the development and promotion of home-like birthing rooms in hospitals).

Health care settings such as self-help clinics arose from the women's health movement, which Marieskind (1975) described as a grass-roots organization dating from about 1970. Drawing parallels to the popular health movement of the mid-19th century, Marieskind saw modern interest in women's health linked to activism for political gains for women. Just as the popular health movement was associated with gaining the vote for women, the 20th century's women's health movement was linked to a progressive, feminist political and economic agenda (Leavitt, 1984). Ruzek (1978) and Marieskind (1975) reported some common features of women's health movement organizations: reduction in hierarchy, changes in the profit-making orientation, increased use of lay workers, involvement of clients in their own care, and commitment to a feminist ideology.

Morgen and Julier (1991) revisited a sample of organizations arising from the women's health movement to document development and change over the decades since the late 1960s. They mailed questionnaires to 144 women's health clinics, advocacy, and education organizations. The authors reported that a significant number of questionnaires were returned, indicating that the organization was no longer in existence (the actual number was not reported). Three quarters of the responding organizations described themselves as focused on prevention or self-care; two thirds identified themselves as ideologically feminist. Commitment to low-income and minority women was high: Most of the organizations served poor and minority women either in excess of or in direct proportion to the percentage of low-income and minority women in their communities. These characteristics conform to much of the original expressed intent of the women's health movement. In contrast to the organizational mission, the organizational structures have tended to change over the decades, from egalitarian staff models (e.g., in some women's health clinics, pay was equal for all workers) to more traditional ranking of workers and from consensus decision making to hierarchical authority. Staff hiring, training, and development continue to reflect feminist principles such as diversity and group solidarity. This study suggests that the women's health movement continues to influence the delivery of health services and that, not without struggle, alternatives to the health business-as-usual continue their work.

TOWARD GENDER-SENSITIVE HEALTH CARE

Women's health care has been described as a "patchwork quilt with gaps" (Clancy & Massion, 1992), reflecting the fragmentation of care that women have experienced and the lack of some health resources women need. Sadly that model remains prevalent in many health care systems. Nonetheless, many have pursued answers to the question: What could gender-sensitive health care look like? Leaders in women's health care have been exploring new models to deliver health care that would be informed by theoretical and conceptual advances related to sex and gender and health care reform efforts, in general. Critics of contemporary health care for women, as well as those concerned with improved health care for men, have advocated gender-sensitive health care. Recommendations to enhance gender sensitivity have emphasized understanding existing gender differences and incorporating these into services. Moreover, some advocates for holistic health care emphasize the importance of integration of the concept of intersectionality in health care, which warrants consideration of factors such as social class, ethnicity, and sexual orientation in addition to gender.

In a recent study of efforts to bring gender sensitivity into health care practice, Celik, Lagro-Janssen, Widdershoven, and Abma (2011) identified opportunities and barriers at the health professional, organizational, and national levels. For health professionals, barriers included gender-sensitive medical curricula and on-the-job training in work places. Opportunities and barriers at the organizational level related to organizational culture and infrastructure in which balance/imbalance between men and women health care professionals shape the consideration of gender with respect to the health professionals as well as patients. Protocols and guidelines used in organizations codify strategies for diagnoses and treatments but may not be based on gender-specific evidence. Finally, policy at organizational as well as national levels is influential in building a gender-sensitive health care system. Such considerations could include the incorporation of efforts to tailor care to local populations, reflecting the realities of everyday life. Celik et al. (2011) advocate mainstreaming gender in ways that reorganize, improve, develop, and evaluate policy in ways that support gender equality perspectives. They note that gender-sensitive health care will require changing systems and structures as well as enhancing the understanding and skills of health professionals.

Each of these efforts has the attendant risks of reproducing the gendered approaches to health care that reinforce gender stereotypes and biases. Gender-neutral or gender-ignorant care is not the goal, but the use of gender-specific theory is evolving to transform care in ways that do not privilege male versus female experiences but do promote gender equity (Im & Meleis, 2001). Gender-tailored or gender-specific interventions are those designed for one gender, reflecting gender as a major factor influencing health. Attention to gender in the scholarship guiding health care as well as the education of health professionals will remain critical in the delivery of gender-sensitive health care for women.

Centers of Excellence in Women's Health

In an effort to model excellence in women's health care, in 1996 the DHHS OWH established the first National Centers of Excellence in Women's Health. By 2009, 18 centers had been developed and designated as part of the national CoEs in Women's Health by the OWH of the DHHS. Seed money funded development of model clinical services for women. Core characteristics of the CoEs included comprehensive, women-friendly, women-focused, women-relevant, integrated multidisciplinary care (Milliken et al., 2001). These centers were envisioned as women-centered sites where primary care would be integrated with reproductive health care and prevention/screening efforts, welcoming to women, sources of health education and information and referrals,

and capable of delivering comprehensive care across the life span. Desirable features were highly visible women providers and staff, atmosphere and environment not threatening or inappropriate to women, and availability of information of particular interest to women. Some of the specific services provided included age-appropriate preventive health services and screening, family planning, gynecologic care, obstetrical care, and care for menopause, mental health issues, breast cancer, osteoporosis, and incontinence. Some centers were established as providing "one-stop shopping," meaning that all services were provided under a single roof/site, whereas others developed as centers without walls. Women's preferences supported both models; for example, some preferred the decentralized without-walls model, as it offered them more choice of providers and more privacy.

Some additional contributions of the CoEs included informational and referral, educational and referral, services of health professionals representing a variety of disciplines, but these are never fully described nor are their contributions to care (Milliken et al., 2001). Some centers contributed culturally appropriate patient education materials and resources in multiple languages to promote informed decision making. CoEs intended to offer flexible scheduling to accommodate multiple demands in women's lives (e.g., as family caregivers, employed workers) and incorporated expanded hours of operation, community-based sites, transportation assistance, and translation services.

Centers were "sold" to academic health centers based on their ability to develop downstream revenues, serving as magnets for women and their families as patients. Much less attractive to these academic health centers were the transformative approach to care and contributions to the educational mission of the institutions. Although many examples are offered of contributions to medical education, there is no mention of the education of the other health professions associated with CoEs (Fife, 2003).

Unique aspects of these CoEs were the integration of research, education, and clinical care in the centers and provision of care for a more diverse population than those receiving care at other women's health centers across the nation (Weisman et al., 1995, 2000). Indeed, the populations cared for by the CoEs included a larger proportion of women of color and more postreproductive age women than in comparison sites (Killien et al., 2000; Mazure, Espeland, Douglas, Champion, & Killien, 2000; Weisman & Squires, 2000). Although the translation of research to care is implied in many of the reports of the CoEs, this terminology was not characteristic.

The CoEs included outreach efforts in their development and found that among the most successful were those that involved existing community groups committed to women's health in their planning (Fife et al., 2001). Among their efforts were partnering with other community groups dedicated to women's health, participation in existing grass-roots efforts within the community, and CoE-initiated efforts. Elements of educational and health care were involved in most efforts. Some examples of community groups were state departments of health, local Native American organizations, minority health coalitions, groups addressing domestic violence, and health alliances.

Grass-roots community programs include city and county health department's efforts to work with women's groups/populations, and CoE-initiated programs developed programs that could be delivered to community groups, such as smoking cessation, sponsorship of a day-long conference on women's health, educational materials for teens, and collaborative mobile breast cancer screening programs with a fully equipped outreach Care-a-Van staffed with bilingual volunteers. Partnership with the YWCA, malls, churches, community centers, domestic violence shelters, food banks, retirement communities and nursing homes, non-English speaking communities, housing assistance/homeless shelters, and community events represented some of multiple efforts to bring health information and screening to communities (Fife et al., 2001).

In addition, the CoEs were committed to incorporating the needs of racial/ethnic minority populations into newer care paradigms (Jackson et al., 2001). Jackson et al. (2001) pointed out that an ideal model of health care for women of color would consider providers of care, content and process of care, and the health care system in which the model operates. They point out that care providers should reflect the diversity of the populations they serve. Absent that diversity, providers need knowledge, attitudes and skills to provide culturally appropriate care to all women, especially underrepresented ethnic groups. As members of multidisciplinary teams (they name the many health disciplines needed), health professionals together collaborate to address complicated social and health care needs of women of color. Content and process of care for women of color should reflect the higher burden of illness, poorer health outcomes, and greater prevalence of risk factors for chronic diseases than other women experience. Life-span approaches for women from adolescence to old age and the integration of prevention, primary care, chronic disease care, reproductive health, and complex psychosocial issues and mental health are needed. Some of the unique services needed include comprehensive risk assessment, community outreach, case management (vs. care or resource management), interpreter services, and health education. Case managers were recommended to bridge women of color and health care institutions and links to community resources. Strategies that include providing transportation, locating facilities in nontraditional settings, and extending operating hours stretch the typical use of resources in academic health centers. Commitment to diversity and social justice will be tested by institutions that take this mission seriously. Creative partnerships with institutions in the community in which the center is located are essential to serving specific populations of women whose vulnerability makes their access to care especially challenging. Some of the centers offered courses focusing on health topics for African American or Hispanic women, and others offered classes to medical students, staff, graduate students in nursing, university employees, and to community volunteers.

Some of the challenges to these centers in academic health centers included the marginalization of faculty who practiced in the centers: because of requirements of practice panel size and hours available in the clinical setting, many providers in these settings were not those in senior academic appointments who were also teaching students and leading research efforts. The metrics for evaluating productivity also pressed providers, and given the practice patterns of women providers who often are sought out by patients for their ability to communicate about their concerns, providers were at risk of being penalized for "lack of productivity." The publications of the CoEs use the cover term *medicine* as they describe the centers and their contributions, obscuring the roles of other health professions in the development of these centers. Consequently, it is impossible to evaluate the impact of all health care professions and their contributions, nor is it possible to track interprofessional practice and education in these centers. Sadly, these centers did not foresee the integration of advanced practice nurses into the mix of providers that is needed to care adequately for women.

The CoEs represented a new model for women's health care in academic health centers that united women's health research, teaching, clinical care, public education and outreach, and career advancement for women in the health sciences (largely focused on medicine vs. other health professions). Based on their first 3 years of experience, Gwinner, Strauss, Milliken, and Donoghue (2000) suggested that this model required transformation from the fragmented set of activities in academic health centers to an integrated system focused around the goal of advancing women's health. Institutional commitment, dedicated professionals, and ability to build on existing resources and bring added value to their institutions were important components.

In an effort to determine whether these new CoEs were truly making different contributions to women's health care, Weisman and Squires (2000) compared the first 12 national CoEs in Women's Heath designated by the DHHS OWH with 56 hospital-based primary care women's health centers that had been identified in the only source of nationally representative data on primary care women's health centers (the 1994 National Survey of Women's Health Centers). Although their analyses revealed similarities of some organizational and clinical attributes of the hospital-based programs that preceded the CoEs, the CoEs demonstrated integration of clinical services with research and medical training in women's health and delivery of services to a more diverse population of women.

In addition to providing some unique features for women, the CoE staff also contributed to the evaluation of health care provided in the centers. Anderson et al. (2001) conducted a qualitative analysis of women's satisfaction with primary care using a panel of focus groups in the National CoE in Women's Health program. Seeking patients' perspectives in an effort to evaluate women's satisfaction with primary care delivered in the CoEs, focus groups of ethnically diverse women ($N = 137$) were conducted nationwide on women's experiences and attributes of health care that they valued. Women revealed holistic concepts of their health, including physical, mental, and emotional dimensions. Women's general view on their health care spanned general, psychological/mental health, social support, roles, reproductive health, childbirth, alternative medicine, and prevention. Dimensions of primary health care important to women included access, office staff service and courtesy, privacy and respect, empathy and empowerment by health care providers, provider skills, care coordination, and environment. Examples of these are given in Table 3.2.

The outcomes led to the creation of a woman-focused health care satisfaction instrument to be used to assess and improve health care delivery (Anderson et al., 2001, 2007; Scholle et al., 2000; Scholle, Weisman, Anderson, & Camacho, 2004). The Primary Care Satisfaction Survey for Women (PCSSW; Scholle et al., 2004) included three dimensions: communication, administration and office procedures (processes), and comprehensiveness. Communication included items such as the professionals' ability to explain things clearly, answer questions in sensitive and caring ways, and take what women said seriously. Care processes (labeled administrative and office procedures) included courtesy of staff, flexible scheduling, provision of privacy, and offers of chances to talk to professionals while dressed (clothes on). Comprehensiveness included items related to care over the previous 12 months, including professional knowledge of women's health issues, interest in mental and emotional health of the woman, health care fitting life stage, and chances to get gynecologic and general health care. The complete scale with individual items is included in Scholle et al. (2004, Table 5, p. 44).

Evaluation of the quality of primary care services provided in 15 of the National CoEs in Women's Health in 2001 incorporated self-reported clinical preventive services and patient satisfaction as indicators of quality of care. Data from more than 3,000 women served by CoE programs were surveyed and compared with quality of care benchmarks from national and local community surveys, including the 1998 Commonwealth Fund Survey of Women's Health, a community sample of women living with a geographical catchment area for three CoEs, and a sample of more than 70,000 women from the 1999 Consumer Assessment of Health Plans Study of commercial managed care plans.

Women in the CoEs were more satisfied with their care and had received more screening tests and counseling services than those in the benchmark studies. The largest effects of CoEs among primary care services were for physical breast examination, mammogram for women 50 and older, and counseling for smoking, domestic violence, and STIs (Anderson et al., 2002).

The evaluation of women's satisfaction with their ongoing primary health care services engaged 1,021 women attending primary care visits with at least one prior visit to the sites (Michigan, Pittsburgh, and Wake Forest) before and immediately after visits. Women were asked about their satisfaction with their visit and health care over the past 12 months. Women's general health, site continuity, and fulfillment of their expectations for care were linked to global ratings of satisfaction through effects on communication, care coordination, and office staff and administration. Care coordination and continuity mediated ratings of care over the past year but day-of-visit ratings were mediated by communication.

The success of these comprehensive clinical programs rested with the support of the leaders of the academic health centers who understood the importance of multidisciplinary programs to the clinical care of women and the education they provided to future providers of women's health care (Milliken et al., 2001). An inquiry to HRSA regarding the CoEs indicated that the OWH no longer certified the centers.

Gender-Sensitive Care in the Veterans Health Administration

Efforts in the U.S. Veterans Health Administration, the largest integrated health care system in the country, have increasingly focused on delivery of gender-sensitive comprehensive primary care to women veterans. Implementation of the Patient Aligned Care Team (PACT)

TABLE 3.2	Dimensions of Primary Health Care Important to Women Receiving Care at National Centers of Excellence in Women's Health Care
DIMENSIONS	**EXAMPLES**
Access	Importance of barriers and supports to using the health care system, e.g., health insurance, understanding how system works
Office staff	Service and courtesy of staff, including receptionist and clerks
Privacy	Respect reflected by securing information and records, privacy when disclosing sensitive information, not feeling "diminished" during examination
Empathy and empowerment	Health care provider skills including awareness and acknowledgement of patients, sensitivity caring attitude, courtesy, communication skills, comfort level and patient trust
Provider skills	Technical skills including knowledge, training, experience
Care coordination	Follow-up, including test results and referrals
Environment	Environment including waiting room, exam room, privacy, gowns provided, room temperature, seating décor, music

Source: Anderson et al. (2001).

initiative to deliver primary care to veterans supports efforts to improve access, continuity, coordination, and comprehensiveness of care that is driven by patients and patient-centered. In a recent examination of how the PACT initiative influences ability to meet the needs of special populations, in particular women veterans, Yano, Haskell, and Hayes (2014) explored challenges for women veterans in obtaining health care and efforts by the VA to provide comprehensive primary care for women. PACT services to provide comprehensive primary care for women veterans is designed to be patient centered, accessible, continuous, coordinating, and delivered in the setting of team-based care. Gender-sensitive comprehensive primary care for women veterans includes providing complete primary care and care coordination by a single primary care provider at one site in a longitudinal relationship to fulfill all primary care needs, including care for acute and chronic illnesses, gender-specific primary care, preventive services, mental health services (e.g., for depression), and coordination of care. Three approved comprehensive primary care clinic models for women veterans have been identified, including:

Model 1: general primary care clinic with one or more designated women's health providers colocated mental health care, efficient referral to specialty gynecology care

Model 2: designated women's health care providers deliver primary care in separate but shared space with readily available or colocated gynecologic and mental health care

Model 3: women's health center with separate, exclusive-use space with a separate entrance, comprising designated women's health providers, with colocated specialty gynecologic, mental health and social work services, and other sub-specialty services (e.g., breast care) in the same location

These three models are being implemented with varying degrees of completeness.

The availability of designated women's health care providers proficient and interested in providing primary care for women veterans in all VA primary care clinics and comprehensive planning for women's health to increase women veterans' quality of care are also included in the expectations for gender-sensitive comprehensive primary care for women veterans. In addition, ensuring safety, dignity, sensitivity to gender-specific needs through ensuring privacy and respecting security needs constitutes an important part of the environment. Using state-of-the-art health care equipment and technology (e.g., for breast imaging and osteoporosis screening) is another expectation, as is the availability of women chaperones for gender-specific exams. Despite these policy changes, challenges remain for women in accessing team care in women's clinics, and designated women's health providers, privacy arrangements, and female chaperones are not universally available. Nonetheless, the VA effort to specify definitions and expectations of gender-sensitive comprehensive primary care for women veterans is a significant contribution to advancing women's health care.

An expert panel of clinicians and social scientists with expertise in women's health, primary care, and mental health rated the importance of tailoring more than 100 aspects of care derived from the IOM definition of comprehensive care and sex-sensitive (gender-sensitive) care as a guide to what aspects of care should be tailored to women veterans (deKleijn, Lagro-Janssen, Canelo, & Yano, 2015). The panel rated more than half of the aspects of care as very to extremely important to tailor to women veterans. Fourteen priority recommendations focused on the importance of design and delivery of services sensitive to trauma histories, adapting to women's preferences and information needs, and sex (gender) awareness and cultural transformation in each aspect of VA operations. Several domains of gender-sensitive comprehensive care were outlined from the first contact, subsequent care, coordination of referrals, health care workforce orientation and training, quality-improvement activities and capacity, gender-specific care (e.g., female reproductive health), gender awareness (clinical understanding and systems of care features), and gender sensitivity. Of note were the definitions guiding these domains, in particular:

Gender awareness—clinical understanding and system of care features ensuring achievement of competencies and processes related to guideline-concordant care for women as well as attention to conditions that are more prevalent in women, present differently, and should be managed differently than those of men

Gender sensitivity—attributes of care reflecting relational and other preferences (e.g., communication style, same-gender clinician, and privacy/safety needs)

Gender-specific care—female reproductive health care (e.g., menopause care and breast and cervical cancer screening)

Consideration of these elements gave priority to delivering reproductive health services tailored to the needs of women veterans, especially gender-specific examinations and management of pelvic and abdominal pain experienced by women with trauma histories; ensuring privacy, safety, dignity, and security of the health care environments; increasing tailoring of care for posttraumatic stress disorder (PTSD), MST, and other forms of sexual violence; tailoring mental health care delivery (e.g., depression and anxiety); implementing employee orientation, training, and education on gender-sensitive comprehensive care; tailoring assessments and screening practices (e.g., breast and cervical cancer and MST screening); tailoring behavioral health interventions (e.g., smoking cessation and addiction treatment); and increasing gender awareness and sensitivity of all VA employees as well as other veterans. In addition, other priorities included retaining women veterans in care by ensuring that continuity of care is with their preferred provider; ensuring practice guidelines, electronic record reminders, and templates are reflective of gender; promoting the use of tailored information letters and adapting the website and call centers to reflect women veterans' preferences and information needs; enhancing marketing and education initiatives to promote the awareness of gender-sensitive comprehensive care in VA settings; tailoring debriefing sessions during military discharge processes to consider women's information and clinical care needs; and tailoring care coordination and navigation between VA and non-VA care (deKleijn et al., 2015).

Despite national efforts to improve women's health services within the Veterans Health Administration, women veterans still underutilize VA health care. A recent assessment indicated that nearly 20% had delayed health care or an unmet need, with younger women experiencing more difficulty in accessing care. Of those who delayed or did not get health care, barriers included unaffordable health care, inability to take time off from work, and transportation difficulties. In addition, being uninsured, not knowing about VA care, having perceptions that VA providers were not gender-sensitive, and having a history of MST predicted delaying or not seeking care (Washington, Bean-Mayberry, Riopelle, & Yano, 2011; Washington, Bean-Mayberry, Mitchell, Riopelle, & Yano, 2011). Military service era was influential in women's health care delivery preferences, with Vietnam era to present veterans using more women's health and mental health care and World War II– and Korean War–era women veterans using more specialty care. Operation Enduring Freedom (OEF), Operation Iraqi Freedom (OIF), and Operation New Dawn (OND) veterans made more health care visits than women of earlier military eras. Health care delivery concerns include location convenience for Vietnam and earlier veterans and cost for the first Gulf War and OEF/OIF/OND veterans. Women of all military service eras rated colocation of gynecology with general health care as important. Ensuring access to specialty services close to home for veterans and access to mental health care reinforce the needs for the integration and coordination of primary care, reproductive health, and mental health care and for the provision of care close to where veterans live (Washington, Bean-Mayberry, Hamilton, Cordasco, & Yano, 2013). The VA recommends designated providers for women in primary care clinics or women's health centers as optimal models for women's primary care. Health care ratings obtained from VA users in a National Survey of Women Veterans indicated that gender-related satisfaction, gender appropriateness of care, and perceptions of VA provider skills were greater in sites adopting these changes. Establishing these optimal care models at sites around the nation is recommended to improve women veterans' experiences with VA care (Washington, Bean-Mayberry, Riopelle, & Yano, 2011). Indeed, the VA roadmap for delivering gender-sensitive comprehensive care for women may serve well as a model for civilian health care settings.

The VA model of care is one that initiated with concerns about veteran health and integrated PACT as an approach to primary care. Gender was not at the center of this model initially but was integrated into the care model while retaining the special concerns about veterans' health. This model exemplifies some elements of intersectionality as discussed by Hankivsky (2012) who alerts us to the possibility of creating additional inequities when using gender as the central point of consideration of health inequities. The importance of considering gender-based inequities as inseparable from other dimensions of womens' places in the social structure (e.g., class, race/ethnicity, sexual orientation, immigration, and ability) will be important for further development of gender-sensitive models of health care. As Havkinsky points out, although gender may be a logical starting place for such considerations, centering sex and gender may prevent or limit the opportunities to learn about other factors affecting life chances, opportunities, and health. Continuing to ask whether gender is the most salient factor as one analyzes the needs and issues of populations will be foundational to identifying important implications of intersectionality. Systematically adopting and applying intersectionality—as Hankivsky (2012) defines it, a "framework for improving understandings of and responses to the complexities of people's lives and experiences"—are a worthy aspirational goals for those envisioning models of gender-sensitive health care.

When both the CoEs and the VA women's health centers were evaluated using comparable key informant surveys, all served urban areas and most had academic partnerships. DHHS CoEs had three times the average caseload as VA centers. Preventive cancer screening and general reproductive services were available at all centers, but DHHS centers offered extensive reproductive services on-site more frequently and VA centers had on-site mental health care more frequently. Although these centers share similar missions and have comparable organization, education, and clinical services, they offered on-site services that differed in relation to the needs of their respective populations (Bean-Mayberry et al., 2007).

Integration of Sexual and Reproductive Health Into Primary Care

Another noteworthy effort has been the proposed integration of SRH care into primary care. A continuing challenge for women accessing comprehensive services has been the fragmentation of SRH—and men face similar challenges (Berg, Taylor, & Woods, 2013; Berg, Shaver, Olshansky, Woods, & Taylor, 2014). In the United States, SRH services are not integrated within a primary health care system of public health and primary care services. Moreover, U.S. national health goals to reduce unintended pregnancies and STIs have not been achieved (U.S. DHHS *Healthy People 2010*, 2000). Two models that could facilitate a coordinated system of sexual and reproductive services within a public and private primary care system in the United States are the WHO (2011) model of SRH services, including standards and provider competencies, and the United Kingdom (UK) model of community SRH standards and clinical competencies within the Royal College of Nursing (2009).

The WHO view of SRH extends beyond maternal–child health care and includes the reproductive health of women and men throughout their life cycles, as well as adolescents. SRH encompasses periods before and beyond reproductive years and is closely associated with sociocultural factors, gender roles, health equity, and respect and protection of human rights. SRH services are envisioned as delivered as a collection of integrated services addressing the full range of SRH needs and must be a part of the existing health care system, coordinating with public health and primary health care and reflecting human rights. WHO recommended a set of core competencies to achieve universal access to integrated SRH within a primary health care system. These are regarded as a minimum package of SRH care all should be able to access regardless of social, physical, and mental status; sex; age; religion; and country.

Thirteen competencies are grouped into four domains:

Domain 1—fundamental basis of competencies builds on SRH provider's knowledge of ethics, human rights; knowledge, behaviors, and attitudes for providing high-quality SRH care include ethical/technical foundation for SRH delivery; considerations of human rights, social values of equity, solidarity and social participation

Doman 2—leadership and management competencies—enabling others and effectively managing primary health care teams to provide quality SRH services

Domain 3—general SRH competencies for health providers—community, health education, counseling, assessment, referral

Domain 4—clinical competencies for SRH provision, including high-quality family planning care; spacing pregnancies; infertility problems; STI and reproductive tract infection (RTI) care; screening/treatment referral for RTIs; comprehensive abortion care; antenatal care; intrapartum care; postnatal care for women/neonates

The UK model is a coordinated system of SRH education, training, and certification for RNs, nurses with advanced training, nurse practitioners, midwives, and nonspecialist physicians working in the National Health Service. Competency-based education, training, and certification in ten areas have been developed and are foundational to this practice. Among these are:

1. Basic SRH services/skill, such as assessment by history and physical exam; problem assessment, risk assessment, and triage; effective communication across cultures, gender, life span, and sexual health; knowledge of basic counseling techniques; empowerment of individuals to make informed decisions; coordination/follow-up/referral; time management; urogynecology lab/specimen preparation; pregnancy testing and counseling; sexual/physical violence prevention

2. Contraception, including knowledge of methods of fertility control and family planning for men and women across the life span, people with disabilities, women after abortion, and difficult-to-reach groups; communication of, patient decision making regarding, and provision and management of fertility control and contraceptive choices; counseling for and management of complex medical/social needs related to contraception and contraceptive requirements and complications resulting from contraceptive failure

3. Unplanned pregnancy care/abortion, including pregnancy diagnostics, pregnancy options counseling and coordination, preabortion and postabortion care for early and later term abortion, medication abortion provision, and aspiration abortion provision by uterine aspiration procedures

4. Women's health/gynecology, such as diagnosis and management of common gynecologic problems; menstrual function/disorders across the life span and basic gynecologic ultrasound exams; managing simple pediatric/adolescent gynecology disorders (e.g., menstrual disorders, fibroids, amenorrhea, nonmenstrual bleeding, congenital abnormalities of the genital tract, and puberty)

5. Assessment of and comanagement of specialty gynecologic problems, such as subfertility problems, infertility diagnostics, gynecologic oncology problems, urogynecology and pelvic floor problems

6. Pregnancy, including diagnosis and management of early pregnancy care and referral, comprehensive antenatal care, labor and delivery/intrapartum care, diagnosis and management of postpartum care and problems for women and or neonates

7. Genitourinary conditions in men (GUM) including assessment, counseling, referral, coordination of care; performing, collecting, interpreting lab tests; diagnosing/managing GUM, including noncomplicated STIs/RTIs, balanitis/urethritis, infertility, and life-span issues

8. Sexual health promotion, including sexual and self-health promotion for women and men; assessing sexual problems with sexual history taking/diagnostics; assessing, managing or referring for sexual assault testing

9. Public health, ethics, and legal competencies, including knowledge of laws regarding family planning, abortion, HIV, violence against women and sexual violence, sex work, and sexuality (sexual orientation and gender identity); health care providers' legal/ethical obligations; element of SRH services and national guidelines, and economic impact and cost of health care options/treatments/prevention

10. Leadership, management, and information technology (IT)/audit competencies, including enabling others or effectively managing teams providing SRH services; knowing national and local SRH policies, standards, and protocols; improving SRH program implementation through evidence and use of technology (Faculty in Sexual and Reproductive Health, 2012; Royal College of Nursing, 2009)

These models of gender-sensitive care attempt to address the need for comprehensive, coordinated, integrated services for women, providing an alternative to the fragmentation of SRH care and primary care or primary health care services. Cappiello and Nothnagle (2013) advocate for a vision in which all women and men in the United States receive high-quality, evidence-based sexual and reproductive care through policy changes that make interprofessional education and training on SRH a priority at federal and state levels (Nothnagle, Cappielllo, & Taylor, 2013).

Gender-Sensitive Counseling and Therapy Models for Women

Another important contribution to women's health care has been the development of mental health counseling and psychotherapy models tailored to women. One form of gender-sensitive health care is relational-cultural therapy (RCT), a form of therapy developed by Jean Baker Miller and her colleagues that recognized and emphasized the central role of relationships as being growth fostering. Several decades ago, in the 1970s, a group of feminist women therapists came together to discuss new ways of understanding psychological growth. The initial group of women consisted of Jean Baker Miller, Irene Stiver, Judith Jordan, Janet Surrey, and Alexandra Kaplan. Miller wrote a groundbreaking book in 1976 with a second edition published in 1986, titled *Toward a New Psychology of Women* (Miller, 1986). This now classic book provides the basic concepts of relational-cultural theory, which is the foundation for RCT. This section of this chapter describes the basic concepts of RCT, followed by a description of the RCT approach that incorporates these basic concepts.

Concepts of Relational-Cultural Theory

At the Stone Center at Wellesley College, a group of women and others studied prevailing theories of psychological development and recognized that these prevailing theories did not explain much of women's experiences (Gilligan, 1982; Gilligan, Rogers, & Tolman, 1991a, 1991b; Jordan, 1997; Jordan, Kaplan, Miller, Stiver, & Surrey, 1991; Miller & Stiver, 1997). The prevailing psychological theories emphasized the importance of separation and individuation as one attains autonomy, which reflects psychological health. Although the scholars at the Stone Center recognized and embraced the importance of a person having agency and a sense of self, they also strongly believed in the need for healthy relationships in order for a person to grow in a psychologically healthy way.

This new approach to understanding women's psychological development was initially referred to as *self-in-relation* theory because it seemed to adequately reflect the notion that individuals develop in relationship to others in their lives. Over time, however, as these feminist scholars continued to study and to learn from one another, they rejected the term *self* and instead shifted their emphasis to relationships and incorporated cultural diversity in an effort to move beyond only the experiences of middle-class White women (who composed this initial group of scholars). They modified how they labeled their theory and began to refer to it as *relational-cultural* theory. Perspectives from women of color, from lesbian women, and from men were actively integrated into the developing theory (Bergman & Surrey, 1997; Coll, Cook-Nobles, & Surrey, 1997; Eldridge, Mencher, & Slater 1997; Rosen, 1997; Tatum, 1997; Turner, 1997; Walker & Rosen, 2004). This approach does not reject the notion of individuation, but it moderates such separateness with connectedness, contributing to a more complex and insightful understanding of adult development, both male and female. "In short, the goal is not for the individual to grow out of relationships, but to grow into them. As the relationships grow, so grows the individual" (Miller & Stiver, 1997, p. 22).

Of great significance is that relational-cultural theory embraces the social context or social determinants of health in recognizing factors that affect psychological growth. The presence of racism, poverty, and lack of access to health care are all examples of social determinants of health that must be understood and addressed in order to foster psychological growth. More recently, scholars at the Stone Center have incorporated current understanding of brain science into relational-cultural theory and RCT. Amy Banks (2006) has written about how neurobiological aspects contribute to interpersonal connections.

Several key factors compose relational-cultural theory. These factors are not mutually exclusive. It is important that they are understood from a holistic perspective in which each factor influences and is influenced by the others.

MUTUALITY

Mutuality refers to the notion of persons experiencing situations together in a simultaneous way. It is important to note that no two persons experience situations in exactly the same way; the key point in mutuality is that experiences do not occur in isolation. Instead, mutuality is characterized by a situation in which two or more persons experience something together, allowing them to share with one another their individual experiences. In this way, each person can better understand the experiences of the others.

AUTHENTICITY

Authenticity is a key concept of healthy relationships and actually reflects the notion that healthy individuals do need a strong sense of self (thus not totally negating the concept of individuation). This concept goes further than simply knowing oneself and having a sense of oneself. Authenticity includes a comfort level in which a person feels safe to share one's authentic, genuine self with others in the relationship.

RECIPROCITY

Similar to mutuality, *reciprocity* refers to a sense of experiencing something together. Different from mutuality, reciprocity emphasizes and highlights the back-and-forth nature of a relationship as opposed to the simultaneity. Similar to mutuality, reciprocity emphasizes the importance of individuals within relationships working together, leading to the understanding of one another as they share back and forth.

EMPATHY

Sharing experiences together and being able to feel what another feels (of course, recognizing that one can never absolutely feel what another is feeling) are key to empathy. *Empathy* describes the process of another person having a sense of sharing experiences of others and being able to express this sense by communicating with and relating to the other person.

CONNECTEDNESS

Connectedness is actually what happens as a result of healthy, growth-fostering relationships. Healthy individuals do not live and function in isolation from others, but instead involve a sense of being a part of another person, whether that be sharing certain ideas and values or sharing certain feelings. Belenky, Clinchy, Goldberger, and Tarule (1997) emphasized connectedness in relation to ways of knowing, with direct reference to women and how women come to know and make meaning of phenomena in their lives. Knowing, making meaning, and developing healthy psychological selves occur within the context of connected relationships with others.

Jean Baker Miller and her colleagues not only developed what they believed were key concepts that defined healthy relationships, but they also identified what occurs as a result of healthy relationships. These results are referred to as the "five good things" and are as follows: (a) zest or well-being, (b) ability and motivation to take action, (c) increased knowledge of self and others, (d) increased sense of worth, and (e) a desire for more connection beyond the current one.

Zest is a sense of well-being that comes from being in a healthy relationship. Both persons in the relationship experience a feeling of energy and passion and feeling that there is a purpose in one's life.

Ability and motivation to take action is the sense of wanting to make constructive changes and having purpose in life. There is a feeling that one can, indeed, be effective in making such constructive changes.

Increased knowledge of self and others refers to the ability to be self-reflective and to also understand the other, to empathize with the other person in the relationship. Such increased knowledge allows for creating and maintaining authenticity within a relationship.

Increased sense of self-worth is a feeling of being worthwhile, of having a place and voice in the world. It is similar to what might be termed in traditional psychology as *increased self-esteem*. It allows one to feel motivated to take action and be able to do so because it is a sense that one does have the wherewithal to be an active member of a group, a community, and a society.

A *desire for more connection* reflects one's continuing desire for ongoing relationships, particularly recognizing the growth-fostering capacity that comes from healthy human connection. This ongoing desire allows greater connection and continuing growth.

RELATIONAL-CULTURAL THERAPY

Judith Jordan aptly describes the guiding foundation, based in relational-cultural theory, for doing RCT. She states that relational-cultural therapists focus on decreasing isolation, increasing one's capacity for self-empathy as well as empathy for others, and appreciating the importance of context and limiting cultural/relational images. Jordan emphasizes that this approach to therapy is guided by an attitude and quality of mutual engagement rather than on any specific intervention techniques (Jordan, 2010).

The relational-cultural therapist works within connections and disconnections. This means that the therapist herself must be aware of any disconnection she is feeling and must stay present in connection with the patient. The relational-cultural therapist also works with empathy. In this case, the therapist must be self-reflective about his or her own feelings that are being aroused in the therapeutic situation. The patient must be aware of the therapist's genuine empathic response(s). This is an example of how a therapeutic relationship, which in many ways is a microcosm of all relationships, is growth fostering for both the patient and the therapist. The therapist also works with relational images. In this case, both the therapist and the patient work together through mutual empathy to deconstruct past relational images that are painful and that limit healthy psychological growth. It is important that the therapist be responsive to the patient in an authentic way, which in turn encourages the patient to feel comfortable and safe to present her authentic self to the therapist. In being responsive, the therapist does not put forth an image of being the authority figure but rather creates a context in the therapeutic relationship in which the therapist is truly authentic and present. Jordan (2010) notes that a judicious use of emotional transparency will help the patient understand her own authentic self and will be comfortable to be authentic in relationships. The therapist must also be aware of and share with the patient the importance and power of the social context. As discussed earlier in this section, the *social context* refers to the social determinants of health, such as racism, poverty, and lack of access to health care.

The process of RCT involves a complex approach that, paradoxically, is not complex at all. It is simply being in relationship with the patient. However, being in relationship is not simple at all. Thus adding to this paradox, this therapeutic approach is most complex as it embraces an authentic involvement in the relationship and in the world itself. Jordan describes how therapists must understand and embrace uncertainty and must live with uncertainty, acknowledging that we all live in an uncertain world. The therapeutic process involves being with the patient in all the complexities this relationship entails.

The efficacy of RCT has been demonstrated in a few studies. Frey (2013) reported on the application of this therapy in June 2004 at the Jean Baker Miller Training Institute. A study conducted by Oakley, Addison, and Piran (2004) used an RCT approach that was time limited and guided by a manual. After collecting and analyzing data at five time points in addition to pretreatment and posttreatment, they found improvement in several outcomes measures, including depression and anxiety, as well as maintenance of these improved outcomes at 3 months and 6 months follow-up. Frey also reported on a study by Tantillo and Sanftner (2003) that compared cognitive behavioral therapy with RCT in a population of women with bulimia. All outcomes, including binge eating and vomiting, were equivalent in both groups, except that the women in the RCT group perceived greater mutuality.

Considerations Related to Risks Associated With Gender-Sensitive Models

The past decades have seen increasing the recognition of biological differences between the sexes and efforts to reduce inappropriate care for women. Increasingly, health care professionals are advised to integrate knowledge of sex and gender differences into treatment plans. Communication in the delivery of health care provides opportunity for creating gender-sensitive encounters, yet evidence suggests that communication also reproduces gender differences. Health care conversations reproduce stereotypical communication styles that reinforce gender bias, convey different attitudes toward treatments for women and men, and convey information that result in gender bias and unequal care. Gender-sensitive care has been proposed as health professionals using competencies in perceiving existing gender differences and incorporating these into treatment. This approach may also run the risk of interjecting preconceived and unconscious assumptions about gender in ways that lead to stereotypical thinking and communication with patients.

A recent analysis of discourse contained in tape-recorded conversations between patients and health professionals revealed different approaches used by female and male patients and health professionals in clinical interactions related to atrial fibrillation (Hedegaard, Ahl, Rovio-Johansson, & Siouta, 2014). Women usually used emotional-oriented statements (e.g., referencing feeling unusual) in describing their health problems, and male patients used performance-oriented statements (e.g., referencing inability to swim the usual distance). Health professionals tended to acknowledge concern for female patients and provide reassurance but downplayed male patients' statements and confirmed their descriptions of performance. Hedegaard et al. concluded that female patients were constructed as fragile and males as competent through gender-stereotypical communication. In an effort to provide gender-sensitive health care, it is possible that assumptions about sex and gender differences in health problems and their manifestations reinforce stereotypes about gender in a context in which the intent is the opposite. The use of open-ended statements or questions by health professionals instead of leading questions that reinforce gender stereotypes allowed conversations to be less influenced by gender stereotypes. Moreover, reflection on the social construction of gender may also prompt awareness of ways in which stereotypes shape health care communications and compromise the equality of treatment.

■ POLICY AND WOMEN'S HEALTH CARE

Dramatic changes in policy related to a U.S. health plan have occurred in the past decade. Along with earlier policy to insure women's reproductive health care, such as that provided by Title X, Medicaid coverage for low-income adults, Medicare coverage for older adults, and Children's Health Insurance Program/s, the ACA has transformed access to health insurance coverage for millions of U.S. women. More than 4 million women enrolled for coverage under the ACA during the first period during which they could do so. An estimated 48.5 million women with individual insurance will receive preventive care without copayment required, and nearly 8.7 million women will gain coverage for maternity services.

Women have unique health care needs that can inform the health care reforms most relevant to them. Among these are women's more complex reproductive health care needs, their experience of greater chronic disease rates, longer life span, more frequent and continuous use of health care over the life span, and higher levels of spending when compared with men (Henry J. Kaiser Family Foundation, 2012). Specific issues related to health care insurance for women include the gaps in insurance coverage and difficulty accessing health care that are attributable to making workforce transitions, being employed in part-time jobs without employee health insurance benefits, and being insured as a dependent: Each of these places women at risk for being unable to obtain needed care. In addition to these factors is the disproportionate number of women who live in poverty or are among the working poor, unable to afford health care and insurance.

Many have looked to the health reform in Massachusetts to understand the impact of increasing health insurance coverage. Women's experience with Commonwealth Care has been studied recently by comparing health care services access, utilization, and cost and health outcomes from Massachusetts before and after the 2006 health care reform. Commonwealth Care eligibility criteria target those with incomes less than 300% of federal poverty level, and Medicaid provides a health safety net for those meeting more stringent eligibility criteria. Two key challenges for women included continuity of coverage (churn) and affordability. Uninsured women in Massachusetts were disproportionately young (18–25 years), Hispanic, and single; less likely to have college degrees; more likely to be unemployed or working part time; and earning low incomes when compared with insured women.

Churn refers to the coverage volatility experienced specifically by low-income women transitioning between Medicaid and subsidized insurance plans as their eligibility status change, with an estimated 16% to 17% experiencing a gap in coverage during their transitions (Fitzgerald, Cohen, Hyams, Sullivan, & Johnson, 2014). Women's vulnerability to churn and gaps in coverage were attributable to their employment patterns, dependent status (they are often insured as dependents of their spouses/partners), and income fluctuations. Churn-related gaps in coverage may lead to transitions in health care providers, as women are required to seek care from different sources, and redundant testing that occurs as new providers repeat tests already done by another provider. Impaired follow-up for health problems, inefficiencies in health record keeping, and disruptive changes in medical care and treatment occur. These consequences are especially worrisome for women with chronic illnesses for whom disease management requires continuity of care from the same health care providers and continuity of medications.

Affordability was also a challenge to women who were covered by Commonwealth Care: Many were paying more than 5% of their incomes in out-of-pocket medical expenses, paying off medical debt, or experiencing problems paying medical bills (Long, Stockley, Birchfield, & Shulman, 2010; Long, Stockley, & Shulmsn, 2011). Women at risk of unmet care needs were in poor to fair health; had incomes 100%

to 299% of federal poverty level; had dependent children; were divorced, separated or widowed; were 26 to 34 years old; and had chronic conditions and physical limitations caused by their health problems. Commonwealth Care worked best for women who were 50 to 64 years of age, had full time employment, had employer-sponsored insurance, and had incomes greater than 500% of the poverty level (Fitzgerald et al., 2014). Evaluation of gender differences in coverage, affordability, and access for women with implementation of the ACA should receive urgent and continued attention.

The Patient Protection and Affordable Care Act

The ACA was enacted into federal law in 2010 and is likely to be the most complex and far-reaching health care legislation since the passage of Medicaid and Medicare in 1965. Its goals are to increase the number of people with access to health insurance, improve the affordability of health insurance and health care services, and improve quality of care (Armstrong, 2015). Implementation is planned over 8 years owing to the complexity of the reform. Anticipated benefits for women include improved access to health insurance coverage, expanded scope of benefits covered by plans, and reduced cost sharing for some services. Although most provisions are not gender specific, the Women's Health Amendment (Section 2713 to Public Health Services Act) mandates coverage without cost sharing for preventive services focused on reproductive health (e.g., contraceptive technology, breast pumps, and breastfeeding counseling).

Women have had access to health insurance coverage before the ACA. Private sector coverage is most often provided through employment-based plans, and public sector sources include Medicare, Medicaid, and state Children's Health Insurance Program (CHIP). Both Medicaid and CHIP provide assistance without the obligation of a premium. A major barrier to insurance coverage is cost. Despite premium payments, women have suffered from limited coverage of services such as prescription contraceptives and maternity care, often treated as exclusions or as preexisting conditions. Coverage of preventive benefits has varied greatly before the ACA under both private and public plans.

Provisions of the ACA expand access to health insurance. These include coverage of adult children up to age 26 years on parents' plans, Medicaid expansion to cover more of the population by raising the income threshold for eligibility, establishing state- or federal-based exchanges or marketplaces that offer individuals options to purchase private insurance that are coupled with tax credits or subsidies for low-income individuals, and supporting policies that include guaranteed issue, prohibition of preexisting conditions, underwriting changes, and individual mandate (Armstrong, 2015). Women with incomes below 133% of the poverty level, including those without children, will be able to access Medicaid coverage in many states. The Medicaid expansion enables coverage for women between the ages of 19 and 64 years, a critical period for women's health.

The ACA expands the scope of benefits covered in insurance plans in significant ways. Plans sold on public and private exchanges are to include essential health benefits, including ambulatory patient services; emergency services; hospitalization; maternity and newborn care; mental health and substance-use disorder (SUD) services, including behavioral health treatment; prescription drugs; rehabilitative and habilitative services and devices; laboratory services; preventive and wellness services; and chronic disease management and pediatric services, including oral and vision care. Maternity and newborn care benefits (prenatal care, labor and delivery, and postpartum care services) and preventive and wellness service benefits are of particular relevance to women.

In addition to the reproductive health provisions, the mental health/SUD services are noteworthy for women. A combination of the Mental Health Parity and Addiction Equity Act and the ACA will extend overall health insurance coverage and the scope of coverage to include mental health and substance abuse benefits (Frank, Beronio, & Glied, 2014). The essential health benefit requirements governing basic coverage include mental health and substance-use services. In addition, Medicaid expansion will cover approximately 65% of newly covered people with mental health disorders and SUDs, and single, childless adults will be eligible for Medicaid, including many who have severe and persistent mental disorders and live in extreme poverty, experience unstable housing, and have co-occurring SUDs. Behavioral health parity means that these services will be covered at parity with medical–surgical coverage. Although this represents transformative change in mental health and SUD services, there remain important areas not covered, including assertive community treatment (ACT), supported employment, supported housing, and long-term residential services. Nonetheless, coverage of mental health and SUD services and parity with medical–surgical care represents significant advancements in health insurance that will serve women well (Beronoio, Glied, & Frank, 2014; Chin, Yee, & Banks, 2014).

Along with passage of the ACA, the National Prevention Council was formed to develop and implement the first national prevention strategy to promote evidence-based interventions to promote health and wellness. The *National Prevention Strategy: America's Plan for Better Health and Wellness* report focused on the importance of quality health care to prevent disease (National Prevention Council, 2011).

An IOM Committee on Clinical Preventive Services for Women (IOM, 2011) focused on closing the gaps in existing preventive services for women. This Committee defined preventive health services to include medications, procedures, devices, tests, education, and counseling that had been shown to improve well-being and/or decrease the likelihood of disease or conditions or to delay them. The Committee reviewed the preventive services recommended by the U.S. Preventive Services Task Force (USPSTF) for women as highly effective, considered the Bright Futures recommendations for girls and adolescents, and recommended eight additional services for inclusion for no-cost coverage (IOM, 2011). See recommended clinical preventive services for women in Table 3.3 and additional recommended services in Table 3.4.

An early provision of the ACA is preventive services without patient cost sharing. These include services rated by the USPSTF as A or B, meaning they are well supported by effectiveness data; immunizations as recommended by the Advisory Committee on Immunization Practices of the Centers for Disease Control and Prevention; preventive care and screening for infants, children, and adolescents endorsed by the HRSA; and preventive care and screening for women that were added under the Women's Health Amendment of the ACA. As the USPSTF adds new recommendations with A or B ratings, they will be added to this list without cost sharing.

The Women's Health Amendment of the ACA (section 2713 to the Public Health Services Act) specifies additional services to be covered without cost sharing as recommended by the IOM (2011). These included: well-woman visits; screening for gestational diabetes; human papillomavirus DNA testing; counseling for STIs; counseling and screening for HIV; contraceptive methods and counseling; breastfeeding support, supplies, and counseling; and screening and counseling for interpersonal and domestic violence. One of the gaps in the ACA is the banning of abortion coverage as an essential benefit.

In addition to these benefits, the ACA included several proposed changes in Medicare affecting benefits for older women. Among these provisions were those that

TABLE 3.3	IOM Committee on Clinical Preventive Services Recommendations for Inclusion in Well-Woman Visits Under the Patient Protection and Affordable Care Act	
PREVENTION/HEALTH PROMOTION	**SCREENING**	**COUNSELING AND INTERVENTIONS**
Pregnancy related	Anemia Bacteriuria Chlamydia Hepatitis B Syphilis Rh incompatibility PPD Suicide History of CVD-related conditions in pregnancy Prenatal care	Breastfeeding Tobacco use Prenatal care
Cancer	BRCA gene Breast cancer Cervical cancer Colorectal cancer	BRCA gene Breast cancer chemoprevention
Chronic illness	BP Diabetes Lipid levels Metabolic syndrome Osteoporosis	Osteoporosis
Substance use		Alcohol misuse Tobacco use Tobacco-use interventions
Healthy behaviors	Eating behaviors Obesity Physical activity levels Preconception care	Healthy diet Obesity Referrals for interventions Preconception care Folic acid supplementation
STIs	Chlamydia < 25 years old CT/GC screen > 25 in high-risk communities GC HIV Syphilis	All STIs counseling for high-risk teens, adults
Mental health	Depression—adolescents, adults	

BP, blood pressure; CT/GC, chlamydia trachomatis/gonococcus; CVD, cardiovascular disease; GC, gonococcus; HIV, human immunodeficiency virus; IOM, Institute of Medicine; PPD, postpartum depression; STIs, sexually transmitted infections.
Adapted from the Institute of Medicine (2011).

TABLE 3.4	Additional Services Recommended by the IOM Committee on Preventive Services for Women
SERVICE	**FOR WHOM AND WHEN**
Screening for gestational diabetes	Pregnant women: 24–28 weeks; first prenatal visit for pregnant women at high risk for diabetes
Human papillomavirus testing—addition of high-risk human papillomavirus DNA testing in addition to cytology testing in those with normal cytology results	Women—30 years of age and no more frequently than every 3 years
Counseling for STIs	Sexually active women—annually
Counseling and screening for human immunodeficiency virus	Sexually active women—annually
Contraceptive methods (full range of FDA-approved methods, sterilization) with patient education and counseling	Women with reproductive capacity—not specified
Breastfeeding support, supplies and counseling; comprehensive lactation support and counseling and costs of renting breastfeeding equipment by a trained provider to ensure successful initiation and duration of breastfeeding	All pregnant women and those in postpartum period—during pregnancy and postpartum
Screening and counseling for interpersonal and domestic violence: involves elicitation of information about current and past violence and abuse in culturally sensitive and supportive manner to address current concerns of safety and other current or future health problems	Women and adolescents—timing not specified
Well-woman visits for recommended preventive services including preconception and prenatal care	Adult women—at least one well-woman preventive care visit annually; several visits may be needed to obtain all necessary recommended preventive services depending on health status, health needs, and other risk factors

FDA, Food and Drug Administration; IOM, Institute of Medicine; STIs, sexually transmitted infections.
Adapted from Institute of Medicine (2011).

would decrease out-of-pocket costs for drugs and preventive services, an annual personalized health plan, and risk assessment; no cost sharing for mammograms, Pap smears, and bone density testing; and some assistance with long-term care costs through voluntary insurance programs. Sadly, many of these were included in the ill-fated Community Living Assistance Services and Supports (CLASS) Act that was intended to include a national voluntary long-term care insurance program that would make it possible for people to purchase government-sponsored insurance during their working years so that if they became unable to care for themselves, they would have access to a cash benefit to purchase services delivered either at home or in a care facility. This act would have begun shifting the financing of long-term care services from a means-tested Medicaid program to an insurance-based system that would be supported by voluntary private contributions (Gleckman, 2011). The United States remains challenged to develop funding for services that older adults, in particular women, will need. Many other countries (e.g., the Netherlands and Japan) offer models of long-term care insurance programs that the United States could emulate.

On the positive side, the ACA codifies the establishment of OWH in major federal agencies, including DHHS, Centers for Disease Control and Prevention, FDA, HRSA, and Agency for Healthcare Research and Quality. These offices establish visible points of accountability for women's health across several federal agencies.

The most controversial provision of ACA has been the contraception mandate, requiring coverage without cost sharing all FDA-approved contraceptive methods, sterilization procedures, and patient education and counseling for all women as prescribed by providers. Over-the-counter contraceptives were also covered if prescribed. Exempted from this requirement were religious employers, and additional accommodations were made for nonprofit organizations affiliated with religious organizations. In a politics-and-religion-trumps-scientific-evidence decision, the U.S. Supreme Court ruled that for-profit firms that object on religious grounds must also be eligible for accommodation, weakening access to contraceptive benefits for women despite scientific data supporting their effectiveness.

Access to at least one annual well-woman visit to obtain recommended preventive services was included in the ACA provisions. More than a single visit may be necessary to complete all preventive screening. Breastfeeding support was also a provision of the ACA, which includes coverage of comprehensive lactation support and counseling, costs of renting or purchasing breastfeeding equipment such as pumps, and workplace requirements to provide time and space for mothers to express milk until the infant is 1 year old.

Another important set of benefits that will improve access for women and girls includes the availability of certified nurse midwives and OB-GYNs regarded as primary care providers; immunization, including the human papillomavirus (HPV) vaccine for women and girls younger than 26 years; allowance of low-income new mothers and newborns to maintain Medicaid coverage beyond the postpartum period; increased support for the reimbursement of certified nurse midwives, birth attendants, and free-standing birth centers; postpartum depression education support services; maternal, infant, and early childhood home visiting programs; and expanded workplace breastfeeding support services. Allowing states to extend eligibility for family planning services to those with incomes below 185% of the poverty level without federal permit process; funding to states to provide evidence-based sex education to reduce teen pregnancy rates and STI incidence; and changes to Medicare to reduce out-of-pocket costs for medications and preventive services are additional provisions.

The ACA has had far-reaching impact on women's health, but there are already erosions of benefits such as seen with accommodation of religious institutions and provisions of contraceptive benefits. The American Academy of Nursing Expert Panel on Women's Health (Berg, Shaver, Olshansky, Woods, & Taylor, 2013) recommended further elaboration beyond the prevention recommendations in the IOM report and the *National Prevention Strategy* report. These include:

Comprehensive health care delivery approaches for preventive services for women

Gender-sensitive and life-span prevention services coordinated in a primary health care system of primary care and public health

Preconception health care as a model of integrative prevention practice

Integration of primary, secondary, and tertiary prevention guidelines in practice

Development and maintenance of a competent workforce to implement prevention services and meet national health goals (Berg et al., 2013)

In addition, the American Academy of Nursing Expert Panel on Women's Health endorsed the IOM (2011) Clinical Preventive Services for Women and strategies for prevention in the *National Prevention Strategies* report. They also advocate the adoption of prevention guidelines that are evidence based; gender sensitive; culturally appropriate; and inclusive of gay, lesbian, and intergender groups. Other areas include mobilizing health professionals to address national health goals and the integration of essential competencies for primary and secondary prevention and clinical management of SRH into professional practice curricula, as well as focusing service improvements on social and structural determinants of preventive services (Berg et al., 2013).

Challenges for the future include those related to the burgeoning population of older women. Gaps in coverage and high out-of-pocket expenses on long-term services continue to affect older women disproportionately. The strong focus on hospital care covered by Medicare has been well established, but rules related to Medicare claims are becoming more stringent about the use of hospital-based services. Coverage of preventive services, such as Pap smears and mammography, came late (1990 and 1991, respectively) in Medicare's history and required a 20% coinsurance payment, leaving women with significant out-of-pocket expenses. The ACA's inclusion of recommended clinical preventive services was significantly broadened by the elimination of cost sharing for highly effective preventive services as recommended by the USPSTF and a personalized health plan with an annual comprehensive risk assessment (well-woman visit). Drug coverage for older women has also been improved under Medicare Part D, and the low-income subsidy of premium and cost-sharing subsidies for beneficiaries have been a significant benefit for women. What remains problematic for older women today is the array of needed care that is not covered: hearing aids, eyeglasses, dental care, extended nursing home stays, or personal care needs. Required co-payments also contribute to high out-of-pocket costs for women whose incomes are marginal. Medicaid coverage provides assistance to an estimated 17% of older women who have Medicare coverage: Dual coverage affords many of these women glasses, vision care, dental care, and hearing aids (dependent on the state of residence), offsetting costs for the poorest of low-income older women. Because women constitute a disproportionate share of those residing in nursing homes and residential care communities, they experience a much greater need than do men for services that Medicare does *not* cover, putting poor women at increased risk for low access to the services they need most. Unpaid and informal caregivers are also predominantly women, and they, too, are not well served by Medicare in its current form. Lack of coverage for services for family members needing care leaves many of the caregivers at financial risk, as they may need to depart from the paid workforce to provide care. Thus an intergenerational disadvantage may be accrued by families in which an older woman requires long-term care services in the United States (Salganicoff, 2015).

■ GLOBAL WOMEN'S HEALTH AND HEALTH CARE

The early decades of the 21st century have been a period of dramatic changes in our consciousness of global issues and globalization. Health and health care have become global issues, as illustrated by the rapid transmission of infectious diseases across international borders, along with the exchange of innovations in health care technology, health care personnel, health information and international collaboration in health professionals' education and research. This rapid change in perspectives has challenged countries around the globe to examine diverse perspectives about health and health care.

Recognizing the importance of girls and women in the world, a recent Lancet Commission on Women and Health studied the complex relations between women and health in our rapidly changing world. The Commission on Women and Health reported that worldwide priorities in women's health have been changing from a narrow emphasis on maternal and child health to a broader framework of SRH and a more encompassing concept of women's health using a life-span framework spanning fetal life to old age (Langer et al., 2015). The Commission examined the roles of women as both users and providers of health care. Providing that they remain healthy throughout life, experience gender equality, and are enabled, empowered, and valued in their societies as caregivers, women make contributions to their own health and that of their families and communities as well as to sustainable development. In an unprecedented analysis, the Commission estimated the financial value of paid and unpaid health care–related contributions women make, often a hidden subsidy to their respective health care systems and societies. They estimated the "value of the invaluable" using data from approximately 52% of the world's population from 32 countries: Contributions approached 2.35% of the gross domestic product for paid work, the equivalent of more than $3 trillion.

Of the many conclusions of the Commission, the most important was that gender-transformative polices were needed to "enable women to integrate their social, biological, and occupation roles and function to their full capacity, and that healthy, valued, enabled, and empowered women will make substantial contributions to sustainable development" (Langer et al., 2015, p. 1). These contributions to health care are especially important given the global complex epidemiological transition, among these the aging of the world's population and increased caregiving needs and demands. Ensuring that women's health needs are met throughout the life span constitutes an important investment in their countries' health and economic well-being related to health care that healthy women will provide.

Around the globe, there are few gender-sensitive policies enabling women to integrate social, biological, and occupational roles; function to their full capacity; and realize their fundamental human rights. A noteworthy exception is Norway and other Nordic countries, where policies support women as well as men during early parenting (e.g., by providing child care so that both women and men can be employed).

The commission concluded its report with four recommendations: value women, compensate women, count women, and be accountable to women. *Valuing women* means ensuring universal access to health care responsive to gender and the life course and ensuring the availability, accessibility, and quality of health services for women's comprehensive needs. Valuing women is reflected in creating gender-responsive policies and programs that reflect an understanding of women, designing programs to reach and benefit women as well as men, and eliminating gender discrimination and promoting gender equality. Recognizing women's paid and unpaid contributions as health care providers requires policies that support their contributions, reduce gender inequality, and empower women. Valuing women implies implementing policies that enable women to integrate their social, biological, and occupational complexities (Langer et al., 2015).

Compensating women includes estimating the value of women's contributions to health care and recompensating their invisible subsidy to health systems and societies. It also includes ensuring equal compensation for equal work in health care as well as in other sectors.

Counting women implies accounting for women in quantification of the health workforce and guaranteeing that sex-disaggregated civil, vital, and health statistics reflect their existence and contributions. Mandating the inclusion of women in research studies and publication of findings that disaggregate sex is another component of counting women, as is counting their contributions to health care. *Being accountable to women* includes the development and implementation of a framework and indicators for women and health, as well as the establishment of mechanisms at global and country levels to ensure accountability for action at any level to influence women and health.

In a recent review of progress toward the 2015 Millennium Development Goals, Meleis (2015) acknowledges the progress in achieving the reduction of maternal and infant mortality rates and increasing primary education for girls but identifies four major barriers that slow progress in meeting the goals for achieving optimal well-being for women. First is the narrow definition of *women's health*, often taken to be synonymous with *reproductive health*, as measured by maternal and infant mortality rates, and the limited access to health care for prenatal and postnatal care and/or family planning services. A life cycle and lifestyle approach that transcends the limits of the reproductive years is needed. Women manage multiple dimensions of health for themselves and their families as well as work inside and outside their homes. Discrimination and gender inequity in compensation challenge women. Moreover, women's longevity may leave them without resources for support as they age and face noncommunicable diseases.

A second barrier is a lack of a coherent theoretical framework for planning and implementing women's health programs, many of which focus on diseases and the reproductive system. Programs that do not accommodate women's multiple roles and the relationship to their environments, social, chemical, and physical, leave women exposed to health-damaging forces that ultimately limit health and development goals. Meleis (2015) recommends that three major concepts frame women's health care programs: equity and equitable care, women's roles, and enabling and empowering environments.

The narrow focus of health professionals' education constitutes another barrier. The narrow definition of *women's health* and lack of consideration of the needs of girls and older women do not prepare health professionals to care accountably for women. Issues that put women at risk for illness and compromised quality of life should be central to a curriculum that also provides integrated interprofessional education and interdisciplinary research programs that reflect gender and sex differences.

Policies and laws fail to support women's lifestyle choices and decisions about their bodies. Inequity for women is reflected in laws related to trafficking daughters to early marriage and servitude and limiting educational opportunities for girls. Laws prohibiting trafficking, circumcision, and mutilation of girls are necessary, as are policies for reporting, educating, preventing, and punishing sexual harassment, abuse, and slavery of women. Laws supporting women's decisions about abortion, family size, and preventing female infanticide are needed.

■ REFERENCES

Albrecht, S., Kelly-Thomas, K., Osbonre, J. S., & Ogbagaber, S. (2011). The SUCCESS program for smoking cessation for pregnant women. *Journal of Obstetric, Gynecologic and Neonatal Nursing, 40*, 520–531.

American Psychiatric Association (APA). (1994). *Diagnostic and statistical manual of mental disorders* (4th ed.). Washington, DC: Author.

American Psychiatric Association (APA). (2013). *Diagnostic and statistical manual of mental disorders* (5th ed.). Washington, DC: Author.

Anderson, R. T., Barbara, A. M., Weisman, C., Scholle, S. H., Binko, J., Schneider, T.,…Gwinner, V. (2001). A qualitative analysis of women's satisfaction with the primary care from a panel of focus groups in the National Centers of Excellence in Women's Health. *Journal of Women's Health, 10*, 637–647.

Anderson, R. T., Weisman, C. S., Camacho, F., Scholle, S. H., Henderson, J. T., & Farmer, D. F. (2007). Women's satisfaction with their ongoing primary health care services: A consideration of visit-specific and period assessments. *Health Services Research, 42*, 663–681.

Anderson, R. T., Weisman, C. S., Scholle, S. H., Henderson, J. T., Oldendick, R., & Camacho, F. (2002). Evaluation of the quality of care in the clinical care centers of the National Centers of Excellence in Women's Health. *Women's Health Issues, 12*, 309–326.

Andrist, L. C., & MacPherson, K. I. (2001). Conceptual models for women's health research: Reclaiming menopause as an exemplar of nursing's contributions to feminist scholarship. *Annual Review of Nursing Research, 19*, 29–60.

Aparasu, R. R. (1999). Visits to office-based physicians in the United States for medication-related morbidity. *Journal of the American Pharmaceutical Association, 39*(3), 332–337.

Armstrong, J. (2015). Women's health in the age of Patient Protection and the Affordable Care Act. *Clinical Obstetrics and Gynecology, 58*, 323–335.

Aslin, A. L. (1977). Feminist and community mental health center psychotherapists' expectations of mental health for women. *Sex Roles, 3*(6), 537–544.

Bachmann, G. A., & Mussman, B. (2015). The aging population: Imperative to uncouple sex and gender to establish "gender equal" health care. *Maturitas, 80*, 421–425.

Banks, A. (2006). *The neurobiology of connection.* Presentation at Summer Training Institute, Jean Baker Miller Training Institute, Wellesley, MA.

Bean-Mayberry, B., Yano, E. M., Bayliss, N., Navratil, J., Weisman, C. S., & Scholle, S. H. (2007). Federally funded comprehensive women's health centers: Leading innovation in women's healthcare delivery. *Journal of Women's Health, 16*, 1281–1290.

Belenky, M. F., Clinchy, B. M., Goldberger, N. R., & Tarule, J. M. (1997). *Women's ways of knowing: The development of self, voice, and mind.* New York, NY: Basic Books.

Berg, J., Shaver, J., Olshansky, E., Woods, N. F., & Taylor D. (2013). A call to action: Expanded research agenda for women's health. *Nursing Outlook, 61*(4), 252.

Berg, J. A., Taylor, D., & Woods, N. F., The Women's Health Expert Panel of the American Academy of Nursing. (2013). Where we are today? Prioritizing women's health services and health policy: A report by the Women's Health Expert Panel of the American Academy of Nursing. *Nursing Outlook, 61*, 5–15.

Berg, J. A., Woods, N. F., Kostas-Polston, E., & Johnson-Mallard, V. (2014). Breaking down silos: The future of sexual and reproductive health care—An opinion from the women's health expert panel of the American Academy of Nursing. *Journal of the American Association of Nurse Practitioners, 26*(1), 3–4.

Bergman, S. J., & Surrey, J. L. (1997). The woman–man relationship: Impasses and possibilities. In J. Jordan (Ed.), *Womens' growth in diversity.* New York, NY: Guilford Press.

Beronoio, K., Glied, S., & Frank, R. (2014). How the Affordable Care Act and Mental Health Parity and Addiction Equity Act greatly expand coverage of behavioral health care. *Journal of Behavioral Health Services & Research, 41*, 410–428.

Boston Women's Health Book Collective. (1974). *Our bodies, ourselves.* Boston, MA: Author.

Boysen, G., Ebersole, A., Canser, R., & Coston, N. (2014). Gendered mental disorders: Masculine and feminine stereotypes about mental disorders and their relation to stigma. *Journal of Social Psychology, 154*, 546–565.

Broverman, I. K., Broverman, D. M., Clarkson, F. E., Rosenkrantz, P. S., & Vogel, S. R. (1970). Sex role stereotypes and clinical judgments of mental health. *Journal of Consultative and Clinical Psychology, 34*(1), 1–7.

Browne, T. K. (2015). Is premenstrual dysphoric disorder really a disorder? *Journal of Bioethical Inquiry, 12*, 313–330.

Cappiello, J., & Nothnagle, M. (2013). SRH Workforce Summit: Now is the time to bring sexual and reproductive health to primary care. *Contraception, 88*, 210–212.

Celik, H., Lagro-Janssen, T. A. L. M., Widdershoven, G. G. A. M., & Abma, T. A. (2011). Bringing gender sensitivity into healthcare practice: A systematic review. *Patient Education and Counseling, 84*, 143–149.

Center for Scientific Review. (2002). *How scientists are selected for study section service.* Retrieved from http://www.csr.nih.gov/events/studysectionservice.htm

Chin, J. L., Yee, B. W. K., & Banks, M. E. (2014). Women's health and behavioral health issues in health care reform. *Journal of Social Work in Disability & Rehabilitation, 13*, 122–138.

Clancy, C. M., & Massion, C. T. (1992). American women's health care: A patchwork quilt with gaps. *Journal of the American Medical Association, 268*, 268–1918.

Coll, C. G., Cook-Nobles, R., & Surrey, J. L. (1997). Building connection through diversity. In J. Jordan (Ed.), *Womens' growth in diversity.* New York, NY: Guildford Press.

Commission on the Social Determinants of Health. (2008). *Closing the gap in a generation: Healthy equity through action on the social determinants of health* (Final report of the commission on social determinants of health). Geneva, Switzerland: World Health Organization.

Coventry, L. L., Bremner, A. P., Jacobs, I. G., & Finn, J. (2013). Myocardial infarction: Sex differences in symptoms reported to emergency dispatch. *Prehospital Emergency Care, 17*, 193–202.

Damoiseaux, V. A., Proost, J. H., Jiawan, V. C., & Melgert, B. N. (2014). Sex differences in the pharmacokinetics of antidepressants: Influence of female sex hormones and oral contraceptives. *Clinical Pharmacokinetics, 53*, 509–519.

Dan, A. J. (Ed.). (1994). *Reframing women's health: Multidisciplinary research and practice.* Thousand Oaks, CA: Sage.

deKleijn, M., Lagro-Janssen, A. L. M., Canelo, I., & Yano, E. M. (2015). Creating a roadmap for delivery gender-sensitive comprehensive care for women veterans. *Medical Care, 53*(Suppl. 1), S156–S164.

Domino, S. E., Bodurtha, J., Nagel, J. D., & the BIRCWH Program Leadership. (2011). Interdisciplinary research career development: Building interdisciplinary research careers in women's health program best practices. *Journal of Women's Health, 20*, 1587–1600.

Ehrenreich, B., & English, D. (1973). *Witches, midwives, and nurses.* Old Westbury, NY: Feminist Press.

Eisenberg, D. M., Davis, R. B., Ettner, S. L., Appel, S., Wilkey, S., Van Rompay, M., & Kessler, R. C. (1998). Trends in alternative medicine use in the United States, 1990–1997: Results of a national follow-up survey. *Journal of the American Medical Association, 280*(18), 1569–1575.

Eisenberg, D. M., Davis, R. B., Ettner, S. L., Appel, S., Wilkey, S., Van Rompay, M., & Kessler, R. C. (1999). Trends in alternative medicine use in the United States, 1990–1997: Results of a national follow-up survey. *Obstetrical and Gynecological Survey, 54*(6), 370–371.

Eldridge, N. S., Mencher, J., & Slater, S. (1997). The conundrum of mutuality: A lesbian dialogue. In J. Jordan (Ed.), *Womens' growth in diversity.* New York, NY: Guilford Press.

Faculty of Sexual and Reproductive Healthcare, Royal College of Obstetricians and Gynecologists. (2012). *Service standards for SRH.* London, UK. Retrieved from www.Fsrh.org/pdfs/ServiceStandards SexualReproductiveHealthcare.pdf

Fankhauser, M. P. (1997). Psychiatric disorders in women: Psychopharmacologic treatments. *Journal of the American Pharmaceutical Association, 37*(6), 667–678.

Federation of Feminist Women's Health Centers. (1991). *A new view of a woman's body*. Los Angeles, CA: Feminist Health Press.

Fife, R. S. (2003). Development of a comprehensive women's health program in an academic medical center: Experiences of the Indiana University National Center of Excellence in Women's Health. *Journal of Women's Health, 12*, 869–878.

Fife, R. S., Moskovic, C., Dynak, H., Winner, C., Vahratian, A., Laya, M. B., …Holaday, L. (2001). Development and implementation of novel community outreach methods in women's health issues: The National Centers of Excellence in Women's Health. *Journal of Women's Health and Gender Based Medicine, 10*, 27–37.

Fisher, S. (1986). *In the patient's best interest*. New Brunswick, NJ: Rutgers University Press.

Fitzgerald, T., Cohen, L., Hyams, T., Sullivan, K. M., & Johnson, P. A. (2014). Women and health reform: How national health care can enhance coverage, affordability, and access for women (examples from Massachusetts). *Women's Health Issues, 24*, e5–e10.

Frank, R. G., Beronio, K., & Glied, S. A. (2014). Behavioral health parity and the Affordable Care Act. *Journal of Social Work in Disability & Rehabilitation, 13*, 31–43.

Frey, L. (2013). Relational-cultural therapy: Theory, research, and application to counseling competencies. *Professional Psychology: Research and Practice, 44*(3), 177–185.

Geller, S. E., Burns, L. R., & Brailer, D. J. (1996). The impact of nonclinical factors on practice variations: The case of hysterectomies. *Health Services Research, 30*(6), 729–750.

Gilligan, C. (1982). *In a different voice: Psychological theory and women's development*. Cambridge, MA: Harvard University Press.

Gilligan, C., Rogers A. G., & Tolman, D. L. (1991a). *Women, girls and psychotherapy*. New York, NY: Guilford Press.

Gilligan, C., Rogers A. G., & Tolman, D. L. (1991b). *Women, girls and psychotherapy: Reframing resistance*. New York, NY: Haworth Press.

Gleckman, H. (2011). Requiem for the CLASS Act. *Health Affairs, 30*, 2231–2234.

Guise, J. M., Nagel, J. D., Regensteiner, J. G., & the Building Interdisciplinary Research Careers in Women's Health Directors. (2012). Best practices and pearls in interdisciplinary mentoring from building interdisciplinary research careers in women's health directors. *Journal of Women's Health, 21*, 1114–1126.

Gwinner, V. M., Strauss, J. F., Milliken, N., & Donoghue, G. D. (2000). Implementing a new model of integrated women's health in academic health centers: Lessons learned from the National Centers of Excellence in Women's Health. *Journal of Women's Health and Gender Based Medicine, 9*, 979–985.

Hammarström, A., Johansson, K., Annandale, E., Ahlgren, C., Alex, L., Christianson, M.,…Berdonk, P. (2014). Central gender theoretical concepts in health research: The state of the art. *Journal of Epidemiology and Community Health, 68*, 185–190.

Hankivsky, L. (2012). Women's health, men's health, and gender and health: Implications of intersectionality. *Social Science & Medicine, 74*, 1712–1720.

Hankivsky, O., Varcoe, C., & Morrow, M. H. (2007). *Women's health in Canada: Critical perspectives on theory and policy*. Toronto, ON: University of Toronto Press.

Hedegaard, J., Ahl, H., Rovio-Johansson, A., & Siouta, E. (2014). Gendered communicative construction of patients in consultation settings. *Women and Health, 54*, 513–529.

Henry J. Kaiser Family Foundation. (2012). *Women's health insurance coverage: Fact sheet*. Menlo Park, CA: Women's Health Policy Program, the Henry J. Kaiser Family Foundation 2012.

Herz, S. (1997). Don't test, do sell: Legal implications of inclusion and exclusion of women in clinical drug trials. *Epilepsia, 38*(Suppl. 4), S42–S49.

Im, E. O., & Meleis, A. I. (2001). An international imperative for gender-sensitive theories in women's health. *Journal of Nursing Scholarship, 33*, 309–314.

Institute of Medicine (IOM). (2001). *Exploring the biological contributions to human health: Does sex matter?* Washington, DC: National Academies Press.

Institute of Medicine (IOM). (2010). *Women's health research: Progress, pitfalls, and promise*. Washington, DC: National Academies Press.

Institute of Medicine (IOM). (2011). *Clinical preventive services for women: Closing the gaps*. Washington, DC: National Academies Press.

Jackson, S., Camacho, D., Freund, K. M., Bigby, J., Walcott-McQuigg, J., Hughes, E.,…Zerr, A. (2001). Women's health centers and minority women: Addressing barriers to care. The National Centers of Excellence in Women's Health. *Journal of Women's Health and Gender-Based Medicine, 10*, 551–559.

Jemmott, L. S., & Jemmott, J. B. III. (1992). Increasing condom-use intentions among sexually active black adolescent women. *Nursing Research, 41*, 273–279.

Jemmott, L. S., Jemmott, J. B., Hutchinson, M. K., Cederbaum, J. A., & O'Leary, A. (2008). Sexually transmitted infection/HIV risk reduction interventions in clinical practice settings. *Journal of Obstetric, Gynecologic, and Neonatal Nursing, 37*, 137–145.

Jemmott, L. S., Jemmott, J. B. III, & O'Leary, A. (2007). Effects on sexual risk behavior and STD rate of brief HIV/STD prevention interventions for African American women in primary care settings. *American Journal of Public Health, 97*, 1034–1040.

Jordan, J. V., Kaplan, A., Miller, J. B., Stiver, I., & Surrey, J. (1991). *Women's growth in connection: Writings from the Stone Center*. New York, NY: Guilford Press.

Jordan, J. V. (1997). *Women's growth in diversity: More writings from the Stone Center*. New York, NY: Guilford Press.

Jordan, J. V. (2010). *Relational-cultural therapy*. Washington, DC: American Psychological Association.

Kaufert, P. A., & Lock, M. (1997). Medicalization of women's third age. *Journal of Psychosomatic Obstetrics and Gynecology, 18*(2), 81–86.

Kazanjian, A., & Hankivsky, O. (2008). Reflections on the future of women's health research in a comparative context: Why more than sex and gender matters. *Women's Health Issues, 18*, 343–346.

Killien, M., Bigby, J. A., Champion, V., Fernandez-Repollet, E., Jackson, R. D., Kagawa-Singer, M.,…Prout, M. (2000). Involving minority and underrepresented women in clinical trials: The National Centers of Excellence in Women's Health. *Journal of Women's Health and Gender-based Medicine, 9*, 1061–1070.

Kirchberger, K., Heier, M., Kuch, B., Wende, R., & Meisinger, C. (2011). Sex differences in patient-reported symptoms associated with myocardial infarction (from the population-based MONICA/KORA Myocardial Infarction Registry). *American Journal of Cardiology, 107*, 1585–1589.

Krieger, N. (2003). Genders, sexes, and health: What are the connections—and why does it matter? *International Journal of Epidemiology, 32*, 652–657.

Langer, A., Meleis, A., Knaul, F. M., Atun, R., Aran, M., Arreola-Omelas, H.,…Frenk, J. (2015). Women and health: The key for sustainable development. *Lancet, 386*(9999), 1165–1210.

Leavitt, J. W. (1984). *Women and health in America*. Madison, WI: University of Wisconsin Press.

Leurent, G., Garlantezec, R., Auffret, V., Hacot, J. P., Coudert, I., Filippi, E.,…LeBreton, H. (2014). Gender differences in presentation, management and inhospital outcome in patients with ST-segment elevation myocardial infarction: Data from 5000 patients included in the ORBI prospective French regional registry. *Archives of Cardiovascular Diseases, 107*, 291–298.

Li, W. W., & Froelicher, E. S. (2010). Predictors of smoking relapse in women with cardiovascular disease in a 30-month study: Extended analysis. *Heart and Lung, 37*, 455–465.

Long, S. K., Stockley, K., Birchfield, L., & Shulman, S. (2010). *The impacts of health reform on health insurance and health care access, use, and affordability for women in Massachusetts*. Boston, MA: Blue Cross Blue Shield of Massachusetts Foundation, Urban Institute.

Long, S. K., Stockley, K., & Shulman, S. (2011). Have gender gaps in insurance coverage and access to care narrowed under health reform? *American Economic Review, 101*, 640–644.

Marieskind, H. I. (1975). The women's health movement. *International Journal of Health Services, 5*(2), 217–223.

Mazure, C. M., Espeland, M., Douglas, P., Champion, V., & Killien, M. (2000). Multidisciplinary women's health research: The National Centers of Excellence in Women's Health. *Journal of Women's Health and Gender Based Medicine, 9*, 717–724.

McBride, A. B., & Mc Bride, W. L. (1983). Women's health scholarship: From critique to assertion. *Journal of Women's Health, 2*, 43–47.

McBride, A. B., & McBride, W. L. (1991). Theoretical underpinning for women's health. *Women and Health, 6*, 37–55.

Meleis, A. (2015). News from the International Council on Women's Health Issues: Barriers to the health of women. *Health Care for Women International, 36*, 965–968.

Miller, J. B. (1986). *Toward a new psychology of women.* Boston, MA: Beacon Press.

Miller, J. B. (2016). *The five good things.* Jean Baker Miller Training Institute. Retrieved from http://www.wellesley.edu/JBMTI/pdf/5goodthings.pdf

Miller, J. B., & Stiver, I. P. (1997). *The healing connection: How women develop relationships in therapy and in life.* Boston, MA: Beacon Press.

Milliken, N., Freund, K., Pregler, J., Reed, S., Carlson, K., Derman, R.,…McLaughlin, M. (2001). Academic models of clinical care for women: The National Centers of Excellence in Women's Health. *Journal of Women's Health and Gender-Based Medicine, 10*, 627–636.

Morgen, S., & Julier, A. (1991). *Women's health movement organizations: Two decades of struggle and change.* Eugene, OR: Center for the Study of Women in Society, University of Oregon.

National Institutes of Health (NIH). (1994). *NIH guidelines on the inclusion of women and minorities as subjects in clinical research.* Bethesda, MD: Office of Research on Women's Health.

National Institutes of Health (NIH) Tracking/Inclusion Committee. (2002, December). Monitoring adherence to the NIH policy on the inclusion of women and minorities as subjects in clinical research: Blue report. Retrieved from http://orwh.od.nih.gov/sexinscience/researchtrainingresources/scor_awards2012-2016.asp

National Prevention Council. (2011). *National prevention strategy: America's plan for better health and wellness.* Washington, DC: U.S. Department of Health and Human Services, Office of the Surgeon General.

Newton, K. M., Buist, D. S., Keenan, N. L., Anderson, L. A., & LaCroix, A. Z. (2002). Use of alternative therapies for menopause symptom: Results of a population-based survey. *Obstetrics and Gynecology, 100*(10), 18–25.

Nothnagle, M., Cappielllo, J., & Taylor, D. (2013). Sexual and Reproductive Health Workforce Project overview and recommendations from the SRH Workforce Summit, January 2013. *Contraception, 88*, 204–209.

Oakley, A., Addison, S., & Piran, N. (2004). *Brief psychotherapy centre for women: Results of a comprehensive two-year outcome study of a brief feminist relational-cultural model.* Poster session at the Jean Baker Miller Training Institute Research Forum, Wellesley, MA.

Paine, L. L., Dower, C. M., & O'Neil, E. H. (1999). Midwifery in the 21st century: Recommendations from the Pew Health Professions Commission/UCSF Center for the Health Professions 1998 Task Force on Midwifery. *Journal of Nurse-Midwifery, 44*(4), 341–348.

Pradel, F. G., Hartzema, A. G., Mutran, E. J., & Hanson-Divers, C. (1999). Physician over-the-counter drug prescribing patterns: An analysis of the National Ambulatory Medical Care Survey. *Annals of Pharmacotherapy, 33*(4), 400–405.

Rosen, W. B. (1997). *The integration of sexuality: Lesbians and their mothers.* In J. Jordan (Ed.), *Womens' growth in diversity.* New York, NY: Guilford Press.

Royal College of Nursing. (2009). *Sexual health competencies: An integrated career and competence framework for sexual and reproductive health nursing across the UK.* London, UK: Royal College of Nursing.

Ruiz, M. T., & Verbrugge, L. M. (1997). A two way view of gender bias in medicine. *Journal of Epidemiology and Community Health, 51*(2), 106–109.

Ruzek, C., Olesen, V., & Clarke, A. (Eds.). (1997). *Women's health: Complexities and differences.* Columbus, OH: Ohio State Press.

Ruzek, S. B. (1978). *The women's health movement: Feminist alternatives to medical control.* New York, NY: Praeger.

Salganicoff, A. (2015). Women and Medicare: An unfinished agenda. *Generations: Journal of the American Society on Aging, 39*, 43–49.

Scholle, S. H., Weisman, C. S., Anderson, R. T., & Camacho, F. (2004). The development and validation of the Primary Care Satisfaction Survey for Women. *Women's Health Issues, 14*, 35–50.

Scholle, S. H., Weisman, C. S., Anderson, R., Weitz, T., Freund, K. M., & Binko, J. (2000). Women's satisfaction with primary care: A new measurement effort from the PHS National Centers of Excellence in Women's Health. *Women's Health Issues, 10*(1), 1–9.

Schulman, K. A., Berlin, J. A., Harless, W., Kerner, J. F., Sistrunk, S., Gersh, B. J., Dube, R.,…Ayers, W. (1999). The effect of race and sex on physicians' recommendations for cardiac catheterization. *New England Journal of Medicine, 340*(8), 618–626.

Schwartz, L. M., Fisher, E. S., Tosteson, A. N., Woloshin, S., Chang, C. H., Virnig, B. A.,…Wright, B. (1997). Treatment and health outcomes of women and men in a cohort with coronary artery disease. *Archives of Internal Medicine, 157*(14), 1545–1551.

Scully, D. (1980). *Men who control women's health.* Boston, MA: Houghton Mifflin.

Scully, D., & Bart, P. (1973). A funny thing happened on the way to the orifice: Women in gynecology textbooks. *American Journal of Sociology, 78*(4), 1045–1050.

Seaman, B. (1972). *Free and female.* Greenwich, CT: Fawcett.

Sechrest, L. (1975). Ethical problems in medical experimentation involving women. In V. Olesen (Ed.), *Women and their health: Research implications for an era.* DHEW HRA 77–3138. Washington, DC: Department of Health, Education, and Welfare.

Shaver, J., Olshansky, E., Woods, N. F., for the Womens' Health Expert Panel of the American Academy of Nursing. (2013) Women's health research agenda for the next decade. A report by the Women's Health Expert Panel of the American Academy of Nursing. *Nursing Outlook, 61*, 16–24.

Tantillo, M., & Sanftner, J. (2003). The relational between perceived mutuality and bulimic symptoms, depression, and therapeutic change in group. *Eating Behaviors, 3*, 349–364.

Tatum, B. D. (1997). Racial identity development and relational theory: The case of Black women in White communities. In J. Jordan (Ed.), *Womens' growth in diversity.* New York, NY: Guilford Press.

Taylor, D., Olesen, V., Ruzek, C., & Clarke, A. (1977). Strengths and strongholds in women's health research. In C. Ruzek, V. Olesen, & A. Clarke, (Eds.), *Women's health: Complexities and differences* (pp. 580–606). Columbus, OH: Ohio State Press.

Taylor, D. L., & Woods, N. F. (1996). Changing women's health, changing nursing practice. *Journal of Obstetric, Gynecologic, and Neonatal Nursing, 25*(9), 791–802.

Taylor, D. L., & Woods, N. F. (2001). What we know and how we know it: Contributions from nursing to women's health research and scholarship. *Annual Review of Nursing Research, 19*, 3–28.

Teitelman, A. M., Tennille, J., Bohinski, J. M., Jemmott, L. S., & Jemmott, J. B. III. (2011). Unwanted unprotected sex: Condom coercion by male partners and self-silencing of condom negotiation among adolescent girls. *Advances in Nursing Science, 34*, 243–259.

Turner, C. W. (1997). Clinical applications of the Stone Center theoretical approach to minority women. In J. Jordan (Ed.), *Women's growth in diversity.* New York, NY: Guilford Press.

United States Reports. (1973). *Roe v. Wade*, 410 U.S. 113.

U.S. Department of Health and Human Services (USDHHS). (2000). *Healthy people 2010: Understanding and improving health.* Washington, DC: U.S. Government Printing Office.

U.S. Department of Health and Human Services (DHHS), Health Resources and Services Administration (HRSA), Office of Women's Health (OWH). (2013). *Women's health curricula: Final report on expert panel recommendations for interprofessional collaborations across the health professions.* Rockville, MD: U.S. Department of Health and Human Services.

U.S. Public Health Services (USPHS). (1992). *Opportunities for research on women's health.* Bethesda, MD: National Institutes of Health.

U.S. Public Health Services (USPHS). (1999). *Agenda for research on women's health for the 21st century: A report of the task forces on the NIH Women's Health Research Agenda for the 21st century.* Bethesda, MD: National Institutes of Health.

U.S. Public Health Services (USPHS). (2010). *Moving into the future with new dimensions and strategies: A vision for 2020 for women's health research.* Bethesda, MD: National Institutes of Health.

U.S. Public Health Services (USPHS). (2015). *Consideration of sex as a biological variable in NIH-funded research.* NOT-OD-15–103. Retrieved from http://grants.nih.gov/grants/guide/notice-files/NOT-OD-15-102.html

U.S. Public Health Services (USPHS) Task Force on Women's Health Issues. (1985). *Women's health: Report of the Public Health Service.* U.S. Department of Health and Human Services. Washington, DC: U.S. Public Health Service.

Walker, M., & Rosen, W. (2004). *How connections heal.* New York, NY: Guilford Press.

Washington, D. L., Bean-Mayberry, B., Hamilton, A. B., Cordasco, K. M., & Yano, E. M. (2013). Women veterans' healthcare delivery preferences and use by military service era: Findings from the National Survey of Women Veterans. *Journal of General Internal Medicine, 28*(Suppl. 2), S571–S576.

Washington, D. L., Bean-Mayberry, B., Mitchell, M. N., Riopelle, D., & Yano, E. M. (2011). Tailoring VA primary care to women veterans: Association with patient-rated quality and satisfaction. *Women's Health Issues, 21*(Suppl. 4), S112–S119.

Washington, D. L., Bean-Mayberry, B., Riopelle, D., & Yano, E. M. (2011). Access to care for women veterans: Delayed healthcare and unmet need. *Journal of General Internal Medicine, 26*(Suppl. 2), 655–661.

Weisman, C. S., Curbow, B., & Khoury, A. J. (1995). The national survey of women's health centers: Current models of women's centered care. *Women's Health Issues, 5*, 103–117.

Weisman, C. S., & Squires, G. L. (2000). Women's health centers: Are the National Centers of Excellence in Women's Health a new model? *Women's Health Issues, 10*, 248–255.

Wennberg, J., & Cooper, M. M. (Eds.). (1999). *The Dartmouth atlas of health care.* Washington, DC: American Hospital Publishing.

Wolf, N. (1997). *Promiscuities: The secret struggle for womanhood.* New York, NY: Random House.

Wood, S. F., Blehar, M. C., & Mauery, D. R. (2011). Policy implications of a new National Institutes of Health Agenda for Women's Health Research, 2010–2020. *Women's Health Issues, 21*, 99–103.

Woods, N. F. (1985). New models of women's health care. *Health Care for Women International, 6*, 193–208.

Woods, N. F. (1992). Future directions for women's health research. *NAACOG's Women's Health Nursing Scan, 6*(5), 1–2.

Woods, N. F. (2000). The U.S. women's health research agenda for the twenty-first century. *Signs: Journal of Women in Culture and Society, 25*(4), 1269–1274.

World Health Organization (WHO). (2010). *Sexual and reproductive health strategic plan 2010–2015 and proposed programme budget for 2010–2011.* Geneva, Switzerland: Author.

World Health Organization (WHO). (2011). *Sexual and reproductive health core competencies in primary care.* Geneva, Switzerland: Author.

Writing Group for the 1996 American Academy of Nursing Expert Panel on Women's Health Issues. (1997). Women's Health and women's health care: Recommendations of the 1996 AAN expert panel on Women's Health. *Nursing Outlook, 45*, 7–15.

Yano, E. M., Bastia, L. A., Bean-Mayberry, B, Eisen, S., Frayne, S., Hayes, P,…Washington, D. L. (2011). Using research to transform care for women veterans: Advancing the research agenda and enhancing research clinical partnerships. *Women's Health Issues, 21*(4S), S73–S83.

Yano, E. M., Bastian, L. A., Frayne, S. M., Howell, A., Lipson, L. R., McGlynn, G., & Fihn, S. D. (2006). Toward a VA women's health research agenda: Setting evidence-based priorities to improve the health and health care of women veterans. *Journal of General Internal Medicine, 21*(Suppl.), S93–S101.

Yano, E. M., Haskell, S., & Hayes, P. (2014). Delivery of gender-sensitive comprehensive primary care to women veterans: Implications for VA Patient Aligned Care Teams. *Journal of General Internal Medicine, 29*(Suppl. 2), S703–S707.

Zachar, P., & Kendler, K. S. (2014). A diagnostic and statistical manual of mental disorders history of premenstrual dysphoric disorder. *Journal of Nervous and Mental Disease, 202*, 346–352.

Zucker, I., & Beery, A. K. (2010). Males still dominate animal studies. *Nature, 465*(7299), 690.

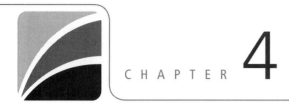

CHAPTER 4

Health Care for Vulnerable Populations

Cheryl L. Cooke • Selina A. Mohammed

Nursing has a long history of providing care to vulnerable populations. Nurse practitioner programs in the mid-1960s were instituted with a focus on training additional primary care providers whose work centered on caring for underserved and vulnerable populations (Van Zandt, Sloand, & Wilkins, 2008). Buerhaus, DesRoches, Dittus, and Donelan (2015) report that in a sample of 1,914 nurse practitioners and physicians whose practices are in primary care, nurse practitioners are more likely to care for racial/ethnic minority patients and patients who were uninsured. Understanding how to best care for vulnerable and underserved women and their families is an essential skill for nurse practitioners. In this chapter, we provide a brief overview describing who vulnerable women are, what their challenges are in society, and how these challenges affect their health. In addition, we discuss the social determinants of health and their effects on vulnerable populations. Finally, we conclude with a discussion on how providers can work with these populations to create solutions that include resilience and increase support in order to improve health outcomes for these women.

De Chesnay and Anderson (2008) describe vulnerability as existing on both individual and aggregate levels. The phrase *vulnerable populations* is used to denote those individuals or communities who experience "stress and anxiety" in any number of realms: sociocultural, environmental, psychological, and physical (De Santis, 2008, p. 275). Women of color, sexual minorities, low-income earners, women with low health literacy, homeless women, substance-using women, immigrants and refugees, and women with physical and/or mental disabilities are examples of vulnerable populations. However, it is important to note that these diverse populations experience vulnerability differently from one another. An example of this can be demonstrated with regard to income inequity. Although both African American and White women may be considered low income and unemployed, African American women will also suffer from the effects of historical racism when attempting to find employment, which can amplify their experience with income inequity, an effect of intersectionality. Intersectionality is a concept that describes how the effects of oppression,

discrimination, and/or racism can build one upon another and heighten their effects in the lives of women, including on their health status. Please refer to Chapter 6 of this text for a more detailed description of this concept.

■ SOCIOCULTURAL FRAMEWORK

Vulnerability and Social Determinants of Health

The social determinants of health are the social and material contexts in which people live, learn, work, and play (Robert Wood Johnson Foundation [RWJF], 2014). Vulnerable populations of women experience the effects of the social determinants of health in unique ways. Consider, for example, income inequality and pregnancy. Income inequality may affect how economically disadvantaged pregnant women access health care services. However, for economically disadvantaged African American women of childbearing years, a group of women with higher rates of preterm birth and low-birth-weight babies, it may also contribute to whether or not that child lives beyond its first year (Mustillo, Krieger, Gunderson, Sidney, & Kiefe, 2004). The outcome of these determinants for vulnerable populations is often captured by the terms *health disparities* and *health inequities*. Although the term *health disparities* has often been used to indicate health differences among all possible groups of people, as noted by Braveman (2014), it was intended to denote worse health among socially disadvantaged and vulnerable groups. In recognition of the relationship between living conditions and health, and the acknowledgment that these living conditions are often caused by societal injustices, the phrase *health inequities* has been increasingly used to move from the systematic health differences adversely affecting vulnerable and disadvantaged groups to a term that more explicitly links identified health differences to deeply rooted social, political, and economic injustices (Braveman et al., 2011; Falk-Rafael & Betker, 2012).

The effects of social determinants and vulnerability may be seen in many aspects of life through higher infant mortality rates, higher rates of interpersonal violence, lack of access to and lower quality of health care services (including substance abuse and mental health treatment), housing instability, socio-economic instability, and reduced life expectancy. The burden, or ability to manage their health successfully, can be greater for these groups of women. Furthermore, the social stigma that accompanies vulnerability is a complication that can limit a woman's ability to improve her health and/or social status.

Benoit, Shumka, and Barlee (2010) describe how social stigma is related to vulnerability in that stigma has been linked to social exclusion, which can be a situation that contributes to lower health outcomes. Individuals are seen as outside of social norms and may be labeled as "different" or "undesirable." This label contributes to negative stereotypes, and often leads to the woman and others identifying her predominantly through these stereotypes. This form of social distancing contributes to labeling and blaming, which leads to a loss of status and discriminatory acts against the woman. We sometimes refer to this as *marginalization*, which occurs when a group's worth is relegated from a more central position to that on the outer edges of society. The effects of marginalization can diminish the social or political impact an individual or a group can exercise to their benefit within society.

Women's Health and Vulnerability: The Challenge of Achieving Optimal Health Status

RACISM AND DISCRIMINATION

Racism and discrimination are deeply embedded in U.S. society. Most of the scientific community now views race as a social construct, rather than a biological marker of difference (Dominguez, 2008; Krieger, 2003). According to American Association of Physical Anthropologists (1996), "There is great genetic diversity in all human populations. Pure races, in the sense of genetically homogenous populations, do not exist in the human species today, nor is there any evidence that they have ever existed in the past" (p. 579). As socially constructed, individuals are understood in terms of racial/ethnic groups through self-identification and as others see that individual. Race can be used as a marker that allows for identifying, separating, and then marginalizing populations, often to their detriment. The term *racism* refers to an organized system categorizing groups of people into "races" in order to distribute goods and resources based on this social ranking (Bonilla-Silva, 1996). *Prejudice* can be defined as "learned prejudgment" about individuals from social groups to which we do not belong (Sensoy & DiAngelo, 2012, p. 28). Discrimination is acting on those prejudgments, to the detriment of nondominant groups (Sensoy & DiAngelo, 2012). Racism and discrimination need to be understood in terms of their structural effects. For example, racist and oppressive acts and behaviors and discriminatory policies within institutionalized social systems, such as education, health care, and economic settings, contribute to the long-term damage that low-income earners, people of color, and sexual minorities experience. Therefore racism must be understood as systems and as a population-level problem rather than as acts, beliefs, or behaviors acted out by problematic people on select individuals (Cooke, Bowie, & Carrère, 2014).

In a review of literature of empirical research on perceived discrimination and health, Williams and Mohammed (2009) found 115 articles in PubMed, during the 3-year period from 2005 to 2007 that empirically examined the association between a measure of perceived discrimination and an indicator of health or health care utilization. Although studies of mental health outcomes (e.g., anxiety and depression, life satisfaction, posttraumatic stress disorder [PTSD], and daily moods) and discrimination tended to dominate this literature, many of these articles also described an association between perceived discrimination and physical health (e.g., poor physical functioning, cardiac conditions, low birth weight, and prematurity).

In addition, links between perceived discrimination and health-seeking behaviors (e.g., delays in seeking treatment, nonadherence to treatment plans, provider trust, and perceptions of the quality of medical encounters) and lifestyle behaviors (e.g., alcohol, tobacco, and substance abuse, as well as risky sexual behaviors) were found (Williams & Mohammed, 2009). These outcomes and their links to perceived discrimination underscore the breadth and depth of how discrimination can negatively affect quality of life and overall health status.

INCOME INEQUALITY AND ITS EFFECTS ON HEALTH

Many of the challenges these particular populations of women face in their journey toward good health and well-being are linked to the effects of discrimination, income inequality, and poor access to care and to the long-term effects of interpersonal violence. Income inequality is deeply connected to poor physical and mental health (Burns, 2015). Low levels of wealth are associated with poor health and health outcomes (Hajat, Kaufman, Rose, Siddiqi & Thomas, 2011), and net worth has been significantly associated with poor/fair health status between and within racial and ethnic groups (Pollack et al., 2013). Thinking about each of these conditions separately and through the lens of different populations of women may provide a greater understanding of the intricacies of how lower social status, health burden, and income disparity all contribute to poorer health outcomes. Each population is faced with different barriers to good health. We describe problems related to income inequality and health inequities and the effects of these problems on specific populations of women.

A by-product of income inequity is food insecurity, an issue that affects the health of low-income women and their families, and may be considered a risk factor for type 2 diabetes (Selingman, Bindman, Vittinghoff, Kanaya, & Kushel, 2007; Seligman, Jacobs, López, Tschann, & Fernandez, 2012). Acute changes in income are related to the severity of food insecurity in some low-income families (Loopstra & Tarasuk, 2013). In a sample of low-income patients from King County, Washington, food insecurity has been linked to depression, poor diabetes control, poor medication adherence, and depression (Silverman et al., 2015).

In low-income earners, some women with diabetes not only experienced issues with food insecurity, but also had transportation problems and at times, lacked the functional ability to put healthy food on the table (Cuesta-Briand, Saggers, & McManus, 2011).

The depth and breadth of income inequality provides a lens through which the provider can see the trade-offs that many patients are forced to make in an effort to meet the basic needs of maintaining food and shelter. The lack of transportation can also limit how a woman participates in her care. An appreciation for the complexities that income inequality adds to a woman's living situation also allows providers to better understand how poor and/or nonadherence to medical treatment or clinic follow-up may occur with this population and also why women in this situation may deem health care a lower priority.

WORKPLACE CHALLENGES AND WOMEN'S HEALTH

Women who are low-income earners are often dealing with workplace problems that can affect their ability to prioritize health care needs. Although women have steadily increased their presence in work that takes place outside of the home, they can often be found working in low-paying jobs that leave them vulnerable to workplace discrimination; lack of access to paid sick days, paid leave, or fair work schedules; challenges with finding high-quality child care; and lack of access to workplace-provided health insurance, retirement benefits, or comprehensive reproductive health services (Ben-Ishai, 2014; National Women's Law Center [NWLC], 2014). Although women encompass one half of all workers, they compose nearly two thirds of the 20 million workers in low-wage jobs in the United States. Low-wage occupations are described by the National Employment Law Project (NELP) as ranging from a median of approximately $7.69 to $13.83 per hour. These jobs include women working as childcare workers, maids, home health aides, and fast-food workers. Women older than 50 years compose 17% of the low-wage workforce, almost three times as numerous as men in their age group (NWLC, 2014). Nearly half of women in the low-wage workforce are women of color, and one third of all low-wage earners are mothers, with 40% of them having family incomes below the poverty level. Many women are working multiple and/or temporary jobs in order to meet their family's economic needs.

In an attempt to find work, low-income women often take positions in harsh work conditions that leave them susceptible to greater health problems. For example, in a study examining social disparities in the burden of occupational exposure, Quinn et al. (2007) found that individuals with lower wages were more likely to report chemical exposure, back pain, repetitive hand motions, and heavy lifting. In addition, there was an excess of exposure to job strain among women compared with men, when gender alone was used to explain exposure reporting.

In addition to working multiple jobs and working in harsh work environments, issues such as lack of high-quality affordable childcare because of volatile and nonstandard work schedules and inconsistent paychecks (e.g., instability in work hours causes a lack of stability in earned income) add additional stressors to these women's lives (Watson &

Swanberg, 2011). Nearly half of low-wage hourly workers lack control in scheduling their work hours and overtime and have no input into starting, quitting, or break times. In addition, 20% to 30% of low-wage hourly workers are required to work overtime with little or no notice. Approximately 25% of part-time, low-wage hourly workers are laid off or have a reduction in their work hours when demand for work is slow (Watson & Swanberg, 2011). These challenges create physical difficulties in maintaining a stable household, as well as adding stress because of income uncertainty.

All of these issues affect the amount of time that low-income women can dedicate to their own self-care. Women in this position are challenged with meeting basic needs versus focusing on health goals. This issue is compounded by the fact that women who suffer from income inequities cannot afford to engage in costly health-promotion behaviors (e.g., gym memberships, yoga classes) and may live in neighborhoods where these amenities do not exist. In addition, physical activity may be further hindered by problems in the built environment, such as lack of sidewalks and a lack of street lighting (DeGuzman, Merwin, & Bourguignon, 2013).

BARRIERS TO CARE IN RURAL COMMUNITIES

Another barrier to care for women is seeking care while living in a rural area. Transportation and long commutes may be an issue for women in rural areas, and limit their ability to seek care in a timely fashion. Lack of health care facilities and women's health specialists in rural communities poses an additional challenge. For example, travel times for mammography and ultrasound-imaging facilities are short for most women. Native American and rural women struggle with longer travel times for breast imaging services (Onega et al., 2014). Living in a rural area can impact both physical and psychosocial functioning, and may do so differentially. For example, Weaver, Himle, Taylor, Matusko, and Abelson (2015) found that non-Hispanic White women living in rural areas had significantly higher odds for lifetime and 12-month major depressive disorder (MDD) and mood disorders than urban African Americans. However, rural African American women had lower rates of lifetime and 12-month MDD than their urban counterparts. These differential outcomes may be indicative of the added burden of race, and the influence of this "difference" while living in an urban setting (Weaver et al., 2015).

Populations of color are also affected by lack of pharmacies in their neighborhoods, which can add to lack of medication adherence for chronic illnesses. Qato et al. (2014) examined the geographic accessibility of pharmacies, exploring the concept of whether pharmacy deserts exist. In Chicago, they found that there were more pharmacy deserts in segregated Black communities, low-income communities, and federally designated medically underserved communities in 2012 than in other areas.

INTIMATE PARTNER VIOLENCE

Intimate partner violence (IPV), also known as interpersonal violence, is a significant issue that affects more than 10 million people in the United States every year (Breiding, Basile, Smith, Black, & Mahendra, 2015). IPV, as defined by the Centers for Disease Control and Prevention (CDC), includes physical and sexual violence, stalking, and psychological aggression (including coercion) by a current or former intimate partner such as a spouse, boyfriend/girlfriend, dating partner, or ongoing sexual partner. Approximately one in four women experience severe physical violence from an intimate partner at some point in her life. One in eleven women has been raped by a current or former partner at some point in her life. It is important to understand that women and sexual minorities not only experience IPV while residing in the same household as their partners, but also experience IPV while living away from the violent partner. Using threats and intimidation around sexual activity, administering drugs or alcohol, and/or taking advantage of a woman while they are unable to consent are all forms of IPV.

People with disabilities experience interpersonal violence at higher rates than people without disabilities, with nearly 1.3 million violent victimizations in 2013 (Harnell, 2015). Rates of serious violence victimization, such as rape and sexual assault, are more than three times higher for persons with disabilities than the age-adjusted rate for persons without disabilities (e.g., with 14 per 1,000 assaults vs. 4 per 1,000 assaults for nondisabled people). Research suggests that women with disabilities report abuse that lasts longer and is more intense than women without disabilities (Violence Against Women, 2015).

Violence during pregnancy may be more common than other problems for which pregnant women are usually screened. Approximately 324,000 pregnant women experience interpersonal violence each year, which is more than likely an underestimate, as most incidents are never reported (American College of Obstetricians and Gynegologists and Centers for Disease Control and Prevention Work Group on the Prevention of Violence During Pregnancy, 2013). Nearly 75% of women receive prenatal care in their first trimester (Osterman, Martin, Matthews, & Hamilton, 2011). These visits represent opportunities for providers to assess for interpersonal violence multiple times throughout a woman's pregnancy. If asked about interpersonal violence, a pregnant woman may be more inclined to report the violence in a desire to protect their child from future abuse (Deshpande & Lewis-O'Connor, 2013) than she might be at other times. However, the reverse is also true: A woman may feel compelled to hide the violence if she has few resources and depends on the perpetrator for economic and social support. Therefore assessment of pregnant women for interpersonal violence is essential and in many events, may be lifesaving for the woman and her child.

Interpersonal violence also has been associated with poor mental health, HIV and other sexually transmitted infections (STIs), and substance abuse. Mental health issues such as depression, anxiety, PTSD, sleep disturbances, and suicidal tendencies are commonly associated with IPV. Findings from systematic reviews and meta-analyses indicate that depression is the most common mental health problem in women experiencing IPV (Mason & Du Mont, 2015; Sabri et al., 2013). Women who have experienced IPV develop HIV and STIs 1.5 to 1.8 times more frequently than women who have not been abused. In addition, women who are abused are almost twice as likely to have an alcohol-use disorder than nonabused women (Mason & Du Mont, 2015).

■ DISCUSSION

What Nurses Can Do

Recognizing the many risk factors of vulnerable women is key to providing support and useful interventions to improve their health. Providers need to view each health encounter as an opportunity to assess women for problems associated with the social determinants of health and the way they interact specifically for each client to affect physical and mental health. There are often multiple problems associated with the social determinants of health in women's lives, and therefore it is important to consider the context within which a woman's health is shaped and maintained.

In the clinic, providers can begin with keen assessments for problems associated with determinants of health such as racial/ethnic discrimination, income inequity, workplace problems, challenges associated with rural living, and issues of interpersonal violence and safety. Once these have been identified as problems the woman is struggling with, appropriate resources must be located and offered. Numerous clinical tools are available to assess women's health, including the CAGE assessment for alcohol use, PHQ-9 to assess for depression, and multiple tools to assess for interpersonal violence available through the CDC (Basile, Hertz, & Back, 2007; Ewing, 1984). Identification of appropriate referrals to social service agencies to assist with applications for programs that provide low-income housing and temporary assistance for needy families (for financial support) is essential. Food security issues can be addressed through federal programs such as the Women, Infant, and Children (WIC) program, local food banks, and an assessment of school meal programs for children.

Women experiencing interpersonal violence and substance-use issues have suggested several ways providers may help them deal with these problems. For example, survivors spoke of working with professionals trained to identify and acknowledge the abuse, and of having safety be recognized as an important intervention. They also suggest that mental health providers focus on both treating the mental illness and exploring the underlying experiences in their lives that have contributed to their current situation and diagnoses and then provide the culturally sensitive care needed for diverse populations (Mason & Du Mont, 2015; Sabri et al., 2013).

Racial and ethnic discrimination must also be addressed, particularly if the provider hopes to better understand the health of women and sexual minorities of color. Understanding the burden of health risks that exists for women of color allows the provider to more closely follow the client and offer a higher level of support. For example, a major predictive risk factor for preterm birth in the United States is being African American. These women are at risk for low-birth-weight babies, preterm labor, and child mortality before first birthdays (Giurgescu, McFarlin, Lomax, Craddock, & Albrecht, 2011). Differences in stressful life events, differences in socioeconomic status (SES), and exposure to racial discrimination and unfair treatment all have an effect on the racial differences in health outcomes (Schulz et al., 2000). Having a sense of the challenges faced by Black women in everyday life, such as unconscious behavior, microaggressions, "daily slights," and overt racism, may allow the provider to work with the client to manage daily stress (Burrow & Hill, 2012; Carter, 2007; Jernigan & Daniel, 2011).

An additional way that women's health providers can improve their understanding of the lives of vulnerable women includes learning the histories of the populations for which they are caring. The experiences of women of color, immigrant women, women with disabilities, and rural women often provide a nontraditional view of life in the United States that may be unfamiliar to providers, who often have a higher SES, who have full access to health care services, and who may not experience racial or ethnic discrimination in their daily lives. Sometimes, this history can be transmitted by working with these populations in nonprofessional situations such as volunteering in disparate communities, participating on health services boards, and attending community functions outside of a provider's own community.

Exploring diverse topics in patient education can be a way to increase the level of trust between a provider and a vulnerable woman. Discussing health topics specific to these clients allows the client to see that the provider is not only interested in the present health problems, but has a more global sense of the woman's world. Being available to women and sexual minorities as a topic expert allows the client and their community to broaden their understandings of health. It also aids the community in building capacity through an increased access to health education and health systems knowledge.

Although invulnerability is the opposite of vulnerability, resilience is also a powerful concept. Vulnerable women are able to demonstrate flexibility and resilience in spite of, and possibly as a result of, experiencing challenging life circumstances. These women are not victims, but rather survivors, of difficult life circumstances. Keeping an open mind about how these women approach their health care needs, and the reasons that they may make certain choices with regard to their health provides another opportunity to create a trusting and safe environment for these populations.

◼ FUTURE DIRECTIONS

A Focus on Social Justice

On a broader level, providers can be involved in patient advocacy and social justice. Providers who engage in advocacy can use their roles to support and champion the rights and interests of their clients (Zolnierek, 2012). This advocacy needs to occur in both the individual and the social realms. Because many root causes and drivers of health stem from social determinants, advocating for a change in social realms and fighting for social justice are imperative to the holistic provision of care. According to Thompson (2014), *social justice* may be defined as:

(a) interventions focused on social, political, economic, and environmental factors that systematically disadvantage individuals and groups; and (b) intervening in the effects of power, race, gender, and class where these and other structural relations intersect to create avoidable disparities and inequities in health for individuals, groups, or communities. (p. E18)

Thus social justice involves examining the ways that patterns of privileges and disadvantage are created and sustained in society, as well as challenging this status quo.

Nurses are in a prime position to advocate for the health of their clients and for social justice. Several nursing and health organizations have charged nurses to engage in social advocacy and social justice. For example, the World Health Organization (WHO) has emphasized the critical role that nurses and other health care providers have in achieving health equity through social justice (WHO, 2008). Viewing the pursuit of health equity as the ethical and moral responsibility of all nurses, the American Association of Colleges of Nursing (AACN) has created a series of *Essentials* documents that nursing schools use to meet accreditation guidelines. The requirement of social justice advocacy in the education of all levels of nursing is evident in these documents (AACN, 1996, 2006, 2008, 2011).

Providers' knowledge of the social determinants of health and participation in activities that promote policy change can significantly improve the lives of their clients. Voting, awareness in changes in health care policy and financing, lobbying activities directed toward issues that affect health and health care, and civic engagement are crucial to eliminating health inequities. Partnerships among clients, providers, communities, and legislative bodies can effect lasting change in the health care system.

◼ REFERENCES

American Association of Colleges of Nursing (AACN). (1996). *The essentials of master's education for advanced practice nursing.* Retrieved from http://www.aacn.nche.edu/education-resources/essential-series

American Association of Colleges of Nursing (AACN). (2006). *The essentials of doctoral education for advanced nursing practice.* Retrieved from http://www.aacn.nche.edu/education-resources/essential-series

American Association of Colleges of Nursing (AACN). (2008). *The essentials of baccalaureate for professional nursing practice.* Retrieved from http://www.aacn.nche.edu/education-resources/essential-series

American Association of Colleges of Nursing (AACN). (2011). *The essentials of master's education in nursing.* Retrieved from http://www.aacn.nche.edu/education-resources/MastersEssentials11.pdf

American Association of Physical Anthropologists. (1996). Biological aspects of race. *American Journal of Physical Anthropology, 101,* 569–570. Retrieved from http://physanth.org/about/position-statements/biological-aspects-race

Basile, K. C., Hertz, M. F., & Back, S. E. (2007). *Intimate partner violence and sexual violence victimization assessment instruments for use in healthcare settings: Version 1.* Atlanta, GA: Centers for Disease Control and Prevention, National Center for Injury Prevention and Control.

Ben-Ishai, L., Matthews, H., & Levin-Epstein, J. (2014). *Scrambling for stability: The challenge of job schedule volatility and child care.* Washington, DC: Center for Law and Social Policy (CLASP).

Benoit, C., Shumka, L., & Barlee, D. (2010). *Stigma and the health of vulnerable women.* Vancouver, Canada: Women's Health Research Network.

Bonilla-Silva, E. (1996). Rethinking racism: Toward a structural interpretation. *American Sociological Review, 62*(June), 465–480.

Braveman, P. (2014). What are health disparities and health equity? We need to be clear. *Public Health Reports, 129*(Suppl. 2), 5–8.

Braveman, P. A., Kumanyika, S., Fielding, J., Laveist, T., Borrell, L. N., Manderscheid, R., & Troutman, A. (2011). Health disparities and health equity: The issue is justice. *American Journal of Public Health, 101*(Suppl. 1), S149–S155. doi:10.2105/AJPH.2010.300062

Breiding, M. J., Basile, K. C., Smith, S. G., Black, M. C., & Mahendra, R. R. (2015). *Intimate partner violence surveillance: Uniform definitions and recommended data elements, version 2*. Atlanta, GA: Centers for Disease Control and Prevention, National Center for Injury Prevention and Control.

Buerhaus, P. I., DesRoches, C. M., Dittus, R., & Donelan, K. (2015). Practice characteristics of primary care nurse practitioners and physicians. *Nursing Outlook*, 63(2), 144–153.

Burns, J. K. (2015). Poverty, inequality and a political economy of mental health. *Epidemiology and Psychiatric Sciences*, 24(2), 107–113.

Burrow, A. L., & Hill, P. L. (2012). Flying the unfriendly skies? The role of forgiveness and race in the experience of racial microaggressions. *Journal of Social Psychology*, 152(5), 639–653.

Carter, R. (2007). Racism and psychological and emotional injury: Recognizing and assessing race-based traumatic stress. *Counseling Psychology*, 35(1), 13.

Cooke, C. L., Bowie, B. H., & Carrère, S. (2014). Perceived discrimination and children's mental health symptoms. *Advances in Nursing Science*, 37(4), 299–314.

Cuesta-Briand, B., Saggers, S., & McManus, A. (2011). "You get the quickest and the cheapest stuff you can": Food security issues among low income earners living with diabetes. *The Australasian Medical Journal*, 4(12), 683–691.

de Chesnay, M., & Anderson, B. (2008). *Caring for the vulnerable: Perspectives in nursing theory, practice and research*. Sudbury, MA: Jones & Bartlett.

DeGuzman, P. B., Merwin, E. I., & Bourguignon, C. (2013). Population density, distance to public transportation, and health of women in low-income neighborhoods. *Public Health Nursing*, 30(6), 478–490.

De Santis, J. (2008). Exploring the concepts of vulnerability and resilience in the context of HIV infection. *Research and Theory for Nursing Practice*, 22(4), 273–287.

Deshpande, N. A., & Lewis-O'Connor, A. (2013). Screening for intimate partner violence during pregnancy. *Reviews in Obstetrics and Gynecology*, 6(3–4), 141–148.

Dominguez, T. P. (2008). Race, racism, and racial disparities in adverse birth outcomes. *Clinical Obstetrics and Gynecology*, 51(2), 360–370.

Ewing, J. A. (1984). Detecting alcoholism. The CAGE questionnaire. *Journal of the American Medical Association*, 252(14), 1905–1907.

Falk-Rafael, A., & Betker, C. (2012). Witnessing social injustice downstream and advocating for health equity upstream: "The trombone slide" of nursing. *Advances in Nursing Science*, 35(2), 98–112.

Giurgescu, C., McFarlin, B. L., Lomax, J., Craddock, C., & Albrecht, A. (2011). Racial discrimination and the black-white gap in adverse birth outcomes: A review. *Journal of Midwifery & Women's Health*, 56(4), 362–370.

Hajat, A., Kaufman, J. S., Rose, K. M., Siddiqi, A., & Thomas, J. C. (2011). Long-term effects of wealth on mortality and self-rated health status. *American Journal of Epidemiology*, 173(2), 192–200.

Harnell, E. (2015). *Crimes against persons with disabilities, 2009–2013—statistical tables*. Washington, DC: U.S. Department of Justice, Bureau of Justice Statistics.

Jernigan, M. M., & Daniel, J. H. (2011). Racial trauma in the lives of Black children and adolescents: Challenges and clinical implications. *Journal of Child and Adolescent Trauma*, 4, 123–141.

Krieger, N. (2003). Does racism harm health? Did child abuse exist before 1962? On explicit questions, critical science, and current controversies: An ecosocial perspective. *American Journal of Public Health*, 93(2), 194–199.

Loopstra, R., & Tarasuk, V. (2013). Severity of household food insecurity is sensitive to change in household income and employment status among low-income families. *Journal of Nutrition*, 143(8), 1316–1323.

Mason, R., & Du Mont, J. (2015). Advancing our knowledge of the complexity and management of intimate partner violence and co-occurring mental health and substance abuse problems in women. *Faculty 1000 Prime Reports*, 7(65). doi: 10.12703/P7-65. Retrieved from http://f1000.com/prime/reports/m/7/65

Mustillo, S., Krieger, N., Gunderson, E. P., Sidney, S., McCreath, H., & Kiefe, C. I. (2004). Self-reported experiences of racial discrimination and Black-White differences in preterm and low-birthweight deliveries: The CARDIA Study. *American Journal of Public Health*, 94(12), 2125–2131.

National Women's Law Center (NWLC). (2014). *Underpaid & overloaded: Women in low-wage jobs*. Washington, DC: National Women's Law Center.

Onega, T., Hubbard, R., Hill, D., Lee, C. I., Haas, J. S., Carlos, H. A.,... Tosteson, A. N. (2014). Geographic access to breast imaging for US women. *Journal of the American College of Radiology*, 11(9), 874–882.

Osterman, M. J. K., Martin, J. A., Matthews, T. J., & Hamilton, B. E. (2011). Expanded data from the new birth certificate data, 2008. *National Vital Statistics Reports*, 59(7). Hyattsville, MD: National Center for Health Statistics.

Pollack, C. E., Cubbin, C., Sania, A., Hayward, M., Vallone, D., Flaherty, B., & Braveman, P. A. (2013). Do wealth disparities contribute to health disparities within racial/ethnic groups? *Journal of Epidemiology and Community Health*, 67(5), 439–445.

Qato, D. M., Daviglus, M. L., Wilder, J., Lee, T., Qato, D., & Lambert, B. (2014). "Pharmacy deserts" are prevalent in Chicago's predominantly minority communities, raising medication access concerns. *Health Affairs (Project Hope)*, 33(11), 1958–1965.

Quinn, M. M., Sembajwe, G., Stoddard, A. M., Kriebel, D., Krieger, N., Sorensen, G.,...Barbeau, E. M. (2007). Social disparities in the burden of occupational exposures: Results of a cross-sectional study. *American Journal of Industrial Medicine*, 50(12), 861–875.

Robert Wood Johnson Foundation (RWJF). (2014). *Social determinants of health*. Retrieved from http://www.rwjf.org/en/our-topics/topics/social-determinants-of-health.html

Sabri, B., Bolyard, R., McFadgion, A. L., Stockman, J. K., Lucea, M. B., Callwood, G. B.,...Campbell, J. C. (2013). Intimate partner violence, depression, PTSD, and use of mental health resources among ethnically diverse black women. *Social Work in Health Care*, 52(4), 351–369.

Seligman, H. K., Bindman, A. B., Vittinghoff, E., Kanaya, A. M., & Kushel, M. B. (2007). Food insecurity is associated with diabetes mellitus: Results from the National Health Examination and Nutrition Examination Survey (NHANES) 1999–2002. *Journal of General Internal Medicine*, 22(7), 1018–1023.

Seligman, H. K., Jacobs, E. A., López, A., Tschann, J., & Fernandez, A. (2012). Food insecurity and glycemic control among low-income patients with type 2 diabetes. *Diabetes Care*, 35(2), 233–238.

Sensoy, O., & DiAngelo, R. (2012). *Is everyone really equal? An introduction to key concepts in social justice education*. New York, NY: Teachers College Press.

Schulz, A., Israel, B., Williams, D., Parker, E., Becker, A., & James, S. (2000). Social inequalities, stressors and self reported health status among African American and white women in the Detroit metropolitan area. *Social Science & Medicine (1982)*, 51(11), 1639–1653.

Silverman, J., Krieger, J., Kiefer, M., Hebert, P., Robinson, J., & Nelson, K. (2015). The relationship between food insecurity and depression, diabetes distress and medication adherence among low-income patients with poorly-controlled diabetes. *Journal of General Internal Medicine*, 30(10), 1476–1480.

Thompson, J. L. (2014). Discourses of social justice: Examining the ethics of democratic professionalism in nursing. *Advances in Nursing Science*, 37(3), E17–E34.

Van Zandt, S. E., Sloand, E., & Wilkins, A. (2008). Caring for vulnerable populations: Role of academic nurse-managed health centers in educating nurse practitioners. *Journal of Nurse Practitioners*, 4(2), 127–131.

Violence Against Women. (2015). WomensHealth.gov. Retrieved from http://www.womenshealth.gov/violence-against-women/types-of-violence/violence-against-women-with-disabilities.html

Watson, L., & Swanberg, J. (2011). *Flexible workplace solutions for low-wage hourly workers: A framework for a national conversation*. Louisville, KY: University of Kentucky.

Weaver, A., Himle, J. A., Taylor, R. J., Matusko, N. N., & Abelson, J. M. (2015). Urban vs. rural residence and the prevalence of depression and mood disorder among African American women and non-Hispanic White women. *Journal American Medical Association Psychiatry*, 72(6), 576–583. doi:10.1001/jamapsychiatry.2015.10

Williams, D. R., & Mohammed, S. A. (2009). Discrimination and racial disparities in health: Evidence and needed research. *Journal of Behavioral Medicine*, 32(1), 20–47.

World Health Organization (WHO). (2008) *Primary health care: Now more than ever*. Retrieved from http://www.who.int/whr/2008/en

Zolnierek, C. (2012). Speak to be heard: Effective nurse advocacy. *American Nurse Today*, 7(10). Retrieved from http://www.americannursetoday.com/speak-to-be-heard-effective-nurse-advocacy

CHAPTER 5

Legal Issues in Women's Health Care

Anna G. Small

The unique facets of women's sexual and reproductive health care are complemented and complicated by legal issues. The legal system, like the health care system, can be challenging to navigate, and health care consumers, providers, and institutions may become overwhelmed when the two intersect. This chapter provides an overview of key legal issues in women's health care so that the reader can navigate the complicated intersection of law and health care.

■ SOCIOCULTURAL CONTEXT

A provider of women's health care should have an understanding for the societal and legal context in which care is provided. At one time, in the not so distant past, access to contraception was seriously limited for most American women. Birth control was illegal in most states; therefore women experienced significant challenges when trying to make choices concerning their fertility. The conversation became: Do married couples, extending to unmarried couples, have the right to decide whether to use contraception while engaging in private acts?

Contraception and a Right to Privacy

Into the 1960s, the state of Connecticut prohibited the use of any drug, medicinal article, or instrument for the purpose of preventing conception (*Griswold v. Connecticut*, 1965). Despite this, Planned Parenthood opened a contraceptive clinic in New Haven, Connecticut, and began to provide birth control to married women. Estelle Griswold, who was the executive director of the clinic, and Dr. Buxton, the medical director of the clinic, were arrested and charged with a misdemeanor related to their work. They appealed their convictions and challenged the validity of the law prohibiting contraception. They were ultimately able to convince the U.S. Supreme Court that the law violated married couples' right to privacy (*Griswold v. Connecticut*, 1965).

The Supreme Court held that married couples had the right to decide whether to use contraception while engaging in private acts. To rule otherwise would be to invade marital privacy. The Court's opinion was significant for two reasons. First, it permitted at least married women to obtain contraception. Second, it established that the right to privacy is a fundamental right even though it is not specifically mentioned in the U.S. Constitution; the right to privacy is in the penumbras of the Constitution. The establishment of privacy as a fundamental right has been the justification for the findings of many courts since that time.

A few years after the landmark case in Connecticut, a Massachusetts case came before the Supreme Court and extended the right to privacy related to contraceptive choice to unmarried women (*Eisenstadt v. Baird*, 1972). The Court held that it was irrational to permit married women the right to use contraception but not to permit unmarried women the same right. Using the equal protection clause of the U.S. Constitution, the Court established that unmarried couples have the same right to contraception as married couples (*Eisenstadt v. Baird*, 1972).

This right to privacy first articulated by the Court in *Griswold* has been relied on by many courts since that time. Citing a right to privacy, the Supreme Court struck down a law prohibiting the distribution of birth control to women younger than 16 years (*Carey v. Population Services*, 1977). In *Moore v. the City of East Cleveland* (1977), it struck down a law prohibiting extended families from living in a single household. In *Roe v. Wade* (1973) the Supreme Court struck down a law prohibiting abortion, and in *Loving v. Virginia* (1967), it struck down a law prohibiting inter-racial marriage. In *Lawrence v. Texas* (2003), the Court struck down laws that attempted to limit consenting adults' right to engage in homosexual sex. All of the decisions in these cases acknowledged that, based on the facts presented, an individual's right to privacy trumps the state's interest in proscribing the behavior in question.

▪ DISCUSSION

The Supreme Court's decisions such as *Griswold* have significance to women's health care because it began to establish a woman's right to control her own fertility, but it also established a "zone of privacy" in which the state has no right to interfere. These concepts have since been extended to permit unmarried women to obtain birth control, live with the relatives they choose, and marry whomever they want and has been used to support the rights of couples to engage in same-sex sexual relationships.

Right to Contraception Today

Most American women take access to contraception for granted. It is interesting to note that the average American woman desires two children and spends approximately 3 years of her life pregnant, in the postpartum period, or trying to get pregnant and, consequently, three quarters of her reproductive life trying not to get pregnant (Publicly Funded, 2015). It is no surprise that access to and funding for contraception is a critical issue in women's health. It is estimated that every year, half of all pregnancies in the United States are unintended and that, by age 45, four in 10 women have had an abortion (Publicly Funded, 2015).

In 2010, $2.37 billion was spent on contraception, 75% of which were Medicaid dollars (Publicly Funded, 2015). The Patient Protection and Affordable Care Act (ACA) contains a "contraceptive mandate," which means that private insurance plans (most often provided through employers) must cover, without co-pay or co-insurance, all forms of contraception approved by the U.S. Food and Drug Administration, including sterilization procedures ("Contraceptive Use," 2015).

There have been legal challenges to this contraceptive mandate, with various employers arguing that they have moral or religious objections to providing contraception to women through employer-sponsored plans. Hobby Lobby, a chain of hobby and craft stores owned by a single extended family, challenged the contraceptive mandate and argued that it violated the family's evangelical Christian beliefs. The case was heard by the Supreme Court, and a closely divided Court opined that it was a violation of the Religious Freedom Restoration Act to require certain closely held corporations to comply with the rules promulgated by the U.S. Department of Health and Human Services intended to implement the contraceptive mandate (*Burwell v. Hobby Lobby Stores, Inc.*, 2014).

The result of the *Hobby Lobby* decision is that women who work for employers who are closely held corporations and who have a religious or moral objection to the contraceptive mandate could have no access to contraception like their counterparts who work for other organizations. The Department of Health and Human Services has recently promulgated new rules that attempt to prevent the expansion of the Supreme Court's decision to companies that are not closely held. In addition, the new rules attempt to provide access to contraception for those women who work for the closely held corporations with objections (The Center for Consumer Information & Insurance Oversight [CCIIO], n.d.). Contraception and other preventive health services will be available to female employees of qualified objecting organizations at no cost to the organization or the women.

Women's Access to Legal Abortion

Abortion, in one form or another, has always been available to women who have had unwanted pregnancies. Before approximately 1880, abortion was unregulated in the United States. Slowly the individual states began to make abortion illegal with limited exceptions. Of course, women still obtained abortions, but because of illegal nature of these abortions, they were frequently unsafe or even self-induced (Our Bodies, Ourselves, 2014).

In 1970, Jane Roe brought suit challenging the constitutionality of the Texas law prohibiting abortion, except in cases where the life of the mother was endangered (*Roe v. Wade*, 1973). Roe stated that she was pregnant and unmarried and wanted to end her pregnancy in an abortion but was prohibited from doing so in violation of her constitutional right to privacy. The Supreme Court found that there was a right to privacy granted by the U.S. Constitution that was not explicit, but rather found in the penumbras of the Constitution. By this, the Court meant that the right to privacy and the freedom to make decisions around reproductive rights is found between the lines or implied in the Constitution.

The Court felt, however, that a woman's right to get an abortion is not unlimited. The states have a compelling interest in imposing certain restrictions on abortion. The Court opined that a "State may properly assert important interests in safeguarding health, in maintaining medical standards, and in protecting potential life" (*Roe v. Wade*, 1973). Thus states have the right to restrict and regulate abortion in the second trimester in "ways that are reasonably related to maternal health" (*Roe v. Wade*, 1973, p. 164). After

> viability, the State in promoting its interest in the potentiality of human life may, if it chooses, regulate, and even proscribe, abortion except where it is necessary, in appropriate medical judgment, for the preservation of the life or health of the mother.

In the early 1970s, viability was considered to occur at approximately 28 weeks of gestation, which corresponds to the beginning of the third trimester of pregnancy.

Although the Supreme Court's written opinion in *Roe v. Wade* acknowledges a woman's right to choose and a woman's right to privacy, it also acknowledges the right of physicians to make these decisions with their patients. The Court stated that during the first trimester, "the abortion decision and its effectuation must be left to the medical judgment of the pregnant woman's attending physician" (p. 163). Additionally, the Court wrote:

> The decision vindicates the right of the physician to administer medical treatment according to his professional judgment up to the points where important state interests provide compelling justifications for intervention. Up to those points, the abortion decision in all its aspects is inherently, and primarily, a medical decision, and basic responsibility for it must rest with the physician. (*Roe v. Wade*, 1973, pp. 165–166)

Although the Court did protect a woman's right to choose, it also showed deference to physician's medical decision making and acknowledged that its decision affected not only the rights of women, but also the rights of physicians to treat their patients as they see fit, preserving the significance of the physician–patient relationship.

Also of interest is that the Supreme Court declined to opine on the definition of personhood or when life begins. Justice Harry Blackmun wrote that since the members of the fields of medicine and philosophy were unable to agree on when life begins, it is a topic the judiciary is not competent to tackle (*Roe v. Wade*, 1973).

The decision in *Roe v. Wade* is significant to women's health care because it has been the law for more than 40 years and women have had the right to choose abortion, with some restrictions, for close to half a century. The decision also has substantial legal significance because the Court protected a right that is not found explicitly stated in the Constitution and with that implied right invalidated laws about abortion in almost every state. Many scholars look at *Roe v. Wade* as having triggered renewed interest in the roll of the courts in interpreting the Constitution.

PROGENY OF *ROE V. WADE*

Roe v. Wade has not permanently resolved the abortion debate, but rather, it has been followed by a significant number of legal cases that have attempted to limit the rights to abortion recognized by the Court. In legal parlance, the cases that come after a landmark case and refine the landmark decision are known as *progeny*. Over time, the Supreme Court has been called on to determine whether states have the right to impose certain restrictions on a woman's right to have an abortion. The Court has upheld some restrictions and struck down others, including those in the following list:

- A husband has no right to interfere in a decision regarding abortion when the decision was made between the wife and her physician. States may not require spousal notification or consent before abortion (*Planned Parenthood of Central Missouri v. Danforth* (1976); *Stenberg v. Carhart*, 2000).
- States may not prohibit specific procedures for used for abortion (i.e., saline amniocentesis and partial birth–abortion; *Planned Parenthood of Central Missouri v. Danforth*, 1976). However, after the federal Partial-Birth Abortion Ban Act of 2003 passed, the Supreme Court upheld its constitutionality and the ban on specific abortion procedures included therein (*Gonzalez v. Carhart*, 2006).
- States may not require that all abortions be performed in hospitals (*Doe v. Bolton*, 1973; *City of Akron v. Akron Center for Reproductive Rights*, 1983; *Planned Parenthood Association of Kansas City, Missouri, Inc. v. Ashcroft*, 1983).
- States may require that all second trimester abortions be performed either in a licensed outpatient clinic or a hospital (*Simopoulos v. Virginia*, 1983).
- Statutes requiring parental notification and consent have been struck down if there is no adequate provision for a judicial bypass. A judicial bypass provides a minor with the procedural option of going to court, generally before a probate judge, and seeking an order that she does not need to notify her parents or that she does not require their consent. Generally, the minor must show that she is mature enough to make the decision about having an abortion or that it is not in her best interest to notify or seek permission from her guardian (*Bellotti v. Baird*, 1979; *City of Akron*, 1983; *Danforth*, 1976; *Hodgson v. Minnesota*, 1990).
- States may impose parental notification and consent requirements on minors when there is an adequate judicial bypass option (*Hodgson*, 1990; *Ohio v. Akron Center for Reproductive Health*, 1990; *Planned Parenthood v. Casey*, 1992).
- States are not required to make public funds available to pay for abortions (*Harris v. McRae*, 1980; *Maher v. Roe,* 1977).
- States may impose a reasonable waiting period before an abortion is performed (24- to 48-hour waiting period is considered reasonable; *Planned Parenthood v. Casey*, 1992).
- The Supreme Court has declined to hear cases that are challenges to states' laws requiring the performance and explanation of an ultrasound before an abortion (Liptak, 2015).

To date, women in the United States have a legal right to choose abortion. Their right to choose is not unfettered, and states may impose reasonable restrictions on abortions as long as the law is designed to protect a compelling state interest. The debate regarding abortion continues and is far from being settled from a legal perspective. Every state's regulations regarding abortions are slightly different, so health care providers should take care to be knowledgeable regarding their state's specific requirements.

Reproductive Technology

Advances in technology and science now permit conception in situations when women were previously unable to conceive. Although the use of these technologies and techniques can be miraculous to a woman who desires a child, the path to motherhood can be fraught with unanticipated legal issues.

IN VITRO FERTILIZATION

In vitro fertilization (IVF) was invented to assist couples who were unable to conceive through traditional biological methods. Louise Joy Brown is considered to have been the first baby born alive as a result of IVF (James, 2013). Her parents, British citizens, had been trying to conceive a child for 9 years but were unable to do so through traditional methods, as her mother suffered from blocked fallopian tubes. In 2010, one of the physicians who developed the IVF technique was awarded the Nobel Prize in Physiology or Medicine for his work. Although IVF brought joy to the Brown family and to millions of other families around the world, some have been critical of the use of IVF because of some of the unintended consequences (James, 2013).

One use of IVF is to permit the screening of certain genetic attributes. Preimplantation genetic testing can be used for a number of reasons that are generally accepted. These include when one or both partners has a history of inheritable genetic disorders, one or both partners is a carrier of a chromosomal abnormality, the mother is of advanced maternal age, or the mother has a history of recurrent miscarriages. In these cases, preimplantation screening can be used to prevent the implantation of an embryo with a devastating condition.

There are, however, a number of preimplantation screening practices that many people find more questionable (Hens et al., 2012). Social sex selection is generally disfavored, as is the practice of creating "savior siblings." Although many consider it acceptable to screen for inheritable conditions, which would be devastating to the newborn, selecting against embryos with genes correlated with late-onset and nonfatal conditions is more problematic. Opponents argue that it is a slippery slope to designer children. The selection for purely cosmetic traits (e.g., eye color, hair color, and skin complexion) is generally considered unethical. In addition, advocates for the rights of the disabled argue that it is inappropriate to value certain lives over the lives of those with specific disabilities (Hens et al., 2012).

OWNERSHIP OF UNUSED EMBRYOS

During the IVF process, a larger number of embryos are created than will be implanted in order to avoid repeating the arduous harvesting process if the initial IVF procedure is unsuccessful. In general, no more than two or possibly three embryos are implanted in order to avoid the health risks of high-level multiples to both woman and fetuses. The embryos that are not immediately implanted are cryo-frozen. Some couples use these additional embryos if no embryos implant, and others use them for subsequent pregnancies. However, there are regularly embryos that remain, and debate has arisen as to what should be done with the embryos.

IVF has furthered the discussion of when life begins. The discussion is, at this point, an ethical and moral one that is not regulated. Courts have generally shied away from a legal determination of when life begins. As the Supreme Court stated:

> We need not resolve the difficult question of when life begins. When those trained in the respective disciplines of medicine, philosophy, and theology are unable to arrive at any consensus, the judiciary, at this point in the development of man's knowledge, is not in a position to speculate as to the answer. (*Roe v. Wade* 1973 , p. 159)

What courts have been forced to address is the ownership of the embryos and even the resultant children. In *Rodgers v. Fasano*, a couple conceived twins through IVF. However, when the twins were born, they were clearly of different racial origins. Genetic testing was done and it became clear that the fertility clinic made a mistake and implanted one of the Fasanos' embryos and one from an unrelated African American couple (*Rodgers v. Fasano*, 2000). A custody battle for the African American child ensued. The court "returned" the African American child to its biological parents and did not grant the Fasanos any visitation because it held that despite Mrs. Fasano acting as an unintentional surrogate, she had no legal right to the resultant child. The court discussed the issue of whether the embryos were persons or property.

In a highly publicized case, two celebrities engaged in a court battle over the right to use embryos after the couple's relationship ended. Nick Loeb publicly discussed the case of ownership of the two embryos created with his former fiancée Sofía Vergara when he published an opinion piece in the *New York Times* (Loeb, 2015). The couple created two female embryos, and Mr. Loeb has filed suit in California seeking permission to have the embryos implanted in a surrogate and then raise the resultant children. Ms. Vergara objects and apparently wants to leave the embryos frozen indefinitely. The issue before the court is either a custody battle over theoretical children or a dispute over ownership of property: the two embryos (*Doe v. Doe*, 2014).

To date, there is no legislation that addresses custody battles over theoretical children. The case filed by Mr. Loeb seeks a form of declaratory relief from the court. In these types of actions, parties seek a determination from a court regarding their legal rights before some irreversible action is taken. Mr. Loeb seeks first to have the court prohibit the company that has stored the embryos from destroying them. Then Mr. Loeb seeks to have the court determine that an agreement he and Ms. Vergara signed, which stated that neither party would use the embryos without the other's consent, is invalid (*Doe v. Doe*, 2014). Although the outcome of this highly public court case has not been resolved, it is not the first case where couples have had to try to battle out in court what will happen to stored embryos and certainly will not be the last time this issue arises.

Some legal scholars have argued that couples who voluntarily agree to have their gametes made into embryos no longer have a property right in the genetic information contained in the gamete. Thus an individual whose genetic information is contained in an embryo intended, or at one time intended, to be implanted via IVF, cannot prevent the implantation by arguing that they do not want to have a genetically related child brought into the world. Like gamete donation, or in unprotected intercourse, once the embryo has formed, property rights in the donor's genetic material is altered (Chan & Quigley, 2007).

Surrogacy Agreements

Some couples turn to surrogacy in order to reproduce. In such an arrangement, there are two women whose health care and legal rights may be at issue: the surrogate and the woman seeking to have a child. A surrogate arrangement may involve a variety of combinations of egg and sperm, making the legal issues even more confounding. A couple seeking to have a child may use their own egg and sperm and have the embryo implanted in a surrogate, or the couple may use a donor egg, donor sperm, or a donor embryo.

Surrogacy has been dealt with in a variety of ways by the states. In some it is considered illegal, whereas others have implemented legislation in an effort to control the commodification of sex, women, childbirth, and children, which can occur during surrogacy (Field, 2014).

One of the first legal cases that arose out of a surrogacy arrangement was *In re Baby M* (1988), when a married couple, William and Elizabeth Stern, contracted with Mary Beth Whitehead for Ms. Whitehead to serve as a surrogate. William's sperm was used to artificially inseminate Ms. Whitehead, so the resultant embryo had half its genetic material from William and half from Ms. Whitehead. Such arrangements are now known as *traditional surrogacy* (Field, 2014). In these arrangements, the surrogate contributes half the genetic material for the baby and carries the baby to term, is compensated for her expenses and efforts, and then agrees to give up her parental rights to the couple contracting for the surrogacy (Field, 2014).

The conflict arose when Baby M was born and Ms. Whitehead refused to give up the child to the Sterns. As the biological father, it was clear that Mr. Stern had at least as much right to the child as Ms. Whitehead. And although the parties had entered into a contract that set forth their arrangement, the New Jersey Supreme Court held the contract was void as a matter of public policy and used the "best interests of the child" standard to determine child custody (*In re Baby M*, 1988). In addition, the court stated the contract was illegal under New Jersey law, which prohibited the exchange of money in connection with adoptions. The court held that Ms. Whitehead was the legal mother of the child and Mr. Stern was the legal father of the child. Ultimately, the court case became a custody battle between Ms. Whitehead and Mr. Stern similar to any child custody case. The court is supposed to consider what custody arrangement is in the best interests of the child and in the case of Baby M, the court held that Mr. Stern should have full custody (*In re Baby M*, 1988).

Since the heart-wrenching case of Baby M, the use of surrogates has grown. Many states have passed laws that govern these arrangements and set forth permissible terms of a surrogacy contract. The legislative intent is to protect the rights of the surrogate as well as the party or parties seeking to have a child. A surrogacy contract is a complicated contract, and a health care provider would be wise to encourage the parties to seek legal advice and counsel. Generally, a legal surrogacy contract will include provisions that permit the health care and basic expenses of the surrogate to be paid by the party seeking to have a baby. It is prohibited, however, to pay a fee to the surrogate for her services. This is intended to prevent surrogacy from becoming an industry, particularly because of the potential abuse of women, which has been reported to occur in some parts of the world (Chan & Quigley, 2007).

With the development of reproductive technology, many surrogacy arrangements are now "gestational surrogacies," in which the surrogate mother has no genetic tie to the resultant child (Field, 2014). These arrangements involve the use of donor eggs, and the courts have analyzed these arrangements in a different manner. One court determined that the birthmother had no parental rights to the resultant child when she had contributed no genetic material to the child. "It is not the role of the judiciary to inhibit the use of reproductive technology when the legislature has not seen fit to do so" (*Johnson v. Calvert*, 1993, p. 787).

Not all states have followed the precedent established by the California court in *Johnson v. Calvert*. Some continue to hold surrogacy contracts void as a matter of public policy and therefore unenforceable. Others have enacted legislation that sets forth the terms and conditions of a valid surrogacy contract, and yet other states have made surrogacy arrangements illegal. Some states distinguish between traditional and gestational surrogacy, and others distinguish between altruistic surrogacy and compensated surrogacy (Field, 2014). The state of New Jersey, the location of the seminal Baby M case, has taken the position that the validity of surrogacy contracts does not depend on whether there is a genetic link between the surrogate and the baby and has permitted at least one woman to retain custody over the twins she carried to term despite having no genetic link to them (Conklin, 2013).

As an example, Florida has legislated surrogacy contracts and requires that the intended parents be married, at least one of the intended parents donate genetic material to the fetus, and a physician has certified that the woman is unable to carry a child to term. The surrogate may not be compensated, but her reasonable expenses may be paid and she can be required to adhere to medical advice about her prenatal health. Once the birth occurs, the intended parents must petition the court to ensure that their parental rights to the child are established and that the terms of the contract were in compliance with the law (Fla. Stat. §742.15).

Other states are "surrogacy" friendly and do not place the same restrictions or requirements on surrogacy arrangements. California, for example, permits the intended parents to obtain a court order before the child's birth, which sets forth that the intended parents are the parents on the birth of the child (Field, 2014). Currently, the "surrogacy market" is centered in Florida and California (Conklin, 2013).

Washington, New York, Michigan, and the District of Columbia have legislation that makes surrogacy contracts illegal (Field, 2014). Despite the legal disfavor of surrogacy in New York, the surrogacy business is thriving, with many couples seeking surrogacy arrangements and multiple agencies set up to match intended parents and surrogates (Conklin, 2013). The contracts regarding the surrogacy are simply executed and carried out in other jurisdictions. Of course, the legal disfavor of the contracts becomes a problem only when the parties no longer agree with the original terms of the contract or some other conflict arises.

Gestational surrogacy is the type that is most commonly practiced today and surrogates are often brought together with couples seeking a surrogate through private agencies, which charge various fees. In addition, if the surrogacy arrangement involves the use of donor eggs, additional parties, and expenses, are involved (Field, n.d.).

The legal rights to a child who is born through the use of reproductive technology is a novel issue for courts to address. Courts have had to address the issue of biological versus legal parenthood. Historically, a woman who bore a child was considered the biological and legal mother. If the woman was married at the time of the birth, the husband was the putative father of the child and was thus considered the legal and biological father (*Michael H. v. Gerald D.*, 1989). With the discovery of DNA and the ability to determine scientifically which man is the biological father of the child, courts have more frequently turned to science to determine paternity rights. However, advancing technologies, which permit the use of donor sperm and donor eggs, further complicate courts' determinations. Biological parenthood may be irrelevant to legal parenthood with, at least in some cases, the biological parents not even desiring parental rights.

Women who serve as surrogates may do so of their free will either out of monetary or altruistic motivation. However, that does not mean that all women who serve as surrogates do so because they want to. Serving as a surrogate can prove to be a profitable way for women to use their bodies without engaging in prostitution or selling their children (Conklin, 2013). Particularly in international surrogacy arrangements, women may feel that it is one of few routes to financial stability. And when the contract goes awry, they may have little, if any, recourse.

Drug Use in Pregnancy

As discussed earlier, courts have yet to weigh in on when life begins, but there have been a line of cases that deals with a woman's right to make decisions during pregnancy when those decisions may be adverse to the interests of the fetus. Prenatal drug use is associated with poor neonatal outcomes and perinatal complications including low birth weight, prematurity, placental abruption, and stillbirth (Hulsey, 2005). Consequently, states have passed laws that permit prenatal testing without consent and laws that are designed to penalize women who engage in prenatal drug use.

In 1996, South Carolina was the first state that prosecuted a woman for illegal drug use in pregnancy on the grounds that it constituted child abuse (Hulsey, 2005). Women were tested for drug use, without consent, in a public hospital in South Carolina. Women who tested positive were arrested, were incarcerated, and faced a prison term of up to 10 years. Several of the women who were arrested under the South Carolina law challenged the law, and the case was ultimately heard by the U.S. Supreme Court, which held that particular law unconstitutional (*Ferguson v. City of Charleston*, 2001). South Carolina continues to have laws that penalize women who use illegal drugs during pregnancy and in 2001 convicted Regina McKnight, whose fetus was stillborn after she used cocaine, of murder. Ms. McKnight was sentenced to 12 years in prison despite having three other minor children. Her sentence was overturned by the South Carolina Supreme Court in 2008 when it ruled that Ms. McKnight did not get a fair trial (Drug Policy Alliance, 2008). A prior appeal of Ms. McKnight failed when the South Carolina Supreme Court held that a pregnant woman who unintentionally heightens the risk of a stillbirth could be found guilty of homicide because of her "extreme indifference to human life" (Drug Policy Alliance, 2008).

Alabama has also been aggressive about removing children from a mother's custody when there is evidence of drug use. The children are often placed with a family member or in foster care under a safety plan that can last for years (Martin, 2015). One woman was evaluated by health care providers during her postpartum hospitalization and evaluated by social services once she went home with the baby. Social services and her physician felt there was no risk to the baby, but within a few weeks she was arrested, charged with a felony punishable with up to 10 years in prison. Alabama has the country's toughest law on prenatal drug use and this woman was alleged to have violated the law when she admitted to taking two, unprescribed, one-half doses of Valium during the last weeks of her pregnancy. The Alabama law can charge a woman with chemical endangerment of her fetus from the earliest weeks of her pregnancy and even if the baby is born completely healthy. A woman charged with a violation of the law not only faces prison time if convicted, but also faces losing custody of her other children (Martin, 2015).

The goal of the laws making drug use during pregnancy a felony has been articulated as forcing women into treatment, not to necessarily incarcerate women or force children into the foster care system. However, critics of the laws state that treating drug addiction as a crime rather than as a disease makes women avoid prenatal care and can interrupt the bonding of a newborn with its mother at a time when the mother is at her most vulnerable (Martin, 2015). Opponents of the laws argue that health care providers should treat all women with compassion and support and avoid stigmatizing women who use drugs (Eggertson, 2013). Loretta Finnegan, MD, a former medical adviser to the Office of Research on Women's Health of the National Institutes of Health, advises using prenatal care as an opportunity to help women with addiction issues and to promote long-lasting meaningful change in the life of a woman and her child. Opponents further urge assisting women during prenatal care with continuing support and assistance into the future in order to effect change (Eggertson, 2013).

Legal Issues in Domestic Violence

Intimate partner violence and other forms of domestic violence are at epidemic proportions in the United States and around the world. One in four women experiences domestic violence in her lifetime (SafeHorizons, 2015). Any women's health care provider must be attuned to the methods for screening for domestic violence and assist his or her patients who are victims. Although men are victims of domestic violence and the incidence of male victims may be underreported, in the United States there are an estimated 10 million cases of domestic violence annually (National Coalition Against Domestic Violence [NCADV], 2015).

A woman's health care provider must be familiar with the social service resources available to aid victims of domestic violence and must also have an understanding of some of the legal issues that surround domestic violence. Domestic violence has significant physical and mental health ramifications. Fifty-six percent of women who experience any partner violence are diagnosed with a psychiatric disorder. A total of 29% of all women who attempt suicide were battered, 37% of battered women have symptoms of depression, 46% have symptoms of anxiety disorder, and 45% experience posttraumatic stress disorder. Additionally, 37% of women's emergency room visits are the result of domestic violence (American Bar Association, 2015). Only 34% of those injured in intimate partner violence receive treatment for their injuries (NCDVA, 2015).

The problems with assisting victims of domestic violence are well documented in the psychosocial literature on the topic. There are a numbers of ways in which the legal system can support such victims, and there are also challenges within this system. It is often overwhelming to a victim to initiate contact with law enforcement, but it is critical to the success of the legal system to obtain a timely and comprehensive police report. Victims are often reluctant to bring law enforcement into the case for a multitude of reasons, but without law enforcement involvement, the perpetrator may not be stopped until it is too late (Colorado Bar Association, 2015). Three of four female homicide victims are killed by a husband or a lover, often with no prior report to law enforcement (CNN, 2015).

Women who are victims of domestic violence may experience long-term health risks as well. According to a study done by the Centers for Disease Control and Prevention, female victims are 80% more likely to suffer a stroke, 70% more likely to have heart disease, 70% more likely to become heavy drinkers, and 60% more likely to become asthmatic than women who are not (Black, 2008). Under the ACA, annual domestic violence screenings are a mandated preventive service (Culp-Ressler, 2013).

Women may not feel supported by law enforcement or the criminal justice system. Not only is it emotionally trying to involve law enforcement, but also in many states domestic battery without permanent injury is only a misdemeanor charge. Women may also be faced with the prospect of losing financial support if their abusive partner is arrests, jailed, or charged (Colorado Bar Association, 2015). Whether or not charges are filed against a perpetrator is determined by the state and not the victim. A state may be less likely to bring charges if the victim is uncooperative and the victim may request leniency for the perpetrator, but the victim cannot unilaterally "dismiss the charges." Cerulli et al. (2015) state that, within the criminal justice system, there are a number of options for those accused of domestic violence. Many jurisdictions have diversion programs for first-time offenders. These programs are similar to probation, and the accused must regularly meet with an officer of the state, attend various classes designed to reduce the incidence of domestic violence, participate in community service, pay court costs, and perhaps pass random drug or alcohol testing. If the accused completes the diversion program successfully, the state agrees to drop the charges.

For those who are not first-time offenders, the accused can enter a plea of guilty or nolo contendere (no contest) in exchange for probation or some other reduction in penalty. The terms of probation are generally similar to those of a diversion program. The difference is that if the accused successfully completes the probation, the charges are not dismissed and if he fails to complete the probation or does not comply with the terms, he may be incarcerated.

Some accused will opt to exercise their rights to a trial. Although anyone accused of a crime in the United States is innocent until proven guilty and has a right to a speedy trial, many accused will waive their right to a speedy trial in order to mount a more comprehensive defense. This may cause the case to drag on for many months, which can be an additional stressor for the victim. The victim will be called to testify at trial, which can be an extremely traumatic experience for her, and she may also be concerned if her children or other relatives were witnesses to the violence and are called to trial. Anyone who receives a subpoena compelling them to testify at trial must comply with the subpoena or face being in contempt of court.

Another way the legal systems attempts to assist victims of domestic violence is through domestic violence injunctions (Nichols, 2013). These are court orders that may be obtained by the victim and order the accused to stay away from the victim as well as generally her place of work and her home. They can be obtained based solely on the accusations of the victim, with no proof required, but these are temporary injunctions, which are effective for a matter of days or weeks when there will be a hearing in front of a judge where both victim and perpetrator have the right to appear and testify. These proceedings are also in open court thus open to the public. The judge may decide whether to make the injunction permanent or dissolve the injunction. Although the injunction may be made "permanent," it is not indefinite, but for a specific period of time, generally no more than a year.

Some jurisdictions have legal services where injunctions can be obtained any day of the week, and there may be volunteers to assist a woman with the paperwork involved. Navigating the judicial system in order to obtain an injunction may be overwhelming, and the victim may need significant support. This support is often available through social services such as women's shelters and other support groups. However, a health care provider should be familiar with what is available so that the victim can be pointed in the right direction.

A woman may have additional legal issues to contend with. She may need to obtain a divorce and negotiate child custody issues, including timesharing and child support. She may have lost her only means of financial support and, because of the psychological effects of domestic violence, may have difficulty making her way through the legal system.

■ FUTURE DIRECTIONS

Improving women's access to care have historically been disproportionately affected by a lack of access to health care and this is in part because of underinsurance or a lack of insurance coverage. The ACA, signed into law on March 23, 2010, by President Barak Obama, has increased Americans' access to care (Blumenthal, Abrams, & Nuzum, 2015). A provision of the law provides for subsidies for Americans purchasing insurance through the Health Care Marketplace and 87% of those using the Marketplace qualify for governmental subsidies. Additionally, a total of 10.8 million Americans have enrolled in Medicaid since ACA's enactment (Blumenthal et al., 2015).

Women benefit from the ACA in very specific ways. Before enactment of all of the ACA provisions, in 2012 a 25-year-old woman could expect to pay 81% more for the same insurance policy offered to her male counterpart ("The ACA is Working for Women," 2015). Additionally, women were more likely to be insured as dependents and therefore more vulnerable to loss of coverage. The ACA provisions make insurance more accessible to women regardless of their status as a dependent. Women are now more likely to be covered and more likely to have better coverage than they did before the ACA ("The ACA is Working for Women," 2015). Even women with Medicare are now able to benefit from various preventive services without having to pay any cost sharing.

The ACA is not the first attempt at expanding coverage for women. Breast and cervical cancers are the leading cancers among women and various government initiatives have been established to increase women's access to screening and treatment for these cancers. Low-income and minority women are at risk for increased mortality and morbidity as well as at risk for not having adequate access to care once screening results are positive (Rosenbaum, 2012). In 1990, Congress established the National Breast and Cervical Cancer Early Detection Program. The program provides grants to states to increase access to breast and cervical cancer screenings for at-risk women. The problem for women participating in the program is that once they have a positive screening test, access to further diagnostic tests and treatment may be unavailable or prohibitively expensive. As a result, in 2000 Congress enacted the Breast and Cervical Cancer Prevention and Treatment Act, which was designed to increase access to follow up care and treatment by permitting states to establish an optional Medicaid program to cover women regardless of income (Rosenbaum, 2012). The ACA ensures that these same women cannot be denied a policy on the private market because of a previous positive screen or treatment through public programs (Rosenbaum, 2012).

As some states opt to expand Medicaid under the ACA, women in expansion states are likely to have greater access to breast and cervical cancer screening and treatment than those in nonexpansion states (Sabik, Tarazi, & Bradley, 2015). Women with health insurance are twice as likely to receive breast and cervical cancer screening and therefore are much more likely to receive timely and appropriate treatment (Sabik et al., 2015).

■ CONCLUSION

A health care provider's advocacy for a woman includes assisting her to navigate the intersection of health care and the law. There are experts in health care law and the provider should be knowledgeable enough to make appropriate referrals to these experts to assist women in their times of legal need.

■ REFERENCES

The ACA is working for women (HHS.gov). (2015). Retrieved from http://www.hhs.gov/healthcare/facts-and-features/fact-sheets/aca-working-women/index.html

American Bar Association. (2015). *Domestic violence statistics*. Retrieved from www.americanbar.org/groups/domestic_violence/resources/statistics.html

Bellotti v. Baird, 443 U.S. 622 (1979).

Black, M. (2008). Adverse health conditions and health risk behaviors associated with intimate partner violence—United States, 2005. *MMWR Weekly, 57*(05), 113–117.

Blumenthal, D., Abrams, M., & Nuzum, R. (2015). The Affordable Care Act at 5 Years (M. Hamel, Ed.). *New England Journal of Medicine, 372*(25), 2451–2458.

Burwell v. Hobby Lobby Stores, Inc., 134 S. Ct. 2751 (2014).

Carey v. Population Services, 431 U.S. 678 (1977).

The Center for Consumer Information & Insurance Oversight (CCIIO). (n.d.). Women's preventive services coverage and non-profit religious organizations. Retrieved from https://www.cms.gov/CCIIO/Resources/Fact-Sheets-and-FAQs/womens-preven-02012013.html

Cerulli, C., Kothari, C., Dichter, M., Marcus, S., Kim, T. K., Wilen, J., & Rhodes, K. V. (2015). Help seeking patterns among women experiencing intimate partner violence. *Violence and Victims, 30*(1), 16–31.

Chan, S., & Quigley, M. (2007, November 8). Frozen embryos, genetic information and reproductive rights. *Bioethics, 21*(8), 439–448.

City of Akron v. Akron Center for Reproductive Rights, 462 U.S. 416 (1983).

CNN. (2015). Domestic (intimate partner) violence fast facts. Retrieved from http://www.cnn.com/2013/12/06/us/domestic-intimate-partner-violence-fast-facts

Colorado Bar Association. (2015). *The challenges and effects of leaving an abusive situation*. Retrieved from http://www.coloradohighschoolmocktrial.org/page.cfm/ID/21090

Conklin, C. (2013). Simply inconsistent: Surrogacy laws in the United States and the pressing need for regulation. *Women's Rights Law Reporter, 35*, 67–94.

Contraceptive Use in the United States. (2015). Retrieved from http://www.guttmacher.org/pubs/fb_contr_use.html

Culp-Ressler, T. (2013). Domestic violence victims tend to suffer from long-term health problems. Retrieved from http://thinkprogress.org

Doe v. Bolton, 410 U.S. 179 (1973).

Doe v. Doe, Case No. SS024581, Superior Court of the State of California, County of Los Angeles. First Amended Complaint filed August 29, 2014.

Drug Policy Alliance. (2008). South Carolina Supreme Court Reverses 20-Year Homicide Conviction of Regina McKnight [Press release]. Retrieved from http://www.drugpolicy.org/news/2008/05/south-carolina-supreme-court-reverses-20-year-homicide-conviction-regina-mcknight

Eggertson, L. (2013). Stigma a major barrier to treatment for pregnant women with addictions. *Canadian Medical Association Journal, 185*(18). doi:10.1503/cmja.109–4653

Eisenstadt v. Baird, 405 U.S. 438 (1972).

Ferguson v. City of Charleston, 532 U.S. 67 (2001).

Field, M. (2014). Compensated surrogacy. *Washington Law Review, 89*, 1155–1184.

Fla. Stat. §742.15.

Gonzalez v. Carhart, 548 U.S. 938 (2006).

Griswold v. Connecticut, 381 U.S. 479 (1965).

Harris v. McRae, 448 U.S. 297 (1980).

Hens, K., Dondorp, W., Geraedts, J., & de Wert, G. (2012). Comprehensive pre-implantation genetic screening: Ethical reflection urgently needed. *Nature Reviews. Genetics, 13*(10), 676–677.

Hodgson v. Minnesota, 497 U.S. 417 (1990).

Hulsey, T. (2005). Prenatal drug use: The ethics of testing and incarcerating women. *Newborn and Infant Nursing Reviews, 5*(2), 93–96.

In re Baby M., 537 A.2d 1227, 1234 (N.J. 1988).

James, S. (2013). Test tube baby Louise Brown turns 35. Retrieved from http://abcnews.go.com/Health/test-tube-baby-louise-brown-turns-35-medical/story?id=19764283

Johnson v. Calvert, 851 P.2d 776, (California, 1993).

Lawrence v. Texas, 539 U.S. 558 (2003).

Liptak, A. (2015, June 16). Supreme Court Refuses to Hear Case on Pre-Abortion Ultrasounds. *New York Times*. Retrieved from http://www.nytimes.com/2015/06/16/us/politics/supreme-court-rejects-north-carolinas-appeal-on-pre-abortion-ultrasounds.html?_r=0

Loeb, N. (2015). Sofía Vergara's Ex-Fiancé: Our Frozen Embryos Have a Right to Live. *New York Times*. Retrieved from http://www.nytimes.com/2015/04/30/opinion/sofiavergaras-ex-fiance-our-frozen-embryos-have-a-right-to-live.html

Loving v. Virginia, 388 U.S. 1 (1967).

Maher v. Roe, 432 U.S. 464 (1977).

Martin, N. (2015). Take a Valium, lose your kid, go to jail. *ProPublica*. Retrieved from https://www.propublica.org/article/when-the-womb-is-a-crime-scene

Michael H. v. Gerald D., 491 U.S 110 (1989).

Moore v. the City of East Cleveland, 431 U.S. 494 (1977).

NCADV. (2015). Domestic violence national statistics. Retrieved from http://www.ncadv.org/learn/statistics

Nichols, A. (2013). Survivor-defined practices to mitigate revictimization of battered women in the protective order process. *Journal of Interpersonal Violence, 28*(7), 1403–1423.

Ohio v. Akron Center for Reproductive Health, 497 U.S. 502(1990).

Our Bodies, Ourselves. (2014). History of Abortion in the United States. Retrieved from www.ourbodiesourselves.org

Planned Parenthood Association of Kansas City, Missouri, Inc. v. Ashcroft, 462 U.S. 476 (1983).

Planned Parenthood of Central Missouri v. Danforth, 428 U.S. 52 (1976).

Planned Parenthood v. Casey, 505 U.S. 833(1992).

Publicly Funded Family Planning Services in the United States. (2015). Retrieved from http://www.guttmacher.org/pubs/fb_contraceptive_serv.html

Rodgers v. Fasano, 715 N.Y.S.2d 19 (N.Y. App. Div. 1st Dep't 2000).

Roe v. Wade, 410 U.S. 113 (1973).

Rosenbaum, S. (2012). Law and the public's health. *Public Health Reports, 127*, 340–344.

Sabik, L., Tarazi, W., & Bradley, C. (2015). State Medicaid expansion decisions and disparities in women's cancer screening. *American Journal of Preventive Medicine, 48*(1), 98–103.

SafeHorizons (2015). Domestic violence: Statistics and facts. Retrieved from http://www.safehorizon.org/page/domestic-violence-statistics-facts-52.html

Simopoulos v. Virginia, 462 U.S. 506 (1983).

Stenberg v. Carhart, 530 U.S. 914 (2000).

CHAPTER 6

Feminist Frameworks for Advanced Practice With Women

Cheryl L. Cooke • Selina A. Mohammed

In the United States, women's health providers are not providing care for just "American" women; they are caring for women and other gendered minorities from disparate countries and living situations. Having a framework that guides understanding of the complexities of women's experiences worldwide provides a broader foundation within which to understand the health needs of these populations. In this chapter, we explore how feminism can guide our thinking about women and how we view and respond to their health care needs. We begin with a discussion of feminism, including feminist theory and inquiry, as background against which to consider concepts central to nursing practice with women. We also examine how knowledge of these theories can be useful in understanding the economic, political, and social situations that contribute to poor health outcomes.

■ WHY FEMINISM IS AN IMPORTANT CONSIDERATION WHEN PROVIDING HEALTH CARE SERVICES

The word *feminism* invokes a variety of responses reflecting confusion and lack of awareness of the large body of feminist theory. It is not uncommon to find women and men who insist they are not "feminists" yet who advocate feminist agendas. For some, feminism conveys threatening images of a social order in which everything is different from the status quo. For others, feminism describes a situation in which gender identity is understood as a notion that imparts equity in political, economic, and social rights. Many definitions of feminism include not only equality for all, but also improvement of the circumstances that underpin inequities, as well as those that maintain cycles of discrimination.

DiEmanuele (2015) suggests that feminist theory is important "because, like any study of injustice, it exposes the illogical format of the arguments that support prejudice and discrimination. Furthermore, it provides a point of

reason—and thus, understanding—for those who are unaffected" (p. 1). In recent years, the role of "feminism" has been challenged in ways that seem focused on dismantling the forward movement in many areas of women's issues, gender identity, and democratic equality. Language that was once used to support the ideals of inclusion and achievement for women and other traditionally marginalized groups is now being appropriated and used to fragment and dismantle groups that have traditionally promoted human rights for one another. For example, since the 1990s, a neoliberal talk-show host consistently refers to feminists as "femi-nazis," or there are websites where young women post pictures with handwritten explanations of why they do not need feminism (e.g., *Merriam-Webster*, n.d.; Rudman, 2012; Women Against Feminism, 2015). Fear-based reactions to our struggle for equality must be met head-on, making it essential to continue to explore how gender is experienced and enacted and how our understandings of it may interfere with achieving optimal health for racial and gendered populations. For example, losses based on both racial and gender group identities continue to contribute to the struggles in pay equity and health disparities (Correa-de-Araujo, 2006; Dey & Hill, 2007). They also contribute to losses in freedom for women and gendered "Others" that have occurred as a result of globalization. These losses ultimately affect health status.

For those unfamiliar, the concept of "Othering," or marking groups as "Other" than dominant, involves power differentials in society that serve to privilege members of dominant society (e.g., men, White people, wealthy people) and marginalize Others (e.g., women, gendered minorities, poor people). This concept describes unequal power relationships between advocates and people who are advocated for, and calls into question who has the right to speak for whom.

This chapter contains historical citations and material from the late 1700s through current times in order to represent the breadth and depth of thought in feminist theory. We briefly explore several prominent feminist theories and concepts that may be considered as supportive of gender-specific health care. Just as there is no single theory that describes health, there is no single definition of feminist theory that covers all situations or gendered groups. Feminists are interested in a wide range of concerns influenced by the particular philosophical, cultural, political, and economic perspectives, from which we view, interact within, interpret, and represent our worlds. As feminist theory is varied and is updated in response to political, social, economic, and environmental changes in our world, we can better understand its history by examining it in "waves" and seeing how these changes built one upon another based on historical change in society. The first wave of U.S. feminism is classically thought of as the events surrounding women's suffrage. The second wave of feminism in the United States began around the late 1960s and centered on organizing women and using feminism as a resource for seeking equality in social organizations. Feminism's third wave, occurring now, responds to several theoretical problems from its second wave, including a focus on narratives and making space for multiple voices and perspectives, and provides a nonjudgmental and inclusive approach in an effort to build political coalitions (Snyder, 2008). Third-wave feminism is committed to increasing the understanding and integration of feminist perspectives from the perspective of gendered identities and developing countries and in the presence of globalization and a globalized world economy, as well as within the postcolonial and neocolonial worlds. The borders of these waves are varied, permeable, and debated, but their historical significance is important in order to understand how the social views and situations of women and other gendered minorities' change over time.

Feminist thought has emerged from a variety of philosophical traditions, including liberal Marxist, psychoanalytic, socialist, existentialist, postmodern, and postcolonial philosophies. In this chapter, we provide an overview of several traditions of feminist philosophical thought. It must be noted that the philosophical traditions on which much of feminist thought are based have disciplinary uses in other areas. For example, Marxist thought is a philosophical tradition that is often used in understanding economic theory but is also useful in understanding the history and subjugation of women in society. The following categories should be considered as a broad guide that underscores the differences in feminist theory, which in many ways reflects the differences in individuals and groups.

■ PERSPECTIVES IN FEMINIST THEORY

Liberal Feminism

Liberal feminists advocate gender justice, with gender equity replacing the politics of exclusion (Tong, 1998). Liberal feminism is exemplified in works such as Mary Wollstonecraft's *A Vindication of the Rights of Woman* (1796) and John Stuart Mill's *On the Subjection of Women* (1878). Liberal feminism often draws on and works within the framework of liberal political theory. The work of the National Organization of Women, in support of equal rights for women, reflects contemporary liberal feminism. Central

to the beliefs of liberal feminists is the assumption that women's subordination is rooted in customary and legal constraints blocking women's entrance to and/or success in the so-called public world. Because society has viewed women as less than men, women have been excluded from many arenas of public life. Liberal feminism seeks to expose these injustices and to develop strategies for enhancing the position of women in society.

Marxist and Socialist Feminism

Marxist feminists, exemplified in some works by Angela Davis (1981, 1989), Catharine MacKinnon (1989), and Iris Young (1990), believe that it is impossible for anyone, especially a woman, to obtain genuine equal opportunity in a class society in which wealth is produced by many people for a powerful few. Marx and Engels were influential voices whose work explored the capitalist economic philosophy that underwrites most of Western political and economic thought and action. Marxist philosophy is also a factor influencing feminist responses to the subjugation of women worldwide. Tracing their works to Engels, Marxist feminists assert that women's oppression originates in the introduction of private property. Beasley (1999) concurs, suggesting that sexual oppression is a form of class oppression. In order to eradicate sexual oppression, Marxist feminists advocate replacing capitalism with a socialist system. In this new system, the means of production would belong to everyone, and women would no longer be economically dependent on men (Beasley, 1999; Tong, 1998).

Radical Feminism

Radical feminists, as exemplified by Mary Daly (1978), Andrea Dworkin (1974, 1976), Gena Corea (1986), and Shulamith Firestone (1970), believe the patriarchal system oppresses women. They advocate that a system characterized by power, dominance, hierarchy, and competition cannot be reformed but must be eradicated. Radical feminist thought suggests that institutions producing and reproducing hierarchy and dominance, especially the family, the church, and the academy (academic institutions), need to be replaced in order to achieve equality. Some radical feminists question the concept of "natural order" in which men are "manly" and women "womanly," with a goal of overcoming whatever negative effects this thinking about biology as destiny has had on women and men. Radical feminists assert that biology, gender (masculinity and femininity), and sexuality (heterosexuality and homosexuality are some forms) are sources of women's oppression (Weedon, 1997). Many radical feminists focus on ways in which gender and sexuality have been used to subordinate women to men. They support reproductive rights as a means of enhancing women's choices. Some advocate escaping the confines of heterosexuality through celibacy, autoeroticism, or lesbianism, emphasizing acceptance of women's own desires (Rich, 1981).

In the 1980s, a political backlash against feminist theory and activism was initiated by conservative forces within the U.S. political landscape, most notably occurring within the Reagan–Bush era of the mid-1980s to early 1990s, and in some ways, this backlash continues today. The backlash criticized the "women's movement" for its support of women's rights, abortion rights, and the movement of women out of the home and into the workplace. Much of the backlash against feminism is centered on what is perceived to be the "radical" aspects of feminist theory, including gender difference and women's sexuality, and serves to undermine the progress of women in society (Rich, 1977, 1981). The results of this backlash against feminism are still being felt through near-constant challenges to the 1973 *Roe v. Wade* court case over abortion rights and the reversal of some affirmative action and other civil rights legislation that benefited women and other marginalized groups. In recent years, these arguments have been appropriated by neoconservatives in the United States and used as politically centered fear tactics to limit equality and self-determination for women in public and private life.

Psychoanalytic Theory and Feminism

Psychoanalytic feminist theorists believe that the centrality of sexuality arises out of Freudian theory and concepts such as the Oedipus complex. Chodorow (1978, 1987, 1994) and Dinnerstein (1976, 1989) exemplify early psychoanalytic, primarily Freudian, feminist thought. Central to their work is the assumption that the root of women's oppression is embedded deeply within their psyche. These theorists recommend dual parenting and dual participation in the work force as means to solve women's oppression. A group of prominent French (and Bulgarian-French, in the case of Kristeva) feminist theorists includes Hélène Cixous (1975, 1991), Luce Irigaray (1974, 1977), and Julia Kristeva (1982), whose work is conducted in critique of Freudian psychoanalysis. These women challenge the theoretical perspectives of Jacques Lacan, a psychoanalyst, whose work furthered that of Freud. The theory presented by the "French feminists" is often conceptualized from both a psychoanalytic and a poststructuralist position (discussed in the following section), and focuses on explorations of subjectivity and agency, abjection, and psychosexual identity formation (Weedon, 1997).

Postmodernism and Feminist Theory

Postmodernism is expressed in feminist theory as a series of theoretical perspectives that view language as constructing our understanding and uses of gender. Much of what is known as postmodern work is conducted from a poststructuralist perspective, a philosophical perspective that heavily relies on the work of Michel Foucault, a French philosopher, whose work critiqued how power and knowledge are constructed and reified. Feminist writings from a poststructuralist perspective critique the ideas of essentialism, the use of power in social relations, and ways that, through the use of language and power, knowledge about the world is produced and legitimated (Butler, 1993, 2000; Weedon, 1997). These orientations involve no single standpoint but do involve several perspectives that can account for the experiences of difference, an aspect of feminist theory that

has been recently approached from postmodern and/or poststructuralist perspectives.

■ EXPERIENCES OF WOMEN OF COLOR, WOMANIST TRADITIONS, AND FEMINIST THEORY

The voices and experiences of women of color are increasingly finding a place within feminist theory. Writers using postmodern, poststructuralist, and critical race theories enable this by calling out the use of metanarratives to describe the lives of women of color as essentially similar to those of White women. For example, as noted by hooks (1999a, 2000), the experiences of African American women are not interchangeable with those of White women. Works by and about African American women challenge us to think about their life experiences and factors affecting their well-being (Collins, 1989, 2000; Crenshaw, 1995; Davis, 1981, 1989, 1991; Dill, 1983, 1987; Gillespie, 1984; Gordon-Bradshaw, 1987; Herman, 1984; hooks, 1984, 1997, 1999b; Lorde, 1984, 1988; Smith, 1982).

The novelist Alice Walker (1983) was first to use the term *womanist,* in which she describes a theory of feminism that explores and advances the issues of African American women in the U.S. context (Taylor, 1998, 2002, 2004, 2005). Womanist traditions offer a feminist theoretical perspective that seeks to encompass the "uniqueness of African American women's experiences" accentuating the similarities and *differences* between African American women's experiences and those of women from other ethnic and racial groups (Banks-Wallace, 2000, p. 36).

In the United States, Latinos are a rapidly growing demographic, representing one seventh of the population. This change in national demographics presents an opportunity for the voices of Latina feminists to emerge and advocate for improvement in health care resource allocation, work conditions, and immigration rights. Works about Latina or Chicana women provide insight into the challenges for women from a burgeoning ethnic minority who experience unique physical, political, and health-related concerns (Anzaldúa, 1987, 1999; Apodaca, 1977; Chavez, Cornelius, & Jones, 1986; del Portillo, 1987; Ginorio & Reno, 1985; Hurtado 1989, 1996; Kelly, Bobo, McLachlan, Avery, & Burge, 2006; Moraga, 1983, 1997; Moraga & Anzaldúa, 1983; Sanchez, 1984; Sánchez-Ayéndez, 1989; Segura, 1989).

Writings about and by Asian Americans, Pacific Islanders, South Asian women, and Native American/First Nations scholars (Chow, 1987; Im, Meleis, & Park, 1999; Johnson et al., 2004; Neufeld, Harrison, Stewart, Hughes, & Spitzer, 2002; Tsutakawa, 1988; Visweswaran, 1994; Woods, Lentz, Mitchell, & Oakley, 1994). Witt (1984), Hale (1985), and Pirner (2005) provide powerful accounts of issues central to women's lives, illustrating points of difference that may help account for health experiences. Their health issues must be understood within the context of traditional family life and hierarchies and within a multigenerational context, as many of these women are first- and second-generation immigrants to the United States. Another important area to consider includes their current work situations and histories, as many of these women engage in unseen labor (i.e., housekeepers, farm workers) and their work exposes them to potential physical and environmental hazards and economic disparities that can complicate their efforts to achieve optimal health.

Queer Theory

Queer theory is part of a resistance movement that describes feminism from lesbian, gay, bisexual, transgendered, and queer (LGBTQ) perspectives with an emphasis of "affinity and solidarity over identity" (Marcus, 2005, p. 196). Queer theory provides an opportunity for understanding gender, offering a lens through which lesbian, gay, and transgendered people understand and interpret their lives within a heteronormativity (Butler, 1993, 2000; Jagose, 1996). As nurses, we want to shrink from language that is disparaging of individuals or groups, but the use of the term *queer* is taken up as an umbrella term "for a coalition of culturally marginal sexual self-identification" LGBTQ studies and theories (Jagose, 1996, p. 1). Queer theory calls on us to question how our discomfort with difference can be directed to work for the good of an often-marginalized group. Using queer theory as a framework for understanding the health challenges of LGBTQ groups, we begin to understand how social identity operates in ways that amplify health issues. For example, lesbian women of childbearing years may be struggling with infertility and have difficulty finding a provider who understands the infertility issues of lesbian women. As the current research exploring the lives and health of the LGBTQ community predominantly focuses on lesbian health issues, additional research underscoring the health of gay, bisexual, and transgendered individuals is necessary (Clear & Carryer, 2001; Ensign, 2001; Glass, 2002; Spinks, Andrews, & Boyle, 2000).

Less prominent but equally as important are feminist theoretical traditions from ecofeminism and feminist liberation theology. Ecofeminism provides a space for feminists to consider the conditions of women within the context of the environment and nature (Griffin, 1978; Haraway, 1989; Sturgeon, 1997). Feminist liberation theologies (Christian, mujerista, and some womanist traditions) provide a theoretical framework for women to use religious and spiritual traditions to enhance their understandings of women's subjugation and oppression (Fulkerson, 1994; Harrison, 1985; Isasi-Diaz, 1993; Isasi-Diaz & Tarango, 1992; Tigert, 2001). With the emergence of ecofeminism, feminist liberation theologies, and queer theory, issues of the ecological, racialized, and gendered experiences of women, communities of color, and LGBTQ communities are gaining theoretical prominence and becoming increasingly legitimized in health and academic communities.

Postcolonial and Transnational Feminist Theories

Postcolonial theory calls into question the history of colonial dominance of the West over other geographical regions and people. As the overarching framework for feminist theory,

transnational feminist theory adds support to the notion of the need for multiple forms of feminism in a postcolonial world (Scott, Kaplan, & Keates, 1997). Postcolonial theory has initiated discussions about the way Western ideas are transmitted into non-Westernized regions; the effects of this transmission, including loss of native languages and traditions; and the Westernization of social structures and institutions. Postcolonial theory offers an opportunity to think and develop strategies that resist contemporary forms of Western colonialism that "undermine and sabotage the self-determining aspirations" of citizens in independent states (Yeatman, 1994, p. 9). In our transglobal environment, the ideals of postcolonialism and transnational feminist theories and movements have become increasingly important.

Postcolonial theory questions the transfer of Western economic strategies and knowledge into more traditional economic systems, often to the economic benefit of the West (sometimes referred to as "the North" in opposition to countries in the Southern hemisphere). Although Western technologies and economic strategies have been useful in some ways to some populations, the effects of these technologies have been detrimental to the social structures, environments, and health of many populations. Another use for postcolonial theory is its provision of a theoretical frame for feminists to critique the effects of transnationalism on the lives of women and children. Finally, recent literature describes nursing itself as a colonized profession (McGibbon, Mulaudzi, Didham, Barton, & Sochan, 2014) and calls for increasing counternarratives that resist subjugation and oppression within the profession.

Issues for women's health providers to consider include the use of child labor and its effects on the family structure, the health effects of transnationalism, and the transfer of health technologies to populations that may not have the infrastructure to support their effective use. Understanding a country's political economy and how it affects the availability of health and social services is another important topic that drives the improvement or deterioration of a population's health outcomes. Postcolonial theories and transnational feminism allow nurses to move between local and global ideas, placing the individual within a more globally oriented response to women's health. In doing so, nurses can work beside women in non-Western counties to deal with the effects of transnationalism, such as inadequate infrastructures, economic and social power, and the subsequent health effects that are accentuated under these conditions.

■ INTERSECTIONALITY

Collins (2000) describes intersectionality as the confluence of oppressions within society. Oftentimes, these expressed oppressions center on race, class, and gender. Intersectionality focuses on how these oppressions are shaped by one another and thus how the sum is greater than its parts. For example, the experience of a Black woman cannot be simply captured by independently examining the experience of being Black or a woman, but needs to be seen in the context of being a Black woman in the historical and social context of today's society.

Crenshaw (1995) is credited with the phrase *intersectionality* as a way of capturing how race, gender, and employment "interact to shape the multiple dimensions of black women's employment experiences" (p. 1244). The notion of intersectionality came into play by Black women, who found that White women's feminism was tied to equality with White men and the Black movement was sexist in the sense that it prioritized Black men's pursuit of equality with White men (Gopaldas, 2013). There was not a space that captured the experience of being both a woman and Black.

Understanding intersectionality involves exploring the concept at both macro and micro levels. The macro level explores the multiple identities of women (e.g., Latina, woman, bisexual) within the context of race, class, and gender. The micro level examines individual identity positions within society in reference to privilege and disadvantage (Gopaldas, 2013). As a health provider, understanding the complexity of how various factors intersect to create a specific experience of wellness and illness is vital to providing excellent care and helping clients achieve optimal health.

■ USING THEORY TO GUIDE PRACTICE

Theory and practice are inextricably linked, each constituting the other. Theory is used to create practice, and practices change as a result of emerging theories. Feminist theory is a fairly new application for nursing research and care. With all new experiences, one has to first learn the tenets of the theory, begin to identify and uncover situations in which the theory is applicable, and ultimately, use the theory to create practice. Feminist theory has spent many years at the margins of theory in nursing, slowly moving toward central positions in research and practice. Nurse researchers and practitioners currently use feminist theory primarily as a framework for conceptualizing issues or as a form of feminist critique of research and practice (Anderson, 2002, 2004; Bunting, 1997; Corbett, 2007; Im, 2000; Im & Meleis, 2001; Johnson et al., 2004; Maxwell-Young, Olshansky, & Steele, 1998; Richman, Jason, Taylor, & Jahn, 2000; Schroeder & Ward, 1998).

Understanding the theoretical background of the struggles around women's and gendered minority rights and recognizing the multiple concerns included in these struggles allow providers to better serve this clientele. In using feminist theory to guide practice, the provider is able to place current struggles in women's and gendered minorities' health into context, particularly when considering determinants of health and the economic, political, and social situations that can contribute to poor health outcomes. Aside from physiological and psychological needs, providers should be involved in issues around safety, esteem, and self-actualization as they pertain to the lives of their clients. A number of problems affecting the health of these populations may be viewed and better understood as a result of using feminist theory and gaining knowledge around the historical complexities of populations. Some of these problems include (a) violence against women and other gendered minorities, (b) social and economic inequities and the effect of these on health, (c) the ways that women's and gendered minorities' health care needs are represented to and by large institutions (e.g., state and federal agencies, insurance plans, and the media) as priorities for funding and research, and (d) how the intermediate disparities of health (e.g., access to primary care, jobs that pay a living wage) contribute to poor health outcomes.

A related issue in feminist practice is the social construction of women and gendered minorities within the health care system. Although a nonhierarchical relationship would be ideal, it is impossible to completely equalize social, political, and historical experiences between providers and their clients. Historically, most providers see themselves as custodians of knowledge, versus seeing this relationship as a shared partnership. At the same time, clients enter the health care interaction as experts of their own bodies and lives, and desire recognition of this expertise by providers.

Validation of the nonrational is another dimension of feminist practice. This orientation allows for multiple competing definitions of problems and many "truths." It emphasizes women's and gendered minorities' ability to reconstruct their own experiences and to find meaning in events that they alone can determine. For example, a woman may perceive that her mastectomy is not a sexual phenomenon, but it raises existential issues for her. The process of problem definition is recognized as subjective. Nonlinear, multidimensional thinking is encouraged (Bricker-Jenkins & Hooyman, 1989; Weedon, 1997). Providers should be attentive to the power relations between themselves and their clients. Practicing from a feminist perspective means being mindful of the ways power relations function and are managed in the health care setting. The analysis and interpretation of subjective and objective data and treatment plans need to be agreed upon by both the provider and the client.

Understanding gender as a social versus biological construction is an important distinction in feminist and nonfeminist perspectives (Allen, Allman, & Powers, 1991; Campbell & Bunting, 1991). In addition, providers working within a feminist framework are concerned with ways to transform the social and health-related conditions that have an impact on their clients' health. It is not enough to describe oppression; it is also important to change the conditions that create and sustain it. This concern gives legitimacy to consciousness-raising, advocacy, and praxis. Praxis references the component of feminist consciousness that leads to social transformation. An awareness of the reality that shapes women's and gendered minorities' lives becomes infused into public values. Reality is renamed according to their experiences. Recognition of the small group as a unit of social change is explicit. Self-help is one means of change but does not substitute for the provision of adequate services from the state. Struggles to implement values, such as egalitarianism, consensus democracy, nonexploitation, cooperation, collectivism, diversity, and nonjudgmental spirituality, are central to feminist practice (Andrist, 1988; Bricker-Jenkins and Hooyman, 1989; Sampselle, 1990). However, consciousness-raising is an ongoing process, often undertaken at some risk, such as exposing previously unstated vulnerabilities, to many of these groups. Facilitating consciousness-raising with women and gendered minorities cannot be abandoned mid-process because this risks leaving them more vulnerable than before the process began. Providing consciousness-raising follow-up support is essential, as it allows the woman who has now recognized her vulnerabilities with the additional support required in order to change them (Wolf, 1996).

Chopoorian (1986) urges us to consider multiple dimensions of environments for human health, a perspective consistent with many feminist theories that link health to social, political, and economic structures as context. Moreover, the emphasis on social relationships, including domination, power, and authority within organizations and families, leads one to examine exploitation of women and gendered minorities and its relationships to their health. Finally, an emphasis on understanding everyday life and its meaning for these populations is consistent with feminist conceptions of the importance of a client's experience.

An ethical feminist practice in nursing understands the category of "woman," "lesbian," "bisexual," and "transgendered" as multiple, shifting, and constantly changing. Nursing practice that understands the complexities of women and gendered minorities, the contexts of their lives, and the multiple and shifting landscape of their health is desirable and attainable. Educating nurses about how these populations' health needs vary and how knowledge of the context of their lives is essential to their developing an ethical feminist practice. Nurses' knowledge about women's and gendered minorities' health problems and the differences in how their health is experienced should be offered through work sites, academic settings, and continuing education offerings that are timely and economically accessible to a wide variety of nursing professionals. Encouraging nurses to further their education in master and doctoral programs translates into improved opportunities for the development of an ethical nursing practice using feminist theory as a central feature of this education. An ethical practice demands attention to intersectionality, reflexive thinking, and self-reflection while avoiding a narcissistic perseveration and self-awareness, and it values local action as a way to influence women's and gendered minorities' health on a global level.

SUMMARY

Emancipatory feminist paradigms orient practice to praxis and facilitate active engagement and participation in the larger society. Being actively engaged and participating in the larger society unites our individual concerns with the concerns for all populations. The goals of feminist practice thus transcend the boundaries of traditional practice in which the client is an individual.

Feminism is an integrative process that helps women and gendered minorities expand their consciousness about health and identity. In this model, the promotion of health is a function of transforming one's life through the expansion of one's consciousness rather than merely engaging in periodic medical checkups (VanderPlatt, 1999). Subjectivity and agency are prominent within a feminist practice. Women and gendered minorities have awareness of themselves and others and the ability to appreciate the complexity of many diverse situations while acting in the own best interest (Beasley, 1999).

In a feminist model, caring occurs in the context of an open and collaborative relationship. Mutual recognition of one another's expertise, sharing of information, and definition of goals in collaboration are the central elements of the process. Information is shared freely between nurses and clients. The nurse as a consultant provides information about the full range of alternatives for health. The clients make prescriptions for their own health based on information about self-care options. They are part of a relationship in which they define and strive for optimal health.

REFERENCES

Allen, D. G., Allman, K. K., & Powers, P. (1991). Feminist nursing research without gender. *Advances in Nursing Science, 13*(3), 49–58.

Anderson, J. M. (2002). Toward a post-colonial feminist methodology in nursing research: Exploring the convergence of post-colonial and black feminist scholarship. *Nurse Researcher, 9*(3), 7–27.

Anderson, J. M. (2004). Lessons from a postcolonial-feminist perspective: Suffering and a path to healing. *Nursing Inquiry, 11*(4), 238–246.

Andrist, L. C. (1988). A feminist framework for graduate education in women's health. *Journal of Nursing Education, 27*(2), 66–70.

Anzaldúa, G. (1987). A feminist framework for graduate education in women's health. *Nursing Inquiry, 4*(4), 268–276.

Anzaldúa, G. (1999). *Borderlands/La Frontera: The New Mestiza.* San Francisco, CA: Aunt Lute Books.

Apodaca, M. L. (1977). The Chicana woman: An historical materialist perspective. *Latin American Perspectives, 4*(1 & 2), 70–89.

Banks-Wallace, J. (2000). Womanist ways of knowing: Theoretical considerations for research with African American women. *Advances in Nursing Science, 22*(3), 33–45.

Beasley, C. (1999). *What is feminism? An introduction to feminist theory.* London, UK & Thousand Oaks, CA: Sage.

Bricker-Jenkins M., & Hooyman, N. (1989). *Not for women only: Social work practice for a feminist future.* Silver Spring, MD: National Association of Social Workers.

Bunting, S. M. (1997). Applying a feminist analysis model to selected nursing studies of women with HIV. *Issues in Mental Health Nursing, 18*(5), 523–537.

Butler, J. (1993). *Bodies that matter: On the discursive limits of sex.* London, UK: Routledge.

Butler, J. (2000). *Gender trouble: Feminism and the subversion of identity.* London, UK: Routledge.

Campbell, J. C., & Bunting, S. (1991). Voices and paradigms: Perspectives on critical and feminist theory in nursing. *Advances in Nursing Science, 13*(3), 1–15.

Chavez, L. R., Cornelius, W. A., & Jones, O. W. (1986). Utilization of health services by Mexican immigrant women in San Diego. *Women & Health, 11*(2), 3–20.

Chodorow, N. (1978). *The reproduction of mothering: Psychoanalysis and the sociology of gender.* Berkeley, CA: University of California Press.

Chodorow, N. (1987). *Feminism and psychoanalytic theory.* New Haven, CT: Yale University Press.

Chodorow, N. (1994). *Feminisms, masculinities, sexualities: Freud and beyond.* Lexington, KY: University of Kentucky Press.

Chopoorian, T. (1986). Reconceptualizing the environment. In P. Moccia (Ed.), *New approaches to theory development* (pp. 39–54). New York, NY: National League for Nursing.

Chow, E. N. (1987). The development of feminist consciousness among Asian American women. *Gender & Society, 1*(3), 284–299.

Cixous, H. (1975). *The Laugh of the Medusa.* London, UK: Oxford University Press.

Cixous, H. (1991). *The book of Promethea.* Lincoln, NE: University of Nebraska Press.

Clear, G. M., & Carryer, J. B. (2001). Shadow dancing in the wings: Lesbian women talk about health care. *Nursing Praxis in New Zealand, 17*(3), 27–39.

Collins, P. H. (1989). The social construction of black feminist thought. *Signs, 14*, 745–773.

Collins, P. H. (2000). *Black feminist thought* (2nd ed.). New York, NY: Routledge.

Corbett, A. M., Francis, K., & Chapman, Y. (2007). Feminist-informed participatory action research: A methodology of choice for examining critical nursing issues. *International Journal of Nursing Practice, 13*(2), 81–88.

Corea, G. (1986). *The mother machine: Reproductive technologies from artificial insemination to artificial wombs.* New York, NY: Harper Collins.

Correa-de-Araujo, R. (2006). Serious gaps: How the lack of sex/gender-based research impairs health. *Journal of Women's Health, 15*(10), 1116–1122.

Crenshaw, K. (1995). Mapping the margins: Intersectionality, identity, politics, and violence against women of color. In K. Crenshaw, N. Gotanda, G. Peller, & K. Thomas (Eds.), *Critical race theory: The key writings that formed the movement.* New York, NY: New Press.

Daly, M. (1978). *Gyn/ecology: The metaethics of radical feminism.* Boston, MA: Beacon Press.

Davis, A. Y. (1981). *Women, race and class.* New York, NY: Vintage Books.

Davis, A. Y. (1989). *Women, culture, and politics.* New York, NY: Random House.

Davis, A. Y. (1991). *A place of rage (Videorecording).* Channel Four Television. New York, NY: Women Making Movies.

Del Portillo, C. T. (1987). Poverty, self-concept, and health: Experience of Latinas. *Women & Health, 12*(3 and 4), 229–242.

Dey, J. G., & Hill, C. (2007). *Behind the pay gap.* Washington, DC: American Association of University Women Educational Foundation.

DiEmanuele, E. (2015). *A comprehensive guide to feminist theory: 20 essential reads.* Retrieved from http://qwiklit.com/2013/10/21/a-comprehensive-guide-to-feminist-theory-20-essential-reads

Dill, B. T. (1983). Race, class, and gender: Prospects for an all-inclusive sisterhood. *Feminist Studies, 9*(1), 131–149.

Dill, B. T. (1987). The dialectics of black womanhood. In S. Harding (Ed.), *Feminism and methodology: Social science issues* (pp. 97–108). Bloomington, IN: Indiana University Press.

Dinnerstein, D. (1976). *The mermaid and the minotaur: Sexual arrangements and human malaise.* New York, NY: Harper & Row.

Dinnerstein, D. (1989). What does feminism mean. In A. Harris & Y. King (Eds.), *Rocking the ship of state: Toward a feminist peace politics* (pp. 13–23). Boulder, CO: Westview Press.

Dworkin, A. (1974). *Woman hating.* New York, NY: Penguin Books.

Dworkin, A. (1976). *Our blood: Prophecies and discourses on sexual politics.* New York, NY: Harper & Row.

Ensign, J. (2001). "Shut up and listen": Feminist health care with out-of-the-mainstream adolescent females. *Issues in Comprehensive Pediatric Nursing, 24*(2), 71–84.

Firestone, S. (1970). *The dialectic of sex: The case for feminist revolution.* New York, NY: Morrow.

Fulkerson, M. (1994). *Changing the subject: Women's discourses and feminist theology.* Minneapolis, MN: Fortress Press.

Gillespie, M. A. (1984). The myth of the strong black woman. In A. M. Jaggar & P. S. Rothenberg (Eds.), *Feminist frameworks: Alternative theoretical accounts of the relations between women and men* (2nd ed., pp. 32–35). New York, NY: McGraw-Hill.

Ginorio, A., & Reno, J. (1985). Violence in the lives of Latina women. *Working Together, 5*(5), 7–9.

Glass, N. (2002). Difference still troubles university environments: Emotional health issues associated with lesbian visibility in nursing schools. *Contemporary Nurse, 12*(3), 284–293.

Gopaldas, A. (2013). Intersectionality 101. *Journal of Social Marketing, 32*(Special Issue), 90–94.

Gordon-Bradshaw, R. H. (1987). A social essay on special issues facing poor women of color. *Women & Health, 12*(3–4), 243–259.

Griffin, S. (1978). *Woman and nature: The roaring inside her.* New York, NY: Harper & Row.

Hale, J. C. (1985). Return to the bear paw. In J. W. Cochran, D. Langston, & C. Woodward (Eds.), *Changing our power: An introduction to women's studies* (pp. 55–60). Dubuque, IA: Kendall/Hunt.

Haraway, D. (1989). *Primate visions: Gender, race, and nature in the world of modern science.* London, UK: Routledge.

Harrison, B. (1985). *Making the connections: Essays in feminist social ethics.* Boston, MA: Beacon Press.

Herman, A. M. (1984). Still . . . small change for black women. In A. M. Jaggar & P. S. Rothenberg (Eds.), *Feminist frameworks: Alternative theoretical accounts of the relations between women and men* (2nd ed., pp. 36–39). New York, NY: McGraw-Hill.

hooks, b. (1984). The myth of black matriarchy. In A. M. Jaggar & P. S. Rothenberg (Eds.), *Feminist frameworks: Alternative theoretical accounts of the relations between women and men* (2nd ed., pp. 369–373). New York, NY: McGraw-Hill.

hooks, b. (1997). *Wounds of passion.* New York, NY: Holt.

hooks, b. (1999a). *Ain't I a woman? Black women and feminism.* Brooklyn, NY: South End Press.

hooks, b. (1999b). *Feminism is for everybody: Passionate politics.* Cambridge, MA: South End Press.

hooks, b. (2000). *Feminist theory: From margin to center.* Brooklyn, NY: South End Press.

Hurtado, A. (1989). Relating to privilege: Seduction and rejection in the subordination of white women and women of color. *Signs, 14*(4), 883–856.

Hurtado, A. (1996). *The color of privilege: Three blasphemies on race and feminism.* Ann Arbor, MI: University of Michigan Press.

Im, E.-O. (2000). A feminist critique of breast cancer research among Korean women. *Western Journal of Nursing Research, 22*(5), 551–565; discussion 566.

Im, E.-O., & Meleis, A. I. (2001). Women's work and symptoms during midlife: Korean immigrant women. *Women & Health, 33*(1–2), 83–103.

Im, E.-O., Meleis, A. I., & Park, Y. S. (1999). A feminist critique of research on menopausal experiences of Korean women. *Research in Nursing & Health, 22*(5), 410–420.

Irigaray, L. (1974). *Speculum of the other woman.* Ithaca, NY: Cornell University Press.

Irigaray, L. (1977). *This sex which is not one.* Ithaca, NY: Cornell University Press.

Isasi-Diaz, A. (1993). *En la lucha/in the struggle: Elaborating a mujerista theology.* Minneapolis, MN: Fortress Press.

Isasi-Diaz, A., & Tarango, Y. (1992). *Hispanic women: Prophetic voices in the church.* Minneapolis, MN: Fortress Press.

Jagose, A. (1996). *Queer theory: An introduction.* New York, NY: New York University Press.

Johnson, J. L., Bottorff, J. L., Browne, A. J., Grewal, S., Hilton, B. A., & Clarke, H. (2004). Othering and being othered in the context of health care services. *Health Communication, 16*(2), 255–271.

Kelly, P. J., Bobo, T. J., McLachlan, K., Avery, S., & Burge, S. K. (2006). Girl World: A primary prevention program for Mexican American girls. *Health Promotion Practice, 7*(2), 174–179.

Kristeva, J. (1980). *Desire in language: a semiotic approach to literature.* New York, NY: Columbia University Press.

Kristeva, J. (1982). *Powers of horror: An essay in abjection.* New York, NY: Columbia University Press.

Lorde, A. (1984). Scratching the surface: Some notes on barriers to women and loving. In A. M. Jaggar & P. S. Rothenberg (Eds.), *Feminist frameworks: Alternative theoretical accounts of the relations between women and men* (2nd ed., pp. 432–436). New York, NY: McGraw-Hill.

Lorde, A. (1988). Age, race, class and sex: Women redefining difference. In C. McEwen & S. O'Sullivan (Eds.), *Out the other side* (pp. 269–276). London, UK: Virago Press.

MacKinnon, C. (1989). *Toward a feminist theory of the state.* Cambridge, MA: Harvard University Press.

Marcus, S. (2005). Queer theory for everyone: A review essay. *Signs, 31*(1), 191–218.

Maxwell-Young, L., Olshansky, E., & Steele, R. (1998). Conducting feminist research in nursing: Personal and political challenges. *Health Care for Women International, 19*(6), 505–513.

McGibbon, E., Mulaudzi, F. M., Didham, P., Barton, S., & Sochan, A. (2014). Toward decolonizing nursing: The colonization of nursing and strategies for increasing the counter-narrative. *Nursing Inquiry, 21*(3), 179–191.

Merriam-Webster (n.d.). Feminazi. Retrieved from http://www.merriam-webster.com/dictionary/feminazi

Mill, J. S. (1878). *The subjection of women.* London, UK: Longmans, Green, Reader & Dyer.

Moraga, C. (1983). A long line of vendidas. In C. Moraga, *Loving in the war years: Lo que nunca pasó por sus labios* (pp. 90–144). Boston, MA: South End Press.

Moraga, C. (1997). *Waiting in the wings: Portrait of a queer motherhood.* Ithaca, NY: Firebrand Books.

Moraga, C., & Anzaldúa, C. (Eds.). (1983). *This bridge called my back: Writings by radical women of color.* New York, NY: Kitchen Table: Women of Color Press.

Neufeld, A., Harrison, M. J., Stewart, M. J., Hughes, K. D., & Spitzer, D. (2002). Immigrant women: Making connections to community resources for support in family caregiving. *Qualitative Health Research, 12*(6), 751–768.

Pirner, D. (2005). "Multiple margins" (being older, a woman, or a visible minority) constrained older women's access to Canadian health care. *Evidence-Based Nursing, 8*(4), 128.

Rich, A. (1977). *Of women born: Motherhood as experience and institution.* London, UK: Virago.

Rich, A. (1981). *Compulsory heterosexuality and lesbian experience.* London, UK: Onlywomen Press.

Richman, J. A., Jason, L. A., Taylor, R. R., & Jahn, S. C. (2000). Feminist perspectives on the social construction of chronic fatigue syndrome. *Health Care for Women International, 21*(3), 173–185.

Rudman, C. (2012). "Feminazi": The history of Limbaugh's trademark slur against women. *Media Matters for America.* Retrieved from http://mm4a.org/1X2SbWb

Sampselle, C. M. (1990). The influence of feminist philosophy on nursing practice. *Image—The Journal of Nursing Scholarship, 22*(4), 243–247.

Sanchez, C. L. (1984). Sex, class and race intersections: Visions of women of color. In B. Brant (Ed.), *A gathering of spirit* (pp. 150–155). New York, NY: Sinister Wisdom.

Sánchez-Ayéndez, M. (1989). Puerto Rican elderly women: The cultural dimension of social support networks. *Women & Health, 14*(3–4), 239–252.

Schroeder, C., & Ward, D. (1998). Women, welfare, and work: One view of the debate. *Nursing Outlook, 46*(5), 226–232.

Scott, J., Kaplan, C., & Keates, D. (1997). *Transitions, environments, translations: Feminisms in international politics.* London, UK: Routledge.

Segura, D. A. (1989). Chicana and Mexican immigrant women at work: The impact of class, race, and gender on occupational mobility. *Gender & Society, 3*(1), 37–52.

Smith, B. (1982). Black women's health: Notes for a course. In R. Hubbard, M. S. Henifin, & B. Fried (Eds.), *Biological woman—The convenient myth* (pp. 227–239). Rochester, VT: Schenkman Books.

Snyder, R. C. (2008). What is third-wave feminism? A new directions essay. *Signs, 34*(1), 175–196.

Spinks, V. S., Andrews, J., & Boyle, J. S. (2000). Providing health care for lesbian clients. *Journal of Transcultural Nursing: Official Journal of the Transcultural Nursing Society, 11*(2), 137–143.

Sturgeon, N. (1997). *Ecofeminist natures: Race, gender, feminist theory and political action.* London, UK: Routledge.

Taylor, J. Y. (1998). Womanism: A methodologic framework for African American women. *Advances in Nursing Science, 21*(1), 53–64.

Taylor, J. Y. (2002). Talking back: Research as an act of resistance and healing for African American women survivors of intimate male partner violence. *Women & Therapy, 25*(3–4), 145–160.

Taylor, J. Y. (2004). Moving from surviving to thriving: African American women recovering from intimate male partner abuse. *Research and Theory for Nursing Practice, 18*(1), 35–50.

Taylor, J. Y. (2005). No resting place: African American women at the crossroads of violence. *Violence Against Women, 11*(12), 1473–1489.

Tigert, L. M. (2001). The power of shame: Lesbian battering as a manifestation of homophobia. *Women & Therapy, 23*(3), 73–85.

Tong, R. (1998). Feminist thought: *A more comprehensive introduction.* Boulder, CO: Westview Press.

Tsutakawa, M. (1988). Chest of kimonos—A female family history. In J. W. Cochran, D. Langston, & C. Woodward (Eds.), *Changing our power: An introduction to women's studies* (pp. 76–83). Dubuque, IA: Kendall/Hunt.

VanderPlatt, M. (1999). Locating the feminist scholar: Relational empowerment and social activism. *Qualitative Health Research, 9*(6), 773–785.

Visweswaran, K. (1994). *Fictions of feminist ethnography.* Minneapolis, MN: University of Minnesota Press.

Walker, A. (1983). *In search of our mothers' gardens.* New York, NY: Harcourt, Brace Jovanovich.

Weedon, C. (1997). *Feminist practice and poststructuralist theory.* Cambridge, MA: Blackwell.

Witt, S. H. (1984). Native women today: Sexism and the Indian woman. In A. M. Jaggar & P. S. Rothenberg (Eds.), *Feminist frameworks: Alternative theoretical accounts of the relations between women and men* (2nd ed., pp. 23–31). New York, NY: McGraw-Hill.

Wolf, D. (1996). *Feminist dilemmas in fieldwork.* Boulder, CO: Westview Press.

Wollstonecraft, M. A. (1796) *A vindication of the rights of woman with strictures on political and moral subjects.* London, UK: Joseph Johnson.

Women Against Feminism. (2015). Retrieved from http://womenagainstfeminism.tumblr.com

Woods, N. F., Lentz, M., Mitchell, E., & Oakley, L. D. (1994). Depressed mood and self-esteem in young Asian, Black, and White women in America. *Health Care for Women International, 15*(3), 243–262.

Yeatman, A. (1994). *Postmodern revisions of the political.* London, UK: Routledge.

Young, I. M. (1990). *Justice and the politics of difference.* Princeton, NJ: Princeton University Press.

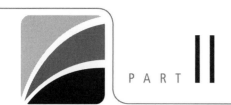

PART II

Health Promotion
and Prevention for Women

Women's Bodies

Elizabeth A. Kostas-Polston • Cara J. Krulewitch

Providing health care to women offers a special opportunity to educate women about their bodies and the intricacies of their female form and functions. Established as the major consumers of health care and the primary gatekeepers of their family's health, women are usually eager to learn about how their bodies work and how to keep them healthy (Hoffman & Johnson, 1995; Pinn, 2003). When given the chance, they often express curiosity about the specifics related to their particular anatomy or physiology. Although a frequently neglected topic in routine health care, women also wonder about their sexuality and their body's ability to experience pleasure.

Discovering that there are unique biological differences about having a female body beyond solely the reproductive system interests many women, as well. Over the past decade, the advanced scientific study of cellular and molecular mechanisms of human biology have uncovered new, significant sex-based differences in physiological functions (Institute of Medicine [IOM] Committee on Understanding the Biology of Sex and Gender Differences, 2001). Being familiar with these discoveries in biological sex differences is important to anyone involved in health care in order to promote a better understanding of the implications for disease prevention and health maintenance of women.

The purpose of this chapter is to highlight key aspects of female anatomy and physiology for those providing health care to women across their life span. The chapter begins with a review of the structural and functional aspects of a woman's anatomy. Next, a brief discussion of the endocrine system and, specifically, the physiological influences of hormone secretion in women's bodies sets the stage for understanding the complexities of women's cyclic rhythms. Finally, a description of initial sexual differentiation and development, pubertal development, and changes occurring during menarche and menopause, as women's bodies mature across their life span, is presented.

■ GENDER DIFFERENCE IN NONREPRODUCTIVE ANATOMY AND PHYSIOLOGY

Sexual dimorphism refers to the condition in which males and females in a species are morphologically different (phenotypic expression; Kirchengast, 2010; *The Free Dictionary*, 2014).

There are differences in a number of body systems in both anatomy and physiology between males and females. A little more than 15 years ago, the IOM evaluated this topic and concluded that (a) sex matters because being male or female is an important variable that results in differences in health and illness that go beyond differences in hormones associated with reproduction, (b) the study of sex differences is evolving into a mature science, and (c) barriers to the advancement of knowledge about sex differences must be eliminated. The IOM made a number of recommendations that sex differences should be evaluated at the cellular level and from the *womb to tomb*. They noted that males and females have different patterns of illnesses and different life spans that raise questions of both biology and environment in these disparities. In many body systems, such as the brain, arguments abound on the influence of phenotypic differences on behavior and abilities (McCarthy, 2016; Pardue & Wizemann, 2001). This section moves away from potential differences in behavior and abilities and focuses on the physical differences that may be observed during a physical examination.

On an average, adult men are about 6 inches taller and weigh about 30 pounds more compared with adult women (Fryar, Gu, & Ogden, 2012). Females have been shown to have 42 % to 68% less absolute strength compared with males (Frontera, Hughes, Lutz, & Evans, 1991) and about 62% of the grip strength of males (Perna et al., 2016).

Variations in lung function can also be observed. Female lungs are smaller in size and weight compared with male lungs that are present throughout life (Carey et al., 2007; Jackson, 2008). Additionally, the conducting airways of adult males are larger than those of adult females, even when lung or body sizes are equivalent (Carey et al., 2007). To this end, Jackson (2008) sought to evaluate sex differences in cardiovascular fitness by evaluating the 2002 to 2007 National Health Examination Survey (NHANES) and found that sex was the strongest predictor of lung function where females have lower levels of VO_2 max (peak oxygen uptake) and cardiovascular fitness across all age groups (Joyner, Barnes, Hart, Wallin, & Charkoudian, 2015).

Similar differences can be found in the integumentary, gastrointestinal (GI), and urinary systems. Female skin is thinner than male skin and has thicker subcutaneous tissues compared with males (Dao & Kazin, 2007). Females tend to deposit fat stores differently from males, with higher stores in the hips and legs compared with the abdomen in males (Jensen, 2002). These differences are amplified in obesity in which increased visceral fat in males contributes to elevated inflammatory cytokines compared with females (Bloor & Symonds, 2014). In the GI system, there are differences in the gut microbiome, in which women have a lower abundance of Bacteroidetes compared with men (Dominianni et al., 2015). Additionally, the liver metabolizes drugs differently in males compared with females. Good examples of this are found in the lower clearance of zolpidem (a sedative) in females compared with males (Greenblatt et al., 2014), leading to a Food and Drug Administration (FDA) warning and different dosing regimens for women compared with men (FDA news release, 2013). It is important to be aware that there may be other similar differences not yet identified. The kidney's ability to conserve water is through the action of vasopressin, a peptide hormone released by the posterior pituitary. The vasopressin receptor that mediates the antidiuretic effect is expressed twice as much in females compared with males (Juul, Klein, Sandström, Erichsen, & Nørgaard, 2011), which may increase the risk of hyponatremia under certain conditions such as open-water swimming (Wagner, Knechtle, Knechtle, Rüest, & Rosemann, 2012).

When it comes to differences in the brain, we do not address the discourse regarding differences in intelligence or behavior; however, we focus our discussion on the demonstrated differences in brain chemistry and structure (deVries & Forger, 2015; deVries & Simerly, 2002; Forger, deVries, & Breedlove, 2015). Differences in the sensory system have also been observed. Females have a higher incidence of dry eye compared with males; this may be attributed to the influence of hormones (Truong, Cole, Stapleton, & Golebiowski, 2014). Pain thresholds also vary; however, the findings present complicated results that still remain mixed. Scientists participating in a National Institutes of Health Consensus Development Conference evaluated the research on sex differences in pain response and found that it varied based on the type of pain that was tested and in some cases, was associated with menstrual cycle influences. Greenblatt et al. (2007) noted that the largest and most consistent findings were for pressure pain and electrical stimulation, whereas the least consistent findings were for thermal pain stimuli. These findings and those of others also demonstrated evidence for sex differences in responsiveness to analgesics, noting that females may respond better to morphine compared with males; however, findings are not as clear for mixed μ- and κ-opioids, such as butorphanol or nalbuphine (Mogil, 2012).

In summary, there are a number of sex differences related to the anatomy and physiology of male and female human beings that should be considered when providing health care to women. These differences affect all body systems.

■ WOMEN'S REPRODUCTIVE ANATOMY AND PHYSIOLOGY

Breasts

Lactation, or the synthesis, secretion and ejection of milk, is the primary function of the breasts. They are also a prominent secondary sex characteristic. Estrogen stimulates maturation of the female breast at puberty through the proliferation and branching of the duct system and full development of the nipples. Proliferation of acini at the ends of the ducts is due to the synergistic action of both progesterone and estrogen (Ellis & Mahadevan, 2013; McGuire, 2016; Pandya & Moore, 2011).

LOCATION

Considered as organs of the integumentary system, breasts are highly specialized variants of sweat (or apocrine) glands, located between the second and sixth ribs and between the sternal and midaxillary lines. About two thirds of the breast lies superficial to the pectoralis major, the remainder to the serratus anterior (Ellis & Mahadevan, 2013).

APPEARANCE

The breasts of healthy women are generally symmetrical in shape and amplitude, although they are often not absolutely equal in size. Breasts are typically measured by both chest circumference and their fullness. What are commonly defined as plural glands are actually two parts of a single, contiguous anatomical breast with a proliferation of a shared nerve, vascular, and lymphatic supply (Porth, 2007). The skin covering the breasts is similar to that of the abdomen. Hair follicles sometimes are noted around the darker pigmented area surrounding the nipple, called the *areola*. Often, women with fair complexions can note a vascular pattern in a horizontal or vertical dimension under the superficial skin of the breast tissue. When present, this pattern is usually symmetrical. The distinguishing difference between male and female breasts is the proliferation and branching of the duct system, glandular epithelium, and nonadipose stroma (Vandenberg, Schaeberle, Rubin, Sonnenschein, & Soto, 2013).

The areolar pigment varies in color from pink to brown, in position on the breast, and in size from woman to woman. The areola surrounds the nipple that is located at the tip of each breast. Several sebaceous glands can be seen on the areola as small elevations that are called *Montgomery's tubercles* to keep the nipple area soft and stretchy. The nipples are more darkly pigmented and usually protuberant because of erectile muscles. Nipple size and shape are highly variable from woman to woman, and the same woman may notice a great deal of variation in the size and shape of her nipples depending on the extent to which they are contracted. The erectile tissue of the nipple is responsive to emotional and tactile stimulation, thus promoting the recreative function of the breasts. Some women have inverted nipples, a condition in which the nipple is dimpled or its central portion is flattened or depressed. A normal nipple that suddenly becomes inverted may indicate the presence of breast cancer (McGuire, 2016, Pandya & Moore, 2011).

Some women have supernumerary nipples, nipples and breasts, or breast tissue. This supernumerary tissue develops along the longitudinal ridges extending from the axilla to the groin, which existed during early embryonic development.

Visible changes in a woman's breast occur in conjunction with her development. Before the age of 10 years, there is little visible distinction between boys' and girls' breasts. At approximately the age of 10 years, the mammary buds appear in girls' breasts. The subareolar mammary tissue is not prominent at this point. The adult breast develops under the influence of estrogen and progesterone. During the transition to adulthood, the prominent subareolar tissue of adolescence recedes into the contour of the remainder of the breast and the nipple protrudes. (See the later section "Puberty" for a more complete description of breast changes that occur during puberty.)

Breast shape and texture are influenced by nutritional factors, heredity, endocrine factors, and hormonal sensitivity in addition to age, muscle tone, and pregnancy. Nodularity, tenderness, and size of the breasts may fluctuate with the menstrual cycle. Usually, women's breasts are smallest during days 4 to 7 of the menstrual cycle, shortly after menstruation. An increase in breast volume, tenderness, heaviness, fullness, and general or nipple tenderness may be experienced just before menstruation.

Short-lived changes of appearance are observed in many women during sexual response, including protuberance of the nipple and increase in breast size. The breasts are highly erogenous organs. They do not merely vary in shape and size with sexual excitement, but there is also a great deal of variation from woman to woman in areas of the breasts perceived as erotic. For example, some women perceive erotic sensations in the areolae, others in the nipple, and still others in the breast tissue near the axilla.

A woman's breasts may also double or triple in size during pregnancy. Striae, engorgement of veins, and increased prominence and pigmentation of the nipple and areolae are common during pregnancy. The glandular tissue of the breast gradually involutes after menopause and fat is deposited. Therefore the breasts of postmenopausal women take on a more flattened contour as they age and appear less firm than before menopause.

A convention useful in describing the appearance of women's breasts during physical examination is a division into four quadrants by vertical and horizontal lines crossing at the nipple (e.g., upper, outer quadrant of left breast). Another landmark, the axillary tail (also called the tail of Spence) is a portion of breast tissue that extends into the axilla. A more precise description of breast landmarks is one that incorporates an analogy to the face of a clock: A lump could be described at 2 o'clock and include the appropriate number of centimeters from the nipple.

COMPONENTS OF BREAST TISSUE

About two thirds of the breast lies on the pectoralis major, overlapping on the serratus anterior, and at its lower end is against the rectus sheath (Ellis & Mahadevan, 2013). There are three main components of tissue in women's breasts: glandular, fibrous, and fatty tissue. Most of the breast is composed of subcutaneous and retromammary (behind the breast) fat. Breast tissue is supported by fibrous tissue, including suspensory ligaments (Cooper's ligaments), extending from the subcutaneous connective tissue to the muscle fascia (Figure 7.1).

An important functional component of the breast is the glandular tissue, which consists of 12 to 25 lobes that terminate in ducts that open on the surface of the nipple. Each lobe is composed of 20 to 40 lobules, each of which contains 10 to 100 alveoli (sometimes called acini).

The alveolus is the basic component of the breast lobule. The hollow alveolus is lined by a single layer of milk-secreting columnar epithelial cells, which are derived prenatally from an ingrowth of epidermis into the mesenchyme between 10 and 12 weeks of gestation. These cells enlarge greatly and discharge their contents during lactation. The individual alveolus is encased in a network of myoepithelial strands and is surrounded by a rich capillary network. The lumen of the alveolus opens into a collecting intralobar (within the lobe) duct through a thin, nonmuscular duct. The intralobar ducts eventually end in the openings in the nipple and are surrounded by muscle cells.

SUPPORTING STRUCTURES

The third and fourth branches of the cervical plexus provide the cutaneous nerve supply to the upper breast and the thoracic intercostal nerves to the lower breast. The perforating branches of the internal mammary artery constitute the chief external blood supply, although additional arterial blood supply emanates from several branches of the axillary artery. Superficial veins of the breast drain into the internal mammary veins and the superficial veins of the lower portion of the neck and from the latter into the jugular vein. Veins emptying into the internal mammary, axillary, and intercostal veins serve deep breast tissue (Pandya & Moore, 2011).

The lymphatic drainage of the breast is of special interest and importance to women because of its role in the dissemination of tumor cells as well as its ability to respond to infection. The lymphatic system of the breast is both abundant and complex. In general, the lymphatics drain both the axillary and internal mammary areas. Lymph from the skin of the breast, with the exception of areolar and nipple areas, flows into the axillary nodes on the same side of the body, whereas the lymph from the medial cutaneous breast area may flow into the opposite breast. The lymph from the areolar and nipple areas flows into the anterior axillary (mammary) nodes.

Lymph from deep within the mammary tissues flows into the anterior axillary nodes but may also flow into the apical, subclavian, infraclavicular, and supraclavicular nodes. Lymph from areas behind the areolae and the medial and lower glandular areas of breast tissue communicates with the lymphatic systems draining into the thorax and abdomen (see Figure 7.1).

The Female Perineum

The diamond-shaped structure bounded by the pelvic diaphragm, symphysis pubis, and coccyx is commonly referred to as the *perineum* (Graziottin & Gambini, 2015). It includes the vulva, clitoris, vaginal orifice, and anus (Hosseinzadeh, Heller, & Houshmand, 2012; Puppo, 2013).

VULVA

The external female genitalia are commonly referred to as the *vulva*. Many of a woman's genital structures can be visualized easily by her with a mirror (Figure 7.2). The configuration of the genitals is strikingly unique to each woman

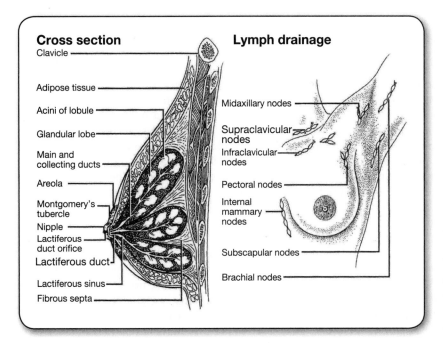

Cross section

Clavicle
Adipose tissue
Acini of lobule
Glandular lobe
Main and collecting ducts
Areola
Montgomery's tubercle
Nipple
Lactiferous duct orifice
Lactiferous duct
Lactiferous sinus
Fibrous septa

Lymph drainage

Midaxillary nodes
Supraclavicular nodes
Infraclavicular nodes
Pectoral nodes
Internal mammary nodes
Subscapular nodes
Brachial nodes

FIGURE 7.1

Components of breast tissue and lymph drainage. Breast tissue is composed of glandular, fibrous, and fatty tissue. Lymph from the skin of the breast flows to the axillary nodes, and lymph from the medial cutaneous area of the breast flows to the opposite breast. Lymph from the areolae and the nipple flows into the mammary nodes.

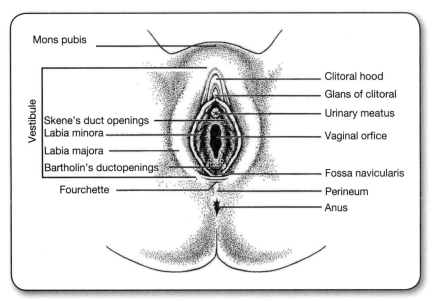

Mons pubis

Vestibule

Skene's duct openings
Labia minora
Labia majora
Bartholin's ductopenings
Fourchette

Clitoral hood
Glans of clitoral
Urinary meatus
Vaginal orfice
Fossa navicularis
Perineum
Anus

FIGURE 7.2
External genitalia.

and highly variable from woman to woman. For example, many paired structures, such as the labia, are not perfectly symmetrical. There are specific anatomical points observed in the external female genitalia; however, as Krissi, Ben-Shitrit, Aviram, and Weintraub (2016) noted, there is wide variation in their anatomical appearance.

Adult female pubic hair is rather coarse, curly, and often darker than the hair on a woman's head. Pubic hair not only covers parts of the vulvar area (mons pubis, labia majora) but may extend upward toward the abdomen and outward onto the inner thighs. The flattened area of pubic hair over the lower abdomen forms the base of an inverted triangle. The triangle is sometimes referred to as the *female escutcheon*. Although this is a somewhat typical pattern, it is not uncommon for healthy women to exhibit variation in this pattern. For example, hair growth may extend up toward the umbilicus in a narrow diamond pattern or back toward the anus. Some women have little pubic hair or a

well-delineated triangular area, whereas others have a prolific hair pattern. As a woman ages, her pubic hair eventually turns gray and thins.

The mons veneris or mons pubis is composed of soft, fatty tissue and lies over the symphysis pubis. The labia majora consist of two larger, raised folds of adipose tissue. The inner surface of the labia majora consists of apocrine (scent), eccrine (sweat), and sebaceous (oil) glands that serve to lubricate as well as stimulate by releasing a classic, female musk scent during sexual arousal. The labia majora are heavily pigmented, and in postpubertal women, their outer surfaces are covered with hair, whereas the inner surfaces are smooth and hairless. In postmenopausal women, the hair on the labia becomes thinner, and the labia and mons appear less full as a result of the loss of fatty tissue.

The labia minora are two very thin folds of inner skin heavily endowed with blood vessels that lie within the labia majora and extend from the clitoris to the fourchette (vaginal outlet). Each of the labia minora divides into a medial and a lateral part. The medial parts join anteriorly to the clitoris to form the clitoral hood (also called prepuce), and the lateral parts join posteriorly to the clitoris. There are more nerve endings in the labia minora than the outer labia majora. There are also more sebaceous glands to lubricate the opening into the vagina (the vestibule) to provide waterproof protection against urine, menstrual bleeding, and bacteria. In some women, the labia minora are completely hidden from view by the labia majora, while in other women the labia minora protrude out from between the labia majora. Frequently, the labia minora are asymmetrical.

The color and texture of the labia minora are highly individual, varying from pink to brown. The clitoral hood covers the clitoris and is believed to protect this extremely sensitive organ from irritation. In some women, the clitoral hood will adhere to the clitoris so that the hood cannot be pulled back very far to reveal the clitoris (Figure 7.3).

The area between the labia minora is called the *vestibule*. It contains both the urethral and vaginal orifices. The hymen, a membranous covering at the vaginal opening, may be intact but more frequently is seen as a ring of small, rounded skin fragments attached to the margins of the vaginal opening. This fluted or ruffled appearance is due to the natural erosion of the hymen from regular childhood activities such as running, jumping, and riding a bicycle. Some women have a more thick and rigid membrane that remains intact even after penile penetration. Approximately one of every 2,000 women has a hymen that must be surgically removed (Hegazy & Al-Rukban, 2012; Stoppard, 2002).

Skene's glands are tiny, clustered paraurethral organs, the ducts of which open laterally and posteriorly to the urethral orifice. Bartholin's glands, located lateral and

slightly posterior to the vaginal introitus, open into the groove between the labia minora and the hymen at the 5- and 7-o'clock positions in relation to the vaginal orifice. Both Skene's and Bartholin's glands are usually not visible, although they are located in tissues that can be visualized, and their openings on the vulva can be seen in some women. These racemose glands serve a lubricating function by secreting mucus. The perineum consists of the tissues between the vaginal orifice and the anus. Beneath the vestibule are two bundles of vascular tissue referred to as the *bulbs of the vestibule* or the *perineal sponge*. These tissues become congested during sexual response (Puppo & Puppo, 2015).

CLITORIS

The various structural components of the clitoris are homologous to similar structures of the male penis (Puppo, 2013). The clitoris, from the Greek word meaning key, has the same number of nerve endings at its tips as the glans of the penis, making it extremely sensitive to tactile stimulation (Puppo, 2013). The clitoris is an external organ that has three erectile sections (glans, body, and crura) lying under the skin. The free part of the clitoris includes the glans located inside of the prepuce, which is formed by the labia minora (Puppo, 2013). The clitoris consists of two corpora cavernosa (cavernous bodies) enclosed in a dense fibrous membrane that is made up of elastic fibers and smooth muscle bundles. Each corpus is connected to the pubic ramus and the ischium. The clitoris is held in place by a suspensory ligament and two small ischiocavernosus muscles that insert into the crura of the clitoris (Masters & Johnson, 1966; Puppo, 2013).

The labia minora are two thin folds of skin that have sebaceous and eccrine glands. They do not have a layer of subcutaneous fat and sit medial to the labia majora. The labia minora have two parts; the first, the lateral parts, form the prepuce of the clitoris, and the second, the medial parts, unite underneath to form its frenulum (Puppo, 2013).

The blood supply to the clitoris emanates from the deep and dorsal clitoral arteries that branch from the internal pudendal artery. The vasculature of the clitoris plays an important role in increasing its size during sexual response.

The length of the clitoral body (consisting of glans and shaft) varies markedly. The size of the clitoral glans may vary from 2 mm to 1 cm in healthy women and is usually estimated to be 4 to 5 mm in both the transverse and longitudinal planes. There is also variation in the position of the clitoris, a function of variation in the points of origin of the suspensory and crural ligaments. The glans is capable of increasing in size with sexual stimulation, and marked vasocongestion increases the diameter of the clitoral shaft (Masters & Johnson, 1966; Puppo, 2013).

The dorsal nerve of the clitoris is the deepest division of the pudendal nerve, and it terminates in the nerve endings of the glans and corpora cavernosa. Pacinian corpuscles, which respond to deep pressure, are distributed in both the glans and the corpora but have greater concentration in the glans and are highly variable. The clitoris is endowed with sensory nerve endings that respond to tactile stimuli as well as pressure. Although afferent stimuli can be received through afferent nerve endings in the clitoral glans and shaft, it is also possible that the clitoris serves as the subjective end

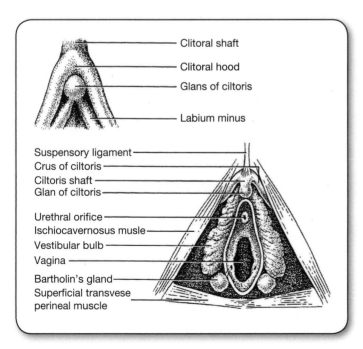

Clitoral shaft
Clitoral hood
Glans of ciltoris
Labium minus

Suspensory ligament
Crus of ciltoris
Ciltoris shaft
Glan of ciltoris
Urethral orifice
Ischiocavernosus muscle
Vestibular bulb
Vagina
Bartholin's gland
Superficial transvese perineal muscle

FIGURE 7.3

The clitoris. The sole purpose of the clitoris is the reception and transformation of sexual stimuli.

Source: Puppo and Puppo (2015).

point or transformer for efferent stimuli from higher neuro-genic pathways (Masters & Johnson, 1966; Puppo, 2013).

VAGINA

Although the vagina can be considered an internal structure, it can be visualized easily with the assistance of a speculum, a light source, and a mirror. The vagina is a musculomembranous canal connecting the vulva with the uterus. It is lined with a reddish pink mucous membrane that is transversely rugated. Under the stratified squamous epithelial lining (much like the skin on the palm of the hand) is a muscular coat that has an inner circular layer and an outer fibrous layer (Figure 7.4).

The vagina is typically a potential rather than a real space, as it is ordinarily an empty, collapsed tube. Although highly distensible, its unstimulated length is approximately 6 to 7 cm anteriorly and 9 cm posteriorly. The vaginal canal inclines posteriorly at about a 45° angle. The cervix is the neck of the uterus and is encased in the vagina anteriorly and superiorly. There is a recessed portion of the vagina adjacent to the cervix, which, together with the cervix, is called the *vaginal fornix*. The fornix has anterior, posterior, and lateral portions.

One of the important physiological functions of the vagina during sexual response is its ability to produce lubrication by means of transudation of mucoid material across its rugated folds. In addition, vaginal lubrication occurs in a rhythmic 90-minute cycle throughout the day and night. The circulatory venous plexus (including the bulbus vestibuli, plexus pudendalis, plexus uterovaginalis, and possibly the plexus vesicalis and plexus rectalis) encircling the vaginal barrel probably provides the circulatory support for vaginal lubrication and a constant natural sloughing of dead epithelial cells. This vaginal discharge is normal and is called *leukorrhea*.

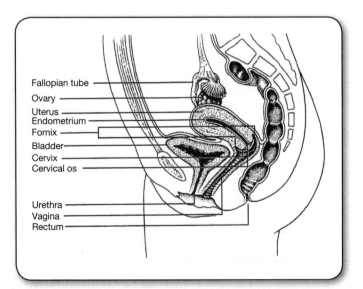

FIGURE 7.4

The internal genitalia. The vaginal canal is a potential rather than a real space and inclines posteriorly at a 45° angle. The cervix pierces the anterior superior wall of the vagina.

In addition to producing lubrication, the vagina demonstrates a remarkable distensive ability during both sexual response and childbirth. Both a lengthening of the vagina and a ballooning of its inner portions have been observed during sexual response (Puppo, 2013). The vascular changes occurring in conjunction with sexual response are profound. The reddish pink hue of the premenopausal woman's vagina changes to a darker purplish vasocongested appearance. In postmenopausal women, the color changes in the vagina, and its expansion during sexual response is less pronounced. As the vagina distends, the rugae become flattened as a result of the thinning or stretching of the vaginal mucosa. The vagina, unlike the clitoris, is not well endowed with nerve endings; although there are deep pressure receptors in the innermost portion, it is primarily in the outer third of the vagina that women report pleasurable sexual sensations (Masters & Johnson, 1966).

CERVIX

Although the cervix might be regarded as an internal structure because it is a part of the uterus, it can be visualized with the aid of a speculum and a light source during a health care provider's examination. The cervix extends from the isthmus of the uterus into the vagina, and it is through the small cervical opening (os) that the uterus and vagina communicate. The cervical os appears as a small closed circle in nulliparous women and may be enlarged or of an irregular shape in parous women. The cervix appears as an oval structure and is usually shiny and pale pink. In postmenopausal women, it may be smaller and less pigmented than in premenopausal women. The stroma (connective tissue forming the supportive framework) of the cervix consists of connective tissue with unstriated muscle fibers as well as elastic tissue.

The stratified squamous epithelium of the outer cervix (the portio) is made up of several layers. The basal layer is a single row of cells resting on a thin basement membrane and is the layer where active mitosis (cell division) is seen. The parabasal and intermediate layers are next. In the intermediate layer are vacuoles containing glycogen. The superficial, keratinized layer varies in thickness in response to estrogen stimulation. The desquamation of this surface layer occurs constantly. The superficial layer contains a large amount of glycogen, as does the intermediate layer. It appears that glycogen plays an important role in maintaining the acid pH of the vagina. Glycogen released by cytolysis of the desquamated cells is acted on by the glycolytic bacterial flora in the vagina, forming lactic acid. In a healthy vaginal ecosystem with a basic pH, the vagina will typically smell salty and slightly musky. Each woman has a unique, characteristic odor that is more noticeable during the hormonal influences associated with ovulation, menstruation, and sexual stimulation (Buy & Ghossain, 2013a).

Just as the endometrium is influenced by the hormonal fluctuations of the menstrual cycle, so is the mucus produced by the secretory cells of the glands in the endocervix (interior cervical canal). This is especially noticeable in premenopausal women. Fluctuations in cervical mucus during the course of the menstrual cycle are discussed later in this chapter.

There is an abrupt transition from the stratified squamous epithelium covering the vagina and the outer surface of the cervix to the tall, glandular columnar cells rich in mucin (proteinaceous mucoid substance) located within the internal cervical canal. This junction between ectocervical cells and endocervical cells is designated as the *transformation zone*. This ever-changing squamocolumnar junction is actually a cellular dividing line where newly forming columnar epithelium in the cervix merge with encroaching stratified epithelium lining. It is an area of increased susceptibility to infection and carcinogens. During a Pap smear to test for cervical cancer, desquamated (exfoliated) cells from the cervix are examined cytologically for cellular abnormalities. For an adequate test, endocervical cells at the squamocolumnar transformation zone, as well as ectocervical squamous cells, must be included.

UTERUS

The uterus is a hollow, pear-shaped organ that is 5.5 to 9 cm long, 3.5 to 6 cm wide, and 2 to 4 cm thick in nulliparous women. The uterus of a parous woman may be 2 to 3 cm larger in any of these dimensions. The uterus is usually inclined forward at a 45° angle from the longitudinal plane of the body. Usually, the uterus is anteverted or slightly anteflexed in position. However, it also may be retroflexed, retroverted, or in a midposition (Buy & Ghossain, 2013b).

The portion of the uterus above the cervix is termed the *corpus* (body) and is constructed of a thick-walled musculature. It is covered with peritoneum on the exterior and lined interiorly with a mucoid surface called the *endometrium*. The body of the uterus is divided into three portions: the fundus, the corpus, and the isthmus. The fundus is the prominence above the insertion of the fallopian tubes, the corpus is the main portion, and the isthmus is the narrow lower portion of the uterus adjacent to the cervix. The uterus is not a fixed organ and can be moved about; for example, during the sexual response cycle, the entire uterus elevates from the true pelvis into the false pelvis.

FALLOPIAN TUBES

Two fallopian tubes, located laterally at either horn of the uterine fundus, run laterally toward the ovaries and are the site for ovum and sperm transport, sperm capacitation, ovum retrieval, fertilization, and embryo transport. Each tube is approximately 10 to 12 cm long. The distal portion of the oviduct is fimbriated; both the middle portion (the ampulla) and the portion of the tube closest to its insertion in the uterus (the isthmus) are extremely narrow. The wider, funnel-shaped ends of the tubes are surrounded by irregular, fingerlike extensions called *fimbriae*. Although not actually attached to the ovary, the fimbriae come into contact with the ovary and are lined with ciliated epithelium that sweep uniformly toward the uterus, acting as a vacuum for any newly released ovum. The outer, serous coat of the oviduct covers a muscular portion consisting of an inner circular layer and a thin, outer longitudinal layer. The mucosal layer, composed of a number of rugae that become more numerous approaching the fimbriated portion, lines the tubes (Houghton & McCluggage, 2013).

OVARIES

The ovaries are paired, almond-shaped, female gonads approximately 3 to 4 cm long, 2 cm wide, and 1 to 2 cm thick. They are located near the pelvic wall at the level of the anterior superior iliac spine. The external ovarian surface has a dull, whitish, opaque appearance. The ovary is composed of three major portions. First, there is an outer cortex lined by a single layer of cuboidal (cube-shaped) epithelium. Through this layer, blood vessels and nerves enter and leave the ovary. Follicles are embedded in the connective tissue of the outer cortex and are either growing or inactive. Second, the central medulla of the ovary is composed of loose connective tissue (stroma), lymphatics, and blood vessels. The ovarian stroma comprises contractile cells, connective tissue cells that provide structural support to the ovary, and interstitial cells that secrete sex steroid hormones (primarily androgens). In addition, the stroma contains the primordial follicles yet to be recruited. Not only do the ovaries release gametes, but they also produce sex steroid hormones—including estrogen, progesterone, and androgens—as well as a number of nonsteroidal factors that regulate the endocrine regulation of ovarian function. The ovary has a rich lymphatic drainage, and an abundant supply of unmyelinated nerve fibers enter the medulla through the rete ovarii (the hilum). The hilum is the point of ovarian attachment to the mesovarium, a peritoneal fold on the posterior surface of the broad ligament (Blaustein, 2013).

At birth, the ovary contains approximately 1 to 2 million germ cells after reaching the acme of follicular formation at 16 to 20 weeks gestation (6 to 7 million oocytes); no new germ cells are ever produced later in life. By the onset of puberty, the total content of germ mass is ultimately reduced through the process of atresia to 300,000 follicles, and only 400 oogonia will achieve ovulation during a woman's reproductive life (Blaustein, 2013; Speroff & Fritz, 2005).

The follicle is the functional unit of the ovary, the source of both the gametes and the ovarian hormones. Each follicle is surrounded by a circular cellular wall called the *theca folliculi*. The theca contains an inner rim of secretory cells (the theca interna) and an outer rim of connective tissue (the theca externa). Within the theca, but separated from it by a layer of thin basement membrane, are the granulosa cells, which in turn surround the ovum. An acellular layer of protein and polysaccharide, the zona pellucida, separates the ovum from the granulosa cells. The theca interna is richly vascularized, although neither the ovum nor the granulosa cells are in contact with any capillaries. The theca and granulosa cells are the primary sex steroid–secreting elements. These cells have receptors for gonadotropins and respond to those released by the anterior pituitary: follicle-stimulating hormone (FSH) and luteinizing hormone (LH).

The development and maturation of the follicle is stimulated by FSH and consists of proliferation of the granulosa cells and the gradual elaboration of fluid within the follicle. Accumulation of the fluid increases rapidly with follicular maturation and causes the follicle to bulge into the peritoneal cavity. As the follicle swells, the ovum remains embedded in granulosa cells (cumulus oophorus), which remain in contact with the theca. As fluid accumulates, the cumulus thins until only a narrow thread of cells connects the ovum with the rim of the follicle. At ovulation, the ovum, surrounded by the corona of granulosa cells (sometimes called the *corona radiata*), while floating in the follicular fluid, ruptures. The ovum and its corona extrude into the peritoneal cavity in a bolus of follicular fluid. This sometimes is perceptible as a crampy sensation, referred to as *mittelschmerz*. After ovulation, ingrowth and differentiation of the remaining granulosa cells fill the collapsed follicle to form a new endocrine structure called the *corpus luteum*. The corpus luteum continues to develop when a pregnancy occurs. When the ovum is not fertilized and dies, the corpus luteum no longer develops and leaves a remnant on the surface of the ovary called a *corpus albicans* (Blaustein, 2013) (Figure 7.5).

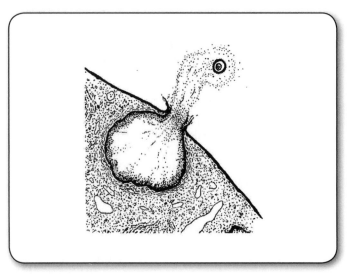

FIGURE 7.5
Ovulation. At ovulation the ovum, surrounded by the corona radiata and floating in the follicular fluid, ruptures into the peritoneal cavity.

Pelvic Supporting Structures

The pelvic floor is described as the complex of interrelated structures that includes the bones, muscles, ligaments, blood vessels, and nerves that support the pelvic organs (Martellucci et al., 2014).

BONY PELVIS

The pelvis is composed of two innominate bones: the sacrum and the coccyx. The innominate bones, in turn, are composed of the ilium, ischium, and pubis. These constitute the hipbones. The pubic bones meet anteriorly at the symphysis pubis, a fibrocartilaginous symphyseal joint. The pubic arch is formed by the inferior borders of the pubic bones and symphysis. The ilium joins with the sacrum posteriorly to form the sacroiliac joint. A woman's pelvis is typically wider and more hollow than a man's because of the flaring of the woman's iliac bones and a curved sacrum (Hosseinzadeh et al., 2012) (Figure 7.6).

MUSCLES

Several sets of pelvic muscles attach to the bony pelvis and can be divided into two main groups: the urogenital triangle and the pelvic floor. These muscle groups both actively and passively support the pelvis and are involved in the voluntary contraction of the vagina and the anus. The layer of muscles that is closest to the skin is called the *urogenital triangle*. Two pairs of long, slender muscles (the ischiocavernosus) run alongside the pelvic outlet and form the two sides of the triangle, with the clitoris at its apex. The superficial transverse perineal muscle extends laterally and forms the base of this triangle. The bulbocavernosus muscles extend from the glans of the clitoris downward under the labia majora, connecting at the perineum, and are shaped like a pair of parentheses. The deep transverse perineal muscle forms a solid triangular base of muscle

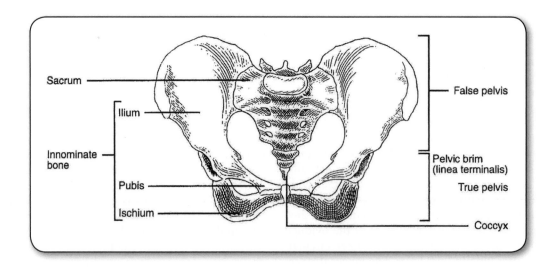

FIGURE 7.6
The bony pelvis. The pelvis is composed of two innominate bones, the sacrum and the coccyx. The innominates are composed of the ilium, the ischium, and the pubis.

immediately behind the open urogenital triangle and is bisected by the vagina and urethra. During orgasm, these muscles all contract simultaneously, compressing the engorged clitoral tissue between them, creating muscle tension and sexual pleasure. Behind the urogenital triangle is the pelvic floor, which is made up of the levator ani muscle (Frye, 1995). The pubococcygeus muscle, part of the levator ani group, has particular significance in women because it is important in sexual sensory function, bladder control, and childbirth—controlling relaxation and extension of the perineum and expulsion of the infant (Hosseinzadeh, Heller, & Houshmand, 2012) (Figure 7.7).

LIGAMENTS

Four pairs of ligaments—cardinal, uterosacral, round, and broad ligaments—provide primary support for the uterus, and the ovarian ligaments and infundibulopelvic ligaments provide ancillary support (Figure 7.8). Overstretching the ligaments is sometimes associated with minor discomfort during strenuous exercise or during pregnancy.

VASCULATURE

The ovarian arteries arise from the abdominal aorta, supply the fallopian tube and ovaries, and ultimately anastomose

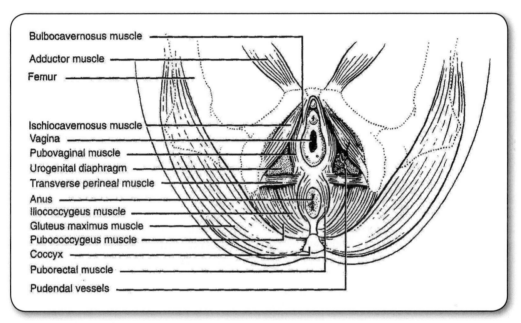

FIGURE 7.7

Pelvic muscles. Several sets of muscles support the pelvic floor. The bulbocavernosus and the pubococcygeus have special significance for sexual function.

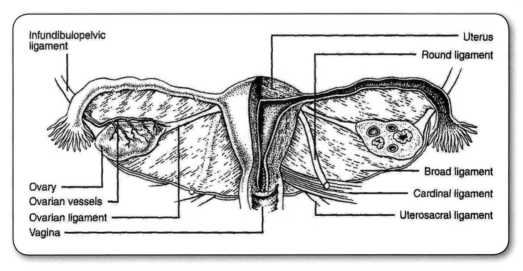

FIGURE 7.8

Ligaments. Four pairs of ligaments support the uterus, tubes, and ovaries. These are the cardinal, uterosacral, round, and broad ligaments.

with the uterine artery. The uterine artery arises from the anterior branch of the hypogastric artery and supplies the cervix and uterus. The vaginal artery arises similarly from the anterior branch of the hypogastric artery. The uterine veins run along the same channels as the uterine artery. The ovarian veins from the vena cava pass through the broad ligament en route to the ovarian hilus (neck of the ovary). On the right, the ovarian vein empties into the inferior vena cava; on the left, it empties into the renal vein.

INNERVATION

The internal genitalia are supplied by autonomic and spinal nerve pathways. The main autonomic supply to the uterus appears to consist of both sympathetic and parasympathetic fibers of the superior hypogastric plexus. The pudendal nerve is the main spinal nerve, providing the source of motor and sensory activation of the lower genital tract.

■ PHYSIOLOGICAL INFLUENCES OF THE ENDOCRINE SYSTEM AND HORMONAL CONTROLS

For adolescent females and adult women, some of the most apparent physical and physiological changes revolve around the influences of female hormones: puberty, menstrual cycles, perimenopause, and menopause. An understanding of these complex processes is crucial for those providing women's health care. The influence of hormones and their impact on a woman's sense of well-being, body image, perception of herself as a woman, reproductive life decisions, and specific health conditions is significant. Women are much more than hormonal, reproductive, and gynecologic beings. However, the relevance of hormonal influences in a woman's life cannot be ignored.

The physical and physiological changes that women experience across the life span are governed by hormonal influences resulting from the communication between the endocrine system and the central nervous system (CNS). Basic knowledge concerning the synthesis and actions of female steroid hormones, other ovarian hormones, and the feedback mechanisms of the hypothalamic–pituitary–ovarian (HPO) axis provides an important understanding of the physical and physiological reproductive and gynecologic changes of adolescence and adulthood.

Hormones, simply defined, are substances produced in special tissues in one part of the body that are released into the blood circulation and travel to target cells in another part or parts of the body, where they exert specific effects. As the field of endocrinology has evolved, it has become apparent that there is great complexity in the communication between hormone-producing tissues and the sites where the homones' effects occur. There are many areas in which this complex communication is not totally understood.

The endocrine system comprises all the glands that secrete hormones (considered as chemical messengers) that are carried by the blood from the glands to target cells elsewhere in the body to elicit systemic biological responses. In addition to discrete organs such as the adrenal or thyroid glands, the definition of *endocrine systems* has been recently expanded to include single cells or clusters of cells that are not anatomically definable as a gland but that can also secrete or produce hormones. The effects of hormones can be either rapid or delayed, or short or long term, depending on their structure and synthesis. A complex feedback system allows for the intricate balance among the hormones secreted and the responses elicited at the level of the target cells throughout the body.

On the target cell (the cell that responds to the presence of the hormone), receptors are the immediate recipients of the chemical messages or information units of hormones. These receptors are structurally organized so that they can specifically recognize and interact with their own cognate hormone, either inside the cell or, more frequently, on the plasma membrane of the cell. All receptors have two essential components: a ligand-binding region that binds the exact hormone for that receptor and an effector region that recognizes the presence of the hormone bound to the ligand region and then initiates the generation of the biological response. As a consequence of the specific receptor–hormone interaction (much like a specific lock and key), a cascade of events, or signal transduction pathways, occurs, and a specific biological response is generated in and, in some instances, around the target cell.

To maintain system precision, receptors have internal physiological regulators to maintain a balance between the extracellular hormone messengers and the number of target cell receptor sites that elicit specific cellular responses. One of these mechanisms is called *downregulation* and has the effect of reducing the number of receptor sites (within target cells) in response to long periods of frequent or intense hormonal bombardment. The other mechanism, *upregulation*, increases the number of receptor sites on the target cell to increase the cell's response to prolonged periods of low concentrations of particular hormones. In other words, if a gland overmanufactures or undermanufactures a particular hormone, the master control gland in the brain notes this from the amount of hormone circulating in the bloodstream and responds by modulating hormone secretion.

As key elements of the CNS, the hypothalamus and pituitary glands are located in the middle of the forebrain on its undersurface, inferior to the third ventricle. Although these structures occupy a very small portion of the brain and account for less than 1% of the brain's weight, the hypothalamus and pituitary function as the master control center for the coordination of both the neural and the endocrine systems (Widmeier, Ruff, & Strong, 2004).

The hypothalamus is responsible for the homeostasis of the interior climate of the body, such as temperature regulation, water balance, and emotional behaviors, in addition to behaviors related to the preservation of the species—hunger, thirst, and reproduction.

The pituitary gland sits in a hollow of the sphenoid bone, just below the hypothalamus. This endocrine gland is attached to the hypothalamus by a stalk that contains nerve filaments and small blood vessels. In adults, the pituitary is composed of two lobes (the anterior and posterior), each of which functions essentially as a distinct gland. The anterior pituitary releases hormones responsible for a wide variety of critical functions, including growth, metabolism, steroid release, breast growth, and milk synthesis, as well as gamete production and sex hormone secretions. These essential bodily capacities are produced by the release of growth hormone (GH), thyroid-stimulating hormone (TSH), adrenocorticotropic hormone (ACTH), prolactin, and two gonadotropic hormones—FSH and LH. The posterior pituitary controls milk let down and uterine contractility as well as water secretion by the kidneys and blood pressure through the release of oxytocin or vasopressin.

The posterior pituitary is an extension of the hypothalamus and communicates through neural connections and electrical messages to release hormones. The anterior pituitary has a unique, localized circulatory connection to the hypothalamus that allows blood to transport special hormones secreted directly from the hypothalamus to the anterior pituitary (hypophysiotropic hormones) to stimulate the release of other, specific hormones of the anterior pituitary.

Of particular importance to the female body is the regulation of the menstrual cycle and the ovaries' ability to produce gametes. This signal transduction pathway is initially stimulated by gonadotropin-releasing hormone (GnRH) secreted by the hypothalamus, which then stimulates the release of FSH as well as LH from the anterior pituitary. FSH and LH are called *gonadotropins* because they stimulate the target cells—ovaries (gonads)—to release steroid hormones estradiol (E2), progesterone, and androgens while a mature egg follicle develops and is subsequently released. The careful monthly orchestration of these various hormonal pathways in the interrelated CNS and endocrine communication system is referred to as the *HPO axis*.

Ovarian Hormones

The ovaries are the primary female reproductive organs. Their two main functions are secretion of female sex hormones and development and release of mature ova. The central part of the ovary, the medulla, is composed of connective tissue, arteries, veins, and lymphatics.

The cortex surrounds the medulla and has approximately one million immature follicles at birth, decreasing through atresia to about 200,000 to 400,000 at puberty. During the reproductive years, the cortex always contains ovarian follicles and ova in varying stages of development.

Four types of cells within the cortex secrete sex hormones: cells of the ovarian stroma, granulosa and theca cells within the ovarian follicles, and cells of the corpus luteum formed from the ruptured follicle after ovulation. All four of these cell types contain receptors for the gonadotropins, FSH, and LH.

Ovarian Steroid Hormones

Sex hormones are steroid hormones. The dominant female sex hormones are estrogen and progesterone produced primarily by the ovaries. Testosterone and other androgens produced by the adrenal glands and ovaries are also present at low levels.

Cholesterol is the precursor for the synthesis of steroid hormones in a process called *steroidogenesis*. The synthesis of estrogen, progesterone, and some androgens begins with the enzymatic conversion of cholesterol within the ovary to the precursor steroid, pregnenolone. The next step in steroidogenesis within the ovaries follows one of two pathways. In one pathway, pregnenolone is converted to 17-hydroxypregnenolone, then to androgen dehydroepiandrosterone (DHEA), and then to another androgen, androstenedione. In the other pathway, pregnenolone is converted to progesterone. Progesterone either enters the circulation as a hormone that acts on target tissues such as the breasts or uterus or undergoes further conversion. This conversion consists of progesterone being converted to 17-hydroxyprogesterone, and then to androstenedione.

ESTROGEN

Estrogen is the overall term used for three similar hormones: estrone (E1), estradiol (E2), and estriol (E3). Estrogen is synthesized by the conversion of androstenedione from either of the two initial pathways. Androstenedione may first be converted within the ovary to the androgen, testosterone. Testosterone is then converted to E2, the most potent of the estrogens in a process called *aromatization*. Androstenedione may also be converted within the ovary to estrone, and testosterone may be converted to estriol (Jones, 2006).

E2 is the most potent and plentiful of the three and is produced primarily by the ovarian follicles and corpus luteum. Most (95%) circulating E2 is derived from the ovaries, with the remaining secreted by the adrenal cortex. E1 is the second most potent and is produced mainly by peripheral adipose conversion of androgens. There is also some synthesis of estrone within the ovary and adrenal glands. E1 is the predominant estrogen produced after the menopause transition. E3 is the weakest of the three estrogens and is primarily a metabolite of E2 and E1. During pregnancy, E3 becomes the predominant estrogen. It is produced in large amounts by the placenta through aromatization of fetal androgens (Jones, 2006; McCance & Huether, 2006).

Estrogen is necessary for the maturation of reproductive organs, development of secondary sex characteristics, closure of long bones after the pubertal growth spurt, and regulation of the menstrual cycle. Estrogen also has an impact on several other organs, including metabolic effects on bones, liver, blood vessels, brain and CNS, kidneys, and skin. Furthermore, estrogen influences many of the maternal physiological adaptations during pregnancy.

PROGESTERONE

Progesterone is produced mainly in the ovaries, with small amounts also secreted by the adrenal glands. During pregnancy, increasing amounts of progesterone are synthesized first by the corpus luteum and then the placenta.

Progesterone and estrogen together influence mammary gland development during puberty and regulate the menstrual cycle. It prepares the endometrium for implantation and is essential for maintaining a pregnancy. Along with estrogen, progesterone influences maternal physiological adaptations during pregnancy.

ANDROGENS

Not all of the androgens produced by the ovary are converted to estrogen or progesterone. Low levels of androgens are present in a woman's circulation coming from the adrenal glands, the ovaries, and the peripheral conversion of circulating androstenedione and DHEA to testosterone. Shortly before the onset of puberty there is a noticeably increased production of adrenal androgens that is referred to as *adrenarche*. This increased androgen production seems to occur independently and does not play a direct role in the initiation of puberty (Jones, 2006). Once puberty starts, there is a rapid increase in androstenedione, as it is then produced by both the adrenal glands and ovaries. Androgens contribute to long bone growth during the pubertal growth spurt, growth of pubic and axillary hair, and activation of sebaceous glands. Androgens also play a role in libido.

Nonsteroidal Ovarian Hormones

Several nonsteroidal hormones are also produced by the ovaries. Inhibin, activin, follistatin, and oocyte maturation inhibitor (OMI) are peptide hormones produced in the ovaries that help modulate ovarian follicular development as well as steroid hormone production. Although inhibin inhibits FSH secretion, it does not inhibit LH secretion. Activin has the opposite effect, enhancing FSH secretion. Inhibin and activin are both present in follicular fluid; however, levels of inhibin are higher than those of activin. Inhibin in the dominant ovarian follicle has a negative feedback on FSH secretion by the anterior pituitary gland. Inhibin and activin also act directly in the ovary to regulate androgen and estrogen production. During pregnancy, inhibin prevents ovulation. With the decreasing number of follicles in perimenopause, there is a decrease in inhibin production, allowing for a small increase in FSH levels. Follistatin also suppresses FSH secretion, probably by binding with activin to inhibit its function. OMI prevents final oocyte maturation until the time of ovulation. This suppression ends within hours of the midcycle LH surge (Breslin & Lucas, 2003; Hatcher & Namnoum, 2004; Jones, 2006).

Insulin-like growth factors (IGF) also play a significant, though not fully understood, role as ovarian regulators. IGFs resemble insulin in structure and function and stimulate cell division and growth in many tissues. The ovaries are a major site for IGF-1 production and action. IGF-1 coordinates ovarian granulosa and theca cell functions and promotes steroidogenesis (Hatcher & Namnoum, 2004; Speroff & Fritz, 2005).

Hypothalamic and Pituitary Reproductive Hormones

The production of estrogen and progesterone is dependent on a mature, intact HPO axis, which involves the secretion of GnRH from the hypothalamus, secretion of LH and FSH by the anterior pituitary gland, negative and positive hormonal feedback systems, and structural integrity of the ovaries.

The hypothalamus is connected to the pituitary gland, which sits within a concave surface in the sphenoid bone. The hypothalamus communicates with the posterior pituitary gland (neurohypophysis) through a nerve tract. The anterior pituitary gland (adenohypophysis) and hypothalamus communicate through a unique hypophyseal portal system.

The mature hypothalamus secretes GnRH in a pulsatile fashion. GnRH does not enter the general circulation; instead it travels through the veins of the hypophyseal portal system directly to the anterior pituitary gland, where it stimulates secretion of FSH and LH. FSH and LH are released in a pulsatile fashion that corresponds with GnRH secretion. FSH and LH enter the general circulation and travel to the ovaries where they influence estrogen and progesterone production.

Circulating levels of estrogen and progesterone exert a feedback effect on the hypothalamic secretion of GnRH and anterior pituitary secretion of FSH and LH. Throughout infancy and early childhood, the hypothalamus is extremely sensitive to negative feedback from low levels of circulating estrogen. GnRH secretion is suppressed by this negative feedback. Hormonal changes begin as the HPO axis matures and becomes less sensitive to low estrogen levels.

■ SEXUAL DIFFERENTIATION AND DEVELOPMENT

Sexual differentiation and development involve a complex series of events that ultimately transform an undifferentiated embryo into a human with a gender identity of female or male. As a result of the complexity of differentiation, one can be born with a genotypic sex that is inconsistent with one's phenotypic sex. Phenotypic sex can be understood as the total perceptible characteristics displayed by an individual under specific environmental circumstances, regardless of the person's genotype. The developmental process of sexual differentiation begins at fertilization with establishment of genetic sex. *Genetic sex* refers to the chromosomal combination from the ovum and sperm, resulting in an XX (female), XY (male), or other combination. *Gonadal sex* refers to the structure and function of the gonads, whereas somatic sex involves the genital organs other than the gonads. *Neuroendocrine sex* refers to the cyclic or continuous production of GnRHs. Although gonadal, somatic, and neuroendocrine sexual differentiation begins before birth, sexual differentiation continues after birth. The development of social, psychological, and cultural dimensions of sexuality, as well as secondary sex characteristics, occurs after birth.

Genetic Sex

Genetic sex is determined at the time of fertilization and is defined by the contribution of an X or Y chromosome from the father. It is interesting to note that, despite the genotype, sexual differentiation will produce a basic female phenotype unless testosterone is present and can be used by the cells of the developing human.

Gonadal Sex

At about 4 to 6 weeks of gestation, germ cells migrate to the site of the fetal gonad. At the sixth week, the gonads are sexually indistinguishable, containing a cortex and medulla layer. If the chromosomal sex is XX, the cortex will differentiate into the ovary, and the medulla will regress; if the chromosomal sex is XY, the medulla will differentiate into a testis and the cortex will regress under the influence of *SRY*, a gene from the sex-determining region of the Y chromosome.

Differentiation of the gonad occurs slightly earlier in male than in female fetuses. At 7 weeks, testicular differentiation begins under the influence of testosterone, which is stimulated by human chorionic gonadotropin (HCG). The ovary differentiates about 2 weeks after testicular differentiation and is identifiable by 10 weeks. By 16 weeks, the oogonia become surrounded by follicular cells, composing the primordial follicle. At 20 weeks gestation, the fetal ovary contains mature compartmentalization with primordial follicles and oocytes, and there are 5 to 7 million germ cells present. Follicular maturation and atresia are already progressing. Approximately one million germ cells remain in the ovary at birth. The oocytes are surrounded by primordial follicles and are arrested in the prophase of the first meiotic (cellular division in which the diploid number of chromosomes is reduced to the haploid) division until the follicle is reactivated at the time of puberty.

Female differentiation is probably linked to a gene on the X chromosome that acts in the absence of androgen. Only one X chromosome is needed for primary ovarian differentiation, explaining why female differentiation may occur in fetuses with XY chromosomes who lack testosterone elaboration at a critical point in development or are unable to use testosterone.

Somatic Sex

The mesonephric (Wolffian duct) and the paramesonephric (Müllerian duct) coexist in all embryos regardless of chromosomal sex. During the third fetal month, one persists and the other disappears. The intrinsic tendency toward feminization produces differentiation of the paramesonephric (Müllerian) system. In the absence of Müllerian inhibiting factor, which inhibits the further development of the Müllerian ducts in male embryos, the paramesonephric system differentiates into the uterine tubes, uterus, and upper vagina.

At the eighth week of gestation, the embryo is bipotential; that is, it can differentiate into either a female or a male. Between 9 and 12 weeks of gestation, the differentiation of external genitalia becomes evident. The urogenital sinus, labioscrotal swellings, and genital tubercle will differentiate into a female pattern in the absence of androgen stimulation and without a Y chromosome. In females, the urogenital folds remain open, developing into the labia minora. The labioscrotal folds differentiate into the labia majora, and the genital tubercle differentiates into the clitoris. The urogenital sinus becomes the vagina and the urethra. The lower vagina is formed as part of the external genitalia. The differentiation of these structures is illustrated in Figures 7.9A and 7.9B.

Fetal endocrine glands are supported by the placenta as well as by the fetal gonads. By the 10th week of gestation, most of the pituitary hormones are apparent. They rise during the first 20 weeks of pregnancy, and then negative feedback mechanisms begin to limit their levels. LH and FSH are apparent at 9 to 10 weeks and peak at about 20 to 22 weeks gestation. FSH stimulates follicular development in females; LH stimulates steroid synthesis in the ovary and later induces ovulation in FSH-primed follicles. Hypothalamic-releasing hormones stimulate ACTH production by about 8 weeks gestation.

■ PUBERTY

Puberty refers to the sequence of events leading to reproductive/sexual maturation and is indicated by the maturation of the genital organs, the development of secondary sex characteristics, and the first occurrence of menstruation in young women. It is a part of the adolescent development process. *Adolescence* refers to all aspects of development, including the physical, psychosocial, and cognitive changes that occur between the ages of 11 and 19 years. The beginning of adolescence is often correlated with the onset of puberty.

A time interval of a decade or more separates birth and puberty. Puberty occurs during the later phases of human growth, long after the initial sexual differentiation. Both growth and differentiation continue during puberty, making it a distinctive part of the life span and requiring complex physiological mechanisms to initiate its occurrence (Plant, 1994; Venturoli, Flamigni, & Givens, 1985). Puberty and the menopausal transition share the characteristic of a transitional period during which a biological series of events culminating in a change in fertility occurs. During puberty, menarche occurs in girls; during the menopausal transition, the final menstrual period occurs in women.

Initiation of Puberty

The initiation of puberty remains poorly understood, although it is recognized that a CNS process must be responsible for its onset. It appears that the HPO axis in girls develops in two definitive stages during puberty. First, early in puberty, gonadotropin secretion gradually increases because of a decrease in the sensitivity of the hypothalamic centers to the negative inhibitory effects of low levels of circulating sex steroids. This can be viewed as a slowly rising set point of decreased sensitivity, resulting in increasing GnRH pulsatile secretions. This in turn leads to increasing gonadotropin production and ovarian stimulation. Second, later in puberty, there is a maturation of the positive feedback response from ovarian estrogen to the anterior pituitary, which stimulates the midcycle surge of LH with subsequent ovulation (Rebar, 2002). This explains why the first few menstrual cycles are anovulatory (for as long as 18 months), although there are frequent exceptions (Speroff & Fritz, 2005).

Current data suggest that the CNS inhibits the onset of puberty until the appropriate time. Thus the neuroendocrine control of puberty is mediated by GnRH-secreting neurons in the hypothalamus, which act as an internal pulse generator. At puberty, the GnRH pulse generator is reactivated or disinhibited, leading to increasing amplitude, frequency, and regularity of GnRH pulses, especially at night (Speroff & Fritz, 2005). Consequently, the hormonal cascade of reproductive processes is triggered— hypothalamic GnRH pulsations stimulate the release of FSH and LH from the anterior pituitary, which then stimulates ovarian steroidal secretions. Just what causes the disinhibition of GnRH is still unknown (Rebar, 2002). It is important to understand that puberty is not merely turned on like a light switch but is rather a functional convergence of all factors. It is more of a concept than an actual focal point of action (Speroff & Fritz, 2005).

Physiological Development and Puberty

Shortly after birth, neonatal FSH and LH levels are still elevated as a result of negative feedback provided by the maternal ovarian hormones during pregnancy. The gonadotropins remain high for approximately 3 months, with resulting transient elevations of E2; FSH and LH then gradually decrease to reach a nadir at 1 to 2 years of age in females. Then, gonadotropin levels begin to rise slightly between 4 and 10 years. Low levels of gonadotropins in the pituitary and circulation during childhood yield little response of the

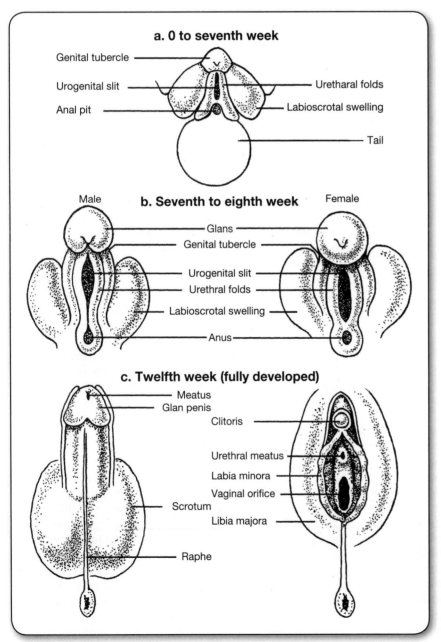

FIGURE 7.9A

(a) External genitalia at 0 to 7 weeks, prior to gender differentiation. (b) As early as weeks 7 and 8 of fetal life, gender differentiation has begun. Before week 6, the embryo appears undifferentiated. (c) By week 12, the external genitalia assume the differentiated appearance. (*continued*)

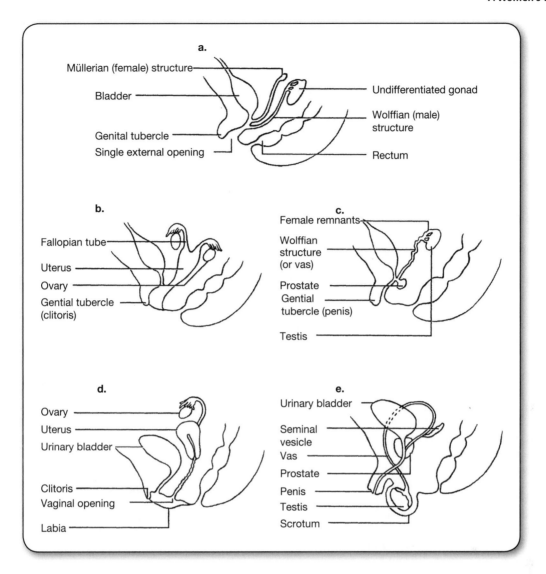

FIGURE 7.9B

(a) Undifferentiated structures; (b) female structure at the third month; (c) male structure at the third month; (d) female mature form; and (e) male mature form.

pituitary to GnRH and maximal hypothalamic suppression. LH pulses appear during infancy, although they are quite irregular. Thus it appears that immaturity of the endocrine systems is not the factor that tempers the onset of puberty. Indeed, all components of the HPO axis below the level of the hypothalamus can respond to GnRH from birth.

Prepubertal Phases

In girls, the first steroids to increase in the circulation from the adrenal cortex are androgens—DHEA, dehydroepiandrosterone sulfate (DHEAS), and androstenedione, which occurs from about 6 to 8 years of age, shortly before FSH begins to rise. Estrogen and LH levels do not begin to increase until 10 to 12 years of age.

During the prepubertal years, three phases are evident: adrenarche, decreases in the suppression of the gonadostat, and amplification of interactions leading to gonadarche. *Adrenarche* refers to the development of pubic and axillary hair and is a function of increased adrenal androgen production. An increase in the size of the inner zone of the adrenal

cortex precedes a classic linear growth spurt by about 2 years. In addition, adrenarche precedes the elevation of estrogens and gonadotropins seen during early puberty and menarche in midpuberty. However, the mechanisms governing adrenarche probably are not the same as those influencing GnRH–pituitary–ovarian axis maturation and gonadarche. Early adrenarche, occurring before 8 years, is not associated with early gonadarche. The mechanisms producing adrenarche remain obscure.

Decreasing repression of the gonadostat refers to the increased responsiveness of the anterior pituitary to GnRH and follicular activity to FSH and LH. Factors that are responsible for derepressing the gonadostat, allowing the hypothalamus and pituitary to become less sensitive to the negative feedback of low levels of estrogens and permitting gonadotropin concentrations to rise, remain uncertain. Sustained elevation of growth GH levels may play a role as the factor responsible for derepressing the gonadostat.

Endogenous GnRH is important in establishing and maintaining puberty. An increasing amplitude and frequency of pulsatile GnRH probably enhances the responses of FSH and LH secretion. GnRH appears to induce cell surface receptors specific for itself and necessary for its action on the surface of gonadotrope cells of the anterior pituitary. Sleep-related pulsations of LH are seen during early puberty. By midpuberty, estrogen enhances LH secretory responses to GnRH (creating positive feedback) and maintains its negative feedback of FSH responses.

Skeletal Growth

GH secretion increases in prepubertal girls. GH is secreted by the anterior pituitary gland and is responsible, along with androgens, for growth of long bones and other tissues. GH needs IGF-I, produced by the liver, to stimulate skeletal growth. Production of IGF-I is regulated by GH, thyroid hormones, and possibly insulin. IGF-I stimulates the target cells that control ossification. IGF-I acts primarily as a local regulator of cell growth and differentiation (Speroff & Fritz, 2005). The growth spurt initiated by these hormones begins at about age 9 years with an increase in both height and fat deposition, and signals the beginning of puberty.

Puberty

A cascade of endocrine events initiated by the release of pulsatile GnRH results in elevated gonadotropin levels and gonadal steroids, with the subsequent appearance of secondary sexual characteristics and, later, menarche and ovulation. Between the ages of 10 and 16 years, the usual sequence includes the appearance of a pulsatile pattern of LH during sleep, followed by pulses of lesser amplitude throughout the day. Increasing levels of E2 result in menarche, and, by the latter part of puberty, the positive feedback relationship exists between E2 and LH that is necessary to stimulate ovulation.

The progression of puberty through a sequence of increased rate of linear growth, breast development, pubarche (onset of pubic hair growth), and menarche occurs over a period of approximately 4.5 years. Usually, the first sign of puberty is acceleration of growth, which is followed by breast budding (thelarche). The growth peak (about 2 to 4 inches within 1 year) usually occurs about 2 years after breast budding. Pubarche usually appears after the appearance of breast budding; axillary hair growth occurs approximately 2 years later. In some girls, pubic hair growth is the first sign of puberty. The growth peak in height occurs about 1 year before menarche. Menarche occurs late in this sequence with a median age of about 12.8 years, after the growth peak has occurred. GH and gonadal estrogen are important factors in the increased growth velocity. In addition, increasing estrogen levels produces breast development, female fat distribution, vaginal and uterine growth, and skeletal growth.

Menarche

Menarche is a function of genetic and environmental influences and occurs between 9.1 and 17.7 years of age, with a mean age of 12.8 years. Improvements in the standard of living and nutrition have produced children who mature earlier than in the past. In cultures that are affluent, menarcheal age has become lower. After menarche, growth slows, with approximately 2.5 inches in height gained after menarche. The age of menarche is correlated for mothers and daughters and between sisters.

Although there have been discussions of a critical weight for menarche to occur (47.8 kg), it is likely that the shift in body composition from 16% to 23.5% fat is a more important factor. The peptide hormone leptin, secreted in adipose tissue, plays a significant role in the relationship between body fat and reproductive function. Leptin acts on the CNS to regulate eating behaviors and energy balance. Leptin levels increase during childhood until the onset of puberty, suggesting that there is a necessary threshold level of leptin (and thus a critical amount of adipose, the source of leptin) for puberty to occur (Garcia-Mayor et al., 1997). Earlier ages of menarche are associated with higher levels of leptin (Matkovic et al., 1997; Speroff & Fritz, 2005). What is also clear is that estrogen secretion, which produces endometrial proliferation, is essential for menarche to occur.

Fertility

A late event in puberty is the development of the positive feedback effects of estrogen on the pituitary and hypothalamus that stimulates the midcycle LH surge necessary for ovulation. For this reason, menstrual cycles are often anovulatory for about 12 to 18 months after menarche. The frequency of ovulation becomes more regular with each menstruation and as girls progress through pubertal changes.

Development During Puberty

The five Tanner (1981) stages are a commonly used indicator of the stage of pubertal development. Based on the assessment of breast and pubic hair growth, it is possible to assess progression through puberty (Figures 7.10A and 7.10B).

In stage 1, a prepubertal stage, there is elevation of the papilla of the breast only. Although the feminine pelvic contour is evident, the breasts are flat. The labia majora are smooth, and the labia minora are poorly developed. The hymenal opening is small, the mucous membranes are dry and red, and the vaginal cells lack glycogen.

In stage 2, there is elevation of the nipple, with a small mound beneath the areola, which is enlarging and beginning to become pigmented. The labia majora become thickened, more prominent, and wrinkled. The labia minora are easily identified because of their increased size, as is the enlarging clitoris. The urethral opening is more prominent, mucous membranes are moist and pink, and some glycogen is present in vaginal cells. Pubic hair first appears on the mons and then on the labia about the time of menarche. The pubic hair is scanty, soft, and straight. There is increased activity of the sebaceous and merocrine sweat glands and in the initial functions of the apocrine glands in the axilla and vulva.

In stage 3, the rapid growth peak has occurred; menarche occurs most frequently during this stage after acceleration of the growth peak. The areola and nipple enlarge, and pigmentation, along with increased glandular size, is more evident. The labia minora are well developed, and the vaginal cells have increased glycogen content. The mucous membranes are increasingly paler. The pubic hair is thicker,

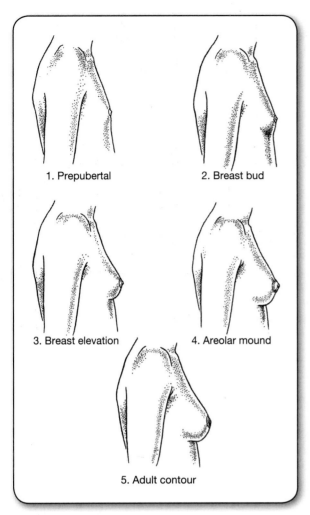

FIGURE 7.10A
Tanner stages for breast development.

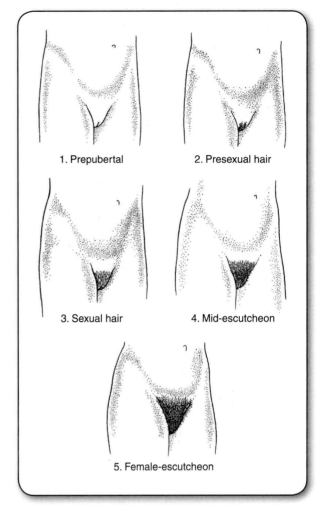

FIGURE 7.10B
Tanner stages for pubic hair development.

coarser, and often more curly at this time. There is increased activity of the sebaceous and sweat glands, with the beginning of acne in some girls along with adult body odor.

In stage 4, the areola project above the plane of the breast, and the areolar glands are apparent. Glandular tissue is easily palpable. Both the labia majora and minora assume the adult structure, and the glycogen content of the vaginal cells begins its cyclic pattern. Pubic hair is more abundant, and axillary hair is present.

In stage 5, the breasts are more mature, with the nipples enlarged and protuberant and the areolar glands well developed. Pubic hair is more abundant and spreads to the thighs in some women or may extend to the umbilicus. Facial hair may increase. Increased sebaceous gland activity of the skin and increased severity of acne may appear.

■ INTERNAL GENITALIA GROWTH AND DEVELOPMENT

Significant changes in a young woman's internal genitalia also occur during puberty. The vagina lengthens to approximately 9 to 10 cm and the vaginal mucosa composed of squamous epithelium thickens. In reproductive-aged women, this membrane is arranged in transverse folds called *rugae*. Before puberty, the vaginal pH is neutral (7). Under the influence of estrogen, lactobacilli in the vagina metabolize glycogen from vaginal epithelial cells, producing lactic acid that decreases the pH level (4–4.5). This acidic environment provides protection from opportunistic pathogens. The vagina does not itself contain any secretory glands. Secretions come from the endocervical glands and from Bartholin's and Skene's glands. Just before menarche, there is a normal increase in the amount of these secretions in the vagina (McCance & Huether, 2006; Seidel, Ball, Dains, & Benedict, 2006).

During puberty, the uterine musculature and vascular supply also increase. The uterus attains its nonpregnant adult size of approximately 5.5 to 8 cm in length and 3.5 to 4 cm in width with muscular walls 2 to 2.5 cm thick. The endometrial lining thickens under the influence of estrogen. Ovaries and fallopian tubes also reach adult size. In females of reproductive age, each ovary is approximately 3 cm long, 2 cm wide, and 1.0 cm thick (Seidel et al., 2006).

■ THE MENSTRUAL CYCLE

Coordination of the Menstrual Cycle

The menstrual cycle requires a complex sequence of physiological events coordinated by the hypothalamus in conjunction with the pituitary, ovary, and uterus and that responds to environmental phenomena.

Major components of the system coordinating the menstrual cycle include the GnRH pulse generator, GnRH released by the hypothalamus, the gonadotropins (FSH and LH) secreted by the pituitary, and estrogen and progesterone produced by the ovary and corpus luteum, respectively. GnRH is released from the hypothalamus in a pulsatile fashion into the pituitary portal circulation. The pituitary gonadotropins respond to the stimulus from GnRH with pulses of LH and FSH released into the peripheral circulation. In response to GnRH and the gonadotropic hormones, the follicles produce E2, and the corpus luteum produces progesterone in response to elevated LH.

This coordinating system can be modulated by many inputs from higher neural centers and peripheral factors influencing the GnRH pulse generator, as well as other hormones. Norepinephrine seems to amplify GnRH secretion, whereas dopamine dampens it. Increased endorphin release inhibits gonadotropin secretion through suppression of the release of GnRH (Speroff & Fritz, 2005).

Ovarian Cycle: The Follicular Phase

The menstrual cycle consists of an ovarian and an endometrial component. The ovarian component is customarily divided into three phases to facilitate discussion: the follicular, ovulatory, and luteal (Figure 7.11). The follicular phase consists of 10 to 14 days of hormonal influence that support the growth of the primordial follicle through the preantral, antral, and preovulatory phases. The primordial follicle consists of the oocyte arrested in the diploid stage of development, in which it still has 46 chromosomes. The initiation of follicular growth does not appear to be dependent on

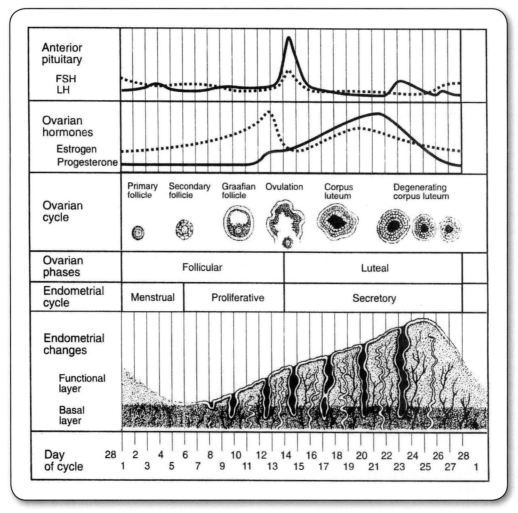

FIGURE 7.11

Coordination of the menstrual cycle.

FSH, follicle-stimulating hormone; LH, luteinizing hormone.

gonadotropins or estrogen. In fact, follicular growth may have begun during the days of the previous luteal phase, when the regressing corpus luteum secretes decreasing amounts of steroids. Indeed, follicles grow continuously, even during pregnancy, ovulation, and anovulation.

During the first few days of the cycle, the follicle that will ovulate is selected and recruited. The mechanism for determining which follicles or how many will grow appears to be the result of two estrogenic actions: a local interaction between estrogen and FSH with the follicle and the effect of estrogen on the pituitary secretion of FSH (Speroff & Fritz, 2005).

Preantral Follicle

A rise in FSH stimulates a group of follicles to grow to the preantral phase (the phase before the antrum is identifiable). During this phase, the zona pellucida appears around the ovum, and the thecal layer begins to organize. The granulosa cells synthesize steroids, producing more E2 than progestins or androgens. The follicle also can convert androgens to estrogens. Activated by FSH, the preantral follicle can generate its own estrogenic microenvironment. FSH can increase the concentration of its own receptors on the granulosa cells, thus inducing the production of E2. Moreover, at low concentrations, androgen enhances its transformation to E2. At higher levels, androgens cause the follicle to produce a more androgenic environment, leading to atresia of the follicle. The follicle's development depends on its ability to convert androgen to estrogen.

Antral Follicle

Accumulation of follicular fluid in the antral follicle provides nurturance in an endocrine microenvironment. Influenced by FSH, E2 becomes the dominant substance in follicular fluid. During the follicular phase, estrogen production occurs by a two-cell, two-gonadotropin mechanism. LH stimulates the theca cells to liberate androgens that are converted to estrogen, and FSH stimulates the granulosa cells to produce E2. Sensitivity to FSH determines the capacity for conversion of androgenic to an estrogenic environment in the follicle.

Selection of the follicle that will ovulate (often called the *dominant follicle*) occurs during cycle days 5 through 7 and requires estrogenic action. By day 7, peripheral E2 levels begin to rise significantly. E2 produces negative feedback that decreases gonadotropin support to other follicles. To survive, the selected follicle must increase its own FSH production. Because the dominant follicle has FSH receptors in the granulosa cells, it can enhance FSH action. These actions effectively allow the selected follicle to increase its own E2 levels and suppress FSH release to other follicles. The theca doubles in vascularity by day 9, producing a siphon for gonadotropins for the selected follicle.

Although the midfollicular increase in E2 levels produces negative feedback to suppress FSH, it exerts a positive feedback on LH. When E2 levels reach a concentration necessary for positive feedback (more than 200 pg/mL sustained for at least 50 hours), the LH surge occurs (Speroff & Fritz, 2005).

Feedback systems involving the pituitary and hypothalamus also enable the selected follicle to control its own development. E2 exerts negative feedback effects at the hypothalamus and anterior pituitary. Progesterone exerts inhibitory feedback at the level of the hypothalamus and positive feedback at the level of the pituitary. FSH is particularly sensitive to E2, whereas LH is sensitive to negative feedback of E2 at low levels and to positive feedback by E2 at higher levels. Progesterone slows LH pulses.

GnRH is secreted in the hypothalamus in a pulsatile fashion that changes in amplitude and duration across the menstrual cycle. During the early follicular phase, GnRH is secreted at approximately 94-minute intervals; in the late luteal phase, it is secreted at 216-minute intervals with a decreased amplitude. In turn, the pituitary releases gonadotropic hormones in a pulsatile fashion.

Preovulatory Follicles

Initiated by the LH surge, the oocyte resumes meiosis, approaching completion of reduction division. E2 concentrations rise to maintain the peripheral threshold necessary for ovulation to occur. LH initiates luteinization of the granulosa cells and the production of progesterone in the granulosa. The preovulatory increase in progesterone facilitates positive feedback of E2 and may be necessary for induction of the midcycle FSH peak. The midcycle increase in local and peripheral androgens deriving from the theca of the nonselected follicles may account for the increased libido some women report at midcycle.

Ovulation

Ovulation occurs about 10 to 12 hours after the LH peak, 24 to 36 hours after the E2 peak. The onset of the LH surge is estimated to occur approximately 34 to 46 hours before the follicle ruptures. LH stimulates the completion of the reduction division in the oocyte (to 23 chromosomes), luteinization of granulosa cells, and synthesis of progesterone and prostaglandins. The continuing rise in progesterone in the follicle up to the time of ovulation may act to end the LH surge. Progesterone also enhances proteolytic enzymes and prostaglandins needed for digestion and rupture of the follicle. Progesterone influences the midcycle rise in FSH, which in turn frees the oocyte from the follicular attachments, converts plasminogen to plasmin (a proteolytic enzyme involved in follicular rupture), and ensures sufficient LH receptors for a normal luteal phase.

Ovarian Cycle: Luteal Phase

The luteal phase is named for the process of luteinization, which occurs after the rupture of the follicle and release of the ovum. The granulosa cells increase in size and take on a yellowish pigment, lutein, from which they were named the corpus luteum, or yellow body. Luteinization involves synthesis of androgens, estrogens, and progesterone. The process of luteinization requires the accumulation of LH receptors during the follicular phase of the cycle and continuing levels of LH secretion. Progesterone acts during this phase to suppress new follicular growth, rising sharply after ovulation with a peak at about 8 days after the LH surge. The length of the luteal phase tends to be more constant than the follicular phase and is consistently close to 14 days from the LH midcycle surge to menses. Luteal phases ranging from 11 to 17 days are considered to be within normal limits. The corpus luteum begins a rapid cessation of activity at about 9 to 11 days after ovulation, and the mechanism triggering this remains unknown. Some speculate that estrogen production and an alteration in prostaglandin concentrations within the ovary are responsible. When pregnancy occurs, the corpus luteum continues to function with the stimulus of HCG, which appears at the peak of corpus luteum function, 9 to 13 days after ovulation. HCG maintains corpus luteum function until approximately the 9th or 10th week of gestation.

Endometrial Cycle

The first portion of the menstrual cycle is dominated by follicular development and secretion and causes proliferation of the endometrium. The first portion of the menstrual cycle is named the *follicular phase* with respect to the ovary and the *proliferative phase* with respect to the endometrium. The second portion of the cycle is influenced by the corpus luteum, and the increasing levels of progesterone evoke secretory changes in the endometrium. The second portion of the menstrual cycle is named the *luteal phase* with respect to the ovary and the *secretory phase* with respect to the endometrium.

Immediately after menstruation, the endometrium is thin, only about 1 to 2 mm thick. Its surface endometrium is composed of low cuboidal cells, the stroma is dense and compact, and the glands appear straight and tubular.

Proliferative Phase

Under the influence of estrogen, the endometrium proliferates and thickens. The endometrium becomes somewhat taller and the surface epithelium becomes columnar. The epithelial lining becomes continuous with the stromal component containing spiral vessels immediately below the epithelial-binding membrane that forms a loose capillary network. Although the stroma is still quite compact, the endometrial glands have become more tortuous. Mitotic activity is evident in both the surface epithelium and the basal nuclei of the epithelial cells lining the endometrial glands. Estrogenic effects are also seen in the secretions of the cervical glands and in the vaginal lining. The variability in the length of this phase of the menstrual cycle is greater than that for the luteal phase. Indeed, the varying number of days of proliferative or follicular phase accounts for the variation in total cycle length.

Secretory Phase

As a result of the developing corpus luteum, progesterone evokes and increases the secretory changes in the endometrium. The surface epithelium is now tall and columnar; the stroma is less compact than earlier in the cycle and is somewhat edematous and vascular. The endometrial glands become increasingly tortuous and convoluted. In addition, by 7 days after ovulation, the spiral vessels are densely coiled. The confinement of the growing endometrium to a fixed structure produces the tortuosity of the glands and spiral vessels.

Implantation usually occurs within 7 to 13 days after ovulation. At this point, the midportion of the endometrium appears lacelike, a stratum spongiosum. The stratum compactum overlies the inner layers of the endometrium and is a sturdy structure.

Premenstrually, the surface epithelium is quite tall, about 8 to 9 mm. The stroma consists of large polyhedral cells. The endometrial glands are very convoluted and serrated, resembling a corkscrew. The lining epithelium of endometrial glands is less well demarcated and smaller because of loss of glycogen into the gland lumen. A large number of lymphocytes and leukocytes are seen, probably as a result of the beginning necrosis of the endometrium.

Menstruation

In the absence of fertilization, implantation, and sustaining HCG, E2 and progesterone levels wane as the corpus luteum ceases to function.

Endometrial growth regresses a few days before the onset of menstruation; at the same time, there is stasis of blood flow to the coiled arteries, with intermittent vasoconstriction. Between 4 and 24 hours before the onset of menstrual bleeding, intense vasoconstriction occurs. The menstrual blood flows from coiled arteries that have been constricted for several hours. Prostaglandins, synthesized in the endometrium as a result of progesterone stimulation, are released and produce more intense vasoconstriction. Dissolving of the endometrium liberates acid hydrolases from the cell lysosomes. The acid hydrolases further disrupt the endometrial cell membranes, completing the process of menstruation. White blood cells migrate through capillary walls, and red blood cells escape into the interstitial space along with thrombin–platelet plugs that appear in the superficial vessels. Leakage and interstitial hemorrhage occur. With increased ischemia, the continuous binding membrane becomes fragmented, and intercellular blood is extruded into the endometrial cavity. The loose, vascular stroma of the spongiosum desquamates. Menstrual flow stops as a result of prolonged vasoconstriction, desquamation of the spongy layer of the endometrium, vascular stasis, and estrogen-induced rebuilding. The lower layer of the endometrium (basalis) is retained, and the stumps of the basal glands and stroma for the ensuing cycle continue to grow from them. The surface epithelium regenerates rapidly and may begin even while other areas are being desquamated.

With menstruation, as much as two thirds of the endometrium is lost. The menstrual flow may last from 2 to 8 days. Menstruation fluid consists of cervical and vaginal mucus as well as degenerated endometrial particles and blood. Sometimes clots may appear in the menstrual fluid. Usually from 2 to 3 ounces of fluid is lost with menses, but the amount of flow is highly variable. Women with more rapid loss experience a shorter duration of flow. Heavier flow and greater blood loss may indicate delayed or incomplete shedding of the endometrium.

Cyclic Changes in Other Organs

In addition to the uterus and ovary, other organs experience cyclic changes. The cervical canal contains about 100 crypts referred to as *columnar glands*; the secretory cells of these crypts secrete mucus into the endocervical canal. The mucus undergoes qualitative and quantitative changes during the menstrual cycle, depending on the hormonal environment. Immediately after menstruation, the mucus is sparse, viscid, and sticky. When examined under a microscope, an abundance of vaginal and cervical cells and lymphocytes can be seen. From about the eighth day of the cycle until ovulation, the quantity and viscosity of the mucus increase. Sometimes an obvious plug of yellow, white, or cloudy mucus of a tacky consistency is present. At midcycle, the mucus is a thin hydrogel containing 2% solids and 98% water. The mucus resembles raw egg white, being clear, stretchy, and slippery. It will stretch without breaking or spin a thread (and is called *spinnbarkheit*). The ability of the mucus to stretch at least 5 to 6 cm has been established as a guideline for determining adequacy of the cervical mucus to support sperm transport. When the midcycle mucus is allowed to dry on a slide, it gives a fern or palm leaf pattern. This pattern is absent after ovulation, during pregnancy, and after menopause. After ovulation, the mucus may again become cloudy, white, or yellow and tacky and may disappear altogether. Women can use the changes in cervical mucus as an indirect index of ovulation.

The cervix itself changes with the menstrual cycle. During the proliferative phase, the os progressively widens, reaching its maximum width just before or at ovulation. At the point of maximum widening, mucus can be seen extruding from the external os. After ovulation, the os returns to a smaller diameter, with the profuse and watery mucus becoming scanty and viscid. These changes are believed to be estrogen induced and are not seen in prepubertal or postmenopausal women or in those whose ovaries have been removed.

The motility of the uterine tubes is greatest during the estrogen-dominant portion of the menstrual cycle. They demonstrate a decreased motility during the progesterone-dominant phase.

Estrogen stimulation leads to cornification of the vagina. After progesterone stimulation, the vaginal epithelium shows an increase in the number of precornified cells, mucous threads, and aggregates of cells.

■ PERIMENOPAUSE

Perimenopause is the transitional period beginning when menstrual cycles become variable and/or when vasomotor symptoms first appear and ending 12 months after the cessation of menses (North American Menopause Society [NAMS], 2007). The average age of onset of perimenopause-related menstrual cycle changes is 46 years with a range from 39 to 51 years. The average duration is 5 years, with a range of 2 to 10 years (Speroff & Fritz, 2005).

Perimenopause brings accelerated follicular loss. Acceleration begins when the number of remaining follicles reaches about 25,000 and continues until there are no functional follicles. As the number of follicles declines there is a decrease in inhibin levels and a corresponding small increase in FSH secretion. In response to the increase in FSH the ovary recruits higher numbers of follicles that only partially develop. This further accelerates follicular loss (NAMS, 2007; Speroff & Fritz, 2005).

With fluctuating changes in E2 synthesis and metabolism, some perimenopausal women experience breast tenderness, migraine headaches, premenstrual mood changes, and bloating, growth of fibroid tumors, and/or vasomotor symptoms. These symptoms may occur while menstrual cycles remain regular. When anovulatory cycles begin to occur, women may experience irregular and heavy/prolonged bleeding. Endometrial thickening under the influence of increased E2 is greater in these anovulatory cycles. There is a lack of progesterone to support the thickened endometrium. Most women do experience some menstrual cycle changes during perimenopause that may include lighter or heavier bleeding, shorter or longer length of bleeding, shorter or longer cycle lengths, or skipped periods (McCance & Huether, 2006; NAMS, 2007).

The majority of perimenopausal women experience some vasomotor symptoms (hot flashes, night sweats). These vasomotor symptoms vary in frequency, intensity, and duration, generally lasting 1 to 5 minutes. Palpitations and feelings of anxiety may accompany the hot flash. Women may experience vasomotor symptoms for a few months to several years before menopause, with an average of 3 to 5 years (NAMS, 2007).

Clinicians should remember that hormonal changes are not the only potential causes for heavy or prolonged uterine bleeding or for vasomotor symptoms. A complete evaluation is necessary. Perimenopausal women and their clinicians must also consider that reproductive capability continues until 1 year after the last menses.

■ MENOPAUSE

Menopause is a normal function of aging that begins as hormonal changes lead to a decrease in ovulation, followed by permanent cessation of menstruation. Between 38 and 42 years of age, ovulation becomes less frequent. Residual follicles have decreased in number from about 300,000 at puberty to a few thousand and are less sensitive to gonadotropin stimulation than earlier in life, are less likely to mature, and produce less estrogen. Menopause occurs when estrogen is insufficient to stimulate endometrial growth so that a woman no longer menstruates (Casper, 2013; Jane & Davis, 2014).

Menopause is defined as a permanent cessation of menstruation for a period of 12 months. Before menopause, women experience a period of changes, referred to *perimenopause*, including irregular menstrual cycles most likely caused by a shortening of the follicular phase as a result of lower E2 secretion. As a woman's cycles become more irregular, vaginal bleeding may occur at the end of a short luteal phase or after an E2 peak without ovulation or corpus luteum formation.

In general, most women do not need to have any hormonal tests done to diagnose menopause. However, in women who have subtle or fluctuating symptoms or who are younger than 45 years when symptoms begin, hormone measurement may be useful and is essential when diagnosing primary ovarian insufficiency. Changes in FSH, E2, inhibin B, and anti-Müllerian hormone (AMH) define the stages of menopause classified by the Stages of Reproductive Aging Workshop (STRAW+1010). STRAW+1010 has identified three stages of menopause: (a) late reproductive phase; (b) menopause transition (perimenopause); and (c) postmenopause. In the late reproductive phase, there are changes in menstrual flow and length and variable FSH and E2. In the perimopause stage, cycle variability persists, FSH is increased, E2 is variable, AMH and inhibin B are low, and symptoms are likely. The postmenopause stage occurs when there is cessation of menstruation, elevated FSH, low E2, AMH, inhibin B and progesterone, and symptoms are more likely (Jane & Davis, 2014). In postmenopausal women, the ovary no longer has active follicles and is associated with the lab findings noted earlier. Androgens are produced by the adrenal cortex and remain the same level as before postmenopause. Occasionally, ovulation occurs after months of amenorrhea and may result in an unintended pregnancy during the menopausal transition. Elevation of both FSH and LH is thought to indicate that pregnancy cannot occur. Nonetheless, to prevent an unwanted conception, women who are experiencing the menopausal transition need to be aware of their fertility status (Baldwin & Jensen, 2013).

Another transition across the life span of a woman is menopause, a complex process of hormonal and anatomical changes that occurs in fluid stages that can be measured by both symptoms and physiological measures. During this time, women can still experience an unintended pregnancy and need support and active listening to receive comprehensive healthcare.

■ SUMMARY

From this discussion, it is evident that certain structures and functions are unique to a woman's body. These are involved in the menstrual cycle, reproduction, and women's sexual response cycles. Women's bodies develop uniquely from the time of conception and early differentiation through pubertal and menopausal transitions. Knowledge of these differences are important when providing health care to women.

■ REFERENCES

Baldwin, M. K., & Jensen, J. T. (2013). Contraception during the peri-menopause. *Maturitas, 76*(3), 235–242.

Blaustein, A. (2013). Human ovary. *Pathology of the Female Genital Tract, 11,* 416.

Bloor, I. D., & Symonds, M. E. (2014). Sexual dimorphism in white and brown adipose tissue with obesity and inflammation. *Hormones and Behavior, 66*(1), 95–103.

Breslin, E., & Lucas, V. (2004). *Women's health nursing: Toward evidence-based practice.* St. Louis, MO: Saunders.

Buy, J. N., & Ghossain, M. (2013a). Embryology, anatomy, and histology of the cervix. In A. Blaustein (Ed.), *Gynecological imaging* (pp. 649–652). Berlin, Heidelberg, Germany: Springer Publishing.

Buy, J. N., & Ghossain, M. (2013b). Anatomy and histology of the uterus body. In J. N. Buy & M. Ghossain (Eds.), *Gynecological imaging* (pp. 589–595). Berlin, Heidelberg, Germany: Springer Publishing.

Carey, M. A., Card, J. W., Voltz, J. W., Arbes, S. J., Germolec, D. R., Korach, K. S., & Zeldin, D. C. (2007). It's all about sex: Gender, lung development and lung disease. *Trends in Endocrinology and Metabolism, 18*(8), 308–313.

Casper, R. F. (2013). Clinical manifestations and diagnosis of menopause. In R. L. Barbieri & W. F. Crowley, Jr. (Eds.), *UpToDate.* Retrieved from http://www.uptodate.com/contents/clinical-manifestations-and-diagnosis-of-menopause

Dao, H., & Kazin, R. A. (2007). Gender differences in skin: A review of the literature. *Gender Medicine, 4*(4), 308–328.

deVries, G. J., & Forger, N. G. (2015). Sex differences in the brain: A whole body perspective. *Biology of Sex Differences, 6,* 15.

deVries, G. J., & Simerly, R. B. (2002). Anatomy, development, and function of sexually dimorphic neural circuits in the mammalian brain. In D. W. Pfaff, A. P. Arnold, A. M. Etgen, S. E. Fahrbach, R. L. Moss, & R. T. Rubin (Eds.), *Hormones, brain, and behavior. Vol. 4: Development of hormone-dependent neuronal systems* (pp. 137–191). San Diego, CA: Academic.

Dominianni, C., Sinha, R., Goedert, J. J., Pei, Z., Yang, L., Hayes, R. B., & Ahn, J. (2015). Sex, body mass index, and dietary fiber intake influence the human gut microbiome. *PloS One, 10*(4), e0124599.

Ellis, H., & Mahadevan, V. (2013). Anatomy and physiology of the breast. *Surgery, 31*(1), 11–14.

The Food and Drug Administration (FDA) News Release. (2013). *FDA requiring lower recommended dose for certain sleep drugs containing zolpidem.* Retrieved from http://www.fda.gov/newsevents/newsroom/pressannouncements/ucm334798.htm

Forger, N. G., deVries, G. J., & Breedlove, S. M. (2015). Sexual differentiation of brain and behavior. In T. M. Plant & A. J. Zelenik (Eds.), *Knobil and Neill's physiology of reproduction* (4th ed., pp. 2109–2155). Amsterdam, The Netherlands: Elsevier. doi:10.1186/s13293-015-0032

The Free Dictionary. (2014). *Sexual dimorphism.* Retrieved from http://www.thefreedictionary.com/sexual+dimorphism

Frontera, W. R., Hughes, V. A., Lutz, K. J., & Evans, W. J. (1991). A cross-sectional study of muscle strength and mass in 45- to 78-yr-old men and women. *Journal of Applied Physiology, 71*(2), 644–650.

Fryar, C. D., Gu, Q., & Ogden, C. L. (2012). Anthropometric reference data for children and adults: United States, 2007-2010. Data From the National Health and Nutrition Examination Survey. *Vital and Health Statistics. 11*(252), 1–48.

Frye, A. (1995). *Healing passage: A midwife's guide to the care and repair of the tissues involved in birth* (5th ed.). Portland, OR: Labrys Press.

Garcia-Mayor, R. V., Andrade, M. A., Rios, M., Lage, M., Dieguez, C., & Casanueva, F. F. (1997). Serum leptin levels in normal children: Relationship to age, gender, body mass index, pituitary-gonadal hormones, and pubertal stage. *Journal of Clinical Endocrinology and Metabolism, 82*(9), 2849–2855.

Graziottin, A. L., & Gambini, D. A. (2015). Anatomy and physiology of genital organs—Women. *Handbook of Clinical Neurology, 130,* 39–60.

Greenblatt, D. J., Harmatz, J. S., Singh, N. N., Steinberg, F., Roth, T., Moline, M. L., … Kapil, R. P. (2014). Gender differences in pharmacokinetics and pharmacodynamics of zolpidem following sublingual administration. *Journal of Clinical Pharmacology, 54*(3), 282–290.

Hatcher, R., & Namnoum, A. (2004). The menstrual cycle. In R. Hatcher, J. Trussell, & A. L. Nelson (Eds.). *Contraceptive technology* (19th ed., pp. 63–72). New York, NY: Ardent Media.

Hegazy, A. A., & Al-Rukban, M. O. (2012). Hymen: Facts and conceptions. *The Health, 3*(4), 109–115.

Hoffman, E., & Johnson, K. (1995). Women's health and managed care: Implications for the training of primary care physicians. *Journal of the American Medical Women's Association, 50*(1), 17–19.

Hosseinzadeh, K., Heller, M. T., & Houshmand, G. (2012). Imaging of the female perineum in adults. *Radiographics: A Review Publication of the Radiological Society of North America, Inc, 32*(4), E129–E168.

Houghton, O., & McCluggage, W. G. (2013). Fallopian tube. In D. C. Allen & R. I. Cameron (Eds.), *Histopathology specimens* (pp. 235–239). London, UK: Springer Publishing.

Institute of Medicine Committee on Understanding the Biology of Sex and Gender Differences. (2001). In T. M. Wizemann & M. L. Pardue (Eds.), *Exploring the biological contributions to human health: Does sex matter?* Washington, DC: National Academies Press.

Jackson, H. (2008). Cardiovascular fitness and lung function of adult men and women in the United States: NHANES 1999–2002. [Thesis]. Fort Worth, TX: University of North Texas Health Science Center. Retrieved from http://digitalcommons.hsc.unt.edu/cgi/viewcontent.cgi?article=1002&context=theses

Jane, F. M., & Davis, S. R. (2014). A practitioner's toolkit for managing the menopause. *Climacteric, 17*(5), 564–579.

Jensen, M. D. (2002). Adipose tissue and fatty acid metabolism in humans. *Journal of the Royal Society of Medicine, 95*(Suppl. 42), 3–7.

Jones, R. (2006). *Human reproductive biology* (3rd ed.). Boston, MA: Elsevier.

Joyner, M. J., Barnes, J. N., Hart, E. C., Wallin, G., & Charkoudian, N. (2015). Neural control of the circulation: How sex and age differences interact in humans. *Comprehensive Physiology, 5*(1), 193–215. doi:10.1002/cphy.c140005

Juul, K. V., Klein, B. M., Sandström, R., Erichsen, L., & Nørgaard, J. P. (2011). Gender difference in antidiuretic response to desmopressin. *American Journal of Physiology. Renal Physiology, 300*(5), F1116–F1122.

Kirchengast, S. (2010). Gender differences in body composition from childhood to old age: An evolutionary point of view. *Journal of Life Science, 2*(1), 1–10.

Krissi, H., Ben-Shitrit, G., Aviram, A., Weintraub, A. Y. From, A., Wiznitzer, A., & Peled, Y. (2016). Anatomical diversity of the female external genitalia and its association to sexual function. *European Journal of Obstetrics, Gynecology, and Reproductive Biology, 196*, 44–47.

Martellucci, J., Bergamini, C., Palla, G., Simoncini, T., Naldini, G., & Valeri, A. (2015). Functional anatomy of the pelvic floor. In J. Martelluci (Ed.), *Electrical stimulation for pelvic floor disorders* (pp. 19–42). London, UK: Springer International Publishing.

Masters, W., & Johnson, V. (1966). *Human sexual response.* Boston, MA: Little, Brown.

Matkovic, V., Ilich, J. Z., Skugor, M., Badenhop, N. E., Goel, P., Clairmont, A., . . . Landoll, J. D. (1997). Leptin is inversely related to age at menarche in human females. *Journal of Clinical Endocrinology and Metabolism, 82*(10), 3239–3245.

McCance, K., & Huether, S. (2006). *Pathophysiology: The biologic basis for disease in adults and children* (5th ed.). St. Louis, MO: Mosby.

McCarthy, M. M. (2016). Multifaceted origins of sex differences in the brain. *Philosophical Transactions of the Royal Society, B371*, 20150106. Retrieved from http://dx.doi.org/10.1098/rstb.2015.0106

McGuire, K. P. (2016). Breast anatomy and physiology. In A. Aydiner, A. Igoi, & A. Soran (Eds.). *Breast disease: Diagnosis and pathology.* (pp. 1–14).

Mogil, J. S. (2012). Sex differences in pain and pain inhibition: Multiple explanations of a controversial phenomenon. *Nature Reviews. Neuroscience, 13*(12), 859–866.

North American Menopause Society (NAMS). (2007). *Menopause practice: A clinician's guide* (3rd ed.). Cleveland, OH: North American Menopause Society.

Pandya, S., & Moore, R. G. (2011). Breast development and anatomy. *Clinical Obstetrics and Gynecology, 54*(1), 91–95.

Pardue, M. L., & Wizemann, T. M. (Eds.) (2001). *Exploring the biological contributions to human health: Does sex matter?* Washington, DC: National Academies Press.

Perna, F. M., Coa, K., Troiano, R. P., Lawman, H. G., Wang, C. Y., Li, Y., . . . Kraemer, W. (2016). Muscular grip strength estimates of the U.S. population from the National Health and Nutrition Examination Survey: 2011–2012. *Journal of Strength & Conditioning Research, 30*(3), 867–874.

Pinn, V. W. (2003). Sex and gender factors in medical studies: Implications for health and clinical practice. *Journal of the American Medical Association, 289*(4), 397–400.

Plant, T. (1994). Puberty in primates. In E. Knobil & J. O'Neill (Eds.), *The physiology of reproduction* (pp. 1763–1788). New York, NY: Raven Press.

Porth, C. M. (2007). *Essentials of pathophysiology: Concepts in altered health states.* Philadelphia, PA: Lippincott Williams & Wilkins.

Puppo, V. (2013). Anatomy and physiology of the clitoris, vestibular bulbs, and labia minora with a review of the female orgasm and the prevention of female sexual dysfunction. *Clinical Anatomy, 26*(1), 134–152.

Puppo, V., & Puppo, G. (2015). Anatomy of sex: Revision of the new anatomical terms used for the clitoris and the female orgasm by sexologists. *Clinical Anatomy, 28*(3), 293–304.

Rebar, R. (2002). Puberty. In J. S. Berek (Ed.), *Novak's gynecology* (13th ed., pp. 805–841). Philadelphia, PA: Lippincott Williams & Wilkins.

Seidel, H., Ball, J., Dains, J., & Benedict, G. (2006). *Mosby's guide to physical examination* (6th ed.). St. Louis, MO: Mosby.

Speroff, L., & Fritz, M. (2005). *Clinical gynecologic endocrinology and infertility* (7th ed.). Baltimore, MD: Lippincott Williams & Wilkins.

Stoppard, M. (Ed.). (2002). *Woman's body: A manual for life.* New York, NY: Dorling Kindersley.

Tanner, J. M. (1981). Growth and maturation during adolescence. *Nutrition Reviews, 39*(2), 43–55.

Truong, S., Cole, N., Stapleton, F., & Golebiowski, B. (2014). Sex hormones and the dry eye. *Clinical & Experimental Optometry, 97*(4), 324–336.

Vandenberg, L. N., Schaeberle, C. M., Rubin, B. S., Sonnenschein, C., & Soto, A. M. (2013). The male mammary gland: A target for the xenoestrogen bisphenol A. *Reproductive Toxicology, 37*, 15–23.

Venturoli, S., Flamigni, C., & Givens, J. (Eds.). (1985). *Adolescence in females.* Chicago, IL: Medical Year Book.

Wagner, S., Knechtle, B., Knechtle, P., Rüst, C. A., & Rosemann, T. (2012). Higher prevalence of exercise-associated hyponatremia in female than in male open-water ultra-endurance swimmers: The "Marathon-Swim" in Lake Zurich. *European Journal of Applied Physiology, 112*(3), 1095–1106.

Widmeier, E., Ruff, H., & Strong, K. (Eds.). (2004). *Vander, Sherman, & Luciano's Human physiology: The mechanisms of body function* (9th ed.). Boston, MA: McGraw-Hill.

CHAPTER 8

Young Women's Health

Catherine Takacs Witkop

Adolescence is a time of significant physical, emotional, social, and cognitive changes, and behaviors and habits developed during this time can have a lasting impact in adulthood. The state of a young woman's health and the decisions she makes during the second and into the third decade of her life can jeopardize her short-term health and long-term well-being. However, on a more positive note, it is precisely during such a formative time that health care providers can provide impactful preventive guidance and services that bolster healthy behaviors and establish the young woman on a trajectory toward health.

This chapter contains an overview of young women's health, beginning with considerations of the demographic characteristics of adolescents in the U.S. population. For the purposes of this chapter, adolescents include those between 10 and 19 years of age. However, where appropriate, issues and services pertaining to young women up to age 25 years will be addressed. Adolescent development occurs in stages and can be affected by numerous factors such as disabilities, race/ethnicity, and the home environment. Furthermore, several contexts, including family, peers, school, community, and the Internet can have an impact on health and development. Health services that adolescents need are driven by challenges in their development and the context in which they live, and health care providers can contribute to the accessibility and quality of care. Finally, the chapter concludes with an outline of the female adolescent visit and consideration of specific conditions and challenges.

■ AN OVERVIEW OF ADOLESCENCE IN THE UNITED STATES

Demographic Characteristics

Adolescents are a large and diverse part of U.S. society. Children ages 10 to 19 years old comprise approximately 14% of the U.S. population (U.S. Census Bureau, 2014). Geographically, adolescents are concentrated in urban and suburban communities, but their percentage of the overall population of the community is greatest in rural areas. They are more ethnically diverse than the general population, with increases in the past decade in the numbers of Hispanic and Asian American adolescents. Estimates suggest that by 2060, the percentage of Hispanic children will be about 34% and children who belong to ethnic/racial "minority" groups will make up 64% of the youth population (Colby & Ortman, 2015).

There are several sources for reliable and comprehensive youth data that are referenced throughout this chapter. Each year, the Annie E. Casey Foundation publishes the *Kids Count Data Book*, intended to highlight key indicators of youth health and assess trends at the state and national level. Sixteen key indicators are measured, and five of these specifically target adolescent health: teen death rate, teen birthrate, high school students not graduating on time, teens who abuse alcohol or drugs, and the percentage of teens not attending school and not working (Annie E. Casey Foundation, 2015). Other than the last indicator, the trend for this decade on the other three key indicators focused on adolescent well-being has been positive. In particular, the teen birthrate has gone from 40 per 1,000 in 2008, to 26 per 1,000 in 2013 (Annie E. Casey Foundation, 2015). The report also highlights ethnic/racial and regional differences in the data. For example, the teen birthrate for Latinos is the highest among the major racial/ethnic groups, at 42 births per 1,000 teenage girls, and regionally, the teen birthrate ranged from 12 per 1,000 adolescents (aged 15–19 years) in Massachusetts compared with 44 per 1,000 in Arkansas (Annie E. Casey Foundation, 2015). This resource is worthwhile for understanding the needs of a provider's adolescent subpopulation.

Another rich source of adolescent health data is collected to support *Healthy People 2020*. This program, launched in 2010 by the Department of Health and Human Services, has the overarching goals of (a) attaining high-quality and longer lives; (b) achieving health equity, eliminating disparities, and improving the health of all groups; (c) creating health-promoting social and physical environments; and (d) promoting quality of life, healthy development, and healthy behaviors across all life stages (U.S. Department of Health and Human Services, 2015). This program tracks approximately 1,200 objectives, which are organized into 42 topic areas. These objectives are national, relying on health agencies at all levels of government, as well as nongovernmental organizations and private sector services. There are 11 adolescent health objectives and several other objectives

BOX 8.1   OBJECTIVES DIRECTLY RELATED TO ADOLESCENT HEALTH FROM *HEALTHY PEOPLE 2020*

AH-1   Increase the proportion of adolescents who have had a wellness checkup in the past 12 months

AH-2   Increase the proportion of adolescents who participate in extracurricular and/or out-of-school activities

AH-3   Increase the proportion of adolescents who are connected to a parent or other positive adult caregiver

AH-4   Increase the proportion of adolescents who transition to self-sufficiency from foster care

AH-5   Increase educational achievement of adolescents and young adults

AH-6   Increase the proportion of schools with a school breakfast program

AH-7   Reduce the proportion of adolescents who have been offered, sold, or given an illegal drug on school property

AH-8   Increase the proportion of adolescents whose parents consider them to be safe at school

AH-9   Increase the proportion of middle and high schools that prohibit harassment based on a student's sexual orientation of gender identity

AH-10 Reduce the proportion of public schools with a serious violent incident

AH-11 Reduce adolescent and young adult perpetration of, and victimization by, crimes.

Other Relevant Objectives

FP-7.1 Increase the proportion of sexually experienced females aged 15 to 44 years who received reproductive health services in the past 12 months

FP-8   Reduce pregnancies among adolescent females (15–17 and 18–19 years)

FP-9   Increase the proportion of adolescents aged 17 years and younger who have never had sexual intercourse (15–17 and 15 years and younger)

FP-10 Increase the proportion of sexually active persons aged 15 to 19 years who use condoms to both effectively prevent pregnancy and provide barrier protection against disease (15–19 years who used a condom at first and last intercourse)

FP-11 Increase the proportion of sexually active persons aged 15 to 19 years who use condoms and hormonal or intrauterine contraception to both effectively prevent pregnancy and provide barrier protection against disease

NWS-5.2 Increase the proportion of primary care physicians who regularly assess body mass index for age and sex in their child or adolescent patients

---

that directly pertain to the health of adolescents, although many others also impact adolescent health (e.g., HIV prevention and screening). The need for these objectives will become clear throughout this chapter as they encourage public health interventions and health services initiatives targeted on the most important current health issues for adolescents. Although many of these evidence-based public health objectives fall outside the scope of influence of the health system, health care providers should be aware of the objectives and attempt to implement as appropriate. Adolescent health care providers should become familiar with the website in which *Healthy People 2020* progress is continually updated (www.healthypeople.gov; see Box 8.1).

■ RISK FACTORS

Risk and Protective Factors

In addition to information on health and well-being, various organizations collect comprehensive data on risk factors that impact the health of adolescents. For example, the Centers for Disease Control and Prevention (CDC), in cooperation with state and local health departments, surveys ninth- through 12th-grade youth in public and private schools with the Youth Risk Behavior Surveillance System (YRBSS). The goals of the survey are to identify health problems in youth, to identify trends in risk-taking behaviors, and to focus the country on adolescent health issues. The YRBSS measures activities that contribute to unintended injuries and violence, tobacco use, alcohol and other drug use, sexual behaviors that contribute to unintended pregnancy and sexually transmitted infections (STIs), unhealthy eating patterns, and physical inactivity (CDC, 2014b). In addition to monitoring these risk behaviors, asthma and obesity rates throughout the United States are followed and reported each year. Data from the 2013 YRBSS are referred to throughout this chapter to understand the most current exposures for U.S. adolescents.

Although risk-taking adolescent behaviors can negatively affect health outcomes, positive factors can counteract the negative factors. Dahlberg and Potter (2001); Hawkins, Kosterman, Catalano, Hill, and Abbott (2005); and others have evaluated both risk and protective factors that impact violence and the use of tobacco, alcohol, and other drugs. Their work has enhanced efforts of school-based and community intervention programs in building strengths and developing skills—in contrast to interventions that focus only on negative outcomes. Community-based programs have been in place for some time, and identifying best practices and effective programs can be a challenge. The

Community Preventive Services Task Force was established by the U.S. Department of Health and Human Services to identify population health interventions that have saved lives, increased life spans, and improved quality of life (Briss, Brownson, Fielding, & Zaza, 2004). The task force produces recommendations (and identifies evidence gaps) to help inform the decision making of federal, state, and local health departments; other government agencies; communities; health care providers; employers; schools; and research organizations. They answer the questions: (a) Which program and policy interventions have been proven effective? (b) Are there effective interventions that are right for my community? (c) What might effective interventions cost; what is the likely return on investment? The task force rates policies and community and school-based interventions based on level of evidence that the interventions are effective, providing policy-makers and other communities with information on effective approaches. It has specifically focused on adolescent health as one of its key topic areas and has addressed a number of issues including alcohol use, alcohol-impaired driving, obesity, high-risk sexual activities, STIs (including HIV), and tobacco use, among many others. Providers of adolescents can better understand community and school-based interventions that have a positive impact on adolescent health by perusing the website of the task force at www.thecommunityguide.org/index.html.

The resiliency model recognizes the ability of youth to buffer themselves from harm and remain healthy even when faced with multiple risk factors. Risk and protective factors are inversely related to each other as they affect health outcomes, and these factors can be identified in the individual, peers, family, school, and community. Youth with multiple risk factors and few protective factors have poorer health outcomes than youth with few risk factors and multiple protective factors. Examples of risk factors are individual lack of school commitment, friends who engage in drug use, family conflict, violence in the school, and community disorganization. Examples of protective factors include an individual's positive social orientation, bonds with friends and within the family, a school's high expectation of youth, and opportunities for youth participation in the community (Hawkins, Smith, & Catalano, 2002). Adelmann (2005) has linked protective factors with positive health behaviors in sixth-grade students: seat belt use, participation in exercise and recreation, quality nutrition intake, and academic achievement. Conversely, his findings reveal that individuals with multiple risk factors had significantly higher negative health behaviors. Barrow, Armstrong, Vargo, and Boothroyd (2007) examined the resiliency of African American adolescents and identified specific protective factors to be fostered: self-efficacy, positive racial/ethnic identity, and commitment to the family and community. In African American youth, the development of ethnic pride was linked with parental influence, self-esteem, and self-control and therefore had a protective impact on risk-taking behaviors (Wills et al., 2007). It is important to identify ways to foster positive factors because African American youth are disproportionately represented in every negative health measure (CDC, 2014a).

School environments and academic connectedness combine to create a strong protective factor for youth. Using social and school connectedness as predictors of future health outcomes, Bond et al. (2007) found that positive social and/or school connectedness in eighth-grade students was associated with positive outcomes (school achievement, mental health, and substance abuse) in the 10th and 12th grades. In addition, they found that having both social and school connectedness was associated with the best outcomes. Youngblade et al. (2007) studied a sample of more than 42,000 adolescents aged 11 to 17 years, from the 2003 National Survey of Children's Health. They concluded that multiple family, school, and community protective factors had a positive influence on youth health behaviors. No single influence in an adolescent's life provides protection from violence, substance abuse, or poor health outcomes, but the individual, family, school, and community all contribute to a strong foundation for positive youth development.

■ ADOLESCENT DEVELOPMENT

Adolescent Stages of Development

During adolescence, development occurs in physical, social, spiritual, and emotional sphere as well as in cognitive and moral spheres. Many theories have been developed to enhance understanding of developmental stages. There are multiple ways to define the boundaries of adolescent development, and there is no consensus between and among researchers, clinicians, parents, and youth themselves. For girls, thelarche marks the first physical sign of pubertal change and is often accompanied by some of the emotional changes of adolescence; this may occur in girls as young as 7 or 8 years old. Considerations for extending adolescence up to 24 or 25 years of age reflect the emerging science on brain development and the tasks of emancipation that extend well into the 20s for some youth (Galvan, Hare, Voss, Glover, & Casey, 2007). Others consider adolescence to run through age 19 years and "young adult" up to age 24 years. In a 2009 National Research Council report on adolescent health services, the committee reviewed a broad range of literature on the topic and generally divided the available evidence into subsets of early adolescence (ages 10–14 years) and adolescence (ages 15–19 years), followed by late adolescence (or early adulthood from ages 20–24 years; National Research Council, 2009). Another accepted breakdown of adolescence ties the stages to schooling: ages 10 to 13 years or middle school, ages 14 to 17 years or high school, and ages 18 to 21 or college, military service, or employment (Neinstein, 2008). Because there are no exact demarcations among stages, this chapter generally refers to early, middle, and late adolescence, as well as young adulthood, without any discrete ages defining the stages.

Each phase of a young woman's development contributes to the foundation for her successful emergence from adolescence and the transition to womanhood. Throughout adolescence, women are seeking independence, identity development, social skills and connections with peers, and body awareness. According to Erickson (1963, 1968), adolescents and young adults must develop their identity to avoid role confusion. In Piaget's (1973) cognitive theory, the adolescent proceeds from concrete operational thinking to formal operational thoughts characterized by abstract thinking. An extension of Piaget's work, Kohlberg's (1981) moral development theory discusses movement from conventional moral reasoning—making judgments based on what is right because of society's regulation—to postconventional morality—making judgments based on universal principles of justice. Carol Gilligan's work developed as a result of her affiliation with Kohlberg and examination of how gender variables challenged the moral development theory. Through further investigation, Gilligan (1982) identified how girls construct moral dilemmas in terms of caring, responsibility, and relationship and not in terms of right, wrong, and rule making. Rew (2005) pointed out that adolescent girls recognize a disparity between care and power and that many choose to abandon the concern for attaining and maintaining power and adopt the concern for caring.

Early Adolescence

The developing characteristics of early adolescence often parallel the rapid physical changes of puberty in most girls. These girls become less interested in family activities and may begin to critique parental influences. The struggle for independence while still being dependent frequently creates family discord and is accompanied by wide mood swings in the young adolescent. A young woman often makes strong attachments to a peer group and experiences the ups and downs of that intensity. She becomes increasingly aware and yet insecure about her body, frequently comparing herself with others. A young woman may be confused about her physical body's impact on others in her social network and in the community. She begins to have sexual feelings and begins to privately question her thoughts and emotions. At this stage in a young woman's development, she is expanding her knowledge, beginning to abstractly process information, fantasize about the future, and daydream about idealistic goals. There is an intense focus on the self, accompanied by an overwhelming self-consciousness that Elkind and Bowen (1979) termed the "imaginary audience."

Middle Adolescence

Middle adolescence is marked by continued withdrawal from the family and increasing conflict at home. Young women also have a heightened interest in peer connections and adopt peer-group norms, which may lead to school and community conflicts as well. Middle adolescence sees involvement in more delinquency, gangs, sports, and clubs as a young woman tries to identify and connect with a peer group. The middle adolescent begins to accept the physical changes of puberty and focuses on developing a personal identity within the peer-group norms in terms of clothing, makeup, and hairstyle. This creative self-expression enhances identity development and body image. During middle adolescence, the invincibility felt by a young woman, and her impression that "it can't happen to me," may lead to poor decision making and risky behaviors.

Late Adolescence

Late adolescence is a time for the young woman to begin the transition to adulthood. If her earlier experiences with independence, peer-group support, and identity development have been empowering, the young woman is well equipped to trust this next phase of her life. If, on the other hand, her early and middle stages of adolescence were complicated by mental illness, an eating disorder, or other chronic problems, the young woman may not be optimally prepared to face the responsibilities and challenges of adult life. The tasks during this phase are to have body acceptance, a clear self-identity, and the ability to critically appraise parents and peers in order to make independent choices.

Physical Development

Before menarche, young women experience dramatic changes in their bodies during a relatively short period, including a deposition of adipose tissue (up to 11 kg of body fat) as well as an increase in height (up to 25 cm), called the *growth spurt* (Tanner, 1962). In addition, premenarcheal girls experience adrenarche (growth of pubic hair, stimulated by androgens), thelarche (breast development stimulated by estradiol), and late in puberty, menarche. Nearly two thirds of girls experience menarche during Tanner's (1981) stage 4 (Brooks-Gunn & Warren, 1985; Brooks-Gunn, Warren, Rosso, & Gargiulo, 1987; Tanner, 1962). Menarche occurs 2 to 2.5 years after breast buds emerge, after the peak height velocity is completed, and at a sexual maturity rating of 3 or 4. The physiological basis of puberty and menarche is discussed more fully in Chapter 7.

In addition to sexual maturation, bone mass or bone mineral density increases. Physical activity level, heredity, nutrition, endocrine function, and medications can positively or negatively affect bone mass in adolescents. Peak bone mass is acquired by early adulthood, so adolescence is a critical time in acquiring bone density necessary for lifelong bone health. Other physical changes of puberty include growth of the internal organs, including the liver, kidneys, and heart. Significant biochemical changes also occur, including changes in serum alkaline phosphatase concentrations, serum ferritin, and erythrocyte mass (Neinstein, 2008). Of all the physical changes associated with puberty, among the most dramatic, unexpected, and misunderstood is the change in adipose mass. On average, girls who mature earlier tend to have higher body mass index (BMI), and slightly shorter girls who mature later tend to be lighter, leaner, and slightly taller when puberty is complete.

In recent years, there has been increasing focus on the developing adolescent brain and its role in social, behavioral, and psychiatric disorders. This work has found that social skills, decision making, and impulsivity are significantly linked to measurable physiological changes in the brain. Nelson, Leibenluft, McClure, and Pine (2005) described the brain's social information processing network and identified three nodes based on function and developmental timing: detection node, affective node, and cognitive-regulatory node. The associations of the adolescent brain's maturation, social inhibition, and risk-taking impulsivity are individualized and remain an area of emerging science (Galvan et al., 2007). A woman's relationship to her body evolves over her life span, and adolescence appears to be a critical period for changes in a young woman's self-concept, body image, physical strength, and emotional well-being (Patton & Viner, 2007).

A growing body of literature (Haudek, Rorty, & Henker, 1999; Hayward et al., 1997; Hayward, Gotlib, Schraedley, & Litt, 1999; Siegel, Yancey, Aneshensel, & Schuler, 1999) indicates that early puberty can be especially challenging for White, Asian, and Hispanic girls. The girls entering puberty before their peers may not be as well prepared for the physical, psychological, and social changes that occur in puberty (Brooks-Gunn, Petersen, & Eichorn, 1985). Early pubertal status has been found to be a predictor of frequent problems seen among adolescent girls (Angold, Costello, & Worthman, 1998; Hayward et al., 1999).

Although few have investigated the implications of pubertal timing for adult functioning, Serepca (1996) examined whether women's objective pubertal timing (their menarcheal age) and subjective timing (perceived timing relative to peers of menarche and breast development) influenced their adult body image and self-esteem. Objective pubertal timing did not differ on any of the body image or self-esteem variables. However, adult women who perceived themselves as early in breast development, compared with their peers, described themselves as heavier and were more preoccupied with being or becoming overweight. They were also less satisfied with their physical appearance than late-maturing women. Late maturers, on both subjective timing measures, reported more positive body-image attitudes than on-time and early maturers. This suggests that perception of relative pubertal development may have lasting implications for women.

A large body of research suggests that early maturing girls are more likely than other girls to exhibit depressive, eating, and delinquent symptoms, as well as general behavior problems (Attie & Brooks-Gunn, 1995; Caspi & Moffitt, 1991; Graber, Brooks-Gunn, Paikoff, & Warren, 1995; Graber, Lewinsohn, Seeley, & Brooks-Gunn, 1997; Hayward et al., 1997; Petersen, Sarigiani, & Kennedy, 1991). In a national probability sample of fifth- to eighth-grade girls, pubertal stage strongly predicted the occurrence of panic attacks and eating disorder symptoms, the frequency of which increased dramatically with advanced pubertal development (Hayward et al., 1999). In these same studies, late-maturing girls demonstrated no consistent pattern of adjustment problems when compared with on-time maturers. Most of the research in this area has been conducted with a subject pool consisting of primarily White middle-class female adolescents. Not all studies have found an association between pubertal status and depression among predominantly White samples. Studies with small sample sizes (less than 110) with multiple predictors using multivariate methods and pubertal status as one variable have not found pubertal status predictive of depression (Brooks-Gunn & Warren, 1989; Paikoff, Brooks-Gunn, & Warren, 1991; Warren & Brooks-Gunn, 1989).

In a growing body of research, African American girls have been found to have higher and more stable self-worth and greater satisfaction with physical appearance compared with White girls (Brown et al., 1998; Doswell, Millor, Thompson, & Braxter, 1998; Parker, Nichter, Nichter, & Vuckovic, 1995; Siegel et al., 1999). This was found despite a higher mean BMI among African American girls (Striegel-Moore & Smolak, 1996). In the first longitudinal study of African American girls (ages 9–14 years) followed more than 5 years, these girls had higher body-image scores and greater tolerance for a higher BMI than White girls. The authors suggested that a reason may be cultural differences in attitude toward physical appearance and obesity among Blacks (Brown et al., 1998). However, Siegel et al. (1999) found that heavier African Americans felt more negatively about their bodies than those who were leaner, suggesting that dominant social norms do also play a role. Exposure to a dominant culture that denigrates different physical features may have an impact on body image among African American young women (Williamson, 1998). Black girls who reported peer pressure were as likely as White girls to be dissatisfied with their weight and try to lose weight by dieting (Schreiber et al., 1996).

Menarche

McDowell, Brody, and Hughes (2007) have analyzed the change in menarche timing over the past century. Data from the 1999 to 2004 National Health and Nutrition Examination Survey (NHANES) on 6,788 women revealed a 0.9-year decline in self-reported age at menarche in all racial/ethnic groups. For women born before 1920, the mean age of menarche was 13.6 years. For women born in 1980 to 1984, the mean age was 12.5 years. To account for this decrease, researchers have suggested multiple related variables, including nutrition status, obesity, race, socioeconomic class, genetic predisposition, and environmental and societal influences (Cesario & Hughes, 2007; Lee et al., 2007).

■ FACTORS INFLUENCING ADOLESCENT DEVELOPMENT

Being Different

Feeling "different" during adolescence can have an impact on the transition from adolescence to adulthood, affecting identity formation, engagement with peers, and self-confidence. All youth experience the feelings of not fitting in or questioning, "Am I normal?" However, these feelings may be intensified in adolescents living outside the dominant norms of society. This section of the chapter examines the impact of disability, chronic illness, race/ethnicity, immigration and refugee status, socioeconomic and family status, and sexual orientation and identity on adolescents.

Disability

Because there is variability in the impact that one or more disabling conditions has on an individual, it is difficult to generalize the effect disability has on the development of an adolescent. Several chronic conditions are more prevalent in adolescents with disabilities and need to be addressed during the visit. For example, the prevalence of obesity in adolescents with disabilities is 17.5%, which is significantly higher than the 13% prevalence in young adults without disabilities (Rimmer, Yamaki, Davis, Wang, & Vogel, 2011). In addition to increased risk for other chronic conditions, obesity also makes self-care and self-transfer (or transfer by others) a greater challenge.

Adolescents with special health care needs often require coordinated care by an experienced health care team. This type of "Medical Home" provides services with a focus on transition to adulthood (for more information, consult www.MedicalHomeInfo.org). The coordination of health services for special needs children in rural areas can have a positive impact on reducing family stress, school absences, and utilization of ambulatory health care (Farmer, Clark, Sherman, Marien, & Selva, 2005). The Medical Home incorporates seven integral elements into the health care of young people and their families:

- Accessible
- Compassionate
- Comprehensive
- Continuous
- Coordinated
- Culturally effective
- Family centered (Medical Home Initiatives for Children With Special Needs Project Advisory Committee, 2004)

Transition services for youth with special health care needs are a requirement of the Individuals with Disabilities Education Act and assist in the preparation of youth to fully participate and be included in adult society by focusing on access to health care, educational and employment transition, social and recreation networks, community living skills, and quality of life (Betz, 2007; Sadof & Nazarian, 2007). In addition to participating in the multidisciplinary team taking care of the patient and being cognizant of the other challenges facing the patient, the health care provider can assist in facilitating the transition to adulthood by treating the young woman with respect, speaking directly to her during the visit (instead of to the caregiver), and if possible, conducting part of the visit, including the examination, without the caregiver present (American College of Obstetricians and Gynecologists [ACOG], 2012). A chaperone should be in the room during the examination, but a positive, dignified experience in which the young adult is treated as such may facilitate her comfort in returning for future visits.

There are additional considerations for the reproductive health visit in adolescent women with disabilities. The rate of sexual abuse among persons with disabilities ranges from 25% to 83% (ACOG, 2012). It is important therefore for the women's health care provider to be aware of this risk and look for possible signs or symptoms of abuse, including significant changes in behavior; depression; sleep disturbances; avoidance or fear of individuals, genders, or situations; refusal to be touched; hints about change in sexual activity; and/or a new understanding of sexual behavior. Physical signs could be bleeding, bruising, or infection of the genitals, rectum, mouth, or breasts; pain with walking or sitting; and nonspecific, unexplained medical problems such as pelvic pain or headaches (ACOG, 2012).

It is important to note that all licensed providers in every jurisdiction in the United States must report suspected sexual or physical abuse of a minor to child protective services. In most jurisdictions, this also applies to young adults with disabilities (ACOG, 2012). If possible, the licensed provider should tell the young woman that reporting will take place, but this needs to be done confidentially and with sensitivity to the patient's circumstances.

Adolescents with disabilities may have menstrual issues that are more complex than the common anovulatory cycles experienced by most young women after menarche. These menstrual cycle abnormalities may result from obesity, thyroid disease (in particular in patients with trisomy 21), medications (antiepileptic and psychiatric medications causing hyperprolactinemia and amenorrhea), or polycystic ovary syndrome (PCOS; more common in teenagers with seizure disorders), among others (ACOG, 2012). Cyclic behavior changes, such as changes in mood around the times of her period, may also be more common in women with disabilities, although making the diagnosis of premenstrual dysphoric disorder (PMDD) can be a challenge, especially with cognitive delays. Seizure disorders are more common in adolescents with disabilities, as are catamenial seizures.

Because of complications with menstrual cycles, menstrual manipulation/suppression is frequently considered in women with disabilities, often at the request of her caregiver (ACOG, 2009). Most contraceptive options are also appropriate for women with disabilities, but unique issues, such as difficulty with inserting a contraceptive ring for adolescents with physical disability or weight gain with medroxyprogesterone acetate (Depo-Provera) in an already obese patient, should be considered before medications are prescribed (ACOG, 2012). Contraceptives should be discussed not only in the context of menstrual suppression, but also in the context of protection against pregnancy. Adolescents with disabilities should not be assumed to be asexual. It is important to know that permanent sterilization in this population is rarely appropriate and introduces significant ethical issues that must be comprehensively addressed. If the patient is deemed competent and she requests sterilization, she may meet the criteria for informed consent. The hospital ethics committee may need to become involved in cases in which sterilization is requested.

Determining the capacity of an adolescent with developmental disabilities to participate in decision making or an informed consent process can be complex. *Incompetency* is a legal determination and must be assessed at a given time and situation before a patient is deemed incompetent. If a legal guardian has been appointed, it is important to understand who can make certain decisions in the adolescent's life. Information on guardianship and consent can be obtained through the National Disability Rights Network (www.ndrn.org).

Chronic Conditions

Although most adolescents are physically healthy when compared with the general population, it is estimated that 12% of adolescents live with a chronic health problem, the most common being diabetes mellitus, asthma, arthritis, epilepsy, and heart disease (Sawyer, Drew, Yeo, & Britto, 2007). Chronic health problems have three characteristics: (a) a biological, psychological, or cognitive basis; (b) expected duration of longer than 12 months; and (c) limitations that require medication, diet, personal assistance, or medical technology; limitations in function in activities or social roles; or the need for medical care or accommodating services that would be unique for the person's age (Sawyer et al., 2007). Youth with chronic conditions often engage in risky behaviors at rates equal to or greater than their same-age peers, putting themselves at even greater risk for negative consequences than their healthy counterparts. Poor medication adherence, pregnancy, and substance abuse can compound chronic health conditions and influence the health status of young women (Sawyer et al., 2007).

Race/Ethnicity

Adolescents and young adults from minority racial/ethnic groups experience inequities in health status and outcomes (Park, Paul Mulye, Adams, Brindis, & Irwin, 2006). Health disparities between African American and White women continue to exist when comparing reproductive health outcomes (infant and maternal mortality, unintended pregnancy, and access to preventive health care; Anachebe & Sutton, 2003). After age 18 years, many young adults have barriers to health insurance and experience low rates of coverage, but Black and Hispanic young adults are most likely to be uninsured (Adams, Newacheck, Park, Brindis, & Irwin, 2007). A study of adolescents in New York State with publicly funded health insurance demonstrated that youth utilized available health services and reduced unmet health needs (Klein et al., 2007). National, state, and community interventions to address racial/ethnic health disparities among youth must focus on improvements in access and the quality of available care.

Immigrant/Refugee

In 2014, 24% of children 17 years of age or younger were first- or second-generation immigrants, and among those children between 5 and 17 years of age, 22% did not speak English at home (although only 5% had difficulty speaking English; Federal Interagency Forum on Child and Family Statistics, 2015). The largest numbers of immigrants come from Mexico, as 30% of the total foreign-born population is from Mexico (Center for Health and Health Care in Schools, 2011).

Because immigrants often lack health insurance and are more likely to live in crowded housing and face food insecurity, immigrant and refugee youth are especially vulnerable in U.S. society (Center for Health and Health Care in Schools, 2011). In a study using data from the 1999 National Survey on American Families, foreign-born noncitizen children were four times more likely than children from U.S.-native families to be without health insurance coverage and to have not visited a mental health specialist in the preceding year (Huang, Yu, & Ledsky, 2006). Foreign-born children were also less likely to have visited a doctor or a dentist in

the previous year and twice as likely to lack a usual source of care (Huang et al., 2006). In a study of parent refugee status and impact on adolescent risk taking, Spencer and Le (2006) found a strong link between parent refugee status and externalizing teen violence in Southeast Asian and Chinese youth. Immigration waves and refugee migration are linked with war and social unrest in the country of origin. Many of these families and youth have been exposed to violence and may have experienced or witnessed torture. A study of Somali and Oromo adolescents revealed a link between the amount of exposure to violent acts and resulting posttraumatic stress, as well as physical, psychological, and social problems (Halcón et al., 2004). The study also identified gender differences among the youth; girls were more likely to report feelings of aloneness, even though they were more likely to be partnered, married, or with their mothers. Yet those same youth often have protective factors that aid in their adjustment to a new country: two-parent and multigenerational households and strong commitment to the family unit (Center for Health and Health Care in Schools, 2011).

Sexual Orientation and Identity

Adolescence is a time for sexual identity development; including sexual orientation. The Guttmacher Institute Report on American Teens' Sexual and Reproductive Health revealed that 8% of females aged 18 to 19 years in 2006 to 2008 reported their sexual orientation as homosexual or bisexual, and 12% reported some same-sex behaviors (any sexual experience; Guttmacher Institute, 2014). There has been an increasing number of studies of lesbian, gay, bisexual, transgender, and questioning (LGBTQ) youth, their sexual identity development, and health risks (Saewyc et al., 2006). As a group, LGBTQ youth experience higher rates of family violence, homelessness, substance abuse, depression, and suicidality than their heterosexual peers. In examining suicidal ideation and suicide attempts among nearly 22,000 adolescents with same-sex experience in the 2004 Minnesota Student Survey, Eisenberg and Resnick (2006) found that lack of supporting and caring environments (including family connectedness, teacher caring, other adult caring, and school safety) was associated with suicidality and that same-sex experience alone was not a predictive variable. Nurses can enhance their communication skills, confront personal bias, and develop cultural competency by using available resources such as the following websites: www.safeschoolscoalition.org, www.pflag.org, and www.glbthealth.org.

Out-of-Home Youth

Out-of-home youth are those adolescents not living in the home of their immediate family or guardian. These can include youth experiencing homelessness with their family or those living with relatives or friends, in foster care, or in detention facilities, as well as runaway youth or unaccompanied minors. Estimating the prevalence of homelessness is a challenge, but in 2013, an annual tally of the homeless conducted by communities throughout the United States included youth younger than 25 years and found that 47,000 youth (unaccompanied individuals younger than 25 years), or 8%

of the homeless population, were "homeless" on the night of the count (National Alliance to End Homelessness, 2014). Youth leave home for a variety of reasons, but neglect and sexual abuse are often triggers and consequently put youth at extreme risk for additional victimization. Homelessness estimates for young adults who are LGBT varied from 6% to 35%, and it is estimated that about 10% of homeless adolescent women were pregnant when homeless (Toro, Dworsky, & Fowler, 2007).

Youth living in foster care may have multiple health and educational needs during adolescence that contribute to barriers to emancipation. Leathers and Testa (2006) surveyed Illinois foster care case workers in charge of 416 youth and found that one third of the youth had barriers to transition: mental health problems, developmental disabilities, or other special needs. Urban youth were receiving fewer services than their rural counterparts, and the more disabled the child with regard to employment, education, or physical health barriers, the less likely he or she was to continue to receive child welfare benefits; the most vulnerable youth were the least likely to receive services beyond the age of 18 years. In an Oregon study of foster care youth in special education compared with other special education students, it was found that foster care youth had lower academic performance and were likely to be maintained in a more restrictive classroom (Geenen & Powers, 2006).

Runaway youth are a transient and ever-changing population. Sanchez, Waller, and Greene (2006) used the 1995 and 1996 National Longitudinal Study of Adolescent Health to identify a data sample of more than 10,000 respondents, ages 12 to 17 years. They reported that during the study year, 6.4% of youth ran away. Girls (7.5%) were more likely than boys to leave home, as were older youth (6.8%), compared with younger adolescents. Youth not living with either parent produced the highest rates of runaway in the previous year at 11.4%, yet 99% of all runaway youth returned "home" within 12 months (Sanchez et al., 2006). Adolescents not living with a biological parent may be living with a grandparent. Grandmothers' experiences as caregivers and their perceived burdens were examined by Dowdell (2004), who found that parental drug abuse was reported as the reason for grandparent caregiving in 80% of cases.

Social Contexts for Adolescent Development

PARENTS

Parental influence is linked to multiple health outcomes in adolescents (Youngblade et al., 2007). Child Trends and the National Adolescent Health Information Center published a summary paper in 2006, *The Family Environment and Adolescent Well-Being: Exposure to Positive and Negative Family Influence*, which cites the following findings from multiple studies:

- More than three quarters of all parents report very close relationships with their adolescent children.
- Many 15-year-olds report difficulty talking to their mothers and fathers about things that really bother them.

- Adolescents who live with two parents are more likely to have parents who know their whereabouts after school.
- Hispanic parents are less likely than White and Black parents to know who most of their adolescent's friends are.
- Foreign-born adolescents are more likely than their native-born peers to eat meals with their family.
- Adolescents with better-educated parents are less likely to be exposed to smoking and heavy drinking by their parents.
- Adolescents whose parents exercise are less likely to be sedentary themselves (Aufausser, Jekielek, & Brown, 2006).

Girls (53%) were more likely than boys (42%) to report that it was difficult or very difficult to communicate with their fathers, and both girls and boys reported less difficulty with their mothers (32%; Aufausser et al., 2006). Positive parental involvement (time together, monitoring whereabouts) influenced an adolescent's health and behavior and was linked with stronger school performance, abstinence from sex and tobacco, and lower rates of delinquency. Negative parental involvement (abuse, alcohol addiction, domestic violence) was linked with poor school performance, delinquency, sexual risk taking, and substance abuse (Aufausser et al., 2006; Pate, Dowda, O'Neill, & Ward, 2007; Power, Stewart, Hughes, & Arbona, 2005; Resnick, Ireland, & Borowsky, 2004; Spencer & Le, 2006). Girls may be more responsive to family involvement and support from parents. One study demonstrated that girls are more likely than boys to abstain or reduce alcohol use when there are high levels of family connectedness, family supervision, and clear messages from parents regarding alcohol use (Sale et al., 2005). In addition, sexually active girls who had mother involvement were more likely to choose more reliable birth control methods and had lower rates of high-risk behavior (Harper, Callegari, Raine, Blum, & Darney, 2004; for additional resources, see www.guttmacher.org). In a study of African American young women, the perception of a good quality parent–adolescent relationship and consistent parental attitudes regarding sex were predictive of higher levels of sexual abstinence in adolescent daughters (Maguen & Armistead, 2006). It is clear that adolescence is a time for parents to remain engaged in their children's lives and to continue to provide guidance and support and to set reasonable boundaries. Other caring adults in young people's lives make vital contributions to the child's well-being as well. Teachers, coaches, religious leaders, neighbors, relatives, and mentors all have essential roles in the lives of youth; communities should support the role of nonparental adults and adolescents to facilitate helpful attachments (Grossman & Bulle, 2006).

SCHOOLS

School environments have an impact on the development of risk and protective factors in adolescents, and positive interventions are linked with positive outcomes into adulthood (Hawkins et al., 2005). Early school connectedness and positive social relationships with peers are predictive of future academic achievement, reduced substance abuse, and improved mental health later in high school (Bond et al., 2007). From the same sample, low levels of school connectedness and/or social connectedness in the 8th grade increased risk of school dropout. Proficient academic skills have also been associated with lower rates of risky behaviors and higher rates of healthy behaviors (CDC, 2014a). School dropout has been linked with multiple risks to health and overall well-being during adolescence and extending into adulthood. High school graduation leads to lower rates of health problems, reduced risk for incarceration, and improved financial stability as an adult (Sum, Khatiwada, & McLaughlin, 2009).

Schools also provide an opportunity for girls to be physically active and to receive health and sex education (Robbins, Gretebeck, Kazanis, & Pender, 2006). In its School Health Profiles, the CDC provides ongoing evaluation of health education, physical education, health services, food services, school policy and environment, and family and community involvement in schools. The CDC also provides useful tools for parents, teachers, and communities to increase physical activity for adolescents (such as that found at www .cdc.gov/healthyyouth/physicalactivity/toolkit/userguide_pa.pdf). Evidence shows that comprehensive sex education programs that provide information about both abstinence and contraception can help delay the onset of sexual activity among teens, reduce their number of sexual partners, and increase contraceptive use when they become sexually active.

COMMUNITIES

Adolescents respond to positive and negative pressure from peers, neighborhoods, families, and schools every day. In addition, young people are continually filtering the powerful media messages that surround them. Youth today have grown up with 24-hour-a-day access to the Internet, television, and other media. In the new millennia, the influence of media on adolescent health requires additional examination. Adolescents need to be aware of Internet safety precautions and use the Internet responsibly. Chow (2004) conducted research on focus groups with a small number of adolescent girls and their response to popular magazines' health-related messages. Young women reported magazine messages were equated with thinness and perfection, and the need for a male companion to provide protection. Adolescents are immersed in media, including cell phones and text messages, the Internet, television, music, and magazines, and the list will continue to expand. The wise health care provider will strive to understand the emerging media influences on young women and encourage the development of skills in media literacy. Media and technology should not be viewed only as evil but should used by health care providers, especially for promoting adolescent health. One study demonstrated that the use of a personalized digital assistant (PDA) at an adolescent wellness visit increased the likelihood of discussions of preventive services and improved the patient's perception of the visit (Olson, Gaffney, Hedberg, & Gladstone, 2009). The CDC has provided a comprehensive overview of technology and its impacts on teens' sexual health, including recommendations for providers to use technology for health promotion and prevention of STIs or other risky sexual behaviors (Kachur et al., 2013).

■ HEALTH SERVICES FOR ADOLESCENTS

Utilization of Health Services

Historically, adolescents have had the lowest rates of utilization of health services among all age groups. Some studies have also shown that when they do present for care, adolescents receive poor-quality health counseling and promotion messages (Ma, Wang, & Stafford, 2005). In recent years, insurance coverage has increased among all groups, including adolescents, and in 2013, 93% of children aged 0 to 17 years had some insurance coverage. Disparities do remain, however, as racial and ethnic minorities are less likely to be insured and to receive health care. Most early adolescents have adequate health insurance but with increasing age are more likely to be uninsured (Adams et al., 2007).

More concerning is the lack of quality care available for adolescents. One potential reason is the lack of a solid model of health care between childhood and adulthood. Because health care providers specializing in pediatrics often are not trained in the rapidly changing needs of adolescents and adult health care providers often do not encourage adolescent patients in their practices, adolescents do not have a true "Medical Home." Health care providers who see the entire spectrum of patients may close this gap somewhat but often do not have comprehensive training in dealing with the complexity of adolescent patients. It was only during the past several decades that the subspecialty of adolescent medicine appeared, likely in response to the increasing proportion of adolescents in the U.S. population, increases in morbidity and mortality in this age group, and understanding of the complex changes in development that occur during this time (Alderman, Rieder, & Cohen, 2003). A significant challenge is the adolescent's concern about confidentiality. Some of the concerns are not founded in reality, and health care providers should ensure that they educate their adolescent patients about confidentiality. However, given the current structure of our health care system and wide variation in public (both federal and state) and private policies and procedures, a young patient's concerns about confidentiality may be appropriate and must be handled with respect and honesty to ensure the maintenance of trust of the adolescent patient.

Consent and Confidentiality

In the United States, rules and regulations regarding adolescent rights to consent for health care vary by state. Consent defines the legal ability to obtain health services, and confidentiality is the ability to choose when to disclose the content of that care. Individual states govern the minor's rights to obtain reproductive health care, mental health services, and substance-abuse assessment and treatment. Reproductive health care can include contraception, sexually transmitted disease and STI assessment and treatment, pregnancy services, and termination of pregnancy care. Defining individual minor's rights in each state is outside the scope of this text, but updated information for each state and the District of Columbia can be found through the Center for Adolescent Health & the Law (www.cahl.org) and the Guttmacher Institute (www.guttmacher.org). Rights to confidentiality and the ability to consent change frequently, and each year there are new attempts by state legislatures to limit or expand the rights of parents/guardians and adolescents. A young woman must understand that there are legal and ethical situations when confidentiality will be broken. If she discloses intent to harm herself or someone else, it is the professional responsibility of the health care provider to break confidentiality and obtain all necessary services to maintain safety for all involved. In addition, if the young woman is a minor and has been assaulted or abused, she is subject to state laws governing child protection (www.childwelfare.gov). It is the health care provider's responsibility to understand and follow the rules in the state where she or he practices. It is important to note that protecting confidentiality in some cases can be a challenge, especially for minors with private insurance, if a medical bill for a procedure or consultation lists the reason for the bill.

The World Health Organization (WHO) has created a framework for adolescent-friendly health care facilities. The main goals are to support adolescent health care that is accessible, acceptable, appropriate, effective, and equitable (Tylee, Haller, Graham, Churchill, & Sanci, 2007). State, national, and international efforts are underway to remove barriers to adolescent health care delivery, improve quality of the services provided, and focus on improving health outcomes. Targeted interventions to promote quality in adolescent health services demonstrate effectiveness. Klein et al. (2001) examined the implementation of the Guidelines for Adolescent Preventive Services into five community and migrant health clinics. They reported improvements in health care provider reporting, and most important, adolescents reported having received positive health counseling messages, comprehensive age-appropriate health screening, and health education materials. Parent involvement can be hampered by language barriers and poor communication between health care providers (Clemans-Cope & Kenney, 2007), but parents have a vital role in the health care and promotion of their children.

A model that was developed in response to adolescents' low utilization of traditional health services and high rates of preventable adverse outcomes is that of school-based health services. The first school-based and school-linked health clinics (SBHCs) were established in the early 1970s with the main goals of reducing soaring teen pregnancy rates and rates of sexually transmitted diseases and STIs. SBHCs have now expanded into comprehensive health services at most clinic sites (Fothergill & Ballard, 1998). An excellent resource is the website for the School-Based Health Alliance available at www.sbh4all.org. There have been multiple benefits demonstrated from SBHCs, including utilization increases in both mental health and physical health services, cost reductions, improved school attendance, and reductions in emergency department utilization among regular users of the clinics (Key, Washington, & Hulsey, 2002). SBHCs are in addition to school nurse services provided in schools. Costello-Wells,

McFarland, Reed, and Walton (2003) reviewed school-based mental health care provided to adolescents in four urban high schools and noted a reduction in barriers to care as well as opportunities for multidisciplinary teamwork on behalf of youth. Even with the advent of expanded services in some schools, gaps remain in linking the most high-risk students with appropriate care (Santor, Poulin, LeBlanc, & Kusumakar, 2006). SBHCs complement community health care and are not intended to replace primary health care providers. SBHCs provide increased access for all adolescents to both medical and mental health services (Juszczak, Melinkovich, & Kaplan, 2003).

■ ASSESSMENT

Health Care Visits for Adolescent Women

With this background, it is easier to comprehend why providing care to an adolescent can be both challenging and incredibly rewarding. Understanding the rapid development during the adolescent years and the factors and contexts that can significantly affect that development allows the health care provider to skillfully approach the encounter with the adolescent patient and hopefully provide the quality care that will improve her or his health and well-being.

The clinician begins by introducing herself or himself, and clarifying the goals of the visit. For the first time in her life, a young woman may present for health care without her parents or guardian. If an adult is present, it is important for a portion of the visit to be with the young woman alone. This can be accomplished by stating, "I am glad you are here for this visit together. Now that she is getting older, it is important for her to have part of this visit by herself. After we have talked together, I will ask you to leave, so she and I have a chance to talk in private." This is also the optimal time to help the young woman and her parent understand her rights to confidentiality and consent. The parent or guardian may also have concerns to address without the adolescent present, and these can be addressed when the parent is out of the exam room. This should be done, however, before the confidential interview with the patient to dispel the perception that confidential information that the patient provides will be shared with the parent.

Preventive health care guidelines for adolescent girls have been developed by national health organizations: *Bright Futures: Guidelines for Health Supervision of Infants, Children, and Adolescents,* sponsored by a collaborative based in the Department of Health and Human Services and the American Academy of Pediatrics (AAP); *Guidelines for Adolescent Preventive Services,* developed by the American Medical Association (AMA); and *Primary and Preventive Health Care for Female Adolescents,* published by the ACOG. National guidelines are utilized to improve the quality of care and to emphasize comprehensive health services, including anticipatory guidance, targeted health screening, immunizations, and physical exam components. *Bright Futures: Guidelines for Health Supervision of Infants, Children, and Adolescents* recommends annual visits for health screening and anticipatory guidance (Hagen, Shaw, & Duncan, 2008).

Bright Futures incorporates a focus on the major morbidities and mortalities of adolescence and therefore emphasizes the importance of risk reduction, injury prevention, pregnancy and sexually transmitted disease prevention, physical growth and development, social and school connectedness, and mental health. National guidelines are reviewed and updated regularly to reflect trends in health indicators and evidence-based research. ACOG also provides guidelines for adolescent care and recommends that the first visit for screening and provision of reproductive preventive health services occur between 13 and 15 years of age, at which time patients may be of early, middle, or late adolescence (ACOG, 2010). This visit can be done as part of the primary care visit, and if training or experience does not allow or the patient prefers to be seen outside of the primary care setting, referral is appropriate for any component of the reproductive health visit that is not covered by the primary health care provider.

The first step in establishing care with adolescents is to create the foundation for a trusting relationship. Making connections is time well spent and requires skill and patience. With an understanding of adolescent development, health status, and health concerns, the health care provider may consider a different approach for the teen patient (e.g., by incorporating motivational interviewing [MI] into the visit). MI is a directive, client-centered counseling style with the goal of eliciting and strengthening motivation for change and evoking plans for changing behavior (Rollnick & Miller, 1995). The purpose of MI is the establishment of a goal-oriented partnership that empowers the client to initiate and actively take responsibility for change. MI does not utilize direct persuasion by a health care provider to resolve conflicts or ambivalence; instead, the health care provider quietly and actively listens. MI recognizes that change is not absolute but fluctuates over time.

MI is well suited for clients who may be more difficult to engage in treatment (e.g., adolescents, substance users, those with high-risk lifestyles). Adolescents' developmental goals are to individuate, experiment, and begin to trust their ability to make health decisions independently. Utilization of MI aids the health care provider in respectful care of the young woman, recognizing her current stage of development and working with her to move toward responsible health care decisions. MI has been adapted to multiple settings other than the field of addiction and substance-abuse treatment, where much of the research has been conducted (Resnicow, Davis, & Rollnick, 2006). One model that has been developed by Miller and Sanchez (1994) is FRAMES, which is an acronym for *f*eedback, emphasis on *r*esponsibility for change, clear *a*dvice to change, *m*enu of options, *e*mpathetic counseling style, and faith in *s*elf-efficacy to change.

It is helpful to look to other theories on adolescent development to guide communication techniques in the clinical setting. Based on the imaginary audience theory of Elkind and Bowen (1979), adolescents are naturally self-conscious about personal discussions. It is useful to preface the discussion with, "I talk with all the young women I see about _____." The natural egocentrism of adolescents and the stages of psychosocial development necessitate careful use of feedback. Feedback that is direct, sincere, and hopeful and that builds on the young woman's protective factors and strengths should be provided. Barriers to effective communication with young women include generalizations and labeling, accusations, blaming, and threats.

Bright Futures (Hagen et al., 2008) recommends that a comprehensive adolescent health history include discussion of the components listed in Box 8.2. Note that these

---

BOX 8.2 COMPONENTS OF COMPREHENSIVE ADOLESCENT HEALTH HISTORY

- Physical development:
  - What changes have you noticed in your body since your last visit?
  - How do you feel about your body and how it is changing?
- Social and emotional development:
  - What do you do for fun in your free time?
  - Do you have a best friend?
  - What are some of the things that make you sad? Angry?
  - What are the four words you would use to describe yourself?
- Health habits:
  - What do you do to stay healthy?
  - What do you do to get exercise and move your body?
  - When was the last time you saw a dentist?
- Nutrition and dietary habits:
  - What and when do you usually eat?
  - How often does your family eat meals together?
  - Do you do things to gain, lose, or manage your weight?

- Safety—car, bike, personal, home, community:
  - Do you wear a seatbelt? Sometimes, rarely, always, never?
  - Do you feel safe in your home?
  - Do you feel safe in your neighborhood?
  - Do you ever carry a weapon?
- Relationships and sexuality:
  - Have you gone out with anyone or started dating?
  - Have you ever had sex before?
  - Do you have sex with males, females, or both?
  - Let's talk about birth control and sexually transmitted diseases.
- Family functioning:
  - Every family is different—how do you get along with the people in your family?
  - Who lives in your home?
- School and/or vocational performance:
  - Where do you go to school? What grade are you in?
  - How are you doing in school? Are you getting any special help in school?
  - Do you have a job?

Source: Hagen, Shaw, and Duncan (2008).

questions should not be asked in the order listed in the box but rather interspersed throughout the interview, as appropriate based on the existing relationship with the patient, her attitude, and her reason for the visit. The questions listed describe the breadth and depth of the interview with the adolescent patient and provide examples of ways to introduce each topic. Particular issues to be discussed are reviewed in depth.

Ginsburg (2007) proposed an acronym that includes protective factors in a young person's life and a review of the person's strengths: SSHADESS (Table 8.1). This tool may also serve as a guide for the health care provider interviewing an adolescent.

General Medical History

Although most teens are healthy without chronic medical conditions, the patient's current and past medical history should be reviewed, including any conditions, medications, and allergies. Family history should be documented or updated in the patient's medical record; in particular, a history of venous thromboembolism; breast, ovarian, colon, or uterine cancer; and other familial gynecologic issues should be noted. Vaccination history also should be reviewed and any missing or indicated vaccinations discussed with the patient (details are given in the following section).

Reproductive Health History

Providing a reproductive health history will likely be a new experience for the patient and her parent. During the initial discussion with the patient and guardian, the provider should explain the difference between a pelvic examination and a Pap test and that the initial visit will not usually require either. Letting the patient know that an internal examination is required only if she has particular concerns will alleviate anxiety that she may have coming into the visit. The health care provider should explain that the first Pap test should be done at age 21. However, at the initial visit, the health care provider should discuss normal pubertal development, appropriate menstrual flow and patterns, and menstrual hygiene. An assessment for menstrual issues such as anovulatory cycles, PCOS, menorrhagia, and dysmenorrhea should be conducted.

The first day of the last menstrual cycle should be considered a "vital sign" in each health assessment for young women. ACOG and AAP developed a document to assist health care providers in the evaluation of the abnormal "vital sign" (ACOG, 2006). The normal cycle is between 21 and 45 days, lasts 7 days or less, and is not excessively heavy (Adams Hillard, 2006).

AMENORRHEA

Primary amenorrhea is defined as no menarche by 14 years of age if there are no secondary sex characteristics,

TABLE 8.1	The SSHADESS Dimensions: Protective Factors and Personal Strengths in Young Persons' Lives
SSHADESS DIMENSIONS	**SAMPLE QUESTIONS/COMMENTS**
Strengths	Tell me some of the things you like best about yourself. Tell me what your friends would say are the best things about you.
School	How is it going for you in school? What are the best and hardest things about school?
Home	How is it going for you at home? What responsibilities or chores do you have in your home?
Activities	What do you like to do with your friends? If you had half a day and could do whatever you wanted, what would you do?
Drugs and substance abuse	At some point in growing up, everyone faces decisions about tobacco, alcohol, and drugs. Do you have friends that smoke or drink?
Emotions and depression	Being healthy is more than being able to run around the track or not having broken bones, but has a lot to do with how we feel about ourselves, how connected we are at home, school, and with our friends. How have you felt over the last couple of months? Do ever think about hurting yourself or dying?
Sexuality	What questions do you have about your body and how it works? If you were with someone you really liked and they wanted to have sex but you did not, what would you do?
Safety	When you are out with your friends, do you feel safe? Do you know how to swim? What would you do if your ride home was drunk or high?

Source: Gingsburg (2007).

no menarche by 16 years old with secondary sex characteristics, no menses for 1 year after achieving sexual maturity stage (SMR) 5, or no menses in any female with the clinical features of Turner's syndrome (Neinstein, 2008). Primary amenorrhea requires an evaluation for potential congenital, hormonal, and genetic etiologies. It is important to complete the evaluation while attending to the emotional and psychological needs of the adolescent. Secondary amenorrhea occurs after menarche when a young woman has no subsequent menses for 6 months or in a regularly menstruating female who has no menses for three cycles (Neinstein, 2008). By conducting a careful history, physical assessment, and standard laboratory tests, the etiology of amenorrhea can be determined. It is essential to rule out pregnancy as the first step in any evaluation.

ABNORMAL UTERINE BLEEDING

In the adolescent, the most common cause of abnormal uterine bleeding is anovulatory cycles. The hypothalamic–pituitary–ovarian (HPO) axis is immature during adolescence and it can take up to 24 months for onset of regular cycles in 55% to 82% of women (Sanfilippo & Lara-Torre, 2009). Irregular cycles can persist in up to 22% of women after 24 months and PCOS should be considered a possible diagnosis. Other etiologies that should be considered are pregnancy, pelvic inflammatory disease, hematologic disorders, endocrine disorders, systemic or chronic illnesses, trauma or abuse, medications, or previously undiagnosed gynecologic pathologies (Emans, Laufer, & Goldstein, 1998). A menstrual calendar is useful for aiding the adolescent in understanding her menstrual cycle and the health care provider in making a diagnosis. Depending on the severity and suspicion for certain etiologies, laboratory assessment may include complete blood count and differential, platelet count, human chorionic gonadotropin, fibrinogen, prothrombin time, partial thromboplastin time, bleeding time, thyroid studies, von Willebrand's factor antigen, Factor VIII activity, Factor XI antigen, Ristocetin C cofactor, and platelet aggregation studies (Sanfilippo & Lara-Torre, 2009) . If the patient is found to have mild (hemoglobin, greater than 11 g/dL) or moderate (hemoglobin, 9–11 g/dL) anemia, iron supplementation should be provided, and combination contraceptives or a progesterone-releasing intrauterine device (IUD) should be considered if contraception is also needed. If severe anemia is found and bleeding symptoms indicate that heavy or frequent menses are the cause, bleeding should be addressed with a contraceptive taper, or the patient should be referred for evaluation and treatment (Sanfilippo & Lara-Torre, 2009).

POLYCYSTIC OVARY SYNDROME

PCOS is a common endocrine disorder with a prevalence of about 4% to 6% of the female population and results in excessive androgens produced by the ovary and possibly adrenal gland. It results in a constellation of signs and symptoms, including hirsutism, irregular menstrual cycles, weight gain or obesity, and acne. A consequence of hyperinsulinemia that could manifest, even in adolescents, is acanthosis nigricans. Because of the similarity of many

of these symptoms with normal puberty, PCOS may be overdiagnosed during adolescence. It is a clinical diagnosis, so laboratory testing is not required, but some have advocated requiring all three Rotterdam diagnostic criteria be present (hyperandrogenism, oligo-ovulation, polycystic ovaries) before diagnosis is made (Agapova, Cameo, Sopher, & Oberfield, 2014). Laboratory testing for hirsutism or evaluation for hyperandrogenism may be indicated. Patients with PCOS may be more at risk of developing metabolic syndrome, which includes (a) increased abdominal fat mass (waist circumference more than 35 inches), (b) increased triglycerides (150 mg/dL or more), (c) decreased high-density lipoproteins (50 mg/dL or less), (d) increased blood pressure (130/85 mmHg or more), and (e) increased plasma glucose (100 mg/dL or more; Sanfilippo & Lara-Torre, 2009).

Because PCOS has future consequences on fertility and overall health, early intervention may help prevent some of the long-term consequences such as insulin resistance, type II diabetes, and cardiovascular disease. Weight loss of about 10% can help restore regular ovulatory cycles in many women, but this may be difficult to accomplish in adolescent women. Combined oral contraceptive pills may help reduce circulating androgens and will usually promote regular withdrawal bleeding. Metformin has been used to address the insulin resistance in PCOS, but its use in adolescence is controversial. Shared decision making is useful in treating adolescents with PCOS, as its treatment relies on both lifestyle changes and possible pharmacologic therapy. Education and discussion of the impact of the symptoms on the patient's life are critical. Helpful resources for young women with PCOS can be found at the website of the Center for Young Women's Health at Children's Hospital in Boston (www.youngwomenshealth.org/index.html). Identification of PCOS, treatment goals, and psychological supports must be developed in a partnership with the adolescent and parents, recognizing the complex emotional and identity development of adolescence.

DYSMENORRHEA

Dysmenorrhea is a common complaint in young women and is usually associated with normal ovulation in the absence of pelvic pathology. Ten percent of young women with dysmenorrhea, however, will experience severe symptoms and may have some pelvic abnormality (Harel, 2006). These women require further evaluation for underlying pathology that may contribute to their cyclic pain.

Endometriosis should be considered in adolescents who have recurrent dysmenorrhea that does not respond to nonsteroidal anti-inflammatory drugs (NSAIDs) or oral contraceptive therapy. It is important to remember that Müllerian anomalies may be associated with endometriosis in 11% to 40% of teenagers with endometriosis and should be considered in the differential diagnosis (Sanfilippo & Lara-Torre, 2009). Adolescents suspected of having endometriosis who continue to have severe symptoms on NSAIDs and/or oral contraceptives may be candidates for laparoscopy and/or gonadotropin-releasing hormone (GnRH) agonist therapy; referral should be made if indicated.

HISTORY OF SEXUAL ACTIVITY

During the confidential visit, the health care provider should assess the patient's history of sexual activity and discuss contraception and STIs. A discussion of sexual and reproductive health is included in the care of all young women regardless of sexual behavior. As seen in the YRBSS from 2013, almost half of all high school students (46.8%) reported having engaged in sexual intercourse, and 15% had four or more sexual partners up to that point. Among those who reported intercourse in the 3 months before the survey, only 59.1% reported using a condom during the last act of intercourse (CDC, 2014b). Each year, the Guttmacher Institute publishes *Facts on American Teen's Sexual and Reproductive Health* (Guttmacher Institute, 2014). This compilation of research on adolescent sexual behavior provides an overview of sexual activity, contraceptive use, access to contraceptive services, rates of STIs, pregnancy, childbearing, and abortion. Similar to YRBSS, this report states that nearly half of all 15- to 19-year-olds in the United States have had sex at least once. At age 15 years, approximately 16% of youth have had sex, and by age 19 years, 71% of teens have engaged in sexual intercourse. Most teens (78% of girls and 85% of boys) report using some form of contraception during their first sexual experience (Guttmacher Institute, 2014). The most common method used by teens is condoms, and most teenaged women (96%) report using them at least once. Teens are at risk of STIs; they represent one quarter of the sexually active population yet account for nearly half of all new STIs.

In addition to asking about voluntary sexual activity, providers should inquire about intimate partner and dating violence, including unwanted or involuntary sexual activity. Between 2006 and 2010, a striking number (11%) of young women aged 18 to 24 years old reported that their first sexual encounter was involuntary. In the 2013 YRBSS, the prevalence of having been forced to have sexual intercourse was 9.1% among White, 11.5% among Black, and 12.2% among Hispanic females. In the 12 months before the survey, 13% of females reported physical dating violence, and 14.4% reported sexual dating violence (CDC, 2014b).

Teen Pregnancy

The Guttmacher Institute reported that each year, nearly 615,000 young women aged 15 to 19 years become pregnant and that in 2010 there were 57 pregnancies per 1,000 young women aged 15 to 19 years. This represents a significant decline from its peak in 1990, thought to be secondary to delays in sexual activity and more consistent use of contraception in those who are sexually active. Pregnancy rates declined for all racial groups from 1990 to 2010, with the sharpest declines among Black teens (56%). However, Black young women continue to have the highest teen-pregnancy rate (100 per 1,000 women aged 15 to 19 years), followed by Hispanics (84 per 1,000) and non-Hispanic Whites (38 per 1,000). Teen pregnancies are largely unplanned (82%). Two thirds of teen pregnancies occur in older adolescents aged 18 to 19 years. The birthrate to teens aged 15 to 19 years dropped 50% from 1991 (62 births per 1,000), to 2011 (31 births per 1,000). Babies born to teens are at

greater risk for health complications, including low birth weight. Teen mothers are also less likely to receive prenatal care or to engage in prenatal care late in their pregnancy. In 2010, 26% of 15- to 19-year-olds ended their pregnancies with abortion, and the primary reasons teens gave for having an abortion included concerns about how a baby would affect their lives, an inability to afford a child, and a feeling of being insufficiently prepared to raise a child at that time in their lives. As of May 2014, 38 states required by law that parents of a minor seeking an abortion are involved in the decision (Guttmacher Institute, 2014).

CONTRACEPTION

Although contraceptives are covered in Chapter 21 of this book, there are some key points to keep in mind when discussing contraceptives with young women. First, it is critical to help the young woman understand her risk of pregnancy with and without various forms of contraception. If she is having sexual intercourse or planning to in the near future, asking her directly if she wants to get pregnant often is the best way to undermine the invincibility many young women feel regarding sexual behavior. Using visual aids, videos, or other tools to clearly illustrate the risk of getting pregnant will likely be more effective than listing types of birth control methods and numbers. A useful handout from the CDC can be accessed at www.cdc.gov/reproductivehealth/unintendedpregnancy/pdf/contraceptive_methods_508.pdf. Furthermore, discussing the patient's preferences and values regarding contraception is critical to ensuring appropriate compliance. Counseling should not be coercive, and using a counseling style that walks the patient through her decision making may be helpful.

Long-acting reversible contraceptions (LARCs) should be a first-line method of birth control for sexually active adolescents, whether nulliparous or parous (Adams Hillard, 2013). This includes both IUDs and implants. When appropriately counseled, young women will choose LARC methods over short-acting contraception, as demonstrated in the prospective CHOICE study in which 62% of adolescents chose LARC methods (63% of the 14- to 17-year-olds chose the implant and 71% of the 18- to 20-year-olds chose an IUD; Mestad, Secura, Allsworth, Madden, Zhao, & Peipert, 2011). Health care providers who do not insert IUDs and/or implants should ensure that information is readily available regarding referral to another provider who does. For health care providers who insert IUDs but are less experienced with providing this service to nulliparous patients, especially adolescents, tips regarding counseling, preprocedure preparation, and insertion are available (ACOG, 2007; Adams Hillard, 2013). All three IUDs currently available on the market (Paragard, Mirena IUD, and Skyla IUD) can be inserted without concern into a nulliparous uterus. Which option is best for an individual patient requires shared decision making, so the patient's concerns and preferences play a role. If LARCs are not desired by the patient, combined oral contraceptive pills, the weekly patch or the vaginal contraceptive ring (placed every 3 weeks) are all effective options for the adolescent, and the type depends on patient preference for dosing.

The availability of emergency contraception, the use of a nonabortifacient, hormonal medication within 72 to 120 hours after unprotected (or underprotected) intercourse, should be discussed with the sexually active adolescent, even if she is on a current contraceptive. Furthermore, barrier methods, such as the male or female condom, should also be highly encouraged for STI prevention, even if the patient is on a reliable form of contraception.

Adolescent decision making regarding sexual behavior, contraceptive use, acquisition of STIs, and pregnancy have lifelong impacts on young women's health, as well as that of their families and communities. Ginsburg (2007) emphasized that providers of adolescent health care services must balance the identification of risky behaviors with the promotion of the independence that teens crave. Both MI and shared decision making are approaches that might resonate with an adolescent struggling with decisions that affect reproductive health. Health care providers can support risk reduction if there is an integration of health promotion, resiliency, and positive youth development during the adolescent health visit.

■ GUIDELINES FOR HEALTH PROMOTION

Other topics of particular concern in young women's health are nutrition, dieting behaviors, eating disorders, mental health, and substance abuse.

Nutrition

Adolescence places new demands on the nutritional status and emerging body image of developing young women. The body has increased demand for calories, protein, calcium, iron, zinc, vitamin C, and folic acid. Normal adolescent eating patterns are a challenge to evaluate, and in contrast to childhood, teens have more meals independent of the family, often skip breakfast, eat frequent snacks, and increase their consumption of convenience foods. In a focus group study examining the eating patterns and beliefs of 203 adolescent boys and girls, Croll, Neumark-Sztainer, and Story (2001) found a high level of knowledge about healthy eating recommendations and identified multiple barriers in their daily routines: lack of time, limited perceived or real availability of healthy food, and lack of understanding or concern about possible health consequences. Eating habits established during the new independence of adolescence are linked with lifelong eating behaviors and may contribute to future health status (Jenkins & Horner, 2005). Food availability and security, family socioeconomic status, and media advertising also play roles in determining food preferences and healthy eating (Taylor, Evers, & McKenna, 2005).

Young women are at particular risk for establishing distorted eating patterns during periods of marked change, especially during the transitions of late adolescence. There are multiple potential contributing factors to eating disorders: biological, familial, environmental, genetic, and social (Emans, 2000). Eating disorders are included in the *Diagnostic and Statistical Manual of Mental Disorders* (5th ed.; *DSM-5*) and include anorexia nervosa, bulimia nervosa, and binge eating disorder (American Psychiatric Association [APA], 2013). The care of young women with disordered eating requires a team of professionals working in collaboration to support the adolescent, her family, and the complex demands of her physical and emotional health.

Overweight and obesity are common issues for young women, have serious implications for long-term health, and have multifactorial etiologies. Female awareness of weight, desire for thinness, and cyclic dieting patterns begin early in life and have been well documented to often start in grade school (Emans, 2000). The CDC (2015b) recommends that all children and adolescents participate in physical activity for at least 60 minutes per day. However, as adolescent girls grow older, they are less likely to participate in vigorous physical activity or participate in school-based physical education. In a North Carolina study of eighth-grade girls, evaluated again in the ninth and 12th grades, a drop from 45% to 34% participation in vigorous exercise over the 4 years was identified. The results also note that eighth-grade participation in exercise was predictive of 12th-grade exercise patterns (Pate et al., 2007). Childhood and early adolescence must be the target of efforts to increase physical activity throughout adolescence and extending into adulthood.

Substance Use and Abuse

This chapter has addressed alcohol and substance abuse in the context of peer, family, and community influences on adolescents. Individual substance use is best understood as a continuum: abstinence, experimental use, regular use, problem use, substance abuse, substance dependency, and secondary abstinence as part of recovery (Knight et al., 1999). Alcohol use among teenage girls is problematic. The 2013 YRBSS survey revealed that 21.1% of high school females reported drinking more than five drinks in a row on at least 1 day in the 30 days before the survey (CDC, 2014b). In addition to the increased risk of addiction, when alcohol is consumed during the adolescent years, it has been shown that teens who use tobacco, alcohol, marijuana, or other drugs are more likely to engage in risky sexual behavior and to have unwanted consequences of sex, such as STIs and unintended pregnancy, than teens who do not use those substances (The National Center on Addiction and Substance Abuse, 2011). Another study showed that women who engage in preconception binge drinking are more likely to have an unplanned pregnancy and to use alcohol and tobacco during pregnancy (Naimi, Lipscomb, Brewer, & Gilbert, 2003).

In terms of drug use, 21.9% of female teens reported current marijuana use in the most recent YRBSS survey (one or more times in the 30 days before the survey; CDC, 2014b). The prevalence of other substance use indicated that asking adolescent patients about substance use during the confidential portion of the health visit is an important part of the health history.

The CRAFFT screening tool developed by Knight et al. (1999) was designed specifically for adolescents and has been validated repeatedly in many different contexts (Connery, Albright, & Rodolico, 2014; see Box 8.3). Other advantages of the CRAFFT tool are its free public access; brevity

BOX 8.3   CRAFFT QUESTIONS

C   Have you ever ridden in a car driven by someone (including yourself) who was high or had been using alcohol or drugs?

R   Do you ever use alcohol or drugs to relax, feel better about yourself, or fit in?

A   Do you ever use alcohol or drugs while you are by yourself, alone?

F   Do you ever forget things you did while using alcohol or drugs?

F   Do your family or friends ever tell you that you should cut down on your drinking or drug use?

T   Have you ever gotten into trouble while you were using alcohol or drugs?

Source: Knight et al. (1999).

(2–3 minutes to complete); availability in many languages; good positive and negative predictive probability for alcohol and drug use, abuse, and dependence; and 74% sensitivity and 96% specificity. A computerized version is now validated that will simplify administration (Knight et al., 2007; Connery et al., 2014). CRAFFT questions are intended for use in developing a partnership with the adolescent and in forming an alliance for future health promotion. Two or more positive answers suggest a significant problem with alcohol or other drugs and necessitate further evaluation. For example, one study has demonstrated its effectiveness in detecting preconception substance use in pregnant young women, 17 to 25 years of age (Chang et al., 2011).

TOBACCO USE

One disadvantage of the CRAFFT tool is that it does not screen for use of tobacco products. It is fortunate that tobacco use by teens in all age groups has been declining since its peak in the late 1990s. This may be the result of legislation to reduce access to tobacco and restrict smoking in public places, of relatively high taxation of tobacco products, and of social marketing campaigns aimed at youth (Evans et al., 2004). However, tobacco use is still prevalent and is associated with higher rates of mental illness and substance abuse (Chang, Sherritt, & Knight, 2005). Furthermore, newer forms of tobacco delivery are becoming more prevalent among teens. The 2013 YRBSS demonstrated that 40% of high school females had ever tried smoking and 15.7% were considered current smokers (smoked a cigarette on at least 1 day during the 30 days before the survey; CDC, 2014b). Electronic cigarettes were not included in the 2013 survey but are a current issue among adolescence, so health care providers should inquire about their use. An appropriate screening technique is to ask if the adolescent ever used cigarettes, other tobacco products, e-cigarettes, and other vaping methods (e.g., hookah), followed by an attempt at quantification (Connery et al., 2014).

Prevention of initiation is the ideal, and the U.S. Preventive Services Task Force (USPSTF) recently recommended that health care providers provide behavioral counseling interventions, including discussion, print materials, or computer applications, to reduce the risk for smoking initiation in adolescents (Moyer, 2013a).

Mental Health

Mental health screening and treatment are integral components in the care of adolescent girls. Women are more likely to experience depression across the life span and, during adolescence, are particularly vulnerable (Garber, 2006). In an examination of gender differences in coping styles by Li, DiGiuseppe, and Froh (2006), depressed young women were more likely to utilize ruminating and emotion-focused coping versus problem-focused and distractive coping skills. Studies have estimated anywhere from one tenth to one half of young adults have been diagnosed with a mental health condition (National Research Council, 2009). The most common diagnoses in the female adolescent population are anxiety and depression. There continue to be health disparities in access to quality mental health services based on race/ethnicity, geography, socioeconomic status, and insurance coverage (Children's Defense Fund, 2003).

During the 12 months before the 2013 YRBSS, 39.1% of females reported feeling so sad or hopeless for 2 or more weeks in a row that they stopped doing a usual activity (CDC, 2014b). Even more alarming, 22.4% of females reported seriously considering attempting suicide, and 10.6% reported having attempted to commit suicide in the 12 months before the survey (CDC, 2014b). Hispanic girls report the highest levels of depression and have attempted suicide at higher rates than Black and White women. Furthermore, among suicidal teens, Hispanic, African American, and Asian American youth are less likely to receive counseling than Whites. This may be related to access, but cultural differences may prevent even those who have access to mental health care from receiving effective, culturally competent care without language barriers (Center for Health and Health Care in Schools, 2011). Health care providers can work within their system and with the community to help facilitate "meaningful access" for immigrants and other adolescents.

Suicide is the third leading cause of death nationally, and in many states it is the second cause of death among adolescents. Suicide screening and prevention are recommended as part of health care for all adolescents. Suicidality is multifaceted and continues to be investigated to provide insights into adolescent mental health and suffering. It is difficult to estimate the prevalence of current clinical diagnoses of mental disorders in adolescents and the impairment of those diagnosed. Young men are more at risk of dying by suicide, whereas young women report higher levels of depression and make more attempts at suicide (CDC, 2014b). Young men typically choose more lethal methods in suicide, such as firearms, hanging, and motor vehicles, resulting in more deaths. Young women tend to choose medication or overdosing; these methods are usually not immediate and allow for help to arrive or be sought.

Finally, bullying is a growing issue for adolescents. In particular, female adolescents are more likely to be victims of cyberbullying than their male counterparts. In 2013, 21% of females reported having been electronically bullied in the 12 months before the survey, higher among White (25.2%) than Black females (10.5%; CDC, 2014b). Being a victim of electronic bullying puts adolescents at increased risk of depression, anxiety, and suicide. Asking the patient about any experiences with bullying, whether physical, verbal, or electronic, is an important part of the adolescent history.

The Physical Examination and Laboratory Screening

The physical examination is a small, but often important, component of the overall assessment of the adolescent patient. *Bright Futures* recommendations (Hagen et al., 2008) include a physical examination for each health supervision visit. The physical examination includes weight, height, BMI, blood pressure, a complete physical examination including dental screening, sexual maturity rating/Tanner staging, and other components to investigate concerning symptoms such as evidence of hirsutism. Vision and hearing screening questions should be completed during each preventive care visit. Vision testing is recommended during each phase of adolescence: early, middle, and late (Hagen et al., 2008). Audiometry is performed based on risk assessment.

PELVIC EXAM

The pelvic exam is no longer an essential part of every young woman's annual examination. With the advent of urine-based sexually transmitted disease and STI screening and the consensus on national cervical screening guidelines, adolescents obtain pelvic examinations based only on risk factors. An internal pelvic examination is generally unnecessary during the first reproductive health visit, but when indicated, the first pelvic examination is an excellent opportunity for health promotion and education about the female body. Providing a clear explanation about the equipment and the procedure, allowing time for the young woman to ask questions, and allowing a friend or family member to be present if desired will reduce her anxiety and increase her cooperation. The patient's developmental status, hymenal opening, and sexual experience should guide the selection of speculum, but generally a Pederson (⅞ inch wide by 4 inches long) or Huffman speculum (½ inch wide by 4¼ inch long) is appropriate (ACOG, 2010). Application of pressure with a single finger to the perineal area may lessen the sensation of the speculum being inserted and may be especially useful for the patient who is not yet sexually active (Sanfilippo & Lara-Torre, 2009). Asking the patient if she has used tampons can assist the provider in determining how comfortable she is with the exam and an estimation of the hymenal opening. Occasionally, during the first pelvic exam, the provider may come across a patient with an imperforate hymen, which will

need to be addressed. Creating a positive experience for the adolescent's first pelvic exam provides the foundation for future preventive gynecologic care. It is also an investment in developing a respectful partnership with the young woman.

SCREENING FOR STIs

All young women who are sexually active (with males, females, or both) must be screened for STIs. Most major organizations recommend screening sexually active young woman aged 24 years or younger annually for chlamydia and gonorrhea (ACOG, 2010; LeFevre, 2014). This test can be completed with a vaginal swab (by patient or by provider), cervical swab, or urine testing using the nucleic acid amplification technique, which may be the most acceptable option to the patient. In September 2006, the CDC released revised recommendations for HIV testing of adults, adolescents, and pregnant women. The new recommendations advise routine HIV screening of all adolescents in health care settings in the United States (Branson et al., 2006). Implementation of these new guidelines and reduction of the barriers to HIV testing are current challenges in ambulatory care settings. In 2014, the USPSTF also released new recommendations on screening for HIV, recommending that all adolescents aged 15 years and older (and younger adolescents who are at increased risk) be screened for HIV (Moyer, 2013b). A one-time screening is recommended, followed by repeated screening for those at increased risk, those engaged in risky behaviors, or those who live in a high-prevalence setting. Syphilis screening is recommended for pregnant adolescents and high-risk youth, including those who have multiple partners; do not use a condom or barrier method; exchange sex for drugs, money, or services; have spent time in jail or detention; are homeless; use intravenous drugs; or have been diagnosed with another STI (CDC, 2015a). Finally, nonjudgmental, risk-reduction counseling appropriate to the individual's developmental age should be provided. This should include counseling about risk behaviors that increase the acquisition of STIs and evidence-based prevention strategies (including abstinence, reduction in numbers of partners, correct condom use; CDC, 2015a). The USPSTF also recommends high-intensity behavioral counseling for all sexually active adolescents to prevent STIs (LeFevre, 2014). Often videos, MI, or other information involving multimedia or social marketing may be more effective.

ADDITIONAL SCREENING

Other screening tests that may be performed as part of the young woman's preventive health visit, based on her history, include screening for anemia, tuberculosis, and dyslipidemia.

Immunizations

Immunizations are an essential and changing part of adolescent preventive health care services. The CDC Advisory Committee on Immunization Practices (ACIP) currently recommends several vaccines for young adolescents aged 11 to 12 years:

- Tetanus-diphtheria-acellular pertussis vaccine
- Meningococcal conjugate vaccine
- Human papillomavirus (HPV) vaccine

As of August 2015, there are three U.S. Food and Drug Administration–approved vaccinations for HPV. See Chapter 32, for further discussion regarding HPV vaccines. The HPV vaccine, bivalent, quadrivalent, or 9-valent, is recommended routinely for females aged 13 to 26 years who have not yet received all doses or completed the vaccination series. Concerns about change in sexual behavior after receiving HPV vaccine have not been substantiated in the literature (CDC, 2015a).

It is recommended that all adolescents, if not previously immunized, receive the following vaccinations:

- Hepatitis B series
- Hepatitis A series
- Polio series
- Measles–mumps–rubella series
- Varicella (chickenpox) series (A second catch-up shot is recommended for adolescents who have previously received only one dose and have no history of chickenpox infection.)

Additional vaccines are recommended for certain adolescents, either because of specific health conditions, exposure to household contacts, or employment that may increase their risk for transmission or infection:

- Influenza
- Pneumococcal polysaccharide
- Hepatitis A

ACIP immunization recommendations are reviewed annually because vaccine-preventable diseases or conditions are identified and vaccine schedules change. The CDC maintains up-to-date immunization schedules at www.cdc.gov/vaccines/schedules/index.html.

Final Discussion With the Patient

Having another discussion with the patient and her parent (after any confidential issues were discussed in the exam room or when with the patient and/or parent alone) will allow the health care provider to discuss the findings of the examination, develop a plan, and answer any additional questions. The health care provider should fully understand and respect any information confidentially shared by the patient as well as any that she would like to share with her parent. Acting as a liaison between the adolescent and the parent can sometimes be helpful, only if the patient has provided permission to do so with confidential issues. Clearly, adolescence is a time of great transition for the young woman seeking care. The visit may be more challenging than providing health care for women at other times in their life, yet the health care provider also has a tremendous opportunity to help set the young woman on a trajectory for healthy behaviors and well-being for the rest of her life.

REFERENCES

Adams Hillard, P. J. (2006). Adolescent menstrual health. *Pediatric Endocrinology Reviews, 3*(Suppl. 1), 138–145.

Adams Hillard, P. J. (2013). Practical tips for intrauterine devices use in adolescents. *Journal of Adolescent Health, 52,* S40–S46.

Adams, S. H., Newacheck, P. W., Park, M. J., Brindis, C. D., & Irwin, C. E. (2007). Health insurance across vulnerable ages: Patterns and disparities from adolescence to the early 30s. *Pediatrics, 119*(5), e1033–e1039.

Adelmann, P. K. (2005). Social environmental factors and preteen health-related behaviors. *Journal of Adolescent Health, 36*(1), 36–47.

Agapova, S. E., Cameo, T., Sopher, A. B., & Oberfield, S. E. (2014). Diagnosis and challenges of polycystic ovary syndrome in adolescence. *Seminars in Reproductive Medicine, 32*(3), 194–201.

Alderman, E. M., Rieder, J., & Cohen, M. I. (2003). The history of adolescent medicine. *Pediatric Research, 54*(1), 137–147.

American College of Obstetricians and Gynecologists (ACOG). (2006). Menstruation in girls and adolescents: Using the menstrual cycle as a vital sign, ACOG Committee Opinion No. 349. *Obstetrics & Gynecology, 108,* 1323–1328.

American College of Obstetricians and Gynecologists (ACOG). (2007). Intrauterine device and adolescents, Committee Opinion No. 392. *Obstetrics & Gynecology, 110,* 1493–1495.

American College of Obstetricians and Gynecologists (ACOG). (2009). Menstrual manipulation for adolescents with disabilities, ACOG Committee Opinion No. 448. *Obstetrics & Gynecology, 114,* 1428–1431.

American College of Obstetricians and Gynecologists (ACOG). (2010). The initial reproductive health visit, Committee Opinion No. 460. *Obstetrics & Gynecology, 116,* 240–243.

American College of Obstetricians and Gynecologists (ACOG). (2012). Reproductive health care for adolescents with disabilities. *Supplement to Guidelines for Adolescent Health Care* (2nd ed.). Washington, DC: American College of Obstetricians and Gynecologists.

American Psychiatric Association (APA). (2013). *Diagnostic and statistical manual of mental disorders* (5th ed.). Arlington, VA: American Psychiatric Publishing.

Anachebe, N. F., & Sutton, M. Y. (2003). Racial disparities in reproductive health outcomes. *American Journal of Obstetrics and Gynecology, 188*(4), S37–S42.

Angold, A., Costello, E. J., & Worthman, C. M. (1998). Puberty and depression: The roles of age, pubertal status and pubertal timing. *Psychological Medicine, 28*(1), 51–61.

Annie E. Casey Foundation. (2015). *Kids count databook.* Baltimore, MD: Annie Casey Foundation. Retrieved from http://www.aecf.org/m/resourcedoc/aecf-2015kidscountdatabook-2015.pdf

Attie, I., & Brooks-Gunn, J. (1995). The development of eating regulation across the life span. In D. Cicchetti & D. J. Cohen (Eds.), *Developmental psychopathology. Vol. 2: Risk, disorder, and adaptation.* New York, NY: Wiley.

Aufausser, D., Jekielek, S., & Brown, B. (2006). *The family environment and adolescent well-being: Exposure to positive and negative influences.* Retrieved from http://nahic.ucsf.edu/downloads/FamEnvironBrief.pdf

Barrow, F. H., Armstrong, M. I., Vargo, A., & Boothroyd, R. A. (2007). Understanding the findings of resilience-related research for fostering the development of African American adolescents. *Child and Adolescent Psychiatric Clinics of North America, 16*(2), 393–413, ix.

Betz, C. L. (2007). Facilitating the transition of adolescents with developmental disabilities: Nursing practice issues and care. *Journal of Pediatric Nursing, 22*(2), 103–115.

Bond, L., Butler, H., Thomas, L., Carlin, J., Glover, S., Bowes, G., & Patton, G. (2007). Social and school connectedness in early secondary school as predictors of late teenage substance use, mental health, and academic outcomes. *Journal of Adolescent Health, 40*(4), 357.

Branson, B. M., Handsfield, H. H., Lampe, M. A., Janssen, R. S., Taylor, A. W., Lyss, S. B., & Clark, J. E. (2006). Revised recommendations for HIV testing of adults, adolescents, and pregnant women in health care settings. *MMWR Recommendations Report, 55*(RR-14), 1–17.

Briss, P. A., Brownson, R. C., Fielding, J. E., & Zaza, S. (2004). Developing and using the Guide to Community Preventive Services: Lessons learned about evidence-based public health. *Annual Review of Public Health*, 25, 281–302.

Brooks-Gunn, J., Petersen, A. C., & Eichorn, D. (1985). The study of maturational timing effects in adolescence. *Journal of Youth and Adolescence*, 14(3), 149–161.

Brooks-Gunn, J., & Warren, M. P. (1985). Measuring physical status and timing in early adolescence: A developmental perspective. *Journal of Youth and Adolescence*, 14(3), 163–189.

Brooks-Gunn, J., & Warren, M. P. (1989). Biological and social contributions to negative affect in young adolescent girls. *Child Development*, 60(1), 40–55.

Brooks-Gunn, J., Warren, M. P., Rosso, J., & Gargiulo, J. (1987). Validity of self-report measures of girls' pubertal status. *Child Development*, 58(3), 829–841.

Brown, K. M., McMahon, R. P., Biro, F. M., Crawford, P., Schreiber, G. B., Similo, S. L.,…Striegel-Moore, R. (1998). Changes in self-esteem in black and white girls between the ages of 9 and 14 years. The NHLBI Growth and Health Study. *The Journal of Adolescent Health: Official Publication of the Society for Adolescent Medicine*, 23(1), 7–19.

Caspi, A., & Moffitt, T. E. (1991). Individual differences are accentuated during periods of social change: The sample case of girls at puberty. *Journal of Personality and Social Psychology*, 61(1), 157–168.

Center for Health and Health Care in Schools. (2011). *Children of immigrant and refugees: What the research tells us*. Retrieved from http://www.healthinschools.org/Immigrant-and-Refugee-Children/Tools-and-Documents.aspx

Centers for Disease Control and Prevention (CDC). (2014a). *Health and academic achievement*. Retrieved from http://www.cdc.gov/healthyyouth/health_and_academics/pdf/health-academic-achievement.pdf

Centers for Disease Control and Prevention (CDC). (2014b). Youth risk behavior surveillance: United States, 2013. *Morbidity and Mortality Weekly Report*, 63(SS-4), 1–168.

Centers for Disease Control and Prevention (CDC). (2015a). Sexually transmitted diseases treatment guidelines. *Morbidity and Mortality Weekly Report*, 64(RR-3), 1–137.

Centers for Disease Control and Prevention (CDC). (2015b). *Youth physical activity guidelines toolkit user guide*. Retrieved from http://www.cdc.gov/healthyyouth/physicalactivity/toolkit/userguide_pa.pdf

Cesario, S. K., & Hughes, L. A. (2007). Precocious puberty: A comprehensive review of literature. *Journal of Obstetric, Gynecologic, and Neonatal Nursing*, 36(3), 263–274.

Chang, G., Orav, E. J., Jones, J. A., Buynitsky, T., Gonzalez, S., & Wilkins-Haug, L. (2011). Self-reported alcohol and drug use in pregnant young women: A pilot study of associated factors and identification. *Journal of Addiction Medicine*, 5(3), 221–226.

Chang, G., Sherritt, L., & Knight, J. R. (2005). Adolescent cigarette smoking and mental health symptoms. *The Journal of Adolescent Health: Official Publication of the Society for Adolescent Medicine*, 36(6), 517–522.

Children's Defense Fund. (2003). *Children's mental health resource kit*. Washington, DC: Author.

Chow, J. (2004). Adolescents' perceptions of popular teen magazines. *Journal of Advanced Nursing*, 48(2), 132–139.

Clemans-Cope, L., & Kenney, G. (2007). Low income parents' reports of communication problems with health care providers: Effects of language and insurance. *Public Health Reports*, 122(2), 206–216.

Colby, S. L., & Ortman, J. M. (2015). Projections of the size and composition of the U.S. population: 2014 to 2060. United States Census Bureau. Retrieved from census.gov/content/dam/Census/library/publications/2015/demo/p25-1143.pdf

Connery, H. S., Albright, B. B., & Rodolico, J. M. (2014). Adolescent substance use and unplanned pregnancy: Strategies for risk reduction. *Obstetrics and Gynecology Clinics of North America*, 41(2), 191–203.

Costello-Wells, B., McFarland, L., Reed, J., & Walton, K. (2003). School-based mental health clinics. *Journal of Child and Adolescent Psychiatric Nursing: Official Publication of the Association of Child and Adolescent Psychiatric Nurses*, 16(2), 60–70.

Croll, J. K., Neumark-Sztainer, D., & Story, M. (2001). Healthy eating: What does it mean to adolescents? *Journal of Nutrition Education*, 33(4), 193–198.

Dahlberg, L. L., & Potter, L. B. (2001). Youth violence. Developmental pathways and prevention challenges. *American Journal of Preventive Medicine*, 20(Suppl. 1), 3–14.

Doswell, W. M., Millor, G. K., Thompson, H., & Braxter, B. (1998). Self-image and self-esteem in African-American preteen girls: Implications for mental health. *Issues in Mental Health Nursing*, 19(1), 71–94.

Dowdell, E. B. (2004). Grandmother caregivers and caregiver burden. *The American Journal of Maternal Child Nursing*, 29(5), 299–304.

Eisenberg, M. E., & Resnick, M. D. (2006). Suicidality among gay, lesbian and bisexual youth: The role of protective factors. *The Journal of Adolescent Health: Official Publication of the Society for Adolescent Medicine*, 39(5), 662–668.

Elkind, D., & Bowen, R. (1979). Imaginary audience behavior in children and adolescents. *Developmental Psychology*, 15(1), 38–44.

Emans, S. J. (2000). Eating disorders in adolescent girls. *Pediatrics International: Official Journal of the Japan Pediatric Society*, 42(1), 1–7.

Emans, S. J., Laufer, M. R., & Goldstein, D. P. (Eds.). (1998). *Pediatric and adolescent gynecology* (4th ed.). Philadelphia, PA: Lippincott Williams and Wilkins.

Erickson, E. (1963). *Child and society* (2nd ed.). New York, NY: W. W. Norton.

Erickson, E. (1968). *Identity, youth and crisis*. New York, NY: W. W. Norton.

Evans, W. D., Price, S., Blahut, S., Hersey, J., Niederdeppe, J., & Ray, S. (2004). Social imagery, tobacco independence, and the truth campaign. *Journal of Health Communication*, 9(5), 425–441.

Farmer, J. E., Clark, M. J., Sherman, A., Marien, W. E., & Selva, T. J. (2005). Comprehensive primary care for children with special health care needs in rural areas. *Pediatrics*, 116(3), 649–656.

Federal Interagency Forum on Child and Family Statistics. (2015). America's children: Key national indicators of well-being. Retrieved from http://www.childstats.gov/americaschildren

Fothergill, K., & Ballard, E. (1998). The school-linked health center: A promising model of community-based care for adolescents. *The Journal of Adolescent Health: Official Publication of the Society for Adolescent Medicine*, 23(1), 29–38.

Galvan, A., Hare, T., Voss, H., Glover, G., & Casey, B. J. (2007). Risk-taking and the adolescent brain: Who is at risk? *Developmental Science*, 10(2), F8–F14.

Garber, J. (2006). Depression in children and adolescents: Linking risk research and prevention. *American Journal of Preventive Medicine*, 31(6, Suppl. 1), S104–S125.

Geenen, S., & Powers, L. E. (2006). Are we ignoring youths with disabilities in foster care? An examination of their school performance. *Social Work*, 51(3), 233–241.

Gilligan, C. (1982). *In a different voice: Psychological theory and women's development*. Cambridge, MA: Harvard University Press.

Ginsburg, K. R. (2007). Viewing our adolescent patients through a positive lens. *Contemporary Pediatrics*, 24(1), 65, 67.

Graber, J. A., Brooks-Gunn, J., & Warren, M. P. (1995). The antecedents of menarcheal age: Heredity, family environment, and stressful life events. *Child Development*, 66(2), 346–359.

Graber, J. A., Lewinsohn, P. M., Seeley, J. R., & Brooks-Gunn, J. (1997). Is psychopathology associated with the timing of pubertal development? *Journal of the American Academy of Child and Adolescent Psychiatry*, 36(12), 1768–1776.

Grossman, J. B., & Bulle, M. J. (2006). Review of what youth programs do to increase the connectedness of youth with adults. *The Journal of Adolescent Health: Official Publication of the Society for Adolescent Medicine*, 39(6), 788–799.

Guttmacher Institute. (2014). Facts on American teens' sexual and reproductive health. Retrieved from http://www.guttmacher.org/pubs/FB-ATSRH.html

Hagen, J. F., Shaw, J. S., & Duncan, P. M. (Eds.). (2008). *Bright futures: Guidelines for health supervision of infants, children, and adolescents* (3rd ed.). Elk Grove Village, IL: American Academy of Pediatrics.

Halcón, L. L., Robertson, C. L., Savik, K., Johnson, D. R., Spring, M. A., Butcher, J. N.,…Jaranson, J. M. (2004). Trauma and coping in Somali and Oromo refugee youth. *The Journal of Adolescent Health: Official Publication of the Society for Adolescent Medicine*, 35(1), 17–25.

Harel, Z. (2006). Dysmenorrhea in adolescents and young adults: Etiology and management. *Journal of Pediatric and Adolescent Gynecology*, 19(6), 363–371.

Harper, C., Callegari, L., Raine, T., Blum, M., & Darney, P. (2004). Adolescent clinic visits for contraception: Support from mothers, male partners and friends. *Perspectives on Sexual and Reproductive Health*, 36(1), 20–26.

Haudek, C., Rorty, M., & Henker, B. (1999). The role of ethnicity and parental bonding in the eating and weight concerns of Asian-American and Caucasian college women. *International Journal of Eating Disorders*, 25(4), 425–433.

Hawkins, J. D., Kosterman, R., Catalano, R. F., Hill, K. G., & Abbott, R. D. (2005). Promoting positive adult functioning through social development intervention in childhood: Long-term effects from the Seattle Social Development Project. *Archives of Pediatrics & Adolescent Medicine*, 159(1), 25–31.

Hawkins, J. D., Smith, B. H., & Catalano, R. F. (2002). Delinquent behavior. *Pediatrics in Review/American Academy of Pediatrics*, 23(11), 387–392.

Hayward, C., Gotlib, I. H., Schraedley, P. K., & Litt, I. F. (1999). Ethnic differences in the association between pubertal status and symptoms of depression in adolescent girls. *The Journal of Adolescent Health: Official Publication of the Society for Adolescent Medicine*, 25(2), 143–149.

Hayward, C., Killen, J. D., Wilson, D. M., Hammer, L. D., Litt, I. F., Kraemer, H. C.,…Taylor, C. B. (1997). Psychiatric risk associated with early puberty in adolescent girls. *Journal of the American Academy of Child and Adolescent Psychiatry*, 36(2), 255–262.

Huang, Z. J., Yu, S. M., & Ledsky, R. (2006). Health status and health service access and use among children in U.S. immigrant families. *American Journal of Public Health*, 96(4), 634–640.

Jenkins, S., & Horner, S. D. (2005). Barriers that influence eating behaviors in adolescents. *Journal of Pediatric Nursing*, 20(4), 258–267.

Juszczak, L., Melinkovich, P., & Kaplan, D. (2003). Use of health and mental health services by adolescents across multiple delivery sites. *The Journal of Adolescent Health: Official Publication of the Society for Adolescent Medicine*, 32(6 Suppl.), 108–118.

Kachur, R., Mesnick, J., Liddon, N., Kapsimalis, C., Habel, M., David-Ferdon, C.,…Schindelar, J. (2013). *Adolescents, technology and reducing risk for hiv, Stds and pregnancy*. Atlanta, GA: Centers for Disease Control and Prevention.

Key, J. D., Washington, E. C., & Hulsey, T. C. (2002). Reduced emergency department utilization associated with school-based clinic enrollment. *The Journal of Adolescent Health: Official Publication of the Society for Adolescent Medicine*, 30(4), 273–278.

Klein, J. D., Allan, M. J., Elster, A. B., Stevens, D., Cox, C., Hedberg, V. A., & Goodman, R. A. (2001). Improving adolescent preventive care in community health centers. *Pediatrics*, 107(2), 318–327.

Klein, J. D., Shone, L. P., Szilagyi, P. G., Bajorska, A., Wilson, K., & Dick, A. W. (2007). Impact of the state children's health insurance program on adolescents in New York. *Pediatrics*, 119(4), e885–e892.

Knight, J. R., Harris, S. K., Sherritt, L., Van Hook, S., Lawrence, N., Brooks, T., . . . Kulig, J. (2007). Adolescents' preference for substance abuse screening in primary care practice. *Substance Abuse*, 28(4), 107–117.

Knight, J. R., Shrier, L. A., Bravender, T. D., Farrell, M., Vander Bilt, J., & Shaffer, H. J. (1999). A new brief screen for adolescent substance abuse. *Archives of Pediatrics & Adolescent Medicine*, 153(6), 591–596.

Kohlberg, L. (1981). *Essays on moral development*. New York, NY: Harper & Row.

Leathers, S. J., & Testa, M. F. (2006). Foster youth emancipating from care: Caseworkers' reports on needs and services. *Child Welfare*, 85(3), 463–498.

Lee, J. M., Appugliese, D., Kaciroti, N., Corwyn, R. F., Bradley, R. H., & Lumeng, J. C. (2007). Weight status in young girls and the onset of puberty. *Pediatrics*, 119(3), e624–e630.

LeFevre, M. L.; U.S. Preventive Services Task Force. (2014). Screening for chlamydia and gonorrhea: U.S. Preventive Services Task Force recommendation statement. *Annals of Internal Medicine*, 161(12), 902–910.

LeFevre, M. L.; U.S. Preventive Services Task Force. (2014). Behavioral counseling interventions to prevent sexually transmitted infections: U.S. PreventiveServices Task Force recommendation statement. *Annals of Internal Medicine*, 161(12), 894–901.

Li, C. E., DiGiuseppe, R., & Froh, J. (2006). The roles of sex, gender, and coping in adolescent depression. *Adolescence*, 41(163), 409–415.

Ma, J., Wang, Y., & Stafford, R. S. (2005). U.S. adolescents receive suboptimal preventive counseling during ambulatory care. *The Journal of Adolescent Health: Official Publication of the Society for Adolescent Medicine*, 36(5), 441.

Maguen, S., & Armistead, L. (2006). Abstinence among female adolescents: Do parents matter above and beyond the influence of peers? *American Journal of Orthopsychiatry*, 76(2), 260–264.

McDowell, M. A., Brody, D. J., & Hughes, J. P. (2007). Has age at menarche changed? Results from the National Health and Nutrition Examination Survey (NHANES) 1999–2004. *The Journal of Adolescent Health: Official Publication of the Society for Adolescent Medicine*, 40(3), 227–231.

Medical Home Initiatives for Children With Special Needs Project Advisory Committee. (2004). Policy statement: Organizational principles to guide and define the child health care system and/or improve the health of all children. *Pediatrics*, 113, 1545–1547.

Mestad, R., Secura, G., Allsworth, J. E., Madden, T., Zhao, Q., & Peipert, J. F. (2011). Acceptance of long-acting reversible contraceptive methods by adolescent participants in the Contraceptive CHOICE Project. *Contraception*, 84, 493–498.

Miller, W. R., & Sanchez, V. C. (1994). Motivating young adults for treatment and lifestyle change. In G. Howard (Ed.), *Issues in alcohol use and misuse by young adults* (pp. 55–82). Notre Dame, IN: University of Notre Dame Press.

Moyer, V. A.; U.S. Preventive Services Task Force. (2013a). Primary care interventions to prevent tobacco use in children and adolescents: U.S. Preventive Services Task Force recommendation statement. *Annals of Internal Medicine*, 159(8), 552–557.

Moyer, V. A.; U.S. Preventive Services Task Force. (2013b). Screening for HIV: U.S. Preventive Services Task Force recommendation statement. *Annals of Internal Medicine*, 159(1), 51–60.

Naimi, T. S., Lipscomb, L. E., Brewer, R. D., & Gilbert, B. C. (2003). Binge drinking in the preconception period and the risk of unintended pregnancy: Implications for women and their children. *Pediatrics*, 111(5, Pt. 2), 1136–1141.

National Alliance to End Homelessness. (2014). *The state of homelessness in America 2014*. Retrieved from http://www.endhomelessness.org/library/entry/the-state-of-homelessness-2014

The National Center on Addiction and Substance Abuse. (2011). *Adolescent substance use: America's #1 public health problem*. *The National Center on Addiction and Substance Abuse at Columbia University*. Retrieved from http://www.casacolumbia.org/addiction-research/reports/adolescent-substance-use

National Research Council. (2009). *Adolescent health services: Missing opportunities*. Washington, DC: National Academies Press.

Neinstein, L. (2008). *Adolescent health care: A practical guide* (5th ed.). Philadelphia, PA: Lippincott Williams & Wilkins.

Nelson, E. E., Leibenluft, E., McClure, E. B., & Pine, D. S. (2005). The social re-orientation of adolescence: A neuroscience perspective on the process and its relation to psychopathology. *Psychological Medicine*, 35(2), 163–174.

Olson, A. L., Gaffney, C. A., Hedberg, V. A., & Gladstone, G. R. (2009). Use of inexpensive technology to enhance adolescent health screening and counseling. *Archives of Pediatrics & Adolescent Medicine*, 163(2), 172–177.

Paikoff, R. L., Brooks-Gunn, J., & Warren, M. P. (1991). Effect of girls' hormonal status on depressive and aggressive symptoms over the course of one year. *Journal of Youth and Adolescence*, 20(2), 191–215.

Park, M. J., Paul Mulye, T., Adams, S. H., Brindis, C. D., & Irwin, C. E. (2006). The health status of young adults in the United States. *The Journal of Adolescent Health: Official Publication of the Society for Adolescent Medicine*, 39(3), 305–317.

Parker, S., Nichter, M., Nichter, M., & Vuckovic, N. (1995). Body image and weight concerns among African-American and White adolescent females: Differences that make a difference. *Human Organizations*, 54, 103–114.

Pate, R. R., Dowda, M., O'Neill, J. R., & Ward, D. S. (2007). Change in physical activity participation among adolescent girls from 8th to 12th grade. *Journal of Physical Activity & Health*, 4(1), 3–16.

Patton, G. C., & Viner, R. (2007). Pubertal transitions in health. *Lancet*, 369(9567), 1130–1139.

Petersen, A. C., Sarigiani, P. A., & Kennedy, R. E. (1991). Adolescent depression: Why more girls? *Journal of Youth and Adolescence*, 20(2), 247–271.

Piaget, J. (1973). *The child and reality*. New York, NY: Grossman.

Power, T. G., Stewart, C. D., Hughes, S. O., & Arbona, C. (2005). Predicting patterns of adolescent alcohol use: A longitudinal study. *Journal of Studies on Alcohol*, 66(1), 74–81.

Resnick, M. D., Ireland, M., & Borowsky, I. (2004). Youth violence perpetration: What protects? What predicts? Findings from the National Longitudinal Study of Adolescent Health. *The Journal of Adolescent Health: Official Publication of the Society for Adolescent Medicine, 35*(5), 424.e1–424.10.

Resnicow, K., Davis, R., & Rollnick, S. (2006). Motivational interviewing for pediatric obesity: Conceptual issues and evidence review. *Journal of the American Dietetic Association, 106*(12), 2024–2033.

Rew, L. (2005). *Adolescent health: A multidisciplinary approach to theory, research, and intervention.* Thousand Oaks, CA: Sage.

Rimmer, J. H., Yamaki, K., Davis, B. M., Wang, E., & Vogel, L. C. (2011). Obesity and overweight prevalence among adolescents with disabilities. *Preventing Chronic Disease, 8*(2), A41.

Robbins, L. B., Gretebeck, K. A., Kazanis, A. S., & Pender, N. J. (2006). Girls on the move program to increase physical activity participation. *Nursing Research, 55*(3), 206–216.

Rollnick, S., & Miller, W. (1995). What is motivational interviewing? *Behavioural and Cognitive Psychotherapy, 23,* 325–334.

Sadof, M. D., & Nazarian, B. L. (2007). Caring for children who have special health-care needs: A practical guide for the primary care practitioner. *Pediatrics Review, 28*(7), e36–e42.

Saewyc, E. M., Skay, C. L., Pettingell, S. L., Reis, E. A., Bearinger, L., Resnick, M.,…Combs, L. (2006). Hazards of stigma: The sexual and physical abuse of gay, lesbian, and bisexual adolescents in the United States and Canada. *Child Welfare, 85*(2), 195–213.

Sale, E., Sambrano, S., Springer, J. F., Peña, C., Pan, W., & Kasim, R. (2005). Family protection and prevention of alcohol use among Hispanic youth at high risk. *American Journal of Community Psychology, 36*(3–4), 195–205.

Sanchez, R. P., Waller, M. W., & Greene, J. M. (2006). Who runs? A demographic profile of runaway youth in the United States. *The Journal of Adolescent Health: Official Publication of the Society for Adolescent Medicine, 39*(5), 778–781.

Sanfilippo, J. S., & Lara-Torre, E. (2009). Adolescent gynecology. *Obstetrics and Gynecology, 113*(4), 935–947.

Santor, D. A., Poulin, C., LeBlanc, J. C., & Kusumakar, V. (2006). Examining school health center utilization as a function of mood disturbance and mental health difficulties. *The Journal of Adolescent Health: Official Publication of the Society for Adolescent Medicine, 39*(5), 729–735.

Sawyer, S. M., Drew, S., Yeo, M. S., & Britto, M. T. (2007). Adolescents with a chronic condition: Challenges living, challenges treating. *Lancet, 369*(9571), 1481–1489.

Schreiber, G. B., Robins, M., Striegel-Moore, R., Obarzanek, E., Morrison, J. A., & Wright, D. J. (1996). Weight modification efforts reported by black and white preadolescent girls: National Heart, Lung, and Blood Institute Growth and Health Study. *Pediatrics, 98*(1), 63–70.

Serepca, R. O. (1996). The implications of pubertal timing for women's body image and self-esteem. *Dissertation Abstracts International: Section B: The Sciences and Engineering, 57*(6-B), 4060.

Siegel, J. M., Yancey, A. K., Aneshensel, C. S., & Schuler, R. (1999). Body image, perceived pubertal timing, and adolescent mental health. *The Journal of Adolescent Health: Official Publication of the Society for Adolescent Medicine, 25*(2), 155–165.

Spencer, J. H., & Le, T. N. (2006). Parent refugee status, immigration stressors, and Southeast Asian youth violence. *Journal of Immigrant and Minority Health/Center for Minority Public Health, 8*(4), 359–368.

Striegel-Moore, R., & Smolak, L. (1996). The role of race in the development of eating disorders. In M. P. Smolak, R. Levine, & R. Striegel-Moore (Eds.), *The developmental psychopathology of eating disorders: Implications for research prevention and treatment* (pp. 259–284), Hillsdale, NJ: Erlbaum.

Sum, A., Khatiwada, I., & McLaughlin, J. (2009). *The consequences of dropping out of high school: Joblessness and jailing for high school dropouts and the high cost for taxpayers.* Boston, MA: Center for Labor Market Studies, Northeastern University. Retrieved from http://www.prisonpolicy.org/scans/The_Consequences_of_Dropping_Out_of_High_School.pdf

Tanner, J. (1962). *Growth at adolescence* (2nd ed.). Springfield, IL: Charles C. Thomas.

Tanner, J. M. (1981). Growth and maturation during adolescence. *Nutrition Reviews, 39*(2), 43–55.

Taylor, J. P., Evers, S., & McKenna, M. (2005). Determinants of healthy eating in children and youth. *Canadian Journal of Public Health/Revue Canadienne de Santé Publique, 96*(Suppl. 3), S20–26, S22.

Toro, P. A., Dworsky, A., & Fowler, P. J. (2007). *Homeless youth in the United States: Recent research findings and intervention approaches.* Retrieved from www.huduser.org/portal/publications/homeless/p6.html

Tylee, A., Haller, D. M., Graham, T., Churchill, R., & Sanci, L. A. (2007). Youth-friendly primary-care services: How are we doing and what more needs to be done? *Lancet, 369*(9572), 1565–1573.

U.S. Census Bureau. (2014). *2014 Population estimates: National characteristics, national sex, age, race and Hispanic origin.* Retrieved from http://www.census.gov/popest/data/index.html

U.S. Department of Health and Human Services, Centers for Disease Control and Prevention. (2015). *Healthy People 2020.* Retrieved from http://www.healthypeople.gov

Warren, M. P., & Brooks-Gunn, J. (1989). Mood and behavior at adolescence: Evidence for hormonal factors. *Journal of Clinical Endocrinology and Metabolism, 69*(1), 77–83.

Williamson, L. (1998). Eating disorders and the cultural forces behind the drive for thinness: Are African American women really protected? *Social Work in Health Care, 28*(1), 61–73.

Wills, T. A., Murry, V. M., Brody, G. H., Gibbons, F. X., Gerrard, M., Walker, C., & Ainette, M. G. (2007). Ethnic pride and self-control related to protective and risk factors: Test of the theoretical model for the strong African American families program. *Health Psychology: Official Journal of the Division of Health Psychology, American Psychological Association, 26*(1), 50–59.

Youngblade, L. M., Theokas, C., Schulenberg, J., Curry, L., Huang, I. C., & Novak, M. (2007). Risk and promotive factors in families, schools, and communities: A contextual model of positive youth development in adolescence. *Pediatrics, 119*(Suppl. 1), S47–S53.

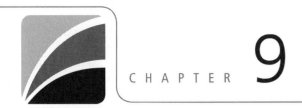

CHAPTER 9

Midlife Women's Health

Nancy Fugate Woods • Judith Berg • Ellen Sullivan Mitchell

Midlife women account for a growing proportion of the U.S. population, but only recently have researchers and clinicians devoted much attention to midlife women's health concerns. During the past three decades, there has been increasing interest in the menopausal transition (MT) as a central feature of midlife women's lives. Although the MT had been a neglected topic in women's health, the changing focus of research about midlife women has provided an important new set of evidence about the transitions in women's bodies that are intertwined with the transitions in their lives. The purposes of this chapter are to (a) define and summarize evidence about women's experiences and perceptions of midlife; (b) review current understanding of the biological changes associated with midlife, with a special emphasis on the MT; (c) characterize symptoms women experience (hot flashes, sleep disruption, mood changes, cognitive changes, pain, and sexual desire changes) and their correlates during MT and postmenopause (PM); (d) explore the relationship of the MT to healthy aging; and (e) propose a program of health promotion and prevention for midlife women.

■ MIDLIFE: DEFINITIONS, PERCEPTIONS, AND TRANSITIONS

Midlife can be defined in a variety of ways, often by using age boundaries, such as 35 to 65 years, to differentiate midlife from younger and older adulthood. Alternatively, definitions can be based on reproductive aging stages using indicators of menstrual cycle changes or hormonal changes (Harlow et al., 2012; Mitchell, Woods, & Mariella, 2000). Women's changing role patterns, using indicators such as a child leaving home or a woman's return to the workplace to designate the beginning of midlife, provides another option, and using women's own perceptions about whether they are in the middle of their lives provides yet another option. Brooks-Gunn and Kirsh (1984) stressed the multidimensional and multidirectional nature of change in midlife, describing the boundaries as fluid and constructed by the society and the individual rather than being determined by chronological age.

Whatever the markers for midlife might be, understanding the context in which women experience midlife is extremely important. Anticipation of midlife by each woman's age cohort (women born at the same time), as well as socialization by other women about what to expect during midlife, contribute to the framework with which women view and interpret the events of midlife. Both anticipated and actual midlife experiences can influence women's notions of health.

Meanings of Midlife

Midlife women from different birth cohorts, those born during different eras, have lived in different worlds (Bernard, 1981); thus it is important to locate women's midlife experiences within the sociopolitical and historical context in which they occur. Contemporary midlife women represent at least two birth cohorts who have had very different lives. Women born during the post–World War II era of the mid-1940s to the mid-1950s an up until the mid-1960s are often termed the *baby boomers* in the United States. These women experienced the women's movement gender revolution of the late 1960s and 1970s in the United States. Women born during the prior decade, from 1935 to 1945, lived their young adult years before the gender revolution and subsequent changes (Coney, 1994). These different experiences are likely to have had an important effect on women who were part of the midlife cohorts engaged in earlier studies, making it important to differentiate their experiences from those of cohorts of midlife women born in prior and later decades.

Neugarten's (1968) work with both midlife women and men studied before and during the 1960s indicated that, for women born before the end of World War II, midlife meant being in control of a complex life. Those who participated in her interviews were socially privileged and recognized their roles as powerful norm-bearers and decision makers. They experienced midlife as a time of heightened sensitivity to their power within a complex social environment. Reassessment of the self was a prevailing theme. Women, compared with men, estimated their age status in the timing of the family life cycle. Launching their children was an important marker of midlife. Changing time perspectives were evident in the interviews with midlife women and men: the time left was of concern. Another aspect of time, the time of one's life, was also a theme in Neugarten's interviews.

Rubin's (1979) classic study *Women of a Certain Age* focused on 160 women who were 35 to 55 years of age when they were studied during the 1970s (born between the 1920s and 1940s). Rubin found that women "of a certain age" struggled with an uncertain identity she labeled the "elusive self." The women Rubin studied were part of a birth cohort that was beginning to be influenced by the women's movement of the 1960s and 1970s. Most had given up the job or careers of their youth for at least 10 years to devote themselves to full-time marriage and motherhood. Nearly 25% were unable to describe who they were. Few described themselves in relation to their work despite their employment. Many described themselves as having two selves, reflecting their difficulty integrating the achieving self with the emotional, intuitive self. Others made a distinction between who they were in relation to being and doing: Their internal identity represented their being, whereas their work represented their doing. For these women, work was what they did, not who they were. Rubin found that these women were not devastated by the "empty nest," the time when their children left home.

The baby boomer cohort born after World War II differentiated itself from women of previous generations by fashioning their lives as individuals. Whereas past generations of women organized their life roles and goals around their family's objectives, baby boomer women now spend more of their lives as single, independent adults, organizing their lives to meet their personal and employment objectives. The baby boomer woman is better educated, lives alone longer than did women of her mother's generation, and participates in the labor force throughout her life regardless of her marital status and the age of her children. She experiences greater financial independence and fertility control than her mother. Marriage and family are no longer the single controlling institutions around which this generation of women organizes their lives, but parenting, partnerships, and caregiving also remain significant components of women's work (McLaughlin, Melber, Billy, & Zimmerle, 1986).

The perceptions and experiences of baby boomer women during their middle years are likely to reflect this dramatic change in their life course. Gilligan (1982a) proposed restoring the missing text of women's development for this cohort rather than simply replacing it with work about men's development. She saw women's middle years as a risky time because of women's embeddedness in relationships, their orientation to interdependence, their ability to subordinate achievement to care, and their conflicts over competitive success. If midlife brings an end to relationships and, with them, a sense of connection for women, then midlife may be a time of despair. Gilligan stressed that the meaning of midlife events for women is contextual, arising from the interaction between the structures of women's thought and the realities of their lives. Women approach midlife with a different history than do men, and they face a different social reality with different possibilities for love and work (Gilligan, 1982a, 1982b).

A study of nearly 500 midlife women (35–60 years in 1986) by the Society for Research on Women in New Zealand (1988) indicated that 80% to 90% had positive attitudes about life, more than 80% had positive attitudes toward their physical appearance and health, and 80% were positive about their futures. Only 14% were unhappy with their daily lives. One third of women reported some stress in their relationships with husbands or partners, such as unemployment, illness, work demands, or finances. Women's experiences with their children were a function of their ages: Of the 35- to 40-year-olds, two thirds found their children stressful, and of the 50- to 60-year-olds, two thirds rated their children not at all stressful.

At the same time that women are experiencing the social transitions associated with parenting responsibilities, they are also experiencing the aging of their bodies. In a series of interviews with a convenience sample of midlife women, Coney (1994) found that signs of aging, such as wrinkles and weight gain, produced grief in some women and no concern in others. Reflections of others' perceptions of aging that included sexist and ageist stereotypes about women, frequently reinforced by mass media, caused some women to be worried about their physical aging. Others were more worried about loss of physical abilities, such as hearing, eyesight, and mobility, and loss of mental powers. Still others felt panicky and negative because they sensed that time was running out for them. The "empty nest" had both positive and negative associations for many of the women Coney studied. Despite negative attitudes toward menopause and aging women, and despite inequities in employment and financial security, midlife women had surprisingly high well-being. They expressed having had achievements and gaining maturity, experience, and confidence that younger women do not have, as well as knowing what they are capable of doing. Having attained some seniority in employment and having launched their children, many women felt freer to concentrate on themselves and decide what they want for the next third of their lives. More secure in their own opinions and beliefs and less afraid of expressing them, the midlife women Coney studied emphasized increasing freedom.

Participants in the Seattle Midlife Women's Health Study (SMWHS)—begun in 1990, when the women were 35 to 55 years of age—responded to these questions: What does "midlife" mean? What events of midlife do women believe are important? Distressing? Satisfying? A particular emphasis of this investigation was to determine whether menopause figured prominently in women's experiences of this part of the life span. Participants' most common image of midlife was getting older (Woods & Mitchell, 1997a). Their emphasis on defining midlife as an age and aging process is consistent with findings from older cohorts of women (Rossi, 1985; Rubin, 1979) and is not surprising, given the youthful value orientation of U.S. society. These women also associated changes of every kind with midlife. They alluded to transitions with respect to their physical bodies, emotions, feelings about being older, outlook on life, relationships, and "change of life." A few referred to their changing health and vulnerability. The notion of midlife as a time of transition is consistent with findings from older birth cohorts of women (Helson & Wink, 1992; Neugarten, 1968). Given the prevalence of life changes among this cohort of midlife women, their emphasis on transitions is not surprising. The centrality of personal achievements and employment in the Seattle women's lives stands in striking contrast to data from older birth cohorts of midlife women. The distinction between images of midlife described by the birth cohort of women Rubin interviewed and those of the women in this study reflect the dramatic changes in lifelong employment patterns women have experienced since the 1970s. The baby boomers did not seem to be trying to figure out what to do with the rest of their lives. They were still juggling the demands of integrating work and family responsibilities. Although emphasis on work-related events and personal goal attainment among this cohort resembled that in studies of men's development (Neugarten, 1968), emphasis on family and health-related events were among those considered most important. Children, spouses, and parents were mentioned frequently as women described the important events of midlife.

Participants in the SMWHS ($N = 508$), with a median age of 41 years at the beginning of the study, reported a variety of stressful or distressing events, which included health problems, deaths, family problems, work-related problems, frustrated goal attainment, and financial problems (Woods & Mitchell, 1997a). Women reported distressing health problems, including their own and those of their parents, with similar frequency. Deaths were also commonly cited as the most distressing event and included the deaths of parents, in-laws, and husbands. Family problems also involved adolescent children, domestic violence, divorce or separation from a spouse, and the ending of relationships. Work problems, including inability to find work, workplace conflicts, and downsizing of workplaces, were also mentioned frequently. Frustrated goal attainment included events such as being unable to finish an academic program on time or having personal time while working on an academic program. Women's financial events included problems such as inability to pay college tuition for a child or afford essentials. When asked to look back over the past 15 years of their study participation and describe the most challenging aspects of their lives, midlife women indicated that most of these events were salient, but only one woman identified menopause as most challenging.

Not surprisingly, the Seattle women's images of midlife and the events they found most important and most stressful reflected their engagement in a broader, more complex world than that of their mothers. No longer focusing only on their roles as mothers and homemakers, contemporary midlife women are attempting to balance the demands of workplace and home, and this is reflected in how they characterized the best and worst of midlife. Unlike Rubin's sample, this sample of midlife women talked freely of their multidimensional selves and the social circumstances that necessitated their viewing themselves differently from their mothers' generation.

A new emphasis on women's preparation for their own aging is evident in both professional and public literature. Sarah Lawrence-Lightfoot (2009) uses the term *third chapter* to designate those years when one is neither old nor young, emphasizing the possibility that these years can be the most transformative time in life. Having courage to challenge ageist stereotypes and creativity to resist old cultural norms (about aging and gender) in combination with curiosity to learn and a spirit of adventure to pursue new passions and experiences are core elements of how one creates the third chapter. In her case

studies, Lawrence-Lightfoot explores the themes of engagement over retreat, labor over leisure, and reinvention over retirement, emphasizing the elements of active engagement, purposefulness, and new learning as themes in the life stories that people write about the third chapter of their lives. Indeed, she emphasizes the power of our stories—new narratives or several narratives—to serve as our maps through this third chapter. Often this period becomes a time of public service and growing toward a new direction. In many ways Lawrence-Lightfoot finds this third chapter as a prime time in life.

In *Composing a Further Life*, Mary Catherine Bateson (2010) introduces a modification to Erik Erickson's model of human development by splitting adulthood into two phases: Adulthood 1 includes the challenge of generation versus stagnation, resulting in the strength of care, and adulthood 2 addresses engagement versus withdrawal, resulting in active wisdom. Bateson's discussion of lifelong learning as part of the developmental processes includes the achievement of receptive wisdom and humility as one resolves the challenges of old age.

Both Lawrence-Lightfoot and Bateson invite us to consider midlife as a period in which we can actively compose a life story or a set of possible stories into which we can live as we age. This theme of creation of our own maps for aging suggests that some of the developmental tasks included in earlier theories need to be revised to accommodate the lengthening life span and women's aspirations for that additional time in one's life.

Contemporary midlife women described midlife similarly to women from earlier birth cohorts with one important exception: the centrality of work and personal achievement in their lives. As women's roles have changed, so have the experiences that women count as important. Personal achievement and work-related events have assumed a central place, along with family events, in how women describe their lives. With a life course that is made more complex than their mothers' by lifelong employment, contemporary midlife women are not wondering what to do with the rest of their lives as much as they are wondering how to juggle the demands of family and work-related responsibilities. In addition, many midlife women are anticipating the next stage of their lives and creating the narratives for their own "third chapter."

Midlife as a Transitional Period

Midlife has earned recognition as a period of developmental transition worthy of study. Indeed, an important area of scholarship related to midlife focuses on multiple types of transitions. Transitions have been identified as periods during which change occurs. One can envision midlife as a transitional period between part of the life span during which reproduction and parenting typically occur, occupying a large component of women's lives (see Chapter 8), and older adulthood, a period focused on adaptation to aging-related changes and ultimately dying (see Chapter 10). During midlife, women experience many types of transitions, including developmental, situational, and health–illness transitions. Although the MT, the period between the late reproductive years when women have regular menstrual periods and the final menstrual period (FMP), is one that has gained the attention of health professionals, other transitions include changes in marital status and parental roles, which may be more salient to some women than menopause, as well as health–illness transitions to experiencing chronic illness. Transitional periods in life create opportunity for adaptation, and these in turn may lead to either positive or negative changes in health status and well-being. Despite emphasis on the negative outcomes of transitions, Smith-DiJulio, Mitchell, Percival, and Woods (2008) found that midlife women experienced well-being during this period. Moreover, women's estimates of their own mastery and satisfaction with social support during this period were important predictors of their well-being. As anticipated, women who experienced negative life events during this period also experienced lower well-being. Experiencing the MT had relatively small effects on well-being.

■ THE MENOPAUSAL TRANSITION

During the 20th century, the term *menopause* was used to refer to the period around the time of the FMP. Women were described as premenopausal, menopausal, or post-menopausal, without specific reference to the time period denoted. In the health sciences the term *menopause* is used to refer to the cessation of menses, the FMP, which is said to have occurred after a woman has ceased menstruating for 1 year (Soules et al., 2001).

The years during which women make the transition to menopause (the MT, the time before the FMP when menstrual periods become irregular) and the first few years after the FMP (early PM) hold great fascination and sometimes frustration for the women experiencing them as well as their health care providers. When midlife women were asked about what they anticipated menopause would be like, the most prevalent theme was uncertainty and mixed feelings (Woods & Mitchell, 1999). These sentiments suggested a need for knowledge about this part of the life span and changing biology.

As women anticipate midlife, menopause is one focus of their concerns. Participants in the SMWHS voiced uncertainty about what to expect menopause would be like, and many had no expectations about the experience, revealing a need for information about this part of the life span (Woods & Mitchell, 1999). Indeed, women defined *menopause* as the cessation of menstrual periods, the end of reproductive capacity, a time of hormonal changes, a new or different life stage, a time of symptoms, a time of changing emotions and changing bodies, and part of the aging process. Of interest is that few defined this period of life as a time of disease risk or one necessitating medical care.

Significant progress has been made in understanding the MT as part of reproductive aging and as it influences women's health during the transition and ultimately their health as they age. Around the globe there have been several longitudinal studies of midlife and the MT: The Massachusetts Women's Health Study (MWHS;

McKinlay, Brambilla, & Posner, 1992), the Study of Women's Health Across the Nation (SWAN; Sowers et al., 2000), the Melbourne Midlife Women's Health Project (Dennerstein, Dudley, Hopper, Guthrie, & Burger, 2000), the Penn Ovarian Aging Study (Freeman et al., 2001), and the SMWHS (Woods & Mitchell, 1997b). Taken together, the results of these studies have contributed to understanding the biological changes that occur during the MT and PM, symptoms women experience, and the influence of the MT on healthy aging. The information in this chapter draws heavily on findings from these studies.

How various U.S. ethnic groups of women define menopause (as used in the popular culture to mean the experiences around the time of the FMP) was unknown until the efforts of investigators for SWAN (Sowers et al., 2000). Results from the multisite study of multiple U.S. ethnic groups indicate widespread differences in women's expectations and experiences as well as areas of similarity across groups. Urban Latina women stressed the primacy of health and the importance of harmony and balance in their lives. They described "menopause" as *el cambio de vida*—something you have to go through. They also stressed that "this time is for me," referring to reorienting and restructuring their lives (Villaruel, Harlow, Lopez, & Sowers, 2002). Conceptions among Japanese American and European American women differed. Change in self-focus, self-satisfaction, and ability to reprioritize values accompanied the transition to menopause. Japanese American women described a metamorphosis from motherhood to nurturing, becoming a more complete human being (Kagawa-Singer et al., 2002). African American women's conceptions of menopause emphasized midlife as a period of developmental changes. They recognized their personal mortality, changing family relationships, and increasing authenticity, re-evaluating life experiences, setting new goals for personal growth, and experiencing greater self-esteem. They emphasized increased self-acceptance and productivity (Sampselle, Harris, Harlow, & Sowers, 2002). Chinese American and Chinese women's conceptions of menopause were inextricably bound with meanings of midlife. For this group, the borders and timing of the MT are ambiguous. The MT represents a natural progression through the life cycle.

Of interest is that expectations of women who have not yet experienced their FMP did not match the experiences of women who had done so. The MT was viewed as a marker for aging. Women believe that it is important to prepare for and manage the MT (Adler et al., 2000), but this belief exists in the context of a lack of access to information and uncertainty about the process.

■ CHANGING BIOLOGY: THE MT AND BEYOND

During the first two decades of the 21st century, efforts to predict the events of the MT culminated in a model for staging reproductive aging. As part of this effort, researchers and clinicians proposed and are testing criteria that women and clinicians can use to anticipate the onset of the MT and PM.

Figure 9.1 includes a model focusing on late reproductive aging through early PM adapted from the Staging Reproductive Aging Workshop + 10 (STRAW+10) held in 2011. (The first STRAW workshop was held 10 years earlier, and results are described in Soules et al. [2001].) The STRAW+10 model is oriented around the FMP, with the time period immediately preceding the FMP labeled the MT and the period immediately following the FMP PM. The MT is divided into two stages: early and late. Criteria used to denote the stages in the STRAW+10 model have been validated using data from several longitudinal studies. The beginning of the early MT is the beginning irregularity of menstrual cycles, with the length of one cycle varying by 7 or more days from the preceding or following cycle. To define the onset of the early MT stage, irregularity was observed to repeat itself at least once during the next 10 bleeding segments (Harlow et al., 2008). The onset of the late MT is denoted by amenorrhea of 60 or more days. For women younger than age 45 years, amenorrhea needs to repeat itself at least once during the next 10 bleeding segments (Taffe et al., 2010). STRAW criteria for staging the MT were validated by the RESTAGE collaboration that compared results from several longitudinal studies of women's menstrual cycles as they approached the FMP (Harlow et al., 2006). Results supported the STRAW recommendations that 60 or more days of amenorrhea be used to define onset of late MT (Harlow et al., 2007) and that early MT onset be defined as a persistent 7 or more days' difference in length of consecutive cycles (Harlow et al., 2008).

STRAW participants divided the reproductive stage into three parts—early, peak, and late—corresponding to women's experience of fertility. The late reproductive stage (stage–3a, just before the MT, was characterized by rising follicle-stimulating hormone (FSH) levels and regular menstrual cycle length, but includes some subtle changes in flow and length of bleeding. Figures 9.2 to 9.4 illustrate the late reproductive and early and late MT stages as indicated by women's menstrual calendars completed by participants in the SMWHS.

STRAW+10 participants divided PM into early and late stages, with the early stage spanning the first 6 years after the FMP based on trajectories of FSH and estradiol. Specific attention focused on the year after the FMP (+1a) and the year after that (+1b), when endocrine changes stabilized. During the last 3 to 6 years of early PM (stage +1c), FSH and estradiol continue to stabilize. Late PM (+2) represents the period during which processes of somatic aging become paramount. STRAW+10 participants also recommended application regardless of women's age, ethnicity, body size, or lifestyle characteristics.

Women's own definitions of the MT, based on their observations of their own experiences, differ from the detailed staging of reproductive aging presented earlier. Women not only observe bleeding, as recorded on menstrual calendars, but also frequently report spotting (bloody discharge that does not require the use of a sanitary napkin or tampon) before, after, and in between episodes of menstrual bleeding and longer and heavier episodes of bleeding (menorrhagia or flooding) that cause them to worry and seek health care. They may define themselves as "in menopause" or "menopausal" based on their bleeding changes, but their definitions may not be consistent with

STAGE	−3a	−2	−1	+1a	+1b	+1c
Terminology	Late Reproductive	Early menopausal transition	Late menopausal transition	Early postmenopause	Early postmenopause	Early postmenopause
Duration	Variable	Variable	1-3 years	1 year	1 year	3-6 years
Menstrual cycle	Subtle changes in amount of flow and length of bleeding	Variable length with persistent difference in consecutive cycles of ≥ 7 days	Amenorrhea ≥ 60 days	Amenorrhea	Amenorrhea	Amenorrhea
				Final menstrual period (FMP)		

FIGURE 9.1

Stages of reproductive aging from late reproductive through early postmenopause.

Adapted from STRAW+10.

Seattle Midlife Women's Health Study
University of Washington
School of Nursing

Late reproductive stage = All segment lengths less than 7 days apart
Bleed-free days after spotting are part of bleeding episode

Year __XXXX____   ID NO___XX____

Day	1	2	3	4	5	6	7	8	9	10	11	12	13	14	15	16	17	18	19	20	21	22	23	24	25	26	27	28	29	30	31
JAN								S	S	B	B	B	B	S	S																
FEB			S	S	B	B	B	S																					■	■	■
MAR	S	S	B	B	B	S	S																				S	S	B	B	B
APR	S																							S	S	B	B				■
MAY																			S		S		B	B	B	S					
JUN														S	B	B	B	S													■
JUL													B	B	B	B	S														
AUG							S		S	B	B	S																			
SEP			S	B	B	B	S	S																							■
OCT		B	B	B	S																			S		B	B	B	B		
NOV	S	S	S																					B	B	B	S	S	S		■
DEC																		S	B	B	B	S	S								

For every day you spot or bleed enter an S or B in the appropriate square. Record a 1, 2, 3 or 4 next to every B day.
(1: light flow, 2: moderate, 3: heavy, 4: very heavy/flooding)
For any month no bleeding or spotting occurs write in NO BLEEDING.
If you forget to record for a month write in FORGOT TO RECORD.

FIGURE 9.2
Menstrual calendar for late reproductive stage.
Adapted from Seattle Midlife Women's Health Study data.

those in the STRAW staging model. *Menopause* is defined as the final day of the FMP. The end of menstruation is marked by the last menstrual period, said to have occurred after women have not menstruated for 1 calendar year (Soules et al., 2001).

Staging reproductive aging provides a useful framework for women to use in anticipating their progress through the MT. It is also useful to clinicians in organizing their understanding of the changing biology around the time of menopause (Santoro et al., 2007).

Reproductive Aging: The MT

In the United States, most women experience their FMP during their late 40s or early 50s, with the median age being 51 to 52 years (Harlow et al., 2006, 2007, 2008; McKinlay et al., 1992; Mitchell & Woods, 2007). Although the FMP occurs only once in a woman's lifetime, the natural MT is a biological process that usually occupies several years of a woman's life, as opposed to being a single occasion (see Table 9.1 for information on ages at and duration of MT stages based on findings from the SMWHS). The early stage of the MT estimated from U.S. women's menstrual bleeding patterns recorded daily on menstrual calendars has been timed to start during the mid-40s and occurred at a median age of 45.5 years for a population of midwestern White women (Treloar, 1981), at 47.5 years as reported in telephone interviews by participants in the MWHS (McKinlay et al., 1992), and 46.6 years based on menstrual calendars obtained from participants in the SMWHS (Mitchell & Woods, 2007; Mitchell et al., 2000). The beginning of the late stage of MT occurred at 49.2 years in the SMWHS. The duration of MT averages 4 to 5 years across the studies but varies widely, with a range of 2 to 7 years and a median of 4.5 years in the Minnesota and 3.5 years in the MWHS samples. The median duration of the early stage was 2.8 years and, for the late stage, 2.3 years in the SMWHS sample (Mitchell & Woods, 2007; unpublished data).

Seattle Midlife Women's Health Study
University of Washington
School of Nursing

Onset Early Menopausal Transition Stage, July 5
Onset = segment lengths 7 or more days apart, repeated within 10 segments
Bleed-free days between bleeding and spotting are part of bleeding episode
No bleeding in November

Year __XXXX___   ID NO___XX____

Day	1	2	3	4	5	6	7	8	9	10	11	12	13	14	15	16	17	18	19	20	21	22	23	24	25	26	27	28	29	30	31
JAN									B	B	B	B																			
FEB			B	B	B	B																							■	■	■
MAR	B	B	B	B																		B	B	B	B						■
APR														B	B	B	B			S	S										■
MAY														S	S	B	B	B													
JUN												B	B	B	B	S															■
JUL				S		B	B	B	B																						
AUG					S	B		B	S																						
SEP		B	B	B		B	S																								■
OCT				B	B	B	B	S																				B	B	B	
NOV																															■
DEC	B	B	B																										B	B	B

For every day you spot or bleed enter an S or B in the appropriate square. Record a 1, 2, 3 or 4 next to every B day.
(1: light flow, 2: moderate, 3: heavy, 4: very heavy/flooding)
For any month no bleeding or spotting occurs write in NO BLEEDING.
If you forget to record for a month write in FORGOT TO RECORD.

FIGURE 9.3
Menstrual calendar illustrating early menopausal transition stage.

Adapted from Seattle Midlife Women's Health Study data.

Endocrine Changes During the MT and Early PM

Irregularity of menstrual periods has been used as an indicator of progression through the MT and is associated with a logarithmic decrease in the number of ovarian follicles as women age. Comparing women aged 45 to 55 years who were menstruating regularly to women having irregular cycles and women who had stopped menstruating, Richardson (1993) found that follicle counts had decreased dramatically among women having irregular cycles and were nearly absent in the postmenopausal group. Although counts of antral follicles are important indicators of ovarian aging, they are not typically used in primary care. Instead, providers often rely on changes in bleeding patterns and cycle regularity as a bases for helping women estimate whether they may be in the MT and at what stage.

STRAW+10 workshop participants reviewed potential indicators of the MT and FMP and recommended further research to identify those with greatest predictive power and clinical utility (Harlow et al., 2012).

The STRAW framework is anchored by changes in menstrual cycle regularity and is useful as a reference point for examining the changes in ovarian (estrogens, progesterone, testosterone, Müllerian inhibiting hormone [MIH], and inhibins) and pituitary (FSH and luteinizing hormone [LH] hormones). An early description of hormonal events of the menstrual cycles of women nearing menopause and those who had experienced their FMP indicated that changes in endocrine levels were complex, not simply declining or increasing over time, and that some women experienced very high estrogen levels in response to increases in FSH before their FMP (Santoro, Brown, Adel, & Skurnick, 1996). These findings are consistent with those of Klein et al. (1996) who found that accelerated follicular development was associated with a monotropic rise in FSH in women between 40 and 45 years who were still cycling. As these women neared the end of regular ovulation, their estradiol levels during the early follicular phases were higher and rose earlier in the follicular phase than was the case in younger women. As reproductive age advanced, their progesterone levels diminished.

Seattle Midlife Women's Health Study
University of Washington
School of Nursing

Onset Late Menopausal Transition Stage, September 14 (Age 50)
Onset = Bleed-free days between segment lengths 60 or more days; repeated within 10 segments if younger than 46
Bleed-free days between bleeding and spotting are part of bleeding episode
SS in February = intermenstrual spotting, not a bleeding episode

Year __XXXX___   ID NO___XX____

Day	1	2	3	4	5	6	7	8	9	10	11	12	13	14	15	16	17	18	19	20	21	22	23	24	25	26	27	28	29	30	31
JAN								B	B	B	B	B		S																	
FEB			B	B	B	S										S	S												■	■	■
MAR																		B	B	B	B	B	S			S					
APR																				S	S	B	S	B		S					■
MAY																		B	B	B	B	B	B	S	S	S	S				
JUN												B	B	B	B	S															■
JUL																														S	B
AUG	B	B																					S	B	B	B	B	S			
SEP													B	B	B	B	B	S	S				B								■
OCT																															
NOV																															■
DEC	B	B	B	B	B	S	S				S																		S	B	B

For every day you spot or bleed enter an S or B in the appropriate square. Record a 1, 2, 3 or 4 next to every B day.
(1: light flow, 2: moderate, 3: heavy, 4: very heavy/flooding)
For any month no bleeding or spotting occurs write in NO BLEEDING.
If you forget to record for a month write in FORGOT TO RECORD.

FIGURE 9.4
Menstrual calendar illustrating late menopausal transition stage.
Adapted from Seattle Midlife Women's Health Study data.

The SWAN, an ongoing multisite longitudinal study of a multiethnic population of U.S. women extending across the MT, was designed to characterize the physical and psychosocial changes that occur during the time of the MT and PM and to observe their effects on later risk factors for age-related diseases and health. SWAN investigators collected data from more than 16,000 women between the ages of 40 and 55 years who were screened from 1995 to 1997. Of these women, 3,302 of them who were between 42 and 52 years of age were enrolled in a longitudinal cohort studied by annual visits and other data-collection efforts for up to 25 years of follow-up, and 900 of these women participated in a daily hormone study. The data being collected in SWAN include ovarian markers, lifestyle and behavior indicators, and markers of cardiovascular and bone health. The results

TABLE 9.1	Duration and Age of Onset of Menopausal Transition Stages											
	EARLY STAGE				**LATE STAGE**				**POSTMENOPAUSE**			
	N	Mean	*SD*	Range	*N*	Mean	*SD*	Range	*N*	Mean	*SD*	Range
Age of onset	121	46.4	3.4	36.6–53.2	130	49.4	2.7	43.1–55.0	114	52.1	2.9	43.7–58.3
Duration (years)	82	2.8	1.5	0.2–6.5	84	2.5	2.7	0.41–7.0	NA	NA	NA	NA

SD, standard deviation.
Adapted from unpublished data from Seattle Midlife Women's Health Study data.

of the SWAN study will make a significant contribution to the understanding of the natural history of the MT (Sowers et al., 2000). The multiethnic SWAN cohort has allowed investigators to explore the variability of endocrine levels with women's racial/ethnic group as well as the stage of the MT.

SWAN investigators found a period of about 4 years when maximal changes occurred in FSH and estradiol; changes in FSH levels preceded those in estradiol. After this period of maximal changes, both FSH and estradiol levels stabilized (Randolph et al., 2003, 2011). The rise in FSH accelerated 2 years before the FMP, and deceleration began immediately before the FMP and stabilized 2 years after the FMP (Randolph et al., 2011), consistent with the findings of Sowers, Zheng, et al. (2008) and the prior findings of Burger et al. from the Melbourne Midlife Women's Health Project (Burger, Dudley, Cui, Dennerstein, & Hopper, 2000; Burger, Dudley, Robertson, & Dennerstein, 2002; Burger et al., 1999). Estradiol levels did not change until about 2 years before the FMP, when they began decreasing and then dropping maximally at the time of the FMP and decelerating to stability about 2 years after the FMP. In obese women, the initial acceleration of FSH occurred slightly later (approximately 5.5 years before the FMP) and was limited compared with the levels for women who were not obese (Randolph et al., 2011). A unique component of the SWAN study was the daily hormone substudy in which Santoro and colleagues found that cycles became anovulatory before the FMP, with declining progesterone levels as women's ovulation occurred more irregularly or stopped (Santoro et al., 2007).

Although the precise cause of cessation of menses is unknown, estradiol levels drop as ovulation occurs less frequently and FSH rises in response to ovarian signals from inhibins and anti-Müllerian hormone (AMH; Burger, Burger, Hale, Robertson, & Dennerstein, 2007; Randolph et al., 2011; Sowers, Zheng, et al., 2008). AMH, produced in growing ovarian follicles, is a direct indicator of ovarian reserve and becomes nondetectable 5 years before the FMP. Inhibin B, produced by small antral follicles, indicates growth of the antral follicle cohort. Inhibin B suppresses FSH secretion by the pituitary and becomes undetectable 4 to 5 years before the FMP (Sowers, Eyvazzadeh, et al., 2008). Dramatic increases in FSH may be responsible for elevated levels of estrogens during the later phase of the MT, producing hyperestrogenism in some women. Dominant follicles continue to produce estradiol and inhibin A, probably as a result of the fall in inhibin B, which allows FSH to rise and stimulate the ovary. As ovulation ceases, the levels of inhibin A fall, reflecting the inability of a dominant follicle to develop (Burger et al., 1999, 2000, 2002).

Current evidence indicates that increasing FSH levels are a useful indicator that the FMP is approaching, but they are not sufficiently specific to diagnose a MT stage, and there is no clear-cut point distinguishing women in the MT within a specified time period compared with those not yet in the MT (Harlow et al., 2006; Randolph et al., 2006). Sustained increases of FSH occur on average 5 to 6 years and LH 3 to 4 years before the FMP (Lenton, Sexton, Lee, & Cooke, 1988; Metcalf, 1988; Randolph et al., 2006). Elevated

gonadotropins have been attributed to both ovarian aging (loss of follicles and therefore reduced estrogen and the reduction in inhibin levels that provide negative feedback to FSH) and the central regulation of aging (decrease in sensitivity to feedback at the hypothalamus and/or pituitary). Wise et al. (2002) have proposed that central regulation of reproductive aging may play a role in the elevated LH and FSH levels occurring during the late reproductive stage and the MT.

In addition to reproductive aging, antral follicle counts (AFCs) may be influenced throughout the life span by exposure to environmental adversity. Bleil et al. (2012) found that women who reported greater levels of perceived stress during their reproductive years (25–35 years) had higher AFCs, a marker of total ovarian reserve. Older women (40–45 years) reporting greater perceived stress had lower AFCs, suggesting that greater stress may enhance reproductive readiness in younger women at the cost of accelerating reproductive aging later in the life span. Bleil hypothesized that environmental adversity promoted the allocation of resources toward greater reproductive readiness by increasing the volume of growing follicles at the cost of depleting more rapidly the ovarian reserve as women aged. Further research is needed to determine whether the effects of stress on ovarian aging would differ under conditions of more extreme stressors.

Androgens

Women produce androgens in both the ovary and adrenal cortex, and current data indicate no difference in metabolic clearance for midlife women regardless of whether they had their FMP. Although the conversion of estrone to estradiol decreased in middle-aged women who continued to menstruate, peripheral aromatization of androstenedione to estrone increased in all women with age regardless of their menopausal status (menstruating to menopausal, and menopausal at both occasions). Women begin producing increasing levels of estrone before FMP (Longcope & Johnston, 1990).

The adrenal gland secretes androgen precursors, including dehydroepiandrosterone sulfate (DHEAS), dehydroepiandroterone (DHEA), androstenedione, and testosterone. Data from the Melbourne Midlife Women's Health Project, a longitudinal study of Australian women during the MT and PM, revealed that testosterone levels remained unchanged during the transition to menopause (from 4 years before FMP to 2 years after), but DHEAS levels decreased as a function of age, not of the MT (Burger et al., 2000). In addition, sex hormone–binding globulin (SHBG) decreased by 43% from 4 years before to 2 years after FMP, with the greatest drop 2 years before FMP. SHBG levels were associated with a drop in estradiol levels over the same period. Free androgen index (FAI), calculated as the ratio of testosterone to SHBG, rose by 80% during the same period, with the maximal change occurring 2 years before the FMP (Burger et al., 2000).

Androgens have also been studied in the SWAN population. Although DHEAS has been found to decline as a function of age, there was a transient rise in DHEAS noted in some SWAN participants during the transition to late perimenopause (the late stage of the MT using the STRAW terminology), followed by a decline during the early PM (Crawford et al., 2009; Lasley et al., 2002). Approximately 85% of women experienced increase in DHEAS between the pre/early MT stage to the late MT/early PM (Crawford et al., 2009). DHEAS provides an important source of estrogen for women during PM because it is converted to estrone. Testosterone levels were stable during the MT in both the Melbroune Midlife Women's Health cohort and the SWAN cohort (Burger et al., 2000; Lasley et al., 2002).

Lasley, Crawford, and McConnell (2011) found that DHEAS, DHEA, and androstenediol increased at their greatest rate and were at peak variability during the years immediately before the FMP when estradiol levels were low. Androstenediol, a prohormone for peripheral conversion to bioactive steroids, acts as a signal transducer in estrogen and androgen receptors. Androsteneiol levels increased fivefold during the time that estradiol levels were decreasing. Lasley et al. proposed that disappearance of inhibin B and rising FSH levels triggered an increase in androstenediol production, producing a transition from estrogenic to androgenic metabolism. SWAN participants produced high levels of androstenediol that were 100 times greater than the levels of estradiol. Lasley et al. (2011, 2013) proposed that the much higher levels of androstenediol, which has lower bioactivity than estradiol, were needed in order to compensate for lower estradiol levels. Although the clinical significance of increasing androstenediol is unknown, the greater concentration of androstenediol coupled with lower estradiol levels during the MT to FMP may contribute to the circulating estrogen pool. These insights may prove valuable in better understanding of endocrine changes during the MT, including the ratio of estrogens to androgens.

Cortisol rose between the early MT stage and late MT stage in the SMWHS, in which assays were obtained multiple times per year (Woods, Carr, Tao, Taylor, & Mitchell, 2006), but no cortisol rise was evident in the annual measures obtained from the SWAN population (Lasley et al., 2002).

Lasley, Crawford, and McConnell (2013) proposed that the wide range of delta-5 steroid production, especially DHEA and androstenediol, may account for the diversity in phenotypes (symptoms and health conditions) observed in women during the MT. The adrenal response to LH may be mediated by LH receptors in the adrenal cortex that may shunt metabolism of pregnenolone to the delta-5 pathway. Whereas older theories attribute the transition to an androgenic from estrogenic transition in metabolism to the disappearance of inhibin B and rising FSH triggering increases in delta-5 (androstenediol) production, current theory suggests that LH stimulates receptors on the adrenal cortex to transition to androgenic metabolism (Lasley et al., 2013). The significance for this metabolic shift for women's experiences of symptoms and health conditions during the MT remains to be investigated.

Data from the multiethnic SWAN study indicate that serum FSH, SHBG, estradiol, testosterone, and DHEAS all are correlated with body mass. Estradiol levels adjusted for body mass do not differ across ethnic groups. Adjusted FSH levels were higher and adjusted testosterone levels were lower in African American and Hispanic women. Thus serum sex steroids, FSH, and SHBG levels vary by ethnicity, but this relationship is highly confounded by ethnic differences in body mass (Randolph et al., 2003).

The MT as a Time of Reregulation

Although some emphasize the physiological dysregulation of the hypothalamic–pituitary–ovarian (HPO) axis functions during the MT, this period in a woman's life may represent a time of reregulation of endocrine function. The ovary produces lower levels of estradiol as the ovarian follicles decrease in number, but the transition is punctuated by higher levels of estradiol in response to increasing levels of FSH. Ovulation ceases and progesterone levels become extremely low or unmeasurable. During the MT, a compensatory response with an increase in peripheral aromatization of the androgen androstenedione to estrone and a time-limited increase in DHEAS occur during the late transition stage. These events may signal a transition from ovarian to ovarian-adrenal metabolism of estrogens, thus supporting reregulation of the HPO axis to a new pattern not dependent on the ovarian production of higher levels of estrogen.

The widespread physiologic effects of estrogens, progesterone, and androgens would warrant compensatory changes in response to their production in order to reregulate the HPO axis, and these alter physiological functioning. The physiological effects of estrogen and progesterone seen in menstruating women change over the course of the MT as estradiol production becomes more variable and eventually diminishes; progesterone production linked to ovulation ceases; testosterone, DHEA, and DHEAS levels remain stable or fluctuate slightly; and androstenediol levels increase dramatically, producing an increasing ratio of estrone to estradiol.

Symptoms During the MT

During midlife, women experience a variety of symptoms, some of which are related to the MT and related endocrine changes and some to aging, as well as a variety of factors influencing symptom experiences across the life span. Hot flashes, sweats, depressed mood, sleep disturbances, sexual concerns or problems, memory symptoms, vaginal dryness, urinary incontinence (UI), and somatic or bodily pain symptoms are among those reported most frequently.

HOT FLASHES

Hot flashes are sudden sensations of heat that usually arise on the chest and spread to the neck and face and sometimes to the arms. They may be accompanied by sweating and flushing in some women (Voda, 1981). Hot flashes and sweats (daytime or nighttime) are often referred to as *vasomotor symptoms.*

Hot flashes occur in an effort to dissipate heat by means of vascular dilation. Voda (1981) characterized the menopausal hot flash from women's own experiences, exploring the question, Who is the woman who has hot flashes and what are the characteristics of the hot flashes? Using data from their daily self-reports, she sought to describe the frequency, duration, trigger, origin, spread, intensity, and method of coping with hot flashes. Voda found that no single pattern characterized women's experiences: Although the majority of hot flashes began on the upper body (e.g., the chest or face), some women noted their hot flashes started in other parts of their body. Hot flashes tended to spread to other areas on the upper body, but for some women spread to the legs and arms or back. On average, a hot flash lasted about 3 minutes. Women distinguished between mild, moderate, and severe hot flashes. They coped with hot flashes in relation to their duration and severity. Internal strategies included ingesting a cold beverage. External strategies involved fanning oneself, showering, or opening a window. Some hot flash triggers included sleep, work activities, recreation and relaxation, and housework. Voda's study emphasized the variability in women's hot flash experiences and how they managed them. In collaboration with Kay and others, Voda extended this work to characterize the experiences of both Mexican American and Anglo women (Kay, Voda, Olivas, Rios, & Imle, 1982). They found that although Anglo women experienced hot flashes negatively, Mexican American women viewed them as positive, a natural part of life, indicating they could no longer have children and meaning they could be confident they would not become pregnant again.

Hot flashes and sweats increase in prevalence as women approach the FMP, with an estimated 33% to 64% of women experiencing hot flashes during the late MT stage (Woods & Mitchell, 2005). Hot flashes have been associated with LH pulses (Casper, Yen, & Wilkes, 1979; Freedman, 2005a), low estradiol (Guthrie, Dennerstein, Hopper, & Burger, 1996; Guthrie, Dennerstein, Taffe, Lehert, & Burger, 2004, 2005; Woods et al., 2007), low inhibin levels (Guthrie et al., 2005), and high levels of FSH (Freeman et al., 2001; Randolph et al., 2005; Woods et al., 2007). SHBG and free estradiol levels were also associated with a lower prevalence of hot flashes (Randolph et al., 2005), and in one study (Overlie, Moen, Holte, & Finset, 2002), androgen levels were associated with a decreased frequency of postmenopausal vasomotor symptoms.

In acute studies in which laboratory stimuli were used to provoke hot flashes, elevations in LH, adrenocorticotropic hormone, and cortisol were closely associated in time with the experience of the hot flash, but no changes were reported in estradiol and FSH levels (Meldrum et al., 1980; Tataryn, Meldrum, Lu, Frumar, & Judd, 1979). In the laboratory, hot flashes were associated with a rise in skin temperature and skin conductance levels, elevated heart and respiratory rate, and reduced blood pH. Lab studies also indicated autonomic nervous system activation, similar to a stress response, in mediating the vasodilation and elaboration of norepinephrine after the hot flash (Freedman, 2005a, 2005b; Freedman & Subramanian, 2005). Potent vasodilators, including calcitonin gene–related peptide, are released during hot flashes but not during exercise or sweating (Thurston, Sutton-Tyrrell, Everson-Rose, Hess, & Matthews, 2008). Although the etiology of hot flashes and the mechanisms stimulating vasodilation remain unclear, most investigators implicate estrogen withdrawal or changing estrogen levels.

SWAN investigators are beginning to characterize the effects of changing estrogen levels on blood vessel structure and function by focusing on the relationship of the MT and associated physiological changes to heart disease risk. Thurston, Sutton-Tyrrell, et al. (2008) found that women who had hot flashes experience lower heart rate variability during hot flashes, suggesting that the parasympathetic nervous system, which helps influence the return to normal heart rate after a stressful experience, may function differently in women with hot flashes than in women who do not have hot flashes. SMWHS participants who experienced a cluster of symptoms including severe hot flashes had higher norepinephrine levels than those experiencing low severity symptoms (Woods, Cray, Herting, & Mitchell, 2012). Thurston, Sutton-Tyrrell, et al. (2008) also found that women who had hot flashes had less expansion of their arteries when blood flow is increased than did women without hot flashes. Others have linked hot flashes to calcification of the aorta as seen in heart disease (Thurston, Christie, & Matthews, 2010; Thurston, Kuller, Edmundowicz, & Matthews, 2010) and increased carotid intima media thickness among midlife women (Thurston, Sutton-Tyrrell, et al., 2011). Women with greater adiposity experience more severe hot flashes (Thurston, Sowers, Chang, et al., 2008; Thurston, Sowers, Sternfeld, et al., 2008; Thurston et al., 2009; Thurston, Santoro, & Matthews, 2011). When hot flashes are measured using physiological monitoring of skin conductance, women with a higher body mass index (BMI) and greater waist circumference had fewer hot flashes, but this was only among older women studied (Thurston, Santoro, & Matthews, 2011). Other evidence indicates that women who experienced hot flashes have higher levels of tissue plasminogen activator (tPA) and Factor VII than those without hot flashes (Thurston, Khoudary, et al., 2011). Taken together, these findings suggest that the role of hot flashes as a marker for subclinical heart disease is worthy of further investigation.

Hot flashes have been linked to both increased FSH and lower estrogen levels and to increased bone turnover during the MT. During the early and late stages of the MT, women with the most frequent hot flashes tended to have higher N-telopeptide levels, a marker of bone loss (Crandall et al., 2011). Moreover, lower estrogen levels as well as higher FSH levels have been associated with higher levels of interleukins (e.g., interleukin-1 beta [IL-1B]), linking both gonadotropins and estrogen to immune response as well as to hot flashes (Corwin & Cannon, 1999).

As Voda (1981) found, hot flashes may be barely noticeable or severe, resulting in a high degree of variability of the experience among women (Smith-DiJulio, Percival, Woods, Tao, & Mitchell, 2007). Thurston, Bromberger, et al. (2008) found that women who were most bothered by hot flashes were those with more negative affect, greater symptom sensitivity, sleep problems, poorer health, longer duration of hot flashes, and younger age and of African American race. Bother related to night sweats was associated with sleep problems and night sweats duration. Hot flashes are sufficiently bothersome to lead many women to seek health care during the MT (Williams et al., 2007, 2008).

Among participants in the SMWHS, hot flash severity increased for women in the late MT stage or early PM. Those who used hormone therapy had a longer duration of the early MT stage, were older at the time of their FMP, had higher levels of FSH, and had more severe hot flashes. Anxiety was also associated with hot flash severity. Older age at entry into the early MT stage and higher urinary estrogen (estrone) levels were associated with decreased hot flash severity. Psychosocial/mood (stress and depressed mood) and lifestyle variables (BMI, activity level, sleep amount, and alcohol use) were not associated with hot flash severity in this study (Smith-DiJulio et al., 2007). In contrast, in daily diary studies, women reported negative affect on the same day and the day after they reported hot flashes, suggesting that negative cognitive appraisal of hot flashes and perhaps other associated symptoms are linked to subsequent experiences of negative affect (Gibson, Thurston, Bromberger, Kamarck, & Matthews, 2011).

BMI (Gold et al., 2004), anxiety (Freeman et al., 2005, 2007), and lifestyle behaviors also have been associated with hot flash severity. As one example, women who smoked reported more severe hot flashes (Gold et al., 2004).

It remains unclear how long hot flashes persist (Woods & Mitchell, 2005). Barnabei et al. (2005) found that between 23% and 37% of participants in the Women's Health Initiative Study who were in their 60s and 11% to 20% in their 70s reported hot flashes. Some Melbourne Midlife Women's Health Project participants reported hot flashes for as long as 10 years after the FMP, although the average duration was 5 years (Col, Guthrie, Politi, & Dennerstein, 2009). Freeman, Sammel, and Sanders (2014) assessed hot flashes annually in 255 women who were followed for 16 years. They found the prevalence increased in each year before the FMP, reaching 46% in the first 2 years after FMP. Hot flashes decreased gradually during the PM and did not return to levels similar to those before the MT until after 9 years after the FMP. One third experienced moderate to severe hot flashes at 10 years or more during the PM. African American women and obese White women experienced a greater risk of hot flashes. Increasing FSH levels before the FMP, decreasing estradiol, and increasing anxiety increased the risk of hot flashes, and higher education levels reduced the risk (Freeman et al., 2014). Avis et al. (2015) reported that SWAN participants experienced a median duration of hot flashes (on more than 6 days in the previous 2 weeks) of 7.4 years. Based on nearly 900 women who experienced a FMP, the median post-FMP persistence was 4.5 years. Women who experienced hot flashes before the MT or in early perimenopause had the longest duration (median: more than 11.8 years), and post-FMP persistence was 9.4 years. Those who were postmenopausal when they first experienced hot flashes had the shortest duration (median: 3.4 years). African American women reported the longest duration of hot flashes compared with other racial/ethnic groups. Factors influencing duration of vasomotor

symptoms were younger age, less formal education, greater perceived stress, higher symptom sensitivity, and higher depressive and anxiety symptoms when hot flashes were first reported.

Analysis of the severity of hot flashes in the SMWHS population indicated an increase in women's age across the spectrum, from age 35 to 60 years. In addition, hot flash severity was associated with lower estrone and higher FSH levels and the late MT stage or early PM. Hot flash severity increased most from 2 years before to 1 year after FMP, declining 3 years after, and was highest during the late stage and all 5 years before FMP (Mitchell & Woods, 2015), consistent with the findings of the SWAN (Randolph et al., 2005) and Penn Ovarian Aging Study (Freeman et al., 2014; Freeman, Sammel, Lin, Liu, & Gracia, 2011). They are also consistent with the relationship between MT stages and PM as described by Freeman et al. (2011). Of interest is the declining severity of hot flashes seen in the SMWHS cohort after 2 years following the FMP. This finding suggests that as the PM progresses, the severity of hot flashes diminishes.

SLEEP SYMPTOMS

An estimated 30% to 45% of women experience disrupted sleep during the MT, with the prevalence of symptoms becoming higher during the late MT stage and early PM (Dennerstein, Lehert, Burger, & Guthrie, 2005). Women believe that awakening during the night is caused by hormonal changes and hot flashes (Woods & Mitchell, 1999) and that hot flashes are correlated with sleep disruption and estrogen levels (Woods et al., 2007), but evidence from a recent study indicates that often women awaken, then have a hot flash (Freedman & Roehrs, 2004).

Shaver was the first to study sleep during the perimenopause using polysomnographic methods in a sleep laboratory, discovering the relationship between sleep problems and ongoing stressful life events and anxiety (Shaver, Giblin, Lentz, & Lee, 1988; Shaver, Giblin, & Paulsen, 1991; Shaver, Johnston, Lentz, & Landis, 2001). Polysomnographic studies of sleep among women during the MT and PM that there was an increase in sleep disruption as women progressed to the PM, as well as psychological distress associated with subjectively experienced symptoms (Shaver et al., 1988; Shaver & Paulsen, 1993). Sleep symptoms have been associated with higher FSH levels during the late reproductive stage and to lower estradiol levels in women who were still cycling (Hollander et al., 2001), but these findings are not consistent across all studies (Woods et al., 2007). When women without hot flashes were monitored overnight, arousals that occurred were associated with sleep disordered breathing and age (Lukacs, Chilimigras, Cannon, Dormire, & Reame, 2004).

Recent findings from a study of relationships between symptoms related to MT and electroencephalogram (EEG) sleep measures indicate that hot flashes were associated with a longer sleep time. Women with higher anxiety symptoms had a longer sleep latency (took more time getting to sleep) and lower sleep efficiency only if they also had hot flashes. Hot flashes and mood symptoms were unrelated to either delta sleep ratio or rapid eye movement (REM) latency (Kravitz et al., 2011). In this same study, elevated beta EEG power in the nonrapid eye movement (NREM) and REM sleep in women during late perimenopause (late MT) and early PM exceeded levels in premenopause (late reproductive stage) and early perimenopause (early MT). Elevated beta EEG power indicated increased arousal and disturbed sleep quality during the late perimenopause (late MT) and early PM (Campbell et al., 2011). These study results suggest that sleep symptoms during the MT may be amenable to symptom management strategies that take into account women's experiences of arousal and their ability to regulate arousal as well as efforts to promote women's general health rather than focusing only on the MT as a causative factor.

Studies of self-reported hot flashes and sleep symptoms indicate that menopause-related factors may have effects on some, but not all, sleep symptoms. SMWHS participants who experienced more severe difficulty going to sleep had several other symptoms such as anxiety, hot flashes, depressed mood, and joint and back pain; reported more stress; were more likely to be in early PM; had a history of sexual abuse; rated their own health more poorly; had lower cortisol levels; and had greater caffeine and less alcohol intake than women who did not have this problem. Age, exercise, estrogen, and FSH were not related to difficulty getting to sleep. On the other hand, women who had more severe awakening during the night were older, more likely to be in the late MT stage or early PM, had higher FSH and lower estrogen (estrone) levels, and reported more severe hot flashes, depressed mood, anxiety, joint pain, backache, perceived stress, poorer overall health, less alcohol use, and history of sexual abuse. Women who had more severe problems with awakening early (and not getting back to sleep) were older; reported more severe hot flashes, depressed mood, anxiety, joint pain, backache, and perceived stress; rated their health more poorly; and had higher epinephrine and lower urinary estrogen levels. Exercise, MT stage, and alcohol use were not related to waking up early (Woods, Smith-DiJulio, & Mitchell, 2010). These findings are consistent with those of other contemporary studies (Ensrud et al., 2008; Kravitz et al., 2009; Pien, Sammel, Freeman, Lin, & DeBlasis, 2008).

Freeman et al. (2014) studied the sleep of participants in the Penn Ovarian Aging Study, who were followed for 16 years. They found that women's sleep before the MT predicted sleep around the time of the FMP: Those who had poor sleep before the MT were at 3.5 times the risk of having poor sleep around the time of the FMP, whereas those who had mild sleep problems were at 1.5 times the risk. There was no relationship of poor sleep and time relative to the FMP among women without poor sleep before the MT. Hot flashes contributed to poor sleep regardless of the sleep status of women before the MT.

Joffe, Crawford, et al. (2013) and Joffe, White, et al. (2013) induced hot flashes measured by skin conductance with a gonadatropin-releasing hormone (GnRH) agonist to determine whether hot flashes induced awakenings measured by polysomnography. The reported frequency of nighttime hot flashes was associated with recorded sleep disturbances, including increasing wake after sleep onset (WASO), awakenings, and early stage sleep. Nighttime hot flashes were also associated with perceptions of increased WASO, awakenings, and scores on the Insomnia Severity Index and Pittsburgh Sleep Quality Index and decreased perceived sleep efficiency. In addition, recorded hot flashes were associated with polysomnography-measured WASO. These findings suggest that hot flashes interrupt sleep during the conditions of the MT.

Recent data on chronic stress and sleep among SWAN participants indicate that women experiencing chronic stress over a period of up to 9 years reported lower subjective sleep quality and insomnia and exhibited increased WASO measured by polysomnography compared with women with low to moderate chronic stress profiles (Hall et al., 2015). These findings, taken together with the relationship between EEG measures of arousal and sleep disruption, suggest an important pathway linking cumulative stress experience and poor sleep during midlife.

DEPRESSED MOOD

Depressed mood symptoms are prevalent among midlife women, with 25% to 29% of women reporting depressed mood during the late MT stage and 23% to 34% during the early PM (Woods & Mitchell, 2005). In some studies, higher FSH and LH levels and increased variability of estradiol, FSH, and LH (within women) were associated with depressed mood symptoms (Freeman et al., 2004; Freeman, Sammel, Lin, & Nelson, 2006), as were lower levels of estradiol (Avis, Crawford, Stellato, & Longcope, 2001; Freeman et al., 2006) and DHEAS (Morrison, Have, Freeman, Sammel, & Grisso, 2001; Schmidt et al., 2002), but other studies show no relationship of depressed mood to endocrine levels (Woods et al., 2008).

Although some would suggest that the MT may be a period of vulnerability to depression, even for women who have no history of it earlier in life (Bromberger et al., 2001, 2003, 2004, 2007; Freeman et al., 2006; Woods et al., 2008), others argue that we are overpathologizing menopause by suggesting that menopause-related depression is a model of biologically induced depression (Judd et al., 2012). The literature about depressed mood in midlife women is complex, and studies use both indicators of depressed mood symptoms, such as the Center for Epidemiologic Studies Depression Scale (CESD) and measures of major depressive disorder, such as the Structured Clinical Interview for *DSM-5* Disorders (SCID). For this reason, it is important to distinguish the results of studies of depressed mood symptoms from those of major depressive disorder.

Studies of depressive symptoms indicate an increase in severity during the MT. Freeman et al. (2006) found that during the early MT stage, women were 1.5 times more likely to have high CESD scores and those in late transition stage were three times more likely to have high CESD scores than women who had not yet begun the MT. In addition, women with a history of depression were at twice the risk of reporting depressed mood during the MT, as were women who had severe premenstrual symptoms, poor sleep, and lack of employment. Those with a rapidly increasing FSH level were less likely to develop depressed mood. Participants in the SMWHS completed the CESD scale annually as a measure of depressed mood symptoms. Age was associated with slightly lower depressed mood (CESD) scores, but being in the late MT stage was associated with more severe depressed mood, although there was no effect of being in the early MT stage or early PM. Hot flash severity, life stress, family history of depression, history of postpartum blues, sexual abuse history, BMI, and use of antidepressants were also individually related to depressed mood. Neither FSH nor estrogen levels were related to depressed mood in this cohort (Woods et al., 2008; Woods, Mariella, & Mitchell, 2006; Woods & Mitchell, 1997b).

Several investigators have suggested that the MT may be a period of vulnerability to the first onset of depressed mood (Bromberger et al., 2007, 2010; Cohen et al., 2006; Freeman et al., 2006). Results of studies of depressed mood symptoms suggest that variability of hormonal levels (estrogen, FSH) and rate of change in FSH are related to depressed mood, although there is no evidence that estrogen levels, themselves are related (Avis, Crawford, et al., 2001; Avis, Stellato, et al., 2001; Avis, Brambilla, McKinlay, & Vass, 1994; Freeman et al., 2006). Although women in the late MT stage are vulnerable to depressed mood, factors that account for depressed mood earlier in the life span continue to have an important influence and should be considered in studies of etiology and therapeutics. Of interest is the potential relationship of androgens to depressed mood: Testosterone rise was associated with depressed mood in a subset of the SWAN study participants (Bromberger et al., 2010), and DHEAS was associated with depressed mood symptoms but not major depression in the Penn Ovarian Aging Study participants (Morrison, Freeman, Lin, & Sammel, 2011).

Bromberger et al. (2009, 2011) made an important distinction between studies of major depressive disorder and depressed mood symptoms, as well as between repeat versus first-onset depressive disorder, during the MT and early PM. Among SWAN participants who responded to a Structured Clinical Interview for *DSM-IV* Axis Disorders (SCID), those in the MT stages (perimenopause) compared with those who had not yet begun the MT or were in the early PM were two to four times more likely to experience a major depressive episode, even when prior depression history, upsetting life events, psychotropic medication use, hot flashes, and serum levels or changes in reproductive hormone levels were taken into account. It is of interest that many of the same predictors of depressive disorder at other parts of the life span were important. Indeed, using the Patient Health Questionnaire (PHQ) to measure depression or the Primary Care Evaluation of Mental Disorders (PRIME-MD), Freeman et al. (2006) found that 11% of the Penn Ovarian Aging Study cohort developed major depression over the 8 years of follow-up. Women in the MT were twice as likely to experience depression as those who had not yet begun the transition and greater variability of estradiol levels was a risk factor for new onset of diagnosed depressive disorder.

In contrast, when Bromberger et al. (2009) considered 266 SWAN participants who had *no* lifetime history of depression and assessed a new onset of depression based

on SCID interviews, she found that 42 (16%) met criteria for new-onset major depression. There was no association between becoming depressed and the MT stages based on either bleeding patterns or reproductive hormones. Instead, women experiencing low role functioning caused by physical health, low social functioning, and anxiety disorder were more likely to experience a first depressive episode during the MT.

Judd et al. (2012) conducted a systematic review of studies of depressed mood and depressive disorder to determine whether depression at the time of menopause might constitute a reproductive-related depressive disorder, the result of a biological response to hormonal change. She concluded there was not sufficient evidence to support depression during the MT as part of a distinctive diagnostic group of reproductive-related depressive disorders and cautioned instead that a more plausible explanation is a biopsychosociocultural model of the processes that may lead to a depressive disorder in midlife. Given the prevalence of depression, clinicians should be alert to the possibility of depression in all of their clinical encounters.

COGNITIVE SYMPTOMS

Women often notice cognitive symptoms such as forgetfulness or difficulty concentrating during midlife, but few rate them as serious, and most attribute these symptoms to changing hormones as well as general aging and life stress (Mitchell & Woods, 2001; Woods, Mitchell, & Adams, 2000). The SWAN reported stage-specific prevalence of forgetfulness ranging from 31% during the late reproductive stage to 42% in PM (Gold et al., 2000). SMWHS participants who experienced more severe difficulty concentrating were slightly older; reported more anxiety, depressed mood, nighttime awakening, perceived stress, and poorer perceived health; and were employed. The best predictors of forgetfulness included slightly older age, hot flashes, anxiety, depressed mood, awakening during the night, perceived stress, poorer perceived health, and history of sexual abuse. MT-related factors were not significantly associated with difficulty concentrating or forgetfulness. Considering women's ages and the context in which they experience the MT may be helpful in understanding women's experiences of cognitive symptoms (Mitchell & Woods, 2011).

Studies of functional changes in memory during the MT indicate that, aside from a period of slightly reduced learning during the MT, there are no significant changes in memory function during this period. The minor slowing of learning during the late MT stage disappears during the early PM (Greendale, 2009; Greendale et al., 2010; Luetters et al., 2007).

PAIN SYMPTOMS

Musculoskeletal and joint aches and pains are a commonly experienced symptom in midlife women (57% of the Melbourne study participants experienced them during the late MT and early PM; Dennerstein et al., 2000). Recent evidence suggests that pain symptoms are influenced by estrogen (Popescu, 2010). In the SMWHS, women experienced a significant increase in back pain during the early and late MT stages and early PM, but estrogen, FSH, and testosterone levels were unrelated to back pain (Mitchell & Woods, 2010). Perceived stress and lower overnight urinary cortisol levels were associated with more severe back pain; a history of sexual abuse and catecholamines did not have a significant effect. Those most troubled by symptoms of hot flashes, depressed mood, anxiety, nighttime awakening, and difficulty concentrating reported significantly greater back pain. Of the health-related factors, having worse perceived health, exercising more, using analgesics, and having a higher BMI were associated with more back pain, but alcohol use and smoking did not have significant effects. Having more formal education was associated with less back pain, but parenting, having a partner, and employment were unrelated. Age was associated with increased severity of joint pain, but MT-related factors, such as stage or hormone levels, were unrelated, as was anxiety. Symptoms of hot flashes, nighttime awakening, depressed mood, and difficulty concentrating were each significantly associated with joint pain, as was poorer perceived health, more exercise, higher BMI, and greater analgesic use. History of sexual abuse was the only stress-related factor significantly related to joint pain severity. Based on these findings (Mitchell & Woods, 2010), which are consistent with those of others (Dugan et al., 2006, 2009; Szoeke, Cicuttini, Guthrie, & Dennerstein, 2008), clinicians working with women traversing the MT should be aware that managing back and joint pain symptoms among midlife women requires consideration of their changing biology as well as their ongoing life challenges and health-related behaviors. Moreover, the relationship between pain and sleep symptoms, including sleep hygiene interventions, should be considered (Mitchell & Woods, 2010).

SEXUAL SYMPTOMS

Changes in sexual desire are troublesome to some women, and these changes become more pronounced in the late MT stage (Avis, Stellato, Crawford, Johannes, & Longcope, 2000; Dennerstein, Randolph, Taffe, Dudley, & Burger, 2002; Dennerstein & Lehert, 2004). Decreased sexual desire was negatively correlated with estradiol levels in one study (Woods et al., 2007), and lower sexual functioning scores in the Melbourne Midlife Women's Health Project were associated with higher FSH levels and lower estradiol levels (Dennerstein et al., 2002). Although there was no relationship with testosterone in the Melbourne study, participants in the Penn Ovarian Aging Study who experienced fluctuations in testosterone levels experienced more problems with sexual desire (Gracia et al., 2004). Painful intercourse (dyspareunia) has been associated with low estradiol levels (Avis et al., 2000), and vaginal dryness has been associated with higher FSH levels and lower testosterone levels (Woods et al., 2007). Vaginal dryness increases in frequency as women progress from the MT to PM; 21% of participants in the Melbourne study reported vaginal dryness during the late MT stage and 47% during early PM (Dennerstein et al., 2000).

SMWHS participants experienced a significant decrease in sexual desire during the late MT stage and early PM (Woods et al., 2010). Those with higher urinary estrone (E1G) and testosterone (T) reported significantly higher levels of sexual desire, whereas those with higher FSH levels reported significantly lower sexual desire. Women using hormone therapy also reported higher sexual desire. Those reporting higher perceived stress reported lower sexual desire, but history of sexual abuse did not have a significant effect. Those most troubled by symptoms of hot flashes, fatigue, depressed mood, anxiety, difficulty getting to sleep, early morning awakening, and awakening during the night also reported significantly lower sexual desire, but there was no effect of vaginal dryness, perhaps because of low prevalence in this cohort. Women with better perceived health reported higher sexual desire, and those reporting more exercise and more alcohol intake also reported greater sexual desire. Having a partner was associated with lower sexual desire. Women's sexual desire during the MT and early PM is related to both biology and the social situation in which she finds herself (Avis, Zhao, et al., 2005; Dennerstein, Lehert, & Burger, 2005; Gracia et al., 2004; Woods et al., 2010).

Longitudinal data about sexual functioning as women experience the MT indicate that the odds of vaginal or pelvic pain increased and sexual desire decreased by late perimenopause (approximation of late MT; Avis et al., 2009). Women used masturbation more frequently during early perimenopause (approximation of early MT) but less during PM. Health, psychological functioning, and the importance of sex were related to each of the sexual function outcomes (self-reports of importance of sex, frequency of sexual desire, arousal, masturbation, sexual intercourse, pain during intercourse, degree of emotional satisfaction, and physical pleasure). Age, race/ethnicity, marital status, change in relationship, and vaginal dryness were associated with sexual functioning. When other factors were considered, the MT was not associated with reported importance of sex, sexual arousal, frequency of sexual intercourse, emotional satisfaction with partner, or physical pleasure.

UI SYMPTOMS

UI symptoms are prevalent among women and appear to increase with age as well as during and after the MT. Approximately 47% of the Melbourne study participants reported being bothered by urinary leakage during the late MT and 53% during early PM (Dennerstein et al., 2000). U.S. data from the National Health and Nutrition Examination Survey (NHANES) indicated that the prevalence of stress urinary incontinence (SUI) peaks in the 50- to 59-year age group, urge urinary incontinence (UUI) peaks in women 80 years and older, and that mixed incontinence is associated with increasing age (Dooley et al., 2008).

Data from the SWAN revealed that nearly 47% of participants reported at least monthly UI at baseline when the cohort was an average age of 45.8 years and an average increase in incidence of 11% per year. The most prevalent type of UI was SUI: 7.6% of women experienced SUI at baseline, and this increased to 15.9% over the course of the study (Waetjen et al., 2007). African American and Hispanic women had the lowest incidence and Whites the highest. Although progression to early and late perimenopause (estimates of STRAW early and late MT stages) from premenopause (STRAW late reproductive stage) was associated with an increase in the incidence of any UI, the transition from the MT stages to PM resulted in a reduced incidence of newly reported UI (approximately half that observed in the late MT stage; Waetjen et al., 2009) Urge incontinence became more prevalent as women progressed to the late MT (Waetjen et al., 2008). Of interest is that estradiol, FSH, testosterone, and DHEA were unrelated to any type of incontinence in the SWAN participants (Waetjen et al., 2011).

Participants in the SMWHS who experienced SUI were more likely to perceive their health as poor, have a history of more than three live births, and were likely to be White. Those experiencing urge incontinence were older, perceived their health as worse, and had a BMI of 30 or higher (Mitchell & Woods, 2013). Women who experienced incontinence reported lower levels of self-esteem and mastery but did not report effects on mood, attitudes toward aging, and menopause on perceived health. MT stage, exercise, estrone, and FSH were not associated with either SUI or UUI (Woods & Mitchell, 2013). Clinicians working with midlife women who experience UI can be alert to the stigmatizing nature of this set of symptoms and to the erosion of self-esteem and sense of control associated with the symptoms.

VULVOVAGINAL SYMPTOMS

Women experience vaginal dryness symptoms as they progress through the MT. Melbourne Midlife Women's Health Project participants reported a progressively increasing prevalence of bothersome vaginal dryness: 3% of women in the reproductive age, 4% in the early MT, 21% in the late MT stage, and 47% who were 3 years PM. Findings from the SWAN cohort indicated women experienced vaginal dryness more frequently as they aged (Gold et al., 2000). Vaginal dryness has been associated with lower estrogen levels in the SMWHS cohort (unpublished data). Vaginal dryness may become more pronounced as women age, and for some, vulvovaginal changes may become bothersome. Some women may also experience vulvovaginal itching, irritation, and burning; vaginal discharge; bleeding after intercourse/penetration; and pain with penetration. Research on vulvovaginal symptoms is focusing on understanding vulvovaginal aging (sometimes referred to as *atrophy*), and some investigators are beginning to study groups of symptoms related to vulvovaginal aging, reflecting their effects on quality of life, including sexual function and interpersonal relationships.

In 2014, the North American Menopause Society and the International Society for the Study of Women's Sexual Health (ISSWSH) terminology consensus conference proposed using the term *genitourinary syndrome of menopause* (GSM), as it is a more accurate, all-encompassing, and publicly acceptable term than vulvovaginal atrophy. GSM is defined as a collection of symptoms and signs associated with a decrease in estrogen and other sex steroids and involving changes to the labia majora and minora, clitoris, vestibule and introitus, vagina, urethra, and bladder. The syndrome may include, but is not limited to, genital symptoms of dryness, burning, and irritation; sexual symptoms of lack of lubrication, discomfort or pain, and impaired function; and urinary symptoms of urgency, dysuria and recurrent urinary tract infections. Women may present with some or all of the signs and symptoms, which must be bothersome and should not be better accounted for by another diagnosis (Portman & Gass, 2014). Research to establish the syndrome versus clusters of symptoms is needed to guide treatment.

Interference With Daily Living and Symptoms

Women indicate that symptoms they experience during the MT and early PM interfere with many aspects of their daily lives (e.g., work, relationships with family and friends; Carpenter, 2001). SMWHS participants rated how they felt each day interfered with their ability to work and their relationships. Hot flashes, depressed mood, anxiety, sleep problems, cognitive and pain symptoms, and perceived health were related individually to work interference, but the most influential factors interfering with work were perceived health, stress levels, depressed mood, and difficulty concentrating. Age was not related to work interference. The most influential factors interfering with relationships were younger age, stress, depressed mood, and difficulty concentrating. MT stage did not affect either type of interference (Woods & Mitchell, 2011).

A Menopausal Syndrome?

Although many assume that there is a "menopausal syndrome" that affects women universally, Avis, Stellato, et al. (2001) found there was no evidence to support this assertion. Findings from the SWAN study revealed that there is no universal menopausal syndrome consisting of a variety of vasomotor and psychological symptoms. Instead, during the MT, women who used hormones and women who had surgical menopause reported more vasomotor symptoms but no more psychological symptoms than did their counterparts. White women reported more psychosomatic symptoms than other ethnic groups, and African American women reported more vasomotor symptoms than other ethnic groups in the SWAN study (Avis, Brockwell, & Colvin, 2005).

The relationships among symptoms any individual woman experiences are important for clinicians to consider. Mitchell and Woods (1996) found that the trajectory of groups of symptoms (e.g., vasomotor symptoms, dysphoric mood, sleep symptoms, and others) changed differently during the MT. The vasomotor symptoms were least reliable across multiple occasions, indicating they were most likely to change across the MT. Avis, Crawford, et al. (2001) and Avis, Stellato, et al. (2001) found that participants in the MWHS experienced multiple types of symptoms: Those who had hot flashes, night sweats, and trouble sleeping also had more depressed mood. Thus Avis proposed a "domino" hypothesis: Depressed mood occurs among women who have vasomotor symptoms and sleep problems related to their changing hormone levels. When the vasomotor and sleep symptoms are taken into account, Avis et al. found that estradiol had no effect on depressed mood.

Despite lack of evidence for a menopausal syndrome, it has become evident that women experience multiple symptoms, with some experiencing multiple severe symptoms. Moreover, researchers studying symptom have identified the importance of studying co-occurring symptoms, or symptom clusters, as a basis for identifying mechanisms that may be common to several symptoms or explain relationships among symptoms. As an example, Joffe and colleagues have found that induced, objectively recorded hot flashes influenced sleep efficiency, creating fragmentation and that perceived hot flashes were associated with perceived poor sleep quality (Joffe, Crawford, et al., 2013; Joffe, White, et al., 2013). In addition, investigators studying symptom clusters are concerned about identifying therapeutics that will maximize effects of an intervention on all or most symptoms and minimize the likelihood that a therapy will have positive effects on one symptom, but exacerbate others (Woods & Cray, 2013).

Cray, Woods, Herting, and Mitchell (2012) identified three clusters of symptoms that women in the SMWHS experienced during the MT and early PM. Among these were clusters of (a) low severity symptoms of all types (hot flashes, mood, sleep disruption, cognitive, pain, and tension symptoms), (b) moderately severe hot flashes with moderate levels of other symptoms, and (c) low-severity hot flashes with moderate levels of all other symptoms (Figure 9.5). The high hot flash cluster versus the low symptom severity cluster was associated with being in the late MT stage as well as with higher levels of FSH, lower levels of estrogen, and higher norepinephrine and lower epinephrine levels. The moderate

severity symptom cluster versus the low severity cluster was associated only with having lower epinephrine levels (Woods et al., 2014). A similar set of symptom clusters has been reported in the Menopause Strategies: Finding Lasting Answers for Symptoms and Health (Ms-FLASH) trial participants, who were selected for their experience of bothersome hot flashes (Woods et al., 2015).

In contrast to a symptom cluster, a syndrome is a pattern of symptoms that is presumably disease specific and results from a common underlying mechanism. It is likely that symptom clusters may be a more useful concept for clinicians caring for midlife women than a menopausal syndrome, which implies a disease. A careful history could elicit from women the symptoms they are experiencing and their impressions of which are related. Knowing the complement of symptoms may help clinicians suggest a tailored therapy regimen (e.g., one that is effective for both hot flashes and sleep disruption).

Symptoms and Culture

There is some evidence that symptoms women report during the MT and PM are a culture-bound phenomenon because women from cultures not influenced by Western medicine reported few symptoms or different symptoms than did Western women. For example, Lock, Kaufert, and Gilbert's (1988) work with Japanese women revealed that their most frequently reported symptom was shoulder pain, not hot flashes. Whether infrequent reporting of hot flashes by Japanese women may be attributable to the high phytoestrogen content in their diets or other features by which culture influences biology remains to be seen.

When considering the relationship of symptoms to the MT, it is important to consider the context in which they occur. Many women juggle multiple obligations for their families, such as parenting adolescent or young adult children, providing caregiving services for their elderly family members, being grandparents, and dealing with employment or the challenges of material stress. The participants in the SWAN study who have trouble paying for basics are at greater risk for nearly every kind of symptom (Gold et al., 2000). Viewing symptoms in the broader context of women's lives may help tailor therapies likely to be most efficacious.

Given the global nature of health care, it is important to focus on women's experiences of menopause in many parts of the world. Although a detailed review of the symptoms women experience around the globe is beyond the scope of this chapter, Sievert (2006) has led research culminating in identification of ways in which diverse populations of women experience menopause. Her work includes a biocultural model in which environment, culture, and biology intersect to influence the expression of symptoms such as hot flashes. Sievert notes that environment prompts consideration of the climate and altitude in which women live their lives and that culture warrants consideration of practices related to marriage, religion, attitudes, medicalization, hysterectomy practices, smoking, reproductive patterns, and diet. Finally, because different populations of the world have different genetic

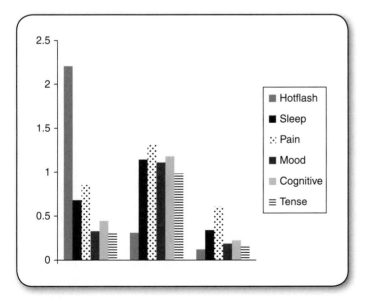

FIGURE 9.5
Symptom clusters during the menopausal transition and early postmenopause.

Adapted from Cray et al. (2012).

characteristics, they also may have differing hormone levels and sweating patterns. Thus variation across populations and the variation within populations of women are complex and together influence women's individual experiences. Indeed, Sievert points out that cross-country comparative studies illustrate the differences between cultures, whereas cross-cultural studies of menopause can facilitate understanding of women's place in society and the influence of social context on symptom experience (Sievert, 2013). In a comparison of symptom experiences across countries, women from different countries report some similar symptoms but may cluster their symptoms differently. For example, expression of somatic with emotional complaints varies across populations, possibly reflecting comfort with expression of emotional symptoms (Sievert & Obermeyer, 2012).

Stress and the MT

Given the nature of symptoms that women experience during the MT, one might ask whether the MT itself is stressful. We found that there was little change in perceived stress as women transitioned from the late reproductive stage to the early and late MT stages and PM. Instead, women who were employed and had a history of sexual abuse and depressed mood experienced greater stress. Those who experienced an improvement in the burdens associated with their roles, more social support, and more adequate incomes reported less stress. Those who appraised aging changes in their bodies as negative and perceived their health as poorer reported higher stress levels (Woods, Mitchell, Percival, & Smith-DiJulio, 2009).

A recent report of chronic stress and sleep in midlife women from the SWAN cohort indicated that upsetting life events assessed annually for up to 9 years were related to women's sleep. Using the Psychiatric Epidemiology Research Interview (PERI) Life Events Scale to assess life events across eight domains (school, work, romantic relationships, children, family, criminal and legal matters, finances, and health), investigators found that relative to women with low or moderate levels of chronic stress, those with high chronic stress had lower sleep quality (Pittsburgh Sleep Quality Index) and were more likely to report insomnia (Insomnia Symptom Questionnaire). They also exhibited increased WASO measured by polysomnography in the home. These results underscore the importance of the cumulation of stress across the life span (Hall et al., 2015).

Exposure to chronic stress appears related to symptom experience during this part of the life span. Clinicians working with women traversing the MT should remain vigilant to the social circumstances of women's lives, focusing on the social as well as endocrine features of this transition. Of interest is that when women who had participated in the SMWHS for 15 years were asked about the most challenging aspect of their lives during this period, only one said that it was the MT (Woods & Mitchell, unpublished).

Well-Being and the MT

Despite the symptoms and experiences of stress during this period, midlife women report high levels of well-being. Although estrone, FSH levels, and hot flash severity had no effect on well-being in the early transition stage, in the late MT stage, they predicted a decrease in well-being, but this decrease did not persist into early PM. The significant variability in women's well-being was affected more by life events and the personal resources available to meet transition demands, such as satisfaction with social support and feelings of mastery, than by the MT (Smith-DiJulio et al., 2008).

■ THE MT AND HEALTHY AGING

Metabolic Changes

Over the past three decades, research about menopause and midlife health has focused on the relationship of the MT to healthy aging, including studies linking dimensions of the MT to health outcomes through metabolic changes affecting bone, muscle, and fat. During the MT and early PM, women experience changes in body composition affecting both lean body mass (bone density and muscle mass) and fat deposition (subcutaneous and intra-abdominal).

Changing Bone

Bone loss accelerates in the late MT and continues in the early PM in both the spine and hip areas. For some women, the decrease in bone mass may progress to osteoporosis. Early studies of the SWAN cohort revealed that, in 2,311 African American and White women followed for 4 years, bone density varied across ethnic groups, with the highest bone mineral density (BMD) levels in African Americans and the lowest in Whites (Finkelstein et al., 2002; Sowers et al., 2003). Dual-energy x-ray absorptiometry testing indicated that, over the 4-year period, women lost 5.6% of the lumbar spine mass as they experienced the MT and PM. Women who experienced surgical menopause lost 3.9% of their bone mass, and those who were in the late MT stage lost 3.2% over 4 years. Serum FSH predicted the 4-year bone loss, with women who had FSH levels of more than 35 to 45 mIU/mL losing the most bone density. Estradiol levels of less than 35 pg/mL were associated with lower BMD, but testosterone, FAI, and DHEAS were not (Sowers et al., 2006).

After further follow-up of SWAN participants that included 5 years before and 5 years after the FMP, Greendale et al. (2012) described the time of onset and offset of BMD loss in relation to the timing of the FMP, age at FMP, BMI, and race/ethnicity in the multiethnic SWAN cohort. Bone loss began 1 year before and slowed 2 years after the FMP in the lumbar spine and femoral neck sites. Bone loss rates occurring between 2 and 5 years PM were lower than those observed from 1 year before to 2 years after the FMP. The cumulative 10-year bone loss was 10.6%, but the majority (7.4%) occurred during the period between 1 year before and 2 years after the FMP. Both greater BMI and African American ethnicity/race were related to lower bone loss, and Japanese or Chinese ancestry was related to higher bone loss rates. These findings provide important confirmation of a period of acute bone loss near the time of the FMP, as reported in earlier studies of smaller and less heterogeneous populations of women. It remains uncertain whether changes in the microarchitecture of bone during this period permanently damages bone (Greendale et al., 2012).

A recent analysis of SWAN data using estimates of bone strength instead of BMD calculated the compression, bending, and impact strength of bone. These, as well as C-reactive protein (CRP), a measure of inflammation, were associated with fracture risk (Ishii et al., 2013).

Muscle

In addition to bone, the fat and muscle components of body composition change with the MT. Sowers et al. (2003, 2006, 2007) assessed body composition in 543 SWAN participants, following them over 7 years by measuring waist circumference and body composition (fat and muscle) using biological impedance measures. Women experienced a 6-year decrease in skeletal muscle mass of approximately 0.23 kg and an absolute cumulative 6-year increase in fat mass of 3.4 kg. The absolute 6-year increase in waist circumference was 5.7 cm. FSH changes were positively correlated with fat mass change. Waist circumference increased until 1 year after the FMP, when it slowed. Fat mass continued to increase after the FMP, with no change in rate (Sowers et al., 2006).

Although most studies of body composition and physical function have involved older postmenopausal women, a recent study examining the contributions of body composition, physical activity, muscle capacity, and muscle quality to physical function performance in midlife women revealed relationships between optimal body composition (lower adiposity and higher lean body mass) and function. Ward-Ritacco, Adrian, Johnson, Rogers, and Evans (2014) assessed body composition using dual-energy x-ray absorptiometry, physical activity indicated by accelerometer (steps/day), and physical function using the Timed Up and Go test, 30-second chair stand test, and 6-minute walk test. Leg strength was measured by isokinetic dynamometry and leg power with the Nottingham Leg Extensor power rig. Muscle quality was calculated as the ratio of leg strength to upper leg lean mass and leg power to total body lean mass. Age and muscle quality (measured as a ratio of muscle power to mass of lower legs) predicted the results of the Timed Up and Go test, a test of speed and agility requiring women to stand from a chair without using their arms and walk 8 feet and return to a seated position. Age and muscle quality calculated with leg strength also predicted results of the chair stand test, a test of endurance estimated by the number of times women could arise from a seated position in 30 seconds. The number of medical conditions,

muscle quality, steps per day (physical activity indicator), and adiposity predicted the results of the timed walk test, a test of gait estimated by the distance covered in 6 minutes of walking. Women who had greater fat mass performed more poorly on the gait measure, although effects were not noted on the measures of endurance or speed and agility in the midlife women. Muscle quality was influential in tests of endurance, gait, and speed and agility. These findings support clinicians' attention to both muscle and fat mass in midlife women, given their potential functional consequences in midlife and old age.

The consequences of loss of skeletal muscle mass may include health outcomes during the postmenopausal period, such as development of sarcopenia, one component of frailty in older adults (Finkelstein et al., 2002; Sowers et al., 2003, 2006). Loss of muscle mass may lead to changes in physical functioning in postmenopausal women, as reflected by the measures of in hand grip, ability to move from a sitting to a standing position, velocity of walking, and perceived physical functioning. Moreover, greater losses have been observed in women with hysterectomy compared with those experiencing a natural menopause (Sowers et al., 2007). The role of muscle in glucose metabolism and physical functioning has not yet been characterized fully in longitudinal studies of the MT. To date, evidence about the influence of changing levels of endogenous estrogen and androgens on muscle function in women during the MT and early PM has not been available from human studies. Studies of frailty in older women in whom multiple low anabolic hormone levels (insulin-like growth factor [IGF-1], free testosterone, DHEAS) have been found, suggesting generalized endocrine dysfunction, emphasize the value of understanding the role of endocrine changes of the MT in the development of sarcopenia and frailty in old age (Cappola, Xue, & Frid, 2009). Physical inactivity, protein intake, and oxidative stress have also been linked to postmenopausal sarcopenia and are modifiable factors that clinicians can consider in promoting the health of midlife women (Maltais, Desroches, & Dionne, 2009).

McClure et al. (2014) examined the influence of inflammatory and hemostatic markers (CRP, plasminogen activator inhibitor type I [PAI-1], tPA, fibrinogen, and Factor VIIc) on physical functioning. They found that higher CRP and tPA were associated with greater limitations in physical functioning. African American women's higher fibrinogen levels were associated with greater physical functioning limitations. The relationship between hemostatic factors and cytokine levels may help account for inflammatory effects on muscle mass and strength.

In addition, El Khoudary et al. (2014) found that reduced estradiol or testosterone was associated with greater physical functioning decline. This is important given that changes in physical function may be a pathway to disability. Moreover, by age 56 to 66 years, nearly 50% of SWAN participant reported limitations in physical functioning, but these levels of function fluctuated, suggesting that interventions may be able to alter functioning levels. Ylitalo et al. (2013) found that higher BMI and arthritis were both associated with the prevalence and onset of limitations in physical functioning.

Fat

With the increasing prevalence of obesity in the United States, understanding changes in fat metabolism during midlife has become increasingly important. Sowers et al. (2007) found that women accumulate an average increase in fat mass of approximately 3.4 kg over a 6-year period. Changes in HPO hormones were related to changing fat metabolism. Increases in FSH have been associated with changes in levels of substances that regulate appetite, fat deposition, and inflammation. Increases of FSH were positively associated with leptin and adiponectin and negatively associated with ghrelin (Sowers, Wildman, et al., 2008).

SWAN data indicate that changes in sex hormones followed changes in waist circumference over a 9-year period during which women were experiencing the MT. Increased waist circumference was associated with subsequent lower SHBG levels, increased testosterone, and lower FSH. Estradiol levels were negatively associated with waist circumference in the early MT but positively associated with waist circumference during the late transition stage. Moreover, estradiol and waist circumference exhibited reciprocal effects. Waist circumference as a marker of weight predicted lower SHBG levels, possibly operating through adiposity-induced hyperglycemia, which may suppress SHBG. Hyperinsulinemia, hyperglycemia, and fatty liver are higher in the presence of greater abdominal fat, thus making it plausible that weight gain lowers SHBG by increasing insulin and glucose and/or by promoting hepatic fat accumulation. Taken together, these findings suggest that weight gain may set in motion endocrine changes during the MT and bear observation for the health promotion of midlife women (Wildman et al., 2012).

Metabolic Syndrome

As changes in both intraabdominal and subcutaneous fat mass occur, women experience changes in lipid patterns, glucose levels and insulin resistance, and thrombotic and inflammatory responses. Collectively, these have been characterized as the metabolic syndrome. As seen in Table 9.2, metabolic syndrome includes several risk

TABLE 9.2	Indicators of Metabolic Syndrome
Abdominal obesity (waist > 35 in)	
Atherogenic dyslipidemia, with triglycerides > 150 mg/dL, HDL < 50 mg/dL, and elevated LDL and small, dense LDL	
Hypertension B/P > 130/85 mmHg	
Fasting blood glucose > 110 mg/dL	
Insulin resistance and glucose intolerance	
Prothrombotic state	
Proinflammatory state	

HDL, high-density lipoprotein; LDL, low-density lipoprotein.

factors for cardiovascular disease (CVD). Many of these risk factors become more prevalent as women complete the MT. Changes in lipid patterns, glucose and insulin, thrombotic and inflammatory processes that compose the metabolic syndrome become more prevalent as women reach the late MT stage and PM.

There is mounting evidence linking endocrine changes during the MT to risk factors for heart disease, including the metabolic syndrome. Higher free androgen and lower SHBG levels are associated with cardiovascular risk factors for women during the MT. Recent evidence suggests that an increasing ratio of testosterone to estrogen is implicated in the development of metabolic syndrome. Women with low SHBG and FAI and high total testosterone at baseline experienced increased risk of metabolic syndrome over 5 years of follow-up. Both the baseline total testosterone:estradiol ratio and its rate of change were associated with the increased incident metabolic syndrome (Torrens et al., 2009).

Lipid Patterns

The SWAN study cohort experienced changing levels of lipids during the late stage of the MT and early PM, consistent with cross-sectional findings from an earlier study (Carr et al., 2000). Total cholesterol, low-density lipoprotein (LDL) cholesterol, trigylcerides, and lipoprotein(a) levels peaked during the late MT and early PM. High-density lipoprotein (HDL) cholesterol also peaked during this period (Derby et al., 2009). Greater increases in ghrelin levels (important in appetite regulation) over the MT were associated with increases in LDL cholesterol (Wildman et al., 2011).

Multiple hormonal changes during the MT and early PM have been implicated in changes in fat deposition and lipid metabolism. In SWAN participants, FSH was associated with increased total cholesterol and LDL cholesterol. Estradiol was associated with increased triglycerides, lower LDL, higher HDL, and higher testosterone was associated with greater BMI and higher triglyceride levels. SHBG was associated with lower waist circumference, BMI, total cholesterol, LDL, and HDL levels. FAI (a measure of bioavailable androgen) was associated with greater waist circumference, BMI, total cholesterol, and triglycerides (Sutton-Tyrell et al., 2005).

A recent report of SWAN data revealed that lower levels of estradiol and SHBG and higher levels of FAI were associated with a higher atherogenic profile of lipoproteins. El Khoudary et al. (2015) found that lower levels of estradiol and SHBG and higher levels of FAI were associated with multiple indicators of a more atherogenic profile of lipoprotein subclasses. Estradiol was negatively related to medium–small LDL particle concentration and positively to HDL particle sizes. SHBG was related negatively to small LDL particle concentration and positively to LDL and HDL particle sizes. FAI was associated negatively with large HDL particle concentration and HDL and LDL particle sizes. These results underscore the important relationship of endocrine metabolism and heart disease risk factors during the MT and PM.

Glucose and Insulin

In another longitudinal study of midlife women, increases in leptin over the MT were associated with greater glucose and insulin and with insulin resistance and also with greater diastolic blood pressure. Larger decreases in adiponectin over the MT were associated with greater increases in insulin and insulin resistance as well as increases in systolic blood pressure and greater decreases in HDL cholesterol (Wildman et al., 2008). FSH levels were associated with increased insulin resistance and lower insulin levels, and testosterone with higher glucose levels. SHBG was associated with lower insulin, glucose, and homeostatic measurement of insulin resistance (HOMA-IR) measures, and free androgen with greater insulin, glucose, and HOMA-IR levels (Sutton-Tyrell et al., 2005).

A report of data from the SWAN cohort indicates that bioavailable testosterone was associated with visceral fat, was a stronger predictor than estradiol, and was similar in effect to SHBG (Janssen et al., 2011). In addition, recent SWAN data implicate the effects of liver fat and insulin resistance in midlife women, indicating that the association between SHBG and insulin were greater among women who had fattier livers (Kavanagh et al., 2013). These data suggest that liver fat and SHBG both have important roles in metabolic risk among midlife women. In addition, cardiovascular fat has been examined in relation to MT status and endogenous sex hormones in the SWAN population. Women in the late MT had approximately 10% more epicardial adipose tissue, 21% more paracardial adipose tissue, and 12% more total heart adipose tissue than those in the late reproductive stage or early MT stages. Aortic perivascular adipose tissue was not associated with the MT stages. Lower estradiol levels were associated with greater paracardial adipose tissue and total heart adipose tissue, and women with the greatest reduction in estradiol had greater volumes of paracardial fat. The role of cardiovascular fat in heart disease during PM remains to be investigated (El Khoudary et al., 2015).

Thrombotic Changes

Studies of hemostatic factors and hormone levels during the MT revealed that both testosterone and estrogen play important roles. Androgens (testosterone and FAI) were positively associated with PAI-1 and tPA. FAI was positively associated with high-sensitivity C-reactive protein (hs-CRP). Lower SHBG levels, which were associated with greater levels of bioavailable testosterone, were also associated with higher levels of PAI-1, hs-CRP, and Factor VIIc (Sowers, Jannausch, et al., 2005). Androgens were strongly associated with fibrinolytic and inflammation markers, even when considering age, body size, smoking, and race/ethnicity in the SWAN cohort (Sowers, Jannausch, 2005; Sowers, Matthews, et al., 2005).

Estrogen was significantly related to some hemostatic factors in the SWAN cohort: Lower estradiol was associated with higher PAI-1 and tPA, but not with fibrinogen, Factor VIIc or hs-CRP. Elevated FSH was related to higher levels of PAI-1, factor VII levels and to lower fibrinogen and hs-CRP. Transitions to PM were not associated with different levels of hemostatic factors. It is possible that endogenous estrogens may be associated with lower CVD risk via fibrinolytic but not coagulation or inflammatory mechanisms (Wildman et al., 2008).

Inflammatory Responses

Changes in intra-abdominal fat metabolism during midlife have been associated with inflammatory markers and adipokines. An increase in intra-abdominal fat from premenopause to PM was correlated positively with the change in serum alpha-amylase (SAA), CRP, tPA, and leptin and negatively correlated with the change in adiponectin (Lee et al., 2009). These are each involved in regulation of fat metabolism, inflammation, and appetite. During the MT, women also experience changing levels of inflammatory markers, including IL-6.

A recent report indicates that there are between-group differences among women who have not yet begun the MT, women in the transition, and women in early and late PM. IL-4 was higher in late postmenopausal women, and IL-2 was higher in women in early PM, as was granulocyte-macrophage colony-stimulating factor (GM-CSF). Age was negatively related to IL-6, but the MT and PM were unrelated. Estradiol was negatively related to IL-6 levels and weakly negatively related to IL-2, IL-8, and GM-CSF (Yasui et al., 2007).

The consequences of changes in inflammatory markers for physical functioning are of interest, given the risk of disability in older women. Recently, McClure et al. (2014) reported that higher levels of tPA-antigen and hs-CRP were associated with subsequent reports of greater limitation in physical functioning in SWAN participants. These findings prompt further consideration of longitudinal changes in inflammatory and hemostatic markers that may help understand and prevent the development of mobility limitations and other types of disability in later life.

Blood Pressure

Changes in blood pressure are of concern because of their relationship to stroke. There is little evidence supporting an effect of the MT on blood pressure. The prevalence of hypertension among the SWAN cohort varies significantly by racial/ethnic group, with Whites, Blacks, Hispanics, Chinese, and Japanese women having respective prevalences of hypertension of 14.5%, 381.%, 27.6%, 12.8%, and 11.0% (Lloyd-Jones et al., 2005). Further research on the evolution of hypertension during the MT is warranted.

Adaptation to Stress

A final set of changes observed in relation to the MT is adaptation to stress. Studies of autonomic nervous system responses across the MT stages and PM have revealed differences in stress response when comparing premenopausal and postmenopausal women. Postmenopausal women exhibited greater increases in heart rate during all laboratory stressors compared with premenopausal women, with a pronounced increase during a speech task stressor deemed to be socially relevant to middle-aged women. Postmenopausal women exhibited greater increases in systolic blood pressure and epinephrine during the speech task, but not in response to other stressors (Saab, Matthews, Stoney, & McDonald, 1989). Subsequent experiments confirmed this effect and demonstrated that women receiving estrogen therapy had an attenuated stress response (Lindheim et al., 1992), but a more recent study with transdermal estrogen in postmenopausal women 52 to 56 years of age revealed that acute transdermal estrogen administration did not attenuate norepinphrine spillover or sympathetically mediate hemodynamic responses (Sofowora, Singh, He, Woods, & Stein, 2005). Recent findings relating chronic stress to sleep disruption in midlife women from the SWAN cohort suggest that increased physiologic arousal as indicated by beta EEG power may be involved (Campbell et al., 2011; Hall et al., 2015). Further research is needed to clarify the relationship of the MT to this marker of arousal and related health effects.

Data from the SWAN study have illuminated characteristics of women's lives that have multisystem, cumulative, burdensome effects on physiological dysregulation, termed *allostatic load*. Investigators modeled effects of race/ethnicity, discrimination, hostlility, socioeconomic status (SES), and perceived stress on allostatic load. They found racial and SES differentials in allostatic load in which African American women and women of lower SES had the highest allostatic load. In addition, among African American women, the indirect effects of increased discrimination and hostility were predictive of a higher allostatic load. For lower income women, the indirect effects of discrimination and hostility were predictive of greater allostatic load, and greater perceived stress was predictive of more rapid increases in allostatic load. For women with lower education, indirect effects through hostility were predictive of a greater allostatic load. These results illuminate complex ways in which race, SES, and psychosocial factors influence allostatic load, suggesting longer term health effects (Upchurch et al., 2015).

■ HEALTH PROMOTION FOR MIDLIFE WOMEN

Health promotion in midlife women includes promoting healthy behaviors to avoid disease plus early detection through regular screening for diseases, with early intervention as a goal. Healthy behaviors include the lifestyle elements of eating healthy foods, engaging in physical activity, and avoiding tobacco use and alcohol or if used at all, using them in moderation. The goal of adopting healthy behaviors is to prevent heart disease, cancer, diabetes, and a number of chronic diseases (Berg, Taylor, & Woods, 2015). The focus of this discussion is on general health-promoting behaviors

and age-appropriate screening practices. Discussion of health promotion and symptom management related to the MT can be found in Chapter 34.

Health-Promoting Behaviors

Health-promoting behaviors can reduce risk factors that play a significant role in disease development for midlife women. These health-promoting behaviors, considered primary prevention, target modifiable risk factors such as overweight and obesity, tobacco use, alcohol overuse, suboptimal nutrition, and sedentary lifestyle or physical inactivity (Stampfer, Hu, Manson, Rimm, & Willett, 2000). *Primordial prevention* is defined as healthy lifestyle behaviors that do not permit the appearance of risk factors. Most urgent among primordial prevention lifestyle habits that do not permit the appearance of risk factors is the lowering of the prevalence of obesity, as it affects blood pressure, lipid profiles, glucose metabolism, inflammation, and atherothrombotic disease progression. With primordial prevention of obesity, healthy eating and physical activity prevent the development of this important risk factor. Physical activity also improves risk factors and has the potential to lower heart rate (Kones, 2011). Of 84,129 midlife women participating in the Nurses' Health Study who had no diagnosis of CVD, cancer, or diabetes at baseline, those who scored in the low-risk range had fewer coronary events. A low-risk profile included women who did not smoke cigarettes, were within the normal weight range (BMI less than 25), maintained a healthy diet (low in transfat and glycemic load; high in cereal fiber, marine n-3 fatty acids, and folate, with a high ratio of polyunsaturated to saturated fats), exercised moderately or vigorously for half an hour a day, and consumed alcohol moderately. Women with this low-risk profile had an incidence of coronary events that was more than 80% lower than that in the rest of the population across the 14 years of follow-up (Stampfer et al., 2000).

Elements of a healthy lifestyle, as defined by the U.S. National Library of Medicine, National Institutes of Health (2013), include the following:

■ Do not smoke or use tobacco
■ Get plenty of exercise
  1. Women who need to lose or keep weight off need at least 60 to 90 minutes of moderate-intensity exercise on most days
  2. For health maintenance, women need at least 30 minutes of exercise a day, 5 days a week
■ Maintain a healthy weight: BMI between 18.5 and 24.9; waist less than 35 inches
■ Get screened and treated for depression if present
■ Women with high cholesterol or triglyceride levels may benefit from omega-3 fatty acid supplements
■ Limit alcohol consumption to no more than one drink per day

Healthy lifestyle behaviors can prevent heart disease, cancer, diabetes, and a number of chronic diseases (Berg et al., 2015).

Coronary Heart Disease

Heart disease is the leading cause of death among U.S. women (Roger et al., 2012). However, adults with low risk factors at midlife have a 70% to 80% lower risk of coronary heart disease (CHD) and CVD mortality (Kurth et al., 2006; Yusuf et al., 2004). Long-term observational studies have noted that an overall healthy lifestyle (prudent diet, not smoking, healthy weight, and physical activity) in midlife may prevent the development of CVD risk factors and CVD events (Chiuve et al., 2014). Health promotion related to reducing modifiable CHD risk factors includes reducing overweight and obesity, eliminating or controlling hypertension, reducing or eliminating dyslipidemia, reducing type 2 diabetes, avoiding tobacco use, and preventing stroke. It is of concern that, in the past two decades, adherence to a healthy lifestyle has deteriorated significantly (Kones, 2011).

OVERWEIGHT AND OBESITY

Disease burden associated with obesity has grown in proportion to the increasing weight of the U.S. population (Centers for Disease Control and Prevention [CDC], 2012). Women are advised to maintain their body weight to less than 25 kg/m^2 (Mosca et al., 2011). The prevalence of obesity increased from 28% to 36% from 1988 to 2006, the consumption of at least five portions of vegetables or fruits was nearly halved, and the level of physical activity also fell while alcohol consumption rose (Kones, 2011). Research findings consistently have identified that a healthy diet is higher in vegetables, fruits, whole grains, low-fat or nonfat dairy, seafood, legumes and nuts; moderate in alcohol; lower in red and processed meat; and low in sugar-sweetened foods and drinks and refined grains (Cespedes & Hu, 2015; U.S. Department of Agriculture [USDA], 2015). Eating a healthy diet is therefore an important aspect of health promotion related to reducing or eliminating overweight and obesity, which can reduce the incidence of CHD and its risk factors as well as type 2 diabetes.

Physical activity has a positive effect on overweight and obesity, producing caloric consumption and regulation of adipose and pancreatic function. Additionally, exercise or physical work improves the capillary system and oxygen supply to the brain, thus enhancing metabolic activity, neuron oxygenation, and neurotropin levels and resistance to stress (Chedraui & Perez-Lopez, 2013; Kaliman et al., 2011). Any health promotion related to reducing overweight and obesity risk factors must include a component of physical activity. The American Heart Association (AHA; 2014a) recommends:

- At least 30 minutes of moderate-intensity aerobic activity at least 5 days per week for a total of 150 minutes
- *Or* at least 25 minutes of vigorous aerobic activity at least 3 days per week for a total of 75 minutes; or a combination of moderate- and vigorous-intensity aerobic activity
- *And* moderate- to high-intensity muscle-strengthening activity at least 2 days per week for additional health benefits (AHA, 2014a, 2014b)

HYPERTENSION

Health promotion related to reducing hypertension, according to the CDC (2013), includes (a) following a health care provider's prescription for medication use; (b) eating a healthy diet low in salt, total and saturated fat, and cholesterol but high in fresh fruits and vegetables; (c) taking a brisk walk three times per day at least 5 days per week; (d) eliminating smoking, and if smoking, quitting as soon as possible. The optimum blood pressure is less than 120/80 mmHg, and guidelines recommend pharmacological treatment of blood pressure of 140/90 mmHg or higher in adults younger than than 60 years. For adults at least 60 years of age, there is strong evidence to support treating hypertension to a goal of less than 150/90 mmHg (James et al., 2014; Mosca et al., 2011). Selecting a diet consistent with current dietary guidelines lowers blood pressure and lipids, which is expected to reduce the risk of CVD in healthy middle-aged and older men and women by one third (Reidlinger et al., 2015).

DYSLIPIDEMIA

Higher-than-normal cholesterol levels can lead to CVD, and lowering cholesterol can reduce women's risk of heart disease and stroke. Health promotion related to lowering cholesterol includes encouraging midlife women to take responsibility for diet management. According to the CDC (2015), eating foods low in saturated fats, trans fats, and cholesterol plus eating foods high in fiber, monounsaturated fats, and polyunsaturated fats can prevent high levels of LDL cholesterol and triglycerides while increasing HDL cholesterol levels. Specific recommendations are:

- Eat less saturated fats from animal products (cheese, fatty meats, and dairy desserts) and tropical oils (such as palm oil)
- Avoid trans fats, which are often found in baked goods (cookies, cakes), snack foods (such as microwave popcorn), fried foods, and margarines
- Limit foods high in cholesterol, including fatty meats and organ meat (liver, kidney)
- Choose low-fat or fat-free milk, cheese, and yogurt
- Eat more foods high in fiber, such as oatmeal, oat bran, beans, and lentils
- Eat a heart-healthy diet that includes more fruits and vegetables and foods low in salt and sugar

Additional health promotion related to lowering cholesterol levels is to exercise at a moderate intensity for at least 2.5 hours each week or get 1.25 hours of vigorous or high-intensity physical activity each week. This can lower LDL and raise HDL. Furthermore, those prescribed cholesterol-lowering medication should take it as prescribed (U.S. Department of Health and Human Services [USDHHS], Office on Women's Health, 2013).

TYPE 2 DIABETES

Type 2 diabetes results from the body's ineffective use of insulin, and more than 90% of people with diabetes worldwide have this form of the disease (World Health Organization

[WHO], 2015). According to the WHO (2015), diabetes can damage the heart, blood vessels, eyes, kidneys, and nerves, resulting in (a) an increased risk of heart disease and stroke (Morrish, Wang, Stevens, Fuller, & Keen, 2001); (b) combined with reduced blood flow, increased nerve damage (neuropathy) in the feet and increased risk of foot ulcers, infection, and possible eventual limb amputation; (c) increased diabetic retinopathy, an important cause of blindness as a result of long-term damage to the small blood vessels in the retina (WHO, 2012); (d) kidney failure (WHO, 2011); and (e) doubled overall risk of dying compared with peers without diabetes (Roglic et al., 2005).

The prevention of type 2 diabetes involves simple lifestyle measures (WHO, 2015):

■ Achieve and maintain a healthy body weight
■ Avoid physical inactivity—get at least 30 minutes of regular, moderate-intensity activity on most days. More physical activity is required for weight control
■ Eat a healthy diet of between three and five servings of fruits and vegetables each day and reduce sugar and saturated fat intake
■ Avoid tobacco use—smoking increases the risk of CVD

Observational studies found that a healthy lifestyle (regular physical activity, moderate alcohol consumption, not smoking, healthy diet, and normal weight range) greatly reduced the risk of developing type 2 diabetes (Glauber & Karnieli, 2013). According to the U.S. Diabetes Prevention Program, the strongest predictor of type 2 diabetes prevention was weight loss. The risk of diabetes was 16% lower for every kilogram of weight lost (Knowler et al., 2009).

TOBACCO AVOIDANCE

Smoking is a major cause of CHD, with the risk associated with number of cigarettes smoked and the duration of smoking. According to the American Lung Association (2013), the gap between men's and women's smoking rates is getting smaller, with the result that women now experience a larger burden of smoking-related diseases than before. Chronic obstructive pulmonary disease (COPD) is more prevalent in smokers, who are almost 13 times more likely to die from it compared with those who have never smoked (USDHHS, 2004). Research has identified that smoking is directly responsible for 80% of lung cancer deaths in women each year, and alarmingly, lung cancer surpassed breast cancer as the leading cause of cancer deaths among women in the United States (USDHHS, 2004).

The major health promotion element for reducing risks associated with smoking is to stop smoking. Many venues, including counseling, nicotine replacement, and pharmacological therapies, are available to help women stop smoking (Turk, Tuite, & Burke, 2009).

STROKE PREVENTION

Stroke is the second leading cause of death worldwide in persons 15 years of age and older (Strong, Mathers, & Bonita, 2007). Stroke cased 5.7 million deaths worldwide in 2005 (Rosamond et al., 2008). The direct and indirect cost of stroke in the United States in 2008 was estimated at \$65.5 billion. It is anticipated that worldwide deaths caused by stroke will rise to 6.5 million in 2015 and 7.8 million in 2030 (Strong, et al., 2007). Stroke is preventable by engaging in healthy lifestyle factors (Chiuve et al., 2014). In addition to healthy lifestyle implementation, the U.S. Preventive Services Task Force (USPSTF, 2009) recommends women aged 55 to 79 years take approximately 75 mg of aspirin per day when the net benefit of ischemic stroke reduction outweighs the increase in risk of gastrointestinal hemorrhage.

STRESS REDUCTION

A common definition of *stress* is when the demands of the stressor threaten to exceed the resources of the individual (Lazarus & Folkman, 1984). Stress has been identified as a major influence upon mood, well-being, behavior, and health. Long-term unremitting stressors can damage health. The relationship between psychosocial stressors and disease is affected by the nature, number, and persistence of stressors as well as by the individual's biological vulnerability (genetics, other constitutional factors), psychosocial resources, and learned patterns of coping (Schneiderman, Ironson, & Siegel, 2005).

Ten healthy habits that can protect from the harmful effects of stress have been recommended by the American Heart Association (2014b). These recommendations include the following: talk with family and friends, engage in daily physical activity, embrace the things you are able to change, remember to laugh, give up bad habits (drink alcohol in moderation, do not smoke), slow down, get enough sleep, get organized, practice giving back, and try not to worry. Incorporating these recommendations and adopting a healthy lifestyle, especially physical activity,—can assist individuals in managing stress more effectively.

Osteoporosis

Osteoporosis is characterized by low bone mass and deterioration of structural bone tissue in aging adults. Women are four times more likely to develop osteoporosis than men (National Osteoporosis Foundation [NOF], 2013). The WHO first convened a group of experts in 1994 to assess fracture risk and its application to screening for postmenopausal osteoporosis. It was this group that first defined osteoporosis using a standardized score, known as a *T-score*, that compared BMD to average values for healthy young women. Categories for diagnosis of osteoporosis based on T-scores are normal (T-score: –1.0 and greater); low bone mass, called *osteopenia* (T-score: between –1.0 and –2.5); osteoporosis (T-score: –2.5 and below; and severe osteoporosis (T-score: –2.5 and below with a history of fracture) (4BoneHealth, 2015). Revised recommendations in 2004 included BMD plus selected risk factors for fracture along with height and weight. A Fracture Risk Assessment Score (FRAX) is calculated to determine a 10-year probability of fracture and is given in two scores: probability of hip fracture and probability for a major osteoporotic fracture, defined as wrist, shoulder, hip, or painful spine fractures (4BoneHealth, 2015).

According to the National Osteoporosis Foundation (2013), 80% of the estimated 10 million Americans with osteoporosis are women. One in two women older than 50 years will break a bone because of osteoporosis. This is attributed to the facts that women tend to have smaller, thinner bones than men and that estrogen decreases sharply when women reach menopause, which can cause bone loss. Approximately 20% of White and Asian American women aged 50 years and older, 10% of Latinas, and 5% of African American women older than 50 years have osteoporosis.

Osteoporosis is a largely preventable disease (Benjamin, 2010). The main controllable determinants of bone health are nutrition, physical activity, weight, smoking cessation, heavy alcohol avoidance, and fall prevention (USDHHS, 2004). The 2004 Surgeon General's Report on Bone Health and Osteoporosis proposed the following seven lifestyle approaches to bone health:

- Eat a well-balanced diet containing the following each day: 6 to 11 servings of grains; three to five servings of vegetables; two to four servings of fruits; two to three servings of dairy or other calcium-rich foods; and two to three servings of meat or beans
- Get adequate calcium intake
- Get recommended intake of vitamin D. Most individuals need 200 IU/d; individuals aged 50 to 70 years need 400 IU/d; and individuals older than 70 years need 600 IU/d. Sunlight and dietary sources of vitamin D are recommended
- Get at least 30 minutes of weight-bearing exercise every day (high impact: stair-climbing, hiking, dancing, jogging, downhill and cross-country skiing, aerobic dancing, volleyball, basketball, gymnastics, weight lifting or resistance training; low-impact weight bearing: walking, treadmill walking, cross-country ski machines, stair-step machines, rowing machines, water aerobics, deep-water walking, low-impact aerobics; nonweight-bearing: lap swimming, indoor cycling, stretching or flexibility exercises, yoga, pilates)
- Maintain a healthy body weight
- Avoid smoking
- Drink alcohol in moderation (for women, one drink per day)

It is also important that midlife women prevent falls. Recommended actions for avoiding falls include (a) exercise regularly, (b) make your home safe (remove things you can trip over, remove small rugs or use tape to keep them from slipping, keep items you frequently use in easy-to-reach cabinets, put grab bars next to your toilet and in the tub and shower, use nonslip mats in the bathtub and on the shower floor, improve lighting in your home, have handrails and lights put in all staircases, wear shoes that give good support and avoid wearing slippers or athletic shoes with deep treads), (c) renew your medicines, and (d) have your vision checked. By implementing these basic recommendations, women will promote their bone health by reducing their risk of falls (CDC, 2004).

Cancer

Cancer cannot be prevented completely, but there are ways to reduce risk. Modifiable risk reduction for breast, cervical, ovarian, and lung cancer has many elements in common. Commonalities include limiting alcohol, being physically active, maintaining a healthy body weight, never smoking or stopping smoking, following recommended dietary guidelines for healthy living, and obtaining recommended screening (Canadian Cancer Society, 2013). Breast and ovarian cancers have additional health-promotion options for women who carry one of the BRCA gene mutations: chemoprevention in the form of selective estrogen-receptor modulators (SERMs) or prophylactic surgery (bilateral mastectomy, bilateral oophorectomy). According to the Canadian Cancer Society (2013), prophylactic mastectomy results in a 90% decrease in breast cancer risk in these high-risk women, and prophylactic oophorectomy can decrease the risk of breast cancer as well as risk of ovarian cancer. Risk reduction and health promotion for midlife women related to cervical cancer is to follow guidelines for Pap smear screening and to adopt lifestyle changes, such as using safer sex practices, stopping smoking, and getting vaccinated when appropriate (American Cancer Society, 2013). Lung cancer risk can be reduced: Do not smoke, stop smoking if you do smoke, avoid secondhand smoke, test your home for radon, avoid carcinogens at work (exposure to toxic chemicals, wear a face mask for protection if toxins do exist), eat a diet full of fruits and vegetables, and exercise most days of the week (Mayo Clinic, 2015).

Depression and Anxiety

The cause of depression and anxiety disorders is not completely clear, but it is known that both are more common in women (National Institute for Mental Health [NIMH], 2013a). Both disorders are thought to be triggered by stressful life events and/or ongoing stressful social conditions. However, there may also be biological, genetic, and psychosocial factors (hormonal balance, brain chemistry, socioeconomic issues, lack of support network, diet, premorbid medical conditions, cognition, personality, and gender; USDHHS, 1999). Often, depression and anxiety occur together, as approximately one half of those diagnosed with a major depression have a coexisting anxiety disorder (USDHHS, 1999). Major depressive disorder is one of the most common mental disorders in the United States, and women are 70% more likely than men to be diagnosed with depression in their lifetime. Depression and anxiety are a leading and increasing cause of disability worldwide, especially for women (Griffiths et al., 2014).

Major risk factors for depression in midlife women include family or personal history of depression, history of postpartum depression, history of or current anxiety disorder, and alcohol and other substance abuse or dependence. Depression may occur concomitantly or as a result of other serious medical illnesses such as heart disease, stroke, cancer, HIV/AIDS, diabetes, or Parkinson's disease (NIMH, 2013b). Many of the risk factors are not modifiable unless associated with lifestyle, such as physical inactivity and obesity, smoking, and intimate partner violence. Savoy and Penckofer (2015) noted that depressive symptoms are an independent risk factor of CVD and they may also negatively affect health-promoting lifestyle behaviors and quality of life in women. Therefore early detection and treatment are key. Signs and symptoms of depression include persistent sad, anxious, or "empty" feelings; feelings of hopelessness or pessimism; feelings of guilt, worthlessness, or helplessness; irritability, restlessness; loss of interest in activities once found pleasurable; fatigue and decreased energy; difficulty concentrating; insomnia, early-morning wakefulness, or excessive sleeping; overeating or appetite loss; thoughts of suicide or suicide attempts; and aches or pains, headaches, cramps, or digestive problems that do not decrease even with treatment (NIMH, 2013b).

Anxiety is often a normal reaction to stress and can be beneficial. When it becomes excessive, the individual may find that the anxiety is not controllable and that it may have negative effects on daily living (NIMH, 2013c). It is known that anxiety disorders and all other mental illnesses are complex and are likely a result of genetic, environmental, psychological, and developmental factors (NIMH, 2013c). Women are 60% more likely to experience an anxiety disorder in their lifetime compared with men. Generalized anxiety is not likely to be related to a specific stressful event. Anxiety disorders commonly occur with other mental or physical illness, including alcohol or substance abuse, and these might mask anxiety symptoms and sometimes heighten them (NIMH, 2013c). There is no specific risk reduction applicable; however, early diagnosis and treatment are key. General lifestyle health promotion, such as optimal diet and nutrition and physical activity, may positively affect anxiety disorders.

Recently, purpose in life has been linked with better mental and physical health. For example, in a nationally representative study of U.S. adults older than 50 years, a higher purpose in life was associated with a higher likelihood of use of preventive health care services (Kim, Strecher, & Ryff, 2014). Several promising interventions have demonstrated that purpose, along with facets of psychological well-being, can be improved (Davidson & McEwen, 2012; Ryff, 2014). Ryff (2014) reviewed a dozen psychiatric intervention studies using cognitive behavioral therapy, meditation, or emotional disclosure and found these all enhance facets of well-being. As people with a higher purpose in life use more preventive health services, it is likely that they will have less of a negative effect on the cost of health care. It would seem prudent to add improving purpose in life to health promotion related to both depression and anxiety disorders.

In a sample of 48,273 Finnish women with a mean age of 45.6 years, physical activity provided a protective effect for later mental health in women. The study suggests that increasing physical activity levels may be beneficial in terms of mental health among midlife and older women (Griffiths et al., 2014).

There are many commonalities in health promotion for disease prevention. Most commonly, experts recommend a healthy lifestyle, as well as primary prevention for diseases that have modifiable risk factors, as primordial. It would be prudent for clinicians to recommend all elements of a healthy lifestyle to their patients and particularly to midlife

women who are more vulnerable to the onset of chronic disease than younger women. In this way, morbidity may be averted or ameliorated.

Health Screening

Health screening is defined as the use of a test or series of tests to detect health risks or preclinical disease in healthy individuals. The purpose is to permit prevention and early intervention (Dans, Silvestre, & Dans, 2011). Health screening is not limited to conducting screening tests, such as Pap smears. Instead, screening must include obtaining personal and family data to determine risk factors, performing a physical examination, and finally conducting screening tests. It should be noted that screening tests do not determine disease presence, and a single test is rarely sufficient to establish a diagnosis (Dans et al., 2011). Often at least two tests in sequence (screening followed by a confirmatory test) are necessary to determine a diagnosis. This approach is practical and generally more economical than using confirmatory tests for screening purposes, as confirmatory tests are usually more accurate but also more expensive. Screening coupled with personal and family history and physical examination data can uncover unrecognized health risks, such as preclinical diabetes, and disease in an asymptomatic stage, such as breast cancer (Dans et al., 2011).

Health screening has been a widely accepted practice in health care, and proponents of screening programs emphasize the potential for early disease detection or assistance in changing unhealthy lifestyles (Hackl, Halla, Hummer, & Pruckner, 2015). However, screening is known to increase health care costs, which may underlie policy decisions to reduce health screening or eliminate it altogether. Recent debate in the literature has raised the issue of potential physical and psychological harm to healthy individuals from health screening and confirmatory testing (Ilic, O'Connor, Green, & Wilt, 2006; Sabbath & Indik, 2006). An example of physical harm is pain or bruising related to a blood draw. Psychological harm usually occurs when an individual tests positive for the condition being screened for, such as a positive finding on mammogram, when being screened for breast cancer (Brewer, Salz, & Lillie, 2007). Confirmatory testing can also cause physical or psychological harm. Therefore it is prudent to weigh the risks and benefits of health screening. Dans et al. (2011) developed the following criteria for evaluating screening strategies: (a) The burden of illness must be high, (b) the tests must be accurate, (c) early treatment should be more effective than late treatment, (d) tests and early treatment must be safe, and (e) the cost of the screening strategy must be justified by the potential benefit. Health care providers would best discuss these issues with their patients and come to a mutual decision about available screening tests.

Despite issues related to health care costs and potential physical or emotional harm, health screening is still considered a valued aspect of health promotion and maintenance. To that end, a number of organizations have made recommendations related to health screening for midlife women (American Academy of Family Physicians: http:www.aafp.org; USPSTF: www.uspreventiveservicestaskforce.org;

TABLE 9.3 | Health Screening Recommendations for Women by the AAFP, USPSTF, HHS, ACOG, and CDC

SCREENING TARGET	AAFP	USPSTF	HHS	ACOG	CDC
Overweight, obesity, and diet/nutrition	Annually; CAV	Screen all adults NRSI	Same as USPSTF	BMI each visit	NRSI
Physical activity	CAV	CAV	CAV	CAV	CAV
Tobacco and alcohol use	CAV	CAV	CAV	CAV	CAV
Depression					
Intimate partner violence	CAV	CAV	CAV	CAV	CAV
Diabetes	Same as USPSTF plus recommendations from American Diabetes Association: all adults 45+ years; all adults with BMI ≥ 25 kg/m^2 and one of following additional risk factors: physical inactivity, first-degree relative with diabetes, high-risk race or ethnicity (Black, Hispanic, Native American, Asian American, Pacific Islander), delivered baby > 9 lb or history of gestational diabetes, high-density lipoprotein cholesterol < 35 mg/dL or triglyceride level > 150 mg/dL, polycystic ovary syndrome, hemoglobin A$_{1c}$ level > 5.7%, impaired glucose tolerance or fasting glucose previously, conditions associated with insulin resistance (obesity, acanthosis nigricans), or history of cardiovascular disease. If results normal, repeat screening in 3 years. Repeat yearly screening if prediabetes, and consider more frequent screening, depending on risk status	Asymptomatic adults with sustained blood pressure (treated or untreated) > 135/80 mm Hg; insufficient evidence to recommend for or against screening adults with blood pressure ≤ 135/80 mmHg. Optimal screening interval is unknown			
Sexually transmitted infections					
CHD: hypertension	CAV	CAV	CAV	CAV	CAV
CHD: dyslipidemia	Same as USPSTF	Screen women 45+ years if at increased risk of CHD; NRSI			
Osteoporosis	Same as USPSTF	Women age 65+ years: DEXA screening Women younger than 65 years: Use WHO Fracture Risk Assessment Tool to risk-stratify	Age 65+ years get DEXA; age 50–65 years ask clinician if bone density test is needed		

(continued)

181

SCREENING TARGET	AAFP	USPSTF	HHS	ACOG	CDC
Cancer: breast	Same as USPSTF	Women age 40–49 years: provider/patient decision; biennial mammography screening beginning at 50 years with insufficient evidence to determine risk/benefit after age 75 years Advise against teaching breast self-examination; insufficient evidence to assess additional benefits/harms of clinical breast examinations in women 40 years and older	Same as USPSTF	Begin annual mammography at age 40 years; clinical breast examinations annually at age 40 years and older	Same as USPSTF
Cancer: ovarian	Routine screening not recommended	Against routine screening			No screening recommendations. Discuss symptoms with clinician
Cancer: cervical	Same as USPSTF	Screen women age 21–65 years with Pap smear q 3 years or, for women 30–65 years who want to lengthen screening interval, screen with combination of Pap smear and human papillomavirus testing q 5 years; recommends against screening in women older than 65 years who have adequate prior screening and are not at high risk; recommends against screening women who have had hysterectomy with removal of cervix and who have no history of a high-grade precancerous lesion		Same as USPSTF	Same as USPSTF
Cancer: colorectal	Same as USPSTF	Screen adults 50–75 years: annual fecal occult blood test; sigmoidoscopy q 5 years plus fecal occult blood q 3 years; colonoscopy q 10 years—all acceptable			Same as USPSTF
Cancer: lung		Age 55–80 years with history of smoking: annual screening with LDCT with 30 pack-year smoking history and currently smoke or have quit within past 15 years; Discontinue when person has not smoked for 15 years or develops health problem that limits life expectancy or ability/willingness to have curative lung surgery			Same as USPSTF

AAFP, American Academy of Family Physicians; ACOG, American College of Obstetricians and Gynecologists; BMI, body mass index; CAV, by convention, screen at all visits; CDC, Centers for Disease Control and Prevention; CHD, coronary heart disease; DEXA, dual-energy x-ray absorptiometry; HHS, U.S. Department of Health and Human Services; LDCT, low-dose computed tomography; q, every; NRSI, no recommendation for screening interval; USPSTF, U.S. Preventive Services Task Force.

Sources: American Diabetes Association (2012), Centers for Disease Control and Prevention (2014a), Centers for Disease Control and Prevention, Division of Cancer Prevention and Control (2014b), http://healthfinder.gov/HealthTopics/Category/doctor-visits/screening-tests/get-your-blood-pressure-checked; http://healthfinder.gov/HealthTopics/Category/ health-conditions-and-diseases/heart-health/drink-alcohol-only-in-moderation; http://rethinkingdrinking.niaaa.nih.gov/IsYourDrinkingpatternRisky/WhatsYourPattern.asp; http://www.healthfinder.gov/ HealthTopics/Category/nutrition-and-physical-activity; http://www.smokefree.gov; Leawood (2003), Moyer (2012), Riley, Dobson, Jones, and Kirst (2013), U.S. Department of Health and Human Services: health-finder.gov (2015), U.S. Preventive Services Task Force (2003, 2015a, 2015b, 2015c).

USDHHS: www.hhs.gov; American College of Obstetricians and Gynecologists: www.acog.org; and CDC: www.cdc .gov). Listed in the following are recommendations for screening midlife women on overweight, obesity, diet and nutrition, physical activity, tobacco and alcohol use, depression, intimate partner violence, diabetes, sexually transmitted infections (including HIV), CHD (hypertension, dyslipidemia), osteoporosis, and cancer (breast, ovarian, cervical, colorectal, and lung). Table 9.3 details recommendations for screening by these organizations. Blank cells in the table occur where organizations have made no specific screening recommendation.

■ REFERENCES

4BoneHealth. (2015). World Health Organization: WHO criteria for diagnosis of osteoporosis. Retrieved from http://www.4bonehealth .org

Adler, S., Fosket, J., Kagawa-Singer, M., McGraw, S., Wong-Kim, E., Gold, E., & Sternfeld, B. (2000). Conceptualizing menopause and midlife: Chinese American and Chinese women in the U. S. *Maturitas, 35,* 11–23.

American Cancer Society. (2013). *Can cervical cancer be prevented?* Retrieved from http://www.cancer.org/cancer/cervicalcancer/ detailedguide/cervical-cancer-prevention

American College of Obstetricians and Gynecologists. (2013). Well-woman care: Assessments & recommendations. *Annual Women's Health Care.* Retrieved from http://www.acog.org

American Diabetes Association. (2012). Standards of medical care in diabetes—2012. *Diabetes Care, 35*(Suppl. 1), S11–S63.

American Heart Association (AHA). (2014a). American Heart Association recommendations for physical activity in adults. Retrieved from http://www.heart.org/HEARTORG/HealthyLiving/PhysicalAcivity/ FitnessBasics/AmericanHeartAssociation-Recomendations-for -Physical-activity-in-Adults_UCM_307976_Article.jsp

American Heart Association. (2014b). Fight stress with healthy habits. Retrieved from https://www.heart.org/HEARTORG/HealthyLiving/ stressManagement/fightStressWithHealthyHabits/fight-Stress-with -Healthy-Habits_ucm_307922_Article.jsp#.V18C7Wwm464

American Lung Association. (2013). *Women and tobacco use.* Retrieved from http://www.heart.org/HEARTORG/HealthyLiving/ PhysicalAcivity/FitnessBasics/AmericanHeartAssociation- Recomendations-for-Physical-activity-in-Adults_UCM_307976_ Article.jsp

Avis, N. E., Brambilla, D., McKinlay, S. M., & Vass, K. (1994). A longitudinal analysis of the association between menopause and depression: Results from the Massachusetts Women's Health Study. *Annual Epidemiology, 4,* 214–220.

Avis, N. E., Brockwell, S., & Colvin, A. (2005). A universal menopausal syndrome? *American Journal of Medicine, 19*(118, Suppl. 12B), 37–46.

Avis, N. E., Brockwell, S., Randolph, J. F., Shen, S., Cain, V. S., Ory, M., & Greendale, G. A. (2009). Longitudinal changes in sexual functioning as women transition through menopause: Results for the Study of Women's Health Across the Nation (SWAN). *Menopause, 16,* 442–452.

Avis, N. E., Crawford, S. L., Greendale, G., Bromberger, J. T., Everson-Rose, S. A., Gold, E. B.,...Thurston, R. C. (2015). Duration of menopausal vasomotor symptoms over the menopause transition. *Journal of the American Medical Association Internal Medicine, 17,* 531–539.

Avis, N. E., Crawford, S. L., Stellato, R., & Longcope, C. (2001). Longitudinal study of hormone levels and depression among women transitioning through menopause. *Climacteric, 4*(3), 243–249.

Avis, N. E., Stellato, R., Crawford, S., Bromberger, J., Ganz, P., Cain V., & Kagawa-Singer, M. (2001). Is there a menopause syndrome?

Menopause status and symptoms across ethnic groups. *Social Science and Medicine, 52*(3), 345–356.

Avis, N. E., Stellato, R., Crawford, S., Johannes, C., & Longcope, C. (2000). Is there an association between menopause status and sexual functioning? *Menopause, 7*(5), 297–309.

Avis, N. E., Zhao, X., Johannes, C. B., Ory, M., Brockwell, S., & Greendale, G. A. (2005). Correlates of sexual function among multi-ethnic middle-aged women: Results from the Study of Women's Health Across the Nation (SWAN). *Menopause, 12*(4), 385–398.

Barnabei, V. M., Cochrane, B., Aragaki, A., Nygaard, I., Williams, R. S., McGovern, P.,...Johnson, S. R.; Women's Health Initiative Investigators. (2005). Menopausal symptoms and treatment-related effects of estrogen and progestin in Women's Health Initiative. *Obstetrics & Gynecology,* 105, 1063–1073.

Bateson, M. C. (2010). *Composing a further life: The age of active wisdom.* New York, NY: Vintage Books.

Benjamin, R. (2010). Surgeon General's perspectives. Bone health: Preventing osteoporosis. *Public Health Reports, 125,* 368–370.

Berg, J., Taylor, D., & Woods, N. (2015). Women at midlife. In E. Olshansky (Ed.), *Women's health and wellness across the lifespan* (pp. 68–95). Philadelphia, PA: Wolters Kluwer.

Bernard, J. (1981). *The female world.* New York, NY: Free Press.

Bleil, M. E., Adler, N. E., Pasch, L. A., Sternfeld, B., Gregorich, S. E., Rosen, M. P., & Cedars, M. I. (2012). Psychological stress and reproductive aging among pre-menopausal women. *Human Reproduction,* 27, 2720–2728.

Brewer, N., Salz, T., & Lillie, S. (2007). Systematic review: The long-term effects of false-positive mammograms. *Annals of Internal Medicine,* 146, 502–510.

Bromberger, J. T., Assmann, S. F., Avis, N. E., Schocken, M., Kravitz, H. M., & Cordal, A. (2003). Persistent mood symptoms in a multiethnic community cohort of pre- and perimenopausal women. *American Journal of Epidemiology, 158*(4), 347–356.

Bromberger, J., Harlow, S., Avis, N., Kravitz, H. M., & Cordal, A. (2004). Racial/ethnic differences in the prevalence of depressive symptoms among middle-aged women: The Study of Women's Health Across the Nation (SWAN). *American Journal of Public Health, 94*(8), 1378–1385.

Bromberger, J. T., Kravitz, H. M., Chang, Y. F., Cyranowski, J. M., Brown, C., & Matthews, K. A. (2011). Major depression during and after the menopausal transition: Study of Women's Health Across the Nation (SWAN). *Psychological Medicine, 41*(9), 1879–1888. doi:10.1017/S003329171100016X

Bromberger, J. T., Kravitz, H. M., Matthews, K., Youk, A., Brown, C., & Feng, W. (2009). Predictors of first lifetime episodes of major depression in midlife women. *Psychological Medicine, 39*(1), 55–64. doi:10.1017/S0033291708003218

Bromberger, J., Matthews, K., Brockwell, S., Schott, L., Gold, E., Avis, N., . . . Randolph, J. F., Jr. (2007). Depressive symptoms during the menopausal transition: The Study of Women's Health Across the Nation (SWAN). *Journal of Affective Disorders, 103*(1–3), 267–272.

Bromberger, J., Meyer, P., Kravitz, H., Sommer, B., Cordal, A., Powell, L.,...Sutton-Tyrrell, K. (2001). Psychological distress and natural menopause: A multi-ethnic community study. *American Journal of Public Health, 91*(9), 1435–1442.

Bromberger, J. T., Schott, L. L., Kravitz, H. M., Sowers, M., Avis, N. E., Gold, E. B.,...Matthews, K. A. (2010). Longitudinal change in reproductive hormones and depressive symptoms across the menopausal transition: Results from the Study of Women's Health Across the Nation (SWAN). *Archives of General Psychiatry, 67,* 598–607.

Brooks-Gunn, J., & Kirsh, B. (1984). Life events and the boundaries of midlife for women. In G. Baruch & J. Brooks-Gunn (Eds.), *Women in midlife* (pp. 11–30). New York, NY: Plenum.

Burger, H., Burger, H. G., Hale, G. E., Robertson, D. M., & Dennerstein, L. (2007). A review of hormonal changes during the menopausal transition: Focus on findings from the Melbourne Women's Midlife Health Project. *Human Reproduction Update, 13*(6), 559–565.

Burger, H., Dudley, E., Cui, J., Dennerstein, L., & Hoppper, J. (2000). A prospective longitudinal study of serum testosterone dehydroepianderosterone sulfate and sex hormone binding globulin levels through the menopause transition. *Journal of Clinical Endocrinology and Metabolism, 85*(8), 2832–2938.

Burger, H., Dudley, E., Hopper, J., Groome, N., Guthrie, J., Green, A., & Dennerstein, L. (1999). Prospectively measured levels of serum FSH, estradiol and the dimeric inhibins during the menopausal transition in a population-based cohort of women. *Journal of Clinical Endocrinology and Metabolism, 84*(11), 4025–4030.

Burger, H., Dudley, E., Robertson, D., & Dennerstein, L. (2002). Hormonal changes in the menopause transition. *Recent Progress in Hormone Research, 57,* 257–275.

Burger, H. G., Cahir, N., Robertson, D. M., Groome, N. P., Dudley, E., Green, A., & Dennerstein, L. (1998). Serum inhibins A and B fall differentially as FSH rises in perimenopausal women. *Clinical Endocrinology, 48*(6), 809–813.

Campbell, J. G., Bromberger, J. T., Buysse, D. J., Hall, M. H., Hardin, K. A., Kravitz, H. M., . . . Gold, E. (2011). Evaluation of the association of menopausal status with delta and beta EEG activity during sleep. *Sleep, 34,* 1561–1568.

Canadian Cancer Society. (2013). *Risk reduction strategies for breast cancer.* Retrieved from http://www.cancer.ca/en/cancer-information/cancer-type/breast/risks/risk-reductionstrategies

Cappola, A. R., Xue, Q. L., & Frid, L. P. (2009). Multiple hormonal deficiencies in anabolic hormone are found in frail older women: The Women's Health and Aging Studies. *Journal of Gerontology. Series A, Biological Sciences and Medical Sciences, 64,* 243–248.

Carpenter, J. S. (2001). The hot flash related daily interference scale: A tool for assessing the impact of hot flashes on quality of life following breast cancer. *Journal of Pain and Symptom Management, 22,* 979–989.

Carr, M. C., Kim, K. H., Zambon, A., Mitchell, E. S., Woods, N. F., Casazza, C. P., . . . Schwartz, R. S. (2000). Changes in LDL density across the menopausal transition. *Journal of Investigative Medicine, 48,* 245–250; *50,* 1947–1954.

Casper, R., Yen, S., & Wilkes, M. (1979). Menopausal flushes: A neuroendocrine link with pulsatile luteinizing hormone secretion. *Science, 205*(4408), 823–825.

Centers for Disease Control and Prevention (CDC). (2004). *Preventing falls among seniors.* Retrieved from http://www.cdc.gov/injury

Centers for Disease Control and Prevention (CDC). (2012). *Overweight and obesity: Adult obesity facts.* Retrieved from http://www.cdc.gov/obesity/data/adult.html

Centers for Disease Control and Prevention (CDC). (2013). *Controlling blood pressure.* Retrieved from http://www.cdc.gov/bloodpressure/control.htm

Centers for Disease Control and Prevention. (2014a). *What screening tests are there?* Retrieved from http://www.cdc.gov/cancer/dcpc/about

Centers for Disease Control and Prevention. Division of Cancer Prevention and Control. (2014b). *What should I know about screening?* Retrieved from http://www.cdc.gov/cancer/dcpc/about

Centers for Disease Control and Prevention (CDC). (2015). *Preventing high cholesterol: Healthy living habits.* Retrieved from http://www.cdc.gov/cholesterol/healthy_living.htm

Cespedes, E., & Hu, F. (2015). Dietary patterns: From nutritional epidemiologic analysis to national guidelines. *American Journal of Clinical Nutrition, 101,* 899–900.

Chedraui, P., & Perez-Lopez, F. (2013). Nutrition and health during midlife: Searching for solutions and meeting challenges for the aging population. *Climacteric, 16*(Suppl. I), 85–95. doi:10.3109/13697137.2013.802884

Chiuve, S., Cook, N., Shay, C., Rexrode, K., Albert, C, Manson, J., . . . Rimm, E. (2014). Lifestyle-based prediction model for the prevention of CVD: The Healthy Heart Score. *Journal of the American Heart Association, 3,* e000954, 1–11. doi:10.1161/JAHA.114.000954

Cohen, L., Soares, C., Vitonis, A., Otto, M., & Harlow, B. (2006). Risk for new onset of depression during the menopausal transition: The Harvard Study of Moods and Cycles. *Archives of General Psychiatry, 63,* 385–390.

Col, N. F., Guthrie, J. R., Politi, M., & Dennerstein, L. (2009). Duration of vasomotor symptoms in middle-aged women: A longitudinal study. *Menopause, 16,* 453–457.

Coney, S. (1994). *The menopause industry: How the medical establishment exploits women.* Alameda, CA: Hunter House.

Corwin, E. J., & Cannon, J. G. (1999). Gonadotropin modulation of interleukin 1 secretion. *Journal of Gender Specific Medicine, 2,* 30–34.

Crandall, C. J., Tseng, C. H., Crawrord, S. L., Thurston, R. C., Gold, E. B., Johnston, J. M., & Greendatle, G. A. (2011). Association of menopausal vasomotor symptoms with increased bone turnover during the menopausal transition. *Journal of Bone and Mineral Research, 26,* 840–849.

Crawford, S., Santoro, N., Laughlin, G. A., Sowers, M. F., McConnell, D., Sutton-Tyrrell, K., . . . Lasley, B. (2009). Circulating dehydroepiandrosterone sulfate concentrations during the menopausal transition. *Journal of Clinical Endocrinology & Metabolism, 94*(8), 2945–2951.

Cray, L., Woods, N. F., Herting, J. R., & Mitchell, E. S. (2012). Symptom clusters during the menopausal transition and early postmenopause: Observations from the Seattle Midlife Women's Health Study. *Menopause, 19*(8), 864–869.

Dans, L., Silvestre, M., & Dans, A. (2011). Trade-off between benefit and harm is crucial in health screening recommendations. Part I: General principles. *Journal of Clinical Epidemiology, 64*(3), 231–239.

Davidson, R., & McEwen, B. (2012). Social influences on neuroplasticity: Stress and interventions to promote well-being. *Nature Neuroscience, 15*(5), 689–695.

Dennerstein, L., Dudley, E. C., Hopper, J. L., Guthrie, J. R., & Burger, H. G. (2000). A prospective population-based study of menopausal symptoms. *Obstetrics & Gynecology, 96,* 351–358.

Dennerstein, L., & Lehert, P. (2004). Modeling mid-aged women's sexual functioning: A prospective, population-based study. *Journal of Sex and Marital Therapy, 30*(3), 173–183.

Dennerstein, L., Lehert, P., & Burger, H. (2005). The relative effects of hormones and relationship factors on sexual function of women through the natural menopausal transition. *Fertility and Sterility, 84*(1), 174–180.

Dennerstein, L., Lehert, P., Burger, H., & Guthrie, J. (2005). Sexuality. *American Journal of Medicine, 118*(12B), 59–63.

Dennerstein, L., Randolph, J., Taffe, J., Dudley, E., & Burger, H. (2002). Hormones, mood, sexuality, and the menopausal transition. *Fertility and Sterility, 77*(Suppl. 4), S42–S48.

Derby, C. A., Crawford, S. L., Pasternak, R. C., Sowers, M., Sternfeld, B., & Matthews, K. A. (2009). Lipid changes during the menopause transition in relation to age and weight: The Study of Women's Health Across the Nation. *American Journal of Epidemiology, 169*(11), 1352–1361.

Dooley, Y., Kenton, K., Cao, G., Luke, A., Durazo-Arvizu, R., Kramer, H., . . . Brubaker, L. (2008). Urinary incontinence prevalence: Results from the National Health and Nutrition Examination Survey. *Journal of Urology, 179,* 656–661.

Dugan, S. A., Everson-Rose, S. A., Karavolos, K., Sternfeld, B., Wesley, D., & Powell, L. H. (2009). The impact of physical activity level on SF-36 Role-physical and Bodily Pain Indices in midlife women. *Journal of Physical Activity and Health, 6,* 33–42.

Dugan, S. A., Powell, L. H., Kravitz, H. M., Everson-Rose, S. A., Karavolos, K., & Luborsky, J. (2006). Musculoskeletal pain and menopausal status. *Clinical Journal of Pain, 22,* 325–331.

El Khoudary, S. R., McClure, C. K., VoPham, T., Karvonen-Gutierrez, C. A., Sternfeld, B., Cauley, J. A., . . Sutton-Tyrrell, K. (2014). Longitudinal assessment of the menopausal transition, endogenous sex hormones, and perception of physical functioning: The study of women's health across the nation. *Journals of Gerontology, Series A, 69*(8), 1011–1017.

El Khoudary, S. R., Shields, K. J., Janssen, I., Hanley, C., Budoff, M. J., Barinas-Mitchell, E., . . . Matthews, K. A. (2015). Cardiovascular fat, menopause, and sex hormones in women: The SWAN Cardiovascular Fat Ancillary Study. *Journal of Clinical Endocrinology & Metabolism, 100,* 3304–3312.

Ensrud, K. E., Stone, K. L., Blackwell, T. L., Sawaya, G. F., Tagliaferri, M., Diem, S. J., . . . Grady, D. (2008). Frequency and severity of hot flashes and sleep disturbance in postmenopausal women with hot flashes. *Menopause, 16*(2), 286–292.

Finkelstein, J., Lee, M., Sowers, M., Ettinger, B., Neer, R., Kelsey, J., . . . Greendale, G. (2002). Ethnic variation in bone density in premenopausal and early perimenopausal women: Effects of anthropometric and lifestyle factors. *Journal of Clinical Endocrinology & Metabolism, 87*(7), 3057–3067.

Freedman, R. R. (2005a). Hot flashes: Behavioral treatments, mechanisms, and relation to sleep. *American Journal of Medicine, 118*(12B), 124–130.

Freedman, R. R. (2005b). Pathophysiology and treatment of menopausal hot flashes. *Seminars in Reproductive Medicine, 23*, 117–125.

Freedman, R. R., & Roehrs, T. (2004). Lack of sleep disturbance from menopausal hot flashes. *Fertility and Sterility, 82*(1), 138–144.

Freedman, R. R., & Subramanian, M. (2005). Effects of symptomatic status and the menstrual cycle on hot flash-related thermoregulatory parameters. *Menopause, 12*, 156–159.

Freeman, E., Sammel, M., Grisso, J., Battistini, M., Garcia-Espagna, B., & Hollander, L. (2001). Hot flashes in the late reproductive years: Risk factors for African American and Caucasian women. *Journal of Women's Health & Gender-Based Medicine, 10*(1), 67–76.

Freeman, E. W., Sammel, M. D., Lin, H., Gracia, C. R., Kapoor, S., & Ferdousi, T. (2005). The role of anxiety and hormonal changes in menopausal hot flashes. *Menopause, 12*, 258–266.

Freeman, E. W., Sammel, M. D., Lin, H., Gracia, C. R., Pien, G. W., Nelson, D. B., . . . Sheng, L. (2007) Symptoms associated with menopausal transition and reproductive hormones in midlife women. *Obstetrics & Gynecology, 110*, 230–240.

Freeman, E. W., Sammel, M. D., Lin, H., Liu, Z., & Gracia, C. R. (2011). Duration of menopausal hot flushes and associated risk factors. *Obstetrics & Gynecology, 117*, 1095–1104.

Freeman, E., Sammel, M., Lin, H., & Nelson, D. (2006). Associations of hormones and menopausal status with depressed mood in women with no history of depression. *Archives of General Psychiatry, 63*(4), 375–382.

Freeman, E. W., Sammel, M. D., Liu, L., Gracia, C. R., Nelson, D. B., & Hollander, L. (2004). Hormones and menopausal status as predictors of depression in women in transition to menopause. *Archives of General Psychiatry, 61* (1), 62–70.

Freeman, E. W., Sammel, M. D., & Sanders, R. J. (2014). Risk of long-term hot flashes after natural menopause: Evidence from the Penn Ovarian Aging Study cohort. *Menopause, 21*, 924–932.

Gibson, C. J., Thurston, R. C., Bromberger, J. T., Kamarck, T., & Matthews, K. A. (2011). Negative affect and vasomotor symptoms in the Study of Women's Health Across the Nation Daily Hormone Study. *Menopause, 18*, 1270–1277.

Gilligan, C. (1982a). Adult development and women's development: Arrangements for a marriage. In J. Giele (Ed.), *Women in the middle years: Current knowledge and directions for research and policy* (pp. 89–114). New York, NY: Wiley.

Gilligan, C. (1982b). *In a different voice: Psychological theory and women's development.* Cambridge, MA: Harvard University Press.

Glauber, H., & Karnieli, E. (2013). Preventing type 2 diabetes mellitus: A call for personalized intervention. *Permanente Journal, 17*(3), 74–79.

Gold, E. B., Block, G., Crawford, S., Lachance, L., FitzGerald, G., Miracle, H., . . . Sherman, S. (2004). Lifestyle and demographic factors in relation to vasomotor symptoms: Baseline results from the Study of Women's Health Across the Nation. *American Journal of Epidemiology, 159*, 1189–1199.

Gold, E. B., Sternfeld, B., Kelsey, J. L., Brown, C., Mouton, C., Reame, N., . . . Stellato, R. (2000). Relation of demographic and lifestyle factors to symptoms in a multi-racial/ethnic population of women 40–55 years of age. *American Journal of Epidemiology, 152*(5), 463–473.

Gracia, C. R., Sammel, M. D., Freeman, E. W., Liu, L., Hollander, L., & Nelson, D. B. (2004). Predictors of decreased libido in women during the late reproductive years. *Menopause, 11*(2), 144–150.

Greendale, G. A. (2009). Effects of the menopause transition and hormone use on cognitive performance in midlife women. *Neurology, 72*, 1850–1857.

Greendale, G. A., Sowers, M. F., Han, W., Huang, M. H., Finkelstein, J. S., Crandall, C. J.,...Karlamangla, A. S. (2012). Bone mineral density loss in relation to the final menstrual period in a multi-ethnic cohort: Results from the Study of Women's Health Across the Nation (SWAN). *Journal of Bone Mineral Research, 27*, 111–118.

Greendale, G. A., Wight, R. G., Huang, M., Avis, N., Gold, E. B., Joffe, H.,...Karamangla, A. S. (2010). Menopause-associated symptom and cognitive performance: Results from the Study of Women's Health Across the Nation. *American Journal of Epidemiology, 171*, 1214–1224.

Griffiths, A., Kouvonen, A., Pentti, J., Oksanen, T., Virtanen, M., Salo, P.,...Vahtera, J. (2014). Association of physical activity with future mental health in older, mid-life and younger women. *European Journal of Public Health, 24*(5), 813–818.

Guthrie, J., Dennerstein, L., Hopper, J., & Burger, H. (1996). Hot flushes, menstrual status, and hormone levels in a population-based sample of midlife women. *Obstetrics & Gynecology, 88*(3), 437–442.

Guthrie, J., Dennerstein, L., Taffe, J., Lehert, P., & Burger, H. (2004). The menopausal transition: A 9-year prospective population-based study. The Melbourne Women's Midlife Health Project. *Climacteric, 7*(4), 375–389.

Guthrie, J., Dennerstein, L., Taffe, J., Lehert, P., & Burger, H. (2005). Hot flushes during the menopause transition: A longitudinal study in Australian-born women. *Menopause, 12*(4), 460–467.

Hackl, F., Halla, M., Hummer, M., & Pruckner, G. (2015). The effectiveness of health screening. *Health Economics, 24*, 913–935.

Hall, M. H., Casement, M. D., Troxel, W. M., Matthews, K. A., Bromberger, J. T., Kravitz, H. M.,...Buysse, D. J. (2015). Chronic stress is prospectively associated with sleep in midlife women: The SWAN Sleep Study. *Sleep, 38*(10), 1645–1654.

Harlow, S., Cain, K., Crawford, S., Dennerstein, L., Little, R., Mitchell, E.,...Yosef, M. (2006). Evaluation of four proposed bleeding criteria for the onset of late menopausal transition. *Journal of Clinical Endocrinology & Metabolism, 91*(9), 3432–3438.

Harlow, S., Mitchell, E., Crawford, S., Nan, B., Little, R., Taffe, J., & ReSTAGE Collaboration. (2008). The ReSTAGE Collaboration: Defining optimal bleeding criteria for onset of early menopausal transition. *Fertility and Sterility, 89*(1), 129–140.

Harlow, S. D., Crawford, S., Dennerstein, L., Burger, H. G., Mitchell, E. S., Sowers, M. F., & ReSTAGE Collaboration. (2007). Recommendations from a multi-study evaluation of proposed criteria for staging reproductive aging. *Climacteric, 10*(2), 112–119.

Harlow, S. D., Gass, M., Hall, J. E., Lobo, R., Maki, P., Rebar, R. W.,...de Villiers, T. J. (2012). Executive summary of STRAW+10: Addressing the unfinished agenda of staging reproductive aging. *Climacteric, 15*, 105–114.

Helson, R., & Wink, P. (1992). Personality change in women from the early 40's to the early 50's. *Psychology and Aging, 7*(1), 46–55.

Hollander, L., Freeman, E., Sammel, M., Berlin, J., Grisso, J., & Battistini, M. (2001). Sleep quality, estradiol levels and behavioral factors in late reproductive age women. *Obstetrics & Gynecology, 98*(3), 391–397.

Ilic, D., O'Connor, D., Green, S., & Wilt, T. (2006). Screening for prostate cancer. *The Cochrane Database of Systematic Reviews, 2006*(3), CD004720.

Ishii, S., Cauley, J. A., Greendale, G. A., Crandall, C. J., Danielson, M. E., Ouchi, Y., & Karlamangla, A. S. (2013). C-reactive protein, bone strength, and nine-year fracture risk: Data from the Study of Women's Health Across the Nation. *Journal of Bone and Mineral Research, 18*, 1688–1698. doi:10.1002/jbmr.1915

James, P., Oparil, S., Carter, B., Cushman, W., Dennison-Himmelfarb, C., Handler, J.,...Ortiz, E. (2014). 2014 evidence-based guideline for the management of high blood pressure in adults: Report from the panel members appointed to the Eighth Joint National Committee (JNC 8). *Journal of the American Medical Association, 311*(5), 507–520. doi:10.1001/jama.2013.284427

Janssen, I., Powell, L. H., Matthews, K. A., Cursio, J. F., Hollenberg, S. M., Sutton-Tyrell, K,...Everson-Rose, S. A. (2011). Depressive symptoms are related to progression of coronary calcium in midlife women: The Study of Women's Health Across the Nation (SWAN) Heart Study. *American Heart Journal, 161*, 1186–1191.

Joffe, H., Crawford. S., Economou, N., Kim, S., Regan, S., Hall, J. E., & White, D. (2013). A gonadotropin-releasing hormone agonist model demonstrates that nocturnal hot flashes interrupt objective sleep. *Sleep, 36*(12), 1977–1985. doi:10.5665/sleep.3244

Joffe, H., White, D. P., Crawford, S. L., McCurnin, K. E., Economou, N., Connors, S., & Hall, J. E. (2013). Adverse effects of induced hot flashes on objectively recorded and subjectively reported sleep: Results of a gonadotropin-releasing hormone agonist experimental protocol. *Menopause, 20*, 905–914.

Judd, F. K., Hickey, M., & Bryant, C. (2012). Depression and midlife: Are we overpathologising the menopause? *Journal of Affective Disorders, 136*(3), 199–211.

Kagawa-Singer, M., Kagawa-Singer, M., Kavanishi, Y., Greendale, G., Kim, S., Adler, S., . . . Wongvipat, N. (2002). Comparison of the menopause and midlife transition between Japanese-American and Euro-American women. *Medical Anthropology Quarterly, 16*(1), 64–91.

Kaliman, P., Parrizas, M., Lalanza, J., Camins, A., Escorihuela, R., & Pallas, M. (2011). Neurophysiological and epigenetic effects of physical exercise on the aging process. *Ageing Research Review, 10*, 475–486.

Kavanagh, K., Espeland, M. A., Sutton-Tyrrell, K., Barinas-Mitchell, E., El Khoudary, S. R., & Wildman, R. P. (2013). Liver fat and SHBG affect insulin resistance in midlife women. The Study of Women's Health Across the Nation (SWAN). *Obesity, 21*, 1031–1038.

Kay, M., Voda, A., Olivas, G., Rios, F., & Imle, M. (1982). Ethnography of the menopause-related hot flash. *Maturitas, 4*, 217–227.

Kim, E., Strecher, V., & Ryff, C. (2014). Purpose in life and use of preventive health care services. *Proceedings of the National Academy of Science USA, 111*(46), 16331–16336. doi:10.1073/pnas.1414826111

Klein, N., Battaglia, D., Fujimoto, V., Davis, G., Bremner, W., & Soules, M. (1996). Reproductive aging: Accelerated follicular development associated with a monotropic follicle-stimulating hormone rise in normal older women. *Journal of Clinical Endocrinology and Metabolism, 81*(3), 1038–1045.

Knowler, W., Fowler, S., Hamman, R., Christophi, C., Hoffman, H., Brenneman, A., . . . Nathan, D. M. (2009). 10-year follow-up of diabetes incidence and weight loss in the Diabetes Prevention Program Outcomes Study. *Lancet, 374*(9702), 1677–1686.

Kones, R. (2011). Primary prevention of coronary heart disease: Integration of new data, evolving views, revised goals, and role of rosuvastatin in management. A comprehensive survey. *Drug Design, Development and Therapy, 5*, 325–380. doi:10.2147/DDDT.S14934

Kravitz, H., Zhao, X., Bromberger, J., Gold, E. B., Hall, M. H., Matthews, K. A., . . . Sowers, M. R. (2009). Sleep disturbance during the menopausal transition in a multi-ethnic community sample of women. *Sleep, 31*, 979–990.

Kravitz, H. M., Avery, E., Sowers, M., Bromberger, J. T., Owens, J. F., Matthews, K. A., . . . Buysse, D. J. (2011). Relationships between menopausal and mood symptoms and EEG sleep measures in a multiethnic sample of middle-aged women: The SWAN sleep study. *Sleep, 34*, 1221–1232.

Kurth, T., Moore, S., Gaziano, J., Kase, C., Stampfer, M., Berger, K., & Buring, J. (2006). Healthy lifestyle and the risk of stroke in women. *Archives of Internal Medicine, 166*, 1403–1409.

Lasley, B., Santoro, N., Gold, E., Sowers, M., Crawford, S., Weiss, G., . . . Randolph, J. (2002). The relationship of circulating dehydroepiandrosterone, testosterone, and estradiol to stages of the menopausal transition and ethnicity. *Journal of Clinical Endocrinology and Metabolism, 87*(8), 3760–3767.

Lasley, B. L., Crawford, S., & McConnell, D. S. (2011). Adrenal androgens and the menopausal transition. *Obstetrics and Gynecology Clinics of North America, 38*, 467–475.

Lasley, B. L., Crawford, S. L., & McConnell, D. S. (2013). Ovarian adrenal interactions during the menopausal transition. *Minerva Gynecology, 65*, 641–651.

Lawrence-Lightfoot, S. (2009). *The third chapter: Passion, risk and adventure in the 25 years after 50*. New York, NY: Sarah Crichton Books.

Lazarus, R., & Folkman, S. (1984). *Stress, appraisal and coping*. New York, NY: Springer Publishing.

Leawood, K. (2003). *Obesity*. American Academy of Family Physicians. www.aafp.org/online/en/home/clinical/exam/obesity.html

Lee, C. G., Carr, M. C., Murdoch, S. J., Mitchell, E., Woods, N. F., Wener, M. J., . . . Brunzell, J. D. (2009). Adipokines, inflammation, and visceral adiposity across the menopausal transition: A prospective study. *Journal of Clinical Endocrinology and Metabolism, 94*(4), 1104–1110.

Lenton, E. A., Sexton, L., Lee, S., & Cooke, I. D. (1988). Progressive changes in LH and FSH and LH: FSH ratio in women throughout reproductive life. *Maturitas, 10*(1), 35–43.

Lindheim, S. R., Legro, R. S., Bernstein, L., Stanczyk, F. Z., Vijod, M. A., Presser, S. C., & Lobo, R. A. (1992). Behavioral stress responses in premenopausal and postmenopausal women and the effects of estrogen. *American Journal of Obstetrics and Gynecology, 167*(6), 1831–1836.

Lloyd-Jones, D., Sutton-Tyrrell, K., Patel, A., Matthews, K., Pasternak, R., Everson-Rose, S., . . . Chae, C. (2005). Ethnic variation in hypertension among premenopausal and perimenopausal women: Study of Women's Health Across the Nation. *Hypertension, 46*(4), 689–695.

Lock, M., Kaufert, P., & Gilbert, P. (1988). Cultural construction of the menopausal syndrome: The Japanese's case. *Maturitas, 10*(4), 317–322.

Longcope, C., & Johnston, C. C., Jr. (1990). Androgen and estrogen dynamics: Stability over a two year interval in peri-menopausal women. *Journal of Steroid Biochemistry, 35*(1), 91–95.

Luetters, C., Huang, M. H., Seeman, T., Buckwalter, G., Meyer, P. M., Avis, N. E., . . . Greendale, G. A. (2007). Menopause transition stage and endogenous estradiol and follicle-stimulating hormone levels are not related to cognitive performance: Cross-sectional results from the Study of Women's Health Across the Nation (SWAN). *Journal of Women's Health, 16*, 331–344.

Lukacs, J., Chilimigras, J., Cannon, J., Dormire, S., & Reame, N. (2004). Midlife women's responses to a hospital sleep challenge: Aging and menopause effects on sleep architecture. *Journal of Women's Health, 13*(3), 333–340.

Maltais, M. L., Desroches, J., & Dionne, I. J. (2009). Changes in muscle mass and strength after menopause. *Journal of Musculoskeletal and Neuronal Interactions, 9*, 186–197.

Mayo Clinic. (2015). *Lung cancer: Prevention*. Retrieved from http://www.mayoclinic.org/disease-conditions/lung-cancer/basics/prevention/con-20025531?p=1

McClure, C. K., El Khoudary, S. R., Karvonen-Gutierrez, C. A., Ylitalo, K. R., Tomey, K., GoPham, T., . . . Harlow, S. (2014). Prospective associations between inflammatory and hemostatic markers and physical functioning limitations in midlife women: Longitudinal results of the Study of Women's Health Across the Nation. *Experimental Gerontology, 49*, 1011–1017. doi:10.1016/jexger 2013.10.016

McKinlay, S., Brambilla, D., & Posner, J. (1992). The normal menopause transition. *Maturitas, 14*(2), 103–115.

McLaughlin, S., Melber, B., Billy, J., & Zimmerle, D. (1986). *The changing lives of American women*. Chapel Hill, NC: University of North Carolina Press.

Meldrum, D., Tataryn, I., Frumar, A., Erlik, Y., Lu, K., & Judd, H. (1980). Gonadotropins, estrogens, and adrenal steroids during the menopausal hot flash. *Journal of Clinical Endocrinology and Metabolism, 50*(4), 685–689.

Metcalf, M. G. (1988). The approach of menopause: A New Zealand study. *New Zealand Medical Journal, 101*(841), 103–106.

Mitchell, E., & Woods, N. (2007). Duration and age of onset of menopausal transition stages. Unpublished data from the Seattle Midlife Women's Health Study.

Mitchell, E. S., & Woods, N. F. (1996). Symptom experiences of midlife women: Observations from the Seattle Midlife Women's Health Study. *Maturitas, 25*(1), 1–10.

Mitchell, E. S., & Woods, N. F. (2001). Midlife women's attributions about perceived memory changes: Observations from the Seattle Midlife Women's Health Study. *Journal of Women's Health and Gender Based Medicine, 10*(4), 351–362.

Mitchell, E. S., & Woods, N. F. (2010). Pain symptoms during the menopausal and early postmenopause: Observations from the Seattle Midlife Women's Health Study. *Climacteric, 13*, 467–478.

Mitchell, E. S., & Woods, N. F. (2011). Cognitive symptoms during the menopausal transition and early postmenopause: Observations from the Seattle Midlife Women's Health Study. *Climacteric, 14*, 252–261.

Mitchell, E. S., & Woods, N. F. (2013). Correlates of urinary incontinence during the menopausal transition and early postmenopause: Observations from the Seattle Midlife Women's Health Study. *Climacteric, 16*(6), 653–662. doi:10.3109/13697137.2013.777038

Mitchell, E. S., & Woods, N. F. (2015). Hot flash severity during the menopausal transition and early postmenopause. *Climacteric, 18*(4), 536–544. doi: 10.3109/13697137.2015.1009436.

Mitchell, E. S., Woods, N. F., & Mariella, A. (2000). Three stages of menopausal transition from the Seattle Midlife Women's Health Study: Toward a more precise definition. *Menopause, 7*(5), 334–349.

Morrish, N., Wang, S., Stevens, L., Fuller, J., & Keen, H. (2001). Mortality and causes of death in the WHO Multinational Study of Vascular Disease in Diabetes. *Diabetologia, 44*(Suppl. 2), S14–S21.

Morrison, M., Have, T., Freeman, E., Sammel, M. D., & Grisso, J. A. (2001). DHEA-S levels and depressive symptoms in a cohort of African American and Caucasian women in the late reproductive years. *Biological Psychiatry, 50*(9), 705–711.

Morrison, M. F., Freeman, E. W., Lin, H., & Sammel, M. D. (2011). Higher DHEA-S levels are associated with depressive symptoms during the menopausal transition: Results from the Penn Ovarian Aging Study. *Archives of Women's Mental Health, 14*, 375–382.

Mosca, L., Benjamin, E., Berra, K., Bezanson, J., Dolor, R., Lloyd-Jones, D.,...Wenger, N. (2011). Effectiveness-based guidelines for the prevention of cardiovascular disease in women—2011 update: A guideline from the American Heart Association. *Circulation, 123*, 1243–1262.

Moyer, V. (2012). Screening for and management of obesity in adults: U.S. Preventive Services Task Force Recommendation Statement. *Annals of Internal Medicine, 157*(5), 373–379.

National Institute for Mental Health. (2013a). *Women and mental health*. Retrieved from http://www.nimh.nih.gov/health/topics/women-and-mental-health/index.shtml

National Institute for Mental Health. (2013b). *Depression*. Retrieved from http://www.nimh.nih.gov/health/topics/depression/index.shtml

National Institute for Mental Health. (2013c). *Anxiety disorders*. Retrieved from http://www.nimh.nih.gov/health/topics/anxiety-disorders/index.shtml

National Osteoporosis Foundation. (2013). *2013 Clinician's guide to prevention and treatment of osteoporosis*. Washington, DC: Author.

Neugarten, B. (1968). The awareness of middle age. In B. Neugarten (Ed.), *Middle age and aging* (pp. 93–98). Chicago, IL: University of Chicago Press.

Overlie, I., Moen, M., Holte, A., & Finset, A. (2002). Androgens and estrogens in relation to hot flushes during the menopausal transition. *Maturitas, 41*(1), 69–77.

Pien, G. W., Sammel, M. D., Freeman, E. W., Lin, H., & DeBlasis, T. L. (2008). Predictors of sleep quality in women in the menopausal transition. *Sleep, 31*, 991–999.

Popescu, A., LeResche, L., Truelove, E. L., & Drangsholt, M. T. (2010). Gender differences in pain modulation by diffuse noxious inhibitory controls: A systematic review. *Pain, 150*(2), 309–318.

Portman, D. J., Gass, M. L.; Vulvovaginal Atrophy Terminology Consensus Conference Panel. (2014). Genitourinary syndrome of menopause: New terminology for vulvovaginal atrophy from the International Society for the Study of Women's Sexual Health and The North American Menopause Society. *Menopause, 21*(10), 1063–1068. doi:10.1097/GME.0000000000000329

Randolph, J., Zheng, H., Sowers, M. R., Crandall, C., Crawford, S., Gold, E. B., & Buga, M. (2011). Change in follicle-stimulating hormone and estradiol across the menopausal transition: Effect of age at the final menstrual period. *Journal of Clinical Endocrinology and Metabolism, 96*, 746–754.

Randolph, J. F., Crawford, S., Dennerstien, L., Cain, K., Harlow, S. D., Little, R., . . . Yosef, M. (2006). The value of follicle-stimulating hormone concentration and clinical findings as markers of the late menopausal transition. *Journal of Clinical Endocrinology and Metabolism, 91*(8), 3034–3040.

Randolph, J. F., Jr., Sowers, M., Bondarenko, I., Gold, E. B., Greendale, G. A.,...Matthews, K. A. (2005). The relationship of longitudinal change in reproductive hormones and vasomotor symptoms during the menopausal transition. *Journal of Clinical Endocrinology and Metabolism, 90*, 6106–6112.

Randolph, J. F., Jr., Sowers, M., Gold, E. B., Mohr, B. A., Luborsky, J., Santoro, N., . . . Lasley, B. L. (2003). Reproductive hormones in the early menopausal transition: Relationship to ethnicity, body size, and menopausal status. *Journal of Clinical Endocrinology and Metabolism, 88*, 1516–1522.

Reidlinger, D., Darzi, J., Hall, W., Seed, P., Chowienczyk, P., & Sanders, T. on behalf of the Cardiovascular disease risk REduction Study (CRESSIDA) investigators. (2015). How effective are current dietary guidelines for cardiovascular disease prevention in healthy middle-aged and older men and women? A randomized controlled trial. *American Journal of Clinical Nutrition, 101*, 922–930.

Richardson, S. J. (1993). The biological basis of the menopause. *Ballière's Clinical Endocrinology and Metabolism, 7*(1), 1–16.

Riley, M., Dobson, M., Jones, E., & Kirst, N. (2013). Health maintenance in women. *American Family Physician, 87*(1), 30–38.

Roger, V., Go, A., Lloyd-Jones, D., Benjamin, E. J., Berry, J. D., Borden, W. B., . . . Turner, M. B.; American Heart Association Statistics Committee and Stroke Statistics Subcommittee. (2012). American Heart Association Statistics Committee and Stroke Statistics Subcommittee. Heart disease and stroke statistics—2012 update: A report from the American Heart Association. *Circulation, 125*, e2–e220.

Roglic, G., Unwin, N., Bennett, P., Mathers, C., Tuomilehto, J., Nag, S., . . . King, H. (2005). The burden of mortality attributable to diabetes: Realistic estimates for the year 2000. *Diabetes Care, 28*(9), 2130–2135.

Rosamond, W., Flegal, K., Furie, K., Greenlund, K., Haase, N., Hailpern, S.,...Hong, Y. (2008). *Circulation, 117*, e25–e3146.

Rossi, A. (1985). *Gender and the life course*. New York, NY: Aldine.

Rubin, L. (1979). *Women of a certain age*. New York, NY: Harper.

Ryff, C. (2014). Psychological well-being revisited: Advances in the science and practice of eudaimonia. *Psychotherapy Psychosomatics, 83*(1), 10–28. doi:10.1159/00035326310

Saab, P. G., Matthews, K. A., Stoney, C. M., & McDonald, R. H. (1989). Premenopausal and postmenopausal women differ in their cardiovascular and neuroendocrine responses to behavioral stressors. *Psychophysiology, 26*(3), 270–280.

Sabbath, A., & Indik, J. (2006). Sudden death on the treadmill. *American Journal of Medicine, 119*, 32–34.

Sampselle, C., Harris, V., Harlow, S., & Sowers, M. (2002). Midlife development and menopause in African American and Caucasian women. *Health Care for Women International, 23*(4), 351–363.

Santoro, N., Brockwell, S., Johnston, J., Crawford, S. L., Gold, E. B., Harlow, S. D.,...Sutton-Tyrrell, K. (2007). Helping midlife women predict the onset of the final menses: SWAN, the Study of Women's Health Across the Nation. *Menopause, 14*(3), 1–9.

Santoro, N., Brown, J. R., Adel, T., & Skurnick, J. (1996). Characterization of reproductive hormonal dynamics in the perimenopause. *Journal of Clinical Endocrinology and Metabolism, 81*, 1495–1501.

Savoy, S., & Penckofer, S. (2015). Depressive symptoms impact health-promoting lifestyle behaviors and quality of life in healthy women. *Journal of Cardiovascular Nursing, 30*(4), 360–372.

Schmidt, P., Murphy, J., Haq, N., Danaceau, M. A., & St. Clair L. (2002). Basal plasma hormone levels in depressed perimenopausal women. *Psychoneuroendocrinology, 27*(8), 907–920.

Schneiderman, N., Ironson, G., & Siegel, S. (2005). Stress and health: Psychological, behavioral, and biological determinants. *Annual Review of Clinical Psychology, 1*, 607–628. doi:10.1146/annurev.clinpsy.1.102803.144141

Shaver, J., Giblin, E., Lentz, M., & Lee, K. (1988). Sleep patterns and sleep stability in perimenopausal women. *Sleep, 11*(6), 556–561.

Shaver, J., & Paulsen, V. (1993). Sleep, psychological distress, and somatic symptoms in perimenopausal women. *Family Practice Research Journal, 13*(4), 373–384.

Shaver, J. L., Giblin, E., & Paulsen, V. (1991). Sleep quality subtypes in midlife women. *Sleep, 14*, 18–23.

Shaver, J. L., Johnston, S. K., Lentz, M. J., & Landis, C. A. (2001). Stress exposure, psychological distress, and physiological stress activation in midlife women with insomnia. *Psychosomatic Medicine, 64*, 793–802.

Sievert, L. (2006). *Menopause: A biocultural perspective*. New Brunswick, NJ: Rutgers University Press.

Sievert, L. L. (2013). Comparisons of symptom experience across country and class. *Menopause, 20*, 594–595.

Sievert, L. L., & Obermeyer, C. M. (2012). Symptom clusters at midlife: A four-country comparison of checklist and qualitative responses. *Menopause, 19*, 133–144.

Smith-DiJulio, K., Mitchell, E. S., Percival, D. B., & Woods, N. F. (2008). Well-being during the menopausal transition and early postmenopause: A within-stage analysis. *Women's Health Issues, 18*(4), 310–318.

Smith-DiJulio, K., Percival, D. B., Woods, N. F., Tao, E. Y., & Mitchell, E. S. (2007). Hot flash severity in hormone therapy users and nonusers across the menopausal transition. *Maturitas, 58*(2), 191–200.

Society for Research on Women in New Zealand. (1988). *The time of our lives: A study of mid-life women*. Christchurch, New Zealand: Christchurch Branch of SRWO.

Sofowora, G. G., Singh, I., He, H. B., Wood, A. J., & Stein, C. M. (2005). Effect of acute transdermal estrogen administration on basal, mental stress and cold pressor-induced sympathetic responses in postmenopausal women. *Clinical Autonomic Research, 15*(3), 193–199.

Soules, M. R., Sherman, S., Parrott, E., Rebar, R., Santoro, N., Utian, W., & Woods N. (2001). Executive summary: Stages of Reproductive Aging Workshop (STRAW). *Climacteric, 4*(4), 267–272.

Sowers, M., Crawford, S., Sternfeld, B., Morganstein, D., Gold, E., Greendale, G., & Kelsye, J. (2000). SWAN: A multicenter, multiethnic community-based cohort study of women and the menopausal transition. In R. Lobo, J. Kelsey, & R. Marcus (Eds.), *Menopause: Biology and pathobiology* (pp. 175–188). San Diego, CA: Academic Press.

Sowers, M., Finkelstein, J., Geendale, G., Donbarenko, I., Cauley, J., Ettinger, B., … & Neer, R. (2003). The association of endogenous hormone concentrations in bone mineral density (BMD) and bone mineral apparent density (BMAD) in pre- and perimenopausal women. *Osteoporosis International, 14*(1), 44–52.

Sowers, M., Jannausch, M., McConnell, D., Little, R., Greendale, G. A., Finkelstein, J. S., … Ettinger, B. (2006). Hormone predictors of bone mineral density changes during the menopausal transition. *Journal of Clinical Endocrinology and Metabolism, 91*(4), 1261–1267.

Sowers, M., Jannausch, M., Randolph, J., McConnell, D., Little, R., Lasley, B., . . . Matthews, K. A. (2005). Androgens are associated with hemostatic and inflammatory factors among women at the mid-life. *Journal of Clinical Endocrinology and Metabolism, 90*(11), 6064–6071.

Sowers, M., Matthews, K., Jannausch, M., Randolph, J., McConnell, D., Sutton-Tyrrell, K., … Pasternak, R. (2005). Hemostatic factors and estrogen during the menopausal transition. *Journal of Clinical Endocrinology and Metabolism, 90*(11), 5942–5948.

Sowers, M., Zheng, H., Tomey, K., Karvonen-Gutierrez, C., Jannausch, M., Li, X., … Symons, J. (2007). Changes in body composition in women over six years at midlife: Ovarian and chronological aging. *Journal of Clinical Endocrinology and Metabolism, 92*(3), 895–901.

Sowers, M. R., Eyvazzadeh, A. D., McConnell, D., Yosef, M., Jannausch, M. L., Zhang, D., … Randolph, J. F., Jr. (2008). Anti-mullerian hormone and inhibin B in the definition of ovarian aging and the menopause transition. *Journal of Clinical Endocrinology and Metabolism, 93*(9), 3478–3483.

Sowers, M. R., Wildman, R. P., Mancuso, P., Eyvazzadeh, A. D., Karvonen-Gutierrez, C. A., Rillamas-Sun, E., & Jannausch, M. L. (2008). Change in adipocytokines and ghrelin with menopause. *Maturitas, 20*, 149–157.

Sowers, M. R., Zheng, H., McConnell, D., Nan, B., Harlow, S., & Randolph, J. F. (2008). Follicle stimulating hormone and its rate of change in defining menopause transition stages. *Journal of Clinical Endocrinology and Metabolism, 93*, 3958–3964.

Stampfer, M., Hu, F., Manson, J., Rimm, E., & Willett, W. (2000). Primary prevention of coronary heart disease in women through diet and lifestyle. *New England Journal of Medicine, 343*, 16–22.

Strong, K., Mathers, C., & Bonita, R. (2007). Preventing stroke: Saving lives around the world. *Lancet Neurology, 6*, 182–187.

Sutton-Tyrrell, K., Wildman, R., Matthews, K., Chae, C., Lasley, B., Brockwell, S., … Torrens, J. (2005). Sex-hormone-binding globulin and the free androgen index are related to cardiovascular risk factors in multiethnic premenopausal and perimenopausal women enrolled in the Study of Women's Health Across the Nation (SWAN). *Circulation, 111*(10), 1242–1249.

Szoeke, C. E., Cicuttini, F. M., Guthrie, J. R., & Dennerstein, L. (2008). The relationship of reports of aches and joint pains to the menopausal transition: A longitudinal study. *Climacteric, 11*, 55–62.

Taffe, J. R., Cain, K. C., Mitchell, E. S., Woods, N. F., Crawford, S. L., & Harlow, S. D. (2010). "Persistence" improves the 60-day amenorrhea marker of entry to late-stage menopausal transition for women aged 40 to 44 years. *Menopause, 17*, 191–193.

Tataryn, I., Meldrum, D., Lu, K., Frumar, A., & Judd, H. (1979). LH, FSH, and skin temperature during menopausal hot flash. *Journal of Endocrinology and Metabolism, 49*(1), 152–154.

Thurston, R. C., Bromberger, J. T., Joffe, H., Avis, N. E., Hess, R., Crandall, C. J., … Matthews, K. A. (2008). Beyond frequency: Who is most bothered by vasomotor symptoms? *Menopause, 15*(5), 841–847.

Thurston, R. C., Christie, I. C., & Matthews, K. A. (2010). Hot flashes and cardiac vagal control: A link to cardiovascular risk? *Menopause, 17*(3), 456–461

Thurston, R. C., Khoudary, S. R., Sutton-Tyrrell, K., Crandall, C. H., Gold, E., Sternfeld, B., … Matthews, K. A. (2011). Are vasomoror symptoms associated with alterations in hemostatic and inflammatory markers? Findings from the Study of Women's Health Across the Nation. *Menopause, 15*, 1044–1051.

Thurston, R. C., Kuller, L. H., Edmundowicz, D., & Matthews, K. A. (2010). History of hot flashes and aortic calcification among postmenopausal women. *Menopause, 17*(2), 256–261.

Thurston, R. C., Santoro, N., & Matthews, K. A. (2011). Adiposity and hot flashes in midlife women: A modifying role of age. *Journal of Clinical Endocrinology and Metabolism, 96*, 1588–1595.

Thurston, R. C., Sowers, M. R., Chang, Y., Sternfeld, B., Gold, E. B., Johnston, J. M., & Matthews, K. A. (2008). Adiposity and reporting of vasomotor symptoms among midlife women: The Study of Women's Health Across the Nation. *American Journal of Epidemiology, 167*(1), 78–85.

Thurston, R. C., Sowers, M. R., Sternfeld, B., Gold, E. B., Bromberger, J., Chang, Y., … Matthews, K. A. (2009). Gains in body fat and vasomotor symptom reporting over the menopausal transition: The Study of Women's Health Across the Nation. *American Journal of Epidemiology, 170*(6), 766–774.

Thurston, R. C., Sowers, M. R., Sutton-Tyrrell, K., Everson-Rose, S. A., Lewis, T. T., Edmundowicz, D., & Matthews, K. A. (2008). Abdominal adiposity and hot flashes among midlife women. *Menopause, 15*(3), 429–434.

Thurston, R. C., Sutton-Tyrrell, K., Everson-Rose, S. A., Hess, R., & Matthews, K. A. (2008). Hot flashes and subclinical cardiovascular disease: Findings from the Study of Women's Health Across the Nation Heart Study. *Circulation, 118*(12), 1234–1240.

Thurston, R. C., Sutton-Tyrrell, K., Everson-Rose, S. A., Hess, R., Powell, L. H., & Matthews, K. A. (2011). Hot flashes and carotid intima media thickness among midlife women. *Menopause, 18*, 352–358.

Torrens, J., Sutton-Tyrell, K., Zhao, X., Mathews, K., Brockwell, S., Sowers, M., & Santoro, N. (2009). Relative androgen excess during the menopausal transition predicts incident metabolic syndrome in midlife women: Study of Women's Health Across the Nation. *Menopause, 16*(2), 257–264.

Treloar, A. E. (1981). Menstrual cyclicity and the pre-menopause. *Maturitas, 3*(3–4), 249–264.

Turk, M., Tuite, P., & Burke, L. (2009). Cardiac health: Primary prevention of heart disease in women. *Nursing Clinics of North America, 44*, 315–325.

U.S. Department of Agriculture (USDA). (2015). Scientific report of the 2015 Dietary Guidelines Advisory Committee. Retrieved from http://www.health.gov/dietaryguidelines/2015-scientific-report/PDFs/Scientific-Report-of-the-2015-dietary-Guidelines-Advisory-Committee.pdf

U.S. Department of Health and Human Services, Substance Abuse and Mental Health Services Administration. (1999). *Mental health: A report of the Surgeon General—executive summary*. Rockville, MD: U.S. Department of Health and Human Services, Substance Abuse and Mental Health Services Administration, Center for Mental Health Services, National Institutes of Health, National Institute of Mental Health.

U.S. Department of Health and Human Services. (2004). *The 2004 Surgeon General's report on bone health and osteoporosis: A report of the Surgeon General*. Washington, DC: HHS, Office of the Surgeon General.

U.S. Department of Health and Human Services: healthfinder.gov. (2015). Get a bone density test: The basics. Retrieved from http://healthfinder.gov/HealthTopics/Category/doctor-visits/screening-tests/get-a-bone-density-test

U.S. Department of Health and Human Services, Office on Women's Health. (2013). *Frequently asked questions.* Retrieved from http://www.womenshealth.gov

U.S. National Library of Medicine, National Institutes of Health. (2013). *Women's health and wellness across the lifespan.* Retrieved from http://nim.nih.gov/medlineplus/ency/article/007188.htm

U.S. Preventive Services Task Force (USPSTF). (2003). Screening for obesity in adults: Recommendations and rationale. *Annals of Internal Medicine, 139*(11), 930–932.

U.S. Preventive Services Task Force (USPSTF). (2009). *Aspiring for the prevention of cardiovascular disease.* Retrieved from http://www.preventiveservicestaskforce.org/uspstf/uspsasmi.htm

U.S. Preventive Services Task Force (USPSTF). (2015a). *Final update summary: Lung cancer: Screening.* Retrieved from http://www.uspreventiveservicestaskforce.org/Page/Document/UpdateSummaryFinal/lung-cancer-screening

U.S. Preventive Services Task Force (USPSTF). (2015b). *Final update summary: Breast cancer: Screening.* Retrieved from http://www.uspreventiveservicestaskforce.org/Page/Document/UpdateSummaryFinal/breast-cancer-screening

U.S. Preventive Services Task Force (USPSTF). (2015c). *Final update summary: Colorectal cancer.* Retrieved from http://www.uspreventiveservicestaskforce.org/Page/Document/UpdateSummaryfinal/colorectal-cancer-screening

Upchurch, D. M., Stein, J., Greendale, G. A., Chyu, L., Tseng, C., Huang, M.,…Seeman, T (2015). A longitudinal investigation of race, socioeconomic status, and psychosocial mediators of allostatic load in midlife women: Findings from the Study of Women's Health Across the Nation. *Psychosomatic Medicine, 77*, 402–412.

Villaruel, A., Harlow, S., Lopez, M., & Sowers, M. (2002). El cambio de vida: Conceptualizations of menopause and midlife among urban Latina women. *Research and Theory for Nursing Practice, 16*(2), 91–102.

Voda, A. M. (1981). Climacteric hot flash. *Maturitas, 3*, 73–90.

Waetjen, E., Johnson, W. O., Xing, G., Wen-Ying, F., Greendale, G. A., & Gold, E. B. (2011). Serum estradiol levels are not associated with urinary incontinence in midlife women transitioning through menopause. *Menopause, 18*, 1283–1290.

Waetjen, L. E., Feng, W. Y., Ye, J., Johnson, W. O., Greendale, G. A., Sampselle, C. M., . . . Gold, E. B. (2008). Factors associated with worsening and improving urinary incontinence across the menopausal transition. *Obstetrics and Gynecology, 111*, 667–677.

Waetjen, L. E., Liao, S., Johnson, W. O., Sampselle, C. M., Sternfield, B., Harlow, S. D., & Gold, E. B. (2007). Factors associated with prevalent and incident urinary incontinence in a cohort of midlife women: A longitudinal analysis of data. Study of Women's Health Across the Nation. *American Journal of Epidemiology, 165*, 309–318.

Waetjen, L. E., Ye, J., Feng, W. Y., Johnson, W. O., Greendale, G. A., Sampselle, C. M., . . . Gold, E. B. (2009). Association between menopausal transition stages and developing urinary incontinence. *Obstetrics and Gynecology, 114*, 989–998.

Ward-Ritacco, C. L., Adrian, A. L., Johnson, M. A., Rogers, L. Q., & Evans, E. M. (2014). Adiposity, physical activity, and muscle quality are independently related to physical function performance in middle-aged postmenopausal women. *Menopause, 21*(10), 1114–1121. doi:10.1097/GME.0000000000000225

Wildman, R. P., Janssen, I., Khan, U. I., Thurston, R., Barinas-Mitchell, E., El Khoudary, S. R.,…Sutton-Tyrrell, K. (2011). Subcutaneous adipose tissue in relation to subclinical atherosclerosis and cardiometabolic risk factors in midlife women. *American Journal of Clinical Nutrition, 93*, 719–726.

Wildman, R. P., Mancuso, P., Wang, C., Kim, M., Scherer, P. E., & Sowers, M. R. (2008). Adipocytokine and ghrelin levels in relation to cardiovascular disease risk factors in women at midlife: Longitudinal associations. *International Journal of Obesity, 32*, 740–748.

Wildman, R. P., Tepper, P. G., Crawford, S., Finkelstein, J. S., Sutton-Tyrrell, K., Thurston, R. C.,…Greendale, G. A. (2012). Do changes in sex steroid hormones precede or follow increases in body weight during the menopause transition? Results from the Study of Women's Health Across the Nation. *Journal Clinical Endocrinology and Metabolism, 97*, E1695–E1704.

Williams, R. E., Kalilani, L., DiBenedetti, D. B., Zhou, X., Granger, A. L., Fehnel, S. E.,…Clark, R. V. (2008). Frequency and severity of vasomotor symptoms among peri- and postmenopausal women in the United States. *Climacteric, 11*, 32–43.

Williams, R. E., Kalilani, L. K., DiBenedetti, D. B., Zhou, X., Fehnel, S. E., & Clark, R. V. (2007). Healthcare seeking and treatment for menopausal symptoms in the United States. *Maturitas, 58*, 348–358.

Wise, P., Smith, M., Dubal, D., Wilson, M., Rau, S., Cashion, A.,…Rosewell, K. (2002). Neuroendocrine modulation and repercussions of female reproductive aging. *Recent Progress in Hormone Research, 57*, 235–256.

Woods, N., Carr, M. C., Tao, E. Y., Taylor, H. J., & Mitchell, E. S. (2006). Increased urinary cortisol levels during the menopausal transition. *Menopause, 13*, 212–221.

Woods, N. F., & Cray, L. (2013). Symptom clusters and quality of life. [Editorial]. *Menopause, 20*, 5–7.

Woods, N. F., Cray, L., Herting, J., & Mitchell, E. S. (2014). Endocrine biomarkers and symptom clusters during the menopausal transition and early postmenopause: Observations from the Seattle Midlife Women's Health Study. *Menopause, 21*(6), 646–652.

Woods, N. F., Hohensee, C., Carpenter, J. S., Cohen, L., Ensrud, K., Freeman, E. W., . . . Otte, J. L. (2015). Symptom clusters among FLASH clinical trial participants. *Menopause, 23*(2), 158–165.

Woods, N. F., Mariella, A., & Mitchell, E. S. (2006). Depressed mood symptoms during the menopausal transition: Observations from the Seattle Midlife Women's Health Study. *Climacteric, 9*(3), 195–203.

Woods, N. F., & Mitchell, E. S. (1997a). Women's images of midlife: Observations from the Seattle Midlife Women's Health Study. *Health Care for Women International, 18*(5), 439–453.

Woods, N. F., & Mitchell, E. S. (1997b). Pathways to depressed mood for midlife women: Observations from the Seattle Midlife Women's Health Study. *Research in Nursing & Health, 20*, 119–129.

Woods, N. F., & Mitchell, E. S. (1999). Anticipating menopause: Observations from the Seattle Midlife Women's Health Study. *Menopause, 6*(2), 167–173.

Woods, N. F., & Mitchell, E. S. (2005). Symptoms during perimenopause: Prevalence, severity, trajectory, and significance in women's lives. *American Journal of Medicine, 118*(Suppl. 12B), 14S–24S.

Woods, N. F., & Mitchell, E. S. (2010). Sleep symptoms during the menopausal transition and early postmenopause: Observations from Seattle Midlife Women's Health Study. *Sleep, 33*, 539–549.

Woods, N. F., & Mitchell, E. S. (2011). Symptom interference with work and relationships during the menopausal transition and early postmenopause: Observations from the Seattle Midlife Women's Health Study. *Menopause, 18*, 654–661.

Woods, N. F., & Mitchell, E. S. (2013). Consequences of incontinence for women during the menopausal transition and early postmenopause: Observations from the Seattle Midlife Women's Health Study. *Menopause, 20*(9), 915–921. doi:10.1097/GME.0b013e318284481a

Woods, N. F., Mitchell, E. S., & Adams, C. (2000). Memory functioning among midlife women: Observations from the Seattle Midlife Women's Health Study. *Menopause, 7*(4), 257–265.

Woods, N. F., Mitchell, E. S., Percival, D. B., & Smith-DiJulio, K. (2009). Is the menopausal transition stressful? Observations of perceived stress from the Seattle Midlife Women's Health Study. *Menopause, 16*(1), 90–97.

Woods, N. F., Smith-DiJulio, K., & Mitchell, E. S. (2010). Sexual desire during the menopausal transition and early postmenopause: Observations from the Seattle Midlife Women's Health Study. *Journal of Women's Health, 19*, 209–218.

Woods, N. F., Smith-DiJulio, K., Percival, D. B., Tao, E. Y., Mariella, A., & Mitchell, E. S. (2008). Depressed mood during the menopausal transition and early postmenopause: Observations from the Seattle Midlife Women's Health Study. *Menopause, 15*, 223–232.

Woods, N. F., Smith-DiJulio, K., Percival, D. B., Tao, E. Y., Taylor, H. J., & Mitchell, E. S. (2007). Symptoms during the menopausal transition and early postmenopause and their relation to endocrine levels over time: Observations from the Seattle

Midlife Women's Health Study. *Journal of Women's Health*, *16*(5), 667–677.

World Health Organization (WHO). (2011). *Global status report on noncommunicable diseases 2010*. Geneva, Switzerland: Author.

World Health Organization (WHO). (2012). *Global data on visual impairments 2010*. Geneva, Switzerland: Author.

World Health Organization (WHO). (2015). Diabetes. Retrieved from http://who.int/mediacentre/factsheets/fs312/en

Yasui, T., Maegawa, M., Tomita, J., Myatani, Y., Yamada, M., Uemura, H.,...Irahara, M. (2007). Changes in serum cytokine concentrations during the menopausal transition. *Maturitas, 56*, 396–403.

Ylitalo, K. R., Karvononen-Gutierrez, C. A., Fitzgerald, N., Zheng, T., Sternfeld, B., El Khoudayr, S. R., & Harlow, S. (2013). Relationship of race/ethnicity, body mass index, and economic strain with longitudinal self-report of physical functioning: The Study of Women's Health Across the Nation. *Annals of Epidemiology, 23*, 401–408.

Yusuf, S., Hawken, S., Ounpuu, S., Dans, T., Avezum, A., Lanas, F., . . . Lisheng, L. (2004). Effect of potentially modifiable risk factors associated with myocardial infarction in 52 countries (the INTERHEART study): Case-control study. *Lancet, 364*, 937–952.

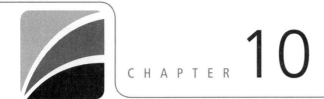

CHAPTER 10

Older Women's Health

Barbara B. Cochrane • Heather M. Young

Our beliefs and assumptions about older women—their capabilities, interests, and goals—influence how we behave toward them. Likewise, our behavior and the care we provide to older women affect their images of themselves. Just as sexism and racism are associated with stereotyping and discrimination simply because of one's gender or skin color, ageism can lead to systematic stereotyping of and discrimination against people because they are old (Ochida & Lachs, 2015; Reyna, Goodwin, & Ferrari, 2007). Getting old is an inevitable and universal process, but personal fears and denial about our own aging can negatively influence our attitudes toward older women. Societal attitudes are not easily changed, but an understanding of aging and older adults' strengths and challenges can increase the effectiveness of the care we provide to this population.

The goal of this chapter is to increase understanding of the multifaceted nature of being an older woman in America today and to serve as a knowledge base for providing appropriate health care. The population of older adults in America is composed mostly of women, many of whom are poor, living alone, and dealing with chronic illness, so most issues of aging and older adults' health can be thought of as women's issues. Although many of the challenges facing older women today are gender based, the context within which these issues arise can be more broadly described as a sociocultural phenomenon in which youth is valued over age and independence is valued over interdependence, regardless of gender.

The term *older women*, as used in this chapter, refers to women 65 years and older. Women's health issues have often focused on reproductive health and the changes associated with menopause, but until recently, women's postmenopausal years have been largely neglected. The lives of older women may span three or four decades (e.g., young old, middle old, oldest old, centenarians), such that this age group encompasses three or more birth cohorts of women who have led diverse lives and experienced a wide variety of challenges and opportunities. As young girls, some of these women experienced the Great Depression, whereas others were born just before Pearl Harbor was attacked. The sociocultural contexts of these older women's lives have been influenced by history and personal experience, changing norms and expectations, and visions and possibilities for the future. These powerful contextual factors

shape individual and collective views of what it means to age well. Topics included in this chapter, therefore, encompass the demographic patterns and social forces that shape older women's lives, age-related changes, key health concerns experienced by older women, and considerations for healthy aging and health promotion.

Over the past two decades, there has been a dramatic increase in evidence related to older women's health and factors that influence health and quality of life. Much of what we know about older women's health comes from long-term, observational studies of men and women, such as the Baltimore Longitudinal Study of Aging, the Framingham Heart Study, the Rancho Bernardo Study, the Seattle Longitudinal Study, and the Health and Retirement Study. Longitudinal studies of women's health have included the Nurses' Health Study and the Women's Health Initiative. All of these studies have followed participants for two or more decades. Some of these studies included only older adults; others enrolled young or midlife adults (and, in some, their children) and followed them through their older adult years. Most of these studies and many others are still ongoing. Analyses of their data will contribute to our understanding of older women's health for many years to come.

■ DEMOGRAPHIC AND ECONOMIC CONSIDERATIONS

Population Trends

The older population in the United States, those 65 years and older, has grown rapidly throughout the 20th century, from 3.1 million in 1900 to 40.3 million in 2010, with projections that this number will more than double to 83.7 million by 2050 (U.S. Census Bureau, 2014). Why this rapid increase? It is a combination of improvements in infant mortality, treatment of infectious diseases, and maturation of a large cohort, the baby-boomer generation. This large segment of the U.S. population was born between 1946 and 1964 and started turning 65 years beginning in 2011. As of the most recent census year in 2010, the percentage of adults 65 years and older made up approximately 13% of the total U.S. population, but they will represent nearly

21% of the total U.S. population by 2050, with the greatest increase occurring between 2010 and 2030 (U.S. Census Bureau, 2014).

In the United States, as in most countries of the world, adult women outnumber adult men (U.S. Census Bureau, 2014). Although male births outnumber female births, men generally have higher mortality rates at every age (National Center for Health Statistics, 2006), so the higher percentage of women compared with men is most pronounced at older ages, reflecting their increased life expectancy. Based on the year 2010 census data, women accounted for 57% of adults 65 years and older and 67% ages 85 years and older (Federal Interagency Forum on Aging-Related Statistics, 2012). Sex differences in life expectancy at age 65 years, however, are declining; they stood at 3.9 years in 1970 and 2.6 years in 2010 (U.S. Census Bureau, 2014).

Economics

The economic status of older women is an important factor in their health status and is influenced not just by current income and poverty rates, but by their Social Security and retirement benefits, relative health care costs, and health care insurance coverage. Although economic trends for older women are rapidly changing as the U.S. economy has changed, and particularly, as more women enter and remain in the workforce full time, women still experience profound economic disadvantages compared with men, in part because of historical differences in life trajectories. For example, men and women in younger cohorts are earning college degrees at about the same rate, but the economic status of the current cohort of older women has been influenced by previous gender gaps in educational opportunity. In 2010, 28% of older men, compared with 18% of older women had attained a bachelor's degree (Federal Interagency Forum on Aging-Related Statistics, 2012).

INCOME AND POVERTY

In each age group of working adults, women earn less than men for comparable work, such that older men who work full time and year round have higher median earnings than older women (Campbell & Pearlman, 2013). To this day, then, more older women than older men will live lives of poverty, regardless of race/ethnicity, geographic residence, age or labor force participation (Administration on Aging, 2014; Callander, Schofield, & Shrestha, 2012; U.S. Census Bureau, 2014). Although poverty rates of older adults in the United States have decreased over the last half century (from 35% in 1959 to 9% in 2010), age and sex disparities still exist (U.S. Census Bureau, 2014). Women still earn less than men for comparable work and have lower total lifetime earnings (U.S. Bureau of Labor Statistics, 2015). This disparity is even more pronounced for racial/ethnic minority women. Latina, American Indian/Alaska Native, and Pacific Islander women in the workforce more commonly receive lower wages, fewer benefits, and no retirement plan (American Association of University Women, 2015). Among adults 65 years and older in 2010, 21% of African American women and 21% of Hispanic women had incomes below the poverty level, compared with 8% of White women and 5% of White men (Federal Interagency Forum on Aging-Related Statistics, 2012). Being older, female, a member of a minority group, and living alone constitutes the greatest risk for poverty.

SOCIAL SECURITY AND RETIREMENT BENEFITS

Initially planned in 1935, Social Security benefits were designed for dependents after the wage earner's retirement, disability, or death. Under the current regulations, Social Security is biased against some older adults and nearly all older women because benefits are still calculated based on pre-1950s family and work structures and more continuous career trajectories (Tamborini & Whitman, 2007; Wright, 2012). Many older women have grown old functioning in the dual role of homemaker and head of household while employed in low- or minimum-wage jobs with much lower lifetime earnings than men. Older women, therefore, are far more likely than older men to be poor on the basis of Social Security and other retirement benefits earned in the workplace. Older women are penalized because they have a career trajectory that has been interrupted by childbearing, child rearing, and care of other family members, including elder care toward the end of their careers. Despite the economic value of this caregiving, spousal Social Security benefits may be limited if the woman's earned income is above a certain minimum level. The disparity in benefits is further widened by women's lower wages for work comparable with their male counterparts', the fact that fewer working women than working men have pensions or save for retirement (in part because their work is more likely to be part time), and dependence on Social Security for a larger share of their retirement income (Hegewisch, Hayes, Milli, Shaw, & Hartmann, 2015).

HEALTH CARE COSTS

Older adults use more health care services than any other age group and make up a significant percentage of the acute care population. These trends are only expected to increase as the baby boomers age. Although there has been a decline in long-term care or nursing home use by older adults over the years, a greater percentage of long-term care residents are women, and more women than men will live their final days in long-term care (Federal Interagency Forum on Aging-Related Statistics, 2012; U.S. Census Bureau, 2014). There are various national and state health programs to which older women may turn, but significant barriers still exist to good health care. In many situations the criteria for employer and supplemental medical insurance coverage are more easily met by men than by women, and women are likely to have greater out-of-pocket expenses for health care over their older adults years, in part because of their increased longevity (U.S. Census Bureau, 2014).

The two major sources of reimbursement for health care used by older women are Medicare and Medicaid. Although most older women have health insurance through Medicare, they still spend the same proportion of out-of-pocket income (15% or more) on health care as they did before the passage of Medicare in 1965, despite recent changes brought on by the Patient Protection and Affordable Care Act (Prospective Payment Assessment Commission, 1989; The Henry J. Kaiser Foundation, 2013). Although some preventive and behavioral counseling services are now covered by Medicare, only about 60% of older adults' health care costs overall are covered (Federal Interagency Forum on Aging-Related Statistics, 2012). These costs are disproportionately borne by women, who have a higher burden of chronic illness but are less likely than men to have Medicare Advantage or supplemental insurance and available family caregivers. The current reimbursement system discriminates against women because of its heavy emphasis on high-technology medical care and acute illness, whereas women with chronic illness and disability have increased needs for long-term services and supports (Hegewisch et al., 2015). Increased out-of-pocket costs for health care therefore become a considerable worry for many older women and may, in fact, limit or prevent their access to care. Each of the potentially reimbursable services has exceptions, copayments, deductibles, and other requirements that place considerable limitations on the coverage overall and cause considerable confusion for older adults. In addition to these restrictions, Medicare does not cover, or covers in extremely limited ways, many important health care services, such as extended long-term care in nursing homes, hearing aids, eyeglasses, dentures, foot care, and outpatient psychotherapy.

Medicare Part D was instituted in 2006 to provide Medicare recipients with coverage for prescription drugs, regardless of income, health status, or prescription drugs used. Although many issues and concerns associated with the implementation of this coverage have been addressed, including a low-income subsidy, there remains a great deal of confusion and concern about appropriate coverage, enrollment periods, and the wide variety of plans and associated formularies and costs. The Centers for Medicare & Medicaid Services (CMS; www.medicare.gov), AARP (www.aarp.org/health/medicare-insurance), and other groups offer helpful online information about this new coverage, as well as searchable databases to identify plans from which to choose, given an individual's current prescription drug needs.

The feminization of poverty among older women, particularly women who live alone and women of color, makes out-of-pocket costs a critical issue that can become untenable for some. Out-of-pocket expenditures for Medicare beneficiaries increase with age, but these costs are higher for older women (approximately $5,036 in 2010) than for older men ($4,327; Salganicoff, 2015). These costs are borne disproportionately by women not only because of their higher burden of chronic illness and need for long-term services and supports, but also because they are less likely to have private insurance and available family caregivers. As the primary source of health care coverage for the poor in America, Medicaid becomes an important health care support for older women, particularly women 85 years and older. Older women are more likely than men to be poor, so Medicaid coverage is both a class and a gender issue, with women representing 68% of those individuals "dually eligible" for both Medicare and Medicaid (Salganicoff, 2015).

■ CONTEXTS OF OLDER WOMEN'S LIVES

Relationships With Family and Friends and Caregiving

Demographic trends for older adults, particularly sex ratios of men to women, help explain why older women are much less likely to be married than older men (44.5% of women 65 years and older compared with 74.5% of men of the same age range; Federal Interagency Forum on Aging-Related Statistics, 2012). Predictably, widowhood is more common than widowerhood, with 35% of men 85 years and older being widowed compared with 73% of women in the same age group (Federal Interagency Forum on Aging-Related Statistics, 2012). Even when older women live alone, their connectedness to other family members and friends is important (Aday, Kehoe, & Farney, 2006; Eshbaugh, 2009) and reflects the importance with which women view their relationships and their self in relation to others (Jack, 1987; Surrey, 1991). With the higher likelihood of being unpartnered with age, close and intimate relationships for older women, many of which are long-term friendships, take on even more importance.

Older women enact many roles in the lives of their families. One of the most important roles is that of a caregiver. Some 60% to 65% of informal caregivers in the home are women (MetLife Mature Market Institute, 2011; National Alliance for Caregiving [NAC], 2009; U.S. Department of Health and Human Services Office of Disability, Aging, and Long-Term Care Policy, 2014). Caregiving prevalence at the household level varies among ethnic groups, with estimates of family caregiving occurring in 19.7% of Asian American, 20.3% of African American, 21.0% of Hispanic, and 16.9% of White households (NAC & AARP Public Policy Institute, 2015). Cultural and generational context shapes both expectations about caregiving and the experience of caregiving, including role and identity, rewards and challenges, and resources and supports (Apesoa-Varano, Tang-Feldman, Reinhard, Choula, & Young, 2015–2016).

Midlife and older women are the most frequent caregivers of aging parents and spouses, with about 25% spending 5 years or more providing care and higher hour caregivers (who spend more than 20 hours a week providing care) spending 10 years or more providing care. This fact is quite extraordinary when one considers the 17 years spent, on average, caring for their own dependent children and the fact that some older women are the primary caregivers for their grandchildren (Ellis & Simmons, 2014). Although midlife women are sometimes described as being in the "sandwich" generation (caring for both their children and their parents), some older adult women may also be providing care for three generations of family members or more.

An extensive literature on caregiving has established both the rewards and strains of this experience, including a sense of meaning, meeting of interpersonal obligations, pleasure in providing care to a loved one, and satisfaction, as well as feelings of burden and emotional stress. The impact of caregiving on the older women is a function of many factors, including vulnerability and strengths, the demands of the care situation, social support, characteristics of the care recipient, the type and quality of the dyad's relationship, and health (Cartwright, Archbold, Stewart, & Limandri, 1994; Chappell & Reid, 2002; MetLife Mature Market Institute, 2011; NAC, 2009; NAC & AARP Public Policy Institute, 2015; U.S. Department of Health and Human Services Office of Disability, Aging and Long-Term Care Policy, 2014; Young, 2003). The physical and emotional demands over a long period can result in negative health outcomes, including increased morbidity and mortality for caregivers (Vitaliano et al., 2002).

Many older women will be the primary providers of end-of-life care for their spouses, and their release from caregiving responsibilities comes with the death of the spouse. However, the death of a spouse, particularly after long-term caregiving, is one of the most significant losses for older women, often requiring great changes in lifestyle (DiGiacomo, Lewis, Nolan, Phillips, & Davidson, 2013). By age 75 years or older, 57% of women are widows, whereas at the same age, only 21% of men are widowed (U.S. Census Bureau, 2014). Given the median age of 59 years for widowhood among women in their first marriage and their life expectancy at that age, many women can expect more than 20 years of widowhood (Kreider & Ellis, 2011; U.S. Census Bureau, 2014). Thus spousal bereavement and widowhood has become almost normative for aging women, and loneliness—the single greatest difficulty experienced by older bereaved spouses—can persist for at least 2 years (Beal, 2006; Powers, Bisconti, & Bergeman, 2014). However, older bereaved spouses also demonstrate an extraordinary degree of resiliency, resourcefulness, and adaptability (Hahn, Cichy, Almeida, & Haley, 2011; see Chapter 18).

Living Arrangements

Older women in every racial/ethnic group, as well as in each age group, because of their increased longevity and fewer available potential partners, are more likely than men to live alone (36% of women compared with 19% of men; U.S. Census Bureau, 2014). However, non-Hispanic White women and African American women are more likely to live alone than Hispanic and Asian women, who are more likely to live with relatives (Federal Interagency Forum on Aging-Related Statistics, 2012). Marital history and number of children may influence these findings, as may cultural variations in beliefs about the care of older relatives or more available extended family members and thus more resources for care (Taylor et al., 2010). Relatives are the main source of assistance for older adults who live alone, but approximately 18% of those who live alone have no one to help them even for a few days.

Nursing homes are the most common institutional setting for older adults, but most women (93%) live in traditional community settings, not in nursing homes, other long-term care facilities, or community housing with special services (Federal Interagency Forum on Aging-Related Statistics, 2012). Relocation to a long-term care facility increases as older adults age; approximately 1% of older adults aged 65 to 74 years live in long-term care facilities, whereas 14% of those 85 years and older live in such facilities (Federal Interagency Forum on Aging-Related Statistics, 2012). Rates of nursing home residence have declined overall in recent years, reflecting both shorter stays in these settings for acute rehabilitation and wider variety of long-term care living arrangements available for older adults. However, the number and percentage of Hispanics and all racial groups except Whites in nursing homes have increased. Older women from racial/ethnic minority groups are more likely than Whites to postpone entering a nursing home, and when they do enter such facilities, they are more likely to have greater functional and cognitive impairments. However, it is possible that biases and prejudices within the long-term care system impede overall access for single women from racial/ethnic minority groups (Young, 2003).

A variety of new living arrangements for older adults is available, including continuing care retirement communities, life care communities, assisted-living residences, and adult day care, along with new models for home care. Many older adults are looking for living arrangements that provide access to high-quality health services but closely resemble ordinary home life, and a "culture change" (e.g., person-centered care, Eden Alternative, Green House) is taking place in long-term care (Baker, 2007; Thomas, 2004; Weiner & Ronch, 2003). Assisted living is the fastest growing sector in long-term care and is increasingly admitting more frail older adults with complex health needs (Cox, 2015; Golant & Hyde, 2008; U.S. Census Bureau, 2014). With an emphasis on independence and choice, assisted living offers a less institutional option than a nursing home and is appealing to many consumers. However, at this time, the assisted-living industry is predominately private pay. These trends in housing offer a wider array of service options for older women, but research regarding the health and well-being outcomes of older adults who live in these settings remains limited (Cox, 2015). In addition, racial/ethnic minority women may actually be experiencing a shift in health disparities, with decreased access to this newer variety of community-based options and, instead, an increased access to nursing homes (Feng, Fenell, Tyler, Clark, & Mor, 2011). There are concerns about both the affordability of these living arrangements and the extent of coordination required to ensure optimal care for older women taking advantage of community-based options.

Rural and Urban Contexts

Although the majority of people 65 years and older live in urban areas, the percentage of older adults in rural areas is slightly higher than in urban areas (17.8% compared with 15.5%; Rural Health Information Hub, 2015). Rural women are more likely to be older than their urban counterparts, given 23% of rural women are 65 years or older compared with 18% of urban women; the percentages of non-Hispanic White and non-Hispanic American Indian/Alaska Native women in rural areas are higher than those from other racial/ethnic groups (Health Resources and Services Administration, 2013). Economic security and access to health care are significant problems for rural residents, many of whom are older adults with chronic illnesses and disabilities. Rural residents have lower average incomes and higher poverty rates than urban residents. They are less likely to have a regular source of health care or sufficient health insurance (Ziller, 2014). Rural older adults living alone are more dependent on Medicaid than their urban-dwelling counterparts, are unlikely to have private insurance, and rely heavily on Medicare. At the same time, they are more likely to have higher rates of chronic illness (little of which is covered by Medicare) and to have limitations in activity as a result of chronic conditions (Young, 2003; Ziller, 2014). In rural settings, community-based resources for managing chronic illness are limited, such that more rural older adults, per capita, reside in nursing homes (National Advisory Committee on Rural Health and Human Services, 2010).

Retirement

Women are less prepared and less likely to retire when they reach retirement age, in large part because of the economic disadvantages related to their work and work-related benefits (U.S. Census Bureau, 2014). However, participation in the labor force is changing, and the gap between men's and women's participation is narrowing considerably. These trends mandate a closer examination of women's adjustment to retirement and the changes in social and personal resources as well as psychological and physical well-being after retirement. To date, most retirement research has focused primarily on men, and studies that have included women do not always examine gender differences (Duberley, Carmichael, & Szmigin, 2014). Most studies of women and retirement focus on the timing of retirement and retirement planning. Reviews of retirement research on women have indicated that because of different life paths and career trajectories, women do not prepare for retirement in the same way that men do, in terms of their decision making or their consideration of risk (Duberley et al., 2014; Simmons & Betschild, 2001). For women, their choices about retirement may be based on being able to contribute to social life more than their productivity. Women report less subjective well-being and satisfaction during retirement than men (Duberley et al., 2014; Quick & Moen, 1998), although this difference is small. Factors that contribute to women's perceptions of a good retirement include good health, fewer years spent in part-time employment, an early retirement, a good postretirement income, volunteer work, as well as more frequent and a greater variety of social activities. As a culture, we lack the societal map for ongoing engagement and meaning after retirement (Friedan, 1993). One of the developmental challenges of late life is determining how one remains involved in connections and activities that are meaningful, despite changes in social networks (Erikson, Erikson, & Kivnick, 1986).

Racial/Ethnic Contexts

Population projections indicate that by the year 2030, the older population will be much more diverse. In 2010, non-Hispanic Whites accounted for 64% of the older population, whereas African Americans, Asians, and Hispanics accounted for 12%, 5%, and 16%, respectively (Hegewisch et al., 2015). These percentages are projected to change by 2050, such that 47% of the older population will be non-Hispanic Whites, and African Americans, Asians, and Hispanics will account for 13%, 8%, and 28%, respectively, along with increasing numbers of immigrant women and older women classified as "other" because they are of two or more races. Currently, 12.4% of older adults are foreign born; immigrant older adults represent considerable diversity in their countries of origin, with wide-ranging languages and cultural traditions (Hayes-Bautista, Hsu, Perez, & Gamboa, 2002; U.S. Census Bureau, 2014). Women from underrepresented racial/ethnic groups will face the greatest challenges with poverty and disease, and it is this segment of the population that is growing the fastest. Among older women living alone in 2010, poverty rates were 12% for non-Hispanic White, about 19% for African American, 17% for Asian, and more than 20% for Hispanic women (U.S. Census Bureau, 2014).

Any consideration of the status of older women of color must be tempered by the fact that accurate information on the demographics of this population has been lacking until recent times (Angel & Hogan, 2004). Zambrana (1988) notes that the undercount of African American and Hispanic populations in the 1970 census led to a political advocacy movement by these groups to obtain more accurate national data. Documentation of the increasing diversity of older adults now challenges the health care system to incorporate greater inclusiveness in its programs and services to meet the varying needs of this changing population.

Lesbian Older Women

With the aging of the population, there are a growing number of older gay, lesbian, and bisexual adults. Although older lesbians may not have revealed their sexual identity publicly during the earlier years of their lives, they have unique health concerns and often remain relatively invisible and underserved within the health care system and by health care researchers (Brotman, Ryan, & Cormier, 2003; Claes & Moore, 2000; Hankivsky et al., 2010; Institute of Medicine, 2011). In the context of societal intolerance for same-sex relationships, older lesbians can face particular challenges in advocating for and participating in decision making for their partners during acute and chronic illness episodes, as well as accessing partner health benefits for their own health care. Lesbian, gay, bisexual, transgender, and queer or questioning (LGBTQ) older women have identified several areas for improvement in health and social services, to address needs for LGBTQ-oriented/friendly legal advice, social events, grief and loss counseling, social workers, and assisted living (Smith, McCaslin, Chang, Martinez, & McGrew, 2010). An increasingly salient issue is effective end-of-life planning, including ensuring legal rights and designated decision makers such as durable powers of attorney, areas where both older LGBTQ adults and health care providers lack adequate preparation (Cartwright, Hughes, & Lienert, 2012; see Chapter 19).

AGE-RELATED PHYSICAL CHANGES

Is the end of life built into its beginning? Several theories of aging focus on aging at a cellular level. For example, the free radical theory of aging suggests that aging is due in part to by-products of oxidative metabolism that attack cellular DNA and result in mutations (Martin, 1992); the thesis of genetic instability refers to faulty copying in dividing cells or the accumulation of errors in information-containing molecules (Kane, Ouslander, & Abrass, 2003). More recently, the study of telomeres—DNA caps on the end of chromosomes, which protect the genetic material and shorten with each replication to a critical point signaling the end of the cell's replicative life—has contributed to our understanding of biological aging and age-related diseases (National Institute on Aging, 2011). For example, longer telomeres in women compared with men are currently being explored as a possible linkage to women's greater longevity (Gardner et al., 2014), and sustained telomere length in cancer cells has been studied as an explanation for the prolonged replication of some cancer cells (Sutphin & Korstanje, 2016).

The Baltimore Longitudinal Study of Aging investigators (U.S. Department of Health and Human Services, 1984) identified six patterns of physical changes that can be viewed as age related: (a) the stability or the absence of significant change with age (e.g., personality); (b) declination with age resulting from age-related illnesses (e.g., arthritis); (c) steady declines in physical function even in the context of general good health (e.g., muscle strength); (d) more precipitous change in function, often associated with disease (e.g., dementia); (e) compensatory change to maintain function (e.g., aerobic capacity); and (f) changes over time that are unrelated to aging but instead reflect more secular trends (e.g., changes in diet resulting from increased processing of foods). Most physical changes of aging are not gender specific, but age-related changes do occur at different rates among individuals, and systems age at different rates within an individual, resulting in the great heterogeneity of aging processes among older adults (Kaeberlein & Martin, 2016).

Cardiovascular

Age-related structural and functional changes in the heart are similar for both older men and women and include increased vascular thickening and resultant stiffness, which correlates with the onset of hypertension in advancing age. Although not strictly a normal change of aging, the effects of lifestyle and heredity on atherosclerotic changes begin fairly early in life and accumulate over time such that most older women and men have some degree of subclinical or clinical coronary heart disease (CHD). (See Chapters 9 and 43 for a discussion on the effect of menopause on heart health.)

Immune Function

Age-related changes in both cell-mediated and humoral immune systems, sometimes described as biological immunosenescence, are often accompanied by an increased incidence of cancer, autoimmune diseases, and infections in older adults (Farley, McLafferty, & Hendry, 2011; Müller & Pawelec, 2016). For example, the reactivation of the herpes zoster virus in older adults is linked to a decline in the immune system with age. In addition, age is a risk factor for many of the cancers that affect older women, such as breast, colorectal, and ovarian cancer (Siegel, Miller, & Jemal, 2016).

Cognition

Cognition refers to the various mental functions—such as thinking, decision making, memory, attention, and problem solving—that are important for gaining, storing, using and expressing knowledge as well as engaging in daily functional activities (Institute of Medicine, 2015). Cognitive aging involves a gradual and dynamic process of changes in cognitive function that occur as a person gets older; these changes involve varying capacities, such as motivation, short- and long-term memory, intelligence, learning and retention of tasks, and other factors that facilitate or impede these capacities. Some abilities decline, whereas others, such as wisdom, remain stable, and yet others, such as knowledge, can improve with age. Some memory impairment may occur as women get older, but dementia, even mild cognitive impairment (MCI), is not considered a part of typical cognitive aging.

Sensory

Presbyopia, a gradual loss of the eyes' focusing ability because of lens changes, results in slightly increased farsightedness and some difficulty with accommodation and is a typical change of aging. Other vision changes, such as glaucoma, cataracts, and age-related macular degeneration are more age-related conditions; they occur more commonly in older adults but not in all (Brodie, 2010). Similarly, presbycusis, a gradual and very slight impairment in hearing, primarily for higher pitched tones, is considered a normal change of aging. Visual and/or hearing impairments have been reported by approximately 15% and 31% of women aged 65 years and older, respectively (Federal Interagency Forum on Aging-Related Statistics, 2012). Unfortunately, the purchase of appropriate corrective devices, such as eyeglasses and hearing aids, for these sensory impairments is a challenge for many older women, who may have insufficient supplemental insurance and income to cover out-of-pocket expenses that are not covered by Medicare.

SELECTED HEALTH ISSUES FOR OLDER WOMEN

Given the diversity of older women's experiences and daily lives, their health issues vary widely. Older women report higher levels of hypertension, asthma, chronic bronchitis and arthritis than men, and their lives are affected by a high risk of heart disease, cancer, and diabetes (Figure 10.1; Federal Interagency Forum on Aging-Related Statistics, 2012). These chronic illnesses cause much of the morbidity that older

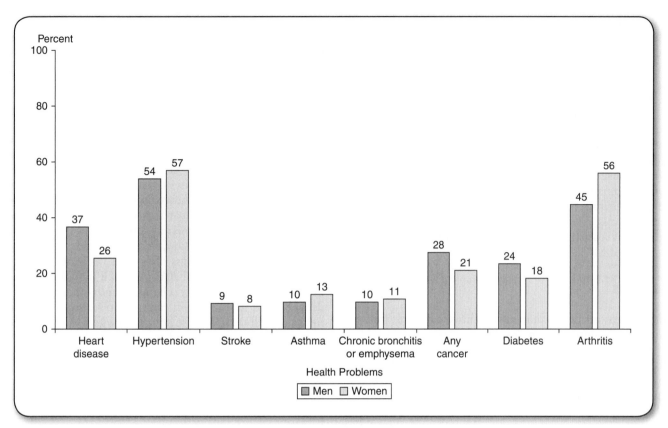

FIGURE 10.1

Percentage of people 65 years and older with selected health problems, by gender, 2009–2010.

Adapted from Federal Interagency Forum on Aging-Related Statistics (2012).

Data Source: Centers for Disease Control and Prevention, National Center for Health Statistics (2010).

women experience, and women's increasing longevity places them at high risk for multiple, concurrent chronic conditions.

Cardiovascular Disease

Clinical manifestations of cardiovascular disease, including hypertension, CHD, and stroke, are known to develop at a later age in women than in men (Institute of Medicine, 2010; Mozaffarian et al., 2016). Unlike men, women are also more likely to be diagnosed with CHD based on having clinical signs and symptoms of angina, rather than myocardial infarction. In addition, women more frequently experience "atypical" myocardial infarction symptoms (e.g., jaw aching, profound fatigue, arm pain without chest discomfort), rather than the more typical substernal chest pain (Canto et al., 2012; DeVon, Ryan, Ochs, & Shapiro, 2008). These findings suggest that there are important differences in the mechanisms of cardiovascular disease development in women compared with men, such as the influence of women's hormonal environment and responses to ischemia at the cellular level (Institute of Medicine, 2010). Strategies for preventing cardiovascular disease focus on the control of risk factors, including controlling smoking, hypertension, high cholesterol, obesity, and diabetes and increasing physical activity (Institute of Medicine, 2010; Mosca, Benjamin, et al., 2011).

Women have a higher prevalence and lifetime risk of stroke than men, primarily because of greater longevity

(Bushnell et al., 2014; Mozaffarian et al., 2016). More important, there is a 16-hour median delay in seeking care from the onset of symptoms, beyond the window of eligibility for thrombolytic treatment. This delay is likely to be related to low awareness of stroke risk factors (e.g., hypertension, hypercholesterolemia, diabetes, migraine with aura, atrial fibrillation, history of pregnancy-related complications, oral contraceptive or postmenopausal hormone therapy, smoking, physical inactivity, obesity) and lack of knowledge about warning symptoms (facial drooping, arm weakness, difficulty with speech, numbness, problems with dizziness or balance, vision symptoms, and severe headache; Bushnell et al., 2014). Because stroke is a leading cause of severe and long-term disability, increasing awareness of early symptoms among older women and management of risk factors are essential efforts. Hypertension is an important risk factor for CHD and stroke, and increases in prevalence among older women, disproportionately affecting African American women (Mosca, Barrett-Connor, & Wenger, 2011).

Cancer

More than 75% of all cancers are diagnosed at age 55 years or older (Siegel et al., 2016). Although breast cancer is diagnosed more frequently in women than any other cancer, lung cancer is the leading cause of cancer death. In recent years, mortality resulting from lung cancer has declined among older men and women, but the rate of decline has been much steeper among older men, a finding that may reflect the fact that cigarette smoking has not declined in women to the extent that it has in men (Siegel et al., 2016; U.S. Census Bureau, 2014). Other leading causes of cancer death in women, besides lung and breast cancer, include colorectal, pancreatic, and ovarian cancer (Siegel et al., 2016). Early detection through regular screening (e.g., mammography, colonoscopy) is critical for minimizing morbidity and mortality. Many older women survive cancer and live with it as a chronic disease. Treatment goals in this phase emphasize symptom management, ongoing monitoring, and optimization of function. Strategies for preventing cancer, similar to preventing cardiovascular disease, focus primarily on lifestyle modification, including healthy eating, physical activity, and weight control (Institute of Medicine, 2015).

Diabetes

Adult-onset or type 2 diabetes mellitus, characterized by a decreased sensitivity to insulin, confers a greater risk for CHD in women than in men (Mosca et al., 2007; Mozaffarian et al., 2016). Obese and overweight older women are at an even greater risk for developing diabetes. However, lifestyle factors, such as healthy eating, physical activity, and weight loss, may improve or even resolve problems with glucose control and obviate the need for medication (Paterson, Thorne, & Dewis, 1998). Currently, prevention and management of diabetes are key areas of nursing research and clinical interventions to decrease morbidity and mortality and enhance quality of life (Amoako, Skelly, & Rossen, 2008; Bond, Burr, Wolf, & Feldt, 2010; Young et al., 2014).

Arthritis

Approximately, 56% of older women report arthritic conditions (Federal Interagency Forum on Aging-Related Statistics, 2012), which may be classified as degenerative or osteoarthritis, with changes in the cartilage of the joint and associated pain, and inflammatory or rheumatoid arthritis, with joint inflammation and stiffness. Medications or surgery can address some of the functional difficulties and pain associated with arthritis, but weight loss and judicious physical activity remain important interventions for arthritis-associated symptoms.

Osteoporosis and Hip Fractures

Hip fractures, usually related to low bone density or osteoporosis, are a major cause of morbidity and mortality in older women, with only 40% of women actually regaining their functional status and independence after diagnosis and treatment of a hip fracture (National Osteoporosis Foundation, 2013) and at least double the mortality compared with women without hip fracture in the first year afterward (LeBlanc et al., 2011). Vertebral fractures may be even more common than hip fractures and can have a marked impact on women's functional health, particularly activities that involve bending and reaching, because of

debilitating back pain, loss of height, and kyphosis. (See Chapters 34 and 35 for a discussion of the effects of menopause on bone health.)

Cognitive Impairment, Alzheimer's Disease, and Related Dementias

MCI, a syndrome distinct from cognitive aging and associated with an increased risk of dementia, is characterized by a measurable change in at least one domain of cognition, without an impact on daily activities (Alzheimer's Association, 2013). Alzheimer's disease (AD) and related dementias are brain disorders characterized by impairments in two or more mental functions, such as memory, language, visual perception, attention, and the ability to reason and solve problems (National Institutes of Health, 2014). Manifestations of dementia can include confusion, behavior and personality changes, and other progressive declines such that a person cannot carry out normal activities of daily living. Because advancing age is the single greatest risk factor for AD, and given the rapid growth of the population aged 85 years and older, the prevalence of AD is expected to grow to nearly 9 million in the United States by 2050 (Plassman et al., 2011). There are some indications that the prevalence of MCI is higher in men than in women; but because of women's increased longevity, the majority of individuals with prevalent dementia are older women, with low cognitive functioning or dementia being an important risk factor for entering a skilled nursing facility (U.S. Census Bureau, 2014).

AD is irreversible, but medical treatment options have been developed that slow its progression, enhance memory, improve functioning, and minimize problem behaviors, such as agitation, sleep disturbances, and wandering. Medications approved to treat AD generally act by inhibiting cholinesterase or lowering glutamate levels in the brain and therefore improving certain cognitive skills and behavioral symptoms (Institute of Medicine, 2010). The long period between diagnosis and death, coupled with generally poor medical insurance coverage, makes the economic and psychological burdens on families of AD victims enormous. Interventions have been developed for families and caregivers of AD patients to enhance caregivers' coping skills and better manage behavioral disturbances (Teri, McCurry, Logsdon, & Gibbons, 2005; Teri et al., 2011; Zarit, Gaugler, & Jarrott, 1999); however, more scientific evidence translated to clinical interventions is needed regarding AD and related dementias in older women (Institute of Medicine, 2010).

Depression

Depression is an important mental health indicator that may represent a recurrent, chronic condition in older adults. Clinically relevant depression affects a higher percentage of older women than men, but it often goes underdiagnosed or undertreated. Women with depressive symptoms often experience high rates of physical illness, functional disability, and greater use of health services (Ayotte, Yang, & Jones, 2010; Barry, Allore, Guo, Bruce, & Gill, 2008). Research on depression in older women has identified important racial/ethnic considerations, including the finding that African American women have higher levels of depression throughout later life, a difference attributable, in part, to both physical health and socioeconomic status (Spence, Adkins, & Dupre, 2011). Medication, counseling and physical activity, ideally in combination, have been effective in treating depression in older adults (Akincigil et al., 2011; Blumenthal et al., 1999; Lavretsky et al., 2011), but insurance coverage restrictions on its treatment can create economic barriers to care for older women who are on fixed incomes.

Urinary Incontinence

Although not a disease, urinary incontinence (UI) has been described as a geriatric syndrome because of its impact on daily life and its prevalence in older adults, which is estimated to be 15% to 65% (depending on the study population). UI increases with age and is higher in frail nursing home residents (Bresee et al., 2014; Wilson, 2006). UI is twice as likely in women as men (Anderson, Davis, & Flynn, 2015). Types of UI include stress (leakage brought on by coughing, sneezing, laughing or straining), urge (associated with overactive bladder syndrome or inability to get to the toilet in time), nocturnal, or a combination of types (Hendrix et al., 2005). Decreased quality of life, depression, social isolation, restricted sexual activity, and falls are frequent consequences of UI (Aguilar-Navarro et al., 2012; Bresee et al., 2014; Hawkins et al., 2011). Transient UI may be an outcome of urinary tract infections, which are frequent among older women, as well as commonly prescribed medications such as antihypertensives and antidepressants (Anderson et al., 2015). In the past, menopausal hormone therapy was recommended as a treatment for UI, but such treatments actually constitute another medication that can increase risk and worsen symptoms of UI in postmenopausal women (Hendrix et al., 2005). Pharmacological treatment with antimuscarinic agents or more invasive treatments, such as surgery, are used for women with severe UI symptoms (Anderson et al., 2015). There is growing evidence of iatrogenic incontinence, induced by the use of catheters and adult diapers for the convenience of staff rather than with the goal of optimal function for the older woman, suggesting careful consideration in initiating physical products to manage continence (Zisberg et al., 2011).

Functional Changes and Frailty

Functional ability is a major determinant of a living situation and the need for supportive services. Acute or chronic illness, injury, or mental health problems can all have an impact on the ability of an older woman to manage instrumental activities of daily living (e.g., doing light housework, doing laundry, preparing meals, grocery shopping, getting around outside, managing money, taking medications, telephoning), as well as basic activities of daily living (e.g., bathing, dressing, getting in or out of bed, getting around inside, toileting, and eating; Federal Interagency Forum on Aging-Related Statistics, 2012). Although disability and functional limitations among older populations are declining, recent estimates are that 15.7 million noninstitutionalized older adults, 59% are older women or have some type of disability; the prevalence increases with advancing age (He & Larsen, 2014).

Older women with severe functional limitations, disability, or multiple comorbid disease conditions may be described as frail, but specific research definitions of frailty have evolved over time. *Frailty* has been described variously as a reaction of older adults to adverse events, increased vulnerability, accumulation of deficits, impaired complexity, and a phenotype or specific geriatric syndrome (Zaslavsky et al., 2013). Fried et al. (2001) defined the frailty phenotype as three or more of the following indicators: shrinking (unintentional weight loss or sarcopenia), poor endurance or self-reported exhaustion, weakness, slow walking speed, and low physical activity. This definition of frailty as a phenotype has been analyzed in research on older adults as being distinct from disability or comorbidity but predictive of profound functional decline and mortality (Fried et al., 2001; Woods et al., 2005). Research on frailty, including its measurement, neurocognitive indicators, other risk factors, biomarkers, as well as trajectories, interventions, and outcomes, is expanding rapidly (Zaslavsky et al., 2013). Our understanding of this phenomenon may one day help prevent its development and minimize its effects on older women's lives.

Elder Mistreatment

Elder mistreatment is a growing, but often hidden, problem in the United States (Fulmer, 2002; Institute of Medicine and National Research Council, 2014). It includes physical, sexual, emotional, and financial or exploitative acts, as well as neglect. These acts may be intentional or unintentional, may occur in the community or institutions, and occur across socioeconomic groups. Risk factors for elder mistreatment include dependency/vulnerability of the elder (e.g., functional impairment), female gender, social isolation, abuser psychosocial problems (e.g., alcohol/substance abuse, mental health issues), and shared living arrangements (Institute of Medicine and National Research Council, 2014). Although there has been an increased awareness of elder mistreatment, research and advocacy have focused on domestic violence of women, so the special problems of older women are sometimes ignored, particularly with regard to long-standing unreported wife abuse, abuse by caregivers, and exploitation and neglect of older women (Fulmer, 2002; Straka & Montminy, 2006). Elder mistreatment is sometimes difficult to identify with certainty, but health care professionals have a responsibility to ensure that it does not go unrecognized, unreported, or untreated. Identification and management of this complex phenomenon, which are best accomplished through interprofessional collaboration, can be challenging (Baker & Heitkemper, 2005).

■ HEALTHY AGING/HEALTH PROMOTION

Healthy aging for older women can involve negotiating a wide variety of challenges and transitions, as well as recognizing and building on various opportunities for growth. It does not necessarily represent a life that is free of chronic illness or functional impairment (Young & Cochrane, 2015). Although some older women live for several decades with excellent health and high function, others with chronic conditions still view themselves as healthy and functional. This latter view is inconsistent with research studies that define *successful aging* as the absence of disability or disease, high cognitive and physical function, and active engagement in life (Rowe & Kahn, 1998). More recently, a phenotype of positive aging focused on physical, social, and emotional functioning has been described in older women and has been found to predict health outcomes, such as decreased mortality, risk of major health conditions or hospitalizations, and risk of dependent living (Woods et al., 2012). Therefore engaging in health promotion and maintenance of function are key goals for many older women, regardless of their current health condition. Lifestyle modifications, including engaging in physical activity, eating a good diet, enhancing safety (e.g. fall prevention), minimizing risk (e.g., vaccinations), and taking an active role in one's health care management, are important components for healthy aging in older women.

Self-Management of Health

To promote personal growth and optimal aging, women need adequate information about their bodies as well as behavioral strategies that ensure a healthy lifestyle. Meeting these goals requires skills in information processing, decision making, integration of change into one's daily life, and action. Older women have been described as health conscious and resilient, and they are actually more likely than older men to have a regular physician, to have seen their physician in the past year, and to seek immediate care if symptomatic (Haber, 2013). With adequate information and skills, and an environment that promotes physical, mental, economic, and social health, older women can be well positioned to maintain independence and achieve late-life health goals. Chronic conditions pose the greatest threat to health, quality of life and functional ability and at the same time are the most amenable to improvement with behavioral health changes, such as healthy eating, activity, reduction of alcohol intake, and smoking cessation. Resources, such as the chronic disease self-management program developed by Lorig and Holman (2003) and technology-enabled coaching (Young et al., 2014), can augment older women's self-management efforts.

■ RECOMMENDED SCREENING

Guidelines for screening for older women are a function of age, risk factors, and multiple comorbidities. Evidence is evolving regarding recommendations. The American Geriatrics Society synthesizes current recommendations and hosts both general and condition-specific current guidelines for care of older adults at the www.GeriatricsCareOnline .org website (American Geriatrics Society, 2014). Federal websites provide detailed information about coverage under Medicare and eligibility for preventive services (www.medicare.gov and www.healthcare.gov). Table 10.1

summarizes current preventive services available through Medicare for older women, and Table 10.2 highlights focus areas for screening and risk assessment for older women.

Health care providers who consistently provide relevant and culturally sensitive information, encouragement, and support for making appointments, as well as a well-timed reminder about the importance of screening and prevention strategies, can have a significant impact on women's adherence to these recommendations, regardless of age or ethnicity (Davisson et al., 2009; Levy-Storms, Bastani, & Reuben, 2004; Lukwago et al., 2003; Palmer, Chhabra, & McKinney, 2011; Todd, Harvey, & Hoffman-Goetz, 2011; Tu et al., 2003).

Physical Activity

There is growing evidence that, with appropriate cautions, the benefits of physical activity in older adults, particularly weight-bearing aerobic exercise such as walking and exercises to improve balance, far outweigh possible risks (U.S. Department of Health and Human Services, 2008). Cardiovascular fitness, insulin resistance, body weight, mobility, bone density, pain, balance, risk of falls, quality of life, depressive symptoms, and cognition have shown improvement in older women who engage in physical activity/exercise, even among those with chronic health conditions or who are very frail (Aoyagi, Park, Park, & Shephard, 2010; de Oliveira, da Silva, Dascal, & Teixeira, 2014; Folta et al., 2009; Heesch, Burton, & Brown, 2011; Kovács, Prókai, Mészáros, & Gondos, 2013; Muir, Ye, Bhandari, Adachi, & Thabane, 2013; Teri et al., 2011; Uusi-Rasi et al., 2015; Wang, Luo, Barnes, Sano, & Yaffe, 2014). Despite these benefits and increased participation in physical activity in the last 20 years among older adults, participation among older women compared with older men remains low; 8% of older women vs. 14% of older men met federal guidelines for regular physical activity (Federal Interagency Forum on Aging-Related Statistics, 2012). Multiple resources, such as the Centers for Disease Control and Prevention's Mall Walking Guide (Belza et al., 2015), are readily available online to program developers and older adults to support innovative, evidence-based physical activity programs and exercises (see Chapter 14).

Healthy Eating

Healthy eating can play an important role in preventing or delaying the onset or morbidity associated with many chronic diseases, such as CHD, cancer, stroke, and diabetes (Federal Interagency Forum on Aging-Related Statistics, 2012). In addition, adhering to recommended dietary guidelines can reduce controllable risk factors for chronic diseases, such as obesity, hypertension, and hypercholesterolemia (Reidlinger et al., 2015). For older women, many of whom tend to gain weight as they age, healthy eating can also be synonymous with good weight control (Du et al., 2010).

Although caloric needs decrease with aging, the need for variety and quality of nutritional intake remains. Older women's diets may be deficient in certain vitamins and minerals, such as vitamin B_{12}, vitamin A, vitamin C,

TABLE 10.1	Screening and Preventive Services for Older Women Under Medicare Coverage	
PREVENTIVE SERVICE	WHAT IS COVERED	WHOM MEDICARE COVERS
Alcohol misuse counseling	Screening and up to four face-to-face counseling sessions/year	All who are not alcohol dependent
Breast cancer	Breast examinations, mammograms, digital technology	Older than 40 years
Cardiovascular screening	Cholesterol, lipid, triglyceride	All
Cervical and vaginal cancer	Pap tests with pelvic examinations	All women
Colorectal cancer	Fecal occult blood test, flexible sigmoidoscopy, screening colonoscopy	Older than 50 years
Depression screening	One per year	All
Diabetes screening	Fasting blood glucose test	At risk
HIV screening	HIV test	At risk
Obesity screening/counseling	Screening and face-to-face counseling	BMI > 30
Osteoporosis	Bone density test	At risk
Tobacco use cessation	Up to eight face-to-face counseling sessions/year	Use tobacco, and not diagnosed with illness caused by tobacco
Vaccinations	Flu/pneumoccal/hepatitis B	All flu/pneumococcal/at risk for hepatitis B

BMI, body mass index.
Source: Centers for Medicare & Medicaid Services (2014).

TABLE 10.2	Screening for Geriatric Health Issues
RECOMMENDATION	FREQUENCY
Falls	Annually
Incontinence	Annually
Cognitive status	If symptomatic
Depression	Annually
Vision	Annually
Hearing	Annually
Nutrition	Obtain weight each visit and height annually; calculate BMI
Mistreatment	Question with clinical suspicion
Safety and preventing injury	Check smoke and carbon monoxide detectors, check water heater temperature, use sun protection, test driving skills, wear seat belts, complete advance directives, and determine health care proxy

BMI, body mass index.
Source: American Geriatrics Society (2014).

vitamin D, calcium, iron, zinc, and other trace minerals (Chernoff, 2005). Factors that influence older women's eating habits include living alone (and not focusing on one's own nutrition or regular meals), lower income (and trying to conserve money by purchasing less expensive processed and fast foods), and chronic disease (with complicated treatment regimens and effects on appetite). Older women who live alone can meet their nutritional needs and minimize social isolation by dining together regularly with friends (Moremen, 2008) (see Chapter 13).

Weight Control

Obesity, described as an epidemic in the United States today, has increased among older women in recent decades (Federal Interagency Forum on Aging-Related Statistics, 2004), yet it is a key modifiable risk factor for disease, morbidity from chronic disease, and death. Obesity is associated with an increased risk of CHD, hypertension, diabetes, some cancers, osteoarthritis, and disability, among other chronic conditions (de S. Santos Machado et al., 2013; Rillamas-Sun et al., 2014; Rolland et al., 2009). Obese older women can derive multiple health benefits from weight loss (Corona et al., 2013; Rossen, Milsom, Middleton, Daniels, & Perri, 2013); however, careful ongoing health assessments are warranted during weight loss to evaluate the impact on lean muscle mass, fracture risk, and other health parameters.

Sleep

Older adults do not always report problems with sleep to their health care providers because the common wisdom has held that sleep disturbances are to be expected as one grows older. However, sleep problems are actually not a normal part of aging (Vitiello, 2009). Although sleep architecture changes—decreased rapid eye movement and slow wave sleep, increased awakenings at night, and a "phase advance" in circadian rhythms (becoming sleepy earlier)—are seen with aging, these changes usually occur before age 65 years and generally have only modest effects on patterns of sleep, such as daytime napping (Vitiello, 2009). Older adults often use sleep management strategies, such as watching television or taking pain medications, which can actually worsen symptoms (Gooneratne et al., 2011). Instead, management of sleep disturbances should include an effort to rule out obstructive sleep apnea and other primary sleep disorders (which can be associated with functional and cognitive declines), promote good sleep hygiene (e.g., establishing a nighttime routine, minimizing exposure to light in the bedroom, not remaining in bed if one is not sleeping), and use cognitive behavioral therapy (Spira et al., 2014; Vitiello, 2009; Yaffe et al., 2011). The use of sleep medications has been associated with a sense of stigma for older women (Walker, Luszcz, Hislop, & Moore, 2012), but such medication can be very effective and should not be avoided. Geriatric pharmacotherapy guidelines for these medications would include a plan to "start low and go slow," because sleep medication can be associated with adverse effects in older adults (e.g., oversedation during the day, falls), cautious monitoring for side effects and drug interactions, particularly if the sleep medication is included on a list of potentially inappropriate medications for older adults (American Geriatrics Society 2015 Beers Criteria Update Expert Panel, 2015).

Prevention of Falls

Because fall-related fractures increase the risk for further decline, the prevention of falls is a top priority. Hip fractures and most other nonvertebral fractures in older women occur because of a fall (North American Menopause Society, 2010), making fall prevention a key safety concern for older women. Falls can have a major impact on women's morbidity and mortality (Hedman, Fonad, & Sandmark, 2013; Yu, Hwang, Hu, Chen, & Lin, 2013). A Cochrane Review of fall-prevention interventions showed that programs likely to be beneficial included multidisciplinary and multifactorial programs with both health and environmental risk factor screening and modification in the community and residential facilities; home hazard assessment and modification, muscle strengthening, and balance retraining programs; and withdrawal of psychotropic medications (Gillespie et al., 2012).

Vaccinations

Because of immune system changes with aging (e.g., immuno-senescence) and an increased prevalence of multiple chronic illnesses, older adults can be particularly vulnerable to infectious conditions, associated profound morbidity with complications, and increased risk of mortality. Therefore older adults are particularly important targets for vaccination. Annual influenza, onetime pneumococcal (after age 65 years), and herpes zoster (after age 60 years) vaccinations are recommended for older adults and are reimbursable by Medicare to guard against these infections and/or minimize their severity and systemic effects (Weinberger & Grubeck-Loebenstein, 2012). Vaccination rates in older adults, however, are inadequate, with 71% of older women and men aged 65 years and older reporting influenza vaccination during the past 12 months and 61% reporting any pneumococcal vaccination (Administration on Aging, 2014).

Medication Management

Prescription drug use has increased dramatically over the years as more and more new medications are introduced. Polypharmacy, or use of multiple medications, can be a significant safety issue for older adults, particularly older women who consume the majority of prescription medications. With the higher number of chronic illnesses with age, the drug burden, along with the potential for drug interactions, increases. Among community-dwelling older adults, 81% take at least one prescription medication, 42% take at least one over-the-counter (OTC) medication, and 49% use a dietary supplement. More important, 29% take at least five prescription medications, and more than half concurrently take more than five prescription, OTC, and dietary supplements. The number of medications increases with age, and women take more than men overall and at least 4% are at risk of major drug–drug interactions (Qato et al., 2008). Certain drugs are generally recognized as being inappropriate for older adults (Fick et al., 2003), yet these continue to be prescribed.

Although polypharmacy has long been a topic of concern in geriatrics, there is increasing evidence of undertreatment of older adults, according to evidence-based guidelines (Simon et al., 2005). The coexistence of multiple diseases (McCormick & Boling, 2005), with sometimes conflicting treatment guidelines, presents challenges for medication management. Increasingly, the foci in health care are on appropriate prescription of medications rather than polypharmacy reduction, ensuring that prescriptions take into consideration age-related changes and evidence-based guidelines and keeping potential drug interactions in mind while attempting to minimize the total medication burden.

Older adults are at particular risk for adverse drug reactions because of age-related changes in pharmacokinetics and pharmacodynamics, resulting in slower excretion and differences in drug metabolism. Adverse drug reactions are the most preventable form of iatrogenic illness, resulting in considerable disability for older adults (Kane et al., 2003). The likelihood of an adverse drug reaction is heightened by inappropriate prescribing, multiple prescribers, or inadequate understanding of the drug indications, administration guidelines, and side effects. Confusion about medication management is greater among older adults who are experiencing mild to moderate memory impairment (which may or may not be a side effect of one or more medications).

Adverse drug events are most commonly related to unintentional overdoses of four major medication classes (warfarin, insulin, oral antiplatelet agents, and oral hypoglycemic agents) and pose a significant cause for hospitalization (Budnitz, Lovegrove, Shehab, & Richards, 2011).

Optimal medication management occurs with appropriate prescription given the goals of the older woman, coupled with evidence-based guidelines that take comorbidities into account. Adherence can be improved by addressing both health literacy and financial considerations, as well as the deployment of enabling technology for reminding and tracking medications.

Social Relationships

Connection with others is core to healthy aging. Women often survive spouses and friends, resulting in changes in their social network, with losses and opportunities to develop new relationships. Women more readily form and nurture relationships and commonly possess skills and abilities to sustain and develop meaningful connections across the life span. Compared with most men, women play a key role in ensuring family connectivity, sustaining friendships over longer periods of time and actively engaging in friendships throughout life.

With changes in work and living situation late in life, women often find themselves actively forming new relationships even in old age. Indeed, 60% of older women have recently made a new close friend (Armstrong, 2000). Older women have active friendship networks, having regular interaction with at least one friend at least weekly, with half having contact daily. Older women have an average social network size of 11.8 friends, with African American women identifying 13.5 friends and White women naming 10.2 friends. Compared to earlier in their lives, more than half had made younger (older than 25 years), cross-generational friends, and several reported their first cross-ethnic friendships (Armstrong, 2000). An important dynamic with age is the change in both family and friendship relationships because of increasing dependence on others for assistance. Differences develop, with friends often providing greater social support and intimacy, while families provide more instrumental support (Siu & Phillips, 2002).

Sexuality

Older women are sexual beings who are capable of meaningful sexual relationships. Normal changes with age generally do not affect women's sexual desires and the ability to experience an orgasm (Addis et al., 2006). Physiological changes associated with lowered estrogen affecting vaginal blood flow can make intercourse uncomfortable. A number of additional factors influence sexual function for older women: established behavioral patterns and preferences, illness, relationship quality, self-esteem, life stressors, and societal values.

Loss of a partner has been reported to be the main reason older women are no longer sexually active (Ginsberg, Pomerantz, & Kramer-Feeley, 2005), and the prevalence of sexual activity declines as widowhood increases with age.

More than 60% of older women between 57 and 64 years are sexually active, 40% among those between 65 and 74 years are active, and less than 20% of women between 75 and 85 years remain active. Among those who are sexually active, approximately half report issues that are bothersome to them, most commonly low desire (43%), difficulty with vaginal lubrication, (39%), and inability to have an orgasm (34%). These concerns are more likely among women with chronic health conditions (Lindau et al., 2007). Discussion of sexual concerns remains limited, with only 22% of women older than 50 years having conversations about their sexuality with health care providers, highlighting the importance of a thorough sexual history to guide possible treatments, such as lubricants, vaginal moisturizers, or estrogen creams to reduce physical discomfort or counseling for issues of relationship quality. If a healthy older woman has remained sexually active, is not inhibited by societal stereotypes and myths against sex with advanced age, and has a partner who has maintained sexual interest and ability to engage in sexual activity, it is likely that she will have continued satisfactory sexual relationships. (See Chapter 19 for a comprehensive life-span discussion of sexuality.)

■ SUMMARY

This chapter focuses on older women and their experiences of aging, shaped by the sociopolitical context of women's lives and the disparities in access to health care and services that are related to gender, race, and class. The economic lives of older women are improving, but their economic disadvantages compared with older men are expected to continue; this is particularly true for women of color who experience the triple effects of gender, age, and ethnicity. The diversity of the older population is growing, and the coming wave of baby boomers represents a challenge for policy makers, private enterprises, families, and health care providers (Young, 2003). As baby boomers attain their eighth decade of life in large numbers, it is highly likely that aging in our culture will be redefined and new solutions and innovations will proliferate in the coming decades.

A woman's experience of aging depends on her personal characteristics and history, access to resources that promote health, and ability to develop strategies for coping with loss and change. Coping with the changes that accompany aging involves some losses that may not be anticipated, but many of the normal psychological and physiological changes that affect older women may be predicted. Improving outcomes for older women starts with primary prevention to improve general health, delay the onset of disability, and increase productivity and well-being; it continues with health promotion to minimize the effects of chronic conditions and optimize quality of life and functional capacity. If women are educated about age-related changes and given time to assimilate and plan for the process of transition from one phase of life to the next, the potential for optimal aging will be enhanced. Sensitivity to the needs and issues of older women and advocacy for appropriate access and service is essential for promoting the health and well-being of this significant population.

■ REFERENCES

Aday, R. H., Kehoe, G. C., & Farney, L. A. (2006). Impact of senior center friendships on aging women who live alone. *Journal of Women & Aging, 18*(1), 57–73.

Addis, I. B., Van Den Eeden, S. K., Wassel-Fyr, C. L., Vittinghoff, E., Brown, J. S., & Thom, D. H.; Reproductive Risk Factors for Incontinence Study at Kaiser Study Group. (2006). Sexual activity and function in middle-aged and older women. *Obstetrics and Gynecology, 107*(4), 755–764.

Administration on Aging. (2014). *A profile of older Americans: 2014.* Retrieved from http://www.aoa.gov/Aging_Statistics/Profile/2014/docs/2014-Profile.pdf

Aguilar-Navarro, S., Navarrete-Reyes, A. P., Grados-Chavarría, B. H., García-Lara, J. M., Amieva, H., & Avila-Funes, J. A. (2012). The severity of urinary incontinence decreases health-related quality of life among community-dwelling elderly. *The Journals of Gerontology. Series A, Biological Sciences and Medical Sciences, 67*(11), 1266–1271. doi:10.1093/gerona/gls152

Akincigil, A., Olfson, M., Walkup, J. T., Siegel, M. J., Kalay, E., Amin, S.,...Crystal, S. (2011). Diagnosis and treatment of depression in older community-dwelling adults: 1992–2005. *Journal of the American Geriatrics Society, 59*(6), 1042–1051. doi:10.1111/j.1532–5415.2011.03447.x

Alzheimer's Association. (2013). 2013 Alzheimer's disease factors and figures. *Alzheimer's & Dementia, 9*(2), 208–245.

American Association of University Women. (2015). *The simple truth about the gender pay gap.* Washington, DC: Author.

American Geriatrics Society. (2014). Clinical guidelines and recommendations. *GeriatricsCareOnline.Org.* Retrieved from http://www.geriatricscareonline.org/ProductStore/clinical-guidelines-recommendations/8/

American Geriatrics Society 2015 Beers Criteria Update Expert Panel. (2015). American Geriatrics Society 2015 updated Beers criteria for potentially inappropriate medication use in older adults. *Journal of the American Geriatrics Society, 63*(11), 2227–2246. doi:10.1111/jgs.13702

Amoako, E., Skelly, A. H., & Rossen, E. K. (2008). Outcomes of an intervention to reduce uncertainty among African American women with diabetes. *Western Journal of Nursing Research, 30*(8), 928–942. doi:10.1177/0193945908320465

Anderson, K. M., Davis, K., & Flynn, B. J. (2015). Urinary incontinence and pelvic organ prolapse. *The Medical Clinics of North America, 99*(2), 405–416.

Angel, J. L., & Hogan, D. P. (2004). Population aging and diversity in a new era. In K. E. Whitfield (Ed.), *Closing the gap: Improving the health of minority elders in the new millenium* (pp. 1–12). Washington, DC: Gerontological Society of America.

Aoyagi, Y., Park, H., Park, S., & Shephard, R. J. (2010). Habitual physical activity and health-related quality of life in older adults: Interactions between the amount and intensity of activity (the Nakanojo Study). *Quality of Life Research: An International Journal of Quality of Life Aspects of Treatment, Care and Rehabilitation, 19*(3), 333–338. doi:10.1007/s11136–010-9588–6

Apesoa-Varano, E., Tang-Feldman, Y., Reinhard, S., Choula, R., & Young, H. (2015–16). Multi-cultural caregiving and caregiver interventions: A look back and a call for future action. *Generations, 39*(4), 39–48.

Armstrong, M. J. (2000). Older women's organization of friendship support networks: An African American-white American comparison. *Journal of Women & Aging, 12*(1–2), 93–108.

Ayotte, B. J., Yang, F. M., & Jones, R. N. (2010). Physical health and depression: A dyadic study of chronic health conditions and depressive symptomatology in older adult couples. *The Journals of Gerontology. Series B, Psychological Sciences and Social Sciences, 65*(4), 438–448.

Baker, B. (2007). *Old age in a new age: The promise of transformative nursing homes.* Nashville, TN: Vanderbilt University Press.

Baker, M. W., & Heitkemper, M. M. (2005). The roles of nurses on interprofessional teams to combat elder mistreatment. *Nursing Outlook, 53*(5), 253–259.

Barry, L. C., Allore, H. G., Guo, Z., Bruce, M. L., & Gill, T. M. (2008). Higher burden of depression among older women: The effect of onset, persistence, and mortality over time. *Archives of General Psychiatry, 65*(2), 172–178.

Beal, C. (2006). Loneliness in older women: A review of the literature. *Issues in Mental Health Nursing, 27*(7), 795–813.

Belza, B., Allen, P., Brown, D. R., Farren, L., Janicek, S., Jones, D. L., ... Rosenberg, D. (2015). *Mall walking: A program resource guide.* Retrieved from http://www.cdc.gov/physicalactivity/downloads/mallwalking-guide.pdf

Blumenthal, J. A., Babyak, M. A., Moore, K. A., Craighead, W. E., Herman, S., Khatri, P.,...Krishnan, K. R. (1999). Effects of exercise training on older patients with major depression. *Archives of Internal Medicine, 159*(19), 2349–2356.

Bond, G. E., Burr, R. L., Wolf, F. M., & Feldt, K. (2010). The effects of a web-based intervention on psychosocial well-being among adults aged 60 and older with diabetes: A randomized trial. *The Diabetes Educator, 36*(3), 446–456. doi:10.1177/0145721710366758

Bresee, C., Dubina, E. D., Khan, A. A., Sevilla, C., Grant, D., Eilber, K. S., & Anger, J. T. (2014). Prevalence and correlates of urinary incontinence among older community-dwelling women. *Female Pelvic Medicine & Reconstructive Surgery, 20*(6), 328–333. doi:10.1097/spv.0000000000000093

Brodie, S. E. (2010). Aging and disorders of the eye. In H. M. Fillit, K. Rockwood, & K. Woodhouse (Eds.), *Brocklehurst's textbook of geriatric medicine and gerontology* (8th ed., pp. 810–821). Philadelphia, PA: Saunders Elsevier.

Brotman, S., Ryan, B., & Cormier, R. (2003). The health and social service needs of gay and lesbian elders and their families in Canada. *The Gerontologist, 43*(2), 192–202.

Budnitz, D. S., Lovegrove, M. C., Shehab, N., & Richards, C. L. (2011). Emergency hospitalizations for adverse drug events in older Americans. *New England Journal of Medicine, 365*(21), 2002–2012.

Bushnell, C., McCullough, L. D., Awad, I. A., Chireau, M. V., Fedder, W. N., Furie, K. L.,...on behalf of the American Heart Association Stroke Council, Council on Cardiovascular and Stroke Nursing, Council on Clinical Cardiology, Council on Epidemiology and Prevention, and Council for High Blood Pressure Research. (2014). Guidelines for the prevention of stroke in women: A statement for healthcare professionals from the American Heart Association/American Stroke Association. *Stroke, 45*(5), 1545–1588. Retrieved from http://stroke.ahajournals.org/content/early/2014/02/06/01.str.0000442009.06663.48

Callander, E. J., Schofield, D. J., & Shrestha, R. N. (2012). Multiple disadvantages among older citizens: What a multidimensional measure of poverty can show. *Journal of Aging & Social Policy, 24*(4), 368–383.

Campbell, C., & Pearlman, J. (2013). Period effects, cohort effects, and the narrowing gender wage gap. *Social Science Research, 42*(6), 1693–1711.

Canto, J. G., Rogers, W. J., Goldberg, R. J., Peterson, E. D., Wenger, N. K., Vaccarino, V.,...Zheng, Z. J.; NRMI Investigators. (2012). Association of age and sex with myocardial infarction symptom presentation and in-hospital mortality. *Journal of the American Medical Association, 307*(8), 813–822.

Cartwright, C., Hughes, M., & Lienert, T. (2012). End-of-life care for gay, lesbian, bisexual and transgender people. *Culture, Health & Sexuality, 14*(5), 537–548.

Cartwright, J. C., Archbold, P. G., Stewart, B. J., & Limandri, B. (1994). Enrichment processes in family caregiving to frail elders. *ANS. Advances in Nursing Science, 17*(1), 31–43.

Centers for Disease Control and Prevention, National Center for Health Statistics. (2010). *National Interview Survey.* Retrieved from http://www.cdc.gov/nchs/nhis.htm

Centers for Medicare & Medicaid Services. (2014). *What Medicare covers.* Retrieved from http://www.medicare.gov/what-medicare-covers/index.html

Chappell, N. L., & Reid, R. C. (2002). Burden and well-being among caregivers: Examining the distinction. *The Gerontologist, 42*(6), 772–780.

Chernoff, R. (2005). Micronutrient requirements in older women. *American Journal of Clinical Nutrition, 81*(5), 1240S–1245S.

Claes, J. A., & Moore, W. (2000). Issues confronting lesbian and gay elders: The challenge for health and human services providers. *Journal of Health and Human Services Administration, 23*(2), 181–202.

Corona, L. P., Nunes, D. P., Alexandre, Tda S., Santos, J. L., Duarte, Y. A., & Lebrão, M. L. (2013). Weight gain among elderly women as risk factor for disability: Health, Well-being and Aging Study (SABE Study). *Journal of Aging and Health, 25*(1), 119–135. doi:10.1177/0898264312466261

Cox, C. B. (2015). *Social policy for an aging society: A human rights perspective*. New York, NY: Springer Publishing.

Davisson, L., Warden, M., Manivannan, S., Kolar, M., Kincaid, C., Bashir, S., & Layne, R. (2009). Osteoporosis screening: Factors associated with bone mineral density testing of older women. *Journal of Women's Health, 18*(7), 989–994. doi:10.1089/jwh.2008.1138

de Oliveira, M. R., da Silva, R. A., Dascal, J. B., & Teixeira, D. C. (2014). Effect of different types of exercise on postural balance in elderly women: A randomized controlled trial. *Archives of Gerontology and Geriatrics, 59*(3), 506–514. doi:10.1016/j.archger.2014.08.009

de S. Santos Machado, V., Valadares, A. L., Costa-Paiva, L. H., Osis, M. J., Sousa, M. H., & Pinto-Neto, A. M. (2013). Aging, obesity, and multimorbidity in women 50 years or older: A population-based study. *Menopause, 20*(8), 818–824. doi:10.1097/GME.0b013e31827fdd8c

DeVon, H. A., Ryan, C. J., Ochs, A. L., & Shapiro, M. (2008). Symptoms across the continuum of acute coronary syndromes: Differences between women and men. *American Journal of Critical Care, 17*(1), 14–24; quiz 25.

DiGiacomo, M., Lewis, J., Nolan, M. T., Phillips, J., & Davidson, P. M. (2013). Transitioning from caregiving to widowhood. *Journal of Pain and Symptom Management, 46*(6), 817–825.

Du, H., van der A, D. L., Boshuizen, H. C., Forouhi, N. G., Wareham, N. J., Halkjaer, J.,...Feskens, E. J. (2010). Dietary fiber and subsequent changes in body weight and waist circumference in European men and women. *American Journal of Clinical Nutrition, 91*(2), 329–336. doi:10.3945/ajcn.2009.28191

Duberley, J., Carmichael, F., & Szmigin, I. (2014). Exploring women's retirement: Continuity, context and career transition. *Gender, Work and Organization, 21*(1), 71–90.

Ellis, R. R., & Simmons, T. (2014). *Coresident grandparents and their grandchildren: 2012.* (Current Population Reports P20–576). Washington, DC: U.S. Census Bureau.

Erikson, E. H., Erikson, J. M., & Kivnick, H. Q. (1986). *Vital involvement in old age: The experience of old age in our time.* New York, NY: W. W. Norton.

Eshbaugh, E. M. (2009). The role of friends in predicting loneliness among older women living alone. *Journal of Gerontological Nursing, 35*(5), 13–16.

Farley, A., McLafferty, E., & Hendry, C. (2011). *The physiological effects of ageing: Implications for nursing practice.* Ames, IA: Wiley-Blackwell.

Federal Interagency Forum on Aging-Related Statistics. (2004). *Older Americans 2004: Key indicators of well-being.* Washington, DC: U.S. Government Printing Office.

Federal Interagency Forum on Aging-Related Statistics. (2012). *Older Americans 2012: Key indicators of well-being.* Washington, DC: U.S. Government Printing Office.

Feng, Z., Fenell, M. L., Tyler, D. A., Clark, M., & Mor, V. (2011). Growth of racial and ethnic minorities in US nursing homes driven by demographics and possible disparities in options. *Health Affairs, 30*(7), 1358–1365. Retrieved from http://content.healthaffairs.org/content/30/7/1358.full.html

Fick, D. M., Cooper, J. W., Wade, W. E., Waller, J. L., Maclean, J. R., & Beers, M. H. (2003). Updating the Beers criteria for potentially inappropriate medication use in older adults: Results of a U.S. consensus panel of experts. *Archives of Internal Medicine, 163*(22), 2716–2724.

Folta, S. C., Lichtenstein, A. H., Seguin, R. A., Goldberg, J. P., Kuder, J. F., & Nelson, M. E. (2009). The Strong Women-Healthy Hearts program: Reducing cardiovascular disease risk factors in rural sedentary, overweight, and obese midlife and older women. *American Journal of Public Health, 99*(7), 1271–1277. doi:10.2105/ajph.2008.145581

Fried, L. P., Tangen, C. M., Walston, J., Newman, A. B., Hirsch, C., Gottdiener, J.,...McBurnie, M. A.; Cardiovascular Health Study Collaborative Research Group. (2001). Frailty in older adults: Evidence for a phenotype. *The Journals of Gerontology. Series A, Biological Sciences and Medical Sciences, 56*(3), M146–M156.

Friedan, B. (1993). *The fountain of age.* New York, NY: Simon and Schuster.

Fulmer, T. (2002). Elder mistreatment. *Annual Review of Nursing Research, 20,* 369–395.

Gardner, M., Bann, D., Wiley, L., Cooper, R., Hardy, R., Nitsch, D.,...Ben-Shlomo, Y.; Halcyon Study Team. (2014). Gender and telomere length: Systematic review and meta-analysis. *Experimental Gerontology, 51,* 15–27.

Gillespie, L. D., Robertson, M. C., Gillespie, W. J., Sherrington, C., Gates, S., Clemson, L. M., & Lamb, S. E. (2012). Interventions for preventing falls in older people living in the community. *The Cochrane Database of Systematic Reviews, 2012*(9), CD007146. doi:1002/14651858.CD007146.pub3

Ginsberg, T. B., Pomerantz, S. C., & Kramer-Feeley, V. (2005). Sexuality in older adults: Behaviours and preferences. *Age and Ageing, 34*(5), 475–480.

Golant, S. M., & Hyde, J. (Eds.). (2008). *The assisted living residence: A vision for the future.* Baltimore, MD: Johns Hopkins University Press.

Gooneratne, N. S., Tavaria, A., Patel, N., Madhusudan, L., Nadaraja, D., Onen, F., & Richards, K. C. (2011). Perceived effectiveness of diverse sleep treatments in older adults. *Journal of the American Geriatrics Society, 59*(2), 297–303. doi:10.1111/j.1532–5415.2010.03247.x

Haber, D. (2013). *Health promotion and aging: Practical applications for health professionals* (6th ed.). New York, NY: Springer Publishing.

Hahn, E. A., Cichy, K. E., Almeida, D. M., & Haley, W. E. (2011). Time use and well-being in older widows: Adaptation and resilience. *Journal of Women & Aging, 23*(2), 149–159.

Hankivsky, O., Reid, C., Cormier, R., Varcoe, C., Clark, N., Benoit, C., & Brotman, S. (2010). Exploring the promises of intersectionality for advancing women's health research. *International Journal for Equity in Health, 9*(5). Retrieved from http://www.equityhealthj.com/content/9/1/5

Hawkins, K., Pernarelli, J., Ozminkowski, R. J., Bai, M., Gaston, S. J., Hommer, C.,...Yeh, C. S. (2011). The prevalence of urinary incontinence and its burden on the quality of life among older adults with Medicare supplement insurance. *Quality of Life Research, 20*(5), 723–732. doi:10.1007/s11136–010-9808–0

Hayes-Bautista, D. E., Hsu, P., Perez, A., & Gamboa, C. (2002). The "browning" of the graying of America: Diversity in the elderly population and policy implications. *Generations, 26*(3), 15–24.

He, W., & Larsen, L. J. (2014). *Older Americans with a disability: 2008–2012.* (American Community Survey Reports ACS-29). Washington, DC: U.S. Government Printing Office.

Health Resources and Services Administration. (2013). *Women's health USA 2013.* Rockville, MD: U.S. Department of Health and Human Services.

Hedman, A. M., Fonad, E., & Sandmark, H. (2013). Older people living at home: Associations between falls and health complaints in men and women. *Journal of Clinical Nursing, 22*(19–20), 2945–2952. doi:10.1111/jocn.12279

Heesch, K. C., Burton, N. W., & Brown, W. J. (2011). Concurrent and prospective associations between physical activity, walking and mental health in older women. *Journal of Epidemiology and Community Health, 65*(9), 807–813. doi:10.1136/jech.2009.103077

Hegewisch, A., Hayes, J., Milli, J., Shaw, E., & Hartmann, H. (2015). *Looking back, looking ahead: Chartbook on women's progress.* Washington, DC: AARP Institute for Women's Policy Research. Retrieved from http://www.aarp.org/content/dam/aarp/ppi/2015/Chartbook-On-Women%27s-Progress.pdf

Hendrix, S. L., Cochrane, B. B., Nygaard, I. E., Handa, V. L., Barnabei, V. M., Iglesia, C.,...McNeeley, S. G. (2005). Effects of estrogen with and without progestin on urinary incontinence. *Journal of the American Medical Association, 293*(8), 935–948.

The Henry J. Kaiser Foundation. (2013). *Medicare's role for older women.* Retrieved from http://kff.org/womens-health-policy/fact-sheet/medicares-role-for-older-women

Institute of Medicine. (2010). *Women's health research: Progress, pitfalls, and promise.* Washington, DC: National Academies Press.

Institute of Medicine. (2011). *The health of lesbian, gay, bisexual, and transgender people: Building a foundation for better understanding.* Washington, DC: National Academies Press.

Institute of Medicine. (2015). *Cognitive aging: Progress in understanding and opportunities for action.* Washington, DC: National Academies Press.

Institute of Medicine and National Research Council. (2014). *Elder abuse and its prevention: Workshop summary.* Washington, DC: National Academies Press.

Jack, D. (1987). Self-in-relation theory. In R. Formanek & A. Gurian (Eds.), *Women and depression: A lifespan perspective* (pp. 41–45). New York, NY: Springer Publishing.

Kaeberlein, M. R., & Martin, G. M. (Eds.). (2016). *Handbook of the biology of aging* (8th ed.). San Diego, CA: Academic Press.

Kane, R., Ouslander, J., & Abrass, I. (2003). *Essentials of clinical geriatrics* (5th ed.). New York, NY: McGraw-Hill.

Kovács, E., Prókai, L., Mészáros, L., & Gondos, T. (2013). Adapted physical activity is beneficial on balance, functional mobility, quality of life and fall risk in community-dwelling older women: A randomized single-blinded controlled trial. *European Journal of Physical and Rehabilitation Medicine, 49*(3), 301–310.

Kreider, R. M., & Ellis, R. (2011). *Number, timing, and duration of marriages and divorces: 2009.* Washington, DC: U.S. Census Bureau.

Lavretsky, H., Alstein, L. L., Olmstead, R. E., Ercoli, L. M., Riparetti-Brown, M., Cyr, N. S., & Irwin, M. R. (2011). Complementary use of Tai Chi Chih augments escitalopram treatment of geriatric depression: A randomized controlled trial. *American Journal of Geriatric Psychiatry, 19*(10), 839–850. doi:10.1097/JGP.0b013e31820ee9ef

LeBlanc, E. S., Hillier, T. A., Pedula, K. L., Rizzo, J. H., Cawthon, P. M., Fink, H. A.,...Browner, W. S. (2011). Hip fracture and increased short-term but not long-term mortality in healthy older women. *Archives of Internal Medicine, 171*(20), 1831–1837. doi:10.1001/archinternmed.2011.447

Levy-Storms, L., Bastani, R., & Reuben, D. B. (2004). Predictors of varying levels of nonadherence to mammography screening in older women. *Journal of the American Geriatrics Society, 52*(5), 768–773.

Lindau, S. T., Schumm, L. P., Laumann, E. O., Levinson, W., O'Muircheartaigh, C. A., & Waite, L. J. (2007). A study of sexuality and health among older adults in the United States. *New England Journal of Medicine, 357*(8), 762–774.

Lorig, K. R., & Holman, H. (2003). Self-management education: History, definition, outcomes, and mechanisms. *Annals of Behavioral Medicine, 26*(1), 1–7.

Lukwago, S. N., Kreuter, M. W., Holt, C. L., Steger-May, K., Bucholtz, D. C., & Skinner, C. S. (2003). Sociocultural correlates of breast cancer knowledge and screening in urban African American women. *American Journal of Public Health, 93*(8), 1271–1274.

Martin, G. (1992). Biological mechanisms of aging. In J. G. Evans & T. F. Williams (Eds.), *Oxford textbook of geriatric medicine* (pp. 41–48). Oxford, UK: Oxford University Press.

McCormick, W. C., & Boling, P. A. (2005). Multimorbidity and a comprehensive Medicare care-coordination benefit. *Journal of the American Geriatrics Society, 53*(12), 2227–2228.

MetLife Mature Market Institute. (2011). *MetLife study of caregiving costs to working caregivers: Double jeopardy for baby boomers caring for their parents.* Retrieved from https://www.metlife.com/assets/cao/mmi/publications/studies/2011/Caregiving-Costs-to-Working-Caregivers.pdf

Moremen, R. D. (2008). Best friends: The role of confidantes in older women's health. *Journal of Women & Aging, 20*(1/2), 149–167. Retrieved from http://offcampus.lib.washington.edu/login?url=http://search.ebscohost.com/login.aspx?direct=true&db=rzh&AN=105755584&site=ehost-live

Mosca, L., Banka, C. L., Benjamin, E. J., Berra, K., Bushnell, C., Dolor, R. J.,...Wenger, N. K.; Expert Panel/Writing Group; American Heart Association; American Academy of Family Physicians; American College of Obstetricians and Gynecologists; American College of Cardiology Foundation; Society of Thoracic Surgeons; American Medical Women's Association; Centers for Disease Control and Prevention; Office of Research on Women's Health; Association of Black Cardiologists; American College of Physicians; World Heart Federation; National Heart, Lung, and Blood Institute; American College of Nurse Practitioners. (2007). Evidence-based guidelines for cardiovascular disease prevention in women: 2007 update. *Circulation, 115*(11), 1481–1501.

Mosca, L., Barrett-Connor, E., & Wenger, N. K. (2011). Sex/gender differences in cardiovascular disease prevention: What a difference a decade makes. *Circulation, 124*(19), 2145–2154.

Mosca, L., Benjamin, E. J., Berra, K., Bezanson, J. L., Dolor, R. J., Lloyd-Jones, D. M.,...Wenger, N. K. (2011). Effectiveness-based guidelines for the prevention of cardiovascular disease in women—2011 update: A guideline from the American Heart Association. *Circulation, 123*(11), 1243–1262.

Mozaffarian, D., Benjamin, E. J., Go, A. S., Arnett, D. K., Blaha, M. J., Cushman, M.,...on behalf of the American Heart Association Statistics Committee and Stroke Statistics Subcommittee. (2016).

Heart disease and stroke statistics—2016 update: A report from the American Heart Association. *Circulation, 133*, e38–e360.

Muir, J. M., Ye, C., Bhandari, M., Adachi, J. D., & Thabane, L. (2013). The effect of regular physical activity on bone mineral density in postmenopausal women aged 75 and over: A retrospective analysis from the Canadian multicentre osteoporosis study. *BMC Musculoskeletal Disorders, 14*, 253. doi:10.1186/1471-2474-14-253

Müller, L., & Pawelec, G. (2016). The aging immune system: Dysregulation, compensatory mechanisms, and prospects for intervention. In M. R. Kaeberlein & G. M. Martin (Eds.), *Handbook of the biology of aging* (8th ed., pp. 408–432). San Diego, CA: Academic Press.

National Advisory Committee on Rural Health and Human Services. (2010). *The 2010 report to the Secretary: Rural health and human services issues.* Retrieved from http://www.hrsa.gov/advisorycommittees/rural/2010secretaryreport.pdf

National Alliance for Caregiving (NAC). (2009). *Caregiving in the US: 2009.* Retrieved from http://www.caregiving.org/data/Caregiving_in_the_US_2009_full_report.pdf

National Alliance for Caregiving (NAC) & AARP Public Policy Institute. (2015). *Caregiving in the U.S. 2015.* Retrieved from http://www.caregiving.org/wp-content/uploads/2015/05/2015_CaregivingintheUS_Final-Report-June-4_WEB.pdf

National Center for Health Statistics. (2006). *Health, United States, 2006 with chartbook on trends in the health of Americans.* Washington, DC: U.S. Government Printing Office.

National Institute on Aging. (2011). *Biology of aging: Research today for a healthy tomorrow.* Retrieved from https://www.nia.nih.gov/health/publication/biology-aging/preface

National Institutes of Health. (2014). *The dementias: Hope through research.* Retrieved from https://www.nia.nih.gov/alzheimers/publication/dementias/introduction

National Osteoporosis Foundation. (2013). *Clinician's guide to prevention and treatment of osteoporosis.* Washington, DC: National Osteoporosis Foundation.

North American Menopause Society. (2010). Management of osteoporosis in postmenopausal women: 2010 position statement of The North American Menopause Society. *Menopause, 17*(1), 24–54.

Ochida, K. M., & Lachs, M. S. (2015). Not for doctors only: Ageism in healthcare. *Generations, 39*(3), 46–57.

Palmer, R. C., Chhabra, D., & McKinney, S. (2011). Colorectal cancer screening adherence in African-American men and women 50 years of age and older living in Maryland. *Journal of Community Health, 36*(4), 517–524. doi:10.1007/s10900-010-9336-4

Paterson, B. L., Thorne, S., & Dewis, M. (1998). Adapting to and managing diabetes. *Image–The Journal of Nursing Scholarship, 30*(1), 57–62.

Plassman, B. L., Langa, K. M., McCammon, R. J., Fisher, G. G., Potter, G. G., Burke, J. R.,...Wallace, R. B. (2011). Incidence of dementia and cognitive impairment, not dementia in the United States. *Annals of Neurology, 70*(3), 418–426. doi:10.1002/ana.22362

Powers, S. M., Bisconti, T. L., & Bergeman, C. S. (2014). Trajectories of social support and well-being across the first two years of widowhood. *Death Studies, 38*(6–10), 499–509.

Prospective Payment Assessment Commission. (1989). *Medicare prospective payment and the American health care system: Report to the Congress.* Washington, DC: Prospective Payment Assessment Commission.

Qato, D. M., Alexander, G. C., Conti, R. M., Johnson, M., Schumm, P., & Lindau, S. T. (2008). Use of prescription and over-the-counter medications and dietary supplements among older adults in the United States. *Journal of the American Medical Association, 300*(24), 2867–2878.

Quick, H. E., & Moen, P. (1998). Gender, employment, and retirement quality: A life course approach to the differential experiences of men and women. *Journal of Occupational Health Psychology, 3*(1), 44–64.

Reidlinger, D. P., Darzi, J., Hall, W. L., Seed, P. T., Chowienczyk, P. J., & Sanders, T. A.; Cardiovascular disease risk REduction Study (CRESSIDA) Investigators. (2015). How effective are current dietary guidelines for cardiovascular disease prevention in healthy middle-aged and older men and women? A randomized controlled trial. *The American Journal of Clinical Nutrition, 101*(5), 922–930. doi:10.3945/ajcn.114.097352

Reyna, C., Goodwin, E. J., & Ferrari, J. R. (2007). Older adult stereotypes among care providers in residential care facilities: Examining the relationship between contact, eduaction, and ageism. *Journal of Gerontological Nursing, 33*(2), 50–55.

Rillamas-Sun, E., LaCroix, A. Z., Waring, M. E., Kroenke, C. H., LaMonte, M. J., Vitolins, M. Z., … Wallace, R. B. (2014). Obesity and late-age survival without major disease or disability in older women. *Journal of the American Medical Association Internal Medicine, 174*(1), 98–106. doi:10.1001/jamainternmed.2013.12051

Rolland, Y., Lauwers-Cances, V., Cristini, C., Abellan van Kan, G., Janssen, I., Morley, J. E., & Vellas, B. (2009). Difficulties with physical function associated with obesity, sarcopenia, and sarcopenic-obesity in community-dwelling elderly women: The EPIDOS (EPIDemiologie de l'OSteoporose) Study. *American Journal of Clinical Nutrition, 89*(6), 1895–1900. doi:10.3945/ajcn.2008.26950

Rossen, L. M., Milsom, V. A., Middleton, K. R., Daniels, M. J., & Perri, M. G. (2013). Benefits and risks of weight-loss treatment for older, obese women. *Clinical Interventions in Aging, 8*, 157–166. doi:10.2147/cia.s38155

Rowe, J., & Kahn, R. (1998). *Successful aging.* New York, NY: Pantheon Books.

Rural Health Information Hub. (2015). *Rural aging.* Retrieved from http://www.census.gov/geo/reference/ua/urban-rural-2010.html

Salganicoff, A. (2015). Women and Medicare: An unfinished agenda. *Generations, 39*(2), 43–50.

Siegel, R. L., Miller, K. D., & Jemal, A. (2016). Cancer statistics, 2016. *CA: A Cancer Journal for Clinicians, 66*(1), 7–30.

Simmons, B. A., & Betschild, M. J. (2001). Women's retirement, work and life paths: Changes, disruptions and discontinuities. *Journal of Women & Aging, 13*(4), 53–70.

Simon, S. R., Chan, K. A., Soumerai, S. B., Wagner, A. K., Andrade, S. E., Feldstein, A. C., … Gurwitz, J. H. (2005). Potentially inappropriate medication use by elderly persons in U.S. Health Maintenance Organizations, 2000–2001. *Journal of the American Geriatrics Society, 53*(2), 227–232.

Siu, O. L., & Phillips, D. R. (2002). A study of family support, friendship, and psychological well-being among older women in Hong Kong. *International Journal of Aging & Human Development, 55*(4), 299–319.

Smith, L. A., McCaslin, R., Chang, J., Martinez, P., & McGrew, P. (2010). Assessing the needs of older gay, lesbian, bisexual, and transgender people: A service-learning and agency partnership approach. *Journal of Gerontological Social Work, 53*(5), 387–401.

Spence, N. J., Adkins, D. E., & Dupre, M. E. (2011). Racial differences in depression trajectories among older women: Socioeconomic, family, and health influences. *Journal of Health and Social Behavior, 52*(4), 444–459.

Spira, A. P., Stone, K. L., Rebok, G. W., Punjabi, N. M., Redline, S., Ancoli-Israel, S., & Yaffe, K. (2014). Sleep-disordered breathing and functional decline in older women. *Journal of the American Geriatrics Society, 62*(11), 2040–2046. doi:10.1111/jgs.13108

Straka, S. M., & Montminy, L. (2006). Responding to the needs of older women experiencing domestic violence. *Violence Against Women, 12*(3), 251–267.

Surrey, J. L. (1991). The "self-in-relation": A theory of women's development. In J. V. Jordan, A. G. Kaplan, J. B. Miller, I. P. Stiver, & J. L. Surrey (Eds.), *Women's growth in connection: Writings from the Stone Center* (pp. 51–66). New York, NY: Guilford Press.

Sutphin, G. L., & Korstanje, R. (2016). Longevity as a complex genetic trait. In M. R. Kaeberlein & G. M. Martin (Eds.), *Handbook of the biology of aging* (8th ed., pp. 3–54). San Diego, CA: Academic Press.

Tamborini, C. R., & Whitman, K. (2007). Women, marriage, and Social Security benefits revisited. *Social Security Bulletin, 67*(4), 1–20.

Taylor, P., Passei, J., Fry, R., Morin, R., Wang, W., Velasco, G., & Dockterman, D. (2010). *The return of the multi-generational family household.* Washington, DC: Pew Research Center.

Teri, L., McCurry, S. M., Logsdon, R., & Gibbons, L. E. (2005). Training community consultants to help family members improve dementia care: A randomized controlled trial. *The Gerontologist, 45*(6), 802–811.

Teri, L., McCurry, S. M., Logsdon, R. G., Gibbons, L. E., Buchner, D. M., & Larson, E. B. (2011). A randomized controlled clinical trial of the Seattle Protocol for Activity in older adults. *Journal of the American Geriatrics Society, 59*(7), 1188–1196. doi:10.1111/j.1532-5415.2011.03454.x

The Centers for Disease Control and Prevention, National Center for Health Statistics. (2010). *National Interview Survey.* Retrieved from http://www.cdc.gov/nchs/nhis.htm

Thomas, W. H. (2004). *What are old people for? How elders will save the world.* Acton, MA: VanderWyk & Burnham.

Todd, L., Harvey, E., & Hoffman-Goetz, L. (2011). Predicting breast and colon cancer screening among English-as-a-second-language older Chinese immigrant women to Canada. *Journal of Cancer Education, 26*(1), 161–169. doi:10.1007/s13187-010-0141-7

Tu, S. P., Yasui, Y., Kuniyuki, A. A., Schwartz, S. M., Jackson, J. C., Hislop, T. G., & Taylor, V. (2003). Mammography screening among Chinese-American women. *Cancer, 97*(5), 1293–1302.

U.S. Bureau of Labor Statistics. (2015). *Highlights of women's earnings in 2014.* (1058). Washington, DC: U.S. Bureau of Labor Statistics.

U.S. Census Bureau. (2014). *65+ in the United States: 2010.* (Current Population Reports P23–212). Washington, DC: U.S. Government Printing Office.

U.S. Department of Health and Human Services. (1984). *Normal human aging: The Baltimore longitudinal study of aging.* Washington, DC: U.S. Government Printing Office.

U.S. Department of Health and Human Services. (2008). *Physical activity guidelines for Americans.* Retrieved from http://health.gov/paguidelines/guidelines

U.S. Department of Health and Human Services Office of Disability, Aging and Long-Term Care Policy. (2014). *Informal caregiving for older Americans: An analysis of the 2011 National Study of Caregiving.* Retrieved from https://aspe.hhs.gov/pdf-report/informal-caregiving-older-americans-analysis-2011-national-health-and-aging-trends-study

Uusi-Rasi, K., Patil, R., Karinkanta, S., Kannus, P., Tokola, K., Lamberg-Allardt, C., & Sievanen, H. (2015). Exercise and vitamin D in fall prevention among older women: A randomized clinical trial. *Journal of the American Medical Association Internal Medicine, 175*(5), 703–711. doi:10.1001/jamainternmed.2015.0225

Vitaliano, P. P., Scanlan, J. M., Zhang, J., Savage, M. V., Hirsch, I. B., & Siegler, I. C. (2002). A path model of chronic stress, the metabolic syndrome, and coronary heart disease. *Psychosomatic Medicine, 64*, 418–435.

Vitiello, M. V. (2009). Recent advances in understanding sleep and sleep disturbances in older adults: Growing older does not mean sleeping poorly. *Current Directions in Psychological Science, 18*(6), 316–320.

Walker, R. B., Luszcz, M. A., Hislop, J., & Moore, V. (2012). A gendered lifecourse examination of sleep difficulties among older women. *Ageing & Society, 32*(Pt. 2), 219–238. doi:10.1017/s0144686x11000201

Wang, S., Luo, X., Barnes, D., Sano, M., & Yaffe, K. (2014). Physical activity and risk of cognitive impairment among oldest-old women. *American Journal of Geriatric Psychiatry, 22*(11), 1149–1157. doi:10.1016/j.jagp.2013.03.002

Weinberger, B., & Grubeck-Loebenstein, B. (2012). Vaccines for the elderly. *Clinical Microbiology and Infection, 18*(Suppl. 5), 100–108.

Weiner, A. S., & Ronch, J. L. (Eds.). (2003). *Culture change in long-term care.* New York, NY: Haworth Press.

Wilson, M. M. (2006). Urinary incontinence: Selected current concepts. *The Medical Clinics of North America, 90*(5), 825–836.

Woods, N. F., Cochrane, B. B., LaCroix, A. Z., Seguin, R. A., Zaslavsky, O., Liu, J., … Tinker, L. F. (2012). Toward a positive aging phenotype for older women: Observations from the women's health initiative. *The Journals of Gerontology. Series A, Biological Sciences and Medical Sciences, 67*(11), 1191–1196. doi:10.1093/gerona/gls117

Woods, N. F., LaCroix, A. Z., Gray, S. L., Aragaki, A., Cochrane, B. B., Brunner, R. L., … Newman, A. B.; Women's Health Initiative. (2005). Frailty: Emergence and consequences in women aged 65 and older in the Women's Health Initiative Observational Study. *Journal of the American Geriatrics Society, 53*(8), 1321–1330.

Wright, R. (2012). Paying for retirement: Sex differences in inclusion in employer-provided retirement plans. *The Gerontologist, 52*(2), 231–244.

Yaffe, K., Laffan, A. M., Harrison, S. L., Redline, S., Spira, A. P., Ensrud, K. E., … Stone, K. L. (2011). Sleep-disordered breathing, hypoxia, and risk of mild cognitive impairment and dementia in older women. *Journal of the American Medical Association, 306*(6), 613–619. doi:10.1001/jama.2011.1115

Young, H. M. (2003). Challenges and solutions for care of frail older adults. *Online Journal of Issues in Nursing, 8*(2), Manuscript 4. Retrieved from http://www.nursingworld.org/MainMenuCategories/ANAMarketplace/ANAPeriodicals/OJIN/TableofContents/Volume82003/No2May2003/OlderAdultsCareSolutions.aspx

Young, H. M., & Cochrane, B. (2015). Healthy aging for women. In E. F. Olshansky (Ed.), *Women's health and wellness across the lifespan* (pp. 95–122). Philadelphia, PA: Wolters Kluwer Health.

Young, H., Miyamoto, S., Ward, D., Dharmar, M., Tang-Feldman, Y., & Berglund, L. (2014). Sustained effects of a nurse coaching intervention via telehealth to improve health behavior change in diabetes. *Telemedicine Journal and E-Health, 20*(9), 828–834.

Yu, W. Y., Hwang, H. F., Hu, M. H., Chen, C. Y., & Lin, M. R. (2013). Effects of fall injury type and discharge placement on mortality, hospitalization, falls, and ADL changes among older people in Taiwan. *Accident; Analysis and Prevention, 50*, 887–894. doi:10.1016/j.aap.2012.07.015

Zambrana, R. (1988). A research agenda on issues affecting poor and minority women: A model for understanding their needs. *Women and Health, 14*(2), 137–160.

Zarit, S. H., Gaugler, J. E., & Jarrott, S. E. (1999). Useful services for families: Research findings and directions. *International Journal of Geriatric Psychiatry, 14*(3), 165–77; discussion 178.

Zaslavsky, O., Cochrane, B. B., Thompson, H. J., Woods, N. F., Herting, J. R., & LaCroix, A. (2013). Frailty: A review of the first decade of research. *Biological Research for Nursing, 15*(4), 422–432.

Ziller, E. (2014). Access to medical care in rural America. In J. C. Warren & K. B. Smalley (Eds.), *Rural public health: Best practices and preventive models* (pp. 11–28). New York, NY: Springer Publishing.

Zisberg, A., Sinoff, G., Gary, S., Gur-Yaish, N., Admi, H., & Shadmi, E. (2011). In-hospital use of continence aids and new-onset urinary incontinence in adults aged 70 and older. *Journal of the American Geriatrics Society, 59*(6), 1099–1104.

CHAPTER 11

Well Woman's Health

Versie Johnson-Mallard • Elizabeth A. Kostas-Polston

The practice of well women's health is not of a reactive health care system that responds to acute and urgent needs, but rather one that nurtures health and well-being (National Women's Law Center [NWLC], 2014; American College of Obstetricians and Gynecologists [ACOG], 2012a). The modern approach to addressing the physical and mental health care needs of women from adolescence to older age is a team approach. Providers of sexual and reproductive health (SRH) services to women range from gynecologic care to geriatric services. Health care professionals nurture the optimal health and well-being of women at significant stages of their lives. This chapter offers suggestions for conducting a SRH physical examination and health history, as well as special considerations for adolescents and older women, and finally an update on age-specific health screening during a well-women visit.

Health care providers educated in primary care specialties, such as family, adult/gerontology, and pediatrics, are knowledgeable to provide SRH care services to women. The U.S. Department of Health and Human Services (DHHS) adopted the Institute of Medicine's (IOM) recommendation that preventive services include one annual well visit at no cost under the 2010 Patient Protection and Affordable Care Act (ACA) to women of all ages (Henry J. Kaiser Family Foundation, 2014; IOM, 2011). As a goal to increase awareness and with funding from Pfizer Inc., the NWLC and the Mary Horrigan Connors Center for Women's Health and Gender Biology at Brigham and Women's Hospital developed resources for consumers, health care providers, and policy makers to help women navigate the SRH preventive services available to them under the ACA (NWLC, 2014). Patients come from varied cultural and socioeconomic backgrounds with a host of personal beliefs regarding their health. Furthermore, patients are surfing the web, reading medical literature and becoming self-educated in Western medicine and alternative and complementary medicine. Women entering the office have thought-out questions and suggestions for their plans of care (Agency for Healthcare Research and Quality [AHRQ], 2016).

■ COMPONENTS OF A WELL-WOMAN VISIT

The well-woman visit is an opportunity to promote health by addressing health concerns and educating women about health risks and disease prevention. During this visit, if language is a barrier for the patient, a qualified, professional translator may be necessary to collect her correct necessary health information.

A woman's health history should be collected while she is clothed. The health care provider should sit at eye level and face the woman. Begin the history with social conversation. Asking sensitive questions in front of family or friends may result in incomplete answers and missed information. Interview your patient alone, if at all possible. If unable to interview the woman alone, attempt to contact her later to fill in any important missing information. The well-woman visit, at minimum, should include:

- Review of health history
- Review of prescription and over-the-counter medications, vitamins, and supplements
- Counseling/education
- Updates on health screening (NWLC, 2014)

Health History

The health history is a fundamental part of the annual visit and may vary depending on age, risk factors, and the woman's and/or her health care provider's preferences (ACOG, 2012a; Conry & Brown, 2015). The best time to begin establishing a relationship with a woman is during your interview to collect her and her family's health history.

An annual visit for an established female patient may consist of:

- Counseling about health maintenance
- Risk assessment
- Body mass index (BMI) assessment
- Screening
- Immunizations

An established patient will require a thorough review and update of her past medical history and social history, as well as a three-generation family history (if known, see Table 11.1). Updating a woman's health history is the opportune time to, together, determine what health care needs may be indicated and how the woman views her personal health. The health history is an investigation of current health, real and potential risk, discovery of knowledge

TABLE 11.1	Components of Patient History
PAST MEDICAL HISTORY	**SOCIAL HISTORY**
■ Medical ■ Medications ■ Allergies ■ Surgery ■ Immunizations	■ Occupation ■ Diet ■ Exercise ■ Tobacco ■ Alcohol ■ Illicit drugs ■ Sexual history ■ Last menstrual period ■ Last Pap smear
FAMILY HISTORY	
■ Mother—HTN, alive ■ Father—healthy, alive ■ Siblings	

HTN, hypertension (high blood pressure).

gaps and is a time to gather information to support any indicated referrals.

Developing a rapport with the woman may decrease any discomfort that might occur when asking personal and oftentimes difficult questions such as drug use, sexual history, and abuse. Asking the question does not imply judgment when asked in a respectful manner and without criticism. Active listening skills, such as leaning forward, nodding, and encouraging further description while saying *tell me more* or *go on*, all indicate interest and serve to instill a sense of trust in the patient–health care provider professional relationship.

It is critical to listen to the woman's response while paying attention to the language and words she uses, as well as her facial expressions and body language. Furthermore, it is important to do everything possible to avoid interruptions while the woman is explaining her concerns and reasons for her health visit. It is very important that the health care provider maintain good eye contact with the woman (not the computer screen) while addressing her. If necessary, the typing of information into the electronic medical chart should be kept to a minimum.

Routine Health Screening

LIPID PROFILE ASSESSMENT

A lipid profile provides health care providers with a risk assessment for morbidity related to coronary heart disease (CHD; Table 11.2). CHD is the most common cause of death in adults in the United States (Bays, Jones, Brown, & Jacobson, 2014). Women considered to be at high risk are those with a family history of premature cardiovascular disease, previous personal history of CHD, a BMI greater than 30, a personal and/or family history of peripheral vascular disease, and diabetes mellitus (Bays, Jones, Brown, & Jacobson, 2014; U.S. Preventive Services Task Force [USPSTF], 2014). The recommended timing for dyslipidemia screening in women ages 20 to 45 years with increased risk for CHD is every 5 years (Fitzgerald, Glynn, Davenport, Waxman, & Johnson, 2015; USPSTF, 2014).

ENDOCRINE SCREENING

The endocrine system is a complex system using hormones that target organs throughout the body. Hormones affect the development of sexual characteristics, fertility, fluid balance, and maintenance of blood pressure (BP). Disorders of the endocrine system are categorized as:

■ Primary disorders: those affecting target organs (e.g., the thyroid or adrenal glands)
■ Secondary disorders: those that affect regulation of target organs (e.g., the pituitary gland)
■ Tertiary disorders: those that arise from the hypothalamus.

Diabetes is the most common endocrine disorder in the United States. Adults with surveilled BP readings greater than or equal to 135/80 mmHg should be screened for diabetes.

Ambulatory BP monitoring is the best method for confirming elevated BP. *Ambulatory monitoring* is defined as measuring BP every 30 minutes over the course of 24 to 48 hours of normal activity. Ambulatory BP monitoring is recommended at intervals of every year for high-risk adults and every 3 to 5 years for those who are at low risk.

Women with a history of gestational diabetes mellitus (GDM) should have lifelong screening for the development of diabetes or prediabetes at least every 3 years. A fasting plasma glucose, 2-hour postload plasma, and hemoglobin A_{1c} (HgA_{1c}) tests are approved for diabetes screening at 3-year intervals. Regardless of the woman's age, glycemic target goals are 80 to 130 mg/dL and less than 7.5% for HgA_{1c} (USPSTF, 2014).

COLORECTAL SCREENING

The goal of colorectal screening in women is to reduce mortality from gastrointestinal system cancer. Colorectal cancer is the third leading cause of cancer death in women. More than 70,000 women develop colorectal cancer and about 24,000 women die from colorectal cancer each year in the United States (ACOG, 2014). ACOG's (2014) recommendation is to begin screening with a colonoscopy at age 50 years. Because of the high mortality risk, African American women should be screened beginning at age 45 years (ACOG, 2014; Rosenbaun & Wood, 2015). The most effective screening interval for colonoscopy is every 10 years. Sigmoidoscopy is recommended every 5 years. It is recommended that high sensitive guaiac and fecal immunochemical testing (noninvasive methods used to detect occult blood in the stool) accompany sigmoidoscopy. The guaiac test requires two samples from each of three consecutive bowel movements at home. It is important to note that a single stool sample collected from a health care provider's rectal examination is not adequate for the detection of colorectal cancer (ACOG, 2014).

SCREENING MAMMOGRAPHY

Breast cancer is the second-leading cause of death from cancer in American women (ACOG, 2011/2014). The

TABLE 11.2	Lipid Profile Components and Levels	
LIPID PROFILE	**COMPONENTS**	**LEVELS**
Total cholesterol	Measures all of the cholesterol	*Desirable:* < 200 mg/dL (5.18 mmol/L) *Borderline high:* 200–239 mg/dL (5.18–6.18 mmol/L) *High:* 240 mg/dL (6.22 mmol/L) or higher
High-density lipoprotein (HDL) cholesterol	"Good cholesterol"; removes excess cholesterol	*Low level, increased risk:* < 50 mg/dL (1.3 mmol/L) for women *Average level, average risk:* 50–59 mg/dL (1.3–1.5 mmol/L) for women *High level, less than average risk:* 60 mg/dL (1.55 mmol/L) or higher
Low-density lipoprotein (LDL) cholesterol	"Bad cholesterol"; deposits excess cholesterol	*Optimal:* < 100 mg/dL (2.59 mmol/L); for those with known disease (ASCVD or diabetes), < 70 mg/dL (1.81 mmol/L) is optimal *Near/above optimal:* 100–129 mg/dL (2.59–3.34 mmol/L) *Borderline high:* 130–159 mg/dL (3.37–4.12 mmol/L) *High:* 160–189 mg/dL (4.15–4.90 mmol/L) *Very high:* < 190 mg/dL (4.90 mmol/L)
Fasting triglycerides	Measures all the triglycerides in all the lipoprotein particles	*Desirable:* < 150 mg/dL (1.70 mmol/L) *Borderline high:* 150–199 mg/dL (1.7–2.2 mmol/L) *High:* 200–499 mg/dL (2.3–5.6 mmol/L) *Very high:* > 500 mg/dL (5.6 mmol/L)

ASCVD, atherosclerotic cardiovascular disease.
Adapted from National Lipid Association (2014).

American Cancer Society (ACS) estimates that in 2016, there will be 249,260 newly diagnosed cases of breast cancer in women and men. Of those newly diagnosed cases, it is estimated that 40,890 American women and men will die (ACS, 2016). It is important to note that although breast cancer is typically associated with women, approximately 1% of all cases are diagnosed in men. Historically, breast cancer screening has included three aspects: (a) breast imaging (e.g., mammography), (b) the clinical breast examination (CBE), and (c) the woman's self-breast screening (monthly breast self-examination [BSE]). The significance and impact that each of these aspects has on the early diagnosis, detection, and prognosis, as well as the appropriate age to initiate and discontinue and the frequency of screening, remain controversial. ACOG (2011/2014) endorses the inclusion of all three aspects in breast cancer screening (Table 11.3). Breast cancer morbidity and mortality can be effectively reduced through screening mammography.

Screening mammography is recommended for women who are not at an increased risk by known genetic workup or personal or family history. Increasing age is the most important risk factor. Known risks include:

■ Family history
■ Breast cancer diagnosis before age 50 years
■ Personal and/or family history of bilateral breast cancer
■ Family history of breast and ovarian cancer
■ Presence of breast cancer in at least one female family member
■ Multiple cases of breast cancer in the family

■ One or more family member with two primary types of *BRCA*-related cancer
■ Ashkenazi Jewish ethnicity
■ History of positive *BRCA* mutations (ACOG, 2011; USPSTF, 2014).

Genetic risk assessment for breast cancer *(BRCA)* mutation testing is a multistep process that includes genetic counseling by trained providers. Interventions in women who are *BRCA* mutation carriers should have early, more frequent, and intensive cancer screening. High-risk women with known *BRCA* mutations should be evaluated for treatment with interventions such as risk-reducing medications (e.g., tamoxifen or raloxifene), and risk-reducing surgery (e.g., mastectomy or salpingo-oophorectomy) (ACOG, 2011; USPSTF, 2014).

Women who have never performed BSE or those with questions about BSE technique should be educated and encouraged to palpate breast tissue and structures monthly so that they become familiar with their breast tissue. Increasing one's awareness as to what her *normal* breast tissue feels like may lead a woman to seek out her health care provider when aberrancies occur.

CERVICAL CANCER SCREENING: PAP TEST

Screening has been successful in lowering morbidity and mortality from cervical cancer and is defined as an internal examination using cytology (Pap test). Cervical cancer screening is age specific and should begin at age 21 years. A Pap test is not recommended on an annual basis

TABLE 11.3	Breast Cancer Screening Recommendations			
PROFESSIONAL ORGANIZATION	**MAMMOGRAPHY**	**CLINICAL BREAST EXAM (CBE)**	**BREAST SELF-EXAM (BSE)**	**BSE AWARENESS**
American College of Obstetricians and Gynecologists	Annually in women ≥ 40 years of age	Every 1–3 years in women aged 20–39 years. Annually in women ≥ 40 years of age.	Consideration when caring for high-risk women	Recommended
American Cancer Society	Annually in women ≥ 40 years of age	Every 1–3 years in women aged 20–39 years. Annually in women ≥ 40 years of age	Optional for women ≥ 20 years of age	Recommended
National Comprehensive Cancer Network	Annually in women ≥ 40 years of age	Every 1–3 years in women aged 20–39 years Annually in women ≥ 40 years of age	Recommended	Recommended
National Cancer Institute	Every 1–2 years in women ≥ 40 years of age.	Recommended	Not recommended	
U.S. Preventive Services Task Force	Age 50–74 years biennially	Insufficient evidence	Not recommended	

Adapted from American College of Obstetricians and Gynecologists (2011/2014).

for any woman at any age. Cytology alone every 3 years is the recommended screening method for women aged 21 to 29 years (ACOG, 2012a; Pascale, Beal, & Fitzgerald, 2016). For women 30 to 65 years of age, cytology and human papillomavirus (HPV; co-testing) every 5 years is the preferred screening method (ACOG, 2012a). High-risk HPV is necessary for the development of precursor lesions and/or cervical cancer. HPV testing alone, for primary screening, is promising in women aged 30 years and older but is not acceptable or recommended at this time (ACOG, 2012a). (See Chapter 32 for detailed information on the association between HPV and cervical cancer.)

For women older than 65 years, no screening is recommended with adequate negative prior screening and no history of moderate or severe cervical intraepithelial neoplasia (CIN, grade 2 or 3) within the past 20 years (ACOG, 2012a). Cervical screening should not be resumed in this age group for any reason (including the introduction of a new sex partner). Furthermore, women with a history of hysterectomy for benign disease do not require cervical screening. However, women older than 65 years of age with a history of CIN2 or 3 should continue to undergo screening (ACOG, 2012a). Any woman with a cervix and a positive history for CIN 2 or 3 or adenocarcinoma in situ should continue to be screened (ACOG, 2012a). Cervical screening practices after HPV vaccination are recommended and should not change.

SRH Examination

CLINICAL BREAST EXAMINATION

CBE was designed to monitor breast size, symmetry, contour, skin color, texture, venous patterns, and lesions

(Table 11.4). The health care provider should begin by inspecting a woman's breasts while noting any dimpling, venous patterns, and symmetry. It is not uncommon for one breast to be slightly larger or smaller. During the CBE and while sitting up, the woman should place her hands on her hips while flexing her pectoral muscles. The health care provider should note any breast changes (e.g., nipple retraction, puckering, and/or changes in vascular patterns). With the woman in the supine position, the health care provider can place a small towel or pillow behind the woman's scapula on the side to be examined. The breast tissue should be distributed by asking the woman to raise her arm above her head. The keys to an effective CBE are examination, palpation, and inspection of the entire breast—from the woman's midchest to the clavicle to the midaxillary areas, as well as the tail of Spence (ACOG, 2012b). It is critical that the health care provider document all findings from the CBE into the electronic medical record. Many electronic medical records also provide the ability to draw or mark areas of concern noted on the CBE onto an electronic diagram. This diagram can then be accessed anytime follow-up is indicated.

PELVIC EXAMINATION

The components of a pelvic examination may vary depending on a woman's age, risks, and assessment findings (Figure 11.1). ACOG (2012b) recommends that a pelvic examination be performed on all women beginning at age 21 years. The decision to collect cervical and/or vaginal

TABLE 11.4	Clinical Breast and Axillae Examination
EXAMINATION	**RECORD ABNORMALITY**
Examine breasts for size, symmetry, contour, skin color and texture, venous patterns, and lesions. Use several positions for inspection: ■ Seated, arms hanging loosely at sides ■ Seated, arms extended over head or flexed behind neck ■ Seated, hands pressed against hips with shoulders rolled forward (or seated, hands pressed together) ■ Seated or standing, and leaning forward from waist	■ Use nipple as center of clock face ■ Draw or mark diagram to depict, size, and location of abnormalities ■ Describe lesion by its clock position ● Distance from nipple ● Relative depth from skin ● Described contour (linear, round, or lobulated) ● Texture (fluctuant, soft, firm, rock hard) ● Mobility (fixed, moble) ● Inflammation, if present (warm, red, tender) ● Associated skin changes (peau d'orange or ulceration)
Nipples Examine nipples for symmerty, direction, countour, color, and texture.	
Breast and Axillae Perform bimanual digital palpation, compressing tissuse between fingers and flat of hand.	
Use palmar finger surface to palpate into axillary hollow for lymph nodes: ■ Palpate medially, anteriorly, and posteriorly.	
Palpate infraclavicular and supraclavicular nodes.	
Continue palpation with woman in supine position. Have her raise one arm behind her head and place small folded towel under shoulder. Use finger pads and push toward chest in systematic pattern. ■ Use light, medium, and deep pressure without lifting fingers. ■ Include tail of Spence.	

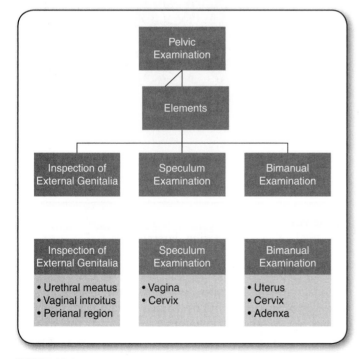

FIGURE 11.1
Pelvic examination.

specimens while performing a pelvic examination for the asymptomatic woman is a shared decision between a woman and her health care provider. Together, they will use sound clinical judgment as a guide to any decision making.

Examination of the external and internal sexual organs is an appropriate component of a comprehensive evaluation of any woman reporting genital symptoms. Women with menstrual disorders, vaginal discharge, infertility, or pelvic pain should undergo a pelvic and bimanual examination. Women presenting with complaints of abnormal uterine bleeding, a change in bowel or bladder function, and/or vaginal discomfort should undergo a pelvic examination (Conry & Brown, 2015; Fitzgerald et al., 2015).

The initial pelvic examination in an adolescent is usually a source of fear. Furthermore, a pelvic examination in a postmenopausal women experiencing atrophic vaginitis and/or vaginal or cervical stenosis can be challenging for the novice health care provider. A woman's hesitancy, concern, and fears may be alleviated by first demonstrating how the speculum works, offering a mirror to reflect the external and internal genitalia, and defining and explaining commonly used medical terminology.

Gloves are worn throughout the pelvic examination, which should begin with the inspection of the soft tissues of the lower and then upper genital tract. With the woman supine and in a lithotomy position and draped, the health care provider should visually inspect the mons and vulva for symmetry and hair quality and growth distribution. It is important to note and later document any piercings, bruising, discharge, rashes, lacerations, and/or tattoos. Next, the health care provider should palpate. To avoid startling the woman and before beginning palpation, the health care provider should inform the woman of the intention to touch her. This is effectively done by first touching the woman's inner thigh and moving up to the labia, then perineum. The health care provider should palpate for lumps and tumors, as well as note any elicited pain. Bartholin's glands are then palpated to look for a cyst or mass. Bartholin's glands are located at approximately the 5 and 7 o'clock positions, in the most distal part of the vagina. The health care provider should note and document any lesions, discharge, erythema, and/or edema.

If indicated, the health care provider should perform a speculum examination and collect specimens for cytology. Using a gentle touch, the health care provider should separate the labia, placing light pressure on the bulbocavernosus muscles, and then insert the speculum (while in the mind's eye, drawing an imaginary line to the woman's rectum) toward the woman's rectum. The selected size of the speculum is based on the size of a woman's vaginal opening. In an adolescent, the Pederson speculum may be appropriate. A Graves speculum is commonly selected for a parous and sexually active woman with a normal BMI. Using a good light source, the health care provider should inspect the walls of the vagina for discharge, erythema, and lesions. The cervix should then be examined for color, shape, discharge, lacerations, polyps, and lesions. A normal cervix is moist, pink, and rounded. Nulliparous women tend to have a closed cervical os. In parous women, the cervix usually appears to have a slit-shaped os. The health care provider should note common cervical variations, which may indicate all of the following: paleness (a possible sign of anemia or menopausal state), bluish (pregnant), or protrusions (polyps). A woman's vaginal discharge should be assessed—noted for odor, color, and consistency. If appropriate, the health care provider should use the appropriate supplies to collect cervical and vaginal specimens. The health care provider should warn the woman that she may feel pressure or fullness during specimen collection and during any manipulation of the cervix. It is not a normal finding for a woman to experience any pain upon cervical and vaginal specimen collection. Health care providers should be careful to follow manufacturers' directions when collecting specimens. Finally, the health care provider withdraws the speculum from the cervix by gently closing the blades before removal from a woman's vagina.

BIMANUAL EXAMINATION

The bimanual examination is performed to determine the size, shape, lie, and location of a woman's uterus and her ovaries. With the woman lying in a lithotomy position and the health care provider standing, the health care provider, with gentle pressure, inserts the index and middle fingers into the woman's vaginal canal (taking care that the thumb does not brush or compress the clitoris or urethra; Figure 11.2). The health care provider's internal finger is then used to palpate the cervix for tenderness/pain, masses, and/or any irregularities. The bimanual examination should not be painful. Cervical motion tenderness (CMT) is an abnormal finding and may indicate ectopic pregnancy, pelvic inflammatory disease, or infections of the cervix. Assessment of the ovaries is accomplished by shifting the internal fingers first to the right and then to the left ovary.

The external hand presses downward toward the internal finger to capture the ovary and uterus (Figure 11.3).

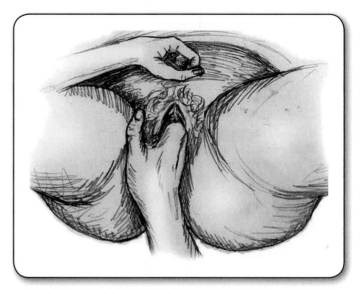

FIGURE 11.2
Bimanual examination, frontal view.

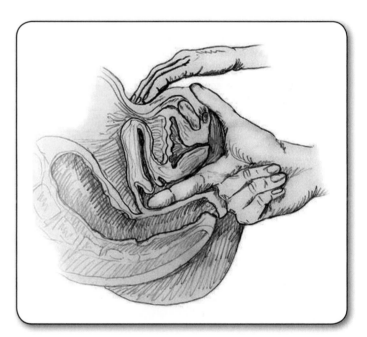

FIGURE 11.3
Bimanual pelvic examination, lateral view.

With the tips of the fingers and with gentle pressure, start at the umbilicus and work down to the symphysis. In obese, prepubescent, and postmenopausal women, the ovaries may not be palpable. When palpable, the ovaries should normally be about 5 cm in diameter, firm, oval, and nontender, depending on phase of a woman's menstrual cycle. The fallopian tubes are not palpable. The ability to palpate the fallopian tubes is an abnormal finding and my indicate, for example, the presence of an ectopic pregnancy.

The health care provider should also assess the uterus for mobility and tenderness. The uterus should be firm, smooth, and nontender. The normal uterus is anterior, pear shaped, and the size of an average women's fist. An enlarged uterus may indicate a pregnancy, fibroid tumors, endometriosis, or carcinoma. The health care provider should estimate the size of a woman's enlarged uterus by weeks of gestation. For example, if the uterus is midpoint between the umbilicus and symphysis pubis, the estimated size of the uterus would be 12 weeks. A uterus that is found to be immobile is an abnormal finding. An immobile uterus may indicate uterine infection, carcinoma, or adhesions.

A cervix positioned toward the anterior canal indicates a retroflexed uterus. A retroverted uterus is not an abnormal finding and does not usually cause health issues for a woman. However, if a woman with a retroverted uterus presents with complaints of pelvic pain, for example, the health care provider should add endometriosis, adhesions, and fibroids to the differential list and rule out pathology (Figure 11.4).

If on evaluation, a woman's uterus and cervix are shifted left or right, this may be an indication of a pelvic mass. Further evaluation with diagnostic imaging (an ultrasound) would be necessary. Palpation of the anterior vaginal fornix (above the cervix) can be used to determine the degree of an anteflexed uterus (Figure 11.5). Palpating the fundus of a woman's uterus down to the posterior fornix supports the finding that a woman's uterus may be retroverted. It is important that the health care provider note if a woman exhibits guarding during the bimanual examination. Guarding is an abnormal finding and is indicative of pain.

RECTOVAGINAL EXAMINATION

A retroverted uterus and adnexal masses can be palpated on rectovaginal examination. The health care provider should first visually examine a woman's external anal area for hemorrhoids, lesions, and/or masses and then ask the woman to bear down. While the woman is bearing down, the health care provider should slowly and carefully, place a gloved and lubricated finger, into the woman's anus, noting the presence of polyps and/or hemorrhoids, as well as the tone of the anal sphincter. It is very important that the health care provider change gloves after performing pelvic and bimanual examinations and before performing a rectovaginal examination. This will avoid cross-contamination (ACOG, 2014).

Special Considerations

THE ADOLESCENT WELL-WOMEN EXAM

Expanding access to primary screening and family planning methods to adolescents improves health outcomes. For the first time in history, the United States is experiencing four decades of low adolescent pregnancy rates (Pascale, Beal, & Fitzgerald, 2016; Sawaya, 2016). Medicaid and the 2010 ACA are posited as part of the reason for these unprecedented low rates. These provisions have allowed significantly improved adolescent access to highly effective methods of birth control (e.g., long-acting reversible contraceptive methods [intrauterine devices and systems and implants]; IOM, 2011). Long-acting reversible contraceptive methods have been proven to be both safe and highly effective in reducing the rates of unintended pregnancy (Richards, 2016).

Adolescents younger than 21 years should not be screened with a Pap test regardless of age at sexual initiation, sexually transmitted infection (STI) history, parity, or other risk factors (ACOG, 2012a). Testing and screening

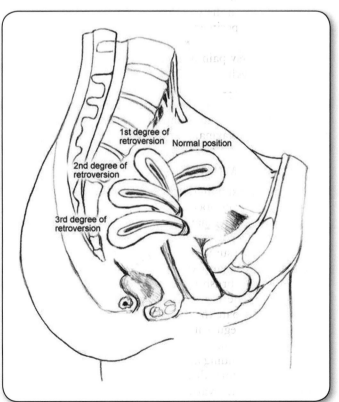

FIGURE 11.5
Degrees of retroversion of the uterus.

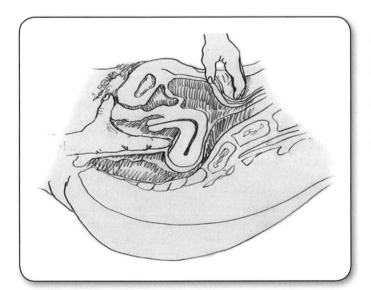

FIGURE 11.4
Retroflexed uterus.

adolescents for HPV infection leads to unnecessary evaluation and overtreatment, which can increase the risk of reproductive problems such as incompetent cervix, stenosis, and/or scarring (ACOG, 2012b). Adolescents who underwent cervical cancer screening (e.g., cervical cytology) and had one or more Pap tests with normal results before the screening guidelines changed should *not* be screened again until they reach age 21 years. Adolescents with a previous abnormal Pap test, followed by two normal tests, should wait until age 21 years to be rescreened (ACOG, 2012a).

Cervical cancer screening every 3 years is recommended for women 21 to 29 years of age. A Pap smear was needed for the prescription of contraceptives, menstrual issues, and screening for and treatment of STIs. Recent evidence supports addressing any of these reproductive health issues regardless of a woman's cervical cancer screening status (ACOG, 2012a). It is not necessary to perform cervical cancer screening in order to provide most contraceptive services (i.e. oral, implants, injections, patches), initiate hormone management of dysmenorrhea or menstrual health, or provide STI screening. Vaginal swabs or urine tests are appropriate, effective alternatives for STI screening.

REPRODUCTIVE AGE

For women in their childbearing years, an annual well-women visit is the perfect opportunity to provide SRH education, immunizations, health screening, and family planning services. Pelvic and bimanual examinations are indicated before procedures such as the insertion of an intrauterine device or system, the fitting of a diaphragm or pessary, and an endometrial biopsy.

One innovative, reproductive health needs measure that came from the Oregon Foundation for Reproductive Health is the One Key Question® Initiative (OKQ; 2012). The OKQ concept was designed to encourage primary care providers to query women about their reproductive health needs. By asking women one question, "Would you like to become pregnant in the next year?" health care providers can support women's preventive reproductive health needs (e.g., pregnancy prevention, preparation for a healthy pregnancy; OKQ, 2012).

MATURE WOMEN

The mature women, defined as 46 to 64 years of age, has special health concerns. By 2020, it is estimated that approximately 20 million American women will be older than 51 years—the mean age for the onset of menopause (Manson & Kaunitz, 2016). Our new generation of health care provider graduates often lack the training and core competencies needed to manage a woman experiencing menopausal symptoms, as well as the necessary knowledge needed to prescribe hormonal treatment (see Chapter 34 for management/treatment guidelines). Inconsistent practice protocols exist based on personal interpretation of the Women's Health Initiative (WHI) study findings and given the many hormonal, bioidentical, *natural,* and complementary and alternative therapies touted as safe and effective.

An annual flu shot, a tetanus booster every 10 years, and screening for hepatitis C are recommended for women older than 65 years (USPSTF, 2014; Figure 11.6). Screening for osteoporosis is recommended for women starting at age 65 years.

Mature women have sexual concerns and sometimes want their health care provider to first address the subject—thereby opening the door to an open and trusting conversation. Age should *not* be a barrier to sexual health topics. Women experience aging differently and should be managed based on a woman's and her health care provider's joint decision making.

■ SUMMARY

Well-women health care provisions have improved preventive health care service for women across their lifetime by promoting a paradigm shift from reactive health care to encouraging health and well-being (Figure 11.7). An annual, well-women visit is a covered benefit under the ACA and by most private insurance and Medicaid plans. With no out-of-pocket cost requirements, private insurance plans, Medicaid, and Title X allow greater access for women to include low-income women who continue to be disproportionately affected by limited information and limited access to preventive care. In 2016, more than 55 million women have access to their choice of safe and efficacious birth-control methods approved by the U.S. Food and Drug Administration (FDA). Well-women visits are a vital element and entry to preventive care, as well as a new paradigm for health care practices. Reproductive health care needs, from adolescence through the reproductive years and into maturity, continue to be managed by health care providers—including specialty and primary care health care providers across a variety of health care disciplines. Nurse practitioners, nurse midwives, physicians, and physician assistants are trained to translate evidence into practice at the point of care, thereby improving the quality of health care delivery and access to comprehensive preventive care.

■ FUTURE DIRECTIONS

Future directions include patient-centered medical homes led by nurse practitioners and other health care professionals. This new wave in health care emphasizes coordination, communication, and the practice of putting women *front and center* as active participants in their health care decision making (Sawaya, 2016). Shared informed decision making has been challenging to implement because of clinic time constraints and patient loads that are needed to meet the economic requirements of health care organizations. This model of health care delivery demands a *huge* paradigm shift, not only in moving to a focus in prevention, but also in the manner in which third-party payers will reimburse health care providers and hospitals, where quality and health outcomes are used to determine reward and monetary compensation. A change of such magnitude will necessitate guidance

FIGURE 11.6

(A) Recommended immunization schedule for adults aged 19 years or older, United States, 2016. (*continued*)

B

VACCINE ▼ / INDICATION ►	Pregnancy	Immuno-Compromising Conditions (Excluding HIV Infection)	HIV Infection CD4+ Count (Cells/µL) < 200	HIV Infection CD4+ Count (Cells/µL) ≥ 200	Men Who Have Sex With Men (MSM)	Kidney Failure, End-Stage Renal Disease, on Hemodialysis	Heart Disease, Chronic Lung Disease, Chronic Alcoholism	Asplenia and Persistent Complement Component Deficiencies	Chronic Liver Disease	Diabetes	Health care Personnel
Influenza[a]	1 dose annually										
Tetanus, diphtheria, pertussis (Td/Tdap)[a]	1 dose Tdap each pregnancy	Substitute Tdap for Td once, then Td booster every 10 yrs									
Varicella[a]		Contraindicated	Contraindicated	2 doses							
Human papillomavirus (HPV), female[a]		3 doses through age 26 yrs									
HPV, male[a]		3 doses through age 26 yrs				3 doses through age 21 yrs					
Zoster		Contraindicated	Contraindicated				1 dose				
Measles, mumps, rubella (MMR)[a]		Contraindicated	Contraindicated								
Pneumococcal 13-valent conjugate (PCV13)[a]						1 dose					
Pneumococcal polysaccharide (PPSV23)					1, 2, or 3 doses depending on indication						
Hepatitis A[a]					2 or 3 doses depending on vaccine						
Hepatitis B[a]						3 doses					
Meningococcal 4-valent conjugate (MenACWY) or polysaccharide (MPSV4)[a]						1 or more doses depending on indication		1 or 2 doses depending on indication			
Meningococcal B (MenB)						2 or 3 doses depending on vaccine					
Haemophilus influenzae type b (Hib)[a]		3 doses post-HSCT recipients only						1 dose			

Legend:

- Recommended for all persons who meet the age requirement, lack documentation of vaccination, or lack evidence of past infection; zoster vaccine is recommended regardless of past episode of zoster
- Recommended for persons with a risk factor (medical, occupational, lifestyle, or other indication)
- No recommendation
- Contraindicated

FIGURE 11.6

(B) Vaccines that might be indicated for adults aged 19 years or older based on medical and other indications.

These schedules indicate the age groups and medical indications for which the administration of currently licensed vaccines is commonly recommended for adults aged 19 years or older, as of February 2016. For all vaccines being recommended on the Adult Immunization Schedule, a vaccine series does not need to be restarted, regardless of the time that has elapsed between doses. Licensed combination vaccines may be used whenever any components of the combination are indicated and when the vaccine's other components are not contraindicated. For detailed recommendations on all vaccines, including those used primarily for travelers or that are issued during the year, consult the manufacturers' package inserts and the complete statements from the Advisory Committee on Immunization Practices (www. cdc.gov/vaccines/hcp/acip-recs/index.html). Use of trade names and commercial sources is for identification only and does not imply endorsement by the U.S. Department of Health and Human Services.

[a] Covered by the National Vaccine Injury Compensation Program.

Recipients of a hematopoietic stem cell transplant (HSCT) should be vaccinated with a 3-dose regimen 6 to 12 months after a successful transplant, regardless of vaccination history; at least 4 weeks should separate doses.

Source: U.S. Department of Health and Human Services, Centers for Disease Control and Prevention (2016).

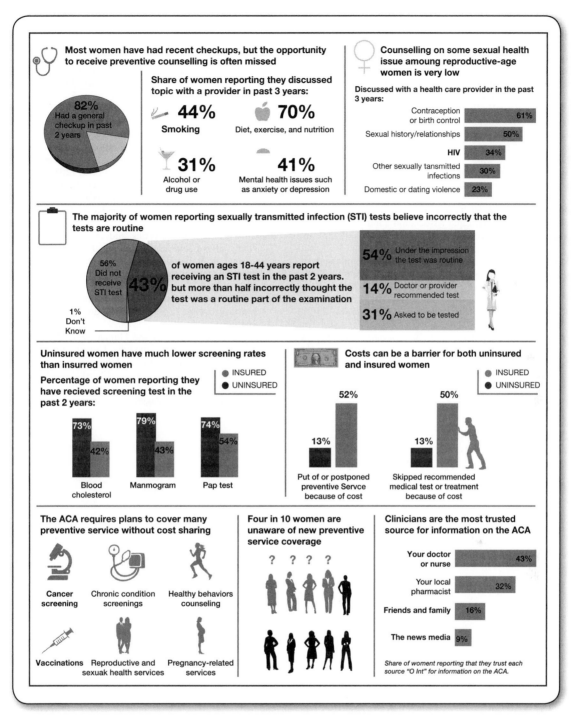

FIGURE 11.7

Preventive services for women and ACA.

ACA, Patient Protection and Affordable Care Act.

for health care providers and women as this new model of health care is incorporated into health care delivery. This is an exciting time to be a health care provider and a woman—the opportunities to help shape these changes are appreciated daily in health care delivery settings. The well-women visit is an opportunity to provide care that is evidence based, has high value, and is woman centered (Sawaya, 2016).

■ REFERENCES

Agency for Healthcare Research and Quality (AHRQ). (2016). *The electronic preventive services selector*. Retrieved from http://epss.ahrq.gov/PDA/index.jsp

American Cancer Society (ACS). (2016). *Cancer facts & figures 2016*. Atlanta, GA: American Cancer Society.

American College of Obstetricians and Gynecologists (ACOG). (2011). Breast cancer screening. Practice bulletin no. 122. *Obstetrics and Gynecology, 118*, 372–82.

American College of Obstetricians and Gynecologists (ACOG). (2011/2014). Breast cancer screening. Practice bulletin no. 122. *Obstetrics and Gynecology, 118*, 372–382.

American College of Obstetricians and Gynecologist (ACOG). (2012a). Screening for cervical cancer. Practice bulletin no. 131. *Obstetrics and Gynecology, 120*, 1222–1238.

American College of Obstetricians and Gynecologist (ACOG). (2012b). *Well-women visit.* Committee opinion no. 534. *Obstetrics and Gynecology, 120*, 421–424.

American College of Obstetricians and Gynecologists (ACOG). (2014). Colorectal cancer screening strategies. Committee Opinion No. 609, 1–7.

Bays, H. E., Jones, P. H., Brown, W. V., & Jacobson, T. A.; National Lipid Association. (2014). National Lipid Association annual summary of clinical lipidology 2015. *Journal of Clinical Lipidology, 8*(Suppl. 6), S1–S36.

Conry, J. A., & Brown, H. (2015). Well-woman task force: Components of the well-woman visit. *Obstetrics and Gynecology, 126*(4), 697–701.

Fitzgerald, T., Glynn, A., Davenport, K., Waxman, J., & Johnson, P. A. (2015). Well-woman visits: Guidance and monitoring are key in this turning point for women's health. *Women's Health Issues, 25*(2), 89–90.

Henry J. Kaiser Family Foundation. (2014). *Women and health care in the early years of the Affordable Care Act: Key findings from the 2013 Kaiser Women's Health Survey.* Retrieved from http://kff.org/womens-health-policy/report/women-and-health-care-in-the-early-years-of-the-aca-key-findings-from-the-2013-kaiser-womens-health-survey

Institute of Medicine (IOM). (2011). *Clinical preventive services for women: Closing the gaps.* Washington, DC: National Academies Press.

Manson, J., E., & Kaunitz, M. A. (2016). Menopause management: Getting clinical care back on track. *New England Journal of Medicine, 374*(9), 803–806. doi:10.1056/NEJMp1514242

National Lipid Association. (2014). Retrieved from https://www.lipid.org/recommendations

National Women's Law Center (NWLC). (2014). *Making the most of well women visits.* Retrieved from http://nwlc.org/issue/health-care-reproductive-rights

One Key Question (OKQ). (2012). *Oregon foundation for reproductive health.* Retrieved from http://www.onekeyquestion.org

Pascale, A., Beal, M. W., & Fitzgerald, T. (2016). Rethinking the well woman visit: A scoping review to identify eight priority areas for well woman care in the era of the Affordable Care Act. *Women's Health Issues: Official Publication of the Jacobs Institute of Women's Health, 26*(2), 135–146.

Richards, C. (2016). Protecting and expanding access to birth control. *New England Journal of Medicine, 374*(9), 801–803.

Rosenbaum, S., & Wood, S. F. (2015). Turning back the clock on women's health in medically underserved communities. *Women's Health Issues, 25*(6), 601–603.

Sawaya, G. F. (2016). Re-envisioning the annual well-women visit. *Obstetrics and Gynecology, 126*(4), 695–696. doi:10.1097/AOG.000000000000001079

U.S. Department of Health and Human Services. (2016). *Recommended adult immunizations schedule: United States–2016.* Atlanta, GA: Center for Disease Control and Prevention.

U.S. Preventive Services Task Force (USPSTF). (2014). *Recommendations for primary care practice.* Retrieved from http://www.uspreventiveservicestaskforce.org/Page/Name/recommendations

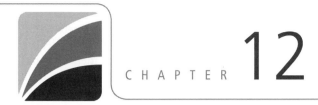

Mental Health

Gail M. Houck

When we seek to learn about "mental health," the literature typically speaks on mental *illness* or mental health *problems*. In fact, a search for literature about the mental health of women leads to numerous articles about depression, particularly postpartum depression. These diagnoses are not insignificant or in any way to be minimized. Yet there must be more to mental health than the absence of mental illness or mental health problems, and mental health is likely more complex than a categorical declaration of its presence. In particular, for women, mental health across the life span must be further understood in the context of enormous sociocultural change over the past six or seven decades. Women born in the years after World War II and the early 1950s, the "leading-edge" or early baby boomers, experienced a more traditional childhood and adolescence, with norms and role expectations that were more constrained and sharply differentiated by gender. In contrast, the "trailing-edge" baby boomer women and subsequent generations (generation X and generation Y or the millennials) have had relative independence from social role constraints with expanded educational and career opportunities. In the face of such dramatic social change, what is mental health for women today as they navigate life's journey without the role models and guides previous generations had?

■ WHO IS A MENTALLY HEALTHY WOMAN?

Interest in mental health or positive psychological health has been renewed in the past decade or so, and when indicated by an absence of psychiatric symptoms, there is an emerging consensus from research findings that psychological health tends to increase across the life span and into old age (Jones & Peskin, 2010). If mental health is more than an absence of psychiatric symptoms, then it is best understood as well-being. The common understanding of well-being entails a sense of happiness and satisfaction (Diener, Suh, Lucas, & Smith, 1999), but this definition perhaps oversimplifies the concept. Rather, well-being is multidimensional in nature, with hedonic and eudaemonic types (Ryan & Deci, 2001).

The hedonic approach to well-being is subjective and includes happiness and life satisfaction (Deiner, 2000).

Happiness is pleasure that is experienced as a rewarding state and is typically accompanied by positive affect, whereas satisfaction is the cognitive judgment or evaluation of life satisfaction (Diener, 2000). Eudaemonic well-being concerns self-realization and meaning and the extent to which one is fully functioning (Ryan & Deci, 2001) and is experienced by having satisfied the basic needs for competence, autonomy, and relatedness (Ryan & Deci, 2000). Accordingly, eudaemonic well-being has multiple dimensions: autonomy, environmental mastery, personal growth, positive relations with others, purpose in life, and self-acceptance (Ryff & Keyes, 1995). These eudaemonic dimensions implicate human development, personal growth, and flourishment (Woods, Rillamas-Sun, et al., 2015) and thereby reflect the grounding of eudaemonic well-being in philosophy and developmental psychology.

In fact, Erikson (1968) theorized that reemerging from each set of developmental existential challenges (he referred to "crisis") provided a greater sense of integration and "an increase in the capacity 'to do well'" (p. 92). This broad conception of the capacity to do well is akin to well-being, and Erickson's theory points to a developmental progression in the psychosocial capacity for the eudaemonic dimensions of well-being. Women's mental health as well-being is hedonic (happiness and satisfaction) and eudaemonic within a developmental context, from adolescence through old age. Thus women's mental health must be defined in accordance with the phases of psychosocial development and their inherent existential challenges, which tend to coalesce around the two themes of self-definition and relatedness (Blatt & Luyten, 2009; Kopala-Sibley, Mongrain, & Zuroff, 2013) or the development of self in relation to others. A central organizing feature of women's development of self is grounded in the ability to establish and maintain relationships (Miller, 2008), and the progression of this psychosocial development should be manifested as women's well-being and mental health.

Overview of Psychosocial Development

Erikson (1963, 1968) articulated a life-span theory of psychosocial development in which individuals must resolve crises linked to specific phases. This means that there are phases linked to age-related physical, cognitive, and emotional development in the given sociocultural context, in which there are salient development issues or what Erikson considered crises. The extent to which these are resolved provides a foundation for subsequent development. Accordingly, the early development of basic trust is central to the development of self in relation to others and is foundational to subsequent capacity for relatedness. In turn, the earliest experiences of autonomy contribute to subsequent identity and definitions of self, as well as the autonomous self in relation to others. These two aspects of development progress simultaneously and influence each other and are ideally integrated into a comprehensive sense of self (Blatt & Luyten, 2009) and into functioning with more maturity and integration (Erikson, 1963, 1968).

Although Erickson positioned the phases and their crises at specific points in the life span, he left room for individual variability in timing of the issues. Even more important for the provider of women's health care is the assumption that the salient developmental crises/issues can arise at any point as a function of psychosocial forces or the challenges of life events. In other words, earlier phases and issues can be revisited in later life, and later issues may become salient earlier if prompted by life circumstances; at all ages, all psychosocial developmental issues can arise. Although this chapter presents the salient developmental issues according to an overall trajectory that describes the typical woman's progression, be mindful that the interaction between individuals and their social environment contributes to individual variations and differences.

Basically, Erikson (1963, 1968) described eight phases of development. In infancy, the organization of attachment in relation to parents is central to the resolution of basic trust versus mistrust, which is foundational to all relationships. In toddlerhood (1–3 years), the resolution of autonomy versus shame lays the groundwork for a balance between self-assertion and self-regulation and for the subsequent resolution of initiative versus guilt in the preschool years (3–6 years), with the salient development of empathy, mutuality, and resilience. During the school-age years (6–12 years), the resolution of industry versus inferiority permits the development of a sense of competence and humility.

Originally, adolescence (12–19 years) was proposed by Erikson (1968) as the salient period for the development of identity versus confusion, during which ideals, values, and beliefs were solidified and roles adopted. Early adulthood (20–25 years) required resolution of intimacy versus isolation as manifested by committed relationships, and adulthood extended from the age of 26 years through 64 years of age, with generativity versus stagnation the central psychosocial development resolved through parenting and other forms of legacy. The final phase entails resolution of integrity versus despair, accomplished through a process of reflective life review.

However, Erikson (1968) noted that there was a prolonged adolescence in industrialized societies during which young adults were permitted to experiment with and explore various roles and identities. This idea laid the groundwork for a theory of emerging adulthood, a phase of development during the late teens through the 20s, made normative in response to the demographic changes in the timing of marriage and childbirth that occurred between the 1970s and the late 1990s (Arnett, 2000). According to Arnett (2000) and researchers who have built on his work, a key feature of emerging adulthood is the opportunity for identity explorations in the three main areas of worldviews, occupation/career, and relationships and involves trying out life possibilities with a progression toward enduring decisions. Emerging adulthood (18–30 years) then delays adulthood to the late 20s/early 30s. Emerging adulthood is now accepted as a developmental phase and a refinement to Erikson's theory of psychosocial development.

This chapter focuses on the postadolescent development of identity and relatedness or self in relation to others. The normative developmental phases of emerging adulthood, young adulthood, midlife, and older adulthood for women are described, including the salient issues and how those may be typically experienced.

■ EMERGING ADULTHOOD

Emerging adulthood is demographically distinct, especially when contrasted with adolescence (Arnett, 2000). Most adolescents up to age 18 years live with one or both parents (97%) or grandparents; only 4% live with extended family or foster parents, and less than 1% live independently (Kreider & Ellis, 2011). Most (approximately 90%), regardless of race/ethnicity, are enrolled in school (Kominski, Elliot, & Clever, 2009), and about 25% of adolescents 15 to 17 years of age are employed full or part time (Fields, 2003). The majority of adolescents are not parents; only 10% of adolescent women become first-time mothers across race/ethnicity, although this percentage includes 19- and 20-year-old women (U.S. Census Bureau, 2012).

By contrast, the demographic status of emerging adults is very difficult to predict on the basis of age. In particular, the residential status of emerging adults may be characterized by a lack of stability. In 1960, 35% of 18- to 24-year-olds lived in the parental home, but that proportion had grown to a little over half in 2014, and among 25- to 34-year-olds, there was an increase from 8% to 12% living in the parental home (U.S. Census Bureau, 2015). Although some of those enrolled in colleges or graduate schools may account for this proportion, many live independently with roommates or in some combination of independent living and reliance on adults (e.g., the dormitory or fraternal living situation) or perhaps alone in an apartment but partially supported by parents. Some may move out of the parental home to work and establish independent living with roommates or, given the rapid expansion of cohabitation in the past few decades, live with a partner (Vespa, Lewis, & Kreider, 2013). Frequent residential changes during emerging adulthood reflect the exploratory nature of this phase, providing a range of living experiences with a variety of people.

The pursuit of higher education is another arena with substantial diversity and change among emerging adults (Arnett, 2000). It is projected that, by 2028, more than half of women 25 years and older will have proceeded to college, across race/ethnicity, although there is variation (62% for

Black and Hispanic women, 86% for Asian women) (Day & Bauman, 2000). As of 2013, nearly one third (31%) of women have earned a bachelor's degree or higher (23% of Black, 16% of Hispanic, 32% of White, and 51% of Asian women; Hegewisch, Hayes, Milli, Shaw, & Hartmann, 2015). In 2011, of those awarded associate and bachelor's degrees, women represented 62% and 57% respectively; they also are 59% of those awarded master's degrees and 52% of those earning a doctorate or professional degree (Hegewisch et al., 2015). Of course, the timing of completion of the degree varies substantially, again pointing up the limited consistency in how emerging adults explore their options.

The median age for marriage among women has increased from 21 years in 1950 to 27 years in 2014 (U.S. Census Bureau, 2015). The proportion of women who are married has declined by about 15%, and the proportion who never married has increased by about 10%. In fact, over a third of generation Y women have never married at 30 years of age (Hegewisch et al., 2015). Birthrates have also declined steadily since 2007 for women 20 to 29 years of age, although at a greater rate for younger women 20 to 24 years old than for those 25 to 29 years old (Hamilton, Martin, Osterman, & Curtain, 2015). This likely represents a delay in childbearing, as the birthrate among 30- to 34-year-old women has steadily increased since 2011 by about 3% to 4% and by 5% in 2014 for women 35 to 39 years of age; the birthrate among women in their early 40s has risen steadily since the 1980s (Hamilton et al., 2015). Across age groups, about 40% are not married at the birth of their first child. Among those women 29 years of age or younger without a college education, about two thirds are married or cohabiting at the birth of their first child, whereas among those 30 years and older, at least three fourths are married or cohabiting (U.S. Census Bureau, 2012). The exploratory phase of emerging adulthood has clearly permitted women to delay marriage and childbearing commitments.

These demographic characteristics, however, have not directly contributed to engaging adults' subjective sense of attaining adulthood. Rather, qualities of character matter: accepting responsibility for one's self, making independent decisions, and becoming financially independent (Arnett, 2000). Settling into these adult responsibilities is a gradual process, accompanied by identity exploration as a key feature, with a cycle of forming commitments, evaluating those commitments, and forming new commitments (Luyckx, Goossens, & Soenens, 2006). Identity explorations occur in the arenas of worldviews, love relationships, and work or career and can be accompanied by risk behaviors in an effort to obtain a wide range of experiences before adulthood (Arnett, 2000).

Identity Exploration and Formation

Identity development is most actively explored during emerging adulthood, with identity status stabilizing once identity-defining commitments have been established and choices made (Kroger, Martnussen, & Marcia, 2010).

These commitments typically include what political and religious beliefs to hold (worldviews), whether and with whom to make a relationship commitment or marry (love relationships), and what career or occupation to pursue (work) (Whitbourne, Sneed, & Sayer, 2009). The identity status model elaborates Erikson's theory about the identity development process and is a means for assessment of the exploration and commitment dimensions of his ideas about identity formation (Marcia, 1966).

The status of identity is based on the defining commitments achieved or decisions made, the degree of identification with those chosen commitments, and the extent of exploration involved to arrive at those identity-defining commitments (Carlsson, Wängqvist, & Frisén, 2015). There are classic questions related to the formation of identity: Who am I? What will I do with my life? What is important to me? The answers may be considered decisions and choices, yet the process of arriving at the self-defining answers that constitute identity formation is not just a cognitive process. "Defining commitments" are transformational choices made about experiences that cannot be fully known ahead of the actual experience. As such, they entail an affective component that extends from personally valued parts of the self, one's uniqueness and preferences, as well as those parts of the self that are tied to highly valued social relationships and groups, such as gender, race/ethnicity, family, and culture (Eccles, 2009). In other words, identity-defining commitments must be "right" and congruent with one's sense of self and of self in relation to others. Thus a process of exploring alternatives, forming commitments, and evaluating those commitments are crucial cyclical dynamics in developing an identity (Luyckx et al., 2006).

The extent of exploration involved to arrive at identity-defining commitments is distinguished in terms of breadth and depth (Luyckx, Soenens, Vansteenkiste, Goossens, & Berzonsky, 2007). Breadth of exploration is the extent to which a young woman considers different identity alternatives. Depth of exploration is an intentional gathering of information relevant to the evaluation of decisions and commitments that are in process or made; in-depth exploration and reevaluation of one's commitments compose an ongoing identity-formation process.

There are four different observable styles linked to the underlying process of identity formation and eventual attainment of an identity status (Kroger et al., 2010). The developmental process may begin with *identity diffusion*, in which there are weak or no identifications and the exploration of options has not occurred or has been constrained. Identity development more normatively begins with *foreclosure*, which is characterized by tentative strong commitments and identifications made in accordance with important childhood figures and little exploration. These early statuses are typically followed by *moratorium*, in which commitments and identifications are weak and various options and alternatives are actively explored. It is expected that the active exploration of alternatives will yield the capacity to make identity-defining decisions and commitments and will thereby result in the status of *identity achievement*.

Most emerging adults experience forward progression rather than regression of identity development to identity achievement: (a) from identity diffusion via foreclosure and moratorium (to identity achievement), (b) from identity diffusion via moratorium, and (c) from foreclosure via moratorium (Carlsson et al., 2015; Kroger et al., 2010). An established identity, through foreclosure or achievement, tends to be more stable (Carlsson et al., 2015). This is especially so if identity is achieved in later emerging adulthood whereas the early decisions and commitments of late adolescence can easily give way to new rounds of exploration as more life situations are encountered and broaden one's range of options (Kroger et al., 2010). Identity-defining commitments are associated with well-being and more positive psychosocial functioning and may be protective against taking risks (Ritchie et al., 2013). However, this holds for identity decisions and commitments that are the right ones for the individual; identity decisions and commitments that are not congruent with one's sense of self have negative consequences (Ritchie et al., 2013).

Thus the nature of exploration before establishing identity-defining commitments is crucial. Active exploration in emerging adulthood is linked to identity achievement and positive well-being (Ritchie et al., 2013). Identity exploration seems to normatively involve some experimentation with risk taking, such as alcohol, driving-related, and sexual risk-taking behavior; the extent and chronicity of the risk behavior separate normative from worrisome trajectories, and should be screened (Ritchie et al., 2013).

Yet an absence of experimentation may reflect personal and/or social constraints on the exploration of alternatives. Those who explore their options in a hesitant, self-critical manner (e.g., foreclosure or diffusion) are more likely to report diminished self-esteem and life satisfaction and lower eudaemonic and psychological well-being. Explorations that are characterized as ruminative in nature, with worry and obsession about making the perfect choice, are also more likely to lead to lower self-esteem and impede identity formation (Ritchie et al., 2013). In these cases, the exploration of alternatives tends to be more broad and less in depth and often linked to intrusive, psychologically controlling or intimidating parenting; such parental control tactics impede rather than facilitate an authentic process of self-exploration for defining identity commitments and, hence, the capacity for identity formation (Luyckx et al., 2007; Perosa, Perosa, & Tam, 2002). These negative outcomes have been found for emerging adult women but are thought to hold across gender (Luyckx et al., 2007).

Continued Identity Development and Developmental Transitions

Mental health in women entails not only identity achievement but how well they are able to cope with challenging developmental transitions beyond emerging adulthood. Transitions present developmental tasks that provide many opportunities, yet are embedded in changing circumstances and uncertainty (Weiss, Freund, & Wiese, 2012). Similar to the process of exploration of identity-defining commitments, the transformation involved in developmental transitions and ongoing identity formation involves not having sufficient knowledge about the subsequent situation to be experienced; one's sense of personal control and well-being are certainly challenged.

A mentally healthy woman has an openness to experience and less traditional gender ideology and expectations, which contributes to self-efficacy and well-being in the context of developmental transitions. For women low in openness to experience, transitional uncertainty is more threatening to their self-efficacy and well-being, and they do not fare as well through developmental transitions. If they in turn hold a traditional gender ideology and attendant expectations, they can avoid uncertainty by restricting developmental options although to do so has other social consequences (Weiss et al., 2012).

Three dimensions of identity have been found to represent the processes of continued identity development and are pertinent to the assessment of how well women cope with future developmental transitions. By the end of the 20s, these dimensions set the path for coping with developmental challenges and women's subsequent identity development or maturation. These include the approach to changing life conditions, meaning making, and development of personal life direction (Carlsson et al., 2015). The *approach to changing conditions of life* concerns a woman's approach to the inevitability that life indeed changes as time goes by. This approach can range from a rigid resistance to change to a capacity and proneness to reformulate and adjust one's identity, perhaps with changes in commitments. *Meaning making* refers to how women create and maintain a sense of identity by reflecting on, and engaging in, discourse about life events and experiences and how these relate to their personal present and future. Women with identity achievement engage in greater narrative processing with more personally meaningful stories. The *development of personal life direction* pertains to how women make decisions about how they want to live their lives, whether they are constrained by social norms and others' expectations or are able to assert themselves and make independent decisions in relation to social norms and expectations from others. That is, choices are made by women with awareness that they are related to and affected by societal and family norms and expectations.

Self-Esteem

Self-esteem has been defined as the evaluation and attitude toward the self and, as such, is perhaps more affective-like in nature, reflecting self-worth or lovability, whereas self-concept is more cognitive in nature and entails self-definition and appraisal of one's strengths and limitations. Positive self-esteem has beneficial effects on mental health and psychosocial functioning, and low self-esteem has detrimental effects and is a central feature of depression, anxiety, and other negative outcomes (Orth, Robins, Trzesniewski, Maes, & Schmitt, 2009; Orth, Trzesniewski, & Robins, 2010; Trzesniewski et al., 2006). As previously noted, emerging adulthood and its inherent transition from adolescence are especially challenging periods given identity exploration. The many alternatives mean changing social environments such as study or living abroad, attending college or vocational school for some period, completing college, searching for and starting a new work position, dating and perhaps developing a more consistent partnership, and moving among various residential arrangements. All of these situations may challenge what might be an otherwise relatively stable self-esteem.

Although children generally begin life with reasonably positive self-esteem, by early adolescence they reveal a steady decline, if not sharp reductions, in self-esteem (Trzesniewski, Donnellan, & Robins, 2003), particularly young women (McMullin & Cairney, 2004). Recently, however, self-esteem was found to slightly increase after high school graduation, with an accelerated increase at about 21 years of age (Wagner, Lüdtke, Jonkmann, & Trautwein, 2013). During emerging adulthood, self-esteem has remarkable continuity, whether high or low (Chung et al., 2014), and remains relatively level throughout adulthood in spite of experiencing the inevitable accomplishments and disappointments of life (Trzesniewski et al., 2003). In fact, self-esteem has a significant prospective impact on real-world life experience, with its link to life-span trajectories of affect and depression and satisfying experiences with relationships and career/occupational status (Orth, Robins, & Widaman, 2012). Higher extraversion, openness to experience, and agreeableness tend to accompany a positive self-esteem in women, and these facilitate adaptive identity exploration (Wagner et al., 2013), as well as social well-being (Hill, Turiano, Mroczek, & Roberts, 2012).

It matters in which domains of self-worth a woman invests. Investing self-worth in one's appearance and approval of others not only hinders self-esteem but also contributes to heightened body surveillance and dissatisfaction with one's own appearance (Overstreet & Quinn, 2012). Instead, deriving self-worth from academic competence, family support, and religious commitment tends to enhance self-esteem and appearance satisfaction. Although women today are more likely to reject traditional gender ideology (traditional roles of housekeeping and motherhood, lower educational and career aspirations), those that do endorse traditional gender ideology are vulnerable to diminished self-efficacy and well-being, even if the ideology provides clear guidelines for behavior and avoids uncertainty and insecurity (Weiss et al., 2012).

An issue related to self-esteem and self-worth is self-promotion. Women have historically been socialized to be modest and to avoid self-promotion, and adherence to the modesty norm is thought to prevent women from achieving the success they might otherwise (Smith & Huntoon, 2014). Violating the modesty norm by engaging in self-promotion triggers discomfort or situational arousal for a fear of backlash; whatever triggers the uncomfortable arousal, research revealed that when a source for any uncomfortable arousal was provided, the result was increased self-promotion success (Smith & Huntoon, 2014). Informing women that such discomfort and arousal can be attributed to gender-based modesty norms will make it possible for them to actively engage in successful self-promotion for their occupation or career. This example of gender norm violation is one of the many subtle dynamics to which women may respond with arousal, even anxiety. It is imperative to explore the dynamics of the situation in which there may have been a norm violation and to identify the source of the arousal or anxiety. Making a reasonable attribution to the cause of the arousal, rather than a diagnosis of anxiety where not warranted, will facilitate women's well-being as we seek to establish new norms.

YOUNG ADULTHOOD

Young adulthood begins in the late 20s or early 30s and extends to the mid-40s that mark middle adulthood or midlife. Identity consolidation is the marker of entry into adulthood (Sneed, Whitbourne, & Culang, 2006) and provides the foundation of the capacity to do well and the basis of self-acceptance and self-esteem (Sneed, Whitbourne, Schwartz, & Huang, 2012). Having established a sense of self and a relational identity, the young adult woman is now ready to form intimacy in close, committed, long-term relationships (Beyers & Seiffge-Krenke, 2010). In other words, identity consolidation and intimacy are closely intertwined and together make possible the transition to the adult roles of employment, committed partnerships, and parenting (Luyckx et al., 2007). Identity and intimacy contribute to well-being in young adulthood and are relatively stable through midlife, with identity being especially core to later well-being (Sneed et al., 2012).

The salient commitments in young adulthood include establishing an occupation or career, forming intimate and long-term relationships or marriage, and becoming a mother. These commitments are important life experiences that are normative and socially desirable during this age period (Arnett, 2000). Developing goals related to these salient commitments during emerging and young adulthood, even with changes in those goals, contributes to greater well-being (Hill, Jackson, Roberts, Lapsley, & Brandenberger, 2011). Although society is less prescriptive about the sequencing and timing of these major life events, those who choose to have an intimate partnership and become parents are typically doing so during young or early adulthood and experience mental health benefits (Jackson, 2004).

Normative Transitions

The normative transition into work is indeed linked to overall life satisfaction (Lee & Gramotnev, 2007). Women, in particular, have been found to experience gains in self-confidence and determination, competence, and effectiveness through involvement in their work; these benefits have held for leading- and trailing-edge baby boomers, although values and women's roles have transitioned substantially between these two cohorts of women (Whitbourne et al., 2009). Nearly half the workforce is now constituted by women, and women's employment has expanded beyond traditional education and health service positions to include managerial and professional occupations (Hegewisch et al., 2015). These circumstances point up the remarkable opportunities and choices available to young women today. Women who establish an occupation or career with a delay in becoming a mother until after 31 years of age (or even the mid-30s or beyond) experience enhanced developmental gains and well-being (Whitbourne et al., 2009). Of course, given the mental health benefits from work, it is not surprising that a transition out of work leads to stress and depression (Lee & Gramotnev, 2007), and such a transition should be recognized as a vulnerability to diminished mental health and well-being for women.

Committed couple relationships are linked to overall life satisfaction (Lee & Gramotnev, 2007; Wade & Pevalin, 2004). Favorable relationship outcomes may be difficult to define, but longitudinal researchers have used a long-term committed relationship as an indicator of relationship success; involvement in a committed relationship is either through marriage or living together with a person of the same or opposite sex (Whitbourne et al., 2009). It seems that intimacy is slowly and steadily enhanced over time for those who delay their commitment to a long-term relationship, whereas those who commit during emerging adulthood tend to peak in their 30s (early adulthood) and experience a continuous decline thereafter (Whitbourne et al., 2009). Relationship commitment is not without adjustments to living together and establishing healthy communication to meet individual needs. Nonetheless, in the absence of dysfunction and violence, relationship commitment points to life satisfaction and well-being. Transitions out of relationships through separation, divorce, or death lead to greater stress and depression and to reductions on all indices of mental health (Lee & Gramotnev, 2007; Wade & Pevalin, 2004). Stress, depression, and mental health disorders are often thought to contribute to the dissolution of a committed relationship, yet when not previously present, rather consistently attend separation and divorce.

The transition to motherhood is a normative life experience that has been consistently linked to diminished well-being (Lee & Gramotnev, 2007). However, motherhood has also been linked to steady growth in a sense of generativity over time, especially if parenthood occurs in the 30s rather than sooner (Whitbourne et al., 2009). By waiting to become mothers until their mid-30s or later, women are able to attain educational goals and establish their occupation or career with some measure of financial security. These women may be less stressed and better able to enjoy their new parenthood status (Benzies et al., 2006). Women with careers who become mothers report higher life satisfaction than those who do not have children (Hoffnung & Williams, 2013). It is likely that the transition to motherhood can be normatively challenging to well-being, but motherhood itself contributes to an overall level of life satisfaction.

The transition to motherhood is a period of adjustment to parenthood, and learning the skills of mothering can be challenging and disorienting under the best of circumstances (Nelson, 2003). Adapting to an infant's temperament, states, and needs and developing responsiveness to cues, cries, and the developmental agenda present multiple demands as the mother recovers from the physiological consequences of childbirth and seeks to establish her identity as a mother. She must adapt to relationship changes with her partner, family, and friends and navigate decisions related to returning to work, the timing of the return, and child care (Nelson, 2003). This process of adaptation to motherhood is similar for adoptive motherhood, although the adoptive mother may have unique concerns, depending on the circumstances of adoption (Fontenot, 2007).

The emotional processing that attends these adaptations and challenges should not be underestimated. The particular challenges of a first-time mother are pointed up by the limited evidence that mental health outcomes are worse for mothers who have multiples first versus those who have a singleton baby before multiples, as well as compared with those who have closely spaced singletons (Wenze, Battle, & Tezanos, 2015). Separate from learning how to mother and developing an identity as a mother, women who have multiples (e.g., twins or triplets) experience worse postpartum and early parenthood mental health outcomes, such as depression, anxiety, and parenting stress, than do mothers of singleton babies; these outcomes are undoubtedly related to the heavier parenting burden and attendant sleep loss and social isolation (Wenze et al., 2015).

Even for mothers of singleton babies, depression in the postpartum period is common, with nearly 20% of new mothers experiencing depression in the first 3 months after the birth of their babies (Werner, Miller, Osborne, Kuzava, & Monk, 2015). Yet, postpartum depression is difficult to predict, with only a third of the women who experience postpartum depression having a history of depression (Robakis et al., 2015). The best predictor of postpartum depression is depression during pregnancy, which may alert care providers to initiate intervention focused on the mother and her infant during maternity care as well as postpartum (Werner et al., 2015), including adolescent mothers (Nicolson, Judd, Thomson-Salo, & Mitchell, 2013).

In turn, optimism and positive expectations during the pregnancy provide protection against postpartum depression, even among those who have a history of mood disorder (Robakis et al., 2015). The key is that the optimism is moderated and not so great as to contrast with or be undermined by the reality of the postpartum mothering experience. Women's health care providers should foster the pregnant woman's "cautious optimism" with realistic expectations, which will more likely shape positive attitudes toward mothering and the mother's feelings of satisfaction and engagement with her infant. Fortunately, most women's experiences do meet or exceed their optimistic expectations rather than bring disappointment, even when they have a history of a mood disorder (Robakis et al., 2015).

Balancing Multiple Identities

In becoming a mother, a woman now typically occupies multiple roles and identities that compete or are in conflict, and paid work presents a major competing role for mothers (Gaunt & Scott, 2014). Whether a woman continues to work after becoming a mother may depend, in part, on the relative salience and centrality of her identities related to her occupation or career and her investment in child care. Perceptions of mothers as irreplaceable primary caretakers and societal ambivalence toward new mothers' employment persist, resulting in substantial variability in the ways mothers distribute their time between paid work and child care (Hoffnung & Williams, 2013). In general, the more central a mother's work identity, the more hours she works for pay and the fewer hours she serves as the sole provider of child care (Gaunt & Scott, 2014). On the one hand, it would seem that the hours in a day that a mother has available for child care would influence the father's or partner's involvement in child care. On the other hand, it is the salience and centrality of her maternal identity that is important, not only to her own involvement, but also to the encouragement or discouragement of the father's or partner's involvement in child care, as well as the balance of their relative share of childcare tasks (Gaunt & Scott, 2014).

In other words, the mother serves as a gatekeeper to her partner's participation in child care. It is a challenge for women to balance their identities for work and motherhood, and they may need help in understanding the ways that their internalized identities and expectations may be guiding their decisions in this regard. Paternal involvement in housework and parenting has expanded (Hegewisch et al., 2015), and the gap between the mother's and the father's hours of child care is much smaller in the face of stronger women's work identities and longer hours in paid work (Gaunt & Scott, 2014). It can be helpful to reflectively explore this issue so that mothers can more consciously make decisions about the balance among work, mothering, and coparenting.

Nurturing Child Development

Mothers change not only in response to transitioning to motherhood, but also in response to learning to nurture their child's developmental needs. The parent–child relationship is conceptualized as a bidirectional and transactional system of influence; in other words, the parent influences the child and the child influences the parent. Although mothers vary in the extent to which they are influenced, Luvmour (2011) found that maternal development typically occurs in five ways as the mother becomes aware of her child's developmental agenda and nurtures her child's developmental imperatives. Notably, each of these developmental changes is related to greater parenting competence (Luvmour, 2011).

First, mothers intentionally seek out and apply child development principles and, by doing so, exercise *personal agency* that both promotes maternal development and is considered a sign of adult development. Mothers begin parenting with family challenges, personal questions, and a need to know how to do things differently. Through self-reflection, gathering knowledge about child development and parenting, and intentionally applying child-development principles in the mother–child relationship and family context, adult development is promoted.

The mother's intentional effort to learn about child development also promotes her cognitive and emotional development. In terms of cognitive development, mothers describe changes in their perspective of self, differentiating from former ways of being and making new meaning of the world. The experience with her child in the course of parenting activates recollections and memories of her own childhood experiences such that she gains new understanding of and derives new meaning from those experiences. Emotional changes and maturation are manifested by a greater awareness of trust, empathy, and affective complexity (i.e., the complexity of greater emotional connectedness, humility, and honesty or authenticity). Attention to the child's developmental needs both currently and for subsequent development involves a conscientious nurturing that in turn enhances trust, empathy, and connectedness.

For many women, changes in a mother's sense of well-being also emerge as she nurtures her child's developmental imperatives. This sense of well-being entails greater self-acceptance, personal strength and confidence, resilience and self-care, open-mindedness, connectedness with self and others, and happiness. When mothers experience this sense of well-being, they described themselves as being in the right place and doing the right thing. Luvmour (2011) found that not all parents attained this sense of well-being; what differentiates those who do from those who do not remains to be understood, but in the meantime, mothers not experiencing a sense of well-being may be vulnerable to parenting stress.

Finally, mothers often experience a positive shift in their quality of being in relationships with others. According to Luvmour (2011), many mothers found that nurturing their child's developmental progression provided opportunities to reexamine, reorganize, and transcend to more complex forms of engagement, not only with their children, but also with others. Many referred to this as the *gaining of wisdom*, but the shift also entailed an improved capacity for emotional presence, insight, and compassion, all improvements for which they experienced gratitude.

In providing care to mothers, it is important to respect and seek to understand the mothering processes and practices of specific cultural groups; the challenge is to differentiate between mothering behaviors that are crucial to children's safety, health, and development and those that are only Western tradition (Koniak-Griffin, Logsdon, Hines-Martin, & Turner, 2006). Careful discernment is required to support maternal competence in the context of her culture and community. A key strategy is to connect mothers with supportive social networks in their communities in order to enhance their psychosocial meanings of motherhood, parenting competence, and social health and well-being (Suplee et al., 2014).

■ MIDDLE ADULTHOOD

Middle adulthood is a rich period in life with many opportunities to gain awareness, especially of one's mortality, to shift priorities, and refine one's identity. As generativity commitments are established and legacy defined, meaning in life and spirituality become salient with the capacity for forgiveness expanded. The complexity of cultural demand, generative desire and commitments, spirituality and beliefs, and concerns and experiences with launching children and caring for parents becomes a part of a woman's *narrative identity*, as she develops her story about her life and what she has done for the next generation as well as its meaning for herself and others (Jones & McAdams, 2013).

Generativity

Early adulthood is the consolidation of identity and the establishment of intimacy, with the careful balancing of personal needs and social demands as a foundation for transitioning to generativity, the commitment to care for future generations, and the contribution to their development and well-being (Jones & McAdams, 2013). Although identity concerns are readdressed and strengthened from emerging to young adulthood through middle adulthood (Beaumont & Pratt, 2011), concerns rest with regard to making lasting, meaningful contributions to the next generation. Having a clear sense of individual identity is necessary for maintaining a sense of life meaning while negotiating intimate connections with others, and facing the tasks of generativity (Erikson, 1980), such as parenting, teaching, coaching, mentorship, and participation in religious, community, and political activities.

Generativity is perhaps a transaction between individuals and their sociocultural environment. A woman's "need to be needed" and desire to leave a legacy may be manifested through a variety of activities: high involvement in parenting; care of aging parents; volunteer activity in her church, her children's school and extracurricular activities, and community organizations; civic or political involvement; leadership; and/or a profession that involves helping or teaching others. Participation in these activities is in turn reinforced by societal expectations regarding adult responsibilities to guide the next generation. The generative desire and societal expectations together contribute to a conscious concern for the next generation, possibly reinforced by a belief in the fundamental worth of humankind, which then becomes translated into commitments to engage in positive actions for the next generation (Jones & McAdams, 2013). Women tend to be more highly generative than men, and their generativity arises from positive family socializing influences (Jones & McAdams, 2013). Generativity is associated with psychological maturity in midlife as well as successful aging in terms of physical functioning and longevity and mental health and well-being (Gruenewald, Liao, & Seeman, 2012; Versey, Stewart, & Duncan, 2013).

The desire to leave a legacy is a feature of generativity that is not entirely selfless and may even reflect an element of narcissism (Newton, Herr, Pollack, & McAdams, 2014). This is likely an adaptive narcissism, which generally tends to diminish from young adulthood through midlife as generativity expands (Hill & Roberts, 2012). Recent findings point to high levels of both generativity and narcissism involved in the highest levels of legacy, which entail both self and other (Newton, Herr, Pollack, & McAdams, 2014). There is a synergy between healthy narcissism and generativity that serves the creation of legacy for future generations.

Identity and Generativity

Generativity, as manifested by generative commitments and actions, is an outgrowth of identity. Given the relative stability of identity formation, as women move into middle age, identity may be better understood as a processing style or way of dealing with identity questions and situations that call for an identity-defining decision (Berzonsky & Kuk, 2000). In middle adulthood, women continue to be faced with experiences and opportunities that require self-examination, a questioning of assumptions and beliefs, an exploration and evaluation of relevant information, and active problem solving. It follows that the identity status from emerging and young adulthood influences the process for addressing the identity questions and decisions encountered in middle adulthood.

Those middle-aged adults who earlier explored alternatives to arrive at identity-defining commitments and decisions (the status of identity achievement) are more likely to have developed an *information-oriented* identity style in which they continue to actively explore and evaluate information relevant to their sense of self and are in turn more engaged in generative commitments and activity. Those with an information-oriented style are especially balanced in terms of intimacy and generativity and are thought to have an integrated character and mature psychological adjustment (Beaumont & Pratt, 2011). Open self-exploration is central to an information-oriented processing style and characterizes psychosocial and mental health.

Those who perhaps reached a foreclosure status and adopted identification and commitment in accordance to important role models are, as middle-aged adults, likely to use a *norm-oriented* process to address identity questions and defining decisions. Those who prefer a norm-oriented process do not engage in self-exploration but rather conform to norms and to the expectations of family and/or significant others. They show some aspects of a psychosocial adjustment in terms of identity certainty but the potential lack of authenticity results in a pseudointimacy and conventional generative commitments and activity (Beaumont & Pratt, 2011).

The statuses of identity diffusion and moratorium both entail weak identifications and commitments, although the patterns of exploration differ. Nonetheless, in middle adulthood, women with weak identifications and low commitment are prone to a diffuse-avoidant way of dealing with identity questions and decisions that essentially involves an avoidance of confronting personal issues and problems, a strategy thought to be self-handicapping. Without self-exploration, they lack self-awareness, which is considered essential for generativity; without a responsiveness to norms or expectations, these individuals fail to even engage in conventional generative commitments and activity. Thus those women who use a diffuse-avoidant style lack maturity and are less psychologically adaptive.

Meaning in Life

Theoretically, people experience the presence of meaning when they comprehend themselves and their social environment with a sense of coherence and understand their unique contributions to life (Dezutter et al., 2013; Steger, Kashdan, Sullivan, & Lorentz, 2008). The presence of meaning is a desirable psychological quality that contributes to enhanced self-esteem and mental health, with less depression, more optimism, and greater life satisfaction (Dezutter et al., 2014; Steger, Frazier, Oishi, & Kaler, 2006). In midlife and late midlife, meaning in life tends to offset concerns about aging, which tend to be exacerbated by life events such as loss of employment, financial insecurity, or illness (Versey et al., 2013). Concerns about aging in midlife hinder successful aging later in terms of active involvement in life and psychological well-being, as well as subjective health (Versey et al., 2013). Thus meaning in midlife portends successful aging with physical and mental health and well-being.

The *search for meaning* refers to people's efforts to establish or increase their understanding of the meaning, purpose, and value of their lives; its importance to human functioning is highlighted by the relationship between the search for meaning and diminished psychological functioning (Steger et al., 2008). Thus the search for meaning may be a solution that is activated by a reduction in or loss of the sense of life's meaningfulness. Those who lack meaning tend to embark on a search for meaning, although this search does not necessarily lead to finding meaning and having its presence.

Since meaning is tied to a comprehension of the self in the world as well as one's unique contributions, it is linked to identity, and its development runs parallel to that of identity (Steger et al., 2006). Accordingly, the development of meaning could be understood in terms of search and presence, much as identity is understood with respect to exploration and commitment. In this way, a pattern of low search and low presence of meaning would be characterized as *meaning diffusion*, low search and high presence would be *meaning foreclosure*, a pattern of high search and low presence would be characterized as *meaning moratorium*, and high search and presence would be *meaning achievement* (Steger et al., 2006). This conceptualization is congruent with research that found a similar conceptualization for the development of spiritual identity (Kiesling, Sorell, Montgomery, & Colwell, 2008). Given that those who experience meaning in their lives are more involved in religious activities (Steger et al., 2006), it seems likely that meaning arises out of the spiritual component of identity.

Spiritual identity is the sense of self that attends to the questions about the nature, purpose, and meaning of life and results in behavior that is congruent with one's core values (Kiesling et al., 2008). Meaning in life, then, is an inherent part of spiritual identity and first becomes salient in adolescence and emerging adulthood as initial decisions and commitments relevant to spirituality are made. Spiritual identity and meaning remain ongoing issues and become especially salient to middle adulthood and the developmental tasks of generativity and leaving a legacy. In their research on spiritual identity, Kiesling et al. (2008) found the spiritual identities to bear a notable similarity to the identity statuses (Marcia, 1966) previously described in this chapter; these spiritual identity statuses are also congruent with the

categories of meaning developmental statuses described by Steger et al. (2006) and again capture patterns of search/exploration and commitments.

Achieved (spiritual) identity is characterized by an exploration of alternatives in religion, beliefs, cultural practices, and perspectives, as well as the intentional choice among options, with identity-defining decisions and commitments made; it is akin to an information orientation with seeking information and engaging in a self-reflective process in response to questions and concerns about identity. It is not surprising that those with achieved identity attained their spiritual identity through intentional choice and expressed that they had found the spirituality right for them (Kiesling et al., 2008). They were able to articulate their spiritual identity and elaborate, with rich imagery, on its modification and evolution. These individuals described the discovery of a new perspective and knowing, a cultivated awareness, and a transformed capacity for being present to others that enhanced intimacy. Their sense of spiritual identity had considerable positive impact on their self-perceptions and self-evaluations, and sense of self-worth; they seemed to be freer to self-critique in the context of greater self-acceptance. Having arrived at a place of ideological and spiritual commitment, they become interested in the heterogeneity of their community, as well as issues of social justice and reconciliation (Kiesling et al., 2008), all of which shape the nature of their generative commitments and legacy contributions.

The *foreclosed (spiritual) identity* is characterized by a strong commitment to particular roles and ideological positions without having explored a range of options and is akin to a norm-oriented approach to dealing with questions and decisions about one's identity. Accordingly, norms and expectations as explicated by family, religious faith, tribalism, and/or ethnicity shape the identity decisions and commitments made, particularly for spiritual identity. For those with a foreclosed spiritual identity, the nature of religious faith exists without making a choice; rather, these individuals feel compelled to sustain their ascribed religious orthodoxy. In essence, living according to these ideas protects these individuals from identity diffusion and from the anxiety of identity choices, provides a sense of belonging in a familial realm and a sense of continuity with their historical self from childhood, and helps them avoid identity decisions regarded as shameful in their social context (Kiesling et al., 2008). Because the spiritual identity was formed in concert with significant others, the expectations of that community continue to hold enormous influences on the sense of self, such that self-expression and authenticity are constrained. There is limited self-reflection or questioning of assumptions and beliefs. Self-perception and self-evaluation are determined by those family members and friends with whom they share their spiritual commitments.

Those individuals in moratorium with respect to spiritual identity have weak identities and weak commitments; there is an exploration of various ideologies and religions without arriving at any commitment or decision. The exploration varies from a tentative, dispersed, and periodic if not impulsive attempt at exploration to a highly intentional, broad, systematic approach. Spirituality is experienced as an expansive and everwidening investigation (Kiesling et al., 2008) although it may also be a way to avoid fear, authenticity, addiction, and philosophical or intellectual rigidity. Whereas serious doubts and questions occur for women in moratorium, with exploration and necessary self-reflectiveness and self-discovery, positive self-worth may be found.

Other work takes a more integrative perspective and attends to the sociocultural context of women's development of spirituality and its links to action for social justice (Tisdell, 2002). From this perspective, experiences and the process of exploration and commitment may be characterized by four overlapping themes (Tisdell, 2002). Accordingly, one theme is that of spiritual development as a spiral process of evolving and reframing spiritual attitudes from one's childhood culture of origin. Significant life experiences often carry personal spiritual experience that can be characterized by the theme of a deepening awareness and honoring of the life force. This latter theme is related to that of the development of an authentic identity; again, spirituality is thought to develop with identity. Finally, many women find that their spirituality compels them to develop a social conscience and to engage in social justice work. The role and relationship of spiritual development to what women view as their authentic identity require attention, and it is important to listen for these themes as women describe their lives. To the extent that spirituality and meaning in life are present and developed, so too may generativity commitments be established and legacy meaningfully formulated.

Forgiveness may develop with spirituality, given the stronger propensity for forgiveness found in middle-aged and older adults, and older women are more readily able to forgive interpersonal conflicts (Silton, Flannelly, & Lutjen, 2013). This propensity to forgive among older adults seems based in values for the integrity of relationships, more constructive and less confrontational strategies, and specific beliefs (spiritual or religious). Forgiveness is an important development as we age, given that it is inversely related to hostility and is thought to actually reduce hostility, and hostility has been rather consistently found to be directly related to poor physical and mental health (Silton et al., 2013). It is posited that attendant hostility with diminished forgiveness contributes to substance use and poor diet, impaired social relations, physiological reactivity, and concomitant changes in the cardiovascular, neuroendocrine, and immune systems (McFarland, Smith, Toussaint, & Thomas, 2012; Silton et al., 2013). Whether it is the development of spirituality or the wisdom of age, or both, that enhances the ability to forgive, there are benefits to physical and mental health and well-being.

The development of a sense of meaning and spirituality is addressed in this section about middle adulthood, as these tend to be more coherent and solidified at this phase of life. Nonetheless, meaning in life first becomes salient in adolescence, and by emerging adulthood, the presence of meaning in life is linked to the most adaptive psychosocial functioning (in short, mental health) whereas the absence of meaning is associated with maladaptive psychosocial functioning (Dezutter et al., 2014).

The correspondence among meaning in life, spirituality, and identity processes cannot be ignored, and therefore a woman's ongoing revision and development of these must be assessed and supported by women's health care providers. The feeling that one's life is meaningful has enormous influence for mental health and well-being and is central to optimal functioning.

The Departure of Children

When children are grown and leave home, the transition has a deep impact on middle-aged parents, no matter how normative the event. The postparental period is also known as the *empty nest*, and families necessarily modify interaction patterns, activities, and relationships. Today, *postparental period* is preferred over the term empty nest, given that the latter has perhaps contributed to a negative view of this phase of life. That negative perception was compounded by the term *empty nest syndrome,* used to describe the depression, loneliness, loss, and identity crisis experienced by some parents when their children became launched. It must be emphasized that this syndrome describes a negative adaptation to the launching phase, in which children transition into emerging adulthood. Together, the launching phase (as children leave home) and the postparental phase (when the last child is launched) take into consideration a transition that occurs over time and may even include the return of young adults to the parental home (Bouchard, 2014).

Given the challenges presented by parenting with respect to diminished marital quality, role equity, and work–family conflicts, it would seem that the launching of children and a postparental status would relieve these difficulties. Certainly, couples have more time and freedom from parenting responsibilities, fewer competing demands between work and parenting, and greater sharing of household responsibilities. Although women may be more likely to leave their committed or marital relationship once their children are launched, they generally experience greater enjoyment and satisfaction with all family relationships, including their partner and adult children, in postparenthood (Bouchard, 2014).

It is to be expected that women experience a sense of loss as they launch their children, with all the poignancy of the first day of kindergarten, graduations, and a move to college. It is also likely that there is ambivalence, with a mix of sadness and relief. It is in the absence of alternative roles with which to build an identity that women experience negative effects on their well-being at this time (Bouchard, 2014). Those who work full time, have meaningful interests, and are engaged in community service activities—in other words, those with an identity in addition to being a mother—tend to experience this transition and postparenthood with greater pleasure. Thus at-home mothers may be more vulnerable to empty nest syndrome.

Caring for Aging Parents

In the face of the launching of children and the postparental time, the death of a parent can exacerbate that loss and contribute to negative effects on women's well-being (Bouchard, 2014). Separate from loss, particularly if the loss is during the launching of children, serving as caregivers for parents yields several challenges as well as positive benefits for women. Providing care to an aging or ill parent is a more common responsibility for a woman in midlife (Hegewisch et al., 2015). Consequently, many women must balance the roles of caregiver and employee and their inherent demands and conflicts. The concurrent demands of caregiving and work are stressful for women, yet they are able to confine the caregiving demands to the family domain, whereas workplace demands exacerbate the caregiving burden (Gordon, Pruchno, Wilson-Genderson, Murphy, & Rose, 2012). Since work has become more central to the identity of women, work-related demands create challenges when caregiving responsibilities intensify. The caregiving activities can be delegated to others in part or in whole in order to reduce the stress and to achieve a better balance between work and caregiving, and emotional support reduces the sense of burden (Gordon et al., 2012). These issues of balance and burden are worth addressing, given that caregiving is a salient experience that influences identity.

There are five ways that adult daughters are affected by the caregiving experience (Pope, 2013). First, women gain awareness of their own aging and potential needs for care when they are older. In particular, if a woman has been focused on parenting and work, the caregiving experience brings about a revised understanding of herself as aging. In some women, this awareness of their own aging provokes aging-related fears and/or a perceived vulnerability to the disease the parent had. The fears tend to be related to some loss of self, particularly independence, and to diminished quality of life rather than death itself.

A third way adult daughters are affected by caregiving for a parent is through the parent offering a point of comparison in terms of their current functioning as well as their future aging. Given that women notably define themselves in relation to others, the caregiving relationship between daughter and parent is especially salient for identity development not only in midlife, but also in older adulthood as well. Another way parental caregiving affects the daughter providing care is through directly learning about the medical and financial aspects of elder care. This acquired knowledge of the realities of family caregiving may explain why women tend to be more pragmatic and proactive in anticipating their own future care needs and therefore to have more formal plans for their future care (Roberto, Allen, & Bleizner, 2001). Finally, caring for a parent offers daughters an example of how to age with respect to attitudes and planning activity. Whether parents provide a positive or negative model, women caregivers can learn from the experience and make choices with respect to their own approach to late life. Whereas the challenges of caregiving for a parent must be assessed and problem-solved, it is equally important to facilitate awareness of the personal and psychological growth and proactive planning for aging that are possible.

■ OLDER ADULTHOOD

Integrity is the salient developmental focus in older adulthood, typically the postretirement years after 65 years of age (Hearn et al., 2012). This eighth and final stage of development in Erikson's psychosocial theory presents the challenge of integrity versus despair (Erikson, 1963, 1968, 1980). This challenge entails a process of life review with an examination of accomplishments, regrets, issues that remain to be addressed, and the meaning of all of these, with eventual reconciliation and acceptance or disappointment and regret. This process requires knowing one's self and one's fit with the ways of one's culture so that there is both an intrapersonal and interpersonal sense of integration. Ideally, one reaches philosophical comprehension of the whole of life with acceptance if not compassion (Hearn et al., 2012). As with the previous developmental periods discussed so far, identity is central to the challenge of integration, with the identity statuses differentiated by intrapersonal characteristics in conjunction with the degree of social engagement.

Quality of life among older adults is a concern for health professionals, policy makers, and researchers, particularly given the growth in the size of this population (Dezutter, Wiesmann, Apers, & Luyckx, 2013). The factors that influence quality of life may vary according to whether a woman is young–old (65–75 years), old–old (75–85 years), or oldest–old (more than 85 years) (Majerovitz, 2006). Several transitions confront older women during these life phases, all carrying a potential sense of loss and a requirement for adaptation to new circumstances of living and social engagement. These transitions include retirement, widowhood, loss of friends and siblings, and relocation, all of which transact with the ongoing development of one's life narrative and the resolution of integrity and attainment of wisdom. Once again, a woman's identity and social relations are concurrent centralities for well-being in older adulthood.

Identity and Integrity

Erikson's model of psychosocial development has come to be better understood as a matrix, not a ladder, in which issues that are associated with earlier phases of development may be revisited throughout life, just as issues typically linked with later adulthood may be confronted at earlier ages (Whitbourne et al., 2009). To some extent, as life circumstances change and evolve, each psychosocial issue likely needs to be reworked in the context of later challenges and life history. The identity processes of assimilation, accommodation, and balance are mechanisms for women to redefine themselves in ways consistent with their experiences in older adulthood (Whitbourne & Skultety, 2006). Identity assimilation is a process by which new experiences are interpreted through the existing identity and a positive sense of self-attribution is retained, whereas the process of accommodation is one whereby the individual makes shifts in identity to accommodate the discrepancies with reality. According to identity process theory, a balance between assimilation and accommodation processes is ideal (Whitbourne & Skultety, 2006) and may help women negotiate the psychosocial challenges of integrity versus despair.

In other words, the exploration and growth around the earlier issues of identity, intimacy, and generativity all contribute to the subsequent psychosocial issue of integrity. The defining characteristics of four integrity statuses have been developed from the work of theorists and researchers (Hearn et al., 2012) and reflect the extent to which the resolution of integrity versus despair has been attained. The four integrity statuses include integrated, pseudointegrated, nonexploratory, and despairing.

Integrated persons are those who have insightful awareness of the self, are positive about themselves, and through their life narratives, can explain the primary influences that formed who they are as a person. Socially mature, they confront their regrets, yet are not overwhelmed by them. Similarly, they confront the challenges of aging and the inability to do as much as they had previously yet accept the sadness, ambiguity, and sense of loss that may attend them. Integrated persons retain their identity commitments, thereby affirming their values, and remain connected to family and friends. In short, they are ego-resilient, and affirm life's worth with curiosity and openness to experience, involvement, and optimism. They are generally content with their lives as lived and with what they have accomplished. Many of these descriptors of integrated persons are much like the indicators of eudaemonic well-being (e.g., personal growth, purpose in life, self-mastery, environmental mastery) that characterize older women, even in the face of challenges to their physical and social functioning (Woods, Cochrane, Zaslavsky, & LaCroix, 2015).

The *pseudointegrated* person is considered partially integrated, owing largely to a lack of self-awareness and a reluctance or unwillingness to engage in self-examination and self-reflection. What is emphasized by the pseudointegrated person is a very successful self-representation, without regrets or uncertainties. They typically have struggled with identity and connections to others, remaining socially immature and even reporting a poor sense of well-being. It is as if the unacceptable aspects of life are completely denied and a pat, satisfactory overall life narrative has been constructed.

Nonexploratory persons are also considered partially integrated but they are characterized by having retained the worldviews and attitudes learned as children, without exploration. In essence, they have a foreclosed identity status that has not evolved over the life course. They are likely to be content and complacent but are not introspective and have engaged in limited, if any, self-examination of values, purpose, or meaning. Thus they stay within their comfort zone of thinking, believing, and feeling without ambiguity, which may have been affirmed by their positive experiences with their career, family, and social life.

The *despairing* person, on reflection, perceives disappointments, missed chances, regrets, and failures as the most salient features of their life narrative. Their pervasive affect is sadness, with a sense of futility and a proneness to negative and depressive feelings. Even if quite self-reflective and able to find some areas of life satisfaction, the result is a dissatisfaction and an insufficient sense of belonging. Being rather closed to new experience and socially immature contributes to a sense that there is not enough time left to find fulfillment.

With integration, a woman ideally reaches philosophical comprehension of the whole of life with acceptance if not compassion (Hearn et al., 2012). This comprehension of the whole of life is akin to a sense of coherence, by which one's situation is perceived as comprehensible, manageable, and meaningful (Dezutter et al., 2013). Those who view their world as comprehensible, manageable, and meaningful can more readily accept their past life, a sign of integrity. Even more important, this sense of coherence is a resource for greater well-being and a buffer against depressive symptoms in older adults. The extent to which women employ a balance of identity processes and have achieved integration and a sense of coherence influence the extent to which they are able to adapt to the transitions inherent in older adulthood. Progress around this psychosocial task needs to be assessed and resources identified for facilitating a life review in order to help older women bring their lives into meaningful and rewarding integration.

Retirement is potentially a challenging transition for women. Historically, retirement was an experience of men and studied as such; most women were employed for financial necessity rather than a career commitment. The differences between men and women in terms of work experience have narrowed and as women have pursued higher education and established careers, retirement has become a transition from those meaningful identity commitments. Previously, those women who spent more time in their work have been more satisfied in retirement; the level of advancement in their career was an influence as it was for men (Whitbourne & Skultety, 2006). What seems clear at the present is that women experience retirement in a more individualized and fragmented way than thought (Duberley, Carmichael, & Szmigin, 2014).

Since the leading-edge baby boomer women have only recently begun to retire, the retirement experience is not well understood for those who chose an occupation or career and integrated that commitment into their identity, perhaps experienced advancement, and now face letting go of aspirations and this identity commitment. Identity processes are likely stimulated by retirement, especially if the woman's occupation or career was salient to her identity and sense of self. Nonetheless, it is important to maintain a sense of self; having a strong self-concept before retirement that is defined beyond the occupational/career role, having the opportunity to practice the occupational/career skills in retirement, and exploring new interests and skills make a difference (Price, 2003).

If a woman's occupation or career carried status, conferred competence, and provided intellectual challenges, then these features likely need to be found in other activities during retirement. Role expansion is one way women substitute the loss of their professional roles with alternative roles (Price, 2003). Succession planning and mentorship with those who are earlier in their same career or taking on roles based on their expertise acquired in their career can serve to ease the transition to retirement and provide an identity commitment that carries a sense of legacy. Alternative sources of identity may be found in recreational activities and other interests, commitments to volunteer work or community organizations, helping friends and neighbors, learning new activities, or paid work (Duberley et al., 2014). By developing new interests and skills and building on previous interests that can now be expanded, retirement can be framed as gaining time for these involvements rather than a loss of work or career (Whitbourne & Skultety, 2006). Establishing a structured schedule to manage this gain in time for these activities is important to providing a sense of purpose and boundaries to excessive demands from family, friends, and organizations (Price, 2003).

To the extent that one's work associates become a primary social network for emotional support, retirement also carries the potential for the loss of emotional support. Of course, much depends on the family and social relationships that provide a context for this transition. The retirement of women can be accelerated by the poor health of a spouse or other family member (Dentinger & Clarkberg, 2002). That circumstance needs to be addressed, since it carries with it the loss of the occupation/career identity commitment, the loss of the emotional support of colleagues, and the potential isolation of caregiving in the face of loss of one's spouse and partner. Again, older women with a history of depression must be considered at risk for a reoccurrence or exacerbation of depression during retirement related to caregiving and the subsequent bereavement process.

Relationship Support

Relatedness as a component of the self does not diminish with aging but is brought forward to older adulthood, perhaps laden with all of the integrated experiences of the life course. Yet how relationships and the social or emotional support they provide influence well-being in older adulthood is not clear-cut. There is a consensus among researchers that social relationships foster cumulative advantage over the life course and contribute to positive health outcomes (Umberson & Montez, 2010), and cross-sectional data support that assertion (Killian & Turner, 2014). Women tend to have larger confidant networks than men (Umberson & Montez, 2010), but findings from the Women's Health Initiative, a longitudinal study of women's aging and health, revealed that social functioning and social resources have only minor effects on well-being in older women (Woods, Cochrane, et al., 2015). It seems that we need to move past assessing social networks in an instrumental sense and examine the quality of intimate, familial relationships and friendships and women's social motivation.

Instrumental support refers to concrete assistance such as transportation and money, whereas *emotional support* refers to relationships that provide empathy, love, care, and understanding (Killian & Turner, 2014). The key is to distinguish between these types of support to better understand what makes a difference in the lives of older adults. Instrumental support can effectively be provided by many social resources in the broader community or in housing communities for older adults. Emotional support, in contrast, is largely derived from one's spouse and family, although a nonfamily network of friends and a mixed or diverse network of family and nonfamily are also important sources of emotional support but are less common as the primary source of support (Killian & Turner, 2014). Those who receive emotional support from a diverse group of family and nonfamily have the advantage of receiving support from a variety of people who may differentially meet their needs.

In addition to the availability of family and friends, social motivation may be of key importance to understanding women's adaptation to changing social circumstances. Social approach and avoidance motives are considered dispositions; approach is characterized as the dispositional anticipation for affiliation, and avoidance is characterized as the dispositional anticipation and fear of rejection (Nikitin, Burgermeister, & Freund, 2012). Such dispositions affect the ability to establish and maintain relationships, thought to be important to mastering the transition from a familiar context to one that is unfamiliar and ambiguous, with new behaviors to be acquired and new social relationships to be established (Nikitin et al., 2012). Establishing and maintaining social relationships has been called out as important to the transitions of retirement, widowhood, and relocation in older adulthood, so it follows that social motives for approach and avoidance would be important as well.

Broadly, research suggests that women who have social approach motivation will more actively seek out social relationships and in turn will be sought out by others. They will tend to perceive more positive social experiences and construe and design their social environment with those who correspond socially. They thereby create an environment that positively and reciprocally influences their social cognitions and behavior in ways that enhance subjective well-being (Nikitin et al., 2012). In contrast, those with social avoidance motivation do not engage in negative behavior but perceive rejection and feel unaccepted; the consequences appear largely cognitive in nature and do, at least initially, contribute to negative expectations and diminished well-being. Cognitive intervention may be of benefit but, even in the absence of direct intervention, research suggests that as a situation becomes more predictable and familiar over time, social connections are made and satisfaction improved (Nikitin et al., 2012).

CAREGIVING

Spouses have been found to be more supportive of an older woman's well-being than any other when the focus is emotional support, and more broadly, it is to family members that she turns to for emotional support more than anyone else (Killian & Turner, 2014). The importance of spousal and family support may be informed, in part, by spousal caregiving that, when needed, is most often provided by available spouses; adult children become caregivers only when spouses are not available (Lima, Allen, Goldscheider, & Intrator, 2008). Unfortunately, late middle-aged couples are more likely to have spousal caregivers who are working full time outside the home, with the implication that they have fewer hours to devote to caregiving activities (Lima et al., 2008).

Other than the available time, the nature of the caregiving experience depends on the nature of the relationship between the woman and her partner; women often hasten retirement when caregiving, contrary to caregiving men and to women who are not caregivers (Dentinger & Clarkberg, 2002). It is thought that women accelerate their retirement in order to spend more quality time with their husbands or partners, which is consistent with findings that couples have higher marital satisfaction when their retirement statuses are congruent (Dentinger & Clarkberg, 2002). The quality of the relationships before caregiving also predicts other consequences to the caregiver. If there has historically been a higher level of marital conflict, women as caregivers will experience an increase in depressive symptoms and diminished happiness (Choi & Marks, 2006). It seems that spousal caregiving may be compromised when intensive personal needs must be provided in a historically strained intimate relationship.

Whether or not the relationship has been strained, women tend to put their own health care needs secondary to the demands of caregiving (DiGiacomo, Lewis, Nolan, Phillips, & Davidson, 2013). In light of their own health issues, the caregiving demands are exacerbated and taxing, yet women tend to not ask for help to manage their caregiving responsibilities and health problems; they quietly endure (DiGiacomo et al., 2013). It is therefore imperative that women's health care providers be sensitive to this dynamic among older women caregivers and necessarily engage around the important health concerns and needs that likely exist.

Becoming a caregiver again challenges a woman's identity. Positioning one's self as a caregiver of one's partner is a salient developmental issue that takes place with a narrative storyline for understanding and framing meaning about one's caregiving activities. Until a woman sees herself as a caregiver, it is difficult to see the challenges involved and engage in her own self-care (O'Connor, 2007). That is, inherent tensions surface between a caregiver's needs and those of their care-receiving partner that challenges the personhood of their partner. Naming the work being done highlights the importance of the availability of a social environment to counter isolation and optimize personal identity and esteem (O'Connor, 2007). Of course, much depends on the perceived changes in the care recipient and hence the caregiver's own identity and the way she perceives herself in the context of the intimate relationship and the sense of closeness (Boylstein & Hayes, 2012).

WIDOWHOOD

Of course, the quality of the relationship with one's spouse/partner mediates the sense of well-being, but the importance of the relationship is underscored by the challenges of widowhood. Widowhood has had noteworthy effects on well-being (Carr & Ha, 2006; Whitbourne & Skultety, 2006; Woods, Cochrane, et al., 2015), although to some extent, these effects likely preceded widowhood if the woman was also her partner's caregiver and she ignored her own needs

for health care and help managing care (DiGiacomo et al., 2013). Those who experience widowhood relatively earlier in older adulthood do return to higher levels of well-being and happiness and considerable life satisfaction (Woods, Cochrane, et al., 2015). Nonetheless, widowhood at the time it occurs is associated with the sadness and grief of loss (Carr & Ha, 2006) and diminished enjoyment of life and happiness, which is offset by a sense of control and resilience (Woods, Cochrane, et al., 2015).

Again, the quality of the relationship should be assessed. On one hand, it could be expected that those with more loving relationships may grieve more intensely, but it has long been thought that those with more conflicted or difficult relationships grieve more deeply the loss of the relationship compounded by the loss of any opportunity to improve and resolve that relationship; evidence points to both occurring (Carr & Ha, 2006). It is difficult to predict the response to widowhood for women moving into older adulthood currently and in the near future, given that women who reached adulthood in the 1970s and beyond have experienced different gender norms than those with whom earlier research was conducted (Woods, Cochrane, et al., 2015) and have had opportunities and choices for relationships and careers that create a different relationship history as a foundation to widowhood. With this scenario, distress may be minimized among future widows (Carr & Ha, 2006).

The nature of the partner's death is also an important factor to consider when assessing the well-being of a woman who has been newly widowed. The opportunity to provide end-of-life care for spouses or partners certainly may allow a preparation for their death and loss and afford a smoother transition to widowhood with the resolution of emotional and practical issues (Carr & Ha, 2006). Yet, the caregiving activities can be stressful, and the nature of the death can leave the care provider with stress and health issues that require attention (DiGiacomo et al., 2013). Of course, much depends on the quality of the relationship before caregiving and the extent to which resolution is reached on the various emotional and practical issues. This latter point holds especially true for those who experience a sudden death, without resolution and closure. Health care providers can play a key role in older women's coping and adjustment with the transition from caregiver to widowhood, especially from a person-centered perspective that is sensitive to the various contextual factors (DiGiacomo et al., 2013).

It is to be expected that older women will experience emotional and psychological distress at the death of a spouse or partner but the research evidence tells us that most women recover over time (Carr & Ha, 2006; Whitbourne & Skultety, 2006; Woods, Cochrane, et al., 2015). Women tend to turn to adult children and their broader range of friendships for emotional support, with positive benefits for their well-being in widowhood. They are much less likely to marry or commit to another relationship, particularly the older they are when widowhood occurs (Hegewisch et al., 2015). This circumstance points to the opportunity to more readily integrate widowhood into one's identity.

Nonetheless, older women with a history of depression will certainly be more vulnerable to depression in the course of bereavement, and health providers need to be alert to this potential in caregiving and soon-to-be widows as well as in those women who were recently widowed (Carr & Ha, 2006). There are community resources for bereavement counseling to facilitate a women's journey through the grief and bereavement process. Private bereavement counselors, hospice providers, community mental health clinics, and senior citizen centers are all potential resources for individual or group-centered bereavement support.

RELOCATION

Widowhood and changes in health status typically lead to an older woman's decision to move out of her home and into the home of a family member or friend or into a community facility (Whitbourne & Skultety, 2006). The quality of this relocation experience depends, to a considerable extent, on whether the woman makes the choice to move or perceives she is "forced" to move, and the fit this decision making and its consequences has for her identity. Diminished physical capacity and physical problems have minor influence on older women's well-being and life satisfaction (Woods, Cochrane, et al., 2015), even if health problems are the reason for moving (Nikitin et al., 2012).

In fact, women 80 years of age and older rate their health as good, very good, or excellent regardless of relatively diminished physical functioning (Woods, Rillamas-Sun, et al., 2015). Furthermore, most of these older women reported moderately high levels of resilience, self-control, and self-mastery but lower levels of environmental mastery (Woods, Rillamas-Sun, et al., 2015). Perhaps diminished environmental mastery is normative if not adaptive for older women if they need to relocate to a new living situation, especially in the context of resilience, self-control, and self-mastery. People who are interpersonally active, planful, and decisive, like those with strong social approach motivation, proactively contribute to a positive social environment and their adaptation during the transition to a new living situation. Even for those who carry a motivation for social avoidance, the outcome appears reasonably positive, with a positive level of well-being and, over just a few months, diminishing negative expectations for and cognitions about rejection and/or lack of acceptance (Nikitin et al., 2012).

The experience of relocation may also be attended by retirement, widowhood, and/or loss of siblings and friends. These compounded experiences create a nexus of loss that needs attention, and health care providers are advised to be sensitive to the experience and avoid pathologizing the pain. The following poetry, *Put Out the Light and Lock the Door* (Brown, 2009), was written by a retired professor who was inspired by her move to a retirement home; she eloquently captures the experience:

Clean out the cabinets, sweep the floor
Pull down the shades, now check once more
Turn off the water, the phone, and the heat
Everything must be left clean and neat.

From this cherished house I now must go
This house where we shared both joy and woe.
This house that bore witness to triumphs and cheers
To music, to laughter, to hopes and to fears

This house where we lived for 30 odd years
This house where we aged with waning powers
This house where you lived out your final hours.

Now as I make the final walk-through
This is the air with memories of you.
Poignantly sad and bitterly sweet
Redolent of happiness and of defeat
Contemplate life, and contemplate death
My heart turns over, and lost is my breath.

The sound of your voice echoes still in the air
The touch of your hand lingers everywhere
Your ghost's at my side as I take my last look
At this house before closing the book
On our good years here as husband and wife.

My leaving now marks the end of that life.
So farewell, my dear ghost, I wish I could stay
But my time is up, and I must away
Put out the light and lock the door
And go forth from this house forever more.

Source: Reprinted from *Reflections, A Collection of Writing and Poetry* by Oregon's Elders (2009) by permission of Margaret Cervenka, Deputy Director.

■ SUMMARY

This chapter takes a psychosocial developmental perspective on women's mental health. The emphasis was on the joint development of identity and relatedness in the normative developmental phases of emerging adulthood, young adulthood, midlife, and older adulthood for women. The salient psychosocial issues were identified and discussed in the context of identity and relationships and the ways those may be typically experienced. Ultimately, women's mental health is reflected in personal integration and well-being, regardless of the life challenges that were encountered. The life journey necessitates psychosocial development, and this is the context in which women's health care clinicians meet women and provide care.

■ REFERENCES

Arnett, J. J. (2000). Emerging adulthood. A theory of development from the late teens through the twenties. *The American Psychologist, 55*(5), 469–480.

Beaumont, S. L., & Pratt, M. M. (2011). Identity processing styles and psychosocial balance during early and middle adulthood: The role of identity in intimacy and generativity. *Journal of Adult Development, 18*, 172–183. doi:10.1007/s10804–011-9125-z

Benzies, K., Tough, S., Tofflemire, K., Frick, C., Faber, A., & Newburn-Cook, C. (2006). Factors influencing women's decisions about timing of motherhood. *Journal of Obstetric, Gynecologic, and Neonatal Nursing, 35*(5), 625–633.

Berzonsky, M. D., & Kuk, L. S. (2000). Identity status, identity processing style, and the transition to university. *Journal of Adolescent Research, 15*, 81–98.

Beyers, W., & Seiffge-Krenke, I. (2010). Does identity precede intimacy: Testing Erikson's theory on romantic development in emerging adults of the 21st century. *Journal of Adolescent Research, 25*, 387–415. doi:10.1177/0743558410361370

Blatt, S. J., & Luyten, P. (2009). A structural-developmental psychodynamic approach to psychopathology: Two polarities of experience across the life span. *Development and Psychopathology, 21*(3), 793–814.

Bouchard, G. (2014). How do parents react when their children leave home? An integrative review. *Journal of Adult Development, 21,* 69–79. doi:10.1007/s10804–013-9180–8

Boylstein, C., & Hayes, J. (2012). Reconstructing marital closeness while caring for a spouse with Alzheimer's. *Journal of Family Issues, 33,* 584–612. doi:10.1177/0192513X11416449

Brown, J. S. (2009). *Put out the light and lock the door: Reflections.* Tigard, OR: Oregon Alliance of Senior and Health Services.

Carlsson, J., Wängqvist, M., & Frisén, A. (2015). Identity development in the late twenties: A never ending story. *Developmental Psychology, 51*(3), 334–345.

Carr, D., & Ha, J. H. (2006). Bereavement. In J. Worell & C. D. Goodheart (Eds.), *Handbook of girls' and women's psychological health* (pp. 387–405). New York, NY: Oxford University Press.

Choi, H., & Marks, N. F. (2006). Transition to caregiving, marital disagreement, and psychological well-being: A prospective U.S. national study. *Journal of Family Issues, 27,* 1701–1722. doi:10.1177/0192513X0291523

Chung, J. M., Robins, R. W., Trzesniewski, K. H., Noftle, E. E., Roberts, B. W., & Widaman, K. F. (2014). Continuity and change in self-esteem during emerging adulthood. *Journal of Personality and Social Psychology, 106*(3), 469–483.

Day, J. C., & Bauman, K. J. (2000). *Have we reached the top? Educational attainment projections of the U.S. population.* Population Division Working Paper No. 43. U.S. Census Bureau, Washington, DC.

Dentinger, E., & Clarkberg, M. (2002). Informal caregiving and retirement timing among men and women: Gender and caregiving relationships in late midlife. *Journal of Family Issues, 23,* 857–879.

Dezutter, J., Waterman, A. S., Schwartz, S. J., Luyckx, K., Beyers, W., Meca, A.,…Caraway, S. J. (2014). Meaning in life in emerging adulthood: A person-oriented approach. *Journal of Personality, 82,* 57–68. doi:10.1111/jopy.12033

Dezutter, J., Wiesmann, U., Apers, S., & Luyckx, K. (2013). Sense of coherence, depressive feelings and life satisfaction in older persons: A closer look at the role of integrity and despair. *Aging & Mental Health, 17*(7), 839–843.

Diener, E. (2000). Subjective well-being. The science of happiness and a proposal for a national index. *The American Psychologist, 55*(1), 34–43.

Diener, E., Suh, E. M., Lucas, R. E., & Smith, H. L. (1999). Subjective well-being: Three decades of progress. *Psychological Bulletin, 125,* 276–302. doi:10.1037/0033–2909.125.2.276

DiGiacomo, M., Lewis, J., Nolan, M. T., Phillips, J., & Davidson, P. M. (2013). Transitioning from caregiving to widowhood. *Journal of Pain and Symptom Management, 46*(6), 817–825. doi:10.1016/S0890–4065(03)00026–4

Duberley, J., Carmichael, F., & Szmigin, I. (2014). Exploring women's retirement: Continuity, context and career transition. *Gender, Work and Organization, 21,* 71–90. doi:10.111/gwao.12013

Eccles, J. (2009). Who am I and what am I going to do with my life? Personal and collective identities as motivators of action. *Educational Psychologist, 44*(2), 78–89. doi:10.1080/00461520902832368

Erikson, E. H. (1963). *Childhood and society* (2nd ed.). New York, NY: W. W. Norton.

Erikson, E. H. (1968). *Identity: Youth and crisis.* New York, NY: W. W. Norton.

Erikson, E. H. (1980). *Identity and the life cycle.* New York, NY: W. W. Norton.

Fields, J. (2003). *Children's living arrangements and characteristics: March 2002.* Current Population Reports, P20–547. Washington, DC: U.S. Census Bureau.

Fontenot, H. B. (2007). Transition and adaptation to adoptive motherhood. *Journal of Obstetric, Gynecologic, and Neonatal Nursing, 36*(2), 175–182.

Gaunt, R., & Scott, J. (2014). Parents' involvement in childcare: Do parental and work identities matter? *Psychology of Women Quarterly, 38,* 475–489. doi:10.1177/0361684314533484

Gordon, J. R., Pruchno, R. A., Wilson-Genderson, M., Murphy, W. M., & Rose, M. (2012). Balancing caregiving and work: Role conflict and role strain dynamics. *Journal of Family Issues, 33,* 662–689. doi:10.1177/0192513X11425322

Gruenewald, T. L., Liao, D. H., & Seeman, T. E. (2012). Contributing to others, contributing to oneself: Perceptions of generativity and health in later life. *The Journals of Gerontology. Series B, Psychological Sciences and Social Sciences, 67*(6), 660–665.

Hamilton, B. E., Martin, J. A., Osterman, M. J., & Curtain, S. C. (2015). Births: Preliminary data for 2014. *National Vital Statistics Reports, 64*(6), 1–19.

Hearn, S., Saulnier, G., Strayer, J., Glenham, M., Koopman, R., & Marcia, J. E. (2012). Between integrity and despair: Toward construct validation of Erikson's eighth stage. *Journal of Adult Development, 19,* 1–20. doi:10.1007/s10804–011-9126–y

Hegewisch, A., Hayes, J., Milli, J., Shaw, E., & Hartmann, H. (2015). *Looking back, looking ahead: Chart book on women's progress.* Research Report, AARP Public Policy Institute. Retrieved from http://www.aarp.org/futureofwork

Hill, P. L., Jackson, J. J., Roberts, B. W., Lapsley, D. K., & Brandenberger, J. W. (2011). Change you can believe in: Changes in goal setting during emerging and young adulthood predict later adult well-being. *Social Psychological and Personality Science, 2*(2), 123–131.

Hill, P. L., & Roberts, B. W. (2012). Narcissism, well-being, and observer-rated personality across the lifespan. *Social Psychological and Personality Science, 3,* 216–223. doi:10.1177/1948550611415867

Hill, P. L., Turiano, N. A., Mroczek, D. K., & Roberts, B. W. (2012). Examining concurrent and longitudinal relations between personality traits and social well-being in adulthood. *Social Psychological and Personality Science, 3*(6), 698–705.

Hoffnung, M., & Williams, M. A. (2013). Balancing act: Career and family during college-educated women's 30's. *Sex Roles, 68,* 321–334. doi:10.1007/s11199–012.0248.x

Jackson, P. B. (2004). Role sequencing: Does order matter for mental health? *Journal of Health and Social Behavior, 45*(2), 132–154.

Jones, B. K., & McAdams, D. P. (2013). Becoming generative: Socializing influences recalled in life stories in late midlife. *Journal of Adult Development, 20,* 158–172. doi:10.1007/s10804–013-9168–4

Jones, J. C., & Peskin, H. (2010). Psychological health from the teens to the 80s: Multiple developmental trajectories. *Journal of Adult Development, 17,* 20–32. doi:10.1007/s10804–009-9075–x

Kiesling, C., Sorell, G. T., Montgomery, M. J., & Colwell, R. K. (2008). Identity and spirituality: A psychosocial exploration of the sense of spiritual self. *Psychology of Religion and Spirituality, 8,* 50–62. doi:10.1037/1941–1022.S.1.50

Killian, T. S., & Turner, M. J. (2014). Latent class typologies for emotional support among midlife and aging Americans: Evidence from the national health and human nutrition examination survey. *Journal of Adult Development, 21,* 96–105. doi:10.1007/s10804–014-9183–0

Kominski, R., Elliot, D., & Clever, M. (2009). *Risk factors for children living in the US, states, and metropolitan areas: Data from the 2007 American community survey 1-year estimates.* Paper presentation. Population Association of America, 2009 Annual Meeting, Detroit, MI. Retrieved from http://www.census.gov/hhes/socdemo/children/data/acs/risk-factors/risk-factors-paper.pdf

Koniak-Griffin, D., Logsdon, M. C., Hines-Martin, V., & Turner, C. C. (2006). Contemporary mothering in a diverse society. *Journal of Obstetric, Gynecologic, and Neonatal Nursing, 35*(5), 671–678.

Kopala-Sibley, D. C., Mongrain, M., & Zuroff, D. C. (2013). A lifespan perspective on dependency and self-criticism: Age-related differences from 18 to 59. *Journal of Adult Development, 20,* 126–141. doi:10.1007/s10804–013-9163–9

Kreider, R. M., & Ellis, R. (2011). *Living arrangements of children: 2009.* Current Population Reports, P70–126. Washington, DC: U.S. Census Bureau.

Kroger, J., Martnussen, M., & Marcia, J. E. (2010). Identity status change during adolescence and young adulthood: A meta-analysis. *Journal of Adolescence, 33,* 683–698. Retrieved from http://dx.doi.org/10.1016/j.adolescence.2009.11.002

Lee, C., & Gramotnev, H. (2007). Life transitions and mental health in a national cohort of young Australian women. *Developmental Psychology, 43*(4), 877–888.

Lima, J. C., Allen, S. M., Goldscheider, F., & Intrator, O. (2008). Spousal caregiving in late midlife versus older ages: Implications of work and family obligations. *The Journals of Gerontology, 63*(4), S229–S238.

Luvmour, J. (2011). Developing together: Parents meeting children's developmental imperatives. *Journal of Adult Development, 18*, 164–171. doi:10.1007/s10804–010-9111-x

Luyckx, K., Goossens, L., & Soenens, B. (2006). A developmental contextual perspective on identity construction in emerging adulthood: Change dynamics in commitment formation and commitment evaluation. *Developmental Psychology, 42*(2), 366–380.

Luyckx, K., Soenens, B., Vansteenkiste, M., Goossens, L., & Berzonsky, M. D. (2007). Parental psychological control and dimensions of identity formation in emerging adulthood. *Journal of Family Psychology, 21*(3), 546–550.

Majerovitz, S. D. (2006). Physical health and illness in older women. In J. Worell & C. D. Goodheart (Eds.), *Handbook of girls' and women's psychological health* (pp. 379–387). New York, NY: Oxford University Press.

Marcia, J. E. (1966). Development and validation of ego-identity status. *Journal of Personality and Social Psychology, 3*(5), 551–558.

McFarland, M. J., Smith, C. A., Toussaint, L., & Thomas, P. A. (2012). Forgiveness of others and health: Do race and neighborhood matter? *The Journals of Gerontology, 67*(1), 66–75.

McMullin, J. A., & Cairney, J. (2004). Self-esteem and the intersection of age, class, and gender. *Journal of Aging Studies, 18*, 75–90. doi:10.1016/j.jaging.2003.09.006

Miller, J. B. (2008). Connections, disconnections, and violations. *Feminism & Psychology, 18*, 368–380. doi:10.1177/0959353508092090

Nelson, A. M. (2003). Transition to motherhood. *Journal of Obstetric, Gynecologic, and Neonatal Nursing, 32*(4), 465–477.

Newton, N. J., Herr, J. M., Pollack, J. I., & McAdams, D. P. (2014). Selfless or selfish? Generativity and narcissism as components of legacy. *Journal of Adult Development, 21*, 59–68. doi:10.1007/s10804–013-9179–1

Nicolson, S., Judd, F., Thomson-Salo, F., & Mitchell, S. (2013). Supporting the adolescent mother–infant relationship: Preliminary trial of a brief perinatal attachment intervention. *Archives of Women's Mental Health, 16*(6), 511–520.

Nikitin, J., Burgermeister, L. C., & Freund, A. M. (2012). The role of age and social motivation in developmental transitions in young and old adulthood. *Frontiers in Psychology, 3*, 366.

O'Connor, D. L. (2007). Self-identifying as a caregiver: Exploring the positioning process. *Journal of Aging Studies, 21*, 165–174. doi:10.1016/j.jaging.2006.06.002

Orth, U., Robins, R. W., Trzesniewski, K. H., Maes, J., & Schmitt, M. (2009). Low self-esteem is a risk factor for depressive symptoms from young adulthood to old age. *Journal of Abnormal Psychology, 118*(3), 472–478.

Orth, U., Robins, R. W., & Widaman, K. F. (2012). Life-span development of self-esteem and its effects on important life outcomes. *Journal of Personality and Social Psychology, 102*(6), 1271–1288.

Orth, U., Trzesniewski, K. H., & Robins, R. W. (2010). Self-esteem development from young adulthood to old age: A cohort-sequential longitudinal study. *Journal of Personality and Social Psychology, 98*(4), 645–658.

Overstreet, N. M., & Quinn, D. M. (2012). Contingencies of self-worth and appearance concerns: Do domains of self-worth matter? *Psychology of Women Quarterly, 36*, 314–325. doi:10.1177/0361684311435221

Perosa, L. M., Perosa, S. L., & Tam, H. P. (2002). Intergenerational systems theory and identity development in young adult women. *Journal of Adolescent Research, 17*, 235–259.

Pope, N. D. (2013). Views on aging: How caring for an aging parent influences adult daughters' perspectives on later life. *Journal of Adult Development, 20*, 46–56. doi:10.1007/s10804–013-9155–9

Price, C. A. (2003). Professional women's retirement adjustment: The experience of reestablishing order. *Journal of Aging Studies, 17*, 341–355.

Ritchie, R. A., Meca, A., Madrazo, V. L., Schwartz, S. J., Hardy, S. A., Zamboanga, B. L.,…Lee, R. M. (2013). Identity dimensions and related processes in emerging adulthood: Helpful or harmful? *Journal of Clinical Psychology, 69*(4), 415–432.

Robakis, T. K., Williams, K. E., Crowe, S., Kenna, H., Gannon, J., & Rasgon, N. L. (2015). Optimistic outlook regarding maternity protects against depressive symptoms postpartum. *Archives of Women's Mental Health, 18*(2), 197–208.

Roberto, K. A., Allen, K. R., & Bleizner, R. (2001). Older adults' preferences for future care: Formal plans and familial support. *Applied Developmental Science, 5*, 112–120. doi:10.1207/S1532480XADS0502_6

Ryan, R. M., & Deci, E. L. (2000). Self-determination theory and the facilitation of intrinsic motivation, social development, and well-being. *The American Psychologist, 55*(1), 68–78.

Ryan, R. M., & Deci, E. L. (2001). On happiness and human potentials: A review of research on hedonic and eudaimonic well-being. *Annual Review of Psychology, 52*, 141–166.

Ryff, C. D., & Keyes, C. L. (1995). The structure of psychological well-being revisited. *Journal of Personality and Social Psychology, 69*(4), 719–727.

Silton, N. R., Flannelly, K. J., & Lutjen, L. J. (2013). It pays to forgive! Aging, forgiveness, hostility, and health. *Journal of Adult Development, 20*, 222–231. doi:10.1007/s10804–013-9173–7

Smith, J. L., & Huntoon, M. (2014). Women's bragging rights: Overcoming modesty norms to facilitate women's self-promotion. *Psychology of Women Quarterly, 38*, 447–459. doi:10.1177/0361684313515840

Sneed, J. R., Whitbourne, S. K., & Culang, M. E. (2006). Trust, identity, and ego integrity: Modeling Erikson's core stages over 34 years. *Journal of Adult Development, 13*, 148–157. doi:10.1007/s10804–007-9026–3

Sneed, J. R., Whitbourne, S. K., Schwartz, S. J., & Huang, S. (2012). The relationship between identity, intimacy, and midlife well-being: Findings from the Rochester Adult Longitudinal Study. *Psychology and Aging, 27*(2), 318–323.

Steger, M. F., Frazier, P., Oishi, S., & Kaler, M. (2006). The meaning in life questionnaire: Assessing the presence of and search for meaning in life. *Journal of Counseling Psychology, 53*, 80–93. doi:10/1037/0022–0167.53.1.80

Steger, M. F., Kashdan, T. B., Sullivan, B. A., & Lorentz, D. (2008). Understanding the search for meaning in life: Personality, cognitive style, and the dynamic between seeking and experiencing meaning. *Journal of Personality, 76*(2), 199–228.

Suplee, P. D., Bloch, J. R., McKeever, A., Borucki, L. C., Dawley, K., & Kaufman, M. (2014). Focusing on maternal health beyond breastfeeding and depression during the first year postpartum. *Journal of Obstetric, Gynecologic, and Neonatal Nursing, 43*(6), 782–791; quiz E51.

Tisdell, E. J. (2002). Spiritual development and cultural context in the lives of women adult educators for social change. *Journal of Adult Development, 9*, 127–140. doi:1068–0667/0400–0127/0

Trzesniewski, K. H., Donnellan, M. B., Moffitt, T. E., Robins, R. W., Poulton, R., & Caspi, A. (2006). Low self-esteem during adolescence predicts poor health, criminal behavior, and limited economic prospects during adulthood. *Developmental Psychology, 42*(2), 381–390.

Trzesniewski, K. H., Donnellan, M. B., & Robins, R. W. (2003). Stability of self-esteem across the life span. *Journal of Personality and Social Psychology, 84*(1), 205–220.

U.S. Census Bureau. (2012). *Statistical abstract of the United States: 2012.* Retrieved from https://www2.census.gov/library/publications/2011/compendia/statab/131ed/2015-statab.pdf

U.S. Census Bureau. (2015). *America's families and living arrangements: 2015.* Retrieved from http://www.census.gov/hhes/families/data/historical.html

Umberson, D., & Montez, J. K. (2010). Social relationships and health: A flashpoint for health policy. *Journal of Health and Social Behavior, 51*, S54–S66.

Versey, H. S., Stewart, A. J., & Duncan, L. E. (2013). Successful aging in late midlife: The role of personality among college-educated women. *Journal of Adult Development, 20*, 63–75. doi:10.1007/s10804–013-9157–7

Vespa, J., Lewis, J. M., & Kreider, R. M. (2013). *America's families and living arrangements: 2012.* Population Characteristics, P20–570. Washington, DC: U.S. Census Bureau.

Wade, T. J., & Pevalin, D. J. (2004). Marital transitions and mental health. *Journal of Health and Social Behavior, 45*(2), 155–170.

Wagner, J., Lüdtke, O., Jonkmann, K., & Trautwein, U. (2013). Cherish yourself: Longitudinal patterns and conditions of self-esteem change in the transition to young adulthood. *Journal of Personality and Social Psychology, 104*(1), 148–163.

Weiss, D., Freund, A. M., & Wiese, B. S. (2012). Mastering developmental transitions in young and middle adulthood: The interplay of openness to experience and traditional gender ideology on women's self-efficacy and subjective well-being. *Developmental Psychology, 48*(6), 1774–1784.

Wenze, S. J., Battle, C. L., & Tezanos, K. M. (2015). Raising multiples: Mental health of mothers and fathers in early parenthood. *Archives of Women's Mental Health, 18*(2), 163–176.

Werner, E., Miller, M., Osborne, L. M., Kuzava, S., & Monk, C. (2015). Preventing postpartum depression: Review and recommendations. *Archives of Women's Mental Health, 18*(1), 41–60.

Whitbourne, S. K., & Skultety, K. M. (2006). Aging and identity: How women face later life transitions. In J. Worell & C. D. Goodheart (Eds.), *Handbook of girls' and women's psychological health* (pp. 370–378). New York, NY: Oxford University Press.

Whitbourne, S. K., Sneed, J. R., & Sayer, A. (2009). Psychosocial development from college through midlife: A 34-year sequential study. *Developmental Psychology, 45,* 1328–1340.

Woods, N. F., Cochrane, B. B., Zaslavsky, O., & LaCroix, A. Z. (2015). *Evaluative well-being in older women.* Paper presentation. Gerontological Society of American 68th Annual Scientific Meeting, Orlando, FL.

Woods, N. F., Rillamas-Sun, E., Cochrane, B. B., LaCroix, A. Z., Seeman, T. E., Tindle, H. A.,...Wallace, R. B. (2015). Aging well: Observations from the Women's Health Initiative Study. *Journal of Gerontology: Medical Sciences, 71*(Suppl. 1), S3–S12. doi:10.1093/gerona/glv054

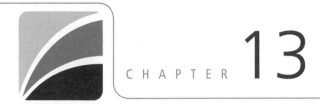
Nutrition for Women

Heather Hutchins-Wiese

Until recently, women's health and subsequent nutrition implications revolved around the reproductive system. Now more research and clinical efforts address a broad spectrum of women's health concerns, especially those unique to or more prevalent in women. With increased life expectancy, women in the United States can live 35 to 40 additional years after childbearing years cease. Those later years can be productive, healthy, and mobile if acute or chronic diseases are prevented or well managed. Lifestyle choices can have a significant role in controlling or modifying the course of diseases, even for those with a genetic predisposition. Of the 10 leading causes of death in women (Table 13.1), nutrition is involved in the etiology or treatment of five of them—heart disease, cancer, stroke, diabetes, and kidney disease (Centers for Disease Control and Prevention[CDC] Office of Women's Health, 2015). This chapter focuses on the contributions of nutrition and dietary behaviors for women throughout the life cycle as well as the prevention and management of selected diseases and conditions that place women at increased risk of mortality and morbidity.

■ THE NUTRIENTS—A BRIEF REVIEW

Food provides the energy needed for biological processes and materials to build and maintain all body cells. These materials are referred to as *nutrients*; each plays a role in ensuring that the biochemical machinery of the human body runs smoothly.

Nutrients are classified into six categories: carbohydrates, lipids, proteins, vitamins, minerals, and water (Table 13.2). Carbohydrates, lipids, and protein are sources of energy and are called macronutrients; vitamins and minerals are micronutrients. Energy released from the macronutrients can be measured in calories—tiny units of energy so small that the typical measure is in kilocalories (kcals) or 1,000 calorie metric units. The basic features of nutrients include:

- Carbohydrates contain carbon, hydrogen, and oxygen combined in small molecules called *sugars* and large molecules represented mainly by starch. Carbohydrates provide 4 kcal/g.
- Lipids (fats and oils) contain carbon, hydrogen, and oxygen (like carbohydrates), but the amount of oxygen is much less. Triglyceride is the main form of fat in food. Fats provide 9 kcal/g.
- Proteins contain carbon, hydrogen, nitrogen, oxygen, and sometimes sulfur atoms, arranged in small compounds called *amino acids*. Chains of amino acids make up dietary proteins. Protein provides 4 kcal/g.
- Vitamins are organic compounds that serve to catalyze or support a number of biochemical reactions in the body.
- Minerals are inorganic compounds (do not contain carbon atoms) that play important roles in metabolic reactions and serve as structural compounds of body tissue, such as bone.
- Water is vital to the body as a solvent and lubricant and as a medium for transporting nutrients and waste. Water is also an inorganic compound, as it does not contain carbon.

Some nutrients the body can make, others it cannot or the amount the body can make is insufficient to meet needs. Therefore it is essential to obtain some nutrients from the foods we eat. Table 13.2 lists essential nutrients that must be consumed from food to meet the body's needs.

As knowledge of nutrition and health continues to expand, the Food and Nutrition Board of the Institute of Medicine updates dietary intake recommendations regularly. The recommendations for individuals are recommended dietary allowances (RDAs) and are scientifically calculated recommendations based on current research to meet the needs of 98% of healthy individuals in a group. When some research, but not enough to make a calculated recommendation, is available, an adequate intake (AI) is developed to cover the needs of all healthy individuals in the groups. The tolerable upper intake level (UL) is the highest level of daily nutrient intake that is likely to pose no risk of adverse health effects to almost all individuals in the general population (Institute of Medicine [IOM]. Panel on Macronutrients & IOM Standing Committee on the Scientific Evaluation of Dietary Reference Intakes, 2005). The RDA, AI, and UL recommendations are for macronutrients, water, vitamins, and elements. Another type of recommendation is a range of intake for macronutrients called the acceptable macronutrient distribution ranges (AMDRs) and includes the essential fats, linoleic acid (LA), and alpha-linolenic acid (ALA), as well as dietary cholesterol, trans fatty acids, saturated fatty acids, and added sugars. The AMDR recommendations do not, however, differentiate between genders. All recommendations are part of what is called the *dietary reference intakes* (DRIs); see Table 13.3 for RDA and AI vitamin and mineral requirements for females and Table 13.4 for the vitamin and mineral UL (U.S. Department of Agriculture, 2016).

Supplements

Approximately two thirds of U.S. noninstitutionalized adults report use of a dietary supplement; 48% to 53% report regular use, with the multivitamin/multimineral supplement being the most common (Dickinson, Blatman, El-Dash, & Franco, 2014). Women report heavier supplement use than men, and supplement use increases with

age for both genders (Dickinson et al., 2014). Health care professionals, including nurses, should screen for use and dose of dietary supplements as well as other complementary and alternative therapies and provide appropriate counseling (or appropriate referrals) on safe and effective use as needed. Screening for supplement use is important because combining supplements and dietary sources of nutrients can provide levels that exceed the UL and pose risk of negative consequences. Additionally, there can be negative interactions between supplements and some medications. The National Institutes of Health Office of Dietary Supplements provides resources for professionals and consumers.

■ REVIEW OF NUTRITIONAL NEEDS THROUGHOUT THE LIFE CYCLE

Infancy and Childhood

The quality and quantity of children's diets are the most constant environmental factors affecting growth and development. Food, feeding, and the satiation of hunger are also important contributors to parent–infant bonding, parent–child interactions, and the child's ability to attend to the environment and learn. Feeding progresses from the newborn's total dependence on breast milk or formula to the preschool girl, who can feed herself, use utensils, make food choices, and communicate clearly regarding hunger and satiety. Food habits developed in childhood can have far-reaching effects on adult nutritional status and eating patterns. Excess weight gain in childhood or adolescence can increase the risk of adult obesity and its related diseases. Inadequate calcium intake in the growing years is an environmental factor that can lead to a reduced bone density in adulthood and elevated risk for osteoporosis later in life. Maternal body size and food intake patterns may even have an impact on an infant and child's health. On the opposite end of the spectrum, malnutrition in the prenatal period or in the early years can have a negative impact on developmental and reproductive abilities later, even in subsequent generations.

Although small body composition differences are seen in boys and girls from about age 6, the nutritional needs do

TABLE 13.1	Leading Causes of Death in Females in the United States, 2013
RANK	**CAUSE OF DEATH**
1	Heart disease[a]
2	Cancer[a]
3	Chronic lower respiratory diseases
4	Stroke[a]
5	Alzheimer's disease
6	Unintentional injuries
7	Diabetes[a]
8	Influenza and pneumonia
9	Kidney disease[a]
10	Septicemia

[a]Causes of death with nutritional implications.
Source: Centers for Disease Control and Prevention Office of Women's Health (2015).

TABLE 13.2	Essential Nutrients					
CARBOHYDRATE	**FAT (LIPIDS)**	**PROTEIN (AMINO ACIDS)**	**VITAMINS**	**MINERALS (MAJOR)**	**MINERALS (TRACE)**	**WATER**
Glucose (or a larger carbohydrate containing glucose)	Linoleic acid (omega-6), alpha-linolenic acid (omega-3)	Histidine, isoleucine, leucine, lysine, methionine, phenylalanine, threonine, tryptophan, valine	Thiamine, riboflavin, niacin, pantothenic acid, biotin, folate, vitamin B_6, vitamin B_{12}, vitamin C, vitamin A, vitamin D, vitamin E, vitamin K	Sodium, chloride, potassium, calcium, phosphorus, magnesium, sulfate	Iron, zinc, iodine, selenium, copper, manganese, fluoride, chromium, molybdenum	Water

TABLE 13.3	DRIs: Vitamin and Mineral RDAs and AI for Healthy, Nonpregnant, Nonlactating Females					
	AGE					
	9–13 Years	14–18 Years	19–30 Years	31–50 Years	51–69 Years	70 Years and Older
Vitamin A (mcg)	600	700	700	700	700	700
Vitamin D (mcg)	11	15	15	15	15	20
Vitamin E (mg)	11	15	15	15	15	15
Vitamin K (mcg)[b]	60	75	90	90	90	90
Vitamin C (mg)	45	65	75	75	75	75
Thiamin (mg)	0.9	1	1.1	1.1	1.1	1.1
Riboflavin (mg)	0.9	1	1.1	1.1	1.1	1.1
Niacin (mg)	12	14	14	14	14	14
Vitamin B$_6$ (mg)	1	1.2	1.3	1.3	1.5	1.5
Folate (mcg)	300	400	400	400	400	400
Vitamin B$_{12}$ (mcg)	1.8	2.4	2.4	2.4	2.4	2.4
Biotin (mcg)[b]	20	25	30	30	30	30
Pantothenic acid (mg)[b]	4	5	5	5	5	5
Choline (mg)[b]	375	400	425	425	425	425
Calcium (mg)	1,300	1,300	1,000	1,000	1,200	1,200
Chromium (mcg)[b]	21	24	25	25	20	20
Copper (mcg)	700	890	900	900	900	900
Fluoride (mg)[b]	2	3	3	3	3	3
Iodine (mcg)	120	150	150	150	150	150
Iron (mg)	8	15	18	18	8	8
Magnesium (mg)	240	360	310	320	320	320
Manganese (mg)[b]	1.6	1.6	1.8	1.8	1.8	1.8
Molybdenum (mcg)	34	43	45	45	45	45
Phosphorus (mg)	1,250	1,250	700	700	700	700
Selenium (mcg)	40	55	55	55	55	55
Zinc (mg)	8	9	8	8	8	8

AI, adequate intake; DRIs, dietary reference intakes; RDAs, recommended dietary allowances.
RDAs are noted in bold.

not differ by gender until puberty. The national DRIs are delineated by gender from 9 years of age.

Adolescence

Adolescence is a dynamic period in human development, with pubertal changes beginning between ages 9 and 11 years in girls. Factors such as body fat percentage and racial/ethnic differences can affect the onset and completion of puberty. Rapid physical growth and the development of secondary sexual characteristics increase the demand for energy and other nutrients. At the same time, tremendous social, cognitive, and emotional growth occurs. There is increased nutritional vulnerability in the teenage years

TABLE 13.4	DRIs: Vitamin and Mineral UL Intakes for All Females					
	AGE					
	9–13 Years	**14–18 Years**	**19–30 Years**	**31–50 Years**	**51–69 Years**	**70 Years and Older**
Vitamin A (mcg)	1,700	2,800	3,000	3,000	3,000	3,000
Vitamin D (mcg)	100	100	100	100	100	100
Vitamin E (mg)	600	800	1,000	1,000	1,000	1,000
Vitamin K (mcg)	ND	ND	ND	ND	ND	ND
Vitamin C (mg)	1,200	1,800	2,000	2,000	2,000	2,000
Thiamin (mg)	ND	ND	ND	ND	ND	ND
Riboflavin (mg)	ND	ND	ND	ND	ND	ND
Niacin (mg)	20	30	35	35	35	35
Vitamin B_6 (mg)	60	80	100	100	100	100
Folate (mcg)	600	800	1,000	1,000	1,000	1,000
Vitamin B_{12} (mcg)	ND	ND	ND	ND	ND	ND
Biotin (mcg)	ND	ND	ND	ND	ND	ND
Pantothenic acid (mg)	ND	ND	ND	ND	ND	ND
Choline (mg)	2	3	3.5	3.5	3.5	3.5
Calcium (mg)	3,000	3,000	2,500	2,500	2,500	2,500
Chromium (mcg)	ND	ND	ND	ND	ND	ND
Copper (mcg)	5,000	8,000	10,000	10,000	10,000	10,000
Fluoride (mg)	10	10	10	10	10	10
Iodine (mcg)	600	900	1,100	1,100	1,100	1,100
Iron (mg)	40	45	45	45	45	45
Magnesium (mg)[a]	350	350	350	350	350	350
Manganese (mg)	6	9	11	11	11	11
Molybdenum (mcg)	1,100	1,700	2,000	2,000	2,000	2,000
Phosphorus (mg)	4,000	4,000	4,000	4,000	4,000	4,000
Selenium (mcg)	280	400	400	400	400	400
Zinc (mg)	23	34	40	40	40	40

DRIs, dietary reference intakes; ND, not determined; UL, upper limit.
[a]UL for magnesium represents pharmacological intake only and does not include intake from food and water.

because of the high nutrient demand, which is affected by lifestyle and food habits, possible use of alcohol and drugs, and special situations such as pregnancy, sports, and excessive dieting or eating disorders (EDs).

Changes in body composition are likely triggers for the initiation of puberty and menarche. Data from the National Health and Nutrition Examination Survey (NHANES) 1999 to 2004 shows that girls, typically prepuberty at age 8 years, have an average body fat percentage of 31, whereas 19-year-old adolescents have an average body fat percentage of 37 (Ogden, Li, Freedman, Borrud, & Flegal, 2011). Because changes in physical growth can occur at different ages in girls, using age as an indicator of nutrient needs is limiting. The use of sexual maturity ratings (or Tanner stages), body composition, and level of physical activity should all be included in the consideration of energy and nutrient needs for the adolescent.

Developing an adult body image is an emotional and cognitive task of adolescent girls that has nutritional implications. The maturing female body, with increased body fat, is in direct contrast to the American culture "ideal" of excessive thinness, reinforced by popular media, fashion, and emphasis on dieting. Thus teenage girls are very dissatisfied with their bodies, frequently attempt weight-loss diets, and are vulnerable for developing EDs (Rohde, Stice, & Marti, 2015; Stice, Marti, & Durant, 2011). Those who rely on unhealthy eating behaviors to lose weight are more likely to have poorer nutrient intake than those who do not (Larson, Neumark-Sztainer, & Story, 2009). Furthermore, unhealthy and disordered eating behaviors tend to remain prevalent as the adolescent becomes a young adult (Neumark-Sztainer, Wall, Larson, Eisenberg, & Loth, 2011).

The other end of the dietary spectrum is childhood and adolescent obesity. Children and adolescents who are overweight are more likely to become obese adults and carry increased risk for chronic health conditions such as diabetes, stroke, heart disease, and certain cancers (Singh, Mulder, Twisk, van Mechelen, & Chinapaw, 2008; Whitlock, Williams, Gold, Smith, & Shipman, 2005). In 2011 and 2012 in the United States, 18% of girls aged 6 to 11 years and 21% of girls aged 12 to 17 years were obese (Ogden, Carroll, Kit, & Flegal, 2014). The high prevalence of obesity highlights the need for dietary monitoring and guidance at a young age (Federal Interagency Forum on Child and Family Statistics, 2015).

NUTRITIONAL NEEDS

Energy needs in adolescent girls are determined by rate of growth, stage of maturation, and physical activity. This individual variability is shown in the DRIs for energy for healthy, active girls compared with sedentary girls: 2,071 versus 1,538 kcal/d (11 years old); 2,368 versus 1,731 kcal/d (15 years old), and 2,403 versus 1,690 kcal/d (18 years old), respectively (IOM Panel on Macronutrients & IOM Standing Committee on the Scientific Evaluation of Dietary Reference Intakes, 2005). Protein needs parallel the growth rate; the typical diet in the United States provides adequate protein and sometimes more than needed. Protein intake becomes a concern when the energy intake is so low that dietary protein is used for energy needs rather than synthesis of new tissue and tissue repair.

Micronutrient needs and their dietary sources are often lacking in the diets of teenage girls. Fruits and vegetables are excellent sources of many vitamins and minerals; additionally, consumption is linked to a reduced risk of cancers and other chronic diseases. Therefore national recommendations are to consume five or more servings of fruits and vegetables daily. A recent comparison of NHANES data from 2003 to 2010 showed that whole fruit consumption increased during that period, whereas fruit juice intake decreased and vegetable intake remained the same; no groups of children met target intakes of vegetables and only 2- to 5-year-olds met goals for fruit intakes (Kim et al., 2014).

Calcium needs are high during puberty and adolescence, with approximately 45% of the adult skeletal mass added between the ages of 9 and 17 years (Weaver & Heaney, 2014). Because the greatest retention of calcium as bone mass occurs in early to middle adolescence, the recommended AI is 1,300 mg for all adolescents aged 9 to 18 years. By comparison, less than 20% of adolescent girls consume that amount, and intake decreases as the adolescent approaches young adulthood (Larson, Neumark-Sztainer, et al., 2009). Sugar-sweetened beverage consumption also has a negative effect on calcium status for this age group because these drinks frequently replace milk. Cola drinks in particular have a high phosphorous content; a low calcium-to-phosphorus ratio may be an added negative impact on bone (Calvo & Tucker, 2013). Thus calcium intake can set the stage early in life for bone health and risk for osteoporosis in later years.

Iron requirements are high in adolescent girls because of the increased muscle mass and blood volume, as well as the iron loss that occurs with menses. The RDAs for iron increase from 8 mg/d in 9- to 13-year-old girls to 15 mg/d in 14- to 18-year-old girls and then increase again as girls enter young adulthood (18 mg/d for 19- to 30-year-old women). National studies have noted that iron consumption is often less than the RDAs in this population (Lytle et al., 2002). Although the incidence of iron deficiency anemia is low, the problem of low iron stores is common.

The need for vitamins and other minerals increases in adolescence but can be met by a well-chosen diet. The risk for marginal or inadequate intakes increases with the omission of fruits and vegetables, skipping meals, cigarette use, ED, chronic diseases, and fad diets. Children and adolescent dietary patterns are influenced by familial factors; the role of family should be addressed to establish healthy eating patterns at an early age.

Young Adulthood

Young adulthood, or the childbearing years, is a time when women create and establish careers, have babies and nurture families, actively participate in their communities, and attempt to balance it all. Nutrient needs are less than in the growing years, yet a variety of factors make achievement of optimal nutrition a challenge for many. These factors include delay in marriage and children and the continuance of the single lifestyle with frequent eating irregularities and poor intake; stressful work and family schedules that leave little time and energy for food shopping and meal preparation; single motherhood (which constitutes the majority of women who have limited food resources); and a lack of basic food knowledge and cooking skills among some young women.

A common complaint of young women is mood changes that accompany the premenstrual period. Numerous diet and lifestyle theories and interventions are proposed to aid in the relief of symptoms of premenstrual syndrome (PMS) and premenstrual dysphoric disorder (PMDD); however, study quality, outcomes, and findings vary. The strongest support is for the use of calcium in the management of PMS. Chasteberry, fruit from the chaste tree, and vitamin B_6

may also be effective (Whelan, Jurgens, & Naylor, 2009). Although evidence is still limited for PMDD, as well as PMS, calcium seems to have the most consistent and robust findings. One should include supplemental and dietary sources of intake when determining total calcium intake for women. Two herbal supplements thought to provide benefit have been found to have no effect on PMS or PMDD symptom are St. John's wort and evening primrose oil (Kelderhouse & Taylor, 2013).

Routine vitamin and mineral supplementation is not generally indicated for healthy young adult women with a well-balanced diet; the exception is for folic acid. Randomized trials have demonstrated the role of folic acid in the prevention of neural tube defects (NTDs), such as spina bifida and anencephaly. Studies have shown that the optimal red cell folate levels for preventing NTDs (906 mmol/L) are achieved from folic acid supplementation, not from diet alone (Shabert, 2004). Because the neural tube closes by day 28 of gestation (before most women realize they are pregnant), folic acid is needed before conception. Therefore, the Centers for Disease Control and Prevention (CDC, 1992) recommends that all women of childbearing years increase their intake of folic acid. One public health measure to address this was the implementation, in 1998, of the addition of folic acid to products made with enriched flour or grain products, such as bread, rice, and pasta. In combination with good dietary sources of folic acid (dark green leafy vegetables, legumes, enriched cereals and grains, orange juice, soy, wheat germ, and almonds and peanuts), women planning a pregnancy should begin a folic acid supplementation of 400 mcg/d (CDC, 1992).

Perimenopause/Menopause

Decreased estrogen production during the menopausal process leads to physiological changes that affect nutritional needs. The loss of estrogen affects the cycle of bone turnover necessary for the maintenance of bone mass in that bone resorption is greater than reformation, resulting in loss of bone mass by the end of the menopausal period and placing women at increased risk of osteoporosis. However, optimal prevention in the early decades (adequate calcium intake and weight-bearing activity) promotes optimal bone density at menopause. Reduced estrogen levels can also have an impact on blood lipids, higher total cholesterol and low-density lipoprotein (LDL) cholesterol levels, and lower high-density lipoprotein (HDL) levels—all negatively affecting cardiovascular health.

The use of natural hormone replacement, namely, soy isoflavones, has grown in popularity, especially in light of the adverse effect of hormone replacement therapy (HRT) (Mangano et al., 2013). Isoflavones are a class of phytoestrogens under the larger umbrella of phytochemicals. Genistein and daidzein are the two most common isoflavones found in soy products. These phytochemicals have weak, nonsteroidal estrogen effects when bound to estrogen receptors and have been studied for effects on menopausal symptoms and related morbidities. Isoflavones in soy may decrease the frequency of hot flashes in menopausal women. A review and meta-analysis of randomized,

controlled studies; however, showed that they had a modest or inconsistent impact on hot flashes (Nelson et al., 2006). A benefit of HRT was prolonged cardiovascular and bone health. When soy proteins were tested in randomized, controlled trials, there was little to no impact on serum lipids (Campbell, Khalil, Payton, & Arjmandi, 2010; Mangano et al., 2013; Wofford et al., 2012). A long-term (1 year), randomized, controlled trial failed to find a benefit for soy protein or isoflavones (together or alone) on bone turnover or bone density (Kenny et al., 2009). Although other studies have looked at different outcomes with varied dosages and sources of soy in different study populations, the evidence as a whole points to a lack of effect of soy, isoflavones, or phytoestrogens for the prevention of bone loss.

TABLE 13.5	Factors With Potential to Impact Nutritional Status in Older Women
FACTOR	**NUTRITIONAL IMPACT**
Decreased lean body mass and strength	Possible increase in protein requirement
Loss of independence and mobility	Limited food access and ability to prepare meals
Decreased energy expenditure, physical activity	Decreased energy requirement, increased need for nutrient-dense diet
Xerostomia (dry mouth)	Chewing and/or swallowing problems, food avoidance
Dysgeusia/hyposmia	Reduced sensory stimulation and appetite changes
Decreased immune function	Possible increased requirement for iron, zinc, and other nutrients
Atrophic gastritis	Increased requirement for folate, calcium, vitamin K, vitamin B_{12}, and iron
Increased blood pressure	Reduced sodium requirement and unprocessed food sources
Menopause	Decreased iron requirement
Reduced skin production and reduced metabolism of vitamin to physiologically active form	Increased requirement for vitamin D and calcium
Increased retention of vitamin A	Reduced requirement for vitamin A
Constipation	Possible increase in fluid and fiber requirements
Depression, social isolation	Poor appetite and limited food intake
Changes in financial status	Possible reduced food access and choices, limited food variety and intake

The Older Woman

As the number of people 65 years and older continues to increase, there is more interest in the health and nutritional needs of this population. With the natural aging process, many physiological, metabolic, and psychosocial changes can alter appetite, digestion, absorption, nutrient requirements, and functional skills needed for food acquisition and preparation (Table 13.5). As women get older, there is increased prevalence of chronic diseases such as heart disease, hypertension, diabetes, and cancer. These conditions may require a modified diet or changes in eating patterns that can be particularly challenging to this population.

The nutritional status of otherwise healthy older adults can deteriorate without much notice; screening tools are commonly used to help health practitioners determine if an older adult is at risk. The American Dietetic Association, the American Academy of Family Physicians, and the National Council on Aging developed the Nutrition Screening Initiative for older adults who live independently (Nutrition Screening Initiative, 1991). The simple screening tool evaluates risk factors such as body weight, living environment, eating habits, and functional status (Box 13.1). Based on the National Screening Initiative results, a more thorough nutritional assessment can be completed and followed by appropriate intervention. This kind of early detection and prevention can be used to promote healthy behaviors and catch early warning signs to reduce hospitalizations and disease.

NUTRITIONAL NEEDS

Energy requirements decrease with age, and although the etiology is multifactorial, it is largely a result of reduced basal metabolic rate and physical activity. Weight gain and an increase in body fat can occur in spite of decreasing dietary intake. Although energy requirements and intake often decrease with age, the requirements for protein, vitamins, and minerals do not decline, and some increase. Therefore it is essential for the older female to choose nutrient-dense foods.

Dietary protein needs may increase in the elderly as a result of diminished protein stores in the declining muscle mass, as well as altered gastrointestinal (GI) function and the presence of acute and chronic diseases. Although the RDA for protein for all adults is 0.8 g/kg/d, evidence indicates that 1.0 to 1.5 g/kg/d may better maintain positive nitrogen balance in older adults (Paddon-Jones et al., 2015). Furthermore, some experts recommend consumption of protein (25 to 30 g) at each meal from a variety of high-quality protein sources along with regular physical activity before or

---

BOX 13.1 CHECKLIST TO DETERMINE YOUR NUTRITIONAL HEALTH

The warning signs of poor nutritional health are often overlooked. To see whether you (or people you know) are at nutritional risk, take this simple quiz. Read the statement below and circle the number in the yes column for those that apply. To find your total nutritional score, add up all the numbers you circled.

	Yes
I have an illness or condition that made me change the kind and/or amount of food I eat.	2
I eat fewer than two meals per day.	3
I eat few fruits, vegetables, or milk products.	2
I have three or more drinks of beer, liquor, or wine almost every day.	2
I have tooth or mouth problems that make it hard for me to eat.	2
I do not always have enough money to buy the food I need.	4
I eat alone most of the time.	1
I take three or more different prescribed or over-the-counter drugs a day.	1
Without wanting to, I have lost or gained 10 pounds in the past 6 months.	2
I am not always physically able to shop, cook, and/or feed myself.	2
Total nutritional score:	

If your total nutritional score is

0 to 2: Good! Recheck your nutritional score in 6 months.

3 to 5: You are at moderate nutritional risk. See what can be done to improve your eating habits and lifestyle. A local office on aging, senior nutrition program, senior citizens center, or health department can help. Recheck your nutritional score in 3 months.

6 or more: You are at high nutritional risk. Bring this checklist next time you see your doctor, dietitian, or other qualified health or social service professional. Talk with them about any problems you have experienced. Ask for nutritional counseling.

Source: Reprinted from Nutrition Screening Initiative (1991). The Nutrition Screening Initiative is a project of the American Academy of Family Physicians, the American Dietetic Association, and the National Council on the Aging, Inc., and is funded in part by a grant from Ross Products Division, Abbott Laboratories Inc.

after the protein-rich meal to prevent the onset or slow the progression of sarcopenia (Paddon-Jones et al., 2015).

The nutritional status of older adults is varied. Age, geographic location, culture, and disease conditions are contributing factors to the heterogeneity of older adult nutrition status. National surveys of food consumption and nutritional status indicate that older adults in the United States are at nutritional risk. With decreased mean energy intakes, nutrients at greatest risk for deficiency are calcium, riboflavin, folate, vitamin B_{12}, vitamin B_6, iron, and zinc (Jain, 2015). Older women have increased needs for vitamins C, D, and the B vitamins as well as calcium, magnesium, and zinc. One nutrient that is often chronically low in older adults is vitamin D, which is necessary for absorption of calcium and phosphorus. In addition to possible limited dietary intake, the skin loses efficiency in converting vitamin D from sunlight. The active form of circulating vitamin D may be reduced in elderly women due to decreased sunlight exposure (especially for the homebound and those in institutions) and diminished conversion of precursors in the liver and kidney. Supplementation of vitamin D should be considered for those at risk—for example, women in long-term care facilities or those living at higher latitudes during winter months. Although providing moderate calcium and vitamin D supplements to healthy elderly is common practice to promote bone health, other nutrients are also important for bone health including protein; vitamins A, C, and K; magnesium; and possibly omega-3 fatty acids.

■ PREGNANCY

Nutritional and lifestyle choices of pregnant women are key contributors to the progression and health of a pregnancy. A pregnancy is considered healthy when the mother is without physiological or psychological pathology and it results in a healthy baby (Kaiser, Campbell, & Academy Positions Committee Workgroup, 2014). The health of mothers and infants is a public health concern as identified in *Healthy People 2020* as a leading health indicator (LHI). LHIs are a group of topics that are determined as high-priority health issues. Women's and infant health is rightly placed as an LHI, for the health of the population is key to future generation's well-being.

Points in history have demonstrated the impact of food deprivation and malnutrition on reproduction. Studies from Russia and the Netherlands during World War II demonstrated a decrease in fertility and an increase in stillbirths, neonatal deaths, and low-birth-weight (LBW) infants (Shabert, 2004). LBW remains a public concern; 8.0% of U.S. newborns are of LBW (National Center for Health Statistics, 2015b). Birth defects and LBW are the number 1 and 2 causes, respectively, of death in U.S. infants (National Center for Health Statistics, 2015a).

The timing and duration of nutritional restriction are significant. During the embryonic stage of fetal development, cells differentiate into three germinal layers. Growth during this time occurs only by an increase in the number of cells.

The fetal stage is the time of most rapid growth. During this time, growth is almost continuous and is accompanied by increases in cell size. Most organ cells continue to proliferate after birth. It is thought that growth in cell size begins at around 7 months gestation and can continue for 3 years after birth. Given this sequence of growth, it is possible to suggest the effects malnutrition might have at different stages of gestation. During the embryonic phase, a severe limitation in nutrients could have teratogenic effects, causing malformation or death. Although malnutrition occurring after the third month of gestation would not generally have teratogenic effects, it could cause fetal growth restriction. During the last trimester, nutritional needs are at a peak as cells increase in both size and number. Poor nutrition in the latter stages of pregnancy affects fetal growth, whereas malnutrition in the early months affects embryonic development and survival.

Maternal size at conception and nutritional history also influence pregnancy outcomes. Prepregnancy body mass index (BMI) is an independent predictor of adverse outcomes of pregnancy, and the prevalence of overweight and obesity in women of childbearing years has nearly doubled since 1976 (Procter & Campbell, 2014). Maternal size is believed to be a controlling factor on the ultimate size of the placenta, which in turn determines the amount of nutrition available to the fetus. Women who have lower prepregnant weights tend to have lighter placentas than women with higher prepregnant weights (Shabert, 2004). Short- and long-term impacts of overweight and overconsumption on maternal health risk include obesity, diabetes, dyslipidemia, and cardiovascular disease (CVD; Procter & Campbell, 2014). Preconception and periconception health care providers should assess the weight status of women who eventually plan to get pregnant in order to promote a normal weight status for optimal health of the mother and child.

Weight Gain During Pregnancy

Gestational weight gain (GWG) follows a typical pattern of little gain in the first, a rapid increase in the second, and a slightly slower rate of gain in the third trimester. Most of the weight gain associated with the products of conception (placenta, fetus, and amniotic fluid) takes place in the second half of pregnancy, whereas maternal stores are laid down very rapidly before midpregnancy then slow down and appear to stop before term. By the time of delivery, the weight gain can be accounted for in the fetus, placenta, amniotic fluid, maternal blood, maternal extracellular fluid, maternal breast and uterus, and maternal fat (Pitkin, 1976). The amount of fat stores gained parallels GWG.

Monitoring weight gain during pregnancy serves to estimate the adequacy of pregnancy progression, including dietary sufficiency. Historically, weight gain in pregnancy was restricted even through the 1960s. The current recommendation for women of normal body weight for height is to gain a total of 25 to 35 pounds. The Institute of Medicine, in 2009, updated guidelines for pregnancy weight gain for subgroups of American women (Table 13.6). The weight

TABLE 13.6	Recommended Total and Rate of Weight Gain During Pregnancy, by Prepregnancy BMI		
PREPREGNANCY BMI	BMI (kg/m²)	TOTAL WEIGHT GAIN RANGE (lb)	RATES OF WEIGHT GAIN[a] IN SECOND AND THIRD TRIMESTER (MEAN RANGE IN lb/wk)
Underweight	< 18.5	28–40	1 (1–1.3)
Normal weight	18.5–24.9	25–35	1 (0.8–1)
Overweight	25.0–29.9	15–25	0.6 (0.5–0.7)
Obese (includes all classes)	≥ 30.0	11–20	0.5 (0.4–0.6)

[a] Calculations assume a 1.1 to 4.4 lb weight gain in the first trimester.

BMI, body mass index.

Source: Institute of Medicine National Research Council (2009).

gain goals are based on prepregnancy BMI, which is weight (in kilograms) divided by height (in meters squared).

Both insufficient and excessive weight gain during pregnancy can affect fetal and maternal outcomes. Poor weight gain is associated with poor fetal growth, LBW, and risk for a preterm delivery (Rasmussen & Yaktine, 2009). Excessive weight gain affects infant growth, increases chances for large-for-gestational-age birth weight and cesarean delivery, as well as associations with the longer term outcome of higher body fatness in childhood (Turner, 2014).

Energy and Macronutrient Needs

ENERGY

As growth requires energy, additional energy above that required for maintenance is needed for pregnancy. RDAs for energy aim to provide optimal weight gain at various stages; meet growth needs of the fetus, placenta, and other maternal tissues; and account for the increased maternal basal metabolism. The RDA for pregnancy includes an additional 340 kcal/d for the second trimester and an additional 452 kcal/d for the third trimester, but this varies with the woman's level of physical activity during her pregnancy. As long as the rate and amount of weight gain are within acceptable limits, the range of energy intake can be quite variable. More energy expenditure for movement is required with increasing body weight, but most pregnant women slow or decrease their activity as pregnancy progresses. Enough energy is needed to protect protein to be used for growth rather than energy expenditure. Caloric restrictions in animals and humans have demonstrated profound negative effects on maternal physiological adjustments and fetal growth and development.

PROTEIN

Dietary protein needs increase during pregnancy to support increases in whole body protein turnover and accumulation of protein for growth of the fetus, uterus, blood volume, placenta, amniotic fluid, and maternal skeletal muscle (IOM Panel on Macronutrients & IOM Standing Committee on the Scientific Evaluation of Dietary Reference Intakes, 2005). The RDA for protein during pregnancy is 71 g/d; this level is 25 g more than the RDA for nonpregnant women.

CARBOHYDRATE

Glucose is the fetus's primary energy source, with an estimated transfer from mother at a rate of 17 to 26 g/d. All glucose transferred to the fetus is utilized by the growing brain by the end of pregnancy (IOM Panel on Macronutrients & IOM Standing Committee on the Scientific Evaluation of Dietary Reference Intakes, 2005). The RDA increases to 175 g/d of dietary carbohydrate for pregnant women.

FAT

Fat is an energy source and also essential for fat-soluble vitamin and carotenoid absorption (Turner, 2014). Intake recommendations for essential n-3 and n-6 fatty acids were determined based on median intakes among pregnant women in the United States, the AI method for estimating nutrient needs. The AI for LA, the essential n-6 fatty acid, is 13 g/d. The AI for ALA, the essential n-3 fatty acid, is 1.3 g/d (IOM Panel on Macronutrients & IOM Standing Committee on the Scientific Evaluation of Dietary Reference Intakes, 2005). The longer chain n-3 fatty acid, docosahexaenoic acid (DHA), accumulates in large amounts in the prenatal and postnatal brain. DHA can be formed from ALA in fetal tissues; therefore ALA can meet essential DHA needs through ALA recommended intakes. DHA intake occurs directly via seafood intake, particularly oily fish. Improved infant and childhood outcomes are associated with maternal seafood consumption (Heppe et al., 2011; Noakes et al., 2012). A balance to meet seafood intake recommendations for a healthy pregnancy while avoiding high methylmercury content can be achieved. The top four sources of high-mercury fish in the United States include tilefish from the Gulf of Mexico, shark, swordfish, and king mackerel. White albacore tuna should be limited to 6 oz/wk for pregnant women. The most commonly consumed fish are low in mercury and include salmon, shrimp, pollock, tuna (light canned), tilapia, catfish, and cod (U.S. Food and Drug Administration, 2014).

Micronutrient Needs

The need for most vitamins and many minerals increases during pregnancy. Many of the water soluble vitamins are used as cofactors in metabolic exchanges and processes essential for growth; therefore needs increase for thiamin, riboflavin, niacin, vitamin B_6, folate, vitamin B_{12}, pantothenic acid, choline, and vitamin C (IOM Food and Nutrition Board, Suitor, & Meyers, 2007). The requirements for fat-soluble vitamins A and D are also increased during pregnancy (Table 13.7). Element needs that increase are iron, magnesium, chromium, copper, iodine, manganese, molybdenum, selenium, zinc, and chloride. Some highlights of vitamins and minerals are given in the following sections, along with their importance during pregnancy.

VITAMIN NEEDS

Vitamin A • The RDA for vitamin A for pregnant women, 770 retinol activity equivalents (RAE), is slightly more than the nonpregnant level. The concern is that excessive intake of vitamin A can be teratogenic. Cases of adverse pregnancy outcomes, such as malformations, have been associated with a daily ingestion of 25,000 IU (7,500 RAE) or more of vitamin A (Rosa, Wilk, & Kelsey, 1986). In addition, epidemiological evidence indicates that the drug isotretinoin (or Accutane, a vitamin A analog used to treat cystic acne) causes major malformations involving craniofacial, central nervous system, cardiac, and thymic changes (Lammer et al., 1985). Use of this drug is contraindicated in pregnancy. Some findings indicate that pregnant women who take vitamin A supplements at levels as low as 2.5 times the RDA increase the risk of delivering a baby with a cranial neural crest defect (Rothman et al., 1995). The Teratology Society (1987) urges that women in their reproductive years be informed that the excessive use of vitamin A shortly before and during pregnancy could be harmful to their babies ("Teratology Society position paper," 1987). It also suggests that manufacturers of vitamin A–containing supplements should lower the maximum amount of vitamin A per unit dosage to 5,000 to 8,000 IU and identify the source of vitamin A. Beta-carotene, a precursor of vitamin A, is not associated with these pregnancy risks.

Vitamin D • The IOM recommendation for vitamin D intake in pregnancy does not differ from nonpregnant women: RDA of 600 IU (15 mcg) and UL of 4,000 IU/d. Vitamin D is necessary for fetal growth and development, particularly of the skeleton and tooth enamel. In 2012, the World Health Organization (WHO) published a guideline for vitamin D intake in pregnant women that applied Cochrane Review methods. The findings suggest that vitamin D supplementation is not recommended during pregnancy for the prevention of pre-eclampsia. Further recommendations state lack of evidence for other maternal or infant outcomes and state that vitamin D supplementation should not be part of routine care of pregnant women (WHO, 2012b). A recent study found that pregnant women supplemented with 2,000 IU (50 mcg)/d improved serum vitamin D status in the mother and infant, preventing vitamin D deficiency in 98% of infants at 8 weeks (March et al., 2015). Maternal supplementation of 400 IU and 1,000 IU prevented vitamin D deficiency in 57% and 84% of infants at 8 weeks, respectively (March et al., 2015). Therefore supplementation up to 2,000 IU (50 mcg)/d may be beneficial to maintain optimum serum 25-hydroxy vitamin D levels. The short- and long-term implications are under investigation.

Folic Acid • Folic acid requirements increase during pregnancy because of augmented maternal erythropoiesis and fetal and placental growth. It is also an essential coenzyme in metabolism and in DNA synthesis. Folic acid deficiency results in megaloblastic anemia. Although it is not as common as iron deficiency anemia, megaloblastic anemia can occur in high-risk women, such as those of low socioeconomic status and those with a multiple pregnancy or chronic hemolytic anemia. Diagnosis may not occur until the third trimester, but biochemical and morphological signs may be seen earlier. Maternal folic acid deficiency in animals is associated with congenital malformations; some evidence in humans suggests an association with pregnancy complications, but well-done studies have not been conducted (Tamura & Picciano, 2006).

The current RDA for folate is 600 mcg for pregnancy, 200 mcg more than the recommendation for nonpregnant women. Synthetic folic acid as a fortified or supplemental source (400 mcg/d), in addition to food forms of folate from a variable diet for women who are capable of becoming pregnant, is recommended (USDA and U.S. Department of Health and Human Services [DHHS], 2010). It is important to note, however, that the tolerable UL of 800 to 1,000 mcg/d from fortified foods and supplements is only double the recommended dose.

The most significant influence of folic acid in pregnancy is its role in preventing NTDs. Randomized clinical trials of several thousand women in Europe in the late 1980s and early 1990s resulted in unequivocal results (Tamura & Picciano, 2006). Good dietary sources of folic acid and supplements are needed before and between conceptions; in fact, the public health recommendations are for "women capable of becoming pregnant" (USDA and DHHS, 2010).

Vitamin B_{12} • Vitamin B_{12} accumulates in the placenta and fetus and is essential for normal blood formation and neurological function. At birth, fetal vitamin B_{12} levels are twice that of the mother. Only new vitamin B_{12} is transferred to the placenta, so supplementation is required for those who limit the intake of meats and meat products. Vegans in particular need supplemental sources of vitamin B_{12}. Deficiency during pregnancy can increase the risk for maternal and fetal megaloblastic anemia, fetal demyelination, and NTDs (Turner, 2014).

TABLE 13.7	DRIs: Vitamin and Mineral RDAs[a] and AI for Pregnant and Lactating Females	
	PREGNANCY	**LACTATION**
Vitamin A (mcg)	**14–18 years: 750**	**14–18 years: 1,200**
	770	1,300
Vitamin D (mcg)	15	15
Vitamin E (mg)	15	19
Vitamin K (mcg)[b]	14–18 years: 75	14–18 years: 75
	90	90
Vitamin C (mg)	**14–18 years: 80**	**14–18 years: 115**
	85	120
Thiamin (mg)	1.4	1.4
Riboflavin (mg)	1.4	1.6
Niacin (mg)	18	17
Vitamin B$_6$ (mg)	1.9	20
Folate (mcg)	600	500
Vitamin B$_{12}$ (mcg)	2.6	2.8
Biotin (mcg)[b]	30	35
Pantothenic acid (mg)[b]	6	7
Choline (mg)[b]	450	550
Calcium (mg)	**14–18 years: 1,300**	**14–18 years: 1,300**
	1,000	1,000
Chromium (mcg)[b]	14–18 years: 29	14–18 years: 44
	30	45
Copper (mcg)	1,000	1,300
Fluoride (mg)[b]	3	3
Iodine (mcg)	220	290
Iron (mg)	27	14–18 years: 10
		9
Magnesium (mg)	14–18 years: 400	14–18 years: 360
	19–30 years: 350	19–30 years: 310
	31–50 years: 360	31–50 years: 320
Manganese (mg)[b]	2	2.6
Molybdenum (mcg)	50	50
Phosphorus (mg)	14–18 years: 1,250	14–18 years: 1,250
	700	700
Selenium (mcg)	60	70
Zinc (mg)	14–18 years: 12	14–18 years: 13
	11	12

AI, adequate intake; DRIs, dietary reference intakes; RDAs, recommended dietary allowances.
[a]DRIs presented for ages 19–30 years and 31–50 years. Unless otherwise indicated, RDAs are noted in bold.

Choline • Large amounts of choline are transferred to the fetus from maternal stores. Therefore, the AI for choline increases to 450 mg/d for pregnant women. Maternal deficiency can negatively affect fetal brain development (Caudill, 2010). Choline intakes may be lower than the recommended intake for many pregnant women. Suggestions for increased dietary intake are needed, as choline is often not included in prenatal vitamin and mineral supplements. Good dietary sources include eggs, salmon, kidney or navy beans, and low-fat milk (Kaiser et al., 2014).

MINERAL NEEDS

Iron • Pregnancy imposes a severe burden on the maternal hematopoietic system. With the natural increase in maternal blood supply in pregnancy, total erythrocyte volume increases by 20% to 30%. Normal hematopoiesis requires a nutritionally adequate diet. To produce hemoglobin, there must be protein to provide essential amino acids and sufficient additional iron. Other vitamins and minerals, such as copper, zinc, folic acid, and vitamin B_{12}, are needed to serve as cofactors in the synthesis of heme and globin. The limiting factor in this synthesis is usually the availability of iron.

Most women require supplemental iron to meet the increased demands during pregnancy. The current recommendation from the WHO is for 30 mg/d of elemental iron (150 mg ferrous sulfate heptahydrate, 90 mg ferrous fumarate, or 250 mg ferrous gluconate). The recommendation is to reduce the risk of LBW, maternal anemia, and iron deficiency (WHO, 2012a). For optimal absorption, the supplement should be taken separately from whole-grain cereals, unleavened whole-grain breads, legumes, tea, and coffee, as these foods and beverages inhibit iron absorption. Citrus, on the other hand, enhances the absorption of nonheme iron (e.g., plant and supplemental iron sources; Kaiser et al., 2014).

Although anemia is a relatively common complication of pregnancy, with 17.4% of pregnant women in industrialized nations presenting with it (Khalafallah & Dennis, 2012), routine supplementation practices have fallen under scrutiny, as the U.S. Preventive Services Task Force (USPSTF) found no studies that evaluated the effects of assessing iron status in pregnant women. Furthermore, they found little evidence that treating low levels has an impact on maternal and infant outcomes (Siu & USPSTF, 2015). The USPSTF recommendation is that there is not enough information on the testing for and routine prescription of iron supplements to healthy pregnant women (Siu & USPSTF, 2015). Furthermore, excessive iron supplementation can retard zinc absorption (Turner, 2014).

Calcium • Calcium deposition in fetal bones and teeth occurs primarily in the third trimester; by the time of a full-term birth, the newborn has accumulated approximately 25 to 30 g of calcium. The current RDA for calcium during pregnancy (1,000 mg/d for adults and 1,300 mg/d for those younger than 19 years) is not an increase over the nonpregnant state because of the increased efficiency of intestinal calcium absorption.

Although available data are insufficient to support routine calcium supplementation for the prevention of osteoporosis in younger women, prenatal nutrition counseling should address dietary strategies to meet calcium needs. Dairy products are an obvious major source of dietary calcium, but other food sources, including calcium-fortified products such as juice and soy milk, contribute. In situations in which dairy products are omitted or restricted in the diet (allergy, lactose intolerance, and veganism) or in which calcium intake is chronically low, calcium supplementation should be considered.

Sodium • Sodium restriction in the diet of pregnant women was standard practice for decades. It is now recognized, however, that healthy pregnant women retain salt normally, and moderate edema appears to be a normal consequence of pregnancy. Fluid retention actually increases the body's need for sodium.

A positive sodium balance occurs in normal pregnancy, resulting from significant changes in renal and hormonal function. The glomerular filtration rate increases by 50% in early pregnancy and remains elevated until late in the third trimester, filtering sodium into the renal tubules. Simultaneously, progesterone produces a salt-losing action in the kidneys, slowing absorption of filtered sodium through the tubules.

To prevent an electrolyte imbalance, the renin–angiotensin–aldosterone system acts as a compensatory mechanism in normal pregnancy. This counterbalances the salt-losing tendencies of progesterone and decreases urinary sodium excretion. The result is that sodium is conserved to meet the needs of the expanded tissue and fluid. Severe sodium restriction can stress the physiological mechanism of sodium conservation, resulting in hyponatremia. Moderation in sodium intake is appropriate for everyone; pregnancy recommendations mirror the nonpregnant population.

Zinc • Zinc has wide-ranging enzymatic, structural, and regulatory functions. Zinc deficiency in pregnancy can cause intrauterine growth retardation, teratogenesis, and embryonic or fetal death (King, 2000). The RDA for zinc during pregnancy is 11 mg/d (12 mg/d for those younger than 18 years), 3 g/d more than the nonpregnant female population. Because iron inhibits zinc absorption, high levels of prenatal iron supplementation may have a negative impact on maternal zinc status. For women taking more than 30 mg/d, supplements of 15 mg/d of zinc and 2 mg/d of copper are recommended (Procter & Campbell, 2014). Good sources of dietary zinc include meat, fish, poultry, dairy products, nuts, whole grains, and legumes. The bioavailability of zinc can be inhibited in vegetarian diets as a result of phytates, fiber, and/or calcium that may inhibit absorption (Kaiser et al., 2014). Therefore the needs of pregnant vegetarians may be higher than those of nonvegetarians.

Alcohol, Artificial Sweeteners, and Caffeine

The teratogenic effects of excessive alcohol consumption are well accepted. In addition to the outcomes of fetal alcohol syndrome and fetal alcohol effects, alcohol use in pregnancy is associated with spontaneous abortion, LBW, and abruptio placentae. As no safe level of alcohol intake in pregnancy can be guaranteed, promoting abstinence before and during pregnancy is recommended. For the health care practitioner inquiring about alcohol intake can sometimes be less threatening when done within the context of a dietary history and usual patterns of food and beverage intake.

Artificial sweeteners used in the U.S. food supply include saccharin, aspartame, and acesulfame-K. Saccharin has been shown to be a weak carcinogen in animals but is not teratogenic. Acesulfame-K is considered safe, but is relatively new in food use, so no long-term studies during pregnancy have been conducted. A product of aspartame metabolism is the amino acid phenylalanine, which can cause brain damage in persons with phenylketonuria. Moderate intake of aspartame in women without phenylketonuria, however, does not increase serum phenylalanine levels high enough to affect the fetal brain. Dietary assessment of pregnant women should include the use of artificial sweeteners, found primarily in soft drinks but also in flavored yogurt, in baked goods, and as a substitute for added sugar. Counseling should encourage the use of nutrient-containing milk and juice or water instead of soft drinks.

Extensive research has been conducted on caffeine's effect on pregnancy outcome, with mixed results depending on study design and population. A large prospective study out of the United Kingdom found that caffeine intake is associated with fetal growth restriction (CARE Study Group, 2008); other studies have had mixed results. Although there is a controversy surrounding the recommendation to eliminate or restrict caffeine intake, women should limit their intake to no more than 200 mg/d (American College of Obstetricians and Gynecologists [ACOG], 2010). In addition to coffee and tea, soft drinks are a major source of caffeine in the United States. The average caffeine content of common beverages are 137 mg in an 8-oz cup of regular coffee, 40 mg in a 1-oz espresso, 48 mg in an 8-oz cup of tea, and 37 mg in 12 oz of cola. Dark chocolate also provides 30 mg caffeine in a 1.45-oz serving (ACOG, 2010).

Diet-Related Problems in Pregnancy

COMMON GI COMPLAINTS

Nausea and vomiting, commonly called *morning sickness*, are reported in 70% to 85% of pregnant women. Standard dietary recommendations for mild nausea include eating frequent, small meals; avoiding offensive odors and spicy or greasy foods; drinking adequate fluids; and getting fresh air (Kaiser et al., 2014). There is limited support for the use of complementary therapies or supplements (typical practices include acupuncture, vitamin B₆, or ginger products) to help alleviate GI symptoms. Rather than a specific diet for managing nausea, pregnant women should be encouraged to eat whatever they tolerate and avoid odors that result in nausea.

For a small percentage of pregnant women, the vomiting can be frequent and severe enough (hyperemesis gravidarum) to affect their nutritional status, resulting in weight loss, decreased nutrient intake, and electrolyte imbalance. These women need medical management and frequently require hospitalization for fluid and electrolyte replacement and possibly nutrition support in severe cases.

Acid reflux, or heartburn, is reported in approximately two thirds of pregnant women (Turner, 2014). Calcium-based antacids have been tested in randomized, controlled trials and are effective for rapid relief of symptoms. Additional, but not empirically tested, common recommendations for heart burn relief include avoiding the supine position for 3 hours after eating; sleeping with an elevated head; eating small, frequent meals; and avoiding greasy and/or spicy foods, as well as tomatoes, highly acidic citrus, carbonated beverages, and caffeine-containing beverages (Kaiser et al., 2014).

Constipation occurs among 11% to 38% of pregnant women and is attributed to the slowed digestive changes of pregnancy or is secondary to iron supplementation (Vazquez, 2010). Adequate fluid and fiber intake recommendations (28 g/d for pregnant women) and regular physical activity can help alleviate constipation.

PREGNANCY-INDUCED HYPERTENSION

The cardinal symptoms of pregnancy-induced hypertension (PIH) are hypertension, proteinuria, and edema, usually occurring after the 20th week of gestation. This condition is unique to pregnancy and resolves only by the termination of the pregnancy. PIH is sometimes referred to as *preeclampsia* and *eclampsia*; the latter is an extension of preeclampsia, with more severity (i.e., seizures and high risk of maternal and infant mortality). PIH, a more appropriate description of this disorder, is most often seen in first pregnancies, obesity, history of preeclampsia, chronic hypertension, older age, and African American race. Criteria for diagnosing PIH include:

- Hypertension: blood pressure of 140/90 mmHg or an increase of 20 to 30 mmHg systolic or 10 to 15 mmHg diastolic above the woman's usual baseline; at least two observations at 6 or more hours apart
- Proteinuria: 500 mg or more in a 24-hour urine collection or random 2+ protein; develops late in the course of PIH
- Edema: significant; usually in hands and face; if left unattended, seizures may occur; can be fatal to either mother or infant

The etiology of PIH is unknown. Nutritional deficiency is suspected; however, because of the socioeconomic and other confounding factors (age, preconception weight, health status, and prenatal care) the etiology remains undetermined. Protein, total energy intake, macronutrient imbalances, omega-3 fatty acids, calcium, sodium, zinc, iron, magnesium, and folate have been studied as potential nutritional triggers; however, definitive findings remain elusive. A basic, healthy diet—including good potassium sources (fruits and vegetables), low-fat dairy products, and high fiber—is associated with a reduced risk of preeclampsia (Frederick et al., 2005). Women at risk for PIH should receive early prenatal care and guidance on following a balanced diet that provides adequate energy and protein.

DIABETES

With the prevalence of overweight and type 2 diabetes mellitus on the rise in the general population, more women are entering pregnancy with diabetes, insulin resistance, or high risk for the development of gestational diabetes. This increases the risk for pregnancy complications and poor birth outcomes.

Pregnancy is a diabetogenic event in which energy needs and fuel requirements are increased. Glucose is the primary fuel, particularly for the growing fetus, who has an uptake rate of glucose at least twice that of an adult. To meet fetal needs, glucose is transferred rapidly from mother to fetus through simple diffusion and active transport. Although glucose crosses the placental barrier, insulin does not, so the fetus is dependent on its own supply for development. Maternal fasting blood glucose levels drop as a result of rapid fetal uptake, which decreases her fasting insulin levels. Even brief fasting can result in the production of ketones, which is an alternative fuel source, but carries the risk of fetal brain damage.

The normal energy metabolism of pregnancy and the maternal–fetal relationship have implications for women with insulin-dependent diabetes mellitus. During the first half of pregnancy, the increased transfer of maternal glucose to the fetus, along with the potential lower food intake because of nausea, may result in reduced insulin requirements. In the second half of pregnancy, the diabetogenic effects of the placental hormones override the continuous fetal drain of glucose, so insulin requirements are increased by as much as 70% to 100% over prepregnant requirements. The risk of ketoacidosis is also increased; pregnant women with diabetes mellitus need frequent monitoring. Because of frequent changes in diet and insulin, these women are best served by a team of professionals, including a skilled registered dietitian.

Diet is critical in the management of pregnant women with diabetes. Increased energy intake is dependent on pre-pregnancy weight, physical activity level, and adequacy of weight gain. It is important to maintain regular meals and snacks, including a bedtime snack to avoid overnight ketonemia. More structured eating schedules and balanced distribution of food in the pregnant state are usually needed to achieve a normoglycemic state. More frequent follow-up visits are need for women with diabetes so that the team can monitor weight gain, blood glucose control, energy and nutrient intake and make adjustments in meal and snack plans or insulin doses as needed.

GESTATIONAL DIABETES

Pregnant women without known prior diabetes should be screened for gestational diabetes between the 24th and 28th weeks of gestation. Two screening options are suggested by the American Diabetes Association ("Standards of medical care in diabetes," 2015); see Table 13.8.

The nutritional recommendations for gestational diabetes are similar to those for preexisting diabetes mellitus, with more frequent prenatal evaluations. Management goals include providing adequate energy and nutrients to support optimum weight gain without episodes of hyperglycemia or ketonemia. Intensive and frequent self-monitoring and health care team evaluations of blood glucose, weight gain, dietary intake and meal and snack timing, and urinary ketones are essential, followed by appropriate adjustments in food intake and meal plans (American Diabetes Association, 2003).

PICA

Pica is the behavior of eating nonfood substances. Although occurring in the broad population, it is most common in pregnant women. Usual substances consumed are clay, starch (laundry starch and chalk), and ice. Pica is associated with a higher incidence of malnutrition because it displaces foods providing needed nutrients. There is a strong link between pica and iron deficiency; it is thought that some of those substances may bind to iron, preventing absorption (Rainville, 1998). Other negative consequences from pica can include intestinal obstruction and toxic levels of heavy metals such as lead.

The reasons for pica are not clearly identified. Culture and tradition passed from generation to generation are important factors. Some reports indicate that women believe these substances relieve nausea, prevent vomiting, relieve dizziness, cure swelling, and stop headaches. Pica behavior is not easy to discourage, but the potentially dangerous consequences should be avoided.

For the practitioner, the immediate need is to identify the pica behavior, which is rarely revealed spontaneously. A dietary intake assessment can address this by asking about cravings or eating unusual substances while obtaining an overall diet pattern. If pica behavior is acknowledged, the practitioner should identify the extent of the amount and frequency, followed by a more thorough dietary and biochemical assessment. The client then can be offered nutrition education regarding the potential harm of the pica behavior, as well as nutritional guidance for strategies to improve her diet for pregnancy.

FOOD SAFETY

Pregnant women should take caution to avoid food-borne illnesses. Bacteria of greatest concern for this special population are *Listeria monocytogenes*, *Toxoplasma gondii*, *Brucella* species, *Salmonella* species, and *Campylobacter jejuni*. Listeriosis, caused by *L. monocytogenes*, can cause premature delivery, stillbirth, or newborn infection. During pregnancy, women should avoid unpasteurized (raw) juices; raw sprouts; and unpasteurized (raw) dairy products, including soft or homemade cheese; and raw or undercooked meat, fish, eggs, and poultry (USDA and DHHS, 2010). Luncheon meat and hot dogs, if consumed, should be heated to steaming hot to kill the *Listeria* organisms (Kaiser et al., 2014).

The U.S. Food and Drug Administration (2014) also recommends that pregnant women avoid eating large fish that accumulate high levels of methylmercury such as shark, swordfish, king mackerel, and tilefish. However, as fatty fish

TABLE 13.8	Strategies for Diagnosing Gestational Diabetes

No uniform approach for GDM diagnosis	
Two options for women not previously diagnosed with overt diabetes	

"ONE-STEP" STRATEGY	"TWO-STEP" STRATEGY

■ 75 g OGTT with PG measurement fasting and at 1 and 2 hours, at 24–28 weeks in women not previously diagnosed with overt diabetes
■ Perform OGTT in the morning after overnight fast (> 8 hours)
■ GDM diagnosis made if PG values meet or exceed:
  ● Fasting: 92 mg/dL (5.1 mmol/L)
  ● 1 hour: 180 mg/dL (10.0 mmol/L)
  ● 2 hour: 153 mg/dL (8.5 mmol/L)
	■ 50 g GLT (nonfasting) with PG measurement at 1 hour (Step 1), at 24–28 weeks in women not previously diagnosed with overt diabetes
	■ If PG at 1 hour after load is ≥ 140 mg/dL (7.8 mmol/L), proceed to 100 g OGTT (Step 2), perform while patient is fasting
	■ GDM diagnosis made when two or more PG levels meet or exceed NDDG-based scores of:
	  ● Fasting: 105 mg/dL (5.8 mmol/L)
	  ● 1 hour: 190 mg/dL (10.6 mmol/L)
	  ● 2 hour: 165 mg/dL (9.2 mmol/L)
	  ● 3 hour: 145 mg/dL (8.0 mmol/L)

GDM, gestational diabetes mellitus; GLT, glucose load test; NDDG, National Diabetes Data Group; OGTT, oral glucose tolerance test; PG, plasma glucose.
Source: American Diabetes Association (2015).

contains healthy omega-3 fatty acids, it should be included in their diets. Up to 12 oz/wk is considered safe, with no more than 6 oz/wk of albacore tuna. Women are also advised to contact their state or local health departments regarding methylmercury or other contaminants in local fish and seafood, as noted (U.S. Food and Drug Administration, 2014).

FOOD TABOOS

Superstitions and taboos about food are as old as human life. Pregnancy seems to be a time of great concern about food taboos, with strong connotation as to what is beneficial or harmful. When these taboos are grounded in ignorance, they can have a deleterious effect on the pregnant woman's diet. Many superstitions have been associated with protein and protein-rich foods, which can be particularly harmful. Some food beliefs in pregnancy center on limiting weight gain in order to have a smaller baby who is easier to deliver. Many food avoidances are rooted in religious or cultural practices that are believed to impart positive qualities in the offspring.

Health care practitioners should remember that a belief does not necessarily imply practice. In our rapidly changing multicultural society, assumptions cannot be made about dietary beliefs and practices based on ethnicity or culture alone. In working with pregnant women who have unhealthy dietary practices based on beliefs or taboos, it is essential to understand and listen to the woman's view, provide explanation and information, and then negotiate.

ADOLESCENT PREGNANCY

Pregnancy in adolescence poses potential physical and psychological risks because adolescence is a period of rapid growth and development with increased nutrient requirements. Teenage girls who become pregnant at a young gynecologic age (the number of years between onset of menses and the date of conception) or who are undernourished at conception have the highest nutritional needs.

It has long been accepted that adolescent girls who are more physiologically mature have no more pregnancy complications than adult women, but a longitudinal study demonstrated that both the young women and their infants are at increased risk (Scholl, Hediger, & Schall, 1997). With increasing maternal weight gains, infant birth weights remained low. Explanations for this disparity include (a) disruption in fetal–placental blood flow associated with the physiology of maternal growth and (b) increases of insulin and growth hormone that enhance maternal fat and weight gain but diminish circulating nutrients available to the fetus. The same longitudinal study of adolescent pregnancies revealed an increased risk of later overweight and obesity. There was deposition of excess subcutaneous fat in central body sites during gestation, which can increase risk for later CVD, type 2 diabetes mellitus, and hypertension (Hediger, Scholl, & Schall, 1997).

Requirements for energy and most other nutrients are the same as those for pregnant adults, individualized according to activity and weight gain. Calcium, phosphorus, and magnesium recommendations are higher than the pregnant adult recommendations (Table 13.7) to reflect the needs of their age cohort. Given teenage girls' typical patterns of dieting, habitual poor food selection, and meal skipping, it can be a challenge to convince pregnant adolescents to consume the nutrient-rich diet needed for a healthy pregnancy. For some young women, limited financial resources and food access create additional barriers. A team that includes social services, nutritional counseling, and other health and community resources best serves pregnant adolescents. A review of enhanced prenatal care interventions for adolescents showed positive pregnancy outcomes (Nielsen, Gittelsohn, Anliker, & O'Brien, 2006).

MULTIPLES PREGNANCY

Energy requirements are in excess of the recommendation for one fetus when the woman is pregnant with multiple fetuses. An estimated 40 to 45 kcal/kg prepregnancy body weight per day is recommended for normal (prepregnancy) weight women. This recommendation equates to 2,364 to 2,659 kcal/d for a woman who was 130 pounds before pregnancy. For underweight women, the estimate is 42 to 50 kcal/kg prepregnancy body weight per day, and 30 to 35 kcal/kg prepregnancy body weight per day is suggested for overweight women. Protein needs are also elevated. The IOM recommends 50 g protein per day above the nonpregnant DRI for protein for the women carrying multiples (Otten, Hellwig, & Meyers, 2006).

Prenatal Nutrition Assessment and Counseling

Nutrition assessment of pregnant women includes a thorough diet and clinical history, anthropometric measures, and laboratory tests. Many factors may place pregnant women at increased nutritional risk (Table 13.9). The presence of one or more of these factors indicates the need for a more intensive nutritional assessment.

Obtaining dietary history is an essential component of the prenatal nutrition assessment, although it is rarely done as part of routine clinical practice. This may result from lack of training and experience, time constraints, or lack of recognition of its value. Several formal tools for collecting extensive dietary information exist, each with strengths and limitations (e.g., 24-hour recall, Food Frequency Questionnaire, and 3-day diet record). Essential diet history information includes food habits (cultural food beliefs, living and cooking facilities, finances or other resources for food), attitudes, folklore, dietary allergies and intolerances, dietary supplement intakes, and lifestyle (physical activity, smoking, and alcohol intake). By combining the evaluation of diet history and usual dietary intake with laboratory results and weight gain, the goals for nutrition counseling can be developed.

Most pregnant women are motivated and receptive to making positive changes in their diets. Nutrition counseling should be individualized, beginning with determination of the woman's nutritional knowledge and reinforcement of already established good food habits. The goals for changes in diet should be clearly identified and include an understandable rationale related to a healthy outcome of pregnancy; for example, more protein is needed not only for the baby's growth, but also for the mother's placenta, uterus, and increased blood. Positive results are more likely when the professional collaborates with the woman (and her partner, if possible) to identify strategies to reach these goals, an example of which might be a vegetarian mother who offers to increase her intake of cheese, tofu, nuts, and milk to get more protein.

Cultural and ethnic food patterns are important for many women and need to be appreciated by health care practitioners. Positive aspects can be reinforced and alternative nutrient sources identified by the client or a nutritionist. The exception is atypical food taboos or beliefs that might have negative nutritional consequences.

◼ LACTATION

Each year, more evidence accumulates to show that breastfeeding is the preferred method for infant feeding, with many benefits for both the infant and mother, including optimal nutrition and immune system enhancement for the infant, reduced risk of sudden infant death syndrome, reduced risk of chronic disease, and reduced infant morbidity and mortality, as well as strong bonding for the mother and child. Benefits for the mother include faster shrinking uterus; reduced postpartum bleeding and delayed ovulation; increased energy expenditure; time and money saved from not purchasing, preparing, and mixing formula; and decreased risk of chronic diseases and postpartum depression (James, Lessen, & American Dietetic Association, 2009). The American Academy of Pediatrics and the Academy of Nutrition and Dietetics have position statements to support exclusive breastfeeding for about 6 months and continued breastfeeding, with the initiation of complementary foods to 1 year (or longer as is mutually

TABLE 13.9	Nutritional Risk Factors in Pregnancy
FACTOR	**SIGNIFICANCE**
Age	The adolescent whose reproductive biological age (chronological age minus menarche age) is less than 3 years. Adolescent pregnancy can be associated with emotional, financial, and educational risks. Advanced age may be associated with high parities. Age of menarche is significant in that it can be delayed by poor nutrition.
Reproductive performance	Short interconceptual periods, particularly when coupled with high parity. Past obstetric history of abortions, poor weight gain, anemia, generalized edema, stillbirth, toxemia, low-birth-weight infants, and premature labor.
Chronic systemic illness	Anemia, thyroid dysfunction, diabetes, chronic infection, malabsorption syndromes, severe psychosocial problems, drugs used to treat these illnesses that may interfere with nutrition.
Weight	Low pregnant weight or low weight (less than 85%) for height, inadequate weight gain during pregnancy, obesity above 120% of standard weight for height.
Atypical eating patterns	Food fads, constant dieting, pica, dietary restrictions based on ethnic or cultural factors.
Substance abuse	Use of tobacco, drugs, or alcohol.
Economic deprivation	Inability to purchase adequate amounts of food to provide needed nutrients; chronic low-level nutritional inadequacy.

desired by mother and infant) (Lessen & Kavanagh, 2015; Section on Breastfeeding, 2012). *Healthy People 2020* has a number of objectives related to breastfeeding initiation and duration. The outcomes from *Healthy People 2010* led to a revision to increase the target goals; see Table 13.10 for specifics (Office of Disease Prevention and Health Promotion, 2015b). Breastfeeding initiation is relatively high but the percentage of women who breastfeed decreases by 3 to 6 months. Barriers to continue breastfeeding include mother's work hours, lack of support (family and professional), changes in health care service delivery, sociocultural factors, inadequate information, and fatigue. It is important to note that this list omits medical rationale for the discontinuation of breastfeeding to focus on the common barriers observed in healthy lactating mothers. Nurses and other professionals who provide prenatal and perinatal care are in a prime position to assist pregnant women with information and counseling regarding the breastfeeding decision and to provide resources and support for those who choose to nurse their infants. Continued support and encouragement is essential during the first few weeks and months of motherhood to continue to breastfeed for the recommended time frames.

From a nutrition perspective, lactation places a greater nutritional demand on a woman than pregnancy does. The DRI of most nutrients are increased (Table 13.7). Milk volume is not affected by the mother's diet; rather, the actions of various hormones in response to physiological changes and infant suckling trigger the initiation and continuation of lactation. The initiation of colostrum, or early milk, is a result of the withdrawal of progesterone in combination with high levels of prolactin (O'Connor & Picciano, 2014). To maintain milk production regular suckling is required, which triggers the hormonal response of prolactin secretion. The hormone oxytocin is also triggered by suckling for milk ejection and let-down (O'Connor & Picciano, 2014).

Time and maternal diet are significant factors in the determination of milk composition, as early milk has a higher composition of nitrogen and total protein, fat-soluble vitamins, phosphorus, sodium, potassium, chloride, and micronutrient minerals but less lactose, total lipids, and water-soluble vitamins; other constituents are similar between early and mature milk (Picciano, 2001). Maternal intake of fatty acids, vitamin B_{12}, thiamin, riboflavin, vitamin B_6, vitamin A, selenium, and iodine, as well as alcohol and caffeine, are reflective from mother's diet to milk. Independent of maternal intake, milk can maintain adequate levels of nutrients when maternal intake is suboptimal by drawing upon maternal stores. However, if a deficiency persists, milk concentrations of the deficient nutrient can also become inadequate. Lipids are the most variable constituents of human milk, which is a rich source of the essential fatty acids LA and ALA, as well as their long-chain polyunsaturated fatty acid (LCPUFA) derivatives, arachidonic acid (AA) and DHA. AA and DHA can be found in some infant formula, as they are major components of the brain, retina, and nervous tissue lipids early in life. Studies have inconclusive evidence for the supplementation of the mother or formula with LCPUFA to enhance infant and child visual acuity or neurodevelopment (Delgado-Noguera, Calvache, Bonfill Cosp, Kotanidou, & Galli-Tsinopoulou, 2015). One of the benefits of breastfeeding is that the infant receives more than nutrients alone from human milk. Some additional components include anti-inflammatory agents, immunoglobulins, antimicrobials, antioxidants, oligosaccharides, cytokines, hormones, and

TABLE 13.10	*Healthy People 2020* Breastfeeding Objective Targets and Recent National Rates		
OBJECTIVE		2020 TARGET RATE (%)	NATIONAL RATE (%)
Increase the proportion of infants who are:			
Ever breastfed (MICH 21.1)		81.9	79.2[a]
Breastfed at 6 months (MICH 21.2)		60.6	49.4[a]
Breastfed at 1 year (MICH 21.3)		34.1	26.7[a]
Breastfed exclusively through 3 months (MICH 21.4)		46.2	40.7[a]
Breastfed exclusively through 6 months (MICH 21.5)		25.5	18.8[a]
Increase the proportion of employers that have worksite lactation-support programs (MICH 22)		38	25[b]
Reduce the proportion of breastfed newborns who receive formula supplementation within the first 2 days of life (MICH 23)		14.2	19.4[a]
Increase the proportion of live births that occur in facilities that provide recommended care for lactating mothers and their babies (MICH 24)		8.1	2.9[b]

MICH, maternal, infant, and child health.
[a]2011 data.
[b]2009 data.
Source: Office of Disease Prevention and Health Promotion (2015b).

growth factors (Chirico, Marzollo, Cortinovis, Fonte, & Gasparoni, 2008).

The recommended energy increase for a breastfeeding mother reflects the production of approximately 750 mL of milk per day but varies with each woman. This assumes exclusive breastfeeding; mothers of infants who receive supplemental infant formula will produce less milk and require less energy. Energy needs are higher if the postpartum woman is also very active or nursing more than one infant. The amount of milk produced usually decreases after 6 months of age as solids are added to the infant's diet. Women who are obese before pregnancy or gain excessive weight during pregnancy may not need much more energy intake. The maternal fat stores accumulated during pregnancy are expected to provide some of the energy for breast milk production in the early months of life.

The postpartum pattern of weight loss during lactation varies greatly from woman to woman. Many will gradually lose 1 to 2 pounds/wk while nursing, whereas others do not. Food intake and physical activity are likely factors in these differing weight patterns. One study of lactating women who were significantly overweight used a diet and exercise program in the first 14 weeks postpartum. Results showed that the women lost about 0.5 kg/wk and that the growth of their infants was the same as those in the control group (Lovelady, Garner, Moreno, & Williams, 2000). These women had an average of 34% body fat, and the diet was reduced by 500 kcal/d. This type of intervention should target significantly overweight or obese women. Normal-weight women who attempt restrictive dieting may be at risk for reduced milk production, as is the case of malnourished women in developing countries. It is generally recommended that breastfeeding women take in at least 1,800 kcal daily (Shabert, 2004).

Early in lactation, primary issues include sore nipples, engorgement, infection, and leaking. Nurses who counsel lactating women should reinforce a varied and healthy diet, urge avoidance of restrictive dieting attempts, and recommend 3,800 mL/d of total liquid for adequate milk production. As women may not automatically feel thirsty to consume that amount, practitioners suggest that the nursing mother drink something each time she sits down to nurse. Consuming 16 oz (1-pint glass or approximately 475 mL) at each of six feedings in a 24-hour period results in an intake of 2,850 mL and requires only an additional 1,000 mL at other times during the day to meet the recommended fluid intake for lactating women.

Breastfed infants as a group tend to grow somewhat slower than do bottle-fed infants. On occasion, a nursing infant may fail to thrive while appearing to nurse adequately. Rather than providing a supplemental bottle right away, possible contributing factors should be thoroughly explored. These include maternal factors (stress, fatigue, use of oral contraceptives or other drugs, smoking, illness, poor diet, and excessive caffeine) and infant factors (poor suck, infrequent feeding, increased energy needs, infection, malabsorption, vomiting, and diarrhea). The health care practitioner can be critical in identifying the contributing factors and working with the mother and infant to find the best strategies to solve the problem.

Nursing mothers are likely to voice other concerns about diet and breastfeeding issues. These include:

1. Vitamin and mineral supplementation for the infant: Vitamin D (400 IU) is recommended.
2. Allergic reaction of the baby to a compound in the breast milk: Most babies tolerate breast milk very well. A minority, however, may demonstrate an adverse reaction to a diet-derived component in breast milk. This is more often seen in highly allergenic families. Cow's milk protein is reported to be the major culprit. If this occurs, lactating women should be advised to avoid the potentially problematic food and assess the infant's behavior in the next few days. If the dietary change is beneficial for the baby, the mother should make sure her own diet is adequate.
3. Contaminants in breast milk: Lactating women are often exposed to a variety of nonnutritional substances that may be transferred to their milk. These substances include drugs, environmental pollutants, viruses, caffeine, and alcohol. Although moderate amounts of many of these agents are believed to pose no risk to nursing infants, some substances provoke concern because of known or suspected adverse reactions (Lawrence & Lawrence, 2005).
4. HIV/AIDS and breast milk: Evidence suggests that the HIV can be transmitted through breast milk. In developed countries, it is recommended that HIV-positive mothers do not breastfeed their infants (Committee on Pediatric AIDS, 2013).

Promotion of Breastfeeding

The decision to or not to breastfeed is usually made during pregnancy. Therefore information and counseling about nursing should be provided to the mother and her partner during prenatal visits, in childbirth classes, and through community programs. Nurses working in a variety of settings can play an important role in providing this education and counseling. Additional knowledge (the specific how-to) and supportive counseling are key to later successful and sustained breastfeeding. The hospital nurse or lactation specialist can provide practical tips and demonstration before the mother and baby go home. Hospitals that adopt the guidelines of the Baby-Friendly Hospital Initiative provide trained staff that initiate breastfeeding in the first half hour of life, offer 24-hour rooming-in, do not give bottles or pacifiers, and provide discharge support or referral for breastfeeding assistance (Baby-Friendly Hospital Initiative, 2012).

The La Leche League International, an educational and support group founded by nursing mothers, is found in most communities. Hospitals with a large obstetrics department often have lactation specialists or other trained nurses available for phone consultation to new mothers. Those with the credentials, such as international board certified lactation consultants (IBCLCs), have completed the International Board of Lactation Consultant Examiners certification process. The national Healthy Mothers, Healthy Babies programs include breastfeeding promotion, as does the Special Supplemental Nutrition Program for Women, Infants, and Children program. Trained peer counselors are available in some community programs; they frequently work with groups who have low rates of breastfeeding, such as low-income women, teens, and minority women.

■ NUTRITION-RELATED CONCERNS OF WOMEN

Obesity and Weight Management

OBESITY PREVALENCE

Obesity is a serious public health concern in the United States and all of North America. Data from 2011 to 2012 show that 34.9% of adults in the United States are obese with a BMI (kg/m^2) of 30 or more (Ogden, Carroll, Kit, & Flegal, 2013). There were no gender differences in the prevalence of obesity as a whole in 2011 to 2012; however, non-Hispanic Black adult women were more obese compared with non-Hispanic Black men (56.6% vs. 37.1%, respectively; Ogden et al., 2013).

DEFINITION OF OVERWEIGHT AND OBESITY

BMI is calculated by dividing a person's weight in kilograms by height in meters squared. For instance, a woman who is 64 inches (1.63 m) tall and weighs 130 pounds (59 kg) has a BMI of 22.3. The use of BMI eliminates the dependence on body frame size. A limitation of BMI is the use in populations with greater muscle tone, as some would be categorized as overweight or obese because of a muscular build. Health risks from excess weight begin when BMI exceeds 25, called *overweight*. *Obesity* is defined by a BMI of 30 or greater (Table 13.11). Obesity can be further categorized as grade 1 (BMI: 30–34.9), grade 2 (BMI: 35–39.9), and grade 3 (BMI: ≥ 40).

Abdominal obesity may be a better predictor than overall obesity for disease risks and causes of mortality. Waist circumference (WC) is the most common and noninvasive measure of abdominal obesity. When used with BMI, the combination is a predictor for increased risk of type 2 diabetes mellitus, hypertension, and CVD; see Table 13.11 for risk assessments. Trends over time have shown increases in BMI for both men and women; the increase in WC should mirror the BMI increases. For women, WC increased at a greater rate than BMI, equating to a significantly larger increase of 2.4 cm for women compared with a 0.2-cm increase observed in men during the same time frame from 1999 to 2001 and 2011 to 2012 (Freedman & Ford, 2015). The possible reasons are unclear, but it is important to note that for women, observing BMI alone may underestimate obesity and disease risk.

CONSEQUENCES OF OBESITY

Obese adults are at increased mortality risk and the risk grows with each obesity category (Flegal, Kit, Orpana, & Graubard, 2013). Controversy lies when determining who is at the lowest mortality risk, those in the normal-weight or overweight BMI category (Hughes, 2013). It is well known that obesity increases the risk of many chronic diseases such as hypertension, coronary heart disease, diabetes mellitus, stroke, gallbladder disease, osteoarthritis, asthma, sleep apnea, and certain cancers (ovarian, breast, endometrial, and colon). Obese women are more likely to present with reproductive dysfunctions resulting from alterations in the hypothalamic–pituitary–ovarian axis, oocyte quality, and endometrial receptivity (Klenov & Jungheim, 2014). More difficult to measure are the emotional consequences of obesity, such as discrimination, low self-esteem, depression, social rejection, and the use of food for consolation and as a coping mechanism. Many women try a variety of dieting regimens to lose weight, which frequently have short-term success, followed by weight gain, so a cyclical pattern persists with no real change in eating and activity patterns.

ETIOLOGY OF OBESITY

Much of normal weight regulation is genetically determined; increased knowledge of specific genes and other markers related to obesity has increased our understanding

TABLE 13.11	BMI Categories and WC Measurements With Associated Disease Risk			
CATEGORY	**BMI (kg/m^2)**	**OBESITY CATEGORY**	**DISEASE RISK[a] RELATIVE TO NORMAL WEIGHT AND WC**	
			Women 88 cm (35 inches) or Less	**Women > 88 cm (35 inches)**
Underweight	< 18.5			
Normal	18.5–24.9			
Overweight	25.0–29.9		Increased	High
Obese	20.0–34.9	I	High	Very high
	35.0–39.9	II	Very high	Very high
Extremely obese	≥ 40.0	III	Extremely high	Extremely high

BMI, body mass index; WC, waist circumference.
[a]Disease risk for type 2 diabetes, hypertension, and cardiovascular disease.
Source: National Heart, Lung, and Blood Institute (2015).

of the process from a genetic basis. The dramatic increase in obesity in the past few decades, however, can be attributed to interactions between our genes and environmental and lifestyle/behavioral choices. The obesogenic environment, where high-fat, energy-dense foods and large portion sizes are palatable, have a low cost, and are easily available in combination with less work-related physical activity and more sedentary behavior in general, has resulted in an imbalance in which there is greater energy in and less energy out, tipping the scale toward a higher body fat mass (Hill, Wyatt, & Melanson, 2000).

The study of hormonal control of food intake and related obesity is an exciting area with new developments on a regular basis. The discovery of leptin fueled research on the genetic basis of obesity; however, research on the adipokine leptin became more complex with each discovery, and it is now far from where it began as an obesity gene. We now know that obese individuals have high circulating leptin levels; however, the issue presents at the receptor level, where obese individuals are more likely than lean individuals to be leptin resistant. Leptin receptors are located at the arculate nucleus of the hypothalamus, and stimulation of these receptors promotes satiety; however, with leptin resistance in obese individuals the signal for satiety is diminished. Gut-derived hormonal signals are also of interest when examining the etiology of obesity. The hormones cholecystokinin, peptide YY, glucogon-like peptide-1, oxyntomodulin, and incretins are gut-derived hormonal signals that promote satiety. Ghrelin is the only gut-derived signal to stimulate appetite.

It must be remembered that genes provide the susceptibility for obesity but do not actually cause it. Weight gain occurs when more energy is consumed than expended. Therefore dietary and activity patterns are key factors in weight changes. It is easy to overconsume with ready food access at home, school, and work; large portions served in eating establishments; and food tied to many social situations. Decreased physical activity plays an even greater role in excess weight gain, as Americans spend more time in sedentary activities such as watching sports instead of participating in them, in front of the computer, and in cars.

WEIGHT MANAGEMENT

Americans spend billions of dollars each year on a multitude of weight-loss efforts, including diet books, commercial weight-loss programs (some providing food), weight-loss and healthy lifestyles classes, exercise programs and equipment, liquid and powdered meal replacements, drugs, herbal products and supplements, acupuncture, hypnosis, and surgery. Despite the high level of resources spent on various weight-loss efforts, the percentage of Americans who are overweight or obese has plateaued at approximately two thirds of the population. Many weight-loss efforts are not successful over time because they have a single narrow treatment focus, appeal to individuals as a new diet but are too restrictive, do not address needed changes in eating and activity behaviors, and/or do not provide information and support. Furthermore, the individual-focused approach to weight management disregards the obesogenic culture we live in. To fully address the obesity epidemic, the physical and social environment must be adjusted to promote a culture change to one that reflects health and wellness.

Most long-term successful weight-management efforts for the individual are neither fast nor flashy. They work over time because they include modifications in food choices, activity, and lifestyle and often also include social support. Dieting alone rarely addresses the weight problem on a permanent basis; behavioral techniques incorporated with weight loss counseling, are a recommended approach at the individual level to promote sustained weight loss (Seagle, Strain, Makris, Reeves, & American Dietetic Association, 2009). Many women trying to lose weight set ideal goals for themselves that are frequently hard to achieve, thus resulting in disappointment and a sense of failure, which colors future attempts. Weight cycling (losing and gaining weight several times over years) is particularly common in overweight women. Many health professionals recommend a gradual reduction in weight with a focus on healthy lifestyle choices, to a level of better overall health if not slimness (Seagle et al., 2009). Obese individuals, with a 5% to 10% weight loss can benefit from improved risk factors including blood glucose, blood pressure, and lipid levels ("Clinical Guidelines," 1998). What is important to emphasize is weight management and strategies to maintain weight loss once it occurs. After the weight is lost, energy requirements, for most people, are permanently lower (Polsky, Catenacci, Wyatt, & Hill, 2014). A return to dietary behaviors before weight loss results in rapid weight regain. What needs to occur after weight loss is consumption of fewer calories or an increase in physical activity compared with before weight loss (Polsky et al., 2014). James O. Hill attempted to quantify the need for less energy after weight loss (Hill, 2009). It was estimated that to maintain a 10% weight loss in an adult with a starting weight of 100 kg would require a permanent caloric deficit of 170 to 250 kcal/d. To maintain a 20% weight loss in the same individual would require a 325- to 480-kcal/d deficit (Hill, 2009). A dedicated and significant behavior change must be maintained to achieve these daily caloric deficits. Therefore strategies that focus on long-term weight management and larger scale cultural changes are needed. An emphasis on healthy lifestyle choices to promote a daily energy deficit of 500 to 1,000 kcal can result in a weight loss of 1 to 2 pounds/wk, assuming moderate physical activity (Seagle et al., 2009). Overall, a sound weight loss diet should:

- Meet nutritional needs—except for energy
- Allow adaptation to individual habits and tastes (emphasize slow and steady weight loss)
- Minimize hunger and fatigue
- Contain common, readily available foods
- Be socially acceptable and incorporated into family meals
- Help promote regular and healthy eating habits (provide enough energy for regular physical activity)

Exercise is a key component in any successful weight-loss weight-maintenance program. A combination of aerobic and resistance training is optimal. The aerobic exercise helps use fat stores for fuel and has positive cardiovascular effects. Strength training increases resting metabolic rate and lean body mass, as well as improves bone density. Exercise alone, without changing diet, can result in slow weight loss. Other benefits of physical activity include stress reduction, a sense of accomplishment, relief of boredom, increased self-control, and improved sense of well-being. Consistency with the exercise program is important in weight management; the activity should be convenient, affordable, pleasant, and relatively easy to do. Many women find classes and group activities to be supportive and reinforcing, but any activity that a woman enjoys should be encouraged (e.g., walking the dog or gardening).

Lifestyle modification in successful weight-management efforts includes analyzing and modifying behaviors relating to weight gain. The use of self-monitoring, problem solving, stimulus control, and cognitive restructuring help implement these changes (Gee, Mahan, & Escott-Stump, 2008). Examples include:

■ Self-monitoring—recording the what, where, and when of food intake, as well as feelings and actions affecting eating, helps identify the settings where eating occurs and the antecedents.
■ Problem solving—defining the eating or weight problem, considering possible solutions, and choosing one to implement, evaluating the outcome, reimplementing that one or trying another, and reevaluating.
■ Stimulus control—altering the environment to minimize the stimuli for eating (e.g., storing food out of sight in the kitchen, slowing the pace of eating by putting down the utensils between bites, avoiding the purchase of "problem" foods).
■ Cognitive restructuring—helping identify and correct the negative thoughts that undermine weight-management efforts. For example, instead of overeating when angry, call a friend or go for a walk; rather than considering a dietary lapse as "blowing my diet," use positive self-talk to continue healthy eating.

Many Americans use commercial weight-loss programs, including Internet-based programs. Some include meal replacement formulas instead of, or with, food. The diets used are generally well balanced, but each program has different components, such as behavior modification and group sessions. In addition, there are always new popular diets in the media—the dietary approach may vary from appropriate to unhealthy. Diets promising fast results with little effort are appealing to those who are overweight but usually have unrealistic expectations and result in feelings of failure. Consumers should be helped to evaluate these popular diets (Gee et al., 2008).

Cardiovascular Disease

Heart disease is the leading cause of death for women in the United States, accounting for one in every four female deaths (Kochanek, Xu, Murphy, Minino, & Kung, 2011), whereas one in three women have some form of CVD (Go et al., 2013). Heart disease is historically thought of as a "man's disease," although nearly the same number of men and women die each year of heart disease in the United States. Much advocacy is placed on heart disease education and prevention for women;

however, only 54% of women recognize that heart disease is their number 1 killer (Mosca, Mochari-Greenberger, Dolor, Newby, & Robb, 2010). The success of other campaigns, such as breast cancer awareness, is partly due to the high rate of survivors who can further support the need for education, early detection, and awareness. The typical onset of heart disease in women is in later years, and the outcome is debilitating or fatal. The risk factors for CVD in women are listed in Table 13.12. Many of these are diet related; most are modifiable by changes in lifestyle. A consensus statement from the American Heart Association provides guidelines for

TABLE 13.12	Classification of CVD Risk in Women
RISK STATUS	**CRITERIA**
High risk (≥ 1 high-risk states)	Clinically manifested CHD
	Clinically manifested cerebrovascular disease
	Clinically manifested peripheral arterial disease
	Abdominal aortic aneurysm
	End-stage or chronic kidney disease
	Diabetes mellitus
	10-year predicted CVD risk ≥ 10%
At risk (> 1 major risk factor)	Cigarette smoking
	SBP > 120 mmHg, DBP > 80 mmHg, or treated HTN
	Total cholesterol > 200 mg/dL, HDL-C < 50 mg/dL, or treated dyslipidemia
	Obesity, particularly central adiposity
	Poor diet
	Physical inactivity
	Family history of premature CVD occurring in first-degree relatives in men < 55 years of age or women < 65 years of age
	Metabolic syndrome
	Evidence of advanced subclinical atherosclerosis
	Poor exercise capacity on treadmill test and/ or abnormal heart recovery after stopping exercise
	Systemic autoimmune collagen-vascular disease (e.g., lupus or rheumatoid arthritis)
	History of preeclampsia, gestational diabetes, or pregnancy-induced hypertension

CHD, coronary heart disease; CVD, cardiovascular disease; DBP, diastolic blood pressure; HDL-C, high density lipoprotein cholesterol; HTN, hypertension; SBP, systolic blood pressure.

preventing CVD in women, including lifestyle factors such as smoking cessation, increased physical activity, dietary intake, weight maintenance and reduction, consumption of omega-3 fatty acids, and stress management (Mosca et al., 2011). See Table 13.13 for specific dietary recommendations.

Osteoporosis

Osteoporosis is a bone disease characterized by low bone strength, predisposing a person to increased risk of fracture. Bone strength reflects the combination of bone density and bone quality. Women are more likely than men to develop the condition, but the prevalence of men with osteoporosis is rising as the male life expectancy increases. The gold standard for bone measurement is dual-energy x-ray absorptiometry (DEXA), which measures body mass to determine bone mineral density (BMD). Osteoporosis is clinically defined as BMD greater than 2.5 standard deviations below the mean peak bone mass in young women for a reference group. *Low bone mass* is defined as a BMD between 1 and 2.5 standard deviations below the mean peak value in young women. Although osteoporosis is a disease of the aging process, the origins develop during the early years of skeletal development and peak bone mass accumulation in childhood and puberty. National surveys indicate that approximately 44 million Americans, mostly women, are affected

by osteoporosis or low bone mass; this number represents 55% of adults older than 50 years (National Osteoporosis Foundation, 2011). Subsequent fracture costs billions in health care dollars. A study of 2002 Medicare data found that fractures cost $14 billion and $2 billion for osteoporotic drug treatment and management (Blume & Curtis, 2011). Nonfinancial losses include requirement of long-term medical care, decreased mobility, and independence, and death.

Osteoporosis can be prevented or delayed by maximizing peak bone mass in the first three decades of life and establishing positive dietary and exercise habits that can sustain the natural bone changes of menopause and aging (American Dietetic Association, 2004). Many nutrients or food components, especially calcium and vitamin D, are linked to bone health. Magnesium, potassium, and vitamin K are also known to have a clearly protective effect on bone health. Nutrients that are likely to have a positive effect on bone health include silicon, strontium, vitamin C, vitamin E, vitamin B_{12}, vitamin B_6, folate, carotenoids, and protein. Omega-3 fatty acids are likely to be beneficial for bone health; however, Mechanistic understanding and conclusive studies remain elusive. Possible negative effects on bone health may be observed with high intakes of sodium, phosphorus, iron, fluoride, and vitamin A (Tucker & Rosen, 2014). Excessive alcohol intake also increases the risk of osteoporosis. It shifts the calcium balance in a negative direction, especially if there is a low dietary intake of calcium.

TABLE 13.13	Specific Dietary Intake Recommendations for Women	
NUTRIENT	**SERVING**	**SERVING SIZE**
Fruits and vegetables	≥ 4.5 cups/d	1 cup raw leafy vegetable, ½ cup cut-up raw or cooked vegetable, ½ cup vegetable juice, 1 medium fruit, ¼ cup dried fruit, ½ cup fresh, frozen or canned fruit, ½ cup fruit juice
Fish	2/wk	3.5 oz, cooked (preferably oily) types of fish
Fiber	30 g/d (1.1 g/10g carbohydrate	Bran cereal, berries, avocado, and so on
Whole grains	3/d	1 slice bread, 1 oz dry cereal, ½ cup cooked rice, pasta, or cereal (all whole-grain products)
Sugar	≤ 5/wk (≤ 450 kcal/wk from sugar sweetened beverages)	1 tablespoon sugar, 1 tablespoon jelly or jam, ½ cup sorbet, 1 cup lemonade
Nuts, legumes and seeds	≥ 4/wk	⅓ cup or 1½ oz nuts (avoid macadamia nuts and salted nuts), 2 tablespoons peanut butter, 2 tablespoons or ½ oz seeds, ½ cup cooked legumes (dry beans or peas)
Saturated fat	< 7% total energy intake	Found in fried foods, fat on meat or chicken skin, packaged desserts, butter, cheese, sour cream, and so on
Cholesterol	< 150 mg/d	Found in animal meats, organ meats, eggs, and so on
Alcohol	≤ 1/d	4 oz wine, 12 oz beer, 1.5 oz 80-proof spirits, or 1 oz 100-proof spirits
Sodium	< 1,500 mg/d	
Trans fatty acids	0	0

Note: The recommended serving amounts are based on a 2,000-kcal diet, and recommendations vary according to individual preference and needs (Lichtenstein et al., 2006).
Note for vitamin D: It is expected that ongoing research regarding the role of vitamin D supplementation in the prevention of cardiovascular disease will shed further light on this issue for future versions of this guideline (Institute of Medicine, 2011).

Optimum calcium intake is essential for bone health in postmenopausal women. Since hormone therapy is currently not indicated for most postmenopausal women, diet becomes more critical. The DRI for calcium increases from 1,000 to 1,200 mg/d for those older than 50 years (Table 13.3). For many women, this level of calcium intake cannot be achieved with diet alone, so supplements are needed. Although calcium supplementation does not have much effect on BMD in the first few years of menopause, it does slow bone loss in the late postmenopausal period (Heaney & Weaver, 2005). Food sources to emphasize include low-fat dairy products, small or canned fish with edible bones, calcium-set tofu, and fortified nondairy milk or juice products. Vitamin D supplementation in combination with calcium is considered the favored dietary treatment for preventing BMD loss and reducing risk of fracture in older adults (Tang, Eslick, Nowson, Smith, & Bensoussan, 2007).

Adequate vitamin D is required for normal bone metabolism because it is integral to calcium absorption. Older persons are more at risk for vitamin D deficiency because their skin is less able to convert sunshine exposure to vitamin D and because there is less exposure for those confined indoors or living in northern climates. Most studies show positive benefits from vitamin D intake. The recommended amounts of this nutrient are increased for older women (see Table 13.3). Epidemiological trials found that a vitamin D intake of 700 to 800 IU can promote a 26% risk reduction in hip fracture and a 23% risk reduction of nonverterbral fractures in adults over age 60 (Bischoff-Ferrari et al., 2005).

Eating Disorders

EDs, which include anorexia nervosa (AN), bulimia nervosa (BN), binge-eating disorder (BED), other specified feeding disorders or EDs, and other unspecified feeding disorders or EDs, are psychiatric and medical conditions described in the *Diagnostic and Statistical Manual of Mental Disorders* (5th ed.; *DSM-5*; American Psychiatric Association [APA], 2013). These conditions are characterized by eating- and feeding-related behavior that results in altered consumption or absorption of food with significant physical and psychosocial consequences (APA & APA *DSM-5* Task Force, 2013). Prevalence of EDs is far more common in females than males with approximately a 10:1 female:male ratio (APA & APA *DSM-5* Task Force, 2013). Most ED onsets occur during adolescence or young adulthood and are more frequently reported in athletes (Ozier, Henry, & American Dietetic Association, 2011). Weight preoccupation, food control, and psychological vulnerability are hallmarks of EDs. Although AN and BN have been identified and treated for many decades, the range of EDs to include recurrent binge eating indicates a wider spectrum. See Table 13.14 for diagnostic criteria for ED.

An ED may be undiagnosed for some time because of the secretive behaviors and sensitive nature of the diseases. Risk factors that may precede diagnosis include female gender, ethnicity, early childhood eating and GI problems, extreme weight and shape concerns, negative self-evaluation, sexual abuse and other traumas, and general psychiatric morbidity (Jacobi, Hayward, de Zwaan, Kraemer, & Agras, 2004). The age of an ED patient is linked to the subclass. The onset of AN is typically during adolescence, but there is an emergence of late onset AN in middle-aged women (Malatesta, 2007). BN can be first observed in adolescence but can continue into adulthood (Ozier et al., 2011). The lifetime prevalence of AN, as characterized in the *DSM-5*, is approximately 1.2% to 2.2% in women and 0.2% in men. The BM prevalence is approximately 0.9% to 2.9% for women and 0.1% to 0.5% for men. The lifetime prevalence of BED is higher at approximately 1.9% to 3.6% among women and 0.3% to 2.0% for men (Smink, van Hoeken, & Hoek, 2012).

ETIOLOGY AND MEDICAL COMPLICATIONS

The etiology of EDs is thought to cover three domains: genetic/biological, psychological, and socioenvironmental; those with a biological predisposition are often triggered by an environmental factor (Bakalar, Shank, Vannucci, Radin, & Tanofsky-Kraff, 2015).

ANOREXIA NERVOSA

A genetic component for AN is indicated by the observation that the disorder is much more common in pairs of identical twins than in pairs of fraternal twins. It is well documented that there is a disturbance in the hypothalamic–anterior pituitary–gonadal axis, but this is likely secondary to malnutrition. The chronic dieting appears to trigger a continuous weight loss and hypometabolic adaptation in vulnerable individuals, leading to a vicious cycle that becomes self-perpetuating.

The medical complications relate primarily to the progressive starvation. These include protein-energy malnutrition, hypoproteinemia, hypokalemia, decreased gastric motility, hypotension, arrested growth, and prolonged reduction of estrogen, which leads to low bone mass and osteoporosis (Ozier et al., 2011). In children and adolescents, normal growth and development may be compromised by pubertal delay, reduction in peak bone mass, and brain abnormalities (Ozier et al., 2011). Serious electrolyte imbalances can occur when vomiting, laxative, or diuretic abuse is present. Muscular weakness, cardiac arrhythmias, and renal impairment may occur. These complications can lead to cardiac and renal damage or to sudden death.

BULIMIA NERVOSA

The etiology theories for BN include addiction, family dysfunction, and cognitive behavioral, sociocultural, and psychodynamic factors (Schebendach, 2008). Depending on the model, different treatment strategies are emphasized. The onset of this disorder is most often seen in the late teens or early 20s, when young women leave home to attend college or to join the workforce. This transitional time in life appears to be a high-risk period for the development of problematic eating behaviors. Since persons with BN are usually in a normal weight range and they are also very secretive, symptoms are more difficult to detect. Most of the medical complications are a result of the inappropriate compensatory behaviors used to counter the binge eating—self-induced vomiting and excessive use of laxatives, diuretics, and enemas.

TABLE 13.14	Diagnostic Criteria for Eating Disorders

Anorexia Nervosa (AN)

A. Restriction of energy intake relative to requirements, leading to a significantly low body weight in the context of age, sex, developmental trajectory, and physical health. *Significantly low weight* is defined as a weight that is less than minimally normal or, for children and adolescents, less than that minimally expected.

B. Intense fear of gaining weight or of becoming fat, or persistent behavior that interferes with weight gain, even though at a significantly low weight.

C. Disturbance in the way in which one's body weight or shape is experienced, undue influence of body weight or shape on self-evaluation, or persistent lack of recognition of the seriousness of the current low body weight.

Coding note: The *ICD-9-CM* code for anorexia nervosa is **307.1**, which is assigned regardless of the subtype. The *ICD-10-CM* code depends on the subtype (see below).

Specify whether:

(F50.01) Restricting type: During the past 3 months, the individual has not engaged in recurrent episodes of binge eating or purging behavior (i.e., self-induced vomiting or the misuse of laxatives, diuretics, or enemas). This subtype describes presentations in which weight loss is accomplished primarily through dieting, fasting, and/or excessive exercise.

(F50.02) Binge-eating/purging type: During the past 3 months, the individual has engaged in recurrent episodes of binge eating or purging behavior (i.e., self-induced vomiting or the misuse of laxatives, diuretics, or enemas).

Specify if:

In partial remission: After full criteria for anorexia nervosa were previously met, Criterion A (low body weight) has not been met for a sustained period, but either Criterion B (intense fear of gaining weight or becoming fat or behavior that interferes with weight gain) or Criterion C (disturbances in self-perception of weight and shape) is still met.

In full remission: After full criteria for anorexia nervosa were previously met, none of the criteria have been met for a sustained period of time.

Specify current severity:

The minimum level of severity is based, for adults, on current body mass index (BM) (see below) or, for children and adolescents, on BMI percentile. The ranges below are derived from World Health Organization categories for thinness in adults; for children and adolescents, corresponding BMI percentiles should be used. The level of severity may be increased to reflect clinical symptoms, the degree of functional disability, and the need for supervision.

Mild: BMI $\geq$ 17 kg/m^2
Moderate: BMI 16–16.99 kg/m^2
Severe: BMI 15–15.99 kg/m^2
Extreme: BMI < 15 kg/m^2

Bulimia Nervosa (BN)

A. Recurrent episodes of binge eating. An episode of binge eating is characterized by both of the following:

1. Eating, in a discrete period of time (e.g., within any 2-hour period), an amount of food that is definitely larger than what most individuals would eat in a similar period of time under similar circumstances.

2. A sense of lack of control over eating during the episode (e.g., a feeling that one cannot stop eating or control what or how much one is eating).

B. Recurrent inappropriate compensatory behaviors in order to prevent weight gain, such as self-induced vomiting; misuse of laxatives, diuretics, or other medications; fasting; or excessive exercise.

C. The binge eating and inappropriate compensatory behaviors both occur, on average, at least once a week for 3 months.

D. Self-evaluation is unduly influenced by body shape and weight.

E. The disturbance does not occur exclusively during episodes of anorexia nervosa.

Specify if:

In partial remission: After full criteria for bulimia nervosa were previously met, some, but not all, of the criteria have been met for a sustained period of time.

In full remission: After full criteria for bulimia nervosa were previously met, none of the criteria have been met for a sustained period of time.

Specify current severity:

The minimum level of severity is based on the frequency of inappropriate compensatory behaviors (see below). The level of severity may be increased to reflect other symptoms and the degree of functional disability.

Mild: An average of 1–3 episodes of inappropriate compensatory behaviors per week
Moderate: An average of 4–7 episodes of inappropriate compensatory behaviors per week
Severe: An average of 8–13 episodes of inappropriate compensatory behaviors per week
Extreme: An average of 14 or mare episodes of inappropriate compensatory behaviors per week

(continued)

TABLE 13.14	Diagnostic Criteria for Eating Disorders *(continued)*

Binge-Eating Disorder

A. Recurrent episodes of binge eating. An episode of binge eating is characterized by both of the following:
   1. Eating, in a discrete period of time (e.g., within any 2-hour period), an amount of food that is definitely larger than what most people would eat in a similar period of time under similar circumstances.
   2. A sense of lack of control over eating during the episode (e.g., a feeling that one cannot stop eating or control what or how much one is eating).
B. The binge-eating episodes are associated with three (or more) of the following:
   1. Eating much more rapidly than normal.
   2. Eating until feeling uncomfortably full.
   3. Eating large amounts of food when not feeling physically hungry.
   4. Eating alone because of feeling embarrassed by how much one is eating.
   5. Feeling disgusted with oneself, depressed, or very guilty afterward.
C. Marked distress regarding binge eating is present.
D. The binge eating occurs, on average, at least once a week for 3 months.
E. The binge eating is not associated with the recurrent use of inappropriate compensatory behavior as in bulimia nervosa and does not occur exclusively during the course of bulimia nervosa or anorexia nervosa.

Specify if:
   In partial remission: After full criteria for binge-eating disorder were previously met, binge eating occurs at an average frequency of less than one episode per week for a sustained period of time.
   In full remission: After full criteria for binge-eating disorder were previously met, none of the criteria have been met for a sustained period of time.

Specify current severity:
The minimum level of severity is based on the frequency of episodes of binge eating (see below). The level of severity may be increased to reflect other symptoms and the degree of functional disability.
   Mild: 1–3 binge-eating episodes per week
   Moderate: 4–7 binge-eating episodes per week
   Severe: 8–13 binge-eating episodes per week
   Extreme: 14 or more binge-eating episodes per week

Other Specified Feeding or Eating Disorder

This category applies to presentations in which symptoms characteristic of a feeding and eating disorder that cause clinically significant distress or impairment in social, occupational, or other important areas of functioning predominate but do not meet the full criteria for any of the disorders in the feeding and eating disorders diagnostic class. The other specified feeding or eating disorder category is used in situations in which the clinician chooses to communicate the specific reason that the presentation does not meet the criteria for any specific feeding and eating disorder. This is done by recording "other specified feeding or eating disorder" followed by the specific reason (e.g., "bulimia nervosa of low frequency").
   Examples of presentations that can be specified using the "other specified" designation include the following:
   1. **Atypical anorexia nervosa:** All of the criteria for anorexia nervosa are met, except that despite significant weight loss, the individual's weight is within or above the normal range.
   2. **Bulimia nervosa (of low frequency and/or limited duration):** All of the criteria for bulimia nervosa are met, except that the binge eating and inappropriate compensatory behaviors occur, on average, less than once a week and/or for less than 3 months.
   3. **Binge-eating disorder (of low frequency and/or limited duration):** All of the criteria for binge-eating disorder are met, except that the binge eating occurs, on average, less than once a week and/or for less than 3 months.
   4. **Purging disorder:** Recurrent purging behavior to influence weight or shape (e.g., self-induced vomiting; misuse of laxatives, diuretics, or other medications) in the absence of binge eating.
   5. **Night eating syndrome:** Recurrent episodes of night eating, as manifested by eating after awakening from sleep or by excessive food consumption after the evening meal. There is awareness and recall of the eating. The night eating is not better explained by external influences such as changes in the individual's sleep-wake cycle or by local social norms. The night eating causes significant distress and/or impairment in functioning. The disordered pattern of eating is not better explained by binge-eating disorder or another mental disorder, including substance use, and is not attributable to another medical disorder or to an effect of medication.

Unspecified Feeding or Eating Disorder

This category applies to presentations in which symptoms characteristic of a feeding and eating disorder that cause clinically significant distress or impairment in social, occupational, or other important areas of functioning predominate but do not meet the full criteria for any of the disorders in the feeding and eating disorders diagnostic class. The unspecified feeding and eating disorder category is used in situations in which the clinician chooses *not* to specify the reason that the criteria are not met for a specific feeding and eating disorder, and includes presentations in which there is insufficient information to make a more specific diagnosis (e.g., in emergency room settings).

INTERVENTION FOR EDs

Persons with EDs are best served by interdisciplinary teams, which include primary care providers, nutritionists, and psychotherapists. These teams should be trained and experienced in working with this population. Settings may include outpatient, day treatment, or psychiatric units; for some patients with AN, a crisis medical state may warrant hospitalization and nutritional rehabilitation, including tube feeding.

NUTRITION ASSESSMENT AND INTERVENTION

In addition to the standard diet history, anthropometric (height, weight, and BMI) indices, and biochemical data, the nutrition assessment (by a specially trained dietitian) should include eating, weight, and body shape attitudes and behaviors, as well as an assessment of behavioral–environmental symptoms such as food restriction, binging, preoccupation, rituals, secretive eating, affect and impulse control, vomiting, other purging, and/or excessive exercise (Ozier et al., 2011). Reported energy intakes may be less than 1,000 kcal/d in young women with AN; caloric intake of those with BN is quite varied. Because of the often limited quantity and variety of food consumed, attention must be given to nutrient adequacy (macronutrients and micronutrients) and fluid and electrolyte balance. Taking the time to determine attitudes, beliefs, and behaviors regarding food and eating is essential to developing appropriate nutrition education and therapy objectives. Some red flags to look for include:

■ Avoidance of certain foods or food groups (e.g., animal foods, all fats, sweets)
■ Preoccupation with food and calorie content
■ Strictly grouping foods as "good" or "bad"
■ Ritualistic eating schedules, preparation, and timing and misconceptions regarding usual portion sizes
■ Certain foods that can trigger a binge episode

Nutrition therapy for AN initially focuses on refeeding to promote a positive energy balance and eventual weight gain. Increments of the caloric prescription are increased slowly, and weight gain goals may be as modest as 1 to 2 lb/wk, with emphasis placed on mutual goal setting between patient and practitioner. The dietary plan should address diet quality, variety of foods consumed, perceptions of hunger and satiety, and potential need for dietary supplements. Psychosocial support and positive reinforcement from caregivers are also essential components of the care plan for individuals with EDs.

For patients with BN, nutrition therapy depends on current weight status. For someone trying to lose weight, a diet plan that does not promote weight gain yet stimulates increased metabolic rate is appropriate. A balanced diet providing DRI of vitamins and minerals eaten at regular meals and snacks will begin to address the cycling periods of restrained eating and binging. The use of self-monitoring techniques, such as keeping a food diary, can sometimes provide a sense of control over eating and help avoid binging. As with other ED patients, mutual goal setting, psychosocial support, and positive reinforcement are important components of the care plan. From the counseling theory standpoint, an approach incorporating cognitive behavioral therapy, interpersonal psychotherapy, or dialectical behavior therapy can be helpful in challenging the erroneous beliefs and thought processes of the person with EDs (Ozier et al., 2011).

Nutrition education, combined with psychotherapy, is key in addressing the long-term outcomes of EDs. The specific nutrition therapy will work best when there is a collaborative relationship between the patient and the nutritionist. Helping the patient separate the food and weight issues from the psychological issues will help ensure more cooperation and progress. Although many of these patients appear to be knowledgeable about nutrition, they have many misconceptions. Nutrition education sessions can include metabolism, energy expenditure, nutrient and energy values of foods, and other topics, but using abstract thinking and a problem-solving process.

MONITORING AND OUTCOME

Regular and ongoing monitoring by appropriate team members is important in the care of ED patients, as these disorders tend to be chronic conditions. Outcome criteria include appropriate weight for height; adequate and balanced food intake; regular menses; realistic understanding of food, weight, and shape; and improved psychological adjustment. Therapy can last for years. Follow-up studies indicate that one third of persons with AN recover fully and the remaining demonstrate lifelong problems with disordered eating (APA, 2006). Although early identification and treatment have significantly reduced mortality from EDs, this population is vulnerable to relapse.

EDs IN PREGNANCY

If a women with a past or lifelong ED becomes pregnant, the health care team needs to screen for signs of active behaviors or depression throughout the pregnancy and postpartum. Postnatal depression is high in women with a history of or a lifelong ED, averaging over 30% (Micali, 2010). Conception and a healthy pregnancy are often a challenge for those with a history of an ED, particularly AN when amenorrhea was long standing. For active BN patients, conception carries an increased risk of miscarriage by two thirds (Micali, 2010). Women with binge-eating disorder who become pregnant are also at higher risk for large-for-gestational-age babies and cesarean section births (Worley et al., 2015). If a woman is able to conceive, the pregnancy is considered high risk because of the psychiatric history. Much emphasis must be placed on appropriate food choices to promote healthy weight gain during pregnancy and a return to a healthy weight after birth while paying sensitive attention to body image issues. Assessment should include questions relating to body weight, eating behaviors, and weight-control behaviors on a regular basis, especially early in pregnancy (Micali, 2010). Recommended assessment questions for pregnant women with a history of EDs can be found in Table 13.15. It is advised for the patient to have regular care visits with a nutritionist specializing in EDs. An interdisciplinary health care team of nurses, obstetricians, and registered dietitians is essential in promoting a healthy pregnancy. Additional prenatal visits are also warranted to closely monitor the growth of the fetus, especially in women with an active or a significant history of AN. Babies of women with active or lifelong AN are more likely to have lower birth weight (Micali,

TABLE 13.15	Antenatal and Neonatal Guidelines, Education, and Learning System (2015)

Screening pregnant women for eating disorders
Assessment questions:

- Ask patients if they have a current/active, past, or lifelong eating disorder
- Ask patients if they have a previous history of amenorrhea or oligomenorrhea
- Determine the patient's BMI category (and educate as needed throughout pregnancy)
- Ask patients about their current views on body weight, shape, and changes resulting from pregnancy
- Ask patients about current dietary and weight-management practices including
  - Does she make herself vomit because she feels uncomfortably full?
  - Does she worry about loss of control over how much she eats?
  - Does she believe she is too fat while others say she is too thin?

BMI, body mass index.
Source: Worley, et al. (2003).

Simonoff, & Treasure, 2007). Postpartum follow-up is also particularly important, as women with active or lifetime EDs often can see an improvement of symptoms during pregnancy but can have severe re-emergence of symptoms postpartum (Worley et al., 2015).

■ NUTRITION AND HEALTH PROMOTION

Nutrition and dietary factors are associated with the major causes of morbidity and mortality in U.S. women; hence, it makes sense that nutrition is a key component of health promotion and disease-prevention efforts. The role of nutrition and diet in promoting health and reducing chronic diseases is documented for many conditions, including diabetes mellitus, CVDs, and some cancers, and for the prevention of LBW (Fitzgerald, Morgan, & Slawson, 2013; Slawson, Fitzgerald, & Morgan, 2013). The national prevention agenda, *Healthy People* (originally published in 1979) is updated each decade with specific health objectives based on priority areas. *Healthy People 2020* includes a variety of health topics; one specific topic is Nutrition and Weight Status with 22 specific nutrition objectives, some with subobjectives to address different age groups. The goal is to meet the stated measurable objectives by the year 2020. See Box 13.2 for a list of the *Healthy People 2020* Nutrition and Weight Status objectives. The topic of Nutrition and Weight Status is of utmost importance to the health of the nation, so it is included as one of the LHIs (Office of Disease Prevention and Health Promotion, 2015a).

Nutrition can be applied to the three levels of disease prevention: primary prevention (aimed at disease risk factors), secondary prevention (screening to detect risk followed by early intervention), and tertiary prevention (treatment and rehabilitation for identified health conditions) (Fitzgerald et al., 2013). An example of primary nutrition prevention is the 5 A Day Program, an education program to encourage people to eat a minimum of five servings of fruits and

vegetables a day. Blood pressure screenings and the Dietary Approaches to Stop Hypertension (DASH) nutrition education program are examples of secondary prevention programs for individuals at risk for hypertension. The DASH diet is high in fruits and vegetables and low in saturated and total fat, with moderate intakes of low-fat dairy. The DASH diet can also be considered a primary prevention for the broad population as well as part of a medical management program for those with identified hypertension. More recent studies have also identified the DASH diet as one that may delay cognitive decline in older adults (Tangney et al., 2014).

The *Dietary Guidelines for Americans* are the current national recommendations for dietary guidance for which nutritional health promotion programs are based upon. The U.S. DHHS and USDA have jointly published the *Dietary Guidelines* every 5 years since 1990 under the National Monitoring and Related Research Act (Public Law 101-445). The *Dietary Guidelines* are based on current scientific and medical knowledge. Current knowledge shows the importance of healthy eating patterns and regular physical activity for good health and for chronic disease risk reduction (U.S. Department of Agriculture & U.S. Department of Health and Human Services, 2015). The *2015–2020 Dietary Guidelines* provides five guidelines followed by recommendations for how individuals can follow the guidelines. (See Box 13.3 for the guidelines and recommendations.) The *2015–2020 Dietary Guidelines* focuses on consumption of a healthy eating pattern within daily caloric needs. To achieve this, choosing foods that are nutrient dense is advised. Nutrient-dense food is one in which the nutrients and other beneficial substances have not been diluted by added solid fats, sugars, or refined starches, or by the solid fats naturally present in the food. Vegetables, fruits, whole grains, seafood, eggs, beans and peas, unsalted nuts and seeds, fat-free and low-fat dairy products, and lean meats and poultry—when prepared with little or no added salt, sugars or fats, or refined starches—are nutrient dense (U.S. Department of Agriculture & U.S. Department of Health and Human Services, 2015).

The *2015–2020 Dietary Guidelines* are in support of a DASH dietary plan or a Mediterranean diet plan. Both diet plans have been associated with positive health outcomes. The USDA also launched the MyPlate campaign with the *2010 Dietary Guidelines for Americans*. The MyPlate icon and message replaced the Food Guide Pyramid, which was active for nearly 20 years from 1992 to 2011. The MyPlate system emphasizes dietary variety from all food groups and portion control using a plate icon to serve as a reminder of healthy eating, but not intended to provide specific messages (Center for Nutrition Policy and Promotion, 2011).

The differing approaches to meet guidelines and recommendations set forth by the DHHS and USDA in the *Dietary Guidelines for Americans* demonstrates the importance of individualized nutrition assessment and plans based on cultural practices and personal preference. Registered dietitians (RDs) as part of a health care team are best suited for developing specific plans with patients and clients to meet health and medical needs. Interprofessional collaborations and communication among RDs, nurses, physicians, and other health care professionals (speech language pathologists, physical therapists, athletic trainers, and/or occupational

BOX 13.2   *HEALTHY PEOPLE 2020* OBJECTIVES FOR THE NUTRITION AND WEIGHT STATUS (NWS) TOPIC

Healthier Food Access

NWS-1   Increase the number of states with nutrition standards for food and beverages provided to preschool-age children in child care

NWS-2   Increase the proportion of schools that offer nutritious foods and beverages outside of school meals

NWS-2.1   Increase the proportion of schools that do not sell or offer calorically sweetened beverages to students

NWS-2.2   Increase the proportion of school districts that require schools to make fruits or vegetables available whenever other food is offered or sold

NWS-3   Increase the number of states that have state-level policies that incentivize food retail outlets to provide foods that are encouraged by the *Dietary Guidelines for Americans*

NWS-4   (Developmental) Increase the proportion of Americans who have access to a food retail outlet that sells a variety of foods that are encouraged by the Dietary Guidelines for Americans

Health Care and Worksite Settings

NWS-5   Increase the proportion of primary care physicians who regularly measure the body mass index of their patients

NWS-5.1   Increase the proportion of primary care physicians who regularly assess BMI in their adult patients

NWS-5.2   Increase the proportion of primary care physicians who regularly assess BMI for age and sex in their child or adolescent patients

NWS-6   Increase the proportion of physician office visits that include counseling or education related to nutrition or weight

NWS-6.1   Increase the proportion of physician office visits made by patients with a diagnosis of cardiovascular disease, diabetes, or hyperlipidemia that include counseling or education related to diet or nutrition

NWS-6.2   Increase the proportion of physician office visits made by adult patients who are obese that include counseling or education related to weight reduction, nutrition, or physical activity

NWS-6.3   Increase the proportion of physician office visits made by all child or adult patients that include counseling about nutrition or diet

NWS-7   (Developmental) Increase the proportion of worksites that offer nutrition or weight management classes or counseling

Weight Status

NWS-8   Increase the proportion of adults who are at a healthy weight

NWS-9   Reduce the proportion of adults who are obese

NWS-10   Reduce the proportion of children and adolescents who are considered obese

NWS-10.1   Reduce the proportion of children aged 2–5 years who are considered obese

NWS-10.2   Reduce the proportion of children aged 6–11 years who are considered obese

NWS-10.3   Reduce the proportion of adolescents aged 12–19 years who are considered obese

NWS-10.4   Reduce the proportion of children and adolescents aged 2–19 years who are considered obese

NWS-11   (Developmental) Prevent inappropriate weight gain in youth and adults

NWS-11.1   (Developmental) Prevent inappropriate weight gain in children aged 2–5 years

NWS-11.2   (Developmental) Prevent inappropriate weight gain in children aged 6 to 11 years

NWS-11.3   (Developmental) Prevent inappropriate weight gain in adolescents aged 12–19 years

NWS-11.4   (Developmental) Prevent inappropriate weight gain in children and adolescents aged 2–19 years

NWS-11.5   (Developmental) Prevent inappropriate weight gain in adults aged 20 years and older

Food Insecurity

NWS-12   Eliminate very low food security among children

NWS-13   Reduce household food insecurity and in doing so reduce hunger

Food and Nutrient Consumption

NWS-14   Increase the contribution of fruits to the diets of the population aged 2 years and older

(continued)

NWS-15	Increase the variety and contribution of vegetables to the diets of the population aged 2 years and older
NWS-15.1	Increase the contribution of total vegetables to the diets of the population aged 2 years and older
NWS-15.2	Increase the contribution of dark green vegetables, red and orange vegetables, and beans and peas to the diets of the population aged 2 years and older
NWS-16	Increase the contribution of whole grains to the diets of the population aged 2 years and older
NWS-17	Reduce consumption of calories from solid fats and added sugars in the population aged 2 years and older
NWS-17.1	Reduce consumption of calories from solid fats
NWS-17.2	Reduce consumption of calories from added sugars
NWS-17.3	Reduce consumption of calories from solid fats and added sugars

NWS-18	Reduce consumption of saturated fat in the population aged 2 years and older
NWS-19	Reduce consumption of sodium in the population aged 2 years and older
NWS-20	Increase consumption of calcium in the population aged 2 years and older

Iron Deficiency

NWS-21	Reduce iron deficiency among young children and females of childbearing age
NWS-21.1	Reduce iron deficiency among children aged 1–2 years
NWS-21.2	Reduce iron deficiency among children aged 3–4 years
NWS-21.3	Reduce iron deficiency among females aged 12–49 years
NWS-22	Reduce iron deficiency among pregnant females

BMI, body mass index.

BOX 13.3 *DIETARY GUIDELINES FOR AMERICANS, 2010: KEY RECOMMENDATIONS*

Balancing Calories to Manage Weight

- Prevent and/or reduce overweight and obesity through improved eating and physical activity behaviors
- Control total calorie intake to manage body weight. For people who are overweight or obese, this will mean consuming fewer calories from foods and beverages
- Increase physical activity and reduce time spent in sedentary behaviors

Foods and Food Components to Reduce

- Reduce daily sodium intake to less than 2,300 mg and further reduce intake to 1,500 mg among persons who are 51 years and older and those of any age who are African Americans or have hypertension, diabetes, or chronic kidney disease. The 1,500 mg recommendation applies to about half of the U.S. population, including children and the majority of adults
- Consume less than 10% of calories from saturated fatty acids by replacing them with monounsaturated and polyunsaturated fatty acids
- Consume less than 300 mg/d of dietary cholesterol
- Keep trans fatty acid composition as low as possible by limiting foods that contain synthetic sources of trans fats, such as partially hydrogenated oils, and by limiting other solid fats
- Reduce the intake of calories from solid fats and added sugars
- Limit the consumption of foods that contain refined grains, especially refined grain foods that contain solid fats, added sugars, and sodium
- If alcohol is consumed, it should be consumed in moderation—up to one drink per day for women and two drinks per day for men—and only by adults of legal drinking age

Foods and Nutrients to Increase

Individuals should meet the following recommendations as part of a healthy eating pattern while staying within their caloric needs.

- Increase vegetable and fruit intake
- Eat a variety of vegetables, especially dark-green and red and orange vegetables and beans and peas
- Consume at least half of all grains as whole grains. Increase whole-grain intake by replacing refined grains with whole grains
- Increase intake of fat-free or low-fat milk and milk products, such as milk, yogurt, cheese, or fortified soy beverages

(continued)

- Choose a variety of protein foods, which include seafood, lean meat and poultry, eggs, beans and peas, soy products, and unsalted nuts and seeds
- Increase the amount and variety of seafood consumed by choosing seafood in place of some meat and poultry
- Replace protein foods that are higher in solid fats with choices that are lower in solid fats and calories and/or are sources of oils
- Use oils to replace solid fats where possible
- Choose foods that provide more potassium, dietary fiber, calcium, and vitamin D, which are nutrients of concern in American diets. These foods increase vegetables, fruits, whole grains, and milk and milk products

Recommendations for specific population groups
Women capable of becoming pregnant

- Choose foods that supply heme iron, which is more readily absorbed by the body, additional iron sources, and enhancers of iron absorption such as vitamin C–rich foods
- Choose 400 mcg/d of synthetic folic acid (from fortified foods and/or supplements) in addition to food forms of folate from a varied diet

Women who are pregnant or breastfeeding

- Consume 8–12 ounces of seafood per week from a variety of seafood types
- Due to their high methylmercury content, limit white (albacore) tuna to 6 ounces/wk and do not eat the following four types of fish: tilefish, shark, swordfish, and king mackerel
- If pregnant, take an iron supplement, as recommended by an obstetrician or other health care provider

Individuals aged 50 years and older

- Consume foods fortified with vitamins B_{12}, such as fortified cereals, or dietary supplements

Building Healthy Eating Patterns

- Select an eating pattern that meets nutrient needs over time at an appropriate calorie level
- Account for all foods and beverages consumed and assess how they fit within a total healthy eating pattern.
- Follow food safety recommendations when preparing and eating foods to reduce the risk of foodborne illnesses

therapists) are key to promote health and well-being for patients.

Several federal food and nutrition programs from the USDA and the DHHS serve the most vulnerable—infants and children, pregnant women, and those with low income. These nutrition programs include the National School Lunch and Breakfast Program (all school-age children can obtain school meals; low-income children receive free or reduced-price meals); Summer Food Service Program (free meals for low-income children at day camps and summer programs); Special Supplemental Nutrition Program for Women, Infants, and Children (low-income pregnant women and children up to 5 years of age who have nutritional risk are provided with nutritious foods, information on healthy eating, and referrals to health care); Head Start and Early Head Start (child-focused child-development program for low-income children from birth to 5 years, pregnant women, and their families); the Older Americans Act Nutrition Program (congregate and home-delivered meals for seniors); and Supplemental Nutrition Assistance Program/SNAP (direct payments in the form of electronic benefits transfer [EBT] to low-income households).

Many national health organizations also provide community-based nutrition prevention programs, including the American Heart Association, American Cancer Society, March of Dimes, American Diabetes Association, and others. Nutrition efforts in health promotion and disease prevention for women are most likely to succeed if they address lifestyle factors, environment, economics (personal and public), and the social and political climates that affect individuals and communities. Partnerships and coalitions among a variety of agencies and organizations can utilize limited resources, even though they take time and energy to develop. Possible partners for promoting good nutrition include public health agencies, primary care providers, schools (early childhood through college), supermarkets, the food industry, agricultural growers and farmers' markets, and print and electronic media.

Nurses working in a variety of settings, including public health, primary care, ambulatory care, school health, and teaching, can have a positive impact on preventive nutrition in the female populations they serve. They are also key team members for initiating nutrition awareness, supporting healthy eating and lifestyle practices, and providing consultation to dietitian and nutritionists when nutrition intervention and counseling are required or requested.

■ REFERENCES

American College of Obstetricians and Gynecologists (ACOG). (2010). ACOG Committee Opinion No. 462: Moderate caffeine consumption during pregnancy. *Obstetrics and Gynecology, 116*(2, Pt. 1), 467–468. doi:10.1097/AOG.0b013e3181eeb2a1

American Diabetes Association. (2003). Gestational diabetes mellitus. *Diabetes Care, 26*(Suppl. 1), S103–S105.

American Diabetes Association. (2015). Standards of medical care in diabetes—2015. *Diabetes Care, 38*(Suppl. 1), S1–S93.

American Dietetic Association & Dietitians of Canada. (2004). Position of the American Dietetic Association and Dietitians of Canada: Nutrition and women's health. *Journal of the American Dietectic Association, 104*(6), 984–1001. doi:10.1016/j.jada.2004.04.010

American Psychiatric Association (APA). (2006). Treatment of patients with eating disorders, third edition. *American Journal of Psychiatry, 163*(Suppl. 7), 4–54. Retrieved from http://www.ncbi.nlm.nih.gov/pubmed/16925191

American Psychiatric Association (APA). (2013). *Diagnostic and statistical manual of mental disorders* (5th ed.). Arlington, VA: American Psychiatric Publishing.

American Psychiatric Association (APA) & American Psychiatric Association (APA) DSM-5 Task Force. (2013). *Diagnostic and statistical manual of mental disorders* (5th ed.). Washington, DC: American Psychiatric Association.

Baby-Friendly Hospital Initiative. (2012). *Baby-friendly USA.* Retrieved from https://www.babyfriendlyusa.org/about-us/baby-friendly-hospital-initiative

Bakalar, J. L., Shank, L. M., Vannucci, A., Radin, R. M., & Tanofsky-Kraff, M. (2015). Recent advances in developmental and risk factor research on eating disorders. *Current Psychiatry Reports*, 17(6), 42.

Bischoff-Ferrari, H. A., Willett, W. C., Wong, J. B., Giovannucci, E., Dietrich, T., & Dawson-Hughes, B. (2005). Fracture prevention with vitamin D supplementation: A meta-analysis of randomized controlled trials. *Journal of the American Medical Association*, 293(18), 2257–2264.

Blume, S. W., & Curtis, J. R. (2011). Medical costs of osteoporosis in the elderly Medicare population. *Osteoporosis International*, 22(6), 1835–1844.

Calvo, M. S., & Tucker, K. L. (2013). Is phosphorus intake that exceeds dietary requirements a risk factor in bone health? *Annals of the New York Academy of Sciences*, 1301, 29–35.

Campbell, S. C., Khalil, D. A., Payton, M. E., & Arjmandi, B. H. (2010). One-year soy protein supplementation does not improve lipid profile in postmenopausal women. *Menopause*, 17(3), 587–593.

CARE Study Group. (2008). Maternal caffeine intake during pregnancy and risk of fetal growth restriction: A large prospective observational study. *British Medical Journal*, 337, a2332. doi:10.1136/bmj.a2332

Caudill, M. A. (2010). Pre- and postnatal health: Evidence of increased choline needs. *Journal of the American Dietetic Association*, 110(8), 1198–1206.

Center for Nutrition Policy and Promotion. (2011). A brief history of USDA food guides. Retrieved from http://www.choosemyplate.gov/sites/default/files/printablematerials/ABriefHistoryOfUSDAFoodGuides.pdf

Centers for Disease Control and Prevention (CDC). (1992). Recommendations for use of folic acid to reduce the number of cases of spina bifida and other neural tube defects. *Morbidity and Mortality Weekly*, 41(1), RR-14; 001.

Centers for Disease Control and Prevention (CDC) Office of Women's Health. (2015). *Leading causes of death in females, United States, 2013 (current listing).* Retrieved from http://www.cdc.gov/women/lcod/2013/index.htm

Chirico, G., Marzollo, R., Cortinovis, S., Fonte, C., & Gasparoni, A. (2008). Antiinfective properties of human milk. *Journal of Nutrition*, 138(9), 1801S–1806S. Retrieved from http://www.ncbi.nlm.nih.gov/pubmed/18716190

Clinical Guidelines on the Identification, Evaluation, and Treatment of Overweight and Obesity in Adults—The Evidence Report. National Institutes of Health. (1998). *Obesity Research*, 6(Suppl. 2), 51S–209S. Retrieved from http://www.ncbi.nlm.nih.gov/pubmed/9813653

Committee on Pediatric AIDS. (2013). Infant feeding and transmission of human immunodeficiency virus in the United States. *Pediatrics*, 131(2), 391–396. doi:10.1542/peds.2012-3543

Delgado-Noguera, M. F., Calvache, J. A., Bonfill Cosp, X., Kotanidou, E. P., & Galli-Tsinopoulou, A. (2015). Supplementation with long chain polyunsaturated fatty acids (LCPUFA) to breastfeeding mothers for improving child growth and development. *The Cochrane Database of Systematic Reviews*, 2015(7), CD007901.

Dickinson, A., Blatman, J., El-Dash, N., & Franco, J. C. (2014). Consumer usage and reasons for using dietary supplements: Report of a series of surveys. *Journal of the American College of Nutrition*, 33(2), 176–182.

Federal Interagency Forum on Child and Family Statistics. (2015). *America's children: Key national indicators of well-being.* Washington, DC: U.S. Government Printing Office.

Fitzgerald, N., Morgan, K. T., & Slawson, D. L. (2013). Practice paper of the Academy of Nutrition and Dietetics abstract: The role of nutrition in health promotion and chronic disease prevention. *Journal of the Academy of Nutrition and Dietetics*, 113(7), 983.

Flegal, K. M., Kit, B. K., Orpana, H., & Graubard, B. I. (2013). Association of all-cause mortality with overweight and obesity using standard body mass index categories: A systematic review and meta-analysis. *Journal of the American Medical Association*, 309(1), 71–82. doi:10.1001/jama.2012.113905

Frederick, I. O., Williams, M. A., Dashow, E., Kestin, M., Zhang, C., & Leisenring, W. M. (2005). Dietary fiber, potassium, magnesium and calcium in relation to the risk of preeclampsia. *Journal of Reproductive Medicine*, 50(5), 332–344.

Freedman, D. S., & Ford, E. S. (2015). Are the recent secular increases in the waist circumference of adults independent of changes in BMI? *American Journal of Clinical Nutrition*, 101(3), 425–431.

Gee, M., Mahan, L. K., & Escott-Stump, S. (2008). Weight management. In L. K. Mahan & S. Escott-Stump (Eds.), *Krause's food & nutrition therapy* (12th ed., pp. 532–562). St. Louis, MO: Elsevier Saunders.

Go, A. S., Mozaffarian, D., Roger, V. L., Benjamin, E. J., Berry, J. D., Borden, W. B., …Turner, M. B.; American Heart Association Statistics Committee and Stroke Statistics Subcommittee. (2013). Heart disease and stroke statistics—2013 update: A report from the American Heart Association. *Circulation*, 127(1), e6–e245.

Grant, R. W., Donner, T. W., Fradkin J. E., Hayes, C., Herman, W. H., Hsu, W. C., …Wexler, D. J. (2015). Standards of medical care in diabetes—2015: Summary of revisions. *Diabetes Care*, 38(Suppl.), S4. doi:10.2337/dc15-S003

Heaney, R. P., & Weaver, C. M. (2005). Newer perspectives on calcium nutrition and bone quality. *Journal of the American College of Nutrition*, 24(Suppl. 6), 574S–581S.

Hediger, M. L., Scholl, T. O., & Schall, J. I. (1997). Implications of the Camden Study of adolescent pregnancy: Interactions among maternal growth, nutritional status, and body composition. *Annals of the New York Academy of Science*, 817, 281–291.

Heppe, D. H., Steegers, E. A., Timmermans, S., Breeijen, H. D., Tiemeier, H., Hofman, A., & Jaddoe, V. W. (2011). Maternal fish consumption, fetal growth and the risks of neonatal complications: The Generation R Study. *British Journal of Nutrition*, 105(6), 938–949.

Hill, J. O. (2009). Can a small-changes approach help address the obesity epidemic? A report of the Joint Task Force of the American Society for Nutrition, Institute of Food Technologists, and International Food Information Council. *American Journal of Clinical Nutrition*, 89(2), 477–484.

Hill, J. O., Wyatt, H. R., & Melanson, E. L. (2000). Genetic and environmental contributions to obesity. *Medical Clinics of North America*, 84(2), 333–346. Retrieved from http://www.ncbi.nlm.nih.gov/pubmed/10793645

Hughes, V. (2013). The big fat truth. *Nature*, 497(7450), 428–430.

Institute of Medicine. (2011). *Dietary reference intakes for calcium and vitamin D.* Washington, DC: National Academies Press.

Institute of Medicine (IOM) Food and Nutrition Board, Suitor, C. W., & Meyers, L. D. (2007). *Dietary Reference Intakes Research Synthesis Workshop summary.* Washington, DC: National Academies Press.

Institute of Medicine (IOM) National Research Council. (2009). Weight gain during pregnancy: Reexamining the guidelines. Washington DC: National Academies Press.

Institute of Medicine (IOM) Panel on Macronutrients & Institute of Medicine (IOM) Standing Committee on the Scientific Evaluation of Dietary Reference Intakes. (2005). *Dietary reference intakes for energy, carbohydrate, fiber, fat, fatty acids, cholesterol, protein, and amino acids.* Washington, DC: National Academies Press.

Jacobi, C., Hayward, C., de Zwaan, M., Kraemer, H. C., & Agras, W. S. (2004). Coming to terms with risk factors for eating disorders: Application of risk terminology and suggestions for a general taxonomy. *Psychological Bulletin*, 130(1), 19–65.

Jain, V. (2015). Micronutrients and the older adult, part 1: Micronutrients of importance to older adults. *The Spectrum* (Winter Supplement), 1–12.

James, D. C., Lessen, R., & American Dietetic Association. (2009). Position of the American Dietetic Association: Promoting and supporting breastfeeding. *Journal of the American Dietetic Association*, 109(11), 1926–1942. Retrieved from http://www.ncbi.nlm.nih.gov/pubmed/19862847

Kaiser, L. L., Campbell, C. G., & Academy Positions Committee Workshop. (2014). Practice paper of the Academy of Nutrition and Dietetics abstract: Nutrition and lifestyle for a healthy pregnancy outcome. *Journal of the Academy of Nutrition and Dietetics*, 114(9), 1447. Retrieved from http://www.ncbi.nlm.nih.gov/pubmed/25699300

Kelderhouse, K., & Taylor, J. S. (2013). A review of treatment and management modalities for premenstrual dysphoric disorder. *Nursing for Women's Health*, 17(4), 294–305.

Kenny, A. M., Mangano, K. M., Abourizk, R. H., Bruno, R. S., Anamani, D. E., Kleppinger, A., …Kerstetter, J. E. (2009). Soy proteins and isoflavones affect bone mineral density in older women: A randomized controlled trial. *American Journal of Clinical Nutrition, 90*(1), 234–242.

Khalafallah, A. A., & Dennis, A. E. (2012). Iron deficiency anaemia in pregnancy and postpartum: Pathophysiology and effect of oral versus intravenous iron therapy. *Journal of Pregnancy, 2012,* 630519.

Kim, S. A., Moore, L. V., Galuska, D., Wright, A. P., Harris, D., Grummer-Strawn, L. M.,... National Center for Chronic Disease Prevention and Health Promotion, Centers for Disease Control and Prevention (CDC). (2014). Vital signs: Fruit and vegetable intake among children—United States, 2003–2010. *MMWR Morbidity and Mortality Weekly Report, 63*(31), 671–676. Retrieved from http://www.ncbi.nlm.nih.gov/pubmed/25102415

King, J. C. (2000). Determinants of maternal zinc status during pregnancy. *American Journal of Clinical Nutrition, 71*(Suppl. 5), 1334S–1343S. Retrieved from http://www.ncbi.nlm.nih.gov/pubmed/10799411

Klenov, V. E., & Jungheim, E. S. (2014). Obesity and reproductive function: A review of the evidence. *Current Opinion in Obstetrics & Gynecology, 26*(6), 455–460.

Kochanek, K. D., Xu, J., Murphy, S. L., Minino, A. M., & Kung, H. C. (2011). Deaths: Final data for 2009. *National Vital Statistics Report, 60*(3), 1–116. Retrieved from http://www.ncbi.nlm.nih.gov/pubmed/24974587

Lammer, E. J., Chen, D. T., Hoar, R. M., Agnish, N. D., Benke, P. J., Braun, J. T.,... Lott, I. T. (1985). Retinoic acid embryopathy. *New England Journal of Medicine, 313*(14), 837–841.

Larson, N. I., Neumark-Sztainer, D., Harnack, L., Wall, M., Story, M., & Eisenberg, M. E. (2009). Calcium and dairy intake: Longitudinal trends during the transition to young adulthood and correlates of calcium intake. *Journal of Nutrition Education and Behavior, 41*(4), 254–260.

Larson, N. I., Neumark-Sztainer, D., & Story, M. (2009). Weight control behaviors and dietary intake among adolescents and young adults: Longitudinal findings from Project EAT. *Journal of the American Dietetic Association, 109*(11), 1869–1877.

Lawrence, R., & Lawrence, R. (2005). *Breastfeeding: A guide for the medical profession* (6th ed.). Philadelphia, PA: Elsevier Saunders.

Lessen, R., & Kavanagh, K. (2015). Position of the academy of nutrition and dietetics: Promoting and supporting breastfeeding. *Journal of the Academy of Nutrition and Dietetics, 115*(3), 444–449.

Lichtenstein, A. H., Appel, L. J., Brands, M., Carnethon, M., Daniels, S., Franch, H. A., ... Wylie-Rosett, J. (2006). Diet and lifestyle recommendations revision 2006: A scientific statement from the American Heart Association Nutrition Committee. *Circulation, 114,* 82–96.

Lovelady, C. A., Garner, K. E., Moreno, K. L., & Williams, J. P. (2000). The effect of weight loss in overweight, lactating women on the growth of their infants. *New England Journal of Medicine, 342*(7), 449–453.

Lytle, L. A., Himes, J. H., Feldman, H., Zive, M., Dwyer, J., Hoelscher, D.,... Yang, M. (2002). Nutrient intake over time in a multi-ethnic sample of youth. *Public Health Nutrition, 5*(2), 319–328. doi:10.1079/PHN2002255

Malatesta, V. J. (2007). Introduction: The need to address older women's mental health issues. *Journal of Women & Aging, 19*(1–2), 1–12. doi:10.1300/J074v19n03_01

Mangano, K. M., Hutchins-Wiese, H. L., Kenny, A. M., Walsh, S. J., Abourizk, R. H., Bruno, R. S.,... Kerstetter, J. E. (2013). Soy proteins and isoflavones reduce interleukin-6 but not serum lipids in older women: A randomized controlled trial. *Nutrition Research, 33*(12), 1026–1033.

March, K. M., Chen, N. N., Karakochuk, C. D., Shand, A. W., Innis, S. M., von Dadelszen, P.,... Green, T. J. (2015). Maternal vitamin D₃ supplementation at 50 mµg/d protects against low serum 25-hydroxyvitamin D in infants at 8 wk of age: A randomized controlled trial of 3 doses of vitamin D beginning in gestation and continued in lactation. *American Journal of Clinical Nutrition, 102*(2), 402–410. doi:10.3945/ajcn.114.106385

Micali, N. (2010). Management of eating disorders during pregnancy. *Progress in Neurology and Psychiatry, 14,* 24–26. Retrieved from http://onlinelibrary.wiley.com/doi/10.1002/pnp.158/pdf

Micali, N., Simonoff, E., & Treasure, J. (2007). Risk of major adverse perinatal outcomes in women with eating disorders. *British Journal of Psychiatry, 190,* 255–259.

Mosca, L., Benjamin, E. J., Berra, K., Bezanson, J. L., Dolor, R. J., Lloyd-Jones, D. M.,... Wenger, N. K. (2011). Effectiveness-based guidelines for the prevention of cardiovascular disease in women—2011 update: A guideline from the American Heart Association. *Circulation, 123*(11), 1243–1262.

Mosca, L., Mochari-Greenberger, H., Dolor, R. J., Newby, L. K., & Robb, K. J. (2010). Twelve-year follow-up of American women's awareness of cardiovascular disease risk and barriers to heart health. *Circulation. Cardiovascular Quality and Outcomes, 3*(2), 120–127.

National Center for Health Statistics. (2015a). *Birth defects or congenital anomalies.* Retrieved from http://www.cdc.gov/nchs/fastats/birth-defects.htm

National Center for Health Statistics. (2015b). *Births and natality.* Retrieved from http://www.cdc.gov/nchs/fastats/births.htm

National Heart, Lung, and Blood Institute. (2015). *Classification of overweight and obesity by BMI, waist circumference and associated disease risks.* Retrieved from https://www.nhlbi.nih.gov/health/educational/lose_wt/BMI/bmi_dis.htm

National Osteoporosis Foundation. (2011). *Facts and statistics.* Retrieved from http://www.iofbonehealth.org/facts-statistics

Nelson, H. D., Vesco, K. K., Haney, E., Fu, R., Nedrow, A., Miller, J.,... Humphrey, L. (2006). Nonhormonal therapies for menopausal hot flashes: Systematic review and meta-analysis. *Journal of the American Medical Association, 295*(17), 2057–2071.

Neumark-Sztainer, D., Wall, M., Larson, N. I., Eisenberg, M. E., & Loth, K. (2011). Dieting and disordered eating behaviors from adolescence to young adulthood: Findings from a 10-year longitudinal study. *Journal of the American Dietetic Association, 111*(7), 1004–1011.

Nielsen, J. N., Gittelsohn, J., Anliker, J., & O'Brien, K. (2006). Interventions to improve diet and weight gain among pregnant adolescents and recommendations for future research. *Journal of the American Dietetic Association, 106*(11), 1825–1840.

Noakes, P. S., Vlachava, M., Kremmyda, L. S., Diaper, N. D., Miles, E. A., Erlewyn-Lajeunesse, M.,... Calder, P. C. (2012). Increased intake of oily fish in pregnancy: Effects on neonatal immune responses and on clinical outcomes in infants at 6 mo. *American Journal of Clinical Nutrition, 95*(2), 395–404.

Nutrition Screening Initiative. (1991). *Report of Nutrition Screening I: Toward a Common View.* Washington, DC.

O'Connor, D. L., & Picciano, M. F. (2014). *Nutrition in lactation.* In A. C. Ross, B. Caballero, R. J. Cousins, K. L. Tucker, & T. R. Ziegler (Eds.), *Modern nutrition in health and disease* (11th ed., pp. 698–711). Baltimore, MD: Lippincott Williams & Wilkins.

Office of Disease Prevention and Health Promotion. (2015a). *Healthy People 2020 leading health indicators.* Retrieved from http://www.healthypeople.gov/2020/Leading-Health-Indicators

Office of Disease Prevention and Health Promotion. (2015b). *Healthy People 2020 topics-objectives.* Retrieved from http://www.healthypeople.gov/2020/topics-objectives/topic/maternal-infant-and-child-health/objectives

Ogden, C. L., Carroll, M. D., Kit, B. K., & Flegal, K. M. (2013). *Prevalence of obesity among adults: United States, 2011–2012.* Hyattsville, MD: National Center for Health Statistics.

Ogden, C. L., Carroll, M. D., Kit, B. K., & Flegal, K. M. (2014). Prevalence of childhood and adult obesity in the United States, 2011–2012. *Journal of the American Medical Association, 311*(8), 806–814. doi:10.1001/jama.2014.732

Ogden, C. L., Li, Y., Freedman, D. S., Borrud, L. G., & Flegal, K. M. (2011 November 9). Smoothed percentage body fat percentiles for U.S. children and adolescents, 1999–2004. *National Health Statistics Report,* (43), 1–7.

Otten, J. J., Hellwig, J. P., & Meyers, L. D. (2006). *DRI, dietary reference intakes: The essential guide to nutrient requirements.* Washington, DC: National Academies Press.

Ozier, A. D., Henry, B. W., & American Dietetic Association. (2011). Position of the American Dietetic Association: Nutrition intervention in the treatment of eating disorders. *Journal of the American Dietetic Association, 111*(8), 1236–1241.

Paddon-Jones, D., Campbell, W. W., Jacques, P. F., Kritchevsky, S. B., Moore, L. L., Rodriguez, N. R., & van Loon, L. J. (2015). Protein and healthy aging. *American Journal of Clinical Nutrition.* doi:10.3945/ajcn.114.084061

Picciano, M. F. (2001). Representative values for constituents of human milk. *Pediatric Clinics of North America, 48*(1), 263–264. Retrieved from http://www.ncbi.nlm.nih.gov/pubmed/11236731

Pitkin, R. M. (1976). Nutritional support in obstetrics and gynecology. *Clinical Obstetrics and Gynecology, 19*(3), 489–513.

Polsky, S., Catenacci, V. A., Wyatt, H. R., & Hill, J. O. (2014). Obesity: Epidemiology, etiology, and prevention. In A. C. Ross, B. Caballero,

R. J. Cousins, K. L. Tucker, & T. R. Ziegler (Eds.), *Modern nutrition in health and disease* (11th ed., pp. 771–785). Baltimore, MD: Lippincott Williams & Wilkins.

Procter, S. B., & Campbell, C. G. (2014). Position of the Academy of Nutrition and Dietetics: Nutrition and lifestyle for a healthy pregnancy outcome. *Journal of the Academy of Nutrition and Dietetics, 114*(7), 1099–1103.

Rainville, A. J. (1998). Pica practices of pregnant women are associated with lower maternal hemoglobin level at delivery. *Journal of the American Dietetic Association, 98*(3), 293–296.

Rasmussen, K. M., & Yaktine, A. L. (Eds.) (2009). *Weight gain during pregnancy: Reexamining the guidelines.* Washington, DC: National Academies Press.

Rohde, P., Stice, E., & Marti, C. N. (2015). Development and predictive effects of eating disorder risk factors during adolescence: Implications for prevention efforts. *International Journal of Eating Disorders, 48*(2), 187–198.

Rosa, F. W., Wilk, A. L., & Kelsey, F. O. (1986). Teratogen update: Vitamin A congeners. *Teratology, 33*(3), 355–364.

Rothman, K. J., Moore, L. L., Singer, M. R., Nguyen, U. S., Mannino, S., & Milunsky, A. (1995). Teratogenicity of high vitamin A intake. *New England Journal of Medicine, 333*(21), 1369–1373.

Schebendach, J. E. (2008). Nutrition in eating disorders. In L. K. Mahan & S. Escott-Stump (Eds.), *Krause's food & nutrition therapy* (12th ed., pp. 563–586). St. Louis, MO: Elsevier Saunders.

Scholl, T. O., Hediger, M. L., & Schall, J. I. (1997). Maternal growth and fetal growth: Pregnancy course and outcome in the Camden Study. *Annals of the New York Academy of Science, 817*, 292–301. Retrieved from http://www.ncbi.nlm.nih.gov/pubmed/9239197

Seagle, H. M., Strain, G. W., Makris, A., Reeves, R. S., & American Dietetic Association. (2009). Position of the American Dietetic Association: Weight management. *Journal of the American Dietetic Association, 109*(2), 330–346. Retrieved from http://www.ncbi.nlm.nih.gov/pubmed/19244669

Section on Breastfeeding. (2012). Breastfeeding and the use of human milk. *Pediatrics, 129*(3), e827–e841. doi:10.1542/peds.2011-3552

Shabert, J. K. (2004). Nutrition during pregnancy and lactation. In L. Mahan & S. Escott-Stump (Eds.), *Krause's food, nutrition and diet therapy* (11 ed., pp. 182–213). Philadelphia, PA: Saunders.

Singh, A. S., Mulder, C., Twisk, J. W., van Mechelen, W., & Chinapaw, M. J. (2008). Tracking of childhood overweight into adulthood: A systematic review of the literature. *Obesity Reviews, 9*(5), 474–488.

Siu, A. L., & U.S. Preventive Services Task Force. (2015). Screening for iron deficiency anemia and iron supplementation in pregnant women to improve maternal health and birth outcomes: U.S. Preventive Services Task Force Recommendation Statement. *Annals of Internal Medicine, 163*(7), 529–536. doi:10.7326/M15-1707

Slawson, D. L., Fitzgerald, N., & Morgan, K. T. (2013). Position of the Academy of Nutrition and Dietetics: The role of nutrition in health promotion and chronic disease prevention. *Journal of the Academy of Nutrition and Dietetics, 113*(7), 972–979.

Smink, F. R., van Hoeken, D., & Hoek, H. W. (2012). Epidemiology of eating disorders: Incidence, prevalence and mortality rates. *Current Psychiatry Reports, 14*(4), 406–414.

Stice, E., Marti, C. N., & Durant, S. (2011). Risk factors for onset of eating disorders: Evidence of multiple risk pathways from an 8-year prospective study. *Behaviour Research and Therapy, 49*(10), 622–627.

Tamura, T., & Picciano, M. F. (2006). Folate and human reproduction. *American Journal of Clinical Nutrition, 83*(5), 993–1016. Retrieved from http://www.ncbi.nlm.nih.gov/pubmed/16685040

Tang, B. M., Eslick, G. D., Nowson, C., Smith, C., & Bensoussan, A. (2007). Use of calcium or calcium in combination with vitamin D supplementation to prevent fractures and bone loss in people aged 50 years and older: A meta-analysis. *Lancet, 370*(9588), 657–666.

Tangney, C. C., Li, H., Wang, Y., Barnes, L., Schneider, J. A., Bennett, D. A., & Morris, M. C. (2014). Relation of DASH- and Mediterranean-like dietary patterns to cognitive decline in older persons. *Neurology, 83*(16), 1410–1416.

Teratology Society (1987). Position paper: Recommendations for vitamin A use during pregnancy. *Teratology, 35*(2), 269–275. doi:10.1002/tera.1420350215

Tucker, K. L., & Rosen, C. J. (2014). Prevention and management of osteoporosis. In A. C. Ross, B. Caballero, R. J. Cousins, K. L. Tucker, & T. R. Ziegler (Eds.), *Modern nutrition in health and disease* (11th ed., pp. 1227–1244). Baltimore, MD: Lippincott Williams & Wilkins.

Turner, R. E. (2014). Nutrition in pregnancy. In A. C. Ross, B. Caballero, R. J. Cousins, K. L. Tucker, & T. R. Ziegler (Eds.), *Modern nutrition in health and disease* (11th ed., pp. 684–697). Baltimore, MD: Lippincott Williams & Wilkins.

U.S. Department of Agriculture. (2016, October 8, 2015). *DRI tables and application reports.* Retrieved from https://fnic.nal.usda.gov/dietary-guidance/dietary-reference-intakes/dri-tables-and-application-reports

U.S. Department of Agriculture (USDA) & U.S. Department of Health and Human Services (DHHS). (2015). *Dietary guidelines for Americans, 2010.* Washington, DC: U.S. Government Printing Office.

U.S. Food and Drug Administration. (2014). *Fish: What pregnant women and parents should know.* Retrieved from http://www.fda.gov/Food/FoodborneIllnessContaminants/Metals/ucm393070.htm

Vazquez, J. C. (2010 August 3). Constipation, haemorrhoids, and heartburn in pregnancy. *British Medical Journal Clinical Evidence,* 1411. Retrieved from http://www.ncbi.nlm.nih.gov/pubmed/21418682

Weaver, C. M., & Heaney, R. P. (2014). Calcium. In A. C. Ross, B. Caballero, R. J. Cousins, K. L. Tucker, & T. R. Ziegler (Eds.), *Modern nutrition in health and disease* (11th ed., pp. 133–149). Baltimore, MD: Lippincott Williams & Wilkins.

Whelan, A. M., Jurgens, T. M., & Naylor, H. (2009). Herbs, vitamins and minerals in the treatment of premenstrual syndrome: A systematic review. *Canadian Journal of Clinical Pharmacology, 16*(3), e407–e429. Retrieved from http://www.ncbi.nlm.nih.gov/pubmed/19923637

Whitlock, E. P., Williams, S. B., Gold, R., Smith, P. R., & Shipman, S. A. (2005). Screening and interventions for childhood overweight: A summary of evidence for the U.S. Preventive Services Task Force. *Pediatrics, 116*(1), e125–e144.

Wofford, M. R., Rebholz, C. M., Reynolds, K., Chen, J., Chen, C. S., Myers, L.,…He, J. (2012). Effect of soy and milk protein supplementation on serum lipid levels: A randomized controlled trial. *European Journal of Clinical Nutrition, 66*(4), 419–425.

World Health Organization (WHO). (2012a). *Guideline: Daily iron and folic acid supplementation in pregnant women.* Geneva, Switzerland: World Health Organization.

World Health Organization (WHO). (2012b). *Guideline: Vitamin D supplementation in pregnant women.* Geneva, Switzerland: World Health Organization.

Worley, L., McKelvey, S., Tariq, S., Yager, J., Lowery, C., & Antenatal and Neonatal Guidelines, Education, and Learning System (ANGELS) Team (2003). *Eating disorders during pregnancy and postpartum.* Board of Trustees University of Arkansas. Retrieved from: http://angelsguidelines.com/guidelines/eating-disorders-during-pregnancy-and-postpartum/

CHAPTER 14

Healthy Practices: Physical Activity

JiWon Choi

Regular physical activity is an essential component of health practices for optimal health. In the U.S. Surgeon General's report on physical activity and health (U.S. Department of Health and Human Services [USDHHS], 1996), physical inactivity was identified as a prevalent nationwide health problem. It also reported on the significant health benefits of moderate-intensity physical activity. The benefits include reduced risk of premature mortality, cardiovascular disease (CVD), colon cancer, and diabetes, as well as enhanced psychological well-being. In 2008, the USDHHS recommended that adults should engage in aerobic exercise at least 150 minutes per week at a moderate intensity or 75 minutes per week at a vigorous intensity. Evaluation of the physical activity level of an individual should be a part of any health assessment, and interventions to maximize physical activity should be included in health care plans.

Physical activity is especially important for women who are at high risk of mortality because of heart disease. Childbearing and childrearing have been identified as common barriers to regular physical activity in women of childbearing age (Cramp & Brawley, 2006), putting them at risk for developing health concerns that can be mediated with exercise. Because women often put their own health needs after those of their family, a focus on the importance of regular physical activity is especially important for women. As beneficial effects of moderate-intensity physical activity is confirmed, active lifestyle during leisure time as well as non-leisure time should be encouraged. Women need to be counseled about how important it is for them to keep their health maximized so they can effectively care for their families.

■ PHYSICAL ACTIVITY, EXERCISE, AND FITNESS

The terms *physical activity, exercise*, and *fitness* are often interchanged, yet they are not the same. *Physical activity* is defined as "any bodily movement produced by skeletal muscle that results in energy expenditure" (Caspersen, Powell, & Christenson, 1985, p. 126). It includes occupational work, household chores, yard work, transportation-related activity, such as walking and biking, leisure-time activity, playing sports, and exercising. Exercise is a subset of physical

activity, which is planned, structured, and repetitive and has the purpose of improving or maintaining physical fitness, physical skills, or health (Caspersen et al., 1985). *Physical fitness* is defined as "a set of attributes that people have or achieve that relates to the ability to perform physical activity" (USDHHS, 1996, p. 21). The attributes can be categorized into health- or performance-related components of physical fitness, depending on their relevance to health or athletic performance. Health-related fitness components are later discussed in detail in the section discussing the assessment of physical fitness.

■ RISK FACTORS AND HEALTH CONSIDERATIONS RELATED TO EXERCISE

Physical Activity and CVD

Numerous studies reported that high levels of physical activity lower the risk of CVD mortality in men and women, even after statistically controlling for the modifiable risk factors (Kannel, Belanger, D'Agostino, & Israel, 1986; LaCroix, Leveille, Hecht, Grothaus, & Wagner, 1996; Paffenbarger, Hyde, Wing, & Steinmetz, 1984). Studies have shown that aerobic exercise produces favorable anatomical and physiological changes, including increased heart size, increased size of coronary vessels, and increased cardiac work capacity. In addition, physical activity influences cardiovascular risk factors, including blood pressure, lipid metabolism, glucose metabolism, and body composition. The role of physical activity on these modifiable risk factors and health outcomes are discussed in the following section.

National surveys have shown that physical inactivity is higher among women than men. The proportion of those who do not meet the 2008 Physical Activity Guidelines was higher among women than men (54.1% vs. 43.9%, age adjusted; Go et al., 2013). Physical activity declines with age and is lower in non-White women than in White women. Both girls and women are reported to participate in leisure-time physical activity, such as sports and recreational activities, less often than their male counterparts (Kimm et al., 2002; Sallis, Prochaska, & Taylor, 2000;

Trost, Owen, Bauman, Sallis, & Brown, 2002). Although women participate in less leisure-time physical activity than men, the reported activity levels are higher when non-leisure time activity such as job, household, or caregiving are considered (Brownson et al., 2000; Eyler et al., 2002; Sternfeld, Ainsworth, & Quesenberry, 1999).

CVD is the leading cause of death, responsible for about one of every three deaths in the United States (Mozaffarian et al., 2015). Among postmenopausal women, CVD is the number 1 cause of death, affecting approximately one of every two women. CVD is a disorder affecting the heart or blood vessels and includes coronary heart disease (CHD), stroke, hypertension, heart failure, and other diseases. The risk factors for CVD can be classified as ones that cannot be controlled and ones that can. Age and family history of early onset of CVD are risk factors that cannot be controlled. Age older than 55 years for females is considered a risk factor. Having a parent or sibling with premature (younger than 55 years of age if male; younger than 65 years of age if female) CVD or death from CVD also increases the risk. The modifiable risk factors include elevated blood pressure, elevated serum total cholesterol (TC) and low-density lipoprotein cholesterol (LDL-C), low serum high-density lipoprotein cholesterol (HDL-C), diabetes mellitus (DM), physical inactivity, and obesity.

Women are also at increased risk for disorders of glucose metabolism and DM as they age. Other important health issues for women that are potentially modified or prevented by exercise include osteoporosis, depression and mood/affective disorders, and menstrual cycle changes and dysfunction. Exercise is also an important factor for women who are pregnant.

■ DIAGNOSTIC CRITERIA

Women who plan to initiate a physical activity program should be screened for the presence of risk factors for various cardiovascular, respiratory, and metabolic diseases, as well as other conditions (e.g., pregnancy, orthopedic injury) that require special attention when developing the exercise prescription. Although exercise testing before initiating a physical activity program is not routinely recommended except for those at high risk, the information obtained from an exercise test is helpful for the development of a safe and effective exercise prescription. Before the exercise testing, an informed consent form should be obtained from the participant. Exercise testing of individuals at high risk should be supervised by a clinician in a setting where emergent care is readily available. Testing of healthy individuals for research purposes may not require clinician supervision. However, all research procedures must be approved by institutional review boards, and a plan for managing emergency events should be in place.

EKG, heart rate, and blood pressure readings are obtained before, during, and after exercise testing. The EKG is monitored to detect any abnormalities in heart rhythm and electrical conductivity. Blood pressure is monitored to determine if any abnormal changes in systolic and diastolic blood pressure occurs as the rate of work progresses from low intensity to maximal or submaximal levels. It is also important to check with the client, asking perceived exertion and observing signs and symptoms during the exercise test, such as chest pain or pressure, unusual shortness of breath, and light-headedness or dizziness.

■ ASSESSMENT

Physical Activity

Because physical activity is a complex set of behaviors, a good measure of it is required in order to provide reliable and valid information on its specific components, including type, intensity, duration, and frequency. Several methods are available for physical activity assessment, including self-report instruments, physiological markers, and motion sensors. Self-reported information, including diaries, logs, or recall surveys is often converted to estimate energy expenditure (i.e., kilocalories [kcal] or kilojoules [kJ]). A total of 1 kcal is the amount of heat required to increase the temperature of 1 kg of water 1°C, and 1 kcal = 4.2 kJ. Because the goal of most self-report instruments is to estimate the energy expenditure attributable to participation in specific types of physical activity, a variety of physiological and mechanical methods can be used to validate the self-reported information by assessing energy expenditure. Physiological methods include direct calorimetry (requiring the participant to remain in a sealed, insulated metabolic chamber) and indirect calorimetry (requiring the participant to wear a mask and to carry a portable equipment for analyzing expired air). Another method of physiologically monitoring energy expenditure is doubly labeled water (requiring the participant to drink a measured amount of water that has been labeled with stable isotopes of hydrogen and oxygen and collect urine over a 7- to 14-day period). Although the use of doubly labeled water is considered the most accurate measure of daily energy expenditure, the lack of information on specific components of physical activity and high cost for the procedure and equipment for analysis for the urine sample make this method infeasible in large-scale studies. A heart rate monitor is a useful tool for helping the participant maintain the optimum heart rate target zone and assess the intensity of physical activity. However, it still lacks other components of physical activity, such as type.

Pedometers are designed to count steps and can measure the distance walked when stride length is programmed into the device. Some pedometers even provide caloric expenditure. They are relatively inexpensive and easy to use. However, they lack information about the intensity of walking. Thus pedometers are accurate for measuring steps but are less accurate for measuring distance and energy expenditure. Accelerometers are also motion sensors that measure movements in terms of acceleration. They operate by detecting accelerations along a given axis, and a single monitor can capture a movement in multiple axes, converting the movement into electrical signals (counts). These counts are used to estimate energy expenditure. Compared with pedometers, accelerometers are considered to provide more accurate and detailed information about the frequency, duration, and intensity of physical activity. However, accelerometers are relatively expensive and do not accurately capture certain types of activities (e.g., stationary biking).

Physical Fitness

The health-related components of physical fitness are cardiorespiratory endurance, body composition, muscular strength, muscular endurance, and flexibility (Caspersen et al., 1985; USDHHS, 1996). The performance-related components of physical fitness are agility, balance, coordination, power, speed, and reaction time (Caspersen et al., 1985). Cardiorespiratory endurance refers to the ability of the circulatory and respiratory systems to supply oxygen to working muscles for an extended time. The best criterion of an individual's cardiorespiratory endurance is the direct measurement of VO_{2max}, the rate of oxygen uptake during maximal exercise (i.e., collection and analysis of expired gas samples). It is expressed in milliliters of oxygen used per kilogram of body weight per minute (mL/kg/min), allowing for meaningful comparisons among individuals with differing body weight. However, the measurement procedure requires expensive equipment, qualified personnel, and a considerable time to administer; thus its use is limited in large epidemiological studies and usual primary care practices.

Alternatively, a number of maximal and submaximal exercise test protocols using the treadmill, cycle ergometer, and bench stepping have been validated to estimate VO_2max without measuring respiratory gases. In addition, performance tests such as distance runs (e.g., 1-mile walk test, 1-mile run test, and 12-minute run test) are devised to predict VO_{2max}. The individual with a higher degree of fitness is expected to walk or run a greater distance in a given period of time or a given distance in less time. Although performance tests may not provide an accurate index of VO_{2max}, they may be useful for clinicians and researchers to establish a baseline of performance and evaluate interventions. Through regular aerobic exercise, people can increase their VO_{2max}.

Body composition is a component of an individual's physical fitness and refers to the relative amount of body fat and lean body mass. Hydrostatic (underwater) weighting is a method used to measure body volume and density from the water displacement. Although it is used as the criterion for assessing percentage of body fat, this method requires time, expense, technical expertise, and the participant's discomfort with being underwater during the procedure. Another method for determining the percentage of body fat is air displacement plethysmography. In this method, body volume is estimated while the client is sitting in a sealed chamber. Compared with hydrostatic weighing, it is quick to administer and requires less client compliance and less technical expertise. However, the equipment is expensive.

Dual-energy x-ray absorptiometry (DEXA) is gaining wide acceptance as a reference method for measuring body composition. This method provides estimates of bone mineral, fat, and lean soft tissue as the x-rays pass through the client. The radiation exposure is minimal, and the method requires minimal client cooperation and minimal technical skill. The major disadvantages of this method are cost and less-than-easy access to the equipment.

Widely used methods for assessing body composition include the body mass index (BMI), waist circumference, and skinfold measurement. BMI is calculated by dividing the weight in kilograms by the height in meters squared. It is a quick and easy method but can be problematic because it does not differentiate between fat and fat-free weight. Waist circumference can alone provide valuable information about disease risk as a measure of regional adiposity (i.e., abdominal obesity; Janssen, Katzmarzyk, & Ross, 2004; National Heart, Lung, and Blood Institute [NHLBI], 1998). Skinfold measurement is the quick, noninvasive, inexpensive method for estimating the percentage of body fat. Commonly used skinfold sites include the abdomen, triceps, chest, midaxillary area, subscapular area, suprailiac area, and thigh.

Muscular strength is the ability of a muscle or a muscle group to generate force, and muscular endurance is the ability of the muscle to continue to perform without fatigue. Tests of muscular strength and endurance include sit-ups, push-ups, bent-arm hangs, and pull-ups. *Flexibility* refers to the range of motion (ROM) available at a joint. As flexibility is specific to each joint of the body, there is no general indicator of flexibility. The criterion method of measuring flexibility is goniometry, which is used to measure the angle of the joint at both extremes in the ROM. Sit-and-reach tests are used to evaluate the flexibility of the hamstring muscles, and the back scratch test is used to assess upper body (shoulder joint) flexibility.

■ GUIDELINES FOR PROMOTING EXERCISE PRESCRIPTIONS

The basic elements of the exercise prescription include frequency (how often), intensity (how hard), time (how long), and type (mode), with the addition of total volume (amount) and progression (advancement) or the FITT-VP principle. The exercise prescription should be made based on the client's characteristics, including age, capabilities, preferences, fitness level, and goals. For details of exercise prescription for healthy populations as well as clinical populations, refer to *ASCM's Guidelines for Exercise Testing and Prescription* by the American College of Sports Medicine (ACSM, 2014).

■ INTERVENTIONS/STRATEGIES FOR RISK REDUCTION AND MANAGEMENT

Physical Activity and Blood Pressure

Several mechanisms are proposed to explain the blood pressure–lowering effects of physical activity. First of all, a bout of physical activity has the immediate and temporary effect of lowering blood pressure through dilation of the peripheral blood vessels. Repeated and regular exercise training induces remodeling of the vasculature of the heart and other blood vessels. Existing arterial vessels are enlarged and new capillaries developed in large muscles. Furthermore, regular exercise training has the ongoing effect of lowering blood pressure by attenuating sympathetic nervous system activity (Pescatello et al., 2004).

Research demonstrates the role of physical activity in the prevention as well as the treatment of hypertension. Longitudinal studies show that high levels of physical fitness are associated with decreased risk of developing hypertension. Barlow et al. (2006) reported that cardiorespiratory fitness, assessed with maximal exercise testing, predicted the incidence of hypertension in 4,884 women observed from 1970 to 1998. Kokkinos et al. (2006) also reported that fitness level was inversely associated with blood pressure in prehypertensive men and women. The effect of participation in multiple short bouts of activity on blood pressure was examined in African American women with prehypertension (130–139/85–89 mmHg) or untreated stage 1 hypertension (140–159/90–99 mmHg). Those who were assigned to an 8-week individualized, home-based lifestyle physical activity program showed a significant reduction in systolic blood pressure (Staffileno, Minnick, Coke, & Hollenberg, 2007). Although the sample size was small, the effectiveness of multiple, short bouts of lifestyle physical activity suggest a potential use of increasing physical activity levels in sedentary women.

A recent systematic review with meta-analysis on the effect of exercise on blood pressure indicated that endurance, dynamic resistance, and isometric resistance training lowers systolic blood pressure and diastolic blood pressure, whereas combined training lowers only diastolic blood pressure (Cornelissen & Smart, 2013). In a small number of studies on isometric resistance training, the effect of isometric resistance training was inconclusive. Based on the current evidence, the exercise prescription in Box 14.1 is recommended for individuals with hypertension (ACSM, 2014).

Physical Activity and Blood Lipids

Because lipids or fats are water-insoluble substances, they need to bind with some other substance to be transported in the blood. Lipoproteins are a group of proteins to which a lipid molecule can attach. Classifications for lipoproteins are based on their size and makeup. The major forms of lipoproteins are LDL-C and HDL-C. The TC content of plasma is a measure of LDL-C, HDL-C, and other lipid components. LDL-C is composed of protein, a small portion of triglyceride (TG), and a large portion of cholesterol. It transports cholesterol and TG in the body to all cells except liver cells and is involved in the development of atherosclerotic plaque in the arteries. On the other hand, the HDL-C is a lipoprotein composed primarily of protein and a minimum of cholesterol or TG. It transports cholesterol from the cells and returns it to the liver to be metabolized. Increased levels of HDL-C help prevent the atherosclerotic process.

Physical activity positively affects lipid metabolism and lipid profiles. The studies have shown increased HDL-C levels and decreased levels of TG, with less consistent reduction in LDL-C and TC (Dishman, Heath, & Lee, 2012). Increased HDL-C and reduced TG levels are often observed after certain exercise thresholds are met (i.e., 15–20 miles/wk of brisk walking or jogging, which produce between 1,200 and 2,200 kcal of energy expenditure per week). TC and LDL-C reductions occur when dietary fat intake is reduced and body weight loss is associated with physical activity (Durstine, Grandjean, Cox, & Thompson, 2002). Although the biological mechanism is not fully understood, physical activity seems to promote the effect of regulatory lipoprotein enzymes on the increased use of TGs as energy. Lifestyle (e.g., diet with reduced fat intake, weight loss) or pharmacological interventions, in addition to physical activity, may be required to maintain normal ranges of lipid and lipoprotein profiles for those with dyslipidemia (Durstine et al., 2002).

A systematic review with a meta-analysis of 35 randomized controlled trials (31 aerobic training and 4 resistance training) conducted in hyperlipidemic and normolipidemic adults found that aerobic exercise training caused small but statistically significant decreases in TC, LDL-C, and TG, with an increase in HDL-C, whereas resistance-exercise training resulted in a statistically significant decrease in LDL-C but without changes for TC, TG, and HDL-C (Halbert, Silagy, Finucane, Withers, & Hamdorf, 1999). However, the authors suggested that the limited effect of resistance training might result from a small number of resistance-training studies. In a randomized, controlled trial with 1,514 and 1,528 healthy men and women, the combination of resistance and aerobic exercise on lipids resulted in greater decreases in TG and LDL-C in men and LDL-C in women when compared with aerobic exercise (Pitsavos et al., 2009). Another systematic review concluded that high-intensity aerobic exercise seems to result in elevated HDL-C, whereas resistance exercise leads to decreases in LDL-C (Tambalis, Panagiotakos, Kavouras, & Sidossis, 2009). These data overall suggest that combining aerobic and resistance activities may have a better effect on lipoprotein in healthy adults than aerobic activities alone. Based on the current evidence, the exercise prescription in Box 14.2 is recommended for individuals with dyslipidemia (ACSM, 2014).

BOX 14.1   EXERCISE PRESCRIPTION FOR INDIVIDUALS WITH HYPERTENSION

Frequency	On most, preferably all, days of the week
Intensity	Moderate intensity (40%–60% of aerobic capacity reserve VO$_2$R[a])
Time	30 minutes of continuous or accumulated physical activity per day
Type	Primarily endurance physical activity supplemented by resistance exercise

[a] VO$_2$R is the difference between the maximum and the resting rate of oxygen consumption.

BOX 14.2 EXERCISE PRESCRIPTION FOR INDIVIDUALS WITH DYSLIPIDEMIA

Frequency	On most, preferably all, days of the week
Intensity	Moderate intensity (40%–75% of VO$_2$R[a])
Time	30 minutes of continuous or accumulated physical activity per day. However, 50–60 minutes of daily exercise is recommended.
Type	Primarily endurance physical activity supplemented by resistance exercise and flexibility exercise

[a] VO$_2$R is the difference between the maximum and the resting rates of oxygen consumption.

BOX 14.3 EXERCISE PRESCRIPTION FOR INDIVIDUALS WITH DIABETES MELLITUS

Frequency	3–7 d/wk
Intensity	40% to < 60% of VO$_2$R[a]; better blood glucose control may be achieved at higher exercise intensities (≥ 60% VO$_2$R)
Time	A minimum of 150 min/wk of exercise at moderate intensity or greater is recommended
Type	Emphasize activities that use large muscle groups

[a] VO$_2$R is the difference between the maximum and the resting rate of oxygen consumption.

Physical Activity and Glucose Metabolism

During physical activity, energy demands for muscular contraction require that more glucose be made available to the muscles. Because glucose is stored in the body as glycogen, primarily in the muscles and the liver, glucose must be freed from its storage and then enters the blood (glycogenolysis). Plasma glucose concentration also can be increased through gluconeogenesis, which uses noncarbohydrate sources such as pyruvate, lactate, and some amino acids to produce glycogen, which is then converted to glucose. Once glucose is delivered to the muscle, insulin facilitates its transport into cells.

Depletion of glycogen stores in both the muscles and the liver stimulates the production of enzymes, which increases non-insulin-dependent uptake of glucose by skeletal muscle (Chibalin et al., 2000; Koval et al., 1999). Exercise has been shown to increase glucose uptake by skeletal muscles, but plasma levels of insulin tend to decline. In addition, the ability of insulin to bind to its receptors on muscle cells increases during exercise, thereby reducing the need for high concentrations of plasma insulin to transport glucose into the cell. However, for the diabetic, special consideration should be given to maintain appropriate blood glucose levels during exercise.

DM is a disease characterized by an elevated blood glucose concentration as a result of defects in insulin secretion and/or an inability to use insulin. Type 1 DM results from severe insulin deficiency, whereas type 2 is caused by insulin-resistant skeletal muscle, adipose tissue, and liver combined with defects in insulin secretion. The management of DM is glycemic control using diet, exercise, and in many cases, medications such as insulin or oral hypoglycemic agents. The beneficial effect of exercise on glucose metabolism is increased insulin receptor activity. Arciero, Vukovich, Holloszy, Racette, and Kohrt (1999) reported that there was a marked increase in glucose disposal after exercise training in obese, hyperglycemic men and women, despite lower insulin levels, indicating that short-term exercise enhances insulin action in individuals with impaired glucose tolerance.

The Diabetes Prevention Program (DPP), a randomized, controlled trial of 3,234 overweight prediabetic adults, found that lifestyle modification aimed at reducing weight by 7% through a low-fat diet and exercise (150 minutes per week) was effective in preventing type 2 DM (Knowler et al., 2002). After 3 years of the intervention, 14% of the group using lifestyle modifications developed diabetes, whereas 29% of the placebo group and 22% of the metformin group (oral hypoglycemic drug) developed diabetes. The lifestyle modification was effective in both men and women across all ethnic groups. These data suggest that interventions aimed at lifestyle modifications can prevent or delay type 2 DM.

Based on the current evidence, the exercise prescription in Box 14.3 is recommended for individuals with DM (ACSM, 2014).

Physical Activity and Bone Health

The type of exercise or activity performed greatly influences skeletal adaptations. Weight-bearing exercise is activity in which the body weight is supported by muscles and bones, thereby working against gravity (e.g., walking, running, resistance training). Nonweight-bearing exercise, in contrast, refers to activity in which the body weight is artificially supported (e.g., stationary cycling, swimming). Weight-bearing activities are more likely to stimulate increased bone mass than nonweight-bearing activities.

Overall, studies suggest that weight-bearing and resistance exercise improve bone mass during childhood and adolescence, increasing or maintaining bone mass through adulthood (Barnekow-Bergkvist, Hedberg, Pettersson, & Lorentzon, 2006; Delvaux et al., 2001). However, cessation of weight-bearing exercise results in a loss of the positive adaptation obtained by training; the increased bone mineral resulting from exercise is lost if exercise is discontinued (Dalsky et al., 1988).

Loss of bone mineral (osteoporosis) is a serious health problem affecting millions of Americans. Clinical problems associated with osteoporosis include greater incidence of fractures and considerable pain from the fractures and curvature of the spine. It is believed that the rapid loss of bone mineral density after menopause is associated with the decrease in estrogen levels. However, postmenopausal women are not the only people at risk for developing osteoporosis and subsequent bone fractures. Young female athletes who experience training-related amenorrhea or menstrual irregularity are at risk for bone loss. Individuals with chronic conditions, such as organ transplantation, autoimmune disease, and seizure disorders, are also at increased risk of osteoporosis as a result of either physical inactivity or drug therapies (e.g., glucocorticoids, antiepileptics). In addition to its positive effect on bone mineral density, exercise may help reduce the risk of fractures by increasing muscular strength and coordination, thereby decreasing the risk of falling (Kemmler, von Stengel, Engelke, Häberle, & Kalender, 2010). Based on the current evidence, the exercise prescription in Box 14.4 is recommended for individuals with osteoporosis (ACSM, 2014):

Physical Activity and Mood and Affect

Some evidence of epidemiological research indicates that physical activity may be associated with reduced symptoms of depression and symptoms of anxiety in men and women (Ross & Hayes, 1988; Stephens, 1988). Similarly, meta-analyses of randomized controlled trials indicate that exercise reduces depressive and anxiety symptoms among people with or without diagnosed depression or anxiety (Ensari, Greenlee, Motl, & Petruzzello, 2015). Some researchers have proposed that exercise induces changes in

neurobiological mechanisms involving elevations in endogenous opioids (e.g., endorphins, enkephalins; Thorén, Floras, Hoffmann, & Seals, 1990) and neurotransmitters (e.g., dopamine, norepinephrine, serotonin; Ransford, 1982) in the brain, which may be associated with elevating mood and reducing pain. Current evidence, however, is limited to explain a biologically plausible explanation for the role of physical activity on mental disorders.

Recently, affect or mood has received more attention as an important determinant of future physical activity. A recent review shows that positive changes in the affective response during moderate-intensity exercise was associated with future physical activity behavior in the small–large effect size range (Rhodes & Kates, 2015). However, the relationship of affective response to exercise with key potential mediators of behavior, such as intention and self-efficacy, were inconclusive. More research is needed to understand the process by which affect may influence behavior. Although exercise is considered to produce the positive changes in affect, overtraining athletes are known to experience mood disturbances in addition to physical symptoms, such as frequent upper respiratory tract infections, muscle soreness, and sleep disturbances (Winsley & Matos, 2011). The optimal exercise program for improving or maintaining mental health has yet to be determined.

Physical Activity and the Menstrual Cycle

Women athletes who perform vigorous exercise training can be placed at high risk for menstrual dysfunction. Low energy availability resulting from exercise and/or dietary restriction is hypothesized to cause disruption to the hypothalamic–pituitary–ovarian (HPO) axis (Plowman & Smith, 2014). Decreased gonadotropin-releasing hormone (GnRH) release from the hypothalamus results in the suppression of the release of pituitary follicule-stimulating hormone (FSH) and luteinizing hormone (LH), which in turn causes attenuated estrogen (estradiol) and progesterone concentration. It has been also proposed that the physical and psychological stress from exercise elevates cortisol levels, resulting in the suppression of the GnRH release and disruption of the normal menstrual cycle.

Menstrual dysfunction can include delayed menarche, shortened luteal phase, anovulation, oligomenorrhea (irregular or inconsistent menstrual cycles), and amenorrhea (complete cessation of menstrual cycle). One of the major concerns with absence of the menstrual cycle is the low levels of circulating estrogen (hypoestrogenia) that may negatively affect bone mass. Almost half of bone mass is attained during adolescence and young adulthood. However, late maturing girls may be at increased risk of failure to reach potential peak bone mass. There is an increased risk of premature bone loss in women with amenorrhea (Ackerman & Misra, 2011).

Physical Activity During Pregnancy and Postpartum

Pregnancy places enormous changes on a woman's body and requires special consideration regarding the amount

---

BOX 14.4 EXERCISE PRESCRIPTION FOR INDIVIDUALS WITH OSTEOPOROSIS

Frequency	Weight-bearing aerobic activities 3–5 d/wk and resistance exercise 2–3 d/wk
Intensity	Moderate intensity (40%–60% of VO_2R^a) for weight-bearing aerobic activities and moderate intensity (60%–80% 1-RM[b], 8–12 repetitions of exercises involving each major muscle group) in terms of bone loading forces
Time	30–60 minutes of combination of weight-bearing aerobic and resistance activities
Type	Weight-bearing aerobic activities and resistance exercise

[a]VO_2R is the difference between the maximum and the resting rates of oxygen consumption.
[b]1-RM: 1-repetition maximum (RM), which is the maximum weight that the individual can lift for a given number of repetitions of an exercise.

and type of exercise for the safety of the fetus and the mother. Overall, substantial evidence indicates that exercise is safe and beneficial for healthy pregnant women (Downs, Chasan-Taber, Evenson, Leiferman, & Yeo, 2012). The benefits include fewer discomforts, less fatigue, and shorter and easier delivery (Artal & Sherman, 1999; Sternfeld, Quesenberry, Eskenazi, & Newman, 1995; Wang & Apgar, 1998). Exercise during pregnancy is also helpful in preventing excessive gestational weight gain (Choi, Fukuoka, & Lee, 2013; Streuling et al., 2011).

In the past, it was recommended that pregnant women limit strenuous exercise by the American College of Obstetricians and Gynecologists (ACOG, 1985). In 2002 however, ACOG revised their recommendation for physical activity for pregnant women in the absence of either medical or obstetric complication, suggesting that pregnant women should adopt the Centers for Disease Control and Prevention and ACSM recommendation for exercise, which is an accumulation of 30 minutes or more of moderate exercise a day on most days of the week (ACOG, 2002).

The U.S. Physical Activity Guidelines suggest that healthy pregnant women should accumulate at least 150 min/wk of moderate-intensity activity. However, pregnant women with cardiovascular, pulmonary, or metabolic disease, as well as those who were physically inactive before pregnancy or who are severely underweight or obese, should seek a health care provider's guidance concerning exercise. The contraindications for exercise during pregnancy are determined by ACOG (2002). In addition, the Physical Activity Readiness Medical Examination (PARmed-X) for pregnancy is a useful tool for screening for potential medical problems and assists with exercise prescription for pregnant women (www.csep.ca/cmfiles/publications/parq/parmed-xpreg.pdf). Maximum exercise testing should be avoided for pregnant women unless it is medically necessary, and it needs to be done under the supervision of a physician (ACSM, 2014).

Because of the demands of pregnancy, certain types of activities are not safe for pregnant women. After the first trimester, pregnant women are advised to avoid supine positions during exercise because the enlarged uterus can apply pressure to the surrounding blood vessels and obstruct venous return leading to decreased cardiac output and orthostatic hypotension. In addition, pregnant women should not participate in activities with a high potential for contact, falling, and trauma. Exercise involving extremes in air pressure such as scuba diving and exercise at altitudes more than 6,000 feet (1,829 m) could be potentially dangerous.

During postpartum, the return to prepregnancy activity should be gradual and based on individual response. There is no evidence to suggest that exercise negatively affects lactation. Findings of studies with lactating women suggest that exercise does not affect breast milk composition and volume or infant growth (Dewey, Lovelady, Nommsen-Rivers, McCrory, & Lönnerdal, 1994; Lovelady, Nommsen-Rivers, McCrory, & Dewey, 1995). In addition, the potential beneficial effects of resistance training on bone mineral density were reported in lactating women (Lovelady, Bopp, Colleran, Mackie, & Wideman, 2009).

FUTURE DIRECTIONS

Women are at increased risk of several conditions that can be effectively modified or prevented with exercise. Partnering with women to identify clear exercise prescriptions that are feasible in their individual lives is critical. More research is needed that focuses on how exercise can further modify or prevent health risks for women and how exercise can be effectively integrated into women's daily life patterns.

REFERENCES

Ackerman, K. E., & Misra, M. (2011). Bone health and the female athlete triad in adolescent athletes. *The Physician and Sports Medicine, 39*(1), 131–141.

American College of Obstetricians and Gynecologists (ACOG). (1985). *Technical bulletin: Exercise during pregnancy and the postnatal period.* Washington, DC: ACOG.

American College of Obstetricians and Gynecologists (ACOG). (2002). Exercise during pregnancy and the postnatal period. ACOG Committee Opinion No. 267. *Obstetrics & Gynecology, 99*(1), 171–173.

American College of Sports Medicine (ACSM). (2014). *ACSM's guidelines for exercise testing and prescription* (9th ed.). Philadelphia, PA: Wolters Kluwer/Lippincott Williams & Wilkins.

Arciero, P. J., Vukovich, M. D., Holloszy, J. O., Racette, S. B., & Kohrt, W. M. (1999). Comparison of short-term diet and exercise on insulin action in individuals with abnormal glucose tolerance. *Journal of Applied Physiology, 86*(6), 1930–1935.

Artal, R., & Sherman, C. (1999). Exercise during pregnancy: Safe and beneficial for most. *The Physician and Sports Medicine, 27*(8), 51–75.

Barlow, C. E., LaMonte, M. J., Fitzgerald, S. J., Kampert, J. B., Perrin, J. L., & Blair, S. N. (2006). Cardiorespiratory fitness is an independent predictor of hypertension incidence among initially normotensive healthy women. *American Journal of Epidemiology, 163*(2), 142–150.

Barnekow-Bergkvist, M., Hedberg, G., Pettersson, U., & Lorentzon, R. (2006). Relationships between physical activity and physical capacity in adolescent females and bone mass in adulthood. *Scandinavian Journal of Medicine & Science in Sports, 16*(6), 447–455.

Brownson, R. C., Eyler, A. A., King, A. C., Brown, D. R., Shyu, Y. L., & Sallis, J. F. (2000). Patterns and correlates of physical activity among U.S. women 40 years and older. *American Journal of Public Health, 90*(2), 264–270.

Caspersen, C. J., Powell, K. E., & Christenson, G. M. (1985). Physical activity, exercise, and physical fitness: Definitions and distinctions for health-related research. *Public Health Reports, 100*(2), 126–131.

Chibalin, A. V., Yu, M., Ryder, J. W., Song, X. M., Galuska, D., Krook, A.,...Zierath, J. R. (2000). Exercise-induced changes in expression and activity of proteins involved in insulin signal transduction in skeletal muscle: Differential effects on insulin-receptor substrates 1 and 2. *Proceedings of the National Academy of Sciences of the United States of America, 97*(1), 38–43.

Choi, J., Fukuoka, Y., & Lee, J. H. (2013). The effects of physical activity and physical activity plus diet interventions on body weight in overweight or obese women who are pregnant or in postpartum: A systematic review and meta-analysis of randomized controlled trials. *Preventive Medicine, 56*(6), 351–364.

Cornelissen, V. A., & Smart, N. A. (2013). Exercise training for blood pressure: A systematic review and meta-analysis. *Journal of the American Heart Association, 2*(1), e004473.

Cramp, A. G., & Brawley, L. R. (2006). Moms in motion: A group-mediated cognitive-behavioral physical activity intervention. *International Journal of Behavioral Nutrition and Physical Activity, 3*, 23.

Dalsky, G. P., Stocke, K. S., Ehsani, A. A., Slatopolsky, E., Lee, W. C., & Birge, S. J. (1988). Weight-bearing exercise training and lumbar bone mineral content in postmenopausal women. *Annals of Internal Medicine, 108*(6), 824–828.

Delvaux, K., Lefevre, J., Philippaerts, R., Dequeker, J., Thomis, M., Vanreusel, B.,...Lysens, R. (2001). Bone mass and lifetime physical activity in Flemish males: A 27-year follow-up study. *Medicine and Science in Sports and Exercise, 33*(11), 1868–1875.

Dewey, K. G., Lovelady, C. A., Nommsen-Rivers, L. A., McCrory, M. A., & Lönnerdal, B. (1994). A randomized study of the effects of aerobic exercise by lactating women on breast-milk volume and composition. *New England Journal of Medicine, 330*(7), 449–453.

Dishman, R. K., Heath, G. W., & Lee, I.-M. (2012). Physical activity epidemiology (2nd ed.). Champaign, IL: Human Kinetics.

Downs, D. S., Chasan-Taber, L., Evenson, K. R., Leiferman, J., & Yeo, S. (2012). Physical activity and pregnancy: Past and present evidence and future recommendations. *Research Quarterly for Exercise and Sport, 83*(4), 485–502.

Durstine, J. L., Grandjean, P. W., Cox, C. A., & Thompson, P. D. (2002). Lipids, lipoproteins, and exercise. *Journal of Cardiopulmonary Rehabilitation, 22*(6), 385–398.

Ensari, I., Greenlee, T. A., Motl, R. W., & Petruzzello, S. J. (2015). Meta-analysis of acute exercise effects on state anxiety: An update of randomized controlled trials over the past 25 years. *Depression and Anxiety, 32*, 624–634. doi:10.1002/da.22370

Eyler, A. E., Wilcox, S., Matson-Koffman, D., Evenson, K. R., Sanderson, B., Thompson, J.,...Rohm-Young, D. (2002). Correlates of physical activity among women from diverse racial/ethnic groups. *Journal of Women's Health & Gender-Based Medicine, 11*(3), 239–253.

Go, A. S., Mozaffarian, D., Roger, V. L., Benjamin, E. J., Berry, J. D., Borden, W. B., ... Turner, M. B.; American Heart Association Statistics Committee and Stroke Statistics Subcommittee. (2013). Heart disease and stroke statistics—2013 update: A report from the American Heart Association. *Circulation, 127*, e6–e245.

Halbert, J. A., Silagy, C. A., Finucane, P., Withers, R. T., & Hamdorf, P. A. (1999). Exercise training and blood lipids in hyperlipidemic and normolipidemic adults: A meta-analysis of randomized, controlled trials. *European Journal of Clinical Nutrition, 53*(7), 514–522.

Janssen, I., Katzmarzyk, P. T., & Ross, R. (2004). Waist circumference and not body mass index explains obesity-related health risk. *American Journal of Clinical Nutrition, 79*(3), 379–384.

Kannel, W. B., Belanger, A., D'Agostino, R., & Israel, I. (1986). Physical activity and physical demand on the job and risk of cardiovascular disease and death: The Framingham Study. *American Heart Journal, 112*(4), 820–825.

Kemmler, W., von Stengel, S., Engelke, K., Häberle, L., & Kalender, W. A. (2010). Exercise effects on bone mineral density, falls, coronary risk factors, and health care costs in older women: The randomized controlled senior fitness and prevention (SEFIP) study. *Archives of Internal Medicine, 170*(2), 179–185.

Kimm, S. Y., Glynn, N. W., Kriska, A. M., Barton, B. A., Kronsberg, S. S., Daniels, S. R.,...Liu, K. (2002). Decline in physical activity in black girls and white girls during adolescence. *New England Journal of Medicine, 347*(10), 709–715.

Knowler, W. C., Barrett-Connor, E., Fowler, S. E., Hamman, R. F., Lachin, J. M., Walker, E. A., & Nathan, D. M.; Diabetes Prevention Program Research Group. (2002). Reduction in the incidence of type 2 diabetes with lifestyle intervention or metformin. *New England Journal of Medicine, 346*(6), 393–403.

Kokkinos, P., Pittaras, A., Manolis, A., Panagiotakos, D., Narayan, P., Manjoros, D.,...Singh, S. (2006). Exercise capacity and 24-h blood pressure in prehypertensive men and women. *American Journal of Hypertension, 19*(3), 251–258.

Koval, J. A., Maezono, K., Patti, M. E., Pendergrass, M., DeFronzo, R. A., & Mandarino, L. J. (1999). Effects of exercise and insulin on insulin signaling proteins in human skeletal muscle. *Medicine and Science in Sports and Exercise, 31*(7), 998–1004.

LaCroix, A. Z., Leveille, S. G., Hecht, J. A., Grothaus, L. C., & Wagner, E. H. (1996). Does walking decrease the risk of cardiovascular disease hospitalizations and death in older adults? *Journal of the American Geriatrics Society, 44*(2), 113–120.

Lovelady, C. A., Bopp, M. J., Colleran, H. L., Mackie, H. K., & Wideman, L. (2009). Effect of exercise training on loss of bone mineral density during lactation. *Medicine and Science in Sports and Exercise, 41*(10), 1902–1907.

Lovelady, C. A., Nommsen-Rivers, L. A., McCrory, M. A., & Dewey, K. G. (1995). Effects of exercise on plasma lipids and metabolism of lactating women. *Medicine and Science in Sports and Exercise, 27*(1), 22–28.

Mozaffarian, D., Benjamin, E. J., Go, A. S., Arnett, D. K., Blaha, M. J., Cushman, M.,...Turner, M. B.; American Heart Association Statistics Committee and Stroke Statistics Subcommittee. (2015). Heart disease and stroke statistics—2015 update: A report from the American Heart Association. *Circulation, 131*(4), e29–322.

National Heart, Lung, and Blood Institute (NHLBI). (1998). *Clinical guidelines on the identification, evaluation, and treatment of overweight and obesity in adults* (NIH publication No. 98–4083). Bethesda, MD: National Institutes of Health, National Heart, Lung, and Blood Institute.

Paffenbarger, R. S., Jr., Hyde, R. T., Wing, A. L., & Steinmetz, C. H. (1984). A natural history of athleticism and cardiovascular health. *Journal of the American Medical Association, 23*, 319–327.

Pescatello, L. S., Franklin, B. A., Fagard, R., Farquhar, W. B., Kelley, G. A., & Ray, C. A.; American College of Sports Medicine. (2004). American College of Sports Medicine position stand: Exercise and hypertension. *Medicine and Science in Sports and Exercise, 36*(3), 533–553.

Pitsavos, C., Panagiotakos, D. B., Tambalis, K. D., Chrysohoou, C., Sidossis, L. S., Skoumas, J., & Stefanadis, C. (2009). Resistance exercise plus to aerobic activities is associated with better lipids' profile among healthy individuals: The ATTICA study. *Quarterly Journal of Medicine, 102*(9), 609–616.

Plowman, S. A., & Smith, D. L. (2014). *Exercise physiology for health, fitness, and performance* (4th ed.). Philadelphia, PA: Wolters Kluwer/Lippincott Williams & Wilkins.

Ransford, C. P. (1982). A role for amines in the antidepressant effect of exercise: A review. *Medicine and Science in Sports and Exercise, 14*(1), 1–10.

Rhodes, R. E., & Kates, A. (2015). Can the affective response to exercise predict future motives and physical activity behavior? A systematic review of published evidence. *Annals of Behavioral Medicine, 49*(5), 715–731.

Ross, C. E., & Hayes, D. (1988). Exercise and psychologic well-being in the community. *American Journal of Epidemiology, 127*(4), 762–771.

Sallis, J. F., Prochaska, J. J., & Taylor, W. C. (2000). A review of correlates of physical activity of children and adolescents. *Medicine and Science in Sports and Exercise, 32*(5), 963–975.

Staffileno, B. A., Minnick, A., Coke, L. A., & Hollenberg, S. M. (2007). Blood pressure responses to lifestyle physical activity among young, hypertension-prone African-American women. *Journal of Cardiovascular Nursing, 22*(2), 107–117.

Stephens, T. (1988). Physical activity and mental health in the United States and Canada: Evidence from four population surveys. *Preventive Medicine, 17*(1), 35–47.

Sternfeld, B., Ainsworth, B. E., & Quesenberry, C. P. (1999). Physical activity patterns in a diverse population of women. *Preventive Medicine, 28*(3), 313–323.

Sternfeld, B., Quesenberry, C. P., Eskenazi, B., & Newman, L. A. (1995). Exercise during pregnancy and pregnancy outcome. *Medicine and Science in Sports and Exercise, 27*(5), 634–640.

Streuling, I., Beyerlein, A., Rosenfeld, E., Hofmann, H., Schulz, T., & von Kries, R. (2011). Physical activity and gestational weight gain: A meta-analysis of intervention trials. *British Journal of Obstetrics and Gynaecology, 118*(3), 278–284.

Tambalis, K., Panagiotakos, D. B., Kavouras, S. A., & Sidossis, L. S. (2009). Responses of blood lipids to aerobic, resistance, and combined aerobic with resistance exercise training: A systematic review of current evidence. *Angiology, 60*(5), 614–632.

Thorén, P., Floras, J. S., Hoffmann, P., & Seals, D. R. (1990). Endorphins and exercise: Physiological mechanisms and clinical implications. *Medicine and Science in Sports and Exercise, 22*(4), 417–428.

Trost, S. G., Owen, N., Bauman, A. E., Sallis, J. F., & Brown, W. (2002). Correlates of adults' participation in physical activity: Review and update. *Medicine and Science in Sports and Exercise, 34*(12), 1996–2001.

U.S. Department of Health and Human Services (USDHHS). (1996). *Physical activity and health: A report of the Surgeon General.* Atlanta, GA: USDHHS, Centers for Disease Control and Prevention, National Center for Chronic Disease Prevention and Health Promotion.

U.S. Department of Health and Human Services (USDHHS). (2008). *Physical activity guidelines for Americans.* Retrieved from www.health.gov/paguidelines/guidelines

Wang, T. W., & Apgar, B. S. (1998). Exercise during pregnancy. *American Family Physician, 57*(8), 1846–1852, 1857.

Winsley, R., & Matos, N. (2011). Overtraining and elite young athletes. *Medicine and Sport Science, 56*, 97–105.

CHAPTER 15

Healthy Practices: Sleep

Carol A. Landis

Sleep is essential for life, health, and well-being. The American Academy of Sleep Medicine (AASM) in collaboration with the Sleep Research Society (SRS) recently published a consensus statement with a recommendation that adults 18 to 60 years of age should obtain *at least* 7 hours of sleep per night (Watson et al., 2015). In a similar fashion, the American Thoracic Society (ATS) published a recent policy statement on the importance of obtaining adequate and good-quality sleep (Mukherjee et al., 2015). They also recommend that adults obtain between 7 and 9 hours of nightly sleep. The Centers for Disease Control and Prevention (CDC) has awarded the AASM a cooperative agreement project called the National Healthy Sleep Awareness Project (2013–2018) (CDC, 2014). The project goals are focused on generating awareness of the growing epidemic of insufficient sleep and subsequent health consequences among children, youth, and adults in the United States. The project is centered on making progress toward meeting the sleep-specific objectives of *Healthy People 2020* (Box 15.1)

The increasing emphasis on advocating and promoting adequate sleep is the result of published CDC reports on the extent of insufficient sleep based on questions about sleep from the national Behavioral Risk Factor Surveillance System Survey of adults in the United States (CDC, 2011). These data reveal that one in three adults reported sleeping less than 7 hours/night and 10% reported not getting enough sleep every day for a month. The problem of daily insufficient sleep is greater among adults aged 18 to 34 years (13.3%) compared with those 55 years or older (7.3%). In the United States and other developed countries, the number of adults and teenagers obtaining recommended amounts of sleep has declined. It has been estimated that adults in modern society sleep more than 2 hours less compared with a 100 years ago before widespread use of electric lighting extended daily activities into the nighttime (1910 = 9 hours; 2002 = 6.9 hours; National Sleep Foundation [NSF], 2010). A recent study of indigenous groups in South America provides data to support the idea that access to electric lights affects sleep duration (de la Iglesia et al., 2015). When participants with access to electricity were compared with those without access, the latter slept about an hour longer, mostly explained by going to bed earlier. Most adults believe that insufficient sleep leads to poor job performance, higher risk for injury, and health problems, yet 50% also believe that severe daytime sleepiness is "normal" (NSF, 2001). The prevalence of insufficient sleep coincides with rising rates of obesity, diabetes, and development of chronic conditions (Mukherjee et al., 2015). Insufficient sleep has been documented to contribute to the development of these conditions, and its role in etiology is an active area of investigation (see section on Sleep Health Promotion).

Obtaining adequate quality sleep is a struggle for many women of all ages. Across the adult life span, women complain about poor sleep to a greater extent compared with men and are at higher risk of developing insomnia (Arber, Bote, & Meadows, 2009). However, investigators from several studies reported that women actually sleep better than men based on objective sleep measures (e.g., with polysomnography [PSG]; Bixler et al., 2009; Redline et al., 2004). In one population-based study of 609 men (49.1 ± 13.8 years) and 715 women (47.0 ± 13.3 years), women showed a higher amount of total sleep time (TST), less stage 1 (of light sleep) and more slow-wave sleep (SWS; Bixler et al., 2009). This paradox could be explained on the basis of a higher prevalence of anxiety and depression in women compared with men because insomnia often occurs in these disorders, yet this does not explain observations of better objectively measured sleep in healthy women. An alternative explanation could be stress exposure, which has been shown to be a significant predictor of insomnia onset in a community-based sample of good sleepers in which women also showed a significantly higher risk for developing insomnia (Pillai, Roth, Mullins, & Drake, 2014). However, these explanations fail to take into consideration the gendered nature of women's lives.

Women's social roles, economic status, and responsibilities, as they endeavor to balance work and family demands, may be an important influence on the assessment of sleep health and sleep problems. An analysis of survey data obtained in 2000 from 8,578 British men and women aged 16 to 74 years revealed that women self-reported significantly more trouble sleeping on at least 4 nights/week compared with men (odds ratio [OR] = 1.49). The odds of poor sleep were reduced by half (OR = 1.27) in models adjusted for age, marital status, socioeconomic factors, worries about life, health status, and mood (anxiety and depression; Arber et al., 2009). In this analysis, four measures of socioeconomic status (not working for pay, income, educational

BOX 15.1   SLEEP-SPECIFIC OBJECTIVES OF *HEALTHY PEOPLE 2020*

- Increasing the proportion of persons with symptoms of obstructive sleep apnea (OSA) who seek medical evaluation
- Reducing the rate of vehicular crashes per 100 million miles traveled that are caused by drowsy driving
- Increasing the proportion of students in grades 9 through 12 who get sufficient sleep
- Increasing the proportion of adults who get sufficient sleep.

Source: U.S. Department of Health and Human Services, Office of Disease Prevention and Health Promotion (2015).

BOX 15.2   SLEEP TERMINOLOGY AND COMMON ABBREVIATIONS

AASM: American Academy of Sleep Medicine
ACT: actigraphy
AHI: Apnea–Hypopnea Index
CBT-I: cognitive-behavioral therapy-insomnia
EDS: excessive daytime sleepiness
ISI: Insomnia Severity Index
MSLT: multiple sleep latency test
NREM: nonrapid eye movement
NSF: National Sleep Foundation
OSA: obstructive sleep apnea
PSG: polysomnography
PSQI: Pittsburgh Sleep Quality Index
REM: rapid eye movement
RLS: restless leg syndrome
SDB: sleep-disordered breathing
SE: sleep efficiency (TST/TIB × 100)
SEM: standard error of the mean
SOL: sleep onset latency
TIB: time in bed
TST: total sleep time
WASO: wake after sleep onset
WHIRS: Women's Health Initiative Insomnia Scale

attainment, and living in rented housing) each showed an independent, statistically significant association with sleep problems. The results from this survey raise doubts about the "primacy" of a biological explanation for poor self-reported sleep among women compared with men. A comprehensive understanding of the gender differences in the prevalence of and risk for sleep problems between women and men will require multidisciplinary and social science studies that take into account the gendered nature of women's multiple roles and responsibilities and how these affect especially time available for sleep. Women are the primary caregivers and managers of family activities and health practices; thus, a careful evaluation of women's sleep, risks for poor sleep quality, and the health consequences of inadequate or insufficient sleep is needed.

■ WHAT IS SLEEP?

Sleep can be defined in multiple ways: a behavioral state, a complex physiological process uniquely distinct from resting, and as a temporary, reversible suspension of consciousness or conscious awareness. Based on PSG data (see Box 15.2 for common sleep terminology), sleep is divided into two main behavioral states: nonrapid eye movement (NREM) and rapid eye movement (REM). NREM sleep is subdivided into three stages based primarily on different frequency and amplitude of electroencephalographic (EEG) and electromyographic (EMG) waveforms, which are called *N1, N2,* and *N3* (AASM, 2007). The criteria for visual scoring of sleep stages were revised in 2007 (AASM, 2007) and NREM stages 3 and 4 were combined into one stage, N3, which represents SWS.

Figure 15.1 is a hypnogram of a night of sleep consistent with that of a young adult. It shows five complete sleep cycles with only two very brief periods of waking during the night. At sleep onset, after a brief waking period, the first sleep cycle begins with a short amount of time spent in

N1 and N2 stages, followed by a longer interval of N3 and a short bout of REM sleep. This first cycle is followed by repeating cycles during which the amount of N3 gradually declines, N2 increases, and the bouts of REM longer, with the longest bout in the early morning before awakening. As one grows older, N3 still predominately occurs during the first half of a night of sleep, but the amount of N3 declines substantially by the fourth and fifth decades, whereas N2 and more frequent brief awakenings increase and bouts of REM become shorter.

Sleep and Wake Regulation

Sleep and wake are highly regulated processes controlled by brain networks. Humans ordinarily are day active, night sleepers. Sleep and wake are under both homeostatic and circadian (*circa dies,* about a day) control (Porkka-Heiskanen, Zitting, & Wigren, 2013). The homeostatic component regulates sleep intensity and duration such that longer intervals of waking are followed by more intense sleep episodes usually of longer duration. Simply put, the longer people are awake, the sleepier they become. The homeostatic drive for sleep rises during the day and dissipates after one falls asleep and throughout a night of sleep. From PSG recordings of sleep-deprived subjects, we know that amounts of both slow wave and REM sleep stages increase after a period of sleep deprivation. The intensity of SWS can be measured by the number of delta waves (frequency from 0.5 to 4 Hz), which is increased substantially in the first NREM period after even one night without sleep.

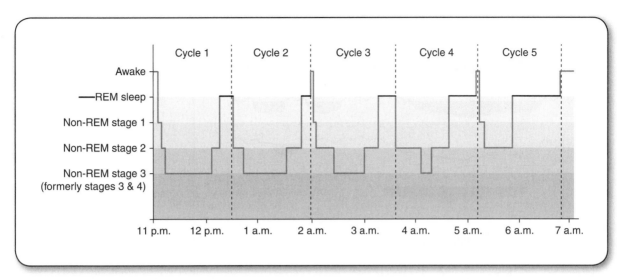

FIGURE 15.1

A typical hypnogram showing sleep stages and cycles in adult sleep.

REM, rapid eye movement.

Image by Luke Mastin. http://www.howsleepworks.com/types_cycles.html.

The timing of sleep and wake is controlled by a circadian clock mechanism located in the suprachiasmatic nucleus (SCN) in the hypothalamus. A "clock mechanism" and genes control the sleep–wake cycle (Zee, Attarian, & Videnovic, 2013). The hypothalamus is considered the master clock or pacemaker for the body, but all cells contain clock genes and show circadian rhythmicity. Clock genes control the timing and distribution of sleep and wake in the daily cycle, and select SCN neurons are thought to operate as an internal alarm clock to actively promote wakefulness (Goel, Basner, Rao, & Dinges, 2013). Circadian rhythms (CRs) persist when people are placed in isolated environments free from external time cues. Light is the main input for synchronizing the SCN to the environment through specific light detectors in the retina (Zee et al., 2013). Physical activity and melatonin, a hormone secreted from the pineal gland, also aid the entrainment of the endogenous clock to the environment. This entrainment is important for both optimal functioning and health. CRs are quite stable in an individual, but variations exist among people, called chronotypes. Some people are morning types, called *larks*, who get up early and function best in morning hours; others are evening types, called *night owls*, who stay up late and function best in evening hours. Some data show that the 24-hour endogenous CR is slightly shorter in women (circa 10 minutes) compared with men, which may contribute to the observation that more women self-report being morning types compared with men (Duffy et al., 2011).

Sleep Patterns Across the Human Life Span

SLEEP CYCLE DEVELOPMENT

Sleep cycle development from infancy to old age is shown in Figure 15.2. Infants have an ultradian sleep–wake rhythm, sleeping in short intervals of time and waking primarily for periodic feeding. By the time children are 4 years of age, they usually have only one nap in the afternoon and by age 10 years, the monophasic pattern of one long sleep episode at night is fully developed. Whether daytime napping continues into adolescence and adulthood is influenced more by volitional choice and culture than by physiology.

NORMATIVE SLEEP VALUES IN ADULTS

Normative sleep values based on PSG are limited because it is expensive to gather such data from a large number of healthy adults and because most data are limited to White participants. A meta-analysis of PSG sleep parameters from 65 laboratory sleep studies using data from 3,533 control participants aged 19 to 102 years revealed that TST and sleep efficiency (SE) declined while wake after sleep onset (WASO) increased (Ohayon, Carskadon, Guilleminault, & Vitiello, 2004). TST ranged from more than 550 minutes (approximately 9.1 hours) in children to less than 350 minutes (less than 5 hours) in adults older than 90 years; WASO ranged from less than 5 minutes in children to more than 80 minutes in adults aged 85 years. The amount of stage N3 or SWS declined after adolescence, and was reduced considerably, whereas N2 stage increased in middle-aged and older adults. The amount of REM sleep as a percentage of recording time is fairly constant. Most changes in sleep occur after 30 years of age and before 60 years of age. Few differences were found between sleep of women and men; however, the magnitude of age effects were attenuated as not all participants had been screened for mental disorders, use of alcohol and other drugs, or sleep disorders such as OSA in all the studies. Of note, no data on race/ethnicity were reported from these data obtained

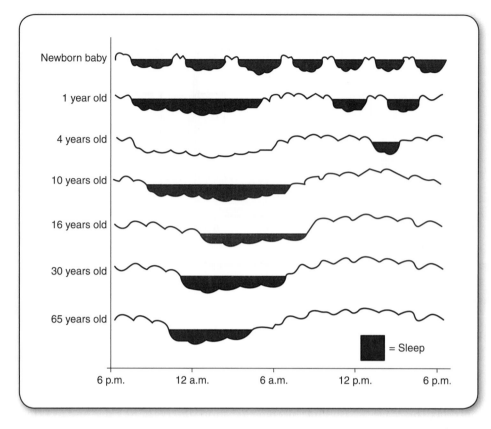

Newborn baby

1 year old

4 years old

10 years old

16 years old

30 years old

65 years old

■ = Sleep

6 p.m.   12 a.m.   6 a.m.   12 p.m.   6 p.m.

FIGURE 15.2
Sleep cycle development.
Image by Luke Mastin. http://www
.howsleepworks.com/need_age.html

from 1967 to 2003. A recent study based on revised AASM scoring criteria (2007) from Austria (Mitterling et al., 2015) in 100 carefully screened White adults 19 to 77 years of age revealed findings similar to those of the meta-analysis: decreased SE, TST, and SWS, although the percentage of WASO increased with a young group (30 years or younger) compared with a group of older adults (60 years or older). No data on gender differences were reported in this study.

Research on normative values for PSG sleep among different racial/ethnic groups is very limited. One narrative review (Durrence & Lichstein, 2006) of four PSG studies comparing sleep in healthy White with African American adults revealed African American participants showed more N1 and N2 stages of sleep and less SWS. One of the studies controlled for sleep disorders and compared laboratory with home sleep and found that although African American adults had lower SWS compared with Whites in both settings, they had more SWS at home compared with the laboratory. Data from the Study of Women's Health Across the Nation (SWAN) PSG home sleep study showed that among a racially diverse group of 368 predominantly premenopausal women, African American women showed on average significantly reduced TST (363.3 minutes [approximately 6 hours]) relative to Whites (393.9 minutes [approximately 6.5 hours]) and Chinese (390.4 [6.5 hours]; Hall et al., 2009). African American women also took longer to fall asleep (sleep onset latency [SOL] – African American, 24.5 minutes; Whites, 4.4 minutes; Chinese,

3.2 minutes); had more WASO (African American, 62.5 minutes; Whites, 47.7 minutes; Chinese, 43.4 minutes); and less percentage of SWS (African American, 2.5%; Whites, 4.4%; Chinese, 3.2%). Both African American and Chinese women had SEs of less than 85% and Pittsburgh Sleep Quality Index (PSQI) scores more than five indicating poor sleep compared with White women. Racial differences persisted after adjustment for socioeconomic status.

Data on self-reported sleep duration yield additional information about differences in sleep among racial/ethnic groups of adults in the United States. The 2007 to 2008 National Health and Nutrition Examination Survey (NHANES) data demonstrate that African American adults have a greater odds of reporting sleep duration of both less than 5 hours (OR = 2.34, p < .002) and less than 6 hours (OR = 1.85, p < .001) compared with Whites (Whinnery, Jackson, Rattanaumpawan, & Grandner, 2014). Hispanics/Latinos and Asians also had higher odds of reporting very short sleep duration (Hispanics/Latino, OR = 2.69, p < .025; Asian, OR = 3.99, p < .002). Those with lower incomes and educational attainment were also more likely to report shorter sleep duration, and these associations remained after controlling for health status. In other studies, African American adults have been more likely to report both short (less than 6 hours) and long (less than 9 hours) hours of sleep (Basner, Spaeth, & Dinges, 2014; Knutson, 2013). Among short sleepers, regardless of sociodemographic characteristics (except those who were unemployed or retired), adults spend time working rather than sleeping; adults working more than one job had the highest odds of sleeping less than 6 hours on weekdays (Basner et al., 2014).

ETIOLOGY AND RISK FACTORS OF SLEEP DISRUPTIONS

Sleep Habits Among U.S. Women

The NSF Sleep in America Poll (NSF, 2007) surveyed 1,003 women 18 to 64 years of age (77% Whites) about their sleep habits and problems. The sample was representative of a typical U.S. household with a telephone. The major findings from the survey revealed that poor sleep affects all aspects of women's lives. Many women were struggling to "do it all" and as a result sacrificed time for sleep as well as healthy practices, such as exercise. Biological as well as many lifestyle factors had an impact on their sleep quality. Sixty percent of the women reported obtaining a good night's sleep only a few times per week. Two thirds of the women reported sleep problems a few nights per week, and 46% reported sleep problems every single night. Working mothers (72%) and single working women (68%) were more likely to experience sleep problems and insomnia symptoms. Other factors associated with nighttime awakenings included noise (39%), child care (20%), and pets (17%). Nearly 50% of women reported that they were the only care providers for children at night. Women also reported excessive daytime sleepiness (EDS) accompanied by (a) experiencing high stress, anxiety, and worries (80%); (b) feeling unhappy or sad (55%), spending less time with friends (39%); (c) being too tired for sex (33%); (d) driving drowsy at least once a month; and (e) being late for work (20%). Some of the women in this survey routinely used prescription antidepressants (12%) or hypnotics (8%), or over-the-counter sleep aids (15%). Compared with women who reported excellent to very good health, women who reported fair to poor health or had a body mass index (BMI) of 30 or above were more likely to experience symptoms of a sleep disorder or had been given a diagnosis of a sleep disorder, missed work because of sleepiness, and use a sleep aid a few nights per week. *The findings in this survey are remarkable in that 80% of the women considered daytime sleepiness as something to accept and to keep going, often by consuming three or more caffeinated beverages per day.* Caffeine is an antagonist for adenosine receptors in the brain, and adenosine is thought to be an endogenous substance underlying the sleep drive that rises during the day (Porkka-Heiskanen et al., 2013). Caffeine has at least a 6-hour half-life, probably longer in older adults, such that caffeinated beverages consumed in the afternoon or early evening may lead to difficulty falling and staying asleep. Thus consumption of caffeine, although an effective countermeasure for daytime sleepiness, eventually may contribute to a vicious cycle of poor sleep, daytime sleepiness, more caffeine consumption, and poor sleep.

SLEEP IN A SOCIAL CONTEXT

Women are vulnerable to limiting sleep time because of work schedules, family routines, and care of children in particular. Data from a recent report from an analysis of the 2011 to 2013 American Time Use Survey (ATUS) provided insights into who provides the majority of "informal" or "nonpaid" care to others, mostly in the form of family obligations to care for children and/or elders living in the same household (Dukhovnov & Zagheni, 2015). The sample of approximately 12,000 persons was designed to be representative of the U.S. population. These analyses revealed that nearly one third of adults in the United States provide informal care to others, and among these, women between the ages of 30 and 50 years made up the highest proportion. Women in the so-called sandwich generation spend more time per day in providing care compared with the general population and the highest proportion of time was spent in parenting, caring for one's children rather than elders. It is important to note that during the stage of life when sleep patterns change the most, women experience high demands on their time in caring for others. Thus it comes as no surprise that women sacrifice sleep time to meet work and family responsibilities.

In U.S. families with at least one school-age child, parents (*n* = 1,103) reported that frequent evening activities and the use of technological devices in the bedroom were associated with fewer hours of sleep, reduced sleep quality, and more complaints of disturbed sleep (Buxton et al., 2015). In this study, more than 90% of parents reported sleep was "very to extremely important," yet 90% of all children did not obtain recommended amounts of sleep. The best predictors for children obtaining recommended amounts of good quality sleep included enforcing rules about limited caffeine intake, not using technological devices in the bedroom, and going to bed at a regular time. Perhaps, not surprising, if parents used technological devices in the bedroom, their children were more likely to use devices in the bedroom.

Women's Sleep During Life Stages

Before mandates from National Institutes of Health that required the inclusion of women in federally funded research studies, many laboratory sleep studies included only men. Today, although studies include men and women participants, the sample size often lacks sufficient power to analyze results based on gender. Nevertheless, beginning with the onset of menarche and continuing throughout life's transitions, women experience changes in reproductive hormones that affect sleep quality and quantity. Gender differences in sleep emerge with the onset of puberty; girls are at higher risk of developing and report more insomnia symptoms after puberty (Hysing, Pallesen, Stormark, Lundervold, & Sivertsen, 2013), and whether the increased risk can be explained primarily on the basis of hormonal changes with puberty is an open question. Sleep complaints are frequently reported during menses, with pregnancy, and during the menopause transition (MT).

MENSTRUAL CYCLE

Scheduling sleep study research in women needs to include documentation of, and preferably control for, where they are in their menstrual cycle. Overall, women are more likely to self-report sleep complaints in the late luteal phase and during menstruation (Kravitz et al., 2005). They complain of trouble falling asleep or long SOL, increased number of awakenings and increased WASO, leading to reduced SE, and in some studies, increased daytime sleepiness (EDS). The odds of reporting trouble sleeping were 29% higher in perimenopause compared with premenopausal women from the SWAN; both groups of women reported more trouble sleeping at the beginning and end of a menstrual cycle. A majority of women (74.5%) reported trouble sleeping for at least 1 night and 19.2% met criteria for chronic insomnia (Kravitz et al., 2005).

A recent PSG study of a small sample of 11 women with insomnia compared with nine controls revealed that both groups showed more awakenings ($p = .003$) and arousals ($p = .025$) per hour of sleep and less percentage of SWS ($p = .024$) during the luteal phase compared with the follicular phase (de Zambotti, Willoghby, Sasson, Colrain, & Baker, 2015). Women with insomnia had shorter sleep duration ($p = .012$), more WASO ($p = .031$), and a lower SE ($p = .034$) than women without insomnia, regardless of menstrual cycle phase. In another PSG study of 33 perimenopausal women aged 43 to 52 years (16 with a clinical diagnosis of insomnia) and 11 premenopausal women without sleep complaints (18–27 years), follicle-stimulating hormone (FSH) levels were positively associated with WASO, number of awakenings and arousals in perimenopausal women ($p < .05$) without sleep complaints independent of age, BMI, and hot flashes (de Zambotti et al., 2015). Similarly, FSH correlated with wakefulness after sleep onset and a light N1 sleep stage in premenopausal women ($p < .05$). However, in perimenopausal women with insomnia, there was no correlation with FSH, but there was with anxiety and depression ($p < .05$). Estradiol did not correlate with sleep in perimenopausal groups but correlated negatively with arousals in premenopausal women ($p < .01$). In summary, sleep is more disrupted in the luteal phase compared with the follicular phase in midlife women. Women with insomnia are more vulnerable to experience poor sleep that may be related to factors intrinsic to insomnia, such as mood disturbances and night-to-night variability, rather than to changing levels of reproductive hormones.

PREGNANCY AND POSTPARTUM

There is evidence of sleep disturbances during pregnancy, both from self-report and from objective sleep measures. Throughout pregnancy there are many changes in physiology associated with hormones, increased body temperature, increased respiratory rate, frequent urination, increased abdominal mass, and vascular load that could contribute to changes in sleep. From the 2007 NSF survey, 24% of women of childbearing age, 40% of pregnant women, and 55% of postpartum women reported obtaining a good night's sleep a few nights a month or less. Most pregnant women in the survey reported obtaining better sleep before pregnancy. Data from a recent Internet survey of 2,427 women showed that across all months of pregnancy, 76% reported poor sleep quality, 38% reported insufficient sleep, 49% reported EDS, and 78% took daytime naps (Mindell, Cook, & Nikolovski, 2015). Based on the Insomnia Severity Index (ISI), 57% reported insomnia symptoms with no differences across months of pregnancy. Frequent urination and inability to find a comfortable sleeping position were also common complaints. Most women fail to sleep through the night by the third trimester of pregnancy and napping during the day becomes more frequent, often to make up for shorter sleep duration, which has been verified with actigraphy (Tsai, Kuo, Lee, Lee, & Landis, 2013). Lower socioeconomic status has been found in association with self-reported poor sleep quality and more fragmented sleep documented with actigraphy during the first trimester (Okun, Tolge, & Hall, 2014).

Changes in PSG-recorded sleep during pregnancy vary, and most studies conducted in the past decade have measured indices of sleep-disordered breathing (SDB) in high-risk women. A recent PSG study compared 27 third-trimester with 21 first-trimester pregnant women, and both with 24 nonpregnant women, in a cross-sectional design. Investigators reported group differences in SE, WASO, number of awakenings, and arousals per hour of sleep (Wilson et al., 2011). Women in the third trimester self-reported worse sleep quality and had statistically significantly more PSG arousals, WASO, and lower TST compared with the other two groups. All women scored in the normal range for depression and anxiety, but nulliparous first- and third-trimester women showed lower SE compared with multiparous women in either trimester.

Pregnant women are at risk for developing sleep disorders besides insomnia. Signs and symptoms of SDB or restless legs syndrome (RLS) may manifest for the first time during pregnancy, so screening is recommended. In the recent Internet survey, symptoms of SDB and RLS were reported by 19% (Berlin Questionnaire) and 24%, respectively (Mindell et al., 2015). The risk of SDB occurs because of changes in physiology, including weight gain, larger neck circumference, nasal congestion, reduced functional residual capacity from diaphragmatic elevation, and reduced oxygen saturation in the supine position from increased ventilation/perfusion mismatch, particularly in the third trimester. The onset of snoring during pregnancy is common and is associated with a higher risk (OR = 2.34) of gestational hypertension and preeclampsia (Dunietz, Chervin, & O'Brien, 2014; Pamidi et al., 2014) and for gestational diabetes (OR = 1.86) (Pamidi et al., 2014). Women who are overweight and obese are at even higher risk of pregnancy-associated SDB. Hypertension during pregnancy is associated with the development of cardiovascular disease (CVD) in later life. Since SDB contributes to the development of CVD (hypertension, myocardial infarction, and stroke) in nonpregnant individuals, SDB during pregnancy may well contribute to cardiovascular morbidity and mortality in older women (Dunietz et al., 2014). Proposed mechanisms for the higher risk of CVD in association with SDB include heightened sympathetic activity, oxidative stress, inflammatory reactions from repeated apneic episodes, and metabolic syndrome. Efforts have been made to predict the presence of SDB in pregnancy with the Berlin Questionnaire and the Multivariable Apnea Risk Index in association with a respiratory disturbance index obtained from PSG, but a BMI of at least 32 kg/m² and tiredness on awakening were the strongest, independent SDB predictors during pregnancy (Wilson et al., 2013). The goal of a study underway, the SDB substudy of the Nulliparous Pregnancy Outcomes Study Monitoring Mothers-to-be (nuMoM2b), is to determine whether SDB during pregnancy is a risk factor for adverse pregnancy outcomes (Facco et al., 2015).

RLS is a common sensorimotor neurological disorder with a prevalence influenced by ethnicity, age, and gender. RLS is associated with unusual "creepy-crawly" sensations in the legs, which are relieved by moving them. Symptoms of RLS can occur at any time of day or night but most often occur when lying quietly after going to bed. In pregnancy, RLS most often is related to iron or folate deficiency, and symptoms often subside with adequate supplementation and/or after birth, but the pathophysiology of RLS in pregnancy is still unclear (Srivanitchapoom, Pandey, & Hallett, 2014). Iron is a cofactor in the synthesis of dopamine, and iron deficiency in the central nervous system is known to lead to RLS. It is quite challenging to treat RLS during pregnancy, as most central nervous system–acting dopaminergic medications routinely used have not been studied in pregnant women, so risks to the fetus are unknown.

Sleep problems have been associated with potential impact on delivery and adverse pregnancy outcomes. As an example, less than 6 hours of sleep during the third trimester, verified with actigraphy, has predicted longer labor duration and is associated with more than four times the likelihood of having cesarean birth (Lee & Gay, 2004). Persistent sleep problems (e.g., poor sleep quality, short sleep duration, sleep disorders) throughout pregnancy have been associated with various adverse pregnancy outcomes (e.g., prenatal depression, gestational diabetes, hypertension, preeclampsia, duration and type of delivery, preterm birth, and low birth weight) across multiple studies (Palagini et al., 2014). Shift work, with disturbed sleep and circadian misalignment, is associated with the development of CVD morbidity and early death (Gu et al., 2015) and could be an occupational hazard for women working during pregnancy. However, a recent meta-analysis indicated a very low risk for preeclampsia, preterm delivery, or other untoward pregnancy outcomes (low birth weight or small-for-gestational-age infants) from shift work (Bonzini et al., 2011).

Most women are sleep deprived during the first postpartum month, and persistent short sleep duration increases the risks for mental and physical morbidity. In the 2007 NSF poll, 42% of women reported that they rarely or never got a good night's sleep and 19% of these women experienced postpartum "blues." Poor sleep quality can predict time to recurrence of postpartum major depression (PPMD), such that over a 17-week interval after delivery for every 1 point elevation in the PSQI global score, the risk of depression recurrence increased 25% among women with a past history of major depression or PPMD (Okun et al., 2011). Weight gain is normal during pregnancy, and failure to return to prepregnancy weight at 1-year postpartum places women at greater risk of midlife obesity compared with women who return to prepregnancy weight (Xiao et al., 2014). Because obtaining less than 5 or 6 hours of sleep per night has been associated with weight gain and obesity in nonpregnant women, postpartum women may be at an even greater risk. In fact, women who continued to self-report sleep an average of at least 5 hours per day at 6 months postpartum had 3.13 greater odds (adjusted) of a weight retention of 5 kg or more at 1 year (Gunderson et al., 2008). Two other studies have shown similar associations but at reduced levels of risk (Xiao et al., 2014). Finding ways for women to increase the amount of sleep they obtain every 24 hours has the potential to enhance women returning to prepregnancy weight.

MIDLIFE, MT, AND EARLY POSTMENOPAUSE

As noted previously, sleep changes the most after age 30 years and before the seventh decade of life (Ohayon et al., 2004). Yet, among studies available for the meta-analysis of PSG findings from control participants in laboratory-based sleep studies, the fewest studies were in this age range. Sleep problems in midlife women are common and cause, as noted in the 2007 NSF survey, significant daytime sleepiness and functional impairments. An increasing number of studies have reported greater amounts of sleep-related daytime sleepiness and fatigue in women compared with men, both in clinic-based and population-based studies, but the reasons for these differences, especially the impact of different gender role and societal expectations, are not well understood (Landis & Lentz, 2006). In general, women report more symptoms than men, are more likely to seek health care, and are overrepresented in general clinic populations such that the prevalence of disorders based exclusively on symptom criteria is much greater in women compared with men. Insomnia is a disorder of symptoms related to initiating and maintaining sleep, as well as waking early in the morning and being unable to fall back to sleep; thus, it is not surprising that the prevalence of insomnia is twofold higher in women compared with men.

The MT • As women transition through menopause, they often complain of insomnia symptoms that are related to hot flashes, but these symptoms are also associated with mood disturbances (anxiety and depression) and perceived stress, and the prevalence of sleep complaints varies widely. One of the central questions in studying sleep during the MT is whether complaints of sleep disturbance are specifically related to menopause per se rather than to the effects of aging, changes in mental health status, or increased perceived stress associated with other life changes commonly experienced during midlife. The overall odds of reporting poor sleep among 67,542 women in a 24-study meta-analysis were significantly higher in all the menopausal stages (perimenopause, postmenopause, and surgical menopause) compared with premenopause (all OR > 1.39, $p <$ .01), with the highest odds after surgical menopause (OR = 2.17, $p <$ .001), despite a large variability of poor sleep symptoms across all the studies (Xu & Lang, 2014). The

OR for postmenopause compared with perimenopause was lower and very small (OR = 1.09). Asian and White women experienced the most disturbed sleep, whereas Hispanic women experienced no sleep changes during the transition. Measures for identifying sleep disturbance varied widely across studies. Based on data from validated questionnaires used in a recent trial focused on treatments for hot flashes, baseline PSQI (mean = 8.23) and ISI (11.6) scores were elevated among healthy women selected for hot flashes, not for sleep disturbance (Ensrud et al., 2012). According to categories of the ISI, 37.6% of the women had mild (8–14), 26.8% had moderate (15–21), and 5.9% had severe (22–28) insomnia. Of note, to be included in this trial, women had to meet the Stages of Reproductive Aging Workshop (STRAW) criteria for the late and early postmenopause stages (Harlow et al., 2012). One limitation of this trial is the failure to screen women for SDB or other sleep disorders using PSG.

Data from at least two longitudinal studies show distinct differences from cross-sectional analyses with respect to sleep disturbance being related specifically to menopause stages. Based on 14-year follow-up data, the prevalence of moderate to severe poor sleep from a retrospective questionnaire completed annually ranged from 28% to 35%, with no relation to the final menstrual period (Freeman, Sammel, Gross, & Pien, 2015). However, women who experienced moderate to severe poor sleep premenopause had greater odds (OR = 3.8) of poor sleep during the transition, whereas women who reported mild sleep disturbance before menopause were 1.5 times more likely to have moderate to severe sleep during menopause. In this analysis, the adjusted odds of experiencing poor sleep if a woman reported hot flashes were increased significantly (OR = 1.79) but independent of baseline sleep reports. Woods and Mitchell (2010) reported that insomnia symptom severity (e.g., difficulty getting to and especially staying asleep and early morning awakening) from annual menstrual diaries was greatest during the late and early postmenopause stages of the transition. Poor sleep also was significantly related to many symptoms (e.g., perceived stress, history of sexual abuse, perceived health, alcohol use, depressed mood, anxiety, and pain). In a review of sleep and menopause, Shaver and Woods (2015) point out that comparing studies of sleep during the MT is quite challenging because of the heterogeneity of samples, inconsistency in screening for sleep disorders, failure to verify menopausal stage, variety of self-report measures used to assess sleep and sleep disturbances, and the relatively few studies of sleep physiology.

The SWAN Sleep Study • An important contribution to understanding the nature and extent of sleep problems during the MT has been derived from the SWAN study of midlife women and the ancillary study of sleep conducted at four of the seven original sites in the United States (Kravitz & Joffee, 2011). Although much of the published data thus far is derived from the first SWAN sleep study in which 67% of the 370 women were in the premenopausal or early perimenopausal stage, the study assessed self-report, behavioral (actigraphy), and PSG measures of sleep. The protocol involved 3 nights of PSG, followed by approximately a month of diary and actigraphic data. The second sleep study involves 2 nights of PSG along with 14 days of diary and actigraphy. Data from this study should permit longitudinal analyses of changes in sleep according to both self-report and physiology as women move through the MT stages (Kravitz & Joffe, 2011). The self-report measure of sleep from the initial SWAN study asked women about problems sleeping (YES, NO) in the previous 2 weeks. Thirty-seven percent of 12,603 women reported sleep problems, and this estimate excludes women on hormones or surgical menopause (Kravitz & Joffe, 2011). The prevalence of sleep problems increased from premenopause to the late phase and early postmenopause in cross-sectional analysis and controlling for age. Among ethnic groups represented, Japanese women reported the lowest (28.2%), and White women reported the highest (40.3%) prevalence; Chinese (31.6%), Hispanic (38%), and African American (35.5%) fell in between the two extremes. In multivariate analysis, vasomotor symptoms (VMSs), psychological symptoms (depression and anxiety), perceived health, pain (arthritis), quality of life, lower income, and marital happiness were associated with sleep problems. In a longitudinal follow-up analysis, three types of insomnia symptoms (trouble falling and staying asleep, early morning awakening) were analyzed if symptoms were present at least three nights each week in the previous 2 weeks. Of the women who transitioned to postmenopause, difficulty staying asleep (analogous to increased WASO) increased the most, from slightly more than 20% before menopause to nearly 50% after menopause. From this longitudinal analysis of data representing a few years, the odds of developing trouble falling asleep or staying asleep on 6 or more nights of 2 weeks increased dramatically (OR ~> 2.5) (Kravitz & Joffe, 2011). These data, albeit representing only a few women in the late MT stage or postmenopause, are consistent with data using prospective diaries reported by Woods and Mitchell (2010).

A distinct advantage of the data derived from the SWAN sleep study was the use of self-report sleep, actigraphy, and at-home PSG measures. Nearly two thirds of the women in this study reported poor sleep quality, with PSQI scores exceeding the cutoff point of greater than 5 (6.6 ± 2.4) (Kravitz & Joffe, 2011). PSG measures of clinical sleep problems showed that 20% of the sample had an Apnea–Hypopnea Index (AHI) of greater than 15/hour of sleep, which is much higher than the 4% reported from a cohort of women of similar age from the initial report of SDB prevalence from the Wisconsin study (Young et al., 1993). An AHI of greater than 15/hour of sleep is used as the clinical cut point for the diagnosis and treatment of OSA, because it is used by Medicare for reimbursement. The overall SWAN AHI mean was 10.4/hour of sleep, indicating a mild form of SDB. In addition, 8% of the women had periodic leg movements associated with EEG arousals of greater than 10/hour of sleep, which is indicative of the periodic limb movement disorder (PLMD) often manifested with complaints of poor sleep or insomnia symptoms.

PSG data can be analyzed to yield estimates of slow versus fast EEG frequencies. Slow or delta frequency is indicative of SWS and is used as a measure of sleep intensity, whereas fast-frequency or beta activity is indicative of the waking state and has been identified as a feature of primary insomnia (Buysse, Germain, Hall, Monk, & Nofzinger, 2011). Higher beta EEG activity could provide an explanation for the increased complaints of poor sleep quality as women transition through the MT. Quantitative analysis of the electroencephalogram from night 2 in the first SWAN sleep study showed that beta frequency power was higher both in NREM and in REM sleep in late and early postmenopausal stages relative to premenopausal and perimenopausal stages, despite no differences in sleep stage amounts (Campbell et al., 2011). However, there were significant covariates, including hot flash frequency, overall health status, and antidepressant drug use that attenuated the association of EEG power with menopausal stage. In another report, cross-sectional analysis revealed higher risk for metabolic syndrome in association with SE and NREM beta power (both OR = 2.1) and AHI (OR = 1.9); all remained significant after adjustment for covariates (Hall et al., 2012). In a subsequent follow-up analysis of 310 women, although the average AHI was similar (8.1/hour) BMI slightly increased and each hour of less sleep time recorded by actigraphy was inversely related to BMI. However, there was no longitudinal association between sleep duration and BMI change for more than 4.6 years (Appelhans et al., 2013).

In general, it is assumed that PSG used at home will be more ecologically valid than the same data obtained in a laboratory setting. In laboratory studies, we usually use the first night as an adaptation night because of the well-known "first night" effect (Heitkemper et al., 2005; Landis, Lentz, Rothermel, Buchwald, & Shaver, 2004). Despite the use of in-home PSG, a first-night effect was observed in the SWAN sleep study with increased TST on nights 2 and 3 and reduced sleep fragmentation compared with night 1 (Zheng et al., 2012). Additional sources of higher night-to-night variability included obesity, past history of smoking, and financial strain. Thus PSG recordings, regardless of setting, may be a source of sleep disruption and overweight; smoking women with financial concerns may be at even higher risk of a "first-night" effect.

Data from the SWAN sleep study from a community sample continue to yield interesting results. Most recently, an analysis of 314 women showed higher pain reports (bodily pain score form the short-form health survey) in association with actigraphically recorded longer sleep duration but with lower SE and self-reported less restful sleep (Kravitz et al., 2015). Women with any pain (n = 211), compared with those without pain (n = 103), were slightly heavier, and were more likely to report taking sleep, antidepressant, and pain medication at sometime during the monthlong study. Regardless of pain, hot flashes occurring at night were associated with higher odds for restlessness, lower SE, and lower odds of feeling rested in the morning.

Postmenopause and Older Women • Sleep complaints are quite common after menopause and among older women. In the 2007 NSF survey, 61% of postmenopausal women

reported insomnia symptoms at least a few nights each week, with 41% reporting the use of some type of sleep aid. This group of women had the highest BMIs, with 36% reporting being overweight and 30% obese. In the self-reported data from the Women's Health Initiative (WHI) (N = 98,705), the frequency of sleep-related symptoms was at least 3 days per week: daytime sleepiness (26%), napping during the day (12%), trouble falling asleep (10%), waking up frequently (40%) with trouble getting back to sleep (15%), early morning waking (18%), and reports of snoring (34%) (Kripke et al., 2001). Minority women (African American, Hispanic, other) reported more trouble falling asleep, more daytime sleepiness, and more naps and snoring compared with White women, but they also reported less nocturnal waking and use of sleep aids. Women who were obese or had a history of depression reported the highest frequency of both short (no more than 5 hours) and long sleep duration (at least 10 hours). In an ancillary study using wrist actigraphy, African American women showed the lowest sleep duration (315 minutes, 5.3 hours) compared with the other racial/ethnic groups, but all groups obtained less than 7 hours of sleep (Kripke et al., 2004). A recent analysis of survival data from 444 women from the original sample of 459 and until 2009 showed that after controlling for chronic conditions such as hypertension, diabetes, myocardial infarction, cancer, and major depression, those who slept less than 300 minutes (5 hours) had a 61% mean survival rate; those who slept more than 390 minutes (6.5 hours) had a 78% mean survival rate, compared with those with a 90% survival rate for actigraphic sleep durations between 300 and 390 minutes (Kripke, Langer, Elliott, Klauber, & Rex, 2011). Many more women slept more than 390 minutes compared to those who slept less than 300 minutes, but these women represented 50 of the 86 deaths that could be verified.

The optimum nighttime sleep duration for older adults is unclear. The recent recommendations for at least 7 hours of sleep for adults (Watson et al., 2015) did not include adults older than 60 years. The meta-analysis of PSG sleep from control participants in laboratory studies showed that for more than age 60 years, the number of studies in which sleep duration was less than 400 minutes far exceeded those reporting more than 400 minutes, or 6.6 hours (Ohayon et al., 2004). A recent elegant laboratory study of sleep propensity comparing healthy young adults (mean 21.9 ± 3.3 years) to a group of healthy older adults (67.8 ± 4.3 years) revealed a reduced capacity for the older adults to sleep during daytime naps as well as at night (Klerman & Dijk, 2008). Sleep duration on average was 1.5 hour shorter in older adults (7.4 ± 0.4, SEM) compared with the young adults (8.9 ± 0.4). This study revealed that older adults were less sleepy in the daytime, an observation that is consistent with self-reported daytime sleepiness previously described in a NSF poll (2002).

Why healthy older adults report lower amounts of daytime sleepiness compared with young adults runs counter to common beliefs and observations of older adults frequently reporting napping or falling asleep while engaged in quiet activities such as watching TV or attending evening concerts or shows. However, many older adults have sleep disorders, such as SDB or PLMD and multiple chronic conditions with comorbid insomnia, which could account for differences unobserved from their healthy counterparts. A recent observational study of actigraphically derived sleep duration in midlife and older adults showed that more frequent napping was associated with shorter subsequent nighttime sleep duration, more daytime sleepiness, more pain and fatigue, and increased cardiovascular risk factors of a higher BMI and a bigger waist circumference (Owens et al., 2010). The prevalence of SDB is known to be much higher in postmenopausal women compared with premenopausal or women in the early stages of the MT. The proportion of elderly women with SDB is nearly equal to that of men. Higher BMIs relative to younger women place postmenopausal women at greater risk for SDB. Observations from the Study of Osteoporotic Fractures in community-dwelling women older than 65 years have provided evidence of significant increased risk of morbidity among those with poor sleep quality or indications of sleep disorders. Among all participants in this study, after 5 years (N = 817, mean age = 87.3 ± 3.3), average actigraphically derived sleep duration was 409.2 ± 66.0 minutes (approximately 6.8 hours), WASO was 65.9 ± 40.4 minutes, and SE was 79.9 ± 9.9% (Spira et al., 2012). In this analysis, 41% developed at least one functional impairment, and those with the shortest TST had an increased risk (OR = 1.93). A subsequent analysis of PSG data from a subset of the participants (N = 302) from two study sites showed that after adjustment for comorbidities and baseline daily function scores, an AHI of greater than 15 increased the risk of functional difficulties (OR = 2.2) compared with women with an AHI of less than 5 (Spira et al., 2014). Data from this study also revealed that older women with short sleep duration or greater WASO are at greater risk for falls (Stone et al., 2008) or depression (Maglione et al., 2014), respectively. However, women in this study who habitually sleep more than 9 hours in 24 hours are at higher risk for dying from CVD compared with women who sleep 8 hours (Stone et al., 2009). Thus older women are at increased risk for poor sleep quality and sleep disorders. Helping women during midlife to develop healthy sleep habits, along with sufficient exercise and weight control, has the potential to assist them to lead healthy lives beyond menopause. In a small study of 30 women and 34 men older than 65 years who had no sleep complaints, diary, actigraphic, and PSG measures revealed relatively satisfactory sleep quality and daytime alertness, with positive correlations among diary-reported sleep measures and physical and mental health quality of life (Driscoll et al., 2008).

Sleep Deficiency

The most common type of sleep deficiency, a concept introduced in the 2011 NIH Sleep Disorders Research Plan (Box 15.3), is voluntary sleep restriction consistent with reports of sleep duration of less than 6 hours nightly sleep. Individuals

---

BOX 15.3   SLEEP DEFICIENCY

Sleep deprivation (DEP-rih-VA-shun) is a condition that occurs if you don't get enough sleep. Sleep deficiency is a broader concept. It occurs if you have one or more of the following:

- You don't get enough sleep (sleep deprivation)
- You sleep at the wrong time of day (i.e., you are out of sync with your body's natural clock)
- You don't sleep well or get all of the different types of sleep that your body needs
- You have a sleep disorder that prevents you from getting enough sleep or causes poor quality sleep

Source: National Heart, Lung, and Blood Institute (2012).

---

simply do not set sleep as a priority and sacrifice time for sleep to other activities. Evidence continues to accumulate that an increasing number of adults in the United States report short sleep duration. Although the average sleep duration reported in a 1985 survey was 7.4 hours compared with 7.18 hours in 2012, the proportion of adults older than 18 years and under 75 years of age reporting no more than 6 hours of nightly sleep increased from 22.3% in 1985 to 29.2% in 2012 (Ford, Cunningham, & Croft, 2015). These proportions are estimated to represent 38.6 and 70.1 million adults, respectively.

HEALTH CONSEQUENCES OF SLEEP DEFICIENCY

There are wide variations in responses to acute sleep deprivation because some individuals appear more sensitive or vulnerable to the effects of sleep loss and others appear resistant. Common responses include increased sleepiness, irritability, lower pain thresholds, difficulty concentrating and other cognitive impairments, poor mood and judgment, attention deficits, and reduced energy and motivation to engage in activities. Maximal physiological sleepiness accumulates quickly after 24 or 48 hours of acute sleep loss. Microsleeps, very short period of sleep, commonly occur. Performance tasks that depend on frontal/parietal lobe function, such as logical reasoning or complex mathematical tasks, seem particularly affected by acute sleep deprivation (Goel et al., 2013). However, a reliable test of sleepiness from sleep loss is a simple psychomotor vigilance test (PVT). This is a valid and reliable test of sustained attention and reaction time to a visual stimulus over a 5- to 10-minute period. Performance on this test deteriorates the longer one stays awake.

Chronic sleep deficiency has been shown to impair immune responses to vaccination, reduce antibody production to the cold virus, produce hyperalgesia, raise circulating levels of proinflammatory cytokines, and increase sympathetic activity (e.g., blood pressure and heart rate; Mullington, Haack, Toth, Serrador, & Meier-Ewert, 2009). Knutson (2013) reviewed the consequences of chronic sleep deficiency with an eye to cardiometabolic disease risk, especially diabetes and CVD. Experimental studies have revealed that sleep restriction of 4 to 5 hours compared with 7 or more hours of time in bed (TIB) over a varying number of consecutive days leads to reduced glucose tolerance and insulin sensitivity, as well as increased caloric intake associated with, and changes in appetite regulation that favors, increased "hunger" (ghrelin) and reduced "satiety" (leptin) hormones. Epidemiological observational studies have shown an increased risk for weight gain and obesity with self-reported short sleep duration. From a meta-analysis of 19 cross-sectional studies in children and 26 cross-sectional studies in adults, the odds of developing obesity (higher BMI) was greater for children (n = 30,002, OR = 1.89) than adults (n = 604,509, OR = 1.55) (Cappuccio et al., 2008). A recent meta-analysis of 12 studies representing 18,720 cases and 70,833 controls revealed increased odds (OR = 1.27) of developing metabolic syndrome with short sleep duration (Xi, He, Zhang, Xue, & Zhou, 2014). Knutson (2013) summarized potential determinants of sleep deficiency as older age, female sex, depression, stress, loneliness, and African American race (compared with Whites). Allostatic load is a concept representing the accumulation of biological disease risk from prolonged or poorly regulated responses to stressors and has been linked to sleep apnea, insomnia, and short sleep duration (Chen, Redline, Shields, Williams, & Williams, 2014). The prevalence of allostatic load was higher among Africans Americans (26.3%) and Hispanics (20.3%) compared with Whites (17.7%). After adjustment for sociodemographic and lifestyle variables, allostatic load was associated with sleep apnea (OR = 1.92), snoring (2.2), and short sleep duration of less than 6 hours (OR = 1.35). Finally, among adults more than 45 years of age, 31% reported sleeping no more than 6 hours and only 4.1% reported sleeping at least 10 hours, but compared with the majority who reported sleeping 7 to 9 hours, both short and long sleep durations were associated with obesity, poor mental health, CVD, stroke, and diabetes (Liu, Wheaton, Chapman, & Croft, 2013). One of the challenges with interpreting these types of data is that it is unknown if the presence of a chronic condition leads to or is the consequence of short or long sleep durations.

Although associations between sleep duration and morbidity are robust, the association between sleep duration and mortality is less clear. Data from a survey of more than 1 million adults showed that both short and long sleep durations were associated with early death (Kripke, Simons, Garfinkel, & Hammond, 1979, cited by Kurina et al., 2013). Other studies have shown a similar U-shaped curve, with a sleep duration of no more than 6 hours and at least 9 hours associated with increased mortality risk. In a critical review of these studies, Kurina et al. (2013) found that two studies supported the association of only short sleep duration and increased mortality risk, 16 supported an association with only long sleep duration, 14 supported a U-shaped effect (both short and

long sleep duration), and 23 found no association at all! Furthermore, the way the survey question was worded had an effect. An association with mortality was more likely to be present if participants were asked to respond to a question about the number of hours they usually sleep versus if they reported their usual bedtime and rise times. There was no association with the latter method of reporting, which required investigators to calculate sleep duration. Self-reported estimates of sleep duration tend to be longer than that measured via actigraphy or PSG. This observation suggests that if people overestimate the amount of sleep they obtain versus what is recorded with actigraphy or PSG, then the proportion of individuals with short duration of less than 6 hours may be higher than current surveys have reported.

Although sleep is variable from night to night and no two nights of sleep are exactly the same, high intra-individual night-to-night variability in sleep duration is associated with poor sleep quality and a common feature of chronic insomnia. As an example, a recent study of variability in sleep duration based on a week of actigraphy in a group of 441 adults showed that high night-to-night variability in sleep duration (e.g., TST), but not SOL or WASO, was associated with lower well-being scores after controlling for age, gender, educational level, and marital status (Lemola, Ledermann, & Friedman, 2013). As has been reported in other studies, African American men and women (n = 128) had lower TST and SE, longer SOL, greater WASO, and greater TST variability compared with White participants (n = 313). They also reported on average higher PSQI sleep quality scores (African American, 8.08 ± 4.4; Whites, 5.8 ± 3.4) and slightly, but significantly higher, general distress, anxiety, and lower life satisfaction scores. Whether race or ethnicity is a defining feature of greater risk for sleep-related morbidity and mortality compared with socioeconomic status, living in impoverished neighborhoods, or educational attainment awaits results from studies yet to be conducted.

◼ DIAGNOSTIC CRITERIA AND RISK FACTORS

Sleep Measures

Sleep indicators fall into three main categories: self-report, behavioral assessments, and sleep physiology (PSG). Self-report measures include daily logs or diaries, sleep quality and hygiene assessments, insomnia, and sleepiness scales, among others (Redeker, Pigeon, & Boudreau, 2015). When comparisons are made among self-report, actigraphy, and PSG, few sleep variables correspond with one another (Buysse et al., 2008). Each category of sleep measure provides a distinctly different dimension of the sleep experience. Self-report is an important indication of one's perception of sleep. Behavioral assessments provide a portrait of rest/activity patterns, especially over time. Finally, PSG enables detection of multiple physiological parameters during sleep that are not subject to recall bias or distortion.

SELF-REPORT MEASURES

Sleep diaries are used routinely in insomnia research and clinical practice (Figure 15.3). An example of a 2-week sleep diary is available to download from the AASM website (http://yoursleep.aasmnet.org/pdf/sleepdiary.pdf).

This type of diary, when completed, provides a visual representation of one's sleep pattern and daily variation in sleep onset, offset, and duration over a 2-week period. Although considered the least accurate measure of sleep compared with actigraphy and PSG, sleep logs and diaries are a necessary and an important component both in research and in clinical sleep medicine. Diaries provide prospective recordings of daily sleep patterns, habits, lifestyle factors, and symptoms affecting sleep quantity and quality. Diaries usually include quantitative assessments of SOL, number of nighttime awakenings, minutes of WASO, TST,

bedtime, and rise time, from which TIB can be determined and SE calculated (TST/TIB × 100). To provide easier comparison across future research studies, sleep investigators have developed a standard sleep dairy for use in research on insomnia (Carney et al., 2012). Diary applications for use on smartphones have been developed and are being used in clinical practice. The Veterans Administration has developed a cognitive behavioral therapy (CBT) for insomnia, called the *CBT-I coach app*, which includes a sleep diary and is designed for use by patients with posttraumatic stress disorder (PTSD) undergoing therapy to help them sleep better (https://mobile.va.gov/app/cbt-i-coach).

Various other types of sleep questionnaires and instruments have been used to measure sleep quality and insomnia symptoms in women (Table 15.1). Because the instruments in Table 15.1 are not capable of establishing

FIGURE 15.3

Self-report diary.

Used with permission from the American Academy of Sleep Medicine (AASM).

TABLE 15.1	Sleep Quality and Insomnia Scales for Use With Women			
SCALE	USE	DESCRIPTION	NOTES	SOURCES
PSQI (Pittsburgh Sleep Quality Index)	Sleep quality	19-item, validated questionnaire with seven subscales	Originally developed as a screening tool for sleep problems in psychiatric disorders	Buysse, Reynolds, Monk, Berman, and Kupfer (1989)
PSQI	Sleep quality	19-item, validated questionnaire with seven subscales	Summary global score of either ≥ 5 or ≥ 8 can be used as a valid measure of poor sleep quality both in research and in clinic populations	Buysse et al. (1989) Smith and Wegener (2003) Carpenter and Andrykowski (1998)
ISI (Insomnia Symptom Inventory)	Insomnia symptom severity: can use to identify insomnia and treatment response	7-item validated questionnaire Score 0–7 = absence of insomnia Score 8–14 = mild insomnia Score 15–21 = moderate clinical insomnia Score 22–28 = severe insomnia	■ Difficulty falling and staying asleep ■ Early wakening ■ Sleep satisfaction ■ Interference with daily functioning ■ Noticeability of improvement ■ Degree of distress attributable to sleep problem	Bastien, Vallières, and Morin (2001) Morin, Belleville, Bélanger, and Ivers (2011)
Insomnia Scale Used in Women's Health Initiative	Insomnia	5-item insomnia rating scale reliability and validity assessed in a very large group of older women representing multiple racial and ethnic groups	Detected sleep disturbances between women taking hormone therapy from placebo and those with mild vs. moderate-to-severe hot flashes	Levine et al. (2003, 2005)

a case definition of insomnia consistent with diagnostic criteria, the Insomnia Symptom Questionnaire was developed to measure chronic insomnia in participants in the SWAN sleep study (Okun et al., 2009). The initial evaluation of this retrospective questionnaire had high reliability and specificity and excellent face validity, but concurrent validity with sleep measures from a prospective diary or PSG (e.g., SOL, WASO, or SE) could not be established. Nevertheless, the questionnaire identified 9.8% of the sample screened for sleep apnea with PSG as meeting criteria for chronic insomnia. This proportion is consistent with epidemiological estimates of chronic insomnia (Ohayon, 2002). Several other self-report instruments that assist with assessing aspects of sleep are also available (Tables 15.2 and 15.3).

BEHAVIORAL ASSESSMENTS

Behavioral assessments are based on visual observation of sleeping behavior via video recordings or in real-time by personal observations. Monitoring body movements with wrist actigraphy provides an objective measure of sleep and wake behavior. Both types of measures are used in clinical sleep medicine. Sleep has certain behavioral characteristics across species: little movement, specific posture, lack of awareness of surrounding environment and, for most, closed eyes.

Although it is easy to observe a person asleep, and video recordings are a routine aspect of a clinical sleep study, it is possible for an individual to "play possum" acting if they are asleep. Using personal real-time observational methods to measure sleep is labor intensive and not likely to be of much use except in hospitals or other types of institutional care.

Actigraphy is based on recordings of body movements with accelerometers placed in small devices, about the size of a typical watch and usually worn on the wrist. Sleep is associated with little movement such that periods of wrist/arm immobility are indicative of sleep, whereas periods with wrist/arm movements are indicative of wake. Sleep and wake episodes are scored with the use of specialized algorithms in commercially available software specific to each type of actigraphic device. Figure 15.4 is a sample of an actigram (Actiware, 5.0, Phillips/Respironics, Inc.) with data obtained over a period of 2.5 weeks from an elderly women (Taibi et al., 2009).

As can be seen from this sample, an actigraph can be worn continuously more than 24 hours for several weeks at a time. These devices are water resistant but not waterproof and are removed for bathing or swimming. The validity of actigraph-derived sleep variables has been established and are most reliable for data obtained from healthy individuals. However, although sensitivity is high for measuring sleep in older women with insomnia, the specificity of measuring WASO with actigraphy is poor relative to PSG (Taibi, Landis, & Vitiello, 2013). Actigraphy will overestimate sleep and underestimate wake behavior in individuals

TABLE 15.2	Self-Report Scales for Sleep Hygiene and Disturbances			
SCALE	**USE**	**DESCRIPTION**	**NOTES**	**SOURCES**
Berlin Questionnaire	Sleep apnea	10-item instrument	Notes snoring, restfulness and patient hypertension	Kang et al. (2013)
STOP-Bang Questionnaire	Sleep apnea	8-item instrument	Identifies presences of risk factors and symptoms for sleep apnea	Vana, Silva, and Goldberg (2013)
Sleep Hygiene Awareness and Practice Scale	Sleep hygiene	Multiple questions that identify common hygiene practices	Identifies awareness of hygiene and hygiene practices	Glovinsky and Spielman (2006)
General Sleep Disturbance Scale	Sleep disturbances	21-item instrument scored 1–7	Identifies common sleep concerns	Lee (1992)
PROMIS (Patient Reported Outcomes Measurement Information System)	Sleep disturbance and wake impairment	Preliminary validity established for both short forms (27 items for sleep disturbance and 16 items for sleep-related impairment) in the PROMIS databank of items	The PROMIS short forms for sleep disturbance and for sleep-related impairment have been found to correlate well with the PSQI and Epworth Sleepiness Scale (ESS) scores	Amedt (2011) Yu et al. (2011)

PSQI, Pittsburgh Sleep Quality Index.

TABLE 15.3	Self-Report Instruments for Measuring Sleepiness			
SCALE	**USE**	**DESCRIPTION**	**NOTES**	**SOURCES**
Epworth Sleepiness Scale (ESS)	Likelihood to doze or fall asleep during typical daily activities (e.g., quietly reading, watching TV, riding in a car, or sitting in traffic waiting for a light to change)	8-item scale	Used most extensively in clinical sleep medicine	Johns (1991, 1992)
Stanford Sleepiness Scale	Level of sleepiness at a given point of time	Eight levels of rating from awake to asleep	Can use at multiple times in a given day	Hoddes, Zarcone, Smythe, Phillips, and Dement (1973)
Karolinska Sleepiness Scale	Level of drowsiness at a given point of time	9-point likert scale	Can use at multiple times in a given day	Akerstedt and Gillberg (1990)

lying quietly in bed awake, which may be one reason that actigraphy is less accurate in measuring SOL (Sánchez-Ortuño, Edinger, Means, & Almirall, 2010) and WASO in insomnia (Taibi et al., 2013). Nevertheless, in conjunction with sleep diaries, increasingly, actigrapy is used in sleep medicine practice as an objective measure of sleep disturbance (Sadeh, 2011), and practice parameters for actigraphy have been published (Morgenthaler et al., 2007).

SLEEP PHYSIOLOGY ASSESSMENTS

PSG is the most accurate, valid sleep measure and remains the gold standard against which other measures of sleep and wake are compared. PSG measures brain waves, muscle tone, eye movements, recordings of heart rate,

respiratory rate, airflow, chest and abdominal muscle, leg movements, oxygen saturation, and exhaled carbon dioxide. PSG is usually conducted in a laboratory setting, but portable equipment can be used in homes or in institutional settings. PSG recordings are the only accurate way to measure sleep stages and cycles. PSG is more expensive; consecutive recordings are often limited to two or three nights in case control studies, but a clinical sleep study usually involves only one recording night. PSG is also used to measure daytime physiological sleepiness in a series of naps, called *multiple sleep latency tests (MSLTs)*. Participants are placed in a quiet bedroom for 20 minutes at 2-hour intervals throughout the day and EEG is recorded. The time from lights out to the first few epochs of sleep is used as a measure of physiological sleepiness. Individuals who are

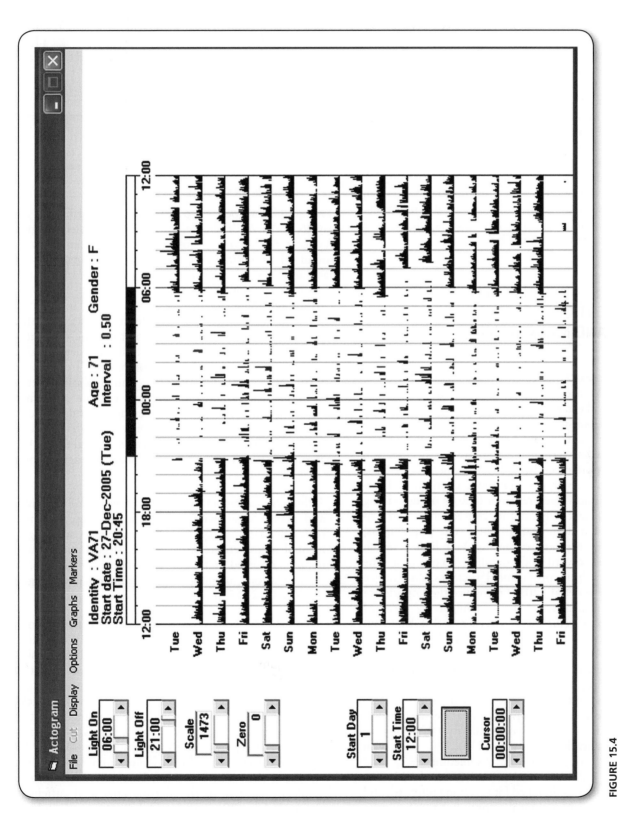

FIGURE 15.4

Actigraphy recording from an elderly woman whose sleep was recorded for 2.5 weeks. The recording begins just before sleep onset on Tuesday evening and continues until the actigraph was removed in the morning on the final day of the recording.

Source: University of Washington, Sleep Research Laboratory.

sleep deprived will often fall asleep within less than 5 minutes. In adults, a cutoff of 10 minutes is used to indicate EDS.

Home-based screening for OSA has gained acceptance with the use of devices such as the Watch PAT 200 (Itamar Medical, Caesarea, Israel), which measures peripheral arterial tone (PAT), pulse oximetry, and heart rate in combination with actigraphy (Yuceege, Firat, Demir, & Ardic, 2013). Although this type of device does not measure EEG, changes in arterial tone, heart rate, and oxygen desaturation are used as indirect indicators of episodes of apnea (pauses in breathing). The Watch-PAT 200 and PSG measures of respiratory events (apnea and hyponeas) have shown reasonably good agreement, especially in adults older than 45 years (Yuceege et al., 2013). OSA occurs because of repeated pauses (apneas) or reductions in airflow (hypneas) that occur frequently during sleep in association with complete or partial airway obstruction. OSA is a common sleep disorder in U.S. adults, with a prevalence of 6% in women and 13% in men, and is associated with significant cardiovascular morbidity (Mukherjee et al., 2015). A clinic sleep study is still required to make a definitive diagnosis of OSA.

■ GUIDELINES FOR HEALTH PROMOTION AND INTERVENTIONS/STRATEGIES FOR RISK REDUCTION AND MANAGEMENT

Modern sleep research has grown substantially since the discovery of REM sleep in the early 1950s. Much of basic sleep research has been oriented toward understanding neurobiological mechanisms and networks that control sleep and wake, describing the consequences of sleep deprivation with the goal of answering questions about the function sleep serves, or more recently, discovering the genetic basis of CRs or sleep phenotypes (duration, continuity, disorders). Current clinical sleep research focuses on describing the extent of deficient sleep and its consequences and primary and comorbid sleep disorders in diverse populations, as well as tests appropriate treatments. Very little research has been oriented toward understanding sleep health. The recent statements from professional societies (Mukherjee et al., 2015; Watson et al., 2015) recognize the importance of sleep health, and recent reviews highlight the perils of inadequate sleep (Cirelli, 2015; Czeisler, 2015; Knutson, 2013; Luyster, Strollo, Zee, & Walsh, 2012).

Buysse (2014) introduced a definition of sleep health (Box 15.4). Inherent in this definition are the dimensions suggested as appropriate for measuring sleep health: satisfaction, alertness, timing, efficiency, and duration. Buysse (2014) developed a scale, SATED, to measure sleep health and recently added a dimension, regularity (D. J. Buysse, personal communication, June 25, 2015). This scale with six items rated "rarely/never = 0," "sometimes = 1," and "usually/always = 2" will yield a total score of "12 = to good sleep health." It is designed for screening purposes and could easily be used in a clinical setting, but psychometric evaluation of the scale has not been published.

> ### BOX 15.4   SLEEP HEALTH
>
> Sleep health is a multidimensional pattern of sleep–wakefulness, adapted to individual, social, and environmental demands, which promotes physical and mental well-being. Good sleep health is characterized by subjective satisfaction, appropriate timing, adequate duration, high efficiency, and sustained alertness during waking hours (Buysse, 2014, p. 12).
>
> *Source*: Buysse, 2014, p. 12.

Sleep Health Promotion

SLEEP HYGIENE PRACTICES

Messages about good sleep practices are well known and easy to find with a simple Internet search (sleep hygiene practices). Box 15.5 contains tips for better sleep organized around 4 Rs for *R*itualizing sleep cues, *R*esisting behaviors that interfere with sleep, *R*elaxing, and *R*egularizing one's sleep–wake rhythm.

Although these practices are well known to sleep scientists and clinicians, many people are unaware of their own habits and practices that are not conducive to good sleep. Furthermore, the empirical basis for sleep hygiene recommendations is largely based on findings from laboratory studies (e.g., caffeine, nicotine, and alcohol). Whether other individual components of sleep hygiene recommendations, such as reducing noise, keeping the bedroom dark and cool, and managing stress, improve sleep has not been well tested (Irish, Kline, Gunn, Buysse, & Hall, 2015). In their review, Irish et al. (2015) summarize practice points for sleep hygiene, as follows:

> Although each recommendation is theoretically sound and plausible, a review of individual sleep hygiene recommendations regarding caffeine use, smoking, alcohol use, exercise, stress, noise, sleep timing, and napping revealed that empirical support for these recommendations in the general population is lacking. (Irish et al., 2015, p. 33)

As noted previously, caffeine is an effective countermeasure for daytime sleepiness. However, from laboratory studies, caffeine consumed before bedtime disrupts sleep in a dose-dependent manner, with the doses of more than 250 mg associated both with self-reported and with actigraphic disrupted sleep, but tolerance may develop quickly (Irish et al., 2015). Fewer studies have examined effects of either reducing caffeine intake or limiting use to morning hours only, as sleep hygiene recommendations suggest. The amounts of caffeine available in some commercial products are large, as shown in Box 15.6. For individuals who are particularly sensitive to the alerting effects of caffeine, a short nap of 15 to 20 minutes midafternoon maybe a better option than consuming a latte or a cappuccino. Irish et al.

BOX 15.5   TIPS FOR BETTER SLEEP

Ritualize Cues for Sleep

- Use your bedroom only for sleep (sexual activity an exception)
- Make the environment quiet, dark, and cool
- Go to bed only when sleepy
- If not asleep in 20 minutes, get up, go elsewhere, read, or do something boring, lie down when drowsy—no longer than 10 to 20 minutes—repeat as necessary

Resist Behaviors Interfering With Sleep

- Avoid heavy meals before bed; have a light snack (mainly starch, some protein, warm drink)
- Avoid strenuous exercise close to sleep (within 2–3 hours); regular daily exercise may help sleep
- Avoid tobacco, alcohol, and caffeine

Relax and Control Tension

- Assume a comfortable posture
- Clear the mind by stopping disturbing thoughts
- Tune out distractions by concentrating on a sound, breathing, a pleasant scene, or sensations
- Practice, practice, practice (15 minutes twice a day)
- Use muscle relaxation, pleasant visual images, and relaxing bodily sensations

Regularize the Sleep–Wake Rhythm

- Define optimal sleep length (the amount of sleep that you need to feel good in the daytime)
- Go to bed consistently at a time that allows achieving optimal sleep length
- Get up at same time every morning no matter the amount of previous night's sleep. (This is an important behavior, as it sets the body's internal "clock.")
- Limit napping to 15 to 20 minutes during the day, especially if nighttime sleep is disturbed

Source: Tips for Better Sleep (2009–2014).

BOX 15.6   EXAMPLES OF CAFFEINE CONTENT IN COMMERCIAL PRODUCTS

Coffee

Dunkin' Donuts coffee with Turbo Shot (large 20 fl oz): 436 mg
Starbucks Coffee (grande, 16 fl oz): 330 mg
Starbucks Coffee (tall, 12 fl oz): 260 mg
Starbucks Caffe Latté, Cappuccino, Caramel Macchiato (grande 16 fl oz): 150 mg
Starbucks VIA House Blend Instant Coffee (1 packet, 8 fl oz): 135 mg
Dunkin' Donuts, or Starbucks Decaf Coffee (16 fl oz): 15–25 mg

Tea

Starbucks Tazo Awake (grande, 16 fl oz): 135 mg
Black tea, brewed for 3 minutes (8 fl oz): 30–80 mg

Soft Drinks (All 12 fl oz)

Pepsi MAX: 69 mg
Mountain Dew: 54 mg
Diet Coke: 47 mg
Seven-Up, Fanta, Fresca, ginger ale, or Sprite: 0 mg

Energy Drinks

5-hour Energy (1.9 fl oz): 208 mg
Monster Energy (16 fl oz): 60 mg
Red Bull (8.4 fl oz): 80 mg

Chocolate Candy and Drinks

Starbucks Hot Chocolate (grande, 16 fl oz): 25 mg
Hershey's Special Dark (1 bar, 1.5 oz): 20 mg
Hershey's Milk Chocolate (1 bar, 1.6 oz): 9 mg

Source: Center for Science in the Public Interest (2012).

(2015) found that napping had minimal adverse effects on nighttime sleep.

For individuals who suffer from chronic insomnia, sleep hygiene instructions alone have not been found very effective but when coupled with CBT, are considered quite effective for improving sleep in adults (Trauer, Qian, Doyle, Rajaratnam, & Cunnington, 2015). Telephone delivery of CBT-I is quite effective for improving sleep and reducing insomnia symptoms in women in the late stage of MT and early postmenopause (McCurry et al., 2016). Results of a clinical trial of older adults with osteoarthritis recruited from a primary care setting showed that those who improved their sleep with the initial treatment of combined CBT-I and CBT for pain intervention showed sustained significant improvements in reduced insomnia symptoms (ISI), improved sleep quality, and pain severity at 18-month follow-up (Vitiello et al., 2014). A self-help–oriented

6-week intervention program was effective in improving sleep quality (PSQI) and insomnia symptoms (ISI) compared with standard sleep hygiene among older adults with comorbid medical conditions (Morgan, Gregory, Tomeny, David, & Gascoigne, 2012). Glovinsky and Spielman's text, *The Insomnia Answer* (2006), provides a personalized program for identifying and managing sleep onset, maintenance, and early morning insomnia symptoms. Glovinsky and Spielman advocate an assessing sleep hygiene practice to assist individuals to identify habits and behaviors that may be disturbing sleep and attending to them, rather than ignoring them, will aid in sleeping better.

EXERCISE EFFECTS ON SLEEP

Among the components of good sleep hygiene practices, evidence for the beneficial effects of regular exercise on sleep seems the most robust. Both regular and, especially, acute bouts of exercise have been shown to improve sleep quality and duration, both by self-report and by PSG measures (Irish et al., 2015). However, data from exercise training of at least 4 weeks' duration has shown mainly improvement in self-reported sleep quality, with limited data available on objective sleep measures. One study comparing a 4-month trial of low-intensity yoga and moderate-intensity walking to control yielded no significant improvement in self-reported sleep quality (PSQI) in 164 middle-aged women (Elavsky & McAuley, 2007). Recent 12-week intervention trials of yoga (Newton et al., 2014) and aerobic exercise (Sternfeld et al., 2014) yielded small, but significant improvements in insomnia symptoms (ISI) compared with usual activity in women with hot flashes; aerobic exercise also was associated with improved sleep quality. Exercise may be quite a beneficial behavior for improving sleep quality (Irish et al., 2015). Exercise is complex, and at present, there are few clear guidelines as to the type, duration, intensity, and timing associated with improving sleep (Irish et al., 2015).

Over the past few years, many technological devices for personal monitoring of physical activity have become commercially available, and many claim that they also monitor sleep. These devices may work well for counting steps, providing estimates of energy expenditure and heart rate, or assisting individuals to reach performance goals, but the ability to monitor sleep accurately is questionable. Many have not undergone reliability or validity testing with PSG or have not been compared with actigraphs that have been validated for sleep.

CONSUMER TECHNOLOGIES FOR SLEEP PROMOTION

Along with technologies for monitoring physical activity, many types of commercial devices have become available and claim to measure sleep with a primary goal of improving it. They aid sleep or wake induction, provide self-guided sleep assessment, entertainment, information sharing, and education about sleep cycle quality or quantity. Most of these devices are readily available over the counter and have not undergone any type of reliability or validity testing. A group of investigators recently evaluated the validity of an application developed for measuring sleep on an iPhone,

compared with laboratory-based PSG (Bhat et al., 2015). They found no correlations between PSG and the application for SE, sleep stages or SOL. Furthermore, an epoch-by-epoch comparison showed low overall accuracy (45.9%), high sensitivity (89.9%), but poor specificity (50%) in detecting sleep. Developers may not be motivated to evaluate the accuracy of their technologies, and despite the presumed inaccuracy of many of them, increasing numbers of individuals are using them. We recently published a review and commentary on some of the most popular devices (Ko et al., 2015). One example of an app "Go! to Sleep" was created by the Cleveland Clinic Sleep Disorders Center and uses a lifestyle-and-sleep habit questionnaire to create a sleep score, tracks this score over time, and provides daily sleep advice to improve one's score (my.clevelandclinic.org/mobile-apps/go-to-sleep-app). Consumer sleep technologies actually have the potential to raise awareness and promote education of about sleep health but may have an unintended consequence of providing inaccurate information about one's actual sleep. The number of devices oriented to monitoring sleep, along with physical activity and nutritional intake, is likely to increase as more and more people rely more and more on technology and the focus of health care becomes more and more oriented toward healthy lifestyles.

■ FUTURE DIRECTIONS

Investigators have begun to seriously study the empirical basis for sleep hygiene practices. More research is needed in naturalistic settings as opposed to the laboratory (Irish et al., 2015). Important questions remain unanswered. At present, unlike physical activity and nutrition, there are no validated public health programs for sleep. Do the following sleep hygiene recommendations (such as keeping a regular sleep and wake pattern; keeping the bedroom quiet, dark, and cool; or avoiding caffeine after lunch) really improve sleep quality and duration? What is an optimal dose of caffeine or alcohol that is associated with good sleep? Do rituals and relaxation exercises before bedtime improve sleep quality and duration? Does reducing caffeine lead to more napping behavior with unintended consequences such as feeling too tired to exercise? What might be the best combination of sleep hygiene practices for various populations? Just as important as studies about the effectiveness of sleep hygiene practices are questions about extending sleep time. Does making more time for sleep actually lead to longer sleep duration and good health outcomes? Do intervention programs fail to assist people to lose weight or sustain weight loss because they are not getting enough sleep? Do community-based walking programs fail to engage and sustain large number of participants because people are just too tired to attend? Among older adults about 50% complain of sleep problems, but 50% do not. Why not? What motivates individuals to obtain adequate sleep? The overall average of sleep duration from a survey in 1985 fell only by approximately 13 minutes, but the number of individuals reporting less than or equal to 6 hours' sleep increased 7%, estimated to represent approximately 31 million in the United States

(Ford et al., 2015). Why are more people sleeping fewer hours? What interventions will work to assist individuals and families to prioritize sleep?

In the United States, a paradigm shift is occurring in health care, from an emphasis on treating medical disorders to preventing them. Simultaneously, in the field of sleep medicine, a paradigm shift is occurring from an emphasis on studies and treatments for sleep disorders to a focus on sleep health and ways to assist people to obtain good, adequate sleep. Perhaps a good starting place is in the home, with families addressing typical household routines. Findings from a recent clinical trial focused on family routines known to influence the growing epidemic of obesity in preschool children yielded positive benefits for sleep duration, although BMI was the primary target (Haines et al., 2013). After a 6-month trial, families (*n* = 62) who received the intervention program (promoting family meals, adequate sleep, limited TV time, and removal of technologies from the child's bedroom through motivational interviewing) reported that their children slept 0.56 hours per day compared with controls (*n* = 59), who slept 0.19 hours per day less. There were no group differences in number of family meals or TVs removed from the child's bedroom, but TV viewing was reduced by 1.06 hours in the intervention group. Children in the intervention group had lower BMIs after the intervention, whereas BMI in control children increased. Families in the study were predominately African American and Hispanic with annual incomes of $20,000 or less. The findings from this study are important, but the authors noted that of the 500 families contacted, only 24% enrolled, and thus the findings are not generalizable. However, bundled lifestyle interventions such as the Healthy Habits, Happy Homes trial hold promise for future prevention studies. Obtaining efficient, restful, satisfying sleep of adequate duration synchronized with one's internal "clock" are key to staying alert throughout the day.

As the 2007 NSF Women and Sleep poll found, far too many women are trying to do it all, perhaps burning the candle at both ends, placing themselves and their families at risk for sleep problems and sleep-related morbidity. Advanced nurse practitioners who are educated about sleep, changes in sleep as women age, and the hazards of inadequate sleep are poised to help improve the sleep of their patients.

■ REFERENCES

Akerstedt, T., & Gillberg, M. (1990). Subjective and objective sleepiness in the active individual. *International Journal of Neuroscience, 52*(1–2), 29–37.

Amedt, J. T. (2011). PROMIS of improved tools for assessing sleep and wake function: Commentary on "development of short forms from the PROMIS sleep disturbance and sleep-related impairment item banks." *Behavioral Sleep Medicine, 10*, 6–24.

American Academy of Sleep Medicine (AASM). (2007). *The AASM manual for the scoring of sleep and associated events: Rules, terminology and technical specifications.* Westchester, IL: Author.

Appelhans, B. M., Janssen, I., Cursio, J. F., Matthews, K. A., Hall, M., Gold, E. B.,…Kravitz, H. M. (2013). Sleep duration and weight change in midlife women: The SWAN sleep study. *Obesity, 21*(1), 77–84.

Arber, S., Bote, M., & Meadows, R. (2009). Gender and socio-economic patterning of self-reported sleep problems in Britain. *Social Science & Medicine, 68*(2), 281–289.

Basner, M., Spaeth, A. M., & Dinges, D. F. (2014). Sociodemographic characteristics and waking activities and their role in the timing and duration of sleep. *Sleep, 37*(12), 1889–1906.

Bastien, C. H., Vallières, A., & Morin, C. M. (2001). Validation of the Insomnia Severity Index as an outcome measure for insomnia research. *Sleep Medicine, 2*(4), 297–307.

Bhat, S., Ferraris, A., Gupta, D., Mozafarian, M., DeBari, V. A., Gushway-Henry, N.,…Chokroverty, S. (2015). Is there a clinical role for smartphone sleep apps? Comparison of sleep cycle detection by a smartphone application to polysomnography. *Journal of Clinical Sleep Medicine, 11*(7), 709–715.

Bixler, E. O., Papaliaga, M. N., Vgontzas, A. N., Lin, H. M., Pejovic, S., Karataraki, M.,…Chrousos, G. P. (2009). Women sleep objectively better than men and the sleep of young women is more resilient to external stressors: Effects of age and menopause. *Journal of Sleep Research, 18*(2), 221–228.

Bonzini, M., Palmer, K. T., Coggon, D., Carugno, M., Cromi, A., & Ferrario, M. M. (2011). Shift work and pregnancy outcomes: A systematic review with meta-analysis of currently available epidemiological studies. *BJOG: An International Journal of Obstetrics and Gynaecology, 118*(12), 1429–1437.

Buxton, O. M., Chang, A. M., Spilsbury, J. C., Bos, T., Emsellem, H., & Knutson, K. L. (2015). Sleep in the modern family: Protective family routines for child and adolescent sleep. *Sleep Health, 1*(1), 15–27.

Buysse, D. J. (2014). Sleep health: Can we define it? Does it matter? *Sleep, 37*(1), 9–17.

Buysse, D. J., Germain, A., Hall, M., Monk, T. H., & Nofzinger, E. A. (2011). A neurobiological model of insomnia. *Drug Discovery Today. Disease Models, 8*(4), 129–137.

Buysse, D. J., Hall, M. L., Strollo, P. J., Kamarck, T. W., Owens, J., Lee, L.,…Matthews, K. A. (2008). Relationships between the Pittsburgh Sleep Quality Index (PSQI), Epworth Sleepiness Scale (ESS), and clinical/polysomnographic measures in a community sample. *Journal of Clinical Sleep Medicine, 4*(6), 563–571.

Buysse, D. J., Reynolds, C. F., Monk, T. H., Berman, S. R., & Kupfer, D. J. (1989). The Pittsburgh Sleep Quality Index: A new instrument for psychiatric practice and research. *Psychiatry Research, 28*(2), 193–213.

Campbell, I. G., Bromberger, J. T., Buysse, D. J., Hall, M. H., Hardin, K. A., Kravitz, H. M.,…Gold, E. (2011). Evaluation of the association of menopausal status with delta and beta EEG activity during sleep. *Sleep, 34*(11), 1561–1568.

Cappuccio, F. P., Taggart, F. M., Kandala, N. B., Currie, A., Peile, E., Stranges, S., & Miller, M. A. (2008). Meta-analysis of short sleep duration and obesity in children and adults. *Sleep, 31*(5), 619–626.

Carney, C. E., Buysse, D. J., Ancoli-Israel, S., Edinger, J. D., Krystal, A. D., Lichstein, K. L., & Morin, C. M. (2012). The consensus sleep diary: Standardizing prospective sleep self-monitoring. *Sleep, 35*(2), 287–302.

Carpenter, J. S., & Andrykowski, M. A. (1998). Psychometric evaluation of the Pittsburgh Sleep Quality Index. *Journal of Psychosomatic Research, 45*(1), 5–13.

Center for Science in the Public Interest. (2012). *Nutrition action health letter.* Retrieved from https://www.cspinet.org/nah

Centers for Disease Control and Prevention (CDC). (2011). Effect of short sleep duration on daily activities—United States, 2005–2008. *Morbidity and Mortality Weekly Reports, 60*, 239–252.

Centers for Disease Control and Prevention (CDC). (2014). *National Healthy Sleep Awareness Project.* Retrieved from http://www.cdc.gov/sleep/projects_partners.html

Chen, X., Redline, S., Shields, A. E., Williams, D. R., & Williams, M. A. (2014). Associations of allostatic load with sleep apnea, insomnia, short sleep duration, and other sleep disturbances: Findings from the National Health and Nutrition Examination Survey 2005 to 2008. *Annals of Epidemiology, 24*(8), 612–619.

Cirelli, C. (2015). *UpToDate. Definition and consequences of sleep deprivation.* Retrieved from www.uptodate.com

Czeisler, C. A. (2015). Duration, timing and quality of sleep are each vital for health, performance, and safety. *Sleep Health, 1*, 5–8.

de la Iglesia, H. O., Fernandez-Duque, E., Golombek, D. A., Lanza, N., Duffy, J. F., Czeisler, C. A., & Valeggia, C. R. (2015). Access to electric light is associated with shorter sleep duration in a traditionally hunter-gatherer community. *Journal of Biological Rhythms, 30,* 342–350. doi:10.1177/0748730415590702

de Zambotti, M., Willoghby, A. R., Sasson, S. A., Colrain, I. M., & Baker, F. C. (2015). Menstrual cycle-related variation in physiological sleep in women in the early menopausal transition. *Journal of Clinical Endocrinology and Metabolism, 100*(8), 2918–2926.

Driscoll, H. C., Serody, L., Patrick, S., Maurer, J., Bensasi, S., Houck, P. R., …Reynolds, C. F. (2008). Sleeping well, aging well: A descriptive and cross-sectional study of sleep in "successful agers" 75 and older. *American Journal of Geriatric Psychiatry, 16*(1), 74–82.

Duffy, J. F., Cain, S. W., Chang, A. M., Phillips, A. J., Münch, M. Y., Gronfier, C.,…Czeisler, C. A. (2011). Sex difference in the near-24-hour intrinsic period of the human circadian timing system. *Proceedings of the National Academy of Sciences of the United States of America, 108*(Suppl. 3), 15602–15608.

Dukhovnov, D., & Zagheni, E. (2015). Who takes care of whom in the U.S.? Evidence from matrices of time transfers by age and sex. *Population and Development Review, 41*(2), 183–206.

Dunietz, G. L., Chervin, R. D., & O'Brien, L. M. (2014). Sleep-disordered breathing during pregnancy: Future implications for cardiovascular health. *Obstetrical & Gynecological Survey, 69*(3), 164–176.

Durrence, H. H., & Lichstein, K. L. (2006). The sleep of African Americans: A comparative review. *Behavioral Sleep Medicine, 4*(1), 29–44.

Elavsky, S., & McAuley, E. (2007). Lack of perceived sleep improvement after 4-month structured exercise programs. *Menopause, 14*(3, Pt. 1), 535–540.

Ensrud, K. E., Joffe, H., Guthrie, K. A., Larson, J. C., Reed, S. D., Newton, K. M.,…Freeman, E. W. (2012). Effect of escitalopram on insomnia symptoms and subjective sleep quality in healthy perimenopausal and postmenopausal women with hot flashes: A randomized controlled trial. *Menopause, 19*(8), 848–855.

Facco, F. L., Parker, C. B., Reddy, U. M., Silver, R. M., Louis, J. M., Basner, R. C.,…Zee, P. C. (2015). NuMoM2b Sleep-Disordered Breathing study: Objectives and methods. *American Journal of Obstetrics and Gynecology, 212*(4), 542.e1–542.e127.

Ford, E. S., Cunningham, T. J., & Croft, J. B. (2015). Trends in self-reported sleep duration among U.S. adults from 1985 to 2012. *Sleep, 38*(5), 829–832.

Freeman, E. W., Sammel, M. D., Gross, S. A., & Pien, G. W. (2015). Poor sleep in relation to natural menopause: A population-based 14-year follow-up of midlife women. *Menopause, 22*(7), 719–726.

Glovinsky, P., & Spielman, A. (2006). *The insomnia answer.* New York, NY: Penguin Group.

Goel, N., Basner, M., Rao, H., & Dinges, D. F. (2013). Circadian rhythms, sleep deprivation, and human performance. *Progress in Molecular Biology and Translational Science, 119,* 155–190.

Gu, F., Han, J., Laden, F., Pan, A., Caporaso, N. E., Stampfer, M. J., …Schernhammer, E. S. (2015). Total and cause-specific mortality of U.S. nurses working rotating night shifts. *American Journal of Preventive Medicine, 48*(3), 241–252.

Gunderson, E. P., Rifas-Shiman, S. L., Oken, E., Rich-Edwards, J. W., Kleinman, K. P., Taveras, E. M., & Gillman, M. W. (2008). Association of fewer hours of sleep at 6 months postpartum with substantial weight retention at 1 year postpartum. *American Journal of Epidemiology, 167*(2), 178–187.

Haines, J., McDonald, J., O'Brien, A., Sherry, B., Bottino, C. J., Schmidt, M. E., & Taveras, E. M. (2013). Healthy Habits, Happy Homes: Randomized trial to improve household routines for obesity prevention among preschool-aged children. *Journal of the American Medical Association Pediatrics, 167*(11), 1072–1079.

Hall, M. H., Matthews, K. A., Kravitz, H. M., Gold, E. B., Buysse, D. J., Bromberger, J. T.,…Sowers, M. (2009). Race and financial strain are independent correlates of sleep in midlife women: The SWAN sleep study. *Sleep, 32*(1), 73–82.

Hall, M. H., Okun, M. L., Sowers, M., Matthews, K. A., Kravitz, H. M., Hardin, K.,…Sanders, M. H. (2012). Sleep is associated with the metabolic syndrome in a multi-ethnic cohort of midlife women: The SWAN sleep study. *Sleep, 35*(6), 783–790.

Harlow, S. D., Gass, M., Hall, J. E., Lobo, R., Maki, P., Rebar, R. W.,…de Villiers, T. J.; STRAW 10 Collaborative Group. (2012). Executive summary of the Stages of Reproductive Aging Workshop + 10:

Addressing the unfinished agenda of staging reproductive aging. *Menopause, 19*(4), 387–395.

Heitkemper, M., Jarrett, M., Burr, R., Cain, K. C., Landis, C., Lentz, M., & Poppe, A. (2005). Subjective and objective sleep indices in women with irritable bowel syndrome. *Neurogastroenterology and Motility, 17*(4), 523–530.

Hoddes, E., Zarcone, V., Smythe, H., Phillips, R., & Dement, W. C. (1973). Quantification of sleepiness: A new approach. *Psychophysiology, 10*(4), 431–436.

Hysing, M., Pallesen, S., Stormark, K. M., Lundervold, A. J., & Sivertsen, B. (2013). Sleep patterns and insomnia among adolescents: A population-based study. *Journal of Sleep Research, 22*(5), 549–556.

Irish, L. A., Kline, C. E., Gunn, H. E., Buysse, D. J., & Hall, M. H. (2015). The role of sleep hygiene in promoting public health: A review of empirical evidence. *Sleep Medicine Reviews, 22,* 23–36.

Johns, M. W. (1991). A new method for measuring daytime sleepiness: The Epworth sleepiness scale. *Sleep, 14*(6), 540–545.

Johns, M. W. (1992). Reliability and factor analysis of the Epworth Sleepiness Scale. *Sleep, 15*(4), 376–381.

Kang, K., Park, K. S., Kim, J. E., Kim, S. W., Kim, Y. T., Kim, J. S., & Lee, H. W. (2013). Usefulness of the Berlin Questionnaire to identify patients at high risk for obstructive sleep apnea: A population-based door-to-door study. *Sleep & Breathing/Schlaf & Atmung, 17*(2), 803–810.

Klerman, E. B., & Dijk, D. J. (2008). Age-related reduction in the maximal capacity for sleep: Implications for insomnia. *Current Biology, 18*(15), 1118–1123.

Knutson, K. L. (2013). Sociodemographic and cultural determinants of sleep deficiency: Implications for cardiometabolic disease risk. *Social Science & Medicine, 79,* 7–15.

Ko, P. T., Kientz, J. A., Choe, E. K., Kay, M., Landis, C. A., & Watson, N. F. (2015). Consumer sleep technologies: A review of the landscape. *Journal of Clinical Sleep Medicine, 11*(12), 1455–1461.

Kravitz, H. M., Janssen, I., Santoro, N., Bromberger, J. T., Schocken, M., Everson-Rose, S. A.,…Powell, L. H. (2005). Relationship of day-to-day reproductive hormone levels to sleep in midlife women. *Archives of Internal Medicine, 165*(20), 2370–2376.

Kravitz, H. M., & Joffe, H. (2011). Sleep during the perimenopause: A SWAN story. *Obstetrics and Gynecology Clinics of North America, 38*(3), 567–586.

Kravitz, H. M., Zheng, H., Bromberger, J. T., Buysse, D. J., Owens, J., & Hall, M. H. (2015). An actigraphy study of sleep and pain in midlife women: The Study of Women's Health Across the Nation sleep study. *Menopause, 22*(7), 710–718.

Kripke, D. F., Brunner, R., Freeman, R., Hendrix, S. L., Jackson, R. D., Masaki, K., & Carter, R. A. (2001). Sleep complaints of postmenopausal women. *Clinical Journal of Women's Health, 1*(5), 244–252.

Kripke, D. F., Jean-Louis, G., Elliott, J. A., Klauber, M. R., Rex, K. M., Tuunainen, A., & Langer, R. D. (2004). Ethnicity, sleep, mood, and illumination in postmenopausal women. *BioMed Central Psychiatry, 4,* 8.

Kripke, D. F., Langer, R. D., Elliott, J. A., Klauber, M. R., & Rex, K. M. (2011). Mortality related to actigraphic long and short sleep. *Sleep Medicine, 12*(1), 28–33.

Kurina, L. M., McClintock, M. K., Chen, J. H., Waite, L. J., Thisted, R. A., & Lauderdale, D. S. (2013). Sleep duration and all-cause mortality: A critical review of measurement and associations. *Annals of Epidemiology, 23*(6), 361–370.

Landis, C. A., & Lentz, M. J. (2006). News alert for mothers: Having children at home doesn't increase your risk for severe daytime sleepiness or fatigue. *Sleep, 29*(6), 738–740.

Landis, C. A., Lentz, M. J., Rothermel, J., Buchwald, D., & Shaver, J. L. (2004). Decreased sleep spindles and spindle activity in midlife women with fibromyalgia and pain. *Sleep, 27*(4), 741–750.

Lee, K. A. (1992). Self-reported sleep disturbances in employed women. *Sleep, 15*(6), 493–498.

Lee, K. A., & Gay, C. L. (2004). Sleep in late pregnancy predicts length of labor and type of delivery. *American Journal of Obstetrics and Gynecology, 191*(6), 2041–2046.

Lemola, S., Ledermann, T., & Friedman, E. M. (2013). Variability of sleep duration is related to subjective sleep quality and subjective well-being: An actigraphy study. *PloS One, 8*(8), e71292.

Levine, D. W., Kripke, D. F., Kaplan, R. M., Lewis, M. A., Naughton, M. J., Bowen, D. J., & Shumaker, S. A. (2003). Reliability and validity of the women's health initiative insomnia rating scale. *Psychological Assessment, 15*(2), 137–148.

Levine, D. W., Dailey, M. E., Rockhill, B., Tipping, D., Naughton, M. J., & Shumaker, S. A. (2005). Validation of the women's health initiative insomnia rating scale in a multicenter controlled clinical trial. *Psychosomatic Medicine, 67*(1), 98–104.

Liu, Y., Wheaton, A. G., Chapman, D. P., & Croft, J. B. (2013). Sleep duration and chronic diseases among U.S. adults age 45 years and older: Evidence from the 2010 Behavioral Risk Factor Surveillance System. *Sleep, 36*(10), 1421–1427.

Luyster, F. S., Strollo, P. J., Zee, P. C., & Walsh, J. K.; Board of Directors of the American Academy of Sleep Medicine and the Sleep Research Society. (2012). Sleep: A health imperative. *Sleep, 35*(6), 727–734.

Maglione, J. E., Ancoli-Israel, S., Peters, K. W., Paudel, M. L., Yaffe, K., Ensrud, K. E., & Stone, K. L.; Study of Osteoporotic Fractures Research Group. (2014). Subjective and objective sleep disturbance and longitudinal risk of depression in a cohort of older women. *Sleep, 37*(7), 1179–1187.

Mastin, L. (2015). *Types and stages of sleep.* Retrieved from http://www.howsleepworks.com/types_cycles.html

McCurry, S. M., Guthrie, K. A., Morin, C. M., Woods, N. F., Landis, C. A., Ensrud, K. E., . . . LaCroix, A. Z. (2016). Telephone delivered cognitive-behavior therapy for insomnia in midlife women with vasomotor symptoms: An MsFLASH randomized trial. *Journal of the American Medical Association-Internal Medicine.* [Epub ahead of print]. doi:10.1001/jamainternmed.2016.1795

Mindell, J. A., Cook, R. A., & Nikolovski, J. (2015). Sleep patterns and sleep disturbances across pregnancy. *Sleep Medicine, 16*(4), 483–488.

Mitterling, T., Högl, B., Schönwald, S. V., Hackner, H., Gabelia, D., Biermayr, M., & Frauscher, B. (2015). Sleep and respiration in 100 healthy Caucasian sleepers: A polysomnographic study according to American Academy of Sleep Medicine standards. *Sleep, 38*(6), 867–875.

Morgan, K., Gregory, P., Tomeny, M., David, B. M., & Gascoigne, C. (2012). Self-help treatment for insomnia symptoms associated with chronic conditions in older adults: A randomized controlled trial. *Journal of the American Geriatrics Society, 60*(10), 1803–1810.

Morgenthaler, T., Alessi, C., Friedman, L., Owens, J., Kapur, V., Boehlecke, B., . . . Swick, T. J.; Standards of Practice Committee; American Academy of Sleep Medicine. (2007). Practice parameters for the use of actigraphy in the assessment of sleep and sleep disorders: An update for 2007. *Sleep, 30*(4), 519–529.

Morin, C. M., Belleville, G., Bélanger, L., & Ivers, H. (2011). The Insomnia Severity Index: Psychometric indicators to detect insomnia cases and evaluate treatment response. *Sleep, 34*(5), 601–608.

Mukherjee, S., Patel, S. R., Kales, S. N., Ayas, N. T., Strohl, K. P., Gozal, D., & Malhotra, A.; American Thoracic Society ad hoc Committee on Healthy Sleep. (2015). An official American Thoracic Society statement: The importance of healthy sleep. Recommendations and future priorities. *American Journal of Respiratory and Critical Care Medicine, 191*(12), 1450–1458.

Mullington, J. M., Haack, M., Toth, M., Serrador, J. M., & Meier-Ewert, H. K. (2009). Cardiovascular, inflammatory, and metabolic consequences of sleep deprivation. *Progress in Cardiovascular Diseases, 51*(4), 294–302.

National Heart Lung, and Blood Institute. (2012). *What are sleep deprivation and deficiency?* Bethesda, MD: National Institutes of Health. Retrieved from www.nhlbi.nih.gov/health/health-topics/ topics/sdd?

National Sleep Foundation (NSF). (2001). An American portrait. *Sleep Matters, 3*, 1–3.

National Sleep Foundation (NSF). (2002). *Sleep in America poll.* Retrieved from http://sleepfoundation.org/sleep-polls

National Sleep Foundation (NSF). (2007). *Sleep in America poll.* Retrieved from http://sleepfoundation.org/sleep-polls

National Sleep Foundation (NSF). (2010). *Sleep in America poll.* Retrieved from http://sleepfoundation.org/sleep-polls

Newton, K. M., Reed, S. D., Guthrie, K. A., Sherman, K. J., Booth-LaForce, C., Caan, B., . . . LaCroix, A. Z. (2014). Efficacy of yoga for vasomotor symptoms: A randomized controlled trial. *Menopause, 21*(4), 339–346.

Ohayon, M. M. (2002). Epidemiology of insomnia: What we know and what we still need to learn. *Sleep Medicine Reviews, 6*(2), 97–111.

Ohayon, M. M., Carskadon, M. A., Guilleminault, C., & Vitiello, M. V. (2004). Meta-analysis of quantitative sleep parameters from childhood to old age in healthy individuals. *Sleep, 27*, 1255–1273.

Okun, M. L., Kravitz, H. M., Sowers, M. F., Moul, D. E., Buysse, D. J., & Hall, M. (2009). Psychometric evaluation of the Insomnia Symptom Questionnaire: A self-report measure to identify chronic insomnia. *Journal of Clinical Sleep Medicine, 5*(1), 41–51.

Okun, M. L., Luther, J., Prather, A. A., Perel, J. M., Wisniewski, S., & Wisner, K. L. (2011). Changes in sleep quality, but not hormones predict time to postpartum depression recurrence. *Journal of Affective Disorders, 130*(3), 378–384.

Okun, M. L., Tolge, M., & Hall, M. (2014). Low socioeconomic status negatively affects sleep in pregnant women. *Journal of Obstetric, Gynecologic, and Neonatal Nursing, 43*(2), 160–167.

Owens, J. F., Buysse, D. J., Hall, M., Kamarck, T. W., Lee, L., Strollo, P. J., . . . Matthews, K. A. (2010). Napping, nighttime sleep, and cardiovascular risk factors in mid-life adults. *Journal of Clinical Sleep Medicine, 6*(4), 330–335.

Palagini, L., Gemignani, A., Banti, S., Manconi, M., Mauri, M., & Riemann, D. (2014). Chronic sleep loss during pregnancy as a determinant of stress: Impact on pregnancy outcome. *Sleep Medicine, 15*(8), 853–859.

Pamidi, S., Pinto, L. M., Marc, I., Benedetti, A., Schwartzman, K., & Kimoff, R. J. (2014). Maternal sleep-disordered breathing and adverse pregnancy outcomes: A systematic review and metaanalysis. *American Journal of Obstetrics and Gynecology, 210*(1), 52.e1–52.e14.

Pillai, V., Roth, T., Mullins, H. M., & Drake, C. L. (2014). Moderators and mediators of the relationship between stress and insomnia: Stressor chronicity, cognitive intrusion, and coping. *Sleep, 37*(7), 1199–1208.

Porkka-Heiskanen, T., Zitting, K. M., & Wigren, H. K. (2013). Sleep, its regulation and possible mechanisms of sleep disturbances. *Acta Physiologica, 208*(4), 311–328.

Redeker, N. S., Pigeon, W. R., & Boudreau, E. A. (2015). Incorporating measures of sleep quality into cancer studies. *Supportive Care in Cancer, 23*(4), 1145–1155.

Redline, S., Kirchner, H., Quan, S. F., Gottlieb, D. J., Kapur, V., & Newman, A. (2004). The effects of age, sex, ethnicity, and sleep-disordered breathing on sleep architecture. *Archives of Internal Medicine, 164*(4), 406–418. doi:10.1001/archinte.164.4.406

Sadeh, A. (2011). The role and validity of actigraphy in sleep medicine: An update. *Sleep Medicine Reviews, 15*(4), 259–267.

Sánchez-Ortuño, M. M., Edinger, J. D., Means, M. K., & Almirall, D. (2010). Home is where sleep is: An ecological approach to test the validity of actigraphy for the assessment of insomnia. *Journal of Clinical Sleep Medicine, 6*(1), 21–29.

Shaver, J. L., & Woods, N. F. (2015). Sleep and menopause: A narrative review. *Menopause, 22*(8), 899–915.

Smith, M. T., & Wegener, S. T. (2003). Measures of sleep: The Insomnia Severity Index, Medical Outcomes Study (MOS) Sleep Scale, Pittsburgh Sleep Diary (PSD), and Pittsburgh Sleep Quality Index (PSQI). *Arthritis & Rheumatism, 49*, S184–S196.

Spira, A. P., Covinsky, K., Rebok, G. W., Punjabi, N. M., Stone, K. L., Hillier, T. A., . . . Yaffe, K. (2012). Poor sleep quality and functional decline in older women. *Journal of the American Geriatrics Society, 60*(6), 1092–1098.

Spira, A. P., Stone, K. L., Rebok, G. W., Punjabi, N. M., Redline, S., Ancoli-Israel, S., & Yaffe, K. (2014). Sleep-disordered breathing and functional decline in older women. *Journal of the American Geriatrics Society, 62*(11), 2040–2046.

Srivanitchapoom, P., Pandey, S., & Hallett, M. (2014). Restless legs syndrome and pregnancy: A review. *Parkinsonism & Related Disorders, 20*(7), 716–722.

Sternfeld, B., Guthrie, K. A., Ensrud, K. E., LaCroix, A. Z., Larson, J. C., Dunn, A. L., . . . Caan, B. J. (2014). Efficacy of exercise for menopausal symptoms: A randomized controlled trial. *Menopause, 21*(4), 330–338.

Stone, K. L., Ancoli-Israel, S., Blackwell, T., Ensrud, K. E., Cauley, J. A., Redline, S., . . . Cummings, S. R. (2008). Actigraphy-measured sleep characteristics and risk of falls in older women. *Archives of Internal Medicine, 168*(16), 1768–1775. doi:10.1001/archinte.168.16.1768

Stone, K. L., Ewing, S. K., Ancoli-Israel, S., Ensrud, K. E., Redline, S., Bauer, D. C.,…Cummings, S. R. (2009). Self-reported sleep and nap habits and risk of mortality in a large cohort of older women. *Journal of the American Geriatrics Society, 57*(4), 604–611.

Taibi, D. M., Landis, C. A., & Vitiello, M. V. (2013). Concordance of polysomnographic and actigraphic measurement of sleep and wake in older women with insomnia. *Journal of Clinical Sleep Medicine, 9*(3), 217–225.

Taibi, D. M., Vitiello, M. V., Barsness, S., Elmer, G. W., Anderson, G. D., & Landis, C. A. (2009). A randomized clinical trial of valerian fails to improve self-reported, polysomnographic, and actigraphic sleep in older women with insomnia. *Sleep Medicine, 10*(3), 319–328.

Tips for better sleep. University of Washington, Center for Research on the Management of Sleep Disturbances. National Institute Nursing Research, NR011400, 2009–2014.

Trauer, J. M., Qian, M. Y., Doyle, J. S., Rajaratnam, S. M., & Cunnington, D. (2015). Cognitive behavioral therapy for chronic insomnia: A systematic review and meta-analysis. *Annals of Internal Medicine, 163*(3), 191–204.

Tsai, S. Y., Kuo, L. T., Lee, C. N., Lee, Y. L., & Landis, C. A. (2013). Reduced sleep duration and daytime naps in pregnant women in Taiwan. *Nursing Research, 62*(2), 99–105.

U.S. Department of Health and Human Services, Office of Disease Prevention and Health Promotion. (2015). *Healthy people 2020*. Washington, DC: Retrieved from https://www.healthypeople.gov/2020/topics-objectives/topic/sleep-health/objectives

Vana, K. D., Silva, G. E., & Goldberg, R. (2013). Predictive abilities of the STOP-Bang and Epworth Sleepiness Scale in identifying sleep clinic patients at high risk for obstructive sleep apnea. *Research in Nursing & Health, 36*(1), 84–94.

Vitiello, M. V., McCurry, S. M., Shortreed, S. M., Baker, L. D., Rybarczyk, B. D., Keefe, F. J., & Von Korff, M. (2014). Short-term improvement in insomnia symptoms predicts long-term improvements in sleep, pain, and fatigue in older adults with comorbid osteoarthritis and insomnia. *Pain, 155*(8), 1547–1554.

Watson, N. F., Badr, M. S., Belenky, G., Bliwise, D. L., Buxton, O. M., Buysse, D.,…Tasali, E. (2015). Recommended amount of sleep for a healthy adult: A joint consensus statement of the American Academy of Sleep Medicine and Sleep Research Society. *Sleep, 38*(6), 843–844.

Whinnery, J., Jackson, N., Rattanaumpawan, P., & Grandner, M. A. (2014). Short and long sleep duration associated with race/ethnicity, sociodemographics, and socioeconomic position. *Sleep, 37*(3), 601–611.

Wilson, D. L., Barnes, M., Ellett, L., Permezel, M., Jackson, M., & Crowe, S. F. (2011). Decreased sleep efficiency, increased wake after sleep onset and increased cortical arousals in late pregnancy. *The Australian & New Zealand Journal of Obstetrics & Gynaecology, 51*(1), 38–46.

Wilson, D. L., Walker, S. P., Fung, A. M., O'Donoghue, F., Barnes, M., & Howard, M. (2013). Can we predict sleep-disordered breathing in pregnancy? The clinical utility of symptoms. *Journal of Sleep Research, 22*(6), 670–678.

Woods, N. F., & Mitchell, E. S. (2010). Sleep symptoms during the menopausal transition and early postmenopause: Observations from the Seattle Midlife Women's Health Study. *Sleep, 33*(4), 539–549.

Xi, B., He, D., Zhang, M., Xue, J., & Zhou, D. (2014). Short sleep duration predicts risk of metabolic syndrome: A systematic review and meta-analysis. *Sleep Medicine Reviews, 18*(4), 293–297.

Xiao, R. S., Kroll-Desrosiers, A. R., Goldberg, R. J., Pagoto, S. L., Person, S. D., & Waring, M. E. (2014). The impact of sleep, stress, and depression on postpartum weight retention: A systematic review. *Journal of Psychosomatic Research, 77*(5), 351–358.

Xu, Q., & Lang, C. P. (2014). Examining the relationship between subjective sleep disturbance and menopause: A systematic review and meta-analysis. *Menopause, 21*(12), 1301–1318.

Young, T., Palta, M., Dempsey, J., Skatrud, J., Weber, S., & Badr, S. (1993). The occurrence of sleep-disordered breathing among middle-aged adults. *The New England Journal of Medicine, 328*(17), 1230–1235.

Yu, L., Buysse, D. J., Germain, A., Moul, D. E., Stover, A., Dodds, N. E., …Pilkonis, P. A. (2011). Development of short forms from the PROMIS™ sleep disturbance and sleep-related impairment item banks. *Behavioral Sleep Medicine, 10*(1), 6–24.

Yuceege, M., Firat, H., Demir, A., & Ardic, S. (2013). Reliability of the Watch-PAT 200 in detecting sleep apnea in highway bus drivers. *Journal of Clinical Sleep Medicine, 9*(4), 339–344.

Zee, P. C., Attarian, H., & Videnovic, A. (2013). Circadian rhythm abnormalities. *Continuum, 19*(1), 132–147.

Zheng, H., Sowers, M., Buysse, D. J., Consens, F., Kravitz, H. M., Matthews, K. A.,…Hall, M. (2012). Sources of variability in epidemiological studies of sleep using repeated nights of in-home polysomnography: SWAN Sleep Study. *Journal of Clinical Sleep Medicine, 8*(1), 87–96.

CHAPTER 16

Genetics and Women's Health

Diane C. Seibert • Elizabeth A. Kostas-Polston

■ OVERVIEW OF THE REACH OF GENETICS AND CLINICAL CARE

Rapid scientific advances are pushing clinicians in all practice communities to become more knowledgeable about genetics. Although the basic tenets of inheritance have been known (and manipulated) since antiquity, the biological mechanisms responsible for an individual's unique characteristics remained shrouded in mystery until very recently. The molecule that forms the foundation for DNA (nucleic acid) was described in 1869 (Dahm, 2008), but nearly a century passed before DNA's precise molecular structure was determined (Pray, 2008), and another 50 years ticked by before the first draft of the human genome was completed in 2003 (Collins, Green, Guttmacher, & Guyer, 2003). Over the past decade, the pace of scientific and technological advances has continued to accelerate, with sequencing speed doubling every 4 months and costs plummeting from hundreds of millions of dollars to just a few thousand dollars during that time (National Human Genome Research Institute [NHGRI], 2013). Researchers are now conducting highly complex Genome-Wide Association Studies (GWASs), combining phenotype, family health history (FHH), and genomics to better explain the development of complex health conditions such as hypertension and diabetes.

Educational leaders across all health care professions are looking for ways to infuse this important (and rapidly evolving) information into curricula effectively, but nursing has the additional challenge of meeting the needs of a professional community that is evolving rapidly as well. This chapter provides an overview of some of the important genomic concepts that all nurses should know but places particular emphasis on the intersection between genomics and women's health.

■ GENETIC AND GENOMIC COMPETENCIES

Virtually every disease has a genetic or genomic component and treatment options increasingly involve genetics in disease prevention, screening, diagnosis, prognosis, and monitoring. In 2005, committed to addressing the practice and knowledge gap in the nursing profession, a panel of nursing leaders, cosponsored by the American Nurses Association (ANA), NHGRI, National Cancer Institute (NCI), and Office of Rare Diseases (ORD), gathered to identify essential genetic and genomic competencies that all registered nurses should have. The following year, *The Essential Nursing Competencies and Curricula Guidelines for Genetics and Genomics* was published. In 2009, an updated version added curricular guidelines for nursing educators to use when creating nursing curricula (Jenkins, 2009). Three years later, an expanded set of genetic/genomic competencies guiding the education of nurses at the graduate level was published. These competencies, the *Essential Genetic/Genomic Competencies for Nurses with Graduate Degrees*, were developed specifically for nurses with advanced degrees, including, but not limited to, advanced practice registered nurses (APRNs), clinical nurse leaders, nurse educators, nurse administrators, and nurse scientists (Greco, Tinley, & Seibert, 2011). None of these documents replaces or recreates existing standards of practice, but rather they incorporate genetic and genomic perspective into nursing education and practice. It is important to note that all three documents were created by consensus, informed by public opinion, and endorsed by more than 30 nursing organizations.

■ SEX, GENDER, AND GENETICS

Genetics plays a role in the majority of the leading causes of death in the United States (Centers for Disease Control and Prevention [CDC], 2015b). Diseases such as cancer, diabetes, and cardiovascular disease are related to epigenetic influences—the complex interactions among shared genes, behaviors, cultures, and environments that influence health and risk (CDC, 2015a; Scheuner, Yoon, & Khoury, 2004).

Biological differences between women and men result from sex determination and differentiation. The sex determination process determines if the female or male sexual differentiation pathway will be followed. Sex differentiation, the development of a given sex, involves many genetically regulated and developmental steps. For example, the

Y chromosome produces testicular differentiation of the embryonic gonad. Gender, usually described as masculinity and femininity, is a social construct and varies across cultures and time. Biological differences between women and men manifest differently when considering health risk. Table 16.1 describes sex and gender influences on health across the life span.

An FHH is an important tool used to identify and prevent or reduce risk. If used properly, it allows the health care provider to take steps toward the early diagnosis and management of disease, as well as make appropriate referrals.

■ WOMEN AS GATEKEEPERS OF FHH AND HEALTH

The collection of an accurate FHH is an essential element of patient assessment, but although most clinicians appreciate how important the FHH is, this important information is rarely collected, updated, or recorded systematically (Welch, Dere, & Schiffman, 2015). Gathering an accurate and complete FHH involves both trust and collaboration; patients have to believe that if they disclose sensitive information, it will be used appropriately, and providers need to ask the right questions at the right time and verify the accuracy of the information they gather. In some families "kinkeepers" play an important role in facilitating family communication (Giordimaina, Sheldon, Kiedrowski, & Jayaratne, 2015) because they maintain and disseminate family health information; although they are not formally recognized, they are often the ones other family members consult when family medical information is needed. It is interesting to note that kinkeepers are often middle-aged women and are more often identified in Caucasian families than in African American or Hispanic American families for reasons that have yet to be completely elucidated (Giordimaina et al., 2015; Thompson et al., 2015). Detailed knowledge of the FHH may be known to these women, not because they are simply curious and ask health-related questions, but because women are often responsible for managing the family's health needs. Nearly half of all working women stay home from work to care for their children when they are ill; 12% of women are the primary caregivers for sick or aging relatives, and nearly one in five women devote more than 40 hours a week caring for ill family members (Ranji & Salganicoff, 2011). It is important to recognize the variety of health care roles and responsibilities that women may play in their families. Female patients may be presenting for care themselves, but they often have the keys to vast stores of information about their family's health, health behaviors, and health risks. Many of these women also bear an inordinate responsibility for the health and well-being of their extended family. They often prepare many of the family meals and influence the amount of exercise their family gets; they contribute to the family's income and often assume responsibility for ensuring that their family members receive necessary preventive health care screenings and interventions (e.g., vaccinations, routine health assessments).

■ FAMILY HISTORY AS A MEANS OF EVALUATING RISK

Family Health History

Inquiring about the health history of one's immediate family is a critical part of collecting an individual's medical history. FHH is the most consistent tool for determining risk factors for human disease across the life span; it reveals diseases (e.g., heart disease, diabetes, cancer, osteoporosis, asthma, hypertension, hypercholesterolemia) that carry significant public health concern (Yoon, Scheuner, & Khoury, 2003; Khoury & Mensah, 2005). It brings to light the complex interactions among shared genes, behaviors, cultures, and environments that influence families' health and disease risk. In fact, the FHH is so important that it has been referred to as the best genetic test available (Genetic Alliance, n.d., 2009; Genetics Home Reference, 2016; Scheuner, Yoon, & Khoury, 2004). Although one's family history cannot be changed, an increased awareness provides health care providers with the opportunity to, for example, personalize and target disease prevention, treatment, and management (Khoury, 2003; U.S. Department of Health and Human Services [USDHHS], n.d.).

Health care providers are armed with a variety of tools for evaluating health risk. The FHH is one such important screening tool. It brings to light epigenetic influences, characterizes trends and patterns of disease that may lead to prevention and treatment, and increases knowledge about health and genetics for individuals and their family members (Genetic Alliance, 2009). As a diagnostic tool, the FHH is used to guide medical decisions about genetic testing and disease risk.

Precision Medicine Initiative

In 2015, the brightest leaders in the United States in science (National Institutes of Health [NIH], 2015) rolled out the Precision Medicine Initiative. This initiative came about as a result of the sequencing of the human genome, improved technologies for biomedical analyses, and new tools for the use of large data sets. The hope is that new scientific evidence will be generated to inform clinical practice. In fact, the overall aim is to integrate this genomic approach for disease prevention and treatment, necessitating a marked paradigmatic shift in the manner in which health care providers currently deliver health care. Overcoming drug resistance, adopting advanced pharmacogenomics (the right drug for the right patient at the right dose), using new targets for prevention and treatment, and using mobile devices to encourage healthy lifestyle behaviors are only but a few of the projected goals. Central to the Precision Medicine Initiative is the FHH.

Contemporary Clinical Practice

In contemporary health care education and training programs, graduate students are taught how to take a thorough

TABLE 16.1	Sex and Gender Influences on Health

MENTAL HEALTH

Females	Males
Twice as likely to experience depression More likely to develop eating disorder, panic disorder, and PTSD Depressed middle-aged women have almost double risk of having a stroke Experience mood symptoms related to hormone changes during puberty, pregnancy, and perimenopause	More likely to show aggressive, impulsive, coercive, and noncompliant behaviors

CARDIOVASCULAR DISEASE

Females	Males
Low-dose aspirin reduces risk of ischemic stroke Blood vessels of a woman's heart smaller in diameter and much more intricately branched Cholesterol plaque may not build up into major artery blockages. Instead, they spread evenly over the entire wall of the artery. This makes diagnosis of artery blockages more difficult Onset of cardiovascular disease later in women	Low-dose aspirin reduces risk of heart attack

OSTEOPOROSIS

Females	Males
More common because of less bone tissue Experience a rapid phase of bone loss because of hormonal changes at menopause	Worse health outcomes postfracture

OSTEOARTHRITIS

Females	Males
More common ≥ 45 years of age Severity significantly worse because of knee and hip anatomy, imbalanced leg muscle strength, and loose tendons and ligaments Black women at greater risk for osteoarthritis complications	More common ≤ 45 years of age

AUTOIMMUNE DISORDERS

Females	Males
80% affected Pain mechanisms in female brain not found in men. Pain associated with irritable bowel syndrome greater in women In animal models, female chromosome set (XX) stimulates development of lupus	Type 1 diabetes and ankylosing spondylitis more common

CANCER

Females	Males
Lung cancer leading cause of death For any given number of cigarettes smoked (when compared with men), appear to be at higher risk of developing lung cancer Breast cancer more common Greater incidence across the life span, and risk increases in seventh decade and beyond	Male teens and young men 55% more likely to die of melanoma Prostate cancer is the leading cause of death More prone to liver cancer

PTSD, posttraumatic stress disorder.
Adapted from Canadian Institutes of Health Research, Institute of Medicine (IOM), National Institute of Arthritis and Musculoskeletal and Skin Diseases (NIAMSD), National Institutes of Health (NIH), National Institute on Drug Abuse (NIDA), NIH Osteoporosis and Related Bone Diseases, National Resource Center (NIH ORBD NRC), World Health Organization (WHO).

family medical history using questions and pedigree collection. It is unfortunate that in clinical practice, time constraints necessitate, at best, an abbreviated collection of family medical history,—oftentimes focusing only on diseases with high prevalence (e.g., heart disease, cancer, hypertension, diabetes; Yoon et al., 2004). The result is an incomplete FHH that is missing critical health information. What is more, the incomplete FHH limits the health care provider's ability to accurately determine health risk as well as to identify potential preventive and treatment measures.

FHH Tools

Because time constraints are a reality, FHH tools have been developed so that patients may complete them before clinic visits. An FHH should reflect the gold standard, a three-generation pedigree (if possible and at minimum) of biological relatives as well as age at diagnosis and age and cause of death of family members. There are many tools available. One such tool, My Family Health Portrait (www.familyhistory.hhs.gov/FHH/html/index.html), is a computerized tool that runs on any web-connected computer or laptop. There is no cost, and once an individual has created a family health portrait, he or she can download the file to his or her personal computer and even share with other family members. This way, family members can share their accurate FHH with their health care providers. This particular tool is part of the U.S. Surgeon General's Family History Initiative (USDHHS, n.d.) that encourages family gatherings to incorporate time to talk about and document health problems that run in families. It is important that the information gathered be reliable, which may require family members checking old health records of loved ones as well as death certificates. Other tools are also available and at no cost.

Genetics, Genomics, and Advanced Practice Nursing

Today, tumultuous changes resulting from advances in biomedical technology are evidenced in all health care disciplines and settings. These advances are redefining the understanding of health and illness and are necessitating changes in education, training, and clinical practice. Advanced practice nurses are positioned to contribute significantly to the genetic and genomic transformation of health care for the purpose of improving clinical outcomes.

For the purpose of defining genomic competencies in advanced nursing practice, the *Essential Genetic and Genomic Competencies for Nurses With Graduate Degrees* (Greco, Tinley, & Seibert, 2011) were developed in 2006 (revised in 2009). These competencies of professional advanced practice nursing are organized under seven topics: (a) risk assessment and interpretation; (b) genetic education; counseling, testing, and results interpretation; (c) clinical management; (d) ethical, legal, and social implications (ELSI); (e) professional role; (f) leadership; and (g) research (Greco et al., 2011). The FHH serves as the clinical starting point (risk assessment and interpretation). Evaluation of the FHH brings to light genetic red flags (reported family health

issues, which become suspect for possible increased health risk; Seibert, 2014). Genetic red flags serve to shape the professional conversation between the health care provider and patient. Genetic and genomic competencies provide a framework to be used in advanced practice nursing.

Pedigrees

FHH data can be captured in several ways: provided in oral communication, written in a narrative, or displayed graphically in a drawing, called a *pedigree*. Pedigrees are particularly useful because they reveal the influence of both heredity and environment on an individual and within a particular family. The pedigree can trace how traits are passed along within a family, and the incidence of a particular characteristic in a family can actually be counted. Standardized symbols (Figure 16.1) can be used to document and communicate of the FHH. Because the FHH constantly evolves, patients should be encouraged to ask about changes in the FHH from their family members, and pedigrees should be reviewed and updated regularly by providers.

The complete pedigree contains information about three generations of family members including first-degree (parents, siblings, and children), second-degree (half siblings, grandparents, aunts, uncles, and grandchildren) and third-degree (cousins) relatives. Whenever possible, data should be recorded electronically to facilitate retrieval, review, and updating.

As time consuming and challenging as collecting an accurate and complete FHH might be, accurately assessing risk to an individual is more difficult because information from disparate (and often multiple) sources must be appraised and synthesized. Several mnemonics have been developed to help clinicians assess genomic risk (Table 16.2).

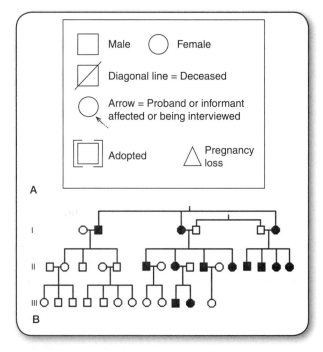

FIGURE 16.1

(A) Common pedigree symbols and (B) three-generation pedigree.

TABLE 16.2	Three Mnemonics for Gathering and Interpreting the FHH
MNEMONIC	**DEFINITION/INTERPRETATION**
SCREEN	Some concern: Do you have any (some) concerns about diseases or conditions that seem to run in your family? Reproduction: Have there been any problems with pregnancy, infertility, or birth defects in your family? Early disease death/disability: Have any members of your family been diagnosed with a chronic disease at an early age, or have members of your family died at an early age? Ethnicity: How would you describe your ethnicity? What country did your ancestors come from? Nongenetic or not necessarily genetic: Are you aware of any nonmedical conditions or risk factors, such as smoking or problem drinking, that are present in your family?
F-Genes	F: Family history: Multiple affected siblings or individuals in multiple generations G: Groups of congenital anomalies E: Extreme or exceptional presentation of common conditions (i.e., early age of onset, condition manifesting in a less-often-affected sex) N: Neurodevelopmental delay or degeneration E: Extreme or exceptional pathology S: Surprising laboratory values
Rule of Too/Two	Too something (tall, short, early, young, many, different) Two of something (tumors, generations, in the family, congenital defects)

FHH, family health history.
Adapted from Genetics in Primary Care Institute. Genetic Red Flags. Available at https://geneticsinprimarycare.aap.org/YourPractice/Family-Health-History/Pages/Genetic%20Red%20Flags.aspx

The first, SCREEN, is used to elicit concerns and/or risk factors regarding a patient's family history; the second, F-GENES, helps stratify clinical features into red-flag categories, and the words *too* and *two* are often used to describe individuals or families with genetic conditions because a particular condition occurs too often, affects too many individuals, or appears in two locations (two primary cancers) or in two generations of family members, and so forth.

Other genetic red flags include disease in the absence of known risk factors, ethnic predisposition to certain genetic disorders, and close biological relationship between parents, such as consanguinity, all of which, if present, raise the index of suspicion that an individual might be at increased risk for developing a particular condition (Arnold & Self, 2012; Borgmeyer, 2005). Referring back to the competencies in the *Essential Genetic and Genomic Competencies for Nurses With Graduate Degrees* (Greco et al., 2011), other questions that might be asked include:

- Is other information (assessment, history, diagnostics) needed to assess her risk?
- Do other family members need to be tested?
- Should a genetic test be offered? If so, which one?
- Is a genetics referral indicated?
- Who will offer posttest counseling and education?
- Assuming a genetic mutation is found, how will clinical care be affected?
- What ELSI issues should be discussed before or after testing?
- Does this case raise any nursing "professional responsibility" concerns?

■ SCENARIOS

This final section contains four examples that provide a brief case narrative, a pedigree, and a glimpse into a health care provider's thoughts as he or she integrates and synthesizes the individual and family health histories with physical examination findings and other clinical data (e.g., laboratory and/or diagnostic testing results) to assess an individual's risk for having (or developing) a particular condition and select an appropriate management strategy.

Scenario 1

JC, a 32-year-old African American female presents for a routine well-woman examination. Her past medical history is significant for three uncomplicated vaginal deliveries and hypothyroidism, which is well managed. She reports no surgeries except for wisdom tooth extraction at age 19. She has no allergies, takes no over-the-counter medications, and regularly takes Synthroid 75 mcg and NuvaRing (contraception). JC is a good historian, providing a thorough FHH (see Figure 16.2).

As you evaluate JC's FHH (Figure 16.2) you immediately notice that she and several other family members have different autoimmune disorders and you suspect that other family members may be at an increased risk for developing autoimmune diseases as well. You also wonder if a gene is involved, whether it may have been inherited from her 72-year-old father, because he, too, has an autoimmune condition. Her mother died relatively young from a stroke, at age 62 years, so family members may share genes that put them at an increased risk for cardiovascular disease, but because the genetics of many complex conditions like autoimmune and cardiovascular disease are unknown, you really cannot evaluate the risk in an empiric way. The National Institutes of Health estimates that 5% to 8% of Americans have an autoimmune disorder, and alterations in immune response are involved in more than 80 human diseases (National Institute of Allergy and Infectious Disease, 2016). Related individuals may not always

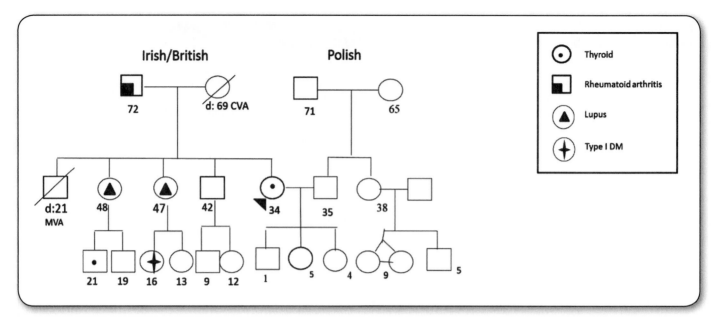

FIGURE 16.2
JC's Family health history.
CVA, cerebrovascular accident; DM, diabetes mellitus; MVA, motor vehicle accident.

develop the same autoimmune disease, and the risk may be greater or smaller depending on the specific disease, but in general, close relatives are more likely to develop related autoimmune disorders. Many genes have been implicated in causing autoimmune disease, primarily genes related to the human major histocompatibility complex (HLA), the most gene-dense region in the human genome, containing around 250 genes, nearly 100 of which are thought to regulate immune function (Goris & Liston, 2012). However, genes associated with the development of autoimmune disease do not usually act in isolation. Environmental exposures and viral infections are common triggers in the development of autoimmune disease. The FHH can be useful in highlighting shared environmental exposures, but in most cases, clear evidence of a specific environmental trigger causing autoimmune disease is absent (Ray, Sonthalia, Kundu, & Ganguly, 2013).

Because those conditions seen in JC's family are so complex, no specific genetic tests are currently available, and no referrals or other diagnostic testing is currently needed. JC should be told that she might be at an increased risk for developing other autoimmune conditions and should be alert to the appearance of unusual symptoms (joint pain, polyuria, polydipsia) and clinicians should carefully assess for early manifestations of other autoimmune conditions.

Scenario 2

DG, a 32-year-old White female presents requesting a genetic test for breast cancer stating she has a "strong family history of breast cancer" (Figure 16.3).

To determine whether she is, in fact, at an increased risk for developing breast cancer compared to other Caucasian women, the FHH is scrutinized for red flags that might

indicate that she is at an increased risk for inherited breast disease (see Figure 16.3):

- Ashkenazi Jewish ancestry (UNKNOWN)
- FH of breast, ovarian, or pancreatic cancer (YES)
- Ovarian cancer at any age (NO)
- FH of breast *and* ovarian or breast *and* pancreatic cancer (NO)
- More than two family members with breast cancer, one at a young age (NO)
- More than three family members with breast cancer at any age (NO)
- Breast cancer in a male relative (NO)
- Breast cancer diagnosed before menopause (≤ 50 years) (NO)
- One or more primary breast cancers in one individual or on the same side of the family (NO)
- Triple negative breast cancer (UNKNOWN)

DC might be at an increased risk for developing breast cancer because she does have two second-degree relatives who have had breast cancer, but she is much more likely to be at "population" (or average) risk because the two affected women are on opposite sides of the family and both developed postmenopausal breast cancer (ages 64 and 59 years). She does not know whether either woman had any genetic testing nor whether either of the tumors were tested for hormone receptor status. She does not think that she has any relatives that were Ashkenazi Jewish, although it is possible as her grandfather was from Poland. Although pieces of information are unknown, DC's FHH is not provocative for inherited breast disease and no further genetic testing for hereditary breast and ovarian cancer (HBOC) genes is indicated at this time.

DC should be reminded, however, that one in every eight women (12.4%) born in the United States will

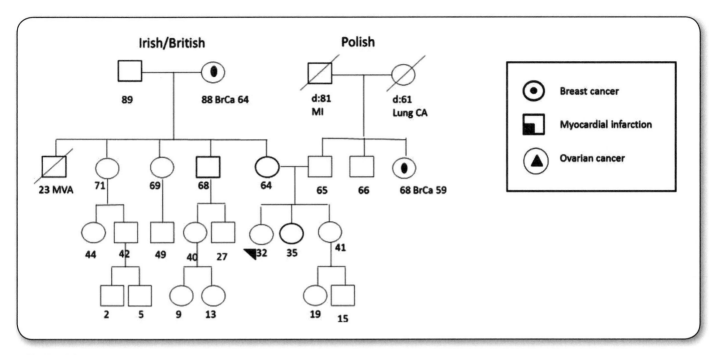

FIGURE 16.3

DG's family health history.

BrCa, breast cancer; CA, cancer; MI, myocardial infarction; MVA, motor vehicle accident.

develop breast cancer at some time during their lifetime. Although current screening recommendations for women at population risk are inconsistent, you should have a conversation with her about when and how often to screen given her FHH, her personal risks (age of menarche and menopause, pregnancy and breastfeeding history, radiation exposure, etc.), and her anxiety about developing breast cancer.

Scenario 3

MB, a 34-year-old Caucasian woman is concerned about developing uterine cancer because her older sister was just diagnosed with it, and was told by *her* doctor that MB should see a genetics specialist. You have known MB for several years, and believe you have a good relationship with her. You last saw her 2 months ago when you started her on oral contraceptive pills after she stopped breastfeeding her son. MB has mild anxiety that is somewhat worse now that she is nearly as old as her father was when he died in a car accident, but is otherwise healthy, has never had any surgery, and takes only combined hormonal birth control pills and multivitamins. Although you have known MB for several years, you have never gathered a detailed, three-generation FHH on her before, and you are surprised at what you learn (see Figure 16.4).

Although you do not know much about hereditary colorectal cancer (CRC) syndromes, you recognize that there are some significant red flags in her FHH.

- Three or more family members have been diagnosed with a CRC-associated cancer (YES)
- One affected family member must have been diagnosed before age 50 (YES)

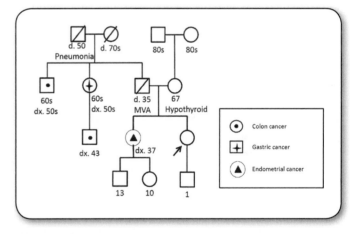

FIGURE 16.4

MB's family health history.

dx, diagnosis; MVA, motor vehicle accident.

- One affected family member must be a first-degree relative to the other two (YES)
- At least two consecutive generations must be affected (YES)

Several family members on MB's paternal side have developed a CRC-syndrome cancer: one first-degree relative (her sister), two second-degree relatives (paternal aunt and paternal uncle), and one third-degree relative (paternal cousin).

SHOULD MB BE OFFERED A GENETIC TEST? IF SO, WHICH ONE?

Genetic testing is appropriate in this case, but the biggest question is what test to order and who to test. The first question to ask is whether any of MB's affected relatives had been tested for a CRC-syndrome mutation; if the family gene is known, MB can be screened for just the familial mutation. If no one in the family has been tested, however, the best person to test is someone with the disease, such as MB's uncle, sister, or cousin because they are still alive. Genetic testing is expensive when the familial mutation is unknown because several genes have to be tested and additional confirmatory tests may also be necessary. Because MB's sister developed a CRC-associated cancer, MB's father likely had the mutation as well, but because he died at a young age, he never manifested the disease.

IS A GENETICS REFERRAL INDICATED?

Although it is certainly possible for a primary care provider to counsel and test MB, this is one of the situations in which it is more appropriate to refer to a genetic professional. Genetic testing can be straightforward and relatively inexpensive when the family mutation is known, but when the mutation is unknown, things become complicated very quickly. This FHH is very likely Lynch syndrome, a hereditary CRC-cancer syndrome, in which mutations in any of five different "mismatch repair" genes have been associated with the development of different cancers (Lindor et al., 2006).

Later, you learn that MB's cousin had genetic tumor testing, which was initially inconclusive but later found to contain a mutation associated with Lynch syndrome and therefore, the family cancer gene was confirmed. Referral to a genetic professional is most appropriate because MB and her family will be offered the time and expertise they need to get their questions and concerns addressed.

DO OTHER FAMILY MEMBERS NEED TO BE TESTED?

There are no other family members on the paternal side who are alive or unaffected except MB's son and typically children are not offered genetic testing for adult onset

disorders, unless a treatment is available that prevents or delays development of disease (Caga-anan, Smith, Sharp, & Lantos, 2012).

IF MB HAS A DELETERIOUS MUTATION, WILL HER CLINICAL MANAGEMENT BE ALTERED?

First, clinicians should be prepared to communicate the increase in risk in a way that MB can understand it. MB may be able to understand statistical risks if they are presented mathematically, but may grasp the concepts better when a more simplistic approach is used to explain risk (e.g., coloring in stick figures). Before risk is discussed, however, a careful review of the literature (or current resources) should be conducted to ensure that the risk numbers being provided are accurate. As knowledge advances, these numbers adjust over time (see Table 16.3).

If MB is found to carry a deleterious familial mutation and has received appropriate genetic counseling, the focus can then shift to reducing risk and identifying clinical manifestations as early as possible. This can be challenging even for oncologists who work with these patients on a daily basis, so the best course of action would be to refer MB and her family to a center specializing in managing people with Lynch syndrome, who can develop a comprehensive management plan that can then be communicated back to the family's primary care providers.

ARE THERE ANY ENHANCED SURVEILLANCE AND/OR RISK REDUCTION OPTIONS FOR MB?

Several screening options are recommended for individuals with Lynch syndrome mutations: annual colonoscopy starting at age 20; upper endoscopy (EGD) annually starting at age 40; annual urinalysis starting at age 30; and endometrial and ovarian cancer symptom education and discussion of prophylactic hysterectomy and oophorectomy by age 40, or when childbearing is complete (Lindor et al., 2006).

TABLE 16.3	Phenotype Variations in Lynch Syndrome	
ASSOCIATED CONDITION	**LIFETIME RISK OF CONDITION**	**NOTES**
Colon cancer	MLH1, MSH2 (43%–82%) MSH6 (20%–44%) PMS2 (15%–20%) EPCAM (75%)	For MLH1, MSH2, and MSH6, risks are lower in women
Endometrial cancer	MLH1, MSH2, and MSH6 (44%) PMS2 and EPCAM: unknown	In 50% of Lynch syndrome women, this is the initial presentation
Gastric cancer	MLH1 and MSH2 (6%–13%)	Highest in males with MSH2 mutation. H. pylori coinfection may raise risk
Ovarian cancer	MLH1 (4%–6%) MSH2 (8%–11%)	30% diagnosed before age 35 years
Bladder cancer	MSH2 > MLH1 Males > Females	Interaction of risks can give dramatic findings, but they are just estimates: Women with MLH1 mutation have 1% risk; men with MSH2 mutation have 27% risk

WHAT ARE THE REPRODUCTIVE IMPLICATIONS?

Because Lynch syndrome is inherited in an autosomal dominant manner, MB should be informed that with each pregnancy the risk for passing the mutation to each child is 50%. Because the familial mutation in MB's family is known, pregestational diagnostic (PGD) testing and prenatal screening would be available to her, but additional counseling from a reproductive geneticist is highly recommended.

WHAT ETHICAL, LEGAL, AND SOCIAL IMPLICATIONS (ELSI) SHOULD BE DISCUSSED BEFORE OR AFTER TESTING?

There are several ELSI in this scenario. Beneficence is applied when MB's increased risk for developing a Lynch-syndrome cancer is identified before the onset of disease. This early recognition of risk offers her the opportunity to discuss options, such as enhanced screening, chemoprevention, or surgery before she develops cancer, improving her longevity as well as the quality of her life. Justice is applied when MB's family members are offered the same counseling and screening services she is. Autonomy is applied when adult family members are offered genetic counseling, testing, and treatment options, but each person has the right to refuse any or all of these interventions. Two ethical constructs, nonmaleficence and privacy, are competing priorities and, depending on the preferences of individual family members, are potentially the most difficult ethical principles to apply evenly. If everyone in MB's family considered to be at increased risk is interested in being counseled and tested, and genetic information is shared freely among family members, then these ethical principles are satisfied; no one is harmed by the information and the concept of privacy, as it relates to carrier status, has been addressed. When *some* but *not all* family members want to know their mutation status, maintaining privacy and minimizing harm becomes more difficult. Finally, Genetic Information Non-Discrimination Act (GINA) insurance and employment protections may apply to some, but not all, family members. MB is protected because she has not been diagnosed with a breast or ovarian cancer, but several of her family members (including her sister) have been diagnosed with cancer, so GINA protections do not apply.

■ SUMMARY

Assessing genetic risk can be complicated, and collecting an FHH can be challenging. The genomic landscape is evolving rapidly, and specialized knowledge is often needed to interpret and translate this information for colleagues, patients, families, and communities. The potential power of genomics to improve health and health care is truly stunning. Very basic information, such as an accurate FHH, can open the door to critical conversations about individual and familial risk, offering the opportunity to make presymptomatic or early diagnoses, choosing the most effective interventions (e.g., pharmacogenomics), increasing communication among family members, and informing reproductive decisions. Everyone on the health care team needs to be fully engaged in working in a community in which genomics features prominently, and partnership with other health care team members (e.g., genetic counselors, medical geneticists, maternal fetal medicine specialists, oncologists, social workers, dietitians, dentists) will be the way health care is delivered in the future.

■ REFERENCES

Arnold, K. M., & Self, Z. B. (2012). Genetic screening and counseling: Family medicine obstetrics. *Primary Care, 39*(1), 55–70.

Borgmeyer C. (2005). Wired for education: aafp takes major cme initiative to the web. *Annals of Family Medicine, 3*(3), 277–278.

Caga-anan, E. C., Smith, L., Sharp, R. R., & Lantos, J. D. (2012). Testing children for adult-onset genetic diseases. *Pediatrics, 129*(1), 163–167.

Centers for Disease Control and Prevention (CDC). (2004). Awareness of family health history as a risk factor for disease—United States, 2004. *MMWR. Morbidity and Mortality Weekly Report, 53*(44),1044.

Centers for Disease Control and Prevention (CDC). (2015a). *Public health genomics: Family health history.* Retrieved from https://www.cdc.gov/genomics/famhistory

Centers for Disease Control and Prevention (CDC). (2015b). *Public health genomics.* Retrieved from https://www.cdc.gov/genomics

Collins, F. S., Green, E. D., Guttmacher, A. E., & Guyer, M. S.; US National Human Genome Research Institute. (2003). A vision for the future of genomics research. *Nature, 422*(6934), 835–847.

Dahm, R. (2008). Discovering DNA: Friedrich Miescher and the early years of nucleic acid research. *Human Genetics, 122*(6), 565–581.

Genetic Alliance (n.d.). *Family health history.* Retrieved from http://www.geneticalliance.org/programs/genesinlife/fhh

Genetic Alliance. (2009). *Understanding genetics: A New York, Mid-Atlantic guide for patients and health professionals.* Retrieved from http://www.ncbi.nlm.nih.gov/books/NBK115563/pdf/Bookshelf_NBK115563.pdf

Genetics Home Reference. (2016). *Why is it important to know my family medical history?* Retrieved from https://ghr.nlm.nih.gov/handbook/inheritance/familyhistory

Genetics in Primary Care Institute (GPCI). (n.d.) *Genetic red flags.* Retrieved from https://geneticsinprimarycare.aap.org/YourPractice/Family-Health-History/Pages/Genetic%20Red%20Flags.aspx

Giordimaina, A. M., Sheldon, J. P., Kiedrowski, L. A., & Jayaratne, T. E. (2015). Searching for the kinkeepers historian gender, age, and type 2 diabetes family history. *Health Education & Behavior, 42*(6), 736–741.

Goris, A., & Liston, A. (2012). The immunogenetic architecture of autoimmune disease. *Cold Spring Harbor Perspectives in Biology, 4*(3), 1–14.

Greco, K. E., Tinley, S., & Seibert, D. (2011). Development of the essential genetic and genomic competencies for nurses with graduate degrees. *Annual Review of Nursing Research, 29*, 173–190.

Greco, K. E., Tinley, S., & Seibert, D. (2011). *Essential genetic and genomic competencies for nurses with graduate degrees.* Silver Spring, MD: American Nurses Association and International Society of Nurses in Genetics.

Jenkins, J. F. (2009). *Essentials of genetic and genomic nursing: Competencies, curricula guidelines, and outcome indicators* (2nd ed.). Silver Spring, MD: American Nurses Association.

Khoury, M. J. (2003). Genetics and genomics in practice: The continuum from genetic disease to genetic information in health and disease. *Genetics in Medicine, 5*(4), 261–268.

Khoury, M. J., & Mensah, G. A. (2005). Genomics and the prevention and control of common chronic diseases: Emerging priorities for public health action. *Preventing Chronic Disease* (serial online). Retrieved from http://www.ncbi.nlm.nih.gov/pmc/articles/PMC1327699

Lindor, N. M., Petersen, G. M., Hadley, D. W., Kinney, A. Y., Miesfeldt, S., Lu, K. H.,...Press, N. (2006). Recommendations for the care of individuals with an inherited predisposition to Lynch syndrome: A systematic review. *Journal of the American Medical Association, 296*(12), 1507–1517.

National Human Genome Research Institute (NHGRI). (2013). *The 10-year anniversary of the Human Genome Project: Commemorating and reflecting* (No. NHGRI2013). Washington, DC: Author. Retrieved from http://www.genome.gov/27555238

National Institute of Allergy and Infectious Diseases. (2016). *Autoimmune diseases.* Retrieved from https://www.niaid.nih.gov/topics/auto immune/Pages/default.aspx

National Institutes of Health (NIH). (2015). *How sex and gender influence health and disease.* National Institutes of Health, Office of Research on Women's Health. Retrieved from orwh.od.nih.gov/resources/sex-and -gender-infographic/images/SexGenderInfographic_11x17_508.pdf

Pray, L. (2008). Discovery of DNA structure and function: Watson and Crick. *Nature Education, 1*(1), 100.

Ranji, U., & Salganicoff, A. (2011). *Women's health care chartbook: Key findings from the Kaiser Women's Health Survey.* Menlo Park, CA: Henry J. Kaiser Family Foundation.

Ray, S., Sonthalia, N., Kundu, S., & Ganguly, S. (2013). Autoimmune disorders: An overview of molecular and cellular basis in today's perspective. *Journal of Clinical & Cellular Immunology.* Retrieved from http://www.omicsonline.org/autoimmune-disorders-an-overview-of -molecular-and-cellular-basis-in-todays-perspective-2155-9899.S10 -003.php?aid=9483

Scheuner, M. T., Yoon, P. W., & Khoury, M. J. (2004). Contribution of Mendelian disorders to common chronic disease: Opportunities for recognition, intervention, and prevention. *American Journal of Medical Genetics Part C: Seminars in Medical Genetics, 125*(1), 50–65.

Seibert, D. C. (2014). Genomics and nurse practitioner practice. *The Nurse Practitioner, 39*(10), 18–28; quiz 28.

Thompson, T., Seo, J., Griffith, J., Baxter, M., James, A., & Kaphingst, K. A. (2015). The context of collecting family health history: Examining definitions of family and family communication about health among African American women. *Journal of Health Communication, 20*(4), 416–423.

U.S. Department of Health & Human Services (USDHHS) (n.d.). *Surgeon General's family health history initiative.* Retrieved from https:// familyhistory.hhs.gov/FHH/html/index.html

Welch, B. M., Dere, W., & Schiffman, J. D. (2015). Family health history: The case for better tools. *Journal of the American Medical Association, 313*(17), 1711–1712.

Yoon, P. W., Scheuner, M. T., & Khoury, M. J. (2003). Research priorities for evaluating family history in the prevention of common chronic diseases. *American Journal of Preventive Medicine, 24*(2), 128–135.

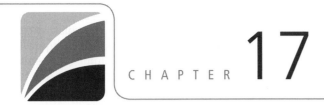

Women and the Workplace

Janice Camp

Work provides a foundation of personal dignity and a source of stability for individuals and their families; good-paying, intellectually rewarding jobs are instrumental in building societal strength and personal resilience, particularly for women. Work often is connected with identity, meaning, and social connection as well as access to medical insurance and retirement benefits. Alternatively, the lack of work, unemployment, or underemployment has been associated with higher rates of illness and low self-esteem (Linn, Sandifer, & Stein, 1985). Work itself may also have deleterious consequences, particularly when that work involves exposure to hazards or injury risks. It is critical that caregivers understand the livelihood of their patients, incorporate that understanding into care plans and treatment strategies, and anticipate and capitalize on opportunities to protect their patients from adverse health outcomes that may be associated with their occupations.

Women have always worked, but in the United States they have increasingly participated in compensated employment. In an agrarian society, most workers were self-employed or worked for family members. The work, while often accompanied by long hours and risky activities, was small scale (one man and one animal, and one woman and one loom). Opportunities for injury and death related to work certainly existed, but most people in agrarian societies died of infectious diseases, poor nutrition, poor sanitation, or war. The Industrial Revolution, starting in the mid-1700s, brought with it an increase in work-related accidents and illnesses. Mechanization and mass production were accelerated by the advent of the steam engine, and people were drawn or enticed off the farms to the new production facilities in small towns or villages, increasing the concentration of workers near these facilities. Machines were built for production and not with the safety of workers in mind. During this time women were increasingly working outside their homes: In fact, women and children were highly desirable, cheap sources of labor and often exploited labor as was the case in the early textile mills.

Work-related injuries reached an all-time high in the late 1800s and early 1900s, which led to investigation into the challenges faced by employed women (Achievements in Public Health, 1900–1999). This ultimately resulted in some protective legislation, restricting women from some forms of work. However, women continued to enter the workforce, and with the production needs associated with World Wars I and II, women were increasingly engaged in hazardous work. The U.S. Army sponsored a comprehensive investigation of the occupational health problems of women, "Women in Industry" (Baetjer, 1946). Dr. Anna Baetjer warned of the reproductive effects for pregnant women of benzene, carbon monoxide, carbon disulfide, lead, mercury, and radiation. After World War II, many women experienced social pressure to leave the workforce; however, by 2015 about 57% of American women were reported to be in the workforce (www.dol.gov/wb/stats/stats-data.htm). Employment is no longer restricted by gender; women find themselves in all workplaces, and many of them are doing hazardous work.

Occupational or workplace health and safety are often placed within a public health framework. Care providers often find the assessment and treatment of work-related injuries similar to the care and treatment of non-work-related illnesses and injuries. Care of a severed finger or broken arm is the same regardless of the precipitating event. However, understanding the population-based model of occupational health as it fits into an overall context of health can assist the care provider in anticipating and preventing similar injuries or illnesses in other members of the community, understand the interaction between workplace exposures and health in general, and help return the patient to an optimal state of wellness. An ecologic or population health model takes a broader perspective and examines the relationship between the biologic characteristics of individuals and their interactions with their peer groups, families, communities, schools, and workplaces, as well as the broad economic, cultural, social, and physical environmental conditions at all levels. An ecological model emphasizes the importance of the social and physical environments that strongly shape patterns of disease and injury, as well as the responses to them over the entire life cycle, providing a broader conceptualization of well-being and not merely the absence of disease (Fielding, Teutsch, & Lester, 2010)

Within the public health framework are the concepts of primary, secondary, and tertiary prevention. Primary prevention seeks to reduce the incidence of disease by altering risk factors or improving resistance through efforts to alter individual or collective behaviors or eliminating or mitigating exposures. Some examples are smoking-cessation programs, drinking-water treatment, or installation of machine guards on saws or punch presses. Secondary prevention includes procedures for the early detection of diseases or early treatment of preclinical forms of diseases to reduce or control disease progression. Examples include mammograms to detect early stage breast cancer, blood lead testing, and surveillance of battery reclamation workers to prevent lead-related disease and symptoms. Tertiary prevention seeks to reduce the impact of diseases or injuries on patient function and well-being; examples here might include quality disability management and return-to-work programs. Providing health care to people who work (about 60% of the American population participate in the labor force) requires incorporating these principles into care strategies and integrating them into workplace health and safety programs.

■ WORKPLACE HAZARDS

When considering health hazards, and hazards to women in particular, one must consider the various types of employment and the hazards related to the activities and tasks in those jobs. Preventing workplace injuries and illness requires anticipation of the possible hazards present, recognition and evaluation of exposures and risks identified, and development of ways to correct or control identified hazards. Anticipation and recognition of hazards is a disciplined analysis of the production facility and activities that includes understanding the production processes, raw materials used, and possible by-products produced. Workplace exposures are typically categorized into chemical, physical, biological, musculoskeletal, and psychosocial.

Chemical Hazards

The use of both natural and synthetic chemicals is pervasive in current manufacturing and commerce; most workers are highly likely to be exposed to some chemical compounds in the course of their employment. The American Chemical Society has more than 100 million unique chemcial substances registered in the Chemical Abstracts Service (CAS) Registry™, of which tens of thousands are in commercial use. The Government Accountability Office (GAO) reports that 1,500 new chemicals are developed each year, though most do not find their way to mainstream use (GAO, 2007). Many new and even existing chemicals have not been fully tested for a range of adverse health outcomes because of the limitations inherent in the U.S. chemical regulatory policy (GAO, 2007; Stephenson, 2009). Although the Environmental Protection Agency is responsible for enforcing the regulations for chemical development under the Toxic Substance Control Act (15 USC (C. 53) 2601–2692) and for protecting the environment and the public from untoward chemical exposures, the U.S. Department of Labor, via the Occupational Safety and Health Administration (OSHA), oversees the use of 450 chemicals in the workplace.

Chemicals in the workplace may be found in a variety of forms: dust (formed from mechanical action), smoke (formed from combustion), fumes (formed from volatilizing metal), mists (water droplets), vapors (evaporate of liquid), gases (particles without defined shape or volume), aerosols (atomized particulate), and liquids. Adverse health effects can occur with acute or chronic exposures to chemicals and can affect any or all body systems (dermal, cardiovascular, neurological, and bone) depending on the composition and molecular makeup of the chemical. Some common chemicals found in the workplace are listed in Table 17.1.

Adverse health effects in response to exposures to chemicals depend on an interaction between the intrinsic toxicity of the chemical, the amount of substance actually delivered (the "dose"), the exposure conditions, and the physiological response of the recipient. The concept of dose is particularly useful when considering the interaction between exposure and the worker. For example, a small person has a higher respiratory rate than a larger person; consequently, they will receive a greater dose with the same exposure. The route of exposure, whether by inhalation, ingestion, or skin contact, will also influence the potential for adverse effects. Some chemicals may be more, or less, biologically available depending on the route of exposure (e.g., asbestos inhaled vs. applied to the skin).

In the workplace, attention is paid primarily to the acute effects of exposure to a single chemical, such as headache, respiratory irritation, or skin rashes, or to the effects of very high concentrations that might lead to loss of consciousness or loss of life. Less attention is paid to health effects related to low-level exposures, exposures to mixtures, or subacute or chronic effects on neurological or reproductive systems. Cancer has been a concern for long-term outcomes in that a growing number of chemicals have been identified as carcinogenic. The International Agency for Research on Cancer (IARC) lists 117 agents known to be carcinogenic to humans and another 361 compounds that are probably or possibly carcinogenic to humans (IARC, 2015). Of additional concern are chemicals that are cocarcinogenic in that the risk of cancer is increased by the interaction between two chemicals, one or both of which may be found in the workplace. An example of this is the greatly increased risk of lung cancer in asbestos-exposed workers who also smoke cigarettes as opposed to asbestos workers who do not smoke. Diet, medications, air pollution, and non-work-related chemicals or activities may also substantially affect the risk of cancer or other adverse health outcomes produced by chemicals found in the workplace.

One example of the interactive effect of workplace and nonworkplace exposures is seen with lead exposures, which occur in occupations such as construction, battery reclamation, and recycling, but also in hobbies such as stain glass construction and shooting activities at firing ranges. Although the Occupational Safety and Health Act (OSHA) workplace allowable limit is of 50 mcg/m³ 8-hour time-weighted average (TWA), there are no regulatory guidelines for limiting exposures for nonwork activities. Women may be uniquely at risk for the effects of lead exposures. The allowable workplace exposure limit does not take into account small-stature workers, pertinent to some women; consequently, these workers may be subjected to a higher dose relative to the same exposure. Furthermore, lead substitutes for calcium in the body and thus accumulates in the

TABLE 17.1	Health Effects of Common Occupational Chemicals		
CHEMICAL	**HEALTH HAZARDS**		**OCCUPATIONS**
	Short Term	**Long Term**	
Asbestos	Respiratory system irritation	Mesothelioma, cancer of lung and pleura, chronic respiratory disease, asbestosis	Shipyard workers, beauticians, textile workers
Anesthetic gases Cycloproprane Divinyl ether Ethyl ether Trichloroethylene Ethyl chloride Vinyl ether Halothane	Reflex depression, cardiovascular depression, respiratory depression, gastrointestinal depression, spontaneous abortions	Hepatoxicity, birth defects	Operating room personnel, day surgery personnel, dental and medical assistants, veterinary personnel, laboratory workers
Acids and alkalis Hydrochloric acid Nitric acid Sulfuric acid Sodium hydroxide Hydrofluoric acid Bleachs	Nose and upper respiratory tract irritation, skin irritation, tissue destruction in large doses	Allergies and sensitization	Laboratory workers, chemical workers, laundry personnel, housekeepers
Beryllium	Respiratory irritation	Sensitiation particularly for genetically suseptible individuals, cancer	Manufacturing of electronics, consumer products, aerospace, defense industry products; some demolition activities
Bisphenol A (BPA)		Low-dose endocrine disruptor that can mimic estrogen, obesity	Plastic manufacturing, used in can liners and some toys
Halogenated hydrocarbons Trichloroethylene *bis* chloro-methyl ether Vinyl chloride Chloroprene Dichlorobromopropane Perchloroethylene (PERC) Carbon tetrachloride Chloroform Polyhalogenated biphenyls (PBBs, PCBs)	Hepatotoxicity, headache, fatigue, nausea and vomiting, dizziness, narcosis, mucous membrane irritation	Liver necrosis, cancer of lung, liver, and skin	Laundry and dry-cleaning personnel, clerical workers, textile finishers, plastics manufacturers, beauticians, cosmetologists, electrical workers, agricultural workers, housekeeping
Organic solvents Benzene Toluene Xylene Triethanolamine Formaldehyde Dimethylformamide Alcohol Acetone Ethylene dioxide (dioxane) Turpentine	CNS depression, bone marrow suppression, liver toxicity, eye and skin irritation, depressed red and white blood cell count	Leukemia, dermatitis, allergies and sensitization, circulatory failure, respiratory arrest, liver and kidney damage	Fire fighters, rubber workers, laboratory workers, research technicians, textile workers, beauticians, cosmetologists, petroleum manufacturers, dry cleaners and laundry workers, housekeers, histology workers
Pesticides	Irritation of the skin and eyes	Nervous system dysfunction, miscarriage, cancer	Agricultural workers, landscapers, wood products manufacturing, pest control, housekeepers

(continued)

TABLE 17.1	Health Effects of Common Occupational Chemicals (*continued*)		
CHEMICAL	HEALTH HAZARDS		OCCUPATIONS
	Short Term	Long Term	
Phthalates	Low-dose endocrine disruptor that can mimic estrogen, obesity	Breast cancer, liver damage	Plastic manufacturing, cosmotologists
Silica	Respiratory or dermal irritation	Silicosis, bronchitis, cancer	Construction, grinding or breaking concrete, stone countertop production
Trace elements Lead Cadmium Mercury Arsenic	Acute respiratory effects, bronchitis, coughing, chest pain, porphyrinuria	Neurological dysfunction, brain damage, cancer, liver and kidney damage, tremor, erethism	Chemical and pesticide workers, battery plant workers, dentists and dental assistants, welders, agricultural workers, paint manufactures, electric workers, seed dressers, firing ranges

CNS, central nervous system.

bone. The lead can mobilize out of the bone during pregnancy potentially affecting the developing fetus. In addition, lead can be tracked home from the workplace if workers do not leave contaminated clothes at work, thus contaminating the home and potentially exposing others in the household. Children are particularly vulnerable to lead exposure in that they can absorb up to 50% of ingested lead, whereas adults absorb less. Workplaces using lead should ensure that they are compliant with the OSHA lead standard (www .osha.gov/SLTC/lead/standards.html).

Physical Hazards

Physical hazards are factors that may cause harm without direct contact with the worker. The most common physical hazards found in the workplace include noise, temperature extremes, ionizing and nonionizing radiation, and vibration.

NOISE

Noise is unwanted sound. Exposure to high sound levels can be stressful and contributes to noise-induced hearing loss. Noise triggers physiological changes in the endocrine, cardiovascular, and auditory systems and interferes with a worker's ability to concentrate and adequately communicate with coworkers. Health and economic impacts of high levels of environmental or community noise have been well documented (Getzner & Zak, 2012).

The pituitary–adrenal axis has a very low threshold for stimulation by noise, estimated to be as low as 68 dB. Activation of the pituitary–adrenal axis leads to increased secretion of adrenocorticotropic hormone (ACTH) and subsequent increase in adrenocortical activity. Thus noise can be considered a nonspecific stimulus capable of inducing ACTH release.

Noise also appears to stimulate the adrenal medulla, resulting in increased urinary excretion of epinephrine and norepinephrine. The cardiovascular response to noise includes peripheral vasoconstriction. It is believed that vasoconstriction in the spiral vessels supplying the organ of Corti is the change probably responsible for noise-induced hearing loss

in humans. Noise exposure in the presence of some chemicals and metals may increase the potential for hearing loss. In addition, animal studies demonstrate that exposure to noise produces decreased placental blood flow, increased incidence of abnormalities in fetal development, and smaller litters.

Noise is measured in decibels (dB) and is typically reported as dBA. OSHA regulates noise levels in the workplace and requires regular measurements of noise levels using specially calibrated instruments. According to OSHA requirements, workers may be exposed to average noise levels of up to 90dBA for no more than 8 hours; however, workers must be enrolled in a hearing conservation program when their 8-hour average noise exposure is at or above 85dBA. Noise levels for typical industrial and community activities include 100 dBA, jet engine at 1,000 feet; 90 dBA, power lawn mower; 80 dBA, garbage disposal; and 60 dBA, normal conversation at about 3 feet.

An initial assessment for noise-induced hearing loss includes an occupational history of exposure to high sound levels, symptom reporting (inability to hear normal conversation at about 3 feet, tinnitus after leaving a noisy environment), and the use of a screening audiogram (Rabinowitz, 2000). Audiograms of work-related hearing loss often indicate as much as a 30-dB loss in speech frequencies, usually around 4,000 Hz. Work-related hearing loss may be temporary, resulting in a "temporary threshold shift" with workers recovering their hearing perception after a period of time away from noisy environments, or it may be permanent, resulting in a "permanent threshold shift." Permanent hearing loss resulting from documented workplace exposures may be compensated through state Workers' Compensation programs.

HEAT

Exposure to hot environments reduces work efficiency and productivity and can be life threatening. With increasing ambient temperatures related to climate change, heat exposure is of particular concern for women living or working in buildings without climate control or who are working outdoors (e.g., agricultural workers). High humidity slows the evaporation process, increasing the potential stress on the body. In addition to agricultural workers, other occupations at risk for heat exposure include laundry and construction workers, fire fighters, hazardous waste workers, and highway flaggers.

Physical exertion decreases the tolerance for heat and interferes with the body's ability to dissipate heat, particularly if evaporation is impeded or slowed. Workers not accustomed to heat exposure may experience compensatory vasoconstriction to the kidney, liver, and digestive organs as the cutaneous vessels dilate. Persons not acclimatized to heat may not perspire efficiently, thus limiting the amount of effective heat dissipation. Underlying chronic health conditions, such as diabetes or cardiovascular disease, and advanced age reduce the body's ability to compensate for exposure to hot environments.

Workers exposed to hot environment can acclimate over a period of a few weeks. Over time, the cutaneous blood vessels are better able to dilate and dissipate body heat; however, unusual and acute spikes in ambient temperature may cause heat stress in even the most acclimated worker. During the acclimatization period, workers should avoid continuous and strenuous work, take frequent rest breaks in a shady area, and stay hydrated (cool drink every 15–20 minutes). Salt supplements are not usually recommended or needed. If the worker is required to wear occlusive clothing (e.g., hazardous waste workers), additional rest breaks and longer acclimatization periods may be needed (www.cdc.gov/niosh/topics/heatstress). The wider variations in ambient temperature that are predicted with progressing climate change will challenge care providers and policy makers to rethink control strategies needed to protect workers in hot environments (Spector & Sheffield, 2014).

IONIZING RADIATION

The principle hazard from ionizing radiation (ultraviolet light, x-rays, gamma rays, or alpha or beta particles) is its ability to pass through biological tissue and excite atoms, changing them to electrically charged ions and damaging DNA. The health effect varies with the type of radiation and the dose received and may range from no noticeable change in organ function to genetic damage or cancer. The health effects associated with radiation exposure have been modeled primarily on a 70-kg male. Exposures to and protection of women should take into account the unique vulnerability of their reproductive role.

Women can be exposed to ionizing radiation in occupations such as dentistry, x-ray technology, radiology, nuclear medicine, quality control in metal industries, nuclear power, or some laboratory or research work. A common form of environmental exposure to radiation is radon gas, found in a variety of geographical areas of the United States and elsewhere. Radon comes from the breakdown of naturally occurring uranium in rocks and soil and can become airborne. Radon has been linked to high rates of lung cancer (www.epa.gov/radon/health-risk-radon).

Symptoms of acute high-dose exposure to ionizing radiation range from burns to "radiation sickness," which is characterized by loss of hair, sore throat, diarrhea, rash, and damage to rapidly proliferating tissues, such as bone marrow. Such an exposure would be expected only in the event of an accidental exposure or ingestion of isotopes of high specific radioactivity. Radiation exposure effects are cumulative with regards to changes in biological tissues, and risk of adverse outcomes increases with continued exposure.

A more insidious form of occupational radiation poisoning comes from long-term exposure to low-level radiation sources or to exposures when proper protective measures are not used. Animal studies suggest that exposure for long periods may produce subcellular tissue damage that can lead to a variety of adverse health outcomes, including cataracts and cancer.

Federal regulations (29CFR 1910:1096) established maximum allowable radiation exposure levels, levels at which no further exposure is permitted until a designated time has elapsed. Protection from the adverse health effects of ionizing radiation includes the use of proper shielding (lead for x-ray or gamma radiation and protective clothing for other forms of radiation such as alpha particles). Persons working in areas where there is a source of radiation should wear personal radiation-monitoring devices for cumulative exposure assessment, and all radioactive chemicals should be appropriately labeled and properly stored and disposed of.

NONIONIZING RADIATION

Nonionizing radiation (also known as *electromagnetic frequency [EMF] radiation*) refers to radiation with enough energy to cause molecules to vibrate but not enough to remove electrons or ionize biological tissue. Electrical fields are characterized by an electrical charge and are easily shielded, whereas moving electrical charges create magnetic fields and are difficult to shield. Common forms of nonionizing radiation include lasers (light amplification by stimulated emission of radiation), ultraviolet light, radio frequency or microwaves, infrared light, and visible light. Common sources of ultraviolet light, the type of nonionizing radiation that presents the greatest health concern, include sunlight, welding, mercury vapor lamps, tanning booths, and black lights. Ultraviolet light does not penetrate deeply, so the eyes and skin are the primary organs of concern related to exposure. Chronic overexposure may lead to cataract and skin cancer. Ultraviolet light is listed as a Group 1 human carcinogen by the IARC. Some nonspecific, vague, and poorly documented symptoms may be related to nonionizing radiation exposure and include increased fatigue, dizziness, headaches, and changes in sensitivity to light and sound.

Occupations or work activities with possible exposure to nonionizing radiation include welders, telecommunication, electricians, glass and steel making, surgical and other lasers, heat lamps, high-voltage power lines, and a wide range of electrical equipment. Exposures can be prevented or mitigated by increasing the distance from the source, as well as using protective glasses, face shields, or goggles and protective clothing. The American Conference of Governmental Industrial Hygienists (ACGIH) has published a consensus standard providing exposure limit guidance to reduce adverse health effects. OSHA and other regulatory agencies have also published permissible exposure limits (PELs) and other guidance for nonionizing radiation and lasers in particular.

Biological Hazards

Work with and around microorganisms, mold allergens, or plant and animal poisons places workers at risk of exposure to potentially harmful infectious agents and associated diseases. Health care and laboratory workers are the primary at-risk professionals; however, workers in public utilities, heating and air conditioning ventilation systems, tattoo parlors, swimming pools, and life guards at public beaches may be at risk as well (Halliday & Gast, 2011).

Musculoskeletal Hazards

Tool design, work station design, and posture requirements for certain jobs frequently require sitting or standing for long periods of time; lifting, pushing or pulling heavy loads; performing highly repetitive movements; or being in awkward postures. These activities can lead to muscloskeletal injuries. Work-related musculoskeletal injuries (injuries that affect bodily movement) account for more than one third of workplace injuries (www.bls.gov/news.release/archives/osh2_11082012.pdf) and the majority of Workers' Compensation claims and time loss. Ergonomic (fitting the work to the worker) programs and interventions such as sit–stand work stations, adjustable table heights, lifting aids, and redesigned production methods and tools can reduce or eliminate musculoskeletal injuries.

Carpal tunnel syndrome is a common musculoskeletal condition that is frequently reported by working women. It presents with pain, tingling, and numbness in the hand along the distribution of the median nerve and is caused by the compression of the nerve in the wrist. Pregnancy, diabetes, and obesity, as well as workplace exposures such as highly repetitive movements, high force, vibration, and awkward postures, may be related to the symptoms. Reducing repetitive movements and using ergonomic supports can prevent carpal tunnel syndrome. Surgery is often proposed as a treatment strategy, but some have found that a long-term benefit from surgical interventions may not be forthcoming (www.lni.wa.gov/ClaimsIns/Files/OMD/MedTreat/CarpalTunnel.pdf).

Effort to regulate hazards related to musculoskeletal injuries was truncated by the U.S. Congress in 2001. OSHA can still issue citations for egregious musculoskeletal hazards under the General Duty Clause (Section 5(a)(1) of the Act; USC Title 29). Because of the medical and retraining costs and effects on productivity of musculoskeletal injuries, many companies voluntarily institute ergonomic programs and provide ergonomic work stations, tools, and training for their workers to prevent musculoskeletal injuries.

Psychosocial Hazards

Workplace stress is probably the major psychosocial hazard faced by American workers. *Work-related stress* can be defined as harmful physical or emotional responses that occur when the requirements of the job do not match the capabilities or resources of the worker. Stress is not all together undesirable; in fact, some stress helps motivate and focus the learning necessary to master new skills and to be productive. Individual coping skills may moderate or accentuate the effects of stressful situation. Some working conditions are considered stressful for nearly all personality types and coping skills, such as:

Task design—heavy workloads with infrequent breaks, long hours, irregular shift work, feeling of lack of control over the work pace

Management and organization—poor communication of organizational culture or goals, poor relationship with supervisor or coworkers, lack of support from coworkers, tight production schedules, inadequate resources, lack of opportunity for growth or advancement

Job expectations—too many responsibilities with too little control, role ambiguity, implementation to new technology or production methods without sufficient training, job insecurity

Work environmental conditions—dangerous or hazardous conditions without control strategies or methods or training to protect oneself, excessive noise, poor housekeeping, poor workstation design, lack of adequate ventilation or light

Most workers can adapt to short-term stresses but may have difficulty compensating for chronic or unresolved stress. Stressful conditions that continue unabated can increase physiological and psychological wear on biological systems and lead to disturbances in sleep patterns, headaches, difficulty in problem solving and maintenance of relationships, and increased risk of injury or illness. There is some suggestion that stressful working conditions interfere with safe work practices and may contribute to absenteeism, tardiness, and staff turnover.

Addressing workplace stress is best done with a two-pronged approach, including organizational change and stress management. To the degree possible, organizational change should be investigated. This might include working with management to adjust workloads, review or modify job expectations, provide adequate training, and improve environmental conditions. Because changing the nature of the work, the organization, or the production process may not be possible, stress-management programs should be instituted. Stress-manangement programs might include education on multiple sources of stress, time-management skills, relaxation exercises, or other personal skills to reduce stress.

Reproductive Hazards

Many women employed in the U.S. workforce are in their childbearing years. According to the Bureau of Labor Statistics (BLS), in 2014, the median age of employed women in the United States was 42 years (www.bls.gov/emp/ep_table_306.htm). In general, healthy women with a normal pregnancy and fetus can work throughout their pregnancy. The fetus is, however, highly vulnerable to exposures that may occur in the mother's workplace, particularly during the first trimester (Selevan, Kimmel, & Mendola, 2000). All parents should be equally watchful for exposures to compounds that can be carried home on clothing or skin, thereby exposing other family members, particularly children, and the home environment. In addition, women should be aware that some compounds, such as lead and some pesticides, can bioaccumulate before pregnancy and affect the developing fetus during gestation. Work-related exposures can precipitate adverse reproductive outcomes in both men and women, including pesticides and environmentally persistent compounds (Kumar, 2004). Companies are prohibited from excluding women from hazardous exposure jobs under Title VII of the 1964 Civil Rights Act. With regard to mitigating exposures to reproductive hazards, the focus should be on making jobs safe for all workers, including women of reproductive age, and on increasing awareness among women and their employers regarding exposures that may affect reproduction and offspring.

Materials that can affect reproduction have several mechanisms of action, including mutagenesis, teratogenesis, and epigenetic transmission. Each is discussed in the following sections.

MUTAGENESIS

Mutagenesis is the process that occurs when chemicals, radiation, or biological agents interact with living cells to cause a change in the genetic material of that cell. The genetic change is called *mutation,* and the substance producing the change, a *mutagen.* Most mutations are harmful and often result in the death of the individual cell. However, mutations may also cause abnormal cell division, which can result in cancer or altered cell function. If a mutation occurs in a germ cell (sperm or egg) before conception, it may be incompatible with life, resulting in infertility of the parent or death of the fetus. Alternatively, mutations in the offspring may also occur, manifesting as congenital defects. It is not known to what extent the rate of mutations is in human cells and to what degree those mutations are increased or influenced by occupational or environmental exposures. It has been suggested that approximately 25% of diseases in the U.S. population have some genetic origin, and up to 30% of spontaneous abortions are found to involve chromosomal aberrations, some of which may be caused by exogenous exposures (Selevan, Lindbohm, Hornung, & Hemminki, 1985; Weselak, Arbuckle, Walker, & Krewski, 2008).

TERATOGENESIS

Teratogenesis is the process that occurs when exposures alter fetal development during gestation to cause fetal death or abnormalities such as cleft lip. Exposures to the fetus generally occur from the mother's blood by way of the placenta, although direct exposures, such as radiation, may also occur. The developing fetus is uniquely sensitive to some chemicals that may not be harmful to the mother. The first trimester (up to 60 days after conception) is thought to be the period of greatest susceptibility to teratogenic insult, although teratogens may affect the fetus to various degrees throughout gestation. There is growing concern that even low-level exposures to the mother can result in fetal anomalies. For example, phthalate exposure may result in male offspring with undescended testacies

or hypospadias. Subtle or dramatic damage to the fetus can also occur with prenatal exposure to a variety of compounds such as thalidomide, some antibiotics, alcohol, lead, and mercury.

EPIGENESIS

Epigenetics is the process by which environmental or external factors regulate the timing, duration, and/or intensity of gene expression. In turn, gene expression may cause variations in phenotypic traits. Some epigenetic changes can be inherited across generations without changing the underlying DNA. External factors are naturally occurring, whereas other factors may be related to lifestyle or various diseases. Recent research suggests that there may be a relationship between epigenetic changes and various health outcomes, such as cancers, immune disorders, and neuropsychiatric disorders. For example, prenatal and early postnatal environmental factors influence the adult risk of developing various chronic diseases and behavioral disorders (Jirtle & Skinner, 2007).

Hazards in Health Care

Health care occupations deserve special mention because they are often heavily populated with women and are notable for the particular hazards associated with this work. Health care workers have a high rate of musculoskeletal injury from patient handling and are at risk for exposures to bloodborne diseases from needlesticks and general exposure to bodily fluids. In addition, they have hazards related to exposure to hazardous drugs, radiation, shift work, and workplace violence.

MUSCULOSKELETAL EXPOSURES IN HEALTH CARE

The health care professions, particularly nurses and other professionals providing direct patient care, have always been at risk for musculoskeletal injury associated with patient handling. With the increasing number of older, sicker, and heavier patients, the risk to these caregivers is even greater.

A study by the Safety and Health Assessment and Research for Prevention program in the Washington State Department of Labor and Industries found that the health care sector had a rate 3.9 times greater for injury than all other industry sectors combined, and nursing staff had the highest back and shoulder injury rates of any occupational group in the state (Silverstein, Howard, Lee, & Goggins, 2006). The medical and time-loss costs to the Workers' Compensation program was considerable, which does not include costs incurred by the employer for turnover and retraining or possible injuries to patients.

In response to this crisis, then-governor Christine Gregoire signed into law the Safe Patient Handling legislation (RCW 70.41.390). This law requires hospitals to implement a safe patient handling program, establish a safe patient handling committee, and purchase lifting aids. Silverstein and others have shown that lifting aids reduce compensable musculoskeletal injury claims in this work group (Evanoff, Wolf, Aton, Canos, & Collins, 2003; Silverstein & Schurke, 2012).

MICROBIOLOGICAL EXPOSURES IN HEALTH CARE

Health care workers are at particular risk of exposure to a variety infectious agents through contact with patient secretions, wounds, excretions, contaminated linens, food trays, and needles. Health effects associated with exposure are wide ranging and can include death. Most health care institutions have well-developed infection-control programs that should include handling of infectious materials. Since 1991, OSHA has enforced the Bloodborne Pathogens Standard (29 CFR 1910.1030), which focuses on hepatitis B and C, HIV, and other potentially infectious materials. In 2000, this law was amended with the Needlestick Safety and Prevention Act to require better needlestick prevention efforts. Together, they require a written exposure control plan, universal precautions, engineering and work practice controls, personal protective equipment (PPE), housekeeping, vaccinations, postexposure follow-up, hazard communication and training, labeling, and recordkeeping. Regular and effective handwashing continues to be one of the primary ways to limit cross-contamination and prevent communicable diseases in health care workers.

With increased and more rapid travel across the globe and changes in vector ranges because of climate change, one can anticipate that health care workers will see more and more varied infectious agents in their patient population (Mills, Gage, & Khan, 2010; Ogden et al., 2006). Global mobility and climate change together will put these frontline workers at risk for new and unanticipated diseases, such as the emergence of the Zika virus in the United States.

HAZARDOUS DRUGS IN HEALTH CARE

Among the hazards faced by some health care workers is mixing, administering, or disposing of hazardous drugs, such as antineoplastic cytotoxic medications, anesthetics, antiviral drugs, and hormones. Chemotherapeutic drugs in particular have been linked to cancers and other health outcomes in the workers mixing and administering these agents (Smith, 2010). The National Institute for Occupational Health and Safety (NIOSH) has developed a list of hazardous drugs (www.cdc.gov/niosh/topics/hazdrug/)

OSHA does not regulate hazardous drug administration, but Washington State adopted a Hazardous Drug Rule in 2012 to address these issues for worker groups such as pharmacists and pharmacy technicians, nurses, physician assistants, physicians, nursing home and home health care staff, housekeeping and environmental services staff, and shipping and receiving personnel (WAC 296–62-500).

According to the Hazardous Drug Rule, employers need to implement a hazardous drug control program, which includes a written program, hazard assessment, high-risk task identification, preventive methods, and employee training. Controls might include biological safety cabinets, laboratory fume hoods, containment isolators, closed system transfer devices, safer sharps devices, and safety interlocks. For some tasks, workers are required to wear PPE

such as gloves, gowns, booties, head coverings, eye protection, and respirators, depending on the compound and the extent of possible bodily contact. This rule may serve as a model for others as a way to protect these health care workers.

WORKPLACE VIOLENCE IN HEALTH CARE

Workplace violence is a concern for all American workers, but violence in health care settings is surprisingly high and disconcerting because of the vulnerability of the patients and the caregiver's commitment to patient safety and well-being. According to the U.S. BLS, in 2000, 48% of nonfatal injuries from work-related violent acts occurred in the health care sector. In 2012, the rate of violence-related injuries and illness was 15 per 10,000 for health care and social assistance versus 4.0 for private industry overall (BLS, 2013).

There are four categories of workplace violence: Type 1, criminal intent such as robbery; Type 2, customer on worker; Type 3, worker on worker; and Type 4, personal relationships such as domestic violence that is perpetrated in the workplace. Although all types can and do occur in the health care settings, Type 3 worker-on-worker violence in the form of bullying; verbal, psychological, or physical abuse; or sexual harassment has received particular attention from occupational health policy makers and professionals (McPhaul & Lipscomb, 2004).

Workplace bullying is the behavior of individuals or groups that includes repeated aggressive acts against a coworker or subordinate that occurs over 6 months or more (Einarsen, Hoel, Zapf, & Cooper, 2003). Workplace bullying can also involve an abuse or misuse of power; it creates feelings of defenselessness and undermines an individual's right to dignity at work. Bullying has also been linked to adverse health outcomes such as sleep disturbances in the victim (Niedhammer, David, Degioanni, Drummond, & Pierre, 2009).

With a few exceptions (Washington State being an exception with the Safety—Health Care Settings law—RCW 49.19), controlling workplace violence is unregulated. However, both NIOSH (www.cdc.gov/niosh/topics/violence/links.html) and OSHA (www.osha.gov/SLTC/etools/hospital/hazards/workplaceviolence/viol.html) publish guidelines to help businesses and health care institutions address and mitigate workplace violence. Universal recommendations note that acknowledging the personal and organizational cost of workplace violence and developing a violence-prevention plan are the first steps toward addressing this problem. A violence-prevention program should include the following elements: evidence of top management commitment in the form of a written statement and resource allocation; employee involvement in violence-prevention committees and follow-up on any actual incidents; worksite analysis, including review of all reports of assaults on employees, strategies for encouraging reporting of incidents, and job hazard analysis to identify high-risk situations or activities; hazard prevention, including adequate staffing, lighting, controlled access to secluded work areas, and alarm systems; and education and training of all personnel to help identify risk factors and control measures. Others continue to work on best practices for providing safe and rewarding workplaces (Lucian Leape Institute, 2013).

Sexual harassment as a form of workplace violence is an unfortunate and all too frequent reality in many workplaces and can be stressful and affect mental and physical health. Although women are often the victim of sexual harassment, men are not immune. Sexual harassment can come in the form of implying job secuity or benefits in return for sexual favors or in the form of a hostile work environment where unwelcome sexual verbal comments, visual images, or psycological harassment is tolerated.

Sexual harassment is a violation of the 1964 Civil Rights Act, which was expanded in 1991 to include gender bias and harassment against both men and women, and includes same-sex harassment. Recommended control strategies are to clearly say "no," document events, and report them to superiors.

SHIFT WORK AND EXTENDED SHIFTS IN HEALTH CARE

Shift work and extended work hours (beyond 8 hr/d) is an integral and accepted practice in the health care industry. Up to 30% of health care workers are engaged in some degree of night shift work. Not only is the health care industry dependent on workers willing to work nonstandard shifts, but globalization has pushed numerous other industries to a 24-hour work cycle, with more employees working nights and rotating shifts.

Shift work and extended hours have been related to increased injury and illness rates, weight gain, fatigue, lower congnitive function, and increased fatality rates (Caruso, Hitchcock, Dick, Russo, & Schmit, 2004). Shift work, particularly night shift, can lead to excessive sleepiness, insomnia, disrupted sleep schedules, depression, irritability, and poor performance. Night shift work may also be related to cancer outcomes (Kolstad, 2008). Not surprisingly, shift work can contribute to challenged personal relationships and difficulty meeting family responsibilities (Rogers, 2008). Strategies for addressing some of the effects of shift work include staying active and consuming caffeinated beverages during waking hours but avoiding them just before sleeping. Sleeping in a dark and quiet environment is advised, as is considering using eye shades and ear plugs. Research suggests that short naps at work when working night shift is an effective strategy for sustaining vigilance, learning, and memory (McDonald et al., 2013).

■ ADDRESSING WORK-RELATED ADVERSE HEALTH OUTCOMES

Occupational Health History

An occupational health history is an invaluable tool for understanding workers' symptoms and designing effective treatment plans. An occupational health history is a chronological list of all the worker's employment with more detail collected to identify occupational exposure to potentially hazardous agents and related health effects. Because work-related illness can present with common symptoms, an occupational health history can help determine whether or not work is a cause or aggravation of adverse health conditions. It helps link health problems to specific workplace exposures or hazards. Also, it can help determine whether or not the patient has the capacity to work and whether or not short- or long-term restrictions are necessary when returning to job tasks.

Assessment forms can be developed for workers/patients to list current and previous jobs or work activities, but more specific information regarding exposures may need to be elicited by interviewing the worker/patient. Some questions to include in developing a structure interview or occupational health history guide include, but are not limited to, those included in Box 17.1.

These questions should be explored for the current and any previous jobs, (including part time or temporary jobs). In addition, the interview should include questions about second or third jobs, hobbies, military service exposures, and work overseas. For an example of an occupational health history form, see Appendix G "Taking an Exposure History" in *Nursing, Health, & the Environment: Strengthening the Relationship to Improve the Public's Health* (Pope, Snyder, & Mood, 1995).

Interpreting the information gleaned from an occupational health history interview may require consultation with occupational health professionals who can assist with selected follow-up questions to better understand workplace

---

BOX 17.1 OCCUPATIONAL HEALTH ASSESSMENT QUESTIONS

What do you do for a living (include the name and address of employer)?

Are you currently employed?

Do you work full time or part time?

In what year and month did you start?

How long is your working day?

Do you work different shifts, and, if so, what is the shift rotation?

What kind of things do you do in a typical working day?

What materials do you work with?

Do you have exposures to chemicals, dust, loud noises, vibration, radiation, biological hazards, or workplace stress?

Are any exposures controlled with ventilation or other controls?

Do you wear special protective clothing?

Do you have any special medical tests because of your work?

If you have health problems, are they better when you are not at work (e.g., on the weekend)?

Does anyone at work have the same health problems?

processes and materials and possible links between exposures and health outcomes. Screening or ongoing surveillance may be required for some exposures covered by OSHA regulations and standards, such as for working with lead or cadmium. Workers with work-related injuries are entitled to Workers' Compensation benefits for medical care, possibly time-loss payments, and/or a disability pension. Application for Workers' Compensation benefits often requires the health care provider to complete necessary forms and refer the patient to the relevant state agency or insurance carrier.

Workers' Compensation

Caring for working populations, particularly injured workers, necessitates a basic understanding of Workers' Compensation programs in the United States. Workers' Compensation is a form of insurance that provides medical benefits, time-loss wage replacement, and disability pension to employees injured in the course of employment. In the event of a fatality, Workers' Compensation programs pay benefits to the immediate family. Workers' Compensation is administered on a state-by-state basis, with a governing board overseeing varying public–private combinations of compensation systems. The benefit award amounts vary widely across the states. Every state except Texas requires employers to carry some form of Workers' Compensation insurance. The Workers' Compensation insurance scheme was the result of the "grand bargain" negotiated between workers and employers over several decades in the United States. In exchange for medical care and time-loss wage replacement in the event of an injury, workers are required to relinquish their right to sue their employer for negligence or for general damages of pain and suffering.

The history of the development of Workers' Compensation is illustrative and helpful in understanding the underpinning of the current systems. There is evidence of "state" compensation for injured workers since ancient times. The laws of the King of Ur-Nammu of ancient Sumeria (2050 BCE) provided compensation for specific work-related injuries. During the feudal Middle Ages, the doctrine of noblesse oblige and the benevolence of the lord of the manor determined whether or not a work-related injury was compensated. The Industrial Revolution brought a gradual change in the relationship between employer (lord of the manor) and workers. Under English common law the principles of contributory negligence (injured worker was some way responsible for the injury), fellow servant (a coworker was in some way responsible for the injury), and assumption of risk (the injured worker knew they were engaged in dangerous or hazardous work) were often used by employers to avoid payment of any compensation to injured workers. Because of the restrictive nature of these legal principles and the lack of preventive measures, injured workers increasingly and successfully sued their employers for negligence.

In the mid- to late 1800s, European countries and the United States were experiencing greater worker unrest over working conditions in the newly industrialized economies. The Prussian chancellor, Otto von Bismarck, facing increasing fatalities from industrialization and increased pressure from left-wing political parties, instituted the Employers' Liability Law of 1871 (social protections for miners and some factory workers) and in 1884 Workers' Accident Insurance (the first modern Workers' Compensation system). The program provided benefits for work-related injuries, including medical care and rehabilitation, and instituted the no-fault (exclusive remedy) system limiting workers' ability to sue. It served as a model for later British and U.S. law.

The U.S. Congress, in response to public pressure and business concerns regarding financial uncertainty and expense of defending lawsuits from injured workers, considered European-style federal Workers' Compensation legislation in the early 1900 but abandoned the effort in lieu of state-level action. Wisconsin was the first state to pass Workers' Compensation legislation in 1911, and Mississippi was the last (1948). The medical community was not particularly supportive of early Workers' Compensation legislation, as reimbursement fees were often regulated.

The current U.S. Workers' Compensation system is a no-fault, state-specific insurance system that is based on Prussian or British models. Employers, with a few exceptions, completely fund the programs by purchasing commercial insurance, setting up a "self-insured" account, or paying into state-managed programs. The goals of the insurance programs are to provide "sure and certain relief" by paying for the financial consequences of treated work-related injuries, compensating the injured for time loss, and paying any temporary or permanent disability benefit that is incurred. Some states allow employers to optionally carry insurance; however, the majority of American businesses carry some form of Workers' Compensation insurance. Notably, some groups (e.g., agriculture, some domestic workers, longshore workers, and railroad workers) are not covered by state Workers' Compensation programs. Some are not covered at all, and others are covered under separate and specific federal compensation programs (Federal Employers Liability Act of 1906; Longshore and Harbor Workers' Compensation Act of 1927).

The definition of *work-related injury* or *illness*, the extent of compensation, the benefit rates, administrative rules and practices, the terms for disability pensions, and caregiver reimbursement schedules are highly variable across the United States and often the source of continued political tension between business and labor groups. Some states permit workers to select their own caregivers, whereas others allow employers to manage care either through "third-party administrators" (TPAs) or through employer-selected caregivers. In addition, the difference between "impairment" (the degree of loss of anatomy or function of a body part or system) and "disability" (degree of impaired ability to perform required work) can be contentious and confusing. The interaction between state Workers' Compensation systems and the Americans with Disabilities Act (1990) and Patient Protection and Affordable Care Act (2010) relative to comprehensive care for injured workers is still evolving. One of the early hopes of the Workers' Compensation scheme was that it would incentivize employers to work to prevent workplace injuries; however, this goal was imperfectly achieved. It was not until the passage of OSHA in 1970 that meaningful prevention efforts in American workplaces were undertaken.

Guidance for the Care Provider

Care of injured workers triggers interactions with insurance carriers, TPAs, claims adjudicators, case managers, employers, and other health care disciplines. In addition to immediate care of the injury or illness, it is important to try to return the injured worker to work as soon as possible and to avoid long-term disability for the benefit of both the worker and the employer. Interacting with a Workers' Compensation system is as legal as it is clinical; unless care providers are familiar with the rules of the state-specific program, they should consult with occupational and environmental health care specialists to navigate the system for the benefit of the patient and best clinical outcomes.

Understanding some terms of use in Workers' Compensation systems is a helpful first step in managing workplace injury and illness care and when referring patients to occupational health care providers. (See Box 17.2 for a definition of terms used.) The relevant state agency that manages Workers' Compensation should be contacted for specifics.

BOX 17.2 WORKERS' COMPENSATION VOCABULARY

Appeals: Workers' Compensation judgments may be appealed in most states to an administrative law judge or administrative board, where the decision is affirmed, modified, or rescinded.

Apportionment: Usually it is used in permanent disability determinations and assigns benefits according to "how much" of a loss is related to separate sources that may not be work-related or be apportioned to different employers. Causation is not apportioned, and the cost of medical care usually is not apportioned. It can also mean division of liability between an employer and a second injury fund that may pay for the portion of a claim attributable to preexisting conditions.

Causation: Identifying the most probable cause of a worker's condition or disability and demonstrating that it arose out of work. For Workers' Compensation purposes "probable cause" is considered to be "more probable than not." Determining legal causation maybe more complicated than medical causation and is often resolved through court proceedings.

Certifying time loss: The health care provider determines whether or not the injured worker is physically able to perform the work described, and if not, the duration of the worker's time loss is "certified" or assigned by the attending care provider.

Compensable injury: An accidental injury arising out of and in the course of employment requiring medical services or resulting in disability or death.

Disability: Disability is the loss of the ability to perform specific jobs or tasks; it represents how an "impairment" combined with the person's age and educational background, vocational background, and other factors affect an injured workers' ability to return to work.

Functional capacity examination: Evaluating a person's specific physical activities (e.g., lifting, bending, pushing, and pulling) and his or her relationship to the ability to perform the specified demands of the job.

Independent medical examination (IME): A medical examination conducted by a health care provider selected by a Workers' Compensation insurer for the purpose of obtaining an expert opinion of the medical condition and treatment of an injured or ill worker and whether the patient has reached maximum benefit ("fixed and stable"). IMEs are conducted for litigation purposes or for closure of a contested Workers' Compensation claim, rather than to provide care.

Impairment: The loss of function of a body part; sometimes confused with disability.

Impairment rating: Health care provider assigns a numerical rating for the type and extent of bodily function that has been lost.

Indemnity benefit: Payments made to an injured or ill worker in an attempt to compensate the employee for lost wages.

Job analysis: When workers are assigned to modified work or are returning to work with a temporary or permanent disability, a job description including an objective assessment of the physical requirements and characteristics of the position should be (and in some states must be) obtained. The job analysis assists the caregiver in relating the job requirements to the worker's physical capabilities.

Latency: Period between exposure and the onset of some occupational diseases; the latent onset of some occupational diseases (e.g., asbestos-related diseases) makes

(continued)

apportioning benefits and obtaining compensation difficult.

Modified work (light duty): The injured worker may not able to return to his or her previous work but is physically capable of temporarily carrying out work of a lighter nature. Workers should be urged to return to modified work as soon as reasonable, as such work is frequently beneficial for body conditioning, staying connected with the social structure of the workplace, and maintaining self-confidence.

Notice of closure: A document sent by the insurer to the injured worker that closes the claim, ends time-loss benefits, or states the extent of disability.

Permanent disability: A determination of "permanent" disability will not be made until the injured worker is considered to be "medically stable." The benefit level for a permanent disability may be based on a regulatory "schedule" or list of compensable conditions or "unscheduled."

Permanent partial disability (PPD): The permanent loss of use or function of any portion of the body may be assigned if physical ability is impaired, even after treatment is completed and the injured worker can still work. Most jurisdictions use a "schedule" (list of body parts that are covered) to assign benefits. Unscheduled (unlisted) conditions may be assigned benefits based on degree of impairment, loss of earning capacity,

continuation of temporary disability benefits, or a combination.

Permanent total disability (PTD): The loss of use or function of a portion of the body that permanently prevents the worker from regularly performing gainful and suitable work.

Third-party administrator (TPA): TPAs conduct Workers' Compensation claims management for self-insured companies. The TPA is accountable to the employer rather than the injured worker and can influence care and claims acceptance and the relationship between the injured worker and the caregiver.

Temporary partial disability (TPD): The injured worker has an impairment but is able to do some type of limited work for a short period of time, and recovery is expected.

Temporary total disability (TTD): The injured worker is unable to do any type of work for a temporary period of time.

Time-loss payments: Compensation paid to an injured worker who loses work time or wages as a result of compensable injury; the compensation level is state specific, but is usually about two thirds of the average monthly wage in the state.

Source: Definitions were obtained from the Oregon and Washington Workers' Compensation websites www.oregonwcd.org and lni.wa .gov/claimsIns.

Disability Prevention

The goal of tertiary prevention is to prevent disability progression and to reduce residual deficits and dysfunction in workers with established disability. Unfortunately, injured workers with compensation claims are at risk of slipping into long-term disability, particularly if they are in the system for 3 months or more (Cheadle et al., 1994). Some injuries are so catastrophic that full recovery is unlikely; however, it has been noted that clinical outcomes for injured workers tend to be worse than those for nonworkers' compensation patients (Wickizer et al., 2011). Chronic disability accounts for less than 20% of the Workers' Compensation claims, but more than 80% of the costs to the system (Cheadle et al., 1994).

Some states have outlined best practices or treatment guidelines for the care of injured workers in an effort to improve the worker health and outcomes and to reduce chronic disability (www.lni.wa.gov/ClaimsIns/Providers/ TreatingPatients/TreatGuide). Efforts to improve the integration of care with strong communication between the injured worker, health care provider, the workplace, and

the Workers' Compensation agency have been suggested to reduce the risk of long-term disability. Others have worked to understand the early issue or conditions that might predict which injured worker might slide into chronic disability. Pain, previous disability with extended time loss, the role of employers in offering modified work, and the influence of caregivers are predictors of chronic disability (Turner et al., 2008). Careful management of chronic pain is an important aspect of care of the injured worker, particularly since early use of opioids (within the first week of injury) has been found to be predictive of chronic disability at 1 year (Franklin, Stover, Turner, Fulton-Kehoe, & Wickizer, 2008).

Supportive claims management is key to assisting the injured worker in regaining function and returning to employment. This might include developing and maintaining good relationships with both the injured worker and the employer, helping with processing paperwork, scheduling and maintaining care appointments, working with care providers to identify work restrictions, negotiating modified work with employers, and facilitating activity coaching. Activity coaching is a treatment strategy for progressively increasing activity under the direction of a professional therapist. Research suggests that financial incentives for caregivers, coupled with care management support, can improve outcomes, prevent disability, and reduce costs for patients and the Workers' Compensation system (Wickizer et al., 2011).

Caring for injured workers can be complicated, time consuming, and at times frustrating: It requires an in-depth understanding of state-specific Workers' Compensation laws and regulations, as well as clinical best practices and workplace issues, in order to return the injured worker to optimal health and to prevent permanent disability. Clinicians are encouraged to collaborate with occupational and environmental health care specialists when providing care to patients with work-related injuries or illnesses.

Controlling Workplace Hazards

Although treating work-related injuries and illness is the most common opportunity practitioners have to deal with occupational health issues, preventing adverse health outcomes related to exposures at work should be the primary strategy. Primary prevention requires the recognition of workplace hazards with a keen understanding of specific production processes, raw materials used, by-products of the production process, available engineering controls, use of PPE, and relevant regulatory guidelines. The standard strategy for controlling workplace exposures is termed the *hierarchy of controls,* a ranking of interventions by first eliminating hazardous materials or operations, substituting hazardous materials for less hazardous ones, instituting engineering controls such as ventilation systems or machine guarding, and exploring administrative controls such as worker rotation through less hazardous jobs. The last control strategy to consider within the hierarchy of controls paradigm is the use of PPE.

Despite their limitations, the use of PPE (respirators, gloves, and occlusive garments) is a frequent strategy used in the workplace or suggested by care providers. However, the use of PPE is limited by the fact that the hazard is not removed, and in some situations the PPE may not be protective enough or may not be permitted by OSHA regulations and may leave the worker poorly or incompletely protected. For example, the use of an air-purifying respirator with a particulate cartridge to protect a worker from a solvent exposure or in an oxygen-deficient atmosphere would be ineffective and inappropriate. When advising workers on the use of PPE, a full understanding of the nature of the hazard is required. In addition, workers need to be medically able to wear the PPE, the PPE must fit properly, and the worker must be trained on its correct use and maintenance. The use of some PPE, such as respirators, requires the development of a written program by the employer, and workers must be trained on the elements of the written program, including how to put on the respirator, care for it, and select the type of respirator relevant to exposures. For more information on the details of helping workers or companies select proper PPE or training on its use and maintenance, an occupational health and safety professional or the NIOSH website (www.cdc.gov/niosh/ppe) should be consulted.

The complete elimination of the hazard is the most permanent and certain solution, and PPE, the least protective and most easily defeated. Incorporating worker-protection concepts into the initial design of the manufacturing process, or Prevention Through Design, is part of a new initiative of the NIOSH and requires not only a recognition of adverse health outcomes associated with a particular process, but also a partnership with designers, engineers, occupational health professionals, and manufacturers to design products with the health of workers and the environment in mind.

The Role of Government in Controlling Workplace Hazards

Historically, the costs of caring for injured workers and even for preventing injuries and illnesses were largely externalized by business and industry. The resulting social costs, as well as pressure from injured workers and their families, motivated government involvement. Most industrialized countries recognized that eliminating and reducing the adverse health effects associated with the production of goods and services require some form of government intervention. Even the most well-meaning company may not have the information or the political will to fully anticipate, evaluate, and control workplace hazards. A high workplace fatality rate in the late 1800s and early 1900s incentivized some states to start state-level safety programs and to initiate Workers' Compensation programs. By 1920, there were 27 state labor departments with industrial hygiene divisions, though few did little more than occasional factory inspections. The social activism and social movements in the 1960s (e.g., voting rights and environmental movement), as well as highly publicized workplace disasters, brought worker health and safety back to the public agenda.

President Lyndon Johnson initiated the first efforts to pass occupational health and safety legislation designed to prevent injuries and illnesses and not just treat them after they had occurred. Distracted by social unrest and the Vietnam War, his efforts failed. Congress took up the effort again after public outcry regarding the death of 68 miners in a mine explosion in West Virginia in 1968. OSHA (Public Law 91:596) was signed into law by Richard Nixon in the end of 1970 (MacLaury, 1994).

The law was far reaching and Congress outlined the lofty goal of "to assure so far as possible every working man and woman safe and healthful working conditions." The law went into effect the following April (April 28, 1971) and established the Occupational Safety and Health Administration in the Department of Labor (OSHA). The law made provisions for each state to develop its own OSHA program and 25 states have done so, though some provide coverage for state employees only. State OSHA plans must have regulations that are at least as effective as the federal OSHA regulations. States that did not develop their own "state plan" are covered by the federal OSHA regulations.

OSHA regulations are wide ranging and include guidance and enforceable standards for both safety and health (www .osha.gov/law-regs.html). In addition to the basic OSHA regulations, there are other regulations that are relevant for occupational health, such as the Workplace Right to Know (requires labeling of chemicals in the workplace and training on their use), community right to know (information available to emergency responders and others on chemicals in use in manufacturing firms in their area). The Workplace Right to Know standard (also known as Hazard Communication Standard, 29 CFR 1910.1200) is particularly useful to caregivers in that it includes the requirement for chemical manufacturers to supply safety data sheets with each shipment of chemicals. Safety data sheets contain information on the chemical properties, handling, precautionary requirements, and known health effects. Users of the chemicals must keep copies of data sheets and make them available to workers and clinicians. Although useful, safety data sheets do not provide information on synergistic or interactive effects and may be incomplete, poorly written, or lacking information on "proprietary compounds." They can help with clinical care, but should be used along with other information about the toxicity of the chemicals in question.

OSHA works to update its regulatory standards, though political pressure has often delayed setting of new standards. Among the OSHA regulations that are frequently referred to are the PELs, which is a listing of several hundred chemicals with their allowable or legal level for exposure to on a daily basis over the course of a working lifetime. PELs are usually designated as 8-hour TWA, short-term exposure limits (STELs; usually 15 to 30 minutes), or ceiling limits and are reported as parts per million or milligrams per cubic centimeter. If workers are exposed to regulated compounds for more than 8 hours, a reassessment of the allowable limits is required. Some state programs may regulate exposures to compounds not regulated by OSHA.

The PELs have been criticized for being set by what industry found to be achievable levels rather than levels related to health outcomes. In addition, political pressure has limited OSHA's ability to update the PEL with new scientific findings; consequently, many of the PELs reflect science and industry control abilities present in the 1960s or 1970s. The OSHA PELs are therefore considered by many occupational health and safety practitioners to be minimal standards.

Since its passage, the Occupational Safety and Health Act has been contentious and has had numerous court challenges to determine congressional intent regarding workplace interventions. Notably are the "Benzene decision" (*Industrial Union Department, AFL-CIO vs. Marshall*) defining "significant risk" when seeking to control exposure to hazardous substances, the "Cotton Dust decision" (*Textile Manufacturers Institute, Inc. v. Donovan*) not requiring OSHA to do a cost–benefit analysis when setting health standards, and the "Barlow decision" (*Marshall v. Barlow's, Inc.*, 436 U.S. 307; 1978) upholding OSHA's right to do workplace inspections with a warrant.

Not only has OSHA met with considerable pressure from business interests, but also Congress has not funded the agency to the level necessary to fully implement its mandate. There are not enough inspectors to review company compliance with state and federal regulations; some companies may never be inspected. To effectively use limited resources, the federal agency and state counterparts often prioritize inspections according to high-risk industries or complaints. Consequently, strategies for preventing workplace injuries and illness rely on the companies themselves and on local occupational safety and health professionals. OSHA also posts directives, fact sheets, and other information to assist employers in complying with regulations. Interestingly, OSHA is responsible for enforcement of whistle-blower provisions of some 20 laws, such as the Sarbanes-Oxley Act, the Patient Protection and Affordable Care Act, and the Food and Drug Administration (FDA) Food Safety Modernization Act, as well as these provisions under the Occupational Safety and Health Act. (Sarbanes-Oxley, also known as the Public Company Accounting Reform and Investor Protection Act or Corporate Auditing Accountability and Responsibility Act, sets requirements for financial accountability and responsibility for corporate boards of directors and management.) Many of the whistle-blower provisions are related to laws that have little to do with occupational health; despite this, OSHA has the responsibility to enforce them.

Other federal agencies such as the Environmental Protection Agency are responsible for implementing other laws that have relevance for workplaces and communities, such as the Toxic Substances Control Act (sets expectations for testing and labeling chemical substances), the Clean Air Act (addresses air pollution), the Clean Water Act (addresses allowable pollution of waterways), the Resource Conservation and Recovery Act (addresses hazardous waste), and the Federal Insecticide, Fungicide, and Rodenticide Act (addresses pesticide use), among others. The regulations associated with these laws are often administered by state as well as the federal agency. Knowledge of the provisions of these regulations is critical in helping clients understand to what protections they are entitled.

In addition to establishing the parameters of the Occupational Safety and Health Administration, the Occupational Safety and Health Act outlined the requirement for a federal agency to conduct research and professional training in the area of occupational health; NIOSH has implemented these requirements. Since its inception, NIOSH has published numerous research findings, reports, criteria documents, guidance documents, and fact sheets on the practice of occupational health and helped establish guidance for state and federal rule making as well as corporate policies to protect worker health (www.cdc.gov/niosh).

Despite political pressures, court decisions, and limited resources, OSHA is landmark legislation and has been largely considered successful (MMWR, 1999). It has incentivized companies to prevent workplace injuries and illnesses, and the workplace fatality rate has dropped from 14,000/yr in 1970 (year of its passage) to around 4,000 today—despite a doubling of the labor force during that time.

International Standards

The United States lags behind many industrialized democracies in the type and level of protection they provide for working people. For example, the European Commission has established a policy on the Registration, Evaluation, Authorization, and

Restriction of CHemicals (REACH; European Commission). Since 2007, the regulations have required manufacturers and importers of chemicals to compile and distribute information on the properties and safe use of their chemicals. Chemicals that cannot be used safely may have restrictions on their use or must be phased out. These regulations place more responsibility than is currently required under U.S. regulations. U.S.-based companies wishing to do business in the EU are required to comply with REACH, and some want to see these regulatory requirements to ultimately be the standard in the United States. Practitioners interested in the understanding of safe chemical compositions and their use may find more current information through the REACH regulations than the U.S. chemical regulations under the Toxic Substances Control Act. OSHA works to maintain some consistency with newer international regulatory developments. Of particular interest for practitioners is the Globally Harmonized System (GHS) of Classification and Labeling of Chemicals to improve the consistency internationally of labeling and training on the use of chemicals.

The World Health Organization (WHO) and the International Labor Organization (ILO) have made workplace health and safety a priority and often exceed the goals of OSHA or U.S.-based businesses. They have shared a definition of occupational health:

The main focus in occupational health is on three different objectives: (i) the maintenance and promotion of workers' health and working capacity; (ii) the improvement of working environment and work to become conducive to safety and health and (iii) development of work organizations and working cultures in a direction which supports health and safety at work and in doing so also promotes a positive social climate and smooth operation and may enhance productivity of the undertakings. The concept of working culture is intended in this context to mean a reflection of the essential value systems adopted by the undertaking concerned. Such a culture is reflected in practice in the managerial systems, personnel policy, principles for participation, training policies and quality management of the undertaking. (GOHNET, 2003; ILO, 2006)

Professional Collaborators

Caring for injured workers and preventing future injuries require a strong collaboration with occupational and environmental health professionals such as occupational and environmental physicians, nurses, industrial hygienists, safety professionals, toxicologists, health physicists, case managers, and vocational rehabilitation counselors. For secondary prevention efforts such as caring for injured workers or managing disability, professional groups such as American Association of Occupational Health Nurses (AAOHN; www.aaohn.org) or the American College of Occupational and Environmental Medicine (ACOEM; www.acoem.org) are helpful collaborators. On the other hand, if primary prevention is the goal, professional groups such as the American Industrial Hygiene Association (AIHA; www.aiha.org), American Conference of Governmental Industrial

Hygienists (ACGIH; www.acgih.org), American Society of Safety Engineers (ASSE; www.asse.org), and Society of Toxicology (SOT; www.toxicology.org) are useful partners.

All of these professional associations develop and publish best practices, guidelines for ethical practice, fact sheets, journals, or other materials on issues related to their practice, and some have developed core curricula to guide practice. They also hold annual meetings, which are useful for professional development and networking. Most have local, state, or regional affiliates and partner with other organizations to develop certification programs as a demonstration of excellence in their discipline.

An important resource developed by the ACGIH is a collection of consensus standards for the use of practicing health and safety experts. The threshold limit values (TLVs) and biological exposure indices (BEIs) are a compendium of information about the levels of a hazard workers can be exposed to day after day without adverse health effects (www.acgih.org/tlv-bei-guidelines/tlv-chemical-substances-introduction). They are reviewed and updated regularly by practicing industrial hygienists and reflect current research on the health effects of chemicals as well as other exposures, such as noise, nonionizing radiation, and vibration. The TLVs incorporate concepts of TWA (or the average exposure over an 8-hour work day, 40-hour work week) and STELs (or short-term exposure averaged over 15 minutes). The TLVs, as well as the PELs, are based on research and case reports of male workers (and largely White male workers); consequently, published allowable exposure levels may not be comparably protective for women. The TLVs are not enforceable but serve as a very useful guidance for occupational health and safety practitioners and others in assessing and controlling workplace hazard.

Unions

No discussion of occupational safety and health is complete without the inclusion of organized labor. Unions were not always supportive of federal legislative effort to protect workers or provide injured workers compensation for injuries, as some union leadership felt it was the union's role to provide health and safety support to its members. Over the years, however, organized labor became a strong advocate for workplace health and safety protections and partnered with many occupational health and safety professionals to oversee implementation of hazard controls. Labor representatives have the right to accompany OSHA inspectors on a site visit and often provide helpful information on work processes and exposures. Unfortunately, with the decline in union membership (about 6% of the private sector workforce and 35% of the public sector workforce [BLS, www.bls.gov/news.release/union2.toc.htm]), the involvement of unions in protecting worker rights and supporting health and safety efforts has also declined. However, among the unions that continue to flourish, many have seen increased involvement of women, who have often stepped into leadership roles (Covert, 2014). If an injured worker is a member of a union, it will be useful for the caregiver to reach out to union representatives for assistance in return-to-work efforts and help in understanding work requirements.

Integrating the Workplace and General Health

Increasingly it has been acknowledged that the work is not, and should not be, isolated from the rest of a worker's life and that the health and safety of people who work should be dealt with holistically. Workplace exposures and stressors have a great influence on the health of the individual and general health. Alternatively, living conditions and the environment contribute to worker health and workplace productivity. To be fully effective in building health and well-being, efforts to prevent workplace injuries and illnesses inside the factory walls must be integrated with promotion of health generally. Early activities in this arena included such activities as vendor-supplied health promotion, smoking cessation, exercise, or weight-loss programs that were offered at the workplace. Others pushed their corporate sustainability commitments beyond being environmentally "green" to incorporating worker health, safety, and well-being into their corporate efforts. NIOSH responded to this goal by developing their Total Worker Health™ program (Schill & Chosewood, 2013) with guidance on integrating workplace illness prevention with health promotion. Evaluation of the effectiveness of these various approaches in improving worker health, safety, well-being, job satisfaction, work–life balance, and productivity is ongoing. Still to be examined is the degree to which workplace-based health promotion programs might divert company resources away from efforts to prevent workplace injuries and illnesses through modification of job tasks, redesign of production processes, or other controls of known hazards. Moreover, there does not appear to be movement on recognizing or changing the environmental conditions, housing, nutrition, or other political policies that contribute to poor health and work-related concerns.

Women are an indispensable part of the American workforce, where many find themselves exposed to hazardous compounds and risky situations. Health care providers have an opportunity to anticipate, evaluate, and control hazards while caring for injuries or illnesses that may occur in the course of work. Even as sociopolitical issues such as worker and business rights, economic demands, and regulatory priorities that are not always compatible with duty to care for patients encroach on the care provider–patient realtionship, supporting and caring for working women is an important and noble calling.

■ REFERENCES

Achievements in Public Health, 1900–1999; Improvements in Workplace Safety—United States. (1900–1999). *Morbidity and Mortality Weekly Report, 48*(22), 461–469.

Baetjer, A. M. (1946). *Women in industry: Their health and efficiency.* U.S. Army. Washington, DC: U.S. Government Printing Office.

Caruso, C. C., Hitchcock, E. M., Dick, R. B., Russo, J. M., & Schmit, J. M. (2004). *Overtime and extended work shifts: Recent findings on illnesses, injuries, and health behaviors.* Cincinnati, OH: NIOSH.

Cheadle, A., Franklin, G., Wolfhagen, C., Savarino, J., Liu, P. Y., Salley, C., & Weaver, M. (1994). Factors influencing the duration of work-related disability: A population-based study of Washington State workers' compensation. *American Journal of Public Health, 84*(2), 190–196.

Covert, B. (2014). How the rise of women in labor could save the movement: A new wave of female labor leaders are winning by thinking big. Retrieved from http://www.thenation.com/article/how-rise-women-labor-could-save-movement.

Einarsen, S., Hoel, H., Zapf, D., & Cooper, C. L. (Eds.). (2003). *Bullying and emotional abuse in the workplace. International perspectives in research and practice.* London, UK: Taylor & Francis.

European Commission. (2015). Retrieved from http://ec.europa.eu/environment/chemicals/reach/reach_en.htm

Evanoff, B., Wolf, L., Aton, E., Canos, J., & Collins, J. (2003). Reduction in injury rates in nursing personnel through introduction of mechanical lifts in the workplace. *American Journal of Industrial Medicine, 44*(5), 451–457.

Fielding, J. E., Teutsch, S., & Lester, B. (2010). Framework for public health in the United States. *Public Health Reviews, 32*(1), 174–189.

Franklin, G. M., Stover, B. D., Turner, J. A., Fulton-Kehoe, D., & Wickizer, T. M. (2008). Early opioid prescription and subsequent disability among workers with back injuries: The Disability Risk Identification Study Cohort. *Spine, 33*(2), 199–204.

Getzner, M., & Zak, D. (2012). Health impacts of noise pollution around airports: Economic valuation and transferability. In J. Oosthuizen (Ed.), *Environmental health: Emerging issues and practice* (Chapter 11, pp. 247-272). Rijeka, Croatia: InTech.

Global Occupational Health Network. (2003). GOHNET newsletter. Issue No. 5, Summer 2003. Geneva, Switzerland: WHO.

Government Accountability Office. (GAO). (2007). *Chemical regulation: Comparison of U.S. and recently enacted European Union approaches to protect against the risks of toxic chemicals.* GAO-07–825. Washington, DC: Author.

Halliday, E., & Gast, R. J. (2011). Bacteria in beach sands: An emerging challenge in protecting coastal water quality and bather health. *Environmental Science & Technology, 45*(2), 370–379.

International Agency for Research on Cancer (IARC). (2015). Retrieved from http://monographs.iarc.fr/ENG/Classification

International Labor Organization. (2006). *R-197 promotional framework for occupational safety and health: Recommendations 2006, No. 197.* Adopted June 15, 2006. Geneva, Switzerland: WHO.

Jirtle, R. L., & Skinner, M. K. (2007). Environmental epigenomics and disease susceptibility. *Nature Reviews. Genetics, 8*(4), 253–262.

Kolstad, H. A. (2008). Nightshift work and risk of breast cancer and other cancers: A critical review of the epidemiologic evidence. *Scandinavian Journal of Work, Environment & Health, 34*(1), 5–22.

Kumar, S. (2004). Occupational exposure associated with reproductive dysfunction. *Journal of Occupational Health, 46*(1), 1–19.

Linn, M. W., Sandifer, R., & Stein, S. (1985). Effects of unemployment on mental and physical health. *American Journal of Public Health, 75*(5), 502–506.

Lucian Leape Institute (2013). Through the eyes of the workforce: Creating joy, meaning, and safer health care. *Report of the Roundtable on the Joy and Meaning of Work and Workforce Safety.* Boston, MA: National Patient Safety Foundation.

MacLaury, J. (1994). *Job safety law of 1970: Its passage was perilous.* Retrieved from http://www.dol.gov/dol/aboutdol/history/osha.htm

McDonald, J., Potyk, D., Fischer, D., Parmenter, B., Lillis, T., Tompkins, L.,…Belenky, G. (2013). Napping on the night shift: A study of sleep, performance, and learning in physicians-in-training. *Journal of Graduate Medical Education, 5*(4), 634–638.

McPhaul, K. M., & Lipscomb, J. A. (2004). Workplace violence in health care: Recognized but not regulated. *Online Journal of Issues in Nursing, 9*(3), 7.

Mills, J. N., Gage, K. L., & Khan, A. S. (2010). Potential influence of climate change on vector-borne and zoonotic diseases: A review and proposed research plan. *Environmental Health Perspectives, 118*(11), 1507–1514.

Niedhammer, I., David, S., Degioanni, S., Drummond, A., & Pierre, P. (2009). Workplace bullying and sleep disturbances: Findings from a large scale cross-sectional survey in the French working population. *Sleep, 32*(9), 1211–1219.

Ogden, N. H., Maarouf, A., Barker, I. K., Bigras-Poulin, M., Lindsay, L. R., Morshed, M. G.,…Charron, D. F. (2006). Climate change and the potential for range expansion of the Lyme disease vector *Ixodes scapularis* in Canada. *International Journal for Parasitology, 36*(1), 63–70.

Pope, A. M., Snyder, M. A., & Mood, L. H. (Eds.). (1995). Taking an exposure history. In *Nursing, health, & the environment: Strengthening the relationship to improve the public's health* (Appendix G). Committee on Enhancing Environmental Health Content in Nursing Practice. Division of Health Promotion and Disease Prevention. Washington, DC: National Academies Press.

Rabinowitz, P. (2000). Noise-induced hearing loss. *American Family Physician, 61*(9), 2749–2756.

Rogers, A. E. (2008). The effects of fatigue and sleepiness on nurse performance and patient safety. In R. G. Hughes (Ed.), *Patient safety and quality: An evidence-based handbook for nurses* (Chapter 40, pp. 509–545). Rockville, MD: Agency for Healthcare Research and Quality.

Schill, A. L., & Chosewood, L. C. (2013). The NIOSH Total Worker Health™ program: An overview. *Journal of Occupational and Environmental Medicine, 55*(Suppl. 12), S8–S11.

Selevan, S. G., Kimmel, C. A., & Mendola, P. (2000). Identifying critical windows of exposure for children's health. *Environmental Health Perspectives, 108*(Suppl. 3), 451–455.

Selevan, S. G., Lindbohm, M. L., Hornung, R. W., & Hemminki, K. (1985). A study of occupational exposure to antineoplastic drugs and fetal loss in nurses. *New England Journal of Medicine, 313*(19), 1173–1178.

Silverstein, B., Howard, N., Lee, D., & Goggins, R. (2006). *Lifting patients/residents/clients in health care: Washington State 2005.* Report to the Washington State Legislature House Commerce and Labor Committee.

Silverstein, B., & Schurke, J. (2012). *Implementation of safe patient handling in Washington state hospitals: Final report to the legislature.* SHARP program, Department of Labor and Industries, Washington State.

Smith, C. (2010). *Lifesaving drugs, deadly consequences: "Secondhand chemo" puts healthcare workers at risk.* Investigate West. Retrieved from http://invw.org/2010/07/09/chemo-main

Spector, J. T., & Sheffield, P. E. (2014). Re-evaluating occupational heat stress in a changing climate. *Annals of Occupational Hygiene, 58*(8), 936–942.

Stephenson, J. (2009). *Chemical regulation: Options for enhancing the effectiveness of the Toxic Substances Control Act.* Statement of John Stephenson, Director, Natural Resources and the Environment, U.S. Government Accountability Office (GAO-09–428T).

Turner, J. A., Franklin, G., Fulton-Kehoe, D., Sheppard, L., Stover, B., Wu, R., ...Wickizer, T. M. (2008). ISSLS prize winner: Early predictors of chronic work disability: A prospective, population-based study of workers with back injuries. *Spine, 33*(25), 2809–2818.

Weselak, M., Arbuckle, T. E., Walker, M. C., & Krewski, D. (2008). The influence of the environment and other exogenous agents on spontaneous abortion risk. *Journal of Toxicology and Environmental Health. Part B, Critical Reviews, 11*(3–4), 221–241.

Wickizer, T. M., Franklin, G., Fulton-Kehoe, D., Gluck, J., Mootz, R., Smith-Weller, T., & Plaeger-Brockway, R. (2011). Improving quality, preventing disability and reducing costs in workers' compensation healthcare: A population-based intervention study. *Medical Care, 49*(12), 1105–1111.

CHAPTER 18

Health Considerations for Women Caregivers

Judith Berg • Nancy Fugate Woods

■ WOMEN AS CAREGIVERS

Women have been the traditional caregivers for their families in most of recorded history. Today, in most nations women are more likely to provide informal care to their families than do men. Informal caregivers provide care or assistance, without pay, to people who are ill or need help with personal activities of daily living (ADL; O'Reilly, Connolly , Rosato, & Patterson, 2008). Current estimates from the American Time Use Survey (ATUS) indicate that nearly one third of the population composes informal caregivers, contributing 1.2 billion hours of unpaid work annually. Women's involvement in caregiving to children is prominent in their 30s, coinciding with their working years, and also during their 50s and beyond, years of grandparenting. In addition, women in their 70s and 80s make noteworthy contributions to spousal care (Duhkovnov & Zagheni, 2015). In the United States, estimates indicate that a majority of caregivers are women, some of whom simultaneously care for aging parents, spouses, children, and more recently, grandchildren. Indeed, the term *sandwich generation* has been used to describe women's position in the middle of aging parents and children needing care. Informal caregiving was valued at $691 billion in 2012, constituting 4.3% of the gross domestic product (GDP) and is predicted to reach $838 billion by 2050 owing to the aging of the population. Nonetheless, informal caregivers usually are not compensated for their services.

How did this arrangement evolve? Sociological studies reveal that caregiving is a product of gender-role socialization, with women being allocated the relational work of families and men the instrumental, external work to generate resources to support the family. That women are "ordered to care" by social convention has been examined by Susan Reverby, who studied the social arrangements that affect women in general and nurses, in particular (Reverby, 1987). Indeed, gender-role socialization expectations are that women will assume responsibility for elder caregiving as well as that for their children. In some societies, the care for family members extends to members of the husbands'

families, increasing the expectations that women will be constantly available as wives, mothers, daughters, and caregivers. Socially constructed arrangements dividing labor in families also extend to women's voluntary contributions of many hours to support community agencies, often viewed as an extension of their family's contributions. In addition, women who do not provide caregiver service to their families may be made to feel guilty about their decisions.

Of consequence for women is that their informal caregiving is contributed as voluntary and without pay. Often women's caregiving work remains hidden and is taken for granted, resulting in the failure of social and health policy makers to consider their contributions to the economy. Many Western countries' health care systems, including home care, rely on women's unpaid work but do not account for their contribution to the GDP. Estimates of the economic value of this unpaid labor in the United States are significant (Duhkovnov & Zagheni, 2015). Moreover, unpaid caregiving often interferes with women accruing retirement benefits such as social security, health care benefits, such as insurance, or other employee benefits, and their absence from the labor force results in their lagging behind men in promotions, salary increases, and the development of skill sets that command higher salaries. Because women are overrepresented in lower paying, lower status occupations, their incomes are often assumed to be discretionary or expendable; thus their willingness to provide caregiving services is assumed to be a "natural" arrangement in families. In turn, the gender disparities in occupational strata are reinforced and are evident even in health care (see Chapter 2).

Lost opportunity costs for women who may need to modify employment commitments or leave their paid work to provide care for their families do not appear in the calculation of the GDP, nor do they afford tax breaks or benefits for women's families. The loss of accrued salary plus social security benefits for women's own retirement and employee benefits packages that include health insurance coverage together are missing from our national calculation. When women are able to re-enter the workforce after providing caregiving, their past absences from work places them in jeopardy because of lost opportunities for training in new skills, reduction of their seniority, or even loss of their jobs, despite the provisions of the U.S. Family and Medical Leave Act. The loss of networking opportunities also removes them from sources of social support, friendship, and professional and occupational information flows and may constrain their friendship networks.

For women who are mothers as well as caregivers, becoming a caregiver increases the demands on relationships, sometimes requiring women to balance the needs of their developing children against the needs of family members, including their spouses or their own parents. An estimated 68% of U.S. women with preschool children are employed, and the absence or low availability of workplace-based child care or leave policies such as in Scandinavian countries complicates the demands they face in providing informal caregiving services (www.dol.gov).

Caregiving experiences punctuate women's life spans. In addition to the assumptions about being the constantly available mother to infants and young children, women are also assumed to be willing and available to provide grand-parenting, spousal care, and parent care. Some may provide care to all of these family members over the course of a lifetime and sometimes simultaneously.

The demand for informal caregivers has increased for a variety of reasons. Among the most pressing is the aging of the population. An estimated 65% of older adults rely on family caregivers, with 30% of these also using formal caregivers. (Family Caregiver Alliance, 2015). In addition, the shortening of hospital stays has resulted in a transfer of health care responsibilities to families earlier in the course of an illness. The use of increased home care technology, such as monitoring devices and even ventilators that can be used in home settings, has shifted many procedures from the health care system to informal caregivers.

In addition to social and economic consequences, recent research findings indicate that caregiving may affect women's health–related behaviors and their health. In this chapter we examine: (a) a framework for considering the factors affecting caregivers' health and health promotion practices; (b) assessment and intervention for caregivers: a review of evidence; and (c) clinical applications of what we know about promoting caregivers' health.

■ FACTORS AFFECTING CAREGIVERS' HEALTH AND HEALTH PROMOTION: A FRAMEWORK

Figure 18.1 provides a framework depicting possible relationships among personal characteristics of the caregiver, caregiver resources, life demands and their relationships to caregiving processes, meaning of caregiving, and health outcomes of caregiving. Each of these components is discussed in this chapter.

Personal Characteristics

Personal characteristics describe people who are the caregivers and include their age, education, personal development, life opportunities, health status, and health-promoting practices as they begin caregiving work (Leveille, Penninx, Melzer, Izmirlian, & Guralnik, 2000). The ages of caregivers in the United States cross the life span: Young adults to the oldest old provide caregiving services. In some circumstances, children and adolescents assume some caregiving responsibilities for family members, sometimes for siblings and parents or grandparents. Middle-aged and older women, including those who are remaining in the workforce, provide the

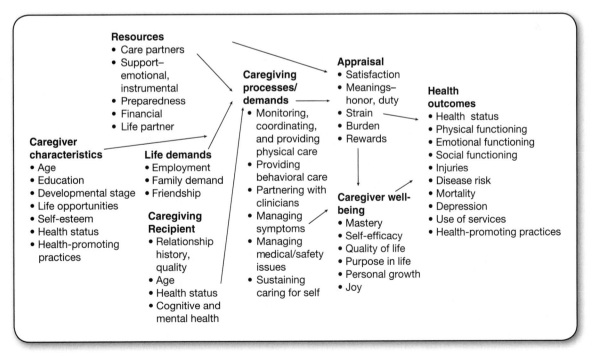

FIGURE 18.1

Factors affecting caregiver's health: Caregiver characteristics, resources, life demands, caregiving recipient, caregiving processes/demands, appraisal, and caregiver well-being influence health outcomes.

majority of the care to U.S. family members. Indeed a recent Behavioral Risk Factor survey indicated that the largest proportion of family caregivers was 50 to 64 years of age, female, Black/non-Hispanic, and married had some college education (Anderson et al., 2013).

A caregiver's education may provide access to information that may be useful in providing caregiver services and obtaining information about the health problem of the person who is the care recipient. The developmental history of the caregiver influences the ability of caregivers to find meaning in the work of caregiving and possible outcomes of caregiving. For example, an adolescent daughter who is caring for a parent might narrow her range of friendships and opt out of continuing school beyond high school and experience the lower income associated with lower educational preparation that persists across her remaining life span. In contrast, an older woman who provides care for a husband may view herself as doing what is consistent with her life stage and personal history.

As women develop health-promoting practices, they may accrue health benefits that sustain their health across their life span. The type of health-promoting practices in which women engage (e.g., physical activity such as walking and eating fresh fruits and vegetables) may become difficult to continue in the face of caregiving demands. Women who are in good health enter caregiving relationships with health advantages, but maintaining their health in the face of caregiving demands may present challenges. Those who assume caregiving in poor health begin this part of their lives having attenuated possibilities for health promotion and illness management, although evidence suggests the possibility for their experiencing well-being despite their health problems.

Life Demands

As women enter caregiving arrangements, they bring with them the complement of roles and responsibilities that characterize their lives. Many perform roles of wife, mother, employee, volunteer, grandparent, or even great-grandparent. The demands of these roles influence not only women's energy levels, but also financial obligations that may be delicately balanced with their incomes and financial reserves. Consequently, the commitment to be a caregiver brings with it financial as well as energy commitments.

Caregiving implies creating or maintaining a relationship with the care recipient. Often the relationship to the person for whom one provides care has been established before the commitment to caregiving is made (Pinquart & Sorenson, 2011). Some women may find themselves caring for family members with whom the relationship does not have a long history, such as in the case of caring for an orphaned young grandchild or a more distant relative with whom there is little opportunity to have developed a relationship. When caregiving results from a family crisis, the demands of new roles may be immediate, as in assuming the care of a young grandchild, and may allow limited time to adapt to new demands (Moore & Rosenthal, 2014; Musil et al., 2010; Musil, Jeanblanc, Burant, Zauszniewski, & Warner, 2013). Also caregiver strain arises from conflicting demands with other roles, including parenting, employment, friendships,

and other volunteer efforts, each of which may have special meanings for the caregiver.

When there is a history of a relationship with the care recipient, the caregiver may be challenged by its nature. Caring for a family member with whom the relationship has been abusive or distant may pose some risk for caregivers. Hodgins, Wuest, and Malcom (2011) found that health outcomes and health promotion for women caregivers were affected by their becoming caregivers because of a sense of duty or obligation and by the quality of their past relationship with the caregiving recipient. Women who had better past relationships were less likely to assume caregiving because of duty or obligation. Indeed, having an abusive parent or partner increased the sense of obligation to provide care for them. Obligation, in turn, influenced caregivers' health such that women who provided care out of a sense of duty had poorer health, including physical, emotional, and relational health and material well-being indicators.

Caregiving Resources

One's ability to provide care for a family member or friend may be enhanced by having access to resources that support the caregiver and her efforts. Among these resources are access to help, including care partners who share the responsibility, provide substitution to afford the caregiver respite and opportunity to engage in valued activities or rest, and instrumental assistance, such as access to information about options in caring for someone who is bedridden or incontinent, as well as providing physical assistance. Access to emotional support, such as provided by a life partner or a close friend, can sustain women in their caregiving efforts. Emotional support in the form of encouraging the caregiver, affirming and valuing the commitment to caregiving, and listening to the expression of feelings can help sustain the emotional energy needed for caregiving as well as support emotional regulation of the caregiver.

Financial resources that support access to respite and instrumental assistance, such as by purchasing home care services, enable caregivers to balance their own personal needs with the care recipient's needs. Long-term care insurance that pays for home care services, as well as other types of health insurance, may contribute to the success of caregiving relationships, but access to these types of insurance benefits are limited. Moreover, these benefits often are associated with one's employment, thus making them inaccessible when a caregiver must resign from employment in order to assume caregiving responsibilities.

Caregiving Processes

At the center of this framework are caregiving processes. What do caregivers do? Despite the impressive contributions of caregivers, there is often limited understanding of the activities in which they engage. Caregiving processes can be described by focusing on meeting the needs of the care recipient for assistance in ADL, such as bathing, dressing, grooming, moving from one place to another, toileting, feeding, and continence care. In addition, caregivers often provide assistance with instrumental ADL (IADL), including conducting financial transactions, such as paying bills; shopping for food and preparing meals; doing housework and laundry; managing transportation; conducting phone conversations; and coordinating and performing medical regimens. What is not included in a simple enumeration of these tasks is the coordination of elements of care: these may include managing multiple caregivers (informal and formal) who may contribute a variety of services; monitoring the care recipient to promote safety and prevent injury, such as falls; anticipating and planning for the needs of the care recipient over a period of time; and maintaining an interpersonal relationship with the care recipient that is appropriate to one's family role, such as wife or mother. Caring for a person with dementia provides some unique challenges, as discussed later in this chapter.

In addition to the informal caregiving activities enumerated earlier, caregivers provide essential health-related services that may include the management of a variety of medications (some with serious side effects), administration of treatments such as the application of dressings or external medications, and performance of prescribed physical activity routines such as those prescribed by a physical therapist. Often the informal caregiver assumes responsibility for identifying health issues, contacting the health care provider about health issues, and communicating about health issues, as well as coordinating health care services for the care recipient (Sadak, Souza, & Borson, 2015).

Many caregivers may assume these responsibilities gradually, providing time to learn best practices. Some, however, assume extensive responsibility for caregiving abruptly, such as at the time of hospital discharge of a family member, and may have little time to prepare for these responsibilities.

■ MEANING OF CAREGIVING

Meanings associated with caregiving vary from feeling that it is an honor to feeling overwhelmed by burden and strain. Caregiver strain and burden are concepts often used to explain the link between caregiving and caregiver health outcomes. Caregiver strain and burden indicate conditions that exist when the emotional or physical health of caregivers is threatened or compromised or when the demands of care outweigh available resources (Given et al., 1992). Caregiver burden has been described in multiple ways, but common to most definitions is the realization that burden is multidimensional. Some differentiate objective indicators of burden, such as the hours devoted to caregiving or the tasks performed, from subjective experiences of burden, such as the impact caregiving has on one's quality of life. Others focus on the perception of burden or strain. Emotional distress may serve as an important indicator of strain or burden, revealing the meaning of the experience to the caregiver. Strain is often expressed as a conflict between two sets of role obligations, such as caregiver–employee, caregiver–parent, caregiver–spouse, and caregiver–friend conflicts. Interventions can be directed at reducing the level of strain or burden as well as reducing the impact of strain or burden on health outcomes (Schumacher, Stewart, & Archbold, 2002).

Not all caregivers experience severe burden or strain. Indeed, many caregivers would describe their experience in positive terms, such as giving them a sense of purpose in life and an opportunity for personal growth and generativity. Despite the emphasis on caregiver burden and related outcomes, such as burnout, researchers have found that caregivers describe a number of rewards they associate with their caregiving situation. *Caregiver satisfaction* has been defined as stable expectation that what one does is a source of personal satisfaction (Lawton, Kleban, Moss, Rovine, & Glicksman, 1989). Others have assessed moments of warmth, comfort, and pleasure in their caregiving situation (Motenko, 1989). Still others have enumerated caregiving events that evoked pleasure, satisfaction, or joy and consider these as uplifts counterbalancing hassles (Kinney & Stephens, 1989).

Picot and Youngblut (1997) developed a scale to assess external (from health care professionals, the care recipient) and internal (personal feelings of achievement and growth) rewards experienced by caregivers. Caregivers who scored high on the rewards scale scored lower on measures of depression and caregiver burden than those who had lower rewards scores. Caregiver rewards were also related to the caregiving context, including the caregiving recipient's needs for help with ADL and IADL deficits and the caregiving situation, including caregiving duration and relationship to the caregiver. Caregivers who provided care to more physically and less instrumentally impaired care recipients enjoyed higher levels of rewards. The increased duration of the caregiving role resulted in lower caregiver rewards. The relationship to the care recipient (e.g., spouse, parents, grandparents) did not influence rewards. Black caregivers perceived higher levels of rewards than Whites, and those with more education reported fewer rewards than those with less formal education. Further understanding of caregiver rewards and ways they are related to the caregiving recipient, characteristics of the caregiver, and the caregiving situation is needed. In addition, exploration of anticipated rewards and potential burden with women who are contemplating assuming caregiving roles may help them clarify their decisions.

■ HEALTH CONSEQUENCES OF CAREGIVING

Anderson et al. (2013) analyzed data from the Centers for Disease Control and the Behavioral Risk Factor Surveillance System (BRFSS) survey to determine effects of caregiving on well-being. Using a question added to the BRFSS in 2009 as a measure of caregiving (whether provided regular care or assistance to friends or family members who have health problems, long-term illness, or disabilities during past month), they derived estimates of caregiving prevalence and its relationship to health. Nearly 20% of BRFSS respondents were caregivers. Caregivers were significantly more likely to be 50 to 64 years of age than younger (18–49 or 65 years and older), female versus male, and non-Hispanic Black versus other racial/ethnic groups; had some college versus college graduate or high school or less education; and were more likely to be married or living with a partner than single, widowed, or some other status.

More caregivers than noncaregivers reported fair or poor health, more frequent physical distress (14 days or more in the last month when physical health interfered with daily activities), more mental distress (14 days or more in the last month when mental health interfered with daily activities), and dissatisfaction with life, despite their having similar access to social support (Anderson et al., 2013). Young caregivers reported more frequent mental distress and more dissatisfaction with life, and older caregivers reported greater likelihood of fair or poor self-rated health or physical distress. These data provide important national estimates of the prevalence and associations of caregiving, with perceptions of the caregiver's health.

■ HEALTH EFFECTS OF CAREGIVING

Caregiving for family members with dementia and other health problems has been associated with caregivers' chronic physical and mental health problems in some studies, particularly when the caregiving is perceived as stressful (Buyck et al., 2011; Fredman, Doros, Cauley, Hillier, & Hochberg, 2010; Goode, Haley, Roth, & Ford, 1998; Gouin, Glaser, Malarkey, Beversdorf, & Kiecolt-Glaser, 2012; Lovell & Wetherell, 2011; Pearlin, Mullan, Semple, & Skaff, 1990; Pinquart & Sorensen, 2003; Roth, Perkins, Wadley, Temple, & Haley, 2009; Schulz et al., 1997; Vitaliano, Zhang, & Scanlon, 2003). Based on these findings, one might anticipate that caregiving would be associated with poor health of caregivers (Ho, Chan, Woo, Chong, & Sham, 2009). In contrast, some studies have revealed the benefits of caregiving for physical health, cognition, and mortality (Bertrand et al., 2012; Brown et al., 2009; Fredman, Doros, Ensrud, Hochberg, & Cauley, 2009; Fredman et al., 2008; O'Reilly et al., 2008; Roth et al., 2013). Caregivers may be more physically robust as a prerequisite for becoming caregivers, especially if they must spend many hours giving care. In addition, the effects of caregiving-related physical activities may build capacity for physical function (Chappell & Reid, 2002; Fredman, Bertrand, Martire, Hochberg, & Harris, 2006; Rosso et al., 2015) and mental health (Goode et al., 1998; Gruenewald, Karlamangla, Greendale, Singer, & Seeman, 2007; Kim & Carver, 2007). Conversely, those whose health worsens may end their caregiving commitments (McCann, Hebert, Bienias, Morris, & Evans, 2004). The "healthy caregiver hypothesis" asserts that not only would healthier adults be more likely to take on caregiving and to remain in that role, but also that the activities of caregiving would promote their health (Fredman, Lyons, Cauley, Hochberg, & Applebaum, 2015).

A recently reported set of analyses from the longitudinal Women's Health Initiative study of 5,600 women aged 65 years and older revealed that there was no difference in the changes observed in grip strength, walking speed, or number of chair stands among older women who were caregivers compared with noncaregivers over a 6-year period but that women who engaged in low-level caregiving, compared with those who did not, had greater grip strength at the first observation (Rosso et al., 2015). Sorting out the effects of caregiving on health versus the influence of the burden of existing chronic disease at the time that older women become caregivers is complex, but the propensity for high-frequency caregivers to have more chronic disease burden at the outset of caregiving, instead of the caregiving demands, may be responsible for higher disease rates observed among these caregivers (Pinquart & Sorensen, 2003). Also, in some studies, women who elected to provide high-frequency caregiving were healthier than those who were noncaregivers or low-frequency caregivers, and this bias toward caregivers being healthier at the outset may be responsible for their continued health during the time they are caregivers. In addition, study results related to the type of caregiving demands will be important in future research. Based on research that investigated caregiver stress, caregivers with greater burden experienced worse physical and mental health and quality of life (Dias et al., 2015; Goode et al., 1998). Understanding caregiver strain or stress and its effects on health may require more careful analysis of the nature of the caregiving activities, such as caregiving for someone with versus someone without dementia. Likewise, understanding the influence of the frequency of caregiving or hours spent in caregiving versus the actual demands of the caregiving situation will be important for future research. Based on findings from the Women's Health Initiative study, Rosso et al. (2015) concluded that caregiving may not have universally negative consequences for caregivers. Indeed, Roth et al. (2015) reexamined the impact of caregiving on mortality risk, confirming that caregivers experience significantly reduced mortality rates compared with noncaregiving counterparts.

Fredman et al. (2015) investigated the relationship between caregiving and mortality, considering the transitions that caregivers make in and out of their roles as well as caregiving intensity. Caregivers were older women with an average age of 81 years who provided care for a spouse or another care recipient who required care because of dementia, frailty or health decline, stroke, or other health problems or who was recovering from fracture or surgery. Caregivers provided assistance with an average of 1.5 ADL and 3.9 IADL tasks, and 38% had been in the role for more than 5 years. Compared with noncaregivers, caregivers experienced a more pronounced reduction in mortality that diminished over time. Caregiving stopped because of the death of the care recipient, transfer of the care recipient to a long-term care facility, move of the care recipient to live with other caregivers, improvement of care recipient's health, or a decline in the caregiver's health. In this same population, an investigation of the effects of caregiving intensity on perceived stress revealed that high-intensity caregivers (those who provided more assistance with ADL and IADL reported the highest levels of stress. Women who assumed caregiving responsibility over the course of the study and those whose levels of caregiving intensity increased both had increasing stress levels (Lyons Cauley, & Fredman, 2015).

Factors that influence the intensity and stress of caregiving may include challenges related to the types of assistance provided, as well as the types of health problems experienced by the care recipients. These may differ when caring for persons with dementia, life-threatening and chronic health problems, end-of-life (EOL) care needs, and care according to the age of the care recipient (e.g., caregiving for one's child vs. one's parent).

POSITIVE CONSEQUENCES OF CAREGIVING

Among the benefits of caregiving was a sense of meaning attributable to caregivers' relationships with the caregiving recipient and their contributions as caregivers to a sense of purpose in life. Opportunities for generativity are linked to theories about aging and human development (e.g., Erickson's description of generativity as central to late-life development). In addition, there may be personal growth related to learning new information and ways of functioning in response to caregiving challenges.

Well-being refers to people's experience of feeling well or positive, as assessed with measures of positive mood, and their evaluations of their lives, as estimated by ratings of the quality of their lives. In addition, eudemonic well-being, as reflected in purpose in life and personal growth, is a commonly used indicator of well-being. Chappell and Reid (2002) assessed the effects of the care recipient's cognitive status, needs for assistance with ADLs, and behavioral problems as they affected caregivers' well-being and estimates of burden. A majority of caregivers and caregiving recipients were women: The average age of caregivers was 51 years (range, 21–85 years), and for caregiving recipients, it was 80 years (range, 65–99 years). Caregivers' well-being was positively related to perceived social support and self-esteem but negatively related to the burden of caregiving and informal hours of care. In contrast to well-being, burden was positively related to the provision of more informal hours of care, lower frequency of getting a break, caregiving recipient behavioral problems and lower self-esteem (Chappell & Reid, 2002). The care recipient's cognitive status and ADL needs were both related to the use of formal services, although neither of these factors directly affected caregiver burden or well-being.

RISK FOR HEALTH PROBLEMS AMONG CAREGIVERS

Who is at greatest risk for negative outcomes of family caregiving? Gonzalez, Polansky, Lippa, Walker, and Feng (2011) examined specific aspects of caregiving that could help identify caregivers who cared for family members with dementia and who who were at risk of ill health and then tailor appropriate interventions for them. They examined effects of providing assistance with ADLs (bathing, dressing, toileting, transferring from bed to chair, continence care, and feeding) as well as IADL (preparing meals, performing housework, doing laundry, handling money, managing transportation, using the telephone, and taking medications). Managing behavior problems such as those included in the Revised Memory-Related Behavior Problem Checklist (Teri et al., 1992) requires caregivers to address depressive behaviors such as crying and acting sad, memory-related problems such as repeating questions and hiding things and then forgetting their location, and disruptive behaviors such as verbal aggression, agitation, and wandering. Informal caregivers who rated their health as fair or poor and who had one or more diagnosed health problems were classified as high risk compared with those without these characteristics (low risk).

Caregivers with low income, depressive symptoms, and high-care demands were more likely to be in the high-risk group of family caregivers (Gonzalez et al., 2011). Providing assistance with bathing, light housework, cooking or preparing meals, and getting around outside was significantly associated with being in the high-risk group of caregivers. Providing assistance in IADL, perceiving high levels of subjective demand, and having higher depression scores were associated with having greater health risks. Having a high income lowered the risk of poor health (Gonzalez, 2011).

Czaja et al. (2009) developed a measure of risk appraisal to screen caregivers of persons with dementia. Among the six areas assessed by this measure were self-care and health behaviors (trouble sleeping, physical health rating), patient problem behaviors (difficulties managing patient ADLs and behavioral problems), burden (feeling stressed because of caregiving responsibilities), depression (feeling sad), social support (satisfaction with support from family and friends), and safety (being at risk because of the caregiver's behavior or impairment). These items can serve as a guide to selecting treatment strategies for caregivers in each area (e.g., self-care), as illustrated by Czaja et al. (2009).

Those who provide both professional and informal caregiving warrant special consideration. Ward-Griffin et al. (2015) studied Canadian nurses who were negotiating professional family care boundaries (double-duty caregivers). They found that nurses providing family care were faced with striving for balance and responding to familial care expectations. They experienced both "reaping the benefits of caregiving," as well as caregiving "taking a toll." Nurses who were double-duty caregivers used multiple strategies to strive for balance: assessing the care situation, advising others about illnesses and treatments, advocating on behalf of their family member, collaborating and cooperating with unpaid and paid caregivers, coordinating family care through delegation to others, and consulting when they needed further knowledge or expertise. Nurses who were family caregivers experienced different situations described as "making it work," "working to manage," and "living on the edge" as they negotiated professional and familial care boundaries. The investigators recommend that the health of nurses and other health professionals who are caregivers for relatives may be at risk if the blurring of professional and family boundaries is not acknowledged. Furthermore, failure to provide adequate resources supporting double-duty caregivers may result in fewer human resources in health care, as some nurses may be lost to practice. Recommendations for policy can be found in Supporting Double-Duty Caregivers: A Policy Brief (www.uwo.ca/nursing/cwg/docs/PolicyBrieffinal.pdf).

ASSESSMENT AND INTERVENTIONS FOR CAREGIVERS: CONTEMPORARY EVIDENCE

Assessment of Caregivers' Health and Fit With Caregiving Demands

Clinicians can provide useful information, emotional support, and coaching to women who are considering assuming the role of a caregiver. An assessment of the caregiver's general health includes an age-appropriate history and physical examination of general health. In addition, advanced practice clinicians can use these tools to appraise the potential demands of caregiving and the caregiver's health status as a basis for planning interventions.

Preparedness or readiness to undertake a caregiving role has been assessed in a variety of ways. Archbold, Stewart, Greenlick, and Harvath (1990) and Archbold et al. (1995) developed an assessment that examines three domains: (a) general preparedness to care for patient's physical and emotional needs; (b) preparedness to handle emergencies, get help, and services; and (c) ability to manage caregiving stress. High scores on the nine-item scale predicted lower role strain among community dwelling caregivers of older patients recently discharged from the hospital (Sherwood et al., 2007) The Caregiver Mastery Scale asks caregivers to rate overload, relational deprivation, economic strains, role captivity, loss of self, caregiving competence, and expressive support. Higher caregiver mastery was associated with a lower number of patient problem behaviors and lower caregiver depression. Gitlin and Rose (2014) assessed caregiver readiness to care for a person with dementia by using a single item that reflects caregiver understanding of behaviors as dementia related and willingness to try strategies to manage behaviors. High caregiver readiness was associated with lower caregiver depression and financial strain despite greater patient cognitive and behavioral burden.

Sadak, Korpka, and Borson (2015) recently reviewed several measures assessing dementia caregiver readiness or activation. Missing from these measures was an assessment of caregiver activation focused on health care for the person living with dementia (Hibbard, Stockard, Mahoney, & Tusler, 2004). They have recently developed and tested a measure for caregiver activation for health care, the Partnering for Better Health–Living With Chronic Illness: Dementia. This 32-item measure reflects seven domains, including ability to (a) recognize and anticipate the day-to-day symptoms and challenges with multiple dimensions of patient health; (b) manage sudden changes in the dimensions of the patient's health, engage health services, and practice self-care; (c) manage the patient's medications; (d) manage day-to-day symptoms and challenges with the patient's health; (e) understand basic aspects of the patient's dementia; (f) recognize sudden/worrisome changes in the dimensions of the patient's health, and (g) advocate for the patient in health care situations. Scores on this scale were related to the caregiver's quality-of-life ratings, as well as other measures of caregiving readiness and stress.

Assessing the caregiving demands and capacity of the potential caregiver is an important basis for determining the caregiver's fit with the demands of the care process. When there is discretion in choosing to be a caregiver (often there is not), an enumeration of the kinds of activities that are required of caregivers can be a useful guide for women. Types of caregiving activities may range from providing assistance with ADL, IADL, and health and health care.

The nature of the caregiving tasks may have different effects on caregivers, and recently developed assessment tools reflect these differences. For example, the Caregiver Demands Scale for use with caregivers of people with cancer (Stetz, 1987) focuses on burden related to meals, intimate care, movement and comfort, medications and treatments, supervision, rest, and acquisition of new skills. Some have employed the Zarit Burden Inventory (1980), an instrument that assesses burden related to health, psychological well-being, finances, social life, and relationship with the patient (Zarit & Zarit, 1986). Others have focused on burden related to self-esteem, lack of family supports, and impact on finances, schedule, and health (Given et al., 1992). Still others have related burden to the frequency, severity, and distress of patient symptoms. A recent review of caregiver measurement instruments focusing on providing care to patients with cancer illustrates the importance of using a multidimensional, valid, reliable, and clinically relevant tool for this type of assessment (Honea et al., 2008). Specific assessment approaches have been developed for caregivers of people with dementia, such as those described earlier. Most of the assessment tools have been developed for research purposes, but some authors advise that use of a brief screening tool or selected subscales of a long instrument may improve clinical applicability (Honea et al., 2008).

Evaluating who is prepared be an informal caregiver can include an assessment of the fit between the demands of caregiving and the potential caregivers' skills, knowledge, and well-being, as well as their physical and emotional capacity. Several of the assessment tools mentioned earlier provide important dimensions to assess and have been tailored to the age and caregiving needs of care recipients. Translating these research instruments to formats useful in practice warrants the attention of researchers.

Interventions for Caregivers

Given the prevalence of informal caregiving, many interventions to support caregivers are being developed and tested. The high prevalence of dementia and its consequences for caregivers have stimulated numerous trials of interventions supporting dementia caregivers. As the population ages and the prevalence of chronic illnesses increases, the need for caregiving for older adults with multiple chronic illnesses problems, such as cancer and heart failure and their associated disabilities, is escalating. In addition, family members provide care for children with chronic illnesses and often provide care for family members at the EOL. Increasingly, grandparents have assumed the role of caregivers to their grandchildren. Research on how to support these diverse populations of caregivers and their unique needs for support will be critical to ensuring the well-being of caregivers and care recipients alike (McGuire, Anderson, Talley, & Crews, 2007).

Interventions for Caregivers of People With Dementia

Caring for a family member with dementia is becoming increasingly common, with more than 15 million unpaid caregivers providing such care (Alzheimer's Association, 2015). Moreover, the estimated value of the care provided by family caregivers for people with dementia was approximately $218 billion in 2014.

Caring for family members with dementia produces many stressors for caregivers, beyond the care recipient's memory and behavior problems, communication challenges, interpersonal conflicts, and role strain; these can precipitate caregiver health problems, compromise well-being, and disrupt social relationships (Black et al., 2010). A recently reported analysis of the National Study of Caregiving indicated that baby boomers who were caregivers for a family member with dementia, when compared with those who were caregivers for family members with other health problems, experienced similar rates of health problems, including high blood pressure and arthritis, and did not differ in how they rated their own health. Significant differences were observed among caregivers for relatives with dementia who provided more help with daily activities, experienced a higher level of caregiving and social activity conflict and more interrupted sleep, and were more likely to feel depressed than caregivers for someone without dementia. Also dementia caregivers were more likely than caregivers providing care for someone without dementia to have engaged paid help, experienced higher caregiving–work conflict, and higher caregiving–other family care (e.g., children) conflict. Outcomes of caregiving included depressed mood, which was increased by caregiving/social activity conflict but lessened by having a higher level of informal support. Caregiving–other family care conflicts were negatively related to how dementia caregivers rated their own health. Being married offset the effects of dementia caregiving on general health. Caregivers for family members without dementia who reported greater levels of interrupted sleep, caregiving–family activity conflict, caregiving–social activity conflict, and less informal support were likely to perceive their own health as poor. Those with more formal education reported lower levels of depressed mood and better perceived health (Moon & Dilworth-Anderson, 2015).

A variety of interventions for informal caregivers have been evaluated, with several Cochrane Reviews available summarizing evidence for their effectiveness. Among these are educational interventions, functional analysis-based interventions for challenging behaviors, cognitive reframing for caregivers, and respite care, among others. Educational interventions for caregivers of people with dementia living in the community include teaching skills for dementia caregiving, such as communication skills, coping and management strategies, information about dementia, and availability of support services. A recent review of seven trials revealed that educational interventions moderately reduced caregiver burden, but in a smaller number of studies, there was a small effect on depression but no effect on the number of transitions of care recipients with dementia to long-term care was observed. Effects of educational interventions on quality of life of the caregiver could not be estimated from the existing studies (Jensen, Agbata Nwando, Canavan, & McCarthy, 2015).

Psychosocial interventions for caregivers of people with dementia often are multicomponent, are tailored to the caregivers and persons with dementia, and have multiple mechanisms of action. Cognitive reframing is an important element of cognitive behavioral therapy (CBT) interventions, often used to reduce stress, depression, and anxiety. In dementia care, cognitive reframing interventions may focus on changing caregivers' beliefs about their care recipient's behaviors and their own performance as caregivers that are maladaptive, self-defeating, or distressing. A Cochrane Review of effects of cognitive reframing interventions for family caregivers of people with dementia examined effects on caregiver stress and mental health. Results indicated a beneficial effect of these interventions on caregiver anxiety, depression, and subjective stress, but no effects were seen on caregiver coping, appraisal of the burden of caregiving, reactions to the behaviors of the person with dementia, or institutionalization of the person with dementia (Vermooji-Dassen, Draskovic, McClery, & Downs, 2011).

Often, interventions focused on helping caregivers manage the challenging behaviors of the person with dementia promote caregiver well-being. A recent study examined the effects of behavioral activation for dementia caregivers that involved scheduling pleasant events and enhancing communications. Behavioral activation and psychoeducational interventions provided more than eight biweekly sessions that led to increased relationship satisfaction and decreased depressed mood for dementia caregivers when compared with the effects of the psychoeducational intervention (Au et al., 2015).

A Cochrane Review of studies of functional analysis-based interventions for challenging behavior in dementia examined the effects of approaches that explore the meaning or purpose of an individual's behavior, extending the activator–behavior–consequences (ABC) approach of behavioral analysis to allow for more than a single explanatory hypothesis for the person's behavior. Often, these interventions are taught to caregivers to manage agitation and aggression. Typically, a therapist develops and evaluates strategies that aid family and staff caregivers to reduce a person's distress and associated challenging behaviors. Analysis of trials that were conducted predominantly in family care settings revealed that functional analysis was one of many components of the care program. Overall, these types of interventions tended to reduce the frequency of challenging behaviors and improve the caregiver reaction, but not their experience of burden or depression. The effects were short lived in these studies (Moniz et al., 2012).

A well-established program of research incorporating functional analysis approaches is the STAR-C program, which has been translated recently for use in community-based settings. Teri et al. (2012) used the ABC approach to behavioral analysis, engaging caregivers in identifying the ABC relationships as a basis for generating problem-solving strategies. The STAR-C program exposes family members to dementia education, effective communication, and implementation of pleasant activities to reduce mood and behavioral disturbances. Strategies to improve their own well-being and reduce adverse reactions to challenging behaviors also are provided in eight weekly sessions in the care recipient's home with four monthly phone calls. In translating the program to a community-based setting, Teri et al. (2012) reduced the intervention to eight weekly sessions. Outcomes included reduction in caregiver depression, burden and reactivity to care recipients' behavior problems, the latter of which was maintained across 6 months. Reductions in depression and better quality of life were important outcomes for care recipients. Caregivers expressed high satisfaction with STAR-C.

Interventions specifically focused on the caregiver often include stress management strategies. Lewis et al. (2009) developed and trialed a stress-busting program (SBP) for caregivers who were providing care for a family member with dementia. The SBP included education, stress management, problem solving, and support delivered in a group setting over 9 weeks. Caregivers experienced improvements in general health, vitality, social function, and mental health and decreases in anxiety, anger/hostility, depression, perceived stress, and caregiver burden. Investigators concluded that when weighed with the potential cost of increased use of acute care and institutionalization of the care recipient, the program was a cost-effective health-promotion strategy for caregivers who manage substantial ongoing stress (Lewis et al., 2009).

Interventions to promote self-care among caregivers have focused on promoting caregiver physical activity and sleep. McCurry, Gibbons, Logsdon, Vitiello, and Teri (2009) found that caregivers for persons with dementia who reported sleep problems at the beginning of a longitudinal study had worse scores on caregiver burden, memory, and measures of quality of life. In addition, sleep quality was reduced by caregiver depression as well as care recipient characteristics, such as amount of assistance needed with ADL. McCurry et al. (2009) studied the effects of standard sleep hygiene, stimulus control, and sleep-compression (limiting time in bed for sleep) strategies, plus education about community resources, stress management, and ABC training to reduce disruptive behaviors. Caregivers' sleep improved immediately after treatment and at 3 months after treatment. King, Baumann, O'Sullivan, Wilcox, and Castro (2002) also studied ways to promote caregiver sleep, comparing a moderate-intensity exercise intervention with a nutrition education attention control condition. Caregivers exercised (walking) for four 30- to 40-minute periods weekly for 1 year. Those who exercised experienced improved sleep and lower systolic blood pressure at the end of the year.

Another important option for some caregivers is the use of respite care, an intervention designed to provide relief to caregivers. A Cochrane Review of intervention studies indicated that there was no difference between the use and the nonuse of respite care in several outcomes, including rates of institutionalization of the person with dementia and caregiver burden. There were few studies available to evaluate, so further evidence is needed about the effects of respite care on caregivers and care recipients, including consideration of the type, duration, and nature of respite services (Maayan, Soares-Weiser, & Lee, 2014).

As indicated earlier, many intervention programs for caregivers of people with dementia incorporate multiple components that reflect the multiple complex needs of both persons in the dyad. Education, emotional support, social network enhancement, and interventions to change the care recipient's behaviors are commonly directed at enhancing caregiver coping efforts and well-being. In some approaches, they are combined with more complex behavioral strategies, such as incorporated in functional analysis approaches of the care recipient's behavior.

Multicomponent interventions present challenges for translation beyond research projects to practice arenas, such as clinical and social service agencies. Gitlin, Marx, Stanlye, and Hodgson (2015) estimate that more than 200 caregiver interventions have been reviewed from 1966 to 2013, but few have been translated into practice. Some of the treatment modalities in the programs that have been evaluated include professional and informal support, psychoeducational interventions, behavior management/skills training, counseling/psychotherapy, self-care/relaxation techniques, and environmental redesign. In addition, care management, specific disease education, skills to manage dependencies in functional ADL, strategies specific to managing behavioral symptoms, and activities to effectively engage patients have been evaluated. Gitlin et al. (2010, 2015) asserts that meaningful benefits to caregivers are often unclear in these studies and that long-term effectiveness, cost-effectiveness, and populations for whom the interventions are most effective remain undefined. Moreover, development and testing of the interventions most often occurs outside of the traditional care systems used for people with dementia. Thus translation of research is of high priority to make programs accessible. Programs that have been evaluated in translational studies include the Skills Care Intervention (Gitlin, Jacobs, & Earland, 2010) that led to the improvement in caregiver knowledge and skills, including their ability to understand memory loss and ways to engage the care recipient; confidence managing behaviors of the care recipient; and self-care. The Resources for Enhancing Alzheimer's Caregiver Health (REACH) program (Nichols, Martindale-Adams, Burns, Graney, & Zuer, 2011) and a version translated by the Veterans Affairs (REACH-VA; Easom, Alston, & Coleman, 2013) improved caregiver burden, depression, impact of depression in everyday life, and frustration, health and confidence in caregiving skills. The Reducing Disability in Alzheimer's Disease (RDAD; Menne et al., 2014; Teri et al., 2012) and STAR Community Consultants (STAR-C; McCurry et al., 2015) programs led to improvements in caregiver strains and reduction of unmet caregiver needs.

Considering all of the interventions that have been translated for care systems or communities, Gitlin et al. (2015) concluded that most have improved caregiver outcomes. Among these outcomes are caregivers' competence, confidence, knowledge, skills, social support, tangible assistance, reaction to care recipient behaviors, caregiver strain, improvement of care recipient activity, positive aspects of caregiving, depression, and self-care. The availability of interventions such as these through community organizations, such as the Alzheimer's Association, Area Agencies on Aging, and others can be a significant resource for caregivers.

Caregiver interventions have been delivered using a variety of media, with many intensive interventions delivered by a professional in the home. Given the difficulty some caregivers experience in arranging respite care for the care recipient, use of approaches that do not require caregivers to leave the home is potentially valuable. An increasing interest in the use of Internet-based interventions for caregivers of people with dementia is evident. The Internet intervention, Mastery Over Dementia (MOD; Blom, Zarit, Zwaaftink, Cuijpers, & Pot, 2015), was evaluated recently in comparison with minimal intervention consisting of e-bulletins. MOD is an innovative guided self-help Internet course designed to reduce caregivers' symptoms of depression and anxiety. MOD was developed using findings from reviews that identified effective face-to-face interventions to diminish caregivers' mental health symptoms, including psychoeducation and active participation of the caregiver, management of behavioral problems, coping strategies, cognitive behavior therapy that included cognitive reframing, and an increase in social support. MOD involved caregivers in eight lessons and a booster session with guidance from a coach, who monitored progress and evaluated homework. The course topics included coping with behavioral problems by solving problems, relaxing, arranging help from others, changing nonhelping thoughts (cognitive restructuring), and communicating with others (assertiveness training). The e-bulletins were provided to the comparison group over a 6-month period. Topics included driving, holiday breaks, medication, legal affairs, activities throughout the day, help with daily routines, safety measures in the home, and possibilities for peer support, but there was no contact with a coach. Effects on depression and anxiety were significantly greater for the Internet course than for the e-bulletins alone.

Interventions for Caregivers of People With Cancer

Cancer represents a life-threatening and life-changing illness for many families, and several interventions for caregivers have been developed and tested. An Oncology Nursing Society–funded recent review of interventions for reducing strain and burden for family caregivers of patients with cancer revealed several categories of useful interventions. Among these were psychoeducational, supportive, psychotherapy, cognitive, and behavioral interventions; massage; healing touch; respite or adult day care; and multicomponent models (Honea et al., 2008).

Psychoeducational interventions include structured programs of information for caregivers that include teaching about the person's disease process, symptom management, psychosocial issues, caregiving resources, coordination of services, and caregiver self-care. These interventions are offered in group formats and may include lectures by people trained to deliver the intervention, opportunity for discussion with other caregivers, and often, written materials for reference. Support may also be part of these interventions.

Supportive interventions focus on building rapport with caregivers and creating opportunities for discussing difficult caregiving issues, successes, and feelings regarding caregiving. Mutual support, among caregivers includes not only emotional support, but also instrumental support such as strategies for caregiving and problem-solving opportunities.

Psychotherapy is another option for caregivers and typically involves individual counseling with a professional related to strategies for managing distress. This service may be particularly valuable for caregivers who have a past conflicted relationship with the care recipient, such as a history of abuse. Cognitive behavioral strategies engage caregivers in learning self-monitoring, addressing negative thoughts and assumptions, promoting problem solving, and encouraging engagement in pleasant experiences.

Caregiving work often includes physical work, and some therapies focus on the caregiver's body. Therapeutic massage uses manipulation of soft tissues to induce relaxation. Healing touch involves noninvasive approaches that use hands to balance human energy fields. Respite care provides services inside or outside of the home and may include assistance with ADL or skilled care with the aim of giving the caregiver time away from caregiving.

An Oncology Nursing Society Putting Evidence Into Practice (PEP) project team concluded that no single intervention could be recommended for nursing practice for caregiver strain or burden based on studies published before their review (up to 2006). Interventions likely to be effective included psychoeducational, psychotherapy, and supportive programs (2008).

A more recent meta-analysis of interventions for family caregivers of people with cancer indicated that several have efficacy on different caregiver outcomes (Northouse, Katapodi, Song, Zhang, & Mood, 2010). Types of interventions included psychoeducational support, skills training, and therapeutic counseling, with some including multiple components. In addition, some trials included content for caregivers that addressed the caregivers' own needs for self-care as well as those of the care recipient. Caregiver outcomes examined included three domains: illness appraisal, coping resources, and quality of life. Interventions in the illness appraisal domain addressed appraisal of caregiving burden, caregiving benefit, and information needs. Small effects of interventions on caregiving burden and caregiving benefit were noted, but large and significant effects of interventions on caregivers' appraisal of their information needs were evident. Interventions in the coping resources domain addressed enhancing active coping strategies, such as problem solving and/or reducing ineffective coping. Persistent moderate effects were evident. In addition, interventions in the coping resources domain focused on increasing self-efficacy, including ability to manage symptoms and provide care, and had small but persistent effects. Interventions in the quality-of-life domain focused on enhancing physical functioning by promoting performance of caregivers' self-care behaviors, such as increasing exercise and improving sleep. These had small but persistent effects. Other quality-of-life interventions that focused on reducing distress and anxiety had small but persistent effects beyond 6 months after intervention. In contrast, interventions did not reduce caregivers' depression. Interventions focused on promoting marital or sexual satisfaction, family support, and couple communication had small, immediate effects, but these did not persist beyond the first few months after intervention. Interventions that focused on social functioning of caregivers led to delayed effects with family members, friends, and peers that did not occur until after 6 months after the intervention (Northouse et al., 2010).

Most of the interventions reviewed by Northouse were delivered jointly or separately to patients and family. Taken together, the results of the studies indicated that multiple outcomes were affected by the interventions, most of which were multidimensional. The timing of different effects varied, likely influenced by the time necessary for caregivers to make changes in order to achieve caregiver benefits, such as those focused on improvement in physical or social function. Sustained effects for some interventions included changes in coping strategies, sense of self-efficacy, and distress/anxiety outcomes. Large effects were observed for increases in knowledge. Limited translation of these interventions to practice settings was noted (Northouse et al., 2010).

Since the Oncology Nursing Society Review was published in 2008, an array of new interventions has been studied for caregivers. Modes of delivery of interventions for caregivers are variable and include in-person individual and group formats, telephonic intervention, online interventions, and interactive health communication technologies (IHCTs) that make use of Internet 2.0/social media types of applications. The emerging use of technology in providing support to caregivers is providing access to an array of new interventions.

IHCTs are being used to deliver psychosocial interventions to couples and families. Badr, Carmack, and Diefenbach (2015) found evidence from a systematic review that incorporating IHCTs in psychosocial interventions with cancer patients and their caregivers was feasible and in some, effective. Of note is the Comprehensive Health Enhancement Support System (CHESS), an extensively studied IHCT with information, support, and coaching components that together facilitate decision making and communication with caregivers (Gustafson et al., 2013). Of the multiple features to provide tailored cancer information are "Ask an Expert," recent news, and resource guide. Support is provided through facilitated bulletin boards, written and video accounts of how other patients and families cope, and interactive tools, including decision-making support, action planning, skills building for easing distress, and journaling. Clinicians are able to receive a report of the patient's health status and questions for the next visit from either the patient or the caregiver. The version of CHESS for lung cancer (CHESS-LC) patients and their caregivers was successful in reducing caregiver burden and negative mood after 6 months use when compared with Internet-only interventions (DuBenske et al., 2014).

CHESS exemplifies an IHCT in a comprehensive interactive system. In addition IHCTs are being developed and tested to facilitate treatment decision making, enhance patient–caregiver communication, and promote lifestyle behavior change (Badr et al., 2015). Nonetheless, of all the caregiver interventions reviewed for cancer care, the multicomponent interventions were rated as most likely to be effective because they use a variety of techniques to reduce burden and thus are able to address a variety of needs. (Honea et al., 2008).

Interventions for Caregivers of People With Chronic Illnesses

Caregiver interventions for those providing care for people who have experienced a chronic illness with consequent disability, such as stroke or congestive heart failure, have also been developed and tested. With the aging of the population and anticipated increased prevalence of complex chronic illnesses requiring caregiver support, these programs will increase in importance.

Stroke often leads to severe and long-term disability for survivors and presents family caregivers with significant challenges. Family caregivers often experience stress, challenges related to rehabilitation, and health concerns for themselves, as well as depression. Recognizing the risk of depression for stroke caregivers as well as stroke survivors, McLennon, Bakas, Jessup, Habermann, and Weaver (2014) investigated perceived task difficulty and life changes among stroke caregivers who experienced mild to moderate depressive symptoms shortly after discharge of the care recipient who had survived stroke. Caregivers with more depressive symptoms reported more difficulty performing tasks and worse life changes. In addition, the gender of the caregivers (female) and their number of chronic illnesses, as well as the effects of survivor mobility and thinking, were associated with depressive symptoms. Among the most difficult tasks were arranging care while away, providing personal care and emotional support, watching and monitoring the stroke survivor, talking with health care providers, assisting with walking, coordinating care, and providing transportation (McLennon et al., 2014).

Despite challenges associated with providing care to stroke survivors, stroke caregivers reported positive aspects of their roles, as revealed by a recent systematic review. Mackenzie and Greenwood (2012) found that perceptions of improvements in the survivor's physical condition, including being able to prevent deterioration and seeing the care recipient being well cared for, were sources of positive experiences. In addition, progress or recovery indicators were sources of pride and satisfaction. Strengthened relationships, feelings of love, and other positive emotions were seen as positive dimensions of caregiving, as was feeling appreciated by the care recipient and the community. These experiences were described as giving meaning to life and reciprocation for past caring. Identifying what was important in life as well as learning new skills and ways of managing difficulties were associated with caregivers' self-esteem and perceptions of strength and mastery. Seeing more positive aspects of caregiving increased over time as caregivers gained more experience (Mackenzie & Greenwood, 2012).

Cheng, Chair, and Chau (2014) conducted a meta-analysis of psychosocial interventions for stroke family, examined effects of psychoeducation and social support groups on caregiver burden, caregiving competency, depression, anxiety, social support, family functioning, physical health, quality of life, satisfaction with the intervention, and use of health services. Limited numbers of studies precluded clear conclusions, but the effects of psychoeducation that focused on improving caregivers' family functioning were small. Training in problem solving and stress coping when offered by telephone may reduce depression and enhance sense of competency of caregivers, but evidence was not sufficient to recommend this approach. Nonetheless, equipping caregivers with caregiving skills was associated with the reduced use of health care resources for stroke survivors (Cheng et al., 2014).

A recently published statement by the American Heart Association and American Stroke Association examined evidence for stroke family caregiver and dyad interventions

(Bakas et al., 2014). Reviewing 17 caregiver intervention studies and 15 caregiver–survivor dyad interventions, investigators focused on determining whether family caregivers and dyad interventions improved stroke survivor and caregiver outcomes, as well as focused on the types of interventions that were most effective. Caregiver outcomes included:

- Preparedness—confidence, self-efficacy, competence, quality of care
- Burden, stress, and strain—task difficulty of care, threat appraisal, and mood
- Anxiety and depression
- Quality of life, including life changes
- Social function—social activity, family functioning
- Coping—confronting, social support, problem solving, optimism
- Service use—health care visits
- Knowledge and satisfaction

The nature of interventions for caregivers included three main categories: skill building, psychoeducation, and support. Skill-building interventions involved processes to facilitate problem solving, goal setting, and communication with health care providers; stress management; hands-on training, such as lifting and assisting with ADL; and communication tailored to the stroke survivor's needs. Psychoeducational interventions focused on providing information such as warning signs of impending stroke, lifestyle changes, and resources, as well as managing survivor emotions, medications and personal care, finances and transportation, and the emotions and health care needs of the stroke survivor. Support interventions included interactions with peers for emotional support and advice, offered through support groups or online discussion forums. A combination of skill building and psychoeducational interventions resulted in positive caregiver outcomes. Psychoeducational interventions alone increased caregiver knowledge, but did not offer improvement in caregiver depression or quality of life. As with interventions for dementia and cancer caregivers, multicomponent approaches appear to be most effective. In addition, offering interventions, both in person as well as via telephone, was associated with more positive effects than either alone, but further investigation is needed of the mode by which the intervention is offered, including the use of Internet-based approaches for this population. Information alone cannot address the complex needs of caregivers (Rodriguez-Gonzalo, Garcia-Marti, Ocana-Colorado, Baquera-De Micheo, & Morel-Fernandez, 2015).

Recommendations with the strongest level of evidence based on this review include interventions with these elements:

- Combining skill building (e.g., problem solving, stress management) with psychoeducational strategies versus interventions with only psychoeducational strategies
- Tailoring or individualizing to the needs of stroke caregivers versus using nontailored approaches
- Delivering information face to face and/or by telephone (Forster et al., 2012)
- Consisting of five to nine sessions

With the growing prevalence of heart failure among older adults, there is an increasing emphasis on interventions for caregivers who are assuming responsibility for their care (Stamp et al., 2015). Investigators have studied the experiences of spouses or partners of people living with advanced heart failure, learning that spouses with higher levels of perceived control had greater levels of well-being and that older spouses enjoyed greater levels of well-being than younger ones. Dracup et al. (2004) recommended that interventions, including information and counseling directed toward enhancing the spouse caregiver's level of control, would be advantageous.

Sullivan et al. (2015) identified three areas of needs among family caregivers of people with heart failure, including competence, compassion, and care of the self. Competence concerns included those related to the ability to perform caregiving tasks safely. Caregivers expressed worry about doing things right, making a serious mistake, and being uncertain about their ability to be a family caregiver. Their descriptions of their concerns included worry about harming the person with heart failure (e.g., giving the wrong medications). They also described vigilance behaviors, such as monitoring activity and dietary restriction, regulating patients' activities, preventing activities, and engaging in anticipatory helping behaviors. In addition, caregivers were concerned about their ability to maintain compassion and provide emotional support to the person with heart failure. A final theme, care of the self, related to caregivers' abilities to juggle multiple responsibilities, obtain personal care for themselves, and have some modicum of escape in which to maintain fitness and well-being (Sullivan et al., 2015). Confidence was an overarching consideration of caregivers in another study and was associated with quality of life in patients and social support of caregivers (Lyons et al., 2015).

In a later study, Imes, Dougherty, Pyper, and Sullivan (2011) conducted in-depth semi-structured interviews with partners of individuals with severe heart failure. They found that the severity of heart failure limited the partner's lifestyle with consequent social isolation and difficulties in planning for the future. Partners were not prepared to manage the disease burden at home in the absence of consistent information and support by health care providers. Moreover, EOL planning was not encouraged by health care providers, nor was it embraced by the patients or partners. Partners focused on symptoms, disease course and duration, dying, and the future as the most difficult for them to manage, and these factors required emotional adaptation on their part. As an example, inactivating an implantable cardiac defibrillator (ICD) at or near the time of death emerged as an issue that needed to be addressed. These investigators suggest the development of multicomponent interventions, such as those for caregivers for people with dementia (e.g., REACH II discussed earlier in this chapter; Imes et al., 2011).

Caregiver intervention trials for heart failure are limited but have included several dimensions. A trial of integrated dyad care compared usual care with a psychoeducational intervention delivered in three modules over a 12-week period through nurse-led, face-to-face counseling, computer-based education, and other written teaching materials (Ågren, Evangelista, Hjelm, & Strömberg, 2012). The modules included cognitive, support, and behavioral components, as well as teaching materials over the three sessions. These addressed topics such as the definition of heart failure, medications, symptom management, and lifestyle modification, as well as direction of care, relationships, and sexual activities. In addition, support components included patients' and partners' need for support and caregiver burden. Behavioral components included intentions, abilities, and self-efficacy related to self-care, barriers to lifestyle modification, and strategies to improve or maintain self-care behavior. There were no significant effects of the interventions on the partners of heart failure patients, but the skill-building and problem-solving education and psychosocial support was effective in enhancing patients' level of perceived control. Additional trials are needed to evaluate the impact of being a family caregiver for heart failure patients.

Interventions for Caregivers of Children With Chronic Illnesses

Parent caregivers of children with chronic and acute illness experience unique sets of challenges as they integrate the roles of parent and caregiver. A recent review of studies on caregivers of children with chronic illness indicated that they report significantly greater parenting stress than do caregivers of healthy children. Greater general parenting stress was related to greater parental responsibility for treatment management but was not related to illness duration and severity across illness populations (Cousino & Hazen, 2013).

In a recent integrative review of nursing research about parenting children with complex chronic conditions (CCCs) spanning 2002 to 2012, Rehm (2013) identified a wide array of impacts of providing care for children with CCCs in the home. Among these were emotional impacts (stress, worry, fear, anxiety, and feelings of being overwhelmed, including depression symptoms) and positive impact (rewards of parenting a child with a CCC, commitment to the child and role in providing care, pride, empowerment, and personal growth in achievements as caregivers, increased empathy for others, and increased closeness to family members). In addition, Rehm identified parental role challenges that included facing conflict between the role as a parent and as a caregiver, difficulty in switching from the affectionate parent to the technical/procedural caregiver, legal barriers to decision making for foster parents, and inadequate preparation for care provision. Family members also reported challenges related to working with health care providers that for some, included changes in their home life when professional providers were always present; constrained communication, affection, privacy, and discipline in the presence of the professional caregivers; negotiations to clarify parental roles versus nursing roles; and lack of clarity of roles for parents and nurses when the child was hospitalized. Another set of themes in this literature was efforts at normalizing family life that were parental efforts to emphasize the normal aspects of life when complete normalization was not possible because of ongoing demands, the intrusiveness of equipment, and stigma. The impact on social relationships and activities families reported included isolation when parents were unable to leave home because of care demands, difficulty arranging child care or respite care because of the child's complex care needs, stigmatizing aspects of the child's

condition, constrained interactions with family and friends, and excursions from home requiring extensive planning and needs for equipment for providing ongoing care. This body of literature also revealed moral implications associated with parenting children with CCCs. Rehm identified parents' concerns about the unfairness of their situations, lack of viable alternatives to home care for children with CCCs, parents' unwillingness to live without their child, and shifts of responsibility and expenses to families from the health care system and society. This extensive review underscores the challenges that face parents who are simultaneously caregivers for children with CCCs.

Kieckhefer et al. (2014) developed and evaluated the Building Family Strengths Program, an educational program provided in the context of a social and supportive environment of parents and facilitators, for parents of children with a variety of chronic health conditions whose children ranged in age from 2 to 11 years. Parents were exposed to seven sessions of a curriculum derived from the Chronic Disease Self-Management Program produced by the Stanford Patient Education Research Center that included an array of topics: impact of living with a childhood chronic illness; emotional dimensions of parenting a child with chronic illness; impact of chronic illness on the child; impact on relationships and family communication; impact on parenting; work with large systems and discovery of resources; skills for effective partnering and shared decision making within the family; and transitions, finding meaning and approaching the future with confidence. These topics were explored using a variety of facilitation techniques, among these brief presentations by cofacilitators related to knowledge, topically structured parent discussions, facilitated peer exchange information and insights, modeling by the co-facilitators providing examples of newly learned skills, and parent development of weekly individualized action plans promoting their practice of the new skills. The intent of these approaches was to honor and encourage the unique support that parents could offer to one another within the context of the curriculum. The processes encouraged parents to practice positive, practical coping strategies and supported them in determining how they could involve their child in developmentally appropriate ways in shared management tasks.

At baseline 56% of parents had high depressive symptoms, which improved significantly when measured 6 months after treatment. In addition, parents experienced improved self-efficacy to manage their child's condition, coping, and family quality of life. Parent–child shared management also increased, but the change was not statistically significant. Most parents completed all or all but one class (86%; Kieckhefer et al., 2014).

A Cochrane Review of psychological interventions for parents of children and adolescents with chronic illnesses, including painful conditions, cancer, diabetes mellitus, asthma, traumatic brain injury, and skin disorders, revealed a limited number of studies. The average age of children in these studies was 14.6 years. Results were analyzed according to disease and by treatment classes that included CBT, family therapy (FT), problem-solving therapy (PST), and multisystemic therapy (MST). Parent behavior and parent mental health outcomes were assessed in relation to the types of therapies. Across all conditions PST led to improved adaptive parenting in families with children with cancer after treatment and improved parent mental health. There were no effects of CBT and limited or no data on FT or MST (Eccleston, Fisher, Law, Bartlett, & Palermo, 2015).

Interventions for Caregivers Providing EOL Care

The aging of populations across the globe has prompted societies to rethink EOL care, with shifting emphasis from cure to palliative care and from institution-based care to care at home, with most approaches dependent on caregiving provided by family members. Palliative care practice has stimulated research about pain and symptom management as well as support for dying individuals and families (see Grady & Gough, 2015; McGuire, Grant, & Park, 2012). Promoting death with dignity has guided the development of new models of care, most of which include family members, in particular, family caregivers.

Caregiver well-being is key to providing palliative/end-of-life (P/EOL) care at home. Williams et al. (2011) noted that efforts to promote caregiver well-being have included grief counseling, educational workshops, and group interventions to provide peer support. Individual countries have created fiscal policy to support P/EOL caregivers, including paid employment leave to care for family members in Canada (Compassionate Care Benefits) and provisions for unpaid leave for some employees in the United States (Family and Medical Leave Act). Caregivers providing P/EOL care face many of the same challenges as those who care for chronically ill family members, including providing for physical care needs; managing complex symptoms; organizing and coordinating care from health professionals and others; acting as a spokesperson, advocate, or proxy; and providing spiritual, emotional, and psychological support. Like other caregivers, P/EOL caregivers experience positive outcomes, as well as burden, strain, and health effects associated with caregiving. Women caregivers tend to experience more demands owing to their multiple roles and strain among them linked to caregiving demands. In addition to stressful roles and role strain, caregivers also experience financial stress, challenges related to lack of family or friendly work environments that allow flexibility and absences to provide care, and lack of available health and social services. McGhan, Loeb, Baney, and Penrod (2013) studied older adult women providing EOL are, identifying several challenges they faced:

- Balancing multiple morbidities of the care recipient that contribute to the complexity of caregiving
- Feeling overwhelmed and exhausted from always being "on" and being unable to deal with their own health issues
- Dealing with personal health issues, such as fitting their own care into EOL care and having less opportunity for outside activities and relationships
- Feeling isolated from family and friends as care demands escalate
- Coordinating care for the care recipient and themselves across systems and multiple health care providers, many of whom focused only on their specialty (McGhan et al., 2013).

Although the population receiving P/EOL care is growing, little is known about the effects of caregiving on caregiver outcomes. Hoefman, Al-Janabi, McCaffrey, Currow, and Ratcliffe (2015) evaluated caregiver outcomes in palliative care, identifying both caregiver experiences of care and caregiver quality of life as important features. Caregiver experiences incorporated into a Carer Experience Scale included caregiver appraisals of the impact of P/EOL care on activities outside of caring, such as socializing, physical activity, and hobbies; support from family and friends, such as personal help in caring or emotional support; assistance from organizations and government, such as help from voluntary groups with respite and practical information; fulfillment from caregiving, such as positive feelings; control over caregiving; and a successful relationship with the care recipient, such as being able to talk and discuss issues without arguing. In addition, the investigators assessed caregiver quality of life by asking caregivers to appraise the extent to which they experienced fulfillment from carrying out care tasks, relational problems with care recipient, problems with their own mental health, problems combining care tasks with their own daily activities, financial problems related to care tasks, support with carrying out care tasks when needed, and problems with their own physical health. Higher negative effects of caregiving experiences were associated with higher negative effects on caregiver quality of life. Lower scores on both were associated with less strain from caregiving, more positive care experiences, and less process utility (reflected in ratings of happiness if all of the caregiving tasks were taken over by another person who would provide all care free of charge at his or her own house).

McGuire et al. (2012) reviewed the literature published between 2006 and 2011 on caregivers providing palliative and EOL care. They found that interventions addressed education and support, including coping skills training; psychoeducational group programs; family meetings; and psychosocial support in the form of visits, educational modules, nurse phone services, and online support. Results supported a need for further development of interventions and studies of their effectiveness for P/EOL caregivers.

Of note is a research program conducted by Hudson and Aranda (2014), the Melbourne Family Support Program. Hudson and Aranda (2014) tested a program of psychoeducational interventions using four psychoeducational interventions, incorporating one-to-one and group format delivery in home and inpatient hospital/hospice settings. Outcomes included family caregivers' preparedness, competence, positive emotions, psychological well-being, and reduction in unmet needs.

In a randomized controlled clinical trial of one-to-one home-based psychoeducation delivered by a nurse, preparedness, competence, rewards, unmet needs, and psychological distress were evaluated. Caregivers were also given a guidebook. Results indicated improvement in preparedness and competence at 2 weeks after the intervention and lessening of psychological distress at 2 months after the patient's death. In an earlier pilot study, positive outcomes were maintained several months after the intervention, and participants reported the positive impact of the program on their lives (Hudson et al., 2008).

Interventions to provide P/EOL caregiver peer support, individual and group counseling, psychoeducation, respite care, and home care are being studied in relation to outcomes, such as caregiver knowledge, personal renewal, community support, and health promotion and prevention of health problems of caregivers. Reduced burden in this population may be associated with efforts to provide caregivers encouragement, assistance, and emotional support, and personal health practices and coping strategies have been enhanced by teaching caregivers coping strategies and health-enhancing behaviors (Williams et al., 2011). Although limited information is available specific to caregivers of children with acute and chronic illness or EOL care, these areas of science are growing. Future research in these areas would be extremely helpful for caregivers whose focus is on children or EOL care, as targeted interventions might provide resources for information, respite care, or additional helpful ways to manage this care.

Health Policy and Caregiving

Policies supportive of family caregivers have been developed. Canada's Compassionate Care Benefits (CCB) offer full-time workers meeting criteria the option to contribute to family caregiving by providing 6 weeks of income support with a 2-week unpaid waiting period before payments begin, with payments of up to 55% of regular earnings, up to a maximum of $457 (Canadian dollars) per week. Job security is ensured for 8 weeks. These benefits can be shared between family members and the benefit can be taken consecutively or broken into shorter periods within a 26-week period. Nonetheless, an interview study of caregivers revealed that the CCB is not sustaining all informal P/EOL caregivers: Gender, income and social status, working conditions, health and social services, social support networks and personal practices, and coping strategies all influenced caregiver burden (Williams et al.,

2011). In the United States, the Family and Medical Leave Act provides support for caregivers that may include their ability to return to their employment when their caregiving is completed, although it does not provide for compensation of employees during the caregiving leave. The impact of the role of the Patient Protection and Affordable Care Act and further development of employment policy for caregivers remains to be evaluated as the population requiring caregiving from family members continues to grow.

◼ NEXT STEPS

Despite many studies of interventions developed for caregivers, the majority have addressed caregiver capacity to provide care (Table 18.1). Fewer efforts have focused on promoting caregiver well-being and health and preventing disease or injury. Missing from most intervention research are studies of the effects of financial strain and the physical challenges of caregiving for caregivers. Given the large number of older caregivers, managing symptoms and comorbidities of both the care recipient and the caregiver warrant increased attention by both researchers and policymakers.

In addition, a new area of investigation in caregiving will focus on multicultural caregiving and interventions that have been culturally tailored to specific populations of caregivers (Apesoa-Varano et al., in press). This effort will provide important perspectives to inform support for caregivers from the diverse cultural backgrounds of North America.

◼ PROMOTING CAREGIVER HEALTH

Assessment of Women Caregivers' Health

Central to clinical assessment of a caregiver's health is the consideration of the woman's age and personal and family

TABLE 18.1	Summary of Interventions for Caregivers	
INTERVENTIONS FOCUSED ON ENHANCING CAREGIVER CAPACITY TO PROVIDE CARE		**INTERVENTIONS FOCUSED ON CAREGIVER WELL-BEING AND HEALTH**
◼ Education: increase knowledge about disease ◼ Caregiving skills ◼ Functional analysis of challenging behaviors (e.g., ABC) ◼ Care coordination		◼ Stress management ◼ Cognitive strategies (e.g., reframing) ◼ Support (e.g., emotional) ◼ Counseling, psychotherapy ◼ Respite care ◼ Massage
INTERVENTIONS DIRECTED AT BOTH CAREGIVER AND CARE RECIPIENT		
◼ Problem solving related to needs of care recipient ◼ Interventions promoting pleasant events ◼ Interventions promoting physical activity ◼ Interventions promoting sleep and regulating activity ◼ Environmental redesign for care recipient (e.g., safety)		◼ Problem solving related to caregiver challenges ◼ Interventions promoting pleasant events ◼ Interventions promoting physical activity ◼ Interventions promoting caregiver sleep ◼ Environmental redesign (e.g., ergonomics of caregiver)

ABC, activator–behavior–consequences.

history. In addition, prevailing literature concludes that caregivers are more likely to experience depressive symptoms and have poorer physical health outcomes compared with noncaregivers (Pinquart & Sorensen, 2003; Schulz & Sherwood, 2008; Vitaliano et al., 2003). In most studies reporting increased risk to health, the poorer health outcomes are linked to stress. However, in a recent analysis of health consequences of caregiving, Roth et al. (2015) noted that caregivers experience symptoms of emotional distress possibly more related to watching a family member struggle with a medical condition and not to the stress of caregiving per se. Also, there is no clear evidence that caregiving presents increased risk for mortality (Roth et al., 2015), but clinicians must consider caregiver age and health status independent of caregiving tasks. Analysis of data from a national epidemiological study that matched caregivers with noncaregivers on multiple confounders that could bias caregiving–mortality association found that caregivers had an 18% survival advantage over a 6-year period compared with the matched noncaregivers (Roth et al., 2013). Certainly there is a prevailing view, despite these more recent findings across larger population-based analyses, that informal caregiving is a stressful obligation that is hazardous to caregivers' health (Administration on Aging, 2012; Carroll, 2013).

It would appear that the caregiver's interpretation of stress or strain associated with caregiving is a key factor. Population-based studies that report negative health consequences from caregiving are for those caregivers who report that their caregiving is stressful. For example, the widely cited interpretation of mortality rates for caregiving spouses of participants in the population-based Cardiovascular Health Study indicates that strained spouse caregivers were 63% more likely to die in the subsequent 4-year follow-up period than the spouses of nondisabled partners (Schulz & Beach, 1999). Of note, however, spouses who provided care but reported no caregiving strain had mortality rates similar to spouses of nondisabled partners (Roth et al., 2015). In a large population-based study, it was found that 44% of spouse caregivers reported no strain (Schulz & Beach, 1999), and in another study, 17% of caregivers reported a lot of strain, and 33% reported no strain (Roth et al., 2009). When *stress* is defined as a relationship between the person and environment that is interpreted by the person as taxing or exceeding personal resources and endangering well-being (Lazarus & Folkman, 1984), it is understandable that caregivers who are confident that they have sufficient resources to manage caregiving situations do not feel stressed (Roth et al., 2015). Alternatively, caregivers might report high levels of stress if they have less-than-adequate information, skills, coping behaviors, help from other family, or formal care resources.

Assessment of Physical and Emotional Health

Because there are conflicting viewpoints on the risks associated with caregiving, clinicians must assess all aspects of a caregiving woman's physical and mental health based on age and individual circumstances. Special attention should be paid to her personal and family health history, relationship to the person receiving care, and the hours per day engaged in caregiving. Screening must encompass cardiovascular disease and pertinent risk factors (hypertension, hypercholesterolemia, smoking, physical inactivity, overweight and obesity, diabetes), osteoporosis, cancer (breast, cervical, and colon), depression and anxiety, menopause transition and/or menstrual issues, and physical abuse by the person receiving care (Berg, Taylor, & Woods, 2015). Attention to all of these factors accommodates potential risks that may or may not be associated with informal caregiving. Moreover, an essential assessment step is to ask the caregiver if she has stress associated with caregiving as well to ask about the rewards she attributes to these activities. See Assessment and Screening of Caregivers' Health in Box 18.1.

There are a number of instruments to measure caregiver burden (Herbert, Bravo, & Preville, 2000), perceived benefits (Beach, Schulz, Yee, & Jackson, 2000), caregiving self-efficacy (Steffen, McKibbin, Zeiss, Gallagher-Thompson, & Bandura, 2007), and perceived social support (Krause, 1995; Krause & Borawski-Clark, 1995). The choice of instrument to use should be determined by the clinical setting and caregiver situation, use, and number of items because some are quite brief and others take more patient time. The assessment scale developed by Picot and Youngblut (1997) to assess external and internal rewards experienced by caregivers may be a useful tool for additional clinical assessment. On

BOX 18.1   ASSESSMENT AND SCREENING OF CAREGIVERS' HEALTH

Physical Health

- Cardiovascular disease
  - Hypertension
  - Hypercholesterolemia
  - Smoking
  - Physical inactivity
  - Overweight and obesity
  - Diabetes
- Osteoporosis
- Cancer
  - Breast
  - Cervical
  - Colon
- Menopause transition or menstrual issues
- Physical abuse

Emotional Health

- Depression
- Anxiety
- Caregiver stress
- Caregiver rewards

this scale, caregivers who scored high on rewards of caregiving scored lower on depression and caregiver burden. This 16-item revised scale is unidimensional and measures the positive consequences of caregiving with acceptable internal reliability consistency (0.8–0.83). Whichever instrument is selected should be intended to determine the caregiver's level of stress and coping, health-promotion practices, and resources, such as social support networks, economic resources, and care respite resources.

Health Promotion

Health promotion for women caregivers is multifaceted and ranges from living a healthy lifestyle, screening for common health conditions encountered as women age, employment, sexuality, accessing economic and respite resources, innovative support services and promoting positive body image and healthy self-esteem. Furthermore, mental health promotion and cultivation of healthy relationships are important aspects of health promotion in women caregivers (Berg et al., 2015) (see Box 18.2).

Living Healthy Lifestyle

Poor lifestyle behaviors include suboptimal diet, physical inactivity, and tobacco use (Mozaffarian et al., 2012). Challenges for women caregivers' healthy lifestyle activities relate to work-related roles, economic stability, health status, and caregiving activities (Moen, 1996; Moen, Dempster-McClain, & Williams, 1992). Multiple role challenges may affect a caregivers' engagement in physical activity and dietary behaviors and these are likely to have a significant effect on her overall healthy lifestyle choices (Berg et al., 2015). Caregivers may neither consider their own health compared with that of the person they take care of nor be encouraged to maintain their own health (Beach & White, 2015). Although there are multiple definitions of maintaining a healthy lifestyle, commonalities include preventing heart disease, cancer, diabetes, and a number of chronic diseases (Berg et al., 2015). The U.S. National Library of Medicine, National Institutes of Health (2013) define behaviors of a healthy lifestyle as:

- Do not smoke
- Exercise. To lose or keep off weight, get moderate exercise for at least 60 to 90 minutes on most days; to maintain health, get at least 30 minutes of exercise per day at least 5 d/wk
- Maintain a healthy weight, which for women is between 18.5 and 24.9 body mass index (BMI)
- Get checked for depression and treated if necessary
- For women with high cholesterol or triglyceride levels, take omega-3 fatty acid supplements
- Drink alcohol in moderation; limit intake to no more than one drink per day

Healthy lifestyle recommendations related to nutrition (Berg et al., 2015) include eat a diet rich in fruits, vegetables, and whole grains:

- Choose lean proteins (chicken, fish, beans, legumes)
- Eat low-fat dairy products
- Avoid sodium (salt) and fats found in fried foods, processed foods, and baked goods
- Eat fewer animal products that contain cheese, cream, or eggs
- Read labels and avoid saturated fats, partially hydrogenated or hydrogenated fats

Culture influences healthy lifestyle choices. In some cultures, engaging in physical activity is not promoted, and it is therefore difficult to motivate caregivers to adopt routine physical activity in these groups of women (Im, Lee, Chee, & Stuifbergen, 2011). Mexican American women place their own health below that of family, so engaging in positive health behaviors take the second place or even the last place (Berg, Cromwell, & Arnett, 2002). Hoffman, Lee, and Mendez-Luck (2012) found that caregiving is associated with poor health behaviors that put baby-boomer caregivers' health at risk in the long term. This may be attributed to caregivers' lack of social support (Ostwald, 2009), or it may be a result of caregiver burden that prevents engagement in health-promotion behaviors (Sisk, 2000).

Discussed previously, screening for physical and emotional health conditions is an important aspect of health promotion. Clinical guidelines related to cardiovascular disease and screening for risk factors (hypertension, hypercholesterolemia, smoking, physical inactivity), osteoporosis, common cancers in women (breast, cervical, colon, and lung), depression and anxiety, and menopause transition and menstrual issues are readily available. Less is understood about health promotion related to employment, sexuality, positive body image and healthy self-esteem, and healthy relationships.

Employment

Evidence suggests that paid employment improves the health of women who have positive attitudes toward employment (Repetti, Matthews, & Waldron, 1989). This may result from social support afforded in a work setting. However, for some women, paid employment may be related to overload or multiple role strain (Repetti et al., 1989) or resultant stress.

BOX 18.2   ELEMENTS OF CAREGIVER HEALTH PROMOTION

- Healthy lifestyle
- Screening for age-appropriate common physical and emotional health conditions
- Employment satisfaction
- Sexuality
- Accessibility of economic and respite resources
- Accessibility to innovative support services
- Promotion of positive body image
- Promotion of health self-esteem
- Promotion of emotional health and well-being
- Cultivation of healthy relationships

Also, there is some evidence that employment can lead to negative health behaviors, such as smoking, increased alcohol use, and more sedentary behavior (Hazuda, Haffner, Stern, & Eifler, 1988; Waldron, 1980). Informal caregivers often leave paid work for periods of time, work part time, or take low-paying jobs (Repetti et al., 1989), contributing to lost income, retirement or health insurance benefits (Berg & Woods, 2009). Therefore employment-related health promotion must weigh the benefits of employment versus role burden and stress. Already working women should be asked about job satisfaction and the number of roles they simultaneously occupy. Women whose employment is stressful might benefit from employment-related counseling and/or conflict resolution training, and clinicians need to have resources available to suggest to these women as a way to reduce situational stress (Berg et al., 2015).

Sexuality

Participation in partnered sexually intimate activities has been linked to increased social support and improvement in well-being (Praire, Scheier, Matthews, Chang, & Hess, 2011). An important aspect of health promotion related to sexuality is to ask women about their sexuality satisfaction and sexual partner. Caregiving women may be caring for their spouses, which may negatively affect engagement in sexual activity and her overall satisfaction with the sexual aspect of her health. This warrants open conversation with the clinician who must have counseling resources to offer. Women in troubled relationships need encouragement to seek counseling related to improving their relationship and self-esteem. It is important that clinicians make sexual assessments part of their routine examinations and be able to discuss sexual matters with their patients in an open and nonjudgmental manner (Berg et al., 2015).

Positive Body Image and Healthy Self-Esteem

Contemporary women are bombarded through the media about societal views of beauty and body image. Caregivers are also constantly reminded of what advertisers view as beautiful, which may underscore a belief that she varies from this image. An essential aspect of health promotion related to body image and self-esteem includes women working to obtain a self-identity independent of the views of others (Pearlman, 1993). One way to develop a self-identity is through assertiveness training, which may also bolster a more positive self-image (McBride, 1990). Apparently, women with values congruent with their behaviors and circumstances report more happiness, satisfaction, and comfort (Howell, 2001), and clinicians are integral to facilitating the process through assessment and counseling referrals as appropriate (American Counseling Association, 2004).

Health Promotion Related to Emotional Health

Caregivers are likely to have higher levels of stress, depression, and psychological distress than noncaregivers (Pinquart &

Sorensen, 2003; Roth et al., 2009, Schulz & Sherwood, 2008). Therefore it is important to assess depression and anxiety in those who report a new onset of symptoms and provide appropriate interventions. The first step in promoting emotional health is to assess for depression and anxiety and, if not present, reassure the caregiver that she does not have these clinical conditions. However, women with depressed mood or who report undue stress from their caregiving activities should be offered resources that may be helpful in alleviating these conditions. Overall, health promotion of emotional health involves all aspects of health promotion already suggested, particularly making healthy lifestyle choices related to nutrition and physical activity (Berg et al., 2015).

Health Promotion Related to Cultivating Healing Relationships

Relationships are key contributors to health. Zender and Olshansky (2015) note that women's relationships with spouses, parents, work colleagues, and friends actually interact with their own personalities and psychological makeup, genetic predispositions, history of relationships, and even physiology to affect health and well-being. Dictionary.com Unabridged (2013) defines *relationship* as a connection, association, or involvement. It is known that women grow toward relationships throughout life, and healthy development hinges on healthy interpersonal relationships (Jordan, Kaplan, Miller, Stiver, & Surrey, 1991). The ways in which relationships affect health are complex and include behavioral, psychosocial, and physiological/biological aspects (Zender & Olshansky, 2015). A greater degree of high-quality social interactions extends the life span; reduces morbidity from cardiovascular disease, depression, recovery from cancer, wound healing, autoimmune diseases, and inflammation-related diseases such as arthritis or kidney disease; improves quality of life; and promotes greater meaning of life for women (Cohen et al., 2007; Fagundes, Lindgren, & Kiecolt-Glaser, 2013; Strating, Suurmeijer, & Van Schuur, 2006; Uchino, 2006).

Health promotion related to relational health includes interventions to improve social engagement, relational capacity, or natural social networks (Cohen & Janicki-Deverts, 2009). One major aspect is to reduce social isolation and loneliness through group or one-on-one interventions. Many of these interventions provide activities and instrumental support by engaging women through active participation (Dickens, Richards, Greaves, & Campbell, 2011). For women caregivers, these interventions are more likely to be obtained through referrals to counseling or by linking caregivers with support groups that hold regular meetings and activities. That in itself affords the caregiving woman with activities that engage her with others.

It is known that relationships are often marred by disconnections and misunderstandings that breed conflict (Zender & Olshansky, 2015). Caregiving situations may involve conflicted relationships with the caregiver and the person or persons being cared for, other relatives and friends who have emotional investment, or health care providers or individuals who represent potential physical or economic resources for the caregiver. Each situation may require a different intervention to promote resolution, thus health care providers assess carefully and then prescribe referral resources that can improve relationship health. These resources may include counseling referrals, support group information, potential economic resources, and respite services.

Caring for Yourself While Caring for Others

Health care providers may overlook the importance of the caregiving woman's need to care for herself and avoid burnout defined as subjective burden related to caregiving. Tips for caring for yourself from Ask Medicare (https://www.medicare.gov/files/ask-medicare-caregiver-support.pdf), include (a) identifying local support services, (b) making connections with others, (c) asking for help, and (d) taking care of personal health through nutrition, regular exercise, and enjoyable activities.

Maslach and Jackson (1982) identified three aspects of burnout among workers in health settings: (a) emotional exhaustion, or loss of emotional resources and a lack of energy to invest in human relationships; (b) depersonalization of the individuals for whom one cares, which refers to a negative and indifferent attitude toward patients; and (c) personal accomplishments, which refer to feelings of self-efficacy and satisfaction in caring for patients. In burnout, a lack of personal accomplishments is the third aspect and may result from emotional exhaustion and depersonalization of patients (Maslach & Jackson, 1982, 1986).

In a study by Ybema, Kuijer, Hagedoorn, and Buunk (2002), higher perceptions of inequity were strongly associated with higher emotional exhaustion and depersonalization, and lower feelings of personal accomplishment. Their findings demonstrated that perceptions of equity or balance in the relationship between patients and their intimate partners are important for preventing caregiver burnout and enhancing positive experiences for the caregiving person. Therefore interventions might best target alleviating perceptions of inequity to reduce potential caregiver burnout (Ybema et al., 2002).

■ INNOVATIVE SUPPORT SERVICES AND RELATED ISSUES

Support services for caregivers do not always fall into the usual categories of physical, emotional, or financial support. Sometimes these services involve "how to" or other means for assisting in caregiving activities or to prevent caregiving burnout. Often the activities of caregiving require education or enlightenment as to how to do something. Support services might be related to demonstrating particular procedures or planning for issues that might come along. Financial issues resources might be related to how to manage money or plan for billing or managing another person's money. Medline Plus at www.nlm.nih.gov/medlineplus is an important website that lists additional resources under the category of related issues.

Related Issues

Resources for caregivers are abundantly available and range from educational to special resources for respite care, financial and legal issues, and skill building. These resources are ever changing, and it is important for clinicians to update their referral and resource lists quite regularly for the benefit of their caregiving patients. Overall, the literature related to caregiving and caregiving resources is growing, probably relative to the increased need for informal caregiving and recognition of caregivers' special needs. However, there are still many unmet needs for informal caregivers, and future research must target those gaps in knowledge, resources, and special assistance to relieve caregiving burden. At the same time, it is important to recognize that some caregivers report their caregiving role provides meaning and gives satisfaction in their lives. From these caregivers, clinicians can learn ways to enhance these in caregivers who report increased burden leading to physical and emotional health issues.

■ REFERENCES

Administration on Aging. (2012). *$1.3 billion to improve the health and independence of America's older adults*. Retrieved from www.acl.gov/NewsRoom/Press_Releases/archive/2012/March/2012_03_02.aspx

Ågren, S., Evangelista, L. S., Hjelm, C., & Strömberg, A. (2012). Dyads affected by chronic heart failure: A randomized study evaluating effects of education and psychosocial support to patients with heart failure and their partners. *Journal of Cardiac Failure, 18*(5), 359–366.

Alzheimer's Association. (2015). *Alzheimer's disease facts and figures*. Alzheimer's and dementia 2015. Retrieved from https://www.alz.org/facts/downloads/facts_figures_2015.pdf

American Counseling Association. (2004). *Midlife and beyond: Issues for aging women*. Retrieved from http://www.redorbit.com/news/health/109713/midlife_and_beyond_issues_for_aging_women

Anderson, L. A., Edwards, V. J., Pearson, W. S., Talley, R. C., Mcguire, L. C., & Andresen, E. M. (2013). Adult caregivers in the United States: Characteristics and differences in well-being, by caregiver age and caregiving status. *Preventing Chronic Disease, 10*, E135. doi:10.5888/pcd10.130090

Apesoa-Varano, E. C., Tang-Feldman, Y., Reinhard, S., Choula, R., & Young, H. M. (in press). Multi-cultural caregiving and caregiver interventions: A look back and a call for future action. *Generations, 39*(4), 39–48. Retrieved from http://www.aarp.org/ppi/issues/caregiving

Archbold, P. G., Stewart, B. J., Greenlick, M. R., & Harvath, T. (1990). Mutuality and preparedness as predictors of caregiver role strain. *Research in Nursing & Health, 13*(6), 375–384.

Archbold, P. G., Stewart, B. J., Miller, L. L., Harvath, T. A., Greenlick, M. R., Van Buren, L.,…Schook, J. E. (1995). The PREP system of nursing interventions: A pilot test with families caring for older members. Preparedness (PR), enrichment (E) and predictability (P). *Research in Nursing & Health, 18*(1), 3–16.

Au, A., Gallagher-Thompson, D., Wong, M. K., Leung, J., Chan, W. C., Chan, C. C.,…Chan, K. (2015). Behavioral activation for dementia caregivers: Scheduling pleasant events and enhancing communications. *Clinical Interventions in Aging, 10*, 611–619.

Badr, H., Carmack, C. L., & Diefenbach, M. A. (2015). Psychosocial interventions for patients and caregivers in the age of new communication technologies: Opportunities and challenges in cancer care. *Journal of Health Communication, 20*(3), 328–342.

Bakas, T., Clark, P. C., Kelly-Hayes, M., King, R. B., Lutz, B. J., & Miller, E. L.; American Heart Association Council on Cardiovascular and Stroke Nursing and the Stroke Council. (2014). Evidence for stroke family caregiver and dyad interventions: A statement for healthcare professionals from the American Heart Association and American Stroke Association. *Stroke, 45*(9), 2836–2852. doi:10/1161/STR .0000000000033

Beach, P. R., & White, B. E. (2015). Applying the evidence to help caregivers torn in two. *Nursing, 45*(6), 30–37. doi:10.1097/01 .nurse.0000464983.54444.80

Beach, S. R., Schulz, R., Yee, J. L., & Jackson, S. (2000). Negative and positive health effects of caring for a disabled spouse: Longitudinal findings from the caregiver health effects study. *Psychology and Aging, 15*(2), 259–271.

Berg, J., Taylor, D., & Woods, N. F. (2015). Women at midlife. In E. Olshansky (Ed.), *Women's health and wellness across the lifespan* (pp. 68–95). Philadelphia, PA: Wolters Kluwer.

Berg, J., & Woods, N. (2009). Global women's health: A spotlight on caregiving. *Nursing Clinics of North America, 44,* 375–384. doi:10.1016/ j.cnur.2009.06.003

Berg, J. A., Cromwell, S. L., & Arnett, M. (2002). Physical activity: Perspectives of Mexican American and Anglo American midlife women. *Health Care for Women International, 23*(8), 894–904.

Bertrand, R. M., Saczynski, J. S., Mezzacappa, C., Hulse, M., Ensrud, K., & Fredman, L. (2012). Caregiving and cognitive function in older women: Evidence for the healthy caregiver hypothesis. *Journal of Aging and Health, 24*(1), 48–66.

Black, S. E., Gauthier, S., Dalziel, W., Keren, R., Correia, J., Hew, H., & Binder, C. (2010). Canadian Alzheimer's disease caregiver survey: Baby-boomer caregivers and burden of care. *International Journal of Geriatric Psychiatry, 25*(8), 807–813.

Blom, M. M., Zarit, S. H., Zwaaftink, R. B., Cuijpers, P., & Pot, A. M. (2015). Effectiveness of an internet intervention for family caregivers of people with dementia: results of a randomized controlled trial. *PLOS ONE, 10*(2), e0116622. doi:10.1371/journal.pone.0116622

Brown, S. L., Smith, D. M., Schulz, R., Kabeto, M. U., Ubel, P. A., Poulin, M.,…Langa, K. M. (2009). Caregiving behavior is associated with decreased mortality risk. *Psychological Science, 20*(4), 488–494.

Buyck, J. F., Bonnaud, S., Boumendil, A., Andrieu, S., Bonenfant, S., Goldberg, M.,…Ankri, J. (2011). Informal caregiving and self-reported mental and physical health: Results from the Gazel Cohort Study. *American Journal of Public Health, 101*(10), 1971–1979.

Carroll, L. (2013, September 5). Alzheimer's extracts a high price on caregivers, 599. NBC News. Retrieved from http://www.today.com/ health/alzheimers-extracts-high-price-caregivers-too-8C11070658

Chappell, N. L., & Reid, R. C. (2002). Burden and well-being among caregivers: Examining the distinction. *The Gerontologist, 42*(6), 772–780.

Cheng, H. Y., Chair, S. Y., & Chau, J. P. (2014). The effectiveness of psychosocial interventions for stroke family caregivers and stroke survivors: A systematic review and meta-analysis. *Patient Education and Counseling, 95*(1), 30–44.

Cohen, S., & Janicki-Deverts, D. (2009). Can we improve our physical health by altering our social networks? *Perspectives on Psychological Science, 4*(4), 375–378.

Cohen, S. D., Sharma, T., Acquaviva, K., Peterson, R. A., Patel, S. S., & Kimmel, P. L. (2007). Social support and chronic kidney disease: An update. *Advances in Chronic Kidney Disease, 14*(4), 335–344.

Cousino, M. K., & Hazen, R. A. (2013). Parenting stress among caregivers of children with chronic illness: A systematic review. *Journal of Pediatric Psychology, 38*(8), 809–828.

Czaja, S. J., Gitlin, L. N., Schulz, R., Zhang, S., Burgio, L. D., Stevens, A. B.,…Gallagher-Thompson, D. (2009). Development of the risk appraisal measure: A brief screen to identify risk areas and guide interventions for dementia caregivers. *Journal of the American Geriatrics Society, 57*(6), 1064–1072.

Dias, R., Santos, R. L., Sousa, M. F., Nogueira, M. M., Torres, B., Belfort, T., & Dourado, M. C. (2015). Resilience of caregivers of people with dementia: A systematic review of biological and psychosocial determinants. *Trends in Psychiatry and Psychotherapy, 37*(1), 12–19. doi:10.1590/2237-6089-2014-0032

Dickens, A. P., Richards, S. H., Greaves, C. J., & Campbell, J. L. (2011). Interventions targeting social isolation in older people: A systematic review. *BMC Public Health, 11,* 647.

Dictionary.com Unabridged. (2013). *Based on the Random House Dictionary.* Random House. Retrieved from http://dictionary .reference.com/browse/relationship

Dracup, K., Evangelista, L. S., Doering, L., Tullman, D., Moser, D. K., & Hamilton, M. (2004). Emotional well-being in spouses of patients with advanced heart failure. *Heart & Lung, 33*(6), 354–361.

DuBenske, L. L., Gustafson, D. H., Namkoong, K., Hawkins, R. P., Atwood, A. K., Brown, R. L.,…Cleary, J. F. (2014). CHESS improves cancer caregivers' burden and mood: Results of an eHealth RCT. *Health Psychology, 33*(10), 1261–1272.

Dukhovnov, D., & Zagheni, E. (2015). Who takes care of whom in the U.S.? Evidence from matrices of time transfers by age and sex. *Population and Development Review, 41*(2), 183–206.

Easom, L. R., Alston G., & Coleman, R. (2013). A rural community translation of a dementia caregiving intervention. *Online Journal of Rural Nursing and Health Care, 13*(1), 66–91.

Eccleston, C., Fisher, E., Law, E., Bartlett, J., & Palermo, T. M. (2015). Psychological interventions for parents of children and adolescents with chronic illness. *The Cochrane Database of Systematic Reviews, 2015*(4), CD009660. doi:10.1002/1461858.CD009660.pub3

Fagundes, C., Lindgren, M., & Kiecolt-Glaser, J. (2013). Psychoneuroimmunology and cancer: Incidence, progression, and quality of life. In B. I. Carr & J. Steel (Eds.), *Psychological aspects of cancer* (pp. 1–11). New York, NY: Springer Publishing.

Family Caregiver Alliance. (2015). *Women and caregiving: Facts and figures.* Retrieved from https://www.caregiver.org/women-and-caregiving -facts-and-figures

Forster, A., Brown, L., Smith, J., House, A., Knapp, P., Wright, J. J., & Young, J. (2012). Information provision for stroke patients and their caregivers. *The Cochrane Database of Systematic Reviews, 2012*(11), CD001919. doi: 10.1002/14651858.CD001919.pube

Fredman, L., Bertrand, R. M., Martire, L. M., Hochberg, M., & Harris, E. L. (2006). Leisure-time exercise and overall physical activity in older women caregivers and non-caregivers from the Caregiver-SOF Study. *Preventive Medicine, 43*(3), 226–229.

Fredman, L., Cauley, J. A., Satterfield, S., Simonsick, E., Spencer, S. M., Ayonayon H. N., & Harris, T. B. (2008). Caregiving, mortality, and mobility decline: The Health, Aging, and Body Composition (Health ABC) Study. *Archives of Internal Medicine, 168*(19), 2154–2162.

Fredman, L., Doros, G., Cauley, J. A., Hillier, T. A., & Hochberg, M.C. (2010). Caregiving, metabolic syndrome indicators, and 1-year decline in walking speed: Results of caregiver-SOF. *Journals of Gerontology Series A: Biological Sciences and Medical Sciences, 65A*(5), 565–572. doi:10.1093/gerona/glq025

Fredman, L., Doros, G., Ensrud, K. E., Hochberg, M. C., & Cauley, J. A. (2009). Caregiving intensity and change in physical functioning over a 2-year period: Results of the caregiver-study of osteoporotic fractures. *American Journal of Epidemiology, 170*(2), 203–210.

Fredman, L., Lyons, J. G., Cauley, J. A., Hochberg, M., & Applebaum, K. M. (2015). The relationship between caregiving and mortality after accounting for time-varying caregiver status and addressing the healthy caregiver hypothesis. *Journals of Gerontology Series A: Biological Sciences and Medical Sciences, 70*(9), 1163–1168. doi:10.1093/gerona/glv009

Gitlin, L. N., Jacobs, M., & Earland, T. V. (2010). Translation of a dementia caregiver intervention for delivery in homecare as a reimbursable Medicare service: Outcomes and lessons learned. *The Gerontologist, 50*(6), 847–854. doi:10.1093/geront/gnq057

Gitlin, L. N., Marx, K., Stanlye, I. H., & Hodgson, N. (2015). Translating evidence-based dementia caregiving interventions into practice: State of the science and next steps. *The Gerontologist, 55*(2), 210–226. doi:10/1093/geront/gnu123

Gitlin, L. N., & Rose, K. (2014). Factors associated with caregiver readiness to use non-pharmacologic strategies to manage dementia-related behavioral symptoms. *International Journal of Geriatric Psychiatry, 29*(1), 93e10.

Gitlin, L. N., Winter, L., Dennis, M. P., Hodgson, N., & Hauck, W. W. (2010). A biobehavioral home-based intervention and the well-being of patients with dementia and their caregivers: The COPE randomized trial. *Journal of the American Medical Association, 304*(9), 983–991.

Gitlin, L. N., Winter, L., Earland, T. V., Herge, E. A., Chernett, N. L., Piersol, C. V., & Burke, J. P. (2009). The tailored activity program to reduce behavioral symptoms in indivudals with dementia: Feasibility, acceptability, and replication potential. *The Gerontologist, 49*(3), 428–439. doi:10.1093/geront/gnp087

Given, C., Given, B., Stommel, M., Collins, C., King, S., & Franklin, S. (1992). The caregiver reaction assessment (CRA) for caregivers to persons with chronic physical and mental impairments. *Research in Nursing and Health, 15*(4), 271–283. doi:10.1002/nur.4770150406

Gonzalez, E. W., Polansky, M., Lippa, C. F., Walker, D., & Feng, D. (2011). Family caregivers at risk: Who are they? *Issues in Mental Health Nursing, 32*(8), 528–536. doi:10.3109/01612840.2011.573123

Goode, K. T., Haley, W. E., Roth, D. L., & Ford, G. R. (1998). Predicting longitudinal changes in caregiver physical and mental health: A stress process model. *Health Psychology, 17*(2), 190–198. doi:10.1037/0278-6133.17.2.190

Gouin, J., Glaser, K. R., Malarkey, W., Beversdorf, D., & Kiecolt-Glaser, J. (2012). Chronic stress, daily stressors, and circulating inflammatory markers. *Health Psychology, 31*, 264–268. doi:10.1037/a0025536

Grady, P. A., & Gough, L. L. (2015). Nursing science: Claiming the future. *Journal of Nursing Scholarship, 47*(6), 512–521. doi:10.1111/jnu.12170

Gruenewald, T. L., Karlamangla, A. S., Greendale, G. A., Singer, B. H., & Seeman, T. E. (2007). Feelings of usefulness to others, disability, and mortality in older adults: The MacArthur Study of successful aging. *The Journals of Gerontology Series B: Psychological Sciences and Social Sciences, 62*(1), 28–37. doi:10.1093/geronb/62.1.p28

Gustafson, D., DuBenske, L., Namkoong, K., Hawkins, R., Chih, M., Atwoods, A. K.,…Cleary, J. F. (2013). An eHealth system supporting palliative care for patients with nonsmall cell lung cancer. *Cancer, 119*(9), 1744–1751. doi:10.1002/cncr.27939

Hazuda, H., Haffner, S., Stern, M., & Eifler, C. (1988). Effect of acculturation and socioeconomic status on obesity and diabetes in Mexican Americans: The San Antonio Heart Study. *American Journal of Epidemiology, 128*(6), 1289–1301.

Herbert, R., Bravo, G., & Preville, M. (2000). Reliability, validity, and reference values of the Zarit Burden Interview for assessing informal caregivers of community-dwelling older persons with dementia. *Canadian Journal on Aging, 19*, 494–507.

Hibbard, J. H., Stockard, J., Mahoney, E. R., & Tusler, M. (2004). Development of the patient activation measure (PAM): Conceptualizing and measuring activation in patients and consumers. *Health Services Research, 39*(4, Pt. 1), 1005–1026. doi:10.1111/j.1475-6773.2004.00269.x

Ho, S. C., Chan, A., Woo, J., Chong, P., & Sham, A. (2009). Impact of caregiving on health and quality of life: A comparative population-based study of caregivers for elderpersons and noncaregivers. *Journals of Gerontology Series A: Biological Sciences and Medical Sciences, 64*, 873–879.

Hodgins, M. J., Wuest, J., Malcolm, J. (2011). Modeling the effects of past relationship and obligation on changes in the health and health promotion of women caregivers of family members with dementia. *Research in Nursing and Health 23*, 440–456.

Hoefman, R., Al-Janabi, H., McCaffrey, N., Currow, D., Ratcliffe, J. (2015). Measuring caregiver outcomes in palliative care: A construct validation study of two instruments for use in economic evaluations. *Quality of Life Research, 24*, 1255–1273.

Hoffman, G., Lee, J., & Mendez-Luck, C. (2012). Health behaviors among baby boomer informal caregivers. *The Gerontologist, 52*(2), 219–230. doi:10.1093/geront/gns003

Honea, N. J., Brintnall, R. A., Given, B., Sherwood, P., Colao, D. B., Somers, S. C., & Northouse, L. L. (2008). Putting evidence into practice: Nursing assessment and interventions to reduce family caregiver strain and burden. *Clinical Journal of Oncology Nursing, 12*, 507–516.

Howell, L. (2001). Implications of personal values in women's midlife development. *Counseling & Values, 46*, 54–65.

Hudson, P., & Aranda, S. (2014). The Melbourne Family Support Program: Evidence-based strategies that prepare family caregivers for supporting palliative care patients. *British Medical Journal Supportive and Palliative Care, 4*, 231–237.

Hudson, P., Quinn, K., Kristjanson, L., Thomas, T., Braithwaite, M., Fisher, J., & Cockayne, M. (2008). Evaluation of a psycho-educational group programme for family caregivers in home-based palliative care. *Palliative Medicine, 22*(3), 270–280. doi:10.1177/0269216307088187

Im, E., Lee, B., Chee, W., & Stuifbergen, A. (2011). Attitudes toward physical activity of white midlife women. *Journal of Obstetric, Gynecologic & Neonatal Nursing, 40*(3), 312–321.

Imes, C. C., Dougherty, C. M., Pyper, R. N., & Sullivan, M. D. (2011). A descriptive study of the partner's experiences of living with severe heart failure. *Heart and Lung, 40*, 208–216.

Jensen, M., Agbata Nwando, I., Canavan, M., & McCarthy G. (2015). Effectivenes of educational interventions for informal caregivers of individuals with dementia residing in the community: Systematic review and meta-analysis of randomized controlled trials. *International Journal of Geriatric Psychiatry, 30*, 130–143.

Jordan, J., Kaplan, A., Miller, J., Stiver, I., & Surrey, J. (1991). *Women's growth in connection: Writings from the Stone Center*. New York, NY: Guilford Press.

Kieckhefer, G. M., Trahms, C. M., Churchill, S. S., Kratz, L., Uding, N., & Villareale, N. (2014). A randomized clinical trial of the Building on Family Strengths Program: An education program for parents of children with chronic health conditions. *Maternal and Child Health Journal, 18*, 563–574.

Kim, Y., Schulz, R., & Carver, C. S. (2007). Benefit-finding in the cancer caregiving experience. *Psychosomatic Medicine, 69*, 283–291.

King, A. C., Baumann, K., O'Sullivan, P., Wilcox, S., & Castro, C. (2002). Effects of moderate-intensity exercise on physiological, behavioral, and emotional responses to family caregiving: A randomized controlled trial. *Journals of Gerontology Series A: Biological Sciences and Medical Sciences, 57*(1), M26–M36. doi:10.1093/gerona/57.1.m26

Kinney, J., & Stephens, M. (1989). Hassles and uplifts of giving care to a family member with dementia. *Psychology and Aging, 4*, 402–408.

Krause, N. (1995). Negative interaction and satisfaction with social support among older adults. *Journals of Gerontology Series B: Psychological Sciences and Social Sciences , 50b*, 59–73.

Krause, N., & Borawski-Clark, E. (1995). Social class differences in social support among older adults. *The Gerontologist, 35*, 498–508.

Lawton, M., Kleban, M., Moss M., Rovine M., & Glicksman, A. (1989). Measuring caregiving appraisal. *Journals of Gerontology Series B: Psychological Sciences and Social Sciences, 44*, 61–71.

Lazarus, R., & Folkman, S. (1984). *Stress, appraisal, and coping*. New York, NY: Springer Publishing.

Leveille, S. G., Penninx, B. W., Melzer, D., Izmirlian, G., & Guralnik, J. M. (2000). Sex differences in the prevalence of mobility disability in old age: The dynamics of incidence, recovery, and mortality. *Journals of Gerontology Series B: Psychological Sciences and Social Sciences, 55*, S41–S50.

Lewis, S. L., Miner-Williams, D., Novian, A., Escamilla, M. J., Blackwell, P. H., Kretzschmar, J. H.,…Bonner, P. N. (2009). A stress-busting program for family caregivers. *Rehabilitation Nursing, 23*, 151–159.

Lovell, B., & Wetherell, M. (2011). The cost of caregiving: Endocrine and immune implications in elderly and non elderly caregivers. *Neuroscience and Biobehavioral Reviews, 35*, 1342–1352. doi:10.1016/j.neubiorev.2011.02.007

Lyons, J. G., Cauley, J. A., & Fredman, L. (2015). The effect of transitions in caregiving status and intensity on perceived stress among 992 female caregivers and noncaregivers. *Journals of Gerontology Series B: Psychological Sciences and Social Sciences, 70*(8), 1–6. doi:10.1093/Gerona/glv001

Lyons, K. S., Vellone, E., Lee, C. S., Cocchieri, A., Bidwell, J. T., d'Agostino, F.,…Riege, B. (2015). A dyadic approach to managing heart failure with confidence. *Journal of Cardiovascular Nursing, 30*, 45, S64–S71.

Maayan, N., Soares-Weiser, K., & Lee H. (2014). Respite care for people with dementia and their carers. *The Cochrane Database of Systemtic Reviews, 2014*(1), Art. No: CD004396. doi:10.1002/14651858.CD004396.pub3

Mackenzie, A., & Greenwood, N. (2012). Positive experiences of caregiving in stroke: A systematic review. *Disability and Rehabilitation, 34*, 1413–1422.

Maslach, C., & Jackson, S. (1982). Burnout in health professions: A social psychological analysis. In G. S. Sanders & J. Suls (Eds.), *Social psychology of health and illness* (pp. 227–251). Hillsdale, NJ: Erlbaum.

Maslach, C., & Jackson, S. (1986). *Maslach burnout inventory*. Palo Alto, CA: Consulting Psychologists Press.

McBride, M. (1990). Autonomy and struggle for female identity: Implications for counseling women. *Journal of Counseling & Development, 69*, 22–26.

McCann, J. J., Hebert, L. E., Bienias, J. L., Morris, M. C., & Evans, D. A. (2004). Predictors of beginning and ending caregiving during a 3-year period in a biracial community population of older adults. *American Journal of Public Health, 94*, 1800–1806.

McCurry, S. M., Gibbons, L. E., Logsdon, R. G., Vitiello, M. V., & Teri, L. (2009). Insomnia in caregivers of persons with dementia: Who is at risk and what can be done about it? *Sleep Medicine Clinics, 5*, 519–526.

McCurry, S. M., Logsdon, R. G., Mead, J., Pike, K. C., LaFazia, D. M., Stevens, L., & Teri, L. (2015). Adopting evidence-based caregiver training programs in the real world: Outcomes and lessons learned from the STAR-C Oregon Translation Study. *Journal of Applied Gerontology, 108*, ii: 0733464815581483. [Epub ahead of print]. doi:10.1177/0744464815581483

McGhan, G., Loeb, S. J., Baney, B., & Penrod, J. (2013). End of life caregiving: Challenges faced by older adult women. *Journal of Gerontological Nursing, 39*, 45–54.

McGuire, D. B., Grant, M., & Park, J. (2012). Palliative care and end of life: The caregiver. *Nursing Outlook, 60*, 351–356.

McGuire, L. C., Anderson, L. A., Talley, R. C., & Crews, J. E. (2007). Supportive care needs of Americans: A major issue for women as both recipients and providers. *Journal of Women's Health, 16*, 784–789.

McLennon, S. M., Bakas, T., Jessup, N. M., Habermann, B., & Weaver, M. T. (2014). Task difficulty and life changs among stroke family caregivers: Relationship to depressive symptoms. *Archives of Physical Medicine and Rehabilitation, 95*, 2484–2490.

Menne, H. L., Bass, D. M., Johnson, J. D., Primetica, B., Kearney, K. R., Bollin, S,…Teri, L. (2014). Statewide implementation of "reducing disability in Alzheimer's disease": Impact on family caregiver outcomes. *Journal of Gerontological Social Work, 57*(6–7), 626–639. doi: 10.1080/01634372.2013.870276

Moen, P. (1996). A life course perspective on retirement, gender, and well-being. *Journal of Occupational Health Psychology, 1*(2), 131–144.

Moen, P., Dempster-McClain, D., & Williams, R. (1992). Successful aging: A life-course perspective on women's multiple roles and health. *American Journal of Sociology, 97*(6), 1612–1638.

Moniz, C. M., Swift, K., James, I., Malouf, R., De Vugt M., & Verhey F. (2012). Functional analysis-based interventions for challenging behavior in dementia. *The Cochrane Database of Systematic Reviews, 2012*(2). Art. No: CD006929. doi:10.1002/14651858.CD006929.pub2

Moon, H., & Dilworth-Anderson, P. (2015). Baby boomer caregiver and dementia caregiving: Findings for the National Study of Caregiving. *Age and Aging, 44*, 300–306. doi:10.1093/aging/aful19

Moore, S. M., & Rosenthal, D. A. (2014). Personal growth, grandmother engagement and satisfaction among non-custodial grandmothers. *Aging and Mental Health, 19*(2), 136–143. doi:10.1080/13607863 .2014.920302.

Motenko, A. (1989). The frustrations, gratifications, and well-being of dementia caregivers. *The Gerontologist, 29*, 166–172.

Mozaffarian, D., Afshin, A., Benowitz, N., Bittner, V., Daniels, S., Franch, H.,…Zakai, N. (2012). Population approaches to improve diet, physical activity, and smoking habits: A scientific statement from the American Heart Association. *Circulation, 126*, 1514–1563.

Musil, C., Jeanblanc, A., Burant, C., Zauszniewski, J., & Warner, C. (2013). Longitudinal analysis of resourcefulness, family strain, and depressive symptoms in grandmother caregivers. *Nursing Outlook, 61*, 225–234.

Musil, C. M., Gordon, N. L., Warner, C. B., Zauszniewski, J. A., Standing, T., & Wykle, M. (2010). Grandmothers and caregiving to grandchildren: Continuity change, and outcomes over 24 months. *The Gerontologist, 51*, 86–100.

Nichols, L. O., Martindale-Adams, J., Burns, R., Graney, M. J., & Zuer, J. (2011). Translation of a dementia caregiver support program in a health care system–REACH VA. *Archives of Internal Medicine, 171*, 353–359. doi:10.1001/archinternmed.2010.548

Northouse, L. L., Katapodi, M., Song, L., Zhang, L., & Mood, D. W. (2010). Interventions with family caregivers of cancer patients: Meta-analysis of randomized trials. A *Cancer Journal for Clinicians, 60*, 317–339. doi:10.3322/caac.20081

O'Reilly, D., Connolly, S., Rosato, M., & Patterson, C. (2008). Is caring associated with an increased risk of mortality? A longitudinal study. *Social Science & Medicine, 67*(8), 1282–1290. doi:10.1016/ j.socscimed.2008.06.025

Ostwald, S. (2009). Who is caring for the caregiver? Promoting spousal caregiver's health. *Family & Community Health, 32*(Suppl. 1), S5–S14. doi:10.1097/01.FCH.0000342835.13230.a0

Pearlin, L. I., Mullan, J. T., Semple, S. J., & Skaff, M. M. (1990). Caregiving and the stress process: An overview of concepts and their measures. *The Gerontologist, 30*, 583–594.

Pearlman, S. (1993). Late mid-life astonishment: Disruptions to identity and self-esteem. In N. D. Davis, E. Cole, & E. D. Rothblum (Eds.), *Faces of women and aging* (pp. 1–23). Binghamton, NY: Haworth Press.

Picot, S. J. F., & Youngblut, J. (1997). Development and testing of a measure of percceived caregiver rewards in adults. *Journal of Nursing Measurement, 5*, 33–52.

Pinquart, M., & Sorensen, S. (2003). Differences between caregivers and noncaregivers in psychological health and physical health: A meta-analysis. *Psychology and Aging, 18*, 250–267. doi:10.1037/0882 –7974.18.2.250

Pinquart, M., & Sorenson, S. (2011). Spouses, adult children, and children-in-law as caregivers of older adults: A meta-analytic comparison. *Psychology and Aging, 26*, 1–14.

Praire, B., Scheier, M., Matthews, K., Chang, C., & Hess, R. (2011). A higher sense of purpose in life is associated with sexual enjoyment in midlife women. *Menopause, 18*(8), 839–844.

Rehm, R. S. (2013). Nursing's contribution to research about parenting children with complex chronic conditions: An integrative review, 2002–2012. *Nursing Outlook, 61*, 266–290.

Repetti, R., Matthews, K., & Waldron, I. (1989). Employment and women's health: Effects of paid employment on women's mental and physical health: *American Psychologist, 44*(11), 1394–1401.

Reverby, S. (1987). *Ordered to care: The dilemma of American nursing, 1850–1945.* New York, NY: Cambridge University Press.

Rodriguez-Gonzalo, A., Garcia-Marti, C., Ocana-Colorado, A., Baquera-De Micheo, M. J., & Morel-Fernandez, S. (2015). Efficiency of an intensive eduational program for informal careivers of hospitalized, dependent patients: Cluster randomized trial. *BMC Nursing, 14*((1), 5). doi:10.1186/s12912–015-0055–0

Rosso, A. L., Lee, B. K., Stefanick, M. L., Kroenke, C. H., Coker, L. H., Woods, N. F., & Michael, Y. L. (2015). Caregiving frequency and physical function: The women's health initiative. *The Journals of Gerontology Series A: Biological Sciences and Medical Sciences, 70*, 210–215. doi:10.1093/gerona/glu104

Roth, D. L., Fredman, L., & Haley, W. E. (2015). Informal caregiving and its impact on health: A reappraisal from population-based studies. *Gerontologist, 55*(2), 309–319. doi:10.1093/geront/gnu177. Epub 2015 Feb 18

Roth, D., Haley, W., Hovater, M., Perkins, M., Wadley, V., & Judd, S. (2013). Family caregiving and all-cause mortality: Findings from a population-based propensity-matched analysis. *American Journal of Epidemiology, 178*(10), 1571–1578. doi:10.l1093/aje/kwt225

Roth, D., Perkins, M., Wadley, V., Temple, E., & Haley, W. (2009). Family caregiving and emotional strain: Associations with quality of life in a large national sample of middle-aged and older adults. *Quality of Life Research, 18*, 679–688. doi:10.1007/ s1136–009-9482–2

Sadak, T., Korpka, A., & Borson, S. (2015). Measuring caregiver activation for health care: Validation of PBH-LCI:D. *Geriatric Nursing, 36*(4), 284–292. doi:10.1016/j.gerinurse.2015.03.003

Sadak, T., Souza, A., & Borson, S. (2015). Toward assessment of dementia caregiver activation for health care: An integrative review of related constructs and measures. *Research in Gerontological Nursing, 9*(3), 145–155. doi:10.3928/19404921–20151019-02

Schulz, R., & Beach, S. (1999). Caregiving as a risk factor for mortality: The caregiver health effects study. *Journal of the American Medical Association, 282*, 2215–2219. doi:10.1001/jama.282.23.2215

Schulz, R., Newsom, J., Mittelmark, M., Burton, L., Hirsch, C., & Jackson, S. (1997). Health effects of caregiving: The caregiver health effects study: An ancillary study of the cardiovascular health study. *Annals of Behavioral Medicine, 19*, 110–116.

Schulz, R., & Sherwood, P. (2008). Physical and mental health effects of family caregiving. *American Journal of Nursing, 108*(Suppl. 9), 23–27. doi:10.1097/001.NAJ.0000336406.45248.4c

Schumacher, K. L., Stewart, B. J., & Archbold, P. G. (2002). Mutuality and preparedness moderate self-efficacy: Reliability and validity studies.

The Journals of Gerontology Series A: Biological Sciences and Medical Sciences, 57(1), P74e–P86.

Sherwood, P. R., Given, B. A., Given, C. W., Schiffman, R. F., Murman, D. L., Eye, A. V.,…Remer, S. (2007). The influence of caregiver mastery on depressive symptoms. *Journal of Nursing Scholarship, 39*(3), 249–255. doi:10.1111/j.1547–5069.2007.00176.x

Sisk, R. (2000). Caregiver burden and health promotion. *International Journal of Nursing Studies, 37*(1), 37–43.

Stamp, K. D., Dunbar, S. D., Clark, P. C., Reilly, C. M., Gary, R. A., Higgins, M., & Ryan, R. M. (2015). Family partner intervention influences self-care confidence and treatment self-regulation in patients with heart failure. *European Journal of Cardiovascular Nursing*, ii. doi:10.1177/1474515115572047

Steffen, A. M., McKibbin, C., Zeiss, A. M., Gallagher-Thompson, D., & Bandura, A. (2007). The revised scale for caregiving the effects of caregiving demand on cancer family caregiver outcomes. *Nursing Research, 56*(6), 425e–433.

Stetz, K. (1987). Caregiving demands during advanced cancer: The spouse's needs. *Cancer Nursing, 10*, 260–268.

Strating, M., Suurmeijer, T., & Van Schuur, W. (2006). Disability, social support, and distress in rheumatoid arthritis: Results from a thirteen-year prospective study. *Arthritis Care & Research, 55*(5), 736–744.

Sullivan, B., Marcuccilli, L., Soan, R., Gradus-Pizio, I., Bakas, T., Jung, M., & Pressler, S. J. (2015). Competence, compassion, and care of the self family caregiving needs and concerns in heart failure. *Journal of Cardiovascular Nursing, 31*(3), 209–214. doi:10.1097/JCN.000000000000241

Teri, L., McKenzie, G., Logsdon, R. G., McCurry, S. M., Bollin, S., Mead, J., & Menne, H. (2012).Translation of two evidence-based programs for training families to improve care of persons with dementia. *The Gerontologist, 52*, 452–459. doi:10.1093/geront/gnr132

Teri, L., Truax, P., Logsdon, R., Uomoto, J., & Al, E. (1992). Assessment of behavioral problems in dementia: The revised memory and behavior problems checklist. *Psychology and Aging, 7*(4), 622–631.

Uchino, B. (2006). Social support and health: A review of physiological processes potentially underlying links to disease outcomes. *Journal of Behavioral Medicine, 29*(4), 377–387.

U. S. National Library of Medicine, National Institutes of Health. (2013). Retrieved from https://www.nlm.nih.gov/medlineplus

Vermooji-Dassen, M., Draskovic, I., McClery, J., & Downs, M. (2011). Cognitive reframing for careers of people with dementia. *The Cochrane Database of Systematic Reviews, Nov 9* (11), Art No. CD005318. doi:10.1002/14651858.CD005318.pub2

Vitaliano, P., Zhang, J., & Scanlon, J. (2003). Is caregiving hazardous to one's health? A meta-analysis. *Psychological Bulletin, 1299*, 46–972. doi:10.1037/e323652004–001

Waldron, I. (1980). Employment and women's health: An analysis of causal relationships. *International Journal of Health Services, 10*, 435–454.

Ward-Griffin, C., Brown, J. B., St-Amant, O., Sutherland, N., Martin-Matthews, A., Keefe, J., & Kerr, M. (2015). Nurses negotiating professional-familial boundaries: Striving for balance within double duty caregiving. *Journal of Family Nursing, 21*, 57–85. doi:10.1177/1074840714562645

Williams, A. M., Eby, J. A., Crooks V. A., Stajduhar, K., Biesbrecht, M., Vuksan, M.,…Allan, D. (2011). Canada's compassionate care benefit: Is it an adequate public health response to addressing the issue of caregiver burden in end of life care? *CMB Public Health, 11*, 335.

Zarit, S., & Zarit J. (1986). *The memory and behavior problem checklist—1987R and The Burden Interview: Instruments and instructions manual*. Pennsylvania, PA: University Park.

Zender, R., & Olshansky, E. (2015). Healing relationships. In E.Olshansky (Ed.), *Women's health and wellness across the lifespan* (pp. 285–308). Philadelphia, PA: Wolters Kluwer.

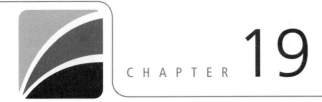

CHAPTER 19

Women's Sexual Health

Elizabeth Kusturiss • Susan Kellogg Spadt

Women have the right to intimate and sexual lives and relationships that are voluntary, desired, pleasurable, and noncoercive. According to the World Health Organization (WHO), "sexual health is not merely the absence of dysfunction, disease and/or infirmity. For sexual health to be attained and maintained it is necessary that the sexual rights of all people be recognized and upheld" (WHO, 2006, p. 5). When women express concerns regarding sexuality and sexual activity, they have the right to expect that advanced practice nurses will provide accurate sexual information, counseling, or therapy. The goal of this chapter is to provide a knowledge base from which nurse practitioners can assess women's concerns about sexual health, provide sexual health care, and make appropriate referrals for their care. This chapter includes a focus on sexuality and sexual health, an updated look at the female sexual response, and sexual development across the life span. Sexual assessment, challenges to female sexual health and sexuality, as well as a thorough discussion on sexual and dysfunction and pain, are also reviewed.

■ SEXUALITY AND SEXUAL HEALTH

According to the Pan American Health Organization and WHO (2006, p. 5):

> Sexuality refers to a core dimension of being human which includes sex, gender, sexual and gender identity, sexual orientation, eroticism, emotional attachment/love, and reproduction. It is experiences or expressed in thoughts, fantasies, desires, beliefs, attitudes, values, activities, practices, roles, relationships. Sexuality is a result of the interplay of biological, psychological, socioeconomic, cultural, ethical and religious/spiritual factors. While sexuality can include all of these aspects, not all of these dimensions need to be experiences or expressed. However, in sum, our sexuality is experienced and expressed in all that we are, what we feel, think, and do.

As a multidimensional construct, female sexuality encompasses a view of oneself as a female and presentation of oneself as a woman, which includes a woman's sexual desire, sexual response, and sexual orientation (Fogel, 2006). A woman's sexuality is a basic part of her life and an important aspect of her health. Few women find that sex has not been important at some time in their lives. Through her sexuality, a woman expresses her identity and her need for emotional and physical closeness with others. A woman's sexuality is present throughout the life span, although the various influences and expressions affecting sexuality may differ over time. One's sexuality is circumscribed by a historic and cultural context and is influenced by traditions, mores, and values. Full development of sexuality depends on the fulfillment of basic human needs such as the desire for contact, emotional expression, intimacy, pleasure, tenderness, and love (WHO, 2006, p. 5). Women express their sexuality differently at different times—alone, with one partner, or with many—and no two women express sexuality in exactly the same way. Expressed positively, sexuality not only can bring much pleasure, but also has the potential to cause great pain. One's sexuality need not be limited by age, attractiveness, partner availability or participation, or sexual orientation.

Dimensions of Women's Sexuality

Sexuality is multidimensional and includes sexual desire, sexual identity, and presentation of self. Women's sexuality can be expressed in a variety of behaviors—including fantasy, self-stimulation, noncoital pleasuring, erotic stimuli other than touch, and communication about needs and desires. It includes the ability to define what is wanted and pleasurable in a relationship.

Sexual desire, or "libido," is interest in sexual expression. For women, the goal of emotional intimacy has a strong influence on sexual desire (Basson, 2000). Although sexual desire has historically been thought of as one's innate spontaneous drive for sexual activity, recent research has changed the way we now view desire in women and places a greater emphasis on intimacy (Basson, 2000). The amount of sexual desire experienced varies from woman to woman and changes across a woman's life span. Sexual desire is learned by experiencing feelings of pleasure, enjoyment, dissatisfaction, or pain during sexual activity. Sexual desire includes interest in sexual activity, which varies in preferred frequency of activity and gender preference for a sexual partner (Fogel, 2006). Sexual desire is, in part, shaped by the culture into which one is socialized (Amaro, Navarro, Conron, & Raj, 2002).

Sexual identity is a form of self-identity, which includes how an individual identifies as female, male, feminine, masculine, or some combination as well as a woman's sexual orientation (Pan American Health Organization & WHO, 2000). This internal framework is constructed over time and enables a woman to develop a self-concept based on her sex, gender, and sexual orientation and to perform socially in regards to her perceived sexual capabilities. This identity is formed in early childhood and evolves throughout a woman's life. A woman's view of herself as female includes her gender identity or internal sense of self as a woman and her feelings of "femaleness." Gender identity enables a woman to organize a self-concept and perform socially in terms of her perceived sex and gender. It contributes to a woman's sense of uniqueness and how she experiences her gender (Pan American Health Organization & WHO, 2000). Gender roles are the behaviors, attitudes, rights, and responsibilities that are associated with each sex. Traditionally, this has been influenced and thought of solely from a biological perspective in that biological females are expected to act out female gender roles. The literature that is more recent suggests that the conceptual framework of gender has changed to include both biological and psychosocial components (Yarber, Sayad, & Strong, 2010). For most women, gender identity is permanent as well as congruent with her sexual anatomy and assigned gender; however, a woman's gender identity may not always be the same as her biological sex. Furthermore, some women experience numerous transitions in their sexual identity as a result of changes in relationships, attractions, and experiences (Farr, Diamond, & Boker, 2014). Studies have shown that women who have sex with women often vary in their sexual identity, sexual behavior, and sexual attraction, and frequently a women's self-described sexual orientation does not align with her sexual behavior in terms of the gender of her partners (Lindley, Walsemann, & Carter, 2013). It is not surprising that the National Health and Nutrition Examination Surveys found 53% of women who had ever had sex with another woman identified as straight or heterosexual (Xu, Sternberg, & Markowitz, 2010). It is imperative that providers do not make assumptions when a woman says she is heterosexual that she in the past or even currently is only having sex with men.

Gender roles are the behaviors, rights, attitudes, and responsibilities that particular cultural groups associate with each sex. *Gender role* is gradually replacing the traditional term *sex role* because the latter term connotes a connection between biological sex and behavior. Gender-role attitude, behavior, and presentation together form a woman's gender role. It is the belief a woman possesses about herself regarding appropriate female personality traits and activities, the actual behaviors a woman manifests, and other's perceptions of her habits and personality (Yarber et al., 2010). Gender-role stereotypes and expectations shape sexual expression. Beliefs about women and men, as well as assumptions regarding appropriate behaviors for both, affect sexual behavior communication patterns and expectations of sexual relationships.

Women's sexuality has been noted to be particularly sensitive to interpersonal, situational, and contextual factors. Women are more likely than men to report that their sexual attractions, behavior, and identities change over time and across situations, often as a result of changes in their relationships or environments. Women are more likely than men to report bisexuality, and women show less stability in their behaviors and attractions than men, thus exhibiting greater sexual fluidity (Farr et al., 2014).

Not long ago, virginity in women until marriage was the norm, and sex outside of marriage was considered immoral. Although conservative religious groups and older Americans may still view all nonmarital sex as sinful, values are shifting today, and nonmarital sex among women in a relational context has actually become the norm. Contraception, legal abortion, and changing gender roles legitimizing female sexuality have helped to lead to the shift from "sin" to acceptance. Although some women report having sex purely for physical release, most women view sex from and within a relational perspective. Although nonmarital sex in women has become the norm the attitude that "bad" women are passionate, experienced, and independent has not entirely changed. Despite changing gender norms, society continues to be hesitant to fully embrace women who are sexually outspoken and experienced (Yarber et al., 2010).

Sexual orientation refers to whom we are sexually attracted to and have the potential for loving. Sexual preferences exist on a continuum ranging from complete orientation to the same sex, through bisexuality, to a complete orientation to the other sex. Sexual practices are not always consistent with sexual orientation. The term *heterosexual* refers to a woman whose sexual orientation is toward members of the opposite gender, whereas a bisexual is a woman whose sexual orientation is toward both genders. The term *lesbian* is generally used for female homosexuals or women whose sexual orientation is toward members of her own gender. The term *queer* is now more widely used by gay scholars and activists who use the term to encompass lesbians, gays, and transgendered individuals (Hyde & DeLamaterm, 2006).

Sexual lifestyles provide the pattern and context for experiencing one's sexuality (Fogel, 2006). Today various types of sexual lifestyles exist and are common for women beyond monogamy and marriage. It is interesting to note that higher levels of sexual satisfaction and pleasure appear to be found in marriage than in singlehood or extramarital relationships. Research reports that married women and men have the highest rates of physical and emotional satisfaction with their partner. The lowest rates of sexual satisfaction have been found in individuals who were neither living with someone nor married—a cohort thought to have the most frequent and satisfying sex. Celibacy is a lifestyle in which women make a conscious choice to abstain from sexual activity. Some women view this choice positively as a means of giving oneself time and energy to devote their attention to other activities, but some may experience nonvoluntary celibacy (e.g., when a woman desires to be in a relationship but is not).

Asexuality refers to a lifestyle in which there is no sexual attraction to males or females or an absence of sexual orientation (Yarber et al., 2010). Asexuality, which has been shown to be more prevalent in women, may be thought of as the absence of sexual behavior, the absence of sexual attraction, self-identification as asexual, or a combination (Van Houdenhove & Gijs, 2014). *Polyamory* has been defined as having emotionally intimate relationships with multiple individuals with sex being permissible, while having an open and honest relationship with one's primary partner or partners who are aware of the other intimate involvements. In polyamorous relationships, individuals are committed to being open about each of the relationships in their lives and should not be synonymous with infidelity. Studies report that polyamory is more prevalent than formerly believed, with up to 33% of lesbian couples identifying as polyamorous. Three types of relationship dynamics exist in the polyamorous community: A woman has one main/primary partner as well as one or more other intimate relationships; a woman has more than one partner with whom she has equally intimate relationships; and last, three or more individuals have intimate relationships with one an other that may or may not include sex (Graham, 2014).

Sexual Health

Current definitions of *sexual health* go beyond issues surrounding sexually transmitted disease and reproduction. Sexual health is the ongoing process of physical, psychological, and sociocultural well-being and is evidenced in the free and responsible expression of sexual capabilities that foster harmonious personal and social wellness, enriching individual and social life (Yarber et al., 2010). Healthy adult sexual behaviors include the ability to appreciate one's own body, affirm that human development includes sexual development and may not always include reproduction or genital sexual experience, express love and intimacy in appropriate ways, identify and live according to one's values, enjoy and express one's sexuality throughout life, seek new information to enhance one's sexuality, prevent sexual abuse, seek early prenatal care and use contraception to avoid unintended pregnancy, and avoid sexually transmitted disease (WHO, 2006). According to the WHO (2006, p. 5):

> Sexual health is a state of physical, emotional, mental and social well-being related to sexuality; it is not merely the absence of disease, dysfunction or infirmity. Sexual health requires a positive and respectful approach to sexuality and sexual relationships, as well as the possibility of having pleasurable and safe sexual experiences, free of coercion, discrimination and violence. For sexual health to be attained and maintained, the sexual rights of all persons must be respected, protected and fulfilled.

Sexual health encompasses the ways we function biologically and our awareness and acceptance of our bodies and behavior. It should allow us to know, understand, and feel at ease in our own bodies. A woman should be comfortable with and aware of her breasts and the appearance, feel, and smell of her vulva, rather than be ashamed. Sexual health has a major impact on a woman's sexual functioning. Stress, minor ailments, and fatigue all affect our sexual interactions, leading to a potential decline in our sexual functioning. Health and sexuality must be recognized as gifts that a woman must care for in order to live both a healthy and a satisfying sexual life (Yarber et al., 2010).

WOMEN'S SEXUAL RESPONSE

A woman's sexual response is highly variable, varying between life stages and different women (Basson, 2008). It is a complex interplay of psychological, physiological, and interpersonal components. Major differences exist in terms of expectations and perceptions of a normal sexual response in women and vary from one culture to another. Expectations vary from highly negative in traditional Asian or African cultures to highly positive in most Western cultures. Religious or traditional cultural beliefs surrounding sex may also commonly play a role in a woman's view of herself as a sexual being and in her response to sexual stimulation. Furthermore, taboos or restrictions regarding sex during pregnancy, menstruation, or menopause can have an impact on a woman's sexual response in many societies (Rosen & Barsky, 2006). Although physiological aspects of the sexual response, such as orgasmic contractions or vasocongestion of the genitals, can be universal in women without sexual dysfunction, the subjective and emotional aspects of sexual response are highly individual and subject to learning and cultural factors.

Various models have been proposed throughout the years to describe the human sexual response. Most recently, traditional models have been reconceptualized to be more representative of women. Masters and Johnson in the 1960s were the first to propose a biological human sexual response cycle based on direct observations of men and women (Kingsberg & Rezaee, 2013). They described the cycle for both men and women as consisting of four stages, which progressed in a linear fashion beginning with excitement, which leads to plateau, orgasm, and finally resolution (Masters & Johnson, 1966). According to this response cycle, each stage had genital and extragenital responses and involved a gradual buildup of sexual tension, which culminated in the release of orgasm. Masters and Johnson were the first researchers to describe the possibility of multiple orgasms in the female response cycle (Rosen & Barsky, 2006). Their model was later modified by Kaplan (1974) in the 1970s, and was represented in a triphasic model, which emphasized desire as the initial and critical phase, which then lead to excitement, followed by orgasm. The introduction to Kaplan's model brought libido into the picture, as it has been viewed until recently as a necessary precursor to the development of adequate excitement and orgasm. Kaplan's model was the basis for the *Diagnostic and Statistical Manual of Mental Disorders*

(3rd ed.; *DSM-III*) and *Diagnostic and Statistical Manual of Mental Disorders* (4th ed.; *DSM-IV*; American Psychiatric Association [APA], 1994) classification system for male and female sexual dysfunction (FSD; Rosen & Barsky, 2006).

Earlier models of the female sexual response focused on a linear biological progression, lacked a focus on psychological or interpersonal issues, and were not reflective of women's actual experiences of sexual response. A newer model, proposed by Basson in 2000, is based on a female-focused circular model, which redefines the phases of the female sexual response and their relationship to one another (Hayes 2011; Rosen & Barsky, 2006). The Basson model included a complex interplay of sexual stimuli, emotional intimacy, psychological factors, and relationship satisfaction and refuted the notion that sexual activities are prompted by a woman's own innate and spontaneous desire or libido (Hayes, 2011; Kingsberg & Rezaee, 2013). Basson noted that women can enter into a sexual scenario from a position of sexual neutrality and commence sexual activity for reasons other than innate desire. Reasons for engaging in sexplay can include emotional reasons (love and commitment), physical reasons (i.e., stress reduction and pleasure), goal-attainment reasons (i.e., revenge and social status), and insecurity reasons (i.e., mate guarding, a sense of duty, or low self-esteem; Basson, 2008). Although noting that spontaneous sexual desire in women is more typical in the early phase of a relationship and less common for sexually content women in long-term relationships, she described "responsive" female desire as an event that is triggered or reactive to incoming sexual stimuli and/or physiological arousal (Basson, 2008; Hayes, 2011). "Responsive sexual desire," Basson posited, could feed back into the cycle, leading to increased arousal. In this updated model, sexual satisfaction with sexual activity (in which orgasm and resolution are not essential) is more representative of a woman's experience. Positive sexual experiences provide further motivation to engage in sexual activity and contribute toward a woman's reasons for allowing sexual stimuli and moving from a sexual-neutral state to a sexual-aroused state (Basson, 2008).

Another essential element in the female sexual response is the disconnect that often exists between a woman's subjective feelings of sexual arousal and the actual physiological changes, such as genital vasocongestion, that have more typically represented sexual arousal. In her research, Basson discovered that subjective arousal does not always correlate with physiological measures of genital congestion and emotions or thoughts have a greater influence on the subjective experience of sexual excitement. Typical women have the ability to experience vaginal lubrication or genital engorgement without the subjective perception of sexual excitement and vice versa (Rosen & Barsky, 2006). Women's experience of arousal is complex and may be better described as a combination of subjective and objective signs. Arousal occurs when the body reacts to stimuli with vulvar swelling, vaginal lubrication, and a heightened sensitivity of the genitalia combined with the subjective experience of feeling excitement and pleasure (Salonia et al., 2010).

■ SEXUALITY ACROSS THE LIFE SPAN

Adolescence

Adolescence (ages 12–19 years) is the social and psychological state that occurs between the beginning of puberty, when the body becomes capable of reproduction, and acceptance into full adulthood (Yarber et al., 2010). It is a time of reorganization of biological, emotional, cognitive, and social functioning (Biro & Dorn, 2005). A primary task of adolescence is establishing a sense of self or identity and, through dating and romantic and sexual experiences, constructing themselves as sexual beings. Developing a healthy sense of sexuality is an essential task in adolescence. During this time, adolescent girls make startling discoveries about their bodies and sex, struggle with self-esteem, develop crushes and begin dating, and often experience their first heartbreak. It is a time that helps define how a woman views herself and as others as sexual people.

The female body undergoes rapid physical changes triggered by the hypothalamus, development of secondary sexual characteristics, increased growth velocity, changes in body composition, and capability of reproduction. Girls typically begin to experience physical changes between 7 and 14 years of age, which include an increase in height, the development of breasts, the growth of underarm and pubic hair, and vaginal mucous secretion, as well as menarche—the average age being 12 years and 4 months (Yarber et al., 2010). These changes are caused by an increase in adrenal androgens, estradiol, thyrotropin, and cortisol (Ponton & Judice, 2004).

The hormonal increase also causes a dramatic increase in sexual interest, including self-exploration through masturbation and partnered sexual activity (Ponton & Judice, 2004). If young girls have not yet begun masturbating before adolescence they will likely begin once the hormonal and physical changes of puberty begin. In a recent study by Robbins et al. (2011), 58% of 17-year-old females had ever masturbated. Most first sexual-partnered interactions in U.S. adolescent females are heterosexual in nature (Zimmer-Gembeck & Helfand, 2007). A recent study looking at sexual activity among female high school students in 2013 reported that 50.7% of high school seniors have had sexual intercourse, with only 51.3% having used a condom (Kann et al., 2014). An estimated 45% of adolescent girls had two or more sexual partners in the previous year (Hall, Holmqvist, & Sherry, 2004). Approximately 50% of teens aged 13 to 16 years engage in oral sex, which they perceive as "risk-free" behavior, as less than 20% use oral protection (i.e., dental dams; Healy, 2008).

For some girls, sexual activity is physically and emotionally satisfying. For others, particularly in cases of abuse or coercion, sex can result in negative emotions such as shame, regret, anger, or disappointment. Adolescent sexuality is defined by a myriad of factors. Internal and external factors interact with a young woman's sexual experiences that are often profound (Foley, Kope, & Sugrue, 2012). One's family and friends, the media, and cultural and ethnic messages play a major role in a young woman's sexuality. Self-esteem, body image, sexual self-concept, and timing of pubertal maturation further affect an adolescent girl's sexual behavior and perceptions. Research has shown that girls with a positive sexual self-concept have more positive attitudes toward sexual expression and sexual experiences (Impett & Tolman, 2006). Early pubertal maturation can be associated with deleterious effects and higher risk of body image concerns, earlier initiation of sex, unprotected intercourse, teen pregnancy, increased depression, and substance use in adolescence (Biro & Dorn, 2005). Adolescents may also face peer pressure to be sexually active, and an additional motivation for sexual activity for girls may be a desire for sexual intimacy rather than a wish for the physical act of intercourse (Chaplic & Allen, 2013).

Adulthood

The transition from adolescence to early adulthood (approximately 20–40 years of age) offers the potential for growth for women if one is aware of and remains open to the opportunities this period brings. In early adulthood, women have a greater understanding of themselves as sexual beings and develop a more mature sexuality. Women establish their sexual orientation, integrate love and sexuality, forge intimate connections, make commitments, make decisions regarding their fertility, and develop a coherent sexual philosophy. The orientation of heterosexual women is often established by adolescence or early adulthood. However, for women who identify as lesbian or bisexual, it may take longer to confirm and accept their sexual orientation. Most are aware of differing societal taboos and can experience much doubt and anxiety.

More recently the prevalence of unmarried adults (never married, divorced, or widowed) has gradually increased, related to women marrying later in adulthood. The result has been women having greater sexual experience, a widespread acceptance of cohabitation, increased unintended pregnancies, increased births and abortions among single women, a rise in single-parent families, and a greater number of separated and divorced women (Yarber et al., 2010). In early adulthood women develop their sexual values and interests, and their "sexual story" begins to take shape. Most women enter into monogamous partnerships, which might mean a decrease in sexual frequency (especially in long-term relationships or because of increasing demands of children; Foley et al., 2012).

Midlife

In middle adulthood (approximately 40–60 years of age), work and family often play major roles in women's lives. Personal time is spent primarily on marital and family matters, which can affect sexual expression by its decreasing intensity, frequency, and significance. Developmental issues that a woman faces in middle adulthood include redefining sex in marital or other long-term relationships, reevaluating sexuality, and accepting the biological aging process (Yarber et al., 2010). Bereavements, economic problems, retirement, children leaving home, divorce, personal illness, and illness

of a partner are all common factors affecting women in midlife that may pose a significant impact on a woman's sexuality (Davis & Jane, 2011).

One of the greatest barriers to a woman's sexuality in midlife is ageism. Our cultures' preoccupation with equating sexiness to youth often leaves the vibrant sexuality of women in midlife socially invisible. This is a time when women may feel sexually unappealing and withdrawn because of the physical changes in their body shape. During this time, women's bodies undergo a number of changes associated with menopause and aging; however, many women in their 40s and 50s continue to be sexually robust and develop increased confidence, which gives them the courage to be more passionate in their sexuality and identity. This is also a time that women find sexually freeing (Foley et al., 2012).

Menopause and adolescence are the two times in a woman's life in which she undergoes dramatic physiological changes, which can have a profound effect on her sexuality. Common sexual difficulties experienced by women in midlife include inability to relax, loss of interest in sex, dyspareunia, arousal difficulties, and anorgasmia. Perimenopause, or the years leading to menopause, is characterized by fluctuating estrogen levels and irregular menses that result in vasomotor symptoms, anxiety, and sleep disturbances, which can negatively impact on a woman's sexual interest and ability to become aroused and/or achieve orgasm (Davis & Jane, 2011). In the United States, the average age of menopause is 51 (Ginsberg, 2006.) It is marked by the cessation of ovarian estrogen production and a decline in estrogen levels, a dominant factor that can affect sexual function (Ginsberg, 2006). This decrease in estrogen affects the urogenital tissues, including the pelvic floor musculature, bladder, urethra, and vagina. Reduced vaginal estradiol alters the microbial environment, predisposing postmenopausal women to vaginal infections and/or urinary tract infections. Up to 45% of postmenopausal women experience symptoms of vaginal atrophy from a decreased elasticity of the vulvovaginal tissues, a thinning vaginal wall, and decreased vaginal lubrication, causing dryness, itching, irritation, burning, and dyspareunia. Women often experience considerable distress related to these symptoms, contributing not only to sexual dysfunction but also to decreased quality of life (Goldstein, Dicks, Kim, & Hartzell, 2013). A more detailed review of vulvovaginal atrophy (VVA) is discussed later in the chapter.

Older Adulthood

Aging is a physiological, psychological, and social transition that often affects a woman's sexuality. Older women have generally been perceived as being undesirable or disinterested in sex. However, this characterization is far from reality for most women (Montemurro & Siefken, 2014). Most women remain sexually active after the age of 50, and the capacity to enjoy sexual activity is not lost with advancing age. Sexual desire and sexual fantasy have been reported in 71% of women 80 to 102 years of age (Maciel & Laganà, 2014). Although research has shown that women are less likely than men to report being sexually active, this has been attributed primarily to health or lack of a partner (Yarber et al., 2010). A study by Waite, Laumann, Das, and Schumm (2009) found that in women aged 57 to 74 years, approximately 63% cited partners' health problems as the reason for sexual inactivity (Montemurro & Siefken, 2014).

Many psychosocial factors affect a woman's sexuality as she ages. As women continue to age, their sexuality becomes less genitally oriented, with a greater focus on the emotional, sensual, and relationship aspects. Chronic illness, hormonal changes, and vascular changes in a woman or her partner can result in decreased sexual activity. After age 60, there is a significant increase in the rate of spousal death. The death of a partner is a critical event in a woman's life and a major causative factor in determining an older woman's sexual interactions. Furthermore, older women may experience difficulty seeing themselves as sexual beings because of culture's association of sexuality, romance, and sexual desires with youth. Social constructions of desirability influence a woman's view of herself as a sexual being. Cultural and social constructs of sexuality frequently influence a woman's perceptions of the physical signs of aging, and losing attractiveness and femininity. If a woman has this negative association she will frequently also have a poor body image and a detrimental effect on sexuality. Conversely, a woman who perceives the aging process in a positive manner with confidence may even experience enhancement of her sexual desire and desirability (Maciel & Laganà, 2014). Although sexual frequency may decrease, intimacy is especially valued and is an essential element for an older woman's well-being (Yarber et al., 2010). Age is not a reliable predictor of the quality and type of intimate relationships, and emotional intimacy typically remains an essential need regardless of a woman's age (Maciel & Laganà, 2014).

Age-related physiological changes in later adulthood can contribute to painful sexual symptoms, and these, in turn, may be associated with reduced sexual desire and activity. Reduced tissue elasticity and thinning of the vaginal tissues may cause irritation or discomfort with penetration, contributing to a reduced desire for sexual activity. Vascular changes associated with sexual arousal and the intensity of muscle contractions with orgasms may diminish (Masters & Johnson, 1966). In addition, loss of fatty tissue of the labia and mons may contribute to tenderness, and these tissues may be easily damaged or abraded with sexual stimulation. Orgasms may decrease in intensity, and in some women, orgasmic contractions become painful. Despite a decrease in sexual response in women with age, sexual function in women decreases at a much slower rate than that in men. With age, caressing and tenderness can become more important in the sexual repertoire than penetration (Dargis et al., 2012).

Body changes may require that women and partners alter how they engage in sexual activity. With aging, adaptations in sexual practices to promote pleasure may include use of water-soluble lubricant and vaginal moisturizers, providing time for increased sexual stimulation to produce arousal, experimenting with different sexual positions to promote comfort, and planning intercourse for times when energy

levels are highest. The highest predictors of sexual satisfaction in women do not relate to sexual frequency or menopausal status but to a woman's sexual self-determination, emotional and physical closeness to her partner, positive communication, and a positive body image (Ringa, Diter, Laborde, & Bajos, 2013).

Childbearing

Pregnancy and childbirth represent a unique period in a woman's life, which involves significant physical, psychological, hormonal, social, and cultural changes that may greatly affect sexuality. These factors may include changes in the couple relationship; planned/unplanned and desired/undesired pregnancy; prior pregnancy, abortion, or miscarriage history; physical and hormonal changes causing poor self-image; mood instability; and difficulty or pain with vaginal intercourse. Sexual dysfunction can become pronounced during this period as a result of these profound physical, emotional, and psychological changes that occur (Johnson, 2011).

A significant decline in female sexual frequency is often found during pregnancy and is related to physical and hormonal changes that occur in each trimester. Fatigue, back pain, dyspareunia, infection, and vulvar varicose veins are physical manifestations common in pregnancy that influence sexual behavior. Increased estrogen, progesterone, and prolactin may cause vomiting, fatigue, weight gain, and breast tenderness, resulting in decreased desire and arousal (Serati et al., 2010). Studies indicate that pregnant women experience decreased clitoral sensation, leading to infrequent or lack of orgasm. Other changes occur in each trimester. Breast tenderness, typically pronounced in the first trimester, can result in a touch that was once pleasurable becoming uncomfortable. Nausea and fatigue and increased vaginal secretions are also common in the first trimester, affecting the desire for intimacy. Although fatigue and many physical manifestations may be present, most women are more physically comfortable in the second trimester, leading to a slight increase in sexual desire and activity. Stress incontinence, hemorrhoids, weight of the partner on the uterus during sex, and subluxation of the sacroiliac joints and pubic symphysis are common during the third trimester, resulting in decreased sexual activity (Johnson, 2011).

Various psychological changes also occur in pregnancy and the postpartum period, often leading to changes in a woman's sexual response, even if the pregnancy is planned and desired. A couple may experience ambivalence about the pregnancy, rather than joy. This is most common during first pregnancies. Factors such as changes in a couple's relationship, anxiety or fear of delivery, low self-esteem, and concerns about body image and health status during pregnancy, as well as negative sequelae (i.e., miscarriage), can contribute to altered sexual desire in women. A growing abdomen may lead to altered self-image, self-confidence, and self-consciousness. As pregnancy progresses, sexual positions, such as female superior, side lying, or rear entry, are often used to accommodate physical limitations. Many fears and myths, including that sexual intercourse results in harm to the fetus, miscarriage, infection, bleeding, and preterm labor, can result in a couple abstaining from sexual intercourse during pregnancy (Johnson, 2011).

The first 6 months after delivery can be a particularly difficult time in terms of a woman's sexuality and quality of life. Postpartum depression, mood changes related to hormonal fluctuations, feelings of being overwhelmed, and altered body image are all common occurrences that can alter desire and the frequency of sex in the postpartum period. Dyspareunia has been reported in 41% to 67% of women within 2 to 3 months after birth and is associated with perineal trauma during delivery. Episiotomy discomfort, decreased lubrication and vaginal dryness resulting from decreased estrogen levels, breastfeeding, and pelvic floor dysfunction all have been linked to dyspareunia after birth. Although vaginal dryness may be experienced by all postpartum women, it is most common in breastfeeding women (Avery, Duckett, & Frantzich, 2000). Furthermore, if fecal and/or urinary incontinence are present after a traumatic vaginal delivery, they can cause further impairment in sexual function (Johnson, 2011).

Infertility

Struggles with infertility and repeated attempts to conceive can compromise sexual self-esteem, expression, activity, and desire. Fertility and virility seem to be inextricably linked in U.S. society. A diagnosis of infertility may negatively affect a woman's sense of sexuality and her self-image and have a profound impact on her relationship. Studies have shown that women with infertility have an increased risk of sexual dysfunction, including decreased arousal, difficulty in achieving or lack of orgasm, and decreased sexual satisfaction (Keskin et al., 2011). Oskay, Beji, and Serdaroglu (2010) found that 61.7% of infertile woman reported sexual dysfunction. In another study, sexual dysfunction was reported in 64% of women with primary infertility and 76% of women with secondary infertility (Keskin et al., 2011). Factors that have been shown to be causative for sexual dysfunction include duration of marriage, partner age, and psychological problems such as depression (Davari Tanha, Mohseni, & Ghajarzadeh, 2014).

Women in treatment for infertility experience sex that is prescribed and planned around ovulation, having little to do with pleasure or sexual desire. Women may experience frustration that their reproductive as well as sexual life is out of their control during infertility treatment. Years of attempting to conceive makes spontaneous sex difficult to maintain and couples often find it difficult to separate spontaneous sex for pleasure from "functional" sex for conception. One or both partners may find themselves avoiding sex because it becomes a vivid reminder of pregnancy (Foley et al., 2012). Women may initiate sexual activity around the time of ovulation, even if they are experiencing low or decreased desire. Male partners can react to the issue of "sex on demand," with reactive impotence— or an inability to perform sexually—especially around the time of ovulation.

■ SOCIOCULTURAL INFLUENCES ON SEXUALITY AND SEXUAL HEALTH

Women experience their sexuality in the context of cultural expectations. Family, society, culture, law, and religion all shape attitudes and behaviors regarding sex. Culture is perhaps the most powerful factor that influences how women behave and feel sexually (Yarber et al., 2010). Sexual norms become institutionalized and are then reinforced by family, religion, education, medicine, media, and government.

Families provide early socialization and shape sexual attitudes, values, and behaviors that contribute to later sexual health or dysfunction. Restrictive family beliefs, such as the belief that expressions of intimacy are shameful, can contribute to a woman's inability to express herself sexually. Poor parent–child interactions can contribute indirectly to sexual problems by decreasing self-esteem and reducing a woman's ability to cope with intimacy (Sheaham, 1989). Messages that sex is something to endure may inhibit sexual expression or enjoyment.

Society defines the behaviors and norms for sexual behavior. Current U.S. cultural values present mixed messages to women: that they are to be sexually responsive but stay within well-defined boundaries. Sex role stereotypes that prescribe "men initiate sexual activity while women exercise control" restrict the range of acceptable behavior for women. Nonmarital sex has become the norm in today's society. This shift is largely because of effective contraception, legal abortion, and changing gender roles legitimizing female sexuality. Women, however, continue to be faced with the dichotomy of fitting into one of two categories: the "good girl" or the "bad girl." The good girl meets current standards of beauty and is a wife and mother who likes sex but not too much. Conversely, the bad girl is sexually free; likes sex too much; asserts her desire to have sex with men, women, or both; acts out the "sexy persona" or defies it; and is too feminine or too masculine in her appearance. This dichotomy affects how a woman views herself as a sexual being (Heasley & Crane, 2003). Social attitudes, beliefs, and values have historically affected and suppressed woman's sexual expression. It was a result of social and political changes in the United States that women gained access to contraception, were able to keep their own names after marriage, or were able to be sexual and single without being condemned as immoral (Heasley & Crane, 2003).

Specific sexual behaviors may be defined as desirable by one cultural group and undesirable by another. A culture's views often differ regarding premarital, extramarital, and marital sex; appropriate sexual positions; accepted sexual activities; and duration of coitus. In part, women form their ideas of what is sexually appropriate and desirable from years of cultural scripting, and these ideas often are the bases of many of the issues women experience in sexual relationships.

Religion also influences sexual attitudes, beliefs, and values and can exert a strong influence throughout a person's life. Religious proscriptions can contribute to sexual concerns or problems. Many religions view sex as something that is acceptable only for procreation and sexual desire as something having a direct connection to immorality and sin. These beliefs may lead to feelings of shame and guilt in women as they experience pleasure and desire (Heasley & Crane, 2003). Accepting or rejecting premarital sex, contraception to prevent pregnancy, and beliefs about monogamy for men and women and condoning or rejecting homosexuality are examples of religious influences in a woman's life.

Laws that regulate and control sexual behavior are common to most societies. Often, periods of societal change are necessary to alter cultural beliefs and change laws. The 1960s and 1970s were pivotal to women's sexuality. During this time, women began to reclaim and redefine their sexuality. Women-centered definitions of sexuality that included sensuality, closeness, mutuality, and relationships emerged during this period.

Rape and Sexual Health

Sexual violence not only violates a woman's rights, but frequently results in a multitude of immediate and long-term health consequences for women (Jina & Thomas, 2013). The lifetime prevalence of attempted or completed rape is estimated to be 20% for women worldwide (Mason & Lodrick, 2013). It has been found that between 6% and 59% of women have experienced sexual violence from their husband or a boyfriend in their lifetime (Dartnall & Jewkes, 2013). When individuals think of rape, most people visualize an image of a stranger attacking a woman in a dark place at knifepoint. In reality, this situation is rare, with most sexual assaults occurring in a private place or in the context of daily lives by someone the woman knows, such as a partner, previous partner, recent acquaintance, or colleague (Jina & Thomas, 2013).

Sexual violence in women has been linked to a myriad of deleterious effects on overall health and sexual functioning. Women with a history of sexual violence have an increased prevalence of sleep, eating, and gastrointestinal disorders; chronic pain; fatigue; fibromyalgia; migraines; chronic pelvic pain; dysmenorrhea; and psychological ramifications, including anxiety, depression, posttraumatic stress disorder (PTSD), and increased suicide attempts. A recent study showed that the prevalence of PTSD ranges from 30% to 94% in survivors of sexual assault (Jina & Thomas, 2013). Sexual violence has been linked to high-risk sexual behaviors such as having unprotected sex, having multiple sexual partners, and having sex while under the influence of alcohol or drugs; these behaviors increase the risk of sexually transmitted infections (STIs) and unintended pregnancy (Jina & Thomas, 2013). In addition, being a victim of sexual assault doubles the chance of developing sexual problems such as difficulty with desire, arousal, and orgasm; and fear of sex; and painful intercourse. PTSD may contribute to a heightened tone and spasm of the pelvic floor muscles, resulting from fear and anxiety, and causing dyspareunia. These findings may manifest relatively shortly after the assault or years later (Postma, Bicanic, van der Vaart, & Laan, 2013).

Women who have been victims of sexual violence may present in a clinical setting with vague complaints such as gastrointestinal distress or bloating. They might manifest a fear of sexual intimacy, history of painful sexual intercourse, infertility, or other reproductive health problems. A high degree of suspicion is required in woman presenting with chronic nonspecific conditions. It has been reported that although victims of sexual assault are frequent consumers of health care, they do not seek care for the sexual violence itself (Jina & Thomas, 2013). This is especially true if a woman has been experiencing symptoms for an extended time. It is imperative that practitioners not only screen for a history of sexual violence, but also have a clear plan for implementing interventions and making appropriate referrals (Jina & Thomas, 2013). Research has shown that directly questioning a woman about past "rape," "trauma," or "abuse" is highly stigmatizing and results in low levels of reporting. Higher levels of reporting have been found when providers question women about behaviorally specific acts such as "being forced into sex against your will" (Dartnall & Jewkes, 2013). Furthermore, it is essential that providers help women recognize that submission, or taking a passive stance, is not the same as consent. Research has shown that many women may submit to sexual intercourse from fear of consequences from resisting or protesting. Women in fear often respond in a passive way, appearing frozen or unable to act. This is vastly different from consent; consent is actively given and actively reinforced, it is not passively assumed. Some women may wrongly assume that if struggle and cries for help did not take place an assault was not committed, which further compounds the shame, guilt, and self-blame a woman feels (Mason & Lodrick, 2013).

■ SEXUAL HEALTH CARE

Assessment

Although there is an increasing public and professional awareness of sexual problems, FSD remains underdiagnosed and undertreated by health care professionals. In fact, most women are pleased or grateful when their health care provider initiates the discussion and believe it is the provider's responsibility to address these sexual health concerns. Studies have shown a number of reasons patients avoid discussing their sexual problems with their health care provider including a lack of opportunity, a sense of embarrassment and shame, the uncertainty of whether sexual problems or concerns are part of health care, a lack of optimism about the outcome of such a discussion, and uncertainty whether sexual dysfunction is truly treatable (Kingsberg & Janata, 2007) Patients question from whom in the health care team they should seek sexual advice. Adding to the burden of the patient is their perception that health care providers are unskilled in sexual problem management and disinterested or reluctant to address their concerns. Health care providers are also disinclined to address or inquire about sexual issues with their patients because of time constraints, deficits in communication skills, an unrealistic fear of offending the patient, concerns regarding adequate reimbursement, lack of available approved treatments, insufficient medical education or training in sexual health, and discomfort and lack of confidence in asking patients sexual questions (Althof, Rosen, Perelman, & Rubio-Aurioles, 2013). Although few providers report taking sexual histories, the providers that do tend to focus on STIs or contraceptive issues rather than sexual function. It is fundamental to the care of women to integrate screening for sexual problems into routine care. Sexual dysfunction is associated with increased anxiety and depression and contributes to decreased interpersonal satisfaction (Sadovsky & Nusbaum, 2006).

> Every person has a right to pursue, receive, and communicate information about sexuality; access reproductive and sexual health care; and to attain the highest level of sexual health. Sexual rights embrace human rights that are already recognized in national laws, international human rights documents and other consensus statements. (WHO, 2006, p. 5)

Establishing rapport and putting patients at ease in a kind and understanding manner is essential when conducting a sexual health history and assessing for any sexual dysfunction. The health care provider sets the tone for the conversation. When the provider is comfortable discussing sexual concerns it helps promote comfort in the patient and puts her at ease. Some providers may benefit from practicing using explicit sexual terminology or topics in order to desensitize themselves. Finding the correct terminology can also be a challenge, as formal words, such as *cunnilingus* or *fellatio*, may not be understood by the patient and the use of slang may be offensive (Kingsberg, 2006). In this instance, asking a woman if she participates or receives "oral sex play" may be more useful. It is essential to ask women direct questions in a empathic, reassuring, but professional and straightforward manner (Althof et al., 2013). Continually monitoring one's own responses for negativity or embarrassment is essential because these feelings are easily conveyed to patients. Body language should also be considered in attempting to put a woman at ease when discussing her sexuality. The provider should sit if possible and provide direct eye contact that gives the patient the impression that her issue is important and worthy of time and attention (Kingsberg, 2006).

Taking a sexual history during a new patient visit is an effective way to begin the conversation, as it sends the message that discussing sexual concerns and functioning is encouraged and appropriate. The sexual history can be obtained in the form of a questionnaire that women complete in the waiting room. This allows the provider to be aware regarding sexual concerns she wishes to discuss. Ideally, a sexual history is taken within a review of systems. The discussion should take place in a private setting, and confidentiality must be ensured. Allowing the woman to be clothed helps eliminate the anxiety, vulnerability, and discomfort that are commonly experienced when sitting in an examination gown (Kingsberg, 2006). Approaching the topic by mentioning the importance of assessing sexual function with all patients, as well as starting with a woman's presenting issue or reproductive stage in relation to her sexual function, is helpful. Normalizing or universalizing techniques beginning the question with "many women..." or "other women

have told me..." can help relieve anxiety in the patient. For example, "Many menopausal women often notice problems with decreased lubrication or discomfort during intercourse. Have you noticed this or any changes in your sexual functioning you would like to discuss?" Most patients are eager to tell their story to a compassionate provider and often do so if they are given the opportunity (Althof et al., 2013). It is therefore indispensable to use open-ended questions when conducting the sexual health history. Closed questions generally follow in order to facilitate gathering specific information such as medical history, menstrual history, and drug reactions. Women may need an explanation for why certain questions are being asked. Beginning with the least-threatening material, such as an obstetric history, and moving to sensitive topics, such as current sexual practices, also respects the need to create a comfortable encounter.

A comprehensive sexual history should include medical, reproductive, surgical, psychiatric, social, and sexual information. As sexual functioning is multifactorial, each domain of function must be assessed in terms of its individual or combined impact. Relevant medical information pertinent for a thorough sexual assessment includes:

- Past medical history
- Current health status
- Reproductive history and current status inclusive of age at menarche, menstrual history, and obstetric history, including spontaneous or induced abortions, history of infertility, contraception history, STI history, age at menopause if pertinent, gynecologic pain, surgeries, and urological functioning
- Endocrine system such as diabetes, androgen insufficiency, estrogen deficiency, and thyroid conditions
- Neurological diseases, such as multiple sclerosis and injuries to the spinal cord, which may impair arousal and orgasm
- Cardiovascular disease, as it has been linked to difficulties with arousal
- Psychiatric illness
- Current use of prescription and over-the-counter medications, as they may contribute to or cause sexual dysfunction

Clarification should be sought when necessary (e.g., to clarify the degree of lubrication present during sexual arousal if pain occurs during sexual intercourse). The woman should be asked to provide a brief description of her present relationship and to rate her relationship with respect to communication, affection, sexual needs met, and sexual communication. Acknowledging that it may be difficult for a woman to discuss the intimate details of her sexual life may also help reassure her and may encourage her to proceed (Althof et al., 2013).

Opportunities for sexual health screening include visits for annual gynecologic examinations, menopause-related concerns, antenatal or postpartum appointments, infertility assessment and treatment, and management of chronic illness and depression. Basic screening for sexual functioning may progress into a more detailed assessment after normalizing the importance of assessing for sexual function. Questioning might begin with, "Are you currently involved in a sexual relationship?" If the woman says that she is, the follow-up might be, "Are you involved in a sexual relationship with men, women, or both?" or "Do you have any sexual concerns or pain with sex?" Another approach may be to simply ask the woman, "Tell me about your partner."

Last, if the woman answers "no" in response to being involved in a sexual relationship, she should be asked, "Are there any sexual concerns you would like to discuss or that have contributed to a lack of sexual behavior?" It is critical that providers do not assume that a woman is heterosexual or behave heterosexually. Although some providers may be concerned that asking about the gender of the patients' partners may not be relevant or may offend, it is imperative. If a woman's partner is assumed to be male and that she is in a heterosexual relationship, she may feel uncomfortable discussing any non-heterosexual behavior (Kingsberg, 2006).

When it is indicated by the woman's health history, her reason for seeking care, her treatment goals, or the need for referral, a physical examination may be performed. The examination may include determination of vital signs and aspects of a general physical examination, particularly abdominal and pelvic. The pelvic examination should include inspection of the external and internal genitalia using specula and bimanual techniques.

Laboratory Studies

Although there are no studies specific to sexual assessment, tests are often indicated when dysfunction is suspected. Vaginal cultures for sexually transmitted diseases should be obtained if there is a history of purulent discharge, postcoital bleeding, or excessive discharge noted at the time of the physical examination; if a bladder infection is suspected or if a woman complains of dyspareunia, a clean-catch urine specimen for culture and sensitivity should be collected.

■ SEXUAL HEALTH CARE INTERVENTIONS

Framework for Intervention

A simple, but effective, framework for providing sexual health care interventions is the Permission, Limited Information, Specific Suggestions, and Intensive Therapy (PLISSIT) model developed by Annon (1976). This approach, which is used by many health care professionals for sexual counseling, comprises four levels of intervention: permission, limited information, specific suggestions, and intensive therapy. As the complexity of intervention levels increases, additional knowledge and skills are needed. All practitioners should be able to provide permission and limited information related to many of the sexual concerns of clients. All advanced practice nurses should be able to intervene at the specific suggestion level. Intensive therapy requires special training, and requires that the patient be referred to experts in the field of sex therapy.

"Permission" is the first step in providing approaching sexual concerns in women. The simple act of asking permission to discuss sexual function conveys respect and

sensitivity toward the patient and gives the implicit message that it is permissible to discuss sexuality either now or in the future. This step involves giving the patient permission to express herself sexually and provides reassurance that her behaviors are "normal" or "okay" (Nusbaum & Hamilton, 2002). Permission is given if the behavior is realistic, is something with which both partners are comfortable, involves no danger or coercion, or causes no harm. Permission involves answering questions about sexual fantasies, feelings, and dreams and may include permission for self-pleasuring (masturbation), initiation of sexual encounters, and the use of fantasy, erotica, and sexual aids such as oils, vibrators, and feathers. Asking about the effect of developmental changes, illness, or lifestyle alterations on sexuality may be ways of giving a woman permission to be a sexual being throughout her life span. Permission giving is particularly helpful for women who are anxious about their sexual adequacy or for clients with sexual dysfunction related to guilt over enjoyment of sexual practices. Examples of interventions at this level are permission to be sexually aroused by normal feelings, to engage in arousing activities such as masturbation and fantasizing, and to have sexual intercourse as often as desired.

"Limited Information" serves the role of providing education and information about anatomy and physiology, the sexual response cycle, myths about relationships, life-cycle changes, and effects of illness on sexuality (Nusbaum & Hamilton, 2002). The information given at this level includes specific facts that are directly related to the woman's area of sexual concern. This level of intervention is helpful in changing potentially negative thoughts and attitudes about specific areas of sexuality and in refuting sexual myths. Any information offered should be immediately relevant and limited in scope. To provide this level of sexual health care, practitioners need to be familiar with a range of sexual behaviors, norms, and forms of expression. This level is particularly useful when women have a sexuality knowledge deficit or anxiety associated with sexual misinformation.

The practitioner can offer "Specific Suggestions" if the patient responds positively. Specific suggestions provide additional information that the patient may or may not choose to use. Although not "prescribing" sexual practices for the patient, the practitioner is offering suggestions that might improve a woman's sexual concern (Nusbaum & Hamilton, 2002). The suggestions do not need to be exotic, complex, or imaginative; usually, they are suggested by the situation. Specific suggestions entail giving direct behavioral suggestions to relieve a sexual problem that is limited in scope or of brief duration. The practitioner and client agree on specific goals, and the clinician offers specific behavioral suggestions that are assessed at a follow-up visit.

Numerous suggestions can be made to clients but are always tailored to individual needs and the particular situation. For example, the practitioner may suggest that many people find the side-lying position to be a pleasurable sexual position for women who may have pain with deep penetration or in those who desire clitoral stimulation during coitus. Additional examples of specific suggestions are use of a water-soluble lubricant or moisturizer to relieve vaginal dryness and to prevent dyspareunia in postmenopausal women; sensate focus exercises (mutual erotic stimulation excluding the genitals) to increase arousal; medication to treat a vaginal infection; and alternative ways of sexual pleasuring (oral–genital contact, mutual masturbation, cuddling, holding, massage) when traditional intercourse is not possible or undesired.

Practitioners should refer the woman for "Intensive Therapy" if the woman's sexual concerns are not fully addressed after offering limited information and specific suggestions and when the problem interferes with sexual expression. This level of intervention is the most complex and should be offered only by professionals with advanced training in sexual counseling and therapy. Referral to a sexual therapist for further assistance is often the appropriate intervention.

■ SEXUAL HEALTH CHALLENGES

Many health-related factors can affect sexual health. Experiencing illness and/or living with specific pathologies, having surgery, becoming disabled, and using medications (both prescription and nonprescription) can have an impact on sexual health. There is a pervasive cultural bias impling that if a woman is disabled or sick, she is no longer a sexual person. Sexuality in the American culture is often only associated with young, healthy, able-bodied women. In addition to coping with feeling "different" from a sexual perspective, women with illness or disability often struggle with changes in their body, self-perception, self-esteem, identity, and social and economic status (Foley et al., 2012).

As seen in Table 19.1, many diseases or health problems have the potential to affect desire, arousal, and orgasm. Similarly, a variety of drugs may affect sexual desire, arousal, and orgasm based on their neuroendocrine, neurovascular, or neurological effects. Treatments that affect the vascular system or that produce nerve damage may also alter sexual function (Basson & Schultz, 2007). Spinal cord injury, vascular damage, neurological damage, and chemotherapy and other medications interfere with genital blood flow or alter feeling in the genitals and impede sexual arousal and orgasm in women. Spontaneous and responsive desire, orgasm, and arousal can be greatly affected by decreasing hormone levels, fatigue, depression, and pain that is often associated with chronic illness (Foley et al. 2012).

Diabetes can cause nerve damage or circulatory problems that cause alterations in sexual functioning. Elevated blood glucose levels often lead to fatigue, resulting in decreased sexual interest. A decrease in vaginal lubrication is also common, and diabetic women have an increased prevalence of dyspareunia. Women with cardiovascular disease often have an overwhelming fear that sex will provoke another heart attack or stroke. They are not only apprehensive about the possibility of another attack, but also fearful of the risks leading to a decrease in arousal and desire. Arthritis is incredibly common in older women and results in difficulties with sexual intimacy because of the pain. General pleasuring of the body, oral sex, and creative sexual positioning allow women with arthritis to experience sexual intimacy with their partner (Yarber et al., 2010).

Cancer in women significantly affects a woman's sexuality. In fact, it has been noted that 30% to 100% of female cancer survivors experience sexual dysfunction. Much of the research on cancer and sexuality has been done with breast cancer survivors; however, emerging literature in gynecologic cancers have reported similar incidences of sexual dysfunction (Dizon, Suzin, & McIlvenna, 2014). Alterations in body image caused by surgery, menopause triggered by chemotherapy, hair loss, pain, and emotional stress make women with cancer more vulnerable to sexual problems. Sexual dysfunctions may result from surgery, radiotherapy, hormone therapy, or chemotherapy. Surgery, such as a mastectomy for breast cancer, or changes in the hormonal milieu, as in the case of an oophorectomy for ovarian cancer, influence a woman's sexuality because of direct anatomic changes. Oophorectomy causes an immediate depletion of estrogen in premenopausal women, resulting in early onset menopause. This leads to symptoms of vaginal atrophy, compromised elasticity, and dryness, all of which can affect the ability of women to engage in sexual intercourse. Hysterectomy often results in direct anatomical changes to the vaginal vault, including fibrosis and vaginal shortening. Mastectomies in women with breast cancer can affect body image and self-esteem, both of which can influence to a woman's sexuality (Dizon et al., 2014). A study by Burwell, Case, Kaelin, and Avis (2006) showed that alterations in body image and perceptions of decreased sexual attractiveness were associated with greater sexual problems and were a negative predictor for sexual activity in cancer patients. Radiotherapy can cause nerve damage, vaginal atrophy, and fibrosis of body areas exposed to radiation, causing obliteration of the vaginal canal in the case of genital radiation. Selective estrogen receptor modulators (SERMs) such as tamoxifen and aromatase inhibitors, which decrease breast tissue exposure to estrogen, frequently can contribute to vaginal dryness, pruritus, and dyspareunia (Cakar, Karaca, & Uslu, 2013). Cytotoxic agents cause fatigue, weakness, nausea and vomiting, and altered body image from hair loss, all of which limit a woman's sexual arousal and interest (Dizon et al., 2014). Providers must be aware of the importance of sexuality for most women, and a diagnosis of cancer does not alter this.

Women with disabilities, whether lifelong or acquired, experience significant challenges to their sexuality (Foley et al., 2012). Women with disabilities are sometimes viewed as asexual by health care providers and the public, and they are not encouraged to express sexual feelings or to be sexually active (Cesario, 2002). A disability of sudden onset often mirrors the grief of a serious illness. Restrictions to a woman's anatomy is shocking initially, and she will need a period to grieve for function that may now be lost. Changes in physical appearance and changes in body image largely affect a woman's sexuality, both in self-concept and in partner responses (Foley et al., 2012). Researchers have found that women with more severe physical impairments experience more sexual depression, less sexual self-esteem, and less sexual satisfaction than those with mild or no impairment and that those with severe physical disabilities engage in sex less frequently. Specific physical effects of a given disability on sexual activity differ with the disability. Women with spinal cord

TABLE 19.1	Potential Effects of Illness, Disease, and Drugs on Sexual Desire, Arousal, and Orgasm	
ILLNESS OR DISEASE	**POSSIBLE EFFECTS ON SEXUAL DESIRE OR AROUSAL**	**POSSIBLE EFFECTS ON ORGASM**
Depression	Low sexual desire in untreated patients; may be linked to sleep disturbance, low self-image, despair, and withdrawal	
Coronary artery disease, myocardial infarction	Frequency of sexual activity often reduced. May be linked to fear of triggering another cardiac event. Comorbid depression may be a factor	
Renal failure	Low desire common in those undergoing dialysis; comorbid depression. Desire may not be triggered because of repeatedly painful sexual episodes caused by estrogen depletion	
Lower urinary tract symptoms, including urinary incontinence	Leakage of urine with vaginal penetration reduces sexual motivation	Orgasm may be delayed or absent
Diabetes	Low desire reported, and difficulty with vasocongestion and lubrication may be a factor	
Hyperprolactinemia	Reduced arousal	Reduced orgasm, dyspareunia
Postmenopause endocrine changes	Vaginal lubrication may be reduced and vasocongestion reduced; may or may not be perceived in relation to sexual desire	Orgasm may be painful
Inflammatory processes		Pelvic inflammatory disease, endometriosis; may perceive pain with orgasm
Bilateral oophorectomy	Loss of ovarian testosterone and androstenedione precursors to estrogen	
Adrenal disease	Lack of precursor sex hormones (androstenedione, DHEA)	
Neurological disease	Direct nerve damage in regions involved in processing sexual stimuli	
Parkinson's disease	Low desire common in women	
Multiple sclerosis	Low desire in conjunction with other sexual dysfunctions more likely with pontine lesions	
Head injury	Direct damage to regions involved in processing sexual stimuli	
Spinal cord injury		Orgasm may be delayed or absent, especially with complete upper motor neuron lesion
Pelvic floor dysfunction		Orgasm delayed or absent
Pelvic nerve damage		Orgasm may be delayed or absent as a result of radical pelvic surgery
Drugs		
Antipsychotics	Low desire, possibly linked to reduced dopamine, increased prolaction, alpha blockade, and muscarinic blockade	Orgasm may be delayed or absent
Antihypertensives	Selective and nonselective beta blockade	
Antidepressants	Stimulate serotonin receptors, including 5-HT$_3$	Selective serotonin reuptake inhibitors may be associated with delayed or absent orgasm

(continued)

TABLE 19.1	Potential Effects of Illness, Disease, and Drugs on Sexual Desire, Arousal, and Orgasm *(continued)*	
ILLNESS OR DISEASE	**POSSIBLE EFFECTS ON SEXUAL DESIRE OR AROUSAL**	**POSSIBLE EFFECTS ON ORGASM**
Antiandrogens	Suppression of GnRH or LH, antagonism of androgens	May be associated with delayed or absent orgasm
Narcotics	Suppression of GnRH	
Antiepileptics	Cytochrome P-450 hepatic enzymes, increased SHBG, decreased testosterone	

DHEA, dehydroepiandrosterone; GnRH, gonadotropin-releasing hormone; LH, leuteinizing hormone; SHBG, sex hormone–binding globulin.
Adapted from Basson and Schultz (2007, Tables 1 and 4); Fogel (2006).

injuries are generally not able to experience orgasm and experience diminished sensations at climax. They are able to experience sensuous feelings in other parts of their bodies and may discover new erogenous areas such as their necks, ears, or thighs. Women with disabilities must overcome the anger that is frequently present if their bodies do not return to their previous sexual function expectations. They must realign their expectations with their actual sexual capabilities in order to establish sexual satisfaction and health (Yarber et al., 2010).

Many medications can alter sexual functioning and cause sexual dysfunctions, including decreased sexual desire, lack of sexual arousal, inadequate lubrication, and delayed or absent orgasm. These effects are summarized in Table 19.1. Depending on the dosage and the individual's mental and physical state, some medications known to inhibit sexual function may also enhance it. Examples of such drugs include the benzodiazepine tranquilizers and chlorpheniramine (Roberts, Fromm, & Bartlik, 1998).

Having a disability or chronic illness does not mean that a woman's sexual life ends. A woman's sexual well-being is a quality-of-life issue, and it is necessary for providers to educate women with physical limitations about their sexuality, including counseling to build self-esteem and combat negative stereotypes. Providers need to give their patients "permission" to engage in sexual activities and suggest new activities or techniques in order for them to be able to have full and satisfying sex lives (Yarber et al., 2010).

Substance use and abuse can have an adverse effect on sexual functioning and sexuality. Sexual dysfunctions can occur with the use of substances such as alcohol, amphetamines, cocaine, opioids sedatives, and tranquilizers (Teets, 1990). As a result of popular culture and media images depicting thin, beautiful, and scantily clad women drinking, the belief that alcohol and sex go together is common. The belief that alcohol is a sexual enhancement is also a popular myth. Alcohol leads to disinhibition, causes decreased lubrication, dulls stimulation, and contributes to sexual risk taking. Similar to alcohol use, most recreational drugs interfere with libido and sexual functioning, including making orgasm difficult. Drug use has been linked to greater risk of acquiring STIs, including HIV. Addiction to various drugs, such as cocaine (especially crack), has contributed to the practice of bartering sex for drugs. This practice has led to the epidemics of STIs and AIDS in many urban areas where condom use is rare (Yarber et al., 2010).

STIs are a significant health issue in the United States, with approximately 19 million new cases occurring each year. Risk factors for STIs in women include not using condoms with male partners, using drugs or alcohol before intercourse, having multiple sex partners, and having concurrent partners. It is important to recognize that although STIs are prevalent in heterosexual women, they are also prevalent in women who identify as gay, lesbian, or bisexual (Lindley, Walsemann, & Carter, 2013). Research has shown that STIs (especially genital herpes and human papillomavirus [HPV]) often have a negative impact on a woman's sexuality. An STI diagnosis has been shown to strongly influence a woman's feelings of sexuality and desirability (Newton & McCabe, 2008b). Women with genital herpes and HPV have been found to be more sexually anxious, more afraid of sex, more concerned about the impression created by their sexuality, and more sexually depressed than women without an STI. In addition, these women have been found to be less sexually satisfied than women without an STI, have lower self-esteem, and have a negative sexual self-concept. Women in a recent study felt their sexual behavior was restricted, and the number of sexual experiences they had was significantly decreased or ceased. This negative impact was found to decrease over time (Newton & McCabe, 2008a). Furthermore, women with genital herpes and HPV in committed relationships have reported that being in relationships buffered them from the shame and stigma of having an STI (Newton & McCabe, 2008a).

The adoption of safer sex practices (see Chapter 30) necessitates altered sexual practices. Women may decide to be celibate to avoid risk, decrease the number of their partners or avoid certain partners, and change or avoid specific sexual activities that increase risk. The risk of sexual coercion may be greater for women in power-imbalanced relationships with men who resist using condoms. Sex roles and sexual double standards may hinder a woman's ability to ask for safer sex practices and contribute to a man's resistance to implementing these practices.

Relationship Issues

Although this belief is changing, women often associate sex with love, and a woman's subjective perception of sexual pleasure is influenced by her perception of her relationship with her partner. Women have reported that their most pleasurable sexual feelings were in response to intercourse with a partner, though their most profound physical sexual responses occurred in response to masturbation (Darling, Davidson, & Jennings, 1991). Although women do report having sex for pure physical release, they typically view sex from a relational perspective and seek emotional connections with partners. For most women, love legitimizes sex. Research has shown that love in conjunction with social rewards, intimacy, commitment, and equity is an important determinant of sexual satisfaction. Communication is the thread that ties sexuality and intimacy. The quality of the communication affects the quality of the relationship, which in turn affects the quality of sex. Sex often serves as the barometer of the relationship: Good relationships tend to consist of satisfying sex, whereas bad relationships tend to consist of unsatisfying sex (Yarber et al., 2010). Sexual communication difficulties can be exacerbated by distrust, feelings of betrayal, and fear of disease when sex has occurred outside of a committed relationship. Sexual dysfunction in one partner may precipitate dysfunction in the other partner; for example, erectile difficulty in a man is sometimes accompanied by lack of vaginal lubrication, orgasmic difficulties, and impaired desire disorders in a female partner.

Loss of a Partner

Loss of a partner can adversely affect opportunities for intimacy as well as sexual expression. Many women define their identity through their relationships; thus loss of a partner can create a loss of the sense of self. Furthermore, the typical image of a widow is that of a grieving woman whose sexual life has ended. Factors that may be related to a woman's sexuality after the loss of a partner are her extramarital sexual experiences, age, and sexual satisfaction in the marriage (Bernhard, 1995). Remarriage is correlated with age. The older a woman is when she loses a partner, the less likely she is to remarry.

■ SEXUAL DYSFUNCTIONS

FSD describes various sexual problems associated with decreased arousal or desire, difficulty with orgasm, and dyspareunia or sexual pain (Shifren, Monz, Russo, Segreti, & Johannes, 2008). Sexual dysfunction in women poses a dramatic impact on quality of life, self-esteem, body image, and interpersonal relationships. Sexual dysfunction is largely underdiagnosed and undertreated. Practitioners are frequently limited in time available to assess sexual problems and in their understanding of the multifactorial nature of sexuality and appropriate treatment options for dysfunction. Although many women are reluctant to discuss sexual problems, as awareness increases in society, women are becoming more comfortable opening up about their sexual difficulties and seeking treatment. The ability of clinicians to have a comprehensive understanding of the evaluation and current diagnostic classification of FSD is essential to the comprehensive care of women (Latif & Diamond, 2013).

Research on FSD documents that sexual dysfunction is a common condition and concern among women in the United States. In a national probability survey of 1,749 women, the U.S. National Health and Social Life Survey estimated that 43% of women reported sexual dysfunction (Laumann, Paik, & Rosen, 1999; Waite et al., 2009). In this survey, a strong association was noted among sexual problems and decreased emotional satisfaction, physical satisfaction, and overall life satisfaction. More recent data from a large cross-sectional population-based survey of 31,581 female adults aged 18 years and older in the United States, the Prevalence of Female Sexual Problems Associated with Distress and Determinants of Treatment Seeking (PRESIDE) study, evaluated the self-reported sexual problems of desire, arousal, and orgasm. Data from this study support earlier research that sexual problems are common among women, with the prevalence of reported sexual problems at 44.2% (Shifren et al., 2008). The most common sexual problem was low desire, with a prevalence of 38.7%, followed by low arousal at 26.1% and difficulty with orgasm at 20.5%. The prevalence of sexual problems increased with age, with 27.2% of women aged 18 to 44 years compared with 44.6% of middle-aged women and 80.1% of elderly women reporting any type of sexual dysfunction. It should be noted that these statistics may be misleading, as the criteria used to assess these data are not those currently used to diagnose sexual dysfunction (Latif & Diamond, 2013).

Women have considerable variation in how they rate the importance of sex, their optimal idea of sexual frequency, their preferred sexual practices, and the amount of stimulation required for arousal and satisfaction. It is important to note that although many women report sexual problems, the problem causes true distress in a smaller percentage of women. The PRESIDE study also evaluated the prevalence of personal distress associated with sexual problems. Although more recent studies have reported increased levels of associated levels of distress, sexually related personal distress was noted in 12% of women. Distress was lowest in women aged 65 years and older (8.9%), intermediate in women aged 18 to 44 years (10.8%), and highest in women aged 45 to 64 years (14.8%), It is important to correlate distressing sexual desire problems with issues such as age, marital/current partner status, poor self-assessed health, current depression, menopause status (natural and surgical menopause), and a history of urinary incontinence and anxiety (Shifren et al., 2008).

The criteria for diagnosis of FSD are classified by the APA's *Diagnostic and Statistical Manual of Mental Disorders (DSM)*. The *DSM* criteria for sexual dysfunctions have evolved throughout the years, reflecting the prevailing thinking of the time of publication. In the *DSM-IV* (APA, 1994), which was used until 2013, the diagnosis of a sexual dysfunction was based on the linear model of human sexual response proposed by Masters and Johnson (1966) and further developed by Kaplan (1974), with the idea that sexual desire was what lead to the initiation of sexual activity. More recent research has questioned the validity of that model because of the strict distinction between different phases of arousal and the linear model proving to be inadequate to explain sexual behavior in women (IsHak & Tobia, 2013). A movement away from the discrete and nonoverlapping phases of sexual function noted in the linear model toward a more circular model more representative of women's sexual response has been recently seen. The linear models have suggested that sexual response is the same for both men and women and that desire always precedes arousal. Basson's (2000) nonlinear model of female sexual response recognizes that female sexual functioning is not as linear as male sexual functioning and is more complex. In this model, women are presumed to have motivations for sexual activity other than physical release. The decision to be sexual may come from a conscious wish for emotional closeness with a partner or as a result of seduction or suggestion from a partner. Sexual neutrality, or being receptive to sexual activity rather than the initiation of sexual activity, is considered to be the normal variant of sexual functioning for women. Basson (2000) points out that sexually healthy women in established relationships may not be aware of spontaneous sexual thoughts and that subjective and physiological sexual arousal can precede desire, negating the assumption that spontaneous desire is always normal in women (Kingsberg & Janata, 2007). This new framework for conceptualizing the female sexual response has led to several proposed changes in the diagnostic criteria of sexual dysfunction (IsHak & Tobia, 2013).

FSD may be lifelong (referring to a sexual problem that has occurred from the first sexual experience) or acquired (referring to a sexual problem that has developed after a time of relatively normal sexual function). FSD is further divided as situational (it is noted only in certain types of situations or stimulation or with certain partners) or generalized (it is not limited to certain situations, partners, or stimulation).

Multiple factors must be considered during the assessment of FSD:

1. Partner factors such as the partner's health status or sexual dysfunction
2. Relationship factors such as poor communication or discrepancies between partners' desire for sexual activity
3. Individual vulnerability factors inclusive of a history of sexual or emotional abuse or a woman's poor body image
4. Cultural or religious factors, which encompass a woman's attitude toward sexuality or inhibitions related to sexual activity and pleasure
5. Medical factors that become relevant to prognosis and treatment

Under the *DSM-IV*, the classification of FSD was divided into four dysfunctions: (a) female desire disorders, including: hypoactive sexual desire disorder and female sexual aversion disorder; (b) female sexual arousal disorder; (c) female orgasmic disorder; and (d) sexual pain disorders, including dyspareunia and vaginismus. In the revised *DSM-5* (APA, 2013), female sexual disorders are reclassified as (a) desire and arousal disorders, (b) genito-pelvic pain/penetration disorder (inclusive of vaginismus and dyspareunia), and (c) female orgasmic disorder. Sexual aversion disorder has been removed from *DSM-5* because of the lack of supporting research (IsHak & Tobia, 2013). The separation of sexual dysfunction caused by a general medical condition from FSD, which is related to psychological causes, has also been removed, noting that most sexual dysfunctions are the result of both psychological and biological factors (Latif & Diamond, 2013). *DSM-5* sexual dysfunctions all require a minimum duration of 6 months, as well as a frequency of experiencing the disorder 75% to 100% of the time. Finally, for appropriate diagnosis, the disorder must cause "significant distress" (IsHak & Tobia, 2013). It has been noted in most surveys that approximately 40% of women do not rate sex as important for their physical or emotional well-being. This has lead to a strong emphasis on distress as a necessary component of the definition of sexual dysfunction in women (Rosen & Barsky, 2006).

Female Orgasmic Disorder

Female orgasmic disorder is characterized by marked delay in, infrequency of, or absence of orgasm and/or in markedly reduced intensity of orgasmic sensations. A wide variability in the type or intensity of stimulation that elicits orgasm has been shown in women. Furthermore, it has been found that subjective descriptions of orgasm are widely varied, which suggests that it is experienced in very different ways, both in various women as well as on different occasions by the same woman. For the diagnosis of female orgasmic disorder to be made, symptoms must be present for a minimum duration of approximately 6 months during approximately 75% to 100% of occasions of sexual activity. This criteria is used to distinguish between transient orgasm difficulties from more persistent orgasmic dysfunction. In addition, clinically significant distress must be present. If FSD symptoms are better explained by another mental disorder, a medical condition, or the effects of a substance/medication, then a diagnosis of FSD would *not* be made. If interpersonal factors, such as intimate partner violence, severe relationship distress, or other significant stressors are present, a diagnosis of female orgasmic disorder would also not be made.

Many women require adequate clitoral stimulation to reach orgasm, and in fact, a relatively small proportion of women report consistently experiencing an orgasm with penile–vaginal intercourse. A woman who experiences orgasm through clitoral stimulation but not with intercourse does not meet the criteria for the diagnosis of a sexual dysfunction. It is important to determine if difficulties with orgasm are the result of inadequate sexual stimulation, in which case education and care would be indicated but a diagnosis would not be made (APA, 2013).

Female Sexual Interest/Arousal Disorder

The diagnostic criteria for female sexual interest/arousal disorder includes lack of or significantly reduced sexual interest/arousal, as manifested by at least three of the following:

1. Absent/reduced interest in sexual activity
2. Absent/reduced sexual/erotic thoughts or fantasies
3. No/reduced initiation of sexual activity and typical lack of response to a partner's attempts to initiate
4. Absent/reduced sexual excitement/pleasure during sexual activity in 75% to 100% of sexual encounters
5. Absent/reduced sexual interest/arousal in response to any internal or external sexual/erotic cues such as visual, written, or verbal
6. Absent/reduced genital or nongenital sensations during sexual activity in 75% to 100% of sexual encounters

It is important to assess interpersonal context when assessing female sexual interest/arousal disorder. A "desire discrepancy," in which a woman experiences lower desire than her partner would not be sufficient for diagnosing this disorder. For the criteria to be met, there must be absence or reduced frequency or intensity of at least three of the six listed indicators for a minimum duration of approximately 6 months. The minimum duration of 6 months is required in order to determine if the symptoms are a persistent problem indicative of dysfunction or a short-term change in sexual interest or arousal, which is common. In order for the diagnosis to be made, clinically significant distress must also accompany the symptoms. Distress may be a result of significant interference in a woman's life and well-being. A diagnosis would also not be made if a lifelong lack of sexual desire is better explained as one's self-identification as "asexual" (APA, 2013).

Genitopelvic Pain/Penetration Disorder

Genitopelvic pain/penetration disorder is diagnosed by persistent or recurrent difficulties in one or more of the following:

1. Vaginal penetration during intercourse
2. Marked vulvovaginal or pelvic pain during vaginal intercourse or penetration attempts
3. Marked fear or anxiety about vulvovaginal or pelvic pain in anticipation of, during, or as a result of vaginal penetration
4. Marked tensing or tightening of the pelvic floor muscles during attempted vaginal penetration

Major difficulty in any one of these symptoms is sufficient to cause clinically significant distress. Therefore a diagnosis can be made on the basis of marked difficulty in only one symptom dimension. All symptom dimensions must be assessed, however, as many woman have more than one symptom.

Marked difficulty having vaginal intercourse or penetration can present as the ability to easily experience penetration in one situation such as tampon insertion or gynecologic examinations, but not in another such as intercourse. If pervasive, pain can cause complete inability to experience vaginal penetration in any situation. Marked pelvic or vulvovaginal pain during penetration attempts or vaginal intercourse indicates that pain occurs in different locations in the genitopelvic area. It is essential to assess the location as well as the intensity of pain. Pain may be characterized as occurring during initial penetration, affecting the vulva (described as "superficial pain"), or it can be felt further into penetration and thrusting, affecting the vagina and the pelvic floor muscles (described as "deep pain"). Pain may be provoked or occurring only with stimulation, unprovoked, or spontaneous or occurs both with provocation and spontaneously. The pain can also persist for a period of time after intercourse has ceased or during urination.

Marked fear or anxiety about pelvic or vulvovaginal pain either in anticipation of or during vaginal penetration is common among women who have regularly experienced pain during sexual intercourse. This is a "normal" reaction and may lead to avoidance of sexual or intimate situations.

Marked tightening or tensing of the pelvic floor muscles with attempted penetration can vary from voluntary muscle guarding to reflexive-like spasm of the pelvic floor in response to fear, anxiety, or anticipation of pain.

Frequently, genitopelvic pain/penetration disorder is associated with other sexual dysfunctions because pain often results in decreased interest, arousal, and avoidance of intimacy. It is critically important to assess pain during the evaluation of any sexual dysfunction in order to determine the role it plays in other dysfunctions (APA, 2013).

In *DSM-IV*, the term *vaginismus* referred to the persistent or recurrent involuntary spasm of the musculature of the outer third of the vagina or persistent difficulty to allow vaginal entry of a finger, a penis, or an object despite a woman's expressed desire to do so (Crowley, Goldmeier, & Hiller, 2009.) Although vaginismus has been removed as a diagnosis from the *DSM-5*, providers should be aware of the terminology, as many continue to use the diagnosis. The decision to remove vaginismus was based on the conclusion that dyspareunia and vaginismus could not be reliably differentiated. This was due in part to a lack of empirical evidence supporting vaginismus as a "vaginal muscle spasm" as well as because of the fact that fear of penetration or pain is commonly found in descriptions of vaginismus (IsHak & Tobia, 2013).

Sexual Pain/Dyspareunia

Sexual pain or dyspareunia is one of the most common complaints seen in general gynecologic practice (Steege & Zolnoun, 2009). In a recent U.S. national sample, approximately 30% of women reported some degree of pain during their most recent sexual experience (Herbenick et al., 2010). Unfortunately, sexual pain is one of the more difficult problems to evaluate, diagnose, and successfully treat. In part, this is because of the multitude of potential etiologies that exist and the fact that many women presenting with dyspareunia do not have one single cause of their pain (Steege & Zolnoun, 2009). In addition, there are few providers capable of properly diagnosing and treating women with sexual pain (Goldstein, Pukall, & Goldstein, 2011).

This is unfortunate in that dyspareunia affects much more than a woman's ability to enjoy sex. It becomes the center of a woman's life, affecting her relationships, sexuality, and self-esteem (Goldstein et al., 2011). Vulvodynia, interstitial cystitis, and endometriosis are three medical conditions in which sexual pain is the primary symptom. These conditions have been found to share common pathogenic factors that magnify sexual pain (Bachmann et al., 2006).

Dyspareunia is the medical term for sexual pain. It refers to persistent or recurrent genital pain that is experienced during or after sexual intercourse (Schultz et al., 2005). It may be attributed to an organic and/or psychological etiology and exists as a symptom stemming from a multitude of painful conditions and disease states (Whitmore, Siegel, & Kellogg-Spadt, 2007). According to Whitmore et al. (2007) the prevalence of dyspareunia varies greatly according to the how it is assessed. When dyspareunia is defined as pain that occurs during or after sexual intercourse, the prevalence among sexually active women has been estimated to be 61% in the general population (Whitmore et al., 2007).

Dyspareunia may occur during initial penetration, throughout the entire act of intercourse, or after intercourse (Whitmore et al., 2007). Women may complain of sexual pain associated with certain positions or may experience the pain with the act of thrusting. Pain may be localized to a specific area of the vulva or vagina or may be generalized and has been described from a sharp and burning pain to a dull ache (Whitmore et al., 2007). Dyspareunia is defined according to when and where the pain occurs related to intercourse. Pain that occurs on initial penetration of the vaginal introitus, once referred to as *superficial, introital,* or *entry dyspareunia,* is now more commonly referred to as *vestibulodynia* (Dhingra, Kellogg-Spadt, McKinney, & Whitmore, 2012; Ferraro, Ragni, & Remorgida, 2008). *Deep dyspareunia* is defined as painful intercourse deep within the vaginal vault (Ferraro et al., 2008).

Vulvodynia

According to Bachmann et al. (2006), vulvodynia is defined as a chronic pain in the vulvar area that has persisted for at least 3 to 6 months without a definable cause. Vulvodynia is a frequent cause of dyspareunia, with the estimated prevalence as high as 15% of all women; however, nearly 50% of women with the condition fail to seek treatment (Harlow, Vitonis, & Gunther Stewart, 2008). In women who do seek medical care, their condition is often misdiagnosed because of a lack of knowledge among health care providers, or because of inconsistent diagnostic criteria (Feldhaus-Dahir, 2011). The International Society for the Study of Vulvovaginal Disease (ISSVD) has classified vulvodynia into generalized (pain throughout the vulvar area) and localized (pain localized to the vulvar vestibule); the latter is referred to as *vestibulodynia.* Vulvodynia is further subdivided into pain that is provoked, occurring with stimuli such as touch, and unprovoked, which is spontaneous and occurs without any stimuli or pressure. Vulvodynia may also be mixed, occurring both spontaneously or with provocation (Feldhaus-Dahir, 2011).

Generalized Vulvodynia

Generalized vulvodynia (GVD) is typically described as a constant burning pain involving much of the vulva and often including the vulvar vestibule (Goldstein et al., 2011). The pain involves both nerve pain and pelvic muscle floor muscle pain produced by overly taut musculature (Goldstein et al., 2011). The structures of the vulva are normal in appearance, and there is no obvious underlying cause (van Lankveld et al., 2010). The etiology of GVD remains elusive, but GVD it most likely occurs from a wide variety of sources and disease processes (Goldstein & Burrows, 2008). Although some women are not able to decipher a trigger for their pain, many report an inciting factor such as having a yeast infection, starting an oral contraceptive (OC) or antibiotic, or sustaining a trauma or having surgery in their pelvic region (Goldstein et al., 2011).

One consensus has emerged regarding the etiology of GVD; however, that generalized unprovoked vulvodynia is described most accurately when it is thought of as a complex regional pain syndrome (CRPS; Goldstein, Marinoff, & Haefner, 2005). Women with vulvodynia, like those with other CRPSs, have enhanced systemic pain perception, a process known as *central nervous system sensitization* (Goldstein et al., 2005). In addition, women with vulvodynia are also more likely to have other CRPSs such as interstitial cystitis and fibromyalgia (Goldstein & Burrows, 2008). This may be explained by another phenomenon known as *wind-up* that is common to CRPS in which there is a "progressively increasing activity in dorsal horn cells of the spinal cord following repetitive activation of primary afferent C-fibers" (Goldstein & Burrows, 2008, p. 33). GVD appears to be a form of neuropathic pain in which women experience a clinical phenomenon called *allodynia,* in which a painful sensation is experienced in response to normal nonpainful stimuli (Goldstein et al., 2011). These women experience hyperalgesia in which stimuli that are known to provoke mild pain create an exaggerated pain response (Schultz et al., 2005). It is unknown what triggers the altered pain response experienced in vulvodynia; however it has been hypothesized that an injury to the pudendal nerve may activate the hypersensitivity. After the injury occurs, the wind-up phenomenon may take place (Goldstein et al., 2011).

Vestibulodynia

Vestibulodynia is the most common cause of dyspareunia in premenopausal women and has been estimated to affect 15% in the gynecologic setting (Landry, Bergeron, Dupuis, & Desrochers, 2008). Vestibulodynia has been defined since 1988 by Friedrich's Criteria as "(1) severe pain upon vestibular touch or attempted vaginal entry, (2) acute pain during cotton swab palpation of the vestibular area, and (3) vestibular erythema" (Landry et al., 2008, p. 155). Recent studies, however, have refuted the third criteria of vestibular erythema as a diagnostic parameter in that many women with vestibulodynia do not present with vestibular erythema (Landry et al., 2008). Vestibulodynia has been referred to by various names, including *vulvar vestibulitis syndrome, localized provoked vulvodynia,* and *provoked vestibulodynia* (Feldhaus-Dahir, 2011). It should be noted, however, that in 2003 the ISSVD stopped using the term *vestibulitis* because the suffix *itis* implied inflammation and consistency in this pathology has not been determined (Haefner, 2006).

Primary vestibulodynia is characterized as pain at first introital touch, regardless of whether the touch is via tampon insertion or sexual debut. Secondary vestibulodynia is pain experienced after an interval of painless intercourse (Goldstein et al., 2005). Vestibulodynia is most often symptomatic during the penetrative phase of sexual intercourse, termed *entry dyspareunia* and may even prohibit penetration (Kellogg-Spadt, Younaitis Fariello, & Safaeian, 2007). The pain may be also be provoked in other situations when pressure is exerted on the vestibule, such as wearing of constrictive clothing, tampon insertion, pelvic examination, bicycle riding, or prolonged sitting (Feldhaus-Dahir, 2011).

Despite the negative impact of vestibulodynia on a woman's ability to have comfortable sexual intercourse, progress surrounding the etiology and treatment has been slow (Landry et al., 2008). The etiology is considered to be multifactorial, and it appears that vestibulodynia is not one disease in itself but rather several underlying conditions that result in a similar set of symptoms (Goldstein et al., 2011). Vulvodynia experts have isolated inflammation, genetic factors, hormonal influences, and psychosocial factors as possible causes (van Lankveld et al., 2010). A possible etiological correlation also has been discussed related to a previous history of recurrent vulvovaginal candidiasis. In addition, a history of OC use has been documented related to vestibulodynia (van Lankveld et al., 2010). It has been noted in recent studies that OCs alter the vaginal epithelium as well as cause vaginal atrophy, which causes pain during intercourse. Interestingly, Harlow et al. (2008) has also noted that women on OCs have significantly lower pain thresholds compared with women not taking OCs. It has been suggested that primary vestibulodynia could be a congenital disorder in which there is a defect in the urogenital sinus during embryological development (Feldhaus-Dahir, 2011). Researchers have also shown an increase in C-afferent nociceptors in the vestibular tissue, which contributes to the hypersensitivity to touch and pain that women with vestibulodynia possess (Feldhaus-Dahir, 2011). Finally, pelvic floor hypertonus is commonly found in women with dyspareunia and vestibulodynia in which the muscle has decreased contractile strength as well as myofascial trigger points that may arise from habitual "clenching" or "tensing" as a defensive reaction to painful penetrative attempts. A vicious cycle of pain leading to further muscle dysfunction has been postulated in high-tone pelvic floor dysfunction, as hypertonus has been thought to activate vulvar mucosal sensitivity (Moldwin & Yonaitis Fariello, 2013).

Impact of Dyspareunia

Dyspareunia is a form of sexual dysfunction that has a significant impact on a woman's sexuality (Ferraro et al.,

2008). Women with vestibulodynia report decreased sexual interest, arousal, satisfaction, and self-esteem. It has been reported that women with deep dyspareunia are less relaxed as well as less fulfilled after sex, have a limited number of intercourse episodes per week, and have less satisfying orgasms (Ferraro et al., 2008). Women often avoid sexual contact and refuse a partner's sexual advances in an attempt to avoid or reduce pain (Sadownik, 2014). Women with vestibulodynia report more negative feelings about sexual contact with their partner. These women are characterized by lower sexual pleasure and a higher degree of erotophobia (van Lankveld et al., 2010).

Women experiencing dyspareunia often feel that physical intimacy becomes an unwelcome physical and emotional challenge (van Lankveld et al, 2010). This often leads to partners of women with dyspareunia feeling helpless, angry, and depressed. They believe their partner is avoiding sex for reasons beyond pain and feel rejected (Goldstein et al., 2011). Therefore, it is essential that such couples discover other ways to be intimate. They must learn that sex involves more than just intercourse and that communicating is a necessary part of a sexual relationship, especially when pain is involved (Goldstein et al., 2011).

Dyspareunia also exhibits a profound impact on a woman's psychological status. It is well documented that feelings of anxiety, depression, and hopelessness are common in women with chronic pain. Higher rates of depression as well as anxiety disorders, including generalized anxiety disorder, simple phobia, obsessive-compulsive disorder, and social phobia, are found in women with dyspareunia (van Lankveld et al., 2010). Unfortunately, even when dyspareunia is resolved, the psychological dysfunction often persists (Goldstein & Burrows, 2008). Although sexual pain is one of the most common complaints in the gynecologic setting, it is never a normal finding. Dyspareunia is often a symptom of a complex multitude of disease states that are poorly understood. In addition, women complaining of sexual pain often have multiple conditions that are related, further exacerbating their pain as well as complicating the diagnosis (Steege & Zolnoun, 2009). It is essential that providers assess for dyspareunia in their practice in that many of these conditions are progressive and detrimental to a women's life. Not only are women with dyspareunia dealing with pain, but also their pain is compounded by the impact it has on their sense of self-esteem, well-being, and relationships (van Lankveld et al., 2010).

Assessing for sexual dysfunction or sexual pain should include a thorough evaluation of the woman's pain (in terms of its quality, quantity, location, duration, and aggravating and relieving factors). A complete medical, surgical, obstetric, gynecologic, and contraceptive history should be collected and should include questions about previous vaginal or pelvic surgeries and pelvic trauma such as rape and sexual abuse. Women should always be questioned about the use of medications, douching, and perineal products such as sprays, deodorants, and sanitary pads. Furthermore, various validated questionnaires have been developed in order to assess sexual dysfunction in women and assist the clinician in establishing a diagnosis. The Brief Sexual Symptoms Checklist for Women (Figure 19.1; Hatzichristou et al., 2010) is a self-report tool that may be

Please answer the following questions about your overall sexual function:

1. Are you satisfied with your sexual function?   ❏ Yes   ❏ No

If no, please continue.

2. How long have you been dissatisfied with your sexual function? _____

3. Mark which of the following problems you are having, and circle the one that is most bothersome:
   ❏ Little or no interest in sex
   ❏ Decreased genital sensation (feeling)
   ❏ Decreased vaginal lubrication (dryness)
   ❏ Problem reaching orgasm
   ❏ Pain during sex
   ❏ Other: _____

4. Would you like to talk about it with your doctor?   ❏ Yes   ❏ No

FIGURE 19.1
Brief sexual symptoms checklist for women.

useful in the primary care setting. It consists of four basic questions regarding the patient's satisfaction with her sexual function, details about specific sexual problems, and willingness to discuss them with a provider.

Other Tools

The Decreased Sexual Desire Screener is a brief questionnaire that was recently found to have a 95% to 96% sensitivity in assessing hypoactive sexual desire disorder (Latif & Diamond, 2013). Although it should be noted that this diagnosis was combined with sexual arousal disorder in the *DSM-5*, the tool may still be beneficial in evaluating a decrease in desire. The Female Sexual Distress Scale is a 12-item scale that focuses on a woman's distress associated with sexual dysfunction. Finally, the Female Sexual Function Index (FSFI) is a 19-item questionnaire that is a brief, multidimensional self-report tool for assessing the key dimensions of sexual function in women (Rosen et al., 2000). This tool assesses sexual functioning in six separate dimensions, including desire, arousal, lubrication, orgasm, satisfaction, and pain, and is the most comprehensive and widely utilized questionnaire in sexual medicine practices (Latif & Diamond, 2013).

Physical examination is necessary to exclude other diagnoses, educate women, and localize the vulvar pain. Women with vulvodynia are often anxious and fearful about the vulvovaginal examination because many have had negative experiences with it. It is helpful and empowering to have the patient observe the examination of the vulva, which can be facilitated by a handheld mirror through which the clinician can review the anatomy of the vulva with the patient. The exam could reveal infection, vaginal atrophy, masses, lesions, pelvic floor muscle dysfunction, deep pelvic pain, or vulvar dermatoses (Latif & Diamond, 2013). During the examination, the vulva should be inspected, examining all surfaces and noting changes in skin color or texture, inflammation and/or lesions. Changes to the vulvar anatomy, such as adherence of the clitoris to the prepuce (i.e., phimosis)

or loss of the labia minora, should be noted and are suggestive of vulvar dermatoses such as lichen sclerosus and/or lichen planus. The vulva should next be palpated with pressure that is light but consistent, using a cotton swab; this is called the *Q-tip test*. In a clockwise manner, beginning at the mons, the examiner moves to the labia majora and perineal and perianal tissue. Throughout the palpation, the patient should be asked if the area being touched is painful. The mons and labia majora are commonly not painful in women with vulvodynia, so beginning the evaluation with these structures can help decrease the fear and anxiety of a painful examination. Still using the cotton swab, the examiner should then palpate the vestibule after separating the labia minora, having the woman identify any painful areas and grade the pain on a scale from 0 to 10. Women with vestibulodynia often believe that the pain is inside the vagina and are often surprised to visualize and learn that the painful area is in fact confined to the vestibule. The internal assessment should be completed by inserting a single digit into the vagina to assess the tone and function of the pelvic floor muscles on the left and right. The clinician should assess the ability of the patient to contract her pelvic floor muscles around the examining finger and then relax that contraction on command. The patient should be asked to characterize the pressure exerted by the examining digit as either causing sensations of pressure or pain. If the patient verifies that pressure on the lateral vaginal wall results in pain, if the examiner feels dramatic tautness of the levator muscles, and/or if a twitch response is elicited (i.e., during muscle palpation, a spasm or twitch is felt by the examiner or the pain the patient feels is referred to another site), the patient likely has pelvic floor muscle hypertonus, which warrants a referral for further evaluation with a physical therapist specializing in the pelvic floor muscles. Last, the bladder, urethra, uterus, and adnexa should be evaluated to rule out pelvic or bladder pathology, both of which can contribute to dyspareunia (Sadownik, 2014).

The first and essential step in treating a woman with dyspareunia is validating that her pain is a real and legitimate condition. It is often very useful to have this discussion in the presence of the patient's partner. Causes of the pain should be discussed, with an emphasis that the etiology is often multifactorial (Sadownik, 2014). A discussion of proper hygiene practices is paramount with all women experiencing vulvar or sexual pain because women might use commercial products that cause irritation and/or damage the skin. Medical treatment of vulvodynia should be individualized, as there is no "one-size-fits-all" approach. Evidence-based topical approaches used in the treatment of pain in the vestibule include hormonal preparations such as compounded estradiol and testosterone cream, cromolyn cream, amitriptyline cream, capsaicin cream, and lidocaine gel. Low-dose oral tricyclic antidepressants such as amitriptyline and nortriptyline, as well as gabapentin and pregabalin, are often used for control of neuropathic pain (Butrick, 2009).

Herbenick et al. (2010) recently concluded that the prevalence of women experiencing pain and difficulty with lubrication is significant. In fact, approximately 54% of women use lubricants because they feel that their vaginal lubrication is insufficient, contributing to increased pain and discomfort with sex. Decreased lubrication is commonly noted in postmenopausal women, breast cancer survivors, lactating women, and women experiencing vulvovaginal pain. Use of lubricants makes sex less painful and more comfortable and is associated with increased sexual pleasure and satisfaction. Given the large number of women who experience painful or uncomfortable sex and feel that vaginal lubrication is insufficient, it is important for clinicians to incorporate questions about vaginal lubrication into any assessment of sexual dysfunction. However, given the potential for lubricants to cause irritation and contribute to discomfort, clinicians should suggest safe and nonirritating options to enhance sexual comfort (Herbenick, Reece, Schick, Sanders, & Fortenberry, 2014).

In women with high-tone pelvic floor musculature, physical therapy is essential in order to reeducate the muscles and facilitate sexual comfort and pleasure. Pelvic floor physical therapy utilizes myofascial release techniques, biofeedback, and electrical stimulation. Vaginal dilators and Thiele massage, or internal massage to the pelvic floor, are frequently used to prepare for sexual penetration in conjunction with precoital analgesics, muscle relaxants, and antispasmodics (Dhingra et al., 2012). Conservative therapies, such as control of chronic constipation and use of topical heat such as warm baths, may be helpful for pelvic floor muscle spasms. Last, trigger point injections to decrease tone in spastic pelvic floor muscles can be used with pharmacotherapy and physical and behavioral therapy (Moldwin & Yonaitis Fariello, 2013).

Referrals for therapy, including both sex therapy and psychotherapy, are frequently utilized in women with sexual dysfunction and especially in women with sexual pain. Both psychotherapy and sex therapy are frequently useful as an adjunct to medical treatment because of the significant psychological impact that vulvodynia has on women. Therapy may be aimed at helping to reestablish a women's self-esteem and self-concept, as well as to help couples learn how to be intimate again after often going through a prolonged stage without any form of intimacy (Sadownik, 2014.)

Genitourinary Syndrome of Menopause/VVA

VVA in menopause related to declining estrogen levels is common and is a frequent cause of sexual dysfunction and pain in this population. Loss of estrogen results in thinning of the vaginal epithelium, loss of collagen, and decreased blood flow in the tissue, leading to decreased lubrication, shortening and narrowing of the vaginal wall, and pale, dry mucosa. Because of the decreased genital perfusion, estrogen deficiency prolongs the time to vaginal vasocongestion, thus contributing to reduced intensity of orgasm (Simon, 2011). VVA is also termed *genitourinary symptom of menopause* (GSM) because estrogen deficiency can affect both the genital system and the lower urinary tract. It is associated with symptoms of vaginal dryness, dyspareunia, vaginal bleeding during or after coitus, burning, itching, irritation, reduced sexual responsiveness, and impaired sexual arousal in the genital system and dysuria, urgency, and frequency in the lower urinary tract (Rahn et al., 2014; Simon, 2011). Approximately half of postmenopausal women in the United States report symptoms of VVA, which causes a significant negative effect on quality of life. Although atrophy-related symptoms are common, only approximately half seek medical care or are offered help by their health care provider (Rahn et al., 2014). Menopausal symptoms, such as hot flashes, typically resolve over time, whereas the symptoms of VVA usually persist or increase without treatment (Portman, Palacios, Nappi, & Mueck, 2014).

Treatment of VVA seeks to restore the vagina and genital tissue to a healthier state and is aimed at alleviating symptoms associated with the estrogen deficiency. First-line treatments include long-acting vaginal moisturizers, lubricants, and vaginal estrogen, as well as continued sexual activity (Portman et al., 2014). Vaginal moisturizers, such as those with polycarbophilic ingredients (Replens) or pH-balanced gels (RepHresh), have been shown to improve vaginal symptoms; however, they have not been shown to have a benefit in histology or sexual function (Simon, 2011). Although systemic estrogen is effective in treating vasomotor symptoms, studies have shown it to provide adequate relief of vaginal dryness in only 40% of women (Portman et al., 2014). Local vaginal estrogen is available in a vaginal cream, ring, or tablet; the vaginal estrogen cream Premarin is also indicated to treat moderate to severe dyspareunia. Local vaginal estrogen cream has been shown to decrease vaginal pH, increase vaginal blood flow and lubrication; improve arousal, orgasm, and sexual satisfaction; and decrease vaginal dryness, pain, and dyspareunia (Simon, 2011). Ospemifene (Osphena) is the first nonhormonal oral alternative to estrogen to treat VVA and dyspareunia. It is a SERM that exerts agonist effects on the vulvovaginal tissue and has been shown to significantly reduce symptoms of vaginal dryness and dyspareunia. Osphemifene is a safe and effective option for the treatment of postmenopausal VVA and is approved by the U.S. Food and Drug Administration (FDA) to treat moderate to severe dyspareunia (Portman et al., 2014).

SUMMARY

When female patients express concerns regarding sexuality and sexual activity, they have the right to expect that advanced practice nurses will provide accurate sexual information, counseling, and/or appropriate therapy. This chapter provided an overview of sexual health and sexual dysfunction and a basis for nurse practitioners to assess women's concerns about sexual health, provide sexual health care, and make appropriate referrals for their care.

REFERENCES

Althof, S. E., Rosen, R. C., Perelman, M. A., & Rubio-Aurioles, E. (2013). Standard operating procedures for taking a sexual history. *The Journal of Sexual Medicine*, 10(1), 26–35.

Amaro, H., Navarro, A. M., Conron, K. J., & Raj, A. (2002). Cultural influences on women's sexual health. In G. M. Wingood & R. J. DiClemente (Eds.), *Handbook of women's sexual and reproductive health* (pp. 71–92). New York, NY: Kluwer Academic/Plenum.

American Psychiatric Association (APA). (1994). *Diagnostic and statistical manual of mental disorders* (4th ed.). Washington, DC: Author.

American Psychiatric Association (APA). (2013). *Diagnostic and statistical manual of mental disorders* (5th ed.). Arlington, VA: American Psychiatric Publishing.

Annon, J. (1976). The PLISSIT model: A proposed conceptual scheme for the behavioral treatment of sexual problems. *Journal of Sex Education and Therapy*, 2(2), 1–15.

Avery, M. D., Duckett, L., & Frantzich, C. R. (2000). The experience of sexuality during breastfeeding among primiparous women. *Journal of Midwifery & Women's Health*, 45(3), 227–237.

Bachmann, G. A., Rosen, R., Pinn, V. W., Utian, W. H., Ayers, C., Basson, R.,...Witkin, S. S. (2006). Vulvodynia: A state-of-the-art consensus of definitions, diagnosis and management. *Journal of Reproductive Medicine*, 51(6), 447–456. Retrieved from http://www.mireproductivemedicine.com

Basson, R. (2000). The female sexual response: A different model. *Journal of Sex & Marital Therapy*, 26(1), 51–65.

Basson, R. (2008). Women's sexual function and dysfunction: Current uncertainties, future directions. *International Journal of Impotence Research*, 20(5), 466–478.

Basson, R., & Schultz, W. W. (2007). Sexual sequelae of general medical disorders. *Lancet*, 369(9559), 409–424.

Bernhard, L. (1995). Sexuality in women's lives. In C. I. Fogel & N. F. Woods (Eds.), *Women's health care* (pp. 475–495). Thousand Oaks, CA: Sage.

Biro, F. M., & Dorn, L. D. (2005). Puberty and adolescent sexuality. *Pediatric Annals*, 34(10), 777–784.

Burwell, S. R., Case, L. D., Kaelin, C., & Avis, N. E. (2006). Sexual problems in younger women after breast cancer surgery. *Journal of Clinical Oncology*, 24(18), 2815–2821.

Butrick, C. W. (2009). Pathophysiology of pelvic floor hypertonic disorders. *Obstetrics and Gynecology Clinics of North America*, 36(3), 699–705.

Cakar, B., Karaca, B., & Uslu, R. (2013). Sexual dysfunction in cancer patients: A review. *Journal of B.U.ON.*, 18(4), 818–823.

Cesario, S. K. (2002), Spinal cord injuries. *AWHONN Lifelines*, 6, 224–232. doi: 10.1111/j.1552-6356.2002.tb00086.x

Chaplic, K. C., & Allen, P. J. (2013). Best practices to identify gay, lesbian, bisexual, or questioning youth in primary care. *Pediatric Nursing*, 39(2), 99–103.

Crowley, T., Goldmeier, D., & Hiller, J. (2009). Diagnosing and managing vaginismus. *British Medical Journey (Clinical Research ed.)*, 338, b2284.

Dargis, L., Trudel, G., Cadieux, J., Villeneuve, L., Préville, M., & Boye, R. (2012). Validation of the Female Sexual Function Index (FSFI) and presentation of norms in older women. *Sexologies*, 21(3), 126–131.

Darling, C. A., Davidson, J. K., & Jennings, D. A. (1991). The female sexual response revisited: Understanding the multiorgasmic experience in women. *Archives of Sexual Behavior*, 20(6), 527–540.

Dartnall, E., & Jewkes, R. (2013). Sexual violence against women: The scope of the problem. *Best Practice & Research. Clinical Obstetrics & Gynaecology*, 27(1), 3–13.

Davari Tanha, F., Mohseni, M., & Ghajarzadeh, M. (2014). Sexual function in women with primary and secondary infertility in comparison with controls. *International Journal of Impotence Research*, 26(4), 132–134.

Davis, S. R., & Jane, F. (2011). Sex and perimenopause. *Australian Family Physician*, 40(5), 274–278.

Dhingra, C., Kellogg-Spadt, S., McKinney, T. B., & Whitmore, K. E. (2012). Urogynecological causes of pain and the effect of pain on sexual function in women. *Female Pelvic Medicine & Reconstructive Surgery*, 18(5), 259–267.

Dizon, D. S., Suzin, D., & McIlvenna, S. (2014). Sexual health as a survivorship issue for female cancer survivors. *The Oncologist*, 19(2), 202–210.

Farr, R. H., Diamond, L. M., & Boker, S. M. (2014). Female same-sex sexuality from a dynamical systems perspective: Sexual desire, motivation, and behavior. *Archives of Sexual Behavior*, 43(8), 1477–1490.

Feldhaus-Dahir, M. (2011). The causes and prevalence of vestibulodynia: A vulvar pain disorder. *Urologic Nursing*, 31(1), 51–54.

Ferraro, S., Ragni, N., & Remorgida, V. (2008). Deep dyspareunia: Causes, treatments, and results. *Current Opinion in Obstetrics & Gynecology*, 20(4), 394–399.

Fogel, C. I. (2006). Sexuality. In K. Schuiling & F. Likis (Eds.), *Women's gynecologic health* (pp. 149–167). Boston, MA: Jones & Bartlett.

Foley, S., Kope, S. A., & Sugrue, D. P. (2012). Sex matters for women: A complete guide to taking care of your sexual self (2nd ed.). New York, NY: Guilford Press.

Ginsberg, T. B. (2006). Aging and sexuality. *The Medical Clinics of North America*, 90(5), 1025–1036.

Goldstein, A., Pukall, C., & Goldstein, I. (2011). *When sex hurts: A woman's guide to banishing sexual pain*. Philadelphia, PA: Da Capo Press.

Goldstein, A. T., & Burrows, L. (2008). Vulvodynia. *Journal of Sexual Medicine*, 5(1), 5–14; quiz 15.

Goldstein, A. T., Marinoff, S. C., & Haefner, H. K. (2005). Vulvodynia: Strategies for treatment. *Clinical Obstetrics and Gynecology*, 48(4), 769–785.

Goldstein, I., Dicks, B., Kim, N. N., & Hartzell, R. (2013). Multidisciplinary overview of vaginal atrophy and associated genitourinary symptoms in postmenopausal women. *Sexual Medicine*, 1(2), 44–53.

Graham, N. (2014). Polyamory: A call for increased mental health professional awareness. *Archives of Sexual Behavior*, 43(6), 1031–1034.

Haefner, H. K. (2006). Report of the international society for the study of vulvovaginal disease terminology and classification of vulvodynia. *Journal of Lower Genital Tract Disease*, 11(1), 48–49. doi:10.1097/01.lgt.0000236962.74136.b9

Hall, P., Holmqvist, M., Sherry, M. A. (2004). Risky adolescent sexual behavior: A psychological perspective for primary care clinicians. *Topics in Advanced Practice Nursing*, 4(1). Retrieved from http://www.medscape.com/viewarticle/467059

Harlow, B. L, Vitonis, A. F., & Gunther Stewart, E. (2008). Influence of oral contraceptive use on adult-onset vulvodynia. *Journal of Reproductive Medicine*, 53(2), 102–110.

Hatzichristou, D., Rosen, R. C., Derogatis, L. R., Low, W. Y., Meuleman, E. J., Sadovsky, R., & Symonds, T. (2010). Recommendations for the clinical evaluation of men and women with sexual dysfunction. *Journal of Sexual Medicine*, 7(1, Pt. 2), 337–348.

Hayes, R. D. (2011). Circular and linear modeling of female sexual desire and arousal. *Journal of Sex Research*, 48(2–3), 130–141.

Heasley, R. & Crane, B. (2003). *Sexual lives: A reader on the theories and realities of human sexualities*. New York, NY: McGraw-Hill.

Herbenick, D., Reece, M., Schick, V., Sanders, S. A., Dodge, B., & Fortenberry, J. D. (2010). An event-level analysis of the sexual characteristics and composition among adults ages 18 to 59: Results from a national probability sample in the United States. *Journal of Sexual Medicine*, 7(Suppl. 5), 346–361.

Herbenick, D., Reece, M., Schick, V., Sanders, S. A., & Fortenberry, J. D. (2014). Women's use and perceptions of commercial lubricants: Prevalence and characteristics in a nationally representative sample of American adults. *Journal of Sexual Medicine*, *11*(3), 642–652.

Hyde, J. S., & DeLamater, J. D. (2006). *Understanding human sexuality.* New York, NY: McGraw-Hill.

Impett, E. A., & Tolman, D. L. (2006). Late adolescent girls' sexual experiences and sexual satisfaction. *Journal of Adolescent Research*, *21*(6), 628–646.

IsHak, W. W., & Tobia, G. (2013). *DSM-5* changes in diagnostic criteria of sexual dysfunctions. *Reproductive System & Sexual Disorders, 2*(2), 122–124. doi:10.4172/2161–038X.1000122

Jina, R., & Thomas, L. S. (2013). Health consequences of sexual violence against women. *Best Practice & Research. Clinical Obstetrics & Gynaecology*, *27*(1), 15–26.

Johnson, C. E. (2011). Sexual health during pregnancy and the postpartum. *Journal of Sexual Medicine*, *8*(5), 1267–84; quiz 1285.

Kann, L., Kinchen, S., Shanklin, S. L., Flint, K. H., Hawkins, J., Harris, W. A., … Zaza, S. (2014). Youth risk behavior surveillance—United States, 2013. Surveillance Summaries. *Morbidity and Mortality Weekly Report, 63*(SS04), 1–168.

Kaplan, H. S. (1974). *The new sex therapy.* New York, NY: Brunner/Mazel.

Kellogg-Spadt, S., Younaitis Fariello, Y., & Safaeian, P. (2007). Treating sexual pain in women. *Advance for Nurse Practitioners, 15*(12), 39–42, 69.

Keskin, U., Coksuer, H., Gungor, S., Ercan, C. M., Karasahin, K. E., & Baser, I. (2011). Differences in prevalence of sexual dysfunction between primary and secondary infertile women. *Fertility and Sterility*, *96*(5), 1213–1217.

Kingsberg, S. A. (2006). Taking a sexual history. *Obstetrics and Gynecology Clinics of North America*, *33*(4), 535–547.

Kingsberg, S. A., & Janata, J. W. (2007). Female sexual disorders: Assessment, diagnosis, and treatment. *The Urologic Clinics of North America*, *34*(4), 497–506, v.

Kingsberg, S. A., & Rezaee, R. L. (2013). Hypoactive sexual desire in women. *Menopause*, *20*(12), 1284–1300.

Landry, T., Bergeron, S., Dupuis, M. J., & Desrochers, G. (2008). The treatment of provoked vestibulodynia: A critical review. *Clinical Journal of Pain*, *24*(2), 155–171.

Latif, E. Z., & Diamond, M. P. (2013). Arriving at the diagnosis of female sexual dysfunction. *Fertility and Sterility*, *100*(4), 898–904.

Laumann, E. O., Paik, A., & Rosen, R. C. (1999). Sexual dysfunction in the United States: Prevalence and predictors. *Journal of the American Medical Association*, *281*(6), 537–544.

Lindley, L. L., Walsemann, K. M., & Carter, J. W. (2013). Invisible and at risk: STDs among young adult sexual minority women in the United States. *Perspectives on Sexual and Reproductive Health*, *45*(2), 66–73.

Maciel, M., & Laganà, L. (2014). Older women's sexual desire problems: Biopsychosocial factors impacting them and barriers to their clinical assessment. *BioMed Research International*, *2014*, 107217.

Mason, F., & Lodrick, Z. (2013). Psychological consequences of sexual assault. *Best Practice & Research. Clinical Obstetrics & Gynaecology*, *27*(1), 27–37.

Masters, W., & Johnson, V. (1966). *The human sexual response cycle.* Boston, MA: Little Brown.

Moldwin, R. M., & Yonaitis Fariello, J. (2013). Myofascial trigger points of the pelvic floor: Associations with urological pain syndromes and treatment strategies including injection therapy. *Current Urology Perspectives*, *4*(5), 409–417. doi:10.1007/s11934–013-0360–71

Montemurro, B., & Siefken, J. M. (2014). Cougars on the prowl? New perceptions of older women's sexuality. *Journal of Aging Studies*, *28*, 35–43.

Newton, D. C., & McCabe, M. P. (2008a). Effects of sexually transmitted infection status, relationship status, and disclosure status on sexual self concept. *Journal of Sex Research*, *45*(2), 187–192. doi:10.1080/00224490802012909

Newton, D. C., & McCabe, M. P. (2008b). Sexually transmitted infections: Impact on individuals and their relationships. *Journal of Health Psychology*, *13*(7), 864–869.

Nusbaum, M. R., & Hamilton, C. D. (2002). The proactive sexual health history. *American Family Physician*, *66*(9), 1705–1712.

Oskay, U. Y., Beji, N. K., & Serdaroglu, H. (2010). The issue of infertility and sexual functioning in Turkish women. *Sexuality and Disability*, *28*, 71–79.

Pan American Health Organization & World Health Organization (WHO). (2000). *Promotion of sexual health: Recommendations for action.* Proceedings of a Regional Consultation convened by Pan American Health Organization, World Health Organization in collaboration with the World Association of Sexology.

Ponton, L. E., & Judice, S. (2004). Typical adolescent sexual development. *Child and Adolescent Psychiatric Clinics of North America*, *13*(3), 497–511, vi.

Portman, D., Palacios, S., Nappi, R. E., & Mueck, A. O. (2014). Ospemifene, a non-oestrogen selective oestrogen receptor modulator for the treatment of vaginal dryness associated with postmenopausal vulvar and vaginal atrophy: A randomised, placebo-controlled, phase III trial. *Maturitas*, *78*(2), 91–98.

Postma, R., Bicanic, I., van der Vaart, H., & Laan, E. (2013). Pelvic floor muscle problems mediate sexual problems in young adult rape victims. *Journal of Sexual Medicine*, *10*(8), 1978–1987.

Rahn, D. D., Carberry, C., Sanses, T. V., Mamik, M. M., Ward, R. M., Meriwether, K. V.,…Murphy, M.; Society of Gynecologic Surgeons Systematic Review Group. (2014). Vaginal estrogen for genitourinary syndrome of menopause: A systematic review. *Obstetrics and Gynecology*, *124*(6), 1147–1156.

Ringa, V., Diter, K., Laborde, C., & Bajos, N. (2013). Women's sexuality: From aging to social representations. *Journal of Sexual Medicine*, *10*(10), 2399–2408.

Robbins, C. L., Schick, V., Reece, M., Herbenick, D., Sanders, S. A., Dodge, B., & Fortenberry, J. D. (2011). Prevalence, frequency, and associations of masturbation with partnered sexual behaviors among US adolescents. *Archives of Pediatrics & Adolescent Medicine*, *165*(12), 1087–1093.

Roberts, L. W., Fromm, L. M., & Bartlik, B. D. (1998). Sexuality of women through the life phases. In L. A. Wallis (Ed.), *Textbook of women's health*. Philadelphia, PA: Lippincott-Raven.

Rosen, R., Brown, C., Heiman, J., Leiblum, S., Meston, C., Shabsigh, R.,…D'Agostino, R. (2000). The Female Sexual Function Index (FSFI): A multidimensional self-report instrument for the assessment of female sexual function. *Journal of Sex & Marital Therapy*, *26*(2), 191–208.

Rosen, R. C., & Barsky, J. L. (2006). Normal sexual response in women. *Obstetrics and Gynecology Clinics of North America*, *33*(4), 515–526.

Sadovsky, R., & Nusbaum, M. (2006). Sexual health inquiry and support is a primary care priority. *Journal of Sexual Medicine*, *3*(1), 3–11.

Sadownik, L. A. (2014). Etiology, diagnosis, and clinical management of vulvodynia. *International Journal of Women's Health*, *6*, 437–449.

Salonia, A., Giraldi, A., Chivers, M. L., Georgiadis, J. R., Levin, R., Maravilla, K. R., & McCarthy, M. M. (2010). Physiology of women's sexual function: Basic knowledge and new findings. *Journal of Sexual Medicine*, *7*(8), 2637–2660.

Schultz, W. W., Basson, R., Binik, Y., Eschenbach, D., Wesselmann, U., & Van Lankveld, J. (2005). Women's sexual pain and its management. *Journal of Sexual Medicine*, *2*, 301–316.

Serati, M., Salvatore, S., Siesto, G., Cattoni, E., Zanirato, M., Khullar, V.,…Bolis, P. (2010). Female sexual function during pregnancy and after childbirth. *Journal of Sexual Medicine*, *7*(8), 2782–2790.

Sheaham, S. L. (1989). Identifying female sexual dysfunction. *Nurse Practitioner*, *14*, 25–26, 28, 30, 32, 34.

Shifren, J. L., Monz, B. U., Russo, P. A., Segreti, A., & Johannes, C. B. (2008). Sexual problems and distress in United States women: Prevalence and correlates. *Obstetrics and Gynecology*, *112*(5), 970–978.

Simon, J. A. (2011). Identifying and treating sexual dysfunction in postmenopausal women: The role of estrogen. *Journal of Women's Health*, *20*(10), 1453–1465.

Steege, J. F., & Zolnoun, D. A. (2009). Evaluation and treatment of dyspareunia. *Obstetrics & Gynecology*, *113*(5), 1124–1136. Retrieved from http://journals.lww.com/greenjournal/pages/default.aspx

Teets, J. M. (1990). What women talk about. Sexuality issues of chemically dependent women. *Journal of Psychosocial Nursing and Mental Health Services*, *28*(12), 4–7.

Van Houdenhove, E., & Gijs, L. (2014). Asexuality: Few facts, many questions. *Journal of Sex & Marital Therapy*, *3*(40), 175–192. doi:10810 .0/0092623.X.2012.751073

van Lankveld, J. J., Granot, M., Weijmar Schultz, W. C., Binik, Y. M., Wesselmann, U., Pukall, C. F.,…Achtrari, C. (2010). Women's sexual pain disorders. *Journal of Sexual Medicine*, *7*(1, Pt. 2), 615–631.

Waite, L. J., Laumann, E. O., Das, A., & Schumm, L. P. (2009). Sexuality: Measures of partnerships, practices, attitudes, and problems in the National Social Life, Health, and Aging Study. *Journals of Gerontology Series B: Psychological Sciences and Social Sciences*, 64(Suppl. 1), i56–i66.

Whitmore, K., Siegel, J. F., & Kellogg-Spadt, S. (2007). Interstitial cystitis/painful bladder syndrome as a cause of sexual pain in women: A diagnosis to consider. *Journal of Sexual Medicine*, 4(3), 720–727.

World Health Organization (WHO). (2006). *Defining sexual health*. Retrieved from http://www.who.int/reproductivehealth/publications/sexual_health/defining_sexual_health.pdf

Xu, F., Sternberg, M. R., & Markowitz, L. E. (2010). Women who have sex with women in the United States: Prevalence, sexual behavior and prevalence of herpes simplex virus type 2 infection—Results from National Health and Nutrition Examination Survey 2001–2006. *Sexually Transmitted Diseases*, 37(7), 407–413.

Yarber, W. L., Sayad, B. W., & Strong, B. (2010). *Human sexuality: Diversity in contemporary America* (7th ed.). New York, NY: McGraw-Hill.

Zimmer-Gembeck, M. J., & Helfand, M. (2007). Ten years of longitudinal research on U.S. adolescent sexual behavior: Developmental correlates of sexual intercourse, and the importance of age, gender, and ethnic background. *Developmental Review, 28*, 153–224.

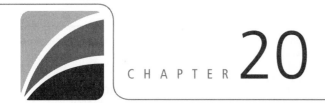
Primary Care of Lesbian, Gay, Bisexual, and Transgender Individuals

Caroline Dorsen • Kathryn Tierney

The reduction of health disparities is a major focus of the U.S. health care agenda, as outlined in *Healthy People 2020* (2016). In the past three decades, research has shown that lesbian, gay, bisexual, and transgender (LGBT) individuals experience significant health care disparities compared with heterosexual and/or cisgender (nontransgender) individuals (Committee on Lesbian, Gay, Bisexual and Transgender Health Issues and Research Gaps and Opportunities; Board on the Health of Select Populations; Institute of Medicine [IOM], 2011). These include decreased access to, and use of, preventive and ongoing health services; increased rates of tobacco, alcohol, and illicit drug use; increased rates of depression, anxiety, and suicidality; increased rates of disordered eating and overweight/obesity; increased rates of sexually transmitted infections (STIs), including HIV; and possibly increased rates and inadequate treatment of cancer and cardiovascular disease (CVD; Committee on Lesbian, Gay, Bisexual and Transgender Health Issues and Research Gaps and Opportunities; Board on the Health of Select Populations; IOM, 2011). Although there are multiple, complex reasons for these disparities, ranging from individual risk behaviors to lack of health care provider (HCP) knowledge, the common thread appears to be the experience of stigma and marginalization and the impact this has on health. In this chapter, we review what is known about the health of LGBT persons and suggest strategies for providing evidence-based care to sexual- and gender-minority patients.

■ REVIEW OF TOPIC

LGBT persons live in almost every, if not every, county in the United States and represent people from all ethnic backgrounds, socioeconomic statuses, and ages. Recent estimates suggest that there are at least 646,000 same-sex U.S. households (Census Bureau, 2011) and that anywhere from 3.8% (Gates, 2006) to more than 10% (Kinsey, Pomeroy, & Martin, 1948) of the U.S. population identifies as LGBT. It is believed that a much higher percentage of people engage in same-sex behaviors but do not identify as LGBT and thus may not be counted in official demographic reports (Committee on Lesbian, Gay, Bisexual and Transgender Health Issues and Research Gaps and Opportunities; Board on the Health of Select Populations; IOM, 2011).

Within the sexual minority community, there are at least four distinct populations (gay, lesbian, bisexual, and transgender), each with its own characteristics, cultures, and health needs (Worthen, 2012). In addition, there are multiple subpopulations based on factors such as age, race, socioeconomic status, and geography that greatly influence the experience of living as a sexual minority in the United States. There is a growing body of literature, however, that examines the common experiences among LGBT individuals, including that which suggests that marginalization and stigma are the common experiential bonds that most LGBT persons share (Committee on Lesbian, Gay, Bisexual and Transgender Health Issues and Research Gaps and Opportunities; Board on the Health of Select Populations; IOM, 2011) and that individual, structural, and societal discrimination and prejudice greatly affect the health behaviors and health outcomes of LGBT persons.

The prevalence of gender dysphoria is unknown. Historically, the transgender population has been so marginalized that it has been essentially ignored. More recently, there have been attempts at determining how many people identify as transgender or have transitioned; however, because the question is complex and because of fear on the part of the community, it has been difficult to get an accurate estimate.

Nurse practitioners (NPs) need to be proactive about asking patients about their sexual orientation and gender identity and personalizing care based on personal risk factors. LGBT persons live and work in every community, and are not easily identifiable by how they look, speak, or act.

Open-ended questions regarding sexual orientation and sexual preferences allow the NP to address specific risk factors as well as incorporate what is known about population level health disparities to improve the health of this vulnerable population.

■ ETIOLOGY

There is no known genetic, social, or hormonal etiology for homosexuality or gender dysphoria. Research to determine these etiologies is ongoing; however, no conclusive evidence exists. How gender identity and sexual orientation are determined is likely related to a combination of nature and nurture, as it is with many human traits. As discussed in this chapter, being homosexual is not a medical disorder, and as such, the etiology or reason for identifying as homosexual is not generally pertinent to providing good clinical care. Likewise, the etiology of one's gender identity may or may not be helpful in providing competent care to people experiencing gender dysphoria. The focus should be solely on the individual's experience and clinical needs.

■ RISK FACTORS

Identifying as LGBT or engaging in same-sex sexual behaviors does not inherently lead to any health problems. NPs, however, need to be cognizant of population-level health issues that disproportionately affect LGBT persons, as well as individual risk factors that may place patients at greater risk than their heterosexual counterparts. LGBT health can be considered from the development/population perspective (i.e., what are the pressing issues for LGBT youth or elders), health risk perspective (i.e., what health risks are important to identify for this person related to behavior, socioeconomical exposure, and family history), and/or a pathology perspective (i.e., what are the major areas of health disparities for LGBT persons). An understanding of these perspectives allows NPs to explore the complexities of LGBT health and translate this knowledge to direct patient care. A more detailed look at the health risks particular to each age group is outlined and suggestions for reducing those risks are reviewed later in this chapter.

The landmark IOM report, *The Health of Lesbian, Gay, Bisexual, and Transgender People: Building a Foundation for Better Understanding* (Committee on Lesbian, Gay, Bisexual and Transgender Health Issues and Research Gaps and Opportunities; Board on the Health of Select Populations; IOM, 2011), concluded that societal stigma has an impact on health from multiple pathways, including the impact of increased stress on lifestyle choices, such as smoking, drinking alcohol, and using illicit drugs, and the newer concept linking increased stress to systemic inflammation, possibly raising the risk of CVD and other chronic health issues.

Research also suggests that fear of negative interactions with HCPs or frank discrimination may decrease access to and use of health care services, including preventative care services and chronic disease management. Similarly, lack of

provider knowledge about LGBT health disparities and how LGBT orientation may impact health can translate to lack of individualized care due to nondisclosure of sexual orientation.

HCPs, including nurses and NPs, often receive little or no training regarding LGBT health care (Lim, Johnson, & Eliason, 2015). Thus conflicted or negative attitudes and lack of knowledge may intertwine to prevent HCPs from providing culturally competent care to LGBT patients. NPs are encouraged to read evidence-based literature on how to best care for this vulnerable population, including the IOM report (Committee on Lesbian, Gay, Bisexual and Transgender Health Issues and Research Gaps and Opportunities; Board on the Health of Select Populations; IOM, 2011).

■ DIAGNOSTIC CRITERIA

Until 1973, homosexuality was considered pathological and was included in the *Diagnostic and Statistical Manual of Mental Disorders* (*DSM*, first edition) of the American Psychological Association. Although gender dysphoria disorders are still listed in the *DSM-5-TR* (2014), the removal of homosexuality as a mental health diagnosis is considered a milestone moment in the history of the LGBT equality movement. Despite these advances, many older LGBT persons may remember a time when their sexual orientation/gender identity was considered pathological and may bear the scars of living in a world that refused to acknowledge a very basic part of their identity. For example, older LGBT persons are more likely than their heterosexual peers to live alone, are not used to having family support in meeting their basic needs, and may feel the need to go back into "the closet" when accessing medical and social services or long-term care for fear of discrimination (Lim & Dorsen, 2014).

Major health organizations and LGBT advocacy groups, such as the IOM and the Fenway Institute, recommend that HCPs ask all patients basic questions about their sexual preference and gender identity during routine assessments. Knowing this information about every patient allows HCPs to tailor episodic and ongoing medical care according to the specific risks and needs of the patient, as well as open a dialogue about whether previous negative interactions with HCPs have influenced the patient's access to, and receipt of, medical care. Providers are encouraged to incorporate simple questions about sexual orientation and gender identity as part of basic patient demographic information and to allow patients to identify in any way that they choose to. For example, a female patient who has sex with other women may or may not identify as gay or may identify as bisexual. Likewise, patients who identify as transgender may or may not be engaged in care to transition from their sex as identified at birth to the sex they identify with as an adolescent or adult. NPs should respect patient choices and assess patients based on risk behaviors and risk factors, rather than on identity labels.

The diagnostic criteria for gender dysphoria are still included in the *DSM-5* (5th ed.; American Psychiatric Association, 2013). A debate is ongoing regarding the usefulness of including gender dysphoria in the *DSM*, but for the time being, it remains a psychiatric diagnosis. The criteria for diagnosis of gender dysphoria are discussed in detail in Chapter 25.

■ ASSESSMENT

Health Disparities

LGBT persons experience health disparities on many of the major U.S. health indicators outlined in *Healthy People 2020*. An easy mnemonic for helping to remember the areas of particular concern for this population is SADCOST (Table 20.1).

LGBT Youth

Although most LGBT adolescents live in supportive environments and experience the normal challenges of the teen years, research suggests that LGBT teens may experience increased rates of school bullying and violence, substance abuse, depression, anxiety and suicidality, risky sexual behavior, and homelessness compared with the general adolescent population (Kann et al., 2011). NPs should be aware that some of these risk factors are ameliorated by the support of parents and/or other influential adults, including teachers and HCPs. Thus asking youth about issues related to their sexual orientation and gender identity, and providing them with a safe space to discuss their concerns, is an essential role for NPs (Bouris et al., 2010).

LGBT in Midlife

During midlife, issues related to accessing preventive care and chronic disease management, having relationships (including marriage equality), and becoming and being parents figure prominently for LGBT persons. Although many of the health care needs of LGBT patients may mirror those of the general population, there is research suggesting that LGBT persons may experience increased rates

of certain acute and chronic illnesses, including cancer and CVD. Patients may come to seek care having had a variety of positive and negative experiences with HCPs and be looking for LGBT-inclusive care (Fredriksen-Goldsen, 2014). NPs can support midlife LGBT patients by asking them their sexual orientation/gender identity; recognizing that the definition of *family* for many LGBT persons may be based not on biology, but rather on "family of choice" in whatever constellation they identify; being sensitive to the possibility of previous stigma and discrimination and the way that this history might affect accessing and receiving health care services; and assessing the possible increased risks for chronic disease, including certain cancers and CVD.

LGBT Elders

Many of the same concerns of older age that affect LGBT persons also affect the general population; these include financial issues, long-term care decisions, and end-of-life issues. However, many concerns are amplified in LGBT populations, including issues related to social isolation caused by rejection by, or disengagement with, families of origin. Decreased rates of reproduction between same-sex partners may lead to isolation later in life, though this trend is changing somewhat with the availability of reproductive technology. There are also some institutional concerns unique to this population. For example, acute care institutions have historically not always allowed LGBT patients to define *family* in an open and inclusive way. This has sometimes led to the exclusion of long-time partners from hospital visitation and care decision making. Although this is quickly changing with the introduction of The Joint Commission's field guide on providing inclusive and welcoming care (The Joint Commission, 2014), some older LGBT persons may be hesitant to identify as LGBT while hospitalized or in long-term care environments because of fear of discrimination. The Supreme Court decision legalizing same-sex marriage in the United States, which inherently gives same-sex spouses certain rights, improves some aspects of health, including the ability to direct medical decision making and access to health care.

■ GUIDELINES FOR HEALTH PROMOTION

STIs and Risky Sexual Behavior

The first, and sometimes only, area that many HCPs equate with LGBT health is increased HIV and STI risk. Risk for HIV and STI depends not on a patient's self-identified sexual orientation (i.e., as lesbian or gay), but rather on individual patient behaviors. For example, although female-to-female transmission of most STIs, including HIV, is rare, many women who identify as lesbian have had sex with male partners in their lifetime, and those who do may be more likely

TABLE 20.1	SADCOST Mnemonic
S	Sexually transmitted infection and risky sexual behavior
A	Attitudes (including those of health care providers)
D	Depression, anxiety, and suicidality
C	Cancer and cardiovascular disease
O	Overweight, obesity, and eating disorders
S	Substance abuse, including alcohol, tobacco, and drugs
T	Trauma and violence

Source: Personal communication (Dorsen, 2015).

to engage in unsafe sex than heterosexual women (Koh, Gómez, Shade, & Rowley, 2005). There are also studies that suggest a particularly high number of HIV infections among transgender women (i.e., people who were labeled as male at birth but now identify as women). One study showed the HIV infection rate among transgender women to be 29 times that of the cisgender population (Herbst et al., 2008).

Depression, Anxiety, and Suicidality

Mental health among LGBT persons is among the most well-researched areas of health in this community. LGBT persons across the life span suffer worse mental health, including depression, anxiety, and suicidality than their heterosexual/cisgender counterparts. Among LGBT youth, there is a three to seven times higher risk of suicide attempt and an increased risk of homelessness (Russell & Joyner, 2001). NPs should be aware of increased risk of mental health concerns and use validated tools, such as the PHQ-2, PHQ-9, or Geriatric Depression Scale, to screen all LGBT patients. Prompt referral to LGBT-inclusive mental health care is of absolute importance. Lists of LGBT and LGBT ally providers are available online, such as the database provided by the Gay and Lesbian Medical Association (www.GLMA.org).

There are no studies testing interventions to decrease rates of depression and suicidality. Educating HCPs, including mental health specialists; creating awareness in school systems and communities; and using available online tools to reach isolated persons are all ways to increase access to care and decrease stigma (IOM, 2011). NPs can help reach patients who are battling depression and anxiety by creating an obviously safe space in their offices with signs and by educating staff, asking open-ended questions regarding feelings of depression and anxiety, and providing appropriate referrals to mental health specialists.

Cancer and CVD

It is unclear whether there is increased risk of cancer or CVD in the LGBT population, although it is widely known that they are among the top causes of death of adults in the United States. What is known is that many LGBT persons may not adhere to clinical health-promotion guidelines that decrease CVD and cancer risk, may have lower rates of early detection via screening and diagnostic tests, and may not receive care until late in the course of the disease (Fredriksen-Goldsen, Kim, Barkan, Muraco, & Hoy-Ellis, 2013).

It is essential to recognize that some of the risk factors for CVD and cancer, such as tobacco use, alcohol use, obesity, and decreased access to care, may be higher for LGBT individuals than the general population. More research is needed to confirm whether these confer increased risk to LGBT patients. NPs should follow the same national guidelines for CVD and cancer screening for LGBT patients as in other individuals.

Overweight, Obesity, and Eating Disorders

Lesbians and bisexual women are more likely to be overweight or obese compared with the general population,

though the reasons for this are not clear (Committee on Lesbian, Gay, Bisexual and Transgender Health Issues and Research Gaps and Opportunities; Board on the Health of Select Populations; IOM, 2011). One factor may be the impact of minority stress and stigma. Knowing the increased risk can help NPs screen for and aggressively treat obesity, which in and of itself can lead to other health issues.

Substance Abuse, Including Alcohol, Tobacco, and Drugs

Rates of tobacco, alcohol, and substance abuse appear to be higher in the LGBT population across the life span compared with the heterosexual population (Committee on Lesbian, Gay, Bisexual and Transgender Health Issues and Research Gaps and Opportunities; Board on the Health of Select Populations; IOM, 2011). Although it is not clear why there is increased use of these substances in this population, it is hypothesized that increased stress related to rejection and marginalization are potential causes. As with all patients, lesbians, bisexual women, and transgender women should be screened for substance abuse. Increasing access to health services, including mental health services, helps decrease the rates of use and ultimately improves the health status of LGBT patients.

Trauma and Violence

LGBT persons are at a significantly increased risk for hate crimes and violence compared with the general population (Committee on Lesbian, Gay, Bisexual and Transgender Health Issues and Research Gaps and Opportunities; Board on the Health of Select Populations; IOM, 2011). Research studies report that anywhere from 10% to 30% of a given sample of LGBT persons have experienced some form of violence based on sexual orientation (Committee on Lesbian, Gay, Bisexual and Transgender Health Issues and Research Gaps and Opportunities; Board on the Health of Select Populations; IOM, 2011). Gay and transgender women also experience domestic violence. Questions regarding safety at home should be part of routine primary care screening at all ages, as it is in the general population.

▣ INTERVENTIONS AND STRATEGIES FOR RISK REDUCTION

No general preventive services guidelines for LGBT persons exist. Therefore NPs must use the existing health-promotion guidelines established for all adolescents and adults and tailor them to individual patients, with a clear understanding of individual risk-taking behaviors, such as smoking or unsafe sexual behaviors, along with an understanding of population-level health inequities. For example, a nuanced understanding of some of the causes of decreased utilization of preventive care services by LGBT persons helps NPs communicate with patients about why they are essential to use and troubleshoot how to access them in a way that is comfortable and safe for the individual. Likewise, understanding structural issues, such as decreased rates of health insurance among LGBT persons, helps NPs work with patients and other providers, such as social workers, to facilitate access to, and use of, health services.

There are areas where NPs may want to consider amending current health-promotion guidelines specifically for the LGBT population. Primary care guidelines for transgender persons include health-promotion information published by the University of California, San Francisco Center of Excellence for Transgender Health (www.transhealth.ucsf.edu) and the World Professional Association for Transgender Health (www.WPATH.org).

■ FUTURE DIRECTIONS

Large population-based studies on the health of the LGBT community have been lacking, in large part because of lack of cultural acceptance of gay, lesbian, and transgender persons (Committee on Lesbian, Gay, Bisexual and Transgender Health Issues and Research Gaps and Opportunities; Board on the Health of Select Populations; IOM, 2011). As cultural acceptance progresses and more HCPs are educated in the particular needs of this population, the health of the community will improve. NPs can help improve the health of LGBT persons by providing a safe space in which they can explore health promotion and educating their peers with current resources. Simply having pamphlets or posters in the waiting room that show same-sex couples, and asking patients about their sexual and gender identities in a nonjudgmental way, can say to patients that they are welcome in a practice.

■ REFERENCES

American Psychiatric Association. (2013). *Diagnostic and statistical manual of mental disorders* (5th ed.). Arlington, VA: American Psychiatric Publishing.

Bouris, A., Guilamo-Ramos, V., Pickard, A., Shiu, C., Loosier, P. S., Dittus, P.,...Michael Waldmiller, J. (2010). A systematic review of parental influences on the health and well-being of lesbian, gay, and bisexual youth: Time for a new public health research and practice agenda. *Journal of Primary Prevention, 31*(5–6), 273–309.

Census Bureau. (2011). *Census bureau releases estimates of same sex married couples.* Retrieved from http://www.census.gov/hhes/samesex

Committee on Lesbian, Gay, Bisexual and Transgender Health Issues and Research Gaps and Opportunities; Board on the Health of Select Populations; Institute of Medicine (IOM). (2011). *The health of lesbian, gay, bisexual, and transgender people: Building a foundation for better understanding.* Washington, DC: National Academies Press.

Dorsen, C. (2016). *Health disparities among LGBT patients: The role of healthcare providers in the college health environment.* [PowerPoint slides]. Retrieved from http://www.njcollegehealth.org/documents/PPCarolineD2016.pdf

Fredriksen-Goldsen, K. I. (2014). Promoting health equity among LGBT mid-life and older adults. *Generations, 38*(4), 86–92.

Fredriksen-Goldsen, K. I., Kim, H., Barkan, S. E., Muraco, A., & Hoy-Ellis, C. P. (2013). Health disparities among lesbian, gay, and bisexual older adults: Results from a population-based study. *American Journal of Public Health, 103*(10), 1802–1809. doi:10.2105/AJPH.2012.301110

Gates, G. J. (2006). *Same-sex couples and the gay, lesbian, bisexual population: New estimates from the American Community Survey.* The Williams Institute on Sexual Orientation Law and Public Policy, UCLA School of Law (p. 10). Retrieved from http://williamsinstitute.law.ucla.edu/wp-content/uploads/Gates-Same-Sex-Couples-GLB-Pop-ACS-Oct-2006.pdf

Gay and Lesbian Medical Association (GLMA). (2006). *Guidelines for care of lesbian, gay, bisexual, and transgender patients.* Washington, DC: Author.

Healthy People 2020. (2016). *Lesbian, gay, bisexual, and transgender health.* Washington, DC: U.S. Department of Health and Human Services, Office of Disease Prevention and Health Promotion. Retrieved from https://www.healthypeople.gov/2020/topics-objectives/topic/lesbian-gay-bisexual-and-transgender-health

Herbst, J. H., Jacobs, E. D., Finlayson, T. J., McKleroy, V. S., Neumann, M. S., & Crepaz, N.; HIV/AIDS Prevention Research Synthesis Team. (2008). Estimating HIV prevalence and risk behaviors of transgender persons in the United States: A systematic review. *AIDS and Behavior, 12*(1), 1–17.

The Joint Commission. (2011). *Advancing effective communication, cultural competence, and patient- and family-centered care for the lesbian, gay, bisexual, and transgender (LGBT) community: A field guide.* Washington, DC: Author.

The Joint Commission. (2014). *Advancing effective communication, cultural competence, and patient- and family-centered care for the lesbian, gay, bisexual, and transgender (LGBT) community: A field guide.* Washington, DC: Author. Retrieved from LGBTFieldGuide.pdf.

Kann, L., Olsen, E. O., McManus, T., Kinchen, S., Chyen, D., Harris, W. A., & Wechsler, H.; Centers for Disease Control and Prevention (CDC). (2011). Sexual identity, sex of sexual contacts, and health-risk behaviors among students in grades 9–12—Youth Risk Behavior Surveillance, selected sites, United States, 2001–2009. *Morbidity and Mortality Weekly Report. Surveillance Summaries, 60*(7), 1–133.

Kinsey, A. C., Pomeroy, W. B., & Martin, C. E. (1948). *Sexual behavior in the human male.* Bloomington, IN: Indiana University Press.

Koh, A. S., Gómez, C. A., Shade, S., & Rowley, E. (2005). Sexual risk factors among self-identified lesbians, bisexual women, and heterosexual women accessing primary care settings. *Sexually Transmitted Diseases, 32*(9), 563–569.

Lim, F., & Dorsen, C. (2014). Older LGBT adults: Social and clinical issues. In M. D. Mezey, B. J. Berkman, C. M. Callahan, T. T. Fulmer, E. L. Mitty, G. J. Paveza, . . . N. E. Strumpf (Eds.). *The encyclopedia of elder care.* New York, NY: Springer Publishing.

Lim, F., Johnson, M., & Eliason, M. (2015). A national survey of faculty knowledge, experience, and readiness for teaching lesbian, gay, bisexual and transgender health in baccalaureate nursing programs. *Nursing Education Perspectives, 36*(3), 144–152. doi:10.5480/14–1355

Russell, S. T., & Joyner, K. (2001). Adolescent sexual orientation and suicide risk: Evidence from a national study. *American Journal of Public Health, 91*(8), 1276–1281.

Worthen, M. G. F. (2012). An argument for separate analyses of attitudes toward lesbian, gay, bisexual men, bisexual women, MtF and FtM transgender individuals. *Sex Roles: A Journal of Research, 68*(11/12), 703–723.

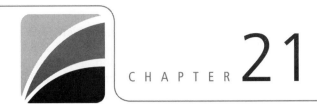

CHAPTER 21

Fertility Self-Management and Shared Management

Richard M. Prior • Heather C. Katz

The journey that led to the development of highly effective, safe, reliable, affordable, and well-tolerated contraceptive options for women has been long, challenging, and is ongoing. The result, however, has been nothing short of a renaissance. By allowing women to control their sexuality and decisions to procreate, they have enjoyed greater freedom to pursue family, economic, and personal goals. An astute provider must gain an understanding of the variables that influence a woman's contraception decisions, her past medical history, and her personal risk factors in order to appropriately filter through the available contraceptive options and provide her the best possible contraceptive solutions. In this chapter, we discuss the variables that contribute to individual choice and the natural, hormonal, barrier, and sterilization contraceptive methods that are widely available in the United States.

■ HISTORICAL AND SOCIAL CONTEXT

No scientific breakthrough has altered as many women's lives so momentously as the development of safe, effective methods for fertility control. Before these methods were available, women suffered chronic illness, fatigue, and even death from unpreventable pregnancy (Cooke & Dworkin, 1979). Multiple pregnancies and unspaced births not only affect women's physical health negatively, but also reduce their economic productivity, leading to increased dependence on others and unfulfilled human potential.

Today, a sexually active woman can affect her physical, educational, socioeconomic destiny—and that of her family and significant others and partners—by choosing to use or not to use contraception. By using a highly effective contraceptive method, she reduces the risk of unplanned pregnancy, which enables her to plan her family along with other aspects of her life. When a woman is able to control her fertility, she gains the opportunity to plan and limit family size or to remain childless.

The ability to prevent or defer childbearing allows a woman to pursue educational opportunities and participate in the labor force. A woman's knowledge that she can, if she wishes, control her childbearing, and society's understanding that women can do so, may broaden her outlook when she considers other life opportunities. Because a planned birth can be integrated into a woman's career or job more readily than an unplanned birth, a planned birth has fewer negative effects on her employment or education. Some women use contraceptive methods successfully to take advantage of educational and employment opportunities. Others are not as successful. Instead, they learn by experience that few events change a woman's life as much as the fear of conception or the reality of an unintended pregnancy.

Margaret Sanger and the Birth Control Movement

In the latter years of the Victorian age, an individual was born who would create a new episode in the contraception drama for U.S. women. Margaret Louise Higgins Sanger, born in Corning, New York, in 1879, dedicated herself to this work after seeing her mother die from tuberculosis and the burden of bearing 11 children and after observing women in New York's Lower East Side die from childbirth or illegal abortions. In 1902, she completed nursing school at White Plains Hospital in New York. Inspired by Emma Goldman, the first nurse to lecture on birth control in the United States, in 1912, Sanger began to publish information about women's reproductive concerns. Her first efforts were a series of articles describing puberty and the functions of a woman's body for the *Call*, a socialist newspaper (Gordon, 1990). These articles were the basis for *What Every Girl Should Know*, a pamphlet published in 1915 and later published as a book (Sanger, 1920a). The first issue of *The Woman Rebel* was published in March 1914. In the same year, Sanger prepared the pamphlet *Family Limitation* and organized a committee called the *National Birth Control League*. She fled to England in October 1914 to avoid prosecution for violating the Comstock Law; federal legislation prohibiting the mailing of obscene material, which included birth control information and devices (Tannahill, 1980). In

England, Sanger met C. V. Drysdale, head of the international birth control movement, and Havelock Ellis, author of *Studies in the Psychology of Sex*. An unfortunate consequence of these meetings was Sanger's introduction to the eugenics movement. That association was to affect views of Sanger's work throughout her life. From England, Sanger went to Holland, where she learned how to fit "pessaries," now known as contraceptive diaphragms, and studied that country's birth control clinic system.

On October 16, 1916, Sanger and her sister Ethel opened the Brownsville Clinic in Brooklyn, New York—America's first birth control clinic. The clinic provided birth control information and education, although both were illegal at the time. From 1916 to 1934, Sanger established birth control clinics, published birth control articles and pamphlets in defiance of the Comstock Law, worked to change birth control laws, organized the American Birth Control League (1921), attended national and international conferences on birth control, lectured around the world, and was jailed more than once for her activities. In 1922, she engaged Dorothy Bocker to run the Clinical Research Bureau. The next year, she hired James F. Cooper to lecture to physicians across the United States about birth control. She smuggled pessaries into the United States through her husband's factory in Canada until 1925, when she convinced two of her supporters to establish the Holland Rantos Company and begin U.S. production. In 1926, she traveled to London, Paris, and Geneva to prepare for a 1927 international meeting, which led to the formation of the International Union for the Scientific Investigation of Population Problems (Himes, 1936). In 1928, she resigned as president of the American Birth Control League but continued to edit the *Birth Control Review* until 1929, when she withdrew from the league and the paper. In April that year, police raided the *Clinical Research Bureau*, because this research was also considered in violation of the Comstock Law, but Sanger did not give up.

The 1930s brought some victories for the birth control movement. In the summer of 1930, the Seventh International Birth Control Conference was held under Sanger's leadership. In 1934, Sanger went to Russia to gather data about the birth control movement there. The next year, she attended the *All India Women's Conference*, met Mohandas Karamchand (Mahatma) Gandhi, and gave 64 lectures across India. The U.S. Congress finally revised the Comstock Act in 1936, redefining obscenity to exclude birth control information and devices. One year later, the American Medical Association resolved that contraception was a legitimate medical service. By 1938, more than 300 clinics were in operation in the United States. In 1939, the American Birth Control League and the Voluntary Parenthood League merged and named Sanger honorary president of what is now Planned Parenthood.

Throughout the 1930s, Sanger continued to promote birth control. In 1952, she persuaded Katherine McCormick, widow of the founder of International Harvester, to fund the research that produced the oral contraceptive (OCs). She also traveled to India to help organize the International Planned Parenthood Federation; the next year in Stockholm, Sanger was elected president of this organization. In 1959, the 80-year-old Sanger attended the International Conference on Population in New Delhi, where she met Prime Minister Nehru. She died in 1966, in Tucson, Arizona (Douglas, 1970; Gordon, 1990; Gray, 1979; Lader, 1955; Marlow, 1979; Sanger, 1920b, 1931, 1938; Sicherman, Green, Kantor, & Walker, 1980).

The New Feminism

Although Sanger was establishing birth control clinics, other U.S. women were working to obtain the right to vote, which they finally gained with the passage of the 19th Amendment in 1920 (Kerber & De Hart, 1995). The suffrage movement reflected women's growing opportunities for paid employment in nursing, teaching, offices, factories, and other fields.

During this period, some advocates saw birth control as a tool; not only for limiting pregnancies, but also promoting social revolution. They believed the solution for many social ills lay in population control (Gordon, 1990). Thus, most birth control advocates were social radicals; some were also socialists or political radicals. After World War I, women returned to work in the home and the birth control movement changed considerably. As health care professionals made birth control an integral part of their practices, they moved it into the mainstream of society. Birth control, which had begun as a radical social movement, shifted decisively into the medical arena, ensuring medical control of contraception (Gordon, 1990).

Recent efforts of feminists to wrest control of reproduction from the hands of medicine have their roots in the birth control movement of the 1920s and 1930s. In 2015, in the United States, the most effective means of contraception—intrauterine devices (IUDs), OCs, hormonal implants, rings, patches, and injectables—remain under physician control. As clinical nurse specialists, nurse practitioners, nurse-midwives, and physician assistants gained prescriptive authority, control of these methods passed to health care professionals other than physicians and into the hands of more women.

Sexual Beliefs and Practices

From the time when the *Kinsey Report* (Kinsey, Pomeroy, Martin, & Gebhard, 1953) revealed that some women masturbated, had premarital sexual experiences, and were orgasmic, the United States public has lived through: (a) the baby boom of the 1950s when many middle-class women returned to or stayed home to raise families; (b) the new wave of feminism of the 1960s beginning with Betty Friedan's *Feminine Mystique* (Friedan, 1963); and (c) the sexual revolution of the 1970s.

Although the feminist movement of the 1960s was gaining momentum, scientists were developing OCs promising freedom from unwanted pregnancy in a pill—a contraceptive method totally disassociated from intercourse. However, physicians controlled this method, as well as abortions (legalized in 1973 with *Roe v. Wade*). To counter medical control of women's bodies, the Boston Women's Health Book Collective published the first edition of *Our Bodies, Ourselves* in 1970, which was a motivation for the rise of women's self-help groups. At the same time, many authors addressed the new sexuality of women, allegedly discovered during the sexual revolution. Thus, although women worked for liberation from feminine stereotypes, they experienced a bombardment of expectations about their sexuality. The role of super woman took on new qualities; not only were United States women expected to be faultless wives, mothers, and career women, but they were also supposed to be able to fulfill all their partners' sexual fantasies. However, the sexual revolution did not relieve women of the burden of contraception. Even today, most sexually active fertile women make most decisions about contraception.

Patterns of Contraceptive Use

During the period of 2006 to 2010, 86.6% of women aged 15 to 44 years reported that they had been sexually active during their lifetimes. Of this group of sexually active women, 99.1% reported that they had experienced some form of contraception. The most commonly used forms reported were the male condom (93.4%) and OCs (81.9%). It is noteworthy that 59.6% had reported using withdrawal, the third most commonly reported method. The average woman uses 3.1 methods of contraception throughout her lifetime (Daniels, Mosher, & Jones, 2013).

At any given moment, 62% of women use contraception. The most commonly used methods include the contraceptive pill (28%) and female sterilization (26%). There are differences by ethnicity, as Whites report higher current contraceptive rates (66%) as compared to Hispanics (60%) or African Americans (54%). White women are significantly more likely to use OCs (21%) as compared to Asians (12%), Hispanics (12%), or African Americans (9.9%; Jones, Mosher, & Daniels, 2012).

Contraceptive Decision Making

From menarche to menopause, women must make decisions about their fertility, including if, how, and when they will regulate it. Women may choose to abstain from heterosexual vaginal intercourse, engage in such intercourse and risk pregnancy, or engage in intercourse and prevent pregnancy by using contraception. Making a decision about contraception is more than selecting among attractive alternatives. It requires strategies and compromises that satisfy personal, social, cultural, and interpersonal needs influenced by constraints, opportunities, values, and norms. When made in cooperation with a health care provider, these characteristics are filtered through the additional variables of medical history and possible contraindications, future health care, and personal goals (such as timing of future pregnancies), and cost.

Deciding to Use Contraception

Decision models assume that individuals' choices are determined by beliefs about their consequences and perceptions of their advantages and disadvantages. Although individuals try to make the best possible choices, they can be hampered by the complexity of a situation, conflicting beliefs

and motives, misinformation, social constraints, and intrapsychic conflicts (Adler, 1979). When making a decision, an individual's values and perceptions of probable outcomes and values are valid, even if they are not objective or consistent with cultural values. Some investigators believe that the decision not to use contraception can be sensible even when pregnancy is not intended. In fact, it may be based on a decision model in which a woman decides that benefits associated with not using a contraceptive outweigh the risks associated with pregnancy (Luker, 1978). Each decision has antecedents and consequences. Antecedents initiate the decision-making process. These are events or incidents that cause doubt, wavering, debate, or controversy. In turn, these lead to a search for options, followed by a gathering of information about these options. Before making a decision, the individual examines and evaluates the feasibility of each option and considers the possible risks and consequences. Consequences are the events or incidents that result from the decision.

When the individual makes a decision, stabilization occurs because the decision ends the doubt, wavering, debate, or controversy. Then the individual may affirm the decision by implementing it, affirm it but postpone implementation, reverse it, or reconsider it and make new decisions as circumstances and desires change. For example, a woman is considering switching from OCs to a barrier device. She may have used other contraceptive methods in the past and probably will consider those along with the numerous choices for barrier contraception. Then she compares the advantages and disadvantages of the various barrier methods with those of other options. After considering the consequences of using a barrier method (such as its use must be linked to intercourse), the necessity of inserting the device in her body, and the need to remove the device in a prescribed time frame, the woman decides to use this contraceptive method. After choosing the particular barrier method, the woman might then consider the consequences of that decision on her relationship with her partner, the need to learn insertion and removal techniques, and other factors unique to her lifestyle and roles.

Before deciding to contracept, a woman must perceive herself as sexually active and at risk for becoming pregnant. A sexual self-concept is strongly correlated with contraceptive use (Winter, 1988). The decision to use contraception is influenced by many factors, such as age, family patterns of health care, advice from a health care provider, the influence of culture (Lethbridge, 1997), socioeconomic status, locus of control, knowledge of pregnancy risks, availability of contraception, approach to risk taking, and relationship with partner (Lethbridge & Hanna, 1997; Mills & Barclay, 2006).

A woman's opinions about contraceptive methods may change with her age, relationships, number of children, plans for future children, and experiences with methods (Grady, Billy, & Klepinger, 2002; Huber et al., 2006; Mathias et al., 2006; Mills & Barclay, 2006). For example, a woman who used a barrier method during the years she was actively planning her family may decide on a tubal ligation when her family is complete. A woman who used OCs during the years she was sure she did not want a pregnancy, may switch to condoms and a spermicide while she prepares to attempt conception. At any time, she may stop using a method because it does not meet her expectations, becomes unavailable, or her situation changes.

Some women manage their fertility regulation without the assistance of a health care provider. These women do not feel a need for educational services or prescription methods. Favorable attitudes toward methods are a prerequisite for contraceptive use and for seeking assistance from a health care provider when a woman believes she needs help choosing a method or accessing a prescription method. The attitudes of health care providers affect women's perceptions of methods, especially when a prescription is required (or other assistance) to procure a birth control method (Bird & Bogart, 2005; Mills & Barclay, 2006; Wysocki, 2006). Sometimes women see a health care provider, obtain a contraceptive method, and then never return. If the prescription expires or the method needs replacement, the woman may discontinue it rather than return to see the health care provider. Still other women switch from one health care provider to another for various reasons. The quality of the interaction between health care providers and their patients can also positively or negatively affect a woman's level of contraceptive use over time (Bird & Bogart, 2005; Mills & Barclay, 2006).

Family Planning Service Settings

Agencies offering family planning services should provide patients free access to current developments through the use of state-of-the-art media. Clinics should be open at convenient hours for all patients. They should welcome a woman, and with her permission, her partner's participation in method selection and educational sessions. The setting should be conducive to teaching and learning. Its waiting and counseling rooms should be large enough to permit various seating arrangements for several persons. To promote teaching and learning, it should have adequate lighting and ventilation. Because individuals have different learning styles and educational backgrounds, health care providers should use various teaching methods, such as one-to-one discussions and group sessions. Women should have access to appropriate and up-to-date educational materials, including those available in print and in the social media, to include "apps" for smartphones and other devices, hands-on displays, and online access (Bird & Bogart, 2005; Tabeek, 2000).

Changing from a technically oriented family planning care delivery system to an educational delivery system with product and nonproduct methods requires fertility awareness education—a basis for all contraception. Increased involvement and control over method selection may increase a woman's use of the method she chooses. The current delivery system of family planning services does not meet the needs of all patients. Drastic change in the system is unlikely, however, unless patients demand more from the system. Patient education may help solve this problem. However, changing the knowledge, attitudes, and behaviors of some family planning health care providers presents a greater challenge. Addressing the role of health care providers in the provision of care will also help to individualize care. Fortunately, most health care providers

are enthusiastic about the future of family planning and are eager to participate in new care delivery systems and to integrate new methods of contraceptive teaching and counseling into their practices (Herrman, 2006; Mills & Barclay, 2006; Tabeek, 2000).

Several types of health care providers offer a range of family planning services, such as counseling, prescribing OCs, the ring or the patch, fitting diaphragms, inserting contraceptive implants or IUDs, administering injectables, and providing family planning education. Health care providers provide these services in private practices; community health centers; hospital-based, public health, and freestanding clinics; and in family planning agencies (Herrman, 2006).

Health care providers' roles range from assisting women with decision making to direct hands-on care. Social workers, counselors with various educational backgrounds, health educators, and lay volunteers also participate in family planning programs. All health care providers bring their personal agendas, biases, values, and cultures to the family planning setting; affecting care delivery and interactions with patients. The style of health care delivery ranges from giving a method to a woman and assuming she will use it to being a partner in the decision-making process.

Health care providers use a variety of interaction styles when caring for women who are making choices about their reproductive health. Health care providers with a paternalistic style assume they know what is best and make decisions for their patients. They commonly use statements beginning with, "I will..." and "You will..." Those with a maternalistic style attempt to influence the woman's choices and gain her acquiescence by stating consequences of an action rather than the alternatives to it. This approach puts the focus on potential outcomes and the effects of the woman's choice on herself or others. Providers using this approach commonly use statements that begin with, "If you don't...then..." Providers using either style of interaction focus on outcomes and attempt to gain adherence with their own predetermined goals.

Health care providers using a participatory style demonstrate respect for a woman's autonomy and ability to make decisions. They focus on the process she uses to reach a decision, presenting alternatives and encouraging her to participate in the decision making. They use statements that begin with "What do you think about...?" or "We can talk about..." The woman's needs and concerns are more likely to emerge in participatory interactions than in maternalistic or paternalistic ones (Schnare & Nelson, 2005; Wysocki, 2006). As Orne and Hawkins (1985) pointed out, "Providers must avoid the temptation to prescribe 'for clients.' Clients must make their own informed choice in collaboration with providers; they should feel supported in their right to choose" (p. 33).

■ CONTRACEPTIVE METHODS

For most women in the United States, fertility regulation is a major concern. Ideally, young women should be taught about their bodies before menarche (the onset of menses), and learn about the developmental changes of puberty and the signs and symptoms of fertility. After menarche, they may begin the journey along the sometimes tortuous path of contraception decision making. During the fertile years, women may decide the number and timing of any pregnancies they choose to have.

Before deciding to use a particular contraceptive method, a woman should weigh the effectiveness against risks (if any), advantages, disadvantages, and adverse effects (Steiner et al., 2006). She should also consider any contraindications that relate to her health history. The effectiveness among contraceptive methods varies considerably. Each method has a theoretical effectiveness (effectiveness under ideal laboratory conditions, which depends solely on the method and not the human user), and use effectiveness (effectiveness under real-life or human conditions, which allows for the user's carelessness or error as well as method failure). Health care providers often use this information when counseling a woman about contraceptive choices and risks. When a woman seeks assistance with family planning, care would ideally include a detailed personal and family health history (Association of Women's Health, Obstetric, and Neonatal Nurses & National Association of Nurse Practitioners in Women's Health, 2002; Hawkins, Roberto-Nichols, & Stanley-Haney, 2008).

The cost of contraception is a significant consideration. For example, some long-acting reversible contraceptive (LARC) methods may be more expensive up front, yet more cost-effective in the long term. A 2015, in-depth analysis calculated costs based on the purchase price of the method, the administration and clinical costs, and costs of failure. This analysis found that IUDs (both copper and progesterone) were the least expensive at around $300 per patient per year. Injections ($432) and patches ($730) were the more expensive per patient-per year options (Trussell, Hassan, Lowin, Law, & Filonenko, 2015). In 2015, some large retailers offer generic combined OCs (COCs) and progesterone only OCs for $4 per month. The 2010 Affordable Care Act mandates that employers provide contraceptive coverage as a part of their employee insurance plans.

Natural Family Planning Methods

Fertility regulation and awareness is the cornerstone and basis for understanding all contraceptive methods; especially the fertility awareness (natural family planning [NFP]) methods. This information assists the woman in knowing when or if she ovulates. Therefore, the health care provider should explore a woman's awareness of her fertility patterns and provide additional information, if needed, before assisting her with the selection of a contraceptive method (Hawkins et al., 2008; Tabeek, 2000). Additionally, some health care providers have taught aspects of fertility awareness to couples who wish to conceive, but are having difficulty (Thijssen, Meier, Panis, & Ombelet, 2014).

Fertility awareness education refers to imparting information about male and female reproductive anatomy and physiology, primary and secondary signs of fertility, and cyclical changes in these signs. All fertility awareness methods use this information, as well as knowledge of female fertile and infertile phases and their relationship to male fertility, and require abstinence from vaginal–penile intercourse during the fertile phase to prevent conception. Because NFP methods are unmodified by chemical, mechanical, or other artificial means, they represent a natural way to regulate fertility (World Health Organization [WHO], 2011).

Evidence from ancient times suggests rudimentary knowledge of periods of relative infertility during the menstrual cycle, as well as at other times in a woman's life. For example, East African women believed that avoiding intercourse for a few days after menstruation would prevent pregnancy (Gordon, 1990). Breastfeeding was recognized as a means to prevent pregnancy and was used by Alaska Natives, Native Americans, and ancient Egyptians (Gordon, 1990). This latter method gained popularity in the 1990s under the title of lactation amenorrhea method (LAM), and is still practiced today (Díaz, 1989; France, 1996; WHO, 2009).

NFP includes cervical mucus, basal body temperature (BBT), and symptothermal and LAMs. Except for LAM, these methods use normal signs and symptoms of ovulation and the menstrual cycle to prevent or achieve pregnancy (Finnigan, 2008). The woman is taught the methods and then asked to observe several cycles to best understand and recognize her fertile and infertile phases.

CERVICAL MUCUS METHOD

The cervical mucus method is based on detecting signs and symptoms of ovulation through consistent observation of the cervical mucus, which is produced by cells in the cervix. Throughout the menstrual cycle cervical mucus changes. Immediately after the menstrual period, cervical mucus is scant and the woman should notice vaginal dryness for a few days. Then mucus is present for a few days, in which the woman should feel vaginal wetness. After this, the mucus becomes clear (as differentiated from milky white, translucent, or creamy color) and slippery or stretchy, similar to raw egg white. The woman should notice increased wetness or a slippery sensation. The peak day of wetness signals ovulation. During ovulation, cervical mucus nourishes sperm, facilitates their passage into the intrauterine cavity, and probably helps select sperm of the highest quality. However, the peak day is only obvious the day after it occurs, when the mucus becomes less slippery and stretchy. After this day, the mucus starts to lose its slippery, stretchy, wet quality, and becomes cloudy and sticky until menses begin.

To use the cervical mucus method, the woman should check her cervical mucus daily, beginning when menstrual bleeding ends or becomes light enough to allow assessment of the mucus. The woman can check her mucus in several ways, depending on her level of comfort with her body. She can wipe a folded piece of toilet tissue across her vaginal opening, and then feel whether the tissue slides across easily or drags, pulls, or sticks. If mucus is present, she can place it between two fingers and check its wetness and stretchiness. These characteristics are referred to as *spinnbarkheit*.

As an alternative, she can check for these characteristics by holding the toilet tissue with both hands and pulling it apart (Finnigan, 2008; Tabeek, 2000).

BBT METHOD

The BBT method is based on the temperature change triggered by the progesterone rise that occurs when the ovum leaves the ovary. To use this method, the woman takes her temperature at the same time every day using a digital basal thermometer; before she eats, drinks, smokes, and/or participates in any physical activity. Then she documents her daily temperature on a chart, noting any variations. During ovulation, the temperature typically rises up to 1° above the preovulatory BBT. To prevent conception, the woman should abstain from intercourse until after 3 days of temperature rise. Infections, illnesses, and other conditions such as fatigue, anxiety, sleeplessness, some medications, use of an electric blanket, and/or a heated waterbed can also increase the body temperature. Therefore, applying the rules for taking and interpreting the BBT are crucial to the effectiveness of this method.

SYMPTOTHERMAL METHOD

The symptothermal method relies on identifying the primary signs of fertility: changes in cervical mucus; BBT; and the position, consistency, and opening of the cervix. Like cervical mucus and BBT, the cervix changes throughout the menstrual cycle. To receive sperm, as ovulation approaches, the cervix becomes softer and changes position to midline and the cervical opening (os) dilates slightly. After ovulation, it reverts to its preovulatory state. While squatting or standing with one foot on a stool or chair, the woman may place a finger in her vagina and feel for position, softness, or firmness.

The symptothermal method also uses observation for secondary signs of fertility: cyclical breast, skin, hair, mood, and energy changes; vaginal aching; spotting; pelvic pain or aching; and *mittelschmerz* (normal, lower abdominal or pelvic pain some women experience during ovulation). By charting primary and secondary signs, the woman detects her fertile phase with great accuracy and can prevent or achieve conception.

A number of devices to predict ovulation are on the market, including an ovulation calculator. The predictions are based on assessment of luteinizing hormone (LH) in urine or saliva. Interactive computer programs also are available to teach fertility awareness methods (Fehring, 2004, 2005; Fehring, Raviele, & Schneider, 2004).

LACTATIONAL AMENORRHEA METHOD

After decades of skepticism in the United States, the LAM is becoming more popular as a fertility awareness method (Arévalo, Jennings, & Sinai, 2003; Fehring, 2004). This method is based on the fact that the length of postpartal amenorrhea is directly affected by the duration of lactation. Postpartal amenorrhea varies among different women and populations. In general, it is shorter than the duration of lactation in populations that use prolonged breastfeeding (Díaz, 1989). In the United States, however, breastfeeding patterns—that is, the duration and amount—vary widely and are affected by women's multiple roles, including that of employee. Introduction of solid food or supplementary formula for the infant, which can be influenced by a woman's sociocultural group and culture of origin, also can affect the duration of amenorrhea by affecting how often a mother breastfeeds. Most important to breastfeeding and amenorrhea is the infant's sucking pattern. Rates of pregnancy with LAM appear comparable to those of other methods (Díaz, 1989; Pérez, Labbok, & Queenan, 1992). Thus, women who plan to breastfeed can be offered information about LAM to consider along with information about other fertility awareness methods.

Several innovations in NFP have resulted from studies of acceptability by couples in many locations around the globe. Arévalo et al. (2003) studied the standard day method of NFP with couples in Bolivia, Peru, and the Philippines. This method requires that users abstain from unprotected intercourse during cycle days 8 through 19. Women follow their cycles using CycleBeads and peak day for mucus. If they choose to, they may also assess other signs such as position of the cervix. CycleBeads was developed by Georgetown University researchers and is an integral part of the standard day method (CycleBeads, 2015; Fehring, 2004; Germano & Jennings, 2006).

ELECTRONIC HORMONAL FERTILITY MONITORING

Electronic hormonal fertility monitors were developed and marketed for the purpose of helping women determine when they are ovulating so they could optimally time intercourse and maximize the opportunity to conceive. The monitors work by detecting the level of LH and estrogen in urine, identifying peak fertility days.

Recently, however, fertility monitors have begun to be used also as a method of avoiding intercourse during fertile periods. One small study compared electronic fertility monitoring as an NFP method to cervical mucus monitoring and found that while both methods were acceptable, the failure rate was lower in the group that used electronic monitoring (Fehring, Schneider, Raviele, Rodriguez, & Pruszynski, 2013). A similar small study found that electronic fertility monitoring was an effective method for avoiding pregnancy in perimenopausal women (Fehring & Mu, 2014).

More research is needed on the feasibility of using electronic fertility monitoring as a standalone strategy for NFP. In time, it may prove to be useful for women who are very comfortable with technology, are uncomfortable with using traditional NFP methods, and/or are looking for confirmation of existing solutions.

■ PRESCRIPTION HORMONAL AND OVER-THE-COUNTER METHODS

There are a multitude of hormonal, barrier methods, and IUDs available to assist women in preventing pregnancy.

Understanding the advantages, disadvantages, cost, and health risks are critical in helping advise a woman on a lasting option and to help manage side effects and other unpleasant symptoms.

Combined OCs

In 1960, the Federal Drug Administration (FDA) ushered in the era of COCs with the approval of the drug Envoid (Christin-Maitre, 2013). Initial research was conducted in the 1950s by Gregory Pincus and was financed by Sanger's colleague Katharine McCormick, who spent $2 million of her own money on the project. COCs have since been extremely popular, as 82% of women of reproductive age identify that they have used them at some point in their life (Daniels et al., 2013) and 28% of women identify that they are currently using them as their primary form of contraception (Jones et al., 2012).

There are significant advantages to COCs that make them a strong birth control option for many women. When taken perfectly, COCs are 99.7% effective at preventing an unintended pregnancy in a year of use (Hatcher, 2011). They offer a quick return to fertility, as women often ovulate within a few cycles of ceasing use. Furthermore, COCs are easy to take, are well tolerated, maintain efficacy when an occasional dose is forgotten, and result in lighter menses. However, it is important to remind patients that COCs provide no protection for sexually transmitted infections (STIs, to include HIV), and for that reason, many women require the addition of a barrier method (e.g., condoms).

The modern COC has two components. The first component, estrogen, provides some contraceptive effect by suppressing the release of follicle-stimulating hormone (FSH) but more importantly stabilizes the endometrium in order to maintain bleeding regularity (Frye, 2006). In the United States, ethinyl estradiol and less commonly mestranol are the synthetic estrogens used in COCs. In the 1960s, Envoid used 150 mg of ethinyl estradiol, which caused a wide variety of unpleasant side effects that included thromboembolic events. Since then, the amount of estrogen contained in COCs has been decreased to less than 35 mg, thereby significantly improving both safety and tolerability (Christin-Maitre, 2013).

The other component of COCs is a synthetic progesterone, which is classified by "generation." Progesterone provides the vast majority of the contraceptive effect by suppressing both the FSH and LH. The result of these altered hormonal conditions is suppression of ovulation, thickening of cervical mucus, and the creation of hormonal conditions within the uterus that are unfavorable for implantation (Frye, 2006). A side effect of the progestin component is androgenization, which can cause acne, hirsutism, and weight gain. Third and fourth generation progestins were developed to be less androgenic and minimize these unpleasant symptoms (Sitruk-Ware & Nath, 2010).

COC pill packs contain both active pills and inert pills. The purpose of the inert pills is to withdraw hormones in order to promote bleeding, as the initial developers believed that women would be reassured by the monthly demonstration of the fact that they are not pregnant. Most monophasic preparations contain a pill that is taken for 21 days followed by 7 days of inert pills that exist only as a daily placeholder until the next round of active pills begins. Multiphasic COCs were developed in the 1980s to lessen side effects by varying the amount of hormones over the course of the first 3 weeks. Multiphasic COCs exist in biphasic, triphasic, and newer quadriphasic regimens.

CONTRAINDICATIONS

Although COCs are very safe, some women are not ideal candidates for their use. It is imperative that health care providers take a detailed medical history before discussing contraceptive options in order to identify conditions that make some women poor candidates or optimal candidates for contraceptive methods. Fortunately, many of the contraindications to COCs do not apply to progesterone-only methods, IUDs, or barrier methods, ensuring that there is a safe and effective option for almost any woman.

The WHO has produced helpful guidelines that identify conditions and states that are contraindications to COCs. These guidelines are available and may be accessed online at no cost (www.who.int/reproductivehealth/publications/family_planning/Ex-Summ-MEC-5/en). Absolute contraindications to COCs include: (a) women who are breastfeeding and less than 6 weeks postpartum; (b) those who are older than 35 years and smoke greater than or equal to 15 cigarettes per day; (c) women with a systolic blood pressure greater than or equal to 160 mmHg; (d) those with vascular disease; (e) those with known heart disease, valvular disease, or stroke; (f) those with current breast cancer; (g) those with a history of diabetes with target end-organ damage; and (h) those with active viral hepatitis, cirrhosis, or liver cancer (WHO, 2009).

Blood pressure must be monitored with each visit, as COCs may raise both the systolic and diastolic blood pressure in some women; although the effect is not usually clinically significant. Negative changes in blood pressure will normalize after cessation of COCs (Chrousos, 2014). Generally, it is considered safe to prescribe COCs to women with normal blood pressures (less than 140/90 mmHg). Women who have well-controlled hypertension, are younger than 35 years, and do not smoke are reasonable candidates for COCs. Women with poorly controlled hypertension and smokers are better candidates for progesterone-only methods, IUDs, or barrier contraception (American College of Obstetricians and Gynecologists [ACOG], 2006).

On occasion, COCs have been known to cause thromboembolic events, such as deep vein thrombosis (DVT) and thromboembolic stroke. Although venous thromboembolism is estimated to occur at a three times higher rate for COC users, the risk is still low (Peragallo Urrutia et al., 2013). COCs should be avoided in women with a history of DVT or pulmonary embolus (PE), those who have prolonged immobilization due to surgery or other conditions, and those with a history of heart disease or stroke (WHO, 2009). Progesterone-only methods are generally safe for use in women with these conditions and are a viable alternative.

Women who have a history of migraines with auras are thought to double their risk of ischemic stroke (ACOG, 2006). Like many other serious COC adverse effects, this risk appears to increase with higher doses of ethinyl estradiol and in women who smoke. Although the risks are low, due to the morbidity associated with ischemic stroke current recommendations are that women who have a history of migraines with auras are prescribed an alternative form of contraception. Women who have a history of migraines without aura, however, are generally considered to be safe to take COCs.

There continues to be a concern over the role of COCs in the development or acceleration of breast cancer. Several meta-analyses have found either no association between COCs and breast cancer, or that the risk is quite small (Nelson et al., 2012). Studies have also demonstrated that there is no increased risk of breast cancer with COC use in women who have the BRAC 1 or 2 gene mutations or with known family histories of breast cancer. Therefore, current recommendations do not include family history of breast cancer as a contraindication of COC use (Cibula et al., 2010).

HEALTH BENEFITS

The use of OCs provides many health benefits that extend beyond contraception. Because OCs tend to stabilize the endometrium, women often experience a lighter menses that benefits women with anemias and heavy or frequent menses. Many women who take COCs (particularly triphasic preparations) experience a significant improvement in acne. COCs have demonstrated effectiveness in decreasing the severity of premenstrual mood symptoms. There is also a decreased incidence of ovarian cancer in women who take COCs, particularly for longer than 10 years of use. Additionally, COC users demonstrate a decrease in the incidence of fibrocystic breasts and endometrial cancers (Schindler, 2013).

ASSISTING PATIENTS WITH THE SELECTION OF COC

Obtaining and understanding a woman's health history and reproductive health goals is the key to selecting a COC. Some newer forms of COCs have nontraditional 21/7 preparations and are useful to help mitigate other health concerns. Women who dislike the inconvenience or symptoms associated with menses may prefer safe, newer preparations that contain 84 active pills and 7 inactive pills, resulting in a period only once every 3 months. This regimen may be particularly attractive to women with menstrual migraines (without auras), menstrual disorders, anemias, and premenstrual symptoms (Jacobson, Likis, & Murphy, 2012). Another newer preparation contains 24 days of active pills followed by 4 days of inert pills, resulting in less unpleasant side effects due to estrogen withdrawal, a lighter menses, and an even lower likelihood of ovulation (Bachmann, Sulak, Sampson-Landers, Benda, & Marr, 2004).

Traditionally, women have been instructed to begin taking COCs on either the first day of menses or the first Sunday after menses begins, known as the *conventional start method*. The advantages of this method are that the days of the week are aligned with those on the pack and establish that the woman is unlikely to be pregnant. Another approach, known as the *quick start method*, has the patient take the medication on the day they are prescribed as long as the health care provider and patient are reasonably sure that the patient is not pregnant. Although studies have shown little difference in the incidence of unintended pregnancies with the quick start method, it provides yet another opportunity for patient choice (Lopez, Newmann, Grimes, Nanda, & Schulz, 2013).

Patients should be encouraged to associate taking their COCs with another daily activity (such as brushing their teeth) in order to develop habit-forming behavior. Those who forget to take one pill should take two the next day. Several smartphone apps exist to help women remember to take their medication and anticipate their periods. Patients who miss two or more pills should continue with the aligned days of the pack and use barrier contraception for the remainder of the cycle. Women who miss pills frequently should explore other types of contraception that do not require daily intervention. Women who miss more than 1 day of triphasic or quadriphasic preparations may benefit from checking manufacturer instructions on product websites.

SIDE EFFECTS

Thirty percent of women who have used COCs have discontinued use due to side effects (Daniels et al., 2013). Therefore, it is important for the health care provider to set expectations and assess and manage side effects with each patient visit to ensure continued use or to partner with the patient to make a change. The most common side effects of COCs include breakthrough bleeding (BTB), nausea, and mild headaches. Most patients simply require reassurance that the side effects will improve after two to four cycles. BTB is a frequent occurrence, and is often due to missed pills. With extended regimens, stopping the pills for 4 days and causing a short withdrawal bleed may prove helpful. Some women will eventually require a formulation with higher doses of estrogen, or, conversely, lower doses of the progestin (Lohr & Creinin, 2006). Headaches are common with all formulations, and may improve with extended regimens (Barr, 2010). Some women may experience melasma (patches of pigmented skin discoloration), which usually dissipates slowly when the medication is stopped.

As a part of patient education, it is important to counsel the patient on the signs and symptoms of serious side effects. The acronym "ACHES" was developed as a mnemonic to help women remember these potential serious adverse effects. Any woman who experiences ACHES should immediately stop taking her COCs and notify her provider. ACHES include:

- Abdominal pain (severe)
- Chest pain (severe), cough, or shortness of breath
- Headaches (severe), dizziness, weakness, or numbness
- Eye problems (vision loss or blurring) or speech problems
- Severe leg pain (calf or thigh)

Contraceptive Patch

The contraceptive patch and the contraceptive ring are estrogen/progesterone combination products that have the same mechanism of action as COCs. The patch and the ring are particularly advantageous to women who find the ritual of remembering a daily medication burdensome. They share the same side effects, risks, contraindications, and noncontraceptive benefits as combined oral products. Both products have a quick return to fertility, as ovulation usually occurs within a few cycles of cessation.

The contraceptive patch was introduced in the United States in 2002. Consisting of a 20 cm² square adhesive patch combining 0.75 mg of ethinyl estradiol with 6 mg of norelgestromin, the product provides a unique alternative to daily dosed COCs (Figure 21.1). With perfect use, the patch is 99.7% effective in preventing pregnancy. With typical use, efficacy falls to 91% (Hatcher, 2011). The patch is theorized to have a slightly higher incidence of thromboembolism than COCs (O'Connell & Burkman, 2007).

USAGE

Applied on the first Sunday after menses, the patch is worn for a week and then replaced for three consecutive weeks. A quick start method similar to COCs is considered an acceptable alternative. On the fourth week, no patch is worn, creating a withdrawal bleed. The cycle is then repeated. The patch is placed on clean skin on any of the following areas: lower abdomen, upper arms, buttocks, and upper torso. The breasts are to be avoided. A patch that partially detaches or becomes completely removed can be reapplied or taped on as long as it has been off for less than 24 hours. A common additional side effect to the patch is skin irritation (WHO, 2011).

There has been concern that some contraceptive products lose effectiveness when used by larger women. The manufacturer of Ortho-Evra (contraceptive patch) recommends caution in using the product in women who weigh more than 198 pounds. Recently a large cohort study found that overweight and obese women were no more likely to be at increased risk of either contraceptive patch or vaginal ring failure (McNicholas et al., 2013). Many experts prefer, however, to recommend an IUD or barrier methods in conjunction with hormonal options to these patients.

Contraceptive Ring

The vaginal contraceptive ring, known in the United States as Nuva-Ring, was approved for use by the FDA in 2001. It is a soft and flexible 54-mm diameter ring that releases 120 mcg/day of etonogestrel and 15 mcg/day of ethinyl estradiol (Figure 21.2) (Brache, Payán, & Faundes, 2013). It is 91% effective in preventing pregnancy with typical use and 99.7% perfect with typical use (Hatcher, 2011). Although other contraceptive rings (to include progesterone-only products) are in development and approved elsewhere in the world, at the time of this writing, only the Nuva-Ring is available in the United States.

USAGE

The contraceptive ring is used very similarly to the contraceptive patch. On the first Sunday after menses, the patient compresses the opposite sides of the ring and inserts it into her vagina. Although the ring can be placed anywhere in the vagina to be effective, it tends to be less apparent to the patient and their partner in the deeper, posterior portion of the vagina. The patient places the vaginal ring on the Sunday following menses and replaces it once a week for a total of 3 weeks. A ring-free fourth week creates a withdrawal bleed (WHO, 2011).

The ring should remain in place at all times throughout the week, to include intercourse. If it falls out, the patient should rinse it with water and put it back in place. If the ring is out of the vagina for more than 3 hours during the

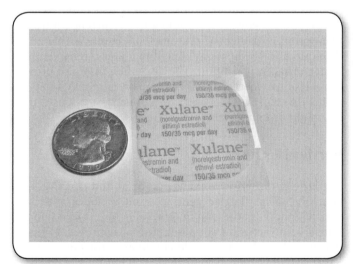

FIGURE 21.1
Contraceptive patch.

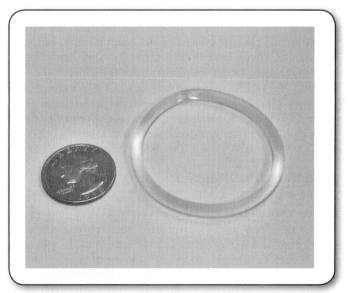

FIGURE 21.2
Contraceptive ring.

first 2 weeks it should be reinserted and a barrier method should be used for the next 7 days. If the ring is out of place for more than 3 hours during the third week, then a new ring should be inserted and a backup barrier method should be used for 7 days (WHO, 2011).

Progesterone-Only Pills

Progesterone-only pills (POPs; also known as "mini-pops") provide an alternative to traditional COCs for women who are not candidates for the estrogen component. POPs' contraceptive efficacy is thought to approximate that of COCs at 91% effective with typical use and 99.7% effective with perfect use (Hatcher, 2011). POPs are most commonly used by lactating mothers who are in the immediate postpartum period and do not wish a long-term progesterone-only solution, such as injectable medroxyprogesterone acetate. Efficacy rates may be lower for women who are not lactating. As there is no estrogen component, breakthrough vaginal bleeding is a common side effect.

USAGE

POPs can be started as quickly as 6 weeks postpartum. It is important to counsel patients so that they understand that POPs lose effectiveness if not taken at the same time every day. A woman who is more than 3 hours late taking her medication should use a backup barrier method for any intercourse following the next 48-hour period (WHO, 2011).

Emergency Contraception

Since the 1970s, both COCs and POPs have been used as emergency contraception (EC). Common reasons for prescribing EC include unprotected intercourse, a mistake in or failure of a contraceptive, or sexual assault. EC is not an abortifacient and does not harm an existing pregnancy.

Dr. Albert Yuzpe pioneered the practice of using two doses of a COC within 72 hours of unprotected sexual intercourse or barrier contraception failure to prevent pregnancy. The *Yuzpe method* used large doses of ethinyl estradiol that often caused unpleasant adverse effects (Li, Lo, & Ho, 2014). Current methods achieve the same results but with more tolerable, lower amounts of hormone. It is believed that the mechanism of action is to prevent or delay ovulation and to thicken cervical mucus.

EC OPTIONS AND USAGE

Any COC could feasibly be used as EC. The *World Health Organization Family Planning Global Handbook* (available free online at http://apps.who.int/iris/bitstream/10665/44028/1/9780978856373_eng.pdf) provides charts with detailed instructions for using almost any existing COC or POP as EC (WHO, 2011). However, if financial resources and availability allow, two FDA-approved commercial products may offer more convenient and potentially efficacious choices.

LEVONORGESTREL

The common, over-the-counter option for EC is levonorgestrel, a progesterone-only product sold in the United States and licensed under the brand Plan B One-Step. This regimen calls for a one 1.5 mg tablet to be taken within 72 hours of unprotected intercourse. Levonorgestrel should not be taken if the patient believes she is pregnant; yet it will not harm an already existing pregnancy. Levonorgestrel is most effective if taken within 48 hours of unprotected intercourse; efficacy decreases at the 48 to 72 hour post-intercourse time period (Hang-Wun, Tsing, & Ho, 2014; Li et al., 2014). Package inserts estimate the product to be around 85% effective in preventing a pregnancy, which otherwise would have occurred. Common side effects include spotting, mild abdominal pain, fatigue, headache, dizziness, and breast tenderness.

ULIPRISTAL

An alternative and arguably more effective prescription-only solution for EC is the progesterone ulipristal acetate (UPA), sold in the United States under the trade name Ella. UPA is to be taken as a single 30 mg dose after unprotected intercourse. The advantage of UPA over levonorgestrel is that it can be taken up to 120 hours after unprotected intercourse. One study demonstrated a failure rate of only 2.1% from 48 to 120 hours after intercourse. The disadvantage of UPA is that it is not available over the counter (Hang-Wun et al., 2014; Li et al., 2014).

COPPER IUD

The copper IUD, being discussed as follows, is also a very effective choice for EC. It is 99% effective as EC and can be placed up to 5 days after the unprotected sexual intercourse event. It has the additional benefit of being the only form of EC that is capable of simultaneously providing a long-term solution (Belden, Harper, & Speidel, 2012). The efficacy of the progesterone IUD has not been tested as EC and is therefore not recommended at this time.

Health care providers should carefully and nonjudgmentally explore the reason(s) that EC was required. This information is *key* to determining if the current contraceptive option is failing for reasons that require a change, or if the situation requires a discussion about a reliable, long-term contraceptive option. The discussion may also provide insight as to whether or not a woman is at risk for pregnancy due to sexual assault. Additionally, a discussion on EC might prompt discussions about risk for STIs.

Barrier Methods

Barrier contraception remains a popular and effective birth control choice. Barrier contraception includes male and female condoms, the diaphragm, and the cervical sponge. Barrier contraception is unique in that it provides (particularly with male and female condoms) protection against STIs. An additional benefit is that many barrier methods (with the exception of diaphragms) are available over the counter at low cost.

MALE CONDOM

The male condom is the oldest, most widely known and most commonly available form of barrier contraception. It is 98% effective at preventing pregnancy when used perfectly and is 82% effective if used typically (Hatcher, 2011). Condoms are arguably the only form of contraception that is primarily managed by the male partner. It is around 90% effective at preventing HIV transmission. The male condom is potentially a good choice for a woman and her partner who cannot or do not wish to engage in hormonal birth control methods.

The correct use of a condom is imperative in order to ensure maximum efficacy. The condom should have at least half an inch of space at the tip of the penis to serve as a reservoir for ejaculation. Immediately upon ejaculating, the male should withdraw from intercourse and the condom should be carefully removed and disposed of. A new condom should be used for any subsequent sexual activity. Condoms can be used with either a water- or silicon-based lubricant—never with an oil-based lubricant as it places the integrity of the condom at risk. Condoms can be used with spermicidal applications. If a condom breaks or spills during sexual activity, health care providers should advise patients to consider EC.

FEMALE CONDOMS

Female condoms provide an alternative to male condoms, and are almost as effective at preventing pregnancy. With perfect use, female condoms are 95% effective and with typical use they are 79% effective in preventing pregnancy (Hatcher, 2011). They are made of a soft plastic film, and are lubricated on both the inside and outside. They are made of two rings, one at the closed end to assist with insertion and one at the open end to keep the condom open (Figure 21.3). They are effective at preventing sexually transmitted disease and are available over the counter. They are, however, a bit more difficult to properly place than a male condom.

Because female condoms are made of plastic, they can be used with any type of lubricant to include those that are oil based. After intercourse, the female condom is removed by twisting the outer ring in order to form a seal, and then gently pulling it out of the vagina. As with the male condom, any contraceptive failures that include breaking or spilling semen into the vagina can be mitigated with EC (WHO, 2011).

DIAPHRAGM

The diaphragm is an older form of barrier contraception that has lost popularity due to newer, well-tolerated, long-acting hormonal contraceptives. It consists of a soft plastic or silicone cap that is placed in the vagina before intercourse in order to cover the cervix (Figure 21.4). It is used with a spermicidal agent to increase efficacy. With perfect use, the diaphragm is 94% effective in preventing pregnancy and with typical use, efficacy declines to 88% (Hatcher, 2011). It requires some dexterity to correctly place the diaphragm before intercourse, which may prove to be a disadvantage to some women.

A visit with a provider who is skilled and experienced in fitting diaphragms is necessary, as there are multiple available sizes. The diaphragm should fit against the vaginal walls, but should not be so tight that it causes discomfort or loose enough to easily dislodge. Women who have a prolapsed uterus are poor candidates due to inadequate diaphragm fitting. A diaphragm must remain in place for at least 6 hours after intercourse, and for no more than 24 hours. Many health care providers suggest that women try a diaphragm while they continue their current method of contraception (WHO, 2011).

CONTRACEPTIVE SPONGE

Another older form of barrier contraception is the contraceptive sponge. It is a one-sized, absorptive polyurethane device that is impregnated with spermicide (Figure 21.5). The Today brand sponge is sold over the counter in the

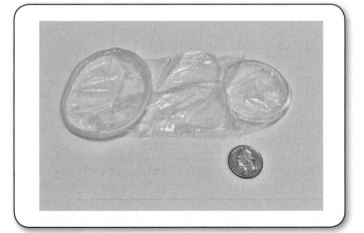

FIGURE 21.3
Female condom.

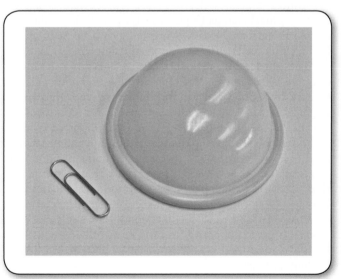

FIGURE 21.4
Diaphragm.

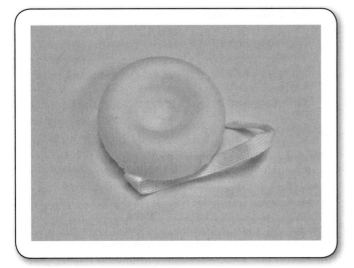

FIGURE 21.5
Contraceptive sponge.

United States and is marketed as an alternative to the condom. The device is moistened with water before placement. The concave portion of the device is placed against the cervix and the opposite side has a loop to use for removing the device after use. The sponge is significantly more effective in nulliparous women than parous women (91% vs. 80% respectively with perfect use and 88% vs. 76%, respectively with typical use; Hatcher, 2011). The sponge should be left in place for at least 6 hours and may be left in place for 24 hours. It does not need to be replaced if there are multiple intercourse sessions within the 24-hour period (Yranski & Gamache, 2008).

■ INJECTABLE CONTRACEPTION

The only injectable form of contraception available in the United States is depot medroxyprogesterone acetate (DMPA), marketed as Depo-Provera. DMPA is available in two formulations: DMPA-IM, given as a deep intramuscular injection, or DMPA-SC, given subcutaneously.

These progestin-only contraceptive injectables are highly effective, safe, convenient, long acting, reversible, and can be used by most women in most circumstances (Jacobstein & Polis, 2014). Since FDA approval for contraceptive use in 1992, DMPA has been used by millions of women. Although women using this progestin-only contraceptive injectable often initially experience irregular bleeding and spotting, long-term DMPA use typically results in amenorrhea. Currently available by prescription only, DMPA usually costs less than $100 per injection. DMPA is safe for most women and most medical conditions and is safe for women of any age, parity, and for women living with HIV. DMPA can be used postabortion or in postpartum breastfeeding mothers.

Because DMPA does not contain any estrogen, it represents a good contraceptive choice for postpartum and lactating women, as well as women who cannot or do not want to take estrogen. DMPA prevents pregnancy primarily through suppression of ovulation. A possible secondary mechanism of action includes thickening of cervical mucus, which decreases sperm penetration, and endometrial atrophy, which prevents implantation (Jacobstein & Polis, 2014).

Both DMPA-IM and DMPA-SC are highly effective. Data from the United States suggest that 0.2% of women with perfect use and 6% of women with typical use of DMPA will experience an unintended pregnancy within the first year of use (Jacobstein & Polis, 2014). It is important to note progestin-only contraceptive injectables are not expected to have lower efficacy in overweight or obese women. Additionally, because DMPA avoids first-pass metabolism, its efficacy is unaffected by a women's use of other medications (Bartz & Goldberg, 2011).

DMPA is available in two formulations: (a) DMPA-IM, 150 mg given as a deep intramuscular injection every 12 weeks; and (b) DMPA-SC, 104 mg given subcutaneously every 12 weeks. Although not FDA approved at this time, the newer subcutaneous dosing could potentially allow for home-based self-administration in the near future (Williams, Hensel, & Fortenberry, 2013).

Usage

DMPA can be started at any time during a woman's menstrual cycle, as long as the health care provider is reasonably sure that the patient is not pregnant (Bartz & Goldberg, 2011). Requiring that a woman needs to be menstruating in order to receive DMPA is an unjustified barrier to care. DMPA can be initiated without a pelvic examination, blood or other lab tests, cervical cancer screening, and/or breast examination (Jacobstein & Polis, 2014).

DMPA-IM is injected into the upper arm or buttock. DMPA-SC can be injected into the upper thigh, upper arm, or abdomen (Jacobstein & Polis, 2014). DMPA has a 14-week duration of action and is recommended to be administered every 12 weeks, thereby providing a 2-week "grace" period for the patient. The possibility of pregnancy should be ruled out in the case of any woman who is more than 2 weeks late for her DMPA injection.

Side Effects

Thorough counseling, patient education, and anticipatory guidance regarding side effects of DMPA are critical. Side effects of DMPA include menstrual disturbances, weight gain, depression, decrease in bone density, allergic reactions, metabolic effects, headaches, nervousness, decreased libido, and breast tenderness (Bartz & Goldberg, 2011).

Menstrual changes occur in almost all women who use DMPA and are the most common cause for dissatisfaction and discontinued use. Bleeding patterns are initially unpredictable, with approximately 70% of women experiencing infrequent but prolonged episodes of bleeding or spotting. Irregular bleeding typically decreases with each reinjection. After the first year of use, close to 50% of women will experience amenorrhea (Bartz & Goldberg, 2011).

Weight gain is commonly reported as a side effect of DMPA and can lead to method discontinuation or reluctance to initiate the method (Beksinska, Smit, Kleinschmidt, Milford, & Farley, 2010). Although weight gain is not consistent for all women, recent studies have shown a 9-pound weight gain with DMPA-IM use, and a 3.5-pound weight gain with DMPA-SC use (Bartz & Goldberg, 2011).

Some women may experience an increase in depression when they use DMPA. However, data are limited and conflicting, and a history of depression is not a contraindication to DMPA use. Long-term DMPA users may develop a decrease in bone mineral density, but this side effect is temporary and reversible on discontinuation of DMPA. Although rare, allergic reactions to DMPA may occur. Some health care providers encourage women to remain in the clinic for 20 minutes after an injection. In addition, women should be asked if they have ever experienced severe itching or redness at the site of a previous DMPA injection site. If so, another DMPA dose should not be repeated (Bartz & Goldberg, 2011).

Because DMPA is an injection, it is not possible to immediately discontinue. Menstrual irregularities, weight gain, depression, allergic reactions, breast tenderness, and headaches may continue until DMPA is cleared from the woman's body, anywhere from 6 to 8 months after her last injection.

Health Benefits

DMPA is associated with certain noncontraceptive benefits, such as a reduction in or elimination of premenstrual symptoms, absence of menstrual bleeding, a reduced risk of pelvic inflammatory disease (PID), a reduced risk of ectopic pregnancy, decreased risk of endometrial cancer, improvement in grand mal seizure control, and hematological improvement in women with sickle cell disease. DMPA-induced amenorrhea may make it a good contraceptive choice for women with menorrhagia, dysmenorrhea, fibroids, and iron deficiency anemia.

Contraindications

There are some conditions where risks may outweigh the benefits. These conditions include cardiovascular disease, women with liver disease, women with a history of breast cancer, and women with unexplained vaginal bleeding before a thorough evaluation. Providing DMPA in these circumstances requires careful clinical consideration (Bartz & Goldberg, 2011). A current diagnosis of breast cancer is the only absolute contraindication to DMPA use.

Women need to be informed of the likely delay in fertility after DMPA use. Return to fertility after a DMPA-IM injection averages between 9 and 10 months, with some studies showing that fertility may not be restored for as long as 22 months (Kaunitz, 1998). DMPA is not the best choice for women who wish to become pregnant within the next 1 to 2 years and should be counseled about alternative contraceptive options.

Serious health issues are rare with DMPA use. However, a woman should immediately contact her health care provider for any of the following warning signs:

- If you think you might be pregnant
- Repeated, very painful headaches
- Depression
- Severe, lower abdominal pain
- Pus, prolonged pain, redness, itching, or bleeding at the injection site
- Any other concerning symptoms

■ CONTRACEPTIVE IMPLANTS

In 1990, the contraceptive levonorgestrel (Norplant) ushered in the era of implantable progestin rods. Norplant consisted of six levonorgestrel containing rods that were inserted into the subdermal layer of the upper, inner arm. It lost popularity when reports about the difficulty in removal of the implant arose (Pushba, Sangita, Shivani, & Chitra, 2011). Although Norplant is no longer being manufactured, there is currently one contraceptive implant available in the United States. It was originally marketed under the brand name Implanon, but has been subsequently marketed as Nexplanon.

Nexplanon

Nexplanon is a hormone-releasing birth control implant for use by women to prevent pregnancy for up to 3 years. Nexplanon is a thin, silicon-free flexible plastic rod, about the size of a matchstick, containing 68 mg of the progestin etonogestrel. The rod slowly delivers an average of 40 mg of etonogestrel every day for at least 3 years, inhibiting ovulation and thickening cervical mucus. The etonogestrel implant is not biodegradable and requires removal either when the patient desires or when the device expires. Nexplanon is reported to be 99.9% effective at preventing pregnancy.

Mechanism of Action

The contraceptive effects of Nexplanon are similar to that of other progestin-containing contraceptives. The progestin etonogestrel, used in Nexplanon, thickens cervical mucus, making it difficult for sperm to penetrate, and it also inhibits ovulation. In addition, this progestin thins the uterine or endometrial lining, which makes it unreceptive to implantation.

Implants are in the top-tier effectiveness category of contraceptives and, like IUDs, offer women a private, low-maintenance, long-acting, and rapidly reversible method of contraception with relatively few side effects. In addition, implants do not interfere with the spontaneity of sex, and can be used by women who want or need to avoid estrogen (Aiken & Trussell, 2014). From a clinical standpoint, their efficacy is indistinguishable from that of sterilization and IUDs (Hatcher, 2011). In addition, a woman's body weight does not appear to play a role in effectiveness

TABLE 21.1	Nexaplanon Use
IMPLANT ADVANTAGES	**IMPLANT DISADVANTAGES**
High effectiveness	Menstrual disturbances
Ease of use	Rare insertion and removal complications
Discreetness	Possible weight gain and other hormone-related adverse symptoms
No adverse effect on acne	Ovarian cysts
Relief of dysmenorrhea	Clinician dependency
Relief of pelvic pain related to endometriosis	No protection against STIs
Few clinically significant metabolic effects	Drug interactions
Reduced risk of ectopic pregnancy	Possible decrease in bone density
No estrogen	Possible increased risk of thromboembolic conditions
Reversibility	
High acceptability and continuation rates	
Cost-effective	

STIs, sexually transmitted infections.
Source: Bartz and Goldberg (2011).

(Table 21.1). Based on current data, an approximate failure rate of Nexplanon is 0.5 to 1 pregnancy/1,000 insertions (Raymond, 2011).

Eligibility Criteria

The vast majority of women are good candidates for Nexplanon. Implants are particularly suitable for women who desire safe, effective, long-term, maintenance-free, reversible contraception. Nexplanon offers women reproductive control, allowing them to postpone a first pregnancy, space pregnancies, or to provide long-term contraception once the desired family size is reached (Pushba et al., 2011). Like other progestin-only contraceptives, implants may be of interest to women who cannot or do not wish to use a contraceptive that contains estrogen.

Nexplanon can be used by teens, nulliparous women, women with multiple sex partners, and women with HIV. However, women who fall into the aforementioned categories should be counseled on the use of barrier methods as Nexplanon does not protect against STIs.

Nexplanon should not be used in women who have:

- Known or suspected pregnancy
- Current or past history of thrombosis or thromboembolic disorders
- Benign, malignant, or active liver disease or liver tumors
- Undiagnosed abnormal genital bleeding
- Breast cancer, history of breast cancer, or other progestin-sensitive cancer
- Women who are taking antiretroviral agents, antiepileptics, and rifampicin. *Pregnancies have been reported in women taking these medications.*
- Allergic reaction to any of the components of Nexplanon

Insertion

A health care provider trained in Nexplanon insertion can perform this minor surgical procedure in the office.

One Nexplanon package consists of a single implant that is 4 cm in length and 2 mm in diameter, which is preloaded into a disposable needle applicator. The rod is typically inserted into the inside portion of the upper arm, in the groove between the biceps and triceps muscles. Local anesthetic can be administered to ease any discomfort with insertion. The rod is then inserted into the subdermal tissue. Insertion deeper than recommended can make removal more difficult (Aiken & Trussell, 2014). Complications of rod insertion are very rare. Infection, bruising, skin irritation, or pain may occur immediately after insertion.

Timing of insertion depends on the woman's recent contraceptive history. If the woman has not used any hormonal contraception in the past month, Nexplanon should be inserted between day 1 and day 5 of the menstrual cycle. If the rod is inserted within 5 days of the start of menses, a backup form of contraception is not needed during the remainder of the cycle. However, if insertion occurs outside of the recommended window, the woman should either abstain from intercourse or use a backup method for the first 7 days after insertion (Raymond, 2011).

Adverse Effects/Symptom Control

Similar to all progesterone-releasing contraceptive methods, Nexplanon causes changes in vaginal bleeding patterns in a large majority of women. These changes vary from amenorrhea, infrequent bleeding, irregular bleeding, or prolonged or frequent bleeding. Although these changes are rarely clinically significant, and many women consider amenorrhea or infrequent bleeding to be a benefit, changes in vaginal bleeding patterns are the most common reason for discontinuation of implant use (Pushba et al., 2011).

The most common complaints related to progesterone-releasing implants are related to the hormonal side effects. These side effects can include weight gain, headache, changes in mood, breast pain, abdominal pain, nausea, loss of libido, ovarian cysts, and vaginal dryness.

Monitoring

Women considering implants should be advised on the advantages, disadvantages, and insertion and removal procedures before use. A user card is included in the Nexplanon packaging. This card should be filled out and given to the patient after insertion so that she will have a record of the location of the implant in the upper arm and when it should be removed.

Pregnancy is extremely rare with the use of Nexplanon. In general, hormonal contraceptives are not dangerous for either the pregnant woman or a developing fetus (Raymond, 2011). If a woman using Nexplanon is found to be pregnant and wishes to continue the pregnancy, the implant should be removed, and no other evaluation or care is needed.

Removal

Before initiating removal of the implant, positive identification of the location of the rod is required. Once the location has been verified, local anesthetic can be injected under the distal end of the rod. The clinician will then push down on the proximal end of the implant to stabilize it, in turn forming a bulge indicating the distal end of the implant. Then, a 2-mm incision can be made from which to remove the rod. The clinician will gently push the implant toward the incision until the tip is visible. Lastly, the clinician will grab the implant with forceps and gently remove it (www.merckconnect.com/nexplanon/insertion-removal.html).

Return to Fertility

Nexplanon prevents pregnancy for up to 3 years and does not interfere with fertility once the rod is removed. In clinical trials, pregnancies occurred as early as 7 to 14 days after the rod was removed. Upon removal, if continued contraception is desired, another form of birth control should be initiated immediately.

■ INTRAUTERINE DEVICES

IUDs or intrauterine systems (IUSs) are small, T-shaped devices made of flexible plastic. In this chapter, the term IUD is used generically in reference to all types of intrauterine contraception unless otherwise noted. An IUD/IUS is inserted into a woman's uterus only by trained health care providers, in this case, for pregnancy prevention. There is one type of IUD available in the United States (copper [ParaGard®]) and two types of hormonal IUSs (Mirena® and Skyla®). Although each works in slightly different ways, none function as abortifacients (Dean & Schwarz, 2011). They are among the most cost-effective contraceptive options available, from $0 to $1,000, depending on IUD/IUS type and the patient's insurance. Although the cost of an IUD might seem high for some, one office visit for an IUD placement can provide anywhere from 3 to 10 years of reliable contraception.

IUDs are one of the most safe, reliable, and cost-effective contraception options available today (Fantasia, 2008). Modern IUDs have an impressive safety record and are safe for most women, including teens, nulliparous women, and HIV-positive women. There are few contraindications to its use (WHO, 2009). They are highly effective and comparable to surgical sterilization and implants (Dean & Schwarz, 2011). IUDs also offer women a private, low-maintenance, long-acting, and rapidly reversible method of contraception with relatively few side effects (WHO, 2009). In addition, IUDs do not interfere with the spontaneity of sex, offer several noncontraceptive health benefits, have high continuation rates, and can be used by women who want or need to avoid estrogen (Dean & Schwarz, 2011). There is no delay in return to fertility with either the copper IUD or the levonorgestrel IUSs.

There are some lingering negative perceptions relating to the IUD that still persist based on first-generation models. In 1970, the Dalkon Shield, a smaller IUD marketed for nulliparous women, was introduced. However, there were multiple reports of serious side effects including infection, septic abortion, perforation of the uterus, heavy bleeding, cramping, ectopic pregnancy, infertility, and death (Fantasia, 2008). Lawsuits as well as the FDA's mandate against the manufacturer of the Dalkon Shield resulted in its removal from the market in the early 1970s. The failure of this IUD was caused in part by a design flaw. The increased risk of pelvic infection appeared to be related to the IUD's multifilament strings, which acted like a wick drawing bacteria from the lower genital tract up into the uterus (Fantasia, 2008). Although these complications were not experienced by users of other IUDs, they caused fear and confusion for both patients and health care providers, essentially leading to the demise of IUD use in the United States.

The current generation of IUDs is much safer and has been engineered to mitigate these and other adverse effects that plagued their first-generation predecessors. However, even today, many factors continue to limit the use of IUDs, including misinformation and a general misunderstanding about the risks of infection, infertility, ectopic pregnancy, as well as a misconception about the mechanisms of action, lack of clinician training, and a lingering fear of litigation (Dean & Schwarz, 2011).

The vast majority of women are good candidates for an IUD. IUDs can be used by teens, nulliparous women, women with multiple sex partners, and women who have had ectopic pregnancies (Dean & Schwarz, 2011). However, IUDs should not be prescribed for women with known pregnancy, an active STI or active PID, in the period immediately after a septic abortion, presenting with unexplained vaginal bleeding, or anatomic abnormalities of the uterus (such as fibroids that disrupt the uterine cavity, a bicornuate uterus, or cervical stenosis).

IUDs appear safe and effective for women who are immunocompromised due to organ transplantation, autoimmune disease, or HIV (Heikinheimo, Lehtovirta, Aho, Ristola, & Paavonen, 2011). They can be used safely in women with cardiac disease and structural heart abnormalities, diabetes, venous thromboembolism, and a history of cesarean section and other cervical surgery (Dean & Schwarz, 2011). The

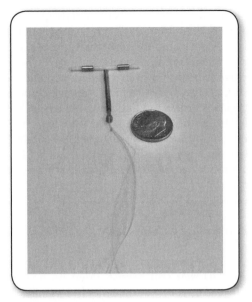

FIGURE 21.6
Copper intrauterine device.

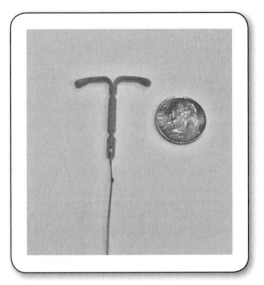

FIGURE 21.7
Levonorgestrel intrauterine system.

IUD should not be newly inserted in a woman with cervical cancer or endometrial cancer, but the method can be continued if the woman desires. IUDs can be used safely in women with a history of breast cancer (Patel & Schwarz, Society of Family Planning, 2012).

Women who are at risk of acquiring STIs should be advised to use condoms, and are generally still good candidates for an IUD (Dean & Schwarz, 2011). If a woman does acquire an infection with chlamydia or gonorrhea, the IUD does not need to be removed. Standard treatment for the woman and her partner is sufficient.

Copper IUDs

The copper T 380 (ParaGard) was developed in the 1970s and approved by the FDA for use in the United States in 1984. It is a T-shaped device with a polyethylene stem and cross arms partly covered by copper wire (see Figure 21.6). It is approved for 10 years of use, although studies indicate effectiveness for up to 12 years (Dean & Schwarz, 2011). The pregnancy rate in women who use the copper IUD is less than 1% in the first year of use (WHO, 2009).

The copper IUD prevents fertilization primarily by creating a spermicidal environment. It causes the uterine endometrium to initiate a foreign body reaction, which results in sterile inflammation and inhibits sperm from reaching the fallopian tube. Additionally, the copper ions permeate the cervical mucus and decrease sperm motility (Arrowsmith, Aicken, Saxena, & Majeed, 2012).

Some women who use a copper IUD complain of heavier, longer, and more uncomfortable menstrual periods. Average monthly menstrual blood loss may be increased by up to 55%. For some, these side effects may decrease over time. These complaints account for two of every 100 women discontinuing use of the copper IUD (Dean & Schwarz, 2011).

Levonorgestrel IUSs

The hormonal IUSs exist in the United States under the brand names Mirena and Skyla. Both levonorgestrel IUSs are made of soft, flexible plastic and contain a hormone-releasing reservoir (see Figure 21.7). Mirena releases 20 mg of levonorgestrel per day, while the Skyla releases 13.5 mg of levonorgestrel per day. Levonorgestrel works by thickening cervical mucus (making it difficult for sperm to penetrate), and also by inhibiting ovulation in some patients (Lewis et al., 2010). In addition, this levonorgestrel thins the uterine or endometrial lining, which reduces or even prevents menstrual bleeding. For this reason, the Mirena IUS can also be used to treat menorrhagia or heavy bleeding (Fraser, 2010).

IUD Insertion Procedure

An IUD can only be inserted by a health care provider who has received special training. Insertion of an IUD may take place at any time during the menstrual cycle, provided the woman is not pregnant. Current preprocedure counseling recommendations for an IUD include warning women of the very low risk of PID in the 20-day postinsertion period. Only women who are symptomatic or those who are at risk for having an STI should be tested before insertion. Women who develop PID can be treated with antibiotics while the IUD is in place. The IUD should only be removed if the patient fails to improve within 72 hours of initiation of antibiotic therapy (Fantasia, 2008).

Before insertion, a bimanual examination is done to determine the uterine position. The procedure to place the IUD begins similar to a Pap smear, with the insertion of a speculum into the patient's vagina. If clinically indicated, a test for chlamydia and gonorrhea can be performed. The cervix is then thoroughly cleansed and sounding of the uterus, with appropriate instrumentation, takes place. The IUD is then inserted through the cervix, into the uterus per manufacturer guidelines, using sterile technique. The IUD threads are made of a monofilament-type string and should be cut at a length to allow the thread to wrap up and around the cervix, approximately 3 cm. The length of the strings should also be noted in the patient's record for future reference. If the threads are cut too short, the woman's partner may complain of discomfort or a poking sensation with intercourse and/or the IUD may be more difficult to reach when removing.

As part of patient education (before discharge), it is important to remind the patient to manually feel for her strings after each menstrual period in order to verify placement of the IUD. If the patient is unable to locate the IUD strings, she should follow-up with her health care provider.

The copper IUD can be placed immediately postpartum. However, for the progesterone-releasing IUSs (Mirena and Skyla), a 6- to 8-week delay should be considered. Earlier placement may result in neonatal exposure to hormones, premature discontinuation of breastfeeding, and a possible risk of perforation during lactation (Dean & Schwarz, 2011).

Adverse Effects

Although adverse effects have significantly decreased since the first-generation models were released, they do still exist. The most common side effect related to IUD use includes change in menstrual patterns. Although not medically harmful, menstrual pattern changes may prove uncomfortable or even unbearable to the patient. Irregular bleeding is common in the first few months of use and is a common reason for discontinuation.

For women using progesterone-releasing IUSs, light bleeding or irregular spotting is to be expected in the early months of use. Once endometrial suppression has been achieved, 25% of women will experience significantly decreased menstrual bleeding while 50% experience amenorrhea or no menstrual bleeding (Fraser, 2010).

The most common complaints related to progesterone-releasing IUSs are related to the hormonal side effects. These side effects can include hirsutism, acne, weight changes, nausea, headache, mood changes, and breast tenderness. These symptoms are the most common reasons for the elective removal of IUSs. Approximately 12% of women prematurely discontinue the use because of hormone-related complaints (Dean & Schwarz, 2011).

Within the first year of IUD use, 2% to 10% of users spontaneously expel the device. Nulliparity, age less than 20 years, menorrhagia, severe dysmenorrhea, and placement immediately postpartum increase the chance of expulsion (Dean & Schwarz, 2011). Although expulsion is not a medical emergency, patients should use a backup method of birth control until they can see their health care provider.

Pregnancy is extremely rare with an IUD in place. However, when a patient does become pregnant, she may be at an increased risk of having an ectopic pregnancy (Dean & Schwarz, 2011). In the rare event of a confirmed pregnancy, the health care provider must make a determination about whether or not the pregnancy is ectopic. If the pregnancy is ectopic, this complication must be managed using best practice standards. If the pregnancy is intrauterine and the device is confirmed to be in the uterus, removal is most often recommended due to increased risk for sepsis, spontaneous abortion, and preterm birth (Fantasia, 2008).

Patient education should include information about checking monthly for the IUD strings as well as signs and symptoms of possible complications, including pain, bleeding, odorous discharge, fever, chills, and missed menses.

Anticipatory counseling about expected menstrual changes is critical. Women who choose a copper IUD need to be counseled that they may experience heavier, longer, and more painful menstrual periods. The use of nonsteroidal anti-inflammatory drugs (NSAIDs) may help with bleeding and pain. Conversely, women using progesterone-releasing IUSs may completely stop having menstrual periods. This is not harmful and does not require any treatment. Women should understand that menstrual periods will return once an IUD/IUS is removed.

IUD Removal

There are numerous reasons and various times when an IUD can or should be removed. These include (Dean & Schwarz, 2011):

- Patient request
- The device reaches its expiration date
- The patient develops a contraindication
- If adverse effects do not resolve

The IUD is removed by securely grasping the threads at the external cervical OS with ring forceps and gently and evenly pulling the IUD out. Asking the patient to bear-down and cough three times can be a useful distraction technique during removal. If significant resistance is met, all removal attempts should cease until it is determined why the IUD is not moving. Once the IUD is removed, it is prudent to show the device to the patient so they are confident that the device has been removed.

◼ STERILIZATION

Sterilization continues to be the most commonly used contraceptive method in the United States. There are two methods of female sterilization available in the United States: transcervical sterilization and tubal ligation. For men and couples who make sterilization decisions together, vasectomy remains an attractive alternative to female methods. There are approximately 700,000 tubal sterilizations and 500,000 vasectomies performed annually (Roncari & Jou, 2011). Advantages of sterilization include its permanence, high rate of efficacy, cost effectiveness, lack of significant long-term side effects, and lack of need for partner adherence.

Permanence may also be viewed as a disadvantage of sterilization. Most women who choose sterilization as their contraceptive method never regret their decision. However, due to relationship changes and other life events, regret is always possible. Women who undergo sterilization before the age of 30 years tend to have a greater risk of regret. Younger women are at greater risk for regret given the longevity of their future fertility and the opportunity for life changes such as divorce, remarriage, or death of a child (Roncari & Jou, 2011). Although sterilization may be reversed with varying degrees of success, it is difficult and expensive.

Transcervical Sterilization

There is currently one FDA-approved transcervical sterilization method that is available in the United States: the Essure® procedure. A similar method (the Adiana® method) was FDA approved, but was later removed from the market by the manufacturer for financial (not safety or efficacy) issues. Advantages of transcervical sterilization include that it can be done in an outpatient/ambulatory setting without general anesthesia, and because it is not considered a surgical procedure may be more cost-effective than tubal ligation.

The Essure contraceptive device consists of a microinsert containing an inner coil of stainless steel and polyethylene terephthalate (PET) fibers and an outer coil of titanium and nickel. It is placed by hysteroscopic guidance in the proximal section of each fallopian tube (Palmer & Greenberg, 2009). The microinsert acts by inducing scar tissue that permanently blocks the fallopian tube within 3 months postinsertion (Saad-Ganem et al., 2014). Tubal occlusion and proper positioning must be confirmed through hysterosalpingogram (HSG; Lorente Ramos, Azpeitia Armán, Aparicio Rodríguez-Miñón, Salazar Arquero, & Albillos Merino, 2015). Placement of the device is contraindicated for patients with known nickel sensitivity. Essure's successful bilateral placement rate is 94.6% (Palmer & Greenberg, 2009).

Health care providers must have the proper training to perform the Essure procedure. In less than 30 minutes, for example, the microinsert can be placed under local anesthesia, without or without sedation, in a properly equipped health care provider's office with appropriately dedicated resources for post-procedure recovery (Roncari & Jou, 2011). It is important to note that successful placement of the inserts is not guaranteed if there is preexisting tubal or uterine scarring. In addition, effectiveness is dependent on growth and formation of tubal scar tissue. A woman must use an alternative form of contraception for at least 3 months following the procedure, until an HSG demonstrates that both tubes are occluded (Lorente et al., 2015).

The most common complications include perforation, improper placement, migration toward the uterine or peritoneal cavity, unintended pregnancy, pain, infection, nickel allergy, and occlusion failure (Adelman, Dassel, & Sharp, 2014). Effectiveness and satisfaction is based on proper placement and follow-up radiographical confirmation of tubal occlusion.

Surgical Sterilization

Tubal ligation sterilization is performed using a laparoscopic approach under general anesthesia. Surgical sterilization for women prevents fertilization by cutting, tying, or clipping the fallopian tubes. Tubal ligation can be done as a planned, laparoscopic procedure in the operating room or as part of a planned cesarean delivery. Surgical tubal sterilization is highly effective with only a 0.5% failure rate (Hatcher, 2011).

Major complications from female tubal sterilizations are uncommon. As with any surgery, there is a risk of hemorrhage, infection, and death from anesthesia-related complications. If the procedure fails and the patient becomes pregnant, the chance that it will be ectopic is considerable (Roncari & Jou, 2011).

Male sterilization, or vasectomy, blocks fertilization by cutting or occluding both vas deferens so that sperm can no longer pass out of the body in the ejaculate (Roncari & Jou, 2011). Male sterilization is not recommended for anyone who is not sure of his desire to end future fertility. Success of a vasectomy must be confirmed through a semen analysis.

Vasectomies are highly effective with only a 0.15% failure rate. A vasectomy is a minor surgical procedure. Fewer than 3% of cases require any follow-up medical attention (Roncari & Jou, 2011). Postoperative complications, such as bleeding or infection as well as failure can occur. The most common complaints after the procedure are swelling of the scrotum, bruising, and minor discomfort. Pain medication and local application of ice are helpful in the immediate post-procedure period.

■ SUMMARY

Modern contraception began with Margaret Sanger's vision to develop long-lasting, effective, safe, highly reliable, and reversible contraception. Current forms of contraception are ever evolving and improving. Today's health care providers must understand the factors that influence a woman's life and contraceptive choices, her medical history, and her personal goals in order to partner with her in selecting contraception that meets both her short-term needs and long-term goals.

■ REFERENCES

Adelman, M. R., Dassel, M. W., & Sharp, H. T. (2014). Management of complications encountered with Essure hysteroscopic sterilization: A systematic review. *Journal of Minimally Invasive Gynecology, 21*(5), 733–743.

Adler, N. (1979). Decision models and population research. *Journal of Population, 2*(3), 187–202.

Aiken, A. A., & Trussell, J. (2014). *Recent advances in contraception*. Retrieved from http://www.ncbi.nlm.nih.gov/pmc/articles/PMC4251416/pdf/medrep-06–113.pdf

American College of Obstetricians and Gynecologists (ACOG). (2006). Use of hormonal contraception in women with coexisting medical conditions (reaffirmed in 2013). *Obstetrics & Gynecology, 107*(6), 1453–1472.

Arévalo, M., Jennings, V., & Sinai, I. (2002). Efficacy of a new method of family planning: The Standard Days Method. *Contraception, 65*(5), 333–338.

Arrowsmith, M. E., Aicken, C. R., Saxena, S., & Majeed, A. (2012). Strategies for improving the acceptability and acceptance of the copper intrauterine device. *The Cochrane Database of Systematic Reviews, 2012*(3), CD008896.

Association of Women's Health, Obstetric, and Neonatal Nurses & National Association of Nurse Practitioners in Women's Health. (2002). *The women's health nurse practitioner: Guidelines for practice and education.* Washington, DC: Author.

Bachmann, G., Sulak, P. J., Sampson-Landers, C., Benda, N., & Marr, J. (2004). Efficacy and safety of a low-dose 24-day combined oral contraceptive containing 20 micrograms ethinylestradiol and 3 mg drospirenone. *Contraception, 70*(3), 191–198.

Barr, N. G. (2010). Managing adverse effects of hormonal contraceptives. *American Family Physician, 82*(12), 1500–1506.

Bartz, D., & Goldberg, A. B. (2011). Injectable contraceptives. In R. A. Hatcher (Ed.), *Contraceptive technology* (20th ed.). Alpharetta, GA: Bridging the Gap Communications.

Beksinska, M. E., Smit, J. A., Kleinschmidt, I., Milford, C., & Farley, T. M. (2010). Prospective study of weight change in new adolescent users of DMPA, NET-EN, COCs, nonusers and discontinuers of hormonal contraception. *Contraception, 81*(1), 30–34.

Belden, P., Harper, C. C., & Speidel, J. J. (2012). The copper IUD for emergency contraception, a neglected option. *Contraception, 85*(4), 338–339.

Bird, S. T., & Bogart, L. M. (2005). Conspiracy beliefs about HIV/AIDS and birth control among African Americans: Implications for the prevention of HIV, other STIs, and unintended pregnancy. *Journal of Social Issues, 61*(1), 109–126.

Brache, V., Payán, L. J., & Faundes, A. (2013). Current status of contraceptive vaginal rings. *Contraception, 87*(3), 264–272.

Christin-Maitre, S. (2013). History of oral contraceptive drugs and their use worldwide. *Best Practice & Research. Clinical Endocrinology & Metabolism, 27*(1), 3–12.

Chrousos, G. P. (2014). Chapter 40: The gonadal hormones & inhibitors. In B. G. Katzung & A. J. Trevor (Eds.), *Basic & clinical pharmacology* (13th ed.). Columbus, OH: McGraw-Hill Education.

Cibula, D., Gompel, A., Mueck, A. O., La Vecchia, C., Hannaford, P. C., Skouby, S. O.,...Dusek, L. (2010). Hormonal contraception and risk of cancer. *Human Reproduction Update, 16*(6), 631–650.

Cooke, C., & Dworkin, S. (1979). *The MS guide to woman's health.* New York, NY: Healthcare Communications.

CycleBeads. (2015). *CycleBeads plan or prevent pregnancy naturally.* Retrieved from http://www.cyclebeads.com

Daniels, K., Mosher, W. D., & Jones, J. (2013). Contraceptive methods women have ever used: United States 1982–2010. *National Health Statistics Reports, 62*, 1–16.

Dean, G., & Schwarz, E. B. (2011). Intrauterine contraceptives. In R. A. Hatcher (Ed.), *Contraceptive technology* (20th ed.). Atlanta, GA: Ardent Media.

Díaz, S. (1989). Determinants of lactational amenorrhea. *Supplement to International Journal of Gynecology and Obstetrics, 1*, 83–89.

Douglas, E. T. (1970). *Margaret Sanger: Pioneer of the future.* New York, NY: Holt.

Fantasia, H. C. (2008). Options for intrauterine contraception. *Journal of Obstetric, Gynecologic, and Neonatal Nursing, 37*(3), 375–383.

Fehring, R. J. (2004). Simple natural family planning methods for breastfeeding women. *Current Medical Research, 15*(1–2), 1–3.

Fehring, R. J. (2005). New low- and high-tech calendar methods of family planning. *Journal of Midwifery & Women's Health, 50*(1), 31–38.

Fehring, R. J., & Mu, Q. (2014). Cohort efficacy study of natural family planning among perimenopause age women. *Journal of Obstetric, Gynecologic, and Neonatal Nursing, 43*(3), 351–358.

Fehring, R. J., Raviele, K., & Schneider, M. (2004). A comparison of the fertile phase as determined by the Clearplan Easy Fertility Monitor and self-assessment of cervical mucus. *Contraception, 69*(1), 9–14.

Fehring, R. J., Schneider, M., Raviele, K., Rodriguez, D., & Pruszynski, J. (2013). Randomized comparison of two Internet-supported fertility-awareness-based methods of family planning. *Contraception, 88*(1), 24–30.

Finnigan, M. (2008). Natural family planning. In J. D. Hawkins, D. Roberto-Nicholas, & J. L. Stanley-Haney (Eds.), *Guidelines for nurse practitioners in gynecological settings* (pp. 27–29). New York, NY: Springer Publishing.

France, M. M. (1996). A study of the lactational amenorrhoea method of family planning in New Zealand women. *The New Zealand Medical Journal, 109*(1022), 189–191.

Fraser, I. S. (2010). Non-contraceptive health benefits of intrauterine hormonal systems. *Contraception, 82*(5), 396–403.

Friedan, B. (1963). *The feminine mystique.* New York, NY: Dell.

Frye, C. A. (2006). An overview of oral contraceptives: Mechanism of action and clinical use. *Neurology, 66*(6, Suppl. 3), S29–S36.

Germano, E., & Jennings, V. (2006). New approaches to fertility awareness-based methods: Incorporating the standard days and two day methods into practice. *Journal of Midwifery & Women's Health, 51*(6), 471–477.

Gordon, L. (1990). *Woman's body, woman's right.* New York, NY: Penguin.

Grady, W. R., Billy, J. O., & Klepinger, D. H. (2002). Contraceptive method switching in the United States. *Perspectives on Sexual and Reproductive Health, 34*(3), 135–145.

Gray, M. (1979). *Margaret Sanger.* New York, NY: R. Marek.

Hang-Wun, R. L., Tsing, S. S., & Ho, P. C. (2014). Emergency contraception. *Best Practice & Research Clinical Endocrinology & Metabolism, 28*, 835–844.

Hatcher, R. A. (2011). *Contraceptive efficacy.* Retrieved from http://www.contraceptivetechnology.org/wp-content/uploads/2013/09/CTFailureTable.pdf

Hawkins, J. W., Roberto-Nichols, D., & Stanley-Haney, J. L. (2008). *Guidelines for nurse practitioners in gynecologic settings* (9th ed.). New York, NY: Springer Publishing.

Heikinheimo, O., Lehtovirta, P., Aho, I., Ristola, M., & Paavonen, J. (2011). The levonorgestrel-releasing intrauterine system in human immunodeficiency virus-infected women: A 5-year follow-up study. *American Journal of Obstetrics and Gynecology, 204*(2), 126.e1–126.e4.

Herrman, J. W. (2006). Position statement on the role of the pediatric nurse working with sexually active teens, pregnant adolescents, and young parents. *Journal of Pediatric Nursing, 21*, 250–252.

Himes, N. E. (1936). *Medical history of contraception.* New York, NY: Schocken.

Huber, L. R., Hogue, C. J., Stein, A. D., Drews, C., Zieman, M., King, J., & Schayes, S. (2006). Contraceptive use and discontinuation: Findings from the contraceptive history, initiation, and choice study. *American Journal of Obstetrics and Gynecology, 194*(5), 1290–1295.

Jacobson, J. C., Likis, F. E., & Murphy, P. A. (2012). Extended and continuous combined contraceptive regimens for menstrual suppression. *Journal of Midwifery & Women's Health, 57*(6), 585–592.

Jacobstein, R., & Polis, C. B. (2014). Progestin-only contraception: Injectables and implants. *Best Practice & Research. Clinical Obstetrics & Gynaecology, 28*(6), 795–806.

Jones, J., Mosher, W., & Daniels, K. (2012). Current contraceptive use in the United States, 2006–2010, and changes in patterns of use since 1995. *National Health Statistics Reports, 60*(18), 1–26.

Kaunitz, A. M. (1998). Injectable depot medroxyprogesterone acetate contraception: An update for U.S. clinicians. *International Journal of Fertility and Women's Medicine, 43*(2), 73–83.

Kerber, L. K., & De Hart, J. S. (1995). *Women's America: Refocusing the past* (4th ed.). New York, NY: Oxford University Press.

Kinsey, A. C., Pomeroy, W. B., Martin, C. E., & Gebhard, P. H. (1953). *Sexual behavior in the human female.* New York, NY: Pocket Books.

Lader, L. (1955). *The Margaret Sanger story.* Garden City, NY: Doubleday.

Lethbridge, D. J. (1997). The influence of culture and socioeconomic status on contraceptive use. In D. J. Lethbridge & K. M. Hanna (Eds.), *Promoting effective contraceptive use* (pp. 51–63). New York, NY: Springer Publishing.

Lethbridge, D. J., & Hanna, K. M. (1997). *Promoting effective contraceptive use.* New York, NY: Springer Publishing.

Lewis, R. A., Taylor, D., Natavio, M. F., Melamed, A., Felix, J., & Mishell, D. (2010). Effects of the levonorgestrel-releasing intrauterine system on cervical mucus quality and sperm penetrability. *Contraception, 82*(6), 491–496.

Li, H. W., Lo, S. S., & Ho, P. C. (2014). Emergency contraception. *Best Practice & Research. Clinical Obstetrics & Gynaecology, 28*(6), 835–844.

Lohr, P. A., & Creinin, M. D. (2006). Oral contraceptives and breakthrough bleeding: What patients need to know. *Journal of Family Practice, 55*(10), 872–880.

Lopez, L. M., Newmann, S. J., Grimes, D. A., Nanda, K., & Schulz, K. F. (2012). Immediate start of hormonal contraceptives for contraception. *The Cochrane Database of Systematic Reviews, 2012*(12), CD006260.

Lorente Ramos, R. M., Azpeitia Armán, J., Aparicio Rodríguez-Miñón, P., Salazar Arquero, F. J., & Albillos Merino, J. C. (2015). Radiological assessment of placement of the hysteroscopically inserted Essure permanent birth control device. *Radiologia, 57*(3), 193–200.

Luker, K. (1978). *Taking chances: Abortion and the decision not to contracept.* Berkeley, CA: University of California Press.

Marlow, J. (1979). *The great women.* New York, NY: Galahad.

Mathias, S. D., Colwell, H. H., Lococo, J. M., Karvois, D. L., Pritchard, M. L., & Friedman, A. J. (2006). ORTHO birth control satisfaction assessment tool: Assessing sensitivity to change and predictors of satisfaction. *Contraception, 74*(4), 303–308.

McNicholas, C., Zhao, Q., Secura, G., Allsworth, J. E., Madden, T., & Peipert, J. F. (2013). Contraceptive failures in overweight and obese combined hormonal contraceptive users. *Obstetrics and Gynecology, 121*(3), 585–592.

Mills, A., & Barclay, L. (2006). None of them were satisfactory: Women's experiences with contraception. *Health Care for Women International, 27*(5), 379–398.

Nelson, H. D., Zakher, B., Cantor, A., Fu, R., Griffin, J., O'Meara, E. S., …Miglioretti, D. L. (2012). Risk factors for breast cancer for women aged 40 to 49 years: A systematic review and meta-analysis. *Annals of Internal Medicine, 156*(9), 635–648.

O'Connell, K., & Burkman, R. T. (2007). The transdermal contraceptive patch: An updated review of the literature. *Clinical Obstetrics and Gynecology, 50*(4), 918–926.

Orne, R., & Hawkins, J. W. (1985). Reexamining the oral contraceptive issues. *Journal of Obstetric, Gynecologic, and Neonatal Nursing, 14*(1), 30–36.

Palmer, S. N., & Greenberg, J. A. (2009). Transcervical sterilization: A comparison of Essure® permanent birth control system and Adiana® permanent contraception system. *Reviews in Obstetrics & Gynecology, 2*(2), 84–92.

Patel, A., & Schwarz, E. B.; Society of Family Planning. (2012). Cancer and contraception. Release date May 2012. SFP Guideline #20121. *Contraception, 86*(3), 191–198.

Peragallo Urrutia, R., Coeytaux, R. R., McBroom, A. J., Gierisch, J. M., Havrilesky, L. J., Moorman, P. G.,…Myers, E. R. (2013). Risk of acute thromboembolic events with oral contraceptive use: A systematic review and meta-analysis. *Obstetrics and Gynecology, 122*(2, Pt. 1), 380–389.

Pérez, A., Labbok, M. H., & Queenan, J. T. (1992). Clinical study of the lactational amenorrhoea method for family planning. *Lancet, 339*(8799), 968–970.

Pushba, B., Sangita, N., Shivani, A., & Chitra, T. (2011). Implanon: Subdermal single rod contraceptive implant. *Journal of Obstetrics and Gynecology of India, 61*(4), 422–425.

Raymond, E. G. (2011). Contraceptive implants. In R. A. Hatcher (Ed.), *Contraceptive Technology* (20th ed.). Alpharetta, GA: Bridging the Gap Communications.

Roncari, D., & Jou, M. Y. (2011). Female and male sterilization. In R. A. Hatcher (Ed.), *Contraceptive technology* (20th ed.). Alpharetta, GA: Bridging the Gap Communications.

Saad-Ganem, A., Alanis-Fuentes, J., López-Ortiz, C. G., Muradas-Gil, L., Quintero-Bernal, P., Palma-Dorantes, J., Charua Levy, E. (2014). Tubal obstruction with an implant inserted by hysteroscopy: A report of 50 cases. *Ginecologi´a y obstetricia de Me´xico, 82*(7), 448–453.

Sanger, M. (1920a). *What every girl should know.* New York, NY: Belvedere.

Sanger, M. (1920b). *Women and the new race.* New York, NY: Truth Publishing.

Sanger, M. (1931). *My fight for birth control.* New York, NY: Dover.

Sanger, M. (1938). *Margaret Sanger: An autobiography.* New York, NY: Dover.

Schindler, A. E. (2013). Non-contraceptive benefits of oral hormonal contraceptives. *International Journal of Endocrinology and Metabolism, 11*(1), 41–47.

Schnare, S. M., & Nelson, A. L. (2005). Evidence based contraceptive choices. *Best Practice & Research Clinical Obstetrics & Gynecology, 20*, 665–680.

Sicherman, B., Green, C. H., Kantor, I., & Walker, H. (1980). *Notable American women: The modern period.* Cambridge, MA: Belknap Press of Harvard University Press.

Sitruk-Ware, R., & Nath, A. (2010). The use of newer progestins for contraception. *Contraception, 82*(5), 410–417.

Steiner, M. J., Trussell, J., Mehta, N., Condon, S., Subramaniam, S., & Bourne, D. (2006). Communicating contraceptive effectiveness: A randomized controlled trial to inform a World Health Organization family planning handbook. *American Journal of Obstetrics and Gynecology, 195*(1), 85–91.

Tabeek, E. (2000). Natural family planning. In J. W. Hawkins, D. Roberto-Nicholas, & J. L. Stanley-Haney (Eds.), *Protocols for nurse practitioners in gynecologic settings* (7th ed.). New York, NY: Tiresias Press.

Tannahill, R. (1980). *Sex in history.* New York, NY: Stein and Day.

Thijssen, A., Meier, A., Panis, K., & Ombelet, W. (2014). 'Fertility Awareness-Based Methods' and subfertility: A systematic review. *Facts, Views & Vision in ObGyn, 6*(3), 113–123.

Trussell, J., Hassan, F., Lowin, J., Law, A., & Filonenko, A. (2015). Achieving cost-neutrality with long-acting reversible contraceptive methods. *Contraception, 91*(1), 49–56.

Williams, R. L., Hensel, D. J., & Fortenberry, J. D. (2013). Self-administration of subcutaneous depot medroxyprogesterone acetate by adolescent women. *Contraception, 88*(3), 401–407.

Winter, L. (1988). The role of sexual self-concept in the use of contraceptives. *Family Planning Perspectives, 20*(3), 123–127.

World Health Organization (WHO). (2009). *Medical eligibility criteria for contraceptive use* (4th ed.). Geneva, Switzerland: Author.

World Health Organization (WHO). (2011). *Family planning: A global update for providers 2011 update.* Geneva, Switzerland: Author.

Wysocki, S. (2006). Effective counseling—At the heart of patient care. *Clinical Issues in Women's Health.* Washington, DC: Nurse Practitioners in Women's Health.

Yranski, P. A., & Gamache, M. E. (2008). New options for barrier contraception. *Journal of Obstetric, Gynecologic, and Neonatal Nursing, 37*(3), 384–389.

CHAPTER 22

Preconception Counseling

Debbie Postlethwaite • Elizabeth A. Kostas-Polston • Kristi Rae Norcross

■ PRECONCEPTION CARE

Preconception care should be a part of preventive health care for all women of reproductive age. Ideally, this care should be delivered in a culturally competent manner. In a 2004 survey, 84% of U.S. women aged 15 to 44 years reported having a health care visit, with only 55% of those reporting that visit to be preventive in nature. These visits afford clinicians opportunities to include preconception health strategies (Centers for Disease Control and Prevention [CDC], 2006). Preconception care is not a specific entity, but has evolved into a health promotion expectation for every clinician caring for women of childbearing age and capacity (CDC, 2002, 2015j; Hobbins, 2003; Johnson et al., 2006). According to the American College of Obstetricians and Gynecologists (ACOG), the challenge of preconception care lies not only in addressing pregnancy planning for women who seek medical care and consultation specifically in anticipation of a planned pregnancy, but also in educating and screening all reproductively capable women on an ongoing basis to identify potential maternal and fetal risks and hazards to pregnancy before and between pregnancy (ACOG, 2005/2015). Preconception care, then, is considered critical to improving the health of the nation. Healthy People 2000 set a target of 60% of clinicians providing age appropriate preconception care. This preconception care goal was removed from *Healthy People 2010* because it was not being measured. The *Healthy People 2020* objectives do set quantifiable goals and address several important contributors of preconception health such as increasing planned pregnancies and increasing folic acid intake by reproductive-age women (Healthy People 2020, n.d.).

Etiology of Pregnancy Intention Status

An unintended pregnancy is defined as a pregnancy that is either mistimed or unwanted at the time of conception (Brown & Eisenberg, 1995; Guttmacher Institute, 2015; Johnson et al., 2006). An example of how pregnancy intention questions are framed either at the onset of a pregnancy or retrospectively is:

At the time of conception was the patient:

■ Wanting to get pregnant? (*planned*)

■ Wanting to get pregnant, but not at this time? (*mis-timed*)
■ Not wanting to become pregnant at all? (*unwanted*)

■ UNINTENDED PREGNANCY

Infant mortality rates (IMR) are important international health indicators that assess the quality of the health of a nation and specifically the health of reproductive-aged women. In 2010, the United States ranked 26th in infant mortality among Organization for Economic Co-operation and Development countries. All things equal, the U.S. IMR ranking remains higher than for most European countries and almost double the IMR for Finland, Sweden, and Denmark (MacDorman et al., 2014). Half of all pregnancies in the United States have been reported as unintended since 1995 (Finer & Zolna, 2011). Births that result from an unintended pregnancy are at higher risk of poor pregnancy outcomes such as birth defects, preterm labor, small for gestational age, maternal mortality, and neonatal death (Finer & Zolna, 2011). Moreover, women at risk of pregnancy in the United States have been reported to be more likely to consume alcohol (10%), tobacco (10%), may be exposed to teratogenic (which may cause birth defects) medications (3%–6%), have chronic diseases such as diabetes (up to 9%), or are classified as overweight or obese (50%; Brown & Eisenberg, 1995; CDC, 2002, 2015j; Johnson et al., 2006; Schwarz et al., 2005, 2007). These exposures are contributed to poor pregnancy outcomes and developmental disabilities. Despite many medical advances of the 20th century, poor pregnancy outcomes continue to be a problem in the United States into the 21st century, partly because of the lack of preconception planning and preconception care. Each year in the United States, 9.6% of babies are born premature. Although the rate has decreased by 8% since 2007, large disparities in risk of preterm birth exist among racial and ethnic groups (CDC, 2015i). When a pregnancy is not planned, there is also an increased chance of exposure to reproductive toxicants at the workplace or in the home (Wilson et al., 2007). Exposure to infectious diseases, such as chlamydia, or inadequate immunization to preventable diseases, such as rubella and hepatitis B, are also more likely when a pregnancy is unintended. There is a greater risk of nutritional deficiencies such as inadequate folic acid, nutritional excesses such as foods high in mercury, and excess caloric intake leading to obesity. In addition to the preconception risks associated with lack of pregnancy planning that result in teratogen exposures and chronic medical conditions, there are social and genetic factors.

For example, a pregnant woman has a 35.6% greater risk of being a victim of violence than a nonpregnant woman (Gelles, 1998). The risk of intimate partner violence increases when the pregnancy is not planned (Miller et al., 2010). Genetic diseases often go unnoticed until a pregnancy is confirmed, when exposure has already occurred (Frye et al., 2011).

Prevalence of Unintended Pregnancy

Pregnancy intention is assessed periodically in U.S. reproductive-age women. This assessment is performed by the National Center for Health Statistics through the use of the National Survey of Family Growth (NSFG). This survey asks women and men about topics related to childbearing, family planning, and maternal and child health. Additionally, the survey asks about pregnancy intention retrospectively for the past pregnancy and for those in the past 5 years. The most recent NSFG data (2006–2010) estimated that 49% (6.4 million) of all pregnancies were unintended, with 37% of births reported as unintended (Mosher, Jones, & Abma, 2012). The United States has held the dubious distinction of having the highest unintended pregnancy rate in the industrialized world for more than a decade. In the 2006 to 2010 NSFG, unintended pregnancies declined among adolescents, college graduates, and the wealthiest women, but increased among poor and less-educated women (Mosher et al., 2012). The proportion of unplanned pregnancies that ended in an elective abortion increased among women aged 20 years and older, but decreased among teenagers, who were now more likely than older women to continue their unplanned pregnancies. The unintended pregnancy rate was highest among women who were aged 18 to 24 years, unmarried, had low income, or were Black or Hispanic (Mosher et al., 2012). The Healthy People 2020 objectives call for an overall reduction in unintended pregnancies in the United States by 30% (CDC, 2015o).

Risk Factors for Unplanned Pregnancy

Almost all women of reproductive age are at risk of an unintended pregnancy and would benefit from preconception health strategies. Let us look more closely at specific subgroups of women at risk. The women exposed to teratogens (substances that may cause birth defects) may be at highest risk of an unintended pregnancy that could result in a poor pregnancy outcome. Teratogens may be prescribed or purchased in the form of over-the-counter medications, environmental reproductive toxicants (hyperthermia, lead, mercury, ionizing radiation), or infectious diseases. A teratogen is a substance, organism, or physical agent capable of causing abnormal development and a teratogen can cause

abnormalities of structure or function, growth retardation, or death of the organism (Dutta, 2015).

It is not always a common practice among clinicians to ask about immediate intention to become pregnant, to assess current risk of pregnancy at the time a medication is prescribed, and/or to assess when the last menstrual period was. In a study reviewing the electronic record data on prescribed medications of 488,175 managed care women aged 14 to 44 years, it was found that at least one potentially teratogenic medication was prescribed for 15.9% of these women (Schwarz et al., 2007). The largest proportion of potentially teratogenic medications was prescribed by internists and family practitioners (48%; Schwarz et al., 2007). Nearly half of the women prescribed a potentially teratogenic medication had no record of sterilization, use of a contraceptive method, or contraceptive counseling during a 2-year period before filling the prescription for the medication. Additionally, there was no statistical difference between women filling a prescription for a potentially teratogenic or a nonteratogenic medication in rates of documented contraceptive counseling (48% vs. 47%, respectively), or of a positive pregnancy test within 3 months after filling the prescription (1.0% vs. 1.4% of prescriptions; Schwarz et al., 2007).

Special Populations of Women Needing Preconception Care Assessment

Women with chronic conditions, such as diabetes, are less likely to plan pregnancies. Chronic conditions that may adversely affect pregnancy include preexisting diabetes mellitus, HIV/AIDS, thyroid disease, seizure disorders, maternal phenylketonuria, and hypertension (ACOG, 2014; Kendrick, 2004; Kim et al., 2005; Postlethwaite, 2003). It is estimated that 8% of women between the ages of 20 and 44 years have undetected diabetes (CDC, 2014). Studies have shown that up to 66% of all pregnancies in women with preexisting diabetes are reported as unintended, despite the fact that they have a two- to threefold risk of birth defects because of inadequate glycemic control at the time of conception (Kendrick, 2004; Kim et al., 2005; Postlethwaite, 2003). In women with HIV infection, there is an increased risk of several major complications, including perinatal morbidity and infection (CDC, 2015e). The most important benefit of pregnancy planning for an HIV-infected mother is the ability to provide medical intervention to minimize the risk of vertical transmission to the neonate (CDC, 2015k). Another example of a chronic medical condition requiring preconceptual attention is thyroid disease. Untreated or inadequately treated thyroid disease may lead to maternal anemia, low birth weight, and impaired brain development of the fetus. High circulating human chorionic gonadotropin (HCG) in the first trimester may result in lowering thyroid-stimulating hormone (TSH) levels, resulting in inadequate levels of circulating thyroid hormones (T3 and T4; American Thyroid Association, n.d.).

CDC adapted the WHO's list of conditions that expose a woman and her fetus to increased risk as a result of unintended pregnancy (WHO, 2014). The CDC created the

United States Medical Eligibility Criteria for Contraceptive Use 2010 (USMEC, 2010), an effective tool to assist clinicians who care for women with chronic medical conditions to promote planned pregnancies by providing safe and effective contraception (CDC, 2010d) (Box 22.1).

Another important subgroup of women at risk of unintended pregnancy is adolescents. Approximately 47% of all high school students report ever having had sexual intercourse (Henry J. Kaiser Family Foundation, 2014a). Teens also report that the most commonly used method of contraception is condoms. However, when asked if they used a condom at last intercourse, 59% sexually active adolescents reported that they had actually used a condom (Child Trends Data Bank, 2014). About one third of all U.S. girls become pregnant before the age of 20 years. Of those resulting in birth, greater than 80% are unintended (CDC, 2015a). U.S. adolescent pregnancy rates are higher than almost every other country in the developed world including Canada, Great Britain, Japan, and Sweden. Teen mothers are more likely to drop out of school and remain single parents, which may contribute to the cycle of poverty as well as contribute to poor birth outcomes (CDC, 2015a; Office of Adolescent Health, 2015). Women with a previous unintended pregnancy constitute another important subgroup. It is estimated that 43% of all U.S. women by 45 years of age will have had an abortion (Guttmacher Institute, 2014; Jones, Frohwirth, & Moore, 2013). More than half of U.S. women (51%) obtaining an abortion report that they were using a method of contraception the month they became pregnant (Guttmacher Institute, 2014; Jones et al., 2013). Births resulting from subsequent unintended pregnancies pose the same or even greater risks for poor pregnancy outcomes resulting from exposure to teratogens, fetotoxins, or adverse social situations such as intimate partner violence, child abuse, and neglect (Dutta, 2015; Gelles, 1998; Miller et al., 2010).

Women of reproductive age are at risk of unintended pregnancy unless they are using long-acting, highly effective, reversible methods of contraception (intrauterine contraception or subdermal implants) or permanent sterilization (www.cdc.gov/reproductivehealth/unintended-pregnancy/contraception.htm). Contraception is a very important component of preconception health because it promotes planned pregnancies. The more effective and less user-dependent the contraceptive method is, the more reliable the method is at reducing the risk of an unintended pregnancy and protecting preconception health (Hatcher et al., 2011).

BOX 22.1   U.S. MEDICAL ELIGIBILITY CRITERIA (USMEC): CONDITIONS ASSOCIATED WITH INCREASED RISK OF ADVERSE HEALTH EVENTS AS A RESULT OF UNINTENDED PREGNANCY

Breast cancer
Complicated valvular heart disease
Diabetes: insulin-dependent; with nephropathy/retinopathy/neuropathy or other vascular disease; or of > 20 years' duration
Endometrial or ovarian cancer
Epilepsy
Hypertension (systolic > 160 mmHg or diastolic > 100 mmHg)
HIV/AIDS
Ischemic heart disease
Malignant gestational trophoblastic disease
Malignant liver tumors (hepatoma) and hepatocellular carcinoma of the liver
Peripartum cardiomyopathy
Schistosomiasis with fibrosis of the liver
Severe (decompensated) cirrhosis
Sickle cell disease
Solid organ transplantation within the past 2 years
Stroke
Systemic lupus erythematosus
Thrombogenic mutations
Tuberculosis

Adapted from CDC (2010d); World Health Organization Medical Eligibility Criteria for Contraceptive Use (4th ed.).

Interventions and Strategies for Risk Reduction and Management

Because at least half of all pregnancies are unintended, many preconception health strategies need to be directed at all women of reproductive age, regardless of intention to become pregnant in the near future. At the same time, preconception health care recommendations should be tailored to the individual woman whenever possible. Some of the recommendations are "passive" and protect preconception health in cases where pregnancies are not planned, while others are more "active" recommendations for women that plan their pregnancies.

PROMOTE PLANNED PREGNANCY

All pregnancies should be planned. Contraception is an essential component of preconception health because it facilitates a planned pregnancy. Adequate contraception is especially important in women exposed to teratogens (prescription medications and other reproductive toxicants), women with chronic conditions (e.g., diabetes), women who have had a previous unintended pregnancy (whether they resulted in a birth or abortion), and all sexually active adolescents. Use the USMEC (2010) to determine which contraceptive methods are safe for women with chronic conditions.

To increase the chances of a planned pregnancy:

- Assess contraception as a *vital sign* before prescribing all medications and when treating women of reproductive age for medical conditions (ACOG, 2006/2015).
- Assist and promote achieving and maintaining a healthy weight or body mass index (BMI).

- Counsel and offer emergency contraception (EC) with every prescription to reproductive-age women who also are using a high-risk or teratogenic medication (ACOG, 2010/2015; see Table 22.1).
- Counsel and offer EC for all women of childbearing age with chronic conditions.
- Promote the use of highly effective methods of contraception when women are exposed to high-risk medications or teratogens (e.g., Food and Drug Administration [FDA] category D or X medications) that cannot be avoided (e.g., statins,

antihypertensives, anticoagulants, anti-seizure medications, isotretinoin).
- Whenever possible, prescribe lower risk or nonteratogenic medications to reproductive-aged women.

■ BIRTH DEFECTS

Birth defects affect about 1% to 3% (one in every 33) babies born in the United States each year. They are the leading cause

TABLE 22.1	D and X Category Medication List

Statins

Atorvastatin—X
Cerivastatin—X
Fluvastatin—X
Lovastatin—X
Pravastatin—X
Simvastatin—X

Anticonvulsants

Carbamazepine—D
Divalproex sodium—D
Mephobarbital—D
Pentobarbital—D
Phenobarbital—D
Phenytoin—D
Secobarbital—D

Benzodiazepines/anxiolytics

Alprazolam—D
Chlordiazepoxide—D
Clonazepam—D
Clorazepate dipotassium—D
Diazepam—D
Estazolam—X
Flurazepam—X
Lorazepam—D
Meprobamate—D
Midazolam—D
Oxazepam—D
Quazepam—X
Temazepam—X
Triazolam—X

Antibiotics

Amikacin sulfate—D
Demeclocycline hydrochloride—D
Doxycycline—D
Gentamicin—D
Minocycline—D
Neomycin sulfate—D
Tobramycin—D

Oncology

Anastrozole—D
Arsenic trioxide—D
Bexarotene—X
Bleomycin sulfate—D
Busulfan—D
Capecitabine—D
Carboplatin—D
Chlorambucil—D
Cisplatin—X
Cladribine—D
Cyclophosphamide—D
Cytarabine—D
Dactinomycin—D
Daunorubicin hydrochloride—D
Docetaxel—D
Doxorubicin—D
Epirubicin—D
Etoposide—D
Exemestane—D
Flurorauracil—X
Goserelin acetate—X
Hydroxyurea—D
Idarubicin hydrochloride—D
Ifosfamide—D
Imatinib mesylate—D
Irinotecan—D
Letrozole—D
Mechlorethamine—D
Melphalan—D
Mercaptopurine—D
Mitomycin—X
Mitoxantrone hydrochloride—D
Paclitaxel—D
Procarbazine hydrochloride—D
Tamoxifen—D
Temozolomide—D
Thioguanine—D
Toremifene—D
Vinblastine sulfate—D
Vincristine sulfate—D
Vinorelbine tartrate—D

Psychiatric

Imipramine—D
Lithium—D
Nortriptyline—D
Paroxetine—D

Cardiology

Amiodarone hydrochloride—D
Atenolol—D
ACE inhibitors—C/D[a]
  Lisinopril
  Benazepril
  Captopril
  Enalapril/Enalaprilat
  Fosinopril
  Moexipril
  Perindopril
  Quinapril
  Ramipril
  Trandolapril

Immunologic agents

Azathioprine—D
Leflunomide—X
Penicillamine—D
Thalidomide—X

Antithyroid medications

Methimazole—D
Propylthiouracil—D
Potassium iodide—D

Gout

Colchicine—D
Colchicine/Probencid—D

Dermatology

Acitretin—X
Isotretinoin—X
Tazarotene—X
Tretinoin (oral)—D

Smoking Cessation

Transdermal nicotine patch—D

Migraine

Dihydroergotamine mesylate—X
Ergotamine—X

Anticoagulants

Warfarin—X

Miscellaneous

Danazol—X
Dienestrol—X
Finasteride—X
Fluoxymesterone—X
Leuprolide acetate—X
Meclofenamate—D
Methotrexate—X
Methyltestosterone—X
Misoprostol—X
Oxandrolone—X
Pamidronate disodium—D
Quinine—X
Raloxifene—X
Ribavirin—X
Testosterone—X

[a]According to the FDA (Food and Drug Administration), angiotensin-converting enzyme (ACE) inhibitor drugs are labeled "pregnancy category C" for the first trimester of pregnancy, and are labeled "pregnancy category D" during the second and third trimesters.
Sources: Briggs and Freeman (2015), Physicians' Desk Reference Staff (2015).

of infant deaths, accounting for more than 20% of all infant deaths and the likelihood of illness and long-term disability (CDC, 2016). Although most birth defects result from genetic, environmental, and lifestyle factors, some may be preventable by improving preconceptual and interconceptual advice, education, and care (ACOG, 2005, 2010; CDC, 2016).

Etiology

When a change to the structure of the body occurs during fetal development, the result is defined as a birth defect. Birth defects can alter the shape or function of one or more parts of the body, causing problems to overall health, how the infant's body develops, and/or how the infant's body works.

Embryo and Organogenesis

The fetus is most susceptible in the first 4 to 10 weeks gestation before most prenatal care is initiated (Figure 22.1).

The embryonic period (up to 8 weeks of gestation) is the most vulnerable time for the development of major morphologic abnormalities of the heart, central nervous system, cranial facial, as well as limb defects. Nutritional, drug, and environmental exposures and infectious agents interrupting normal cell organization and differentiation can cause birth defects (King et al., 2015). The dark gray in the schematic in Figure 22.1 (primarily in the embryonic period) represent when the major congenital anomalies occur to the most vital organs such as the central nervous system, heart, eyes, limbs, and ears. The period when the major organ systems are forming is referred to as organogenesis, which primarily occurs between 17 and 56 days after conception. When there is exposure of great magnitude in the first 2 weeks, it is most likely to result in an early spontaneous abortion (see first two columns). Exposure(s) to toxic substances in the embryonic period (up to 8 weeks gestation) have traditionally been considered teratogens, whereas exposures after 8 weeks are usually referred to as fetotoxins (represented by the shaded light blue bars). Fetotoxins are substances

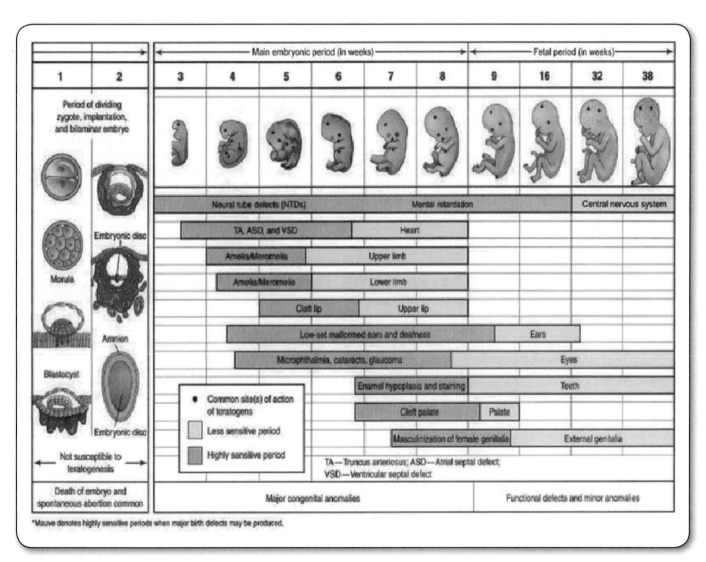

FIGURE 22.1
Embryo and organogenesis.
Source: Moore and Persaud (1998).

that cause no structural changes like those that occur in the embryonic stage of development, but are toxic to the fetus and can impair normal growth and function (Dutta, 2015). Examples of fetotoxins include:

■ Nicotine
■ Cocaine (both teratogen and fetotoxin)
■ Amphetamines
■ Angiotensin-converting enzyme inhibitors (ACE-I; antihypertensive, both teratogenic and fetotoxic) (King et al., 2015)

Teratogen and fetotoxins are dependent on the following elements (Dutta, 2015):

■ Genotype susceptibility (genetically coded information of the individual)
■ Timing of exposure (determines whether teratogen or fetotoxin)
■ Specific mechanism (such as gene mutation)
■ Manifestation (dependent on stage of development exposure occurs)
■ Agent (drug, disease, or environmental agent)
■ Dose effect (from no effect to lethal)

Because of greater physiologic vulnerability in the preconception and early gestational periods, many exposures (medications, nutritional deficiencies, other toxic substances) put women at risk of birth defects that are preventable.

Prescription Medications That Increase the Risk of Birth Defects

Because of the number of unplanned pregnancies, development of the fetus can be affected by prescription medications that may be harmful even before the pregnancy is confirmed. It is estimated that women of reproductive age in the United States receive 11.7 million prescriptions for potentially teratogenic (Class D or X medications) each year (Andrade et al., 2006; FDA, 2014; Schwarz et al., 2005). It is also estimated that U.S. women using Class D or X medications receive contraceptive counseling on less than 20% of ambulatory care visits (FDA, 2014; Schwarz et al., 2005) and approximately 6% of U.S. pregnancies are exposed to potentially teratogenic, Class D or X medications (FDA, 2014; Lee et al., 2006; Schwarz, 2007).

Assessment of Risk of Prescribed Teratogens

To assist health care providers to determine the safety of medication use during pregnancy, the U.S. FDA developed a drug classification system (FDA, 2014; see Table 22.2). Although not perfect, this classification system provides guidance about medication safety use during pregnancy and during exposure through breastfeeding. In some cases the medication is classified as potentially more dangerous in certain gestational periods than in others. In other words, a medication may be classified as D in the first trimester and C in the second and third trimester. For example, ACE-I (common antihypertensive medication) are classified as C in the first trimester and D in the second and third trimesters. For many years, health care providers were encouraged to change women from ACE-I to a different antihypertensive once pregnancy was diagnosed. In 2006, a landmark study published in the *New England Journal of Medicine* (Cooper et al., 2006) showed that infants exposed to ACE-I only in the first trimester had a significantly greater risk (RR: 2.71) of congenital anomalies than infants with no ACE-I exposure. Investigators concluded that because of the increased

TABLE 22.2	FDA Drug Classification System
CATEGORY	**INTERPRETATION**
A	Adequate, well-controlled studies in pregnant women have not shown an increased risk of fetal abnormalities to the fetus in any trimester of pregnancy.
B	Animal studies have revealed no evidence of harm to the fetus; however, there are no adequate and well-controlled studies in pregnant women. *Or* animal studies have shown an adverse effect, but adequate and well-controlled studies in pregnant women have failed to demonstrate a risk to the fetus in any trimester.
C	Animal studies have shown an adverse effect and there are no adequate and well-controlled studies in pregnant women. *Or* no animal studies have been conducted and there are no adequate and well-controlled studies in pregnant women.
D	Adequate well-controlled or observational studies in pregnant women have demonstrated a risk to the fetus. However, the benefits of therapy may outweigh the potential risk. For example, the drug may be acceptable if needed in a life-threatening situation or serious disease for which safer drugs cannot be used or are ineffective.
X	Adequate well-controlled or observational studies in animals or pregnant women have demonstrated positive evidence of fetal abnormalities or risks. The use of the product is contraindicated in women who are or may become pregnant.

FDA, Food and Drug Administration.
Source: Food and Drug Administration (2014).

rates of congenital anomalies found in the exposed group, ACE-I cannot be considered safe and should be avoided in first trimester (Cooper et al., 2006).

Before prescribing or recommending a medication to a reproductive-aged woman, it is advisable to check the FDA pregnancy risk drug classification system as well as other medication safety sources. Not all medication safety sources are in agreement, so it is usually safe for health care providers to make recommendations based on the highest risk assigned, or to prescribe an alternative medication with a lower risk level whenever possible.

Commonly Prescribed D and X Medications for Females of Reproductive Age

Please note that these are general classifications and many medications fall into a variety of drug classes. Table 22.1 is a list of a combination of D and X medications (Briggs & Freeman, 2015; Micromedex, 2007; Physicians' Desk Reference Staff, 2015). As these references are not in 100% agreement, Table 22.1 may differ from some health care provider practices. When preparing Table 22.1, the list of commonly prescribed medications, the highest risk category among the three sources was selected and noted in the table. This list is not exhaustive.

Interventions and Strategies for Risk Reduction and Management

It is imperative, then, that all clinicians caring for women taking class D and X medications provide reliable and efficacious contraception as well as accurate preconception risk information at the time of prescribing. Because the use of potentially teratogenic medications is at times necessary to maximize the health of women of reproductive age, clinicians must engage women in shared decision making around the use of contraception when these medications are prescribed, and improved drug-labeling systems should be developed. Given the high rate of unintended pregnancies (Brown et al., 1995), even with the use of reliable and effective contraception (Hatcher et al., 2011), it is critical that women understand exposure to teratogens and any potential dangers to a pregnancy. One simple step is to promote timely access to emergency contraception when prescribing a potential teratogen to women of reproductive age (ACOG, 2010/2015).

■ PRECONCEPTION HEALTH AND LIFESTYLE RISKS

Smoking

ETIOLOGY

Tobacco products and smoke contain more than 7,000 chemicals, including formaldehyde, cyanide, and nicotine. Nicotine produces serious side effects and is addictive.

Smokers are exposed to carbon monoxide that constricts blood vessels, which in turn decreases oxygen levels in the blood (CDC, 2015f).

PREVALENCE

In the United States and in other industrialized countries, 18% of women smoked in the 1990s. The proportion of women who report smoking during pregnancy has dropped substantially since the 1990s, to 9% in 2013 (MacDorman et al., 2014). However, there are disparities in smoking rates by race/ethnicity and by maternal education (Tong et al., 2011). Smoking has been found to be fetotoxic by reducing fetal oxygenation by decreasing placental blood flow. Although there are no safe levels of smoking in pregnancy, the fetotoxic effects are dose related. Preterm birth, low birth weight, and other adverse perinatal outcomes associated with maternal smoking in pregnancy can be prevented if women stop smoking before or during early pregnancy (CDC, 2015m).

INTERVENTIONS AND STRATEGIES FOR RISK REDUCTION AND MANAGEMENT

Health care providers should promote smoking cessation before pregnancy even with women with low-level exposures. Only 20% of smokers are successful in stopping once they are pregnant (ACOG, 2011). Because the rate of successful smoking cessation is low, it is recommended that smoking is assessed at every encounter within the health care system (ACOG, 2011). The March of Dimes promotes a 5- to 15-minute, 5-step counseling approach called "The 5 A's" (March of Dimes, 2008). The clinician can perform this approach during routine preconception or prenatal visits. This approach has been shown to improve smoking cessation rates among pregnant women by at least 30% (March of Dimes, 2008). Studies suggest that certain factors make it more likely that a woman will be successful in her efforts to quit smoking during pregnancy. These include:

- Attempting to quit in the past
- Having a partner who does not smoke
- Getting support from family or other important people in her life
- Understanding the harmful effects of smoking (ACOG, 2011)

Smoking and alcohol cessation interventions have been demonstrated to be effective in certain populations, but have been shown to be less effective with persons at highest risk (e.g., injection-drug users and multiple substance users) (U.S. Department of Health and Human Services [USDHHS], 2007).

Alcohol Use

ETIOLOGY

Alcohol is an organic solvent and acts as a neurotoxicant when consumed or by crossing the placenta (Day et al., 2013; Hamilton et al., 2014). Prenatal exposure to alcohol can damage the developing fetus and is the *leading preventable cause* of birth defects and intellectual and neurodevelopmental disabilities (Williams & Smith, 2015). Besides fetal alcohol syndrome (FAS), alcohol consumed in pregnancy can also lead to low-birth-weight infants, miscarriages, and stillbirths (Moore et al., 2014; O'Connor, 2014). Fetal alcohol spectrum disorder (FASD) covers a range of impairments from severe, such as Karli's FAS, to mild. Its effects can include impaired growth, intellectual disabilities and such neurological, emotional, and behavioral issues as attention deficit hyperactivity disorder (ADHD), vision problems, and speech and language delays. These disabilities last a lifetime—there is no cure, only early intervention treatment, which can improve a child's development. FASD is also sometimes characterized by a cluster of facial features: small eyes, a thin upper lip and a flat philtrum (the ridge between the nose and upper lip).

PREVALENCE

Although the prevalence of FAS in the United States during the 1980s and 1990s was reported as 0.5 to 2 cases per 1,000 live births, recent studies aggressively diagnosing FASD have reported FAS rates and FASD estimates of 6 to 9 cases and 24 to 48 cases per 1,000 children (or up to 5%), respectively, while continuing to consider these rates underestimates (May & Gossage, 2001; May et al., 2009, 2014). There is *no safe time* during pregnancy to *drink any amount of alcohol* (May & Gossage, 2001; May et al., 2009; May et al., 2014; Williams & Smith, 2015). Often, irreversible harm occurs before a woman realizes that she is pregnant. The CDC analyzed data from the 2006–2010 Behavioral Risk Factor Surveillance System (BRFSS) survey for women aged 18 to 44 years and found almost 50% of childbearing age (i.e., aged 18–44 years) use alcohol, and 15% of women who drink alcohol in this age group binge drink (CDC, 2012a). The BRFSS also reported that 7.6% of pregnant women used alcohol (CDC, 2012a). Women who binge drink are more likely to have unprotected sex and multiple sex partners (Substance Abuse and Mental Health Administration, 2006), thus increasing the risk of unintended pregnancy (CDC, 2015c) and sexually transmitted infections (STIs; CDC, 2015c; DeSimone, 2010).

INTERVENTION AND STRATEGIES FOR RISK REDUCTION AND MANAGEMENT

Health care providers should promote cessation or limiting of alcohol use especially in reproductive-aged women. Fetal alcohol syndrome and other alcohol-related birth defects can be prevented if women cease intake of alcohol before conception and throughout a pregnancy and while breastfeeding (March of Dimes, n.d.; Moore et al., 2014; O'Connor, 2014). This includes beer, wine, wine coolers, and hard liquors. Provide nonjudgmental support and appropriate chemical dependency referrals to promote alcohol cessation and recovery.

It is important to educate patients so that they understand the implications of drinking during pregnancy.

- Alcohol-related birth defects and developmental disabilities are completely preventable when pregnant women abstain from alcohol use.
- Neurocognitive and behavioral problems resulting from prenatal alcohol exposure are lifelong.
- Early recognition, diagnosis, and therapy for any condition along with the FASD continuum can result in improved outcomes for the child.
- During pregnancy:
  - No amount of alcohol intake should be considered safe.
  - There is no safe trimester to drink alcohol.
  - All forms of alcohol, including beer, wine, and liquor, pose similar risk.
  - Binge drinking poses dose-related risk to the developing fetus.

Recreational Drugs

ETIOLOGY

Recreational drugs interrupt the way the brain's cells communicate through neurotransmission. The exact response, whether dampened or stimulated by a drug, varies greatly depending on which neurotransmitters are affected. During the early stages of drug use, the effects wear off with the drug; however with chronic abusers, long-term changes in cell-to-cell communication result (National Institute on Drug Abuse [NIDA], 2007; Substance Abuse and Mental Health Services Administration, 2014).

PREVALENCE

According to a 2005 U.S. national survey on drug use, nearly 4% of pregnant women have been found to use illicit drugs such as marijuana, cocaine, ecstasy, other amphetamines, and heroin (CDC, 2006; March of Dimes, n.d.). It is often difficult to delineate what adverse perinatal outcomes are attributed to specific illicit drugs because of inherent impurities in street drugs, and because of multiple drug, smoking, and alcohol use in some women.

INTERVENTION AND STRATEGIES FOR RISK REDUCTION AND MANAGEMENT

When screening for smoking, or other sensitive subjects, frame the questions for building trust and for the purpose of improving health. The following are some examples to assist the clinician.

Framing Statement:
"Because smoking, alcohol, and recreational drug use have become so mainstream, I have started to ask all my patients routinely about it."

Indirect Question:
"*Have* you and your friends tried any recreational drugs in the past?"

Direct Question:

"In the past 1 to 3 months, have you taken any recreational drugs such as marijuana, speed, cocaine, ecstasy, or heroin?"

Affirmation:

"Thank you for sharing this information with me today. Would you be interested in learning more about the health effects to you should you become pregnant? Are you interested in a drug cessation program?"

Provide nonjudgmental support and provide appropriate referrals for drug use cessation.

Reproductive and Developmental Toxicants at Home and at Work

ETIOLOGY

Reproductive toxicants can affect both men and women's fertility, result in teratogenic effects during pregnancy, increase pregnancy loss (spontaneous abortions and fetal death), and contribute to developmental delays and learning disabilities in children (Association of Reproductive Health Professionals [ARHP], 2010). Toxic substances that can affect men's and women's fertility and childbearing include: (a) neurotoxicants such as lead, mercury, and organic solvents (degreasers); (b) endocrine disruptors such as polychlorinated biphenyls (PCBs, found in old electrical transformers, hydraulic systems, welding equipment, broken fluorescent light fixtures), polybrominated diphenyl ethers (PCBEs, flame retardants), dioxins (waste incineration, backyard fires), and phthalates (used in plastics, cosmetics, and pesticides); and (c) thyroid toxicants such as perchlorate (dry-cleaning solution). These substances may contribute to neurobehavioral and cognitive disorders, reproductive abnormalities, thyroid dysfunction, and other adverse health effects if exposure occurs during the prenatal period, infancy, childhood, and adolescence.

PREVALENCE

About 17% of children in the United States now suffer from one or more learning, behavioral, or developmental disabilities (National Environmental Trust, 2000). There has been a dramatic increase in these developmental disabilities in the past 25 years (National Environmental Trust, 2000). The relationship between exposures to toxic substances and this increase is unknown, but many researchers speculate that these increases in chronic health conditions are associated with exposures to toxicants in the work and home environment (National Environmental Trust, 2000). Toxic substances such as lead, mercury, organic solvents, ionizing radiation (x-ray), and chemotherapeutic drugs have been associated with adverse pregnancy outcomes including spontaneous abortion, low birth weight, and birth defects (Lassi et al., 2014; National Environmental Trust, 2000; Postlethwaite, 2003). It is thought that the earlier the exposure after conception and the greater the magnitude of exposure, the greater the risk of a lethal outcome. When toxicant or teratogen exposures occur from conception to Day 14 postconception, there is a much higher rate of spontaneous abortion. The magnitude of the

exposure depends on several factors: (a) active metabolites within the chemical or substance, (b) duration of exposure, (c) fat solubility of chemical or substance, (d) placental transfer of substance or chemical, (e) maternal disease (e.g., epilepsy or diabetes), and/or (f) genotype of fetus. Some chemicals are commonly thought to be toxic to the fetus without supporting evidence. Although these chemicals are known as respiratory and skin irritants, they have not been associated with harm to the fetus (Lassi et al., 2014; National Environmental Trust, 2000; Postlethwaite, 2003; see Box 22.2).

Workplace Toxicant Exposures

ASSESSMENT OF RISK

If a woman reports concerns about possible exposures to potential toxicants at work or symptoms she believes are associated to her work environment such as symptoms of dizziness or nausea, she should take the following steps (OSHA, n.d.):

1. Request a Material Safety Data Sheet (MSDS) from her employer. The MSDS is a document prepared by the manufacturer that contains information about the hazards of working with a given product or material and how to work safely with that material. All U.S. employers are required by law in most states to make available and to provide training on the health hazards of toxicants used in the workplace and how to protect against harmful exposures, including those that pose a risk to reproduction and pregnancy (Lassi et al., 2014; OSHA, n.d.).
2. The employee should report her concern about a possible exposure and resulting injury or illness to her employer.
3. Call the local or regional hazard evaluation service (contact Environmental Protection Agency for more information; OSHA, n.d.).
4. If injury or illness has resulted from toxicant exposures in the workplace, consult and refer to an

---

BOX 22.2   COMMON CHEMICALS UNLIKELY TO HARM A FETUS

Ammonia
Chlorine
Hydrochloric acid
Nitric acid
Sulfuric acid
Sodium hydroxide
Glutaraldehyde (Cidex)
Potassium hydroxide
Sodium hypochlorite (bleach)
Asbestos
Fiberglass
Silica

Adapted from Department of Health Services, Hazard Evaluation System and Information Service (2007).

occupational medicine specialist for further evaluation and treatment (Lassi et al., 2014; OSHA, n.d.).

INTERVENTION AND STRATEGIES FOR RISK REDUCTION AND MANAGEMENT

- Encourage planned pregnancies to mitigate risks.
- Encourage all reproductive-aged women and men to find out about environmental and workplace hazards *before* pregnancy.
- If employers and employees follow the MSDS recommendations and the workplace is made safe for all employees, then the workplace is safe for pregnancy.
- Remind couples that male exposure also has potential for harm and that harm, caused by reproductive toxicants, can occur through all developmental stages. Whenever possible it is best to prevent or minimize exposure as much as possible.
- Do not eat or drink in the same area when working with toxicants.
- Avoid exposure to toxicants, especially during preconception or during pregnancy.
- Provide adequate ventilation and use proper protective equipment (e.g., gloves) when handling toxicants.
- Avoid "take home" exposures by showering/changing to clean clothing before entering the home.
- Use only cold tap water for cooking and drinking. Run the water for at least 30 seconds before use to help reduce lead exposure from old plumbing.

■ COMMON PREVENTABLE BIRTH DEFECTS

Neural Tube Defects

Neural tube defects (NTD) are the most common preventable birth defect and are associated with a nutritional deficiency in folic acid or food folate (a type of B vitamin; CDC, 2015h, 2015b; Rasmussen et al., 2008).

ETIOLOGY

The neural tube develops in the first 4 weeks of pregnancy, often before many women even know they are pregnant. Inadequate closure of the neural tube results in an NTD, specifically spina bifida or anencephaly. Babies with anencephaly will result in either a stillborn birth or a neonatal death. Unlike anencephaly, which is 100% fatal, 80% of babies born with spina bifida survive (CDC, 2015h, 2015b; March of Dimes, n.d.). The average lifetime cost for caring for a child with spina bifida is around $532,000, with some costs ranging more than $1,000,000 (CDC, 2015h, 2015b; March of Dimes, n.d.). These costs do not take into account the physical and emotional costs to the family. Research has shown that getting enough folic acid before and during pregnancy can prevent most NTDs.

PREVALENCE

Each year in the United States, there are more than 4,000 pregnancies or 2,500 to 3,000 births (1/1,000 births) affected by NTDs, which include both spina bifida (when the fetal spine column does not close causing paralysis below the affected area), and anencephaly (when most of the brain does not develop; CDC, 2015h, 2015b; March of Dimes, n.d.).

ASSESSMENT OF RISK OF NTD

Obesity, diabetes, and convulsant disorders as well as certain medications have been shown to increase the risk of NTDs by interfering with folic acid absorption (CDC, 2015d; Rasmussen et al., 2008). Obesity has been shown to double the risk of NTDs, despite the use of folic acid, but weight loss before pregnancy may reduce NTD risk (Rasmussen et al., 2008).

HEALTH PROMOTION

Folic acid has been shown to reduce the risk of NTDs by 50% to 70% (CDC, 2015d; March of Dimes, n.d.). In order to reduce the risk of NTDs, CDC recommends that all women of childbearing age, who are capable of becoming pregnant, take in 400 micrograms folic acid each day—even those not trying to get pregnant. The easiest way to obtain adequate folic acid is by consuming a diet filled with folate rich foods (dark leafy greens, legumes, broccoli, and asparagus), with foods fortified with folic acid (such as cereals, pasta, and bread), and/or by taking a daily multivitamin (CDC, 1992).

INTERVENTIONS AND STRATEGIES FOR RISK REDUCTION AND MANAGEMENT

Adequate folic acid has been shown to reduce the risk of NTDs by two thirds (CDC, 1992; CDC, 2015h; CDC, 2015b; CDC, 2015d; March of Dimes, n.d.; Rasmussen et al., 2008). Synthetically produced folic acid has twice the bioavailability as food folate. Consumption of folic acid fortified foods produced in the United States are estimated to add 100 micrograms of folic acid per day to the average person's dietary intake of essential nutrients. Almost all multivitamins that contain 100% of the recommended dietary allowances (RDA) will contain at least 400 micrograms of folic acid (CDC, 1992).

■ CHRONIC MEDICAL CONDITIONS AS TERATOGENS

Chronic medical conditions may affect the quality of preconception health. These include medical conditions such as hypertension, obesity, diabetes, HIV/AIDS, cardiovascular diseases (CVDs), systemic lupus, seizure disorders, thyroid disease, and chronic depression. Some of these medical conditions may increase the risk of congenital malformations and they may also require the use of medications that may be teratogenic (e.g., ACE-I, some anticonvulsants, some antidepressants; ACOG, 2013a; American Diabetes Association [ADA], 2013; CDC, 2014c, 2014d).

Diabetes Mellitus

One of the best examples of a medical condition increasing risk is diabetes mellitus. Since the advent of insulin, there has been dramatic improvement in maternal–fetal health outcomes in all areas except for congenital anomalies (ADA, 2013; CDC, 2014b; Kendrick, 2004; Kim et al., 2005; Postlethwaite, 2003).

ETIOLOGY

These malformations occur by the seventh week of gestation and are primarily caused by inadequate glycemic control. Inadequate maternal glycemic control leads to hyperglycemia, hyperketonemia, hypoglycemia, excess somatomedin inhibitor (insulin-like growth factors), deficiency of arachadonic acid (essential fatty acid), and excess oxygen free radicals. Deficiency in arachadonic acid and excess free radicals can lead to embryonic malformations (Kendrick, 2004; Postlethwaite, 2003).

Despite these known risks, diabetic women are less likely to plan their pregnancies compared with the general population (34%–41% vs. 51%; Kendrick, 2004; Kim et al., 2005; Mills, 2010; Postlethwaite, 2003). In one national study, women with diabetes were asked if they recalled receiving counseling about the importance of glycemic control before a pregnancy and about receiving contraceptive counseling in order to plan their pregnancy. Fifty-two percent reported they received information about the importance of glycemic control before pregnancy and only 37% recalled any family planning advice (Kim et al., 2005).

PREVALENCE

The frequency of congenital anomalies ranges from 4.9% to 10% in infants born to insulin-dependent diabetic mothers (IDDM; Kendrick, 2004; Kim et al., 2005; Mills, 2010; Postlethwaite, 2003). This is a two- to threefold increase in birth defects among women with IDDM (6%–9% vs. 2%–3%) and twice the risk of spontaneous abortion over the risk to nondiabetic mothers (Kendrick, 2004; Kim et al., 2005; Mills, 2010; Postlethwaite, 2003). Malformations linked to IDDM account for 30% to 50% of perinatal deaths, and primarily involve the central nervous system: anencephaly, spina bifida, holoprosencephaly (10-fold increase); cardiac anomalies: ventricular septal defects, transposition of the great vessels (fivefold increase); and sacral agenesis or caudal dysplasia (200- to 400-fold increase) (Kendrick, 2004; Postlethwaite, 2003).

ASSESSMENT OF RISK

Initial laboratory testing includes assessment of hemoglobin (HGB) A1C and a random albumin-to-creatinine ratio (ACR). If the ACR is elevated, a 24-hour microalbumia level should be collected and evaluated. Increased HGB A1C levels that are greater than or equal to 3 standard deviation (SD) above the normal level (greater than or equal to 6.3%) significantly elevate a woman's risk of spontaneous abortions and congenital malformations. In addition, health care providers need to assess celiac and vitamin B_{12} levels because of autoimmunity risk. Dipstick elevated proteinuria levels should be further evaluated with a 24-hour urine protein level.

HIV/AIDS

ETIOLOGY

HIV attacks the immune system CD4 cells, preventing natural immunity, and resulting in increasing viral load levels from undetectable at 40 to 75 copies per milliliter of blood to millions of copies. Through contact with blood and body fluids, labor, prechewing baby's food, and sharing needles, razors or drug equipment, HIV is transmitted. When there is a coexisting STI, such as herpes simplex virus (HSV) or hepatitis, HIV is three to five times more likely to spread. With viral loads as low as 3,500 copies, HIV transmission risk exists (CDC, 2015k). Acquired immune deficiency syndrome (AIDS) diagnosis is confirmed with viral loads by laboratory testing (CDC, 2015k) or by AIDS-defining conditions found at *Mortality and Morbidity Weekly Report* (MMWR; CDC, 2008).

PREVALENCE

About 80% of the estimated 270,000 U.S. women with HIV are reproductive-age women (CDC, 2015e; Henry J. Kaiser Family Foundation, 2014b). In patients with HIV infection, there is an increased risk of perinatal morbidity and infection transmission (CDC, 2008; 2015e; Henry J. Kaiser Family Foundation, 2014b). The number of HIV affected women in the United States that gave birth increased by 30%, from 6,000 to 7,000 in 2000 to 8,700 in 2006 (CDC, 2015e). Risk of transmission of HIV to infants of infected mothers has been reduced to less than 1% in women taking antiretroviral medication during pregnancy as recommended (CDC, 2015k, 2015e). HIV is disproportionately greater in African American children in the United States (CDC, 2015e; Henry J. Kaiser Family Foundation, 2014b).

ASSESSMENT OF RISK

One of the most important benefits of pregnancy planning for an HIV-infected mother is being able to provide medical intervention to minimize the risk of vertical transmission to her baby. Both the USMEC (CDC, 2010d) and the World Health Organization's *Medical Eligibility Criteria for Contraceptive Use* (WHO-MEC; WHO, 2014) recommend universal screening of all men and women of reproductive age before pregnancy and at the onset of prenatal care. If an individual is a known HIV/AIDS carrier, then the use of two methods of contraception (barrier protection plus a more effective method) is recommended to prevent an unplanned pregnancy and HIV transmission (CDC, 2010d; WHO, 2014). When HIV is detected early in pregnancy, the risk of HIV transmission from an HIV-positive mother to the fetus and newborn can be reduced to 2% or less (CDC, 2015k, 2015d). Risk reduction may be achieved through universal screening, early detection, early treatment, delivery by cesarean section, and avoidance of breastfeeding

(CDC, 2008, 2010d, 2015e, 2015k; Henry J. Kaiser Family Foundation, 2014b; WHO, 2014).

Chronic Hypertension

ETIOLOGY

Hypertensive disorders complicate 5% to 10% of pregnancies (ACOG, 2015). Hypertensive risks presented in pregnancy are related to treatment (e.g., ACE-I and beta blockers such as Atenolol, which pose teratogenic risks), and adverse sequela such as maternal and infant morbidity and mortality (e.g., superimposed preeclampsia, premature delivery, placental abruption, and stillbirth), and a long-term risk of maternal CVD (ACOG, 2013a, 2015; Hutcheon et al., 2011).

PREVALENCE

Hypertension is the most common medical disorder of pregnancy, is reported to complicate up to one in ten gestations, and affects an estimated 270,000 women in the United States every year (ACOG, 2015; CDC, 2015e; Henry J. Kaiser Family Foundation, 2014b; National High Blood Pressure Education Program Working Group, 2000). Preeclampsia complicates 3% of all pregnancies (ACOG, 2013a, 2015; Hutcheon et al., 2011; National High Blood Pressure Education Program Working Group, 2000).

ASSESSMENT

In 2013, ACOG released new guidelines for the diagnosis and management of hypertension in relation to pregnancy. Hypertension is classified as chronic (before pregnancy), gestational (after 20 weeks gestation), preeclampsia (elevated blood pressure with proteinuria or any of listed severe features), and chronic with superimposed preeclampsia. Assessment of blood pressure greater than or equal to 160 systolic or greater than or equal to 110 diastolic on two evaluations, greater than 4 hours apart; elevated liver enzymes alanine aminotransferase/aspartate aminotransferase (ALT/AST); urine protein and creatinine ratio; creatinine; thrombocytopenia (platelets < 100,000); pulmonary edema or new onset cerebral or visual disturbances, are essential to rule out severe features associated with preeclampsia (ACOG, 2013a). Preconception counseling focuses on lifestyle modifications and management or elimination of comorbidities before conception for decreasing risk. In future pregnancies ensure folic acid supplementation and consider low-dose aspirin for women who experience preeclampsia (CDC, 2014c). Dietary modifications regarding salt, vitamin A, vitamin E, and calcium supplementation demonstrated no effect on risk in the U.S. pregnant population; however, consideration can be offered for women for low-dose aspirin after the first trimester to decrease risk of adverse perinatal outcomes and preeclampsia (ACOG, 2013a). Finally, women who experienced a preterm birth because of preeclampsia have increased risk of later life CVD. Annual visits for blood pressure evaluation, cholesterol, fasting glucose, and BMI are recommended by ACOG (2013a).

Phenylketonuria

ETIOLOGY

Phenylketonuria (PKU) is another example of a chronic disease that can act as a potent teratogen. PKU is an autosomal recessive disease causing a deficiency in phenylalanine hydroxylase (American Academy of Pediatrics Committee on Genetics, 2001). This deficiency prevents phenylalanine from being metabolized into tyrosine after the intake of proteins (American Academy of Pediatrics Committee on Genetics, 2001).

PREVALENCE

In the United States, about 1 in 10,000 to 15,000 infants are born with PKU each year. If identified and treated, intellectual and developmental disabilities in infants can be prevented. Left untreated, high levels of phenylalanine can lead to microcephaly and developmental delays in 75% to 90% of babies exposed (American Academy of Pediatrics Committee on Genetics, 2001; Levy & Ghavami, 1996; March of Dimes, 2013).

ASSESSMENT

PKU testing has been standard for many years in all newborns born in the United States. Females born with PKU must maintain strict dietary control throughout their reproductive years to limit their levels of phenylalanine. A level above 20 mg/dL may cross the placenta and cause embryonic and fetal damage, for example, fetal growth retardation, microcephaly, psychomotor handicaps, and congenital heart defects (American Academy of Pediatrics Committee on Genetics, 2001; Levy & Ghavami, 1996; March of Dimes, 2013).

Pregnancy and Chronic Medical Conditions

Chronic medical conditions can stress and therefore negatively impact a woman's pregnancy. Additionally, a woman's pregnancy may stress a woman's chronic health condition, leading to exacerbation. Chronic medical conditions include heart disease, systemic lupus, rheumatoid arthritis, seizure disorders, and psychiatric conditions (e.g., depression, psychosis). Women with these and other chronic medical conditions should receive expert advice (from a high-risk perinatologist) in anticipation or when planning pregnancy.

INTERVENTIONS AND STRATEGIES FOR RISK REDUCTION AND MANAGEMENT

All pregnancies in women with chronic medical conditions should be planned.

DIABETES

■ Promote glycemic control and highly effective contraception in all women with preexisting diabetes to reduce the increased risk of birth defects.

- The two- to threefold increase in the prevalence of birth defects among infants of women with type 1 and type 2 diabetes is substantially reduced through proper management of diabetes.
- Screen all women annually for diabetes mellitus with prior gestational diabetes mellitus (GDM).
- Before conception, promote the use of highly effective reversible contraception until glycemic control is achieved.

HYPOTHYROIDISM

- The dose of Levothyroxine®, for treatment of hypothyroidism, will need to be adjusted during early pregnancy. This is necessary to ensure proper neurologic development of the fetus (American Thyroid Association, 2013).

HEART DISEASE AND HYPERTENSION

- Avoid prescribing ACE-I, Atenolol, and statins in reproductive-aged women whenever possible.
- Reevaluate cardiovascular function before a planned pregnancy.
- Promote the use of appropriate contraception to facilitate a planned pregnancy.
- Follow U.S. and WHO medical eligibility criteria (CDC, 2010d; WHO, 2014) for women with known CVD.
- Help women be realistic about their pregnancy risks and the consequences of aging and heart disease.

MATERNAL PHENYLKETONURIA

- Adverse outcomes can be prevented when afflicted mothers adhere to a low-phenylalanine diet before conception and continue throughout pregnancy (American Academy of Pediatrics Committee on Genetics, 2001; Levy & Ghavami, 1996; March of Dimes, 2013).
- Check phenylalanine levels frequently during reproductive years.

HIV/AIDS

- Preexposure prophylaxis (PREP) and postexposure prophylaxis (PEP) medications reduce the risk of high-risk exposure groups.

Infectious Diseases as Teratogens

Infectious diseases may also act as teratogens when exposure occurs in the immediate preconception period and/or during pregnancy. Examples of infectious diseases that may be teratogenic or fetotoxic include toxoplasmosis gondii, HIV, syphilis, rubella, varicella, cytomegalovirus (CMV), parvovirus, and herpes. The common acronym that describes screening for most of these congenital infections is known as TORCH screening. TORCH, which stands for *Toxoplasma gondii*; *o*ther viruses (syphilis, HIV, measles, and more); *r*ubella (German measles); *c*ytomegalovirus; and *h*erpes simplex, is a screening test.

ETIOLOGY

TORCH and other congenital infections may cause damage to the central nervous system and other organs leading to mental retardation, microcephaly, learning disabilities, eye and hearing defects, cardiac anomalies, gastrointestinal anomalies, and damage to the liver and spleen (CDC, 2000, 2010b, 2012b, 2014d, 2015n).

PREVALENCE

TORCH infectious agents affect 1% to 3% of all live births and are among the leading causes of neonatal morbidity and mortality (Neu et al., 2015).

ASSESSMENT

It is recommended that all women of reproductive age know their immune status for rubella and varicella before pregnancy (CDC, 2000, 2014d; Medline Plus, 2014; Neu et al., 2015).

Toxoplasmosis

ETIOLOGY

The single-cell protozoan parasite called *Toxoplasma gondii* causes this rare disease. Toxoplasmosis is commonly transmitted in cat feces and through consumption of raw and undercooked meat, and rarely congenital or contracted through organ transplant. After eating infected rodents, cats shed the parasite oocytes in their feces (either in the litter box or outside in the soil) for up to 3 weeks (CDC, 2013, 2015n). The period of highest risk of acquiring primary toxoplasmosis infection is 10 to 24 weeks gestation.

PREVALENCE

In the United States, toxoplasmosis is considered to be a leading cause of death attributed to foodborne illness. In fact, one in five adults older than 12 years have been infected and carry the *Toxoplasma* parasite. Ironically, though, few have symptoms because their immune system is intact, thereby keeping the parasite from causing illness (CDC, 2013, 2015n).

ASSESSMENT

After determining precise exposure date, serological testing for immunoglobulin G (IgG) and immunoglobulin M (IgM) is routinely used; however, parasites directly observed in bodily fluids can be used to make the diagnosis (CDC, 2015n). With congenital transmission, the amniotic fluid can be tested for *Toxoplasma*-infected DNA (CDC, 2015n).

HEALTH PROMOTION

Risk reduction for transmission of toxoplasmosis can be achieved through good hand washing; washing of vegetables; proper cleaning (hot soapy water) and handling of cutting boards during food preparation; avoidance of handling cat feces, changing cat litter, and/or avoiding dirty cat litter boxes; and wearing gloves when gardening. High-risk women are screened via laboratory testing (CDC, 2013, 2015n).

Varicella

ETIOLOGY

The greatest risk period for malformations caused by varicella (chicken pox) infection is within the first 6 to 18 weeks of gestation (CDC, 2014a). There is also a risk of varicella infection to the newborn if infection occurs in late pregnancy near delivery. Varicella infection is not only dangerous to the growing fetus. Up to 20% of pregnant women who become infected with varicella develop pneumonia. Pneumonia acquired as a result of a varicella infection is associated with a maternal mortality rate of as high as 40% (CDC, 2014a).

PREVALENCE

Most women (between 85% and 95%) will be immune to varicella before pregnancy. Approximately 1.5% of infants will acquire congenital varicella syndrome if a nonimmune pregnant woman contracts the virus during the first 28 weeks of pregnancy (American Academy of Pediatrics and the American College of Obstetricians and Gynecologists, 2012).

ASSESSMENT AND MANAGEMENT

Verification of varicella immunity is determined by laboratory testing, proof of previous vaccination, or health care provider confirmation of infection. Women who are rubella nonimmune and not pregnant should receive the varicella vaccine. During routine obstetric care, it is standard of care to screen all pregnant women for immune status. Those who are nonimmune receive the varicella vaccine after delivery.

Parvovirus B-19

ETIOLOGY

Parvovirus B-19 (also called fifth disease) is commonly known as erythema infectiosum. The virus is transmitted through sputum, saliva, and nasal secretions. The initial mild symptoms of fever, headache, and runny nose present for 80% of those affected followed with a characteristic rash on the cheeks ("slap cheek") from 4 to 14 days following exposure. By the time the rash appears, the virus is no longer infectious (CDC, 2012b).

Parvovirus B-19 can infect the fetus before birth. Although no birth defects have been reported as a result of fifth disease, it may cause the death of an unborn fetus (CDC, 2012b; March of Dimes, 2012). If acquired in the first trimester (rare), parvovirus B-19 can contribute to spontaneous abortion. Although rare (less than 5% of pregnant women are infected with parvovirus B-19), if exposed during the second trimester, the risks of severe fetal anemia, hydrops fetalis, and stillbirth are significantly increased (CDC, 2012b; March of Dimes, 2012).

PREVALENCE

In the general population, 50% of women are immune to parvovirus B-19; therefore, the mother–baby pair are already protected. The risk of fetal death is 5% to 10% if the mother becomes infected.

ASSESSMENT

Pregnant women who have not previously had fifth disease should avoid contact with patients who are actively infected. Individuals are contagious during the mild symptoms before the rash or joint pain and not contagious during the rash or "slapped cheek" appearance (CDC, 2012b; March of Dimes, 2012).

Rubella

ETIOLOGY

Rubella (German or three-day measles) is a viral infection spread through coughing and sneezing of an infected person. In approximately half of those infected, following fever symptoms, a facial rash spreads to the rest of the body lasting 2 to 3 days (CDC, 2000, 2014d). Lack of rubella immunity appears to be associated with a generation of young people who were born too late to acquire rubella immunity through natural infection, yet too early to receive vaccine mandated by school entry laws. The lack of immunity has also been associated with foreign-born women of mostly Hispanic descent, especially those with little or no access to immunization programs (CDC, 2000). Congenital rubella syndrome consists of multiple severe anomalies: eye defects resulting in vision loss or blindness, hearing loss, heart defects, mental retardation, and occasionally movement disorders, all of which frequently result in miscarriage or stillbirth.

PREVALENCE

Rubella exposure within the first 8 weeks of gestation will cause congenital rubella syndrome in ~85% of exposed pregnancies (CDC, 2014d). The highest rates (up to 90%) are associated with infections occurring during the first trimester (CDC, 2014d). Birth defects caused by maternal rubella infection, after 20 weeks gestation, are rare (CDC, 2014d). Additionally, adolescents and young women aged 12 to 19 years have the lowest immunity (CDC, 2014d).

ASSESSMENT

Titers for rubella are standard of care with each pregnancy. Laboratory testing is done for the purpose of assessing a pregnant woman's immunity status.

Cytomegalovirus

ETIOLOGY

CMV is prevalent in the excretions of infants and toddlers as well as of adults who are immunosuppressed (e.g., those undergoing organ transplant, HIV positive). Women working in health care settings with immunosuppressed patients or those working in childcare should be screened before a planned pregnancy as they are at greater risk of contracting CMV (CDC, 2010b). Although the CMV IgG antibody test determines whether a person has been infected, the CMV IgM and IgG avidity tests determine whether the infection is recent or not. It is important to note that these tests are not always commercially available and are not always accurate (CDC, 2010b).

CMV is a member of the herpes virus group, which also includes herpes simplex types 1 and 2, varicella-zoster virus (chickenpox), and Epstein–Barr virus (infectious mononucleosis; CDC, 2010b).

PREVALENCE

CMV is common among adults and infects between 40% and 85% of adults by 40 years of age. Annually, one child in 150 is born and is affected by a CMV infection (CDC, 2010b).

ASSESSMENT AND HEALTH PROMOTION

Because it is so pervasive, routine screening is not currently recommended. Instead, *meticulous hand washing* should be stressed to prevent transmission of CMV in health care and childcare settings.

Herpes

ETIOLOGY

There are two types of HSV: type 1 (usually oral pharyngeal in origin) and type 2 (usually genital in origin). There is a greater likelihood of subclinical viral shedding with type 2 than with type 1 HSV (CDC, 2015l).

PREVALENCE

With most neonatal herpes infections, there is a 30% to 50% transmission rate to the newborn (CDC, 2015l). Acquiring a primary herpes outbreak in the genital area late in pregnancy and/or near delivery carries greater risk of fetal diagnosis with congenital herpes.

ASSESSMENT AND MANAGEMENT

Women with a history of genital herpes lesions (type 1 or type 2) should inform their health care provider before or at the first prenatal visit. Pregnant women with a history of herpes will be given prophylactic treatment for HSV suppression, beginning at 36 weeks gestation. Routine serologic testing for HSV remains controversial. We currently have no immunizations for HIV, CMV, toxoplasmosis, parvovirus, and/or HSV. Prevention of transmission, appropriate screening, and awareness of the importance of screening high-risk populations are essential.

INTERVENTIONS AND STRATEGIES FOR RISK REDUCTION AND MANAGEMENT

Assess immunization status on all women of reproductive age.

- *Rubella seronegativity.* Rubella vaccination provides protective seropositivity and prevents congenital rubella syndrome.
- *Human papillomavirus (HPV)*
  - Assess need for quadrivalent HPV vaccine before pregnancy.
  - Vaccinate all women younger than 26 years old.
- *Hepatitis B (HBV)*
  - Screen for exposure and vaccinate to prevent exposure during pregnancy.
- *Varicella immune status*
  - Check for seronegativity and vaccinate in women with no history of chicken pox or if their status is in question.

Routinely offer and encourage effective contraception after administration of vaccines.

Screen for STI Exposure Before Pregnancy

Early STI screening and treatment may prevent associated adverse outcomes in pregnancy. STIs are strongly associated with ectopic pregnancy, infertility, and chronic pelvic pain, resulting in fetal death or substantial physical and developmental disabilities, including mental retardation and blindness.

- Screen all women younger than 26 years old annually for *Chlamydia trachomatis* and *Neisseria gonorrhoeae* (CDC, 2015l).
- Ask about HSV exposure with women and partners, and consider serologic screening (controversial) and prophylactic treatment near delivery in women with positive partners.
- Screen for HBV and vaccinate before pregnancy if a woman is negative. Prevention of HBV infection in women of childbearing age prevents transmission of infection to infants. HBV screening and vaccination also eliminate risk of sequela, which includes possible hepatic failure, liver carcinoma, cirrhosis, and death (CDC, 2015l).
- Screen all women for HIV before pregnancy. If HIV infection is identified before pregnancy, timely antiretroviral treatment can be administered, and women (or couples) should be given additional information, which is known to prevent mother-to-child transmission (CDC, 2015l).
- Encourage safe sex practices for reducing STI risk as part of preconception care. *Safe sex* includes abstinence, mutual masturbation, dry kissing, hugging, body massage, and condom use with intercourse and/or oral sex.

Risk of Preconception Overweight and Obesity

ETIOLOGY

Preconception obesity leads to greater risk of NTDs, gestational diabetes, gestational hypertension, and difficult management of labor resulting in operative deliveries (ACOG, 2013b/2015, 2013c/2015). Postpartum obesity elevates the risks for recurrent medical problems with each subsequent pregnancy.

PREVALENCE

Obesity and diabetes are epidemic in the United States. More than half of U.S. women are overweight and one third of them are considered obese (CDC, 2014e). Diabetes affects 9.1 million or 8.9% of women aged 20 years and older and it is estimated that one third go undiagnosed (ADA, 2013). The prevalence of diabetes is two to four times higher in women that are of Black, Hispanic, Latin American, American Indian, or Asian/Pacific Islander decent (ADA, 2013). In women of reproductive age, 2% to 5% of women will develop gestational diabetes, which may result in a greater risk of developing type 2 diabetes (ADA, 2013). It is estimated that obesity can also lead to a greater risk of NTDs, despite the recommended 400 mcg daily intake of folic acid likely because of lower circulating blood levels (ACOG 2013b/2015, 2013c/2015; ADA, 2013; CDC, 2014e; Rasmussen et al., 2008).

MANAGEMENT AND HEALTH PROMOTION

Weight loss before pregnancy was also shown to reduce risks of NTDs in overweight women (CDC, 2014c, 2014e; Rasmussen et al., 2008). Women avoiding consumption of carbohydrates for weight loss purposes are at risk of folic acid deficiency; low-carbohydrate diets usually limit folate fortified carbohydrate-rich foods (e.g., breads, cereals, pasta; ACOG, 2014; CDC, 2015d). Being either over or underweight may also contribute to difficulty with conception because of an increased risk of infrequent ovulation or anovulation.

INTERVENTIONS AND STRATEGIES FOR RISK REDUCTION AND MANAGEMENT

BMI and Weight Management for All Women Regardless of Age • Women who are over- or underweight may have a difficult time conceiving and are at a greater risk of NTDs despite folic acid supplementation (ACOG, 2014; CDC, 2015d). Women who lose weight before pregnancy can reduce their risk of NTDs; however, women on low-carbohydrate diets are at a greater risk of inadequate folic acid intake (ACOG, 2014; CDC, 2015d). Maternal obesity increases the risk of preterm delivery, diabetes, cesarean section, and hypertensive and thromboembolic disease (ACOG, 2013b/2015, 2013c/2015, 2014; CDC 2014e).

Lead and Mercury

ETIOLOGY

Lead and mercury are widespread in the environment. The most common source of mercury is from the burning of wastes contaminated with inorganic mercury and the burning of fossil fuels, primarily coal. Methyl mercury is formed from inorganic mercury through anaerobic organisms in aquatic environments. The natural food chain in aquatic environments results in higher levels of methyl mercury in larger predator fish, leading to human exposure from consumption of seafood. Lead and mercury are neurotoxicants and may also harm the kidneys of a developing fetus (Boucher et al., 2012; CDC, 2010c). Exposure to heavy metals, such as lead and mercury, during pregnancy are potentially harmful to a developing fetus.

PREVALENCE

Mercury and lead levels among pregnant women vary by race and ethnicity. Mean lead levels in U.S. pregnant women are generally low (less than 5 mcg/dL; CDC, 2010a). In the United States, there is no standard for blood mercury levels in pregnant women, although blood mercury levels greater than 5.8 mcg/L have raised concerns (Boucher et al., 2012; CDC, 2004; U.S. Environmental Protection Agency [USEPA], 2015). There appears to be a negative relationship between prenatal lead and mercury exposure and fetal growth and neurodevelopment (Boucher et al., 2012; CDC, 2004; CDC, 2010a; USEPA, 2015).

When testing mercury and lead levels in pregnant women, a single blood lead test may not reflect cumulative lead and/or mercury exposure. Therefore, results from a single blood test may not be sufficient to establish the full nature of the developmental risk to the fetus. Repeat testing may be necessary (CDC, 2004, 2010c; USEPA, 2015).

MANAGEMENT

FDA and EPA recommend that all pregnant women avoid swordfish, shark, tilefish, and king mackerel, and should limit consumption of other seafood to a maximum of 12 ounces per week (FDA, 2016). Methyl mercury is removed from the body naturally, but may take more than a year to return to safe levels once they have become high. Therefore, all women who could become pregnant should also follow the same recommendations (FDA, 2016). To avoid excessive lead exposure from old plumbing, use only bottled or cold tap water for cooking or drinking and let the tap run for at least 30 seconds before using. Lead is also used in paint found on pottery, especially terra cotta. Always recommend lead-free pottery or clear glass for baking or reheating (CDC, 2010c; USEPA, 2015).

Testing lead levels is important. The CDC recommends counseling on supplemental calcium, iron, and prenatal vitamins for levels greater than or equal to 5 mg/dL (CDC, 2010c). A thorough investigation of both occupational and home-risk factors, conducted by the local health department, is indicated for levels greater than or equal to 15 mg/dL. Treatment through chelation for lead levels greater than or equal to 45 mg/dL is also recommended (CDC, 2010c). Mercury levels are tested in the first morning urine preferably; blood levels can be assessed as early as 3 days after exposure (CDC, 2010c).

Bacteria

ETIOLOGY

Listeriosis is a foodborne infection caused by the bacterium *Listeria monocytogenes*. Listeria monocytogenes is found in soil and water. Animals carry the bacterium without appearing ill and contaminate foods, such as meat and dairy products, as well as vegetables from manure used as fertilizer (CDC, 2015g). Unlike most foodborne bacteria, listeria can grow at refrigerator temperatures. Listeria is most frequently found in nonpasteurized cheeses (e.g., feta, brie, camembert, and blue-veined cheeses, some white Mexican cheeses, and panela); hot dogs, lunch meat (unless reheated until steaming hot); refrigerated pates and meat spreads; refrigerated smoked seafood (e.g., salmon, trout, whitefish, cod, tuna, or mackerel), as well as other unpasteurized milk-containing products (CDC, 2015g).

Symptoms of listeriosis include flu-like symptoms (e.g., stiff neck, fever, muscle aches, nausea, diarrhea), and if infection spreads to the central nervous system, symptoms may include headache, stiff neck, confusion, loss of balance, or convulsions. Infected pregnant women may experience only mild, flu-like symptoms. There is no screening test for listeriosis. In suspected cases, listeriosis is confirmed with blood and cerebral spinal fluid cultures. Once confirmed, prompt intravenous antibiotic treatment is recommended. If diagnosed and treated quickly, the likelihood of transmission to the fetus may be minimized. Even so, prompt treatment is not a guarantee of fetal survival (CDC, 2015g).

PREVALENCE

Listeriosis is recognized as a serious public health problem in the United States because it affects an estimated 2,500 persons each year. Those infected become seriously ill, and approximately 500 die from the infection (CDC, 2015g). Pregnant women are 20 times more likely to contract listeriosis (CDC, 2015g). Approximately one third of all cases of listeriosis occur during pregnancy. Spontaneous abortion, stillbirth, premature delivery, and/or infection of the newborn are negative health outcomes associated with listeriosis infection during pregnancy (CDC, 2015g).

INTERVENTIONS AND STRATEGIES FOR RISK REDUCTION AND MANAGEMENT

Prevention of exposure to listeria is the best way to prevent (CDC, 2015g; FDA, 2016). Prevention of listeriosis can be achieved by:

- Avoiding unpasteurized dairy containing foods
- Thoroughly cooking all meats before eating
- Washing all vegetables before eating
- Good hand washing and washing all knives and cutting boards after handling uncooked foods
- Storage of uncooked meats separately from all other foods
- Consumption of all ready to eat and perishable foods as soon as possible (CDC, 2015g; FDA, 2016)

■ GENETICS

The Risk of Genetic Anomalies and the Role of the Family History

ETIOLOGY

Mutations in single genes (monogenetic), multiple genes (multifactorial inheritance disorders), combination genes and environment, or damaged chromosomes can cause genetic anomalies (Manipalviratn, Trivax, & Huang, 2013; National Human Genome Research Institute [NHGRH], 2015). The mother or father may pass on genetic abnormalities to the infant. Genetic abnormalities occur when a gene becomes flawed because of a mutation. In some cases, a gene or part of a gene may be missing. These defects occur at fertilization and are mostly nonpreventable. A particular genetic defect may be present throughout a family history of one or both parents. Before a planned pregnancy, it is optimal to know about family history for inherited diseases and congenital anomalies. In this multicultural world, it is also important to know whether partners planning pregnancies are related by blood (consanguineous), such as first cousins. Marrying a first cousin is preferred in some cultures and religions (e.g., Muslims). Consanguinity is common, especially in people originating from North Africa, the Middle East, and large parts of Asia (Abbas & Yunis, 2014; Bennett et al., 2002).

PREVALENCE

In the United States, approximately 1 out of every 33 babies is born with a birth defect, of which many are related to genetics (Manipalviratn et al., 2013). In regard to consanguinity, worldwide, about 10.4% of all marriages are among relatives (Abbas & Yunis, 2014; Bennett et al., 2002).

INTERVENTIONS AND STRATEGIES FOR RISK REDUCTION AND MANAGEMENT

Cultural sensitivity and a nonjudgmental attitude to consanguineous couples are essential to foster good working relationships between the medical profession and communities where consanguineous marriage is more common (Postlethwaite, 2009).

Assessment of family medical history for three to four generations back is recommended for those individuals with a known history of genetic conditions as well as recommended for screening consanguineous couples (Abbas & Yunis, 2014; Bennett et al., 2002; USDHHS, n.d.). Some genetic conditions are more common in certain ethnic backgrounds. For instance, women of Southeast Asian or Mediterranean background should be tested for hemoglobin E/beta thalassemia. If a woman or her male partner has any Black/African American background, she should be tested for sickle cell disease. Whites (non-Hispanic) should be tested for cystic fibrosis. Eastern European Jewish (Ashkenazi) background couples should be tested for Tay-Sachs disease, Canavan disease, and familial dysautonomia (Abbas & Yunis, 2014; Bennett et al., 2002).

Inherited Medical Conditions

If a woman, her partner, or any close family member (children, parents, sisters/brothers, aunts/uncles) have a history of genetic/birth defects or inherited conditions, they should be referred for genetic counseling. Genetic counselors will obtain a family history, screen, and test pregnant women as determined appropriate.

The following medical conditions should be evaluated by a genetic counselor for possible genetic predisposition:

- NTDs (e.g., spina bifida, anencephaly)
- Down syndrome
- Mental retardation
- Bleeding disorder (e.g., hemophilia)
- Muscular dystrophy, other muscle/nerve disorder
- Cystic fibrosis
- Tay-Sachs
- Sickle cell anemia
- Polycystic kidney disease
- Heart defect at birth
- Cleft lip/palate

Genetic Counseling Before Planning a Pregnancy

INTERVENTIONS AND STRATEGIES FOR RISK REDUCTION AND MANAGEMENT

Preconception counseling should include a review of personal, family, and medical health history. The U.S. Surgeon General has developed an Internet-based tool, My Family Health Portrait (familyhistory.hhs.gov/FHH/html/index .html), in which individuals can create their family health history. This tool can assist families in organizing their family tree while identifying common diseases that may run in their family. It is also an effective way pregnant women can provide their family health history to their health care provider who then can identify risk of disease. This tool is available in different languages (USDHHS, n.d.).

Pregnant women and their family members should be encouraged to gather and write down familial health problems. To learn about their family history, pregnant women should ask questions, talk about family history at family gatherings, and even review information on death certificates and family medical records. If possible, they should collect information about their grandparents, parents, aunts and uncles, nieces and nephews, siblings, and children. Important information includes (a) major medical conditions (e.g., heart disease, stroke, cancer, diabetes, Alzheimer's, obesity, blindness, deafness); (b) age of disease

onset; (c) age and cause of death; (d) history of infertility, miscarriages, stillbirths, and/or infant deaths; (e) history of birth defects, learning disabilities, and/or mental retardation; and (f) ethnic background. Pregnant women with a family history of a genetic disorder(s) should be referred for genetic counseling.

ASSESS FAMILY MEDICAL AND GENETIC RISKS BEFORE PREGNANCY

- Provide culturally sensitive family history and genetic screening.
- Refer for genetic counseling with family history of specific medical conditions and thorough ethnicity-based screening.

Intimate Partner Violence

ETIOLOGY

Intimate partner violence (IPV) is a preventable public health problem that affects millions of women regardless of age, economic status, race, religion, ethnicity, sexual orientation, or educational background. IPV includes overpowering a partner to physical and psychological abuse, sexual violence, and reproductive coercion (ACOG, 2012). Physical abuse can include throwing objects, pushing, kicking, biting, slapping, strangling, hitting, beating, threatening with a weapon, and/or use of a weapon against the victim. Psychological abuse is targeted at decreasing a woman's self-worth and can include harassment, verbal abuse (e.g., name calling, degradation, blaming, threats, stalking, and isolation). The abuser will oftentimes isolate the woman from her family and friends as well as leave the woman without food, money, and/or transportation. Sexual violence can range from unwanted kissing, touching, and/or fondling to sexual coercion and rape. Reproductive coercion involves the control of a woman's reproductive health. In these situations, the abuser may (a) disrupt a woman's effort at contraception, (b) intentionally expose the abused woman to STIs (including HIV), and/or (c) control the outcome of a pregnancy, for example, force the woman to have an abortion or injure in a way that causes a miscarriage (ACOG, 2012).

IPV has been linked to early parenthood, severe poverty, overwhelming emotional distress, perpetrator problem drinking/drug use, and unemployment (National Institute of Justice [NIJ], 2007). The consequences of IPV in pregnancy result in later entry to prenatal care and poor pregnancy outcomes such as preterm labor, low-birth-weight babies, fetal trauma, unhealthy maternal behaviors (e.g., inadequate diet, substance abuse, inadequate exercise), as well as peripartum and postpartum depression and difficulty breastfeeding (Rodriguez et al., 2008; Zink, 2007).

PREVALENCE

IPV (also referred to as domestic violence) includes physical, sexual, and/or emotional abuse by a current or ex-intimate partner, and can occur in women of any educational background, ethnicity, culture, religion, sexual preference, or socioeconomic status. It is estimated that 1.5 million women in the United States are victims of IPV annually with about 5.2% of pregnant women affected (Rodriguez et al., 2008; Zink, 2007). In one international study, associations were noted between a greater risk of unintended pregnancy and IPV (Pallitto & O'Campo, 2004). Fifty-five percent of respondents had had at least one unintended pregnancy, and 38% had been physically or sexually abused by their current or most recent partner (Pallitto & O'Campo, 2004). The adjusted odds of having had an unintended pregnancy were significantly elevated if a woman had been physically or sexually abused (odds ratio, 1.4; Tjaden & Thoennes, 2000a, 2000b). Female victims of IPV have a 50% to 70% increase in gynecologic, central nervous system related, and stress-related problems, with women sexually and physically abused most likely to report problems (Campbell et al., 2002). In many cases, the recurrent presenting complaints of women who are experiencing IPV include depression, which is two to four times more prevalent, and alcohol dependence, which is close to three times more prevalent than the general population (Campbell et al., 2002).

INTERVENTIONS AND STRATEGIES FOR RISK REDUCTION AND MANAGEMENT

Screening for Intimate Partner Violence Recommendations • Although women of all ages may be subjected to IPV, it is most prevalent among women of reproductive age. Health care providers are in a unique position to assess and provide support for women subjected to IPV. USDHHS (2013) has recommended that IPV screening and counseling be a part of women's preventive health visits (Institute of Medicine [IOM], 2011). Health care providers must not rule out the possibility of IPV with women who present with injuries, somatic complaints without diagnosis (e.g., chronic pain, fatigue, headache, neurologic symptoms), gastrointestinal pain, pelvic pain, STIs, depression, anxiety, insomnia, and/or multiple or erratic visits with a series of vague complaints. Screening for IPV may be difficult for many clinicians.

Screening for IPV should occur at new patient visits, during annual examinations, and at various other times when a woman presents for health care. Screening in the pregnant woman begins at the first prenatal visit, and at least one time per trimester (ACOG, 2013a). Screening should be conducted privately. Health care providers should avoid questions that use stigmatizing terms (e.g., abuse, rape, battered, violence; see Box 22.3).

Health care providers should:

- Screen women for IPV in a private and safe setting with the woman alone
- When appropriate, use a professional language interpreter only
- At the beginning of the assessment, offer a framing statement to show that screening is done universally; not because IPV is suspected
- Inform the woman of the confidentiality of the discussion as well as any state law disclosure mandates
- Incorporate IPV screening into the woman's routine medical history

---

BOX 22.3   EXEMPLAR INTIMATE PARTNER VIOLENCE SCREENING QUESTIONS

Introducing or Framing Question

"Unfortunately, violence is a problem for many women. Because it affects health and well-being, I ask all my patients about it..."

"Because violence is so common in many women's lives, I have begun asking about this routinely."

Indirect Inquiry

"How are things at home?"

Direct Inquiry

"Do you ever feel physically or emotionally threatened or hurt by your intimate partner?"

"Have you been hit, kicked, punched, or otherwise hurt by someone in the past year? If so, by whom?"

"Do you feel safe in your current relationship?"

"Is there a partner from a previous relationship who is making you feel unsafe?"

After receiving a response about the risk of IPV, the next step is to offer an affirmation to the woman:

"I am so glad you shared this with me."

"This can have a significant effect on your health."

"There are resources available to help you."

If IPV is confirmed, the next step is to assess safety:

"Is it safe for you to go home today?"

"Is there someplace you can go that you feel safe?"

Adapted from American College of Obstetricians and Gynecologists (2012).

- Identify community resources for women affected by IPV

Screening at periodic intervals, including during well-woman visits and prenatal care visits, can improve the lives of women who experience IPV. Preventing the lifelong consequences associated with IPV can have huge impact on the reproductive, perinatal, and overall health of women.

■ REFERENCES

Abbas, H. A., & Yunis, K. (2014). The effect of consanguinity on neonatal outcomes and health. *Human Heredity*, 77(1–4), 87–92.

Alcoholism: Clinical & Experimental Research. (2008, September 15). Women Who Binge Drink At Greater Risk Of Unsafe Sex And

Sexually Transmitted Disease. *ScienceDaily, 15*. Retrieved from www .sciencedaily.com/releases/2008/09/080904215613.htm

American Academy of Pediatrics Committee on Genetics. (2001). Maternal phenylketonuria. *Pediatrics, 107*(2), 427–428.

American Academy of Pediatrics and the American College of Obstetricians and Gynecologists. (2012). *Perinatal infections*. In *Guidelines for perinatal care* (4th ed., pp. 411–414). Washington, DC: American College of Obstetricians and Gynecologists.

American College of Obstetricians and Gynecologists (ACOG). (2005/2015). *The importance of preconception care in the continuum of women's health care*. Number 313. Retrieved from http://www.acog .org/Resources-And-Publications/Committee-Opinions/Committee -on-Gynecologic-Practice/The-Importance-of-Preconception-Care-in -the-Continuum-of-Womens-Health-Care

American College of Obstetricians and Gynecologists (ACOG). (2006/2015). *Menstruation in girls and adolescents: Using the menstrual cycle as a vital sign*. Committee Opinion No. 651. *Obstetrics & Gynecology, 126*(6), 1328.

American College of Obstetricians and Gynecologists (ACOG). (2010/2015). *Emergency contraception*. Committee Opinion No. 152. *Obstetrics & Gynecology, 126*(3), 685–686.

American College of Obstetricians and Gynecologists (ACOG). (2011). *Smoking cessation during pregnancy: A clinician's guide to helping pregnant women quite smoking*. Chapel Hill, NC: University of North Caroline.

American College of Obstetricians and Gynecologists (ACOG). (2012). *Intimate partner violence*. Committee Opinion No. 518. Retrieved from http://www.acog.org/-/media/Committee-Opinions/Committee -on-Health-Care-for-Underserved-Women/co518.pdf?dmc=1%26ts= 20150112T2118022948

American College of Obstetricians and Gynecologists (ACOG). (2013a). *Hypertension in pregnancy. Obstetrics and Gynecology, 122*(5), 1–100.

American College of Obstetricians and Gynecologists (ACOG). (2013b/2015). *Obesity in pregnancy*. Committee Opinion No. 548. *Obstetrics & Gynecology, 126*(6), 1321–1322.

American College of Obstetricians and Gynecologists (ACOG). (2013c/2015). *Weight gain during pregnancy*. Committee Opinion No. 549. Retrieved from https://www.acog.org/-/media/Committee -Opinions/Committee-on-Obstetric-Practice/co548.pdf?dmc=1&ts= 20160123T1902298227

American College of Obstetricians and Gynecologists (ACOG). (2014). Preconception and interconception care. In *Guidelines for women's health care: A resource manual* (4th ed., pp. 381–398). Washington, DC: ACOG.

American College of Obstetricians and Gynecologists (ACOG). (2015). *First-trimester risk assessment for early-onset preeclampsia*. Committee Opinion No. 638. *Obstetrics & Gynecology, 126*(3), 689.

American Diabetes Association (ADA). (2013). *Living with diabetes before pregnancy*. Retrieved from http://www.diabetes.org/living -with-diabetes/complications/pregnancy/before-pregnancy.html

American Thyroid Association (2013.). *Thyroid disease and pregnancy*. Retrieved from http://www.thyroid.org/thyroid-disease-pregnancy

Andrade, S. E., Raebel, M. A., Morse, A. N., Davis, R. L., Chan, K. A., Finkelstein, J. A.,...H. Gurwitz, J. (2006). Use of prescription medications with a potential for fetal harm among pregnant women. *Pharmacoepidemiology and Drug Safety, 15*(8), 546–554.

Association of Reproductive Health Professionals (ARHP). (2010). The links between environmental exposures and reproductive health. *Clinical Proceedings*, 1–28.

Bennett, R. L., Motulsky, A. G., Bittles, A., Hudgins, L., Uhrich, S., Doyle, D. L.,...Olson, D. (2002). Genetic counseling and screening of consanguineous couples and their offspring: Recommendations of the national society of genetic counselors. *Journal of Genetic Counseling, 11*(2), 97–119.

Boucher, O., Jacobson, S. W., Plusquellec, P., Dewailly, E., Ayotte, P., Forget-Dubois, N.,...Muckle, G. (2012). Prenatal methylmercury, postnatal lead exposure, and evidence of attention deficit/hyperactivity disorder among Inuit children in Arctic Québec. *Environmental Health Perspectives, 120*(10), 1456–1461.

Briggs, G. G., & Freeman, R. K. (2015). *Drugs in pregnancy and lactation* (10th ed.). Philadelphia, PA: Wolters Kluwer Health.

Brown, S. S., & Eisenberg, L. (1995). *The best intentions: Unintended pregnancy and the well-being of children and families*. Washington, DC: National Academies Press.

Campbell, J., Jones, A. S., Dienemann, J., Kub, J., Schollenberger, J., O'Campo, P.,...Wynne, C. (2002). Intimate partner violence and physical health consequences. *Archives of Internal Medicine, 162*(10), 1157–1163.

Centers for Disease Control and Prevention (CDC). (1992). *Recommendations for the use of folic acid to reduce the number of cases of spina bifida and other neural tube defects*. Retrieved from http://www.cdc.gov/mmwr/preview/mmwrhtml/00019479.htm

Centers for Disease Control and Prevention (CDC). (2000). Measles, rubella, and congenital rubella syndrome—United States and Mexico, 1997–1999. *Morbidity and Mortality Weekly Report, 49*(46), 1048–1059.

Centers for Disease Control and Prevention (CDC). (2002). *Safe motherhood: Promoting health for women before, during and after pregnancy*. Washington, DC: U.S. Department of Health and Human Services.

Centers for Disease Control and Prevention (CDC). (2004). Blood mercury levels in young children and childbearing aged women: United States, 1999–2002. *Morbidity and Mortality Weekly Report, 53*(43), 1018–1020.

Centers for Disease Control and Prevention (CDC). (2006). Recommendations to improve preconception health and health care—United States: A report of the CDC/ATSDR Preconception Work Group and the Select Panel on Preconception Care. *Morbidity and Mortality Weekly Report, 55*(No. RR-6), 1–23.

Centers for Disease Control and Prevention (CDC). (2008). Appendix A: AIDS-defining conditions. *Morbidity and Mortality Weekly Report, 57*(No. RR10), 9.

Centers for Disease Control and Prevention (CDC). (2010a). Blood lead and mercury levels in pregnant women in the United States, 2003–2008. *NCHS Data Brief*, (52), 1–8.

Centers for Disease Control and Prevention (CDC). (2010b). *Cytomegalovirus (CMV) and congenital CMV infection*. Retrieved from http://www.cdc.gov/cmv/clinical/index.html

Centers for Disease Control and Prevention (CDC). (2010c). *Guidelines for the identification and management of lead exposure in pregnant and lactating women*. Retrieved from http://www.cdc.gov/nceh/lead/ publications/LeadandPregnancy2010.pdf

Centers for Disease Control and Prevention (CDC) (2010d). US medical eligibility criteria for contraceptive use, 2010. *Morbidity and Mortality Weekly Report, 59*(No. RR-4), 1–86.

Centers for Disease Control and Prevention (CDC). (2012a). Alcohol use and binge drinking among women of childbearing age—United States, 2006–2010. *Morbidity and Mortality Weekly Report, 61*(28), 534–538.

Centers for Disease Control and Prevention (CDC). (2012b). *Parvovirus B-19 and fifth disease*. Retrieved from http://www.cdc.gov/parvo virusB19/references.html

Centers for Disease Control and Prevention (CDC). (2013). *Parasites— Toxoplasmosis (Toxoplasma infection)*. Retrieved from http://www .cdc.gov/parasites/toxoplasmosis

Centers for Disease Control and Prevention (CDC). (2014a). *Chickenpox and pregnancy*. Retrieved from http://www.cdc.gov/vaccines/adults/ rec-vac/pregnant.html

Centers for Disease Control and Prevention (CDC). (2014b). *National diabetes statistics report: Estimates of diabetes and its burden in the United States*. Retrieved from http://www.cdc.gov/diabetes/pubs/ statsreport14/national-diabetes-report-web.pdf

Centers for Disease Control and Prevention (CDC). (2014c). *Preconception health and health care*. Retrieved from http://www.cdc.gov/ preconception/careforwomen/immunization.html

Centers for Disease Control and Prevention (CDC). (2014d). *Rubella (German measles, three-day measles)*. Retrieved from http://www.cdc .gov/rubella/about/index.html

Centers for Disease Control and Prevention (CDC). (2015a). *About teen pregnancy: U.S. teen pregnancy outcomes by age, race, and Hispanic ethnicity*. Retrieved from http://www.cdc.gov/teenpregnancy/about/ index.htm

Centers for Disease Control and Prevention (CDC). (2015b). *Birth defects: Data and statistics*. Retrieved from http://www.cdc.gov/ncbddd/ birthdefects/data.html

Centers for Disease Control and Prevention (CDC). (2015c). *Fact sheets: Excessive alcohol use and risks to women's health*. Retrieved from http://www.cdc.gov/alcohol/fact-sheets/womens-health.htm

Centers for Disease Control and Prevention (CDC). (2015d). *Folic acid: Birth defects count*. Retrieved from http://www.cdc.gov/ncbddd/birthdefectscount/faq-folic-ntd.html

Centers for Disease Control and Prevention (CDC). (2015e). *HIV among pregnant women, infants, and children*. Retrieved from http://www.cdc.gov/hiv/risk/gender/pregnantwomen/facts

Centers for Disease Control and Prevention (CDC). (2015f). *Information for health care providers and public health professionals: Preventing tobacco use during pregnancy*. Retrieved from http://www.cdc.gov/reproductivehealth/maternalinfanthealth/tobaccousepregnancy/providers.html

Centers for Disease Control and Prevention (CDC). (2015g). *Listeria (Listeriosis)*. Retrieved from http://www.cdc.gov/listeria/index.html

Centers for Disease Control and Prevention (CDC). (2015h). *National Center on Birth Defects and Developmental Disabilities (NCBDDD)*. Retrieved from http://www.cdc.gov/ncbddd/aboutus

Centers for Disease Control and Prevention (CDC). (2015i). *National prematurity awareness month*. Retrieved from http://www.cdc.gov/features/prematurebirth

Centers for Disease Control and Prevention (CDC). (2015j). *Preconception health and health care: Information for health professionals*. Retrieved from http://www.cdc.gov/preconception/hcp

Centers for Disease Control and Prevention (CDC). (2015k). *Pre-exposure prophylaxis (PrEP)*. Retrieved from http://www.cdc.gov/hiv/basics/prep.html

Centers for Disease Control and Prevention (CDC). (2015l). *Sexually transmitted diseases treatment guidelines, 2015*. Retrieved from http://www.cdc.gov/mmwr/preview/mmwrhtml/rr6403a1.htm

Centers for Disease Control and Prevention (CDC). (2015m). *Tobacco use and pregnancy*. Retrieved from http://www.cdc.gov/reproductivehealth/tobaccousepregnancy

Centers for Disease Control and Prevention (CDC). (2015n). *Toxoplasmosis (Toxoplasma infection)*. Retrieved from http://www.cdc.gov/parasites/toxoplasmosis/gen_info/pregnant.html

Centers for Disease Control and Prevention (CDC). (2015o). *Unintended pregnancy prevention*. Retrieved from http://www.cdc.gov/reproductivehealth/unintendedpregnancy

Centers for Disease Control and Prevention (CDC). (2016). *Birth defects: Data & statistics*. Retrieved from http://www.cdc.gov/ncbddd/birthdefects/index.html

Child Trends Data Bank. (2014). *Condom use: Indicators on children and youth*. Retrieved from http://www.childtrends.org/wp-content/uploads/2012/07/28_Condom_Use.pdf

Cooper, W. O., Hernandez-Diaz, S., Arbogast, P. G., Dudley, J. A., Dyer, S., Gideon, P. S.,...Ray, W. A. (2006). Major congenital malformations after first-trimester exposure to ACE inhibitors. *New England Journal of Medicine, 354*(23), 2443–2451.

Day, N. L., Helsel, A., Sonon, K., & Goldschmidt, L. (2013). The association between prenatal alcohol exposure and behavior at 22 years of age. *Alcoholism, Clinical and Experimental Research, 37*(7), 1171–1178.

Department of Health Services, Hazard Evaluation System and Information Service. (2007). *If I'm pregnant, can the chemicals I work with harm my baby?* Richmond, CA: Department of Health Services, Hazard Evaluation System and Information Service.

DeSimone, J. (2010). *Binge drinking and risky sex among college students*. American Association of Wine Economists (AAWE) Working Paper, No. 59, 1–39.

Dutta, S. (2015). Human teratogens and their effects: A critical evaluation. *International Journal of Information Research and Review, 2*(3), 525–536.

Food and Drug Administration (FDA). (2014). *Content and format of labeling for human prescription drug and biological products: Requirements for pregnancy and lactation labeling*. Federal Register, 79(No. 233), 72063–72103.

Food and Drug Administration (FDA). (2016). *Food safety for moms-to-be*. Retrieved from http://www.fda.gov/food/resourcesforyou/healtheducators/ucm081785.htm

Finer, L. B., & Zolna, M. R. (2011). Unintended pregnancy in the United States: Incidence and disparities, 2006. *Contraception, 84*(5), 478–485.

Frye, D., Brookshire, G. S., Brookshire, A., LaGrave, D., & Brasington, C. K. (2011). Practice guidelines for communicating a prenatal or post-natal diagnosis of Down syndrome: Recommendations of the National Society of Genetic Counselors. *Journal of Genetic Counseling, 20*(5), 432–441.

Gelles, R. J. (1998). Violence and pregnancy: Are pregnant women at greater risk of abuse? *Journal of Marriage and the Family, 50*(3), 841–847.

Guttmacher Institute. (2014). *Facts on induced abortion in the United States*. Retrieved from www.guttmacher.org/pubs/fb_induced_abortion.html

Guttmacher Institute. (2015). *Unintended pregnancy in the United States*. Retrieved from https://www.guttmacher.org/pubs/FB-Unintended-Pregnancy-US.html

Hamilton, D. A., Barto, D., Rodriguez, C. I., Magcalas, C. M., Fink, B. C., Rice, J. P.,...Savage, D. D. (2014). Effects of moderate prenatal ethanol exposure and age on social behavior, spatial response perseveration errors and motor behavior. *Behavioural Brain Research, 269*, 44–54.

Hatcher, R. A., Trussell, J., Nelson, A. L., Cates, W., Jr., Kowal, D., & Policar, M. (2011). *Contraceptive technology* (20th ed.). New York, NY: Ardent Media.

Healthy People 2020. (n.d.). *Understanding maternal, infant, and child health: Preconception health status*. Retrieved from http://www.healthypeople.gov/2020/topics-objectives/topic/maternal-infant-and-child-health

Henry J. Kaiser Family Foundation. (2014a). *Sexual health of adolescents and young adults in the United States*. Retrieved from http://kff.org/womens-health-policy/fact-sheet/sexual-health-of-adolescents-and-young-adults-in-the-united-states

Henry J. Kaiser Family Foundation. (2014b). *Women and HIV/AIDS in the United States*. Retrieved from http://kff.org/hivaids/fact-sheet/women-and-hivaids-in-the-united-states

Hobbins, D. (2003). Full circle: The evolution of preconception health promotion in America. *Journal of Obstetric, Gynecologic, and Neonatal Nursing, 32*(4), 516–522.

Hutcheon, J. A., Lisonkova, S., & Joseph, K. S. (2011). Epidemiology of pre-eclampsia and the other hypertensive disorders of pregnancy. *Best Practice & Research. Clinical Obstetrics & Gynaecology, 25*(4), 391–403.

Institute of Medicine (IOM). (2011). *Clinical preventive services for women: Closing the gaps* (pp. 71–141). Washington, DC: National Academies Press.

Johnson, K., Posner, S. F., Biermann, J., Cordero, J. F., Atrash, H. K., Parker, C. S., . . . Curtis, M. G. (2006). Recommendations to improve preconception and health care in the United States: A report of the CDC/ATSDR Preconception Care Work Group and the Select Panel on Preconception Care. *Morbidity and Mortality Weekly Report, 55*(RR-06), 1–23.

Jones, R. K., Frohwirth, L., & Moore, A. M. (2013). More than poverty: Disruptive events among women having abortions in the USA. *The Journal of Family Planning and Reproductive Health Care/Faculty of Family Planning & Reproductive Health Care, Royal College of Obstetricians & Gynaecologists, 39*(1), 36–43.

Kendrick, J. M. (2004). Preconception care of women with diabetes. *Journal of Perinatal & Neonatal Nursing, 18*(1), 14–25; quiz 26.

Kim, C., Ferrara, A., McEwen, L. N., Marrero, D. G., Gerzoff, R. B., & Herman, W. H.; TRIAD Study Group. (2005). Preconception care in managed care: The translating research into action for diabetes study. *American Journal of Obstetrics and Gynecology, 192*(1), 227–232.

King, T. L., Brucker, M. C., Fahey, J. O., Kreibs, J. M., Gegor, C. L., & Varney, H. (2015). *Varney's midwifery* (5th ed.). Burlington, MA: Jones & Bartlett Learning.

Lassi, Z. S., Imam, A. M., Dean, S. V., & Bhutta, Z. A. (2014). Preconception care: Caffeine, smoking, alcohol, drugs and other environmental chemical/radiation exposure. *Reproductive Health, 11*(Suppl. 3), 1–12.

Lee, E., Maneno, M. K., Smith, L., Weiss, S. R., Zuckerman, I. H., Wutoh, A. K., & Xue, Z. (2006). National patterns of medication use during pregnancy. *Pharmacoepidemiology and Drug Safety, 15*(8), 537–545.

Levy, H. L., & Ghavami, M. (1996). Maternal phenylketonuria: A metabolic teratogen. *Teratology, 53*(3), 176–184.

MacDorman, M. F., Mathews, T. J., Mohangoo, A. D., & Zeitlin, J. (2014). International comparisons of infant mortality and related factors: United States and Europe, 2010. *National Vital Statistics Reports, 63*(5).

March of Dimes. (n.d.). *Birth defects and other health conditions.* Retrieved from www.marchofdimes.org

March of Dimes. (2008). *Preconception during pregnancy: Smoking during pregnancy.* Retrieved from http://208.74.202.108/printableArticles/19695_1171.asp

March of Dimes. (2012). *Fifth disease and pregnancy.* Retrieved from http://www.marchofdimes.org/pregnancy/fifth-disease-and-pregnancy.aspx

March of Dimes. (2013). *PKU (phenylketonuria) in your baby.* Retrieved from http://www.marchofdimes.org/complications/phenylketonuria-in-your-baby.aspx

Manipalviratn, S., Trivax, B., & Huang, A. (2013). Genetic disorders and sex chromosome abnormalities. In A. H. Decherney (Ed.), *Current Diagnosis & Treatment* (67–96). New York, NY: McGraw-Hill.

May, P. A., Baete, A., Russo, J., Elliott, A. J., Blankenship, J., Kalberg, W. O.,…Hoyme, H. E. (2014). Prevalence and characteristics of fetal alcohol spectrum disorders. *Pediatrics, 134*(5), 855–866.

May, P. A., & Gossage, J. P. (2001). Estimating the prevalence of fetal alcohol syndrome. A summary. *Alcohol Research & Health: The Journal of the National Institute on Alcohol Abuse and Alcoholism, 25*(3), 159–167.

May, P. A., Gossage, J. P., Kalberg, W. O., Robinson, L. K., Buckley, D., Manning, M., & Hoyme, H. E. (2009). Prevalence and epidemiologic characteristics of FASD from various research methods with an emphasis on recent in-school studies. *Developmental Disabilities Research Reviews, 15*(3), 176–192.

Medline Plus. (2014). *TORCH screen.* Retrieved from www.nlm.nih.gov/medlineplus/ency/article/003350.htm

Miller, E., Jordan, B., Levenson, R., & Silverman, J. G. (2010). Reproductive coercion: Connecting the dots between partner violence and unintended pregnancy. *Contraception, 81*(6), 457–459.

Mills, J. L. (2010). Malformations in infants of diabetic mothers. *Birth Defects Research. Part A, Clinical and Molecular Teratology, 88*(10), 769–778.

Moore, K. L., & Persaud, T. V. N. (1998). *The developing human: Clinically oriented embryology* (6th ed.). Philadelphia, PA: W. B. Saunders. Retrieved from https://www.researchgate.net/profile/Dana_Barr/publication/5625928/figure/fig2/Fig-2-Critical-periods-in-human-development-from-Moore-KL-Persaud-TVN-The.png

Moore, E. M., Migliorini, R., Infante, M. A., & Riley, E. P. (2014). Fetal alcohol spectrum disorders: Recent neuroimaging findings. *Current Developmental Disorders Reports, 1*(3), 161–172.

Mosher, W. D., Jones, J., & Abma, J. C. (2012). Intended and unintended births in the United States: 1982–2010. *National Health Statistics Reports* (No. 55), 1–28.

National Environmental Trust. (2000). *Polluting our future: Chemical pollution in the US that affects child development and learning.* Retrieved from https://www.csu.edu/cerc/documents/PollutingOurFuture.pdf

National High Blood Pressure Education Program Working Group. (2000). Report of the National High Blood Pressure Education Program Working Group on High Blood Pressure in Pregnancy. *American Journal of Obstetrics & Gynecology, 183*(1), S1–S22.

National Human Genome Research Institute (NHGRH). (2015). *Frequently asked questions about genetic disorders.* Retrieved from http://www.genome.gov/19016930

National Institute of Justice (NIJ). (2007). *Causes and consequences of intimate partner violence.* Retrieved from http://www.nij.gov/topics/crime/intimate-partner-violence/pages/causes.aspx

National Institute on Drug Abuse (NIDA). (2007). *Impact of drugs on neurotransmission.* NIDA Notes. Retrieved from http://www.drugabuse.gov/news-events/nida-notes/2007/10/impacts-drugs-neurotransmission

Neu, N., Duchon, J., & Zachariah, P. (2015). TORCH infections. *Clinics in Perinatology, 42*(1), 77–103.

Occupational Safety & Health Administration (OSHA). (n.d.). *Hazard communication standard: Safety data sheets.* Retrieved from https://www.osha.gov/Publications/OSHA3514.html

O'Connor, M. J. (2014). Mental health outcomes associated with prenatal alcohol exposure: Genetic and environmental factors. *Current Developmental Disorders Reports, 1*(3), 181– 188.

Office of Adolescent Health. (2015). *Trends in teen pregnancy and childbearing.* Retrieved from http://www.hhs.gov/ash/oah/adolescent-health-topics/reproductive-health/teen-pregnancy/trends.html

Pallitto, C. C., & O'Campo, P. (2004). The relationship between intimate partner violence and unintended pregnancy: Analysis of a national sample from Colombia. *International Family Planning Perspectives, 30*(4), 165–173.

Physicians' Desk Reference Staff (PDR). (2015). *Physicians' desk reference* (69th ed.). Montvale, NJ: Thomson PDR.

Postlethwaite, D. (2003). Preconception health counseling for women exposed to teratogens: The role of the nurse. *Journal of Obstetric, Gynecologic, and Neonatal Nursing, 32*(4), 523–532.

Postlethwaite, D. A. (2009). Reproductive health. *A provider's handbook on culturally competent care, women's health* (1st ed.). Oakland, CA: Kaiser Permanente.

Rasmussen, S. A., Chu, S. Y., Kim, S. Y., Schmid, C. H., & Lau, J. (2008). Maternal obesity and risk of neural tube defects: A metaanalysis. *American Journal of Obstetrics and Gynecology, 198*(6), 611–619.

Rodriguez, M. A., Heilemann, M. V., Fielder, E., Ang, A., Nevarez, F., & Mangione, C. M. (2008). Intimate partner violence, depression, and PTSD among pregnant Latina women. *Annals of Family Medicine, 6*(1), 44–52.

Schwarz, E. B., Maselli, J., Norton, M., & Gonzales, R. (2005). Prescription of teratogenic medications in United States ambulatory practices. *American Journal of Medicine, 118*(11), 1240–1249.

Schwarz, E. B., Postlethwaite, D. A., Hung, Y. Y., & Armstrong, M. A. (2007). Documentation of contraception and pregnancy when prescribing potentially teratogenic medications for reproductive-age women. *Annals of Internal Medicine, 147*(6), 370–376.

Substance Abuse and Mental Health Services Administration. (2006). *Results from the 2013 National Survey on Drug Use and Health: Summary of national findings.* NSDUH Series H-48, HHS Publication No. (SMA) 14–4863. Rockville, MD: Author.

Tjaden, P., & Thoennes, N. (July, 2000a). *Extent, nature, and consequences of intimate partner violence: Findings from the National Violence Against Women Survey.* Washington, DC: U.S. Department of Justice; Publication No. NCJ 181867.

Tjaden, P., & Thoennes, N. (2000b). *Full report of the prevalence, incidence, and consequences of violence against women: Findings from the National Violence Against Women Survey.* Publication No. NCJ183781. Washington, DC: U.S. Department of Justice.

Tong, V. T., Dietz, P. M., England, L. J., Farr, S. L., Kim, S. Y., D'Angelo, D., & Bombard, J. M. (2011). Age and racial/ethnic disparities in prepregnancy smoking among women who delivered live births. *Preventing Chronic Disease, 8*(6), A121.

U.S. Department of Health and Human Services (USDHHS). (2007). Alcohol and tobacco. *Alcohol Alert, 71*, 1–6.

U.S. Department of Health and Human Services (USDHHS). (n.d.). *My Family Health Portrait: A tool from the surgeon general.* Retrieved from https://familyhistory.hhs.gov/FHH/html/index.html

U.S. Department of Health and Human Services (USDHHS). (2013). *Affordable Care Act rules on expanding access to preventive services for women.* Retrieved from http://www.hhs.gov/healthcare/facts-and-features/fact-sheets/aca-rules-on-expanding-access-to-preventive-services-for-women/index.html

U.S. Environmental Protection Agency (USEPA). (2015). *Mercury compounds.* Retrieved from http://www3.epa.gov/airtoxics/hlthef/mercury.html

Williams, J. F., & Smith, V. C.; Committee on Substance Abuse. (2015). Fetal alcohol spectrum disorders. *Pediatrics, 136*(5), e1395–e1406.

Wilson, R. D., Johnson, J. A., Summers, A., Wyatt, P., Allen, V., Gagnon, A., …Society of Obstetricians and Gynecologists of Canada. (2007). Principles of human teratology: Drug, chemical, and infectious exposure. *Journal of Obstetrics and Gynaecology Canada: JOGC = Journal D'obste´Trique Et Gyne´Cologie Du Canada, 29*(11), 911–926.

World Health Organization (WHO). (2014). *Medical eligibility criteria for contraceptive use* (5th ed.). Geneva, Switzerland: WHO Press.

World Health Organization Medical Eligibility Criteria for Contraceptive Use (WHO MEC). (2010). *Medical eligibility criteria for contraceptive use* (4th ed.). Geneva, Switzerland: World Health Organization.

Zink, T. (2007). The challenge of managing families with intimate partner violence in primary care. *Primary Care Companion to the Journal of Clinical Psychiatry, 9*(6), 410–412.

CHAPTER 23

Prenatal Care and Anticipating Birth

Lisa L. Ferguson

■ PRENATAL CARE

Maternal mortality in 1920 was 690 per 100,000 births and dropped to eight per 100,000 births in 2008. Cunningham et al. (2010) attribute this decline in maternal mortality to prenatal care. Prenatal care was designed to decrease the morbidity and mortality of mothers and infants alike (Cunningham et al., 2010; Lockwood & Magriples, 2015). This is achieved by early and accurate dating of gestational age, early risk identification, continued monitoring of maternal and fetal well-being, recognition of problems with appropriate interventions, and patient education (Lockwood & Magriples, 2015). Prenatal care provides opportunities for education to assist the new mother and family in adjusting to the physical changes of pregnancy as well as the psychological adjustments required in an expanding family unit.

This chapter discusses prenatal care of the pregnant woman and her fetus. Common discomforts of pregnancy are introduced and described, and the etiology, risk factors, and treatment discussed. The structure and composition of clinic visits are defined to include screening tests, fetal well-being monitoring strategies, and patient education topics. Finally, medical conditions affecting pregnancy are outlined with strategies to manage them and points at which referral is necessary.

Discomforts of Pregnancy

NAUSEA AND VOMITING

Nausea and vomiting of pregnancy (NVP) are complaints shared by nearly 70% of women in the United States (Einarson, Piwko, & Koren, 2013). Undertreatment of NVP frequently results because of the conviction that nausea and vomiting are an expected course of pregnancy, the fear of medications harming the fetus, or the historical lack of effective pharmacological management (Niebyl & Briggs, 2014). As a result, pregnant women often experience negative impact on their quality of life (QoL) as well as adding to the economic burden on society in increased health care costs and loss of work productivity.

The cause of NVP is unclear; however, multiple theories have been proposed. Rapid rises in hormone concentrations such as estrogen and human chorionic gonadotropin (hCG); delayed or dysrhythmic gastric motility; *Helicobacter pylori* infection; and mental/emotional disturbances and stress response are all thought to contribute to nausea and vomiting in pregnancy (Smith, Refuerzo, & Ramin, 2015; Thomson, Corbin, & Leung, 2014).

Pregnancy-related risk factors include hydatidiform mole, multiple gestation, and history of previous NVP. Nonpregnancy associated causes encompass a history of nausea and vomiting while taking estrogen-derived medications, the absence of a multivitamin regimen before pregnancy, and a history of gastroesophageal reflux disease (GERD; Taylor, 2014; Thomson et al., 2014).

There are no clear diagnostic criteria for NVP, thus the diagnosis is determined by clinical presentation. Average onset of NVP is between 5 and 9 weeks of gestation and usually resolves by 20 weeks (Niebyl & Briggs, 2014; Smith et al., 2015; Thomson et al., 2014). Although symptoms may only occur in the morning, they frequently take place throughout the day. Symptoms can include "nausea, gagging, retching, dry heaving, vomiting, odor and/or food aversion" (Niebyl & Briggs, 2014, p. S31).

Initial evaluation begins with a review of weight, orthostatic blood pressure measurements, heart rate, and a urinalysis. Comparing the weight from this visit to that of the last visit reveals any weight loss sustained by the patient. Orthostatic blood pressure, heart rate, and specific gravity of the urine can indicate hydration status and need for possible IV fluids. Ketosis confirms lack of adequate food intake and must be addressed if present.

A thorough patient history related to the symptoms is paramount in determining the difference between pregnancy and nonpregnancy-related causes of nausea and vomiting. Obtain and document from the patient the onset, timing, severity, aggravating and alleviating factors, and appearance of the vomitus (Niebyl & Briggs, 2014). Emesis should not contain bile or blood if pregnancy is the cause. Often, NVP is elicited by motion, heartburn, certain foods and odors. Ask about fever, abdominal pain, change in bowel habits, headache, neck stiffness, and changes in vision (Niebyl & Briggs, 2014). What has she tried to alleviate the nausea and vomiting herself?

Physical examination encompasses assessing for signs of dehydration, such as skin turgor and mucous membrane quality; evaluation of skin and sclera color for signs of jaundice; auscultation of bowel sounds; palpation of the abdomen for masses (other than a gravid uterus), distention, elicited pain, and hepatosplenomegaly; and evaluating for costovertebral angle tenderness (CVAT).

Simple interventions such as changes in diet, avoidance of triggers, and complementary and alternative therapies should be first-line treatment for NVP (Smith et al., 2015). If her prenatal vitamin or iron preparation are contributing to nausea and vomiting, reassure her that they may be safely discontinued until her symptoms abate. She may also substitute a children's chewable vitamin that contains folic acid (FA). Encourage the patient to discover what foods she can tolerate and build her menu around these items. Avoiding things such as coffee, spicy, acidic, or high fat foods, and fried foods may be helpful. Protein-containing foods have proven to decrease nausea and should be consumed before rising from bed (Jednak et al., 1999). Several small meals, every 1 to 2 hours, should be ingested slowly throughout the day. Chilled, transparent, sour, and carbonated beverages are easier to tolerate in small amounts between meals and snacks. With a lack of research into the efficacy of diet changes on NVP, surveys given to affected women who did make dietary adjustments described moderate relief of their symptoms (Ebrahimi, Maltepe, & Einarson, 2010).

Many things may act as triggers for nausea and vomiting and should be identified and avoided. Odors such as foods, perfumes, and chemicals; optical or physical motion such as flashing lights and driving; rapid positional changes; excessive heat; and left-side lying after eating can elicit NVP (Smith et al., 2015). Efficacy of this simple technique has not been well studied.

Vitamin B_6 improves mild to moderate nausea when 25 mg is taken orally every 6 to 8 hours (Smith et al., 2015). Over-the-counter (OTC) antihistamines, such as meclizine, dimenhydrinate, and diphenhydramine, have been shown to be both safe and effective in significantly reducing nausea and vomiting in pregnancy (Smith et al., 2015). Table 23.1 contains dosing recommendations for these medications. The combination of vitamin B6 and the antihistamine doxylamine is modestly effective for symptom relief and is available both OTC (in the form of half a tablet of Unisom and the vitamin as recommended previously) and

as a prescription medication. This regimen is recommended by the American College of Obstetricians and Gynecologists (ACOG) as first-line pharmacotherapy for NVP (ACOG, 2004).

Acupressure, a mode of treatment used in Chinese medicine, has demonstrated the ability to decrease the sensation of nausea. Devices using this technique, such as SeaBands, are available in most drug stores and are easy to use (Why Seabands?, 2013). Systematic review of available research suggests that acupressure significantly reduces nausea in NVP (Lee & Frazier, 2011). Sucking on peppermint candy or consuming ginger in the form of supplements, biscuits, tea, or candy can reduce the symptoms of nausea (Smith et al., 2015; Thomson et al., 2014). Ginger capsules containing 250 mg taken by mouth four times daily are recommended. Ginger is more effective than placebo and as effective as vitamin B_6 in reducing NVP (Ding, Leach, & Bradley, 2013).

Second-line therapy can be considered in women with NVP refractory to first-line treatments. This includes the dopamine antagonists promethazine, prochlorperazine, and metoclopramide and the serotonin antagonist ondansetron (Smith et al., 2015). Metoclopramide, promethazine, prochlorperazine, and ondansetron are equally efficacious in treatment of NVP (Archer, Steinvoort, Larson, & Oderda, 2014; Smith et al., 2015). Table 23.2 demonstrates recommended dosages for these medications.

One possible risk reduction strategy is to ensure the patient is taking a daily prenatal vitamin before conception. Continuing appropriate management of preexisting GERD may forestall nausea and vomiting in some women with this condition.

HEARTBURN

Up to 85% of women describe symptoms of heartburn during pregnancy and 50% have symptoms beginning in the first trimester (Clark, Dutta, & Hankins, 2014). These symptoms have adverse effects on a pregnant woman's QoL and capability to work (Law, Maltepe, Bozzo, & Einarson, 2010; Naumann, Zelig, Napolitano, & Ko, 2012).

Heartburn manifests as many symptoms such as retrosternal pain or burning, indigestion, regurgitation, belching, and the taste of acid in the mouth (Clark et al., 2014; Malfertheiner, Malfertheiner, Kropf, Costa, & Malfertheiner, 2012). These symptoms are similar to those

TABLE 23.1	Antihistamine Dosing
Diphenhydramine	25–50 mg by mouth every 4–6 hours
Meclizine	25 mg by mouth every 4–6 hours
Dimenhydrinate	25–50 mg by mouth every 4–6 hours

TABLE 23.2	Dopamine and Serotonin Antagonist Dosing
Prochlorperazine	5–10 mg by mouth or IM every 6 hours
	25 mg rectally twice daily
Metoclopramide	10 mg by mouth or IM every 6–8 hours
Promethazine	12.5–25 mg by mouth, rectally, or IM every 4 hours
Ondansetron	4–8 mg every 8 hours

IM, intramuscular.

of myocardial infarction and panic attack and, therefore, must be differentiated from those diagnoses.

Decreased lower esophageal sphincter (LES) pressure is caused by increased progesterone, the growing uterus increasing intra-abdominal pressure, abnormal gastric emptying, and delayed small bowel transit (Clark et al., 2014; Phupong & Hanprasertpong, 2014). Estrogen and progesterone decrease the LES tone by 50% (Clark et al., 2014; Naumann et al., 2012).

Although the majority of pregnant women experience heartburn, there are risk factors that make this discomfort more likely. A prior history of heartburn will almost certainly guarantee its occurrence in pregnancy. Elevated pre-pregnancy body mass index (BMI), multiparity, advancing gestational age, and Caucasian ethnicity all increase the risk of heartburn in pregnancy (Naumann et al., 2012; Phupong & Hanprasertpong, 2014).

There are no existing diagnostic criteria for heartburn, it is diagnosed based on the clinical picture (Phupong & Hanprasertpong, 2014). Physical exam is typically normal; however, some patients may experience mid-epigastric pain (MEP) with or without palpation. History can reveal retrosternal pain, often characterized as a burning sensation; frequent burping; regurgitation of acid or stomach contents into the esophagus or mouth; or a "bad" acidic taste in the mouth. Patients may report they have tried OTC antacids such as TUMS or Maalox with or without relief.

Making the same dietary changes as are recommended in NVP can help decrease its occurrence. Lifestyle changes including elevating the head of the bed (helps diminish gastric secretion and reflux), chewing gum (stimulates saliva, helps neutralize acid), and not eating late at night are all ways to help eliminate this pregnancy discomfort (Phupong & Hanprasertpong, 2014).

OTC preparations can be used to enhance the self-management of heartburn in pregnancy. Three classes of medications that are available without a prescription and can be used safely in pregnancy are antacids, histamine-2 antagonists (H-2 blockers) and proton pump inhibitors (PPIs). Aluminum, calcium, and magnesium-containing antacids neutralize stomach acid. Histamine-2 receptor antagonists work to reduce acid production in the stomach by the parietal cells. PPIs stop the production of acid in the stomach by the proton pumps. One final OTC preparation, Gaviscon, is an alginate-based reflux suppressant and in one study showed an efficacy of 91% (Strugala et al., 2012).

Beginning pregnancy with a healthy BMI is one way to mitigate heartburn. Good medical management of heartburn before pregnancy may reduce its severity during the gestational period.

BACK PAIN

Musculoskeletal discomfort is a common complaint in pregnancy with back pain constituting the majority of those complaints. Low back pain during or after pregnancy contributes to driving up health care costs. In Scandinavian countries, one fifth of women who are pregnant take up to 7 weeks of sick time during their pregnancies as a result of back pain. Of women who experience back pain in their first pregnancy, 94% will have back pain in succeeding

pregnancies and two thirds of these women become temporarily disabled and are on leave from work (George et al., 2013).

In pregnancy, low back pain is caused by the enlarging uterus pulling the abdomen and spine forward, straining the supporting back muscles. It can also occur because the gravid uterus is exerting pressure on the nerve roots, causing sciatica. Professions requiring lifting, pushing, pulling, sitting, and twisting for long periods of time increase the risk of incurring low back pain. Other risk factors include obesity, increasing age, cigarette smoking, depression/anxiety, tall height, and decreased abdominal and spinal muscular strength.

There are no diagnostic criteria for back pain in pregnancy. The diagnosis is based on the symptoms described by the patient. To ensure there are no other physiologic causes of back pain, exploration of symptomatology and a physical exam should be done. Questions should focus on the following: onset of symptoms (abrupt or gradual); prior history of back pain and its course; history of back surgery; history of recent fall, motor vehicle accident, or other trauma; any heavy lifting, to include lifting of children; or recent fever or chills. Characterize the pain using OLDCAART: onset; location; duration; characteristic of pain; aggravating, associated, and relieving factors; and treatments done. Inspect the skin of the back for signs of bruising or trauma. Palpate the area of concern for any masses that may indicate possible muscle spasms.

Stretching exercises can be recommended for low back pain, especially in early pregnancy. Yoga is safe in pregnancy and can help strengthen back muscles. A maternity belt or band can be used to support the gravid uterus, thus relieving stress on the back muscles. These garments are readily available at department stores, maternity shops, and places such as Target and Walmart. Wearing shoes with low (not flat) heels and good arch support helps ease back pain. Using a board under a too-soft mattress can relieve back pain as can sitting in a chair with good back support or a pillow in the small of the back. Heat, cold, and massage are alternative methods to ease back pain. Tylenol may be recommended in the lowest dose that provides relief, using no more than 4 g in 24 hours. Referral for physical therapy can be given for those whose symptoms interfere with their ability to work and perform activities of daily living (ADL).

PELVIC PAIN

Pelvic pain is described in one fifth of pregnant women and becomes worse as the pregnancy advances, affecting work, ADL, and sleep (Pennick & Liddle, 2013). Many times, the etiology is musculoskeletal; however, more serious causes such as ectopic pregnancy, appendicitis, and spontaneous abortion (SAB) need to be ruled out.

In pregnancy, pelvic pain can be attributed to the stretching of any of the supporting structures in the pelvis, including the round ligaments. As the gravid uterus enlarges, it puts additional weight and therefore stress on the supporting apparatus. Ligaments resist stretching and, as a result, cause symptoms of pain such as burning, stabbing, pinching, or soreness. Other structures of the abdomen and pelvis are tested as well as the ligaments. Muscles must stretch to accommodate the growing uterus and occasionally result in a widening of the gap between the diastasis recti. The symphysis pubis begins to relax because of the effects of the hormone relaxin at about 10 to 12 weeks of gestation. Rearrangement of the pelvic organs can trigger pain and is self-limiting. Other causes of pelvic pain, which require immediate attention, are infection, appendicitis, ectopic pregnancy, ovarian mass, ovarian torsion, and SAB. Nonemergent sources of pelvic pain in pregnancy may also come from the bowels. Gas passing through the intestines can cause significant pain, as well as constipation. Advancing gestational age is the highest risk factor for pelvic pain related to pregnancy.

The clinical picture supplies the diagnosis. A history of bowel movements, recent diet, travel outside of the country, and exposure to illnesses should be elicited. Again, OLDCAART is used to assess the pain. Auscultation for bowel sounds can differentiate between gastrointestinal (GI) and other causes of pelvic pain. Palpation of the abdomen and pelvis can localize the pain and reveal any abnormal masses that may be present. A pelvic exam must be performed to detect any abnormal masses not palpable externally. Note the color and consistency of the cervical discharge and the condition of the cervix itself. Collection of a wet prep and specimen for chlamydia and gonorrhea testing is done at this time. During both external and internal palpation, distract the patient with conversation unrelated to her pain. If she is distractable, the etiology is unlikely to require a surgical response. Severe and exquisite pain requires further evaluation. An emergent ultrasound (U/S) can rule out ectopic pregnancy, ovarian masses, and ovarian torsion. It can also inform of the viability of the pregnancy if it is beyond 8 weeks.

Treat any signs of infection. The presence of numerous white blood cells in the wet prep, with or without mucopurulent discharge, warrants treatment for chlamydia and gonorrhea to protect both the mother and the fetus. Treatment of infections is discussed further in this chapter. Tylenol is the only OTC medication that can be prescribed for pain in pregnancy. If pain is severe enough for anything stronger, a referral to an OB/GYN is necessary. Most of the time, education and reassurance is all that is needed to ease the fear of pelvic pain in pregnancy. The pregnant woman should be given anticipatory guidance about how the growing uterus will affect her body. If she is aware there is a normal cause, the pain can be better understood and tolerated.

SLEEP DISTURBANCE

In 2013, Nodine and Matthews, through a literature review, described three sleep disorders in pregnancy: breathing-related sleep disorders, restless legs syndrome (RLS), and insomnia. Interrupted sleep is common in pregnancy, affecting up to 97% of women. This has traditionally been thought of as a common discomfort of pregnancy and not much effort has been put into its treatment. New research has associated sleep disturbance with negative outcomes in pregnancy, thus increasing the need for effective management strategies of these complaints.

Breathing-related sleep disorders include snoring, upper airway resistance syndrome, and obstructive sleep apnea (OSA). Diagnosis of these conditions requires a sleep study done overnight in a sleep lab. Hormonal and physiologic adaptations in pregnancy contribute to these conditions as well. Weight gain and an enlarging gravid uterus cause a rising level of the diaphragm and less space for lung expansion. The swelling of mucous membranes by the action of estrogen can lead to nasal congestion and restricted pharyngeal area. As it has been well established that these disorders are linked to hypertension in adults, increasing evidence supports an association between breathing-related sleep disorders and gestational hypertension and preeclampsia. Management of these disorders is related to the extent of the condition. For simple upper airway resistance, nasal strips have been shown to be efficacious in the nonpregnant population. Other recommendations include regulation of weight gain, elevation of the head, refraining from sleeping in the supine position, and limited ingestion of sedatives and alcohol. Efficacy of these interventions has not been evaluated in pregnancy. Management of OSA relies on continuous positive air pressure (CPAP) which is well tolerated, safe, and effective in pregnancy.

Approximately 30% of women who are pregnant experience RLS, which contributes to sleep deprivation and fatigue during waking hours (Nodine & Matthews, 2013). Diagnosis of RLS is made through data collected from a sleep history and must include all four of the following International Classification of Sleep Disorders (ICSD)-2 criteria: a strong urge to move the legs, usually accompanied by discomfort; the urge to move and discomfort occur during inactivity; movement such as stretching or walking immediately relieves the symptoms, but they recur with subsequent inactivity; and symptoms occur primarily in the evening/night (Nodine & Matthews, 2013). Iron or folate deficiencies are well-known causes of RLS, a condition which is exacerbated during pregnancy. Management strategies include sleep hygiene and lifestyle changes; massage and acupuncture; treatment of folate and iron deficiencies; and medications such as codeine, gabapentin, and zolpidem. As with any opioid, codeine should be used with caution and as a last resort for severe symptoms.

More than 80% of women suffer from insomnia at some time in their pregnancy, with complaints more prevalent in the third trimester (Nodine & Matthews, 2013). Consequences of insomnia consist of daytime sleepiness, irritability, decreased energy levels, adverse moods, increase in work accidents, car mishaps, and sick leave time. Late pregnancy insomnia has been shown to increase pain perception in labor, increase labor time, and increase rates of operative deliveries. Discomforts of pregnancy, such as back pain, nocturia, active fetal movement, breast tenderness, and leg cramps contribute to insomnia. Increases in estrogen and progesterone decrease the rapid eye movement sleep stage, increase release of cortisol (which increases arousal), and change nocturnal breathing patterns. Diagnosis is made using a sleep history and careful documentation in a sleep diary. Management of insomnia involves sleep hygiene and lifestyle changes; acupuncture; relaxation techniques such as yoga and massage; light therapy; treatment of depression; and medications such as codeine, zolpidem, diphenhydramine, and doxylamine. Again, codeine should be a last resort and used carefully in pregnancy.

SHORTNESS OF BREATH

Shortness of breath (SOB) is experienced by 60% to 70% of women during pregnancy. For the majority of women, this is a common discomfort. However, a small percentage of pregnancies can be affected by other disorders that manifest as dyspnea and must be evaluated to ensure the health and safety of the mother and fetus (Weinberger, 2015).

The onset of SOB is gradual, begins in the first or second trimester, increases in frequency in the second trimester, and stabilizes in the third trimester. It is not associated with exercise, coughing, wheezing, or pain, and is at its worst with sitting. A careful history and auscultation of the lungs will guide diagnosis. The etiology is not well known, but is likely caused by progesterone-mediated hyperventilation. Increased blood volume and cardiac output, physiologic anemia, and changes in respiratory physiology also contribute to dyspnea in pregnancy. Evaluation of dyspnea must be accomplished to differentiate between dyspnea of pregnancy and other underlying conditions such as peripartum cardiomyopathy, asthma, anemia, pulmonary embolism or edema, amniotic embolism, and preeclampsia/eclampsia.

Discussion of normal physiologic changes in pregnancy and reassurance will help the patient understand this process and reduce anxiety related to this normal discomfort of pregnancy. Advice to minimize SOB during pregnancy can include not overeating and taking frequent breaks when exercising.

Clinic Visits

INITIAL VISIT

The initial visit should occur before 10 weeks gestation to allow for recommended screening to be performed and provide early identification of risk factors that may negatively affect the pregnancy. This is an optimum time to deliver health and safety information, offer anticipatory guidance, and answer patient questions, for both first-time mothers and multiparous women.

A complete history should take place at this visit and include personal, family, and father of the baby (FOB) information. Obtain demographic data such as patient name, birth date, race, address and phone number, emergency contact information, marital status, occupation, education, primary language spoken, and FOB name and phone number. Document prior pregnancies by including gravida, full term, premature, induced abortion, SAB, ectopic, multiple births, and living children. Record menstrual history with date of last menstrual period (LMP), whether known, approximate, or unknown. Continue with a description of how many days between cycles, age of onset of menses, whether a birth control method was used at the time of conception, and the date of the first positive pregnancy test. Gather a history of prior pregnancies, noting date of delivery, gestational age, length of labor, birth weight of infant, type of delivery, whether anesthesia was used or not, place of delivery,

whether it was a preterm delivery, and list any complication of the pregnancy and/or deliveries.

It is essential to complete a comprehensive medical history of the patient and family. Although not exhaustive, Table 23.3 lists items to be included in this history. There are many patient history templates that can be used in gathering these data. ACOG offers an obstetrical history and antepartum record for sale on their bookstore website, listed in the web resources in this book's ancillary materials. The March of Dimes has made available free tablet-based software that provides screening and risk assessment of the pregnant patient. The questionnaire is quite thorough and can be downloaded from www.nchpeg.org.

Risk assessment incorporates genetic/hereditary, environmental, occupational, and recreational exposures that may pose a risk to the pregnancy. Genetic and hereditary risk factors are considered within the medical history,

TABLE 23.3	Patient and Family Medical History
Cardiovascular Disease	**Blood Dyscrasias**
Hypertension	Anemia
Arrhythmia	Thrombophilia
Congenital anomalies	
Thromboembolic disease	**Infectious Diseases**
	Herpes
Endocrine Disorder	Gonorrhea
Diabetes, including gestational	Chlamydia
Thyroid	HIV
	Syphilis
Gastrointestinal Disease	
Hepatitis	**Gynecologic History**
Gallbladder	Diethlylstilbesterol (DES)
Inflammatory bowel	exposure
	Abnormal Pap history and
Kidney Disease	treatment
Pyelonephritis	Genital tract disease or
Urinary tract infections	procedures
Congenital anomalies	
	Substance Use
Neurologic/Muscular Disorders	Alcohol
	Tobacco
Seizures	Illicit or recreational drugs
Aneurysm	
Arteriovenous malformation	**Other Indicators**
Headaches	Breast disorders
	Cancer
Psychiatric Disorders	Mental retardation
Eating disorder	Birth defects/genetic
Depression, including postpartum	disorders
Psychosis	Trauma/violence/abuse
	Blood transfusion
Autoimmune Disorder	Surgical procedures
Lupus	Hospitalizations
Rheumatoid arthritis	Allergies
	Medications
Pulmonary Disease	Nutrition
Asthma	
Tuberculosis	

but occupational, environmental, and recreational factors are not always explored there. The type of work the patient performs and the work environment can give clues to hazards she may not be aware of. A factory worker may be exposed to elevated noise and vibration levels or be required to do heavy lifting. Health care and child care workers risk exposure to infectious diseases. Cosmetologists work with chemicals that may be breathed in or absorbed through the skin. The location and type of housing a person dwells in can also contribute to unforeseen dangers such as airborne toxic chemicals and lead. Some hobbies and recreational activities can be dangerous. Sky and underwater diving are contraindicated in pregnancy. Any contact sport should be avoided. Painting, soldering, glass fusing, and welding all produce fumes, which should be well ventilated or avoided altogether. Modifiable risk factors include smoking, drug and alcohol use, and dangerous sports or activities. A discussion about smoking, drug, and alcohol cessation is warranted if these are current risk factors. Make appropriate referrals for assistance in discontinuing these behaviors.

The physical exam performed on the initial visit is similar to a well-woman exam (see Chapter 11). Vital signs are examined at every prenatal visit, before the exam, and include height, weight, temperature, respiratory rate, blood pressure, and pulse. Auscultate lung and heart sounds and a heart murmur may be appreciated. A grade II systolic ejection murmur is the physical manifestation of increased plasma volume and cardiac output and is normal in pregnancy. Palpate the thyroid for nodules; a slight increase in size typically occurs. Perform a gentle breast exam as the breasts and nipples can be very tender. Palpate the abdomen for masses; assess for CVAT. Conduct a pelvic exam, beginning with visual evaluation of the vulva. Examine for lesions, abnormal discharge, and varicosities. Palpate for masses and lymphadenopathy. Insert a speculum, noting the condition of the vaginal walls. Examine the cervix for masses, blood, and discharge. The cervical os should be closed, although in a multiparous woman, it may be gaping. This is the opportunity to take samples for a Pap smear and human papillomavirus (HPV) testing if indicated, wet prep, and testing for chlamydia and gonorrhea. Gently remove the speculum and insert two lubricated fingers into the vagina. Abdominally palpate the gravid uterus and determine its size. Palpate the adnexa for masses and tenderness. It is not necessary to search for fetal heart tones (FHT). Before 10 to 12 weeks of gestation, heart tones are not audible with a portable Doppler. The timing and elements of subsequent prenatal visits are listed in Table 23.4.

Laboratory tests usually done in addition to those gathered during the physical exam include urinalysis with culture and sensitivity, urine pregnancy test, serum rubella and varicella titers, complete blood count, ABO/Rh and antibody screen, rapid plasma reagin (RPR), HIV, hepatitis B&C, sickle cell screen, and other labs as indicated by the patient's history. A history of a first-degree relative with diabetes, patient BMI in the obese category, or a prior diagnosis of gestational diabetes warrants an early 1-hour glucose tolerance test (1°GTT). Laboratory tests performed during later visits are listed in Table 23.5.

Continued physical activity or activity begun early in the prenatal course contributes to decreased weight gain and better delivery outcomes. Any physical activity that does not involve contact such as walking, jogging, swimming, and cycling can be a part of an exercise program for the pregnant woman. Care must be taken when engaging in these activities as the center of gravity changes with increased uterine size, and the hormones relaxin and progesterone loosen the body's tendons and ligaments, rendering the patient prone to tripping. The heart rate should be kept below 140 bpm. Safety devices appropriate to the activity, such as eye protection and helmets, should be used. Sexual activity can continue during pregnancy, as long as there is no risk of preterm labor. A well-balanced diet is essential in fueling both the mother and the growing fetus. Avoid shark, swordfish, king mackerel, white or albacore tuna, and tilefish, which contain high levels of mercury. Eat no more than 12 oz of other fish and shellfish weekly. Avoid eating unpasteurized milk and soft cheeses; hot dogs, deli, and luncheon meats (unless cooked to steaming hot); and raw meat and eggs. The craving for unusual substances such as chalk, clay, laundry detergent, laundry starch, and others is called pica. Discourage the ingestion of these substances and ask the patient to inform you if she is having these cravings as they may be manifestations of iron deficiency.

Discuss the care plan with the patient. Visits will be every 4 weeks until 28 weeks. Talk to her about nausea and vomiting, heartburn, and dizziness that she may experience and strategies to treat them. Let her know you will offer her fetal aneuploidy screening at her next two visits, depending on her risk factors. Warning signs that should be discussed are bleeding and abdominal pain. She should not be experiencing any vaginal bleeding and should be evaluated either in the office or the nearest emergency room (ER) if bleeding occurs. Persistent abdominal pain should also be evaluated to rule out appendicitis or an ectopic pregnancy.

Patient vaccination status, ideally, is determined during preconceptual counseling. Often, women do not avail themselves of this service and may not be sufficiently protected from certain diseases. All women should be immunized against influenza during the recommended season. The flu is most dangerous to the young, the elderly, and pregnant women. No live vaccines are given during pregnancy because of their teratogenic effects.

Iron and FA supplementation are necessary to both maternal and fetal health. Often times, the mother cannot tolerate iron early in pregnancy because of constipation and/or nausea and vomiting. Some clinicians will recommend chewable children's vitamins to help decrease these side effects. OTC ducosate sodium is helpful in reducing constipation. If iron is not at all tolerated because of nausea and vomiting, taking it can be suspended until NVP subsides.

10 TO 12 WEEKS

At this and each subsequent visit, the following data should be obtained and assessed: patient weight, blood pressure, pulse, and FHT; signs of depression and domestic violence; and iron and FA intake. After the initial pelvic exam, there is no need to do another one unless there are signs of infection, bleeding, or abdominal pain/contractions. If a first

TABLE 23.4	Elements of Prenatal Visits							
PRENATAL VISIT	**INITIAL VISIT**	**10 TO 12 WEEKS**	**16 TO 18 WEEKS**	**22 WEEKS**	**28 WEEKS**	**32 WEEKS**	**36 WEEKS**	**38 TO 41 WEEKS**
History	Complete	Update	Update	Update	Update	Update	Update	Update
Physical Exam								
Complete	*							
BP	*	*	*	*	*	*	*	*
Weight	*	*	*	*	*	*	*	*
Pelvic/cervix exam	*							*
Fundal height	a		*	*	*	*	*	*
Fetal heart rate/position		*	*	*	*	*	*	*
Labs								
Hct or Hgb	*				*			
ABO/Rh	*							
ABS	*	If indicated			If indicated			
Pap smear		If indicated						
GTT					*			
Fetal aneuploidy screen		Offer b	Offer					
CF screen	Offer							
Urinalysis/culture	*							
Urine protein	*							
RPR	*				c			
Rubella titer	*							
GC/CT	*				c			
Hep B	*							
HIV	*				d			
Group B strep							*	
Psychosocial								
Barriers to care	*		*			*		
Housing	*		*			*		
Nutrition	*		*			*		
Smoking	*		*			*		
Substance abuse	*		*			*		
Depression	*	*	*	*	*	*	*	*
Safety	*	*	*	*	*	*	*	*

aBimanual exam.
bFirst trimester screen 11 to 14 weeks.
cRetest in third trimester if high risk.
dSome states require third trimester screen.

ABO/Rh, blood types A, B, AB, and O/rhesus blood type + or −; ABS, amniotic band syndrome; BP, blood pressure; CF, cystic fibrosis; GC/CT, gonorrhea/chlamydia trachomatis; GTT, glucose tolerance test; Hct or Hgb, hematocrit or hemoglobin; Hep B, hepatitis B; RPR, rapid plasma reagin.

TABLE 23.5	Laboratory Tests Performed During Clinic Visits
VISIT	**TEST**
Weeks 10–18	Fetal aneuploidy screening
Week 28	Rh antibody testing and RhoGAM (if not received this pregnancy); 1-hour glucose tolerance test (GTT); chlamydia/gonorrhea testing if high risk
Week 36	GBS
Weeks 28–36	HIV

GBS, group beta streptococcus.

TABLE 23.6	Weight Gain Goals in Pregnancy
BMI	**RECOMMENDED WEIGHT GAIN (LB)**
< 20	28–40
20–26	25–35
26.1–29	15–25
> 29	< 15

BMI, body mass index.

trimester fetal aneuploidy screen is desired or necessary by history, blood can be drawn between 11 and 14 weeks (Driscoll & Gross, 2009). An U/S is also done during this period to measure the fetal nuchal translucency (NT) or the amount of fluid behind the fetal neck, present in all fetuses. An excessive amount of fluid can be an indication of an aneuploidy. The serum analysis and U/S must be evaluated together in order to give a positive screen.

Preterm labor is not a concern at this stage of pregnancy. If an SAB is to occur, there exists neither the means to stop it or the ability to save the fetus. Generally, the age of viability is considered somewhere between 23 and 24 weeks. Discussion about the approximate size of the fetus and how big it will be at the next visit is appropriate. Anticipatory guidance about NVP, if this has not already been discussed, should be given. Open a dialogue on breastfeeding with the patient. The longer she has to learn and think about it, the more prepared and willing she will be to attempt it. Let her know what physiological changes she will be experiencing, such as skin changes, soft tissue swelling, physiologic anemia, weight gain, increased breast size and sensitivity, alterations in taste, and cravings.

Review lab results from the initial visit with the patient. Anticipatory guidance about the need for RhoGAM and its timing should be done if applicable. If the patient began this pregnancy with an elevated BMI or excessive weight is an issue, ask about current eating habits and review normal weight gain in pregnancy with her. A woman with a healthy BMI will gain between 25 and 35 pounds in pregnancy. Table 23.6 depicts weight gain goals for pregnancy. Emphasize that exercise is important to maternal/fetal health and delivery of the baby. Review any modifiable risk factors identified at the initial visit.

16 TO 18 WEEKS

A second trimester fetal aneuploidy screen, also known as the quad screen, can be done between 15 and 22 weeks of gestation. Maternal blood is drawn and using demographic data such as age, weight, gestational age, and race, serum factors are analyzed and the risk of aneuploidy calculated

and reported. A fetal anatomic survey is performed after 18 weeks of gestation and reports normal versus abnormal fetal anatomy.

A common concern for mothers at this stage of pregnancy is fetal movement. Quickening is the first time a mother can feel her fetus moving. This feeling can be described as bubbles, gas, or flutters. The time when quickening occurs varies with each individual and pregnancy. It can begin as early as 16 weeks to as late as 22 weeks. Reassurance that with good FHT, the absence of fetal movement is not concerning, is often enough to satisfy an anxious mom. Discuss any lab results from the last visit and follow up on modifiable risk factors. Ensure the patient is taking prenatal vitamins and FA; review nutrition in pregnancy.

22 WEEKS

Beginning with this visit, measure the fundal height. This is done with a disposable measuring tape, marked in centimeters. The zero point of the tape is placed and held on the upper edge of the symphysis pubis and pulled taut over the abdomen until the fundus is palpated. The measurement recorded is known as the fundal height and is usually within 2 cm of the estimated gestational age (EGA). Three or more centimeters greater or less than the EGA warrants an U/S to observe fetal growth.

Preterm labor education and prevention continue at this visit. Signs of preterm labor, prevention strategies, and when to seek emergency care should be discussed with the patient. Anticipatory guidance about expected body changes and fetal growth is appropriate during this visit as well. Discussion about how this family unit plans to integrate the coming new member should begin. Exploring emotions, changes in couple relationship, daily schedules, parental responsibilities, and expectations has likely already begun. Encourage continued evaluation of these topics to help ease the transition to parenthood and a new family dynamic. Continue to inquire about modifiable risk factors and attempt to mitigate any that exist. Suggest considering and enrolling in breastfeeding and childbirth education classes. Prepare the patient for the hospital stay by discussing items to bring, length of stay, and hospital policies such as number of people allowed in the delivery room, use of recording devices, and presence of children.

28 WEEKS

At this visit, a 1°GTT is ordered to screen for gestational diabetes. The only instruction for testing is that the patient needs to be fasting for the first blood draw. Inform the patient that if the test is abnormal, she will be sent for a 3°GTT that will diagnose whether she is affected by gestational diabetes. Anti-D immune globulin is given to women who are Rh(D) negative. If needed, Tdap (tetanus, diphtheria, and pertussis) vaccination is ideal for the infant if given between 27 and 36 weeks.

Continue preterm labor education and prevention, physiology of pregnancy, modifiable risk factor, and fetal growth discussions. Hospital preregistration and tour of the labor and delivery (L&D) unit can relieve some of the burden of delivery day. Discuss plans for work, such as plans to stop work before delivery, how long maternity leave will be, and even the possibility of no longer working after delivery. Teach the patient the rationale behind and how to do fetal kick counts. Give guidance on when she should seek emergency care if she is not feeling fetal movement.

32 WEEKS

Warning signs related to preeclampsia and eclampsia are given at this visit. Educate on acceptable travel restrictions for the upcoming weeks. Continue preterm labor education and prevention, physiology of pregnancy, modifiable risk factors, and fetal growth discussions.

Prompt the patient to begin considering what type of contraception she desires after delivery, where she will obtain child care, and who will be her pediatrician. Introduce the possibility of an episiotomy during delivery and reassure her about her continued ability to participate in and enjoy sex. This is also an opportunity to inform her about changing sexuality for her, her partner, and their relationship. If lab results from the last visit have not been reviewed, it can be done during this visit. Mothers with prior cesarean sections may want to discuss their desire for a vaginal birth for this pregnancy. A referral to an obstetrician will help inform her of this possibility.

36 WEEKS

At this visit, some providers will begin cervical examinations to determine the readiness for delivery. Others will not do a sterile vaginal exam unless there is an indication there will be cervical change. The fewer vaginal exams, the less likely it is to introduce infection. Leopold's maneuvers are performed during the examination to confirm fetal position. If there is any doubt of the presenting part of the fetus, a quick look with an U/S can offer confirmation. A culture of the vagina and anus is taken for group beta streptococcus (GBS) screening. In some states a third trimester HIV test is mandatory and can be done at this visit. If the patient is high risk, a repeat gonorrhea/chlamydia trachomatis (GC/CT) and RPR is recommended at this time.

Loss of the mucous plug can occur at any time, but is more likely to occur between now and delivery. Discussion that this is not a sign of imminent delivery is appropriate. Continue preterm labor education and prevention, physiology of pregnancy, modifiable risk factors, and fetal growth discussions. Introduce education about routine postpartum care and management of late pregnancy symptoms. Reiterate observing for symptoms of preeclampsia and give L&D warnings. Postpartum depression can occur as early as late third trimester; the patient should be aware of these signs and when she should seek emergency care.

38 TO 41 WEEKS

A sterile vaginal exam for cervical dilatation can be performed at this visit if the patient desires. At term, some providers will offer to "strip" or "sweep" the membranes in an attempt to induce labor. Other providers will offer advice for natural ways to induce labor. Semen contains prostaglandins, a hormone used to ripen the cervix. Intercourse, if comfortable at this point, can bring about labor. Some recommend rides down bumpy roads, drinking raspberry leaf tea, and eating borscht, based on anecdotal reports. None of these methods have been proven to bring about labor.

Discuss postpartum vaccinations for the mother, postterm pregnancy management, and breastfeeding. Preeclampsia warnings should continue to be given along with L&D warnings. Discuss GBS results and, if positive, antibiotic use in labor. Advise patient that this would be an ideal time to learn infant cardiopulmonary resuscitation (CPR) and recommend resources for classes.

POSTPARTUM (4–6 WEEKS)

Vital signs, weight, height, and BMI calculation are examined. The patient will want a baseline postpregnancy weight to evaluate her weight loss efforts. A depression screening tool such as the Edinburgh Postpartum Depression Screen (EPDS) should be administered to assess the extent, if any, of postpartum depression. A score of 12 or greater warrants referral to a mental health professional. History at this visit should include information about the delivery: infant sex and weight, EGA at time of delivery, hours of labor, type of delivery, whether anesthesia was used, and complications, if any, of the delivery. Document current state of vaginal bleeding (i.e., has her bleeding stopped, has her menses returned). A full well-woman exam is done as a postpartum exam with a few additions. The breasts are examined for redness, excessive warmth, hard, painful masses, and cracked nipples. Assess breastfeeding success and refer as needed to a lactation consultant for any breastfeeding problems. During the pelvic exam, assess the perineum for healing of any tears and/or repairs that may have been done and document. Chart any lochia that is present. Evaluate that the uterus has nearly or fully involuted. If the patient had GDM, a 6-week postpartum 2-hour GTT should be ordered to evaluate normalization of glucose tolerance.

As long as any lacerations are healed, it is okay to resume intercourse at this time. Determine the type of contraception desired, and education the patient on its use. Postpartum depression is possible up until 6 months after delivery. The mother should be aware of signs and notify her provider if any of these are present. Optimally, the infant's pediatrician will be evaluating the mother for postpartum depression at the well-baby visits.

Medical Conditions During Pregnancy

ASTHMA

Asthma is seen often in pregnancy as it is a common disease among younger females, affecting 4% to 8% of all pregnancies (Cunningham et al., 2010). Asthma in pregnancy follows the rule of thirds: one third of affected women will get better, one third will remain the same, and one third will get worse. This disease should be carefully monitored in pregnancy, as it increases the chances of SAB, vaginal hemorrhage, preeclampsia, hypertension, and prematurity (Schatz & Weinburger, 2015).

Asthma is usually a preexisting condition in which the patient is either on medication or has not been affected by the symptoms since childhood. New-onset asthma can be diagnosed with history of sudden onset when exposed to a trigger with wheezing, coughing, and/or dyspnea. Auscultation of the lungs will reveal global, high-pitched expiratory wheezing. In severe attacks, tachypnea, tachycardia, and use of accessory muscles may also be appreciated. Pulmonary function tests are used to evaluate suspected asthma. Spirometry measures forced expiratory volume in one second (FEV_1) and forced vital capacity (FVC). A decrease in the FEV_1/FVC below normal demonstrates airflow obstruction. The measured FEV_1 compared with normal predicted value describes the degree of airflow limitation. Bronchodilator response can be assessed with repeat spirometry 10 to 15 minutes after administration of a rapid-acting bronchodilator, two to four puffs. A 12% or greater increase in FEV_1 with an absolute rise in FEV_1 of a minimum of 200 mL indicates a positive response.

Initial management of asthma consists of identifying and avoiding triggers, monitoring peak expiratory flow rate (PEFR) twice daily, and education about recognizing when to seek emergency care. Pharmacological therapy may be required in pregnancy and is a stepwise approach as recommended by the Working Group on Asthma and Pregnancy of the National Asthma Education Program. Table 23.7 describes this recommended therapy. Acute exacerbations of asthma not relieved by self-treatment require immediate medical attention.

DIABETES

Diabetes affected nearly 6% of females in the United States in 2011 (Centers for Disease Control and Prevention [CDC], 2013). It is thought that the rate of diabetes has increased because of the poor Western diet and lack of exercise in the population. Certain ethnic groups tend to have higher rates, such as Hispanics and Native Americans (Akkerman et al., 2012). Lower socioeconomic status contributes because patients may not be able to afford lean meats, fresh fruits, and vegetables. Women who have preexisting diabetes must be counselled and carefully monitored during pregnancy. Some women may develop diabetes during pregnancy caused by the change in carbohydrate metabolism. Untreated diabetes in pregnancy results in stillbirth, macrosomia, increased

TABLE 23.7	Pharmacological Management of Asthma in Pregnancy
SEVERITY	**THERAPY**
Mild intermittent	Inhaled beta-agonist such as albuterol as needed
Mild persistent	Low-dose inhaled corticosteroid such as budesonide Other safe choices: cromolyn, leukotriene antagonists, or theophylline
Moderate persistent	Low-dose inhaled corticosteroid such as budesonide and long-acting beta-agonist such as salmeterol (preferred) OR Medium-dose inhaled steroids and long-acting beta-agonist if needed Other safe choices: low-dose (or medium if needed) inhaled steroids and theophylline or leukotriene antagonists
Severe persistent	High-dose inhaled corticosteroids and long-acting beta-agonist and oral steroids if needed Other safe choices: high-dose inhaled corticosteroids and theophylline and oral steroids

cesarean delivery rates, birth trauma, and infant hypoglycemia, and exposes the child to future risks of childhood obesity, gestational diabetes mellitus (GDM), diabetes mellitus (DM) type 2, and metabolic syndrome (Federico & Pridjian, 2012).

Autoimmune destruction of pancreatic beta-cells results in complete insulin deficiency and is known as DM type 1 (DM1). This form of diabetes is responsible for about 5% to 10% of the disease (American Diabetes Association, 2014). Risk factors for DM1 are genetic predisposition and ill-defined environmental factors.

Type 2 DM (DM2) is characterized by insulin resistance and relative insulin deficiency. The etiology of DM2 is unknown, likely multifactorial, and does not involve beta-cell destruction. This form accounts for 90% to 95% of all of diabetes. Risk factors include genetic predisposition, history of gestational diabetes, hypertension, hyperlipidemia, obesity, increased age, and lack of exercise (American Diabetes Association, 2014).

Insulin resistance is a normal physiological occurrence in pregnancy that begins in the second trimester. When the pancreas cannot overcome this resistance, gestational diabetes (GDM) occurs (Petraglia & D'Antona, 2014). The incidence of GDM is between 1% and 14% of all pregnancies (American Diabetes Association, 2014). Women are at increased risk for GDM if they have a personal history of GDM; Hispanic, African or Native American, South or East Asian, or Pacific Islander; first-degree relative with diabetes; BMI of greater than 30; age greater than 25; delivery of a baby more than 9 pounds; unexplained fetal loss or infant with birth defect; maternal birth weight greater than 9 pounds; glucosuria; and medical conditions associated with diabetes such as polycystic ovary syndrome, metabolic syndrome, glucocorticoid use, or hypertension (Coustan & Jovanovic, 2015).

Although 90% of women who are pregnant carry at least one risk factor for impaired glucose tolerance, nearly 3% to 20% of women diagnosed with GDM have no risk factors (Coustan & Jovanovic, 2015). As a result, screening for gestational diabetes is routinely done between 24 and 28 weeks of gestation in women who are at low or no risk of diabetes. For women who carry GDM risk factors, an early GTT should be performed during the first trimester. Diagnosis of GDM can be made based on serum glucose testing. A 1°GTT consists of a 50-g glucose-containing liquid administered orally irrespective of last oral intake. At 1-hour post-ingestion, serum glucose is measured and patients with results equal to or greater than 140 mg/dL are scheduled for a 3°GTT. The American College of Obstetricians and Gynecologists (ACOG) recommends a threshold of 135 mg/dL for patients who are ethnically at higher risk for diabetes (American Diabetes Association, 2014). In a 3°GTT, the patient drinks a 100-g glucose-containing liquid after an initial fasting blood draw. Every hour after ingestion of the glucose, blood is taken and the serum glucose level evaluated. Table 23.8 describes the diagnostic criteria required to diagnose GDM from a 3°GTT. A diagnosis of overt diabetes can be made with results of fasting glucose levels of 126 mg/dL or greater.

Risk reduction for gestational diabetes focuses on the overweight or obese patient. Weight loss and increased physical activity, during and before pregnancy, have both been demonstrated to reduce the risk of GDM in several observational studies (Artal, 2015; Coustan & Jovanovic, 2015). A healthy diet can lead to weight loss and, therefore, decrease GDM risk. The efficacy of exercise and healthy diet in reducing GDM risk increases when these two interventions are combined (Artal, 2015).

Women who have DM1 must be counselled before pregnancy and carefully monitored during the gestational period. Tight glucose control is key to a healthy pregnancy with positive outcomes. Establishing normal blood glucose levels before conception is the first step. Diet and exercise can help maintain this normal equilibrium along with correct insulin dosing. These women are typically managed with insulin therapy by an obstetrician or maternal–fetal medicine physician.

Women with DM2 and GDM must also monitor their blood glucose levels. This is done four times daily (fasting and 1–2 hours postprandial), documented, and brought to the provider for evaluation. Goals for glycemic control should be 90 to 99 mg/dL fasting, less than 140 mg/dL 1-hour postprandial, and 120 to 127 mg/dL 2 hours postprandial (Federico & Pridjian, 2012). Treatment modalities for GDM are similar to those used for risk reduction. Dietary restriction and moderate-intensity physical activity are recommended, although carbohydrate restricting that results in ketosis starvation is to be avoided (Federico & Pridjian, 2012). For those women who cannot maintain glycemic control with lifestyle interventions, referral to an obstetrician for initiation of oral glyburide, metformin, or insulin therapy is recommended.

Women with preexisting diabetes and those with poorly controlled GDM undergo regular antepartum fetal testing because of the higher risk of fetal death. U/S for fetal growth starts at 28 weeks of gestation and is reevaluated every 3 to 4 weeks. Beginning at 32 to 34 weeks of gestation, bi-weekly to weekly biophysical profile (BPP) and nonstress testing (NST) is performed. The frequency of this testing increases to twice weekly beginning at 36 weeks until delivery.

HYPERTENSION

Hypertension (HTN) is one of the most common medical conditions seen in pregnancy, affecting 5% to 10% of total pregnancies, and is the second leading cause of maternal death in the United States (Cunningham et al., 2010; National High Blood Pressure Education Program Working Group on High Blood Pressure in Pregnancy, 2000). This disease is a major factor in the incidence of stillbirths and the morbidity and mortality of the neonate. Hypertension in pregnancy contributes to the occurrence of abruption placentae, acute renal failure, cerebral hemorrhage, disseminated intravascular coagulation, and hepatic failure. Etiology of hypertensive disorders in pregnancy is not well known and is likely multifactorial. Risk factors for hypertension include obesity, advancing age, race, family history,

TABLE 23.8	Diagnostic Criteria: GDM Using the 3-Hour GTT			
	PLASMA OR SERUM GLUCOSE LEVEL[a]		**PLASMA LEVEL**[b]	
	mg/dL	**mmol/L**	**mg/dL**	**mmol/L**
Fasting	95	5.3	105	5.8
One hour	180	10.0	190	10.6
Two hours	155	8.6	165	9.2
Three hours	140	7.8	145	8.0

GDM, gestational diabetes mellitus; GTT, glucose tolerance test.
Adapted from (a) Coustan and Jovanovic (2015) and (b) the National Diabetes Data Group (1979).

decreased adult nephron mass, high sodium diet, physical inactivity, excessive alcohol intake, diabetes, dyslipidemia, certain personality traits, and depression (Basile & Bloch, 2014).

The National High Blood Pressure Education Program Working Group on High Blood Pressure in Pregnancy (2000) classifies the hypertensive diseases affecting pregnancy as follows: gestational hypertension, preeclampsia and eclampsia syndrome, preeclampsia syndrome superimposed on chronic hypertension, and chronic hypertension.

By definition, gestational hypertension is "blood pressure elevation detected for the first time after midpregnancy without proteinuria" (National High Blood Pressure Education Program Working Group on High Blood Pressure in Pregnancy, 2000, p. S3). This elevation is either systolic blood pressure (SBP) equal to or greater than 140 mmHg or diastolic blood pressure (DBP) equal to or greater than 90 mmHg. If preeclampsia syndrome does not manifest and blood pressure returns to normal before 12 weeks postpartum, the diagnosis is transient hypertension of pregnancy. However, if the blood pressure remains elevated after 12 weeks postpartum, chronic hypertension is the diagnosis (National High Blood Pressure Education Program Working Group on High Blood Pressure in Pregnancy, 2000). Management of gestational hypertension is dictated by severity, gestational age, and whether or not preeclampsia is present. Pharmacologic treatment is begun when SBP reaches 160 mmHg or greater. Methyldopa is generally the first-line therapy used by most providers. If the patient cannot tolerate the sedative side effects or blood pressure cannot be maintained below 160 mmHg systolic on methyldopa, labetalol, nifedipine, and hydralazine may be safely used. Diuretics are not used because of the risk of decreased plasma volume in the mother. Angiotensin-converting enzyme (ACE) inhibitors, angiotensin II receptor blockers (ARBs), and direct renin inhibitors are absolutely contraindicated in pregnancy. See Table 23.9 for dosing schedules related to these antihypertensives in pregnancy.

Preeclampsia affects every organ system with reduced perfusion associated with vasospasm and initiation of the coagulation cascade. It is diagnosed when the patient with gestational hypertension also presents with proteinuria (greater than or equal to 0.3 g of protein in a 24-hour urine specimen). Complaints of headache, visual disturbances, and epigastric or right upper quadrant pain in the presence of gestational hypertension without proteinuria should lead the clinician to be highly suspicious of preeclampsia. Laboratory studies such as liver enzymes and platelet count should be monitored with this diagnosis (Table 23.10). Risk factors for preeclampsia include previous history of preeclampsia or chronic hypertension, diabetes, collagen vascular, renal vascular, or renal parenchymal disease, obesity, gestation of multiples, age greater than 35 years, and African American race (National High Blood Pressure Education Program Working Group on High Blood Pressure in Pregnancy, 2000; Cunningham et al., 2010). There are no prevention strategies that have proven effective in reducing the incidence of preeclampsia. Eclampsia is diagnosed with the onset of seizures in a preeclamptic patient. Management and treatment of the patient with preeclampsia should be referred to an obstetrician.

Preeclampsia superimposed on chronic hypertension offers a poorer prognosis than either chronic hypertension or preeclampsia alone. This hypertensive disorder can be difficult to recognize, but because of its prognosis, a high degree of suspicion is warranted. The chronic hypertensive pregnant woman garners close monitoring for and early treatment of preeclampsia.

Chronic hypertension is defined as hypertension existing before pregnancy or is diagnosed before 20 weeks of gestation (Cunningham et al., 2010). Women with chronic hypertension require prenatal counseling and lifestyle modification in order to prepare for a safe and healthy pregnancy. Patients may remain on prepregnancy pharmacotherapy as long as the medication is not contraindicated for pregnant women. DBP should be maintained below 90 mmHg in these patients.

Monitoring for fetal well-being in hypertensive pregnant women is essential in producing positive birth outcomes. Accurate dating must be performed in the event that early delivery is required. A baseline fetal measurement should also be obtained to monitor growth. An U/S done between

TABLE 23.9	Hypertensive Treatment in Pregnancy	
MEDICATION	**DOSE/TIMING**	**SIDE EFFECTS**
Methyldopa	250 mg 2–3 times daily; increase every 2 days as needed (maximum dose: 3 g daily)	Slow onset of action, sedative effect, mild antihypertensive
Labetalol	100 mg twice daily, may increase as needed every 2–3 days by 100 mg twice daily (titration increments not to exceed 200 mg twice daily) until desired response is obtained	Dizziness, fatigue, nausea
Nifedipine	30–90 mg once daily as sustained release tablet, increase at 7- to 14-day intervals, maximum dose 120 mg/d	Nausea, heartburn, headache, dizziness, peripheral edema
Hydralazine	10 mg 4 times daily for the first 2 to 4 days; increase to 25 mg 4 times daily for the balance of the first week; further increase by 10 to 25 mg/dose gradually (every 2 to 5 days) to 50 mg 4 times daily (maximum: 300 mg daily in divided doses)	

TABLE 23.10	Hypertensive Lab Tests in Pregnancy
LABORATORY TEST	**COMMENT**
Hemoglobin and hematocrit	
Platelet count	
Urine protein	24-hour urine specimen for initial testing
Serum creatinine	
Serum uric acid	
Serum transaminase	
Serum albumin, lactic acid dehydrogenase, blood smear, and coagulation profile	For severe preeclampsia

18 and 20 weeks gestation will provide these data and growth can be followed through fundal height assessment. If fetal growth restriction is suspected, NST and BPP should be implemented.

BLEEDING IN PREGNANCY

Although alarming to the mother, bleeding is quite common throughout pregnancy (Norwitz & Park, 2014). Despite its frequent occurrence, bleeding in pregnancy must be evaluated when it occurs.

First trimester vaginal bleeding often does not have a known etiology. Evaluation is directed toward a definitive diagnosis, if there is one, and elimination of serious pathology. A history of the current episode of bleeding is gathered, including the onset, duration, and characteristics of bleeding (pad count, clots, and size of clots); associated symptoms such as lightheadedness, pain, and/or cramping; and passage of tissue. Prior obstetric and medical history should contain past ectopic pregnancies or miscarriages, pelvic inflammatory disease, current use of an intrauterine device (IUD), medication use, and blood dyscrasias. Obtain a serum hCG, Rh(D) typing with antibody screen, and hematocrit or hemoglobin level. Vital signs can often point to the severity of bleeding; evaluate for tachycardia, hypotension, orthostatic hypotension, and dizziness.

Physical evaluation begins with checking FHT in a gestation of greater than 10 to 12 weeks. Detection of a fetal heartbeat with a portable Doppler is reassuring of fetal well-being. Inability to locate the FHT at this gestation or greater requires further evaluation with an obstetric ultrasound. Examine the vulva for presence of blood, clots, and tissue. Insert a speculum to evaluate the vaginal walls and cervix. Look for tears, lesions, warts, abnormal discharge, and polyps. Remove any tissue visible in the vault or extruding from the cervix. All recovered tissues, whether brought in by the patient or removed by the clinician, are sent to pathology for evaluation for products of conception. Take and send specimens for chlamydia/gonorrhea testing and perform a wet prep. Visible lesions of the cervix warrant a

Pap smear. An open cervical os indicates impending abortion. Perform a bimanual exam for estimation of gestational age, presence of uterine and/or adnexal masses and pain, and palpate the internal cervical os to estimate the amount of dilatation, if any.

An obstetric U/S can help direct treatment of the woman with bleeding in pregnancy. If the pregnancy is determined to be nonviable because of lack of cardiac activity, an abortion is likely. Refer to the section on SAB for further information. An ectopic pregnancy may be detected via U/S; this is discussed in one of the following sections. Evaluation of the wet prep may reveal a large amount of white blood cells, yeast, or trichomonads. Treatment of these findings is outlined in the Vaginal Infections and STIs section. If no etiology has been found for bleeding, the patient should be reassured that the cause of bleeding is likely nothing that will jeopardize her or the baby. Regardless of the etiology, all Rh(D) negative women who bleed in pregnancy require anti-D immune globulin for protection against alloimmunization.

ECTOPIC PREGNANCY

Implantation of the blastocyst outside of the uterine cavity, known as an ectopic pregnancy, occurs in about 2% of all pregnancies, and results in 6% of deaths related to pregnancy (Cunningham et al., 2010). Until definitively excluded, all bleeding and pelvic pain in early pregnancy is thought to be an ectopic pregnancy.

Tubal damage related to sterilization, corrective surgery, or prior ectopic pregnancy gives the highest risk for an ectopic pregnancy. Other risk factors are failed contraceptive method, IUDs, prior genital/pelvic infection, smoking, prior cesarean section, multiple sex partners, history of abortion, infertility, and assistive reproductive technology.

Clinical presentation of ectopic pregnancy is diverse and is contingent on rupture of the gestation. Signs and symptoms include pelvic pain, vaginal bleeding, abdominal or pelvic tenderness. Severe sharp, stabbing, or tearing lower abdominal/pelvic pain, cervical motion tenderness, bulging of the vaginal cul-de-sac, dizziness, syncope, and neck or shoulder pain indicate a ruptured ectopic pregnancy. Frequently, women will have very elusive or no signs or symptoms of an ectopic pregnancy. Vital signs may be normal or pulse may be tachycardic and blood pressure may drop.

History concentrates on risk factors and the characteristic of bleeding and pain. A serum beta-hCG, blood typing with antibody screening, and a hematocrit must be drawn. Physical exam includes blood pressure for postural changes, abdominal palpation for tenderness and distention, speculum exam to assess bleeding, bimanual exam of the uterus for size and careful examination of the adnexa for masses and tenderness, and check for cervical motion tenderness.

Diagnosis is made using a combination of the beta-hCG levels and transvaginal ultrasound (TVUS). The U/S may reveal a frank ectopic pregnancy, an adnexal mass suggestive of an ectopic pregnancy, an intrauterine pregnancy (IUP), or no sign of pregnancy at all. Management of a frank ectopic or adnexal mass is left to the obstetrician. An

IUP with bleeding and or pain should follow the work-up for vaginal bleeding and pelvic pain. If there is no ultrasonographic evidence of a pregnancy with levels of beta-hCG equal to or greater than 2 mIU/mL, the diagnosis of pregnancy of unknown location is made with scheduled serial beta-hCG and TVUS performed under the supervision of an obstetrician. As in all cases of vaginal bleeding in an Rh(D) negative woman, ensure anti-D immune globulin is administered.

SPONTANEOUS ABORTION

Also known in lay terms as a miscarriage, a spontaneous abortion (SAB) is the premature delivery of a fetus before the age of viability. SAB incidence is highest in the first trimester with 80% occurring during this time.

Chromosomal anomalies are responsible for 55% of these early pregnancy failures (Cunningham et al., 2010). Other causes include teratogens, uterine anomalies, maternal infections, hypothyroidism, diabetes, radiation, and thrombophilias. Increased risks for SAB are advanced maternal age, a history of SAB, smoking, moderate to high alcohol use, high caffeine intake, and cocaine use.

A woman having an SAB generally presents with either vaginal bleeding and cramping or with absent FHT, via portable Doppler, in a pregnancy with an established presence of FHT. The history concentrates on the presenting symptoms and gestational age. Baseline beta-hCG and hematocrit are drawn, along with blood typing and antibody screen. A pelvic exam is performed to assess the amount of bleeding, search for fetal tissue, and assess the condition of the cervical os. Bimanual exam determines the size of the uterus and gentle probing of the internal cervical os reveals whether it is open or not. TVUS is completed in order to detect cardiac activity, first seen at about 5.5 to 6 weeks of gestation. The presence of a gestational sac with its EGA, yolk sac, and fetal pole are also components of the TVUS report.

There are five categories of SAB based on the dilatation of the internal cervical os and the whereabouts of the products of conception. A threatened abortion is one in which there is still fetal cardiac activity, the internal cervical os is closed, but the mother is suffering from vaginal bleeding. This bleeding may or may not be accompanied by pelvic pain or cramping. Watchful waiting is the intervention used in this instance. Most cases of vaginal bleeding in a threatened abortion subside and the pregnancy advances normally. In a missed abortion, the cervical os is closed and the products of conception are retained in the uterus. There may or may not be vaginal bleeding and pelvic pain in this type of abortion. Inevitable abortion is characterized by vaginal bleeding, pelvic cramping, and a dilated cervical os. Often, products of conception can be seen or felt in the os. Management of the missed and inevitable abortion can be expectant, medical, or surgical, based on the preference of the mother. In an incomplete abortion, the internal cervical os remains open while some or all products of conception remain in the uterus. Management of this type of SAB tends to be more conservative. An internal os that is open for prolonged time periods can result in uterine infection and retained products may produce hemorrhage. In a hemodynamically stable woman with a closed os, a period of expectant management of 3 to 4 weeks can be used. If products are not expelled or hemorrhage occurs, immediate surgical management is performed. In a woman with an open cervical os that does not close within 1 to 2 hours of observation, surgical evacuation is recommended (Cunningham et al., 2010; Tulandi & Al-Fozan, 2014). In addition to the aforementioned management strategies, if the patient is Rh(D) negative, anti-D immune globulin should be administered.

VAGINAL INFECTIONS AND STIs

The same vaginal infections and STIs that affect any woman and discussed in Chapter 29 can affect a pregnant woman. Etiology, risk factors, diagnostic criteria, assessment, and patient education remain the same. There are a few medication restrictions in pregnancy for treatment of vaginal infections and STIs, which are discussed here.

Yeast infections pose no danger to mother or fetus if left untreated, but can be quite uncomfortable for mom. Intravaginal imidazoles for 7 days is safe in pregnancy as well as 100,000 units of nystatin intravaginally for 14 days (obtainable from a compounding pharmacy). Terconazole has not been well studied in pregnancy and safety information regarding this treatment in pregnancy is minimal. Fluconazole should be avoided in pregnancy as it has been demonstrated to produce birth defects in women who took high doses of the drug in the first trimester of pregnancy (Sobel, 2015).

Asymptomatic bacterial vaginosis (BV) was once treated to prevent preterm labor in pregnant women; however, ACOG no longer recommends this as routine practice as it has no effect on decreasing the incidence of preterm labor in infected women (ACOG, 2012a). The three treatment options for BV in pregnancy are metronidazole 500 mg orally twice daily for 7 days, metronidazole 250 mg orally three times daily for 7 days, or clindamycin 300 mg orally twice daily for 7 days. The CDC has removed its recommendation for restriction of metronidazole in the first trimester; however, some clinicians still avoid its use in early pregnancy (Sobel, 2015).

Maternal infection with syphilis can cause fetal infection at any stage, although it is uncommon before 18 weeks of gestation (Cunningham et al., 2010). This can lead to preterm labor, fetal demise, and neonatal infection. Treatment for the pregnant woman is the same as benzathine penicillin G treatment for the nonpregnant woman. Infection discovered in the second trimester warrants referral to a maternal–fetal medicine specialist for sonographic evaluation of the placenta and fetus (Workowski & Berman, 2010). Treatment in the latter half of pregnancy can result in preterm labor and/or fetal distress if treatment triggers a Jarisch–Herxheimer reaction. Patient education should include seeking care for contractions, decreased fetal movement, and fever.

Gonorrhea in pregnancy can result in preterm labor, premature rupture of membranes, chorioamnionitis, and postpartum infection and affects all stage of pregnancy. Treatment is the same as that for nonpregnant women with the exception of doxycycline, which is contraindicated in pregnancy (Cunningham et al., 2010).

Chlamydial infection in pregnancy does not carry the risk of abortion or preterm delivery, but vertical transmission to the fetus can cause pneumonia and ophthalmia neonatorum. Treatment with azithromycin, amoxicillin, or erythromycin is safe in pregnancy at the same doses as for nonpregnant patients (Cunningham et al., 2010).

Primary herpes simplex virus (HSV) infection in the first half of pregnancy and recurrent infection near delivery offer the least risk for neonatal transmission of the disease. Risk is highest with primary infections close to delivery. That being said, treatment for outbreaks during pregnancy and prophylactic treatment beginning at 36 weeks gestation for any HSV-infected woman will provide shortened course of disease manifestation and prevent outbreaks near time of delivery. Acyclovir and valacyclovir are the only antivirals safe in pregnancy (Cunningham et al., 2010).

Genital warts, caused by the HPV, tend to grow in number and size during pregnancy and may prevent vaginal delivery by blocking the vaginal outlet. Although rare and benign, vertical transmission of HPV to the neonate can cause juvenile-onset recurrent respiratory papillomatosis. Because transmission risk is so low, the current recommendation is not to deliver infants of affected mothers via cesarean section unless the vaginal outlet is blocked, preventing vaginal delivery. Treatment of genital warts in pregnancy is limited to trichloracetic acid (TCA) or bichloracetic acid (BCA) weekly, cryotherapy, laser ablation, or surgical excision (Cunningham et al., 2010).

The care of the woman who has HIV in pregnancy, whether diagnosed previously or during pregnancy, can be complicated and is best done in consultation with a physician who has experience in treating this disease. Treatment is advised for all pregnant women infected with HIV as it decreases the risk of transmission to the fetus. If the patient is already on highly active antiretroviral therapy (HAART), she may remain on it as long as it is successful in suppressing the viral load and the treatment does not contain efavirenz (a teratogen) (Cunningham et al., 2010). Newly diagnosed pregnant women will need counseling to decide on the best course of HAART for them.

HYPEREMESIS GRAVIDARUM

Although nausea and vomiting is a common discomfort of pregnancy, when it is severe and recalcitrant to antiemetic therapy and dietary modification, it can adversely affect both mother and fetus. Hyperemesis gravidarum is severe prolonged nausea and vomiting resulting in weight loss, dehydration, and ketosis (Miller & Gilmore, 2013). Complications from this illness include rapid, excessive weight loss, esophageal rupture, Mallory–Weiss tears, hypoprothrombinemia, renal failure, and Wernicke encephalopathy (a neurologic condition resulting from thiamin deficiency that requires immediate treatment to prevent death) (So, 2015).

Elevated or rapidly increasing levels of hormones of pregnancy seem to be the cause of hyperemesis gravidarum. A woman is at increased risk for this complication with prior history of hyperemesis, a GI illness, nonsmoker, race other than Caucasian, hyperthyroidism, current or prior molar pregnancy, multiple gestation, depression or psychiatric disorder, younger age, female fetus, or diabetes (Cunningham et al., 2010; Graham, Devarajan, & Datta, 2014).

Diagnosis is based on clinical picture and laboratory results. Other underlying illnesses should be ruled out using the same work-up as recommended in NVP discussed earlier in this chapter. A weight loss of 10% or greater, ketonuria, and a urine specific gravity of greater than 1.030 are laboratory indicators of hyperemesis. Treatment involves hospitalization with IV rehydration, thiamine supplementation, IV antiemetics or corticosteroids, and in some cases, parenteral nutrition therapy (Miller & Gilmore, 2013).

ANEMIA

Anemia is defined as a drop in hemoglobin levels less than 11 g/dL (hematocrit less than 33%) in the first and last trimesters and less than 10.5 g/dL (hematocrit less than 32%) in the second (Bauer, 2014). This blood condition causes fatigue, dizziness, mild dyspnea, and weakness (Freil, 2014). In pregnancy, anemia increases the risk for venous thromboembolism, preterm delivery, and postpartum infections in the mother (Bauer, 2014; Freil, 2014; Cunningham et al., 2010).

Hematologic changes in pregnancy are responsible for creating physiologic anemia of pregnancy (Bauer, 2014). As the plasma volume increases, red blood cell production also increases, but at much smaller volume. This disproportion is at its height during the second trimester. Iron requirement in pregnancy is near 1,000 mg for a singleton gestation. With iron deficiency affecting nearly 8 million childbearing aged women in the United States, most pregnancies begin with lower iron stores than needed for support of both the mother and fetus (Cunningham et al., 2010).

Replacement of iron stores is accomplished with daily oral iron preparations, which contain 200 mg of elemental iron. Iron can cause nausea and constipation, further complicating normal discomforts of pregnancy. Ducosate sodium 100 mg twice daily will avert constipation and iron may be avoided if NVP is an issue, but should be reinstated as soon as tolerated by the patient. In a patient with severe iron deficiency anemia who cannot tolerate oral iron, parenteral therapy is given. Blood transfusion for anemia is rarely recommended.

Prepregnancy administration of iron supplements can build iron stores and decrease the incidence of iron deficiency anemia in pregnancy. Supplementation should begin 3 months before conception.

SICKLE CELL TRAIT AND DISEASE

Worldwide, 300 million people have sickle cell trait; it affects people of African, Mediterranean, Middle Eastern, Indian, and Hispanic descent (Vichinsky, 2015). Sickle cell trait does not confer sickle cell disease; however, pregnant women with this carrier condition do require prenatal counseling and increased monitoring during pregnancy. Sickle cell disease, on the other hand, increases the risk of complications for both mother and fetus. Because of the seriousness of these complications, care of the pregnant woman with sickle cell disease is best left to an experienced obstetrician.

Women with sickle cell trait are at twice the risk for asymptomatic bacteriuria and urinary tract infections (UTIs) than nonaffected pregnant women (Cunningham et al., 2010). Urinalysis should be conducted during each trimester and a symptom history obtained at each visit. History, physical, and diagnostic criteria are discussed in the next section.

URINARY TRACT INFECTIONS

The most common bacterial infection in pregnancy affects the urinary tract, and if not treated can evolve into a serious medical complication, pyelonephritis. Bacteriuria, if left untreated, can increase the risk of preterm delivery, low-birth-weight infant, and gestational hypertension (Cunningham et al., 2010; Hooton & Gupta, 2015). Many pregnant women have bacteriuria and are unaware of its presence. Others will complain of the same symptoms experienced by nonpregnant women.

Etiology of urinary tract infections (UTIs) in pregnancy is the same as in nonpregnant women. The gravid uterus exerting pressure on the bladder and relaxation of smooth muscles leading to dilatation of the ureters may assist in movement of bacteria from the bladder to the kidney, increasing the risk of pyelonephritis. Women with diabetes, sickle cell trait, and sickle cell disease are at increased risk for cystitis (Hooton & Gupta, 2015).

Often, a woman will have no complaints at the visit, but a dip of her urine will demonstrate the presence of bacteria. This is known as asymptomatic bacteriuria (ASB) and, as 25% of infected women will progress to UTIs, is treated as a UTI (Cunningham et al., 2010). Patients with frank UTIs present with painful urination. Frequency and urgency are normal physiologic changes in pregnancy and, while may be a presenting symptom, may not be helpful in diagnosis. A history of these symptoms includes timing, characteristics of dysuria, characteristics of the urine, number of times the restroom is used, how many nighttime visits occur, and presence of back or flank pain. The physical exam comprises two elements: suprapubic tenderness and CVAT. Suprapubic tenderness makes the diagnosis of cystitis more likely, but should not preclude empiric treatment if absent. The presence of CVAT accompanied by temperature greater than 100.4 is suspicious for pyelonephritis and requires referral and work-up. Diagnosis is made based on symptoms and/or urinalysis with a culture for sensitivity. A urine specimen is obtained for a urine dip, and a positive nitrite and/or leukocyte reading is indicative of a UTI. A urinalysis will reveal pyuria and bacteriuria. Most clinicians will treat a pregnant patient with complaints of a UTI, whether or not the urine dip is suspicious for infection.

Treatment using a 3-day regimen is 90% effective in curing bacteriuria (Cunningham et al., 2010). Nitrofurantoin 100 mg twice daily for 7 days is used as typical treatment in pregnancy. See Table 23.11 for other pharmacologic treatment options.

MULTIFETAL GESTATION

With advancements in infertility treatments, multifetal gestations have risen sharply in the United States in the past

TABLE 23.11	Oral Pharmacological Management of Cystitis in Pregnancy			
SINGLE-DOSE TREATMENT	**3-DAY TREATMENT**	**OTHER OPTIONS**	**TREATMENT FAILURE**	**SUPPRESSIVE THERAPY**
Amoxicillin 3 g	Amoxicillin 500 mg tid	Nitrofurantoin 100 mg qid for 10 days	Nitrofurantoin 100 mg tid for 21 days	Nitrofurantoin 100 mg at bedtime until delivery
Ampicillin 2 g	Ampicillin 250 mg tid	Nitrofurantoin 100 mg bid for 7 days		
Cephalosporin 2 g	Cephalosporin 250 mg tid	Nitrofurantoin 100 mg q hr for 10 days		
Nitrofurantoin 200 mg	Ciprofloxacin 250 mg bid	Amoxicillin 500 mg tid for 7 days		
Trimethoprim-sulfamethoxazole 320/1,600 mg	Levofloxacin 250 mg q day			
Fosfomycin 3 g	Nitrofurantoin 50 to 100 mg qid or 100 mg bid			
	Trimethoprim-sulfamethoxazole 160/800 mg bid			

bid, twice a day; q, every; qid, four times a day; tid, three times a day.

25 years (Cunningham et al., 2010). This creates an increased burden on the health care system and society because of the cost of premature births, long-term disability care, and maternal morbidity (Cunningham et al., 2010). Maternal deaths, preeclampsia, and postpartum hemorrhage risk are doubled and the risk of fetal malformation rises with multifetal gestation. Because of the increases in both maternal and fetal risks, multifetal pregnancies are considered high risk.

Outside of assisted reproductive therapy (ART), multifetal pregnancies result from either the splitting of one fertilized ovum or the fertilization of multiple separate ova. Risk factors for dizygotic (two fertilized ova) twinning include black race, maternal history of twins, increased parity, conceiving within 1 month of cessation of oral contraceptive use, obesity, height 65 inches or greater, increasing maternal age, and good nutrition (Chasen & Chervenak, 2015; Mandy, 2013; Cunningham et al., 2010). The only reliable method to diagnose multifetal pregnancy is with ultrasonography (Chasen & Chervenak, 2015). At any time during the pregnancy, demonstration of size greater than dates, based on initial bimanual exam or fundal height measurement, warrants ultrasound examination. Once identified, these high-risk pregnancies should be referred to an obstetrician.

OBESITY

In 2014, Ogden, Carroll, Kit, and Flegal reported the 2012 prevalence of obesity in women aged 20 years and greater was 36.1%. Therefore, more than one third of patients who are pregnant may present as obese. According to the CDC, obesity is defined as a BMI of 30 kg/m^2 or greater (CDC, 2012).

Obesity in pregnancy carries multiple maternal and perinatal risks. Antepartum dangers include gestational diabetes, pregnancy-associated hypertension and/or preeclampsia, postterm pregnancy, multifetal pregnancy, UTIs, OSA, miscarriage, and venous thromboembolism. Problems in labor consist of dysfunctional labor, cesarean section, shoulder dystocia, and both spontaneous and medically indicated preterm delivery. Threats to the fetus and infant are congenital anomalies and death. Postpartum risks involve postpartum infection and postpartum hemorrhage (Cunningham et al., 2010; Nuthalapaty & Rouse, 2014).

Before conception, obese women should lose weight to decrease their BMI below 30 kg/m^2, thus mitigating some of the risks obesity brings to pregnancy. Losing weight during pregnancy is not recommended. Limiting weight gain in pregnancy is a management strategy that can reduce associated risks. Cunningham et al. recommend gaining no more than 15 to 20 pounds (Cunningham et al., 2010). Meal planning and exercise work together to control weight gain in pregnancy. An early or first trimester GTT can discover an unknown diabetic condition and give providers an opportunity for early intervention. First and second trimester ultrasounds confirm gestational age, number of fetuses, and congenital defects. Routine monitoring of blood pressure will detect the onset of pregnancy-associated hypertension (Nuthalapaty & Rouse, 2014).

Obese women who have had bariatric surgery should wait 12 to 18 months after surgery to become pregnant. If gastric banding was performed, the bariatric provider should monitor the pregnant woman throughout her pregnancy for the need for band adjustments. Nutritional and vitamin deficiencies can be a problem in a patient who has had bariatric surgery and monitoring for these conditions in pregnancy is extremely important (Cunningham et al., 2010).

IUD IN SITU

Although failure rates in women who use IUDs or intrauterine systems (IUS) range from 0.2% to 0.8%, pregnancy still does occur. An IUD in situ constitutes a threat to the pregnancy and must be removed.

The majority of the time, pregnancy with IUD use occurs because of a malpositioned device or the pregnancy was undetected before insertion. Risk factors include noncompliance with abstinence before insertion and inexperienced inserting provider. The risk of SAB is higher with the IUD in place, although removing the device does not guarantee there will not be a subsequent pregnancy loss.

Generally, the patient is aware that she has an IUD in place. An ultrasound is performed to understand the position of the device in relation to the pregnancy. The patient is counselled on the risks for removal of the IUD with a current pregnancy versus the risks of leaving the IUD in situ. If the strings are visible, the IUD can be removed from the uterus or endocervical canal and disposed of. The patient should be counseled that some bleeding is normal, but she should return if she soaks two pads in an hours' time, over 2 hours (Tulandi & Al-Fozan, 2014).

■ FUTURE DIRECTIONS

Reducing the Number of Prenatal Visits

Typical prenatal care provides 16 prenatal appointments for an uncomplicated pregnancy that lasts at least 41 weeks. The National Institute of Health and Care Excellence (NICE) proposes a decreased schedule that offers 10 visits for first-time mothers and seven visits for multiparous women. This new schedule is supported by a systematic review of randomized trials that compared the outcomes of programs with four to nine appointments to programs with 13 to 14 appointments. The findings revealed that decreased number of appointments was not associated with statistically significant increase in maternal death, preterm delivery, or small for gestational age deliveries. However, there was an increase in perinatal mortality in low- to middle-income women with the decreased appointment program. Furthermore, mothers were found to be less satisfied with fewer visits. These findings prompted a shift in focus to establish which prenatal care elements are evidence based and create a program that includes these components in a manner that is tailored to patient risks (Lockwood & Magriples, 2013).

NONINVASIVE FETAL TESTING

Fetal aneuploidy testing has historically relied on maternal blood tests for screening and either chorionic villi sampling or amniocentesis for confirming diagnosis. Screening via maternal serum required multiple markers, resulting in expensive and very time-consuming testing. Newer technology has allowed the ability to analyze samples for anomalous DNA in days, more accurately than ever before. Results can be obtained at a gestation as early as 10 weeks, 1 week after sample submission, with an ability to detect 98% of Down syndrome cases and a less than 0.5% false-positive rate (ACOG, 2012b).

GROUP PRENATAL VISITS

For first time mothers and women who have had babies alike, as long as the pregnancy is progressing normally without any complications, group prenatal care can provide more patient education and improved outcomes. Centering Healthcare Institute developed CenteringPregnancy as a vehicle to provide prenatal care, highlighting education and support, to help decrease preterm births by 33% (Garretto & Bernstein, 2014). This form of prenatal care gives the provider the opportunity to provide education while encouraging family member participation, support among group members, and self-reliance. Typical total time spent on prenatal care over the course of a pregnancy is roughly 2 hours (Garretto & Bernstein, 2014). With CenteringPregnancy, about 20 hours are devoted to education in health promotion and self-management, performing prenatal examinations, and fostering peer support. This model does not affect provider productivity and allows for more in-depth discussion of pregnancy-related issues.

■ REFERENCES

Akkerman, D., Cleland, L., Croft, G., Eskuchen, K., Heim, C., Levine, A.,...Westby, E. (2012). *Routine prenatal care* (15th ed.). Bloomington, MN: Institute for Clinical Systems Improvement.

American College of Obstetricians and Gynecologists (ACOG). (2004). Practice bulletin 52: Nausea and vomiting of pregnancy. *Obstetrics and Gynecology, 103,* 803–815.

American College of Obstetricians and Gynecologists (ACOG). (2012a). *Practice bulletin 130: Prediction and prevention of preterm birth.* Retrieved from http://www.mhpa.org/_upload/ACOGPracticeBulletin No130_PredictionandPreventionofPretermBirth_Oct2012.pdf

American College of Obstetricians and Gynecologists (ACOG). (2012b). *Committee opinion 545: Noninvasive prenatal testing for fetal aneuploidy.* Retrieved from http://www.acog.org/-/media/Committee -Opinions/Committee-on-Genetics/co545.pdf?dmc=1&ts=201503 22T1046348656

American Diabetes Association. (2014). Diagnosis and classification of diabetes mellitus. *Diabetes Care, 37*(Suppl. 1), S81–S90.

Archer, M., Steinvoort, C., Larson, B., & Oderda, G. (2014). *Antiemetics drug class review* (Final report, March 2014). Salt Lake City, UT: University of Utah College of Pharmacy.

Artal, R. (2015). The role of exercise in reducing the risks of gestational diabetes mellitus in obese women. *Best Practice & Research. Clinical Obstetrics & Gynaecology, 29*(1), 123–132.

Basile, J., & Bloch, M. J. (2014). *Overview of hypertension in adults.* Retrieved from http://www.uptodate.com/contents/overview-of-hyper tension-in-adults?source=machineLearning&search=risk+factors+for+ hypertension&selectedTitle=1~150&sectionRank=1&anchor=H6#H6

Bauer, K. A. (2014). *Hematologic changes in pregnancy.* Retrieved from http://www.uptodate.com/contents/hematologic-changes-in -pregnancy?source=search_result&search=anemia+in+pregnancy&sel ectedTitle=1~150

Centers for Disease Control and Prevention (CDC). (2012). *Defining overweight and obesity.* Retrieved from http://www.cdc.gov/obesity/adult/ defining.html

Centers for Disease Control and Prevention (CDC). (2013). *Number (in millions) of civilian, noninstitutionalized persons with diagnosed diabetes, United States, 1980–2011.* Retrieved from http://www.cdc.gov/ diabetes/statistics/prev/national/figpersons.htm

Chasen, S. T., & Chervenak, F. A. (2015). *Twin pregnancy: Prenatal issues.* Retrieved from http://www.uptodate.com/contents/twin -pregnancy-prenatal-issues?source=see_link

Clark, S. M., Dutta, E., & Hankins, G. D. (2014). The outpatient management and special considerations of nausea and vomiting in pregnancy. *Seminars in Perinatology, 38*(8), 496–502.

Coustan, D. R., & Jovanovic, L. (2015). *Diabetes mellitus in pregnancy: Screening and diagnosis.* Retrieved from http://www .uptodate.com/contents/diabetes-mellitus-in-pregnancy-screening -and-diagnosis?source=search_result&search=gdm+risk+factor&selec tedTitle=1~52

Cunningham, F. G., Leveno, K. J., Bloom, S. L., Hauth, J. C., Rouse, D. J., & Spong, C. Y. (2010). *Williams obstetrics.* New York, NY: McGraw-Hill.

Ding, M., Leach, M., & Bradley, H. (2013). The effectiveness and safety of ginger for pregnancy-induced nausea and vomiting: A systematic review. *Women and Birth: Journal of the Australian College of Midwives, 26*(1), e26–e30.

Driscoll, D. A., & Gross, S. (2009). Clinical practice. Prenatal screening for aneuploidy. *New England Journal of Medicine, 360*(24), 2556–2562.

Ebrahimi, N., Maltepe, C., & Einarson, A. (2010). Optimal management of nausea and vomiting of pregnancy. *International Journal of Women's Health, 2,* 241–248. Retrieved from http://www.ncbi.nlm .nih.gov/pmc/articles/PMC2990891

Einarson, T. R., Piwko, C., & Koren, G. (2013). Prevalence of nausea and vomiting of pregnancy in the USA: A meta analysis. *Journal of Population Therapeutics and Clinical Pharmacology, 20*(2), e163– e170. Retrieved from http://europepmc.org/abstract/med/23863545

Federico, C., & Pridjian, G. (2012). An overview of gestational diabetes. In D. Bagchi & N. Sreejayan (Eds.), *Nutritional and therapeutic interventions for diabetes and metabolic syndrome* (pp. 195–207). doi:10.1016/B978–0-12-385083-6.00016–4

Freil, L. A. (2014). *Anemia in pregnancy. The Merck manual, professional edition.* Retrieved from http://www.merckmanuals.com/professional/ gynecology_and_obstetrics/pregnancy_complicated_by_disease/ anemia_in_pregnancy.html?qt=anemia&alt=sh

Garretto, D., & Bernstein, P. S. (2014). CenteringPregnancy: An innovative approach to prenatal care delivery. *American Journal of Obstetrics and Gynecology, 210*(1), 14–15.

George, J. W., Skaggs, C. D., Thompson, P. A., Nelson, D. M., Gavard, J. A., & Gross, G. A. (2013). A randomized controlled trial comparing a multimodal intervention and standard obstetrics care for low back and pelvic pain in pregnancy. *American Journal of Obstetrics and Gynecology, 208*(4), 295.e1–295.e7.

Graham, A., Devarajan, S., & Datta, S. (2014). Complications in early pregnancy. *Obstetrics, Gynaecology and Reproductive Medicine, 25*(1), 1–5.

Hooton, T. M., & Gupta, K. (2015). *Urinary tract infections and asymptomatic bacteriuria in pregnancy.* Retrieved from http://www .uptodate.com/contents/urinary-tract-infections-and-asymptomatic -bacteriuria-in-pregnancy?source=search_result&search=bacteriuria+ in+pregnancy&selectedTitle=1~150

Jednak, M. A., Shadigian, E. M., Kim, M. S., Woods, M. L., Hooper, F. G., Owyang, C., & Hasler, W. L. (1999). Protein meals reduce nausea and gastric slow wave dysrhythmic activity in first trimester pregnancy. *American Journal of Physiology, 277,* G855–e861. Retrieved from http://www.uptodate.com/contents/treatment-and-outcome-of- nausea-and-vomiting-of-pregnancy/abstract/5?utdPopup=true

Law, R., Maltepe, C., Bozzo, P., & Einarson, A. (2010). Treatment of heartburn and acid reflux associated with nausea and vomiting during pregnancy. *Canadian family physician Médecin de Famille Canadien, 56*(2), 143–144.

Lee, E. J., & Frazier, S. K. (2011). The efficacy of acupressure for symptom management: A systematic review. *Journal of Pain and Symptom Management, 42*(4), 589–603.

Lockwood, C. J., & Magriples, U. (2013). *Prenatal care (second and third trimesters)*. Retrieved from http://www.uptodate.com/contents/prenatal-care-second-and-third-trimesters

Lockwood, C. J., & Magriples, U. (2015). *Initial prenatal assessment and first trimester prenatal care*. Retrieved from http://www.uptodate.com/contents/initial-prenatal-assessment-and-first-trimester-prenatal-care

Malfertheiner, S. F., Malfertheiner, M. V., Kropf, S., Costa, S.-D., & Malfertheiner, P. (2012). A prospective longitudinal cohort study: Evolution of GERD symptoms during the course of pregnancy. *BioMed Central Gastroenterology, 12*(131). Retrieved from http://www.biomedcentral.com/1471–230X/12/131

Mandy, G. T. (2013). *Neonatal outcome, complications, and management of multiple births*. Retrieved from http://www.uptodate.com/contents/neonatal-outcome-complications-and-management-of-multiple-births?source=search_result&search=multifetal+pregnancy&selectedTitle=1~150

Miller, L., & Gilmore, K. (2013). Hyperemesis, gastrointestinal and liver disorders in pregnancy. *Obstetrics, Gynaecology and Reproductive Medicine, 23*(12), 359–363.

National Diabetes Data Group. (1979). Classification and diagnosis of diabetes mellitus and other categories of glucose intolerance. *Diabetes, 12*, 1039–1057.

National High Blood Pressure Education Program Working Group on High Blood Pressure in Pregnancy. (2000). Report of the national high blood pressure education program working group on high blood pressure in pregnancy. *American Journal of Obstetrics and Gynecology, 183*(1), S1–S22.

Naumann, C. R., Zelig, C., Napolitano, P. G., & Ko, C. W. (2012). Nausea, vomiting, and heartburn in pregnancy: A prospective look at risk, treatment, and outcome. *Journal of Maternal-Fetal & Neonatal Medicine, 25*(8), 1488–1493.

Niebyl, J. R., & Briggs, G. G. (2014). The pharmacologic management of nausea and vomiting of pregnancy. *Journal of Family Practice, 63*(Suppl. 2), S31–S37.

Nodine, P. M., & Matthews, E. E. (2013). Common sleep disorders: Management strategies and pregnancy outcomes. *Journal of Midwifery & Women's Health, 58*(4), 368–377.

Norwitz, E. R., & Park, J. S. (2014). *Overview of the etiology and evaluation of vaginal bleeding in pregnant women*. Retrieved from http://www.uptodate.com/contents/overview-of-the-etiology-and-evaluation-of-vaginal-bleeding-in-pregnant-women?source=search_result&search=bleeding+in+pregnancy&selectedTitle=1~150

Nuthalapaty, F. S., & Rouse, D. J. (2014). *The impact of obesity on female fertility and pregnancy*. Retrieved from http://www.uptodate.com/contents/the-impact-of-obesity-on-female-fertility-and-pregnancy?source=search_result&search=sleep+loss+in+pregnancy&selectedTitle=2~150

Ogden, C. L., Carroll, M. D., Kit, B. K., & Flegal, K. M. (2014). Prevalence of childhood and adult obesity in the United States, 2011–2012. *Journal of the American Medical Association, 311*(8), 806–814.

Pennick, V., & Liddle, S. D. (2013). Interventions for preventing and treating pelvic and back pain in pregnancy. *Cochran Database of Systematic Reviews, 2013*(8). doi:10.1002/14651858.CD001139.pub3

Petraglia, F., & D'Antona, D. (2014). *Maternal endocrine and metabolic adaptation to pregnancy*. Retrieved from http://www.uptodate.com/contents/maternal-endocrine-and-metabolic-adaptation-to-pregnancy?source=see_link

Phupong, V., & Hanprasertpong, T. (2014). Interventions for heartburn in pregnancy (Protocol). *The Cochrane Database of Systematic Reviews, 2014*(11). doi:10.1002/14651858.CD011379

Schatz, M., & Weinberger, S. E. (2015). *Management of asthma during pregnancy*. Retrieved from http://www.uptodate.com/contents/management-of-asthma-during-pregnancy?source=search_result&search=asthma+in+pregnancy&selectedTitle=1~150

Smith, J. A., Refuerzo, J. S., Ramin, S. M. (2015). *Treatment and outcome of nausea and vomiting of pregnancy*. Retrieved from http://www.uptodate.com/contents/treatment-and-outcome-of-nausea-and-vomiting-of-pregnancy?source=search_result&search=nausea+and+vomiting+in+pregnancy&selectedTitle=1~77

So, Y. T. (2015). *Wernicke encephalopathy*. Retrieved from http://www.uptodate.com/contents/wernicke-encephalopathy

Sobel, J. D. (2015). *Candida vulvovaginitis*. Retrieved from http://www.uptodate.com/contents/candida-vulvovaginitis?source=search_result&search=vaginal+infections+in+pregnancy&selectedTitle=1~150

Strugala, V., Bassin, J., Swales, V. S., Lindow, S. W., Dettmar, P. W., & Thomas, E. C. (2012). Assessment of the safety and efficacy of a raft-forming alginate reflux suppressant (liquid gaviscon) for the treatment of heartburn during pregnancy. *ISRN Obstetrics and Gynecology, 2012*, 481870.

Taylor, T. (2014). Treatment of nausea and vomiting in pregnancy. *Australian Prescriber, 37*(2), 42–45. Retrieved from http://www.australianprescriber.com/magazine/37/2/issue/202.pdf#page=6

Thomson, M., Corbin, R., & Leung, L. (2014). Effects of ginger for nausea and vomiting in early pregnancy: A meta-analysis. *Journal of the American Board of Family Medicine, 27*(1), 115–122.

Tulandi, T., & Al-Fozan, H. M. (2014). *Spontaneous abortion: Management*. Retrieved from http://www.uptodate.com/contents/spontaneous-abortion-management?source=see_link&anchor=H5#H5

Vichinsky, E. P. (2015). *Sickle cell trait*. Retrieved from http://www.uptodate.com/contents/sickle-cell-trait?source=search_result&search=sickle+cell+trait+pregnancy&selectedTitle=1~63

Weinberger, S. E. (2015). *Dyspnea during pregnancy*. Retrieved from http://www.uptodate.com/contents/dyspnea-during-pregnancy?source=search_result&search=shortness+of+breath+in+pregnancy&selectedTitle=1~150

Why Seabands? (Manufacturer webpage). (2013). Retrieved from http://www.sea-band.com/why-seaband

Workowski, K. A., & Berman, S.; Centers for Disease Control and Prevention (CDC). (2010). Sexually transmitted diseases treatment guidelines, 2010. *Recommendations and Reports: Morbidity and Mortality Weekly Report, 59*(RR-12), 1–110.

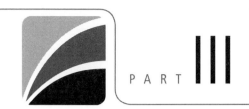

PART III

Managing Symptoms and Women's Health Considerations

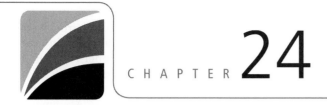

CHAPTER 24

Breast Health Considerations

Deborah G. Feigel • Kathleen Kelleher

Clinical evaluation of the breast, indications for screening and diagnostic imaging, and appropriate follow-up of findings are major issues in women's health care for patients and health care providers. Meticulous attention to examination techniques, referral for screening and diagnostic testing, and close attention to follow-up of referrals are essential for optimizing breast health through early identification of disease and the minimization of patient nonadherence and provider liability. Early detection and treatment of breast cancer is the ultimate purpose of screening and breast health care.

■ DEFINITION AND SCOPE

Anatomy

The breast is an enlarged and modified sweat gland made up of ducts and lobules. The mature breast borders the second rib or clavicle superiorly, the lateral edge of the sternum medially, the sixth rib inferiorly, and the mid-axillary line laterally. Breast tissue extends into the axillary tail of Spence. Blood is supplied from the internal mammary and lateral thoracic arteries and drains into the axillary, internal mammary, or intercostal veins. The breast lymphatics drain centrally to the axillary nodes and less often to the internal mammary or supraclavicular nodes. Muscles that surround and support the breast include the pectoralis major, pectoralis minor, serratus anterior, and latissimus dorsi.

The pigmented nipple, surrounded by the areola at the center of the breast, becomes more prominent at puberty. It enlarges and pigmentation increases during pregnancy due to increased vascularity. Montgomery tubercles, the openings of small pimple-like sebaceous glands called Montgomery glands, are located on the surface of the areola and provide lubrication during lactation. Each nipple has multiple openings for milk ducts. Each duct connects to a lactiferous sinus which then branches into a lobe containing a network of ducts and lobules. There are 12 to 18 lobes arranged around the nipple like the spokes on a wheel. The lobules end in terminal ductal lobular units (TDLUs) where milk is produced and most cancers originate. The lobule is the functional unit of the breast and consists of terminal ducts and acini. Each lobe contains an independent ductal system that transfers milk to the nipple. Milk collects in the lactiferous sinuses for breastfeeding. The breast is composed of epithelial and stromal tissue. The epithelial component consists of the ductal and lobular units. The stroma composes most of the tissue in the nonlactating breast and is made up of fibrous connective tissue and fat. Cooper's ligaments are made up of stromal tissue and attach to the skin and the fascia of the pectoralis major muscle suspending and supporting the breast parenchyma.

Breast Development

Breast development starts from the hormonal changes that begin at puberty. Estrogen stimulates the development of ducts and connective tissue. Lobes, which form after ovulation begins, are thought to be a result of progesterone secretion. Breast development stages are known as Tanner phases (1–5). Phase 1 consists of elevation of the nipple with no palpable glandular tissue or pigmentation of the areola. In phase 2, glandular tissue develops under the areola, and the nipple and breast project as a single mound. Phase 3 is marked by palpable glandular tissue and the increase in size and pigmentation of the areola. During phase 4, there is enlargement of the areola that forms a secondary mound above the level of the breast. Phase 5 is the final phase. During this phase, the breast assumes a smooth contour with no projection of the areola and nipple (Osborne & Boolbol, 2015).

Life-Cycle Variations

Young women tend to have dense breast tissue due to a larger amount of stroma and parenchyma compared to fat. Estrogen and progesterone stimulation during the menstrual cycle causes enhanced ductal and stromal proliferation resulting in fullness, nodularity, and tenderness. With the onset of menses, the decline in hormone levels cause proliferation to regress, improving breast tenderness and nodularity. Days 3 to 10 in the cycle are optimal for self-breast examination (SBE) and clinical breast examination (CBE) for accuracy and patient comfort. Pregnancy results in marked ductal and lobular proliferation that increases over the course of the pregnancy, making a CBE at the first prenatal visit an important baseline examination. After the discontinuation of breastfeeding, epithelial breast tissue regresses and the ratio of adipose tissue to parenchyma increases. In perimenopause, ductal and lobular elements regress and are replaced by adipose tissue, a process known as involution. Recent research suggests that incomplete postmenopausal involution in breast tissue may contribute to increased breast cancer risk (Milanese et al., 2006). In the postmenopausal breast, the stromal and epithelial tissue regresses and is replaced with adipose tissue; however, genetic predisposition and exogenous hormone therapy influence this process resulting in considerable variation in postmenopausal breast tissue density and nodularity.

■ BENIGN BREAST CONDITIONS

Abnormal Breast Development

Breast development before 8 years of age is known as premature telarche. This usually occurs in the first 2 years of life without other signs of puberty. It is bilateral and usually resolves without treatment in 3 to 5 years. If accompanied by other signs of puberty, before 8 years of age, it is known as precocious puberty. Precocious puberty is usually idiopathic but work-up by a pediatrician or endocrinologist is recommended.

Abnormal breast growth in adolescents such as amastia (congenital absence of the breast), Poland's syndrome (congenital absence of both the breast and pectoralis muscle), or trauma resulting in damage to the breast bud (e.g., chest-tube placement in infancy is a common cause) usually requires mammoplasty after the age of 16 years (when breast development is usually completed). Juvenile gigantomastia and hormonal or medication-induced macromastia often cause physical and emotional distress and can be treated with elective breast reduction.

Breast growth in adolescents can be uneven leading to breast asymmetry, which can be distressing. Young women often need reassurance that small differences in size are normal and may resolve with time. Major asymmetry is uncommon but may require surgical intervention if emotional distress is severe.

Polythelia, or accessory nipple tissue, is a frequently encountered congenital abnormality and can occur anywhere along the "milk line" from the axilla to the groin. Accessory mammary tissue, or polymastia, is also seen, most frequently in the axilla. This tissue may enlarge or function during pregnancy and lactation, even producing milk if associated with an accessory nipple.

Elective Breast Surgery

Once breast development is complete, women may elect to undergo elective surgery to change the appearance of their breasts. Women with significant breast asymmetry, very small, or very large breasts may have difficulty finding clothes that fit well or may wish to change their appearance for a variety of reasons.

Women with very large breasts may suffer from back pain, neck pain, shoulder grooving, and difficulty in exercising. Breast reduction (reduction mammoplasty) is often performed to lessen the physical and emotional effects of breast hypertrophy. Women need to be counseled in depth about potential risks and long-term effects. Asymmetry, significant scarring, fat necrosis, and infection may occur; however, most patients are very relieved and pleased with the results.

Breast enlargement or augmentation mammoplasty is performed by a plastic surgeon. During this procedure, an implant is placed behind the breast tissue or pectoralis muscle through a periareolar, inframammary, or transaxillary incision. Risks include contracture, infection, hematoma, and possible mammographic distortion. Implants will likely need replacement every 10 to 15 years. Mammograms in women with implants are more difficult to perform and require additional views to image all breast tissue. MRI can be used to evaluate breast implants for rupture. Decreased sexual pleasure may occur due to firmness and loss of nipple sensation. To date, there has been no reliable scientific data linking silicone implants to connective tissue diseases, and implants do not appear to increase the risk of breast cancer.

Mastopexy is performed to improve ptosis or raise sagging breasts. As a result of this procedure, scarring may be extensive and women should be counseled that ptosis may recur.

Patients undergoing elective breast surgery should follow surgical instructions carefully. A preoperative mammogram and a new baseline mammogram 6 months after surgery is usually recommended for women older than 30 years or for those women who have significant family histories for breast disease. It is important to note that breast surgery alters the mammographic appearance of breast tissue.

Breast Pain

Mastalgia can be cyclical or noncyclical and may present unilaterally or bilaterally. Mastalgia that occurs cyclically is usually considered normal and is related to hormonal stimulation of the breast during the menstrual cycle. Causes of noncyclical breast pain include large cysts, infection, benign and malignant masses, inflammatory breast cancer, hormone therapy, macromastia, ductal ecstasis, and hidradenitis supportiva. Diet and lifestyle causes of breast pain, such as caffeine, smoking, high fat diets, and iodine deficiency, have also been proposed, but not firmly established. Breast examination in women with breast pain should include a careful examination while assessing for signs suggestive of malignancy, such as a mass, asymmetry, skin changes, and/ or bloody nipple discharge. All areas of the breast including the axilla and supraclavicular and infraclavicular spaces should be examined in both sitting and supine positions. Palpation of the breast away from the chest wall with the patient sitting or in a sidelying position can help to differentiate parenchymal pain versus a chest wall etiology. Palpation of the ribs and musculature posterior to the breast mound can reproduce the pain. Mammograms and ultrasound (U/S) for focal pain should be performed. Any breast pain that occurs with redness and inflammation needs immediate evaluation to rule out inflammatory breast cancer. Persistent localized breast pain should also be referred for evaluation to rule out occult malignancy. Once breast disease is eliminated as a cause, reassurance is often the only treatment indicated. Some women anecdotally note slight relief with less caffeine, but this has not been reproduced reliably in clinical trials. Breast and chest wall pain can be treated conservatively with oral and/or topical over-the-counter nonsteroidal anti-inflammatory drugs (NSAIDs), application of ice or heat, and good support or sports bras. For severe pain, a variety of medications are available, including danazol, bromocriptine, low-dose oral contraceptives, and tamoxifen. Except for low-dose oral contraceptives, women with severe breast pain should be treated by breast specialists due to significant risk and side effect profiles associated with these other prescription medications.

Infections

Mastitis is an infection of the breast tissue that usually occurs in lactating women, but can occur infrequently in nonlactating women. Treatment with antibiotics and analgesics is indicated. If untreated, an abscess can result that usually requires surgical incision and drainage. Any breast infection not responding rapidly to antibiotic treatment should be referred to a specialist to rule out inflammatory breast cancer. Nonlactational abscesses may be more common in women who smoke, have inverted nipples, or implanted foreign bodies (such as nipple piercings). Infection of sebaceous glands and cysts may also be encountered.

Mondor's Disease

Superficial thrombophlebitis or Mondor's disease is uncommon. This condition usually results from trauma, surgery, or pregnancy, but can be spontaneous. The palpable thrombosed vein is usually linear and tender. Treatment consists of analgesics and warm compresses and does not require anticoagulation.

Nipple Discharge

Breast discharge is usually benign and may be caused by high prolactin levels, medications, or breast stimulation. History and examination should determine if the discharge is spontaneous or induced, from one duct or multiple ducts, and from one or both breasts. The discharge should be described as serous, sero-sanguinous, bloody, brown, clear, milky, green, or blue black. Frequency and amount should be documented.

Galactorrhea occurs in nonlactating women and may be caused by medications (commonly estrogens, antihypertensives, antidepressants, and antipsychotics). Galactorrhea usually is spontaneous, ample in amount, is from both breasts and from multiple ducts. Pregnancy testing should be performed if the patient is of childbearing age and prolactin levels should be obtained. Prolactin levels more than 20 ng/mL are abnormal and may indicate the presence of a pituitary adenoma or prolactinoma. Prolactin should be drawn early in the morning and should precede breast examination or any breast stimulation. An MRI or CT scan of the brain is used to evaluate the pituitary gland if prolactin levels are elevated. Other causes of galactorrhea include hypothyroidism, renal disease, and Forbes–Albright syndrome.

Pathological breast discharge is characterized as spontaneous, usually unilateral, and comes from a single duct. Persistent discharge and discharge that is sero-sanguinous, brown, or contains gross blood is worrisome and requires further evaluation to rule out malignancy. Bloody nipple discharge can occur in pregnancy due to increased vascularity. Intraductal papilloma, a benign condition that is rarely palpable, is the most common cause of bloody discharge. Breast discharge can be checked for blood with a Hemoccult card. It is important to note that absence of blood *does not rule out malignancy*. Discharge can be placed on a slide and fixed for cytological analysis; however, this is not widely recommended as a negative test is usually nondiagnostic, and a result of atypical cells may not necessarily indicate malignancy. Ductography of the breast and/or ductal lavage is sometimes used to evaluate breast discharge; however, evidence of its diagnostic value and clinical application has been mixed. Surgical removal of the duct is the standard treatment for bloody and pathological discharge.

Masses

PUBERTY/ADOLESCENCE

A normal breast bud, or mammary tissue growth at puberty, may feel like a retroareolar mass. Most breast masses in adolescence are fibroadenomas that feel smooth and rubbery on palpation, or cysts that often feel like marbles. These masses should be imaged with U/S to rule out suspicious features and should be followed carefully in adolescents and young women. Palpable masses in young women should be referred to a specialist for evaluation unless clearly benign, and biopsy should be considered if there are any suspicious clinical or imaging features. Occasionally, fibroadenomas can become very large and should be referred for surgical excision. Most fibroadenomas are benign, but can uncommonly consist of abnormal stromal hyperplasia, which then is classified as a benign or malignant phyllodes tumor. Phyllodes tumors arise from the stromal or fibrous supportive tissue, are similar in character to sarcomas, and are very rare. Treatment usually consists of wide local excision only.

Adults

A breast mass in an adult woman should be considered *cancer until proven benign*. Most masses are found by women or their partners incidentally or on SBE, and also detected by a clinician on CBE. Common masses include fibroadenomas, cysts, fibrocystic nodules and ridges, lipomas, and carcinoma. If the area in question matches symmetrically in the opposite breast, it is probably an individual finding particular to the patient, and should be referred for imaging (usually mammograms and targeted

U/S) as well as to a surgeon breast specialist if not clearly benign. Evaluation of a mass in a menstruating woman should include a thorough examination before and after menses. If the mass persists, a mammogram and targeted U/S, in all women older than 30 years, should be done. In women younger than 30 years of age, a breast mass can initially be evaluated by U/S alone. Mammogram and/or breast MRI may also be indicated.

U/S can help to determine whether a breast mass is a simple cyst, complex cyst, solid, or normal glandular tissue. Simple fluid-filled cysts may be followed without intervention, while complex cysts and solid masses may need further evaluation by aspiration, biopsy, or serial imaging follow-up. Once women have reached menopause, many palpable masses are potentially malignant. Careful evaluation is indicated, including history, date of onset, how it was discovered, practice of SBE, location, size, character, and any recent changes. Mammograms and U/S should always be performed; MRI may also be indicated.

There are multiple conditions within the breast that are found by women and their clinicians, which may be asymptomatic or result in nodularity, pain, and/or masses. Cystic breast changes are the most common due to parenchymal hormonal stimulation and cyst formation. These changes usually decrease after menopause without exogenous estrogen stimulation. Fibrocystic changes are too common to be called a disease; this common condition ranges from harmless changes in tissue, to changes that are associated with an increased risk of cancer. There is a broad group of tissue changes comprising benign breast disease, which generally fall into two categories: proliferative and nonproliferative lesions. Generally, nonproliferative lesions do not increase the risk of breast cancer, while proliferative lesions are associated with varying degrees of increased cancer risk (Table 24.1).

Nonproliferative lesions include cysts, metaplasia, adenosis, papillomas, fibroadenomas, fibrosis, and ductal ectasia. A single papilloma is a benign lesion that often occurs in the subareolar breast tissue, but can be present anywhere in the ductal system. It is the most common cause of bloody or serous nipple discharge. Papillomas are usually not palpable and are usually not seen on mammography. Multiple papillomas, or papillomatosis, is considered a proliferative lesion. Fibroadenomas are benign tumors of the stroma, are often palpable, and can be seen on mammograms and U/S. Ductal ectasia is a dilated, thickened, and tortuous duct(s). Other benign breast conditions include galactoceles, hematomas, fibroadenolipomas, lipomas, neurofibromas, tubular adenomas, sarcoidosis, diabetic mastopathy (typically seen in women with type 1 diabetes with associated retinopathy and neuropathy), and fat necrosis. Fat necrosis usually results from trauma and may feel like small firm nodules that can be difficult to differentiate from a malignancy. The presence of oil cysts on a mammogram is indicative of this condition.

Proliferative lesions associated with a small increase in risk include ductal hyperplasia without atypia, sclerosing adenosis, papillomatosis, complex fibroadenomas (fibroadenomas-associated proliferative changes, sclerosing adenosis, or papillary apocrine changes), and radial scar. Radial scar is a benign lesion found on mammography, which is not related to trauma or previous surgery. The cause is unknown. This finding usually requires a biopsy to differentiate it from carcinoma. Atypical ductal hyperplasia (ADH), atypical lobular hyperplasia (ALH), and lobular carcinoma in situ (LCIS) are proliferative lesions associated with a moderate increased risk of breast cancer. ADH can be associated with malignancy. ALH and LCIS can be associated with neighboring malignancy as well. Complex lesions containing atypia are also seen, such as atypical Papilloma, columnar alteration with atypia, or fibroadenoma associated with atypia. Referral to a surgeon for excision is necessary for all atypical lesions to exclude the possibility of breast cancer; however, most lesions will not be associated with malignancy and are considered "markers" for increased risk of cancer in either breast.

Skin Changes

Many benign skin changes can occur on the breast skin, including moles, skin tags, keloids, inclusion cysts, and sebaceous cysts. Any lesions that have changed or have an irregular appearance need prompt referral to a dermatologist for evaluation and possible biopsy. Skin retraction or dimpling is a sign of breast cancer, often advanced, but can also be associated with benign processes such as scar tissue from previous surgery. Redness or inflammation with or without peau d'orange (orange peel skin) may indicate an infection or inflammatory breast cancer.

Nipple Changes

Nipple fissures can occur in lactating women. Cleanliness, the application of lanolin, and air drying are preventive. Nipple shields and/or a referral to a lactation consultant may also be helpful. Any scaling, eczematous changes, redness, erythema, a recurring scab, and/or nonhealing area on the nipple requires prompt referral to rule out Paget's disease, a rare form of breast cancer that presents in the nipple.

■ BREAST ASSESSMENT

Clinical Breast Examination

Average risk women should have a CBE every 3 years in their 20s to 30s, and every year for women aged 40 years

TABLE 24.1	Approximate Relative Risk of Breast Cancer Associated With Benign Breast Disease and Atypia
BREAST PATHOLOGY RESULTS	**RELATIVE RISK (RR)**
Nonproliferative changes	1–2 times increase in RR
Proliferative changes	2 times increase in RR
Atypia	4 times increase in RR

and older. CBE is an effective diagnostic skill, often related to the experience and training of the examiner. Between 5% and 10% of masses are found during clinical examination. CBE may detect 3% to 45% of masses that mammography misses. The average amount of time required to perform a good CBE is 6 to 8 minutes. This time is challenged by the discomfort and embarrassment that some patients experience during a breast examination, particularly those who are young or have a history of physical or sexual abuse. A good examination needs to cover all breast tissue including the axilla. Breast awareness should be discussed with the patient with advice to report changes to her health care provider. A CBE involves visual inspection of the breasts with the woman sitting with arms at her sides, raised over head, and with shoulders hunched and her hands at waist height to evaluate any visible dimpling, puckering, or skin changes. Palpation of the entire breast (from the clavicle to the inframammary crease vertically, and the sternum to the mid-axillary line horizontally) and axilla is done with the patient sitting and supine. Supraclavicular and axillary nodes are best evaluated in the sitting position. The effectiveness of SBE has been questioned and various health agencies have ambivalent or conflicting recommendations regarding this practice. SBE may result in increased benign biopsies and psychological distress. Although recommendations are mixed, SBE or breast awareness continues to be advocated by most breast cancer organizations and clinicians. The accuracy of the practice varies with the skill of the patient. A study conducted in China found that there was no difference in breast cancer mortality rates between women who did SBE and those who did not (Thomas, 2002). Until further data are available, breast awareness continues to play an important role for younger women who are not having other screening tests and it is important for all women to monitor their own health. Women can be advised that performing SBE may result in identification of benign processes but also early detection of a malignancy. Early detection and treatment is associated with increasing survival of patients diagnosed with breast cancer. Any patient presenting with an abnormal finding should have a complete medical and breast history, including documentation of risk factors for breast cancer. A current mammogram is mandatory and a thorough CBE must be performed. Clinical examination must correlate with diagnostic findings (concordance); mammograms do not have 100% sensitivity and may miss some lesions. A negative mammogram in the presence of a clinical palpable mass *does not rule out breast cancer*.

CBE, breast imaging, and needle biopsy are referred to as "the triple test." If the triple test indicates a benign process, the likelihood of error is small; however, if there is any clinical concern, even with negative imaging, or if the patient may be nonadherent or have difficulty returning, further evaluation by a specialist should be immediate (Bleicher, 2015).

Liability and Documentation

Breast care is a critical area of patient care and a potential liability. Patient presentation, history, physical examination, all testing, and follow-up plans and visits must be documented in detail ("if it is not documented then it did not take place"). Meticulous patient education throughout the diagnostic process and follow-up is important to prevent unrealistic patient expectations, facilitate early diagnosis, and help prevent loss to follow-up and liability.

Diagnostic Testing

MAMMOGRAM

Mammography continues to be the gold standard for breast cancer screening, but has a false negative rate of 10% to 15%, with a slightly higher rate in younger women. Therefore, mammography cannot exclusively rule out cancer (Bleicher, 2015). Patients should be made aware of the shortcomings of mammography screening so as to eliminate the unrealistic expectation that a normal mammogram means there is no possibility of malignancy. False positives may also occur; 5% to 10% of all screening examinations are reported as abnormal and 80% to 90% of women with abnormal results do not have breast cancer (ACS, 2015). All mammography facilities should be accredited by the American College of Radiology. Facility certification can be verified at www.acr.org.

Types of Mammograms • Mammograms are ordered as (a) screening, a routine mammogram on a patient without a problem or as (b) a diagnostic examination in a patient with a breast complaint or abnormal examination. The screening mammogram consists of two standard views of each breast: the medial–lateral–oblique (MLO) and the cranio-caudal (CC). Diagnostic mammograms usually include more views than a four-view screening mammogram (90° medial-lateral [ML], spot compression, or magnification views). Diagnostic mammograms are indicated when a screening mammogram is abnormal, a patient has a history of breast cancer or a high-risk benign lesion, or has a new palpable mass. Diagnostic mammography is best performed with a radiologist on site, so that additional views can be taken if indicated. U/S or sonogram is usually indicated for any abnormal density or mass seen on the mammogram and for any palpable abnormality. Mammography is digital (similar to a digital camera), or analog (like a regular camera with the image printed on film). Both modalities are certified by the American College of Radiology. Digital mammography is more effective in women with dense breast tissue. Density is determined by the radiologist and is included in the report. Computer-assisted detection (CAD) is a computer program that aids the radiologist when reading digital breast films. CAD may, at best, be equivalent to double read (two radiologists) mammograms, and may lead to increased patient callbacks for additional imaging as well as more benign breast biopsies (false positives). Findings on mammograms can include nodules, asymmetry, densities, or calcifications. Mammography is the only reliable tool available for the detection of breast microcalcifications that may indicate early, therefore potentially curable, ductal carcinoma in situ (DCIS). Breast calcifications are detected commonly on screening mammograms and are most often benign and classified accordingly without any additional workup. In women with indeterminate (possibly malignant calcifications) on screening studies, additional mammogram views, such as ML and micro-focus magnification views are usually obtained to determine the need for short-term (usually 4–6 months) follow-up or biopsy.

Women may be puzzled and alarmed by calcifications and ask if they should discontinue their calcium supplements or dairy intake, and/or request a biopsy. They should be reassured that calcifications are common, most are noncancerous and related to benign tissue changes, and have no relationship to calcium intake. Worrisome calcifications are usually those that are very small (micro) and are new or increased, with a clustered or branching pattern. These patterns of calcification need further exploration to determine if a biopsy is indicated to rule out early malignancy. A breast biopsy using the mammogram to guide the biopsy (an "image-guided" biopsy) is known as a stereotactic biopsy.

Women should be given yearly prescriptions for mammograms beginning at age 40 years and follow-up should be meticulously tracked. More than seven major health organizations have recommendations on age to start and frequency of mammography. Most suggest starting at age 40 years and then repeating every 1 to 2 years (Mahon, 2007). Women with significant risk factors should have their first baseline mammogram at age 35 years or earlier if there is an abnormal examination finding or very significant family history. Furthermore, they should consider seeing a breast specialist for guidance. Health care providers need to review each patient's history individually before deciding on frequency and initiation.

The American College of Radiology Breast Imaging Reporting and Data System (BI-RADS) is a standardized reporting system resulting in an assessment of findings and recommendations. Mammogram reporting is as follows:

- BI-RADS 0: Needs additional imaging evaluation and/or earlier mammograms for comparison
- BI-RADS 1: Negative
- BI-RADS 2: Benign findings
- BI-RADS 3: Probably benign finding; short interval follow-up suggested
- BI-RADS 4: Suspicious abnormality; biopsy should be considered
- BI-RADS 5: Highly suggestive of malignancy; appropriate action should be taken
- BI-RADS 6: Known biopsy-proven malignancy; appropriate action should be taken (D'Orsi, 2005)

ULTRASOUND

U/S or sonogram is an adjunct diagnostic method for a clinical breast examination and/or mammogram and can assess the nature of a mammographic nodule, density, or palpable mass. It is also helpful in dense breasts. U/S should be ordered for further evaluation of mammographic findings and of any palpable mass, even in the setting of a normal mammogram. U/S is not helpful in diagnosing or clarifying calcifications. It is used as guidance for core breast biopsies, fine needle aspiration (FNA), and cyst aspiration. Its low specificity and high false positive rate means the use of U/S, in the general population, is uncertain. There is no evidence to screen asymptomatic women with this modality (Mahon, 2007).

MAGNETIC RESONANCE IMAGING

Breast MRI is a costly examination that may be very helpful in assessing high-risk patients or those with very dense breast tissue, and is an adjunct to standard breast imaging. Breast MRI images breast tissue using a magnet, not ionizing radiation. A breast MRI can cost much more than $1,200, making it a substantially more expensive test than mammograms and U/S. The cost of a breast MRI may not be covered by health insurance and usually requires preauthorization. Breast MRI may be indicated in women who are newly diagnosed with breast cancer to rule out occult locally advanced disease, multifocal disease (more than a single tumor), and contralateral disease (cancer in the opposite breast; Mahon, 2007).

MRI may also be helpful in high-risk women. The American Cancer Society (ACS) recently published guidelines for MRI screening in high-risk women (ACS, 2015). The ACS recommends MRI screening in women (a) with a documented breast cancer (BRCA) 1 or 2 mutation; (b) with an untested blood relative of a BRCA mutation carrier; (c) with a 20% to 25% or greater lifetime risk of breast cancer based on accepted risk calculation models; (d) who have received chest radiation (such as for lymphoma) between ages 10 and 30 years; and (e) with several other less common genetic abnormalities involving genetic mutations in gene TP53 (Li-Fraumeni syndrome), and PTEN (Cowden and Bannayan–Riley–Ruvalcaba syndromes) and their first-degree relatives (ACS, 2015). MRI is also indicated when findings are indeterminate after a conventional imaging work-up, for evaluation of the effect of neoadjuvant chemotherapy, and when evaluating the local extent of disease in patients with known cancer (Saslow, 2007).

BIOPSY

Patients who are found to have a suspicious palpable mass or suspicious density or calcifications on mammogram or U/S need to have breast tissue sampled for an accurate diagnosis. The goal of any method of biopsy is to remove as little tissue as possible, and to make the diagnosis with as little trauma as possible and with as close to 100% accuracy as possible. Biopsies can be performed in multiple ways. The simplest is FNA, which may or may not require local anesthesia. When performing FNA, a small gauge needle is inserted into the abnormal area and the cells that are sheared off are fixed on a slide and analyzed. If the abnormality is a cyst, the fluid can be sent for cytology. Aspiration should resolve a cyst and it should not reoccur. If it does not disappear or if it reoccurs, further assessment is required. FNA does not allow for histological (tissue) examination; instead, FNA consists only of examination of the cells placed on the slide. FNA performed with image guidance tends to be more accurate than without. A negative FNA does not rule out malignancy.

A core needle biopsy (CNB) can be performed under mammogram (stereotactic), U/S, or MRI guidance for almost any abnormality, and without imaging guidance for a palpable mass. It is performed with a large gauge needle to obtain tissue "cores" following injection of a local anesthetic. CNB provides breast tissue for architecture and histology and can usually rule out breast cancer if the histology is concordant (makes sense) with the imaging. Stereotactic CNB is performed using the mammogram as a guide. A three-dimensional mammographic image is obtained with the patient in a prone, sitting, or sidelying position and a computer helps the radiologist or surgeon guide the needle placement. CNB is performed in a radiology department under a radiologist's guidance. If findings from a core biopsy are inconclusive (not concordant), a surgical biopsy may be required.

An MRI-guided CNB is done when the lesion is best visualized or only seen on an MRI. The same CNB technique is used as described earlier, except that the biopsy must be approached from the lateral breast, making biopsies in the medial breast somewhat more challenging. In most image-guided biopsies a small surgical marker is placed at the site of the biopsy to provide guidance for the surgeon, if surgery is necessary or to provide a reference area for future mammographic evaluation.

SURGICAL BIOPSY

Incisional biopsy removes a piece of the mass and is used for diagnosis alone. Excisional biopsy of a palpable mass (removing the entire lump) is also done for diagnosis, but may also serve as treatment (e.g., removing the lump). Cancer treatment is usually not accomplished with excisional biopsy alone.

If a lesion is nonpalpable (such as with calcifications), and is seen on a mammogram or U/S, it must be localized for the surgeon before excision. This is accomplished by the radiologist placing a thin surgical wire through or next to the site (wire localization) to guide the surgeon. Placement is confirmed by mammogram and the surgeon removes the tissue around the wire. The specimen removed is x-rayed to confirm that the correct tissue was obtained. For the purposes of diagnosing a breast abnormality, wire localization has largely been replaced in tertiary care and cancer centers where patients have access to CNB. Core biopsy allows diagnosis and cancer surgery planning without a surgical procedure for diagnosis alone. Excisional biopsy is necessary with lesions that cannot be reached with CNB (such as a very far posterior lesion), vague lesions where risk of a false negative is higher, in patients without access to CNB, and for discordant CNB histology (e.g., the mammogram is highly suspicious for cancer but the biopsy shows completely normal breast tissue).

The majority of CNBs performed are found to be benign. Those that are cancerous will almost always require surgery (the biopsy only samples the area and does not remove it completely). Additional surgery is required to obtain clear margins when excisional biopsy has been performed leaving residual cancer in the breast. Surgical evaluation of the lymph nodes may also be necessary. Bruising and slight tenderness are very common after CNB and surgical biopsy. A good support bra, ice, and over-the-counter analgesics are usually all that are required for pain relief. Small hematomas often occur, but large hematomas are not uncommon. If a patient requires anticoagulation for a medical reason, consultation with the patient's primary physician is indicated regarding the suspension of therapy before biopsy and or surgery.

■ BREAST CANCER

Breast cancer is the most common female malignancy and the second leading cause of cancer death in women (lung cancer is the first; ACS, 2015). One in eight women will develop breast cancer in her lifetime and risk increases with age. It was estimated that 231,840 cases of invasive breast cancer, 62,530 in situ breast cancers, and about 40,000 deaths would occur in the United States in 2015. Furthermore, of all the cases estimated in 2015 for breast cancer, 2,360 were estimated to occur in men (ACS, 2015). The cause of most breast cancer is unknown and is probably multifactorial. Breast tumors are most often sporadic while a small portion is attributed to inherited familial syndromes. Hormone therapy and radiation may also be causative. Dietary fat intake and body weight have been studied, but have not been shown to be causative (Willett et al., 2015).

Breast cancer can develop anywhere in the breast, and anywhere there is breast tissue, including the axilla and in the inframammary crease. Breast cancer may be present for 5 years or more before it becomes palpable and begins in the terminal ductal lobular unit. Noninvasive or in situ breast cancer that is contained within the ducts is known as DCIS. DCIS is most often treated by wire-localized lumpectomy followed by radiation; however, debate is ongoing about optimal treatment. Some patients with DCIS will eventually develop invasive carcinomas but it is impossible to predict which patients will advance or not (ACS, 2015). LCIS is not considered a malignancy or noninvasive cancer, but is a marker for increased risk of future breast cancer in either breast.

Invasive cancer breaks through the basement membrane of the duct or lobule, thereby gaining access to blood vessels and the lymphatic system, giving it the ability to spread outside of the breast. Biopsy and surgery establish the type and extent of disease.

Risk Factors for Developing Breast Cancer

1. The *number one risk factor* for breast cancer is being female.
2. *Age* is the second most significant risk factor.
3. *Family history of breast cancer*, particularly in first-degree relatives (parent, sibling, and child), increases risk; however, only 5% to 10% of breast cancer is classified as hereditary. Inherited breast cancer involves the BRCA 1 or BRCA 2 tumor suppressor genes. Mutations of these genes result in an increased risk of cancer at an earlier age, in both breasts, and an increased risk of ovarian cancer. Males can carry these genes and may have an increased risk of early prostate and male breast cancer. Many mutations have been identified and are inherited from either the maternal or paternal side in an autosomal dominant manner. Carriers of BRCA 1 have a 65% chance of developing breast cancer by age 70 years, and BRCA 2 carriers a 45% chance (Antoniou et al., 2003). Screening an MRI and/or consideration of prophylactic/preventive mastectomy and/or oophorectomy

may be recommended. Genetic counseling should be conducted and is often advised before genetic testing due to medical, ethical, psychosocial, legal, and privacy issues. Other genetic disorders that may predispose women to breast cancer include Li-Fraumeni syndrome, Cowden syndrome, Bannayan–Riley–Ruvalcaba syndrome, and Peutz-Jeghers syndrome (Garber & Offit, 2005). Genetic counselors play an essential role in decision making related to this type of testing, together with the patient's other health care providers who need to assist the patient with decisions as testing has become more available. Probability tools to evaluate the need for genetic testing in women at potential risk are used. Careful selection is important due to cost and ethical issues including possible insurance discrimination, although national legislation has made this practice illegal. The results may often have a strong emotional impact on a patient and family members who may require supportive intervention.

4. *Reproductive factors* such as age at menarche (less than 12 years), menopause (greater than 55 years) and first birth (later or no children = increased risk), and long-term exogenous hormone exposure are factors in increased breast cancer risk. The Women's Health Initiative reported that women without a uterus, who used exogenous estrogen alone, did not have an increased risk for developing breast cancer at 8 years of follow-up (Ravdin et al., 2007). Findings did support an increase in breast cancer risk in women with a uterus who used exogenous estrogen and progesterone in combination at 4 years of therapy (Rossouw et al., 2007). Oral contraceptives do not seem to increase risk (Willett et al., 2015).

5. *Ethnicity*: Breast cancer incidence is higher in White women but risk of death from breast cancer is higher in minority women (ACS, 2015). Later identification, more aggressive and hormone-negative tumors, and shorter time to recurrence are factors lending to this difference. Racial disparities may exist in treatment and access to screening (Centers for Disease Control [CDC], 2012). Incidence for African American women younger than 35 years is twice the rate for young White women and the mortality rate is three times higher (ACS, 2015). African American women have fewer mammograms than Caucasian women of the same socioeconomic status (ACS, 2015; CDC, 2012). Caregiving responsibilities are often described as impediments to annual screening. Patients might be asked about their ability to follow through on recommended testing by their health care provider. Latinas have lower breast cancer rates but tend to be diagnosed later, possibly contributing to more aggressive disease. Asian women have lower risk; however, the risk increases after immigration to the United States (Willett et al., 2015).

6. *Previous breast biopsies and history of ADH, ALH, or LCIS*: Atypical hyperplasia is associated with a fourfold increase in relative risk of breast cancer (Degnim et al., 2007). LCIS is not considered as a noninvasive cancer and is a marker for increased risk

of future breast cancer in either breast. DCIS confers a significantly elevated risk of associated and future invasive breast cancer and is usually managed similarly to invasive carcinoma (described later in this chapter).

7. *Exposure to ionizing radiation*: Radiation treatment to the chest, for conditions such as lymphoma and benign thyroid disease, increases risk (Willett et al., 2015).

8. *Alcohol intake*: Women who consume more than one to two alcoholic beverages per day have a higher risk of breast cancer than those who do not. Alcohol may impact endogenous estrogen levels (Willett et al., 2015).

9. *Obesity*: Recent evidence suggests obesity may be a risk factor, particularly in postmenopausal women (Willett et al., 2015). Weight loss has the potential to change breast cancer incidence, morbidity, and mortality (Gucalp, Morris, Hudis, & Dannenberg, 2015).

10. *Breastfeeding*: Studies show a probable protective benefit of breast feeding (Willett et al., 2015).

There is no scientific evidence that breast implants, abortions, or deodorants cause or increase the risk of breast cancer (Willett et al., 2015).

Risk Assessment

The known risk factors that place a woman at greater risk of developing breast cancer need to be considered to individualize patient care. Clinical tools, such as the Gail model and Claus model (discussed later in this chapter) are used in assessing breast cancer risk and can assist health care providers in their practice. Women who are identified to have increased risk should be closely followed with yearly mammograms (age appropriate), early CBE, possibly screening breast MRI (as per ACS guidelines), and be encouraged to perform regular SBE.

Risk Modification

In addition to very close clinical and radiologic monitoring of women who have been determined to be at increased risk, modification and reduction of risk should be considered and discussed. Most risk factors are not modifiable (e.g., age, family history, age at first childbirth), while others are modifiable lifestyle choices, which are not easily or realistically changed (e.g., alcohol consumption). Risk modification should include a discussion about, for example, avoidance or reduction in alcohol intake, and either reduction in dosage or the possibility of eliminating hormone therapy. Surveillance Epidemiology and End Results (SEER), a program of the National Cancer Institute, data supports women stopping or not starting hormone replacement therapy (HRT; CDC, 2007). Publication of findings from the Women's Health Initiative (WHI) in 2002 was likely a contributing factor for the observed national decrease in breast cancer rates in subsequent years (Ravdin et al., 2007; Rossouw, 2002). No solid data exist supporting increased physical activity and reduced fat intake as a means for decreasing breast cancer risk; however, there is a trend suggesting that these actions may be helpful. Women who lowered their dietary fat in the WHI had a lower incidence of hormone-receptor–positive breast cancer (Prentice et al., 2006). Weight gain before and after menopause is associated with increased risk. Encouraging patients to lose excess weight for the purpose of decreasing breast cancer risk may motivate improvement in diet and exercise levels (Eliassen, Colditz, Rosner, Willett, & Hankinson, 2006). A healthy diet and exercise are also overwhelmingly beneficial in reducing the risk of heart and vascular disease, both of which contribute to the death of four times more women than breast cancer each year in the United States.

Chemoprevention

A woman's breast cancer risk can be assessed with the use of a breast cancer risk model. Several models are available and easily accessible. The Gail model is available on a disk from the National Cancer Institute (www.cancer.gov) or online at www.cancer.gov/bcrisktool. This model can underestimate risk in women with a possible genetic predisposition to breast cancer because it does not calculate for second-degree affected relatives, early age at diagnosis, and family history of ovarian cancer. The Claus model estimates risk solely based on family history, ages at cancer diagnosis, and patient age. It does not identify individual breast cancer risk but predicts the probability of finding a BRCA mutation. BRCAPro (among other models) predicts risk of carrying a BRCA mutation based on family history (available at www.southwestern.edu). The IBIS or Tyrer-Cuzick model (www.ems-trials.org/riskevaluator) assesses more family members than only first degree, and also incorporates hormone use, menarche, and family incidence of ovarian cancer. There is no perfect model to assess risk in any one patient and genetic counselors often use several models to assess risk.

Myriad Genetics also has a tool that predicts for BRCA mutations and is available online through Myriad and can be downloaded (www.myriad.com). In women suspected of carrying a mutation, a referral for genetic counseling is highly recommended. Women with a greater than or equal to 1.67% 5-year risk of developing breast cancer, based on the Gail model, should consider medication to reduce breast cancer risk (chemoprevention; Vogel, 2006). Tamoxifen, a selective estrogen receptor modulator (SERM) that is also used for treatment of breast cancer, has been shown to reduce the risk of breast cancer by up to 49% over 5 years in this population of women at increased risk for developing breast cancer (Vogel, 2006). The SERM raloxifene has been shown to have a similar preventive effect with fewer risks (Vogel, 2006). Raloxifene has been approved by the Food and Drug Administration (FDA) for breast cancer risk reduction. Breast cancer treatment drugs called aromatase inhibitors (AIs), such as anastrazole, letrozole, and exemestane, by reducing estrogen levels, show promise in reducing breast cancer risk and risk of recurrence by 50%, but may lessen bone density (Rimawi & Osborne, 2015).

Tamoxifen and raloxifene have potentially significant risks and side effects. Some women who would benefit from risk-reduction medication have opted not to, due to fear of complications or underestimation of benefits (Rimawi & Osborne, 2015). Health care providers need to be familiar with assessing breast cancer risk and discussing prevention options in high-risk patients; or referring patients to a breast specialist, genetic counselor, or medical oncologist for careful consideration of preventive medications. Careful consideration of risks and benefits are essential as there are risks associated with these medications (Gradishar & Cella, 2006). Women are frequently not made aware of their risk status and therefore not afforded the opportunity to participate in discussions that can lead to informed decisions about preventive treatment options (Salant, Ganschow, Olopade, & Lauderdale, 2006). High-risk women considering risk-reduction drug therapy are best referred to and monitored by a specialist.

Surgical Prophylaxis

In women who have a very significant lifetime risk of breast cancer (such as BRCA mutation carriers), prophylactic mastectomy can be considered. Prophylactic mastectomy is performed by a surgeon and/or plastic surgeon, and reduces the woman's lifetime risk of breast cancer by more than 90%. The emotional toll of this type of surgery and the physical changes that will result need to be thoroughly discussed with the patient by her surgeon.

Types of Breast Cancer

Malignant changes usually occur in the ducts or lobules of the breast. Approximately 80% of breast cancers originate in the ducts and most of the remaining 20% in the lobules. Noninvasive breast cancer is classified as DCIS. DCIS is further classified by growth pattern and architecture, which includes comedo, noncomedo, solid, cribiform, micropapillary, and papillary types. DCIS is a breast cancer precursor at its earliest and the most curable stage and is comprised of a neoplastic lesion confined to the ducts and lobules of the breast. DCIS is often discovered by abnormal calcifications seen on a mammography and now accounts for up to 20% of newly diagnosed breast cancers.

Ideal local therapy (surgery and/or radiation) for treatment of DCIS is currently being debated. The goal of treatment for DCIS involves reducing the risk of a recurrent ipsilateral or contralateral breast cancer. It is generally agreed on that DCIS should be treated by wide surgical excision (lumpectomy and related procedures) or by mastectomy if extensive. Radiation to the breast following excision (breast conservation therapy [BCT]) is currently considered standard of care; however, controversy exists in the breast cancer treatment community on how much treatment for DCIS is required. Studies have been done or are underway using tumor characteristics and genetics to determine risk stratification and thus determine which patients may benefit from surgery alone (Hughes et. al., 2009). However, risk stratification to determine treatment is not being performed outside of the clinical trial setting. Systemic therapy such as tamoxifen does reduce the risk of ipsilateral or contralateral breast cancers in patients treated with BCT and estrogen-receptor–positive tumors (Wapnir et al., 2011). The 2013 National Comprehensive Cancer Network (NCCN) guidelines recommend women with estrogen-receptor-positive tumors consider the addition of tamoxifen after BCT and in women undergoing surgical excision alone. The incidence of DCIS is increasing; this is thought to be due to better mammographic imaging and biopsy techniques, and more women having mammograms. Although DCIS is an early and most likely curable breast cancer, it is still a difficult and stressful diagnosis as most women consider DCIS no different from invasive cancers when initially diagnosed. Clinicians can be helpful by supporting and reassuring patients and referring them to support groups and or reliable resources (Nekhlyudov, Kroenke, Jung, Holmes, & Colditz, 2006).

Invasive or infiltrating breast cancer is ductal or lobular in origin. Invasive ductal carcinoma (IDC) is the most common form of breast cancer. It begins in the duct, grows into the surrounding tissue, and has the ability to spread outside of the breast by lymphatics or blood vessels. It is the most common type of breast cancer and usually presents as a palpable mass or as an abnormal nodule or density on a mammogram and/or U/S. Medullary, tubular, and mucinous carcinomas are less common types of ductal carcinoma. Treatment is initially surgical with wide excision (lumpectomy, partial mastectomy, segmentectomy, quadrantectomy) or mastectomy, with surgical evaluation of the lymph nodes for spread of the cancer. Radiation to the remaining breast tissue, after lumpectomy, is performed to reduce the risk of cancer recurrence in the breast and may be indicated after mastectomy in certain patients deemed at high risk for local cancer recurrence. Antihormonal therapy in hormonally responsive cancers (tamoxifen, AIs) and/or chemotherapy are frequently recommended as additional therapy.

Inflammatory breast cancer is an aggressive form of breast cancer that presents as swelling, redness, warmth, and possibly *peau d'orange* (orange peel) of the breast skin due to blocked lymph drainage from cancer within the dermal lymphatic system. This can mimic mastitis, but is usually not painful or accompanied by fever or leukocytosis. *Any patient with breast inflammation treated with antibiotics that does not completely resolve should be referred to a breast cancer specialist or surgeon immediately.* Initial treatment is often with chemotherapy and/or radiation followed by surgery.

Paget's disease is an uncommon presentation of ductal carcinoma that infiltrates the nipple causing changes that range from a rash, itching, redness, flaking, bleeding, or a recurrent scab or nonhealing sore. Diagnosis is made by breast examination, mammogram, and a nipple biopsy. Mastectomy is the recommended treatment, although less invasive surgery has been explored and used.

Infiltrating or invasive lobular carcinoma (ILC) makes up about 5% to 10% of breast cancers (Li, Anderson, Daling, & Moe, 2003). The cancer cells originate in the lobules, invade the surrounding tissue and can spread via the lymph channels or bloodstream. Lobular carcinoma is more likely to be multicentric or multifocal (two or more separate tumors) and bilateral than IDC. It can also be more difficult to identify on mammography and CBE because it tends to more closely mimic the texture and mammographic appearance of normal breast tissue. As a result, it is often more advanced when detected compared with IDC.

Other cancers are found in the breast including phyllodes tumor, angiosarcoma, and lymphoma, as well as metastatic cancers from other sites in the body that are rare.

Breast Cancer in Pregnancy

Breast cancer that occurs in pregnancy is rare (ACS, 2015). Although rare, when diagnosed, breast cancer is often advanced as the breast undergoes extensive, normal, physiological changes readying for lactation making CBE and breast awareness more difficult and less effective. Treatment depends on trimester and stage of malignancy at diagnosis. Patients in their first trimester need to decide on mastectomy or lumpectomy, and radiation therapy is delayed until after delivery leading to an increase in the risk of recurrence. Patients in their second and third trimesters experience less of a delay in time to delivery, so lumpectomy is a better option. Pregnant women with more advanced disease may be started on chemotherapy in their second or third trimester but there is little data regarding fetal safety or long-term consequences available (Litton & Theriault, 2015). Some patients who are diagnosed with advanced breast cancer may opt for pregnancy termination but this is a very personal decision that must be made by a fully informed patient (Litton & Theriault, 2015). Breast cancer in pregnancy is a crisis for both the pregnant woman and her family, and a supportive oncology team is needed.

Breast Cancer Staging

The stage of breast cancer helps to determine adjuvant or additional treatments. Stages 1 to 4 are a combination of the size of the tumor (T), lymph node involvement (N), and distant metastasis (M; Harris, 2015), spread outside of the breast and lymph nodes to other parts of the body, most commonly to the bone, lung, liver, and brain.

Axillary lymph node involvement is the most important prognostic indicator. If malignant cells are found in lymph nodes, there is an increased risk of metastasis. Pathology is described as negative, microscopic (few cells), gross (visible malignancy in the node), and will describe whether extracapsular extension from the lymph node is present. Traditionally, evaluation of lymph nodes involve axillary lymph node dissection (ALND), which removes most of the affected nodal and fatty tissue in the axilla. This procedure may result in loss of sensation or pain under the arm, and, more troubling, lymphedema. Lymphedema occurs in up to 20% of patients who have ALND (DiSipio, Rye, Newman, & Hayes, 2013) and can be chronic and difficult to manage. Axillary sentinel lymph node biopsy (SLNB), a less invasive procedure, is associated with lower rates of lymphedema, 5% to 6% (DiSipio et. al., 2013). Blue dye and/or a radioisotope are injected and used to map the lymph node basin drainage of the breast, identifying the first or sentinel node(s) that a cancer would spread to if it is going to spread. The surgeon then removes the node(s) for histological evaluation and analysis. This procedure is used in invasive breast cancer but not usually in DCIS unless it is high grade or extensive. If positive nodes are found on SLNB, and ALND is usually indicated. Tables 24.2 and 24.3 describe tumor staging and nomenclature.

TUMOR GRADE

Tumor grade is not part of the staging system, but plays an important part in decision making about adjuvant treatment. Grade is based on the degree of cell abnormality compared to normal ductal or lobular cells and is classified as grade 1, 2, or 3. Table 24.4 describes cytological and histological attributes for each tumor grade.

TABLE 24.2	TNM Staging
Stage 0	Tis, N0, M0
Stage 1	T1, N0, M0
Stage 2	T1, N1, M0 T2, N1 or 2, M0 T3, N0, M0
Stage 3	T1, 2, 3 or 4; N2, M0 T3, N1, M0
Stage 4	Any T, N3, M0 Any T, Any N, M1

is, in situ; T, tumor; TNM, tumor, node, metastasis.
Adapted from NCCN.org

BIOLOGIC MARKERS

Tumor markers are used to determine prognosis and treatment. Estrogen and progesterone receptors on cancer cells mediate the cells' response to estrogen and progesterone. About 75% of breast cancers express one or both of these receptors that indicate a tumor should respond to hormonal therapy (www.breastcancer.org). HER2 is an oncogene, which is overexpressed in 18% to 20% of invasive cancers, is more aggressive, and indicates a poorer prognosis, especially if lymph nodes are positive (Mahon, 2007). Herceptin is a targeted biological therapy specific for the overexpressed HER2 protein. Studies have shown great promise in reducing cancer recurrence and possibly mortality in HER2-positive cancers (Romond et al., 2005). Genetic evaluation of the tumor is also being used to help predict a tumor's response to endocrine and chemotherapy. The most common profiles used are the 21-gene recurrence score, MammaPrint, and the Risk of Recurrence score.

SURGICAL MARGINS

When breast cancer is removed surgically, a margin of normal tissue around it is removed as well. This margin is important in gauging the risk of leaving tumor behind in the breast and therefore risk of local recurrence. Clear or negative margins are the gold standard for adequate tumor excision with the amount of gross margin (not microscopic) varying by institutional practice (Moran et al., 2014). When tumor sections are examined microscopically the entire tumor is inked externally for margin reference. "No tumor on ink" is the widely accepted standard for excision (2013 SSO/ASTRO guidelines, surgonc.org).

TABLE 24.3	Tumor Staging Nomenclature		
T STAGE (SIZE OF TUMOR IN CENTIMETERS)	N: NODAL STATUS	M: PRESENCE OF METASTASIS	STAGE
Tis (DCIS)	N0 = Negative	M0 = Negative	0 = In situ carcinoma
T1 = 2 cm or less	N1 = Positive	M1= Positive	1 = Invasive tumors ≤ 2 cm in size with negative nodes and no distant metastasis
T2 = 2–1.5 cm	N2/3 = Positive nodes outside axillary nodes (e.g., supra and/or infraclavicular)		2 = Any tumor with positive lymph nodes is stage 2 or above
T3 > 5 cm	N2/3 = Positive nodes outside axillary nodes (e.g., supra and/or infraclavicular)		3 = Any T4 tumor or tumors > 5 cm with positive lymph nodes
T4 = Locally advanced breast cancer			4 = Any size tumor with any lymph node status but with distant metastasis

DCIS, ductal carcinoma in situ; Tis, tumor in situ.
Adapted from NCCN.org.

TABLE 24.4	Tumor Grade
Grade 1 tumors	■ Ductal/lobular cells normal in appearance ■ Well differentiated ■ Slower growing than higher grade tumors
Grade 2 tumors	■ Ductal/lobular cells abnormal in appearance ■ Moderately differentiated
Grade 3 tumors	■ Ductal/lobular cells very abnormal in appearance ■ Poorly differentiated ■ Faster growing than lower grade tumors

Adapted from Harris (2015).

Treatment

Breast cancer is a complex heterogeneous disease and its management is tailored to the individual woman's cancer and to her preferences. Surgical and adjuvant therapy options are based on many factors, including tumor size and characteristics, tumor stage, biological markers, comorbidities in the patient, and genetic profiling of the tumor. The field of breast cancer research is rapidly expanding, leading to frequent changes in standard treatment. Breast cancer treatment is a topic too broad to cover in detail in this chapter. What follows is a comprehensive overview for the nonspecialized health care provider.

SURGERY

Surgery continues to be the mainstay of breast cancer treatment. Surgical options are decided based on the extent of the cancer and patient preference. The majority of women newly diagnosed with breast cancer are surgically amenable to BCT/lumpectomy and radiation. Breast conserving surgery consists of lumpectomy, partial mastectomy, quadrantectomy, segmentectomy, or wide local excision with examination of the lymph nodes in invasive disease (SLNB and/or ALND). Reexcision is performed for positive or close margins. The amount of tissue removed varies but can be up to one quarter or more of the breast. Lymph node positivity usually has no bearing on whether a woman can have BCT. Radiation to the remaining breast tissue to reduce the risk of recurrence is usually indicated as standard of care in invasive cancer and DCIS, but this recommendation can vary based on the tumor type, size, margins, and patient comorbidities (Darby et al., 2011; Early Breast Cancer Trialists' Collaborative Group [EBCTCG], 2011).

When tumors are large (compared to breast size), multicentric, or a patient does not have access to or cannot receive radiation therapy, mastectomy may be indicated over BCT. Modified radical mastectomy is removal of the breast and axillary lymph nodes and is indicated for node positive disease clinically or on SLNB. Simple or total mastectomy removes the entire breast with no lymph nodes and may be done in DCIS, invasive cancer (performed with SLNB that is negative), or prophylactically for women at high risk. Skin-sparing techniques and nipple-sparing

surgery are being performed in certain subsets of women to aid in breast reconstruction. Surgical assessment of each individual patient, breast size, lesion size, and so on, helps to determine the use and may result in a better cosmetic outcome (Mehrara, 2015). Breast reconstruction is an option for most patients and can be done at the time of mastectomy or as a delayed operation. Radical mastectomy includes removing the breast, chest wall muscles, and all nodes and is rarely performed except in the case of very advanced local disease. For women who are judged to be good candidates for BCT, the choice of treatment options is up to the patient, with guidance from her surgeon and other breast cancer providers (Harris & Morrow, 2015).

BREAST RECONSTRUCTION

Breast reconstruction may be done at the time of mastectomy, later, or not at all depending on patient preference. Breast care providers make recommendations individually tailored to the patient's needs and desires, keeping in mind the best cancer operation for treatment. Patients may have less distress over the loss of a breast with immediate reconstruction. Some patients are not good candidates for immediate reconstruction. When postmastectomy chest wall radiation is required, there may be increased risk for surgical complications due to impaired wound healing, fibrosis, or infection. If the need for radiation cannot be determined before mastectomy, delayed reconstruction is preferable (Mehrara, 2015).

Breast reconstruction is accomplished in many ways, with continued advances in the field. The most common reconstruction begins with the insertion of a tissue expander that is placed under the pectoralis muscle, and saline is injected gradually over a few months to stretch the overlying muscles and skin. The expander is then replaced with a permanent saline or silicone implant. Silicone implants may provide a more natural-looking reconstruction than saline implants. Implant reconstruction requires less extensive surgery and less hospital time than tissue reconstruction, but usually involves a second procedure to insert the permanent implant and/or reconstruct the nipple areolar complex. Implants have a more youthful contour with less droop (ptosis) than a natural breast; therefore some patients will elect plastic surgery on the opposite breast to uplift, augment, or reduce the remaining breast for symmetry. Federal law dictates that this surgery and reconstruction be covered by health insurance plans. Implants do have the risk of capsular contracture in which scar tissue around the implant tightens, resulting in distortion. Radiation to the implant increases the risk of contracture and implants should be evaluated for replacement after 8 to 10 years.

TISSUE RECONSTRUCTION

Native tissue reconstruction or "tissue flaps" require more extensive surgery and hospital time but can result in a more anatomical cosmetic appearance. Tissue from the back (latissimus flap), abdomen (transverse rectus abdominis muscle [TRAM] flap), or buttock (gluteal flap) is used to form a breast or create a pocket for an implant. Diabetics and women who smoke are often discouraged from this option as circulatory changes may affect healing. A latissimus flap involves moving an oval section of skin, muscle, fat, and blood vessels from the back, below the shoulder blade, through a tunnel made under the skin of the underarm. A TRAM flap takes tissue from the transverse rectus abdominis muscle. A section of fat, muscle, and skin is tunneled under the skin up to the breast, or can be attached with microvascular surgery to blood vessels in the chest wall (a "free flap"). A "tummy tuck"-type closure is performed at the donor site. TRAM flaps have a significant complication rate including partial to complete loss of the flap, fat necrosis, and weakening of the abdominal wall resulting in hernias or back pain. Gluteal flaps harvest gluteal muscle, skin, and fat, which is transferred and attached to the chest wall with microvascular surgery. Morbidity can also be significant and donor site asymmetry can be a distressing problem. Variations of these surgical procedures are common and the field is rapidly advancing with newer, less invasive, and innovative techniques.

Women can choose a breast form or prosthesis instead of reconstruction. Prostheses have been improved and are lighter and more comfortable than earlier models. The American Cancer Society, the Breast Cancer Network of Strength, Komen for the Cure®, and other local societies often provide financial assistance for patients (see www.acs.org, www.y-me.org, and ww5.komen.org/BreastCancer/FinancialResources.html).

SURGICAL COMPLICATIONS

The risk of any surgical procedure involves risks related to anesthesia, infection, bleeding, comorbidities, pain, and other potentially unforeseen complications. One of the most difficult (for patient and provider) breast surgery complications is lymphedema. Any disruption in lymph drainage following ALND dissection or SLNB biopsy results in an increased risk for development of lymphedema of the arm, although the risk is smaller with SLNB. Lymphedema, once it has developed, is very difficult to treat and can be very debilitating. All patients should be educated about this condition, how to avoid it, and what to watch for as warning signs. Arm measurements can diagnose the condition early and are important in follow-up care. Women with axillary nodal involvement by tumor and/or who receive axillary nodal radiation are at the highest risk. Other risks include obesity and injury or infection in the arm since surgery (McLaughlin, 2015). Lymphedema of the breast can also occur following BCT and is a similarly difficult-to-manage complication. All women who have surgery for breast cancer should be educated about this risk. Symptoms may include a sensation of tightness or swelling under the arm that may extend down the entire arm (this is often confused with postoperative disruption of the sensory intercostal brachial nerve, which should be differentiated). Treatment includes elastic sleeves, complex decongestive physiotherapy (CDP) to encourage collateral lymphatic drainage (patients with congestive heart failure [CHF] or blood clots need to have medical clearance for this procedure) or daily massage. If lymphedema is chronic, infections and loss of arm function can occur.

Women should avoid any injuries or infection in the surgical arm. Antibiotics should be prescribed as needed. Injections, vaccinations, venipuncture, intravenous (IV) lines, and blood pressure readings are best administered, accessed, and/or obtained from the unaffected arm when possible. Many other recommendations are made to prevent lymphedema, including (a) using electric razors for axillary hair removal; (b) avoiding manicures; (c) wearing gloves during gardening or contact with chemicals; (d) avoidance of constrictive clothing or jewelry; and (e) wearing a compression sleeve on airplanes. Although suggested, there is little strong scientific evidence to support these recommendations. Bioimpedance spectroscopy (BIS) is currently being used to detect lymphedema early, when treatment is most effective. This technology is used in clinical assessment of symptoms associated with unilateral lymphedema. Specifically, the technology measures resistance to electrical current while comparing fluid compartments between a patient's affected and nonsurgical side. L-Dex®, marketed by ImpediMed, is one such system (international.l-dex.com).

RADIATION THERAPY

Radiation is almost always advised after lumpectomy for invasive breast cancer to reduce the risk of recurrence in the remaining breast tissue, and usually advised after lumpectomy for DCIS (EBCTCG, 2011). Radiation therapy after mastectomy is sometimes indicated to reduce the risk of recurrence in the chest wall or axilla. Radiation after mastectomy is indicated if the tumor is more than 5 cm, involves the skin or chest muscle, involves multiple axillary nodes, and in advanced nodal involvement, such as supraclavicular nodes and nodes with extension of tumor into the surrounding tissue.

Radiation to the breast is usually administered as a standard total dose, which is administered as fractionated small doses in short sessions, 5 days a week, for 4 to 6 weeks (to add up to the total dose at the end of treatment). CT planning and small tattoos guide the angle of the beam to help prevent injury to the heart, lungs, and other normal tissues. Fatigue and skin irritation (sometimes severe) are the most troubling side effects. The breast skin may become more pigmented, may thicken, become edematous or fibrous, and may shrink or enlarge following completion of therapy. These changes usually lessen with time.

Radiation may also be delivered to the lumpectomy site and is known as partial breast radiation (PBR). PBR is delivered in three ways: (1) by placement of small catheters containing radioactive material in the tumor bed (brachytherapy); (2) by a balloon applicator temporarily inserted into the excisional cavity into which radioactive beads are inserted (MammoSite®; Harris, 2015); or (3) as external radiation beams directed at the tumor site. The advantage over standard radiation therapy is that PBR can be delivered in much less time, usually a few days. A large national clinical trial, National Surgical Adjuvant Breast and Bowel Project (NSABP) B39, is currently underway to help evaluate the effectiveness of PBI compared to standard radiation therapy (www.NSABP.pitt.edu/B-39.asp), but PBI is currently available as an option in most large U.S. cities.

CHEMOTHERAPY

The decision to recommend chemotherapy depends on many factors including the size of the tumor, biological markers, lymph node status, metastasis if present, and increasingly, tumor genetics. Chemotherapy is not given for DCIS. Patients with invasive cancer determined to be at significant risk for cancer recurrence are usually treated.

Chemotherapy is prescribed by a medical oncologist. Many chemotherapy agents work by interfering with cells that are rapidly dividing (hair follicles, bone marrow, intestinal tract cells) and can result in hair loss, nausea, mouth sores, changes in taste and/or smell, and gastrointestinal (GI) disturbances. Premature menopause can also result. Agents are often used in combination or can be used alone. Herceptin may be administered in combination with chemotherapy for HER2-positive disease.

Dosages and regimens of chemotherapy, known as protocols, vary based on tumor profiles, tumor response, and patient comorbidities. There are many other chemotherapeutic agents that can be used in early, advanced, recurrent, or metastatic disease. Chemotherapy is most often used in the adjuvant setting, after surgery, but can be given as neoadjuvant therapy, before surgery. Chemotherapy drugs are given intravenously, often via a port device, which is removed when treatment is completed; in some cases, it is given orally.

Chemotherapy is almost always a frightening and challenging experience for patients. The risk of serious adverse effects is not small, although it is better managed or prevented with pre- and postchemo medication combinations. Breast cancer is the most common indication for chemotherapy among women in the United States and chemotherapy accounts for the largest number of serious adverse events among treatment options. Adverse effects include infection, fever, neutropenia, thrombocytopenia, anemia, constitutional symptoms, dehydration, electrolyte disorder/s, nausea, emesis, diarrhea, deep vein thrombosis (DVT), and pulmonary embolus (PE). Patients will be better prepared to make informed treatment decisions if counseled about the possible risks associated with each type of recommended chemotherapy.

Antihormonal and biological therapies (such as Herceptin) also carry the risk of potentially serious complications. The benefits and risks of any therapy should be fully disclosed to all breast cancer patients by a medical oncologist using the best information available to allow informed decision making. Multigene diagnostic tests, such as Oncotype or MammaPrint, may be used to determine recurrence risk before deciding on the need for chemotherapy (Harris, 2015).

HORMONAL THERAPY

Hormonal therapy is often recommended alone or in addition to chemotherapy in hormone-receptor-positive invasive breast cancer. Tamoxifen is the most commonly prescribed antihormonal agent and works by binding to a cell's receptors to block the usage of estrogen and progesterone. The AIs letrozole, exemestane, and anastrazole disrupt the production of aromatase, which is needed to synthesize estrogen.

Tamoxifen, an AI, or a sequential combination is generally used for treatment. The majority of AIs cannot be used in pre- or perimenopausal women. At this time, tamoxifen, an AI, is the only antihormonal agent that can be used in premenopausal women.

BIOLOGICAL THERAPY

Herceptin targets the overexpressed HER2 protein in HER2-positive breast cancer. It targets cancer cells more specifically, and therefore has fewer side effects than chemotherapy. Herceptin increases the risk of serious cardiotoxicity CHF and possibly arrhythmias (4% or less of patients based on most data; Aspita & Perez, 2015). Many new biological agents are being used and tested in clinical trials.

CLINICAL TRIALS

Many clinical trials are available for women undergoing breast cancer treatment. The purpose of a clinical trial is to identify a new treatment technique or drug that will be better at treating the cancer than standard therapy. Participants should never receive any treatment in a clinical trial that is less than standard of care. All of the recent advances in radiation techniques, biological, chemo, and antihormonal therapy, and in tumor genetic profiling, have come to fruition as a result of patient participation in clinical trials. Current clinical trials are available at www.cancer.gov/clinicaltrials.

ALTERNATIVE TREATMENTS

Alternative therapies in treating breast cancer have not been well studied, but are available. Their effectiveness is unknown and most cancer specialists do not recommend them as a sole treatment option. Complementary and integrative medicine consist of vitamins, herbs, special diets, and spiritual healing. Until further research is available, complementary and integrative therapy should only be recommended in addition to conventional therapy and under the direction of an oncologist.

Breast Cancer Patient Support and Education

Patients going through breast cancer diagnosis and treatment are almost always apprehensive, frightened, and confused. Answering questions and lowering barriers to good patient, oncologist, and surgeon communication can be very helpful. There are many excellent breast cancer websites, literature, and peer-to-peer patient support networks available to assist patients in decision making. Women should be encouraged to access and use these resources for themselves and for family members.

SUPPORT DURING TREATMENT

Women should be advised to finish any dental work before chemotherapy, as they are more prone to infection during treatment. Nausea is treated preventively with medication. Fatigue is a common problem that may not readily resolve, leading to patient frustration and depression. Vomiting, diarrhea, mouth ulcers, and throat soreness can be troublesome but are usually controllable with medication. Hair loss is very common and can be emotionally and physically painful. Women describe the feeling of hair coming out as uncomfortable and are advised to have it cut short as soon as it starts to fall out to lessen the discomfort. Wigs and specially made head coverings in many styles are available.

During chemotherapy bone marrow suppression occurs and avoidance of infections is extremely important. Women should be counseled to stay out of large crowds, wash their hands often, practice careful oral hygiene, get plenty of rest, and keep any cuts or scratches clean. Exposure to sexually transmitted infections should be minimized. Eating a healthy diet is important to minimize weight gain that often occurs during chemotherapy; however, some dietary restrictions may be advised by the oncologist, such as avoiding soft cheeses, deli meats, and salad bars because these foods and sites may have bacteria that can impact an immunocompromised patient. Chemotherapy patients can gain 5 to 15 pounds and possibly more with longer treatment and with prednisone therapy. The reasons for creeping weight gain and stalled weight loss during cancer treatment are unknown, but may be related to the sudden onset of menopause, changes in metabolism, less physical activity during recovery due to fatigue, snacks to lessen nausea, and increased appetite from steroids. Muscle mass can also decrease during chemotherapy leading to fat increases.

Patients should be encouraged to fend off unwanted pounds with careful diet and exercise including careful weight training with specialized instruction for cancer patients and aerobic exercise as tolerated. Sessions with a nutritionist and trainer can be very helpful.

A premenopausal woman's menstrual periods may stop during chemotherapy and may not restart, leading to premature menopause. However, pregnancy may still occur even after long periods of amenorrhea and birth control should be discussed with women during this time. Nonhormonal methods of contraception and control of menopausal symptoms (e.g., vasomotor symptoms) are indicated in this population.

In young women who may want to start or add to their family after treatment, protection of ovarian function with medication or egg harvesting may be a viable option. Referral to a reproductive endocrinologist is important to discuss all reproductive options. Pregnancy after breast cancer should be a decision made by the patient and her oncologist and obstetrician and should be considered high risk (Ruddy & Ginsburg, 2015).

Follow-Up Care

EMOTIONAL IMPACT

Four times more women die of heart disease than from breast cancer in the United States, but women tend to fear the risk of breast cancer much more. Survivors of breast cancer go on to live healthy and productive lives, but the trauma of the diagnosis and the difficulty of some treatment combinations can result in mild to severe psychological distress and often lasting physical effects. Psychosocial concerns of survivors include fear of recurrence, fatigue, trouble sleeping,

pain, body image disruption, sexual dysfunction, intrusive thoughts about illness and persistent anxiety, feelings of vulnerability, and concerns about mortality. The experience of breast cancer has several phases, each with its own issues. Diagnosis, treatment, completing treatment, reentry, survivorship, recurrence, and palliation for advanced cancer all need to be dealt with along with socioeconomic factors, cultural issues, availability of support, access to care, and the presence of other illnesses or life crises (Hewitt, Herdman, & Holland, 2004).

Patients who have survived cancer have gone through difficult and challenging times and may struggle with depression, physical changes, changes in their sexual relationship, changes in libido, and fear of recurrence, and often require time, empathy, and reassurance. Posttraumatic stress disorder (PTSD)-like syndromes are not unusual. It is important to assess coping mechanisms, psychological adjustment to cancer, perceived family support, and to refer for psychological assessment and counseling as appropriate. Patient participation in peer support groups is often of benefit. Providers may benefit from reading patient narratives to more fully understand the challenge of cancer (Trillin, 1981).

Breast cancer survivors have a higher risk of developing another breast cancer, so follow-up and annual mammograms are very important. Some survivors experience gaps in care, which may be due to fear of recurrence and dread of repeated treatment (Snyder et al., 2009). Providers caring for breast cancer survivors need to be aware of previous treatments to design posttreatment care plans while coordinating with the medical oncologist. Many survivor programs are being designed and implemented to address surveillance and the wide range of needs and issues that survivors face.

Women recovering well following treatment for early breast cancer may be discharged from an oncologist's care, but should have close follow-up care that should include history, physical examination, review of systems (recurrence can often show up subtly, such as nagging back or abdominal pain), bone density testing, mammograms, and any other testing based on an oncologist's or survivor clinic's recommendations. Follow-up testing is dependent on the extent of disease and treatments received.

RECURRENT BREAST CANCER

Local recurrence (in the breast or chest wall) or regional recurrence (in the lymphatics) of breast cancer is a distressing event for cancer survivors, but is often salvageable with additional surgery. In the case of recurrence after BCT, mastectomy is indicated because radiation cannot be performed again and likely will not affect overall cure or survival. Chest wall recurrence after mastectomy is much more problematic and may require radiation, extensive surgery, and/or possibly chemotherapy.

Distant recurrence of breast cancer in the body is traumatic and emotionally challenging for all survivors. Newer therapies have led to better treatment responses and control of disease. Many clinical trials are available for women who have progressive disease on standard therapy, using new drugs, drug combinations, and innovative therapies.

SURVIVORSHIP

Although more than 40,000 women in the United States died of breast cancer in 2015, mortality has been decreasing by approximately 2.4% per year (ACS, 2015). There are more women living with and surviving breast cancer today than ever before and 80% to 90% of women are diagnosed with early stage tumors or localized disease (ACS, 2015). Incidence of breast cancer had been slowly and steadily increasing until 2002, when a substantial drop in new cases was noted. Today, women diagnosed with early breast cancer are thought to have close to a 90% chance of survival (ACS, 2015). New therapies are extending the lives of women with recurrent or advanced disease. As health care providers, it is essential to educate women about risks, screening, prevention, and new therapies available for treatment to continue to advance survivorship and continue the favorable trends that are being realized in breast cancer care.

■ REFERENCES

American Cancer Society (2015). *Facts and figures 2015*. Atlanta, GA: American Cancer Society.

Antoniou, A., Pharaoh, P., Narod, S., Risch, H., Eyfjord, J., Hopper, J.,…Easton, J. (2003). Average risks of breast and ovarian cancer associated with BRCA 1 or BRCA 2 mutations detected in case series unselected for family history: A combined analysis of 22 studies. *American Journal of Human Genetics*, 72(5), 1117–1130.

Aspita, A., & Perez, E. (2015). Side effects of systemic therapy: Neurocognitive, cardiac and secondary malignancies. In J. Harris, M. Lippman, M. Morrow, & C. Osborne (Eds.), *Diseases of the breast* (pp. 692–703). Philadelphia, PA: Wolters Kluwer.

Bleicher, R. (2015). Management of the palpable mass. In J. Harris et al. (Eds.), *Diseases of the breast* (pp. 29–37). Philadelphia, PA: Wolters Kluwer.

Breastcancer.org. (2015). *Cancer Statistics*. Retrieved from http://www .breastcancer.org/symptoms/understand_bc/statistics

Centers for Disease Control and Prevention (CDC). (2012). Vital signs: racial disparities in breast cancer severity—United States 2005–2009. *Morbidity and Mortality Weekly Report*, 61(45), 927.

Darby, S., McGale, P., Correa, C., Taylor, C., Arringada, R., Clarke, M.,…Peto, R. (2011). Effect of radiotherapy after breast conservation surgery on 10 year recurrence and 15 year breast cancer death: Meta-analysis of individual patient data for 10,801 women in 17 randomized trials. *Lancet, 378*(9804), 1707–1716.

D'Orsi, C. (2005). Reporting and communication. In L. Bassett (Ed.), *Diagnosis of diseases of the breast* (pp. 111–123). Philadelphia, PA: Elsevier.

Degnim, A. C., Visscher, D. W., Berman, H. K., Frost, M. H., Sellers, T. A., Vierkant, R. A.,…Hartmann, L. C. (2007). Stratification of breast cancer risk in women with atypia: A Mayo cohort study. *Journal of Clinical Oncology: Official Journal of the American Society of Clinical Oncology*, 25(19), 2671–2677.

DiSipio, T., Rye, S., Newman, B., & Hayes, S. (2013). Incidence of unilateral arm lymphoedema after breast cancer: A systematic review and meta-analysis. *The Lancet. Oncology*, 14(6), 500–515.

Early Breast Cancer Trialists' Collaborative Group (EBCTCG). (2011). Effect of radiotherapy after breast conserving surgery on 10-year recurrence and 15-year breast cancer death: Meta-analysis of individual patient data for 10,801 women in 17 randomized trials. *Lancet, 378*(9804), 1707–1716.

Eliassen, A. H., Colditz, G. A., Rosner, B., Willett, W. C., & Hankinson, S. E. (2006). Adult weight change and risk of postmenopausal breast cancer. *Journal of the American Medical Association, 296*(2), 193–201.

Garber, J., & Offit, K. (2005). Hereditary cancer predisposition syndromes. *Journal of Clinical Oncology*, 23, 276–292.

Gradishar, W. J., & Cella, D. (2006). Selective estrogen receptor modulators and prevention of invasive breast cancer. *Journal of the American Medical Association*, 295(23), 2784–2786.

Gucalp, A., Morris, P., Hudis, C., & Dannenberg, A. (2015). Implications of obesity in breast cancer. In J. Harris, M. Lippman, M. Morrow, & C. Osborne (Eds.), *Diseases of the breast* (pp. 700–714). Philadelphia, PA: Wolters Kluwer.

Harris, J. (2015). Staging of breast cancer. In J. Harris, M. Lippman, M. Morrow, & C. Osborne (Eds.), *Diseases of the breast* (pp. 495–503). Philadelphia, PA: Wolters Kluwer.

Harris, J., & Morrow, M. (2015). Breast conserving therapy. In J. Harris, M. Lippman, M. Morrow, & C. Osborne (Eds.), *Diseases of the breast* (pp. 514–535). Philadelphia, PA: Wolters Kluwer.

Hewitt, M., Herdman, R., & Holland, B. (2004). *Meeting the psychosocial needs of women with breast cancer*. Washington, DC: National Academies Press.

Hughes, L. L., Wang, M., Page, D. L., Gray, R., Solin, L. J., Davidson, N. E.,…Wood W. C. (2009). Local excision alone without irradiation for ductal carcinoma in situ of the breast: A trial of the Eastern Cooperative Oncology Group. *Journal of Clinical Oncology*, 27(32), 5319.

Li, C. I., Anderson, B. O., Daling, J. R., & Moe, R. E. (2003). Trends in incidence rates of invasive lobular and ductal breast carcinoma. *Journal of the American Medical Association*, 289, 1421–1424.

Litton, J., & Theriault, R. (2015). Breast cancer during pregnancy and subsequent pregnancy in breast cancer survivors. In J. Harris, M. Lippman, M. Morrow, & C. Osborne (Eds.), *Diseases of the breast* (pp. 855–863). Philadelphia, PA: Wolters Kluwer.

Mahon, S. (2007). *Breast cancer*. Pittsburgh, PA: Oncology Nursing Society.

McLaughlin, S. (2015). Lymphedema. In J. Harris, M. Lippman, M. Morrow, & C. Osborne (Eds.), *Diseases of the breast* (pp. 590–601). Philadelphia, PA: Wolters Kluwer.

Mehrara, B., & Ho, A. (2015). Breast reconstruction. In J. Harris, M. Lippman, M. Morrow, & C. Osborne (Eds.), *Diseases of the breast*. Philadelphia, PA: Wolters Kluwer.

Milanese, T. R., Hartmann, L. C., Sellers, T. A., Frost, M. H., Vierkant, R. A., Maloney, S. D.,…Visscher, D. W. (2006). Age-related lobular involution and risk of breast cancer. *Journal of the National Cancer Institute*, 98(22), 1600–1607. doi:10.1093/jnci/djj439

Moran, M., Schnitt, S., Guiliano, A., Harris, J., Khan, S., Horton, J., . . . Morrow, M. (2014). American Society for Radiation Oncology Consensus Guideline on Margins for Breast Conserving Surgery with whole breast irradiation in stages I and II invasive breast cancer. *International Journal of Radiation Oncology Biology Physics 88*(37), 553–564.

National Cancer Institute. www.cancer.gov

Nekhlyudov, L., Kroenke, C. H., Jung, I., Holmes, M. D., & Colditz, G. A. (2006). Prospective changes in quality of life after ductal carcinoma-in-situ: Results from the Nurses' Health Study. *Journal of Clinical Oncology: Official Journal of the American Society of Clinical Oncology*, 24(18), 2822–2827.

Osborne, M., & Boolbol, S. (2015). Breast anatomy and development. In J. Harris, M. Lippman, M. Morrow, & C. Osborne (Eds.), *Diseases of the breast* (pp. 3–14). Philadelphia, PA: Wolters Kluwer.

Prentice, R. L., Caan, B., Chlebowski, R. T., Patterson, R., Kuller, L. H., Ockene, J. K.,…Henderson, M. M. (2006). Low fat dietary pattern and risk of invasive breast cancer: The Women's Health Initiative Randomized Controlled Dietary Modification Trial. *Journal of the American Medical Association*, 295, 629–642.

Ravdin, P. M., Cronin, K. A., Howlader, N., Berg, C. D., Chlebowski, R. T., Feuer, E. J.,…Berry, D. A. (2007). The decrease in breast-cancer incidence in 2003 in the United States. *New England Journal of Medicine*, 356(16), 1670–1674.

Rimawi, M., & Osborne, C. (2015). Adjuvant systemic therapy: Endocrine therapy. In J. Harris, M. Lippman, M. Morrow, & C. Osborne (Eds.), *Diseases of the breast* (pp. 619–634). Philadelphia, PA: Wolters Kluwer.

Romond, E. H., Perez, E. A., Bryant, J., Suman, V. J., Geyer, C. E., Jr., Davidson, N. E.,…Wolmark, N. (2005). Trastuzumab plus adjuvant chemotherapy for operable HER2-positive breast cancer. *New England Journal of Medicine, 3531*, 673–684.

Rossouw, J. E., Anderson, G. L., Prentice, R. L., LaCroix, A. Z., Kooperberg, C., Stefanick, M. L.,…Ockene, J.; Writing Group for the

Women's Health Initiative Investigators. (2002). Risks and benefits of estrogen plus progestin in healthy postmenopausal women: Principal results from the Women's Health Initiative randomized controlled trial. *Journal of the American Medical Association, 288*(3), 321–333.

Ruddy, K., & Ginsburg, E. (2015). Reproductive issues in breast cancer survivors. In J. Harris, M. Lippman, M. Morrow, & C. Osborne (Eds.), *Diseases of the breast* (pp. 1155–1162). Philadelphia, PA: Wolters Kluwer.

Salant, T., Ganschow, P., Olufunmilayo, I., & Lauderdale, D. (2006). "Why take it if you don't have anything?" Breast cancer risk perceptions and prevention choices at a public hospital. *Journal of General Internal Medicine, 21,* 779–785.

Saslow, D. (2007). American Cancer Society guidelines for breast screening with MRI as an adjunct to mammography. *A Cancer Journal for Clinicians, 57,* 75–89.

Snyder, C. F., Frick, K. D., Kantsiper, M. E., Peairs, K. S., Herbert, R. J., Blackford, A. L.,...Earle, C. C. (2009). Prevention, screening, and surveillance care for breast cancer survivors compared with controls: Changes from 1998 to 2002. *Journal of Clinical Oncology: Official Journal of the American Society of Clinical Oncology, 27*(7), 1054–1061.

Thomas, D. B., Gao, D. L., Ray, R. M., Wang, W. W., Allison, C. J., Chen, F. L.,...Self, S. G. (2002). Randomized trial of breast self-examination in Shanghai: Final results. *Journal of the National Cancer Institute, 94*(19), 1445–1457. doi:10.1093/jnci/94.19.1445

Trillin, A. S. (1981). Of dragons and garden peas: A cancer patient talks to doctors. *New England Journal of Medicine, 304*(12), 699–701.

Vogel, V. G. (2006). Effects of tamoxifen vs raloxifene on the risk of developing invasive breast cancer and other disease outcomes. The NSABP Study of Tamoxifen and Raloxifene (STAR) P-2 Trial. *Journal of the American Medical Association, 295*(23), 2727–2741. doi:10.1001/jama.295.23.joc60074

Wapnir, I. L., Dignam, J. J., Fisher, B., Mamounas, E. P., Anderson, S. J., Julian, T. B.,...Wolmark, N. (2011). Long-term outcomes of invasive ipsilateral breast tumor recurrences after lumpectomy in NSABP B-17 and B-24 randomized clinical trials for DCIS. *Journal of the National Cancer Institute, 103*(6), 478–488.

Willett, W., Tamimi, R., Hankinson, S., Hazra, A., Eliassen, A., & Colditz, G. (2015). Nongenetic factors in the causation of breast cancer. In J. Harris, M. Lippman, M. Morrow, & C. Osborne (Eds.), *Diseases of the breast* (pp. 211–267). Philadelphia, PA: Wolters Kluwer.

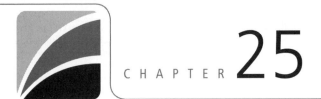

CHAPTER 25

Caring for the Transgender Patient

Kathryn Tierney • Caroline Dorsen

Gender identity is the internal sense of being male or female (Coleman et al., 2012). For most of the population, gender identity is congruent with the physical genitalia with which they are born, but when there is incongruence between the individual's gender identity and the natal sex there can be significant distress (WPATH, 2011). Treatment of gender dysphoria is often aimed at relieving that discomfort using changes in gender expression, hormone therapy, and/or gender-affirming surgery. Taking care of individuals who are transgender requires special attention to terminology and consideration of the effect of various treatments on the physical anatomy in terms of acute risks and long-term health maintenance.

■ DEFINITION/SCOPE

Gender dysphoria is the discomfort a person experiences when physical sex or assigned gender is not congruent with their gender identity (Coleman et al., 2012). It may be impossible to accurately determine the number of individuals who experience gender dysphoria at any given time because gender is fluid and self-determined. Historically, estimates have been made by studying the use of the diagnostic codes for gender identity disorder and gender dysphoria, rates of gender-affirming surgery, or applications for legal gender change (Institute of Medicine [IOM], 2011; Zucker & Lawrence, 2009). However, these particular measures are certain to underestimate the true prevalence because of inconsistencies in coding, lack of access to health care providers or surgeons, and limited access to legal gender marker changes because of state and local laws. In addition, terminology used to describe gender dysphoria or gender transition is not ubiquitous in the community and this can lead to underreporting. For instance, a woman who has transitioned from male to female may not consider herself transgender once she presents full time as female, having completed what she defines as her transition. Complicating the issues with terminology is the fact that many people who experience gender dysphoria are hesitant to participate in studies given the violence the community has endured historically (Grant et al., 2011).

The definitions associated with gender and gender identity are largely dependent on culture. Table 25.1 provides a glossary of terms related to gender identity. Not all people who are gender nonconforming will subscribe to all or any of these descriptions. It is important to use terminology with all patients that will allow individuals to explore their gender within the context of their physical and mental health in a safe environment. Moreover, it is essential to ascertain each individual person's particular gender identity and how they relate this identity to their health. Using the person's preferred name and preferred pronoun is essential in creating a meaningful patient–provider relationship. This will help the provider to determine the interventions that will be most effective at improving health and sense of well-being.

Nurse practitioners encounter both transwomen and transmen in their practice. Each group has distinct health needs based on existing physical structure and hormones and/or surgery used to transition to the preferred gender.

■ ETIOLOGY

There is no clear etiology for the incongruence between intrinsic sense of gender and natal sex (Gooren, 2006). On the one hand, it has long been assumed that gender dysphoria was purely psychiatric in nature and was considered a mental illness. On the other hand, more recent biological theories posit that because the brain and genitals develop at different points in time there is the possibility of having a brain that is predisposed to identify with one gender being born with genitals normally associated with other gender. This assumes that gender is binary, though it is more likely that gender, and its relationship to culture, is more of a continuum.

Though the diagnostic criteria for gender dysphoria are still established by the *Diagnostic and Statistical Manual of Mental Disorders* (5th ed.; *DSM-5*; American Psychiatric

TABLE 25.1	Glossary of Terms Related to Gender Identity
Sex	The term applied at birth as male or female, usually based on the physical appearance of the external genitalia
Gender identity	An individual's intrinsic sense of being male, female, or an alternative gender
Transgender	An umbrella term that describes an individual whose gender identity does not necessarily correspond to the sex they were assigned at birth
Gender dysphoria	The sense of incongruence between assigned sex and gender identity
Transwoman	Biologic male whose expressed gender is female
Transman	Biologic female whose expressed gender is male
Cisgender	An individual for whom biologic and expressed gender are the same

Source: World Professional Association for Transgender Health (2011).

Association [APA], 2013), it is now understood that a person's gender identity, whether or not it is consistent with natal sex, is not a disorder (Coleman et al., 2012). The discomfort associated with the incongruence can certainly lead to enough distress to cause other more serious disorders such as depression or anxiety; however, gender dysphoria itself is a variant of biology that is outside what our society considers normal.

■ SYMPTOMS

Gender dysphoria can range from mildly disconcerting to profoundly disruptive. Someone who identifies with one gender may choose activities, roles, or actions more commonly associated with that gender. The incongruence comes both at a personal level when that identity does not match the abilities or presentation of the physical body and at a social or interpersonal level when there is confusion or discomfort when the person does not follow gender-specific, culturally, or socially determined norms. Symptoms include depression, anxiety, and body dysphoria, as well as the desire to fulfill cultural roles or expectations of the other gender. Puberty is an especially challenging time for many people with gender dysphoria given the rapid changes in body and development of secondary sex characteristics of the natal gender, which is often in direct opposition to the person's internal sense of gender identity (Wallien & Cohen-Kettenis, 2008).

BOX 25.1 *DSM-5* DIAGNOSTIC CRITERIA FOR GENDER DYSPHORIA

A. Marked incongruence between one's experienced/expressed gender and assigned gender, of at least 6 months' duration, as manifested by two or more of the following indicators:
 1. A marked incongruence between one's experienced/expressed gender and primary and/or secondary sex characteristics (or, in young adolescents, the anticipated secondary sex characteristics)
 2. A strong desire to be rid of one's primary and/or secondary sex characteristics because of a marked incongruence with one's experienced/expressed gender (or, in young adolescents, a desire to prevent the development of the anticipated secondary sex characteristics)
 3. A strong desire for the primary and/or secondary sex characteristics of the other gender
 4. A strong desire to be of the other gender (or some alternative gender different from one's assigned gender)
 5. A strong desire to be treated as the other gender (or some alternative gender different from one's assigned gender)
 6. A strong conviction that one has the typical feelings and reactions of the other gender (or some alternative gender different from one's assigned gender)
B. The condition is associated with clinically significant distress or impairment in social, occupational, or other important areas of functioning, or with a significantly increased risk of suffering, such as distress or disability (APA, 2013)

Source: American Psychiatric Association. (2013). *Diagnostic and statistical manual of mental disorders DSM-V-TR* (5th ed., text rev.). Washington, DC: Author. P. 452 (302.85 F64.1)

■ EVALUATION/ASSESSMENT

Gender dysphoria is classified both by the *DSM-5* and the ICD-9 coding system. Box 25.1 contains the criteria for diagnosis according to the *DSM-5*. Although an argument can be made against use of an umbrella term to describe a diverse population of people who experience some level of incongruence between their gender identity and their natal sex, having a clear set of diagnostic criteria and coding allows for more consistent health care, insurance coverage, and the ability to secure grant funding for future research.

Current guidelines require that a person seeking medical or surgical gender transition must undergo some type of mental health evaluation in order to start hormone therapy or have gender-affirming surgery. Mental health providers are typically involved in making or confirming the diagnosis of gender dysphoria. Individuals participate in therapy to assist in personal acceptance of their gender identity, as well as how to relate to family members and friends during the process of gender transition. The decision of whether or not to start hormone therapy is based on informed consent, however, leaving open the option of diagnosis and treatment at the level of the prescriber.

The criteria for starting hormone therapy are listed in Box 25.2. Informed consent must be completed such that the patient is aware of the potential reversible and irreversible side effects of hormone therapy. Any existing mental or pertinent physical illnesses must be reasonably well controlled before starting hormones. It is important to note that mental illness itself is not a contraindication to medical or surgical gender transition (Coleman et al., 2012).

The role of the nurse practitioner will be to facilitate the diagnosis of gender dysphoria in patients presenting with those symptoms, and to determine the health care needs of those individuals who have started or completed the transition process. For transmen this means determining the need for pelvic exams and Pap smears, as well as evaluation of existing breast tissue. For transwomen, this may involve evaluation of the neovagina, as well as screening and treatment of breast tissue. It is also essential that the nurse practitioner assess each person for management of other diagnoses that could affect long-term health and well-being such as hypertension or diabetes.

■ TREATMENT/MANAGEMENT

Gender dysphoria can be alleviated in multiple ways. The method is often driven by the individual's desires and access to health care and support. This transition can include, but is not limited to, social transition through gender expression, hormone therapy, surgical alteration, and/or legal name and gender changes (Coleman et al., 2012). Hormone therapy has been found to have the effect of decreasing depression and improving self-esteem (Gorin-Lazard et al., 2013). Although they could be very important treatment modalities, hormone therapy and surgical options are not always available to the individual because of financial, social, or safety concerns. The goal of any treatment is to alleviate or minimize the distress caused by the incongruence of physical appearance and gender identity.

Coleman et al (2012) and the Endocrine Society (Hembree et al., 2009) provide the standards of care and treatment for individuals with gender dysphoria. These guidelines are flexible and are meant to provide a framework for providers to give compassionate and competent care. They are important resources to guide not only the diagnosis of gender dysphoria, but also the treatment along an adaptable continuum to meet the needs of the individual undergoing transition. Not all individuals will elect to use any or all of the options available for medical or surgical transition. Treatment and preventative screenings must be tailored to the patient's physical and emotional needs.

Transwomen

The mainstay of hormone therapy for transwomen transitioning from male to female is estrogen (Coleman et al., 2012; Hembree et al., 2009). Use of exogenous estrogen suppresses testosterone production and leads to changes in the body that are more consistent with female characteristics. Typical estrogen preparations and doses are listed in Box 25.3. Expected effects of estrogen therapy include breast tissue development, redistribution of fat in a more female-type pattern, softening of the skin, decrease in the frequency of spontaneous erections, and decrease in testicular volume (Hembree et al., 2009). Potential side effects of estrogen therapy include deep vein thrombosis or pulmonary embolism, liver enzyme changes, cholelithiasis, hyperprolactinemia, and migraines (Hembree et al., 2009).

Other medications, such as spironolactone and finasteride, may also be used for their anti-androgen effects. Progesterone is used at the discretion of the prescriber given that it is suspected to increase risk of breast cancer, cardiac events, and depression (Rossouw et al., 2002). Progesterone has not been shown to have significant clinical benefit in terms of modifying body shape or breast tissue growth and should be used with caution (Wierckx, Gooren, & T'Sjoen, 2014).

■ BOX 25.2   CRITERIA FOR STARTING HORMONES

1. Persistent, well-documented gender dysphoria
2. Capacity to make a fully informed decision and to consent for treatment
3. Age of majority in a given country
4. If significant medical or mental health concerns are present, they must be reasonably well controlled

Source: Hembree et al., 2009.

BOX 25.3   HORMONE REGIMENS

Transwomen

Oral estradiol: 2–6 mg daily
Transdermal estradiol: 0.1–0.4 mg twice weekly
Parenteral estradiol valerate or cypionate: 5–20 mg every 2 weeks or 2–10 mg every week

Transmen

Parenteral testosterone: cypionate or enanthate 100–200 mg every 2 weeks or 50–100 mg every week
Transdermal testosterone: gel 2.5–10 g/d or patch 2.5–7.5 mg/d

Source: Coleman et al., 2012.

Health assessment and evaluation by the nurse practitioner include breast exam, assessment of risk of cardiac disease and stroke, and risk of osteoporosis. Breast exams are performed at the same intervals as recommended for natal-born females (Hembree et al., 2009). Risk of cardiac disease and stroke should be modified with lifestyle changes and medication according to current guidelines (Hembree et al., 2009). Decisions to screen or treat for osteoporosis should be made based on age, hormone use, history of gonad removal, and other known risk factors for bone loss such as smoking and alcohol intake. Particular attention should be paid to the transwoman who has undergone orchiectomy but is not taking hormone therapy given the lack of sex steroids to protect bone health.

Though hormone therapy is typically the most accessible treatment option available, many transwomen will also elect to have some form of gender-affirming surgery. Surgical options include mammoplasty, vaginoplasty, orchiectomy, penectomy, clitoroplasty, and vulvoplasty. If the woman has undergone removal of the testicles, the exogenous estrogen dose is typically lowered, and all other anti-androgen therapy is discontinued. Other feminizing surgeries that do not modify the genitalia are also available, such as laser hair removal and facial feminizing surgery.

Feminizing hormone therapy for at least 12 months is recommended before breast augmentation surgery to improve aesthetic outcomes (Coleman et al., 2012). There is no difference in recommendations for evaluation of breast symptoms or disease in transwomen who have undergone breast augmentation compared with natal-born females. Special attention should be paid to women who have undergone a procedure commonly referred to as "pumping" in which highly viscous preparations of mineral oil or silicone oil are injected into the breasts, hips, buttocks, or other areas to create a body contour associated with the female body. Injecting preparations of silicone oil that were not designed to be injected into subcutaneous tissue can cause devastating effects on the person's health including migration of the oil, changes in skin color, deformity, and death (Christensen, 2007). Referral should be made to a knowledgeable surgeon for consideration of treatment if the woman has undergone this procedure.

Vaginoplasty is the surgical construction of a vaginal canal; orchiectomy and penectomy are performed at the time of the surgery. The neovagina can be lined either by inverting the penile skin or by using a section of the colon. In the case of using the penile skin, preventative screenings must include assessment for risk of human papillomavirus (HPV) and cancer; cytology testing is not recommended, however, the tissue should be examined annually for signs of HPV (Center of Excellence for Transgender Health, 2011). Colonic neovagina should be evaluated by vaginoscopy, a procedure similar to a colonoscopy, to evaluate the tissue for colon cancer.

The prostate gland is typically not removed during gender-affirming surgery. Screening for prostate cancer with the prostate specific antigen (PSA) can be difficult because of the risk of false negative when the person is taking estrogen (Wenisch et al., 2014). If the woman has had a vaginoplasty, the most sensitive screening for prostate cancer is a digital exam through the neovagina. The prostate is typically smaller because of the use of estrogen and may be more difficult to evaluate by the usual digital rectal exam.

There should be a discussion regarding fertility and reproduction with the individual before starting medical transition if possible (Coleman et al., 2012). Cryopreserving sperm before starting estrogen therapy is preferable if the person has access to the procedure and/or the funds to have it cryogenically preserved given the risk of infertility after long-term estrogen therapy (Lübbert, Leo-Rossberg, & Hammerstein, 1992; Schulze, 1988). Once hormone therapy is initiated, and presuming the individual has not had an orchiectomy, it is possible to withdraw cross-gender hormones in order to restore fertility. The level of fertility and how long it takes to produce viable sperm is likely person specific and may be related to the length of time the individual has been taking estrogen.

Transmen

The mainstay of treatment for transmen transitioning from female to male is testosterone (Hembree et al., 2009). Testosterone is available as an injectable oil suspension or a transdermal preparation in the form of creams, gels, or patches. Typical doses of each preparation of testosterone are available in Box 25.3. Use of testosterone leads to a more phenotypic male presentation by both suppressing estrogen and exerting its own effects on the body. Testosterone causes dropping of the voice, increased muscle mass, increased facial and body hair growth, and cessation of menses (Hembree et al., 2009). Side effects of testosterone therapy can include acne, increased liver enzymes, vaginal atrophy, and erythrocytosis (Hembree et al., 2009). Other medications to aid in transition are rarely used, though progesterone is sometimes used to suppress menses. Finasteride or other 5 alpha-reductase inhibitors may be used for male-pattern baldness. Testosterone cream may be used on the clitoris to increase clitoromegaly. It is important to avoid using alcohol-based medications on this area, and the dose used must be subtracted from the total dose (Center of Excellence for Transgender Health, 2011).

The target serum testosterone level is the upper quartile of age-matched natal males (Hembree et al., 2009). Increasing the level above recommended targets increases risks of side effects from testosterone, including erythrocytosis and liver dysfunction. It is also important to review with individuals using testosterone therapy that abnormally high testosterone levels will have the adverse effect of aromatization to estrogen, which will lead to more feminizing effects and menstruation if they have an intact uterus. There is no documented clinical benefit to increasing testosterone levels above the age-matched natal normal.

Surgical options for transmen include mastectomy, hysterectomy, oophorectomy, metoidioplasty, phalloplasty, and scrotoplasty. The most common procedures are mastectomy and metoidioplasty given their low complexity and low cost compared with other procedures. Phalloplasty, especially, is a complex, expensive surgery and is not performed routinely in the United States; transmen seeking this procedure must travel abroad. Not all individuals will opt for any or all available surgeries. It is of utmost importance to ascertain what, if any, procedures the person has undergone so that the provider can anticipate and treat any issues with the existing structures.

The nurse practitioner can be an invaluable participant in the health care of transmen. Particular attention must be paid to coaching individuals through potentially painful exams, especially of the pelvis. Pelvic exams can be anxiety producing as well as physically uncomfortable. Trust between the provider and the patient is essential in promoting preventative care and appropriate treatment of any acute issues. Cervical cytology and pelvic exam should be performed according to current recommendations for natal females based on past exams and risk of HPV (Potter et al., 2015). It is important to alert the pathologist reading the cytology sample that the individual is taking testosterone in order to account for the atrophy seen in the tissue. It is unclear if testosterone therapy affects risk of polycystic ovarian syndrome (PCOS; Ikeda et al., 2013). Obesity, dyslipidemia, and insulin resistance must be managed aggressively; however, there is no clear evidence that testosterone therapy increases ovarian cysts or risk of ovarian cancer. Any vaginal bleeding that cannot be explained by high or low levels of testosterone should be evaluated with transvaginal ultrasound (U/S); however, routine use of U/S in an asymptomatic individual is not recommended (Unger, 2014). Vaginal atrophy can occur once testosterone therapy has been initiated and is caused by estrogen deficiency. The treatment in the transmale is the same as for cis-gendered females, with attention to using the lowest dose of estrogen possible. The low dose of estrogen used for this treatment should not affect testosterone levels or rate of masculinization.

Mammograms for transmen should be performed according to current recommendations for natal females if the individual has not undergone mastectomy. It is not necessary to have a mammogram before surgery if the person would not otherwise be considered appropriate for screening (Hembree et al., 2009).

■ FUTURE DIRECTIONS

The science of caring for the transgender individual is rapidly growing and improving. It is unfortunate that because of the lack of cultural acceptance historically, research is still nascent. Experts in clinical practice have provided a significant information base from which clinicians can draw when caring for those who are gender nonconforming. Nurse practitioners have the opportunity to provide a much-needed service to a historically marginalized group of people. As more and more providers are able to compassionately and competently care for transgender individuals and research and experience lead to more advanced understanding and improved surgical procedures, the health of the individuals and the community will improve.

■ REFERENCES

American Psychiatric Association (APA). (2013). *Diagnostic and statistical manual of mental disorders* (5th ed.). Arlington, VA: American Psychiatric Publishing.

Center of Excellence for Transgender Health. (2011). *Primary care protocol for transgender patient care*. San Francisco, CA: University of California, Department of Family and Community Medicine.

Christensen, L. (2007). Normal and pathologic tissue reactions to soft tissue gel fillers. *Dermatologic Surgery: Official Publication for American Society for Dermatologic Surgery, 33*(Suppl. 2), S168–S175.

Coleman, E., Bockting, W., Botzer, M., Cohen-Kettenis, P., DeCuypere, G., Feldman, J. (2012). Standards of care for the health of transsexual, transgender, and gender-nonconforming people, version 7. *International Journal of Transgenderism, 13*(4), 165–232.

Gorin-Lazard, A., Baumstarck, K., Boyer, L., Maquigneau, A., Penochet, J. C., Pringuey, D.,...Auquier, P. (2013). Hormonal therapy is associated with better self-esteem, mood, and quality of life in transsexuals. *The Journal of Nervous and Mental Disease, 201*(11), 996–1000.

Gooren, L. (2006). The biology of human psychosexual differentiation. *Hormones and Behavior, 50*(4), 589–601.

Grant, J. M, Mottet, L. A., Tanis, J., Harrison, J., Herman, J. L., & Keisling, M. (2011). *Injustice at every turn: A report of the national transgender discrimination survey*. Washington, DC: National Center for Transgender Equality and National Gay and Lesbian Task Force.

Hembree, W. C., Cohen-Kettenis, P., Delemarre-van de Waal, H. A., Gooren, L. J., Meyer, W. J., Spack, N. P.,...Endocrine Society. (2009). Endocrine treatment of transsexual persons: An Endocrine Society clinical practice guideline. *Journal of Clinical Endocrinology and Metabolism, 94*(9), 3132–3154.

Ikeda, K., Baba, T., Noguchi, H., Nagasawa, K., Endo, T., Kiya, T., & Saito, T. (2013). Excessive androgen exposure in female-to-male transsexual persons of reproductive age induces hyperplasia of the ovarian cortex and stroma but not polycystic ovary morphology. *Human Reproduction, 28*(2), 453–461.

Institute of Medicine (IOM). (2011). *The health of lesbian, gay, bisexual, and transgender people: Building a foundation for better understanding*. Washington, DC: National Academies Press.

Lübbert, H., Leo-Rossberg, I., & Hammerstein, J. (1992). Effects of ethinyl estradiol on semen quality and various hormonal parameters in a eugonadal male. *Fertility and Sterility, 58*(3), 603–608.

Potter, J., Peitzmeier, S. M., Bernstein, I., Reisner, S. L., Alizaga, N. M., Agenor, M., Pardee, D. J. (2015). Cervical cancer screening for patients on the female-to-male spectrum: A narrative review and guide for clinicians. *Journal of General Internal Medicine, 30*(12), 1857–1864.

Rossouw, J. E., Anderson, G. L., Prentice, R. L., LaCroix, A. Z., Kooperberg, C., Stefanick, M. L.,...Ockene, J.; Writing Group for the Women's Health Initiative Investigators. (2002). Risks and benefits of estrogen plus progestin in healthy postmenopausal women: Principal results from the women's health initiative randomized controlled trial. *Journal of the American Medical Association, 288*(3), 321–333.

Schulze, C. (1988). Response of the human testis to long-term estrogen treatment: Morphology of Sertoli cells, Leydig cells and spermatogonial stem cells. *Cell and Tissue Research, 251*(1), 31–43.

Unger, C. A. (2014). Care of the transgender patient: The role of the gynecologist. *American Journal of Obstetrics and Gynecology, 210*(1), 16–26.

Wallien, M. S., & Cohen-Kettenis, P. T. (2008). Psychosexual outcome of gender-dysphoric children. *Journal of the American Academy of Child and Adolescent Psychiatry, 47*(12), 1413–1423.

Wenisch, J. M., Mayr, F. B., Spiel, A. O., Radicioni, M., Jilma, B., & Jilma-Stohlawetz, P. (2014). Androgen deprivation decreases prostate specific antigen in the absence of tumor: Implications for interpretation of PSA results. *Clinical Chemistry and Laboratory Medicine, 52*(3), 431–436.

Wierckx, K., Gooren, L., & T'Sjoen, G. (2014). Clinical review: Breast development in trans women receiving cross-sex hormones. *Journal of Sexual Medicine, 11*(5), 1240–1247. doi:10.111/jsm.12487

Zucker, K. J., & Lawrence, A. A. (2009). Epidemiology of gender identity disorder: Recommendations for the standards of care of The World Professional Association for Transgender Health. *International Journal of Transgenderism, 11*(1), 8–18. doi:10.1080/15532730902799946

CHAPTER 26

Sexual Health Problems and Dysfunctions

Candi Bachour • Candace Brown

Sexuality is basic to the human condition, and women rate sexuality as an important quality-of-life issue. The Centers for Disease Control and Prevention (CDC) notes that the World Health Organization (WHO, 2006) defines *sexual health* as:

> A state of physical, emotional, mental and well-being. In relation to sexuality; it is not merely the absence of disease, dysfunction, or infirmity. Sexual health requires a positive and respectful approach to sexuality and sexual relationships, as well as the possibility of having pleasurable and safe sexual experiences, free of coercion, discrimination, and violence. (WHO, 2006)

Healthy sexual function with a partner nurtures the relationship, whereas sexual dysfunction may cause relationship disharmony with untoward repercussions to both partners. Healthy sexual functioning improves self-image and increases the motivation to take care of health concerns and adopt a healthier lifestyle. Studies suggest that less than one half of patients' sexual concerns are recognized by their clinicians, who are mostly unaware of the nature and severity of the sexual concerns of their patients (American College of Obstetricians and Gynecologists, 2003).

The clinician's role in assessing sexual dysfunction, initiating treatment, and making appropriate referrals is critical because women view their sexuality as an important quality-of-life issue that frequently is affected by reproductive events. Moreover, gynecologic disease processes and therapeutic interventions can potentially affect sexual response.

■ NORMAL SEXUAL RESPONSE

Sexual Response Cycle

Most clinicians are aware of the traditional human sexual response cycle of Masters and Johnson (1987) and Kaplan

(1988). This cycle depicts a linear sequence of discrete events, including desire, arousal, plateau of constant high arousal, peak intensity arousal and release of orgasm, possible repeated orgasms, and then resolution.

Neither the stimuli to which the response occurs nor the nature of the "cyclicity" is evident in this traditional model as applicable to the female sexual response. The usefulness of this model in depicting women's sexuality is limited by the following conditions: women are sexual for many reasons—sexual desire, as in sexual thinking and fantasizing, may be absent initially; sexual stimuli are integral to women's sexual responses; the phases of women's desire and arousal overlap; nongenital sensations and a number of emotions frequently overshadow genital sensations in terms of importance; arousal and orgasm are not separate entities; the intensity of arousal (even if orgasm occurs) is highly variable from one occasion to another; orgasm may not be necessary for satisfaction; the outcome of the experience strongly influences the motivation to repeat it; and dysfunctions may overlap (e.g., desire and arousal disorders, orgasm and arousal disorders).

An alternative sexual response model that depicts an intimacy-based motivation integral to sexual stimuli and the psychological and biological factors that govern the processing of those stimuli (e.g., determining the woman's arousability) has been suggested by Basson (2002). If sexual arousal is experienced, provided the stimuli continue, the woman remains focused, and the sexual arousal is enjoyed, she may be driven by sexual desire to continue the experience for the sake of the sexual sensations (as well as her emotional desire to be closer to her partner). A psychologically and physically positive outcome heightens her emotional intimacy with her partner, thereby strengthening the "motor" or "power" behind her sexual response cycle. Any "spontaneous" desire (i.e., the traditional sexual thinking, conscious sexual wanting and fantasizing) may augment the intimacy-based cycle. Spontaneous desire is particularly common early in relationships or when partners have been apart and is sometimes related to the menstrual cycle.

Physiology of Normal Sexual Response

Although there are still large gaps in the understanding of female sexual function, sex steroids and neurotransmitters in the central and peripheral nervous systems appear to play a significant role (Clayton, 2007). In the central nervous system (CNS), the neurotransmitter dopamine appears to modulate sexual desire. In addition, dopamine, along with norepinephrine, increases the sense of sexual excitement and the desire to continue sexual activity (Clayton, 2007). Increasing levels of serotonin can diminish the effects of both dopamine and norepinephrine, whereas melanocortins, small protein hormones, may have a stimulatory effect on dopamine (Clayton, 2007). Estrogen and testosterone function may, at least in part, be modulated by the effects of serotonin activity in the hypothalamus and associated limbic structures (Clayton, 2007). Other hormones also are involved in CNS modulation of sexual behavior. These include oxytocin, which may enhance sexual receptivity and orgasmic response (Clayton, 2007). Conversely, the pituitary hormone prolactin negatively influences the sexual excitement phase and is inversely related to dopamine function (Clayton, 2007).

In the periphery, sex hormones are important mediators of genital structures and function (Clayton, 2007). Nitric oxide (NO) and vasoactive intestinal peptide (VIP) are implicated in engorgement of clitoral tissue following sexual stimulation; however, adequate levels of estrogen and free testosterone are needed in order for NO to stimulate vasocongestion. Peripheral serotonin has negative effects on vasocongestion, NO function, and sensation. Prostaglandin E and cholinergic fibers also induce vasocongestion.

Women's sexual arousal often has been equated with vaginal lubrication. This unconscious reflex organized by the autonomic nervous system in response to mental or physical stimuli that are recognized as sexual is only one aspect of sexual arousal. In addition to "genital arousal," women may also experience cognitive arousal, or the feeling of being "turned on." Subjective sexual arousal is a product of the following components: mental sexual excitement—proportional to how exciting the woman finds the sexual stimulus and context; vulvar congestion—direct awareness (tingling, throbbing) is highly variable; pleasure from stimulating the engorging vulva; vaginal congestion—the woman's direct awareness is highly variable; pleasure from stimulating congested anterior vaginal walls and Halban's fascia; increased and edified lubrication—wetness usually is not directly arousing to the woman; vaginal nonvascular smooth muscle relaxation—the woman usually is unaware of this; pleasure from stimulating nongenital areas of the body; and other somatic changes—blood pressure level, heart rate, muscle tone, respiratory rate, and temperature.

■ SEXUAL DYSFUNCTION

Pathophysiology of Sexual Dysfunction

Problems with female sexuality have traditionally been presumed to be mainly the result of psychological factors, in part because women have a much more intimacy-based sex drive when compared with men. However, in many cases, psychological and physical problems are interrelated.

Etiology and Prevalence

Population surveys highlight the fact that female sexual disorders are highly prevalent. Comparison among countries is problematic because different definitions and methodologies are employed in different surveys. The National Health and Social Life Survey that was conducted in 1992 involved personal interviews with a probability sample of the United States population between the ages of 18 and 59 years (Berman & Bassuk, 2002). The survey found that 43% of women reported significant sexual complaints lasting several months in the preceding year. The most common concern was lack of sexual interest (reported by 33% of women), followed by difficulty reaching orgasm (24%) and problems with lubrication (19%).

In 2007, a population-based study found that relationship factors were more important to low desire than age or menopause, whereas physiological and psychological factors were more important to low genital arousal and low orgasmic function than relationship factors (Hayes et al., 2008). Sexual distress was associated with both psychological and relationship factors.

Risk Factors

Numerous risk factors are associated with sexual dysfunction in women. Women may have certain medical conditions or take medications that place them at increased risk of sexual dysfunction. In addition, those women with a history of sexual or physical abuse or those with relationship difficulties are at increased risk. Finally, different cultural backgrounds, where there may be conflicts with personal or family values as well as societal taboos and inadequate education, place women at risk of sexual dysfunction.

MEDICAL CONDITIONS

Numerous medical conditions are associated with sexual dysfunction (Bachmann & Avci, 2004; Berman & Bassuk, 2002; Box 26.1). Women with spinal cord injuries may experience an orgasmia. Complete spinal cord injuries involving sacral segments result in an inability to achieve physiological genital vasocongestion. An incomplete injury, however, can leave a woman with a degree of physiological lubrication in the case of sensory preservation at the T11 to L2 dermatomes (Sipski, Alexander, & Rosen, 1997).

Female sexual dysfunction may be the result of peripheral vascular or cardiovascular diseases, hypertension, and high blood cholesterol levels (Bachmann & Avci, 2004; Berman & Bassuk, 2002). Insufficient blood flow resulting from arterial diseases may cause vaginal wall and clitoral smooth muscle fibrosis, which result in vaginal dryness and dyspareunia (Berman & Bassuk, 2002). Blunt trauma and surgical disruption may lead to a decrease in vaginal and clitoral blood flow, resulting in sexual dysfunction (Berman & Bassuk, 2002).

BOX 26.1   MEDICAL CAUSES OF FEMALE SEXUAL DYSFUNCTION

Neurological Problems

- Spinal cord injuries

Cardiovascular Disease

- Hypertension
- Hypercholesterolemia
- Peripheral vascular disease

Cancer

- Ovarian cancer
- Endometrial cancer
- Breast cancer

Urogenital Disorders

- Stress and urinary incontinence
- Uterine prolapse

Hormonal Loss or Abnormalities

- Natural and surgical menopause
- Diabetes mellitus
- Hyperprolactinemia
- Hypothyroid and hyperthyroid states

Adapted from Bachmann and Avci (2004).

Gynecologic malignances may cause abnormal bleeding and abdominal discomfort before the diagnosis, which may stop women from engaging in any type of sexual activity. Additionally, radiation and chemotherapy used in gynecologic cancer treatment may have adverse effects on vaginal elasticity and thickness of the vaginal wall, causing dyspareunia and problems with sexual arousal (Cartwright-Alcarese, 1995). The adverse effects of cancer therapies are not limited to physiological effects. Malignancies coexist with psychological and social difficulties and may impair self-image and decrease sexual desire. This issue is particularly important in conditions that may impair self-image, such as having a mastectomy or hair loss after chemotherapy.

Hormonal changes associated with menopause and aging, such as estrogen/androgen depletion, often cause important physical and psychological adverse effects on sexual function. Estrogen depletion often leads to dyspareunia, sleep disturbances, mood swings, and depression. The thinning of the vaginal epithelium, atrophy of the vaginal wall smooth muscle, and elevated pH changes in the vagina may ultimately result in vaginal dryness and pain during intercourse. Urogenital disorders, characterized by stress and/or urge incontinence (see Chapter 28), may also affect a woman's level of comfort during sexual activity for fear of leakage.

Androgen depletion is associated with muscle wasting, mood changes, and loss of sexual motivation, including a decrease in libido and a diminution in sexual fantasy (Bachmann, Bancroft, & Braunstein, 2002). Approximately 45% of all women report a decrease in sexual desire after menopause (Laumann, Paik, & Rosen, 1999). Several studies have looked at this issue, especially in the surgically menopausal population, and consistently find an association between sexual interest and androgens. At physiological replacement levels, androgen use should not result in masculinizing side effects. Hirsutism, voice deepening, adverse lipid changes, and skin changes have been the key concerns in using androgens in women with loss of sexual desire. These adverse events are infrequent with low-dose regimens.

Because several studies report improved sexual function in postmenopausal women after estrogen and androgen therapy, the use of these gonadal hormones will continue to increase as more women present to their clinicians with sexual complaints (Buster et al., 2005; Sarrel, Dobay, & Wiita, 1998; Sherwin, 1991; Shifren et al., 2000).

Other hormonal imbalances that may affect sexual functioning include diabetes mellitus, hyperprolactinemia, and hypothyroid and hyperthyroid states (Bachmann & Avci, 2004).

MEDICATIONS ASSOCIATED WITH SEXUAL DYSFUNCTION

The most common medications associated with female sexual dysfunction are selective serotonin reuptake inhibitors (SSRIs; Box 26.2). Delay or absence of orgasm with reduced sexual desire occurs in up to 70% of women taking SSRIs (American College of Obstetricians and Gynecologists, 2003; Phillips, 2000). In general, any antidepressants that interfere with serotonergic pathways (nonselectively), such as SSRIs, or with acetylcholine pathways, such as tricyclic antidepressants, induce sexual dysfunction. In contrast, antidepressants that impact dopaminergic and (central) noradrenergic receptors, or selective hydroxytryptamine 5-HT$_{1A}$ and 5-HT$_{2C}$ receptors, are not likely to reduce sexual response (American College of Obstetricians and Gynecologists, 2003; Phillips, 2000). Therefore, those antidepressants least likely to interfere with sexual response include non-SSRI antidepressants, such as nefazodone (Serzone), mirtazapine (Remeron), bupropion (Wellbutrin), venlafaxine (Effexor, at doses of 150 mg or lower), duloxetine (Cymbalta), and buspirone (BuSpar; American College of Obstetricians and Gynecologists, 2003; Phillips, 2000). A newly approved medication, vortioxetine (Brintellix), has multimodal activity as both a 5-HT$_{1A}$ receptor agonist and a 5-HT$_3$ antagonist and was found to have relatively low sexual side effects when compared with placebo (Boulenger, Loft, & Olsen, 2014). This may provide an alternative to the traditional SSRI; however, head-to-head studies are needed to verify this agent's utility.

Other centrally acting medications, including psychoactive substances, such as antipsychotics, barbiturates, and benzodiazepines, and codeine-containing opiates may

BOX 26.2   MEDICATION-INDUCED SEXUAL DYSFUNCTION

Psychoactive Medications

- Antipsychotics
- Barbiturates
- Benzodiazepines
- Selective serotonin reuptake inhibitors (SSRIs)
- Tricyclic antidepressants

Anticholinergics

- Antihistamines

Antihypertensives

- Beta-blockers
- Centrally acting (clonidine, methyldopa)
- Diuretics

Antilipid Medications

- Hormones
- Oral contraceptives
- GnRH agonists
- Medroxyprogesterone
- Selective estrogen receptor modulators (SERMs)

Adapted from American College of Obstetricians and Gynecologists (2003); Phillips (2000).

affect sexual function (American College of Obstetricians and Gynecologists, 2003; Phillips, 2000). Opinion varies as to whether anticonvulsants are associated with low sexual desire. Many women can take anticonvulsants for diseases other than epilepsy without experiencing sexual side effects. Anticholinergic agents, which interfere with acetylcholine function, such as antihistamines, also impair sexual response (American College of Obstetricians and Gynecologists, 2003; Phillips, 2000).

Antihypertensives that penetrate the blood–brain barrier, such as beta-blockers and centrally acting antihypertensives, as well as diuretics, may reduce sexual desire (American College of Obstetricians and Gynecologists, 2003; Phillips, 2000). However, calcium channel blockers and angiotensin-converting enzyme (ACE) inhibitors are generally not considered to have sexual side effects. Other cardiovascular agents, such as antilipemics, may also induce sexual problems (American College of Obstetricians and Gynecologists, 2003; Phillips, 2000).

Agents, which interfere with the hypothalamic-pituitary-ovarian axis, such as gonadotropin-releasing hormone agonists, like leuprolide (Lupron), are likely to induce sexual

problems. A subgroup of women using oral contraceptives reported low sexual desire, which may be caused by reduced free testosterone production and an increased serum level of sex hormone–binding globulin, which also may cause low sexual desire in some women receiving estrogen therapy. Progestins, such as medroxyprogesterone, may also induce sexual dysfunction by their negative effects on the mood (Phillips, 2000). Some estrogen agonist/antagonists may have estrogen antagonistic activity in the vagina. Thus, raloxifene (Evista), tamoxifen (Soltamox), and phytoestrogens may exacerbate vaginal dryness and dyspareunia (American College of Obstetricians and Gynecologists, 2003; Phillips, 2000).

PSYCHOLOGICAL FACTORS ASSOCIATED WITH SEXUAL DYSFUNCTION

Several psychological factors can negatively affect sexual function. Relationship problems can interfere with a woman's interest in sexual expression and undermine her enjoyment of sexual experiences. A woman's cultural and religious background may affect how she views sexual activities, and interpersonal factors, such as depression, stress, substance use, or sexual trauma, can affect how the woman is able to interact and emotionally connect with others.

Interpersonal Factors • Low libido frequently accompanies women with major depression. Women who report mood changes, sleep disturbance, fatigue, decreased concentration, low self-esteem, reduced interest in activities, decreased energy and motivation, and appetite or weight changes may improve in sexual function if their depression is effectively treated (Box 26.3).

Women who are under tremendous stress often feel they do not have time to engage in sexual activity and may view it as just "another responsibility." Those who work full time, take care of children, and carry the majority of responsibility for domestic activities may hold resentment toward their partner. In addition, assuming the role of "mother" and "wife" in heterosexual relationships may reduce a woman's feeling of being sexual, in both her eyes and in those of her partner. Increasing ways to reduce stress, such as increased partner assistance with responsibilities and having "date nights" may improve sexual response.

Although alcohol and other recreational substances may temporarily produce a "disinhibiting" effect on women who are anxious about sexual activity, and subsequently improve responsivity, chronic substance abuse impairs sexual function.

Many researchers report a relationship between sexual abuse during childhood and female sexual dysfunction. Many of these studies, however, have been limited by both small numbers and by the omission of comparison groups. The lack of a comparison group is relevant because of the high percentage of women who, during routine gynecologic care, report sexual problems (Nusbaum, Gamble, Skinner, & Heiman, 2000). Of 412 women seen in a sexual dysfunction clinic with their husbands, sexual dysfunction was diagnosed in 182 of the women (Sarwer & Durlak, 1996). Of women who had experienced childhood abuse, 63% had

BOX 26.3   PSYCHOLOGICAL CAUSES OF FEMALE SEXUAL DYSFUNCTION

Interpersonal

- Depression/anxiety
- Stress
- Alcohol/substance abuse
- Previous sexual or physical abuse

Relationship

- Relationship quality and conflict
- Lack of privacy
- Partner performance and technique

Sociocultural

- Conflict with religious, personal, or family values
- Societal taboos
- Inadequate education

Adapted from Bachmann and Avci (2004).

BOX 26.4   SEXUAL HISTORY

- History of present illness
- Typical encounter
- Current medications
- Past medications
- Current medications
- Medical history
- Social history
- Psychiatric history
- Family history
- Developmental and sexual history
- Relationship history
- Stressors
- Psychiatric examination
- Mental status
- Physical problems or limitations
- Current diagnoses
- Specifiers of the diagnosis (e.g., is it acquired or lifelong, situational, or generalized?)

female sexual dysfunction and 37% did not. Of the women without any history of abuse, 48% had sexual dysfunction. Abuse involving penetration or violence was specifically related to adult sexual dysfunction.

Other psychological factors commonly affect sexual response in women. These may include negative sexual experiences, including fear of a likely unsatisfactory or painful outcome; decreasing self-image; potent nonsexual distractions (e.g., baby); lack of physical privacy; feelings of shame; lack of education regarding sexual anatomy and physiology; embarrassment; partner sexual dysfunction; lack of safety from pregnancy and sexually transmitted infection; and fear of physical safety.

Relationship Factors • Perhaps the most common contributor to sexual dysfunction in women is a nonfunctional relationship with her partner. A variety of factors may contribute to this, including poor communication skills, infidelity, control issues, partner substance abuse, and parental conflicts. A woman will often seek sex therapy in order to improve the relationship, whereas if she and her spouse attended relationship therapy, her sexual function would most likely improve.

Lack of privacy, due to the presence of children or relatives living with a couple, may also affect a woman's comfort level in engaging in sexual activity. Additionally, any partner dysfunction can reduce a woman's motivation to be sexual. Commonly, this includes erectile dysfunction, premature ejaculation in male partners, and desire or orgasm difficulties in female partners.

Sociocultural Factors • Women who were raised in a very strict religious background, where sexual activity before marriage was considered wrong, may find it difficult to automatically transition into feeling sexual once she gets married. If she received the message that sex was "dirty," she may find it very difficult to think of it as an "act of love" in a committed relationship. Moreover, some cultures encourage a woman to have sex only as a function of performing "wifely duties" and that a respectable woman should not enjoy the pleasures of sex. Finally, many women may not have received any education about sex, including basic knowledge of female and male anatomy, and a woman's sexual response.

EVALUATION/ASSESSMENT

History • A comprehensive sexual history is the first step in establishing the diagnosis of a female sexual disorder. Sexual inquiry is aimed at exploring the areas of the woman's concerns, moving from general to more specific areas.

Box 26.4 identifies the components of a thorough sexual history. Questions that are asked during the history of the present illness include chief sexual complaints (in the woman's own words) and eliciting information on the onset, duration, precipitating factors, and other sexual complaints. The clinician attempts to determine whether the symptoms are situational (occur in only one setting) or are generalized (present in all settings) and whether they are lifelong (have always been present) or acquired (there was a time when there was normal sexual functioning). The clinician determines the woman's and her partner's explanation for the symptoms because patients often add significant insight into the cause of the problems. It is important to know why the woman is seeking treatment now, the amount of distress, and the woman's motivation for seeking treatment, as these factors may affect her interest in and ability to follow the therapy plan. Information is elicited on the type of previous treatment and its success.

Women are asked to describe a typical sexual encounter. This allows the woman to "tell her story" and to feel heard. The typical encounter discussion evaluates all phases of sexual response (including desire, arousal, orgasm) and pain. The frequency and types of sexual activity are determined along with which partner initiates the activities. It is important to keep in mind that women often do not "initiate" sexual activity, rather their desire is more related to their "receptivity" to their partner. The significance of contextual factors, such as time of day, location, fatigue, privacy, atmosphere, and foreplay are elicited. These factors can often be addressed by providing techniques in which to increase sexual stimulation. Fantasies can give information on sexual desire and normal sexual thoughts; however, they are often difficult to elicit at an initial interview and should not be prompted. It is preferable for the woman to spontaneously disclose information about her sexual fantasies because it is important that she feels comfortable discussing these thoughts. Both the woman's and her partner's response to the symptoms are determined because they may involve misinterpretation and lead to communication difficulties.

Current medications are identified to determine any drug-induced sexual dysfunction. Past medications are recorded to determine previous response and assess if a change in medications is required.

A thorough medical history, including a history of illnesses, surgeries, and neurological problems; head, eyes, ears, nose, and throat (HEENT) disorders; and endocrinologic, respiratory, cardiovascular, gastrointestinal, and genitourinary disorders, is obtained to determine illness-induced contributory factors. The woman's last menstrual period, childbirth history, date of last Pap smear, serum laboratory testing, mammogram, and bone density test are determined. Any history of allergies is identified, in case a medication is prescribed. A personal and family history of illnesses such as hypertension, cardiovascular disease, cerebrovascular accidents, and cancer are ascertained, as prescribing hormone therapy will depend on these factors.

The psychiatric history includes any previous treatment, hospitalizations, and suicide attempts. Women are questioned about previous or present psychotherapy, marital therapy, or sex therapy. Response to current and previous antidepressants is determined, as well as the presence of smoking, alcohol use, and substance use. A family history of psychiatric illness is also important in determining the presence of risks factors, and in selecting proper antidepressants based on a family member's response.

Areas to be discussed during the family history include ethnicity, religion, parental interactions (demonstration of affection among family members and toward the woman), individual relationships with each parent (role modeling), and sibling relationships. Cultural factors, such as views of sexuality (premarital sex, masturbation, and sexual roles) and their negative connotations, are also assessed. Women who have been raised in strict religious settings may feel uncomfortable about having sex after marriage when it was unacceptable before marriage. They may also have inadequate sexual education. Women who have not observed parents who were affectionate, or who divorced early on, may not have had appropriate role models. Selection of mates may be based on maladaptive relationships with parental figures.

The development and sexual history includes childhood, adolescent, and adult categories. Childhood history includes any losses, number of friends, family role, sexual knowledge, and sexual abuse. Early childhood experiences may have a long-term effect on self-esteem and comfort with one's sexuality. Adolescent areas include response to puberty, body image, masturbation, onset of sexual activity, and descriptions of dating and any rape. Poor body image may carry over into adulthood and affect a woman's ability to feel "sexy." Feelings of guilt about masturbation are elicited. Adult areas cover college and occupations. A higher level of education may predict whether a woman will be a good candidate for individual therapies as described as follows.

Relationship history concentrates on the current relationship, including partner description, conflicts, loss of trust or fidelity, communication problems, control issues, and intimacy. Conflicts often surround control issues, such as decisions regarding finances, parenting, and household responsibilities. It is important to determine whether the couple feels comfortable displaying nonsexual affection or if all types of affection have been abandoned. The number of children are identified and whether there are any conflicts regarding parenting. Previous relationships, including first major relationships and previous marriages and relationships (including lesbian, bisexual, and transgender relationships), are ascertained. Previous relationships can determine whether there is a pattern of choosing partners who are unlikely to be candidates for meaningful, long-term relationships, which may be addressed in individual counseling (see Chapter 19).

Any stressors are identified, such as relationship, work, illness, parenting, financial, and loss or deaths. Determining which stressors were present at the onset of sexual dysfunction can identify the relationship between these factors and the onset of sexual disturbance.

The psychiatric examination includes assessment of speech, thought process, judgment, insight, mood, and affect. The clinician determines whether the woman is euthymic, depressed, anxious, irritable, hypomanic, or labile. Mental status includes the woman's appearance, orientation, concentration, intellect, and memory (see Chapter 16). These observational skills can determine the presence of a psychiatric disorder and its contribution to sexual symptoms.

Based on this information, the clinician will make an initial diagnosis and specify whether the condition is lifelong or acquired type, due to psychological or combined factors, and whether the condition is generalized or situational.

Physical Examination • Physical examination is crucial for diagnosing some sexual disorders. For example, with chronic dyspareunia, a very careful genital examination is performed, especially of the introitus, because in most cases of dyspareunia, the pain is introital. Careful detailed inspection for vulvar atrophy or dystrophy or posterior fourchette scars (often facilitated by allowing the woman to see the examination using a mirror) and testing for allodynia around the hymenal edge with a cotton swab are needed. Resting vaginal tone and voluntary muscle contraction can be assessed approximately by the examining finger(s) and/ or with the use of perineometry. Tenderness, often focal from pressing on the deep levator ani ring, can be checked along with pain and discomfort by palpating the uterus and adnexa. Fixed retroversion can be determined, along with any nodularity suggestive of endometriosis. Bladder and urethral sensitivity can be assessed by palpating the anterior vaginal wall (see Chapter 28).

The role of the detailed physical examination for orgasmic disorder is less obvious when the disorder has been lifelong. Nevertheless, it can reassure the woman to know that the results of her physical examination are normal. In cases of acquired female orgasmic disorder, especially in the presence of neurologic disease, the examination is important and requires additional neurologic testing. Cold sensation from the clitoris can be detected by using a cold water-based lubricant. This modality of sensory testing is clinically more relevant to orgasm potential than the use of touch. The motor aspect of the orgasm reflex (i.e., pudendal nerves S2 through S4) can be checked by asking the woman to voluntarily contract the muscles around the vagina or the anus or both.

Pelvic examinations for women with low libido or difficulty with arousal may have limited usefulness unless sexual pain is present. A general physical examination for acquired loss of desire or arousal is reasonable, although clues to any systemic illness usually would be found in the history.

On the other hand, pelvic examination and testing of vaginal pH and wet prep evaluation of vaginal secretions are helpful in eliminating common vaginal infections such as yeast, *Trichomonas*, and bacterial vaginitis. Vaginal, cervical, and vulvar swabs for culture may be indicated in women with chronic dyspareunia. Dyspareunia associated with vulvar atrophy is readily diagnosed during a pelvic examination.

DIFFERENTIAL DIAGNOSES

The classifications of female sexual dysfunction have been defined by the International Consensus Development Conference on Female Sexual Dysfunction (Basson, 2005; Basson, Berman, & Burnett, 2000). The consensus conference panel built on the existing framework of the WHO *International Classification of Disease-10* (ICD-10; WHO, 1994) and the *Diagnostic and Statistical Manual of Mental Disorders, Fourth Edition* (DSM-IV) of the American Psychiatric Association (1994). The former *DSM-IV* classifications were expanded to include psychogenic and organic causes of desire, arousal, orgasm, and sexual pain disorders. An essential element of the *DSM-IV* and the newer *Diagnostic and Statistical Manual of Mental Disorders, Fifth Edition* (DSM-5; APA, 2013) diagnostic system is the personal distress criterion, meaning that a condition is considered a disorder only if it creates distress for the woman experiencing the condition. The current *DSM-5* now combines sexual desire, specifically hypoactive sexual desire disorder (HSDD), and female sexual arousal disorder (FSAD) into one category— sexual interest arousal disorder (SIAD; Box 26.5).

BOX 26.5   FEMALE SEXUAL DYSFUNCTION CATEGORIZED ACCORDING TO THE *DSM-IV* AND *DSM-5* CRITERIA

DSM-IV

- Sexual desire disorders (sexual desire/interest disorders)
  - Hypoactive sexual desire disorder
  - Sexual aversion disorder
- Sexual arousal disorder
- Orgasmic disorder
- Sexual pain disorders
  - Dyspareunia
  - Vaginismus
- Noncoital sexual pain disorders
- Sexual dysfunction due to a general medical condition
- Substance-induced sexual dysfunction
- Sexual dysfunction not otherwise specified
- Paraphilias
- Gender identity disorder

DSM-5 Changes

- Sexual desire disorder and sexual arousal disorder combined
  - Sexual interest arousal disorder (SIAD)
  - Sexual aversion removed
- Orgasmic disorder
- Sexual pain disorders (dyspareunia and vaginismus combined)
  - Genito-pelvic pain/penetrative disorder
- Noncoital sexual pain disorders (sexual dysfunction due to a general medical condition removed)
- Gender dysphoria
  - Gender identity disorder removed

Adapted from American Psychiatric Association (1994, 2013).

Sexual Desire Disorder • *Sexual aversion disorder* is defined as "the persistent or recurrent phobic aversion to and avoidance of sexual contact with a sexual partner, which causes personal distress" (Basson, 2005; Basson et al., 2000, p. 809). It is often the case that a woman's sexual aversion is the result of past sexual trauma or sexual abuse (Rosen, 2000). It is difficult to assess the frequency of this disorder because the data on prevalence do not distinguish this dysfunction from HSDD or the newer classification of SIAD.

Sexual Interest Arousal Disorder • As previously stated, hypoactive sexual desire disorder and FSAD have now been combined into one classification—SIAD. Due to SIAD being a newer disorder in the *DSM-5*, its prevalence is unknown; however, HSDD was reported in up to 30% of women (Laumann et al., 1999). SIAD criteria are met when a women experiences at least three symptoms for at least 6 months, including lack of interest in sexual activity; reduced or absent fantasies and/or erotic thoughts; lack of initiation and receptivity to sexual activity; diminished pleasure during sexual activity; diminished or absent desire during a sexual encounter; and a reduction in sexual sensations both genital and nongenital (APA, 2013).

For women who are both pre- and postmenopausal, problems achieving adequate lubrication during sexual stimulation may be present; however, the prevalence of the problem is higher in the postmenopausal population. A woman's perception of personal distress or deficiency remains crucial to the diagnosis of sexual interest arousal disorder, as well as other sexual disorders (Basson, 2005).

Data generated by a National Health and Social Life Survey (NHSLS) study indicated that 20% of women experience lubrication problems with sexual exchange (Laumann et al., 1999). Other research reports that a high percentage (44.2%) of postmenopausal women who have a low estrogen level have lubrication problems during vaginal penetration, which may lead to dyspareunia and postcoital bleeding (Rosen, 2000). Androgens also appear to play a role in the maintenance of sexual arousal and the treatment of diminished sexual arousal; however, they do not appear to significantly affect vaginal lubrication.

Problems with SIAD can have a purely psychological component or also may be in conjunction with medical treatments that cause reduced blood flow to the vagina or clitoris. These include pelvic surgery, trauma to the pelvic floor, radiation therapy, or medications such as gonadotropin-releasing hormone agonists (Berman & Goldstein, 2001).

Orgasmic Disorder • *Orgasmic disorder* is defined as "the persistent or recurrent difficulty, delay in, or absence of attaining orgasm following sufficient sexual stimulation and arousal, which causes personal distress" (Basson, 2005; Basson et al., 2000, p. 890). This condition is usually further subdivided into either primary or secondary. Primary orgasmic disorder refers to a woman's inability to achieve an orgasm under any circumstances. A secondary orgasmic disorder most often refers to an inability to reach climax only during intercourse; orgasm can otherwise be achieved either with masturbation or during sexual foreplay. Inability to have orgasm via intercourse is common, occurring in approximately one third of women, and is only problematic if it distresses the woman. Trauma to pelvic nerves resulting from pelvic surgery or trauma to pelvic organs may be associated with this disorder. Implicit in this definition is an acceptance that a woman does not have a release during her experience of arousal and this lack of release is distressing to her.

Studies of the general population and sex therapy clinic populations indicate that the prevalence of female orgasmic disorder ranges from 24% to 37% (Laumann et al., 1999; Spector & Carey, 1990). Although the incidence is reported

to be significantly higher in single women and postmenopausal women, there seems to be no differences when populations are compared by race, socioeconomic status, and educational or religious background (Laumann et al., 1999).

Sexual Pain Disorders • *Dyspareunia* is defined as "recurrent or persistent genital pain associated with sexual intercourse" (Basson, 2005; Basson et al., 2000, p. 890). When looking at both pre- and postmenopausal populations, 14.4% of all women report pain during sexual activity (Bachmann et al., 2002). This percentage appears to increase with the onset of menopause, where up to 34% of postmenopausal women report pain during coital exchange (Rosen et al., 1993). The rise in prevalence may be the result of vaginal irritation from diminished moisture and loss of vault elasticity (Rosen, 2000). Like the other female sexual disorders, dyspareunia has both physical and psychological components. Women with previous sexual trauma or assault may experience pain during coitus in the absence of a physical cause. A lack of foreplay may result in sparse lubrication, which can lead to vaginal irritation. In addition to estrogen lack, several health conditions such as diabetes mellitus, scleroderma, and other connective tissue conditions increase the prevalence of coital pain. Vulvar vestibulitis and hymenal tags can cause localized pain during penetration that may be triggered by cotton swab probing during the gynecologic examination. Deep penetration pain may be the result of gynecologic problems, such as pelvic adhesions, pelvic inflammatory disease, ovarian pathologies, and/or a retroverted uterus. Pathologic conditions involving adjacent structures such as bowel, bladder, and pelvic floor musculature may also cause deep penetration pain. Sexual pain disorders have been reported in 10% to 15% of women (Rosen, 2000).

Vaginismus is defined as "recurrent or persistent involuntary spasm of the musculature of the outer third of the vagina that interferes with vaginal penetration, and causes personal distress" (Basson, 2005; Basson et al., 2000, p. 890). It may be generalized or situational. Generalized vaginismus is characterized by involuntary vaginal spasms, which occur in all situations. Situational vaginismus refers to a dysfunction that is apparent only in a specific situation, such as vaginismus that is triggered by intercourse and not with insertion of a tampon. In sex therapy clinics, 15% to 17% of women report vaginismus (Spector & Carey, 1990). It is worth noting that vaginismus and dyspareunia have now been collapsed into a single diagnostic category—*genito-pelvic pain/penetration disorder* per the new *DSM-5* classification system (APA, 2013).

Genito-pelvic pain/penetration disorder criteria are met when a woman experiences difficulty with at least one of the following: vaginal penetration; pain with vaginal penetration; fear of vaginal penetration or fear of pain during vaginal penetration; or pelvic floor dysfunction (APA, 2013). This new *DSM-5* classification combines dyspareunia and vaginismus due to similarities between the two conditions. Due to the lack of research on this condition, this chapter reviews pertinent information on the conditions as separate entities.

Other Sexual Pain Disorders • Noncoital sexual pain disorder is the new category of sexual pain disorders that was added to the *DSM-IV* classification system after the 1998 International Consensus Development Conference (Basson, 2005; Basson et al., 2000). It is described as recurrent or persistent genital pain induced by noncoital sexual stimulation. This category, with a wide variety of etiologies including infections, genital trauma or mutilation, and vulvodynia, recognized that pain may occur during oral- and manual-stimulation sexual activities and is still part of the *DSM-5* (Rosen, 1993). Vulvodynia is listed under "other sexual pain disorders," because nonsexual activities such as exercising, bike riding, or sitting for a long duration of time can also trigger the symptoms. This condition, which is highly prevalent and poorly understood, is defined by the International Society of the Study of Vulvovaginal Disorders as "chronic vulvar discomfort with feelings of rawness, burning, stinging, and irritation" (Moyal-Barraco & Lynch, 2004, p. 774). Subtypes of vulvodynia include generalized (involving the whole vulvar area) and localized (involving the vestibule, or outer vagina), and may be spontaneous or provoked. Provoked vestibulodynia (PVD; previously known as vulvar vetibulitis) is the most common subtype of localized vulvodynia. PVD is associated with burning that is secondary to pressure on the vestibule and/or penetration during sexual activity. In PVD, vaginal penetration is often painful or simply impossible for most women with this condition. The etiologies and a variety of treatment options are still under investigation. Women with vulvodynia may see several clinicians and undergo a range of treatments before receiving the correct diagnosis. In addition to psychological reasons, factors such as injury to the pelvic floor nerves and muscles, long-term oral contraceptive use, diets high in oxalate, and trauma may contribute to its symptoms.

DIAGNOSTIC STUDIES

Psychometric Tests • Tools that are available to evaluate female sexual disorders such as the Brief Index of Sexual Functioning for Women (BISF-W), the Derogatis Interview for Sexual Functioning (DISF/DISF-SR), and the Female Sexual Function Index (FSFI) are multidimensional self-report instruments that are standardized to meet basic psychometric criteria of reliability and validity (Derogatis, 1994; Rosen et al., 2000; Taylor, Rosen, & Leiblum, 1994). These questionnaires have historically been used for research and not for clinical practice, however, use in clinical practice is increasing.

Laboratory Tests • If a medical etiology is implicated, laboratory values (complete blood count with differential [CBC + diff], complete metabolic panel [CMP], thyroid-stimulating hormone [TSH], cholesterol panel [high-density lipoprotein cholesterol, HDL-C; low-density lipoprotein cholesterol, LDL-C], follicle-stimulating hormone [FSH], estradiol, dehydroepiandrosterone sulfate [DHEA-S], serum sex hormone-binding globulin [SHBG], total and free testosterone) are in order. The need for performing a Pap smear and mammogram are determined, particularly if hormone therapy is being considered.

Other currently available laboratory investigations are of limited value. Estrogen status usually is detected by history and examination, although there may be occasions when assessment of estradiol levels is needed. Significantly, more women with an estradiol level of less than 50 pg/mL report vaginal dryness, dyspareunia, and pain compared with women with an estradiol level of more than 50 pg/mL. Prospective records of coital behavior and concomitant steroid analysis revealed that women with an estradiol level of less than 35 pg/mL reported reduced coital activity (American College of Obstetricians and Gynecologists, 2004). FSH testing during perimenopause is of limited value, given the marked fluctuations.

Testosterone levels are insensitive and inaccurate unless the dialysis method is used. However, when the history suggests that the concern is loss of androgen production, the testosterone level is assessed by the best method available to ensure that it is not high normal or high. It is more important to obtain either the free testosterone or percent free testosterone level rather than the total testosterone level, because SHBG binds with testosterone and the total testosterone level does not reflect the amount of testosterone free to act on androgen receptors. Typically, when the free testosterone level is in the lower quartile of the normal range for the specific lab used, the woman may benefit from androgen therapy (Bachmann et al., 2002). However, a woman needs to be adequately estrogenized before testosterone therapy, and if she is naturally menopausal, progesterone is added to prevent endometrial hyperplasia in women who have a uterus.

When infertility or oligomenorrhea is present, prolactin levels are measured to account for low desire. When signs or symptoms of thyroid disease are present, TSH levels are measured.

TREATMENT/MANAGEMENT

Based on information gathered primarily during the history, the clinician will make an initial diagnosis and specify whether the condition is lifelong or acquired type, due to psychological or combined factors, and whether the condition is generalized or situational. The clinician will also identify an initial plan, such as requesting another patient visit, partner visit, or couple visits. If medical etiology is implicated, laboratory values are assessed (see section "Diagnostic Studies"). The clinician determines whether the woman would benefit from medications or if she needs to be referred to another professional.

Self-Management Measures • Women are provided information and education about normal anatomy, sexual function, and normal changes of aging, pregnancy, and menopause. To enhance stimulation and eliminate routine, the clinician encourages use of erotic materials (videos and/or books); suggests self-pleasuring to maximize familiarity with pleasurable sensation; encourages communication during sexual activity; recommends use of vibrators; discusses varying positions, times of day, or places; and suggests making a "date" for sexual activity. Distraction techniques are also discussed, including encouraging erotic or nonerotic fantasy; recommending pelvic muscle contracting and relaxation (similar to Kegel exercise) with intercourse; and recommending use of background music and videos or television. The clinician recommends sensual massage, sensate-focus exercises (sensual massage with no involvement of sexual areas), where one partner provides the massage and the receiving partner provides feedback as to what feels good (aimed to promote comfort and communication between partners), and oral or noncoital stimulation, with or without orgasm. To minimize dyspareunia, the clinician recommends sexual positions including female superior or side lying for control of penetration depth and speed and use of lubricants, topical lidocaine, and warm baths before intercourse.

Psychological Treatment • There are many reasons for a reduction in sexual function, particularly desire, in couples who have been together for a long time. In general, the infatuation of courtship feeds the flames of desire; as the infatuation dies down, the intensity of the passion diminishes, as well as when a marriage matures, other concerns of the partners, such as earning a living, making a home, and raising a family become more pressing, absorbing some of the energy that had previously been channeled into romance. Gradually, the roles of wage earner and domestic worker take primacy over the role of lover. Finally, the fatigue and stress of work, child rearing, household duties, medical problems, and substance abuse may dampen sexual desire.

Psychological factors that reduce sexual desire after marriage are related to attitudes toward oneself, sex, and one's partner. For instance, self-doubts involving a sense of inadequacy or a fear of failure can carry over into sexual activities.

Some women whose physical appearance does not measure up to their ideal may feel ashamed or self-critical, and they may avoid lovemaking. A woman may dislike the size of her breasts or the shape of her thighs. Fearing that she does not appear womanly—that she lacks sex appeal—this woman may engage in a self-deprecation that interferes with the spontaneous expressions of her sexual drive.

Interpersonal problems between partners are a frequent source of trouble in a woman's sex life. One of the most obvious problems is a discrepancy in couple preferences—when, where, how, how long, and how often they have sexual activity. Conflicting desires about timing, frequency, or variety of sex activity can breed resentment, anxiety, or guilt. These unpleasant emotions can then interfere with their sexual contacts.

A medley of attitudes toward a woman's partner can encroach on her sexual feelings. For instance, if she believes that her mate is using her, does not care about her feelings, or is undeserving, she may experience an automatic inhibition of her sexual desire.

Many dysfunctional psychological thoughts can be corrected through cognitive therapy. Box 26.6 provides a list of negative thoughts about sex that represent cognitive distortions. These thoughts occur in many women during sex, and they interfere with sexual desire and satisfaction. These ideas, which generally reflect attitudes about herself, her mate, or sex in general, can be corrected by using cognitive

therapy (Beck, 1988). Cognitive therapy focuses on how the woman and her partner perceive each other and the way they communicate, miscommunicate, or fail to communicate. The cognitive approach is designed to remedy distortions and deficits in thinking and communication. The essence of cognitive therapy consists of exploring with the woman and her partner their unrealistic expectations, self-defeating attitudes, unjustified negative explanations, and illogical conclusions. Cognitive therapy helps correct these negative thoughts, attitudes, and misinterpretations, and couples often find that their sexual desire can once again become active.

Complementary and Alternative Medicines

Herbal Remedies and Over-the-Counter Supplements. The passage of the 1994 Food and Drug Administration (FDA) Dietary Supplement Health and Education Act (DSHEA) allowed for the expanded availability of androgenic substances. Androgenic dietary supplements do not require regulatory review and have thus not undergone formal trials for efficacy and safety. DHEA and androstenedione are the two major androgen supplements currently available, although there are a growing number of "pro-androgen" supplements being introduced to the marketplace either through the Internet or in stores without prescriptions.

BOX 26.6   NEGATIVE THOUGHTS DURING SEX

Thoughts About Self

- Parts of my body are not attractive.
- My body is not sexy enough.
- I am not good at this.
- I won't reach a climax.
- I won't satisfy my partner.

Thoughts About Partner

- You're in too much of a hurry.
- You're only interested in your own pleasure.
- You're too mechanical.
- I wonder what you're thinking.
- I'm afraid I'll let you down.
- How long is this going to take?
- That doesn't feel good but I'm afraid to tell you.
- You're trying too hard; I wish you'd relax.
- If only this weren't so important.
- I'm not really enjoying this.
- This is all you're interested in.

Adapted from American College of Obstetricians and Gynecologists (2004).

Compounds that are made up of "generally recognized as safe" substances require no formal regulatory review. One such product, Zestra for women, is an oil that contains natural botanical ingredients (borage seed oil, evening primrose oil, special extracts of angelica, coleus forskohlii, antioxidants, and vitamin E) with natural fragrances (Fourcroy, 2003). Before the market entry of Zestra, the sponsor conducted a small, randomized, double-blind, crossover study in 20 women, of whom 10 had FSAD (Ferguson et al., 2003). The study reported statistically significant improvements compared to placebo in levels of arousal, desire, satisfaction, and sexual pleasure (irrespective of SSRI use for some study participants). Zestra is meant to be applied (0.5–1 mL) with general massage to the external female genitalia, clitoris, labia, and vaginal opening at least 3 to 5 minutes before vaginal intercourse for enhanced sexual experience. A similar and larger multicenter randomized, placebo-controlled study of 200 women was conducted by the sponsor to further evaluate the efficacy of Zestra for mixed female sexual dysfunction (FSD). The study found similar results reporting improvements compared to placebo for arousal, desire, and treatment satisfaction (Ferguson, Hosmane, & Heiman, 2010).

ArginMax is a proprietary nutritional supplement consisting of extracts of ginseng, ginkgo, damamiana, arginine, and vitamins and minerals. In a 4-week, placebo-controlled study, women receiving ArginMax reported an improvement in sexual desire, clitoral sensation, and satisfaction with their overall sex life, a reduction of vaginal dryness, and an increase in frequency of sexual intercourse and orgasms without any significant adverse effects (Ito, Trant, & Polan, 2001). Oral products that contain high doses of l-arginine need to be used with caution in women with histories of oral and/or genital herpes, due to a potentiating effect. In addition, ginseng is used with caution in women with poorly controlled hypertension. More stringent scientific studies are needed for this interesting combination of supplements.

Mechanical Devices • The Eros-Clitoral Therapy Device, a small handheld mechanical device that increases blood flow to the clitoris, labia, and vagina by creating a vacuum over the clitoris, is the only FDA-approved mechanical device for the treatment of female sexual dysfunction. Clinical trials suggested that it improves genital sensation, lubrication, ability to experience orgasm, and sexual satisfaction (Billups et al., 2001). This device requires a prescription. The recommended use is three or four times a week, independent of sexual intercourse for tissue-conditioning effects or before intercourse. Eros therapy can be used as monotherapy or as adjunctive therapy such as with estrogen and/or testosterone therapy.

Pharmacotherapeutics

Hormone Therapy. Estrogen and androgen therapy may play a key role in the treatment of peri- and postmenopausal women. Estrogen therapy is helpful in relieving dyspareunia and may be helpful in treating arousal disorders by decreasing coital pain and improving clitoral sensitivity, arousal, and libido (Sherwin, 1991). However, estrogen therapy alone may not provide adequate relief of problems related to sexual function other than for dyspareunia and lubrication complaints.

Conditions resulting in low testosterone levels in women such as aging, oophorectomy, ovarian failure, adrenal insufficiency, and corticosteroid use may adversely affect sexual motivation. Symptoms of androgen insufficiency may include fatigue, decreased well-being, and decreased sexual desire (Bachmann et al., 2002). Although testosterone replacement has not yet been approved by the FDA for low libido in postmenopausal women, it has been shown to improve sexual function in some postmenopausal women (Buster et al., 2005; Sarrel et al., 1998; Shifren et al., 2000).

No guidelines for testosterone replacement therapy for women with disorders of desire and consensus of "normal" or "therapeutic" levels of testosterone therapy exist. Many clinicians are concerned about the lack of safety data on the role of testosterone in breast cancer and on hepatic side effects; however, hepatocellular damage or carcinoma are rare at prescribed dosages (American College of Obstetricians and Gynecologists, 2004) and the development of breast cancer has not been reported clinically (Slayden, 1998).

The side effects of testosterone, which occur in 5% to 35% of patients, include lower levels of HDL-C, acne, hirsutism, clitoromegaly, and voice deepening (Slayden, 1998). However, these side effects on lipoprotein levels are rarely significant if estrogen and testosterone are coadministered; moreover, most other side effects are reversible with discontinuation of testosterone or a dosage adjustment (Geldfand & Wiita, 1997). Before starting testosterone therapy, clinicians need to establish a baseline of acne, hirsutism, and other androgenic signs and counsel women about potential androgenic changes.

Before initiating testosterone treatment, clinicians discuss the potential and theoretic risks and the individual risk and benefit assessment with the woman. In general, women with current or previous breast cancer, uncontrolled hyperlipidemia, liver disease, acne, or hirsutism should not receive testosterone therapy.

Treatment guidelines are provided in Box 26.7. Women need to understand that testosterone is not approved by the FDA for the treatment of desire disorders in women before initiating therapy.

Compounded Bioidentical Hormones. Compounded drugs are agents that are prepared, mixed, assembled, packaged, or labeled as a drug by a pharmacist (American College of Obstetricians and Gynecologists, 2005). Unlike drugs that are approved by the FDA to be manufactured and sold in standardized dosages, compounded medications often are custom made for a patient according to a clinician's specifications. One category of compounded products is referred to as "bioidentical hormones"; however, there is confusion over what this term implies. Bioidentical hormones are plant-derived hormones that are biochemically similar or identical to those produced by the ovary or body.

The steroid hormones most commonly compounded include dehydroepiandrosterone, testosterone, pregnenolone, progesterone, estrone, estradiol, and estriol (American

BOX 26.7   ANDROGEN THERAPY FOR TREATMENT OF FEMALE ANDROGEN INSUFFICIENCY[a]

Screening

- Baseline testosterone levels[b] (free and total), estradiol levels,[c] DHEA-S,[d] baseline fasting lipid profile, baseline liver enzyme levels, mammography, Pap smear

Initiate Therapy[e]

- Combination product (*Covaryx* or *Covaryx HS*, generic esterified estrogen and methyltestosterone, off-label testosterone gel [*Testim*])[f]
- Testosterone gel (*Testim*) 1% (5 g/5 mL tube); apply ½ mL *qod–qd*[g]
- DHEA 25 mg one capsule PO*hs*
- Compounded testosterone vanishing cream[h]

Reevaluation at 3 Months

- Repeat androgen levels, DHEA-S, estradiol, fasting lipid profile, liver enzyme levels

Monitor Symptoms and Side Effects

Continued therapy

- Taper to lowest effective dose
- Monitor lipid levels, liver enzyme levels once or twice yearly
- Routine Pap smear and mammography screenings

[a]These are recommendations; no evidence-based protocols are available on androgen therapy for the treatment of women with desire disorders.

[b]Many authors recommend that total levels remain in "normal" range for premenopausal women.

[c]Metabolic pathway of testosterone metabolism ends with estradiol.

[d]Dehydroepiandrosterone sulfate (DHEA).

[e]None of these medications is labeled by the U.S. Food and Drug Administration (FDA) for treatment of desire disorders.

[f]Combination product formerly known as *Estratest* is now under the brand name *Covaryx*.

[g]The FDA recently required labeling of topical testosterone products regarding the potential risk of inadvertent secondary exposure to children via contact with the treated patient.

[h]Use in conjunction with consultation with compounding pharmacist.

DHEA, dehydroepiandrosterone; DHEA-S, dehydroepiandrosterone sulfate.

Adapted from Phillips (2000).

College of Obstetricians and Gynecologists, 2005). Biochemical hormones are available with various routes of administration, including oral, sublingual, and percutaneous, or as implants, injectables, and suppositories. Examples of compounded hormones include Biest and Triest preparations. The name Biest (biestrogen) commonly refers to an estrogen preparation based on a ratio of 20% estradiol and 80% estriol on a milligram-per-milligram basis. A similar preparation, Triest (triestrogen), usually contains a ratio of 10% estradiol, 10% estrone, and 80% estriol. It is important to note that these ratios are not based on each agent's estrogenic potency, rather they are based on the milligram quantity of the different agents added (Boothby, Doering, & Kipersztok, 2004).

Currently, there is no scientific evidence to support claims of increased efficacy or safety for bioidentical hormones. Purchases of compounded hormones are not typically reimbursed by insurance companies. Additionally, the FDA has approved a bioidentical progesterone (micronized) and many forms of bioidentical estradiol, which are manufactured by pharmaceutical companies and available through traditional pharmacies.

Sildenafil (Viagra). An elective inhibitor of phosphodiesterase 5 (PDE-5), sildenafil (Viagra) blocks the activity of PDE-5, causing the accumulation of 3′,5′-cyclic guanosine monophosphate in the corpora cavernosa, which in turn leads to muscle relaxation (Fourcroy, 2003). Sildenafil has been prescribed to millions of men for treatment of sexual dysfunction.

Several recent studies report on clinical trials of sildenafil in women. Trials suggested that sildenafil may partially reverse sexual dysfunction in women with spinal cord injuries (Sipski, Rosen, Alexander, & Hamer, 2000) and improve arousal frequency, sexual fantasies, sexual intercourse, and orgasm (Caruso, Intelisano, Lupo, & Agnello, 2001). Sildenafil also provides an improvement in vaginal lubrication and clitoral sensitivity (Kaplan, 1999). Additional clinical trials have found that sildenafil is effective for female sexual dysfunction caused by SSRIs, and it provides an improvement in sexual function of patients with antidepressant-induced sexual dysfunction in both women and men (Shen, Urosevich, & Clayton, 1999). This finding was not supported by another clinical trial that reported sildenafil did not improve the sexual response among women with female sexual arousal disorder (Basson, McInnes, Smith, Hodgson, & Koppiker, 2002). However, sildenafil treatment is well tolerated and no serious adverse effects have been reported in women. As with men, women who are using nitrates or have cardiovascular disease should not be prescribed PDE-5 inhibitors.

Future Medications for Management • There are at least eight major pharmaceutical therapeutic paths being pursued for treatment of female sexual disorders. These include androgens, dopaminergic agonists, flibanserin, melanocortin-stimulating hormone, adrenoceptor antagonists, prostaglandins, ospemifene, and tibolone. Most of these agents have been previously studied in men for either male androgen deficiency or male erectile disorder.

Androgens. Phase III studies are being conducted using transdermal testosterone patches for treating naturally and surgically menopausal women with low sexual desire. Several clinical trials involving women with low libido who had undergone bilateral oophorectomy and hysterectomy found testosterone therapy beneficial, especially in regard to sexual motivation (Buster et al., 2005; Shifren et al., 2000). It is estimated that more than 4 million prescriptions are written off-label yearly, and postmenopausal women with HSDD may benefit from transdermal testosterone therapy (Davis & Braunstein, 2012). Side effects of testosterone have included hair growth and acne and safety has been documented in short-term randomized controlled trials; however, trials in longer duration are needed to assess long-term risks such as cardiovascular effects.

Phase II to III studies evaluating testosterone gel products for female sexual dysfunction are underway (Fourcroy, 2003). Transdermal gel is thought to represent an improvement over transdermal delivery by patches because it offers more dosage flexibility, less irritation potential, and a better cosmetic appearance. One such product, Libigel (Biosante Pharmaceuticals, Inc., Lincolnshire, IL), a transdermal testosterone gel for postmenopausal women with HSDD, is currently being evaluated for long-term cardiovascular risks, breast cancer risk, and general safety outcomes (White et al., 2012). These long-term risks remain unknown and previous studies have reported high placebo response and high rates of androgenic side effects during short-term use. Additional randomized, placebo-controlled studies are needed to elucidate risks versus benefits along with efficacy for these products.

Dopaminergic Agents. The use of dopaminergic agents was found to have a stimulatory effect on sexual behavior in some patients with Parkinson's disease (Fourcroy, 2003). Moreover, patients who received bupropion (Wellbutrin) for the treatment of SSRI-induced sexual adverse events reported experiencing an increase in libido (Gitlin, Suri, Altshuler, Zuckerbrow-Miller, & Fairbanks, 2002). Dopamine appears to be a "prosexual" or "activating" neurotransmitter, while serotonin is an inhibitor (Fourcroy, 2003).

A sublingual formulation of a nonselective D1 and D2 dopamine receptor agonist apomorphine has been approved in Europe and is awaiting registration in the United States for the treatment of erectile dysfunction (Fourcroy, 2003). Unconfirmed rumors suggest the development of an apomorphine product for female sexual dysfunction. An intranasal formulation of apomorphine for the treatment of both male and female sexual dysfunction is also being developed.

Flibanserin. Flibanserin is a drug that has been shown to have inconsistent effects for treating depression in animal models. It is a serotonin 5-HT$_{1A}$ agonist and a 5-HT$_{2A}$

antagonist (Borsini et al., 2002). These subtype receptors of serotonin are thought to be related to libido. Phase III trials have investigated the efficacy of flibanserin in treating low sexual desire in premenopausal women. Three large randomized trials compared flibanserin and placebo, with 2,310 randomized to flibanserin and 1,238 randomized to placebo (Derogatis et al., 2012; Katz, 2013; Thorp, Simon, & Dattani, 2012). Improvements in desire were found in the number of satisfying sexual events, level of sexual desire on FSFI domain, and reduction of stress related to the low desire (Derogatis et al., 2012; Katz, 2013; Thorp, Simon, & Dattani, 2012). After a recent and third review, the FDA has approved flibanserin (Addyi) as the first FDA-approved treatment for HSDD (Gellad, Flynn, & Alexander, 2015). Because of the risk of severe hypotension and syncope when combined with alcohol, the drug is being released with a risk evaluation and mitigation strategy (REMS) program requiring prescribers to be certified. Additionally, a black box warning has been added due to this interaction (Gellad et al., 2015). Common side effects include dizziness, nausea, fatigue, and somnolence (Derogatis et al., 2012; Katz, 2013; Thorp, Simon, & Dattani, 2012; 9%–12% in flibanserin group vs. 3%–8% in placebo group), and women are consulted before any treatment decision is made (Thorp, Palacios, Symons, Simon, & Barbour, 2014).

α-Melanocyte-Stimulating Hormone. Recent findings indicate that effects on sexual dysfunction may be stimulated through melanocortin receptors in the brain. A nasally administered analogue of α-melanocyte–stimulating hormone, namely PT-141, was recently found to be effective in a small group of premenopausal women in improving both low sexual arousal and libido in an at-home setting (Diamond et al., 2006). Research suggests that it works through a mechanism involving the central nervous system.

α-Adrenoceptor Antagonists. Phentolamine is a combined α$_1$- and α$_2$-adrenoceptor antagonist that was originally approved for the treatment of pheochromocytoma-induced hypertension and norepinephrine-related dermal necrosis (Fourcroy, 2003). The effects of oral phentolamine 40 mg daily were assessed in a placebo-controlled, pilot study of six postmenopausal women with lack of lubrication or subjective arousal during sexual stimulation (Rosen, Phillips, Gendrano, & Ferguson, 1999). Mild improvements in subjective (self-reported) arousal and objective (measured) changes in vaginal blood flow were observed.

Prostaglandins. This class of drug is perceived to have an effect in improving arousal by relaxing the vaginal arterial smooth muscle and increasing vaginal secretions (Fourcroy, 2003). A placebo-controlled study of 79 postmenopausal women with sexual arousal disorders investigated local application of the prostaglandin alprostadil at 100 mcg and 400 mcg and compared this to placebo. Alprostadil 400 mcg resulted in a significant improvement over placebo in genital tingling and lubrication associated with sexual arousal, and in subjective reports of sexual arousal and satisfaction with arousal following visual sexual stimulation (Heiman et al., 2006). The women receiving alprostadil 400 mcg reported significantly greater changes from the baseline of genital warmth, tingling, level of sexual arousal, satisfaction with sexual arousal, and sexual satisfaction than those receiving 100 mcg alprostadil or placebo. Alprostadil is also being explored in phase II studies for premenopausal women (Fourcroy, 2003).

Tibolone. Tibolone is a selective tissue estrogenic activity regulator (STEAR) that has not been approved by the FDA due to the risk of recurrent breast cancer and stroke (Bundred et al., 2012). Tibolone has metabolites with estrogenic, androgenic, and progestagenic properties and randomized trials have shown improvement in sexual function for postmenopausal women receiving tibolone when compared to estradiol taken orally or transdermally (Cayan, Dilek, Pata, & Dilek, 2008; Nijland, 2008). Further studies are needed to assess the safety and efficacy of tibolone for treating female sexual dysfunction in postmenopausal women.

Ospemifene. Up to 15% of women treated with estrogen therapy for dyspareunia do not have symptom relief and may need alternative treatment (McLendon, Clinard, & Woodis, 2014). Ospemifene is the first FDA-approved medication for treating moderate to severe dyspareunia associated with vulvovaginal atrophy. Ospemifene (Osphena) is a selective estrogen receptor modulator (SERM) with estrogenic activity in the vagina, and no studies have shown significant effects on the endometrium or breasts (McLendon et al., 2014; Wurz, Kao, & DeGregorio, 2014). To date, five phase III clinical trials have been conducted, which focused on efficacy, treatment for dyspareunia and vaginal dryness, and long-term safety and efficacy data. All studies included postmenopausal women aged 40 to 80 years, and the most common side effect was hot flushes (McLendon et al., 2014; Wurz, Kao, & DeGregorio, 2014). An extension study lasting a total of 52 weeks compared 30-mg and 60-mg doses to placebo and found no clinically significant adverse events (Simon, Lin, Radovich, & Bachmann, 2013). Ospemifene (60 mg daily) may be a safe alternative for treating dyspareunia due to atrophy in postmenopausal women who cannot or would prefer not to use a vaginal estrogen product.

Referrals • Typical reasons for referring a patient are listed in Box 26.8. In these instances, referral to a psychiatrist, psychologist, psychiatric nurse practitioner, sex therapist, or sexual medicine practice specialist may be in order. The best way to determine the location of a qualified certified sex therapist is to go to the website of the American Association of Sex Educators, Counselors, and Therapists (AASECT; www.AASECT.org).

Considerations for Special Populations • Different sexual concerns affect a woman during the reproductive life span. During childhood, sexual abuse may leave a permanent effect on a woman's sense of sexuality and trust in sexual partners. During adolescence, special concerns relate to her response to puberty, menstruation, and her body image.

BOX 26.8   REASONS TO REFER A WOMAN WITH SEXUAL COMPLAINTS

- If she has a complex history, including both physical and psychological symptoms
- If she has not responded to traditional therapy (e.g., antidepressants)
- If it appears there are major relationship issues (e.g., infidelity)
- If there is a history of sexual abuse or domestic violence
- If multiple medical conditions are present with coexisting medications
- If the clinician does not have adequate knowledge in treating sexual disorders
- If the clinician does not have adequate time or desire to treat sexual disorders

---

A pregnant woman may avoid sexual activity due to fear of placing the fetus at risk, although there is little evidence to advise against coitus unless there are strong contraindications (Brown, Bradford, & Ling, 2009). Childbirth also brings about a change in the sexual relationship. Dyspareunia and breastfeeding, in particular, may affect a woman's level of sexual activity. Education by a clinician in regard to pregnancy, childbirth, and lactation is essential in assisting couples through this rewarding, yet often stressful period of their lives.

Postmenopausal women have to cope with both physical and psychological changes that may affect their sexuality. Dyspareunia from vaginal atrophy, body image concerns, and attitudes about the appropriateness of sex may affect sexual activity.

Certain subgroups of women may feel alienated from sexuality as portrayed in the media. These include women from different cultural and ethnic backgrounds, those raised in restrictive religious environments, women in lesbian (or same-sex) relationships, and women with physical disabilities. Transgendered women, who have female genitalia and identify themselves as male ("gender identity disorder"), may particularly suffer from societal discrimination. Counseling by a knowledgeable and nonjudgmental clinician is essential.

■ FUTURE DIRECTIONS

Many women experience sexual dysfunction. Medical conditions, psychosocial factors, medications, or a combination of factors can cause sexual dysfunction. A comprehensive history is always necessary and physical examination is needed in selective cases to identify the type and cause(s) of the sexual dysfunction so that an effective management plan can be developed. Multiple management options exist, and in cases when the response is not satisfactory to the woman or the complexity level is high, referral to a specialist is warranted. Multiple new therapies are being evaluated that may be of use for women in the near future.

■ REFERENCES

American College of Obstetricians and Gynecologists. (2003). Sexuality and sexual disorders. In R. Basson (Ed.), *Clinical updates in women's health Sexuality and sexual disorders* (pp. 22–32). Washington, DC: American College of Obstetricians and Gynecologists.

American College of Obstetricians and Gynecologists. (2004). Hormone therapy: Sexual dysfunction. *American Journal of Obstetrics and Gynecology, 104*, S85.

American Psychiatric Association. (1994). *Diagnostic and statistical manual of mental disorders* (4th ed.). Washington, DC: Author.

American Psychiatric Association. (2013). *Diagnostic and statistical manual of mental disorders* (5th ed.). Arlington, VA: American Psychiatric Publishing.

Bachmann, G., Bancroft, J., Braunstein, G., Burger, H., Davis, S., Dennerstein, L., . . . Traish, A. (2002). Female androgen insufficiency: The Princeton consensus statement on definition, classification, and assessment. *Fertility and Sterility, 77*, 660.

Bachmann, G. A., & Avci, D. (2004). Evaluation and management of female sexual dysfunction. *Endocrinologist, 14*, 337.

Basson, B., Berman, J. R., Burnett, A., Derogatis, L., Ferguson, D., Fourcroy, J., . . . Whipple, B. (2000). Report of the International Consensus Development Conference on Female Sexual Dysfunction: Definitions and classifications. *Journal of Urology, 163*, 888–893.

Basson, R. (2002). A model of women's sexual arousal. *Journal of Sex & Marital Therapy, 28*, 1.

Basson, R. (2005). Women's sexual dysfunction: Revised and expanded definitions. *Canadian Medical Association Journal, 172*(10), 1327–1333.

Basson, R., McInnes, R., Smith, M. D., Hodgson, G., & Koppiker, N. (2002). Efficacy and safety of sildenafil citrate in women with sexual dysfunction associated with female sexual arousal disorder. *Journal of Women's Health & Gender-Based Medicine, 11*(4), 367–377.

Beck, A. (1988). *Love is never enough.* New York, NY: Harper and Row.

Berman, J. R., & Bassuk, J. (2002). Physiology and pathophysiology of female sexual function and dysfunction. *World Journal of Urology, 20*(2), 111–118.

Berman, J. R., & Goldstein, I. (2001). Female sexual dysfunction. *The Urologic Clinics of North America, 28*(2), 405–416.

Billups, K. L., Berman, L., Berman, J., Metz, M. E., Glennon, M. E., & Goldstein, I. (2001). A new non-pharmacological vacuum therapy for female sexual dysfunction. *Journal of Sex & Marital Therapy, 27*(5), 435–441.

Boothby, L. A., Doering, P. L., & Kipersztok, S. (2004). Bioidentical hormone therapy: A review. *Menopause, 11*(3), 356–367.

Borsini, F., Evans, K., Jason, K., Rohde, F., Alexander, B., & Pollentier, S. (2002). Pharmacology of flibanserin. *CNS Drug Reviews, 8*(2), 117–142.

Boulenger, J. P., Loft, H., & Olsen, C. K. (2014). Efficacy and safety of vortioxetine (Lu AA21004), 15 and 20 mg/day: A randomized, double-blind, placebo-controlled, duloxetine-referenced study in the acute treatment of adult patients with major depressive disorder. *International Clinical Psychopharmacology, 29*(3), 138–149.

Brown, C. S., Bradford, J., & Ling, F. W. (2009). Sex and sexuality in pregnancy. In J. J. Sciarra (Ed.), *Gynecology and obstetrics* (Vol. 2). Philadelphia, PA: Lippincott Williams & Wilkins.

Bundred, N. J., Kenemans, P., Yip, C. H., Beckmann, M. W., Foidart, J. M., Sismondi, P., . . . Kubista, E. (2012). Tibolone increases bone mineral density but also relapse in breast cancer survivors: LIBERATE trial bone substudy. *Breast Cancer Research, 14*(1), R13.

Buster, J. E., Kingsberg, S. A., Aguirre, O., Brown, C., Breaux, J. G., Buch, A., . . . Casson, P. (2005). Testosterone patch for low sexual desire in surgically menopausal women: A randomized trial. *Obstetrics and Gynecology, 105*(5, Pt. 1), 944–952.

Cartwright-Alcarese, F. (1995). Addressing sexual dysfunction following radiation therapy for a gynecologic malignancy. *Oncology Nursing Forum, 22*(8), 1227–1232.

Caruso, S., Intelisano, G., Lupo, L., & Agnello, C. (2001). Premenopausal women affected by sexual arousal disorder treated with sildenafil: A double-blind, cross-over, placebo-controlled study. *BJOG: An International Journal of Obstetrics and Gynaecology, 108*(6), 623–628.

Cayan, F., Dilek, U., Pata, O., & Dilek, S. (2008). Comparison of the effects of hormone therapy regimens, oral and vaginal estradiol, estradiol + drospirenone and tibolone, on sexual function in healthy postmenopausal women. *Journal of Sexual Medicine, 5*(1), 132–138.

Clayton, A. H. (2007). Epidemiology and neurobiology of female sexual dysfunction. *Journal of Sexual Medicine, 4*(Suppl. 4), 260–268.

Davis, S. R., & Braunstein, G. D. (2012). Efficacy and safety of testosterone in the management of hypoactive sexual desire disorder in postmenopausal women. *Journal of Sexual Medicine, 9*(4), 1134–1148.

Derogatis, L. R. (1997). The Derogatis Interview for Sexual Functioning (DISF/DISF-SR): An introductory report. *Journal of Sex & Marital Therapy, 23*(4), 291–304.

Derogatis, L. R., Komer, L., Katz, M., Moreau, M., Kimura, T., Garcia, M., . . . Pyke, R.; VIOLET Trial Investigators. (2012). Treatment of hypoactive sexual desire disorder in premenopausal women: Efficacy of flibanserin in the VIOLET Study. *Journal of Sexual Medicine, 9*(4), 1074–1085.

Diamond, L. E., Earle, D. C., Heiman, J. R., Rosen, R. C., Perelman, M. A., & Harning, R. (2006). An effect on the subjective sexual response in premenopausal women with sexual arousal disorder by bremelanotide (PT-141), a melanocortin receptor agonist. *Journal of Sexual Medicine, 3*(4), 628–638.

Ferguson, D. M., Hosmane, B., & Heiman, J. R. (2010). Randomized, placebo-controlled, double-blind, parallel design trial of the efficacy and safety of Zestra in women with mixed desire/interest/arousal/orgasm disorders. *Journal of Sex & Marital Therapy, 36*(1), 66–86.

Ferguson, D. M., Steidle, C. P., Singh, G. S., Alexander, J. S., Weihmiller, M. K., & Crosby, M. G. (2003). Randomized, placebo-controlled, double blind, crossover design trial of the efficacy and safety of Zestra for Women in women with and without female sexual arousal disorder. *Journal of Sex & Marital Therapy, 29*(Suppl. 1), 33–44.

Fourcroy, J. L. (2003). Female sexual dysfunction: Potential for pharmacotherapy. *Drugs, 63*(14), 1445–1457.

Geldfand, M. M., & Wiita, B. (1997). Androgen and estrogen androgen hormone replacement therapy: A review of the safety literature, 1941 to 1996. *Clinical Therapeutics, 19*, 383.

Gellad, W. F., Flynn, K. E., & Alexander, G. C. (2015). Evaluation of flibanserin: Science and advocacy at the FDA. *Journal of the American Medical Association, 314*(9), 869–870.

Gitlin, M. J., Suri, R., Altshuler, L., Zuckerbrow-Miller, J., & Fairbanks, L. (2002). Bupropion-sustained release as a treatment for SSRI-induced sexual side effects. *Journal of Sex & Marital Therapy, 28*(2), 131–138.

Hayes, R. D., Dennerstein, L., Bennett, C. M., Sidat, M., Gurrin, L. C., & Fairley, C. K. (2008). Risk factors for female sexual dysfunction in the general population: Exploring factors associated with low sexual function and sexual distress. *Journal of Sexual Medicine, 5*(7), 1681–1693.

Heiman, J. R., Gittelman, M., Costabile, R., Guay, A., Friedman, A., Heard-Davison, A., . . . Stephens, D. (2006). Topical alprostadil (PGE1) for the treatment of female sexual arousal disorder: In-clinic evaluation of safety and efficacy. *Journal of Psychosomatic Obstetrics and Gynaecology, 27*(1), 31–41.

Ito, T. Y., Trant, A. S., & Polan, M. L. (2001). A double-blind placebo-controlled study of ArginMax, a nutritional supplement for enhancement of female sexual function. *Journal of Sex & Marital Therapy, 27*(5), 541–549.

Kaplan, H. S. (1988). *The illustrated manual of sex therapy* (2nd ed.). New York, NY: Psychology Press.

Kaplan, S. A., Reis, R. B., Kohn, I. J., Ikeguchi, E. F., Laor, E., Te, A. E., & Martins, A. C. (1999). Safety and efficacy of sildenafil in postmenopausal women with sexual dysfunction. *Urology, 53*(3), 481–486.

Katz, M., DeRogatis, L. R., Ackerman, R., Hedges, P., Lesko, L., Garcia, M., & Sand, M.; BEGONIA trial investigators. (2013). Efficacy of flibanserin in women with hypoactive sexual desire disorder:

Results from the BEGONIA trial. *Journal of Sexual Medicine, 10*(7), 1807–1815.

Laumann, E. O., Paik, A., & Rosen, R. C. (1999). Sexual dysfunction in the United States: Prevalence and predictors. *Journal of the American Medical Association, 281*(6), 537–544.

Masters, W. H., & Johnson, V. E. (1987). *Human sexual response.* Boston, MA: Little Brown.

McLendon, A. N., Clinard, V. B., & Woodis, C. B. (2014). Ospemifene for the treatment of vulvovaginal atrophy and dyspareunia in postmenopausal women. *Pharmacotherapy, 34*(10), 1050–1060.

Moyal-Barraco, M., & Lynch, P. F. (2004). 2003 ISSVD terminology and classification of vulvodynia: A historical perspective. *Journal of Reproductive Medicine, 49,* 772.

Nijland, E. A., Weijmar Schultz, W. C., Nathorst-Boös, J., Helmond, F. A., Van Lunsen, R. H., Palacios, S.,…Davis, S. R.; LISA study investigators. (2008). Tibolone and transdermal E2/NETA for the treatment of female sexual dysfunction in naturally menopausal women: Results of a randomized active-controlled trial. *Journal of Sexual Medicine, 5*(3), 646–656.

Nusbaum, M. R., Gamble, G., Skinner, B., & Heiman, J. (2000). The high prevalence of sexual concerns among women seeking routine gynecological care. *Journal of Family Practice, 49*(3), 229–232.

Phillips, N. A. (2000). Female sexual dysfunction: Evaluation and treatment. *American Family Physician, 62*(1), 127–36, 141.

Rosen, R., Brown, C., Heiman, J., Leiblum, S., Meston, C., Shabsigh, R., …D'Agostino, R. (2000). The Female Sexual Function Index (FSFI): A multidimensional self-report instrument for the assessment of female sexual function. *Journal of Sex & Marital Therapy, 26*(2), 191–208.

Rosen, R. C. (2000). Prevalence and risk factors of sexual dysfunction in men and women. *Current Psychiatry Reports, 2*(3), 189–195.

Rosen, R. C., Phillips, N. A., Gendrano, N. C., & Ferguson, D. M. (1999). Oral phentolamine and female sexual arousal disorder: A pilot study. *Journal of Sex & Marital Therapy, 25*(2), 137–144.

Rosen, R. C., Taylor, J. F., Leiblum, S. R., & Bachmann, G. A. (1993). Prevalence of sexual dysfunction in women: Results of a survey study of 329 women in an outpatient gynecological clinic. *Journal of Sex & Marital Therapy, 19*(3), 171–188.

Sarrel, P., Dobay, B., & Wiita, B. (1998). Estrogen and estrogen-androgen replacement in postmenopausal women dissatisfied with estrogen-only therapy. Sexual behavior and neuroendocrine responses. *Journal of Reproductive Medicine, 43*(10), 847–856.

Sarwer, D. B., & Durlak, J. A. (1996). Childhood sexual abuse as a predictor of adult female sexual dysfunction: A study of couples seeking sex therapy. *Child Abuse & Neglect, 20*(10), 963–972.

Shen, W. W., Urosevich, Z., & Clayton, D. O. (1999). Sildenafil in the treatment of female sexual dysfunction induced by selective serotonin reuptake inhibitors. *Journal of Reproductive Medicine, 44*(6), 535–542.

Sherwin, B. B. (1991). The impact of different doses of estrogen and progestin on mood and sexual behavior in postmenopausal women. *Journal of Clinical Endocrinology and Metabolism, 72*(2), 336–343.

Shifren, J. L., Braunstein, G. D., Simon, J. A., Casson, P. R., Buster, J. E., Redmond, G. P.,…Mazer, N. A. (2000). Transdermal testosterone treatment in women with impaired sexual function after oophorectomy. *New England Journal of Medicine, 343*(10), 682–688.

Simon, J. A., Lin, V. H., Radovich, C., & Bachmann, G. A. (2013). One-year long-term safety extension study of ospemifene for the treatment of vulvar and vaginal atrophy in postmenopausal women with a uterus. *Menopause, 20*(4), 418–427.

Sipski, M. L., Alexander, C. J., & Rosen, R. C. (1997). Physiologic parameters associated with sexual arousal in women with incomplete spinal cord injuries. *Archives of Physical Medicine and Rehabilitation, 78*(3), 305–313.

Sipski, M. L., Rosen, R. C., Alexander, C. J., & Hamer, R. M. (2000). Sildenafil effects on sexual and cardiovascular responses in women with spinal cord injury. *Urology, 55*(6), 812–815.

Slayden, S. M. (1998). Risks of menopausal androgen supplementation. *Seminars in Reproductive Endocrinology, 16*(2), 145–152.

Spector, I. P., & Carey, M. P. (1990). Incidence and prevalence of the sexual dysfunctions: A critical review of the empirical literature. *Archives of Sexual Behavior, 19*(4), 389–408.

Taylor, J. F., Rosen, R. C., & Leiblum, S. R. (1994). Self-report assessment of female sexual function: Psychometric evaluation of the Brief Index of Sexual Functioning for Women. *Archives of Sexual Behavior, 23*(6), 627–643.

Thorp, J., Palacios, S., Symons, J., Simon, J., & Barbour, K. (2014). Improving prospects for treating hypoactive sexual desire disorder (HSDD): Development status of flibanserin. *Journal of Obstetrics & Gynaecology, 121*(11), 1328–1331.

Thorp, J., Simon, J., Dattani, D., Taylor, L., Kimura, T., Garcia, M.,… Pyke, R.; DAISY Trial Investigators. (2012). Treatment of hypoactive sexual desire disorder in premenopausal women: Efficacy of flibanserin in the DAISY study. *Journal of Sexual Medicine, 9*(3), 793–804.

White, W. B., Grady, D., Giudice, L. C., Berry, S. M., Zborowski, J., & Snabes, M. C. (2012). A cardiovascular safety study of LibiGel (testosterone gel) in postmenopausal women with elevated cardiovascular risk and hypoactive sexual desire disorder. *American Heart Journal, 163,* 27–32.

World Health Organization. (1994). *International statistical classification of diseases and related health problems (ICD-10).* Geneva, Switzerland: WHO.

World Health Organization. (2006). *Defining sexual health: Report of a technical consultation on sexual health* (pp. 28–31). Geneva, Switzerland: Author. Retrieved from http://www.who.int/reproductive health/publications/sexual_health/defining_sexual_health.pdf

Wurz, G. T., Kao, C. J., & DeGregorio, M. W. (2014). Safety and efficacy of ospemifene for the treatment of dyspareunia associated with vulvar and vaginal atrophy due to menopause. *Clinical Interventions in Aging, 9,* 1939–1950.

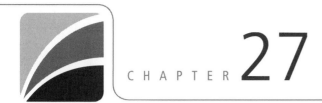

CHAPTER 27

Vulvar and Vaginal Health

Robert Gildersleeve

Vaginal and vulvar issues related to abnormalities of dermatologic and anatomic origin can be neoplastic or non-neoplastic. Understanding both typical and atypical female genitalia is important in identifying and managing vulvar and vaginal problems for women and expands the clinician's previously established foundation of basic science, embryology, anatomy, infectious disease, genetics, physiology, and pathophysiology, as well as other fields of study.

It is important to first consider anatomic and embryologic development because it can lead to a more intuitive understanding of disease. This is the case with Müllerian abnormalities, such as vaginal septum or septate uterus. Once the developmental process is known, the malformations are recognized as missteps in development. This knowledge can also facilitate recollection of related issues that may require investigation, such as renal collecting system abnormalities in the case of uterine malformation. Knowledge of anatomic location is imperative to understanding the function of these structures (e.g., periurethral glands), and therefore the goal of treatment: return to normal function with a minimal possibility of untoward consequences.

■ EMBRYOLOGY AND ANATOMY

Development plays a crucial role in understanding the histologic, anatomic, and functional nature of disease. Comprehension of the tissue's embryologic origin allows a more complete understanding of how and why disease develops and progresses, and how it can be effectively managed. Even with limited exposure to the specific clinical problem, observation, examination, and clinical correlation are greatly enhanced with good comprehension of anatomic development.

Anatomic variation becomes more intuitive when developmental processes are also understood, especially in the case of paramesonephric (Müllerian) defects of the fallopian tubes, uterus, and vagina. Vaginal development progresses from both endoderm and ectoderm. The distal two thirds of the vagina is derived from the urogenital sinus (ectoderm; Koff, 1933). The proximal one third is derived from the paramesonephric ducts (Figure 27.1). In females,

the paramesonephric ducts complete their development as the mesonephric (wolffian) ducts regress (Fu Yao, 2002). Structures derived from these parallel ductal systems form either male or female internal reproductive organs based on the appropriate creation and recognition of genetic signals. Paramesonephric-derived structures include the fallopian tubes, uterus, cervix, and proximal third of the vagina.

External Features

Some features of the external genitalia can be difficult to appreciate on examination in healthy women. It can be difficult to locate specific epithelial glands until they become swollen, as with a cyst. Recognizing the normal locations of glands, folds, ducts, nerves, and other structures facilitates determination of the possible causes of problems. In the case of external anatomy, diagrams provide the most effective way both to display these features and to define the terms used in describing their location (Figures 27.1–27.2). Clinical terminology is used to follow a disease course or to describe a disease process to a colleague. This allows more specific localization of findings.

The mons pubis and labia majora are readily visible on inspection of the female genitalia. Both contain adnexal structures of hair and sebaceous glands. The perineal body between the vagina and anus lacks these structures. The perineum (perineal body) is crucial to normal anatomic orientation of the vagina. It forms and maintains the outermost support structure for pelvic organs. Obstetric injuries to this area are frequently associated with loss of support and prolapse of the uterus, bladder, and rectum (Ashton-Miller & DeLancey, 2007; Maher & Baessler, 2006; Monnerie-Lachaud, Pages, Guillot, & Veyret, 2001). On separation of the labia majora, the prepuce, clitoris, labia minora, and urethra become apparent. In Figure 27.2, note the location of Bartholin's and Skene's glands because they can play important roles in abnormalities. At the distal vagina (near the introitus or opening), the hymen or its remnants can be seen. There are multiple anatomic variations that are customary with most genital structures, especially the labia and hymen. There is rugation of the vagina. The most proximal portion of the vagina (nearest the cervix) is known as the fornix, further divided into lateral, anterior, and posterior

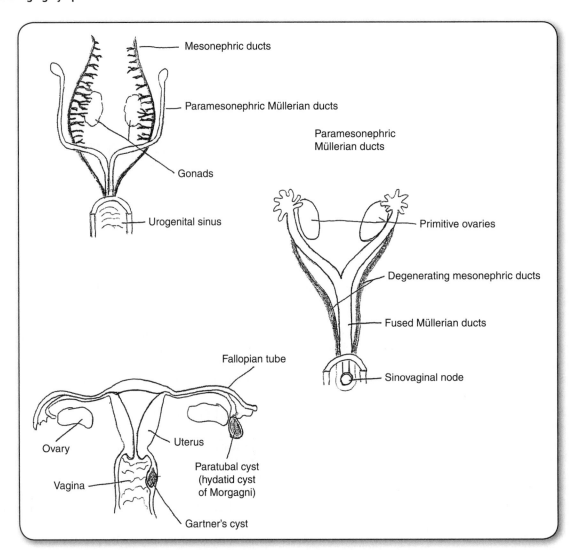

FIGURE 27.1

Embryologic development of ducts.

Adapted from Kaufman, Faro, and Brown (2004).

fornices. The normal configuration of the closed vagina varies (Barnhart et al., 2006). Some published studies have described the closed vagina as having an "H" (Figure 27.3) or butterfly shape (Fielding et al., 1996; Fielding, 1998). This configuration is attributable to lateral support of the vagina from the pelvic sidewalls. Support defects are indicated by loss of rugation and protrusion of the vagina around the speculum from any direction. Examination is performed dynamically, moving the speculum so that defects can be seen along any surface. There are five surfaces of the vagina: apex, two sidewalls, anterior surface (bladder), and posterior surface (rectum). The apex is supported predominantly by the uterosacral and cardinal ligament complexes. The lateral sidewalls are attached to the arcus tendineus fasciae pelvis via endopelvic fibroelastic connective tissue. The anterior and posterior walls are composed of more fibroelastic connective tissue, forming a septum between the vagina and both the bladder and rectum, respectively (Ashton-Miller & DeLancey, 2007; DeLancey, 1992; Maher & Baessler, 2006; Monnerie-Lachaud et al., 2001; Mostwin, Genadry, Sanders, & Yang, 1996; Muir, Aspera, Rackley, & Walters, 2004).

Internal Features

BONY STRUCTURES

The skeletal framework in which the female genitalia reside is composed of four bones: pubis, ilium, ischium, and sacrum (Figure 27.4; Netter, 2006; Standring, 2008; Stenchever, Droegmueller, Herbst, & Mischell, 2007). The pelvic outlet is bordered by the pubis anteriorly, the ilium and ischium laterally (the ischial tuberosities composing the most inferior portion), and the sacrum posteriorly. The pubis has a joint in the midline at the pubic symphysis. This can become markedly tender during pregnancy because the joint loosens and becomes more mobile, attributable to the effects of progesterone and the increasing pressure from the growing fetus. The iliac bones contain the femoral joints laterally. Their broad surfaces (also known as the allae, or wings) allow muscles of the back, legs, and abdomen to attach externally, and the anatomy of the pelvic floor to develop internally. The three-dimensional muscular structures of the pelvis and hip play an important role in both form and function of the pelvis. Although the spatial relationships are

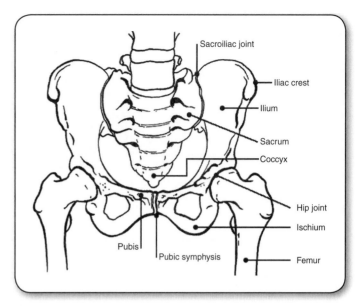

FIGURE 27.4
Pelvic bones.

Adapted from Gabbe, Niebyl, and Simpson (2007).

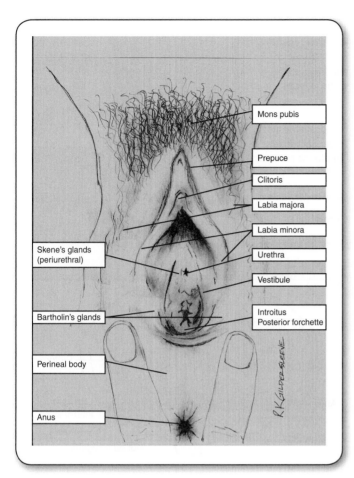

FIGURE 27.2
External female genitalia.

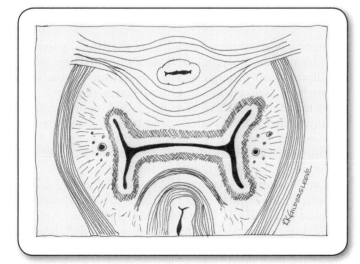

FIGURE 27.3
Cross section of vaginal shape, a crude H.

complicated to visualize, they are important because they impact sciatic pain, urinary stress incontinence, and pelvic organ prolapse, as well as other disorders.

The ischial tuberosities are the bony arcs on which body weight rests when sitting; they supply additional surface area for muscular attachment and add depth to the pelvis. The sacrum is the most inferior portion of the spine. An internally concave, arcing triangular shape, it forms the back wall of the pelvis. The sacral promontory is the ridge protruding anteriorly from the sacrum at the pelvic inlet, and is readily palpable in women of average weight. However, deep palpation can cause discomfort because of pressure on the abdominal structures, such as the aorta and large and small bowel.

MUSCULATURE

The musculature of the pelvis is relatively large and complex in its three-dimensional architecture. They are described as superficial and deep muscles with the external vulva and vagina as the reference point. Viewed in lithotomy position, superficial muscles are those nearest the distal, or outermost, vagina (Figure 27.5). An alternative approach is to view the bowl of muscle that comprises the pelvic floor from inside the pelvis, which facilitates visualizing the relationships of pelvic organs internally (Figure 27.6).

Superficial muscles of the pelvis are between the skin and the urogenital diaphragm. The urogenital diaphragm is a triangular region bounded by the pubis anteriorly and the ischial tuberosities laterally. The muscles attach from the ischial tuberosities to the pubis. The bulbospongiosus muscles surround the vagina from the perineal body to the pubis. Transverse perineal muscles span from the perineal body to the ischial tuberosities laterally. Posteriorly, the perineal body comprises the external and internal anal sphincters (Figures 27.6 and 27.7; Netter, 2006; Standring, 2008; Stenchever et al., 2007).

The levator ani (levator plate) consists of four deep muscles that form the pelvic floor. These muscles extend from the pubis to the coccyx (pubococcygeus), form a hammock around the rectum initiating at the pubis

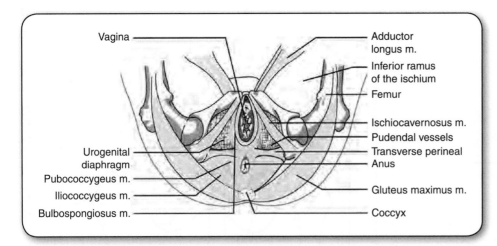

FIGURE 27.5
Pelvic triangle.

m, muscle.
Source: Helen and Secor (2015).

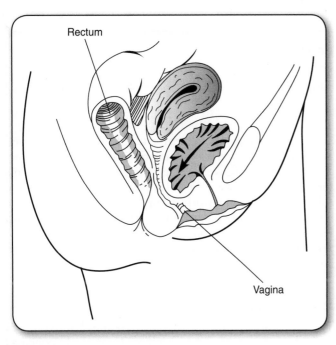

FIGURE 27.6
Pelvic viscera.

Source: Secor and Fantasia (2012).

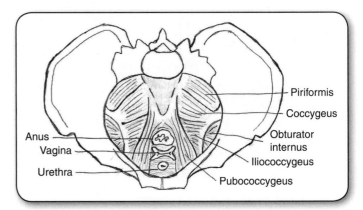

FIGURE 27.8
Pelvic floor musculature.

Adapted from Gabbe et al. (2007).

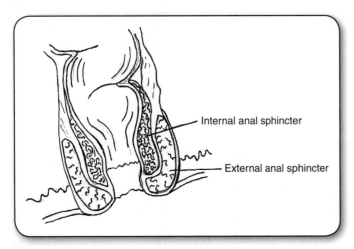

FIGURE 27.7
Anatomy of the anus and rectum.

Adapted from Wilson (2005).

(puborectalis), and then extend from the lateral pelvis to the sacrum (iliococcygeus and coccygeus). They create an elliptical gap through which the urethra, vagina, and rectum pass, known as the genital hiatus (Figure 27.8). These muscles function to keep the genital hiatus closed in healthy women. Defects attributable to age-related changes and obstetric trauma have been implicated in pelvic floor dysfunction. This can lead to urinary incontinence and pelvic organ prolapse, highlighting the importance of their anatomic function (Ashton-Miller & DeLancey, 2007; DeLancey, 1992; Maher & Baessler, 2006; Monnerie-Lachaud et al., 2001; Mostwin et al., 1996; Muir et al., 2004). Lateral support to the vagina is provided through attachments to the arcus tendineus fasciae pelvis, also known as "the white line" (Pit, De Ruiter, Lycklama A Nijeholt, Marani, & Zwartendijk, 2003). This is located at the juncture of the lateral levator muscles and the medial aspect of the internal obturator muscle.

INNERVATION

The vulva and vagina are predominantly innervated by the pudendal nerve (Figure 27.9). This nerve originates from S2 to S4 and provides motor and sensory supply to

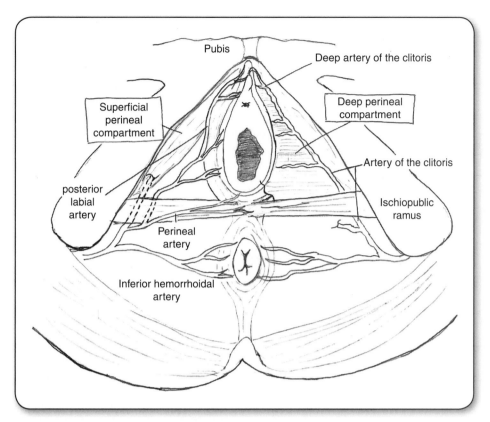

FIGURE 27.9
Vascular supply and innervation of the perineum.
Adapted from Gabbe et al. (2007).

the majority of the vulva and lower vagina as well as the muscles of the anal sphincter, which form the posterior perineal body (Netter, 2006; Standring, 2008; Stenchever et al., 2007). Other prominent nerves include the ilioinguinal and posterior femoral cutaneous. The local dermatomes are illustrated in Figure 27.10. The vagina has two different sources of innervation, as would be expected considering embryologic development. The proximal one third of the vagina receives sympathetic (T11–L5) and parasympathetic innervation (S2–S4) from the uterovaginal and hypogastric plexi, and the pudendal nerve innervates the distal two thirds (Figures 27.9 and 27.11; Krantz, 1958).

VASCULAR SUPPLY

The vascular supply to the lower genital tract is similar in anatomy to the nervous supply; hematologic and nervous supplies are tethered throughout the body as neurovascular bundles. The pudendal artery is a branch of the anterior division of the internal iliac artery. The distribution of the pudendal artery is the same as that of the pudendal nerve, serving nearly the entirety of the vulva, perineal body, and anus, as well as the distal vagina (Netter, 2006; Standring, 2008; Stenchever et al., 2007). The vaginal artery is a branch of the internal iliac artery and serves the remainder of the vagina (Figures 27.9 and 27.12).

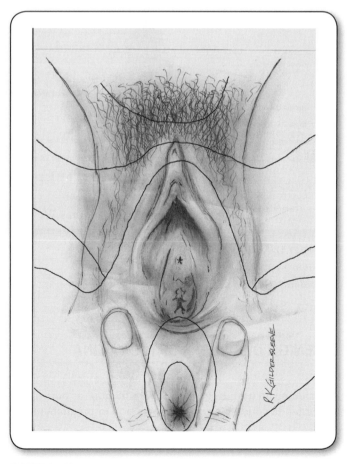

FIGURE 27.10
Vulvar dermatomes.

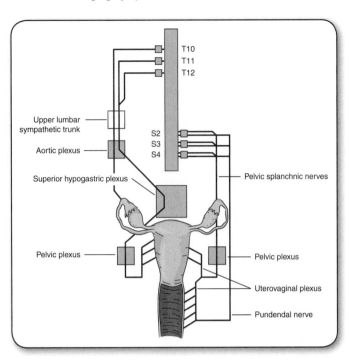

FIGURE 27.11

Innervation of internal genitalia.

Adapted from Gabbe et al. (2007).

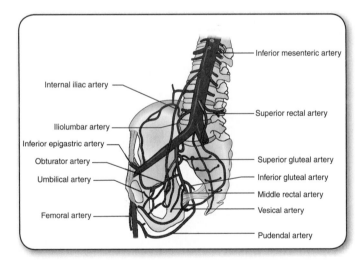

FIGURE 27.12

Vascular supply of pelvis.

Adapted from Gabbe et al. (2007).

■ BENIGN DISORDERS OF THE VAGINA

Considered anatomically, the vagina functions as both a sexual organ (a conduit allowing conception of pregnancy) and an obstetric organ (a conduit allowing for delivery). There is a broad range of anatomic variation, the parameters of which become more apparent with clinical experience. The length and shape of the labia minora, the development of the clitoris and its hood, the amount of fullness provided by adipose tissue in the labia majora, and the structure of the hymen all vary notably among typical women. A number of benign conditions can be recognized on inspection. Management for these conditions is based on the severity of the woman's symptoms. Thus, if not bothersome to the woman, treatment may not be necessary. Decisions regarding treatment follow the shared decision-making model that fully engages the woman.

Vaginal Septa

ETIOLOGY

Embryologic development of the vagina provides an explanation for the variety of septa that can occur. Transverse septa can arise from incomplete dissolution of the vaginal plate where the urogenital sinus tissue, derived from the ectoderm, meets the paramesonephric ducts, derived from the endoderm. Hematocolpos (an accumulation of blood in the vagina) can develop if the septum (or imperforate hymen) is complete enough to impede menstrual flow. Longitudinal septa are derived from incomplete fusion of the paramesonephric ducts. Instead of dissolution of the medial portions of the two paramesonephric ducts through a process called apoptosis, or programmed cell death, a persistent central wall dividing left from right, either in part or completely, develops. Longitudinal septa can occur anywhere through the uterus, cervix, or vagina. Longitudinal septa in the vagina are recognized as Müllerian abnormalities (Figure 27.13), prompting further evaluation of the uterus, tubes, kidneys, and renal collecting systems. These Müllerian abnormalities may have important implications for fertility, and can be associated with renal and urinary collecting duct abnormalities as well as cervicothoracic somite dysplasias (malformations of the vertebral bodies) in 15% to 30% of patients (Oppelt et al., 2006).

EVALUATION/ASSESSMENT

Vaginal septa commonly present in the adolescent population as amenorrhea or dysmenorrhea in those who have recently undergone menarche (Nazir, Rizvi, Qureshi, Khan, & Khan, 2006). Complaints may include low abdominal pain, vaginal pain, or cramping without any vaginal blood loss. However, unusual presentations have been reported, such as an inability to void (due to the vaginal and pelvic masses in a case of complicated Müllerian abnormality; Kleinman & Chen, 2012). Septa can be visualized on examination as a sometimes tense, discolored, membranous bulge in the mid

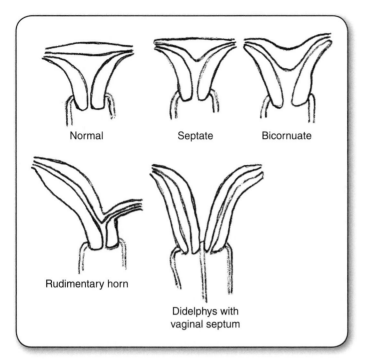

FIGURE 27.13

Illustration of Müllerian abnormalities.

Adapted from Fu Yao (2002).

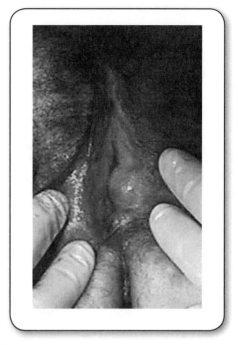

FIGURE 27.14

Bartholin's duct cyst.

Adapted from Kaufman et al. (2004).

to upper vagina. Examination of the vagina is done carefully, or the presence of parallel vaginal canals can easily be overlooked, even when the clinician has been alerted to a previously identified anomaly. This is true of both speculum and digital examinations. In gynecology, frequent palpation is more sensitive than inspection.

TREATMENT/MANAGEMENT

Excision can be performed for complete resolution. It is notable that the pressure developed behind the septum can be considerable and can result in rather forceful extrusion of blood on incision. The pressure contained within the uterus and vagina helps to explain the symptoms described by patients in these instances. Additional investigation is indicated to assess the extent of the Müllerian abnormality, which can be considerable and involve multiple systems (Schutt, Barrett, Trotta, & Stovall, 2012). The adolescent girl with trouble voiding had Herlyn–Werner–Wunderlich syndrome, an unusual malformation of uterus didelphys, unilateral blind vaginal pouch with ipsilateral renal agenesis.

Bartholin's Duct Cyst

ETIOLOGY AND EVALUATION/ASSESSMENT

The Bartholin's ducts typically drain into the vaginal introitus posteriolaterally. They can become occluded, leading to Bartholin's gland cyst, or infected, resulting in Bartholin's gland abscess (Figure 27.14). Bartholin cysts are found in about 3% of asymptomatic women based on an MRI study (Berger, Betschart, Khandwala, Delancey, & Haefner, 2012). A Bartholin's abscess has been found to be both mono and

polymicrobial and similar in constitution to normal vaginal flora. *Escherichia coli* were found to be the most common infectious agent in one study, though only 61% of cases were culture positive (Kessous, 2013).

TREATMENT/MANAGEMENT

Self-Management Measures • Cysts are best managed conservatively with frequent applications of warm compresses, soaking in a warm tub, and using sitz baths (Lashgari & Curry, 1995). These measures allow for dissolution of the blockage or spontaneous rupture, and resolution of the cyst. Massage of the area may help with expression of accumulated fluid, which is tested for infection.

Surgical Intervention • If the cyst persists or becomes significantly symptomatic because of size or abscess formation, incision and drainage is indicated. Traditional management is stab incision after administration of local anesthetic at the introitus. Placement of the incision is near the hymenal ring to mimic the anatomic location of drainage as closely as possible. A Word catheter is inserted and maintained for at least 3 weeks (Word, 1968). This time frame allows adequate time for the epithelium to completely cover the newly created passageway. Recurrent cysts are treated with marsupialization, again at the vaginal introitus, not the vulvar epithelium. Marsupialization is the surgical creation of an outlet to the duct (Figure 27.15). The key feature of marsupialization is careful identification of the gland's epithelial lining and suturing it to the epithelium of the vaginal introitus. This ensures a continued avenue for drainage, making recurrent problems extremely unlikely (10% or less; Blakey, Dewhurst, & Tipton, 1966). Most marsupializations can be performed in

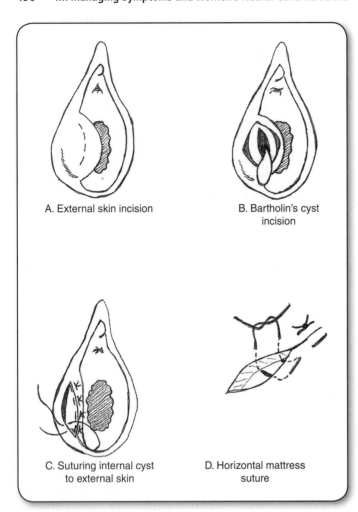

A. External skin incision

B. Bartholin's cyst incision

C. Suturing internal cyst to external skin

D. Horizontal mattress suture

FIGURE 27.15

Diagram of marsupialization.

Adapted from Kaufman et al. (2004).

the office using local anesthesia. However, an especially large cyst or abscess can be so painful that deep sedation or general anesthesia becomes necessary. The success of marsupialization and ablative techniques, such as carbon dioxide laser vaporization or alcohol sclerotherapy, makes complete excision of Bartholin's gland unwarranted in almost all situations (Cobellis, 2006; Fambrini et al., 2008). Not only is it a painful, extensive, and difficult dissection, it can also be complicated by refractory hemorrhage or fistula (Zoulek, Karp, & Davila, 2011). Systematic review has not identified a clearly superior method of management (Wechter, Wu, Marzano, & Haefner, 2009); therefore, clinical discretion is employed. Broad-spectrum antibiotics are administered if cellulitis is present, taking into consideration that methicillin-resistant staphylococcal species were found in 64% of vulvar abscesses in one trial (Thurman, Satterfoeld, & Soper, 2008).

Skene's Duct Cyst

ETIOLOGY AND EVALUATION/ASSESSMENT

Less common than Bartholin's duct cysts, Skene's duct cysts are anterior and lateral in location, along the labia minora.

Known also as the periurethral gland, providing an accurate description of its location, Skene's gland can become occluded, leading to increasing pressure and swelling. This can elicit pain because of either tense tissue or infection. Differential diagnosis must also include urethral diverticulum, leiomyoma, vaginal wall inclusion cyst, urethral prolapse, urethral caruncle, and less commonly, malignancy or Gartner's duct cyst (Tunitsky, Goldman, & Ridgeway, 2012).

TREATMENT/MANAGEMENT

Self-Management Measures • Management is similar to that employed when treating Bartholin's duct cysts. Attempts at nonsurgical resolution employ modalities such as warm compresses and soaking in warm baths as well as manual expression via massage. Expressed material is tested for infection.

Surgical Intervention • When the clinician is confident of the correct diagnosis or has been referred to a specialist for evaluation and management, surgical resolution may be appropriate. If self-management is not successful, or if pain is so prominent that conservative management is untenable, incision and drainage can be performed in the office setting after the administration of a local anesthetic (Hopkins, & Snyder, 2005; Stenchever et al., 2007).

Mesonephric (Gartner's) Duct Cyst

ETIOLOGY AND EVALUATION/ASSESSMENT

Gartner's duct cysts are thin-walled, fluid-filled remnants of the incompletely reabsorbed mesonephros (Figure 27.1). In the male, the mesonephros would have formed the epididymis, and vestigial portions of this system in women can produce cystic structures in the lateral vagina, usually in the proximal two thirds. These can vary in depth, with some being found superficially. Although some Gartner's cysts may be membranous in appearance, others may be palpable as soft, subtle distortions through an otherwise normal appearing vaginal mucosa. These are usually 1 to 3 cm in diameter; however, they can be broader as well (Hopkins & Snyder, 2005; Stenchever et al., 2007). The vast majority of times, these cysts are asymptomatic, and treatment is not required. Rarely, they can produce dyspareunia, mechanical blockade (e.g., of tampons), or complaints of pain in the vagina. They can lead to symptoms and perhaps even urethral diverticula, which has been reported in pregnancy (Iyer & Minassian, 2013).

TREATMENT/MANAGEMENT

If intervention is needed, marsupialization is the preferred method (Binsaleh, Al-Assiri, Jednak, & El-Sherbiny, 2007); however, anatomic location will determine the proper procedure to perform. Urethral diverticula are excised, for example.

Non-Neoplastic Conditions of the Vagina

The distinction between non-neoplastic and neoplastic disease can be clarified by identifying the location of the changes on pathologic specimens. The term "histologic" refers to microscopically viewed tissue in an undisturbed orientation (such as a cervical biopsy). This is distinguished from "cytologic," wherein a sampling of cells is viewed microscopically without the benefit of tissue structure (e.g., a smear of cervical cells). If the cellular changes are confined to their correct location in the tissue structure (usually by a basement membrane, Figure 27.16), the sample is considered non-neoplastic (benign). Alternatively, if cellular changes are apparent in tissues adjacent to or distant from the correct structural location, the specimen is considered to be neoplastic (malignant). For example, abnormal appearing squamous epithelial cells that are contained by their basement membrane are non-neoplastic; they have not infiltrated the dermis (Figure 21.17). Once they have broken that barrier, however, they have become invasive, or malignant.

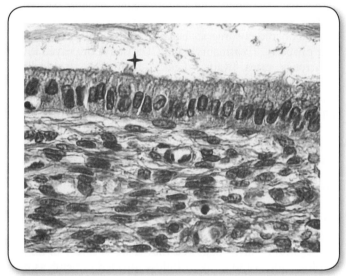

FIGURE 27.16
Normal histology of ectocervix.

Source: http://screening.iarc.fr/atlashisto_detail.php?flag=0&lang=1&Id=000 03816&cat=B3

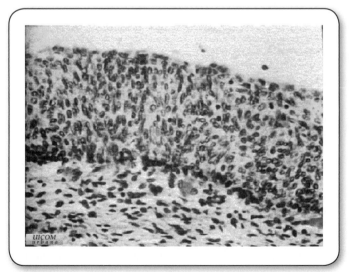

FIGURE 27.17
Carcinoma in situ of the cervix.

Source: www.med.illinois.edu/m2/pathology/PathAtlasf/WWW_images/ V2435.html

One entity that becomes unavoidable in dealing with non-neoplastic (and neoplastic) disease of the lower genital tract is human papillomavirus (HPV). HPV is discussed in detail in Chapter 32; however, a few points are emphasized here.

Some varieties of the more than 120 different types of HPV presently identified have been designated as "high-risk type" viruses. These are the types that are deemed causative of dysplasia of the cervix, vagina, and vulva (Clifford, Smith, Plummer, Muñoz, & Franceschi, 2003). Dramatic accumulation and implementation of knowledge regarding the nature of HPV infection and the dysplasia it causes is currently underway. The results of initial inoculations of women in the general public using type-specific HPV vaccine are now being reviewed. Clinical trials have displayed nearly 100% efficacy in protecting against infection by these virus types (Harper et al., 2004; Munoz et al., 2010; Villa et al., 2005). Among the four virus types covered by the quadrivalent vaccine are the most common high-risk types present today (HPV virus types 16 and 18). These two virus types are associated with almost 75% of cervical cancers. The vaccine is engineered to produce virus-like particles (VLPs), which stimulate recognition of the virus and initiate an immune response. The VLPs contain no genetic material, and thus cannot cause infection. Together with the VLPs for types 6 and 11, which prevents low-grade dysplasia and genital warts attributable to these viruses, the quadrivalent vaccine will hopefully reduce the incidence of cancer, just as it has proved to decrease the antecedent preinvasive diseases of the cervix, vagina, vulva, as well as anal disease in homosexual men (Palefsky, 2011). Careful follow-up and epidemiologic studies will be required to measure the actual outcomes; however, optimism seems reasonable at the present time. Although pathologic conditions of the cervix will be most dramatically affected by this vaccine, it will also reduce vaginal and vulvar dysplasias.

VAGINAL INTRAEPITHELIAL NEOPLASIA

Etiology and Evaluation/Assessment • Vaginal intraepithelial neoplasia (VAIN) is analogous to cervical dysplasia; however, it is far less prevalent. Dysplasia in the lower genital tract is essentially a "field effect." Infection with HPV can lead to cellular changes in the epithelium of any genital tissue. Viral DNA can incorporate itself into cellular DNA and then alter cellular controls, creating a preinvasive condition. Lesions can be visualized within the vagina as whitened plaques on occasion; however, VAIN is most frequently first detected with cervical cytologic screening. Although abnormalities are most commonly cervical, not all abnormal Pap smears will have a cervical origin; sampling of the cervix via spatula or brush cannot avoid the collection of epithelial cells from the vagina as well. The epithelia of the vagina and vulva have been similarly exposed to HPV and are therefore at risk of dysplastic change as well. The discrepant incidence of disease that occurs at the cervix is related to the special physiology of the squamocolumnar junction. Rapid turnover of cells in this region leads to the increased likelihood of abnormal growth. Dysplastic epithelial changes in the vagina progress slowly and are described similarly to those in the cervix, denoted as VAIN I to III.

Presentation is most common with concurrent or preceding cervical dysplasia (cervical intraepithelial neoplasia [CIN]). Patients are largely asymptomatic; however, some do exhibit manifestations such as irritation, discharge, or bleeding.

Diagnostic Studies • Identification most likely results from an abnormal cytologic smear. Cytologic smears are not site-specific biopsies; cells are collected from the vagina, ectocervix, endocervix, and possibly even the endometrium. Cytologic smears are interpreted by viewing cells without the benefit of the tissue structure surrounding them. Taken out of context, it is especially important to provide historical information to the pathologist to make evaluation more accurate and useful clinically. For example, all of the following situations can alter the appearance of cells microscopically: the woman is postmenopausal, menstruating, or receiving estrogen therapy; the woman has a history of cervical dysplasia or cancer or has concurrent infection; or the sample is a smear of the vaginal apex after removal of the cervix. As stated previously, identification is most likely to occur because of an abnormal cytologic smear. Importantly, sampling of the vaginal apex in women who have undergone hysterectomy with a history of CIN II or greater remains important because VAIN II or greater will develop in as many as 7.4% of cases (González Bosquet et al., 2008; Schockaert, Poppe, Arbyn, Verguts, & Verguts, 2008).

Once abnormal cytology has been discovered, colposcopic examination is used as the most effective means of investigating the extent of disease and selecting sites for biopsy. Shiller's iodine stain is helpful in assessing the margins of the lesion. In women who have normal cervical colposcopy, special care is taken to view the proximal third of the vagina, where most vaginal lesions are located (Murta, Neves Junior, Sempionato, Costa, & Maluf, 2005). Multifocal disease is the rule with VAIN. Thus, meticulous examination of the entire vaginal canal is imperative, because skip lesions (islands of tissue abnormality in separate locations in the vagina) are frequently present (Desaia & Creasman, 2007). Biopsy sites are selected to include the most concerning locations. Local anesthesia, either topical or injectable, is used for vaginal biopsy procedures because they are significantly more painful than cervical biopsy procedures.

Treatment/Management • Management has taken many forms, including close clinical observation (for regression of low-grade lesions), excision, topical chemotherapy, laser vaporization, and cryoablative therapy (Buck & Guth, 2003; Caglar, Hertzog, & Hreshchyshyn, 1981; Cardamakis, 1998; Desaia & Creasman, 2007; Diakomanolis, Rodolakis, Boulgaris, Blachos, & Michalas, 2002). Excision can be highly effective; however, the risk of vaginal stenosis (narrowing) is significant when areas of tissue are removed. Chemotherapy with 5-fluorouracil (5-FU) versus laser ablative therapy has shown comparable results. However, 5-FU can cause profound irritation when used for prolonged courses. There are numerous protocols attempting to minimize the caustic effects, with varying degrees of success. Basically, it still remains a fairly noxious, nonspecific treatment. Laser can also be painful during the healing process. There are no perfect treatment options. However,

the distribution of the laser's ablative effect is easier to control, which may limit the indiscriminant irritation of 5-FU contamination that is frequently external to the vulva. Imiquimod topical treatment has also shown promise used in low-dose weekly treatments for 3 to 9 weeks (Buck & Guth, 2003). Imiquimod can also be associated with irritating symptoms, but is well tolerated by most patients. Risk factors for recurrence following laser vaporization include age less than 49 years and a disease classification of VAIN III (Kim, 2009).

Reports of the use of cavitational ultrasonic surgical aspiration (CUSA) are encouraging (Robinson, Sun, Bodurka-Bevers, Im, & Rosenshein, 2000), albeit limited. This technology uses ultrasonic energy to lyse tissue via the generation of vacuoles within cells, and then aspirates the debris. There is a preferential destruction of cells with higher water content, therefore leaving vascular structures spared. It is effectively used in liver, neurologic, and gynecologic oncology surgeries because of this unique and desirable property. Treatments using CUSA have displayed lower recurrence rates (Rader, Leake, Dillon, & Rosenshein, 1991). It also allows for easily directed effects with the handheld aspirator, leaving little collateral damage to surrounding tissues from thermal injury (Hambley, Hebda, Abell, Cohen, & Jegasothy, 1988; Thompson, Adelson, Jozefczyk, Coble, & Kaufman, 1991). Whatever treatment modality is selected, it is considered carefully with the woman because progression to invasive cancer is a possibility, especially with VAIN II and III lesions.

There is no clear consensus on follow-up regimens for VAIN due to its low prevalence and therefore limited understanding of the natural history of the disease. Recent investigations have suggested that there is safety in annual cytology and colposcopy to follow affected patients as progression seems unlikely and resolution is very likely (Zeligs et al., 2013).

■ NEOPLASTIC VAGINAL DISEASE

Squamous Carcinoma

ETIOLOGY

Although squamous cell carcinoma of the vagina is the most common form of vaginal cancer (approximately 85% of cases), malignancies of the vagina are extremely rare (Wu et al., 2008). There are between 1,000 and 2,000 cases of vaginal carcinoma diagnosed in the United States annually, with 65% to 95% being of squamous type (Ries, Melbert, Krapcho, 2008; Siegel, Ma, Zou, & Jemal, 2014). Incidence and survival vary on the basis of race and ethnicity, with African American and Hispanic women as well as women of Asian Pacific Island descent having both increased disease rates and decreased survival rates as compared to women of other ethnicities (Shah, Goff, Lowe, Peters, & Li, 2009; Wu et al., 2008). The association with HPV is strong, and suggests viral etiology in the majority of cases (Creasman, Phillips, & Menck, 1998; Sugase & Matsukura, 1997). The type of HPV found most commonly in cancers of the cervix, vagina, and vulva is slightly variable. In cancers of the cervix and vagina, the two most commonly encountered subtypes were 16 and 18. However, in vulvar cancers the two most common HPV subtypes were 16 and 33 (Insinga, Liaw, Johnson, & Madeleine, 2008; Smith, Backes, Hoots, Kurman, & Pimenta, 2009). The vast majority of disease is located in the proximal half of the vagina. Identification of cancer is most likely to occur with cytologic screening (Pap smear). A small minority of patients will present with bleeding, typically preceded by vaginal discharge (Eddy, Marks, Miller, & Underwood, 1991; Manetta, Gutrecht, Berman, & DiSaia, 1990). Lymphatic distribution from the proximal half of the vagina will mimic the distribution of cervical disease to the iliac lymph nodes, ascending to the aortic lymph nodes. Dissemination from the distal half of the vagina is usually to the inguinal lymph nodes; however, there is far less predictability about the pattern of distribution for lesions in the distal vagina (Creasman et al., 1998; Sugase, & Matsukura, 1997).

EVALUATION/ASSESSMENT AND DIAGNOSTIC STUDIES

Examination includes cytologic studies of the cervix and vagina in the event a lesion is not visible. Biopsy is imperative if lesions are seen. Promulgation could be via local invasion or via dissemination through the lymph-vascular space. Distribution to the paracolpos or pelvic organs can present with urinary tract symptoms if the lesion is located anteriorly. Similarly, posterior lesions can be symptomatic through the rectum; however, they are more commonly asymptomatic. Examination and investigation of metastasis does not overlook any of the possible sites of drainage. Recommended studies include cystoscopy, computer-aided tomography (or intravenous pyelogram), chest x-ray, and colonoscopy (or sigmoidoscopy). There is emerging evidence that sentinel lymph node evaluation can be useful in making treatment decisions in affected patients (Hertel et al., 2013).

TREATMENT/MANAGEMENT

Squamous cell carcinoma is usually managed with radiation, predominantly internal radiation; however, with bulkier disease external radiation is used to shrink the tumor before placement of intracavitary devices (Leung & Sexton, 1993). There are circumstances when surgical resection can be used, such as stage I disease of the proximal vagina; however, surgical intervention is contraindicated when the disease has metastasized or extended to the pelvic sidewalls. In these cases, pelvic exenteration (removing everything in the pelvis: bladder, reproductive organs, and rectum) would be ineffective. Decisions regarding treatment are individualized because no absolute consensus exists for all situations. In part, this may be due to the rarity of this disease entity.

Survival is closely related to stage of disease. Approximate estimates of 5-year survival rates are as follows: stage 0, 96%; stage I, 73%; stage II, 58%; and stages III to IV, 36% (Creasman et al., 1998). Recurrence is a particularly disheartening occurrence, resulting in a 5-year survival rate of approximately 10% (Eddy et al., 1991; Manetta et al., 1990; Peters, Kumar, & Morley, 1985).

Adenocarcinoma

ETIOLOGY

Adenocarcinoma of the vagina is also a rare entity; however, an increase in its incidence occurred in the generation following diethylstilbestrol (DES) use. DES was predominantly used during the 1940s and 1950s in high-risk pregnancies to reduce fetal loss, with some use continuing through the 1970s. Observant clinicians recognized the common history in a number of women identified with adenocarcinoma of the cervix and vagina, and DES was implicated as the causative factor (Herbst & Scully, 1970). DES-exposed women have approximately a 1% chance of developing a cervical or vaginal adenocarcinoma by age 24 years. Age of diagnosis heavily favors the early to mid twenties. Approximately 60% to 70% of cases of adenocarcinoma of the vagina during the late 20th century were associated with DES exposure. The incidence has dropped precipitously following the decline in the use of DES (shifted later in time by approximately 20 years). Adenocarcinoma has been noted to arise in the context of a variety of conditions (Lee, Park, Lee, Kim, & Seo, 2005; McCluggage, Price, & Dobbs, 2001; Tjalma & Colpaert, 2006). These represent rare occurrences and do not appear to indicate changing disease incidence; rather, they suggest heightened scrutiny and study of the disease. History of endometriosis is an example of a condition that can lead to the development of adenocarcinoma of the vagina, even after hysterectomy has been performed in postmenopausal women (Nomoto et al., 2010).

EVALUATION/ASSESSMENT AND DIAGNOSTIC STUDIES

Carcinomas typically present with abnormal uterine bleeding in young women. Friable adenomatous tissue replacing more substantial squamous epithelium leads to irregular vaginal bleeding. Visual examination reveals the abnormal epithelium and prompts biopsy. Clinical findings include a glandular, velvety appearing vaginal epithelium, similar to vaginal adenosis (Figure 27.18), a "cock's comb" cervix

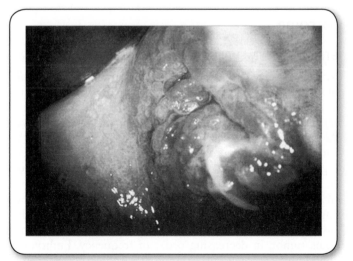

FIGURE 27.18

Vaginal adenosis.

From Hammes and Laitman (2003).

(transverse ridges on the cervix), and hooding of the cervix by the anterior vagina. Biopsy is needed for diagnosis.

TREATMENT/MANAGEMENT

Management strategies include radical hysterectomy (removing much more of the supporting tissue lateral to the uterus [parametria] than standard hysterectomy), partial or complete vaginectomy, and radiation therapy. In very advanced disease, exenteration is a consideration. In very limited disease, it is possible to perform local excision and use limited radiation therapy to preserve function and fertility without a marked increase in recurrence risk (McNall et al., 2004). Referral to a gynecologic oncology specialist is necessary.

Melanoma

ETIOLOGY AND EVALUATION/ASSESSMENT

Melanoma is an extremely rare disease entity that can occur in the vagina. Melanoma has a remarkably poor prognosis in comparison to other vaginal cancers, with reported 5-year survival rates below 15% (Buchanan, Schlaerth, & Kurosaki, 1998; Peters et al., 1985). Recent accumulation of data from the Surveillance, Epidemiology, and End Result (SEER) registry that identified about 200 patients with vaginal melanoma found 2- and 5-year survival rates of 24% and 15% (despite 46% of cancers diagnosed as stage 1; Kirschner, Kidd, Dewees, & Perkins, 2013). Presentation is most common with vaginal bleeding and/or mass. This is most frequently visualized as a polypoid nodularity on clinical examination (Gupta, Malpica, Deavers, & Silva, 2002).

TREATMENT/MANAGEMENT

Treatment can vary from exenteration (i.e., hysterectomy and vaginectomy) to wide local excision. Adjuvant therapies include radiation and chemotherapy. None of these is significantly effective with advanced disease.

Sarcoma

ETIOLOGY AND EVALUATION/ASSESSMENT

Sarcoma is also extremely rare and occurs more commonly in pediatric age groups than other gynecologic cancers, although the average age at diagnosis in the SEER registry data was 54 years. Of 4,000 vaginal cancers found over 22 years, 221 were sarcomas. Survival at 5 years was 89% for stage I disease and 47% for stage II disease, suggesting aggressive tumor behavior (Ghezelayagh, Rauh-Hain, & Growdon, 2015). Diagnosis is made with the biopsy of suspicious lesions, typically a bulky lesion in the upper vagina. Types of sarcoma include leiomyosarcoma, rhabdomyosarcoma, mixed Müllerian sarcoma, and endodermal sinus tumor, in decreasing order of frequency. Embryonal rhabdomyosarcoma (also known as sarcoma botryoides) is found in girls younger than 8 years of age. It is recognized because of its "bunch of grapes" appearance—a soft multiloculated mass occasionally protruding from the vagina.

Leiomyosarcoma has been reported most commonly in the perimenopausal years.

TREATMENT/MANAGEMENT

Treatment is based primarily on conservational surgery (sparing the uterus and vagina) and, for embryonal rhabdomyosarcoma, chemotherapy. Survival rates in the pediatric age group can reach 90% in low-stage disease; however, metastatic disease will diminish survival rates to about 25% (Breneman et al., 2003; Peters et al., 1985).

■ BENIGN DISORDERS OF THE VULVA

The prevalence of vulvar disorders favors the postmenopausal patient population; however, they can be present at any age. Most commonly they present innocuously with mild symptoms and subtle, slow onset. This subtle presentation, occurring primarily in postmenopausal women, who too often have their gynecologic health neglected, undoubtedly leads to delayed diagnosis. Besides causing prolonged discomfort for the woman, it may also result in advancing severity of disease, including advancement from benign to malignant disease. Attention is paid to the most trivial complaints. Besides a careful examination of the vulva, a review of systems is employed to elicit symptoms not reported by the woman. Perhaps the most important characteristic for a clinician during this process is a well-developed suspicious instinct, always considering that malignant and premalignant diseases are a possibility.

Current classification of vulvar dermatoses by the International Society for the Study of Vulvovaginal Disease (ISSVD) is based on histologic characteristics of disease state (Lynch, Moyal-Barrocco, Bogliatto, Micheletti, & Scurry, 2007). The rationale for altering the nomenclature from previous definitions is to streamline the use of appropriate therapeutic interventions based on biopsy results (Lynch & Micheletti, 2006; Moyal-Barracco & Lynch, 2004; Sideri et al., 2005). The offending dermatosis, once histologically classified (Box 27.1), is referenced to the various diseases that most commonly present within that category. Then the clinician can focus on the differential diagnoses via both pathologic and clinical information to select appropriate treatment (Voet, 1994).

However, the clinical diagnosis is not based on biopsy results alone. If a clinician is fairly certain of the diagnosis after an office examination, therapy is instituted (Lorenz, Kaufman, & Kutzner, 1998). If the biopsy is performed and a diagnosis is likely, again therapy is initiated. The classification becomes useful when no diagnosis is reached definitively, either by clinical examination or by histologic evaluation. In this event, the new system would simplify the diagnostic dilemma. When managing vulvar disease it is especially important to monitor results of therapy to ensure resolution or improvement. If therapy is initiated and the condition is refractory, the selected diagnosis and the course of therapy is reconsidered. Liberal use of biopsy (and rebiopsy) is employed to verify diagnostic accuracy. The capacity to recognize specific conditions on inspection evolves with experience and training. Some examples of common

BOX 27.1   2006 ISSVD CLASSIFICATION OF VULVAR DERMATOSES (2016 UPDATE): PATHOLOGIC SUBSETS AND THEIR CLINICAL CORRELATES

Spongiotic Pattern

Atopic dermatosis
Allergic contact dermatitis
Irritant contact dermatitis

Acanthotic Pattern (Formerly Squamous Cell Hyperplasia)

Psoriasis
Lichen simplex chronicus
  Primary (idiopathic)
  Secondary (superimposed on lichen sclerosus, lichen planus, or other vulvar dermatoses)

Lichenoid Pattern

Lichen sclerosus
Lichen planus

Dermal Homogenization/Sclerosus Pattern

Lichen sclerosus

Vesiculobullous Pattern

Pemphigoid, cicatricial type
Linear IgA disease

Acantholytic Pattern

Hailey-Hailey disease
Darier's disease
Papular genitocrural acantholysis

Granulomatous Pattern

Crohn's disease
Melkersson–Rosenthal syndrome

Vasculopathic Pattern

Aphthous ulcers
Behçet's syndrome
Plasma cell vulvitis

Adapted from Lynch, Moyal-Barracco, Scurry, and Stockdale (2016). Retrieved from the 2016 update of the ISSVD terminology http://3b64we1rtwev2ibv6q12s4dd.wpengine. netdna-cdn.com/wp-content/uploads/2016/03/CURRENT-ISSVD-TERMINOLOGY-AND-CLASSIFICATION-OF-VULVAR-DISEASES_CLINICAL-DIAGNOSIS.pdf

disease variations are provided in the following sections. The 2016 update of the ISSVD terminology can be useful in understanding diseases and their clinical phenotypes (Lynch et al., 2016).

Lichen Sclerosus

ETIOLOGY AND EVALUATION/ASSESSMENT

Similar to many vulvar dystrophies, lichen sclerosus presents with pruritus, irritation, burning, and dyspareunia. Although it can occur at any age, it is most common in postmenopausal women. The association between lichen sclerosus and autoimmune disease has been identified, with one study showing a 30% correlation between a lichen sclerosus diagnosis and an autoimmune disorder (Cooper, Ali, Baldo, & Wojnarowska, 2008). Considered from another perspective, lichen sclerosus confers a relative risk of 4.7 for having concomitant extragenital psoriasis (Eberz, Berghold, & Regauer, 2008). External genitalia can appear atrophic as the skin is thin, and the labia and clitoris can lose their normal architecture. The anatomy of these structures becomes blunted, smoothing contours and blurring normal anatomic borders, dramatically so with advanced disease (Figure 27.19). Vulvar epithelium becomes pallorous, shiny,

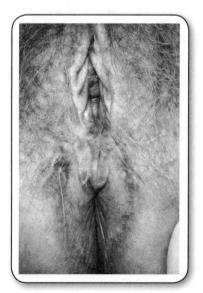

FIGURE 27.19
Lichen sclerosus.
Adapted from Habif (2004).

and crinkly (often described as a parchment paper appearance). Distribution is symmetric across the vulva, labia, and perineum and extends perianally frequently. Diagnosis can be made with inspection on most occasions.

TREATMENT/MANAGEMENT

Self-Management Measures • Self-care includes avoiding all possible irritants, which is extremely important for any woman who has lichen dystrophy or any other vulvar dystrophy. Several regimens are used. Box 27.1 presents one possible regimen. It is important that the clinician employ a short interval for follow-up and reassessment.

Pharmacotherapeutics • Empiric therapy is usually initiated based on clinical examination. Follow-up examination is within a few weeks to ensure improvement. Any doubts about diagnosis are resolved with biopsy. Treatment has evolved from testosterone cream to clobetasol 0.05% cream, a potent corticosteroid (Lorenz et al., 1998). Review of effective treatments has suggested that clobetasol propionate, mometasone furoate, and pimecrolimus are effective treatments for genital lichen sclerosus (Chi, Kirtschig, Baldo, Lewis, Wang, & Wojnarowska, 2012). Symptoms will show only modest improvement when topical estrogen is employed. There are many variations in recommended treatment regimens, the common principles being frequent application early in treatment and then titration to a sufficient maintenance dose to control symptoms. One treatment regimen is suggested in Table 27.1. Although complete resolution can be achieved, women will frequently have recurrent symptoms and require repeated courses of therapy. Changing to a low-potency steroid is advisable for maintenance therapy. Prolonged use of topical steroids, especially high-potency steroids, can lead to epithelial atrophy and tissue fragility.

Topical immunomodulator medications are being used more frequently and are displaying encouraging results. Use of tacrolimus (Protopic) and pimecrolimus (Elidel) creams or ointments has resulted in favorable regression of disease and improvement in symptomatology with extended courses of therapy (6–24 weeks of twice-daily application; Hengge et al., 2006; Virgili, Lauriola, Mantovani, & Corazza, 2007). One case report used psoralen (Oxsoralen) with ultraviolet-A (UVA) light to treat extragenital lichen sclerosus that was refractory to other treatment modalities (Valdivielso-Ramos, Bueno, & Hernanz, 2008). A well-conducted study comparing clobetasol to tacrolimus found the former significantly more effective in treating vulvar lichen sclerosus (Funaro, Lovett, Leroux, & Powell, 2014).

TABLE 27.1	Suggested Clobetasol Treatment Regimen for Lichen Sclerosus
TIME PERIOD	**FREQUENCY OF ADMINISTRATION**
Weeks 1–6	Daily
Week 7: resolution (maintenance)	2–3 times per week

Hyperplastic Squamous Vulvar Conditions

ETIOLOGY, EVALUATION/ASSESSMENT, AND DIFFERENTIAL DIAGNOSES

Conditions related to squamous overgrowth generally present with raised, whitened epithelium. Intense pruritus is a hallmark of change and may lead to the histologic changes of thickening and acanthosis (hyperkeratosis and thickened malpighian ridges, respectively). The most notable diagnosis among these is lichen simplex chronicus; however, other similar appearing acanthotic dermatoses, as noted in the 2006 ISSVD classification system, are considered (Box 27.1). The patient's accompanying history may include insatiable itching. This pruritus may exacerbate, or even be the source of, the hyperplasia. Excoriations can result, complicating appearance as well as intensifying symptoms to include pain. Examination shows thickened whitened areas diffusely distributed over the vulva. Distribution tends to be on the labia majora, from clitoris to anus, bilaterally. Excoriations may be present as a result of the trauma of scratching.

TREATMENT/MANAGEMENT

In addition to self-care that employs a strict perineal regimen (Box 27.1), treatment is with potent corticosteroids. Similar to other dermatoses, newer immunomodulators are showing promise (Goldstein, Parneix-Spake, McCormick, & Burrows, 2007). Approximately 83% of women have exhibited complete resolution of disease using pimecrolimus (Elidel) 1% cream, and 16% improvement of pruritus has been reported in one small trial (Kelekci et al., 2008). Investigation into alternative methods, such as focused ultrasound treatments, has been reported; however, clobetasol (Betanate) remains the preferred medication (Li et al., 2007; Lorenz, 1998). Clinical resolution may require as long as 8 weeks; therefore additional medication to mitigate pruritus, such as nonsedating antihistamines, is necessary.

Lichen Planus

ETIOLOGY

Lichen planus is a disease that is systemic and immunologically mediated (Cooper, Dean, Allen, Kirtschig, & Wojnarowska, 2005). It results in vulvar and vaginal disease in the majority of patients. Its cause is unknown. Presentation can be in the mucosa of the oral, nasal, and anal cavities as well as the scalp, nails, and skin of the body. Chemical, infectious, or physical irritants are known to cause exacerbations. Malignancy has been reported in association with lichen planus (Chiu & Jones, 2011).

SYMPTOMS AND EVALUATION/ASSESSMENT

Mild to severe degrees of pruritus is the typical presenting complaint. In more advanced or erosive disease, burning and pain become more dominant complaints. Examination can show a variety of different findings, including erythema, or violet changes with reticular or erosive patterns;

synechiae; loss of architecture; and even ulcers. The vaginal erosions or ulcerations can lead to obliteration of the vagina (Lotery & Galask, 2003). Examination also focuses on the oral mucosa, which may provide confirmation of diagnosis. With significant epithelial damage and erosion, a sometimes copious malodorous discharge can occur.

TREATMENT/MANAGEMENT

Self-Management Measures • Management first attempts to identify and remove any noxious stimuli, including meticulous care of the perineum (Box 27.1) and the use of sitz baths.

Pharmacotherapeutics • Potent topical steroid creams are also used and there are occasions when systemic steroid use becomes necessary. As always, biopsy is needed for persistent or suspicious lesions. Treatment can result in resolution; however, refractory disease is common. With prolonged use of topical steroids, about 75% of women will show some improvement (Cooper & Wojnarowska, 2006). Immunosuppressive medications, such as systemic or topical cyclosporine (Cicloral, Gengraf), have been employed in difficult cases (Al-Hashimi et al., 2007; Campos-Domínguez et al., 2006). There also is evidence of improvement from the immunomodulatory effects of photopheresis (also known as extracorporeal photochemotherapy) in oral lichen planus (Marchesseau-Merlin et al., 2008). This is a process of administering psoralen (a light-activated medication) and then exposing the blood extracorporeally to ultraviolet light. Remission has been seen in a number of case reports; however, relapse in treatment-free intervals frequently occurs. Although photopheresis has not yet been used in the treatment of genital lichen planus, it may pose a potential treatment option in the future. Use of Apremilast, a phosphodiesterase-4 inhibitor that decreases production of tumor necrosis factor alpha, thus reducing inflammation, has been reported to show success in suppressing disease, although larger studies are needed to clarify its effectiveness and role in care (Paul, Foss, Hirano, Cunningham, & Pariser, 2013).

Lichen Simplex Chronicus

ETIOLOGY

Lichen simplex chronicus (LSC), also referred to as neurodermatitis, is a chronic hypertrophic condition caused by persistent itching and repetitive scratching. The original source of the irritation is not always clear, but the disease occurs more frequently in women with atopic histories, or can follow persistant infections (Boardman, Botte, & Kennedy, 2005; Rimoin, Kwatra, & Yosipovitch, 2013). The chronic itch-scratch cycle leads to marked erythema, edema, and lichenification (thickening) of the skin, appearing leathery in advanced cases. LSC has also been associated with malignancy uncommonly (Tiengo et al., 2012).

TREATMENT/MANAGEMENT

Goals of treatment are to break the itch-scratch cycle and attempt to determine the underlying cause of the symptoms, treating if an etiology can be identified (e.g., chronic yeast identified with culture). Scratching at night is a common problem, not only affecting sleep, but also taking away conscious control over scratching. Use of medication to enhance sleep is frequently helpful until symptoms are better controlled. Medications employed include high-potency topical steroid for relief of symptoms and hypertrophy (clobetasol), or an immunomodulator, such as pimecrolimus (Elidel) 1% cream (Boardman et al., 2005; Goldstein & Parneix-Spake, 2006; Rimoin et al., 2013).

Vulvar Squamous Intraepithelial Lesions

ETIOLOGY

Vulvar squamous intraepithelial lesions (SIL), formerly known as vulvar intraepithelial neoplasia (VIN) is another disease related to HPV infection most commonly (Bonvicini et al., 2005; Hillemanns & Wang, 2006). Terminology has been changed to improve pathologic accuracy and reflect the benign nature of VIN I (now known as low-grade squamous intraepithelial lesion [LSIL]), currently thought of as HPV-related condyloma (Wilkinson, Cox, Selim, & O'Connor, 2015). HPV-16 seropositive individuals are almost five times as likely to develop vulvar SIL as naïve subjects (Smith et al., 2009). Analogous to preinvasive disease of the cervix and vagina, it is far less common than cervical disease, yet slightly more common than vaginal disease. Risk factors are the same as those for cervical disease, including multiple sexual partners, a history of sexually transmitted infections (STIs), and tobacco use. Interestingly, vulvar SIL and CIN have been identified as synchronous lesions (Pai, Pai, Gupta, Rao, & Renjhen, 2006). The most commonly affected age groups have historically been perimenopausal and postmenopausal women. This appears to be shifting to the fourth decade of life (Jones & Rowan, 1994; before 1980, vulvar SIL was mostly seen in women 60–69 years old) and may be the result of the increasing prevalence of high-risk types of HPV (Baldwin et al., 2007). Progression of VIN III to invasive cancer was once considered to be in the range of 5% (Campion & Singer, 1987; Ferenczy, 1992; Hørding, Junge, Poulsen, & Lundvall, 1995; Woodruff, 1991). VIN II and III are now referred to as high-grade squamous intraepithelial lesion [HSIL]. Because the HPV infection and cellular changes occur as a "field effect," vulvar cancer increases the risk of cervical dysplasia as well (de Bie et al., 2009). There is a significant potential that the natural history of the disease has changed. Not only has the population affected become younger, advancing disease has also been reported in relatively short intervals (within 5 years) in untreated subjects, and in an alarming 87% of 113 affected women studied over an 8-year period (Baldwin et al., 2007; Buscema & Woodruff, 1980; Crum, Liskow, Petras, Keng, & Frick, 1984; Jones & Rowan, 1994). VIN also can arise in the context of vulvar dermatoses and was formerly referred to as differentiated type VIN (VIN usual, basaloid, warty, or mixed types; Chiu & Jones, 2011; Tiengo et al., 2007). Current terminology should mimic that of cervical diseases using LSIL or HSIL. This nomenclature was adopted at a consensus conference attended by a number of professional organizations in 2012, the ISSVD being one.

SYMPTOMS, EVALUATION/ASSESSMENT, AND DIAGNOSTIC STUDIES

Presenting symptoms are usually mild irritation, pruritus, and occasionally areas of cracks or sores that do not heal. Examination is methodical and meticulous. Findings can range from hypopigmented or hyperpigmented skin to erythematous, thickened, or whitened regions (Figure 27.20). Distribution can be anywhere from the clitoral hood to the anus, most commonly in the inferior labia and perineum. Colposcopic examination is frequently useful to view affected areas. There exists some evidence that acetic acid and toluidine blue may make affected areas more readily identifiable; however, they are not very specific to high-grade VIN. They therefore can lead to extensive regions of vulvar epithelium appearing abnormal, few of which would merit aggressive treatment. Consequently, acetic acid and toluidine blue are best used to guide possible areas of biopsy, highlighting those areas that are the most concerning in appearance and for which biopsy will aid in determining the severity of disease. Good clinical judgment and intraoperative pathologic evaluation of surgical margins are the best guides to determining the extent of disease and amount of resection (treatment) necessary.

TREATMENT/MANAGEMENT

Although it is a reasonable and common clinical practice to treat presumptively once for "yeast" or other infection (such as bacterial vaginosis), it is important to note that self-diagnosis is far from accurate and that continued "infection" may actually indicate VIN.

In addition to careful perineal care (Box 27.2), management is either via excision or by ablation (most commonly laser, cryotherapy, or even chemotherapy). Excision is preferable because it yields a surgical specimen that can be evaluated for invasive disease, thereby providing the opportunity to ensure no invasion following treatment (Penna, Fallani,

Fambrini, Zipoli, & Marchionni, 2002). It is notable, however, that use of imiquimod topical cream to stimulate the immune system has shown some promise (it stimulates the body to produce interferon alfa, interleukin-12, and tumor necrosis factor 2α). Evidence suggests a suppressed cellular immune response in the tissues of VIN patients, adding biological plausibility to the therapy (van Seters et al., 2008). This opens opportunities to treat low-grade (and possibly moderate- or even high-grade) disease medically, providing a means to avoid more invasive, aggressive therapies (Le, Hicks, Menard, Hopkins, & Fung, 2006; van Seters et al., 2007). Recommendations from the National Cancer Institute (NCI) have been changed based on this accumulating evidence. The NCI now considers imiquimod first-line therapy for VIN I to III (van Seters et al., 2008). Regression is possible with VIN I, and observation with frequent reevaluation (via colposcope) remains the most reasonable management plan in patients deemed responsible, and therefore likely to follow-up as prescribed. Persistent lesions after 12 to 20 weeks of therapy may require surgical excision (American College of Obstetricians and Gynecologists [ACOG] Committee Opinion Number 509, 2011). Also available in the treatment lexicon is cidofovir, a selective inhibitor of viral DNA polymerase. Reports exist showing some favorable results, although it has not enjoyed widespread use in clinical practice (Calista, 2009; Koonsaeng et al., 2001).

Excision and ablation are used for higher grade disease (VIN II to III) unresponsive to medical management. Although these are effective management strategies, they do have negative consequences. For example, ablative therapies tend to be very uncomfortable during the healing process; in addition, excision can be disfiguring and lead to painful scarring. Efforts at reconstruction have been employed with some success (Thomas, 1996). This is useful especially in circumstances that require large areas of excision. It is wise to excise all areas of high-grade dysplasia completely, because recurrence and even dissemination to any newly grafted areas are more common if margins of resection are positive for high-grade changes. Aggressive management has been proven beneficial, with rates of invasive carcinoma reduced

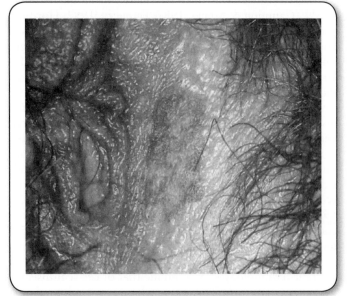

FIGURE 27.20
Vulvar intraepithelial neoplasia, hyperpigmented.

BOX 27.2   SIMPLE PERINEAL CARE REGIMEN

- Limit use of underwear whenever possible (air exposure is good)
- When underwear are worn, use 100% cotton
- Do not use soaps, deodorants, or powders on the vulva (wash only with water; a gentle soap is used for the rest of the body; use only unscented toilet tissue and sanitary products)
- Avoid abrading the skin (rinse after urination, pat the vulva dry with a soft cotton towel after voiding or bathing)
- Avoid commercial vaginal lubricants

to less than 4% (Jones, & Rowan, 1994). Patients with HPV infection, high-grade (II–III) lesions of VIN, and multifocal disease are at elevated risk for recurrence and merit careful surveillance (Hillemanns, Wang, Staehle, Michels, & Dannecker, 2006; Küppers, Stiller, Somville, & Bender, 1997). As with any immunocompromised patient, disease related to infectious etiology will be more problematic. Thus HIV-positive patients need more frequent follow-up to ensure disease state stability (Abercrombie & Korn, 1998).

Vulvodynia

ETIOLOGY

Vulvodynia is a condition of pain and inflammation affecting the introitus posteriorly at the vulvar vestibule (localized), or over the vulva more diffusely (generalized; Bachmann, 2006; Haefner et al., 2006). It is further classified as provoked or unprovoked. Although there is some evidence that these are unlikely to be two distinct entities, they are more likely points in a continuum of the vulvar pain syndrome (Edwards, 2004). Localized vulvodynia was formerly referred to as vulvar vestibulitis.

Although the etiology is unclear, vulvodynia is considered a chronic pain syndrome involving three interrelated physiologic systems (vestibular/vulvar mucosa, pelvic floor musculature, and central nervous system pain pathways) as well as psychosocial and relational factors (Brotto, Basson, & Gehring, 2003; Edwards, 2003; Graziottin & Brotto, 2004; Lundqvist & Bergdahl, 2005). A centralized neurologic component to this pain syndrome was suggested in one study in which subjects with vulvodynia were tested against pain-free controls for response to vulvar and peripheral pressure. Vulvodynia subjects displayed significantly lower pain thresholds in both locations versus controls (Giesecke et al., 2004).

EVALUATION/ASSESSMENT

The hallmark of vulvodynia is vulvar pain in the absence of a discrete lesion that might cause the pain. Pain is typically characterized as irritating, raw, and burning. Self-reported dyspareunia and stinging pain are strongly associated with vulvodynia (Petersen, Kristensen, Lundvall, & Giraldi, 2009). It limits sex and even tampon use (suggested as an outcome measure for vulvodynia research; Foster et al., 2009). Gross inspection may show no notable findings. However, there have been cases of treatment success after colposcopic examination has implicated chronic candidal infection (Pagano, 2007). In the case of localized vulvodynia (vulvar vestibulitis), there is typically erythema of the vestibule, and on closer inspection small erythematous lesions can be seen (Figure 27.21). Examination includes applying pressure to these lesions in a very specific manner (for instance, with a cotton-tipped applicator). Classically, these areas of erythema will be exquisitely sensitive to touch, indicating what is defined as provoked disease. Similarly, generalized vulvodynia may also be provoked or unprovoked, classified based on history and physical examination. Vulvodynia has been linked to other pelvic pain syndromes such as interstitial cystitis (Peters, Girdler, Carrico, Ibrahim, & Diokno, 2008).

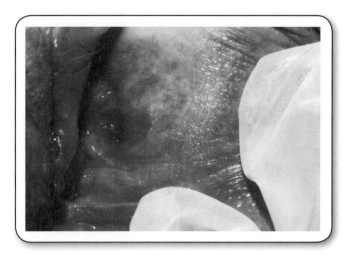

FIGURE 27.21

Vulvar vestibulitis.

Reprinted with permission from Libby Edwards, MD, Chief of Dermatology at Carolinas Medical Center, Charlotte, North Carolina.

TREATMENT/MANAGEMENT

The complexity of the disease suggests that the treatment approach is multifaceted; no single treatment will work for all patients. Treatment needs to be understood as a process.

Self-Management Measures • One of the most practical approaches is a perineal care regimen (Box 27.1) to remove any potential source of noxious stimuli (Hartmann, Strauhal, & Nelson, 2007; Welsh, Berzins, Cook, & Fairley, 2003). Lubrication for intercourse should employ natural oils rather than commercial lubricants that may exacerbate pain.

Complementary and Alternative Medicine • Frustration and despair are common in patients with vulvodynia because only about 1 in 10 patients per year will have symptomatic remission (Reed, Haefner, Sen, & Gorenflo, 2008). In addition, the impact on self-esteem, sexual identity, and relationships can be dramatic. Compounding this is the fact that qualified and experienced specialists may be difficult to find. Thus consideration must be given to counseling, psychotherapy, sex therapy, and cognitive behavioral therapy as well as medical or surgical approaches (Stockdale & Lawson, 2014).

Pharmacotherapeutics • Medical therapy can involve addressing pain pathways by using drugs, such as amitriptyline (Elavil), gabapentin (Neurontin), or pregabalin (Lyrica; Harris, Horowitz, & Borgida, 2007; Reed, Caron, Gorenflo, & Haefner, 2006). Superficial symptomatic management employs topical anesthetics, such as viscous lidocaine; in addition, tricyclic antidepressants administered orally or compounded for topical use may be considered. Similarly, gabapentin has also been formulated for use topically with favorable results (Boardman, Cooper, Blais, & Raker, 2008). Pelvic rehabilitation with physical therapy and biofeedback techniques may address some of the issues associated with pelvic muscular involvement (Graziottin & Brotto, 2004; refer to vaginismus in Chapter 21). Refractory cases will at times progress to surgical excision of the affected area. There is even a report of the use of botulinum toxin (Botox) in combination with surgical excision for a refractory case of severe vulvodynia (Gunter, Brewer, & Tawfik, 2004).

■ NEOPLASTIC VULVAR DISEASE

Squamous Carcinoma

ETIOLOGY

The vast majority of vulvar carcinomas (greater than 85%) are of squamous type. The natural history of vulvar carcinoma initiation is not completely clear; there is some limited evidence that it can develop in the context of intraepithelial neoplasia. The average age of presentation for patients with in situ disease is 45 to 50 years; however, invasive disease is found most commonly in the 65- to 70-year age group. Evidence suggests that incidence rates may be increasing and the age of onset may be decreasing; these trends need to be clarified over time (Hampl, Deckers-Figiel, Hampl, Rein, & Bender, 2008). Incidence rates of invasive vulvar cancers are about one third lower in African American and Hispanic women relative to White women (Saraiya et al., 2008). HPV has been associated with vulvar carcinoma (Bonvicini et al., 2005; Madeleine et al., 1997). HPV-16 specifically has been implicated in increasing the risk of invasive disease about threefold (Madeleine et al., 1997). Interestingly, the relative risk of in situ disease is significantly higher, ranging from 3.6 to 13 in some studies. This is supported by the fact that HPV infection is more common in women with vulvar HSIL (80% to 90%) than it is in women with vulvar carcinoma (30% to 75%). Although the explanation for this discrepancy has yet to be elucidated absolutely, it may be age related. Younger patients (aged 30–59 years) tend to have cancers linked to HPV infection, smoking, STIs, and early sexual debut, frequently as young teenagers. Older patients (aged 60–89 years) may have histories more aligned with vulvar inflammation or dystrophy and only infrequently have HPV exposure (Jones, Crandon, & Sanday, 2013). Recent studies support the supposition that there are paths to vulvar carcinoma other than through HPV infection (Andersen, Franquemont, Williams, Taylor, & Crum, 1991; Kurman, Toki, & Schiffman, 1993; Toki et al., 1991).

SYMPTOMS, EVALUATION/ASSESSMENT, AND DIAGNOSTIC STUDIES

Presenting symptoms tend to be long-standing pruritus, irritation, bleeding, or nodularity. Not only do these chronic symptoms indicate processes that are likely to develop slowly through time, they also alert all clinicians caring for women to the potential for malignancy or other pathologic processes. The scenario of delayed treatment occurs all too common, and can be attributed only partially to patients. Very frequently do women seek care for vulvar complaints and treatments are proffered for extended periods without referral or biopsy-proven histologic diagnosis. Any clinician performing cervical cytologic screening tests is diligent

in vulvar examination and review of systems. Biopsy is required for all suspicious lesions (discolorations, papules, ulcers, thickened regions, and lesions refractory to usual treatments; Figure 27.22). If the diagnosis is uncertain, biopsy is needed. Areas of bleeding, pruritus, or tingling merit special attention, because these are common presenting features of vulvar dystrophy and carcinoma.

The majority of vulvar cancers arise in the labia majora (Burke et al., 1995). As stated previously, they tend to develop and grow slowly. It is not uncommon, despite a long history of a vulvar "sore," to be unable to identify metastasis. Lymph nodes are positive in about one third to one half of all vulvar cancers staged (Hacker, 2009). When metastasis has occurred, its pattern through the lymphatics is very predictable. Integral to understanding clinical evaluation and surgical staging is the knowledge of the lymphatic drainage of the vulva. Generally, distribution is superficial to the ipsilateral inguinal femoral nodes and then deep to the obturator and pelvic iliac nodes (de Hullu et al., 2000). Rarely, deep nodes can be positive without evidence of disease at the superficial femoral nodes. Although ipsilateral dissemination is typical for most tumors that are lateral of midline, for example, in the mid-labia, tumors located near the clitoris or perineum can present with positive nodes to either side. Distant spread of disease is possible via a hematogenous route, most commonly arising in the lung.

TREATMENT/MANAGEMENT

Management is by wide local excision and staging lymph-node biopsy of either one or both inguinal regions, depending on the location of the primary lesion and the extent of distribution (de Hullu et al., 2000). Options exist for lymph-node staging because of the predictable pattern of spread. Lymph-node sampling from the inguinofemoral region is the traditional method; however, some clinicians are opting for sentinel node biopsy in an effort to reduce the need for extensive dissection (Johann, Klaeser, Krause, & Mueller, 2008). Inguinofemoral node status is the most significant prognostic indicator in vulvar cancer (Woelber et al., 2009). Efforts are made to preserve the clitoris and labia if possible; however, complete excision of disease is the

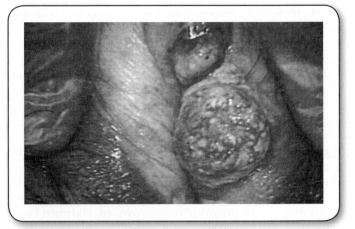

FIGURE 27.22

Vulvar squamous cancer.

principal objective. Liberal use of intraoperative frozen section to confirm tumor-free margins is preferred. Disease that is especially close to the urethra and/or anus presents additional difficulty in surgical management. Outcomes of treatment are very encouraging with early stage disease. Five-year survival rates in stage I and II disease are approximately the same at about 90%. Survival rates diminish with advancing stage. Stage III and IV survival rates range from 60% to 20% (Saraiya et al., 2008; Tantipalakorn, Robertson, Marsden, Gebski, & Hacker, 2009; Woelber et al., 2009). Use of radiotherapy for cancers is most common in unresectable disease, or with International Federation of Gynecology and Obstetrics stage III or IV disease where survival is improved with adjuvant therapy (Gaffney et al., 2009). There is some evidence that the use of preoperative neoadjuvant chemotherapy in especially advanced tumors can make surgical resection more feasible, with less extensive resection required (Aragona et al., 2012). This could possibly allow for preservation of critical structures that would otherwise be included within the margins of the resection.

Melanoma

ETIOLOGY AND EVALUATION/ASSESSMENT

Following squamous carcinoma, melanoma is the second most common malignancy of the vulva. However, it is rare, accounting for only 5% of vulvar cancers. Lesions usually develop from nevi, most commonly on the labia minora. Pigmented lesions of the vulva are most commonly junctional nevi. These can be multifocal, and all pigmented lesions merit biopsy, usually via excision. Melanoma has presented in the teen years and continues to present into the ninth decade. It can be either nodular or diffuse. Lesions appear as brown, blue, or even black pigmentations; occasionally, these are ulcerations or papular nodules.

TREATMENT/MANAGEMENT

Stage and prognosis are based on the depth of invasion. The constructs used to define this are the Breslow depth (in millimeters) or Clark's classification (invasion depth defined by tissue type: epidermis, papillary dermis, reticular dermis, subcutaneous tissue; Verschraegen et al., 2001; Wechter et al., 2004). Clark's level I and II imply invasion into the papillary ridges of the epidermis and are treated only by wide local excision (equivalent to Breslow depth correlate would be approximately 0.76 mm of invasion). Greater Breslow depths are treated with wide local excision coupled with lymph node dissection. Distribution of the disease is similar to that of squamous cancers, with dissemination to the inguinal lymph nodes preceding invasion of the pelvic nodes. The predictability of nodal spread has led to the evaluation of sentinel lymph-node sampling, similar to that in breast cancers or cutaneous melanomas. Results suggest that this is a reliable means of evaluating the stage and guiding the treatment modalities. Classification based on the American Joint Committee on Cancer (AJCC) for cutaneous melanoma seems to apply to the vulva as well (Seifried et al., 2014).

Survival is nearly 100% at 5 years if Clark's level is I or II. When the tumor is more deeply invasive, survival is dependent on regional nodal metastasis. Dissemination to inguinal nodes decreases the survival rate to less than 30%, compared with greater than 60% 5-year survival if these lymph nodes are negative. Patients with the disease to the pelvic nodes have a fairly dismal likelihood of survival (Verschraegen et al., 2001; Wechter et al., 2004). Using AJCC categories, patients with stage 0–II had a significantly better melanoma specific survival (5-year survival = 63.6%, $n = 59$) compared with those with stage III disease (5-year survival = 0%, $n = 12$, $p < 0.001$; Seifried et al., 2014). Treatment has been attempted with adjuvant chemotherapy and irradiation. However, no useful protocols have yet been identified to extend survival. Efforts have been reported to marginally improve survival with biochemotherapy; however, its usefulness has not been demonstrated in a prospective manner. Gene therapy is another option being investigated and may hold promise in the future.

Adenocarcinoma

ETIOLOGY AND EVALUATION/ASSESSMENT

Arising in Bartholin's glands, sweat glands, or as Paget's disease, adenocarcinoma of the vulva is a rare entity (Finan & Barre, 2003; Kokcu, Cetinkaya, Aydin, & Kandemir, 2004; López-Varela, Oliva, McIntyre, & Fuller, 2007). Most occur in postmenopausal women. Therefore, any enlargement in Bartholin's glands in this population are treated with the utmost suspicion. Presentation can be with mass, dyspareunia, or ulceration.

TREATMENT/MANAGEMENT

Surgical intervention (wide local excision or radical vulvectomy and inguinal lymphadenectomy) in combination with regional radiotherapy is the typical treatment modality. Pelvic node dissection has only been indicated in the event of positive regional nodes. Spread to regional lymph nodes significantly diminishes the likelihood of survival. The average overall 5-year survival rate in one study was 67% (Cardosi, 2001). Adjuvant radiation therapy has improved survival to as high as 86% with wide local excision and to 78% with radical vulvectomy (Balat, Edwards, & Delclos, 2001). Alternatives to surgical management are with radiation or chemoradiation alone. These have demonstrated 5-year survival rates of about 66% and thus represent reasonable treatment options for select patients (Finan & Barre, 2003). Intestinal, sweat gland, and mammary-type tumors have been reported as well as metastatic disease from appendix or other sites. Intestinal types may confer significant risks of colon cancer (Cormio et al., 2012). Mammary types may respond well to excision and hormonal treatments, similar to primary breast cancers (Benito et al., 2012).

Basal Cell Carcinoma

ETIOLOGY AND EVALUATION/ASSESSMENT

As with other locations in the body, basal cell carcinoma are slow-growing, well-circumscribed pearly lesions. Basal cell carcinoma typically exhibits features of central umbilication, telangiectasia, pink plaque, and perhaps ulceration (DeAmbrosis, Nicklin, & Yong-Gee, 2008). There are, however, reports of more atypical phenotypes (Suda & Kakinuma, 2006). Women complain of pruritus and occasional intermittent bleeding. In a series of six case studies, the average age at diagnosis was 76 years and pruritis was the most common complaint, with symptoms present for 13 to 24 months before treatment (Mulvany, Rayoo, & Allen, 2012).

TREATMENT/MANAGEMENT

Excision is usually sufficient treatment because lymphatic invasion, while reported, is extremely rare (de Giorgi, Salvini, Massi, Raspollini, & Carli, 2005; Mateus et al., 2001; Pisani, Poggiali, De Padova, Andreassi, & Bilenchi, 2006). Although the clinical course is usually fairly benign with identification and excision, basal cell carcinoma has been responsible for disease-related mortality on rare occasions (Feakins & Lowe, 1997).

Paget's Disease

ETIOLOGY, EVALUATION/ASSESSMENT, AND DIAGNOSTIC STUDIES

Another condition that arises elsewhere in the body and occurs in the vulva is Paget's disease. Characterized by erythematous, well-demarcated lesions along with areas of indurated, excoriated thickening, it presents with pruritus and pain in older women, remote from menopause. In up to 20% of cases it can be associated with an underlying adenocarcinoma; therefore, it is important for the clinician to conduct the clinical examination with a level of suspicion and to perform adequate biopsy of the area, which may be an indication for fine-needle aspiration (MacLean, Makwana, Ellis, & Cunnington, 2004; Tebes, Cardosi, & Hoffman, 2002).

TREATMENT/MANAGEMENT

Treatment is usually with full-thickness wide local excision (MacLean et al., 2004; Tebes et al., 2002). However, radiation therapy has been successful in cases of in situ disease or poor surgical candidates (Moreno-Arias, Conill, Sola-Casas, Mascaro-Galy, & Grimalt, 2003). In some cases, complete resolution has been obtained with the use of imiquimod cream (Hatch & Davis, 2008). Clear margins are achieved by using frozen section evaluation liberally. Unfortunately, recurrent lesions are not uncommon, even when negative margins have been obtained.

Sarcoma

ETIOLOGY AND EVALUATION/ASSESSMENT

Sarcomas of the vulva are even more rare than cases of melanoma, basal cell carcinoma, and Paget's disease. These will be symptomatic and occur earlier in life (about age 40 years). Types include rhabdomyosarcoma, which has a poor prognosis attributable to early metastasis and rapid growth; as well as leiomyosarcoma, which grows less quickly and is not known for distant metastasis early in the disease process. Other histological variants include fibrosarcoma and epithelioid sarcoma.

TREATMENT/MANAGEMENT

Treatment measures include wide local excision or vulvectomy, depending on the clinical presentation of the lesion (Ulutin, Zellars, & Frassica, 2003). Sarcomas of the vulva are characterized by rapid growth, high metastatic potential, frequent recurrences, aggressive behavior, and high mortality rate (Chokoeva et al., 2015).

■ FUTURE DIRECTIONS

There are numerous conditions that affect the health and well-being of the vulva and vagina. It can take years of practice for the clinician to recognize the conditions presented in this chapter and incorporate them into the lexicon of existing disease states. Initial conservative therapy is often reasonable, such as following a strict perineal care regimen; however, biopsy will be needed for clear diagnosis to guide management in many instances. Referral to a specialist is suggested when the woman's symptoms are not resolving, when diagnosis is uncertain, and when specialty care intervention is needed. Added research on less invasive diagnostic techniques and treatment modalities are ongoing and will shape the future of identifying and treating these conditions.

■ REFERENCES

Abercrombie, P. D., & Korn, A. P. (1998). Vulvar intraepithelial neoplasia in women with HIV. *AIDS Patient Care and STDs, 12*(4), 251–254.

ACOG Committee Opinion Number 509. (2011). Management of vulvar intraepithelial neoplasia. *Obstetrics & Gynecology, 118*(5), 1192–1194.

Al-Hashimi, I., Schifter, M., Lockhart, P. B., Wray, D., Brennan, M., Migliorati, C. A.,...van der Waal, I. (2007). Oral lichen planus and oral lichenoid lesions: Diagnostic and therapeutic considerations. *Oral Surgery, Oral Medicine, Oral Pathology, Oral Radiology, and Endodontics, 103*(Suppl.), S25.e1–S25.e12.

Andersen, W. A., Franquemont, D. W., Williams, J., Taylor, P. T., & Crum, C. P. (1991). Vulvar squamous cell carcinoma and papillomaviruses: Two separate entities? *American Journal of Obstetrics and Gynecology, 165*(2), 329–335; discussion 335.

Aragona, A. M., Cuneo, N., Soderini, A. H., Alcoba, E., Greco, A., Reyes, C., & Lekmann, S. (2012). Tailoring the treatment of locally advanced squamous cell carcinoma of the vulva. *International Journal of Gynecological Cancer, 22*(7), 1258–1263.

Ashton-Miller, J. A., & DeLancey, J. O. (2007). Functional anatomy of the female pelvic floor. *Annals of the New York Academy of Sciences, 1101,* 266–296.

Bachmann, G. A., Rosen, R., Pinn, V. W., Utian, W. H., Ayers, C., Basson, R.,...Witkin, S. S. (2006). Vulvodynia: A state-of-the-art consensus on definitions, diagnosis and management. *Journal of Reproductive Medicine, 51*(6), 447–456.

Balat, O., Edwards, C. L., & Delclos, L. (2001). Advanced primary carcinoma of the Bartholin gland: Report of 18 patients. *European Journal of Gynaecological Oncology, 22*(1), 46–49.

Baldwin, P., Nicholson, A., Alazawi, W., Moseley, R., Coleman, N., & Sterling, J. (2007). Viral and cytogenetic profile of vulval intraepithelial neoplasia. *Journal of Reproductive Medicine, 52,* 112. Abstract.

Barnhart, K. T., Izquierdo, A., Pretorius, E. S., Shera, D. M., Shabbout, M., & Shaunik, A. (2006). Baseline dimensions of the human vagina. *Human Reproduction, 21*(6), 1618–1622.

Benito, V., Arribas, S., Martínez, D., Medina, N., Lubrano, A., & Arencibia, O. (2012). Metastatic adenocarcinoma of mammary-like glands of the vulva successfully treated with surgery and hormonal therapy. *Journal of Obstetrics and Gynaecology Research, 39*(1), 450–454.

Berger, M. B., Betschart, C., Khandwala, N., Delancey, J. O., & Haefner, H. K. (2012). Incidental Bartholin gland cysts identified on pelvic magnetic resonance imaging. *Obstetrics & Gynecology, 120*(4), 798–802.

Binsaleh, S., Al-Assiri, M., Jednak, R., & El-Sherbiny, M. (2007). Gartner duct cyst simplified treatment approach. *International Urology and Nephrology, 39*(2), 485–487.

Blakey, D. H., Dewhurst, C. J., & Tipton, R. H. (1966). The long term results after marsupialization of Bartholin's cysts and abscesses. *Journal of Obstetrics and Gynaecology of the British Commonwealth, 73*(6), 1008–1009.

Boardman, L. A., Botte, J., & Kennedy, C. M. (2005). Recurrent vulvar itching. *Obstetrics & Gynecology, 105*(6), 1451–1455.

Boardman, L. A., Cooper, A. S., Blais, L. R., & Raker, C. A. (2008). Topical gabapentin in the treatment of localized and generalized vulvodynia. *Obstetrics and Gynecology, 112*(3), 579–585.

Bonvicini, F., Venturoli, S., Ambretti, S., Paterini, P., Santini, D., Ceccarelli, C.,…Musiani, M. (2005). Presence and type of oncogenic human papillomavirus in classic and in differentiated vulvar intraepithelial neoplasia and keratinizing vulvar squamous cell carcinoma. *Journal of Medical Virology, 77*(1), 102–106.

Breneman, J. C., Lyden, E., Pappo, A. S., Link, M. P., Anderson, J. R., Parham, D. M.,…Crist, W. M. (2003). Prognostic factors and clinical outcomes in children and adolescents with metastatic rhabdomyosarcoma—A report from the Intergroup Rhabdomyosarcoma Study IV. *Journal of Clinical Oncology: Official Journal of the American Society of Clinical Oncology, 21*(1), 78–84.

Brotto, L. A., Basson, R., & Gehring, D. (2003). Psychological profiles among women with vulvar vestibulitis syndrome: A chart review. *Journal of Psychosomatic Obstetrics and Gynaecology, 24*(3), 195–203.

Buchanan, D. J., Schlaerth, J., & Kurosaki, T. (1998). Primary vaginal melanoma: Thirteen-year disease-free survival after wide local excision and review of recent literature. *American Journal of Obstetrics and Gynecology, 178*(6), 1177–1184.

Buck, H. W., & Guth, K. J. (2003). Treatment of vaginal intraepithelial neoplasia (primarily low grade) with imiquimod 5% cream. *Journal of Lower Genital Tract Disease, 7*(4), 290–293.

Buck, H. W., & Guth, K. J. (2003). Treatment of vaginal intraepithelial neoplasia (primarily low grade) with imiquimod 5% cream. *Journal of Lower Genital Tract Disease, 7*(4), 290–293.

Burke, T. W., Levenback, C., Coleman, R. L., Morris, M., Silva, E. G., & Gershenson, D. M. (1995). Surgical therapy of T1 and T2 vulvar carcinoma: Further experience with radical wide excision and selective inguinal lymphadenectomy. *Gynecologic Oncology, 57*(2), 215–220.

Buscema, J., & Woodruff, J. D. (1980). Progressive histobiologic alterations in the development of vulvar cancer. *American Journal of Obstetrics and Gynecology, 138*(2), 146–150.

Caglar, H., Hertzog, R. W., & Hreshchyshyn, M. M. (1981). Topical 5-fluorouracil treatment of vaginal intraepithelial neoplasia. *Obstetrics and Gynecology, 58*(5), 580–583.

Calista, D. (2009). Topical 1% cidofovir for the treatment of vulvar intraepidermal neoplasia (VIN1) developed on lichen sclerosus. *International Journal of Dermatology, 48*(5), 535–536.

Campion, M. J., & Singer, A. (1987). Vulval intraepithelial neoplasia: Clinical review. *Genitourinary Medicine, 63*(3), 147–152.

Campos-Domínguez, M., Silvente, C., de la Cueva, P., González-Carrascosa, M., Lecona, M., Suárez, R., & Lázaro, P. (2006). [Erythrodermic lichen planus pemphigoides]. *Actas Dermo-Sifiliográficas, 97*(9), 583–586.

Cardamakis, E., Kourounis, G., Dimopoulos, D., Avaraki, M., Ginopoulos, P., Stathopoulos, E., … Mantou, H. (1998). Treatment of vaginal intraepithelial neoplasia (VAIN) with interferon alpha-2a, CO2 laser, vaporisation and isotretinoin. *Cancer Detection and Prevention, 22*(Suppl. 1). Retrieved from http://www.cancerprev.org/Journal/Issues/22/101/19/2963

Cardosi, R. J., Speights, A., Fiorica, J. V., Grendys, E. C., Hakam, A., & Hoffman, M. S. (2001). Bartholin's gland carcinoma: A 15-year experience. *Gynecologic Oncology, 82*(2), 247–251.

Chi, C., Kirtschig, G., Baldo, M., Lewis, F., Wang, S., & Wojnarowska, F. (2012). Systematic review and meta-analysis of randomized controlled trials on topical interventions for genital lichen sclerosus. *Journal of the American Academy of Dermatology, 67*(2), 305–312.

Chiu, T., & Jones, R. W. (2011). Multifocal multicentric squamous cell carcinomas arising in vulvovaginal lichen planus. *Journal of Lower Genital Tract Disease, 15*(3), 246–247.

Chokoeva, A., Tchernev, G., Cardoso, J., Patterson, J., Dechev, I., Valkanov, S.,…Wollina, U. (2015). Vulvar sarcomas: Short guideline for histopathological recognition and clinical management. Part 2. *International Journal of Immunopathology and Pharmacology, 28*(2), 178–186.

Clifford, G. M., Smith, J. S., Plummer, M., Muñoz, N., & Franceschi, S. (2003). Human papillomavirus types in invasive cervical cancer worldwide: A meta-analysis. *British Journal of Cancer, 88*(1), 63–73.

Cobellis, P. L., Stradella, L., De Lucia, E., Iannella, I., Pecori, E., Scaffa, C.,…Colacurci, N. (2006). Alcohol sclerotherapy: A new method for Bartholin gland cyst treatment. *Minerva Ginecologica, 58*(3), 245–248.

Cooper, S. M., & Wojnarowska, F. (2006). Influence of treatment of erosive lichen planus of the vulva on its prognosis. *Archives of Dermatology, 142*(3), 289–294.

Cooper, S. M., Ali, I., Baldo, M., & Wojnarowska, F. (2008). The association of lichen sclerosus and erosive lichen planus of the vulva with autoimmune disease: A case-control study. *Archives of Dermatology, 144*(11), 1432–1435.

Cooper, S. M., Dean, D., Allen, J., Kirtschig, G., & Wojnarowska, F. (2005). Erosive lichen planus of the vulva: Weak circulating basement membrane zone antibodies are present. *Clinical and Experimental Dermatology, 30*(5), 551–556.

Cormio, G., Carriero, C., Loizzi, V., Gizzi, F., Leone, L., Putignano, G.,…Selvaggi, L. (2012). "Intestinal-type" mucinous adenocarcinoma of the vulva: A report of two cases. *European Journal of Gynaecological Oncology, 33*(4), 433–435.

Creasman, W. T., Phillips, J. L., & Menck, H. R. (1998). The National Cancer Data Base report on cancer of the vagina. *Cancer, 83*(5), 1033–1040.

Crum, C. P., Liskow, A., Petras, P., Keng, W. C., & Frick, H. C. (1984). Vulvar intraepithelial neoplasia (severe atypia and carcinoma in situ). A clinicopathologic analysis of 41 cases. *Cancer, 54*(7), 1429–1434.

DeAmbrosis, K., Nicklin, J., & Yong-Gee, S. (2008). Basal cell carcinoma of the vulva: A report of four cases. *The Australasian Journal of Dermatology, 49*(4), 213–215.

de Bie, R. P., van de Nieuwenhof, H. P., Bekkers, R. L., Melchers, W. J., Siebers, A. G., Bulten, J.,…de Hullu, J. A. (2009). Patients with usual vulvar intraepithelial neoplasia-related vulvar cancer have an increased risk of cervical abnormalities. *British Journal of Cancer, 101*(1), 27–31.

de Giorgi, V., Salvini, C., Massi, D., Raspollini, M. R., & Carli, P. (2005). Vulvar basal cell carcinoma: Retrospective study and review of literature. *Gynecologic Oncology, 97*(1), 192–194.

de Hullu, J. A., Hollema, H., Piers, D. A., Verheijen, R. H., van Diest, P. J., Mourits, M. J.,…van Der Zee, A. G. (2000). Sentinel lymph node procedure is highly accurate in squamous cell carcinoma of the vulva. *Journal of Clinical Oncology: Official Journal of the American Society of Clinical Oncology, 18*(15), 2811–2816.

DeLancey, J. O. (1992). Anatomic aspects of vaginal eversion after hysterectomy. *American Journal of Obstetrics and Gynecology, 166*(6, Pt. 1), 1717–1724; discussion 1724.

Desaia, P. J., & Creasman, W. T. (2007). *Clinical Gynecologic Oncology* (7th ed.). St. Louis, MO: Mosby.

Diakomanolis, E., Rodolakis, A., Boulgaris, Z., Blachos, G., & Michalas, S. (2002). Treatment of vaginal intraepithelial neoplasia with laser ablation and upper vaginectomy. *Gynecologic and Obstetric Investigation, 54*(1), 17–20.

Eberz, B., Berghold, A., & Regauer, S. (2008). High prevalence of concomitant anogenital lichen sclerosus and extragenital psoriasis in adult women. *Obstetrics and Gynecology, 111*(5), 1143–1147.

Eddy, G. L., Marks, R. D., Miller, M. C., & Underwood, P. B. (1991). Primary invasive vaginal carcinoma. *American Journal of Obstetrics and Gynecology, 165*(2), 292–296; discussion 296.

Edwards, L. (2003). New concepts in vulvodynia. *American Journal of Obstetrics and Gynecology, 189*(Suppl. 3), S24–S30.

Edwards, L. (2004). Subsets of vulvodynia: Overlapping characteristics. *Journal of Reproductive Medicine, 49*(11), 883–887.

Fambrini, M., Penna, C., Pieralli, A., Fallani, M. G., Andersson, K. L., Lozza, V., ...Marchionni, M. (2008). Carbon-dioxide laser vaporization of the Bartholin gland cyst: A retrospective analysis on 200 cases. *Journal of Minimally Invasive Gynecology, 15*(3), 327–331.

Feakins, R. M., & Lowe, D. G. (1997). Basal cell carcinoma of the vulva: A clinicopathologic study of 45 cases. *International Journal of Gynecological Pathology: Official Journal of the International Society of Gynecological Pathologists, 16*(4), 319–324.

Ferenczy, A. (1992). Intraepithelial neoplasia of the vulva. In M. Coppelson (Ed.), *Gynecologic oncology* (pp. 443–463). Edinburgh, London: Churchill Livingstone.

Fielding, J. R., Griffiths, D. J., Versi, E., Mulkern, R. V., Lee, M. L., & Jolesz, F. A. (1998). MR imaging of pelvic floor continence mechanisms in the supine and sitting positions. *American Journal of Roentgenology, 171*(6), 1607–1610.

Fielding, J. R., Versi, E., Mulkern, R. V., Lerner, M. H., Griffiths, D. J., & Jolesz, F. A. (1996). MR imaging of the female pelvic floor in the supine and upright positions. *Journal of Magnetic Resonance Imaging, 6*(6), 961–963.

Finan, M. A., & Barre, G. (2003). Bartholin's gland carcinoma, malignant melanoma and other rare tumours of the vulva. *Best Practice & Research. Clinical Obstetrics & Gynaecology, 17*(4), 609–633.

Foster, D. C., Kotok, M. B., Huang, L. S., Watts, A., Oakes, D., Howard, F. M., ...Dworkin, R. H. (2009). The tampon test for vulvodynia treatment outcomes research: reliability, construct validity, and responsiveness. *Obstetrics and Gynecology, 113*(4), 825–832.

Fu Yao, S. (2002). *Pathology of the uterine cervix, vagina, and vulva* (2nd ed.). Philadelphia, PA: Elsevier Science, copyright 2002.

Funaro, D., Lovett, A., Leroux, N., & Powell, J. (2014). A double-blind, randomized prospective study evaluating topical clobetasol propionate 0.05% versus topical tacrolimus 0.1% in patients with vulvar lichen sclerosus. *Journal of the American Academy of Dermatology, 71*(1), 84–91.

Gabbe, S., Niebyl, J., & Simpson, J. L. (2007). *Obstetrics: Normal and problem pregnancies* (5th ed.). St Louis, MO: Elsevier Mosby.

Gaffney, D. K., Du Bois, A., Narayan, K., Reed, N., Toita, T., Pignata, S., ...Trimble, E. L. (2009). Patterns of care for radiotherapy in vulvar cancer: A Gynecologic Cancer Intergroup study. *International Journal of Gynecological Cancer: Official Journal of the International Gynecological Cancer Society, 19*(1), 163–167.

Ghezelayagh, T., Rauh-Hain, J. A., & Growdon, W. B. (2015). Comparing mortality of vaginal sarcoma, squamous cell carcinoma, and adenocarcinoma in the surveillance, epidemiology, and end results database. *Obstetrics & Gynecology, 125*(6), 1353–1361.

Giesecke, J., Reed, B. D., Haefner, H. K., Giesecke, T., Clauw, D. J., & Gracely, R. H. (2004). Quantitative sensory testing in vulvodynia patients and increased peripheral pressure pain sensitivity. *Obstetrics and Gynecology, 104*(1), 126–133.

Goldstein, A. T., & Parneix-Spake, A. (2006). Pimecrolimus cream 1% for treatment of vulvar lichen simplex chronicus. *Journal of Obstetrics & Gynecology, 107*(4), 54S–55S.

Goldstein, A. T., Parneix-Spake, A., McCormick, C. L., & Burrows, L. J. (2007). Pimecrolimus cream 1% for treatment of vulvar lichen simplex chronicus: An open-label, preliminary trial. *Gynecologic and Obstetric Investigation, 64*(4), 180–186.

González Bosquet, E., Torres, A., Busquets, M., Esteva, C., Muñoz-Almagro, C., & Lailla, J. M. (2008). Prognostic factors for the development of vaginal intraepithelial neoplasia. *European Journal of Gynaecological Oncology, 29*(1), 43–45.

Graziottin, A., & Brotto, L. A. (2004). Vulvar vestibulitis syndrome: A clinical approach. *Journal of Sex & Marital Therapy, 30*(3), 125–139.

Gunter, J., Brewer, A., & Tawfik, O. (2004). Botulinum toxin a for vulvodynia: A case report. *Journal of Pain: Official Journal of the American Pain Society, 5*(4), 238–240.

Gupta, D., Malpica, A., Deavers, M. T., & Silva, E. G. (2002). Vaginal melanoma: A clinicopathologic and immunohistochemical study of 26 cases. *American Journal of Surgical Pathology, 26*(11), 1450–1457.

Habif, T. P. (2004). *Clinical dermatology* (4th ed.). St. Louis, MO: Elsevier.

Hacker, N. F. (2009). Vulvar cancer. In J. S. Berek, N. F. Hacker, (Eds.), *Practical gynecologic oncology* (5th ed., pp. 553–596). Philadelphia, PA: Lippincott Williams & Wilkins.

Haefner, H. K., Collins, M., Davis, G. D., Edwards, L., Foster, D. C., Hartman, E. D., ...Lynch, P. J.; Vulvodynia. ACOG Committee Opinion: No 345. (2006). Vulvodynia guideline. *Journal of Lower Genital Tract Disease 2005, 9*(1), 40–51.

Hambley, R., Hebda, P. A., Abell, E., Cohen, B. A., & Jegasothy, B. V. (1988). Wound healing of skin incisions produced by ultrasonically vibrating knife, scalpel, electrosurgery, and carbon dioxide laser. *Journal of Dermatologic Surgery and Oncology, 14*(11), 1213–1217.

Hammes, B., & Laitman, C. J. (2003). Diethylstilbestrol [DES] update: Recommendations for the identification and management of DES-exposed individuals. *Journal of Midwife Womens Health, 489*(1), 19–29.

Hampl, M., Deckers-Figiel, S., Hampl, J. A., Rein, D., & Bender, H. G. (2008). New aspects of vulvar cancer: Changes in localization and age of onset. *Gynecologic Oncology, 109*(3), 340–345.

Harper, D. M., Franco, E. L., Wheeler, C., Ferris, D. G., Jenkins, D., Schuind, A., ...Dubin, G.; GlaxoSmithKline HPV Vaccine Study Group. (2004). Efficacy of a bivalent L1 virus-like particle vaccine in prevention of infection with human papillomavirus types 16 and 18 in young women: A randomised controlled trial. *Lancet, 364*(9447), 1757–1765.

Harris, G., Horowitz, B., & Borgida, A. (2007). Evaluation of gabapentin in the treatment of generalized vulvodynia, unprovoked. *Journal of Reproductive Medicine, 52*(2), 103–106.

Hartmann, D., Strauhal, M. J., & Nelson, C. A. (2007). Treatment of women in the United States with localized, provoked vulvodynia: Practice survey of women's health physical therapists. *Journal of Reproductive Medicine, 52*(1), 48–52.

Hatch, K. D., & Davis, J. R. (2008). Complete resolution of Paget disease of the vulva with imiquimod cream. *Journal of Lower Genital Tract Disease, 12*(2), 90–94.

Helen, A. C., & Secor, R. M. (2015). *Advanced health assessment of women clinical skills and procedures* (3rd ed.). New York, NY: Springer Publishing.

Hengge, U. R., Krause, W., Hofmann, H., Stadler, R., Gross, G., Meurer, M., ...Gollnick, H. (2006). Multicentre, phase II trial on the safety and efficacy of topical tacrolimus ointment for the treatment of lichen sclerosus. *British Journal of Dermatology, 155*(5), 1021–1028.

Herbst, A. L., & Scully, R. E. (1970). Adenocarcinoma of the vagina in adolescence. A report of 7 cases including 6 clear-cell carcinomas (so-called mesonephromas). *Cancer, 25*(4), 745–757.

Hertel, H., Soergel, P., Muecke, J., Schneider, M., Papendorf, F., Laenger, F., ...Hillemanns, P. (2013). Is there a place for sentinel technique in treatment of vaginal cancer? *International Journal of Gynecological Cancer, 23*(9), 1692–1698.

Hillemanns, P., & Wang, X. (2006). Integration of HPV-16 and HPV-18 DNA in vulvar intraepithelial neoplasia. *Gynecologic Oncology, 100*(2), 276–282.

Hillemanns, P., Wang, X., Staehle, S., Michels, W., & Dannecker, C. (2006). Evaluation of different treatment modalities for vulvar intraepithelial neoplasia (VIN): CO(2) laser vaporization, photodynamic therapy, excision and vulvectomy. *Gynecologic Oncology, 100*(2), 271–275.

Hopkins, M. P., & Snyder, M. K. (2005). Benign disorders of vulva and vagina. In M. G. Curtis & M. P. Hopkins (Eds.), *Glass's office gynecology* (6th ed., pp. 417–426). Baltimore, MD: Lippincott Williams & Wilkins.

Hørding, U., Junge, J., Poulsen, H., & Lundvall, F. (1995). Vulvar intraepithelial neoplasia III: A viral disease of undetermined progressive potential. *Gynecologic Oncology, 56*(2), 276–279.

Insinga, R. P., Liaw, K. L., Johnson, L. G., & Madeleine, M. M. (2008). A systematic review of the prevalence and attribution of human papillomavirus types among cervical, vaginal, and vulvar precancers and cancers in the United States. *Cancer Epidemiology, Biomarkers & Prevention: A Publication of the American Association for Cancer Research, Cosponsored by the American Society of Preventive Oncology, 17*(7), 1611–1622.

Iyer, S., & Minassian, V. A. (2013). Resection of urethral diverticulum in pregnancy. *Obstetrics & Gynecology, 122*(2, Pt. 2), 467–469.

Johann, S., Klaeser, B., Krause, T., & Mueller, M. D. (2008). Comparison of outcome and recurrence-free survival after sentinel lymph node biopsy and lymphadenectomy in vulvar cancer. *Gynecologic Oncology, 110*(3), 324–328.

Jones, I. S., Crandon, A., & Sanday, K. (2013). Squamous cell carcinoma of the vulva. *Journal of Lower Genital Tract Disease, 17*(3), 267–272.

Jones, R. W., & Rowan, D. M. (1994). Vulvar intraepithelial neoplasia III: A clinical study of the outcome in 113 cases with relation to the later development of invasive vulvar carcinoma. *Obstetrics and Gynecology, 84*(5), 741–745.

Kaufman, R. H., Faro, S., & Brown, D. (2004). *Benign diseases of the vulva and vagina* (5th ed.). St. Louis, MO: Elsevier Mosby.

Kelekci, H. K., Uncu, H. G., Yilmaz, B., Ozdemir, O., Sut, N., & Kelekci, S. (2008). Pimecrolimus 1% cream for pruritus in postmenopausal diabetic women with vulvar lichen simplex chronicus: A prospective non-controlled case series. *Journal of Dermatological Treatment, 19*(5), 274–278.

Kessous, R., Aricha-Tamir, B., Sheizaf, B., Shteiner, N., Moran-Gilad, J., & Weintraub, A. Y. (2013). Clinical and microbiological characteristics of Bartholin gland abscesses. *Obstetrics & Gynecology, 122*(4), 794–879.

Kim, H. S., Park, N. H., Park, I. A., Park, J. H., Chung, H. H., Kim, J. W.,…Kang, S. B. (2009). Risk factors for recurrence of vaginal intraepithelial neoplasia in the vaginal vault after laser vaporization. *Lasers in Surgery and Medicine, 41*(3), 196–202.

Kirschner, A. N., Kidd, E. A., Dewees, T., & Perkins, S. M. (2013). Treatment approach and outcomes of vaginal melanoma. *International Journal of Gynecological Cancer, 23*(8), 1484–1489.

Kleinman, J. T., & Chen, B. (2012). Trouble voiding in an adolescent girl. *Obstetrics & Gynecology, 120*(4), 944–947.

Koff, A. K. (1933). Development of the vagina in the human fetus. *Contributions to Embryology, 24*(140), 59–91.

Kokcu, A., Cetinkaya, M. B., Aydin, O., & Kandemir, B. (2004). Primary-adenocarcinoma of Bartholin's gland: A case report. *European Journal of Gynaecological Oncology, 25*(5), 651–652.

Koonsaeng, S., Verschraegen, C., Freedman, R., Bossens, M., Kudelka, A., Kavanagh, J.,…Snoeck, R. (2001). Successful treatment of recurrent vulvar intraepithelial neoplasia resistant to interferon and isotretinoin with cidofovir. *Journal of Medical Virology, 64*(2), 195–198.

Krantz, K. E. (1958). Innervation of the human vulva and vagina: A microscopic study. *Obstetrics and Gynecology, 12*(4), 382–396.

Küppers, V., Stiller, M., Somville, T., & Bender, H. G. (1997). Risk factors for recurrent VIN. Role of multifocality and grade of disease. *Journal of Reproductive Medicine, 42*(3), 140–144.

Kurman, R. J., Toki, T., & Schiffman, M. H. (1993). Basaloid and warty carcinomas of the vulva. Distinctive types of squamous cell carcinoma frequently associated with human papillomaviruses. *American Journal of Surgical Pathology, 17*(2), 133–145.

Lashgari, M., & Curry, S. (1995). Preferred methods of treating Bartholin's duct cyst. *Contemp Obstetrics & Gynecology, 40*, 38–42.

Le, T., Hicks, W., Menard, C., Hopkins, L., & Fung, M. F. (2006). Preliminary results of 5% imiquimod cream in the primary treatment of vulva intraepithelial neoplasia grade 2/3. *American Journal of Obstetrics and Gynecology, 194*(2), 377–380.

Lee, K. S., Park, K. H., Lee, S., Kim, J. Y., & Seo, S. S. (2005). Adenocarcinoma arising in a vaginal Müllerian cyst: A case report. *Gynecologic oncology, 99*(3), 767–769.

Leung, S., & Sexton, M. (1993). Radical radiation therapy for carcinoma of the vagina–impact of treatment modalities on outcome: Peter MacCallum Cancer Institute experience 1970–1990. *International Journal of Radiation Oncology, Biology, Physics, 25*(3), 413–418.

Li, C., Bian, D., Chen, W., Zhao, C., Yin, N., & Wang, Z. (2007). Evaluation of squamous hyperplasia and lichen sclerosus after focused ultrasound treatment. *Journal of Reproductive Medicine, 52*, 116.

López-Varela, E., Oliva, E., McIntyre, J. F., & Fuller, A. F. (2007). Primary treatment of Bartholin's gland carcinoma with radiation and chemoradiation: A report on ten consecutive cases. *International Journal of Gynecological Cancer: Official Journal of the International Gynecological Cancer Society, 17*(3), 661–667.

Lorenz, B., Kaufman, R. H., & Kutzner, S. K. (1998). Lichen sclerosus. Therapy with clobetasol propionate. *Journal of Reproductive Medicine, 43*(9), 790–794.

Lotery, H. E., & Galask, R. P. (2003). Erosive lichen planus of the vulva and vagina. *Obstetrics and Gynecology, 101*(5, Pt. 2), 1121–1125.

Lundqvist, E. N., & Bergdahl, J. (2005). Vestibulodynia (former vulvar vestibulitis): Personality in affected women. *Journal of Psychosomatic Obstetrics and Ggynecology, 26*(4), 251–256.

Lynch, P. J., & Micheletti, L. (2006). The demise of dystrophy: A history of the evolving terminology. *CME Journal of Gynecologic Oncology, 10*, 142–146.

Lynch, P. J., Moyal-Barrocco, M., Bogliatto, F., Micheletti, L., & Scurry, J. (2007). ISSVD classification of vulvar dermatoses: Pathologic subsets and their clinical correlates. *Journal of Reproductive Medicine, 1*, 3–9.

Lynch, P. J. Moyal-Barracco, M., Scurry, J., & Stockdale, C. (2016). *Journal of Lower Genit Tract Disorders, 16*(4), 339–344. Retrieved from http://3b64we1rtwev2ibv6q12s4dd.wpengine.netdna-cdn.com/wp-content/uploads/2016/03/CURRENT-ISSVD-TERMINOLOGY-AND-CLASSIFICATION-OF-VULVAR-DISEASES_CLINICAL-DIAGNOSIS.pdf

MacLean, A. B., Makwana, M., Ellis, P. E., & Cunnington, F. (2004). The management of Paget's disease of the vulva. *Journal of Obstetrics and Gynaecology: The Journal of the Institute of Obstetrics and Gynaecology, 24*(2), 124–128.

Madeleine, M. M., Daling, J. R., Carter, J. J., Wipf, G. C., Schwartz, S. M., McKnight, B.,…Galloway, D. A. (1997). Cofactors with human papillomavirus in a population-based study of vulvar cancer. *Journal of the National Cancer Institute, 89*(20), 1516–1523.

Maher, C., & Baessler, K. (2006). Surgical management of posterior vaginal wall prolapse: An evidence-based literature review. *International Urogynecology Journal and Pelvic Floor Dysfunction, 17*(1), 84–88.

Manetta, A., Gutrecht, E. L., Berman, M. L., & DiSaia, P. J. (1990). Primary invasive carcinoma of the vagina. *Obstetrics and Gynecology, 76*(4), 639–642.

Marchesseau-Merlin, A. S., Perea, R., Kanold, J., Demeocq, F., Souteyrand, P., & D'Incan, M. (2008). Photopheresis: An alternative therapeutic approach in corticoresistant erosive oral lichen planus. *Annales de Dermatologie et de Vénéréologie, 135*(3), 209–212.

Mateus, C., Fortier-Beaulieu, M., Lhomme, C., Rochard, F., Castaigne, D., Duvillard, P., & Avril, M. F. (2001). Basal cell carcinoma of the vulva: 21 cases. *Annales de dermatologie et de vénéréologie, 128*(1), 11–15.

McCluggage, W. G., Price, J. H., & Dobbs, S. P. (2001). Primary adenocarcinoma of the vagina arising in endocervicosis. *International Journal of Gynecological Pathology: Official Journal of the International Society of Gynecological Pathologists, 20*(4), 399–402.

McNall, R. Y., Nowicki, P. D., Miller, B., Billups, C. A., Liu, T., & Daw, N. C. (2004). Adenocarcinoma of the cervix and vagina in pediatric patients. *Pediatric Blood & Cancer, 43*(3), 289–294.

Monnerie-Lachaud, V., Pages, S., Guillot, E., & Veyret, C. (2001). [Contribution of pelvic floor MRI in the morphological and functional analysis of pre- and postoperative levator muscle in patients with genital prolapse]. *Journal de Gynécologie, Obstétrique et biologie de la reproduction, 30*(8), 753–760.

Moreno-Arias, G. A., Conill, C., Sola-Casas, M. A., Mascaro-Galy, J. M., & Grimalt, R. (2003). Radiotherapy for in situ extramammary Paget disease of the vulva. *Journal of Dermatological Treatment, 14*(2), 119–123.

Mostwin, J. L., Genadry, R., Sanders, R., & Yang, A. (1996). Anatomic goals in the correction of female stress urinary incontinence. *Journal of Endourology/Endourological Society, 10*(3), 207–212.

Moyal-Barracco, M., & Lynch, P. J. (2004). 2003 ISSVD terminology and classification of vulvodynia: A historical perspective. *Journal of Reproductive Medicine, 49*(10), 772–777.

Muir, T. W., Aspera, A. M., Rackley, R. R., & Walters, M. D. (2004). Recurrent pelvic organ prolapse in a woman with bladder exstrophy: A case report of surgical management and review of the literature. *International Urogynecology Journal and Pelvic Floor Dysfunction, 15*(6), 436–438.

Mulvany, N. J., Rayoo, M., & Allen, D. G. (2012). Basal cell carcinoma of the vulva: A case series. *Pathology, 44*(6), 528–533.

Munoz, N., Kjaer, S. K., Sigurdsson, K., Iversen, O. E., Hernandez-Avila, M., Wheeler, C. M.,…Haupt, R. M. (2010). Impact of human papilloma-virus (HPV)-6/11/16/18 vaccine on all HPV-associated genital diseases in young women. *Journal of National Cancer Institute, 102*, 325–339.

Murta, E. F., Neves Junior, M. A., Sempionato, L. R., Costa, M. C., & Maluf, P. J. (2005). Vaginal intraepithelial neoplasia: Clinical-therapeutic analysis of 33 cases. *Archives of Gynecology and Obstetrics, 272*(4), 261–264.

Nazir, Z., Rizvi, R. M., Qureshi, R. N., Khan, Z. S., & Khan, Z. (2006). Congenital vaginal obstructions: Varied presentation and outcome. *Pediatric Surgery International, 22*(9), 749–753.

Netter, F. (2006). *Atlas of human anatomy* (4th ed.). Philadelphia, PA: Rittenhouse Book Distributors Inc.

Nomoto, K., Hori, T., Kiya, C., Fukuoka, J., Nakashima, A., Hidaka, T.,...Takano, Y. (2010). Endometrioid adenocarcinoma of the vagina with a microglandular pattern arising from endometriosis after hysterectomy. *Pathology International, 60*(9), 636–641.

Oppelt, P., Renner, S. P., Kellermann, A., Brucker, S., Hauser, G. A., Ludwig, K. S.,...Beckmann, M. W. (2006). Clinical aspects of Mayer-Rokitansky-Kuester-Hauser syndrome: Recommendations for clinical diagnosis and staging. *Human Reproduction, 21*(3), 792–797.

Pagano, R. (2007). Value of colposcopy in the diagnosis of candidiasis in patients with vulvodynia. *Journal of Reproductive Medicine, 52*(1), 31–34.

Pai, K., Pai, S., Gupta, A., Rao, P., & Renjhen, P. (2006). Synchronous vulvar intraepithelial neoplasia (VIN) of warty type and cervical intraepithelial neoplasia (CIN): Case report. *Indian Journal of Pathology & Microbiology, 49*(4), 585–587.

Palefsky, J. M., Giuliano, A. R., Goldstone, S., Moreira, E. D., Aranda, C., Jessen, H.,...Garner, E. I. (2011). HPV vaccine against anal HPV infection and anal intraepithelial neoplasia. *New England Journal of Medicine, 365*(17), 1576–1585.

Paul, J., Foss, C. E., Hirano, S. A., Cunningham, T. D., & Pariser, D. M. (2013). An open-label pilot study of Apremilast for the treatment of moderate to severe lichen planus: A case series. *Journal of the American Academy of Dermatology, 68*(2), 255–261.

Penna, C., Fallani, M. G., Fambrini, M., Zipoli, E., & Marchionni, M. (2002). CO_2 laser surgery for vulvar intraepithelial neoplasia. Excisional, destructive and combined techniques. *Journal of Reproductive Medicine, 47*(11), 913–918.

Peters, K., Girdler, B., Carrico, D., Ibrahim, I., & Diokno, A. (2008). Painful bladder syndrome/interstitial cystitis and vulvodynia: A clinical correlation. *International Urogynecology Journal and Pelvic Floor Dysfunction, 19*(5), 665–669.

Peters, W. A., Kumar, N. B., & Morley, G. W. (1985). Carcinoma of the vagina. Factors influencing treatment outcome. *Cancer, 55*(4), 892–897.

Petersen, C. D., Kristensen, E., Lundvall, L., & Giraldi, A. (2009). A retrospective study of relevant diagnostic procedures in vulvodynia. *Journal of Reproductive Medicine, 54*(5), 281–287.

Pisani, C., Poggiali, S., De Padova, L., Andreassi, A., & Bilenchi, R. (2006). Basal cell carcinoma of the vulva. *Journal of the European Academy of Dermatology and Venereology, 20*(4), 446–448.

Pit, M. J., De Ruiter, M. C., Lycklama A Nijeholt, A. A., Marani, E., & Zwartendijk, J. (2003). Anatomy of the arcus tendineus fasciae pelvis in females. *Clinical Anatomy, 16*(2), 131–137.

Rader, J. S., Leake, J. F., Dillon, M. B., & Rosenshein, N. B. (1991). Ultrasonic surgical aspiration in the treatment of vulvar disease. *Obstetrics and Gynecology, 77*(4), 573–576.

Reed, B. D., Caron, A. M., Gorenflo, D. W., & Haefner, H. K. (2006). Treatment of vulvodynia with tricyclic antidepressants: Efficacy and associated factors. *Journal of Lower Genital Tract Disease, 10*(4), 245–251.

Reed, B. D., Haefner, H. K., Sen, A., & Gorenflo, D. W. (2008). Vulvodynia incidence and remission rates among adult women: A 2-year follow-up study. *Obstetrics and Gynecology, 112*(2, Pt. 1), 231–237.

Ries, L. A. G., Melbert, D., Krapcho, M., Stinchcomb, D. G., Howlader, N., Horner, M. J., ... Edwards, B. K. (Eds.). (2008). *SEER cancer statistics review, 1975–2005.* Bethesda, MD: National Cancer Institute.

Rimoin, L. P., Kwatra, S. G., & Yosipovitch, G. (2013). Female-specific pruritus from childhood to postmenopause: Clinical features, hormonal factors, and treatment considerations. *Dermatologic Therapy, 26*(2), 157–167.

Robinson, J. B., Sun, C. C., Bodurka-Bevers, D., Im, D. D., & Rosenshein, N. B. (2000). Cavitational ultrasonic surgical aspiration for the treatment of vaginal intraepithelial neoplasia. *Gynecologic Oncology, 78*(2), 235–241.

Saraiya, M., Watson, M., Wu, X., King, J. B., Chen, V. W., Smith, J. S., & Giuliano, A. R. (2008). Incidence of in situ and invasive vulvar cancer in the U.S., 1998–2003. *Cancer, 113*(Suppl. 10), 2865–2872.

Schockaert, S., Poppe, W., Arbyn, M., Verguts, T., & Verguts, J. (2008). Incidence of vaginal intraepithelial neoplasia after hysterectomy for cervical intraepithelial neoplasia: A retrospective study. *American Journal of Obstetrics and Gynecology, 199*(2), 113.e1–113.e5.

Schutt, A. K., Barrett, M. R., Trotta, B. M., & Stovall, D. W. (2012). Perioperative evaluation in Herlyn-Werner-Wunderlich syndrome. *Obstetrics & Gynecology, 120*(4), 948–951.

Secor, R. M. C., & Fantasia, H. C. (2012). *Fast facts about the gynecologic exam for nurse practitioners.* New York, NY: Springer Publishing.

Seifried, S., Haydu, L. E., Quinn, M. J., Scolyer, R. A., Stretch, J. R., & Thompson, J. F. (2014). Melanoma of the vulva and vagina: Principles of staging and their relevance to management based on a clinicopathologic analysis of 85 cases. *Annals of Surgical Oncology, 22*(6), 1959–1966.

Shah, C. A., Goff, B. A., Lowe, K., Peters, W. A., & Li, C. I. (2009). Factors affecting risk of mortality in women with vaginal cancer. *Obstetrics and Gynecology, 113*(5), 1038–1045.

Sideri, M., Jones, R. W., Wilkinson, E. J., Preti, M., Heller, D. S., Scurry, J., ...Neill, S. (2005). Squamous vulvar intraepithelial neoplasia: 2004 modified terminology, ISSVD Vulvar Oncology Subcommittee. *Journal of Reproductive Medicine, 50*(11), 807–810.

Siegel, R., Ma, J., Zou, Z., & Jemal, A. (2014). Cancer statistics, 2014. *CA: A Cancer Journal for Clinicians, 64*(1), 9–29.

Smith, J. S., Backes, D. M., Hoots, B. E., Kurman, R. J., & Pimenta, J. M. (2009). Human papillomavirus type-distribution in vulvar and vaginal cancers and their associated precursors. *Obstetrics and Gynecology, 113*(4), 917–924.

Standring, S. (Ed.). (2008). *Gray's anatomy: The anatomical basis of clinical practice* (40th ed.). Philadelphia, PA: Churchill Livingstone.

Stenchever, M. A., Droegmueller, W., Herbst, A. L., & Mischell, D. (2007). *Comprehensive gynecology* (5th ed.). St. Louis, MO: Mosby.

Stockdale, C. K., & Lawson, H. W. (2014). 2013 vulvodynia guideline update. *Journal of Lower Genital Tract Disease, 18*(2), 93–100.

Suda, T., & Kakinuma, H. (2006). Erosive velvety lesion on the vulva–vulvar basal cell carcinoma. *Archives of Dermatology, 142*(3), 385–390.

Sugase, M., & Matsukura, T. (1997). Distinct manifestations of human papillomaviruses in the vagina. *International Journal of Cancer, 72*(3), 412–415.

Tantipalakorn, C., Robertson, G., Marsden, D. E., Gebski, V., & Hacker, N. F. (2009). Outcome and patterns of recurrence for International Federation of Gynecology and Obstetrics (FIGO) stages I and II squamous cell vulvar cancer. *Obstetrics and Gynecology, 113*(4), 895–901.

Tebes, S., Cardosi, R., & Hoffman, M. (2002). Paget's disease of the vulva. *American Journal of Obstetrics and Gynecology, 187*(2), 281–283; discussion 283.

Thomas, S. S., Chenoy, R., Fielding, J. W., Rollason, T. P., Jordan, J. A., & Bracka, A. (1996). Vulvoperineal reconstruction after excision of anogenital multifocal intraepithelial neoplasia ("MIN"). *British Journal of Plastic Surgery, 49*(8), 539–546.

Thompson, M. A., Adelson, M. D., Jozefczyk, M. A., Coble, D. A., & Kaufman, L. M. (1991). Structural and functional integrity of ovarian tumor tissue obtained by ultrasonic aspiration. *Cancer, 67*(5), 1326–1331.

Thurman, A. S., Satterfoeld, T. M., & Soper, D. E. (2008). Methicillin-resistant *Staphylococcus aureus* as a common cause of vulvar abscesses. *Obstetrics and Gynecology, 112*, 538–544.

Tiengo, C., Deluca, J., Belloni-Fortina, A., Salmaso, R., Galifi, F., & Alaibac, M. (2012). Occurrence of squamous cell carcinoma in an area of lichen simplex chronicus: Case report and pathogenetic hypothesis. *Journal of Cutaneous Medicine and Surgery, 16*(5), 350–352.

Tjalma, W., & Colpaert, C. (2006). Primary vaginal adenocarcinoma of intestinal type arising from a tubulovillous adenoma. *International Journal of Gynecological Cancer, 16*(3), 1461–1465.

Toki, T., Kurman, R. J., Park, J. S., Kessis, T., Daniel, R. W., & Shah, K. V. (1991). Probable nonpapillomavirus etiology of squamous cell carcinoma of the vulva in older women: A clinicopathologic study using in situ hybridization and polymerase chain reaction. *International Journal of Gynecological Pathology: Official Journal of the International Society of Gynecological Pathologists, 10*(2), 107–125.

Tunitsky, E., Goldman, H. B., & Ridgeway, B. (2012). Periurethral mass: A rare and puzzling entity. *Journal of Obstetrics & Gynecology, 120*(6), 1459–1464.

Ulutin, H. C., Zellars, R. C., & Frassica, D. (2003). Soft tissue sarcoma of the vulva: A clinical study. *International Journal of Gynecological Cancer: Official Journal of the International Gynecological Cancer Society, 13*(4), 528–531.

Valdivielso-Ramos, M., Bueno, C., & Hernanz, J. M. (2008). Significant improvement in extensive lichen sclerosus with tacrolimus ointment and PUVA. *American Journal of Clinical Dermatology, 9*(3), 175–179.

van Seters, M., Beckmann, I., Heijmans-Antonissen, C., van Beurden, M., Ewing, P. C., Zijlstra, F. J.,...KleinJan, A. (2008). Disturbed patterns of immunocompetent cells in usual-type vulvar intraepithelial neoplasia. *Cancer Research, 68*(16), 6617–6622.

van Seters, M., van Beurden, M., ten Kate, F. J. W., Ewing, P. C., Kagie, M. J., Meijer, C. J. M.,... Helmerhorst, T. J. M. (2007). Effectiveness of imiquimod 5% cream in women with high grade vulvar intraepithelial neoplasia: Final results of a randomized, controlled trial. *Journal of Reproductive Medicine, 52*, 137. Abstract.

van Seters, M., van Beurden, M., ten Kate, F. J., Beckmann, I., Ewing, P. C., Eijkemans, M. J.,...Helmerhorst, T. J. (2008). Treatment of vulvar intraepithelial neoplasia with topical imiquimod. *New England Journal of Medicine, 358*(14), 1465–1473.

Verschraegen, C. F., Benjapibal, M., Supakarapongkul, W., Levy, L. B., Ross, M., Atkinson, E. N.,...Legha, S. S. (2001). Vulvar melanoma at the M. D. Anderson Cancer Center: 25 years later. *International Journal of Gynecological Cancer: Official Journal of the International Gynecological Cancer Society, 11*(5), 359–364.

Villa, L. L., Costa, R. L., Petta, C. A., Andrade, R. P., Ault, K. A., Giuliano, A. R.,...Barr, E. (2005). Prophylactic quadrivalent human papillomavirus (types 6, 11, 16, and 18) L1 virus-like particle vaccine in young women: A randomised double-blind placebo-controlled multicentre phase II efficacy trial. *The Lancet. Oncology, 6*(5), 271–278.

Virgili, A., Lauriola, M. M., Mantovani, L., & Corazza, M. (2007). Vulvar lichen sclerosus: 11 women treated with tacrolimus 0.1% ointment. *Acta Dermato-Venereologica, 87*(1), 69–72.

Voet, R. L. (1994). Classification of vulvar dystrophies and premalignant squamous lesions. *Journal of Cutaneous Pathology, 21*(1), 86–90.

Wechter, M. E., Gruber, S. B., Haefner, H. K., Lowe, L., Schwartz, J. L., Reynolds, K. R.,...Johnson, T. M. (2004). Vulvar melanoma: A report of 20 cases and review of the literature. *Journal of the American Academy of Dermatology, 50*(4), 554–562.

Wechter, M. E., Wu, J. M., Marzano, D., & Haefner, H. (2009). Management of Bartholin duct cysts and abscesses: A systematic review. *Obstetrical & Gynecological Survey, 64*(6), 395–404.

Welsh, B. M., Berzins, K. N., Cook, K. A., & Fairley, C. K. (2003). Management of common vulval conditions. *The Medical Journal of Australia, 178*(8), 391–395.

Wilkinson, E. J., Cox, J. T., Selim, M. A., & O'Connor, D. M. (2015). Evolution of terminology for human-papillomavirus-infection-related vulvar squamous intraepithelial lesions. *Journal of Lower Genital Tract Disease, 19*(1), 81–87.

Wilson, S. F. (2005). *Health assessment for nursing practice* (3rd ed.). St. Louis, MO: Elsevier.

Woelber, L., Mahner, S., Voelker, K., Eulenburg, C. Z., Gieseking, F., Choschzick, M.,...Schwarz, J. (2009). Clinicopathological prognostic factors and patterns of recurrence in vulvar cancer. *Anticancer Research, 29*(2), 545–552.

Woodruff, J. D. (1991). Carcinoma in situ of the vulva. *Clinical Obstetrics and Gynecology, 34*(3), 669–676.

Word, B. (1968). Office treatment of cyst and abscess of Bartholin's gland duct. *Southern Medical Journal, 61*(5), 514–518.

Wu, X., Matanoski, G., Chen, V. W., Saraiya, M., Coughlin, S. S., King, J. B., & Tao, X. G. (2008). Descriptive epidemiology of vaginal cancer incidence and survival by race, ethnicity, and age in the United States. *Cancer, 113*(Suppl. 10), 2873–2882.

Zeligs, K. P., Byrd, K., Tarney, C. M., Howard, R. S., Sims, B. D., Hamilton, C. A., & Stany, M. P. (2013). A clinicopathologic study of vaginal intraepithelial neoplasia. *Obstetrics & Gynecology, 122*(6), 1223–1230.

Zoulek, E., Karp, D. R., & Davila, G. W. (2011). Rectovaginal fistula as a complication to a Bartholin gland excision. *Obstetrics & Gynecology, 118*(2, Pt. 2), 489–491.

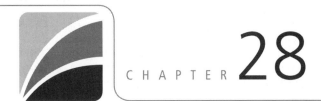

CHAPTER 28

Perimenstrual and Pelvic Symptoms and Syndromes

Candy Wilson • Regina A. McClure • Elizabeth A. Kostas-Polston

Menstruation has a symbolic meaning within all cultures. Attitudes and beliefs about menstruation are culturally defined and typically handed down from mother to daughter. It is postulated that milestones experienced by women, such as menarche, pregnancy, and menopause, contribute to bodily based experiences that bring women in closer contact with the realities about their body to develop a language for talking about any illness (Charteris-Black & Seale, 2010). Socialization about menstruation contributes to individual appraisal of perimenstrual symptoms.

Well-woman examinations provide an excellent opportunity for health care providers to educate women about normal hormonal changes and remedies to ameliorate symptoms within the normal expectation. However, for some women, the hormonal changes associated with menstruation or uterine structural abnormalities bring extreme pain, emotional changes, and/or excessive blood loss that negatively influence their lives. This chapter provides an overview of the etiology, symptoms, evaluation, and management of abnormal uterine bleeding (AUB), amenorrhea, premenstrual syndrome, menstrual headaches, and dysmenorrhea.

■ FEDERATION OF GYNECOLOGY AND OBSTETRICS NOMENCLATURE AND PALM-COEIN CLASSIFICATION SYSTEM

In April 2011, the International Federation of Gynecology and Obstetrics (FIGO) published an international consensus report and new FIGO nomenclature and PALM-COEIN classification systems for abnormalities of menstrual bleeding (Munro, Critchley, Broder, & Fraser, 2011). These new recommendations came about for a variety of reasons. For example, experts felt that the old FIGO nomenclature (e.g., dysfunctional uterine bleeding, menorrhagia, menometrorrhagia, metrorrhagia, oligomenorrhea) was not useful in helping clinicians delineate etiology and clinical management. Furthermore, terms were poorly defined and used inconsistently among health care providers in the United States and abroad. Regarding classification, experts determined that there existed a wide spectrum of potential causes of abnormal menstrual bleeding and that a new classification system would lend itself to greater clinical and scientific utility (Madhra, Fraser, Munro, & Critchley, 2014). For example, if a woman was diagnosed with endometrial hyperplasia and ovulation dysfunction with no other abnormalities, she would be categorized as AUB $P_0 A_0 L_0 M_1$-$C_0 O_1 E_0 I_0 N_0$. Recognizing that the full notation might be cumbersome, the full notation can be abbreviated: AUB – M;O (American College of Obstetricians and Gynecologists [ACOG], 2012). Although the new FIGO nomenclature and PALM-COEIN classification systems were announced in 2011, many health care providers continue to use the old terminology. This chapter introduces and utilizes the new nomenclature and classification system (Figure 28.1).

■ MENSTRUAL CYCLE

In order to address abnormal perimenstrual conditions, it is important to first understand the normal menstrual physiology. Normal cyclic uterine bleeding is dependent on the complex interaction among the hypothalamus, the anterior lobe of the pituitary gland, and the ovaries. Increasing estrogen levels secreted by the follicles within the ovaries result in proliferation of the endometrium. Following ovulation, the corpus luteum continues to produce estrogen, but more importantly, the corpus luteum becomes the source of progesterone. Together these hormones stabilize the endometrium and prepare it for implantation of a blastocyst, should fertilization occur. If fertilization and implantation do not occur, the corpus luteum degenerates and the resulting drop in hormone levels lead to withdrawal bleeding. An intact coagulation pathway is also important in the regulation of normal menstruation. For example, deficiency of platelets or abnormal platelet function can result in profound changes in the menstrual cycle (e.g., heavy bleeding of longer duration). Usual menstrual flow begins every 24 to 38 days with regularity (cycle-to-cycle variation 2–20 days)

FIGURE 28.1

PALM-COEIN abnormal uterine bleeding classification.

Adapted from Munro, Critchley, Broder, and Fraser (2011).

and lasts 4 to 8 days. The average volume of menstrual blood loss is approximately 5 to 80 mL (Fritz & Speroff, 2011; Hartmann et al., 2013). A structural menstrual history aids in the assessment of the patient.

■ ABNORMAL UTERINE BLEEDING

Definition and Scope

ACOG has defined AUB as bleeding that occurs from the uterine corpus that is abnormal in regularity, volume, frequency, or duration, and occurs in the absence of pregnancy (ACOG, 2000/2013/2015). AUB is any bleeding disturbance that occurs between menstrual periods, excessive and/or prolonged (Black, Moore, & Fraser, 2013). Altered menstrual patterns or volume of menses blood flow are some of the greatest concerns for premenopausal women seeking health care and severely affect physical and mental quality of life (Lobo, 2012; Matteson, Raker, Clark, & Frick, 2013). It is estimated that 56.2 million nonpregnant women between the ages of 18 and 50 years annually seek health care for AUB (Matteson et al., 2013). Approximately 20% to 30% of women will experience AUB during their reproductive years and a significant number will require emergent care (Matteson, Raker, Pinto, Scott, & Frishman, 2012). AUB can cause illness burden that negatively influences quality of life, work productivity, and finances (Matteson et al., 2013). AUB may be acute or chronic and associated with heavy menstrual bleeding (HMB) or intermenstrual bleeding (IMB; ACOG, 2000/2013/2015; see Table 28.1).

HEAVY MENSTRUAL BLEEDING

HMB is the most common complaint of AUB (Singh et al., 2013) and is designated by the acronym AUB/HMB. Clinical

TABLE 28.1	Issues Affecting QOL in Women With AUB
ISSUE	**DESCRIPTION OF THE ISSUE**
Irritation and inconvenience	Related irritation and inconvenience of unscheduled and/or heavy bleeding episodes.
Bleeding-associated pain	Affected by severe cramping pain during heavy bleeding episodes.
Self-conscious about odor	Concerned that other people could be offended by perceived odor during menstrual bleeding.
Social embarrassment	Embarrassing episodes involving staining clothing and/or furniture because of heavy flow of blood clots and/or unpredictable menstrual bleeding.
Ritual-like behavior	Described routines and practices aimed at avoiding all circumstances where she could find herself in an embarrassing situation where clothes could be stained in a public: ■ Carry hygiene products at all times. ■ Try to anticipate/predict bleeding episode. ■ Avoid social activities. ■ Schedule activities according to availability and proximity to bathroom.

AUB, abnormal uterine bleeding; QOL, quality of life.
Adapted from Matteson, Munro, and Fraser (2011).

definitions of HMB include the psychosocial aspect. HMB is defined as excessive menstrual blood loss, which interferes with a women's physical, emotional, social, and quality of life (QOL; National Institute for Health and Care Excellence [NICE], 2007).

Chronic HMB (formally known as *menorrhagia*) is defined as AUB that has occurred for 6 months, as compared with acute, which is defined as an episode of bleeding that can be emergent requiring immediate intervention to prevent excessive blood loss. Intermenstrual bleeding (formally known as *metrorrhagia*) is defined as bleeding that randomly occurs between defined predictable menstrual patterns (Munro, Critchley, Broder, et al., 2011). Terminology previously used to describe AUB was based on Greek and Latin words, leading to ambiguity in meaning and usage. Therefore, women's health experts recommended changing the terminology.

INTERMENSTRUAL BLEEDING

IMB refers to AUB that occurs at any time during the menstrual cycle other than during normal menstruation. According to the FIGO nomenclature, IMB is designated by the acronym AUB/IMB. It is oftentimes difficult to differentiate IMB from irregular, frequent periods. Similar to AUB/HMB, AUB/IMB is a symptom, not a diagnosis, and warrants follow-up evaluation (Table 28.2).

TABLE 28.2	Symptoms of AUB	
CHARACTERISTIC	**TERMINOLOGY (ABBREVIATION)**	**DESCRIPTION**
Disturbances of heaviness of flow	Heavy menstrual bleeding (HMB)	Excessive menstrual blood loss, which interferes with women's physical, emotional, social, and material QOL, and which can occur alone or in combination with other symptoms
	Heavy and prolonged menstrual bleeding (HPMB)	Less common and is important to make a distinction from HMB as may have different etiologies and respond to different therapies
	Light menstrual bleeding	Based on woman's complaint
Disturbances of regularity (normal variation +2 to 20 days)	Irregular menstrual bleeding (IrregMB)	A range of varying lengths of bleeding-free intervals exceeding 20 days within one 90-day reference period
	Absent menstrual bleeding (amenorrhea)	No bleeding in a 90-day period
Disturbances of frequency (normal every 24–38 days)	Infrequent menstrual bleeding	Bleeding at intervals > 38 days apart (1–2 episodes in a 90-day period)
	Frequent menstrual bleeding	Bleeding at intervals < 24 days apart (more than 4 episodes in a 90-day period)
Disturbance of duration of flow (normal 3–8 days)	Prolonged menstrual bleeding	Describes menstrual blood loss, which exceeds 8 days in duration
	Shortened menstrual bleeding	Menstrual bleeding less than 3 days in duration
Irregular, nonmenstrual bleeding	Intermenstrual bleeding (IMB)	Irregular episodes of bleeding, often light and short, occurring between otherwise fairly normal menstrual periods
	Postcoital	Bleeding postintercourse
	Premenstrual and postmenstrual spotting	Bleeding that may occur on a regular basis for 1 or more days before or after the recognized menstrual period
Bleeding outside reproductive age	Postmenopausal bleeding (PMB)	Bleeding occurring more than 1 year after the acknowledged menopause
	Precocious menstruation	Bleeding occurring before 9 years of age
Acute AUB	Acute AUB	An episode of bleeding in a reproductive-aged woman, who is not pregnant, that is of sufficient quantity to require immediate intervention to prevent further blood loss
Chronic AUB	Chronic AUB	Bleeding that is abnormal in duration, volume, and/or frequency and has been present for most of the past 6 months

AUB, abnormal uterine bleeding; QOL, quality of life.
Adapted from Singh et al. (2013).

ETIOLOGY AND COMPONENTS OF PALM-COEIN CLASSIFICATION SYSTEM

Menstrual bleeding that causes a woman to alter her lifestyle or causes anxiety warrants a thorough history, assessment, and physical evaluation to determine the etiology and any indicated intervention(s) (ACOG, 2012; Singh et al., 2013). Pregnancy is the primary reason for AUB. Health care providers should consider gynecologic structural defects or systemic sources as possible causes of AUB, once pregnancy has been ruled out. FIGO developed a classification system that delineates the nine categories that cause AUB (Munro, Critchley, & Fraser, 2011). This classification is known by the acronym PALM-COEIN: Polyp (AUB-P), Adenomyosis (AUB-A), Leiomyoma (AUB-L), Malignancy and Hyperplasia (AUB-M), making up the PALM portion of the acronym; and Coagulopathy (AUB-C), Ovulatory disorders (AUB-O), Endometrial (AUB-E), Iatrogenic (AUB-I), and Not yet classified (AUB-N), making up the COEIN portion of the acronym. PALM describes structural causes that can be identified

by visualization and/or histopathology. COEIN describes sources that are not defined by imaging or histopathology (Figure 28.1).

Polyps (AUB-P) • Polyps are hyperplastic overgrowths of endometrial glands and stroma that project from the surface of the endometrium and are usually found by ultrasound (U/S; usually saline infusion ultrasonography) and/or hysteroscopic examination (with or without histopathology; Munro, Critchley, & Fraser, 2011). Endometrial polyps are a source for AUB, IMB, or postmenopausal bleeding. Polyps can also contribute to fertility issues or pregnancy complications. Furthermore, up to 35% of women with polyps do not experience AUB. In these cases, polyps are usually discovered incidentally. For women with symptoms, the symptoms do not necessarily correlate with the size, location, and/or number of polyps present (Salim, Won, Nesbitt-Hawes, Campbell, & Abbott, 2011; Smith & Netter, 2008). Premenopausal women with AUB and polyps are less likely to be diagnosed with an endometrial neoplasia as compared with menopausal women with polyps (Lee, Kaunitz, Sanchez-Ramos, & Rhatigan, 2010). It is thought that polyps produce local inflammation, which in turn contributes to AUB and infertility (El-Hamarneh et al., 2013; Lieng et al., 2010). Though the exact cause remains unknown, genetic factors may contribute to the development of endometrial polyps. Risk factors for the development of endometrial polyps include age, hypertension, obesity, and Tamoxifen use. Conflicting evidence exists as to whether increased estrogen and progesterone receptor concentrations contribute to the development of polyps. Polyps less than 1 cm often regress in size within a year, as compared with polyps that are 1.5 cm or greater. Polyp regression may be associated with isolated events of HMB and cramping, followed by the resumption of normal menstruation (Salim et al., 2011).

Adenomyosis (AUB-A) • Adenomyosis is a benign condition of the uterus and is defined by the presence of endometrial glands and stroma within the myometrium (Naftalin et al., 2014). About 1% to 15% of premenopausal women have adenomyosis (Black et al., 2013; Smith & Netter, 2008). The typical patient is a parous woman in her 40s (Black et al., 2013). The pathophysiologic connection between adenomyosis and AUB remains unclear (Fritz & Speroff, 2011; Munro, Critchley, & Fraser, 2011). Women with adenomyosis are most likely to experience AUB and dysmenorrhea. Furthermore, adenomyosis and leiomyomas often coexist (Black et al., 2013).

Leiomyomas (AUB-L) • Uterine leiomyomas (fibroids) are benign neoplasms that develop from uterine smooth muscle and can grow into enlarged pelvic masses that cause AUB and pelvic pain (Fritz & Speroff, 2011). Age is the most common risk factor, with a lifetime risk in women older than 45 years being more than 60%. Leiomyomas are located on the uterus or cervix and any number of fibroids can be present at one time. The size and site affects the symptoms experienced. There are three types of fibroids based on location: intramural, serosal, and submucosal. The most common fibroid, intramural, develops within the myometrium. Serosal fibroids arise from the external surface of the uterus. Submucosal fibroids develop near the inner surface of the endometrium and are likely to cause HMB and infertility (Black et al., 2013).

The etiology of fibroids is unknown, but several correlates have been identified including: African or Caribbean ethnicity, overweight, nulliparous, polycystic ovary syndrome (PCOS), diabetes, hypertension, and a family history of fibroids (Black et al., 2013). Hormone levels associated with pregnancy promote fibroid growth, whereas during menopause, when hormone levels decrease fibroids tend to shrink. Fibroids can also undergo pathological changes including hyaline degeneration, cystic degeneration, calcification, infection (abscess formation), and necrobiosis. Most leiomyomas are asymptomatic and less than 1% are leiosarcomas (cancerous; Fritz & Speroff, 2011).

Malignancy and Premalignant Conditions (AUB-M) • AUB-M includes both premalignant and malignant lesions. Atypical hyperplasia and malignancy are relatively uncommon in premenopausal women (Munro et al., 2011). AUB is the *primary* symptom of endometrial neoplasia. Risk factors for atypical hyperplasia or endometrial cancer include advanced age, nulliparity with a history of infertility, obesity, polycystic ovaries, a family history of endometrial or colon cancer, and/or a history of Tamoxifen use (Fox, 2012).

Coagulopathy (AUB-C; Systemic Disorders of Hemostasis) • Coagulopathy is defined as a spectrum of systemic hematologic disorders that impede the blood's ability to coagulate, potentially triggering AUB (Munro, 2011). Although the relationship between coagulopathy and AUB is unclear, platelet dysfunctions, rare clotting factor deficiencies, and/or low platelets are commonly associated with AUB (Black et al., 2013; Munro, Critchley, Broder, et al., 2011). One example of a coagulopathy that causes AUB is von Willebrand disease. Von Willebrand disease is a genetic hemorrhagic disorder caused by a missing or defective clotting protein (von Willebrand factor), which leads to impaired primary hemostasis. Approximately 13% of women who present with complaints of extended and extensive vaginal bleeding (AUB) will be diagnosed with von Willebrand disease (Munro & Lukes, 2005). When collecting a thorough structured patient history, health care providers have a high probability of diagnosing bleeding disorders (see Table 28.3).

Ovulatory Disorders (AUB-O) • Ovarian dysfunction (formerly classified as *dysfunctional uterine bleeding* [DUB]), produces a progesterone deficient/estrogen dominant state that produces an irregular, often infrequent, and unpredictable menstrual flow that ranges from absent or minimal to excessive (Sweet, Schmidt-Dalton, Weiss, & Madsen, 2012). Endocrine conditions (e.g., PCOS, uncontrolled diabetes mellitus, thyroid disorders, hyperprolactinemia) interfere with the hypothalamic–pituitary–ovarian (HPO) axis, and can lead to ovulatory dysfunction (ACOG, 2013; Munro, Critchley, Broder, et al., 2011; Sweet et al., 2012). In addition, AUB-O can result from mental stress, obesity, anorexia,

TABLE 28.3	Structured History to Screen for Coagulopathies (AUB-C) or Disorders of Systemic Hemostasis

1. Heavy menstrual bleeding since menarche?
2. One of the following:
   - ■ Postpartum hemorrhage?
   - ■ Surgical-related bleeding?
   - ■ Bleeding associated with dental work?
3. Two or more of the following symptoms:
   - ■ Bruising 1–2 times/month?
   - ■ Epistaxis 1–2 times/month?
   - ■ Frequent gum bleeding?
   - ■ Family history of bleeding symptoms?

Note: Consider coagulopathy testing for the following criteria: (a) heavy menstrual bleeding since menarche, (b) one item from Item 2, or (c) two or more items from Item 3.
Source: Munro et al. (2011).

weight loss, and/or extreme exercise (Munro, Critchley, Broder, et al., 2011). Gonadal steroids or drugs that affect dopamine metabolism, such as phenothiazines and tricyclic antidepressants, may contribute to anovulation by raising prolactin levels (Munro, Critchley, Broder, et al., 2011).

Endometrial Causes (AUB-E) • When a woman's ovaries are producing predictable and cyclic menstrual patterns, yet she is experiencing AUB, this is highly suggestive of an abnormality that resides in the endometrium (Munro, Critchley, Broder, et al., 2011). AUB originating in the endometrium is usually related to some combination of inflammatory disorders, infection, or disruptions of angiogenesis (Munro, Critchley, Broder, et al., 2011). At present, diagnostic tests are not available for detection of abnormalities related to endometrial homeostasis (Fox, 2012).

Iatrogenic (AUB-I) • Gynecologic and nongynecologic interventions can be the source of AUB-I. Iatrogenic causes include contraceptive use (e.g., intrauterine devices/systems, medroxyprogesterone injections, progestin-only birth control pills, etonogestrel implants), and treatment with exogenous gonadal steroids (e.g., estrogens, progestins, androgens) and systemic agents that affect blood coagulation or ovulation. Abnormal bleeding (unscheduled) after initiation of a contraceptive method containing gonadal steroids is not unusual for the first 3 to 6 months. Anticoagulants and tricyclic antidepressants can cause AUB-I.

Not Classified (AUB-N) • AUB-N is reserved for entities that are poorly defined and not well understood or studied (e.g., arteriovenous malformation [AVM], myometrial hypertrophy; Munro, Critchley, Broder, et al., 2011). Complications related to undiagnosed pregnancy, genital tract trauma, foreign bodies in the reproductive tract, and cigarette smoking are thought to be possible sources of AUB-N (Black et al., 2013).

Risk Factors

Many of the risk factors were discussed in the earlier section. Women with AUB are more likely to be younger, White, and obese than women without AUB (Matteson et al., 2013). The family history, particularly the history of a woman's mother or sister, can provide great insight into potential cause(s) for AUB.

Symptoms

ACOG has suggested that health care providers use the menstrual cycle differentiating between normal and abnormal menstrual bleeding (ACOG, 2015a). Abnormal bleeding patterns often precipitate a visit to a health care provider's office for evaluation and work-up. Symptoms of abnormal bleeding may include: (a) bleeding heavier or for more days than normal, (b) soaking feminine hygiene products in 2 hours or less (often, but not always, *bleeding through* hygiene products onto clothing), (c) bleeding between periods, (d) bleeding after intercourse,

(e) spotting anytime in the menstrual cycle, and/or (f) bleeding after menopause (ACOG, 2012). Women who present with abnormal menstrual bleeding may also experience symptoms of anemia (e.g., pale skin, fatigue, shortness of breath, and headache; Lopez, Cacoub, Macdougall, & Peyrin-Biroulet, 2015), and/or symptoms of thyroid, pancreas, or pituitary disorders. In all cases, it is important to determine whether the abnormal menstrual bleeding is of clinical significance.

Evaluation/Assessment

Diagnosis of AUB requires a detailed history, thorough physical examination, appropriate laboratory tests, and diagnostic imaging. Determination of laboratory and diagnostic imaging should be individualized.

MEDICAL HISTORY

A woman's medical history is perhaps the single most important tool used when evaluating AUB. Detailed information regarding intermenstrual intervals, duration of bleeding, volume, and the onset of abnormal menstrual bleeding can provide essential clues about possible etiology and can help guide determination of diagnostic imaging. When collecting a woman's medical history, it is important to consider other factors (e.g., age, weight, previous menstrual patterns, and other medical problems). Predictable cyclic menses, even though heavy in nature, are generally associated with ovulation (Fritz & Speroff, 2011).

In contrast, ovarian dysfunctional bleeding is usually irregular and unpredictable, variable in amount and duration, and most often observed in adolescents and perimenopausal women as well as in obese women and those with PCOS. Regular cycles that are increasing in amount and/or duration of bleeding or chronic, AUB/IMB superimposed on regular cycling may be associated with uterine structural lesions such as polyps or myomas (Singh & Belland, 2015). The most common cause of a sudden departure from regular, predictable cycles is a complication of pregnancy (Fritz & Speroff, 2011). If a woman presents with AUB/HMB from menarche or gives a history of frequent epistaxis (bleeding gums with brushing of teeth), or past episodes of excessive bleeding from trauma or surgery, she should be suspect for a coagulation disorder (Table 28.3; Matteson, Munro, & Fraser, 2011). It is important to note that adolescents who present with a hemoglobin (Hgb) of less than 10 g/dL and/or require a blood transfusion have an increased risk (20%–30%) for a coagulopathy. Women with endometrial hyperplasia or adenocarcinoma often have a history of anovulation with long-term unopposed estrogen exposure. When obtaining a woman's medication history, it is important that the health care provider ask about prescription medications, over-the-counter (OTC) vitamins, and herbal remedies that may contribute to or cause AUB (e.g., warfarin, heparin, nonsteroidal anti-inflammatory drugs [NSAIDs], hormonal contraceptives, gingko, ginseng, motherwort; ACOG, 2012).

Blood loss greater than 60 to 80 mL per menstrual cycle is typically associated with anemia (ACOG, 2010; Fritz & Speroff, 2011). A woman's subjective assessment of her menstrual blood loss does not correlate with laboratory analysis for the diagnosis of anemia (Schumacher et al., 2012). The current recommendation for assessing the impact of AUB involves a two-part approach: a structured menstrual history and a symptoms impact element (Matteson et al., 2011; Table 28.4).

PHYSICAL EXAMINATION

A systematic approach to the physical examination is an important and necessary component of the initial assessment. Any time a woman presents complaining of significant vaginal bleeding, it is critical to evaluate her vital signs to establish whether immediate medical or surgical intervention is indicated. Acute AUB/HMB should be managed promptly (e.g., medication, blood transfusion) and systematically to minimize morbidity (Singh et al., 2013). If hemodynamically stable, the woman's medical history will inform her physical examination. A head-to-toe assessment is required to help determine the cause for and the effects of the AUB. For example, obesity, hirsutism, acne, and acanthosis nigricans of the neck may be signs of PCOS and metabolic syndrome; and a thyroid nodule may be a sign of thyroid disease. Additionally, bruising and petechia of the mucous membranes may be physical signs of a coagulopathy, such as von Willebrand disease or idiopathic thrombocytopenia. It is also very important for the health care provider to establish whether the AUB is uterine and not from another source(s) (e.g., gastrointestinal [GI], genitourinary tract [GU]). A speculum examination should be performed to assess for cervical and/or vaginal lesions (ACOG, 2012). Uterine size, shape, and consistency may indicate pregnancy as a source of AUB. A bimanual exam may be consistent with an enlarged uterus with irregular contours indicating the presence of uterine myomas, adenomyosis, or endometriosis, and the presence of uterine tenderness may indicate endometritis or pelvic inflammatory disease (PID).

Differential Diagnoses

Ovarian dysfunction is typically the source of AUB at the extremes of childbearing age groups (adolescents and perimenopausal women). Anovulatory menstrual patterns are sporadic in timing and volume and can be related to hormonal contraceptive use, pregnancy, and pelvic infection. Ovulatory patterns are usually predictable (within a few days) and typically increase in volume of blood loss over months or years. Ovulatory patterns of AUB include structural lesions and endometrial hyperplasia. The most common AUB differential diagnoses across a woman's life span are provided in Table 28.5.

Diagnostic Studies

LABORATORY TESTING

In reproductive-aged women, it is always important to rule out pregnancy as a possible cause of AUB, even if the patient has had a tubal ligation or denies sexual activity. Cervical cytology to evaluate for cervical neoplasia as well as cervical cultures to rule out sexually transmitted infections (STIs) may also be indicated. If the health care provider suspects thyroid disease, thyroid function tests should be obtained (Singh et al., 2013). Hypothyroidism is commonly associated with AUB (ACOG, 2012).

Along with a structured medical and family history uptake, a complete blood count and platelets are recommended to exclude anemia and thrombocytopenia. Furthermore, ACOG (2012) recommends testing for von Willebrand disease in all patients (particularly adolescents) with excessive bleeding without any apparent cause, or with any bleeding that does not respond to medical treatment. Von Willebrand disease is the most common inherited blood disorder and is a result of a defect in von Willebrand factor, a protein necessary for normal thrombus formation at the site of vascular injury (Matteson et al., 2011). It is especially prudent to screen those adolescents with heavy bleeding onset at menarche for a coagulation disorder, such as von Willebrand disease. Consultation with a hematologist is recommended if a coagulation disorder is suspected. Coagulopathy laboratory testing includes: (a) prothrombin time (PT) (international normalized ratio [INR]) and partial thromboplastin time (PTT) (fibrinogen or thrombin time are optional), (b) von Willebrand-ristocetin cofactor activity, and (c) von Willebrand factor antigen, Factor VIII (ACOG, 2013; Munro, Critchley, Broder, et al., 2011).

To establish ovulatory dysfunction as a cause of the AUB, basal body temperature evaluation and luteal phase serum progesterone levels should be evaluated to determine ovulatory status. A progesterone level greater than 3 ng/mL would be an indication that ovulation has occurred. The best time to test a woman's progesterone level is 1 week before her expected menstrual cycle (Fritz & Speroff, 2011). Determining the luteal phase of a menstrual cycle may be difficult in women diagnosed with AUB. Endometrial sampling, an expensive and invasive procedure that can establish whether the endometrium is secretory (indicating ovulation), is generally not necessary to determine ovulation. Once ovulatory dysfunction has been established, a thyroid-stimulating hormone (TSH) level should be evaluated to rule out thyroid disorders. A prolactin level should also be considered. If the prolactin level is elevated, it should be repeated as a fasting blood test (ACOG, 2013). Liver or renal function studies are only indicated in women with signs and symptoms or a current history of systemic disease.

DIAGNOSTIC TESTING

Ultrasonography and MRI • Transvaginal ultrasonography (TVUS) should be the first-line imaging modality for women presenting with AUB (Singh et al., 2013). In adolescents, transabdominal ultrasonography (TAUS) may be more appropriate (ACOG, 2012). For premenopausal women, U/S should be performed between days 4 and 6 of the menstrual cycle (ACOG, 2011). The use of TVUS for evaluation of a woman's endometrial echo-complex thickness is helpful when determining which women should undergo endometrial sampling. When ruling out polyps as the source

TABLE 28.4	Elements of a Structured Menstrual History	
I. FOUR CRITICAL DIMENSIONS		
1. Frequency	Frequent	< 24 days
	Normal	24–38 days
	Infrequent	> 38 days
2. Regularity of menses, cycle-to-cycle variation more than 12 months	Absent	No bleeding
	Regular	Variation ± 2–20 days
	Irregular	Variation < 20 days
3. Duration of flow	Prolonged	> 8.0 days
	Normal	4.5–8.0 days
	Shortened	< 4.5 days

4. Volume assessment
- Number of menstrual products used per period
- Use of more than one menstrual product simultaneously
- Use of incontinence pads
- Frequency of changing menstrual products at times of heaviest flow
- Size and number of blood "clots"
- Soaking through/staining of clothing
- Frequency of changing menstrual products at night

II. DIAGNOSTIC MODULE

Ask questions and take a medical history to develop a list of differential diagnoses and finally the final diagnosis.

Structural abnormalities?[a]	Intermenstrual spotting?
	Postcoital bleeding?
	Pelvic pain (severity and treatment)?
	Pelvic pressure?
Underlying hemostatic disorder?[b,c]	
Ovulatory dysfunction?[d]	Bleeding regularity?
	Weight changes?
	Exercise habits?
Endometrial dysfunction?[e]	Bleeding dimensions?
	History of gonorrhea, chlamydia, and/or PID?

III. SYMPTOM IMPACT MODULE

Incorporate questions that address menstrual bleeding that are meaningful to women (e.g., social embarrassment, fear of social isolation, and QOL).

Bleeding questions

- Change in menstrual pattern
- Number of menstrual products (pads or tampons or both) on the heaviest day
- Frequency of menstrual products (pads or tampons or both) used at night
- Rate of change of products at time of heaviest flow
- Information about blood clots

(continued)

TABLE 28.4	Elements of a Structured Menstrual History (continued)

Social embarrassment

- Bleeding through clothes
- Bleeding onto furniture
- Bleeding onto sheets
- Bleeding through her clothes while not at home
- Need to change clothes when not at home

Fear of social embarrassment

- Questions about anxiety
- Questions about depression
- "I worry about…"

Avoidance behavior

- Missing work
- Changing social plans
- Canceling activities that require leaving the house
- Extra clothes at work
- Extra menstrual products at all times

[a] Targeted medical history → Polyps, hyperplasia, and cancer can be associated with intermenstrual spotting and postcoital bleeding; leiomyomas can be associated with increased pelvic pressure, urinary pressure, and constipation; and adenomyosis can be associated with pelvic pain.
[b] Consider incorporating a validated screening questionnaire.
[c] Targeted medical history → Severe infection, liver disease, leukemia. Women with a positive screen should be considered for further laboratory evaluation and referral to a hematologist.
[d] Targeted medical history → Thyroid disease, prolactin disorders, medications that can affect ovulation
[e] Targeted medical history → Medication use (e.g., DMPA, oral contraceptive pills, tranquilizers, psychotropic medications, copper intrauterine device)
DMPA, depo-medroxyprogesterone acetate; PID, pelvic inflammatory disease; QOL, quality of life.
Adapted from Matteson, Munro, and Fraser (2011).

TABLE 28.5	Common Differential Diagnoses by Age	
AGE GROUP	**DIFFERENTIAL DIAGNOSIS**	
13–18 years	Persistent anovulation because of immature/ dysregulation of HPO axis	
	Hormonal contraceptive use (often inconsistent use)	
	Pregnancy	
	Pelvic infection	
	Coagulopathies	
	Tumors	
19–39 years	Pregnancy	
	Structural lesions (e.g., leiomyomas or polyps)	
	Anovulatory cycles (PCOS)	
	Hormonal contraceptive use	
	Endometrial hyperplasia	
	Endometrial cancer (less common, but can occur)	
40 years to menopause	Anovulatory bleeding because of declining ovarian function	
	Endometrial hyperplasia or carcinoma	
	Endometrial atrophy	
	Leiomyomas	

HPO, hypothalamic–pituitary–ovarian; PCOS, polycystic ovary syndrome.
Adapted from ACOG (2012).

of a woman's AUB, TVUS may not be an effective screening tool as small polyps may be undetectable. It is important for health care providers to note that when attempting to rule out adenomyosis, a negative U/S evaluation is not conclusive (Munro, Critchley, Broder, et al., 2011). TVUS criteria for findings that may be consistent with adenomyosis (AUB-A) include: (a) globular uterine configuration, (b) poorly defined endometrial-myometrial junction, (c) myometrial echogenic linear striations, (d) thickening of the myometrium, (e) asymmetry of the anterior–posterior myometrial thickness, (f) irregular myometrial cystic spaces, and (g) heterogeneous myometrial echo texture (Brosens, de Souza, Barker, Paraschos, & Winston, 1995). TVUS and magnetic resonance imaging (MRI) may help to differentiate ovulatory abnormal menstrual bleeding from anatomic causes such as uterine myomas, adenomyosis, or endometrial polyps (Munro, Critchley, & Fraser, 2011; Naftalin et al., 2014).

Saline Infusion Sonohysterography • Excessive menstrual bleeding associated with myomas usually correlates with the location and size of a myoma. Intramural myomas that obstruct the uterine vasculature contribute to excessive cyclic bleeding. Saline infusion sonohysterography (SHG) assists in the diagnosis of discrete uterine abnormalities such as submucosal fibroids (Singh et al., 2013). SHG involves infusion of sterile saline through a small catheter into the uterine cavity (ACOG, 2013). This diagnostic test allows for precise assessment of the endometrial cavity, to include measurements of the thickness of the endometrium. In peri- and postmenopausal women presenting with AUB, the risk of endometrial hyperplasia and endometrial cancer is remote when the endometrial thickness is less than 4 or 5 mm (Fritz & Speroff, 2011). In premenopausal woman, the thickness count of their endometrium will vary depending on the timing of the U/S and the woman's menstrual cycle. During the proliferative phase, the thickness can range from 4 to 8 mm as compared with the secretory phase, when it may range from 8 to 14 mm (ACOG, 2013).

Aspiration Biopsy and Dilation and Curettage • Health care providers should consider obtaining endometrial tissue samples from women with a family history of hereditary nonpolyposis colorectal cancer syndrome (Singh et al., 2013). As postmenopausal bleeding (PMB) is the *most common presenting symptom* for endometrial carcinoma, any bleeding after 12 months of complete amenorrhea warrants immediate evaluation. There are two procedures used to obtain endometrial tissue for histologic evaluation: aspiration biopsy (e.g., endometrial biopsy) and dilation and curettage (D&C; Gungorduk et al., 2014). Aspiration biopsy of the endometrium should be performed in women older than or equal to 40 years of age presenting with AUB. Moreover, aspiration biopsy should be performed in women in all age groups with a history of 2 to 3 years of untreated, anovulatory bleeding, especially if they are obese and/or have not responded to medical treatment (Fritz & Speroff, 2011). Endometrial tissue is collected by using a straw-like device with a plunger that the health care provider gently pulls back on after she or he gently inserts into the uterus. Pulling back on the plunger creates a suction, which allows for collection of the endometrial sample. Before inserting the catheter, using sterile technique, the health care provider measures the depth of the uterus to avoid perforation. Endometrial aspiration is an office procedure that requires no or minimal analgesic or anxiolytic medication. In anticipation of this procedure, women may be counseled to take OTC NSAIDs, as directed by the manufacturer. Office endometrial biopsy should be the *first line assessment* of the endometrium (Singh et al., 2013). A blinded biopsy provides 100% specific and positive predictive value (PPV), however, falls short in sensitivity and negative predictive value (NPV; Salim et al., 2011). Therefore, if an endometrial biopsy is negative and the woman's AUB persists and/or the endometrial biopsy specimen is considered inadequate, then further diagnostic testing is indicated (e.g., hysteroscopy; ACOG, 2013). Women should be referred for further evaluation if:

- There is a history of repeated or persistent irregular or intermenstrual bleeding, or if risk factors for endometrial carcinoma are present
- Cervical cytology is abnormal
- Pelvic examination is abnormal
- There is significant pelvic pain unresponsive to simple analgesia
- Failure of first-line treatment after 6 months (Black et al., 2013)

Aspiration biopsy and surgical D&C have been shown to be equally successful in diagnosing endometrial pathologies (Gungorduk et al., 2014). Unfortunately, focal pathologies can elude both sampling techniques as the health care provider blindly conducts both (Gungorduk et al., 2014; Kazandi et al., 2012).

Hysteroscopy Directed Endometrial Sampling • Although an invasive procedure, hysteroscopy with guided biopsy is the *gold standard* for diagnosis of intrauterine pathology (e.g., endometrial polyps; Salim et al., 2011). Hysteroscopy permits full visualization of the endometrial cavity and endocervix, and is useful when verifying the diagnosis and when less-invasive procedures such as aspiration biopsy, TVUS, and SHG are inadequate (ACOG, 2013). Targeted biopsy samples collected via hysteroscopy improve the sensitivity of endometrial cancer diagnosis to 99.5% (ACOG, 2013). Hysteroscopy can be performed in the office or operating room (ACOG, 2013).

Treatment/Management

MEDICAL MANAGEMENT

Acute AUB • The method of treatment for acute AUB depends on clinical stability, overall acuity, suspected etiology of the bleeding, desire for future fertility, and underlying medical problems (ACOG, 2013; Black et al., 2013; Singh et al., 2013). Management of acute AUB is targeted at controlling the episode of heavy bleeding and reducing menstrual blood loss in future menstrual cycles. Intravenous (IV) conjugated equine estrogen is the only U.S. Food and Drug Administration (FDA) approved treatment for acute AUB. In situations of acute AUB, surgical management may be the choice of treatment, although medical management is the preferred initial treatment.

A category of drug therapy that is an effective treatment for chronic AUB is antifibrinolytic drugs. Although the research is limited, antifibrinolytics reduce bleeding in women with AUB by 30% to 55% (Lethaby, Farquhar, & Cooke, 2000; Lukes et al., 2010). Although not indicated for women with acute AUB, tranexamic acid (an antifibrinolytic) has been shown to reduce bleeding in surgical patients, limiting the need for blood transfusion (James et al., 2011). James et al. (2011) recommend the use of tranexamic acid (oral or IV) for acute AUB. Additionally, intrauterine tamponade with a 26F Foley catheter infused with 30 mL of saline solution appears to successfully control bleeding (Hamani, Ben-Shachar, Kalish, & Porat, 2010; James et al., 2011).

Once hemodynamically stable, multiple, long-term treatment options are available for use. Hormonal management is the recommended, first-line medical treatment. In addition to IV conjugated equine estrogen, combined oral contraceptives (COCs) (monthly or extended cycling), progestin therapy (oral or intramuscular), the levonorgestrel intrauterine system, tranexamic acid, and NSAIDs are all recommended therapies. Medical therapy using COCs or cyclic progesterone therapy is the mainstay of treatment for ovulatory dysfunctional bleeding. Health care providers should add progestin or transition women who have received IV conjugated equine estrogen to COCs. Long-term unopposed estrogen therapy is contraindicated as it increases a woman's risk of endometrial hyperplasia and carcinoma. Contraindications to hormone therapy must be considered before prescribing. Health care providers should consult with the *U.S. Medical Eligibility Criteria for Contraceptive Use* (Centers for Disease Control and Prevention [CDC], 2010) to determine which women are eligible for treatment with hormone therapy. It is important to remember that estrogen-containing contraceptives are contraindicated for women older than 35 who smoke or who have a history of thromboembolic disease. Progesterone hormonal options are ideal for these women.

A shared treatment goal with realistic expectations that includes discussion about anticipated side effects improves a woman's satisfaction and the likelihood of her continuation of treatment. It is also important for the health care provider to remember that unless the underlying problem is corrected, similar episodes of AUB are likely to recur (ACOG, 2013; Fritz & Speroff, 2011).

A hematologist should follow women with known or newly diagnosed coagulopathies. Desmopressin has been shown to be effective in treating acute AUB in women with von Willebrand disease. Desmopressin can be administered via intranasal inhalation, intravenously, or subcutaneously (Kadir, Lukes, Kouides, Fernandez, & Goudemand, 2005). Desmopressin is contraindicated in women with massive hemorrhage who are receiving IV fluid resuscitation as it may result in fluid overload (James et al., 2011). What is more, fluid retention and hyponatremia have been linked to Desmopressin therapy (James et al., 2011). In women with von Willebrand disease, treatment with recombinant factor VIII and von Willebrand factor may be required to control severe hemorrhage (ACOG, 2009). Because of the known effect on platelet aggregation and other interactions with drug therapies that might affect liver function and the production of clotting factors, women with known bleeding disorders or platelet function abnormalities should avoid NSAIDs (Kadir et al., 2005).

Chronic AUB

Combined Hormonal Treatments. The amount of abnormal bleeding that a woman is experiencing along with an assessment of her complete blood count (CBC) will determine her initial treatment regimen. On determination of hemodynamic stability, a low-dose, monophasic oral contraceptive may be used (one pill twice daily). Bleeding should markedly slow or stop within 24 to 48 hours, although the treatment regimen should continue for 5 to 7 days. If the woman presents with mild anemia, iron therapy (dietary intake and/or iron supplementation) is needed in conjunction with the low-dose contraceptive. If the woman presents with severe anemia, the health care provider should consider inpatient management to allow for IV high-dose estrogen and possible blood transfusion (ACOG, 2013).

To prevent heavy withdrawal bleeding on discontinuation of this twice-daily regimen, the woman can take the COC daily until the package of pills is completed. Withdrawal bleeding can be expected within a few days after the last active pill. A maintenance therapy of a low-dose COC should be prescribed and initiated. Over time, COCs have been shown to reduce menstrual blood flow by 60% when compared with a woman's natural cycle (Singh et al., 2013).

Occasionally, women who are taking COCs on a regular basis may experience AUB, such as irregular bleeding. Once the health care provider has confirmed that the irregular bleeding is not because of missed pills, she or he may consider changing the COC formulation to one with a higher progestational and androgenic effect, with lower estrogen. It can take up to 3 months to determine if the change in COC formulation was effective in resolving the irregular bleeding.

Although it has not been studied for effectiveness in resolving AUB, combined estrogen-progestin contraception with either the vaginal ring (NuvaRing) or the transdermal patch (Ortho Evra) has also been determined to be appropriate for maintenance therapy (Singh et al., 2013). Extended cycling and continuous use of oral contraceptives, the contraceptive patch, or the vaginal ring all appear to have reduced both the amount of blood loss per cycle and the number of bleeding episodes per year when compared with regular, monthly regimens with a pill-free week allowing for a withdrawal bleed (Singh et al., 2013).

Nonsteroidal Anti-Inflammatory Drugs. There is a progressive increase in levels of prostaglandins in the endometrium throughout the menstrual cycle, with very high concentrations noted in the menstrual endometrium. NSAIDs inhibit prostaglandin synthesis via the inhibition of the enzyme cyclooxygenase. Although the exact mechanism of action is not understood, it appears that the end effect is a reduction of menstrual blood loss, when compared with placebo. The most commonly used NSAIDs are naproxen (550 mg, orally, on the first day of menses; then 275 mg daily thereafter) and mefenamic acid (500 mg, 3 times daily for 5 days). Treatment should be initiated one day before the onset of menses and continue for 3 to 5 days or until bleeding stops (Singh et al., 2013). Both naproxen and mefenamic acid have been shown to decrease blood loss by approximately 20% to 40% (Singh et al., 2013). Although helpful, NSAIDs do not appear to be as effective as tranexamic acid, danazol, or the levonorgestrel-releasing intrauterine system (LNG-IUS; Lethaby, Duckitt, & Farquhar, 2013). Contraindications to NSAIDs include hypersensitivity, preexisting gastritis, and peptic ulcer disease (Singh et al., 2013; see Table 28.6).

Progestin-Only Methods. Progestin-only methods are available for women who prefer nonestrogen methods or have a contraindication to combined hormonal contraceptives. After a thorough work-up and confirmation of the source of the AUB, the health care provider should consider the LNG-IUS as a possible means of AUB treatment. The LNG-IUS is a progestin-releasing intrauterine system/device that has two FDA approved indications: (1) as a method of contraception, and (2) for the treatment of AUB/HMB. This 32-mm device administers 20 mcg of levonorgestrel (LNG) daily to the endometrium, resulting in endometrial atrophy, thereby reducing mean uterine vascular density. Systemic side effects are minimal because of the low concentration of LNG that is absorbed into the systemic circulation (0.4–0.6 nmol/L). The LNG-IUS is FDA approved for 5 years

TABLE 28.6	NSAIDs and COX-2 Inhibitors Commonly Used for Primary Dysmenorrhea	
DRUG	**TRADE NAME**	**RECOMMENDED DOSAGE**
Ibuprofen	Advil, Motrin	400 mg every 4–6 hours
Naproxen	Aleve	220 mg every 8–12 hours
Naproxen	Anaprox	Initially 550 mg, then 550 mg every 12 hours or 275 mg every 6–8 hours
Naproxen	Naprelan	1 g once daily
Naproxen	Naprosyn	Initially 500 mg, then 500 mg every 12 hours or 250 mg every 6–8 hours
Diclofenac	Cataflam	50 mg every 8 hours
Meclofenamate	Meclomen	50–100 mg every 4–6 hours for up to 6 days starting with menstrual flow
Mefenamic acid	Ponstel	Initially 500 mg, then 250 mg every 6 hours (take with food)
Celecoxib	Celebrex	Initially 400 mg, then 200 mg twice daily

COX-2, cyclooxygenase-2; NSAIDs, nonsteroidal anti-inflammatory drugs.

of continuous, intrauterine use. Studies have suggested that women who have a LNG-IUS inserted have similar bleeding outcomes as women who have had an endometrial ablation (Singh et al., 2013). In the first few months after insertion, many women reported intermenstrual spotting, but the spotting was resolved after a few months with up to 80% of women becoming amenorrheic by 1-year postinsertion (Singh et al., 2013). The LNG-IUS is more effective than oral medication at reducing menstrual flow. Women using the LNG-IUS reported a significant improvement in their QOL with minor adverse effects (Lethaby, Hussain, Rishworth, & Rees, 2015). Side effects reported included breast tenderness, bloating, weight gain, and ovarian cysts (Lethaby et al., 2015). Health care providers should consider the LNG-IUS as a first-line therapy for appropriate candidates with AUB that is not associated with anatomic abnormalities of the uterus. The 3-year LNG-IUS contraceptive, a smaller system/device measuring 28 mm, releases 14 mcg of LNG daily. This smaller device is not FDA approved for AUB/HMB.

Some women prefer not to use the intrauterine system and instead opt for another type of progesterone therapy.

Women who chose an oral progestin agent for menstrual control and contraception must be counseled about the importance of taking the pill at the same time each day. It is important to note that few women experience reduced menstrual blood loss when using the progesterone-only pill (POP) for contraception (Singh et al., 2013).

Injected progestin, depo-medroxyprogesterone acetate (DMPA), is both a contraceptive and has been used to treat AUB/HMB. DMPA works by suppressing ovulation and ovulatory steroidogenesis, thereby reducing the estrogen-mediated stimulation of the endometrium, leading to endometrial atrophy (Singh et al., 2013). The first few months of treatment, women can expect unpredictable and irregular spotting and bleeding. Approximately 50% of women will experience amenorrhea by 1 year of continued use. Other side effects include breast tenderness, nausea, weight gain, mood disturbances, and a small reduction in bone mineral density that reverses once the medication has been discontinued. Health care providers should use caution when using DMPA in women with a history of depression.

Estrogen Therapy. When AUB/HMB is associated with a thin, denuded endometrium, as seen in adolescent girls and perimenopausal women, treatment should include high-dose estrogen therapy. High-dose estrogen therapy successfully stops heavy bleeding by promoting endometrial growth to cover the fragile, denuded endometrial surfaces. Estrogen is given either IV or orally, depending on the amount of abnormal menstrual bleeding. IV conjugated estrogen (Premarin) is given 25 mg, IV, every 4 hours until the menstrual bleeding subsides. If high-dose oral therapy is administered, 1.25 mg conjugated estrogen or 2 mg micronized estradiol is given by mouth, every 4 to 6 hours for 24 hours, then tapered to a once daily dose for 7 to 10 days (Fritz & Speroff, 2011). Both regimens are effective means for stopping bleeding, and should be followed by treatment with either a progestin or COC for the purpose of stabilizing the endometrium and providing a regular menstrual cycle (Singh et al., 2013). High-dose estrogen is contraindicated in women with a past history of thrombosis and/or with a family history of spontaneous thromboembolism (Fritz & Speroff, 2011).

Danazol. Danazol, a derivative of testosterone, has been shown to be effective in reducing heavy menstrual blood loss, but the androgenic side effects (e.g., weight gain, acne, hirsutism) tend to be an issue for most women. Danazol inhibits ovarian steroid genesis through suppression of the pituitary–ovarian axis and reduces blood losses by up to 80%. The prescribed regimens range between 100 mg and 400 mg daily, in divided doses. Danazol and gonadotropin-releasing hormone agents (GnRH) agonists have considerable side effects and are considered as treatment only after medical and/or surgical treatments have failed and/or are contraindicated (Singh et al., 2013).

GnRH Agonists. GnRH agents suppress pituitary secretion of follicle stimulating hormone (FSH) and luteinizing hormone (LH), creating a hypoestrogenic, menopausal-like state. Cessation of menstruation usually occurs within 3 to 4 weeks after administration. GnRH agonist treatment has most commonly been used to treat the symptomatology associated with adenomyosis, leiomyomas, or endometriosis, or as pretreatment before surgery for abnormal menstrual bleeding. GnRHs can be administered intramuscularly, subcutaneously, or intranasally. Menopausal symptoms such as hot flashes and vaginal dryness are common side effects. The most significant disadvantage to GnRH agonists is rapid bone demineralization that increases the risk of osteoporosis. Because of this serious side effect, it is recommended that treatment be limited to no more than 6 months (Singh et al., 2013). Another disadvantage of GnRH therapy includes the possibility of regrowth of previously treated uterine leiomyomas once therapy has been discontinued (Black et al., 2013).

Antifibrinolytics. Women with AUB/HMB have elevated endometrial levels of plasminogen activators with more local fibrinolytic activity as compared with women with normal menstrual loss. Antifibrinolytics cause a degradation of blood clots. They have been shown to be effective in reducing blood flow volume by 40% to 60% as compared with NSAID and luteal-phase progestins (Singh et al., 2013). The primary issue with antifibrinolytic use is the associated GI side effects as well as increased risk of intermenstrual bleeding. There is no evidence that antifibrinolytic therapy increases the risk of thromboembolic disease, even in high-risk women (Singh et al., 2013).

SURGICAL MANAGEMENT

The need for surgical treatment is based on a woman's hemodynamic stability, severity of bleeding, contraindications to hormonal management, a failed response to medical management, and underlying medical condition(s) (ACOG, 2013). Surgical interventions include D&C, myomectomy, endometrial ablation, uterine artery embolization, and hysterectomy. Surgical intervention is chosen based on the hemodynamic stability of the woman and her desire for future fertility. Uterine artery embolization and endometrial ablation have been shown to successfully control acute AUB (Bowkley, Dubel, Haas, Soares, & Ahn, 2007; Nichols & Gill, 2002).

Operative Hysteroscopy • In cases in which structural abnormalities are the cause of acute AUB, surgical procedures such as hysteroscopy with D&C, polypectomy, and/or myomectomy may be indicated. Operative hysteroscopy is primarily used to treat intra cavity lesions such as submucosal fibroids and endometrial polyps (Salim et al., 2011). This is a quick, safe, and effective outpatient procedure. It is important to remember that D&C without hysteroscopy is inadequate for evaluation of uterine disorders and has been shown to only temporarily reduce abnormal bleeding (Bettocchi et al., 2001). Surgical intervention for polyps is usually reserved for polyps greater than 1 cm; smaller polyps often spontaneously regress (Salim et al., 2011).

Myomectomy, or removal of intramural or subserosal uterine leiomyomas (fibroids), is the procedure of choice for women who have symptomatic leiomyomas and wish to preserve their fertility. The type of surgical procedure chosen (e.g., hysteroscopy, laparoscopy, or laparotomy) is dependent on the number, size, and location of the leiomyomas. Leiomyomas reoccur within 5 years in up to 60% of myomectomy cases (Black et al., 2013).

Uterine Artery Embolization • Uterine artery embolization is another treatment option for symptomatic leiomyomas (including heavy bleeding). This is a minimally invasive procedure whereby using local anesthesia, a small catheter is inserted through the femoral artery and then guided into the uterine artery through x-ray imaging. The uterine artery is then occluded with embospheres, polyvinyl alcohol particles, coils, or gel foam, resulting in necrosis and shrinkage of the leiomyoma(s). Uterine artery embolization is not recommended for large leiomyomas or in women who desire to retain their fertility.

Hysterectomy • As a last resort in women who do not respond to medical treatment, hysterectomy (the definitive treatment for controlling heavy bleeding) may be necessary. The procedure can be performed vaginally, laparoscopically, or abdominally depending on the woman's diagnosis and the etiology of the AUB. Hysterectomy is a major procedure that requires hospitalization, several weeks of recovery, and is associated with significant morbidity and even mortality.

Endometrial Ablation • Endometrial ablation should be considered only as a last resort and in cases in which the woman does not desire future fertility. Furthermore, it is critical to rule out endometrial carcinoma as the cause of the acute AUB before performing an endometrial ablation. Endometrial ablation is a less-invasive procedure and an alternative to hysterectomy for treatment of AUB. There are several ablation techniques available including thermal balloon, circulated hot fluid, cryotherapy, radiofrequency electrosurgery, and microwave energy. These newer technologies treat the endometrial cavity globally rather than ablating the endometrium section by section, as was done with rollerball electrosurgery or laser. Randomized controlled trials (RCTs) indicate that endometrial ablation has been associated with positive patient satisfaction, even without the occurrence of amenorrhea, following the procedure (Singh et al., 2013). As a result, bleeding is controlled in 87% to 97% of women and more than 80% require no additional surgery for up to 5 years after ablation (Singh et al., 2013). When preparing the patient for ablation, it should be emphasized that the goal of the procedure is to reduce menstrual bleeding and not to induce amenorrhea (see Table 28.7).

SELF-MANAGEMENT

Options for self-management of AUB are dependent on etiology. Lifestyle changes may be helpful (e.g., exercise, weight loss, stress management). Women who are overweight or obese may experience an improvement or cessation of their symptoms with as little as a 10 to 15 pound weight loss (www.acog.org/Patients/FAQs/Polycystic-Ovary-Syndrome-PCOS). Regular exercise is one means for weight loss.

TABLE 28.7	Recommended Preoperative Checklist for Global Endometrial Ablation

- Document failure, refusal, or intolerance to medical management
- Confirm that patient does not desire future pregnancy
- Establish a plan for contraception
- Exclude endometrial hyperplasia or malignancy with a tissue sample
- Perform adequate endometrial imaging to exclude a lesion that would preclude the use of global endometrial ablation

Adapted from Sharp (2006).

Women with diabetes should be counseled on the importance of maintaining their blood sugars in normal range.

INTEGRATIVE MEDICINE

Although acupuncture is used for various gynecologic concerns, research on AUB and fibroids is limited (Smith & Carmady, 2010; Zhang, Peng, Clarke, & Liu, 2010). In one study, acupuncture was proven effective in reducing the size of one patient's myoma, resulting in resolved anemia and a subsequent pregnancy (Habek & Akšamija, 2014). In an animal model study, researchers reported improved ovarian function in rats with induced PCOS who were later treated with electroacupuncture (Maliqueo et al., 2015).

In a meta-analysis of 38 RCTs, treatment with Guizhi Fuling Formula (consisting of five herbs—*Ramulus Cinnamomi, Poria, Semen Persicae, Radix Paeoniae Rubra* or *Radix Paeoniae Alba,* and *Cortex Moutan*) reduced uterine fibroids when used either alone or with mifepristone. To date, no serious adverse events have been reported. It should be noted, however, that the authors of the meta-analysis reported the methodological quality of the RCTs as overall poor (Chen et al., 2014).

■ AMENORRHEA

Definition and Scope

Amenorrhea is the absence or cessation of menstruation and can be further defined as primary or secondary, depending on the woman's presentation. Primary amenorrhea is defined as no menses by age 14 years associated with the absence of the development of secondary sexual characteristics, or no menses by age 16 years even in the presence of normal secondary sexual characteristics (Fritz & Speroff, 2011). Secondary amenorrhea is defined as the absence of menses for a period of three cycles, or 6 months in a woman with previously normal menstruation (Fritz & Speroff, 2011). There are many underlying diseases and disorders that can result in amenorrhea (Box 28.1).

Etiology

The usual cause of amenorrhea is physiological (e.g., pregnancy, lactation). In the case of lactation, milk production relies on a rise in prolactin, which inhibits GnRH release thereby preventing normal ovarian stimulation. On cessation of lactation, menses typically return within weeks (Black et al., 2013). There are numerous causes for amenorrhea and many are rare.

Primary amenorrhea is often caused by chromosomal irregularities that lead to ovarian insufficiency (e.g., Turner syndrome) or anatomic abnormalities (e.g., Müllerian agenesis). Disorders arising from the hypothalamus, anterior pituitary, ovary, and genital tract make up the pathological causes of amenorrhea. Pathologic causes of secondary amenorrhea most commonly are the result of PCOS, hypothalamic amenorrhea, hyperprolactinemia, or primary ovarian insufficiency.

HYPOTHALAMIC DISORDERS

Impairment of the GnRH pulsatile secretion occurs from reversible conditions such as weight loss–related amenorrhea, stress-related amenorrhea, and exercise-related amenorrhea. In these conditions, a *functional hypothalamic amenorrhea* (FHA) results, which is characterized by low or normal levels of FSH and LH, normal prolactin levels, normal imaging of the pituitary fossa, and low estrogen.

Regular menstruation requires an endocrine balance and is dependent on healthy weight parameters with healthy levels of fat storage. The two body states that can affect the menstrual status include unhealthy weight loss (loss of body weight of 10%–15% typically seen in aggressive calorie-restrictive diets) and strenuous physical training (e.g., athletes). The sequela of such a high-intensity exercise regimen may result in an unhealthy state known as the *female athlete triad.* The prevalence is unknown as athletic women may not present with the three criteria: (a) disordered eating, (b) amenorrhea, and (c) osteoporosis (Matzkin, Curry, & Whitlock, 2015).

PITUITARY DISORDERS

High prolactin levels from pituitary disorders can cause secondary amenorrhea. About 40% of prolactin-secreting tumors originate in the anterior pituitary. One third of women with this type of tumor complain of galactorrhea. Antidopaminergic effects from medications can cause an elevation in prolactin levels, thereby leading to amenorrhea. These medications include phenothiazines, antihistamines, butyrophenones, metoclopramide, cimetidine, and methyldopa.

In rare circumstances, severe obstetric hemorrhage and subsequent hypotension can permanently damage the anterior pituitary. This rare necrosis of the anterior pituitary is referred to as Sheehan's syndrome. Sheehan's syndrome may be a source of secondary amenorrhea.

OVARIAN DISORDERS

Genetic syndromes, autoimmune disorders, ovary removal or destruction, and neoplasms commonly precipitate ovarian disorders. Premature ovarian failure (POF) is defined as the cessation of ovarian function before the age of 40 years. POF is characterized by amenorrhea and an increase in

BOX 28.1   MAJOR CAUSES OF AMENORRHEA

Disorders of the Outflow Tract

Congenital
  Complete androgen resistance
  Imperforate hymen
  Müllerian agenesis
  Transvaginal vaginal septum
Acquired
  Intrauterine synechiae (Asherman's syndrome)
  Cervical stenosis

Primary Ovarian Insufficiency

Congenital
  Gonadal dysgenesis (other than Turner syndrome)
  Turner syndrome or variant
Acquired
  Autoimmune destruction
  Chemotherapy

Pituitary

Autoimmune disease
Cocaine
Cushing syndrome
Empty sella syndrome
Hyperprolactinemia
Infiltrative disease (e.g., sarcoidosis)
Medications
  Antidepressants
  Antihistamines
  Antihypertensives
  Antipsychotics
  Opiates

Other pituitary or central nervous system tumor
Prolactinoma
Sheehan syndrome

Central Nervous System Disorders (Hypothalamic Causes)

Eating disorder
Functional (overall energy deficit)
Gonadotropin deficiency (e.g., Kallmann syndrome)
Infection (e.g., meningitis, tuberculosis, syphilis)
Malabsorption
Rapid weight loss (any cause)
Stress
Traumatic brain injury
Tumor

Other Endocrine Gland Disorders

Adrenal disease
Adult-onset adrenal hyperplasia
Androgen-secreting tumor
Chronic disease
Constitutional delay of puberty
Cushing syndrome
Ovarian tumors (androgen producing)
Polycystic ovary syndrome (multifactorial)
Thyroid disease

Physiologic

Breastfeeding
Contraception
Exogenous androgens
Menopause
Pregnancy

Adapted from Klein and Poth (2013).

gonadotropin levels that result in a hypoestrogenic state. POF affects approximately 1% of all women and is usually nonreversible. Turner syndrome is the most common genetic syndrome associated with POF. Autoimmune disorders, such as systemic lupus erythematosus (SLE) and myasthenia gravis (MG), cause autoimmune oophoritis. Although extremely rare (occurs in only approximately 4% of women) it can lead to POF. Other causes of amenorrhea include surgical removal, destruction by radiation, and/or infection of the ovaries. Although ovarian neoplasms are rare, in such cases, excessive levels of estrogen and testosterone are produced.

POLYCYSTIC OVARY SYNDROME

PCOS affects 5% to 10% of childbearing-aged women and is associated with approximately 75% of all anovulatory disorders causing infertility. Often women will complain of light or infrequent periods. On U/S, a woman's ovaries may appear enlarged and contain many small fluid-filled structures just under the ovarian capsule, which are often not *true* cysts. The polycystic ovary has an increased ovarian stroma, which may lead to abnormal endocrine properties. Although approximately 25% of women will have PCOS-appearing ovaries on U/S, only a small percentage will develop true PCOS.

Women with PCOS have elevated pituitary and ovarian hormone levels, specifically, an abnormally elevated LH level and absence of the LH surge. Estrogen and FSH levels are often normal and because of alterations in the feedback process, the result is an increased LH:FSH ratio. Ovarian secretion of testosterone, androstenedione, and dehydroepiandrosterone (DHEA) is also elevated, and prolactin levels, too, are elevated.

Pathogenesis of PCOS • The cause of PCOS is unknown; however, there is evidence pointing to both genetic predisposition and lifestyle. The hallmark signs of PCOS are abnormalities in androgen biosynthesis and insulin resistance. Insulin resistance lends itself to obesity and hyperlipidemia, both of which increase the risk of a woman developing a noninsulin-dependent diabetes and metabolic syndrome.

The ovary produces the primary androgens, testosterone and androstenedione, whereas the adrenal glands produce DHEA. In the case of a woman with PCOS (abnormalities in androgen biosynthesis and insulin resistance), the production of androgens is significantly increased by insulin and insulin-like growth factors. This production cannot be suppressed by adrenal steroids; however, it can be suppressed by GnRH agonists.

PCOS is clinically diagnosed by inclusion of two of the following three criteria: (a) light and/or irregular menses, or amenorrhea; (b) on examination, physical evidence of hyperandrogenism; and (c) cystic appearing ovaries on U/S examination.

UTERINE CAUSES

Scarring of the endometrium resulting from trauma and/or infection, leading to the development of endometrial adhesions, can also cause amenorrhea. This condition is known as Asherman's syndrome. Asherman's syndrome is often caused by severe postpartum hemorrhage that requires dilation and sharp curettage, resulting in some endometrial damage and adhesions.

HIDDEN MENSTRUATION

Cervical stenosis can obstruct or block menstrual flow, leading to amenorrhea. Stenosis can occur from infection as well as surgical procedures (e.g., D&C, elective abortions), which lead to an obstruction of the outflow tract. Hidden menstruation can also be caused by an imperforate hymen and transverse vaginal septum (Fritz & Speroff, 2011).

Risk Factors

As with many other perimenstrual symptoms and syndromes, risk factors for amenorrhea depend on etiology. The defining characteristic in determining differentials and final diagnosis(es) is whether the woman has ever experienced menstruation. As with any form of AUB, a detailed history of a woman's medical and family history is warranted as often there is genetic predisposition.

Symptoms

Amenorrhea is the absence or cessation of menstruation. Menstruation usually begins within 2 years of thelarche, or breast budding. As an aside, although most adolescents begin menstruating by 16 years of age, the onset of puberty has fallen substantially across the developed world. This is attributed to improved nutrition and access to preventive health services (Bellis, Downing, & Ashton, 2006). Secondary amenorrhea occurs in women who have previously experienced menstruation, yet have not menstruated for at least 6 months. It is important for health care providers to consider amenorrhea as a symptom of a systemic condition. As such, evaluation and assessment of the woman experiencing amenorrhea is critical.

Evaluation/Assessment

A thorough history and physical examination is the first step when working-up a women presenting with amenorrhea.

HISTORY

The amenorrheic woman's history should include information regarding her growth and development, specifically changes of puberty such as breast development and pubic hair growth. The beginning of breast development signals estrogen stimulation. She should be asked about physical and emotional signs of cyclic hormonal changes (e.g., breast tenderness, mood changes). Cyclic abdominal pain may be a sign of outflow tract obstruction such as an imperforate hymen. It is also important to inquire about eating habits, exercise patterns, changes in body weight, drug use, prescription medications, current or previous acute or chronic illnesses, presence of emotional stress, as well as to conduct a comprehensive family history. Changes in hair growth, skin, and/or frequency of headaches should be noted. Headaches, if associated with galactorrhea and visual disturbances, may indicate a pituitary tumor (Klein & Poth, 2013; Practice Committee of the American Society for Reproductive Medicine, 2008).

PHYSICAL EXAMINATION

In the majority of cases, the physical examination is normal, but occasionally it may provide additional clues that point to the possible cause of the woman's amenorrhea. Anthropomorphic measurements, or the growth chart, may substantiate a delay in menses as just a constitutional delay of growth and puberty. An elevated body mass index (BMI), especially if associated with truncal obesity, may be a sign of PCOS or Cushing's disease. Furthermore, skin changes such as acanthosis nigricans, acne, and hirsutism also suggest PCOS, whereas purple striae suggest Cushing's disease. Tanner staging will provide insight. Breast development is an excellent indictor of ovarian estrogen production. Dysmorphic features, such as a webbed neck, widely spaced nipples, or short stature, may indicate Turner syndrome. When examining the breasts, any galactorrhea should be noted. If only a vaginal pouch is present with absent or sparse pubic hair, androgen insensitivity syndrome (AIS) should be considered, whereas the same findings with normal pubic hair may be suggestive of Müllerian agenesis (congenital absence of a vagina and abnormal or absent uterine and fallopian tube development). It is important to note that breast development is normal with both AIS and Müllerian agenesis (Klein & Poth, 2013; Practice Committee of the American Society for Reproductive Medicine, 2008).

Differential Diagnoses

ANATOMICAL ABNORMALITIES

Müllerian agenesis, a congenital malformation, is a common cause of primary amenorrhea. It is manifested in women with normal breast and pubic hair development, with no visible vagina, and other congenital malformations such as defects in the urinary tract and fused vertebrae. Imperforate hymen and a transverse vaginal septum may obstruct menstrual flow, yet women may experience cyclic premenstrual changes and complain of pelvic pain. In women presenting with Müllerian agenesis, the physical examination will be consistent with a normal vaginal opening, shortened vagina, no cervix, and a palpable bloody mass (hematocolpos).

In rare instances, AIS, testicular feminization or male pseudo hermaphroditism will cause amenorrhea. Women with AIS will have normal breast development, sparse or absent pubic and axillary hair, and a blind vaginal pouch. Furthermore, they may have 5-alpha reductase deficiency, which is characterized by partially virilized genitalia. Laboratory analysis of serum testosterone will be consistent with what a normal value would be in a male. This is because of the contrast in genotype and phenotype (gonadal sex = male, contrasting phenotype = female). Women with this syndrome should be referred to a specialist for follow-up care.

Cervical os stenosis may occur following cervical procedures. Symptoms include worsening dysmenorrhea or prolonged light staining or spotting after menses. Amenorrhea can occur on rare occasions. U/S evaluation may reveal a hematometra (blood retained in the uterus).

Secondary amenorrhea is a symptom of Asherman's syndrome. This syndrome is iatrogenic; it is caused by uterine instrumentation during gynecologic or obstetric procedures that in turn cause intrauterine adhesions that obstruct or obliterate the uterine cavity. Administering an estrogen/progesterone challenge test in a woman with Asherman's syndrome will result in a no withdrawal bleed.

PRIMARY OVARIAN INSUFFICIENCY

Ovarian disorders can cause primary or secondary amenorrhea. Primary ovarian insufficiency is characterized by follicle depletion or dysfunction that leads to impaired ovarian function. Ovarian insufficiency is diagnosed in women less than 40 years of age with a history of amenorrhea or light, infrequent periods and elevated FSH measured on two separate occasions, 1 month apart. Women who desire fertility should be referred to a reproductive endocrinologist, early in their medical care, for counseling regarding egg donation or in vitro fertilization (IVF). Approximately 5% to 10% of women diagnosed with ovarian insufficiency conceive and deliver a pregnancy. Hormone therapy may be indicated to help reduce vasomotor symptoms experienced because of ovarian insufficiency. Health care providers should consider prevention of osteoporosis by prescribing weight-bearing exercises, supplemental calcium (1,200 mg/daily), and vitamin D (800 IU/daily).

Primary ovary insufficiency has been attributed to chromosomal abnormalities, fragile X permutations, autoimmune disorders, radiation therapy, and chemotherapy. For example, Turner syndrome has unique physical characteristics including a webbed neck, a low hairline, cardiac defects, and lymphedema. Women who present with short stature and amenorrhea are suspect for Turner syndrome and so should undergo genetic testing (e.g., karyotype analysis). An endocrinologist and/or genetics counselor may need to be consulted. A genetic counselor will complete a family history consisting of a three-generation pedigree, and will appropriately counsel and recommend further genetic testing that may be warranted. Autoimmune disorders should be evaluated by determining thyroid function and adrenal autoantibodies.

HYPOTHALAMIC AND PITUITARY CAUSES

For proper functioning, the ovaries require hormonal stimulation from the hypothalamus and pituitary. Stress, weight loss, excessive exercise, and/or disordered eating negatively influence the function of the HPO axis, thereby decreasing ovarian function that leads to a reduction in the availability of estrogen. As a result, laboratory tests will reveal low or low-normal levels of serum FSH, LH, and estradiol. However, these results can fluctuate. Women with a reduced calorie intake should be evaluated for eating disorders, fad diets, and malabsorption syndromes (e.g., celiac disease). Treatment involves nutrition support and education. A bone density measurement may be necessary to evaluate a woman's bone health. It may be necessary to prescribe OTC calcium and vitamin D supplements. Although COCs will restore regular menses, they will not correct bone loss or protect bone health. Bisphosphonates are not helpful in this population of women.

Diagnostic Studies

A pregnancy test should be the first step in the laboratory evaluation. The most common cause of secondary amenorrhea is pregnancy. After ruling out pregnancy, the health care provider should collect a CBC and comprehensive metabolic panel. The work-up for amenorrhea is a three-step process.

STEP ONE

This step includes a serum prolactin level, TSH, FSH, and a progestational challenge test (Table 28.8). If the woman's history or physical examination is suggestive of a hyperandrogenic state, consider ordering a serum free and total testosterone, and DHEA concentration. If galactorrhea is present, imaging of the sella turcica may be indicated, particularly if the prolactin level is elevated (Box 28.2).

Although hypothyroidism is an infrequent cause of amenorrhea, it is easy to diagnose and menstrual cycles resume promptly with thyroid hormone replacement therapy. The purpose of the progestational challenge test is to evaluate the level of endogenous estrogen present as well as to assess for any outflow tract abnormalities. A withdrawal bleed should occur within 2 to 7 days after conclusion of the challenge test. A positive bleed indicates the presence of a reactive endometrium and a functioning outflow tract. A diagnosis of anovulation is confirmed if a woman's prolactin and TSH levels are normal. If galactorrhea is not present, no further evaluation is necessary. No withdrawal bleeding indicates either an outflow tract abnormality or inadequate estrogen stimulation of the endometrium.

TABLE 28.8	Progestational Challenge Test and Estrogen/Progestin Challenge Test	
DRUG	**DOSING**	**DURATION**
Parenteral progesterone in oil	200 mg, intramuscularly	Single dose
Micronized progesterone	300 mg, orally	Daily for 5 days
Medroxyprogesterone acetate (Provera)	10 mg, orally	Daily for 5 days

BOX 28.2   CAUSES OF GALACTORRHEA

Prolactin-secreting pituitary tumor
Medications
    Phenothiazine derivatives
    Opiates
    Diazepam
    Tricyclic antidepressants
    Amphetamines
Hypothyroidism
Excessive estrogen (e.g., oral contraceptives)
Nipple stimulation
Thoracotomy scars
Cervical spinal lesions
Herpes zoster
Stress
Hypothalamic lesions
Other prolactin-secreting tumors (e.g., lung and renal tumors; uterine leiomyoma)
Severe renal disease

Adapted from Speroff and Fritz (2005).

STEP TWO

Step two of the diagnostic work-up involves administering a second round of the estrogen/progestin challenge test (Table 28.8). In the absence of a withdrawal bleed, a validating second estrogen/progestin challenge is recommended. After the second test, the woman will have either a withdrawal bleed or not. No withdrawal bleeding indicates an outflow tract abnormality. U/S is indicated to determine if a uterus is present; an MRI or laparoscopy of the pelvis may be necessary for confirmation of the diagnosis. In women with a normal uterus, but an imperforate hymen or a transvaginal septum, outflow tract obstruction may be confirmed as the cause. A positive withdrawal bleed indicates a problem with either the HPO axis or the ovary.

STEP THREE

During step three, the gonadotropin assay (FSH and LH) is drawn and sent for laboratory analysis. There should be a delay of 2 weeks between the conclusion of step two and the beginning of step three, as administration of the estrogen/progestin challenge test may cause an artificial alteration in gonadotropin levels. Elevated FSH (greater than 20 IU/L) and LH (greater than 40 IU/L) suggest ovarian dysfunction, whereas normal or low levels of FSH (less than 5 IU/L) and LH (less than 5 IU/L) suggest a pituitary or hypothalamic abnormality. When the gonadotropin levels are found to be elevated, they are repeated to confirm that they are not transient. In the case of normal or low levels of gonadotropins, MRI of the sella turcica is indicated to rule out a pituitary tumor. A normal MRI indicates a hypothalamic cause of amenorrhea. It is important to note that all women younger than the age of 30 years diagnosed with ovarian dysfunction based on elevated gonadotropins must be further evaluated with a karyotype. The presence of mosaicism (an individual with at least two cell lines such as 45,X/46,XY) with a Y chromosome requires removal of the gonads because of a significant increase in the risk of malignancy.

Elevated gonadotropins associated with amenorrhea and hypoestrogenism may indicate a menopausal state. On average, menopause occurs at 50 years of age and is a result of depletion of ovarian follicles. Menopause that occurs before age 40 years is considered to be POF. As with menopause, POF places a woman at risk of osteoporosis and heart disease. POF has also been associated with autoimmune disorders, of which hypothyroidism is the most common (Black et al., 2013). Other less common autoimmune disorders include Addison's disease and diabetes mellitus (DM). A fasting glucose and antibodies testing for 21-hydroxylase should be included in the woman's work-up. POF may also be the result of alkylating chemotherapy and radiation of the pelvic area. Approximately 50% of women diagnosed with POF experience intermittent ovarian function. As such, elevated gonadotropins are not always indicative of infertility status, and conception remains a possibility.

Normal or low FSH and LH levels along with normal imaging studies is consistent with hypothalamic amenorrhea. This is a diagnosis of exclusion and is associated with suppression of GnRH below its critical range and disruption in the normal HPO axis. The most common causes for this type of amenorrhea are excessive weight loss (frequently associated with an eating disorder), strenuous exercise, and/or stress. A rare cause of hypothalamic amenorrhea is an inherited genetic disorder, Kallmann syndrome. This syndrome results in deficient secretion of GnRH and is also associated with anosmia (inability to smell; Fritz & Speroff, 2011; Klein & Poth, 2013; Practice Committee of the American Society for Reproductive Medicine, 2008).

Additional evaluation includes U/S to determine whether there are any anatomical reproductive abnormalities. If a pituitary tumor is suspect, MRI should be conducted (Klein & Poth, 2013).

Treatment/Management

MEDICAL MANAGEMENT

Treatment should be directed at the cause of a woman's amenorrhea and individualized to meet her needs. A woman desiring to achieve pregnancy will be managed differently from a woman wanting only to reestablish a normal menstrual cycle or needing hormone therapy (HT) for symptoms of hypoestrogenism.

For women with PCOS, oral contraceptives or cyclic administration of progestational agents will establish regular withdrawal bleeding and help to maintain a normal endometrium. Oral contraceptives also have the additional benefit of lowering free testosterone levels, thereby decreasing the symptoms of hyperandrogenism. For women with insulin resistance, insulin-sensitizing agents (e.g. Metformin) have been shown to improve ovulatory function. Still others may desire conception and need induction of ovulation in order to conceive.

Patients with POF may need HT to address vasomotor symptoms and to prevent osteoporosis. If the amenorrhea is associated with an eating disorder, weight gain generally restores normal menstruation. In many cases, women with severe eating disorders will require the intervention of a psychologist or psychiatrist who specializes in the management of these conditions. Women diagnosed with conditions such as hyperprolactinemia or outflow tract abnormalities must be referred to specialists for treatment and management (e.g., endocrinologist, surgeon).

SELF-MANAGEMENT

If amenorrhea is confirmed to be a symptom of PCOS, protecting the woman's endometrium from hyperplasia by establishing regular menstrual cycles, treating her androgenic signs and symptoms, and decreasing her insulin resistance are all of critical importance. If she is overweight or obese, weight-reduction strategies may be helpful in restoring normal menstruation, decreasing insulin resistance, and lowering androgen levels. In cases where the woman's amenorrhea is a symptom of the female athlete triad, she will need to be counseled on eating healthy meals with plenty of calories and calcium to maintain healthy bone mass. Women with PCOS that suffer with hirsutism and acne may benefit from visiting an aesthetician to improve healthy skin. Topical OTC acne products and a skin care regimen should be discussed and a referral provided to a dermatologist as needed.

INTEGRATIVE MEDICINE

Women with chronic health complaints are higher users of integrative techniques; however, there is limited evidence regarding efficacy. Furthermore, integrative treatments are oftentimes cost prohibitive. Although limited, various treatments for PCOS have been reported. For example, in one small study (Smith & Carmady, 2010), acupuncture was used to treat PCOS. Another small study demonstrated that acupuncture treatments improved all circulating hormones as compared with a physical therapy program in women with PCOS (Johansson et al., 2013). In a meta-analysis conducted by researchers, herbal medicine treatments for PCOS appeared to be beneficial for improving amenorrhea and hyperandrogenism (Arentz, Abbott, Smith, & Bensoussan 2014).

■ PREMENSTRUAL SYNDROME AND PREMENSTRUAL DYSPHORIC DISORDER

Definition and Scope

PREMENSTRUAL SYNDROME

Dr. William Dewees of the University of Pennsylvania first identified premenstrual syndrome (PMS) in 1843. During that time, PMS was referred to as the *melancholies of menstruation*. Dewees theorized that the uterus controlled the female body and was able to modify disease (Taylor, 2005). The exact cause of this highly complex, psychoneuroendocrine disorder remains a mystery. PMS is the cyclic recurrence of symptoms that occur in the luteal phase of the menstrual cycle, are variable in intensity and effect on daily life, and cease shortly after the onset of menstruation (ACOG, 2014). PMS symptoms negatively affect a woman's QOL. Approximately 85% of women experience one or more PMS symptom before and/or during their menses. It is estimated that of these women, approximately 32% meet the criteria for PMS (Borenstein, Chiou, Dean, Wong, & Wade, 2005; see Table 28.9).

PREMENSTRUAL DYSPHORIC DISORDER

Up to 3% to 5% of women suffer from premenstrual dysphoric disorder (PMDD), a more severe form of PMS, with significant impairment in a woman's individual, family, social, and occupational activities (Braverman, 2007; Gillings, 2014). PMDD is defined by the American Psychiatric Association (APA) as the "cyclic recurrence of severe, sometimes disabling changes in affect—such as mood lability, irritability, dysphoria, and anxiety—that occur in the luteal phase of a woman's menstrual cycle and subside around or shortly thereafter the onset of menses" (ACOG, 2014, p. 610). The primary distinction between PMS and PMDD is that the symptoms of PMDD are severe and interfere with a woman's ability to function, as comparable with other mental disorders (e.g., major depressive episode, general anxiety disorder; see Table 28.10).

Etiology

The etiologies of PMS and PMDD are not known. Although estrogen and progesterone levels have been found to be normal in women with PMS and PMDD, it has been postulated that there may be an underlying neurobiological vulnerability to normal fluctuations of these hormones (ACOG, 2014).

TABLE 28.9	Commonly Reported Symptoms and Diagnostic Criteria for PMS

PHYSICAL SYMPTOMS

Food cravings
Bloating and weight gain
Swelling of hands and feet
Fatigue
Gastrointestinal symptoms
Headache
Breast engorgement and tenderness
Abdominal cramps

PSYCHOSOCIAL SYMPTOMS

Anxiety
Depression
Hostility
Irritability
Panic attacks
Paranoia
Violence toward self or others
Social withdrawal
Angry outbursts
Crying spells
Poor concentration

Premenstrual syndrome can be diagnosed if a woman reports at least one of the physical symptoms and psychosocial symptoms during the 5 days leading up to her menses for three menstrual cycles.

Symptoms are relieved within 4 days of the onset of menses, without recurrence until at least cycle day 13.

The symptoms are present in the absence of any pharmacologic therapy, hormone ingestion, or drug or alcohol use.

The symptoms occur reproducibly during prospective recording of two menstrual cycles.

The woman exhibits identifiable dysfunction in social, academic, or work performance.

Sources: American College of Obstetricians and Gynecologists (2014), Chandru, Indusekhar, and O'Brien (2011), Mortala, Girton, and Yen (1989).

TABLE 28.10	Diagnostic Criteria for Premenstrual Dysphoric Disorder

At least five symptoms must be present in the final week before the onset of menses, improve within a few days after the onset of menses, and be minimal or absent in the week following menses.

1. One or more of the following symptoms must be present:
   - Marked affective lability (mood swings, feeling suddenly sad or tearful, or increased sensitivity to rejection)
   - Marked irritability, anger, or increased interpersonal conflicts
   - Marked depressed mood, feelings of hopelessness, or self-deprecating thoughts
   - Marked anxiety, tension, or feelings of being keyed up/on the edge (or both)
2. One or more of the following symptoms must additionally be present (making for a total of five symptoms when combined with symptoms for aforementioned Item 1):
   - Decreased interest in usual activities (work, school, and friends)
   - Difficulty concentrating
   - Lethargy, easy fatigability, or marked lack of energy
   - Marked change in appetite, overeating, or food cravings
   - Hypersomnia or insomnia
   - Sense of being overwhelmed or out of control
   - Physical symptoms (breast tenderness, swelling, joint or muscle pain, bloating, weight gain)

Symptoms should be documented by prospective daily ratings during at least two symptomatic cycles.

Symptoms are associated with clinically significant distress or interference with woman's social, academic, or work performance, or relationships with others.

The symptoms are not an exacerbation of symptoms of another disorder (major depressive disorder, panic disorder, persistent depressive disorder, or personality disorder).

The symptoms are not attributable to the physiologic effects of a substance (pharmacologic therapy, hormone ingestion, or drug or alcohol use).

Adapted from American College of Obstetricians and Gynecologists (2014); American Psychiatric Association (2013).

Risk Factors

Although PMS affects reproductive-aged women, those with severe symptoms tend to be in their late thirties (Shah et al., 2008). Sociocultural factors influence a woman's experiences with menstruation. Interestingly, reported symptoms of PMS vary according to geographic location, marital status, parity, education, and occupation (Shah et al., 2008). For example, women in Western cultures have been socialized to expect uncomfortable symptoms before menstruation (Fritz & Speroff, 2011). There is also a relationship between menstrual symptoms experienced by mothers and daughters, as well as between sisters, suggesting that responses to menstruation may be learned (Gillings, 2014). It has been hypothesized that PMS has a high heritability and is based on evolutionarily preservation of the species by improving fertile partner matches (Gillings, 2014).

Symptoms

There are more than 200 symptoms attributed to PMS (Table 28.9; ACOG, 2000/2013/2015; ARHP, n.d.; Chandru, Indusekhar, & O'Brien, 2011). Symptoms vary in character and intensity from woman to woman and may differ in the same woman from cycle to cycle. Symptoms include, and are not limited to, depression, angry outbursts, irritability, crying spells, anxiety, confusion, social withdrawal, poor concentration, insomnia, breast tenderness, food cravings, bloating and weight gain, headaches, swelling of hands and feet, fatigue, GI symptoms, and abdominal pain. It is important for health care providers to note that depression and anxiety disorders are the most common conditions that overlap with PMS. Determining whether depression and anxiety are symptoms of PMS or separate conditions will be guided by a woman's medical history. For example, the health care provider should inquire as to whether the symptoms of depression and anxiety are present all month, as well as whether or not symptoms are more pronounced just before and during menstruation. The key to diagnosis of PMS is the timing of the symptoms and not the symptoms themselves (Fritz & Speroff, 2011).

Evaluation/Assessment

There are two components to diagnosing PMS. The first is one of exclusion; the health care provider must rule out other medical and psychiatric etiologies. The second component is evidence via a woman's completed calendar that supports true modulation of symptoms severe enough and impairing her QOL. It is critical that the calendar be generated prospectively for 2 to 3 calendar months. Several symptom diary charts are available to aid in the timing of the symptoms of PMS (Fritz & Speroff, 2011). Health care providers, through collection of a careful history, physical examination, and laboratory testing, should be able to rule out medical and psychiatric diagnoses. There are two established guidelines for the diagnosis of PMS and PMDD (Tables 28.9 and 28.10).

Differential Diagnoses

Any condition that results in cyclic mood or physical changes should be included in the differential diagnoses of PMS and PMDD. Several different diagnoses are considered when working a woman up for PMS and/or PMDD. There are three major categories of diagnoses:

1. Medical problems (e.g., angina, asthma, chronic fatigue syndrome, cyclic mastalgia, diabetes, endometriosis, genital herpes, menstrual-associated migraine, endocrine disorders, GI conditions, neurologic disorders, substance abuse, thyroid disorders)
2. Psychiatric disorders (e.g., anxiety, depression, personality disorder, psychosis, bipolar affective disorders, posttraumatic stress disorder)
3. Premenstrual exacerbations of medical and/or psychiatric conditions (ARHP, n.d.)

Diagnosis of PMS or PMDD is based on exclusion of any of these conditions.

Diagnostic Studies

The diagnosis of PMS or PMDD is not easy, nor can it be made in one office visit. What is more, women often present with symptomology because they have seen their mother or sister suffer from symptoms of PMS or PMDD. On completion of her premenstrual symptom diary (2–3 consecutive months), the woman will follow-up with her health care provider. Although there are no recommended laboratory tests or diagnostic imaging, the health care provider should run a variety of tests for ruling out other pathology. For example, a chemistry profile, CBC, and TSH may be part of the initial testing. Further testing will be based on the woman's history

and physical examination. PMS and PMDD are most often diagnoses of exclusion.

Treatment/Management

The overall goals of treatment for either PMS or PMDD are to reduce symptoms, restore normal function, and optimize the woman's overall health. The approach to treatment is based on the specific symptom or constellation of symptoms and their severity. In most cases, treatment options should be approached in a three-step process: (1) supportive therapy, which includes a complex carbohydrate diet, aerobic exercise, nutrition supplements, and spironolactone; (2) administration of selective serotonin reuptake inhibitors (SSRIs), anxiolytic agents (for women who do not respond to SSRIs); and (3) hormonal ovulation suppression with oral contraceptives or GnRH agents (ACOG, 2014).

SELF-MANAGEMENT MEASURES

The first self-management measure that a woman newly diagnosed with PMS or PMDD should be counseled about is lifestyle change. It is critical that the woman understand the importance of her role in managing symptoms. Lifestyle change includes diet and physical activity. The strongest evidence for effective PMS interventions include calcium supplementation, the use of the diuretic spironolactone, COCs that contain drospirenone (an analog of spironolactone), and cognitive behavioral therapy (CBT) (Nevatte et al., 2013). Drug therapy should be considered for women with severe symptoms and/or those with who fail or do not respond well to supportive therapy. SSRIs, the recommended initial drug of choice, have been found to be very effective when treating both PMS and PMDD (ACOG, 2014). Treatment with anxiolytic alprazolam is also effective in women whose symptoms are not relieved by any of the aforementioned treatment interventions.

Diet and Exercise • For women with mild to moderate PMS, lifestyle changes, such as regular aerobic exercise, three to four times a week, particularly during the luteal phase of the menstrual cycle, and nutritional changes (reducing caffeine, salt, alcohol, and a diet rich in complex carbohydrates) may be helpful. Although the evidence supporting these interventions comes from epidemiologic studies rather than randomized trials, there is little risk or cost to the woman, and anecdotal experience has shown that when implemented, they decrease the severity of PMS symptoms in some women (ARHP, n.d.; Chandru et al., 2011).

Vitamin and Mineral Supplements • Dietary supplements have been studied in RCTs with conflicting results (Braverman, 2007; Chandru et al., 2011). Calcium as a nutritional supplement has showed the most promise. It appears to improve mood as well as several somatic symptoms such as water retention, food cravings, and pain. Although the exact biological mechanism with respect to PMS is not well understood, increased calcium levels improve the regulation of calcium homeostasis (Nevatte et al., 2013). An added benefit of calcium is improvement of bone density (Bertone-Johnson et al., 2005). For treatment of PMS, calcium 600 mg by mouth twice a day is recommended.

The role of vitamin B$_6$ (pyridoxine), a cofactor in serotonin and dopamine metabolism, in the treatment of PMS is unclear. Studies have shown that taking vitamin B$_6$ in doses of up to 100 mg/d may be of modest benefit (Chandru et al., 2011). Vitamin B$_6$ can also be found in a wide variety of foods including fortified cereals, beans, meat, poultry, fish, and some fruits and vegetables. It is important to counsel women about the danger associated with exceeding vitamin B$_6$ supplementation of 100 mg/d, specifically, symptoms of peripheral neurotoxicity (Chandru et al., 2011). It is recommended to discontinue supplemental B$_6$ if no improvement in symptomology is observed.

Researchers have reported mixed results for treatment with magnesium and vitamin E, and treatment with soy isoflavones have been proven to be noneffective (Nevatte et al., 2013). Studies have shown superior efficacy for essential fatty acids that contain linoleic acid, gamma-linoleic acid, oleic acid, and vitamin E in improving PMS when compared with placebo (Nevatte et al., 2013). Data are conflicting regarding the benefit of evening primrose oil; it appears to be most beneficial for cyclical mastalgia (ARHP, n.d.; Chandru et al., 2011; Nevatte et al., 2013).

Mind/Body Therapies • Mind/body therapies (MBTs) are based on the emerging scientific evidence that thoughts and feelings affect normal physiology as well as physical health (Girman, Lee, & Kligler, 2003). The goal is to help women learn to cope with premenstrual symptoms, including stress. Mind/body approaches vary widely and include interventions such as psychotherapy (e.g., individual counseling, psychoeducational group therapy), massage, reflexology, hypnotherapy, biofeedback, guided imagery, yoga, and relaxation training. Most of the evidence regarding mind/body approaches for PMS is limited, but since many of these methods teach coping strategies for reducing stress or increasing relaxation, there is still strong rationale for including them in the treatment of PMS (Girman et al., 2003). The International Society for Premenstrual Disorders reported positive benefits of CBT (Nevatte et al., 2013). This therapy may benefit by reframing negative and irrational thinking and increasing coping skills. Even though the use of fluoxetine was superior for treating anxiety related to PMS, CBT was weakly superior as compared with placebo for the remaining symptoms (Nevatte et al., 2013).

Psychoeducational group therapy may be especially helpful. This is a unique opportunity for women to not only learn about their disorder, but to be afforded the opportunity to meet with other women who share similar experiences. This shared experience has been shown to reduce the sense of isolation that many women who suffer from PMS feel. Over time, many women are empowered by the support and their increased knowledge about PMS, and as a result of therapy, develop new behaviors and strategies to help reduce symptoms of PMS (ARHP, n.d.; Nevatte et al., 2013).

Complementary and Alternative Medicine • Referral to an acupuncturist may provide some relief from symptoms. Some research shows promise, though not definitive, in ameliorating PMS symptoms (Cho & Kim, 2010; Jang, Kim, & Choi, 2014; Kang, Jeong, Kim, & Lee, 2011). True acupuncture techniques are tailored to the individual woman's need and therefore make interventional research design more challenging. Jang, Kim, and Choi (2014) reported in their systematic review that acupuncture and herbal medicine improved symptoms by 50%.

Herbal Preparations. Chasteberry (*Vitex agnus-castus*) is used by medical herbalists to treat female hormonal disorders and is considered a hormone modulator (British Herbal Medicinal Association [BHMA], 1996). This herb has been reported to improve PMS symptoms when taken daily (20 mg/d; Braverman, 2007), especially those such as irritability, anger, mood swings, headaches, and breast fullness (Chandru et al., 2011). One study involving 1542 women with PMS reported 33% of the patients had total relief of symptoms with an additional 57% reporting partial relief (Taylor, Schuiling, & Sharp, 2006). German health authorities have approved the use of chasteberry for PMS, irregularities of the menstrual cycle, and mastodynia (breast pain/tenderness). Chasteberry is contraindicated in pregnancy and during lactation.

Agnolyt®, a commercially available chasteberry, has few reported side effects and is sold in most health food stores. No other evidence of improvement in PMS symptoms has been reported when using other herbal preparations (e.g., black cohosh, ginko biloba, kava, or oil of evening primrose; BHMA, 1996). It would follow that St. John's wort (*hypericum pefortum*), because of its SSRI-like effects, would be a logical choice for treating PMS symptoms. In one small study, 19 women with PMS were treated with St. John's wort. At the conclusion of the study, women reported at least a 50% reduction in symptom severity (Taylor et al., 2006). The use of St. John's wort in women with PMS has yet to be studied using an RCT study design. It is important that health care providers note that St. John's wort induces enzyme systems, such as cytochrome P450 (which, when activated, increases the rate at which many drugs are cleared from the bloodstream, thereby reducing their efficacy; Taylor et al., 2006).

PHARMACOTHERAPEUTICS

Hormonal Therapy • Even though hormonal changes that occur with the menstrual cycle are not a causative factor for PMS or PMDD, they can produce mood changes and/or other physical symptoms in susceptible women. Some have postulated that within the central nervous system (CNS) is a mechanism that determines susceptibility. For this reason, it has been proposed that eliminating the menses, using hormonal contraception, for example, is often effective. Continuous use of COCs or DMPA may help decrease symptoms that are not relieved by nonpharmacological interventions, although study results evaluating the effects of oral contraceptives and PMS have been mixed (ARHP, n.d.; Braverman, 2007). Contraceptives that contain drospirenone and ethinyl estradiol have been FDA approved for the treatment of PMDD in women who choose to use an oral contraceptive as their method of contraception (Lopez, Kaptein, & Helmerhorst, 2012). GnRH analogs have generally reduced both physical and psychological symptoms; however, because of their negative effects on bone density, use for longer than 6 months is not recommended. Progesterone therapy has not demonstrated consistent positive outcomes (Ford, Lethaby, Roberts, & Mol, 2012). Topical progesterone has not been studied because other routes of administration have not been shown to be beneficial for reduction of PMS symptoms (Fritz & Speroff, 2011). GnRH agonists and surgical oophorectomy have also been shown to be effective in treating women with PMS or PMDD (ACOG, 2014).

Selective Serotonin Reuptake Inhibitors • For women with severe PMS or PMDD, SSRI pharmacotherapy should be considered. Numerous RCTs have shown that almost all SSRIs are superior to placebo in improving premenstrual emotional and physical symptoms (Freeman, Sammel, Lin, Rickels, & Sondheimer, 2011; Shah et al., 2008). The effect of SSRI therapy is rapid, with symptom improvement generally seen within 24 to 48 hours (Braverman, 2007). This differs from the treatment of depression or anxiety, where it may take 4 to 6 weeks to see the maximum effect suggesting a different mechanism of action for the treatment of symptoms of PMS or PMDD. Benefits of intermittent SSRI therapy include fewer adverse side effects and less cost to the woman. Intermittent therapy can be started at the beginning of the luteal phase of the menstrual cycle (e.g., 2 weeks before the expected menstrual period) or on the first day that the woman experiences her initial symptoms. With either regimen, the drug is discontinued within 1 to 3 days after the first day of menses. In a meta-analysis, intermittent SSRI dosing was found to be less effective than continuous dosing (Shah et al., 2008). Other antidepressants, such as clomipramine (Anafranil) and desipramine (Norpramin), are considered second-line therapies for PMS or PMDD and are less well tolerated. Alprazolam (Xanax), a short-acting benzodiazepine, with anxiolytic and antidepressant properties, has been shown to be more effective that placebo, but should be used with caution because of the risk of tolerance and dependence. SSRIs are generally well tolerated, but may be associated with side effects such as GI symptoms (nausea), insomnia, fatigue, headache, dry mouth, dizziness, tremor, and sweating. These side effects generally resolve within a few weeks after initiation, and may not be much of an issue given the recommended short-term, intermittent dosing. Long-term, continuous dosing may be associated with decreased libido and delayed orgasm. SSRI therapy will most likely be necessary through menopause. Most women will experience a recurrence of symptoms when discontinuing the SSRI (Shah et al., 2008). It is important to note that although there are a number of successful therapeutic interventions available for the treatment of PMS, they by no means replace the health care provider–female patient relationship.

■ MENSTRUAL MIGRAINES

Definition and Scope

Migraines are predominately a female disorder. Several female reproductive milestones correlate with a change in migraine frequency or type, thereby implicating sex hormones in the pathogenesis of migraines (Sacco, Ricci, Degan, & Carolei, 2012). Migraines occur in 34.5% of adult women and 20.1% of men (Pakalnis & Gladstein, 2010). Headache disorders that occur relative to menstrual cycles are called catamenial migraine (Mathew, Dun, & Luo, 2013). There are two types: pure menstrual migraines (migraines that occur only during menstruation) and menstrual-related migraines (which occur regularly with menstruation, but also occur during other days of the month; Mathew et al., 2013). The International Classification of Headache Disorders (ICHD-3 beta) provides diagnostic criteria for the two most common menstrual-related headaches: migraine without aura and menstrual-related migraine without aura (Headache Classification Committee of the International Headache Society, 2013). Menstrual migraine can occur from estrogen fluctuations, either from a naturally occurring menstrual cycle or from the withdrawal of exogenous progestogen provided by COCs or cyclical hormone therapy, which make management strategies differ (Headache Classification Committee of the International Headache Society, 2013). Collaboration with a neurologist is appropriate and encouraged in women with ongoing menstrual migraines.

Etiology

Throughout the reproductive years, menstruation is one of the most significant events related to the occurrence of migraine attacks. The greatest incidence is during the 5-day window that begins 3 days before onset, and continues through the first 3 days of menstruation. Migraine without aura appears to be associated with estrogen withdrawal, whereas migraine with aura is associated with high estrogen levels. Differences may be related to a woman's ability to metabolize estrogens, or to a polymorphism in her genes encoding for sex hormones, their receptors, or metabolites of the hormonal pathways (Sacco et al., 2012).

Estrogen and progesterone influence the pain-processing networks and the endothelium involved in the pathology of migraine (Sacco et al., 2012). These hormones are present in the CNS by passively crossing the blood-brain barrier. Estrogens affect the cellular excitability of the cerebral vessels. Furthermore, there are interrelationships between estrogens and brain neurotransmitters such as serotonin, norepinephrine, dopamine, and endorphins. Estrogen increases serotonergic tone. Peak estrogen levels are associated with a significant decrease in magnesium levels that affects the N-methyl-D-aspartate (NMDA) channel opening (Sacco et al., 2012). Prostaglandins also play a role in the development of menstrual migraine. Systemic circulation of prostaglandins can lead to throbbing headache, nausea, and vomiting. Estrogen facilitates the glutaminergic system, thereby potentially enhancing neural reactivity, which in turn is modulated by progesterone (Sacco et al., 2012).

Risk Factors

Menstrual-related migraine has repeatedly been found to be longer in duration, more disabling, and less responsive to acute therapy. Studies have shown that women may experience their first migraine with the initiation of COCs. In women with a history of migraines, COC use may cause a worsening of frequency and severity, or no change in migraine occurrence. In COC users, migraines are more likely to be worse during the pill-free week (Sacco et al., 2012). Menstrual migraine is often comorbid with other conditions such as dysmenorrhea, irregular cycles, ovarian cysts, endometriosis, and heavy menstrual bleeding (Calhoun, 2012).

Symptoms

Migraines are typically unilateral, pulsating in quality with moderate to severe pain, and interfere with a woman's QOL. Often, the headache is aggravated by light (photophobia) or sounds (phonophobia). Typically, headaches last 4 to 72 hours and last longer than a migraine with aura. Attacks of menstrual migraine (MM) are associated with nausea and vomiting as compared with nonmenstrual headaches without aura (Mathew et al., 2013; Sacco et al., 2012). It has been long established that there is a strong correlation between PMS and MM.

Auras are described a visual, sensory, or speech disturbances. Visual symptoms are described as flickering lights, spots, or lines and/or negative features such as loss of vision. Sensory symptoms can include positive features, such as pins and needles, and/or negative features such as numbness. Auras usually occur within 60 minutes before headache onset (Mathew et al., 2013).

Evaluation/Assessment

Gathering a thorough medical history is the first step in the assessment of a woman presenting with migraine headache. It is important to assess if the migraines occur at other times than just during menstruation. Women who suffer with migraines without aura tend to have attacks that last longer in duration and are accompanied by nausea as compared with women with nonmenstrual migraines (Vetvik, Benth, MacGregor, Lundqvist, & Russell, 2015). When evaluating and assessing women with migraines, health care providers should pay special attention to the woman's vascular and neurological examination (Table 28.11). Bajwa and Wootton (2016) refer to the mnemonic *SNOOP* when assessing and examining a patient. This mnemonic helps to triage patients who present with emergent cases.

- *Systemic symptoms*, illness, or condition (e.g., fever, weight loss, cancer, pregnancy, immunocompromised state including HIV)
- *Neurologic symptoms* or abnormal signs (e.g., confusion, impaired alertness)
- *Onset that is new or sudden*
- *Other associated condition* or features (e.g., head trauma, illicit drug use, or toxic exposure; headache awakens patient from sleep, headache is worse with Valsalva maneuver or is precipitated by a cough, exertion, or sexual activity)
- *Previous headache history* with headache progression or change in attack frequency, severity, or clinical features

TABLE 28.11	History and Examination for the Chief Complaint of Menstrual Migraine
HISTORY	**PHYSICAL EXAMINATION**
Age at onset	Obtain blood pressure and pulse
Aura or prodromal symptoms	Assess for bruit at neck, eyes, and head
Frequency of headaches	Palpate the head, neck, and shoulders
Location and radiation of pain	Assess temporal and neck arteries
Associated symptoms	Palpate the spine and neck muscles
Family history of migraines	Cranial nerve assessment
Precipitating and relieving factors	
Ability to engage in activities with migraine	
Ask about relationship between food and alcohol	
Previous treatment and response to treatment	
Any recent change in vision	
Any recent trauma	
Changes in sleep, exercise, weight, or diet	
Changes in method of birth control	
Association with environmental triggers	
Effects of menstrual cycle and exogenous hormones	

Adapted from Bajwa and Wootton (2016).

Differential Diagnoses

Several differential diagnoses could be added to a working differential list for a chief complaint of migraine. Researchers have reported characteristics of stress-related anxiety or depression in women who suffer with migraines without aura (Parashar, Bhalla, Rai, Pakhare, & Babbar, 2014). Tension-type headaches can occur anytime during the month irrespective of menstrual cycle, present bilaterally with a pressing or tightening quality, are not aggravated by routine physical activity, and do not accompany nausea, vomiting, or photophobia (Headache Classification Committee of the International Headache Society, 2013). Sinus congestion accompanying menstruation can precipitate sinus pressure and headache. Any new onset of headache should be worked up for a number of possible serious disorders.

Diagnostic Studies

The diagnostic work-up for a new onset menstrual migraine is the same as with any other new onset headache. Women presenting with a positive *SNOOPS* should be triaged into an emergent care category. The choice for brain imaging is MRI as it is more sensitive in the detection of edema, vascular lesions, and other intracranial pathology. When there is concern that the woman has presented with a thunderclap headache (a headache that is severe and sudden onset), a CT scan can also be performed. A thunderclap headache is oftentimes a symptom of subarachnoid hemorrhage (SAH) that is associated with a very high mortality rate. Should a person survive SAH, they are usually left with a high degree of morbidity and residual impairment. Laboratory analysis will be guided by a woman's physical examination and the health care provider's working differential. It is common, especially in cases of new onset headache, that a spinal tap and CSF analysis and testing is conducted.

Treatment/Management

Women who experience migraines only during menstruation respond more positively to hormone prophylaxis (Headache Classification Committee of the International Headache Society, 2013) as compared with those with nonmenstrual-related migraines (Tepper, 2013). Treatment is triaged into three levels of care: (1) acute treatment (during the attack), (2) mini-prevention (preventive maintenance during the menstrual window), and (3) long-term prevention (daily preventive treatment used throughout the month; Tepper, 2013).

SELF-MANAGEMENT

Not all women experience the same triggers that can induce a migraine. Notable migraine triggers include stress, lack of sleep or jet lag, food additives, alcohol, odd or strong smells, hunger or dehydration, highly caffeinated beverages, medication overuse, bright lights and loud sounds, changes in weather, hormones, physical activity, and foods. Avoiding triggers such as the weather is impractical and can become restrictive. What is more, health care provider recommendation to avoid triggers is not evidence based. Rather, some have suggested that health care providers counsel women to *cope with* rather than *avoid* triggers, as avoidance may further sensitize women to headache precipitating factors (Hoffman & Recober, 2014). Avoiding triggers can become a significant stressor. Health care providers should individualize patient recommendations and women with menstrual headaches should use common sense when balancing trigger avoidance and coping strategies (Hoffman & Recober, 2014). Referring the patient with ongoing symptoms of menstrual migraine is encouraged.

INTEGRATIVE MEDICINE

Acupuncture is performed routinely for the prevention and treatment of migraines, despite the lack of strong evidence (Zhang et al., 2010). There is limited existing evidence regarding the relationship between vitamin supplementation and decrease in migraine incidence. Newman and Yugrakh (2014) reported that magnesium 360 mg/d, beginning on day 15 of the menstrual cycle and continued until menstruation, reduced the number of headache days, pain, and distress. Riboflavin (200 mg or 400 mg/d) is thought to be effective in treating migraine (Newman & Yugrakh, 2014). There is ongoing research examining whether vitamins B_6, B_9, and B_{12}, E, and C play a role in treating migraines (Shaik & Gan, 2015).

PHARMACOTHERAPEUTICS

Regardless of whether menstrual or nonmenstrual-related migraine, treatment strategies are the same, with the addition of mini-prophylaxis and hormonal manipulation for treatment of menstrual migraines (Pakalnis & Gladstein, 2010). There are three general treatment strategies for menstrual migraine management: acute, mini-prevention (before and during), and long-term prevention. Women with irregular cycles are not good candidates for mini-prevention strategies because of the unpredictability of their menses (Calhoun, 2012). One strategy for women with irregular cycles is to have the woman use basal body temperature or to use an ovulation predictor kit to evaluate when ovulation will occur.

Nonsteroidal Anti-Inflammatory Drugs • NSAIDs are the oldest class of migraine treatments that effectively block prostaglandin synthesis by inhibiting the enzyme cyclooxygenase, enhancing adrenergic transmission by increasing norepinephrine release and suppressing inflammation that decreases central sensitization (Mathew, Dun & Luo, 2013). NSAIDs initiated 5 to 7 days before the onset of menstruation may decrease or eliminate the migraine (Tepper, 2013).

Triptans • Triptans are effective short-term prophylactic treatment for menstrual migraine (Hu, Guan, Fan, & Jin, 2013). The triptans are selective serotonin receptor agonists that interfere with migraine pathogenesis and are effective in relieving any associated neurovegetative symptoms (e.g., changes in sleeping patterns, mood, and appetite; Hu et al., 2013). The three most commonly used triptans are frovatriptan, naratriptan, and zolmitriptan. Triptans have been found to be more effective than placebo in preventing menstrual migraines and reduce their frequency (when treating 2–3 days before the onset of menstruation). Triptans and other adjunctive therapies, such as NSAIDs, estradiol, and topirmatate, are thought to increase the effectiveness by reducing or aborting menstrual migraines (Hu et al., 2013; Tepper, 2013).

Hormonal Therapies • The use of COCs may have differing effects on menstrual migraines. COCs are contraindicated in women who experience migraine attacks with aura. For some women, migraine with aura may present with the initiation of COCs. In this case, COCs should be discontinued.

Migraine Without Aura. There are several approaches to providing a sustained level of estrogen throughout the month by prescribing supplemental estradiol (e.g., hormonally active pills, transdermal application using a menstrual suppression strategy). These approaches are associated with overall reduction in migraine severity and frequency. Estrogen supplementation provided during menstruation includes: (a) oral (1 mg/d), (b) gel (1.5 mg/d), or (c) patch (moderate to high dose) delivery systems (Tepper, 2013).

Migraine With Aura. According to the *U.S. Medical Eligibility Criteria for Contraceptive Use 2010*, prescribing considerations for women with migraines are delineated by those with and without aura (CDC, 2010). COCs should *not* be prescribed for women suffering from migraine with aura as they may lead to further vascular risk such as stroke and SAH. The ideal treatment for migraine with aura is a nonhormonal method, with the copper intrauterine device (IUD; a long-acting reversible contraception [LARC] method) preferred.

■ DYSMENORRHEA

Definition and Scope

Dysmenorrhea is the most common gynecologic condition among reproductive-aged women and occurs in 45% to 95% of menstruating women (Kural, Noor, Pandit, Joshi, & Patil, 2015). Dysmenorrhea is an underdiagnosed condition consisting of painful menstruation. It often goes undiagnosed because many women dismiss the symptoms as a normal part of menstruation. More than one half of women who menstruate have some pain for 1 to 2 days each month (ACOG, 2015b). Although mild discomfort during menstruation is widely experienced by most women, actual dysmenorrhea is cyclic pain that prevents normal activity and requires medication (ACOG, 2015b). The pain is characterized as cramping or *labor-like* pain that begins with or just before the onset of menses and generally lasts for 2 to 3 days. The pain may be experienced in the lower abdomen and lower back and may radiate into the inner aspects of the thighs. There are two types of dysmenorrhea. An excess of prostaglandins leading to painful uterine muscle activity causes primary dysmenorrhea. Primary dysmenorrhea is associated with ovulatory cycles and does not usually occur until later in adolescence. It is estimated that 14% to 26% of adolescents have pain severe enough to cause them to miss school and work (ACOG, 2015b). Secondary dysmenorrhea is caused by a disorder of the reproductive tract (e.g., adenomyosis, endometriosis, PID, cervical stenosis, leiomyomas, and polyps); secondary dysmenorrhea tends to get worse over time (ACOG, 2015b).

Etiology

Primary dysmenorrhea is caused by excessive secretion of uterine prostaglandins, specifically prostaglandin F_2 ($PGF_{2\alpha}$), released from the endometrium during the menses. $PGF_{2\alpha}$ induces uterine contractions that can lead to uterine hypoxia. During the luteal phase of the menstrual cycle, declining levels of progesterone cause lysosomes to release a phospholipase enzyme, which in turn hydrolyzes cell membrane phospholipids to generate arachadonic acid.

Arachadonic acid serves as a precursor for the synthesis of prostaglandins. Prostaglandin synthesis is mediated by two isoforms of cyclooxygenase (COX-1 and COX-2), enzymes that convert arachadonic acid to several metabolites, including $PGF_{2\alpha}$. Higher concentrations of $PGF_{2\alpha}$ have been found in the menstrual fluid of women with dysmenorrhea (ACOG, 2015b). Intensity of menstrual cramps has been found to be directly related to the amount of $PGF_{2\alpha}$ released. The association between $PGF_{2\alpha}$ and dysmenorrhea is supported by three observations: (1) in anovulatory cycles without dysmenorrhea, menstrual fluid concentration of prostaglandins is not elevated; (2) intravenous injection of $PGF_{2\alpha}$ causes uterine cramps and pain; and (3) medications that inhibit prostaglandin secretion relieve dysmenorrhea (ACOG, 2015b). $PGF_{2\alpha}$ can also cause nausea, vomiting, diarrhea, headache, and dizziness, symptoms that are frequently associated with primary dysmenorrhea. Along with $PGF_{2\alpha}$, the uterus also produces prostaglandin E_2 (PGE_2), which has been implicated as a cause of primary menorrhagia, as it is a potent vasodilator and inhibitor of platelet aggregation (Beckmann et al., 2014).

Risk Factors

The scope and risk factors of primary dysmenorrhea are not fully understood. The most widely accepted reason of primary dysmenorrhea is the overproduction of uterine prostaglandins. Risk factors that are associated with primary dysmenorrhea include higher BMI, extreme ends of the reproductive years, and nulliparity. Menstrual and family history include early age of onset of menses, longer and heavier menstrual flow, and family history of dysmenorrhea. Lifestyle behaviors that have been linked to primary dysmenorrhea include smoking and alcohol consumption. The copper IUD may also be associated with increased menstrual pain, whereas the LNG-IUS tends to decrease menstrual pain. The most common causes of secondary dysmenorrhea have accompanying AUB associated with endometriosis, adenomyosis, or fibroids.

Symptoms

Primary dysmenorrhea usually begins early in the reproductive years and has a clear and predictable pattern, beginning before or at the start of menstruation. The pain typically lasts 8 to 72 hours and is most severe on the first day of menstruation. Systemic symptoms include nausea, vomiting, diarrhea, fatigue, and insomnia because of the pain (Beckmann et al., 2014). Secondary dysmenorrhea is often caused by endometriosis, but other causes include adenomyosis, leiomyomas, and PID. The initiation of the pain pattern can start anytime, but typically presents greater than 2 years after menarche. Often it is accompanied by AUB/HMB or AUB/IMB (Beckmann et al., 2014).

Evaluation/Assessment

HISTORY

Primary dysmenorrhea is a diagnosis of exclusion. A complete history and physical examination are needed to make an accurate diagnosis. A thorough history should include questions to determine when the pain occurs, how the patient treats the pain, if there are associated symptoms, how contraceptives affect the pain, and if the pain becomes more severe over time (ACOG, 2015b). The onset of primary dysmenorrhea in close proximity to menarche and the timing of the pain in relationship to the menses are key diagnostic features of primary dysmenorrhea. A contraceptive history should be obtained to rule out if an IUD, for example, may be the cause of menstrual pain. The onset of pain is typically the first day of menses, peaks in severity during the first 2 days of the menstrual cycle, and then decreases thereafter. Patients may also experience nausea, vomiting, diarrhea, and headache during these painful cycles.

A detailed medical history should reveal symptoms related to underlying gynecologic abnormalities, in turn informing the etiology of a woman's secondary dysmenorrhea. A woman diagnosed with adenomyosis, leiomyomata, or polyps may present with AUB/HMB with combined dysmenorrhea (Beckmann et al., 2014). Pelvic heaviness or changes in abdominal shape may suggest large leiomyomata or intra-abdominal neoplasia, whereas infection is usually associated with chills, malaise, and fever (Beckmann et al., 2014). Secondary dysmenorrhea accompanied by report of infertility raises the possibility of endometriosis or chronic PID (Beckmann et al., 2014).

PHYSICAL EXAMINATION

The physical examination of a symptomatic woman with dysmenorrhea is directed at discovering possible causes (Beckmann et al., 2014). Primary dysmenorrhea can only be diagnosed when the physical examination does not reveal pelvic diseases or other gynecologic abnormalities. Assessment may reveal generalized pelvic tenderness focused more in the area of the uterus than the adnexa, no palpable abnormalities of the uterus, and no abnormalities on speculum or abdominal examination (Beckmann et al., 2014). In some instances, diagnostic imaging may be indicated to rule out pelvic abnormalities and definitively diagnose primary dysmenorrhea.

The physical examination of patients with secondary dysmenorrhea varies depending on the causative pathology. Leiomyomata may cause pelvic asymmetry or irregular enlargement of the uterus. Findings on bimanual exam usually include an irregular-shaped immobile uterus, with either a firm or rubbery solid consistency (Beckmann et al., 2014). Although adenomyosis can only be definitively diagnosed by histologic examination, physical examination may reveal a uterus that is tender, symmetrically enlarged, and "boggy" (Beckmann et al., 2014). Endometriosis should be suspected when there are painful nodules in the posterior cul-de-sac and restricted motion of the uterus. If infection is suspected, a cervical culture should be collected and sent for ruling out STIs (*Neisseria gonorrhoeae* and *Chlamydia trachomatis*). More invasive procedures, such as laparoscopy, may be needed to make a confirmatory diagnosis.

Differential Diagnoses

In most cases, the final diagnosis can be reached by careful history and physical examination; in some instances,

a diagnostic laparoscopy may be needed for histological confirmation. Conditions to consider include processes outside the uterus (e.g., endometriosis, tumors, adhesions, and nongynecologic causes), those within the myometrium (e.g., adenomyosis, myomas), and conditions within the endometrium (e.g., myomas, endometrial polyps, infection, intrauterine contraceptive devices, cervical stenosis). When the patient continues to experience pain between menstrual periods, these conditions may be the source of her chronic pelvic pain.

Treatment/Management

The goal of treatment is to reduce the menstrual pain so that the woman's health and QOL improve. Once diagnosed, approaches to treatment and management include pharmacologic, nonpharmacologic, and surgical interventions.

INTEGRATIVE MEDICINE

Magnesium has been used to relieve primary dysmenorrhea although the ideal dose, type of magnesium (e.g., magnesium oxide, magnesium carbonate), and dosing regimen have not been clarified. Vitamin B_1 (100 mg daily) and vitamin E (100 mg daily) have been shown to reduce menstrual pain more effectively than placebo, although the evidence for their efficacy is limited (Tseng, Chen, & Yang, 2005). One study noted that adolescents who drank 2 teacups of rose tea 1 week before the onset and through the 5th day of their menses, reported less menstrual pain and distress at 1, 3, and 6 months, when compared with controls (Tseng et al., 2005).

Although there is no solid evidence to support it, there are studies to support the use of exercise as a way to reduce the severity of dysmenorrhea. A Cochrane Review of seven RCTs showed that high-frequency transcutaneous electrical nerve stimulation (TENS) is more effective for relieving menstrual pain when compared with the placebo group (Schiøtz, Jettestad, & Al-Heeti, 2007). Acupuncture has been shown to be somewhat effective in alleviating dysmenorrhea (ACOG, 2000/2013/2015). There is not enough evidence to recommend herbal and dietary therapies for dysmenorrhea, however, many home remedies may provide a certain level of relief for some women.

PHARMACOTHERAPEUTICS

Acetaminophen and NSAIDs are the most commonly prescribed medications for treatment of primary dysmenorrhea. When taken as prescribed, they are often very effective in providing pain relief. NSAIDs reduce pain by inhibiting prostaglandin synthesis and by their direct CNS analgesic effect. They reduce the amount of prostaglandins that the body makes and lessen their effect. For optimal efficacy, it is best to start NSAIDs 1 to 2 days before the anticipation of the onset of menses/pain, as their effectiveness for treating pain appears to decrease once menses has begun. Women are counseled to take both medications *as needed,* although if pain control is poor, the woman may benefit from regularly scheduled doses. Because of a long-standing history of safety and efficacy, OTC availability, and relative low cost, NSAIDs have become the treatment of choice for primary dysmenorrhea. Although adverse side effects occur infrequently with intermittent use of NSAIDs, health care providers should be aware that there is always a possibility and that therapy should discontinue. Women with coagulopathies, asthma, aspirin allergy, liver damage, peptic ulcer disease, or stomach disorders should not take NSAIDs (ACOG, 2000/2013/2015).

Cyclooxygenase inhibitors (COX-2 inhibitors), such as celecoxib, have been found to be effective in treating dysmenorrhea, although no studies have shown they are any better than naproxen. In the recent past, COX-2 inhibitors were becoming the NSAIDs of choice because of their specific and targeted action to treat dysmenorrhea. However, because of serious health and safety concerns, including life-threatening cardiovascular and GI adverse effects, they now are rarely used (Beckmann et al., 2014).

COCs containing estrogen and progestin can be used to treat dysmenorrhea in women who do not desire childbearing and who may not be able to tolerate NSAID therapy. By suppressing ovulation and stabilizing estrogen and progesterone levels, COCs lower the level of endometrial prostaglandins and reduce spontaneous uterine activity. COCs can be taken cyclically in the traditional 28-day schedule, or for more extended periods of time allowing for longer intervals between menses (Beckmann et al., 2014). Oftentimes dysmenorrhea can be completely eliminated by the continuous use of hormonal contraceptives (Beckmann et al., 2014). Hormonal contraceptives, as long as not contraindicated, may be given for more than 6 to 12 months. Many women continue to experience pain-free menses even after discontinuation of hormonal treatment. The pill, the patch, and the vaginal ring are options, along with progestin-only methods like the DMPA injection or an implantable intrauterine system (LNG-IUS). Oral contraceptives and NSAIDs are known to have a synergistic effect on menstrual pain caused by primary dysmenorrhea (Beckmann et al., 2014). They can be taken together to achieve pain relief, or alone.

Women who do not respond to acetaminophen, NSAID, and/or hormonal contraceptive therapy should be reevaluated for abnormalities associated with secondary dysmenorrhea. For conditions such as adenomyosis and when the woman wishes to preserve fertility, a definitive treatment plan may not be an option. Instead, a symptomatic treatment plan of analgesics or menstrual cycle modification may be most appropriate (Beckmann et al., 2014).

SURGICAL THERAPY

In women who do not respond to medical therapies, surgery may be indicated for definitive treatment. The type of surgical procedure is dependent on the underlying cause of pain as well as if fertility is desired. Laparoscopic uterosacral ligament division and presacral neurectomy may be indicated, although this is considered a conservative surgical therapy. There are, however, significant intraoperative risks, including injury to adjacent vascular structures and chronic constipation, which limit this as an option (Beckmann et al., 2014). A partial or total hysterectomy may eventually be required for treatment of adenomyosis, endometriosis, or residual pelvic infection that has not been responsive to medical treatments or even conservative surgical therapies.

■ FUTURE DIRECTIONS

The menstrual cycle is a natural process for women. However, the cyclic changes or structural anomalies can produce ill-effects and negatively impact women's lives. Management of the disorders covered in this chapter is an evolving science. Early recognition through genetic identification can tailor patient management of these conditions.

■ REFERENCES

American College of Obstetricians and Gynecologists (ACOG). (2000/2013/2015). *Management of abnormal uterine bleeding associated with ovulatory dysfunction.* ACOG Practice bulletin No. 136. *Obstetrics and Gynecology, 115,* 206–218. doi:10.1097/AOG.0b013e3181cb50b5

American College of Obstetricians and Gynecologists (ACOG). (2009). *von Willebrand disease in women.* Committee Opinion No. 451. *Obstetrics and Gynecology, 114,* 1439–1443.

American College of Obstetricians and Gynecologists (ACOG). (2010). *Noncontraceptive uses of hormonal contraceptives.* ACOG Practice bulletin No. 110. *Obstetrics & Gynecology, 115,* 206–218. doi:10.1097/AOG.0b013e3181cb50b5

American College of Obstetricians and Gynecologists (ACOG). (2012). *Diagnosis of abnormal uterine bleeding in reproductive-aged women.* ACOG Practice bulletin No. 128. *Obstetrics and Gynecology, 120,* 197–206. doi:10.1097/AOG.0b013e318262e320

American College of Obstetricians and Gynecologists (ACOG). (2013). *Management of acute abnormal uterine bleeding in nonpregnant reproductive-aged women.* ACOG committee opinion No. 557. *Obstetrics & Gynecology, 122,* 176–185. doi:10.1097/01.AOG.0000431815.52679.bb

American College of Obstetricians and Gynecologists (ACOG). (2014). Premenstrual syndrome. In *Guidelines for women's health care: A resource manual* (4th ed., pp. 607–613). Washington, DC: American College of Obstetricians and Gynecologists.

American College of Obstetricians and Gynecologists (ACOG). (2015a). *Menstruation in girls and adolescents: Using the menstrual cycle as a vital sign.* Committee Opinion No. 651. *Obstetrics & Gynecology, 126,* e143–e146.

American College of Obstetricians and Gynecologists (ACOG). (2015b). *Frequently asked questions gynecologic problems (FAQ 046) dysmenorrhea: Painful periods.* Retrieved from http://www.acog.org/Patients/FAQs/Dysmenorrhea-Painful-Periods

American Psychiatric Association (APA). (2013). *Diagnostic and statistical manual of mental disorders* (5th ed.). Arlington, VA: American Psychiatric Publishing.

Arentz, S., Abbott, J. A., Smith, C. A., & Bensoussan, A. (2014). Herbal medicine for the management of polycystic ovary syndrome (PCOS) and associated oligo/amenorrhoea and hyperandrogenism: A review of the laboratory evidence for effects with corroborative clinical findings. *BMC Complementary and Alternative Medicine, 14,* 511.

Association of Reproductive Health Professionals (ARHP). (n.d.). *Managing premenstrual symptoms.* Retrieved from http://www.arhp.org/Publications-and-Resources/Quick-Reference-Guide-for-Clinicians/PMS

Bajwa, Z. H., & Wootton, R. J. (2016). *Evaluation of headache in adults.* UpToDate. Retrieved from http://www.uptodate.com/contents/evaluation-of-headache-in-adults

Beckmann, C. R. B., Ling, F. W., Herbert, W. N. P., Laube, D. W., Smith, R. P., Casanova, R.,…Weiss, P. M. (2014). *Obstetrics and gynecology* (7th ed.). Baltimore, MD: Lippincott Williams & Wilkins.

Bellis, M. A., Downing, J., & Ashton, J. R. (2006). Adults at 12? Trends in puberty and their public health consequences. *Journal of Epidemiology and Community Health*, 60(11), 910–911.

Bertone-Johnson, E. R., Hankinson, S. E., Bendich, A., Johnson, S. R., Willett, W. C., & Manson, J. E. (2005). Calcium and vitamin D intake and risk of incident premenstrual syndrome. *Archives of Internal Medicine*, 165(11), 1246–1252.

Bettocchi, S., Ceci, O., Vicino, M., Marello, F., Impedovo, L., & Selvaggi, L. (2001). Diagnostic inadequacy of dilatation and curettage. *Fertility and Sterility*, 75(4), 803–805.

Black, K., Moore, P., & Fraser, I. S. (2013). *Gynaecological disorders*. In I. Symonds & S. Arulkumaran (eds.), *Essential obstetrics & gynaecology* (pp. 233–263). Oxford, UK: Elsevier.

Borenstein, J., Chiou, C. F., Dean, B., Wong, J., & Wade, S. (2005). Estimating direct and indirect costs of premenstrual syndrome. *Journal of Occupational and Environmental Medicine/American College of Occupational and Environmental Medicine*, 47(1), 26–33.

Bowkley, C. W., Dubel, G. J., Haas, R. A., Soares, G. M., & Ahn, S. H. (2007). Uterine artery embolization for control of life-threatening hemorrhage at menarche: Brief report. *Journal of Vascular and Interventional Radiology*, 18(1, Pt. 1), 127–131.

Braverman, P. K. (2007). Premenstrual syndrome and premenstrual dysphoric disorder. *Journal of Pediatric and Adolescent Gynecology*, 20(1), 3–12.

British Herbal Medicinal Association (BHMA). (1996). *British Herbal Pharmacopoeia*. Bristol, UK: British Herbal Medicine Association.

Brosens, J. J., de Souza, N. M., Barker, F. G., Paraschos, T., & Winston, R. M. (1995). Endovaginal ultrasonography in the diagnosis of adenomyosis uteri: Identifying the predictive characteristics. *British Journal of Obstetrics and Gynaecology*, 102(6), 471–474.

Calhoun, A. H. (2012). Current topics and controversies in menstrual migraine. *Headache*, 52(Suppl. 1), 8–11.

Centers for Disease Control and Prevention (CDC). (2010). US medical eligibility criteria for contraceptive use, 2010. *Morbidity and Mortality Weekly Report*, 59(No. RR-4), 1–86.

Chandru, S., Indusekhar, R., & O'Brien, S. (2011). Premenstrual syndrome. In R. W. Shaw, D. Leusley, & A. Monga (Eds.), *Gynaecology* (4th ed., pp. 391–404). Oxford, UK: Elsevier.

Charteris-Black, J., & Seale, C. (2010). *Gender and the language of illness*. New York, NY: Palgrave Macmillan.

Chen, N. N., Han, M., Yang, H., Yang, G. Y., Wang, Y. Y., Wu, X. K., & Liu, J. P. (2014). Chinese herbal medicine Guizhi Fuling formula for treatment of uterine fibroids: A systematic review of randomised clinical trials. *BMC Complementary and Alternative Medicine*, 14, 2.

Cho, S. H., & Kim, J. (2010). Efficacy of acupuncture in management of premenstrual syndrome: A systematic review. *Complementary Therapies in Medicine*, 18(2), 104–111.

El-Hamarneh, T., Hey-Cunningham, A. J., Berbic, M., Al-Jefout, M., Fraser, I. S., & Black, K. (2013). Cellular immune environment in endometrial polyps. *Fertility and Sterility*, 100(5), 1364–1372.

Ford, O., Lethaby, A., Roberts, H., & Mol, B. W. J. (2012). Progesterone for premenstrual syndrome. *The Cochrane Database of Systematic Reviews*, 2012(4). doi:10.1002/14651858.CD003415.pub2

Fox, K. E. (2012). Management of heavy menstrual bleeding in general practice. *Current Medical Research and Opinion*, 28(9), 1517–1525.

Freeman, E. W., Sammel, M. D., Lin, H., Rickels, K., & Sondheimer, S. J. (2011). Clinical subtypes of premenstrual syndrome and responses to sertraline treatment. *Obstetrics and Gynecology*, 118(6), 1293–1300.

Fritz, M. A. & Speroff, L. (2011). *Clinical gynecologic endocrinology and infertility*. Philadelphia, PA: Wolters Kluwer.

Gillings, M. R. (2014). Were there evolutionary advantages to premenstrual syndrome? *Evolutionary Applications*, 7(8), 897–904.

Girman, A., Lee, R., & Kligler, B. (2003). An integrative medicine approach to premenstrual syndrome. *American Journal of Obstetrics and Gynecology*, 188(Suppl. 5), S56–S65.

Gungorduk, K., Asicioglu, O., Ertas, I. E., Ozdemir, I. A., Ulker, M. M., Yildirim, G.,...Sanci, M. (2014). Comparison of the histopathological diagnoses of preoperative dilatation and curettage and Pipelle biopsy. *European Journal of Gynaecological Oncology*, 35(5), 539–543.

Habek, D., & Akšamija, A. (2014). Successful acupuncture treatment of uterine myoma. *Acta Clinica Croatica*, 53(4), 487–489.

Hamani, Y., Ben-Shachar, I., Kalish, Y., & Porat, S. (2010). Intrauterine balloon tamponade as a treatment for immune thrombocytopenic purpura-induced severe uterine bleeding. *Fertility and Sterility*, 94(7), 2769.e13–2769.e15.

Hartmann, K. E., Jerome, R. N., Lindegren, M. L., Potter, S. A., Shields, T. C., Surawicz, T. S., & Andrews, J. C. (2013). *Primary care management of abnormal uterine bleeding: Comparative effectiveness review No. 96*. (Prepared by the Vanderbilt Evidence-based Practice Center under Contract No. 290-2007-10065 I.) AHRQ Publication No. 13-EHC025-EF. Rockville, MD: Agency for Healthcare Research and Quality. Retrieved from www.effectivehealthcare.ahrq.gov/reports/final.cfm

Headache Classification Committee of the International Headache Society. (2013). The international classification of headache disorders (3rd ed., beta version). *Cephalalgia*, 33(9), 629–808.

Hoffman, J., & Recober, A. (2014). Migraine and triggers: Post hoc ergo propter hoc? *Current Pain and Headache Reports*, 17(10), 1–11.

Hu, Y., Guan, X., Fan, L., & Jin, L. (2013). Triptans in prevention of menstrual migraine: A systematic review with meta-analysis. *Journal of Headache and Pain*, 14, 7. doi:10.1186/1129-2377-14-7

James, A. H., Kouides, P. A., Abdul-Kadir, R., Dietrich, J. E., Edlund, M., Federici, A. B.,...Winikoff, R. (2011). Evaluation and management of acute menorrhagia in women with and without underlying bleeding disorders: Consensus from an international expert panel. *European Journal of Obstetrics, Gynecology, and Reproductive Biology*, 158(2), 124–134.

Jang, S. H., Kim, D. I., & Choi, M. S. (2014). Effects and treatment methods of acupuncture and herbal medicine for premenstrual syndrome/premenstrual dysphoric disorder: Systematic review. *BMC Complementary and Alternative Medicine*, 14. doi:10.1186/1472-6882-14-11

Johansson, J., Redman, L., Veldhuis, P. P., Sazonova, A., Labrie, F., Holm, G.,...Stener-Victorin, E. (2013). Acupuncture for ovulation induction in polycystic ovary syndrome: A randomized controlled trial. *American Journal of Physiology. Endocrinology and Metabolism*, 304(9), E934–E943.

Kadir, R. A., Lukes, A. S., Kouides, P. A., Fernandez, H., & Goudemand, J. (2005). Management of excessive menstrual bleeding in women with hemostatic disorders. *Fertility and Sterility*, 84(5), 1352–1359.

Kang, H. S., Jeong, D., Kim, D. I., & Lee, M. S. (2011). The use of acupuncture for managing gynaecologic conditions: An overview of systematic reviews. *Maturitas*, 68(4), 346–354.

Kazandi, M., Okmen, F., Ergenoglu, A. M., Yeniel, A. O., Zeybek, B., Zekioglu, O., & Ozdemir, N. (2012). Comparison of the success of histopathological diagnosis with dilatation-curettage and Pipelle endometrial sampling. *Journal of Obstetrics and Gynaecology: The Journal of the Institute of Obstetrics and Gynaecology*, 32(8), 790–794.

Klein, D. A., & Poth, M. A. (2013). Amenorrhea: An approach to diagnosis and management. *American Family Physician*, 87(11), 781–788.

Kural, M., Noor, N. N., Pandit, D., Joshi, T., & Patil, A. (2015). Menstrual characteristics and prevalence of dysmenorrhea in college going girls. *Journal of Family Medicine and Primary Care*, 4(3), 426–431.

Lee, S. C., Kaunitz, A. M., Sanchez-Ramos, L., & Rhatigan, R. M. (2010). The oncogenic potential of endometrial polyps: A systematic review and meta-analysis. *Obstetrics and Gynecology*, 116(5), 1197–1205.

Lethaby, A., Farquhar, C., & Cooke, I. (2000). Antifibrinolytics for heavy menstrual bleeding. *The Cochrane Database of Systematic Reviews*, 2000(4). Art No. CD000249. doi:10.1002/14651858.CD000249

Lethaby, A., Duckitt, K., & Farquhar, C. (2013). Non-steroidal anti-inflammatory drugs for heavy menstrual bleeding. *The Cochrane Database of Systematic Reviews*, 2013(1), CD000400.

Lethaby, A., Hussain, M., Rishworth, J. R., & Rees, M. C. (2015). Progesterone or progestogen-releasing intrauterine systems for heavy menstrual bleeding. *The Cochrane Database of Systematic Reviews*, 2015(4), CD002126.

Lieng, M., Istre, O., & Qvigstad, E. (2010). Treatment of endometrial polyps: A systematic review. *Acta Obstetricia Et Gynecologica Scandinavica*, 89(8), 992–1002.

Lobo, R. A. (2012). Abnormal uterine bleeding. In R. A. L. Gretchen, M. Lentz, D. M. Gershenson, & V. L. Katz (Eds.), *Comprehensive gynecology* (6th ed., pp. 805–814). Philadelphia, PA: Elsevier Mosby.

Lopez, A., Cacoub, P., Macdougall, I. C., & Peyrin-Biroulet, L. (2015). Iron deficiency anemia. *Lancet*, 387(10021), 907–916. doi:10.1016/S0140-6736(15)60865-0

Lopez, L. M., Kaptein, A. A., & Helmerhorst, F. M. (2012). Oral contraceptives containing drospirenone for premenstrual syndrome. *The*

Cochrane Database of Systematic Reviews, 2012(2). doi:10.1002/14651858.CD006586.pub4

Lukes, A. S., Moore, K. A., Muse, K. N., Gersten, J. K., Hecht, B. R., Edlund, M.,...Shangold, G. A. (2010). Tranexamic acid treatment for heavy menstrual bleeding: A randomized controlled trial. *Obstetrics and Gynecology, 116*(4), 865–875.

Madhra, M., Fraser, I. S., Munro, M. G., & Critchley, H. O. (2014). Abnormal uterine bleeding: Advantages of formal classification to patients, clinicians and researchers. *Acta Obstetricia Et Gynecologica Scandinavica, 93*(7), 619–625.

Maliqueo, M., Benrick, A., Alvi, A., Johansson, J., Sun, M., Labrie, F.,...Stener-Victorin, E. (2015). Circulating gonadotropins and ovarian adiponectin system are modulated by acupuncture independently of sex steroid or ß-adrenergic action in a female hyperandrogenic rat model of polycystic ovary syndrome. *Molecular and Cellular Endocrinology, 412*, 159–169.

Marsh, C. A., & Grimstad, F. W. (2014). Primary amenorrhea: Diagnosis and management. *Obstetrical & Gynecological Survey, 69*(10), 603–612.

Mathew, P. G., Dun, E. C., & Luo, J. J. (2013). A cyclic pain: The pathophysiology and treatment of menstrual migraine. *Obstetrical & Gynecological Survey, 68*(2), 130–140.

Matteson, K. A., Munro, M. G., & Fraser, I. S. (2011). The structured menstrual history: Developing a tool to facilitate diagnosis and aid in symptom management. *Seminars in Reproductive Medicine, 29*(5), 423–435.

Matteson, K. A., Raker, C. A., Clark, M. A., & Frick, K. D. (2013). Abnormal uterine bleeding, health status, and usual source of medical care: Analyses using the Medical Expenditures Panel Survey. *Journal of Women's Health (2002), 22*(11), 959–965.

Matteson, K. A., Raker, C. A., Pinto, S. B., Scott, D. M., & Frishman, G. N. (2012). Women presenting to an emergency facility with abnormal uterine bleeding: Patient characteristics and prevalence of anemia. *Journal of Reproductive Medicine, 57*(1–2), 17–25.

Matzkin, E., Curry, E. J., & Whitlock, K. (2015). Female athlete triad: Past, present, and future. *Journal of the American Academy of Orthopaedic Surgeons, 23*(7), 424–432.

Munro, M. G., Critchley, H. O., Broder, M. S., & Fraser, I. S.; FIGO Working Group on Menstrual Disorders. (2011). FIGO classification system (PALM-COEIN) for causes of abnormal uterine bleeding in nongravid women of reproductive age. *International Journal of Gynaecology and Obstetrics: The Official Organ of the International Federation of Gynaecology and Obstetrics, 113*(1), 3–13.

Munro, M. G., Critchley, H. O., & Fraser, I. S.; FIGO Menstrual Disorders Working Group. (2011). The FIGO classification of causes of abnormal uterine bleeding in the reproductive years. *Fertility and Sterility, 95*(7), 2204–2208, 2208.e1.

Munro, M. G., & Lukes, A. S.; Abnormal Uterine Bleeding and Underlying Hemostatic Disorders Consensus Group. (2005). Abnormal uterine bleeding and underlying hemostatic disorders: Report of a consensus process. *Fertility and Sterility, 84*(5), 1335–1337.

Naftalin, J., Hoo, W., Pateman, K., Mavrelos, D., Foo, X., & Jurkovic, D. (2014). Is adenomyosis associated with menorrhagia? *Human Reproduction, 29*(3), 473–479.

National Institute for Health and Care Excellence (NICE). (2007). *Heavy menstrual bleeding: Assessment and management.* London, UK: RCOG Press.

Nevatte, T., O'Brien, P. M., Bäckström, T., Brown, C., Dennerstein, L., Endicott, J.,...Consensus Group of the International Society for Premenstrual Disorders. (2013). ISPMD consensus on the management of premenstrual disorders. *Archives of Women's Mental Health, 16*(4), 279–291.

Newman, L. C., & Yugrakh, M. S. (2014). Menstrual migraine: Treatment options. *Neurological Sciences, 35*(Suppl. 1), S57–S60. doi:10.1007/s10072-014-1743-3

Nichols, C. M., & Gill, E. J. (2002). Thermal balloon endometrial ablation for management of acute uterine hemorrhage. *Obstetrics and Gynecology, 100* (5, Pt. 2), 1092–1094.

Pakalnis, A., & Gladstein, J. (2010). Headache and hormones. *Seminars in Pediatric Neurology, 17*, 100–104. doi:10.1016/j.spen.2010.04.007

Parashar, R., Bhalla, P., Rai, N. K., Pakhare, A., & Babbar, R. (2014). Migraine: Is it related to hormonal disturbances or stress? *International Journal of Women's Health, 6*, 921–925.

Practice Committee of American Society for Reproductive Medicine. (2008). Current evaluation of amenorrhea. *Fertility and Sterility, 90*, S219–S225. doi:10.1016/j.fertnstert.2008.08.038

Sacco, S., Ricci, S., Degan, D., & Carolei, A. (2012). Migraine in women: The role of hormones and their impact on vascular diseases. *Journal of Headache and Pain, 13*(3), 177–189.

Salim, S., Won, H., Nesbitt-Hawes, E., Campbell, N., & Abbott, J. (2011). Diagnosis and management of endometrial polyps: A critical review of the literature. *Journal of Minimally Invasive Gynecology, 18*(5), 569–581.

Schiøtz, H. A., Jettestad, M., & Al-Heeti, D. (2007). Treatment of dysmenorrhoea with a new TENS device (OVA). *Journal of Obstetrics and Gynaecology: The Journal of the Institute of Obstetrics and Gynaecology, 27*(7), 726–728.

Schumacher, U., Schumacher, J., Mellinger, U., Cerlinger, C., Wienke, A., & Endrikat, J. (2012). Estimation of menstrual blood loss volume based on menstrual diary and laboratory data. *BMC Women's Health, 12*, 24. doi:10.1186/1472-6874-12-24

Shaik, M. M., & Gan, S. H. (2015). Vitamin supplementation a possible prophylactic treatment against migraine with aura and menstrual migraine. *BioMed Research International.* Retrieved from http://dx.doi.org/10.1155/2015/469529

Shah, N. R., Jones, J. B., Aperi, J., Shemtov, R., Karne, A., & Borenstein, J. (2008). Selective serotonin reuptake inhibitors for premenstrual syndrome and premenstrual dysphoric disorder: A meta-analysis. *Obstetrics and Gynecology, 111*(5), 1175–1182.

Sharp, H. T. (2006). Assessment of new technology in the treatment of idiopathic menorrhagia and uterine leiomyomata. *Obstetrics & Gynecologists, 108*, 990–1003.

Singh, S., Best, C., Dunn, S., Leyland, N., Wolfman, W. L., Leyland, N.,... Clinical Practice—Gynaecology Committee; Society of Obstetricians and Gynaecologists of Canada. (2013). Abnormal uterine bleeding in pre-menopausal women. *Journal of Obstetrics and Gynaecology Canada: JOGC = Journal D'obsteTrique Et GyneCologie Du Canada, 35*(5), 473–479.

Singh, S. S., & Belland, L. (2015). Contemporary management of uterine fibroids: Focus on emerging medical treatments. *Current Medical Research and Opinion, 31*(1), 1–12.

Smith, C. A., & Carmady, B. (2010). Acupuncture to treat common reproductive health complaints: An overview of the evidence. *Autonomic Neuroscience: Basic & Clinical, 157*(1–2), 52–56.

Smith, R. P., & Netter, F. H. (2008). *Netter's obstetrics and gynecology.* Philadelphia, PA: Saunders Elsevier.

Speroff, L., & Fritz, M. A. (2005). *Clinical gynecologic endocrinology and infertility* (7th ed.). Philadelphia, PA: Lippincott Williams & Wilkins.

Sweet, M. G., Schmidt-Dalton, T. A., Weiss, P. M., & Madsen, K. P. (2012). Evaluation and management of abnormal uterine bleeding in premenopausal women. *American Family Physician, 85*(1), 35–43.

Taylor, D. (2005). Perimenstrual symptoms and syndromes: Guidelines for symptom management and self-care. *Advanced Studies in Medicine, 5*, 228–241.

Taylor, D., Schuiling, K. D., & Sharp, B. A. (2006). Menstrual cycle pain and discomforts. In K. D. Schuiling & F. E. Likis (Eds.), *Women's gynecologic health.* Boston, MA: Jones & Bartlett.

Tepper, D. E. (2013). Menstrual migraine. *Journal of Head and Face Pain, 2014*, 403–404. doi:10.111/head.12279

Tseng, Y. F., Chen, C. H., & Yang, Y. H. (2005). Rose tea for relief of primary dysmenorrhea in adolescents: A randomized controlled trial in Taiwan. *Journal of Midwifery & Women's Health, 50*(5), e51–e57.

Vetvik, K. G., Benth, J. Š., MacGregor, E. A., Lundqvist, C., & Russell, M. B. (2015). Menstrual versus non-menstrual attacks of migraine without aura in women with and without menstrual migraine. *Cephalalgia: An International Journal of Headache, 35*(14), 1261–1268.

Zhang, Y., Peng, W., Clarke, J., & Liu, Z. (2010). Acupuncture for uterine fibroids. *The Cochrane Database of Systematic Reviews, 2010*(1), CD007227. doi:10.1002/14651858.CD007221.pub2D007221.pub2

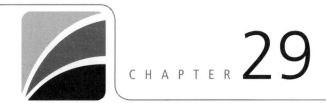

CHAPTER 29

Urologic and Pelvic Floor Health Problems

Richard S. Bercik • Cherrilyn F. Richmond

Urologic and pelvic floor health problems, including issues such as prolapse, urinary incontinence (UI), interstitial cystitis (IC), and urinary tract infections (UTIs), can significantly reduce quality of life (QOL) for women. Accurate identification and management are critical to prevent untoward sequelae and to sustain high QOL.

■ PELVIC ORGAN PROLAPSE

Pelvic relaxation disorders (also referred to as pelvic organ prolapse) is the term used to describe clinical manifestations of damaged or weakened support mechanisms in the female pelvis. Pelvic organ prolapse includes disorders of the anterior vaginal compartment (cystocele and urethrocele), the posterior vaginal compartment (rectocele), the apical compartment (uterus or posthysterectomy vaginal vault), the rectovaginal space (enterocele), and the perineum (Weber et al., 2000).

Women who experience pelvic organ prolapse have symptoms that can be mild to severe and can alter their QOL. Evaluation of the problem, degree of bother, and possibilities for management are individualized for each woman.

Etiology

An understanding of the anatomy of pelvic support is essential to understanding pelvic organ prolapse and its management. Pelvic organ support is maintained by a combination of pelvic musculature and connective tissue. The uterosacral and cardinal ligaments comprised mostly of smooth muscle, vascular elements, and loosely organized collagen fibers are responsible for uterine and apical support. They merge with the ring of pericervical fascia either posteriorly (uterosacral) or laterally (cardinal). These are the main structures of uterine support as the round ligaments do not contribute in any significant way to uterine support (DeLancey, 1994). The anterior endopelvic fascia extends distally from the pericervical ring to the perineal membrane and laterally to the arcus tendineus fascia pelvis (ATFP; Weber & Walters, 1997). The lateral margin of the vagina is attached to the sidewall at the ATFP, which extends from the ischial spine anteriorly to the pubovesical ligament (DeLancey, 1994). Anterior compartment prolapse can occur either from defects in these attachments (paravaginal defect) or disruption of the vaginal muscularis (central cystocele; Ashton-Miller & DeLancey, 2007).

Posteriorly, a true fascial layer has been identified between the rectum and vagina; this layer has been identified not only in adult cadavers, but also in newborns and is derived from mesenchymal differentiation (Ashton-Miller & DeLancey, 2007). Posterior prolapse results from defects in this layer which can occur laterally, centrally, or in combination. Enteroceles form because of a defect in the superior portion of this layer (Lukacz & Luber, 2002; Segal & Karram, 2002). The levator muscle complex is also integral to maintaining pelvic organ support. Composed of the puborectalis, pubococcygeus, and iliococcygeus muscles, this complex forms a sheet of muscular support for the pelvic viscera (Ashton-Miller & DeLancey, 2007; DeLancey et al., 2007). This structure extends from pelvic sidewall to sidewall and encircles the urethra, vagina, and rectum establishing the genital hiatus. Enlargement of the genital hiatus occurs during vaginal childbirth, and while it will often approach predelivery diameters postpartum, residual changes persist after delivery. With aging, time, abdominal pressures, and hypoestrogenic conditions the levator is prone to further loss of tone and resultant pathologic widening of the genital hiatus. When this occurs pelvic organ prolpase often results, as connective tissue support can no longer compensate for levator muscle weakness.

Definition and Scope

Prevalence of pelvic organ prolapse disorders increases with age, so that as the population older than 65 years continues to increase so will the demand for the evaluation and management of pelvic organ prolapse. Approximately 200,000 women undergo more than 300,000 inpatient procedures for pelvic organ prolapse in the United States each year, and one in nine American women will have a surgical procedure for pelvic organ prolapse or UI throughout their lifetime (MacLennan, Taylor, Wilson, & Wilson, 2000).

Pelvic organ prolapse is generally considered a disorder that occurs in White, parous, postmenopausal women; however, these preconceptions have been proven false. Although pelvic organ prolapse affects all women, exact incidence is difficult to establish because the dividing line between normal parous support and pelvic organ prolapse is difficult to define. Some degree of descent occurs in most women who have experienced vaginal childbirth, and yet the vast majority of these women have no symptoms.

Pelvic organ relaxation is commonly seen in about 50% of parous women and 40% of women aged 45 to 85 years can have stage 2 prolapse (Deger, Menzin, & Mikuta, 1993; Rortveit et al., 2007). Formal graded pelvic examinations (pelvic organ prolapse quantification [POPQ]) performed on a population of gynecologic patients revealed that 2.6% of the women had stage 3 prolapse (within 1 cm of introitus) and none had stage 4 prolapse (Drutz & Alarab, 2006).

The rate of vaginal vault prolapse after hysterectomy is reported to range from 0.5% to 1.5% (Swift et al., 2005). Aging of the population will further increase the number of women affected; it has been estimated that by the age of 80 years, approximately 11% of the female population will have had a corrective procedure for either pelvic organ prolapse or UI (Swift et al., 2005).

In 1999, the International Continence Society published a consensus statement on standardizing terminology related to lower urinary tract function (Weber et al., 2001). In general, pelvic organ prolapse is defined as descent of the pelvic structures to a degree which interferes with organ function, causes distress (emotional or physical) to the patient, creates a life-threatening condition, or significantly interferes with everyday activity. Pelvic organ prolapse is described by the location of key anatomical structures, in relation to fixed points such as the ischial spines and the hymenal ring. Physical examination is the main tool to describe the affected segments and the points of maximal prolapse. Terms such as cystocele, rectocele, and enterocele are avoided because of their lack of descriptive quality. Preferably, terms such as "anterior vaginal wall," "posterior vaginal wall," "vaginal apex," and "genital hiatus" are used in conjunction with standardized measurements. Nine specific points or measurements comprise the POPQ. Listed here are the pelvic relaxation disorders (with their previously used terminology).

ANTERIOR VAGINAL WALL PROLAPSE

Anterior vaginal wall prolapse (previously referred to as cystocele) is the inferior and ventral displacement of the anterior vaginal wall (and possibly bladder) caused by an anterior pelvic support defect. This may be because of a midline (central) defect in the vesicovaginal connective tissue or a lateral (paravaginal) defect, which involves a detachment of the vagina from the ATFP.

HYPERMOBILE URETHRA

Hypermobile urethra (previously referred to as urethrocele) is a significant downward rotation (more than 35°) of the distal anterior vaginal wall caused by a defect in the suburethral connective tissue and pubourethral (pubovisceral) ligaments.

APICAL VAGINAL PROLAPSE

Apical vaginal prolapse (previously referred to as enterocele) results in uterine prolapse, or if the uterus is absent, vaginal cuff prolapse. A defect in uterosacral and cardinal ligament support (type I) is thought to be the mechanism for this prolapse.

POSTERIOR VAGINAL WALL PROLAPSE

Posterior vaginal wall prolapse (previously referred to as rectocele) is the ventral and superior displacement of the posterior vaginal wall (and possibly the distal rectum and anus) caused by a defect in the rectovaginal connective tissue.

Risk Factors

Gender, aging, and childbirth are the most significant risk factors for pelvic organ prolapse. Prolonged labor followed by cesarean delivery does not protect a woman from pelvic relaxation (Gimbel et al., 2003; Jelovsek, Maher, & Barber, 2007). Nulliparity protects against pelvic organ prolapse only until menopause. As nulliparous women progress further beyond menopause, the incidence of pelvic organ prolapse continues to rise and probably equals that of a parous female at age 75 years (Richter, 2006). Twenty percent of the Women's Health Initiative population had some degree of pelvic organ prolapse (Jelovsek et al., 2007).

Modifiable risk factors include weight, smoking status, avoidance of constipation, and maintaining good physical conditioning. Therefore, it is possible for lifestyle interventions to reduce the lifetime risk for pelvic organ prolapse. These interventions include avoiding constipation, avoiding chronic heavy lifting, avoiding chronic coughing associated with smoking, maintaining a healthy weight, and maintaining the strength of the striated muscles of the pelvic floor. Examples of nonmodifiable factors include congenitally acquired connective tissue abnormalities, aging, and menopause (Jelovsek et al., 2007; Nieminen, Huhtala, & Heinonen, 2003; Nygaard, Bradley, & Brandt, 2004; Tegerstedt, Miedel, Maehle-Schmidt, Nyrén, & Hammarström, 2006).

Symptoms

Symptoms of pelvic organ prolapse are varied and at times nonspecific. Usually, symptoms are related to the degree of prolapse and the predominant compartment affected (Santaniello et al., 2007). Patients with vaginal prolapse often do not complain of any symptoms until the prolapse has progressed to stage 3 (i.e., the leading point of prolapse is within 1 cm of the vaginal introitus). At this point, patients often complain of a vaginal protrusion or bulge first noticed while bathing (Burrows, Meyn, Walters, & Weber, 2004; Digesu, Chaliha, Salvatore, Hutchings, & Khullar, 2005).

Stage 1 and 2 prolapse may have few to no symptoms. At this stage, the leading point of prolapse is not yet 1 cm beyond of the hymenal ring. Early symptoms of stage 1 and 2 prolapse include lower back pain, pelvic heaviness or fullness, vaginal pain, and pain during intercourse. Urinary complaints may include urinary urgency, hesitancy, and UI or anorgasmia during sexual activity. Rectal frequency and urgency alternating with bouts of constipation are common. In general, symptoms worsen with increased physical activity and/or prolonged standing (Drutz & Alarab, 2006; Fitzgerald et al., 2006; Richter et al., 2007).

Stage 3 prolapse consists of the leading point of prolapse to be more than 1 cm beyond the hymenal ring but not yet completely prolapsed. At this point, patients will often complain of being able to feel the organs descending into or beyond the vagina. Often patients are unable to engage in sexual activity at this point. There is difficulty using tampons and pain with sitting or prolonged walking as the vaginal protrusion progresses. Symptoms of obstructive urination often worsen at this stage so that incomplete bladder emptying, postvoid dribbling, excessive straining to void, or the need to manually reduce the prolapse to void ("digital splinting") might arise. Similarly, symptoms associated with obstructive defecation might be problematic at this point. Constipation, rectal straining, and need to digitally splint to defecate can occur (Drutz & Alarab, 2006; Kahn et al., 2005; Mouritsen & Larsen, 2003; Swift et al., 2005; Weber & Richter, 2005). Symptoms associated with this stage are often quite distressing to the patient, prompting the patient to seek treatment.

Stage 4 prolapse consists of complete prolapse of one or more vaginal components. After hysterectomy this consists of complete vaginal eversion with enterocele. Pain is often present because of mucosal drying, erosion, and ulceration combined with persistent rubbing of the prolapse as the patients perform everyday activity. Symptoms of obstructive voiding worsen so that urinary retention is usually present. Advanced cases may result in urinary retention with urethral obstruction or ureteral blockage resulting in hydroureter, hydronephrosis, and subsequent renal damage. These patients may require an indwelling bladder catheter or learn to perform clean intermittent self-catheterization (CISC). Urinary infection risk is increased and at times urosepsis may be the presenting symptom.

Women with advanced pelvic organ prolapse often do not complain of UI. They may have a normal urethral continence mechanism, but also may have occult stress incontinence (also labeled potential or masked stress urinary incontinence [SUI]). This occurs because urethral kinking increases urethral resistance leading to obstruction which then masks an incontinent urethral mechanism. Recent data indicate that this may occur in as many as 33% of patients with advanced pelvic organ prolapse (Burrows et al., 2004; Davis & Kumar, 2005).

Evaluation/Assessment

HISTORY

In addition to obtaining a history regarding symptoms of urinary, defecatory, and sexual dysfunction, a complete history is needed to determine possible medical comorbidities. Measures of the impact of symptoms on the patient's QOL also must be completed.

Obstetric history, including a review of pregnancies and deliveries, is essential. Include route of delivery, number of deliveries, length of labor and second stage, birth weights, operative deliveries, episiotomy with or without laceration, and presence of any postpartum incontinence (anal and urinary). If applicable, a thorough review of perimenopause and menopause-related symptoms and history is completed. Specifically, time since the last menstrual period, a timeline of menopause-related symptoms and problems associated with vaginal atrophy (e.g., pain, dryness, discharge, and dyspareunia) are considered. The medical history must be complete and specifically address the presence of diabetes, any neurological disorders, changes in mental status, and medications. Surgical history with specific questions regarding hysterectomy (route and indication), oophorectomy, any vaginal surgery, prior surgery for pelvic organ prolapse and/or UI must also be complete. Social history includes caffeine and alcohol intake, occupation, marital status, sexual activity, and living environment. The last item, living environment, is particularly important for the geriatric patient; for example, physical obstruction to bathroom facilities is problematic. Finally, family history with attention to pelvic organ prolapse, urinary or fecal incontinence, collagen diseases, and early menopause should be documented.

Many patients with pelvic organ prolapse do complain of UI. In general, detecting UI by history has a high sensitivity but low specificity. It is further complicated by the fact that 10% to 30% of patients with stress UI also have overactive bladder UI. In patients with pure stress UI symptoms, 65% to 90% will have stress UI on urodynamic testing. If urge incontinence, enuresis, and sensory urgency are present, 80% to 85% will have overactive bladder identified on urodynamic testing (Helström & Nilsson, 2005; Fitzgerald & Brubaker, 2002; Reena, Kekre, & Kekre, 2007). Historical items to obtain are in Box 29.1.

PHYSICAL EXAMINATION

The physical examination includes a general examination to identify any undiagnosed cardiac, pulmonary, gastrointestinal, or other disorders. Pelvic examination includes close inspection of the vulva and vagina with attention to potential epithelial lesions (see Chapter 27). Any ulcers or suspicious lesions should be biopsied. Evaluation of the genital hiatus (introitus) is done both at rest and with straining. Note the thickness of the perineal body and look for a "dovetail" sign indicating a nonintact external anal sphincter. During the digital rectal examination assess external anal sphincter tone (four grades; see Box 29.2).

A focused neurological examination is performed, including evaluation of sensory function of the sacral

BOX 29.1   HISTORY FOR UI

Severity

1. How often do "accidents" occur?
2. Do you leak urine when you cough, laugh, or sneeze?
3. Do you wear pads/protection?
4. If yes, how many pads/day?
5. Does this problem interfere with your social life or work?

Infection, Malignancy

1. Do you have a history of bladder or kidney infections?
2. Do you have pain or discomfort on urination?
3. Have you ever had blood in your urine?

Voiding Dysfunction

1. Is the urine stream slow or intermittent?
2. Do you have to strain to get the urine out?
3. After urination, do you have dribbling or a sensation that your bladder is still full?

Urge/Detrusor Instability

1. Do you ever have an uncomfortable need to rush to the bathroom to urinate?
2. If yes, do you ever have an "accident" before you reach the toilet?
3. How many times during the day do you urinate?
4. How many times do you get up from sleep to urinate?
5. When in a hurry or under stress, do you feel an urgent need to urinate?
6. Have you had any episodes of wetting the bed?
7. Do you ever have leakage during intercourse?

BOX 29.2   SPHINCTER TONE GRADING

1. No squeeze felt
2. Squeeze felt minimally around finger
3. Squeeze felt less than 50% finger circumference
4. Squeeze felt more than 50% finger circumference and held for longer than 2 seconds

BOX 29.3   PELVIC ORGAN PROLAPSE QUANTIFICATION MEASUREMENTS

1, 2. Two along the anterior wall
3, 4. Two along the posterior
   5. Location of the cervix (or cuff if uterus is absent)
   6. Location of the posterior fornix
   7. Size of the genital hiatus
   8. Thickness of the perineal body
   9. Total vaginal length

reflex (contraction of external anal sphincter noted when stroking of the labia majora or clitoris [also referred to as the "anal wink"]).

The speculum examination focuses on vaginal support. Inspect the lateral vaginal fornices looking for obliteration of sulci, indicating a paravaginal defect. Note the presence or absence of vaginal rugae. Smooth vaginal epithelium points to a fascial defect in that area. Split speculum examination, using only the posterior blade, is very helpful in determining what compartment is prolapsing. Depression of the posterior wall aids inspection of the anterior compartment and splinting a prolapsed anterior vaginal wall will allow for visualization of a posterior defect. Bimanual pelvic examination includes assessment of levator tone both at rest and with contraction. During rectal examination, palpation of the anal sphincter is done to determine any defects. Additionally, the patient is asked to contract the anal sphincter to assess tone (Box 29.2).

The examiner must determine the point of maximal prolapse for each vaginal compartment. This can be done in one of several ways. Traction may be applied at the point of prolapse; this is only possible with uterine prolapse. Examining the patient while she stands and bears down (Valsalva maneuver) will usually confirm the full extent of prolapse. This is readily performed by having the patient place one foot on a low stool while the examiner palpates the vaginal walls during the maneuver. It is helpful to have the patient confirm that the extent of the protrusion seen by the examiner is as extensive as that which she has experienced. The patient may use a small handheld mirror to view the protrusion during this process. This examination is especially important if the supine examination is not consistent with the woman's history.

The International Continence Society approved a standard system to measure pelvic organ prolapse. The POPQ system evaluates nine measurements (see Box 29.3).

The POPQ system has many advantages. It is easily learned, is a standardized approach using the introitus as a reference point, and is reproducible from observer to observer (Chiarelli, Brown, & McElduff, 1999; Kelly, 2003). While evaluating the prolapse, clinicians should, at a minimum, measure the points along the anterior wall, the posterior wall, and the cervix that prolapse the furthest. The reference for these points is the hymenal ring, which is considered "zero" location. Points proximal to the hymen

dermatomes, perineal area, and the lower extremities. Motor function of the lower extremities, including extension and flexion of the hip, knee, and ankle, and inversion/eversion of each foot is also assessed. Be sure to check the patellar and ankle reflexes, as well as the bulbocavernosus are designated negative, while those beyond the hymen are positive. For example, a cervix that advances to 1 cm proximal to the hymen is at –1 position, while if it were 3 cm beyond the hymen, the prolapse would be designated +3. Points of maximal prolapse for the anterior and posterior vaginal walls can also be so documented. These measurements provide a standard system to quantify the degree of prolapse (Muir, Stepp, & Barber, 2003; Weber et al., 2001).

Diagnostic Studies

LABORATORY EVALUATION

Urinalysis and culture and sensitivity to rule out UTI are performed on all patients. Consider blood urea nitrogen (BUN), creatine, estimated glomerular filtration rate (eGFR), calcium, and glucose if there is any suspicion of renal compromise. Urine cytology is performed for patients older than 50 years of age who have irritative bladder symptoms (e.g., urgency, frequency) or hematuria with a negative urine culture. Cytology has a sensitivity of 40% to 50% and specificity greater than 90%. Referral for cystoscopy is indicated for acute onset of irritative symptoms without infection, positive cytology, or unexplained hematuria with a negative culture. Microscopic hematuria with three or greater red blood cells (RBCs) per high power field on a properly collected specimen should be investigated (Ghibaudo & Hocke, 2005).

CLINICAL TESTING

All patients should be screened for UTI, have their postvoid residual (PVR) measured, and have simple cystometric studies done. The PVR is measured within 15 minutes of voiding (measure voided volume). This can be done by bladder catheterization or by using a dedicated ultrasound unit configured for bladder volume measurement. There is no mutually agreed on volume that constitutes an abnormal PVR. Most investigators agree that less than 50 mL is normal and that greater than 200 mL is abnormal. The International Continence Society (ICS) states that the PVR should be less than 25% of the total bladder volume (PVR/PVR+ voided volume less than 0.25; Chiarelli et al., 1999; Helström & Nilsson, 2005; Mouritsen, 2005).

Simple cystometric evaluation includes retrograde filling of the bladder in 50-mL increments with room temperature saline. This can be done with a 50-mL irrigation syringe and catheter. To perform a simple cystometry, after the patient has voided and the volume has been recorded, place the patient in the supine position. The patient is then catheterized and the PVR noted. The catheter is left in place and a 60-mL bulb syringe is attached to the end of the catheter. Remove the bulb from the top of the syringe and begin filling it with 50 mL of fluid. Record the volume at which the patient first has the sensation of bladder filling (S1), the first urge to void (S2), and the maximum volume of filling that the patient is able to tolerate (S3). Look for sudden elevation of the fluid level in the syringe that may indicate bladder spasm. Normal ranges for S1, S2, and S3 are 90 to 150 mL, 200 to 300 mL, and 300 to 600 mL, respectively. Once the bladder is full, have the patient cough and observe

for stress incontinence. If negative, repeat this maneuver while reducing any anterior prolapse in order to identify occult stress incontinence. The clinician should be careful to avoid urethral compression while doing this. Finally, measuring voiding time and voided volume is a simple way to screen for voiding disorders. Average flow should be greater than 10 mL/sec. Reduced flow rates may indicate a voiding dysfunction, which is an indication for follow-up, complex, multichannel, urodynamic studies.

URODYNAMICS

Urodynamic testing is not necessary in all patients, but there are certain situations when it can be particularly helpful. When occult UI is identified and surgical correction is planned for presumed stress UI, it is important to confirm with urodynamic testing which type of incontinence is present. This ensures that surgery is appropriate. Conversely, it can be useful to repeat urodynamics postoperatively if surgical correction has failed to diagnose new reasons for incontinence. Urge symptoms may be exacerbated postoperatively because of manipulation of the bladder. Alternatively, nerve injury could contribute to a neurogenic component of urinary voiding dysfunction. The desire to understand the etiology of incontinent episodes is also sufficient indication for urodynamic testing.

There are multiple components of urodynamic testing. Cystometry is the study of the bladder pressures and volumes during both the filling and storage phase. A simple office version (see simple cystometry described earlier) or a computerized multichannel cystometry can be performed. Indications for multichannel cystometry are found in Box 29.4.

A pressure flow study evaluates bladder function by correlating pressure and flow during voiding. This study (also referred to as a CMG-Uroflow) is helpful when evaluating voiding dysfunction.

Uroflometry is the study of urinary flow rates. A normal urinary stream should rise quickly but steadily. Flow should then be maintained at a constant rate for a period, followed

---

BOX 29.4 INDICATIONS FOR MULTICHANNEL CYSTOMETRY

1. Mixed incontinence symptoms
2. Symptoms of overactive bladder not responsive to therapy
3. Inconclusive simple cystometry results
4. Recurrent incontinence
5. Neurological signs/symptoms
6. Urinary retention
7. Continuous leakage
8. Low volume stress UI or workup before surgery for UI
9. Previous radiation therapy or radical surgery
10. Previous anti-incontinence surgery

by a brisk, but not abrupt decline in flow. Simple uroflow can be done by measuring the voiding time and voided volume to obtain an average flow rate. This rate should be greater than 10 mL/sec for females older than 65 years and 12 mL/sec for woman of ages 45 to 65 years. Maximum flow (Q max) can be obtained by electronic (complex) uroflow measurements and should be 20 to 35 mL/sec. Complex uroflow is indicated if symptoms of obstructed voiding are present or simple uroflow is abnormal.

EMG measures the muscle activity of the external urethral sphincter using surface or needle electrodes placed close to or into the sphincter. EMG may be helpful when evaluating women with neurogenic bladder but does not add significant information for routine evaluation of UI.

A urethral pressure profile is necessary to determine the presence or absence of intrinsic sphincter deficiency (ISD). A urodynamic pressure catheter is pulled through the urethra from the bladder neck to the urethral meatus, and the urethral pressures are continuously recorded. Alternatively, urethral pressures can be measured in the lumen at rest, during coughing or straining, and during voiding. Urethral closure pressure (UCP) is urethral pressure minus vesical pressure. UCP less than 20 cm H_2O indicates ISD while greater than 30 cm H_2O is considered normal.

IMAGING STUDIES

In general, imaging studies are not clinically indicated for pelvic organ prolapse. One exception is stage 4 anterior prolapse or complete vaginal eversion (Barber, Lambers, Visco, & Bump, 2000; Jelovsek et al., 2007; Ross, 1996). In such instances, ureteral obstruction with consequent hydroureter and/or hydronephrosis can occur. Renal sonography or IVP can identify this consequence of advanced prolapse and are certainly indicated if the renal indices (serum BUN and creatinine) are elevated. Although both static and dynamic MRI techniques, including defecography, have been used to evaluate pelvic organ prolapse, no normative values for these studies have been determined, and therefore the International Continence Society does not consider their use essential. MRI defecography may be helpful when clinical symptoms and clinical examination do not correlate.

QOL ASSESSMENTS

Through the use of validated QOL questionnaires pre- and posttreatment measures may be collected. Examples of these QOL tools include the Pelvic Floor Distress Inventory (PFDI), Pelvic Floor Impact Questionnaire (PFIQ), and the Prolapse Quality of Life Questionnaire (P-QOL; Barber, 2007; Digesu et al., 2005; Jelovsek & Barber, 2006; Ross, 1996). These tools can be time consuming and may not be applicable in general practice. Short versions of several of these tools have been developed and validated, and can be used in clinical practice. The PFDI-20 consists of 20 questions and the PFIQ-7 consists of seven questions. Both tools are valid and reliable, and are used to assess the impact of pelvic relaxation on QOL in women (Barber, Walters, & Cundiff, 2006). The PISQ 12 (Female Sexual Function Index and the Sexual History Form 12) has been demonstrated to accurately measure the effect of pelvic organ prolapse on the patient's sexual function (Price, Jackson, Avery, Brookes, & Abrams, 2006).

Multiple studies have documented the impact of pelvic organ prolapse on the patient's perceived QOL. It is no surprise that pelvic organ prolapse negatively affects QOL, sexual function, and perceived body image (Barber, Walters, & Bump, 2005). The more advanced prolapse affects sexual and bowel function more so than urinary function. Patients with stage 2 prolapse report more distress related to UI than patients with stage 3 and 4 prolapse. Patients with posterior vaginal prolapse report higher overall distress especially as related to bowel function and fecal incontinence (Fitzgerald et al., 2007). Apical vaginal prolapse (cervix and uterus, or vaginal apex if uterus is absent) has more impact on sexual function and dyspareunia than either the anterior or posterior compartment defects. Finally, patients with more advanced prolapse are more likely to feel self-conscious and less likely to feel physically attractive, sexually attractive, or feminine (Barber et al., 2005).

Treatment/Management

Treatment consists of both nonsurgical and surgical modalities. Nonsurgical treatment includes pelvic floor muscle therapy (PFMT), medications, and pessary use. Treatment is generally dictated by symptoms and/or functional impairment. When prolapse is severe enough to cause urinary obstruction, ureteral compromise, vaginal erosion, or severe vaginal infection, treatment is certainly mandated. Otherwise, the patient's comfort, preferences, and QOL are factored into any treatment plan.

PELVIC FLOOR MUSCLE THERAPY

PFMT is often recommended to women with stage 1 and 2 vaginal prolapse. PFMT involves a concentrated exercise regimen of 6 to 12 weeks led by either a knowledgeable and appropriately trained physical therapist, nurse practitioner, or other appropriate staff member. This exercise regimen involves instructing the patient in the correct methods to isolate and contract the muscles of the pelvic floor. Although PFMT will not reverse anatomic derangements, it may alleviate many of the symptoms of pelvic organ prolapse including urinary/fecal urgency, frequency, and incontinence (Jelovsek & Barber, 2006; Kammerer-Doak, 2009). Multiple observational studies have indicated subjective relief for patients treated with PFMT (Blackwell, 2003; Bruch & Schwandner, 2004; Goode et al., 2003; Lagro-Janssen, Smits, & van Weel, 1994; Lamers & van der Vaart, 2007; Rosenbaum, 2007). Pelvic floor muscle rehabilitation (PFMR) and electrical stimulation (ES) therapy and/or pessary therapy are indicated measures if a woman's QOL is affected and she does not wish to have surgery or desires to delay surgery, is not a good candidate for surgery, has failed surgery, or wishes to have more children (Jelovsek & Barber, 2006). A recent randomized trial for stage 1 and 2 pelvic organ prolapse indicated that PFMR may actually improve the anatomic derangement and reduce the degree of prolapse in nearly half of the patients undergoing treatment (Sampselle, 2003).

PELVIC FLOOR MUSCLE REHABILITATION AND ELECTRICAL STIMULATION

The pelvic floor musculature provides support to maintain the position and function of the pelvic organs. When weakened, it loses its ability to adequately support these structures. In addition, sphincters that surround the urethra and anus also lose strength and tone and may not close tight enough to prevent leakage. This often occurs with activities that increase intra-abdominal pressure. PFMR is targeted toward the levator ani, which consists of the pubococcygeus, the puborectalis, the ileococcygeus, and the coccygeus muscles. Strengthening of these muscle groups is an integral part of PFMR/ES (Hagen, Stark, Glazener, Sinclair, & Ramsay, 2009; Hagen, Stark, Maher, & Adams, 2006; Jelovsek & Barber, 2006).

The muscle fiber type is determined by the nerve fiber supplying it. Slow twitch striated muscle fibers (tonic, type 1) sustain activity, whereas fast twitch striated muscle fibers (phasic, type 2) are involved in bursts of activity. In asymptomatic women, the PFM are approximately 30% fast fibers and 70% slow fibers. A muscle contraction must be:

- Greater than that of its ordinary everyday activity in order to increase in force
- Longer lasting to increase the endurance capability

A digital, vaginal examination helps the provider determine the degree of muscle levator ani strength and is recorded and graded as in Table 29.1.

The exercise program will consist of squeezing and holding the levator ani muscle contraction. The average mmHg pressure generated and the maximal time in seconds for maintaining a contraction for each patient is determined at baseline and recorded as the baseline contractile strength and time. The goal for these intervals is to hold each contraction for 10 seconds and then to relax the muscle for 10 seconds. However, in patients who are unable to hold the contraction for 10 seconds at baseline, the study is performed using their baseline contractile time in seconds. Patients perform squeeze–hold–relax repetitions until fatigue of the muscle is noted (fatigue is defined as not being able to hold the contraction for the baseline time in seconds or a drop from the peak contraction strength). Once a patient's muscle begins to fatigue, she is instructed to perform two additional repetitions for her home therapy. This exercise program is used to develop strength and endurance (instructions for doing Kegel exercises are available at www.webmd.com/women/tc/kegel-exercises-topic-overview), under visual video computerized observation and instruction by the provider with a PFMR unit. The patient's maximum pelvic muscle strength contraction for the endurance exercise is measured in mmHg.

The patient is either able or not able to contract and relax muscles when instructed. An appropriate or inappropriate response will be obtained. The contractions will be graded as nonexistent, weak, moderate, or strong, and the average will be measured in mmHg of duration. With the patient performing the directed squeezing and relaxing of the pelvic-floor muscles, the duration of contraction (in seconds) and the number of repetitions are recorded.

The patient is encouraged through detailed and explicit instruction on how to perform and improve the PFM

TABLE 29.1	Muscle Strength Scale
STRENGTH	**DESCRIPTION**
None	No discernible muscle contraction, pressure and/or displacement of examiner's finger
Flicker	1/5 Trace but instant contraction < 1 second, very slight compression of examiner's finger
Weak	2/5 Weak contraction or pressure with or without elevation/lifting of examiner's finger, held for > 1 second but < 3 seconds
Moderate	3/5 Moderate contraction or compression of examiner's finger with or without elevation/lifting of finger, held for at least 4 to 6 seconds, repeated three times
Firm	4/5 Firm contraction with good compression of examiner's finger with elevation/lifting of finger toward the pubic bone, held for at least 7 to 9 seconds, repeated four to five times
Strong	5/5 Unmistakably strong contraction and grip of examiner's finger with posterior elevation/lifting of finger, held for at least 10 seconds, repeated four to five times

function. Fast twitch exercises are done to decrease urinary urges and prevent leakage. With this exercise, the fast twitch or short muscle fibers are strengthened. The patient's maximum pelvic muscle strength contraction for fast twitch exercise is measured in mmHg. The average strength of the fast twitch contraction is measured if the short muscle fiber develops weak, moderate, or strong amplitude.

The next portion consists of electrical stimulation. The vaginal probe is kept in the vagina and electrical stimulation is initiated for stress UI patients. –50 Hz are used for 15 minutes, with a pulse of 5 seconds on and 5 seconds off. A similar pattern is used for urge UI and overactive bladder patients, except that a frequency of 12.5 Hz is selected. The stimulation regimen used is an alternating 50 Hz and 12.5 Hz every other week for mixed UI. The electrical stimulation level is measured in uv/ma. Toleration of the stimulation is evaluated because electrical stimulation will be maintained during therapy based on the patient's tolerance. Management of the patient involves instructing her to continue the prescribed exercise at home. For home therapy, the patient will be prescribed exercise repetitions based on their endurance and muscle fatigue. All patients will need to do exercises three times per day, 7 days/week in a sitting, standing, and lying position.

NEUROLOGIC STIMULATION THERAPY

Electrical stimulation devices to treat UI are taught to stimulate the pelvic muscles indirectly via electrodes, vagina sensor or probe, and acupuncture needle or directly such as intravesical stimulation implant. This therapy can be used in combination with Kegel exercises or alone.

Electrical stimulation is typically used in PFMR to stimulate the pelvic nerves to enhance the contractile response. Electrical stimulation works via the model of neuromodulation, which remodels the neuronal reflex loop by stimulating afferent nerve fibers of the pudendal nerve that influence this reflex loop. By this method of inhibiting bladder reflex contraction and using high-intensity stimulus for short duration (15 minutes), the bladder spasm is reduced or the detrusor muscle is "calmed." Electrical stimulation has also been shown to strengthen the pelvic muscle and structural support of the urethra and the bladder neck. Thus, we hypothesize that combined therapy with PFMR and electrical stimulation should provide patients with an optimal combination for improving UI symptoms.

Intone • Intone is a prescriptive medical device that provides noninvasive treatment for overactive bladder (OAB)/mixed UI. The device combines Kegel exercises and electrical stimulation via voice guided instruction to be used at home. It requires 12 minutes therapy per day for about 3 months. The insertion unit can be inflated in the vagina for a snug fit to accommodate different size vaginal calibers. The sensor within the insertion unit measures pelvic muscle strength. The stimulation unit in the device uses biphasic wave forms to ensure patient comfort and to prevent skin irritation, alternating between 12 and 50 Hz (Barber et al., 2007).

Percutaneous Tibia Nerve Stimulation • Percutaneous tibia nerve stimulation (PTNS) or neuromodulator is the stimulation of nerves that enervate the bladder indirectly. The theory of neurologic stimulation therapy is that stimulation of the nerves can stimulate pelvic muscle contractions and/or detrusor contractions. The initial studies of neurologic stimulation therapy focused on the sacral nerve. Although sacral nerve stimulation can improve the symptoms of incontinence, the procedures to implant these devices are somewhat invasive. Therefore, PTNS was developed. This procedure delivers retrograde access to the sacral nerve plexus via electrical stimulation of the posterior tibial nerve. PTNS involves a needle electrode being inserted into the posterior tibial nerve at the medial malleolus of the ankle to a depth of 3 to 4 cm. The electrode is then connected to a handheld nerve stimulator, which sends an electrical impulse to the nerve. This nerve impulse is then transmitted to the sacral plexus, which regulates the control of bladder and PFMs. The maximum treatment intensity is determined by slowly increasing the stimulus until the patient's great toe begins to curl. The level at which the patient's toe curls is determined to be the maximum intensity for treatment. The most common side effects are local and related to placement of the electrode. They include minor bleeding and bruising, mild pain, tingling, and inflammation of the skin. To date there have been no serious adverse events reported in any of the observational studies or clinical trials regarding PTNS. In the clinical trials, which have systematically assessed adverse effects, overall rates of bruising, bleeding, discomfort, and leg tingling have been low, although not all studies have reported the exact percentages (Davis et al., 2012; Guralnick, Kelly, Engelke, Koduri, & O'Connor, 2015; Peters et al., 2013).

PESSARY THERAPY

Pessary therapy is an integral part of the management of pelvic organ prolapse (Dannecker, Wolf, Raab, Hepp, & Anthuber, 2005; Kincade et al., 2005). Pessaries are especially helpful for women who are medically unable to undergo surgery or wish to avoid a surgical procedure. Pessaries are made of silicone, soft plastic, rubber, and clear plastic and may have a bendable, metal form, which allows contouring for the patient's anatomy. Most modern pessaries are made of silicone as this material is less likely to discolor, less likely to fracture from repeated cleaning, and seems to be less allergenic than rubber.

Indications include the need for vaginal support, UI, and incompetent cervix in pregnancy. Pessaries are often chosen when a patient has medical comorbidities rendering surgery dangerous or the patient desires an alternative to surgery. Pessaries may also be used preoperatively to identify occult UI or to hasten healing of atrophic, inflamed, or eroded vaginal epithelium before surgery.

Pessary fitting is accomplished through trial and error. Figure 29.1 shows many of these devices. In general, the type of pessary used is determined by the stage of prolapse, the main compartment affected, and the size of the genital hiatus (introitus). Active pelvic or vaginal infections must be treated before pessary use. If significant vaginal atrophy or epithelial drying or erosion is present, then a course of vaginal estrogen will be required before pessary placement.

For stage 1 or 2 prolapse, the following devices may be used: (a) ring (with or without support); (b) dish (with or without urethral bolster); and (c) Hodge (with or without support). The ring and dish pessaries are placed in a manner similar to diaphragm placement. One edge is placed under the symphysis pubis and the other edge in the posterior fornix. These pessaries are often not retained in the patient who has had a total hysterectomy. Once placed, the ring and dish pessary should rest in the anterior compartment of the vagina. For this reason, they are both very helpful for anterior vaginal wall prolapse (cystocele). Both of these pessaries are usually easy for a patient to remove and reinsert. The Hodge pessary requires advanced knowledge for proper placement. It usually has one edge resting behind the cervix with the other edge against the perineum. The Hodge is often difficult for a patient to remove and reinsert on her own.

Stage 3 anterior and apical prolapse may be treated by the dish or ring, but often these are not retained and larger volume pessaries are needed. Examples of these are the donut and Gellhorn devices. The donut pessary has a much thicker, rounded edge and occupies more space within the vagina than the ring or dish. This pessary is helpful when the introitus is very wide. Because of its size, this pessary precludes sexual activity and therefore sexually active patients need to learn how to remove and reinsert the device. Insertion is generally accomplished by aligning the long axis of the device with the introitus and with steady firm pressure (and lubrication) placing the pessary into the distal vagina. Once in the vagina, the provider rotates the pessary 90° and advances it into the proximal portion of the vagina.

The Gellhorn device is "T"-shaped and has a flat discoid section with a stem. The stem can range between 2 and 4 cm and the disc between 1 and 3 inches. This pessary is meant

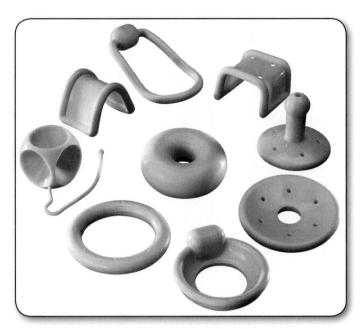

FIGURE 29.1

Pessaries are available in a wide variety of configurations and sizes. Clinicians should be familiar with at least one type of pessary used to treat each stage of pelvic organ prolapse.

Source: Courtesy of Cooper Surgical, Inc.

to have the disc against the upper apex or cervix and the stem against the perineum. It is inserted by aligning the flat disc vertically against the introitus and then slowly pushing it into the distal vagina. Once proximal to the hymen, the device is rotated so that the stem is facing the provider. The device is then further inserted into the upper vagina. Once in place, the provider must ensure that the disc does not cause undue pressure against the vaginal epithelium. A finger should be easily inserted between the pessary and the vaginal wall along the entire 360° of the disc. This device generally precludes sexual activity because it is quite difficult for a patient to remove and reinsert (Kaaki & Mahajan, 2007).

Stage 4 prolapse usually requires larger volume pessaries. The aforementioned donut and Gellhorn pessaries may be attempted. When these are not retained, a cube or inflato-ball pessary may be used. The first pessary is cube shaped and has concavities on each surface so that it will create suction to stay in place. It is compressible so that its volume can be reduced for insertion by squeezing together its sides. Once in the vagina, it will expand slightly and stay in place. Again one must be sure that the device does not cause pressure to the vaginal epithelium. The cube pessary is difficult for a patient to remove.

The inflato-ball pessary has the advantage that it can be inflated and deflated for insertion and removal. This allows a patient with advanced prolapse to remove the device at night and to potentially be sexually active. The device comes with a bulb similar to a sphygmometer, which attaches to a stem with a valve. The deflated ball is placed into the vagina and the patient inflates it until it is retained and is comfortable. The valve is opened for deflation and removal. Ideally, a patient will remove this device every night and reinsert in the morning. This will help to prevent vaginal infection and erosion.

After fitting, the patient remains in the office to ambulate in order to ensure retention of the pessary. This may prevent repeat visits for the patient for whom the initial device is too small or not the right shape. The patient should also demonstrate the ability to void before leaving. When appropriate, the patient should be instructed on how to remove and reinsert the device. Have the patient return within 1 week to examine the vagina for any signs of irritation, erosion, or infection. At this and subsequent visits, the provider must carefully look for signs of excess pressure against the vaginal walls, such as erosion, laceration, or granulation tissue. The device must also be inspected to be sure it is intact. Vaginal irrigation with iodine or chlorhexidine gluconate may be used if secretions are excessive. Once pessary therapy is established, regular visits at 2- to 3-month intervals are recommended. Unless contraindicated, a maintenance schedule of vaginal estrogen therapy is instituted to prevent erosion of the vaginal epithelium (Cundiff et al., 2007; Nygaard et al., 2004; Powers et al., 2006). With larger pessaries, or when a patient does not regularly remove the device, it is common for the patient to develop a malodorous vaginal discharge caused by a change in the bacterial environment of the vagina. Commonly, anaerobic bacteria may overgrow the normal flora. In these instances, intermittent use of antibiotic vaginal creams (e.g., metronidazole- or clindamycin-containing preparations) may be used for patient comfort.

Complications associated with pessary use include vaginal discharge and odor, vaginal bleeding, urinary retention, constipation, and rarely vaginal fistula because of erosion into a proximate organ (Dannecker et al., 2005). A recent survey of 104 pessary users showed that 70% of the women were satisfied or more than satisfied with pessary therapy and 20% were unable to continue pessary use, mostly because of repeated expulsion of the pessary (Powers et al., 2006). The patient should be informed to notify the provider immediately should she develop vaginal bleeding, abdominal pain, urinary or bowel retention, or signs of UTI.

The most common reasons for discontinuing pessary use include a persistent vaginal discharge, worsening UI, pain, recurrent vaginal erosions, failure to provide support, and inability to retain the pessary in the vagina.

PHARMACOTHERAPEUTICS

Local estrogen therapy is a mainstay of therapy in the postmenopausal patient who has no contraindication to its use. Increased vascularity and collagen content of the vaginal mucosa may explain diminution of symptoms in women with early-stage vaginal prolapse (Bernier & Jenkins, 1997; Hanson, Schulz, Flood, Cooley, & Tam, 2006; Maito, Quam, Craig, Danner, & Rogers, 2006; North American Menopause Society, 2007). Local estrogen therapy is generally prescribed with pessary usage to reduce the risk of erosion of the vaginal mucosa. Added vaginal lubrication and moisture may aid in the placement and removal of a pessary. Local estrogen therapy may increase the biomechanical strength of vaginal tissue, and, while not reversing anatomic derangement, does ameliorate many of the symptoms caused by early-stage pelvic organ prolapse (Castelo-Branco, Cancelo, Villero, Nohales, & Juliá, 2005; Suckling, Lethaby, & Kennedy, 2006).

Vaginal estrogen preparations are available as creams, suppositories, or an estradiol-impregnated silicone ring placed in the vagina. When using either a cream or suppository form, it is common to have a short period of treatment induction followed by a maintenance schedule. With use of the ring, no induction schedule is employed and the ring is simply placed intravaginally for up to 90 days (Hsu, Chen, Delancey, & Ashton-Miller, 2005).

A typical initial schedule of cream would be to place 1.0 to 2.0 g of conjugated equine estrogen cream (Premarin) or 2.0 to 4.0 g of estradiol vaginal cream (Estrace) in the vagina nightly for 1 to 4 weeks. After repeat vaginal examination, a maintenance schedule would usually employ 0.5 to 1.0 g of Premarin or 1.0 to 2.0 g of Estrace cream one to two times per week. A similar schedule may be used with the estradiol vaginal suppositories (Vagifem). Although the absorption of estrogen into the bloodstream is much less with vaginal preparations than with oral or transdermal products, the clinician must pay attention to the same precautions and contraindications associated with systemic use (Dezarnaulds & Fraser, 2003; Maito et al., 2006; Weber, Walters, Schover, & Mitchinson). Pregnancy, undiagnosed vaginal bleeding, active liver disease, porphyria, an active thromboembolic disorder or a past thromboembolic disorder associated with estrogen use, an estrogen sensitive malignancy (e.g., breast, endometrium), or prior hypersensitivity to estrogen are all absolute contraindications to estrogen use. Relative contraindications include history of thromboembolic disorder not associated with pregnancy or estrogen use, prior history of estrogen-sensitive neoplasm, gallbladder disease, benign hepatic adenoma, and untreated hypertension or diabetes.

Patients are typically placed on therapy for 3 to 6 months. Long-term maintenance treatment may be needed, especially if a pessary is used. In those cases, regular monitoring at 3- to 6-month intervals is necessary and should include endometrial biopsy if abnormal uterine bleeding should occur. All forms of vaginal estrogen performed similarly when comparing efficacy to relieve symptoms of atrophy, but the estradiol ring may cause fewer side effects such as abnormal bleeding and breast pain and a lower likelihood of endometrial hyperplasia (Hsu et al., 2005). Multiple studies revealed greater ease of use and patient satisfaction with the estradiol ring than with vaginal cream (Hsu et al., 2005).

SURGICAL MANAGEMENT

Surgery for pelvic organ prolapse includes vaginal, abdominal, and laparoscopic (with or without robotic technology) procedures (often in combination). Surgery often involves correction of multiple defects. Anterior and apical defects can be approached through one of the previously mentioned routes, while posterior defects are usually corrected via the vaginal route. The aim of surgery is to relieve symptoms, restore normal function, and create a durable repair (Carlström, Karlgren, Furuhjelm, & Ryd-Kjellén, 1982; Martin et al., 1984).

Repair of Anterior Defects • Proper correction of a cystocele depends on identification of the defect causing the prolapse. As previously mentioned, defects may be central or lateral (paravaginal). The standard anterior colporrhaphy with midline plication of endopelvic connective tissue is a vaginal procedure that only corrects a central defect. Unfortunately, recurrence of anterior prolapse is common and may be as high as 40% for standard colporrhaphy (Maher, Baessler, Glazener, Adams, & Hagen, 2007). Paravaginal repair attempts to reattach the lateral vagina to the ATFP and can be completed either abdominally (most common), laparoscopically, or vaginally. Laparoscopic and vaginal paravaginal defect repairs require advanced surgical skills and can be quite difficult to complete. The long-term success of paravaginal repair is not known (Committee on Practice Bulletins-Gynecology, American College of Obstetricians and Gynecologists, 2007). When both central and lateral defects exist, the surgeon faces a difficult dilemma (Diez-Itza, Aizpitarte, & Becerro, 2007).

Complications of anterior colporrhaphy include failure (20%–50%), infection (3%–5%), de novo urgency-frequency syndrome (5%–25%), and less commonly dyspareunia, vaginal stenosis, and urinary retention or incontinence (Maher et al., 2007; Morse et al., 2007). Complications of paravaginal defect repair also include urgency-frequency syndrome, urinary retention, and possible recurrent posterior prolapse.

In the past 10 years, surgical mesh augmentation for the correction of anterior defects has become more common. Initial reports described the attachment of mesh by suture to the ATFP bilaterally. Highest success rates seem to be with the use of permanent material. Long-term success rates are not known, but short-term failures (2 years) have been reported as low as 5%. Complications related to mesh use include infection, induration, and mesh exposure. Mesh exposure (also referred to as erosion or extrusion) occurs in 3% to 9% of patients and is generally easily managed. Symptoms include vaginal discharge and bleeding. Most exposures are reversed with local estrogen treatment alone. If not, then excision of exposed mesh with reapproximation of the vaginal epithelium is easily accomplished (Daneshgari, Moore, Frinjari, & Babineau, 2006; de Tayrac, Deffieux, Gervaise, Chauveaud-Lambling, & Fernandez, 2006; Maher & Baessler, 2006; Naumann & Kolbl, 2006; Sergent et al., 2007).

Repair of Vaginal Apical Prolapse • Surgical procedures for vaginal apical prolapse include abdominal, vaginal, laparoscopic, or combined approaches. The "gold standard" of therapy is the abdominal sacral colpopexy (Moen, 2004; Weber & Richter, 2005). This procedure has the lowest long-term failure for all procedures described with a success (no apical prolapse) of 78% to 100%. The mean reoperation rate for pelvic organ prolapse for this procedure is 4.4% (Salomon et al., 2004). As an abdominal procedure, it entails longer operative time, lengthier hospitalization, higher blood loss, and higher rates of bowel and ureter complications than procedures completed through the vaginal approach. Long-term complications include UI, voiding dysfunction, and erosion of vaginal mucosa overlying mesh material (mesh erosion). Sacrocolpopexy using laparoscopic and robotic surgery techniques has been introduced to avoid the problems associated with the abdominal approach. The initial results are very promising with cohorts of patients with 2 to 5 years of follow-up recently being published (Hilger, Poulson, & Norton, 2003; Klauschie, Suozzi, O'Brien, &

McBride, 2009; North, Hilton, Ali-Ross, & Smith, 2010; Nygaard et al., 2004). Studies to date indicate that these repairs are as durable as their abdominal counterparts.

Vaginal approaches for the surgical correction of apical prolapse have usually entailed either a sacrospinous ligament fixation or uterosacral ligament suspension (which may also be done laparoscopically) to secure the vaginal apex into the hollow of the sacrum. Both procedures may be done either at the time of hysterectomy or for posthysterectomy vault prolapse. The long-term success rates of these procedures generally are lower than abdominal or laparoscopic approach apical support surgeries. These procedures generally require less postoperative analgesia, a shorter hospital stay, and less recovery time than the abdominal approach (Carlström et al., 1982; Dietz et al., 2007; Maher et al., 2004; Misraï et al., 2008; Patel, O'Sullivan, & Tulikangas, 2009; Weber & Richter, 2005).

Repair of Posterior Defects • The traditional vaginal approach to posterior defects involves the midline plication of the rectovaginal connective tissue. Although recurrence is less common than with anterior procedures, dyspareunia may occur in as many as 38% of the patients undergoing these procedures. In the past 10 years, a "site-specific" repair has gained favor for correction of posterior defects. This repair involves the identification and repair of specific defects in the rectovaginal fascia. These defects may occur in multiple configurations and the repair should succeed in repairing all defects while reattaching the fascia to the perineal body. To date, no studies have confirmed long-term superiority of either approach (Abramov et al., 2006; Karram et al., 2001; Paraiso, Barber, Muir, & Walters, 2006; Silva et al., 2006).

Obliterative Procedures • Partial and complete colpocleisis involve the partial or complete obliteration of the vaginal cavity. Partial colpocleisis (LeFort procedure) involves denuding large sections of the vaginal epithelium followed by suturing together the anterior and posterior vaginal walls. This is often done in combination with an anti-incontinence procedure, levator plication, and/or perineorrhaphy. Complete colpocleisis removes the vaginal epithelium in its entirety. Recurrence rates range from 0% to 10%. These procedures are reserved for older patients who do not wish to retain vaginal function and whose medical comorbidities preclude an extensive reparative procedure (Ghielmetti, Kuhn, Dreher, & Kuhn, 2006; Glavind & Kempf, 2005; Hullfish, Bovbjerg, Gibson, & Steers, 2002; Wheeler et al., 2005).

COMPLICATIONS ASSOCIATED WITH VAGINAL MESH PROCEDURES

In 2008 and then again in 2011, the U.S. Food and Drug Administration (FDA) released two bulletins regarding possible complications associated with the use of mesh in pelvic floor surgery. The alerts essentially dealt with vaginal approach procedures using mesh for both prolapse and UI treatment. Subsequent to these alerts there has been a rapid increase in product liability lawsuits surrounding these

TABLE 29.2	Complications Associated With Vaginal Mesh Procedures
Dyspareunia	
Partner dyspareunia	
Pelvic pain	
Voiding dysfunction, for example, urinary incontinence, urinary retention, OAB	
Mesh erosion/exposure	
Bladder injury	
Rectal injury	
Infection	
Vaginal discharge	
Vaginal bleeding	
Recurrent UTI/cystitis	
Recurrent vaginitis	
Neuralgia	
Pudendal nerve damage	
Obturator nerve damage	
Groin pain	

OAB, overactive bladder; UTI, urinary tract infection.

procedures. The conditions associated with these devices are listed in Table 29.2, although this is not a comprehensive list. When evaluating patients with these conditions or symptoms who have had a vaginal mesh procedure for either prolapse or incontinence, it is imperative to document the timeline and severity of these conditions as they relate to prior surgeries. The examination should document specific locations of vaginal/genital pain, tenderness, visible mesh, bands or tightness in the vagina, and muscular pain or tightness. The provider might consider referral to a physician or center with expertise treating mesh complications.

FUTURE DIRECTIONS

Pelvic organ prolapse is quite common and affects millions of women. Pelvic organ prolapse includes a variety of conditions and symptoms may range from none to total vaginal prolapse with urinary/fecal obstruction. The clinician should systematically approach the patient in order to determine the extent of anatomic derangement, the level of functional impairment, and the appropriate management strategies for the patient. The woman's expectations and desires must be factored into all treatment decisions. A realistic description of any treatment success must be relayed to the woman so that she can make a truly informed decision. Future study is aimed toward identifying procedures that are less invasive and have greater long-term success.

■ PAINFUL BLADDER SYNDROME/ INTERSTITIAL CYSTITIS

Painful bladder syndrome/interstitial cystitis (PBS/IC) is a disorder characterized by bladder pain of variable severity, lasting over a protracted period. It can affect women or men, but is more common in women. The diagnosis and treatment of PBS/IC are controversial, similar to other enigmatic medical conditions of unknown origin that are difficult to treat.

Definition and Scope

Definitions of PBS/IC have widely varied over the past few decades and are continuing to evolve. Before 2002, IC was defined in research settings according to the criteria of the National Institute for Diabetes and Diseases of the Kidney (NIDDK); however, the NIDDK criteria were too restrictive for general use, so in 2002 the ICS published new recommendations for definition of the painful bladder disorders (Abrams et al., 2002; MacLennan et al., 2000). The ICS defines PBS as a clinical syndrome (i.e., a complex of symptoms) consisting of "suprapubic pain related to bladder filling, accompanied by other symptoms, such as increased daytime and nighttime frequency in the absence of proven infection or other obvious pathology" (Oravisto, 1975; Wein, Hanno, & Gillenwater, 2010). By comparison, the term "interstitial cystitis" is reserved for patients who have PBS symptoms and who also demonstrate "typical cystoscopic and histological features" during bladder hydrodistension (Tomaszewski et al., 2001).

The International Society for the Study of Bladder Pain Syndrome (ESSIC) proposed another system. The diagnosis of bladder pain syndrome (BPS), distinct from PBS, is based on the presence of pain related to the urinary bladder and accompanied by at least one other urinary symptom. Diseases that cause similar symptoms need to be excluded and cystoscopy with hydrodistension and biopsy (if indicated) should be performed. The ESSIC suggests avoiding the term IC, and instead using the term BPS, followed by a grade denoting severity of cystoscopic appearance and severity of biopsy findings (if performed; van der Merwe et al., 2008). Further refinement of terminology is likely during the coming years.

Because of variable diagnostic criteria, reported prevalence rates for PBS/IC vary widely. Population-based studies report prevalence rates of 10 to 865 cases per 100,000 women (Clemens, Meenan, O'Keeffe Rosetti, et al., 2005; Clemens, Meenan, Rosetti, Gao, et al., 2005). A survey of participants in the United States Nurses' Health Studies suggested a prevalence of 52 to 67 cases per 100,000 women (Curhan, Speizer, Hunter, Curhan, & Stampfer, 1999). The prevalence of physician-diagnosed PBS/IC in a managed care population was 197 cases per 100,000 women and 41 per 100,000 men, but the prevalence of PBS/IC symptoms in the same population was much higher, at 11% of women and 5% of men (Clemens, Meenan, O'Keeffe Rosetti, et al., 2005; Clemens, Meenan, Rosetti, Gao, et al., 2005).

The estimated clinical prevalence is highest in reports by researchers who believe that many, or even most, women with chronic pelvic pain may actually have IC, as well as those who think that many men with lower urinary tract symptoms or prostatitis also may have IC and those who use somewhat nonspecific symptom questionnaires to make the diagnosis (Clemens, Meenan, O'Keeffe Rosetti, et al., 2005; Clemens, Meenan, Rosetti, Gao, & Calhoun, 2005; Jones & Nyberg, 1977; Nickel, Teichman, Gregoire, Clark, & Downey, 2005). The "true prevalence" of PBS/IC will only be established when agreement is reached about diagnostic criteria and a gold standard is available for its diagnosis.

Etiology

Little is known about the etiology and pathogenesis of PBS/IC. Ongoing and future research will likely demonstrate that patients currently grouped together under the umbrella diagnosis of PBS/IC actually suffer from several distinct conditions with distinct etiologies. Several pathogenic mechanisms have been proposed to explain the clinical phenomena, and it is accepted that any of several inciting factors may lead to the clinical manifestation of PBS/IC.

Many studies have documented that patients with IC have urothelial abnormalities present in bladder biopsies (Graham & Chai, 2006; Hurst et al., 1996; Slobodov et al., 2004). Importantly, it is not known whether these urothelial abnormalities represent primary or secondary phenomena (i.e., whether the bladder abnormalities are secondary to another process that is yet unrecognized). These abnormalities include altered bladder epithelial expression of HLA Class I and II antigens, decreased expression of uroplakin and chondroitin sulfate, altered cytokeratin profile (toward a profile more typical of squamous cells), and altered integrity of the glycosaminoglycan (GAG) layer (Graham & Chai, 2006; Hurst et al., 1996; Slobodov et al., 2004). In addition, the expression of interleukin-6 and P2X3 ATP receptors is increased, and activation of the nuclear factor-kB (*NFkB*) gene is enhanced (Graham & Chai, 2006; Hurst et al., 1996; Slobodov et al., 2004).

The GAG layer normally coats the urothelial surface and renders it impermeable to solutes; thus, defects in this layer may allow urinary irritants to penetrate the urothelium and activate the underlying nerve and muscle tissues (Parsons, 2007). This process may promote further tissue damage, pain, and hypersensitivity. Bladder mast cells may also play a role in the propagation of ongoing bladder damage after an initial insult.

Antiproliferative factor (APF) may also have a pathogenic role in the generation of PBS/IC symptoms. APF is a glycopeptide that is produced by the urothelium of IC patients, but not by controls without IC (Mouritsen & Larsen, 2003). APF may affect urothelial activity through altered production of growth factors and other proteins involved in urothelial growth and function.

It is likely that neurologic upregulation with central sensitization and increased activation of bladder sensory neurons during normal bladder filling plays a role in the generation and maintenance of PBS/IC symptoms (Nazif, Teichman, & Gebhart, 2007). This increased sensitivity may be present in the bladder itself, or may be because of increased activity and new pathways within the central nervous system. Animal models suggest that hypersensitivity in bowel and other pelvic organs may be responsible for sensitization of the bladder (Ustinova, Fraser, & Pezzone, 2006). Similar alterations in neural pathways may be responsible for the tenderness that is present in PBS/IC patients. It is also possible that the increase in visceral (bladder) sensitivity is secondary to a primary somatic injury that has sensitized central pathways that overlap with afferents from the bladder.

Risk Factors

Studies have consistently found that PBS/IC is more common in women with a female : male ratio typically reported as 4.5 to 9 females to one male (Ashton-Miller & DeLancey, 2007; DeLancey et al., 2007; Swift et al., 2005). The mean age of diagnosis is probably about 42 to 45 years, although symptoms have been recognized in children (Close et al., 1996; Koziol, Clark, Gittes, & Tan, 1993). A greater concordance of IC among monozygotic than dizygotic twin pairs suggests a genetic susceptibility to IC (Warren, Keay, Meyers, & Xu, 2001).

In a population-based study, PBS/IC was associated only with depression in men. In women, it was associated with depression, history of UTIs, chronic yeast infections, hysterectomy, and use of calcium channel blockers or cardiac glycosides. Use of thyroid medications or statins showed an inverse association (Hall et al., 2008).

Symptoms

The presentation of PBS/IC is variable, but there are many common clinical features. All patients with PBS/IC have pain, which is associated with bladder filling and/or emptying, and usually accompanied by urinary frequency, urgency, and nocturia (O'Leary, Sant, Fowler, Whitmore, & Spolarich-Kroll, 1997; Bogart, Berry, & Clemens, 2007; Teichman & Parsons, 2007). The pain that is thought to be of bladder origin is usually described as being suprapubic or urethral, although patterns such as unilateral lower abdominal pain or low back pain with bladder filling are common. The severity of pain ranges from mild burning to severe and debilitating.

Increased urinary frequency arises because the pain of bladder filling is partially or completely relieved by voiding, so patients prefer to maintain low bladder volumes. Clinically, it is useful to ask patients why they void frequently to help distinguish PBS/IC from other causes of frequency. As an example, patients with overactive bladder syndrome void frequently to avoid urinary urge incontinence, whereas in PBS/IC they void frequently to avoid discomfort.

Affected patients may also describe chronic pelvic pain that is distinct from their bladder pain, as well as other ongoing, distinct pain symptoms. These patients often carry several diagnoses, such as irritable bowel syndrome (another visceral pain syndrome), dysmenorrhea, endometriosis, vulvodynia, migraine, or fibromyalgia. They may also describe exacerbation of their PBS/IC symptoms during times when other pain symptoms are at their worst (e.g., "flares" of PBS/IC when irritable bowel syndrome is symptomatic).

The character of symptoms may vary from one day to the next in a single patient. Exacerbation of PBS/IC symptoms may occur after intake of certain foods or drinks (e.g., strawberries, oranges, beer, and coffee), or during the luteal phase of the menstrual cycle, stressful times, or after activities such as exercise, sexual intercourse, or being seated for long periods of time (e.g., a plane trip) (Koziol, 1994).

In severe disease, urinary frequency of as many as 60 voids daily may occur, with associated disruptions of daytime activities, and of sleep (Koziol, 1994). Patients may describe sitting on the toilet for hours at a time in order to let urine dribble from their bladders more or less continuously so that bladders remain as empty as possible and pain is minimized. Associated disruption of home and work life, avoidance of sexual intimacy, and chronic fatigue and pain predictably result in some degree of worsening of QOL in all affected patients. In surveys, 50% of patients reported being unable to work full time, 75% described dyspareunia, 70% reported sleep disturbance, and 90% reported that PBS/IC affected their daily activities (Koziol, 1994).

The majority of patients describe symptoms that are of gradual onset, with worsening of discomfort, urgency, and frequency over a period of months (Koziol, 1994). A smaller subset of patients describe symptoms that are severe from their onset. Symptoms of PBS/IC begin suddenly, with some patients able to name the exact date on which symptoms began. In other patients, symptoms begin after an apparently uncomplicated UTI or surgical procedure, episode of vaginitis or prostatitis, or after a trauma, such as a fall onto the coccyx. In hindsight, these "sentinel events" have often been empirically diagnosed and treated, and usually are themselves somewhat enigmatic (Koziol, 1994).

Evaluation/Assessment

A thorough history and physical examination of patients with PBS/IC is of critical importance in making a diagnosis, and also in treatment planning. Identifying and clarifying symptoms often can assist with ruling out other possible differential diagnoses and will provide information to guide the treatment plan. On observation, many patients will be tearful and appear fatigued and/or depressed. Variable tenderness of the abdominal wall, hip girdle, soft tissues of the buttocks, pelvic floor, bladder base, and urethra is almost universally present, probably because of sensitization of afferent nerve fibers in the dermatomes (thoracolumbar and sacral) to which the bladder refers.

In some women, adequate speculum and bimanual examination cannot be conducted because of exquisite tenderness of the pelvic tissues. Pelvic ultrasound can be helpful for assessing the pelvic organs in these patients. It is

> ## BOX 29.5 DIFFERENTIAL DIAGNOSES TO CONSIDER IN PAINFUL BLADDER SYNDROME/INTERSTITIAL CYSTITIS
>
> - Bladder stones (urolithiasis)
> - Carcinoma of the bladder in situ
> - Gynecologic disorders (endometriosis, ectopic pregnancy, fibroids, ovarian tumor)
> - Inflammation of the bladder (caused by chronic low-grade bacterial cystitis, cyclophosphamide cystitis, tuberculosis cystitis, radiation cystitis)
> - Kidney disease (renal tuberculosis)
> - Neurological disorders (multiple sclerosis)
> - Pelvic floor dysfunction (PFD)
> - Prostatitis (men)
> - Sexually transmitted diseases (STDs; e.g., genital herpes, chlamydia)
> - Surgical adhesions
> - Urethrocele (bladder hernia into the vagina) or cystocele (tissue growth around the urethra)
> - Urinary tract infection

important to remember that allodynia (perception of non-noxious stimuli, such as light touch, as being noxious or painful; Koziol, 1994) can be present in any patient who has been in chronic pain. Allodynia may make it impossible to perform an adequate pelvic examination in the awake patient. In this situation, clinicians may choose to begin empiric treatment for PBS/IC, and to defer full examination until either symptoms have improved to the point where examination is possible, or until symptoms have failed to respond to usual therapies and the diagnosis must be revisited.

DIFFERENTIAL DIAGNOSES

Several diseases and conditions have symptoms similar to PBS/IC. They may be ruled out, diagnosed instead of IC, or found to be coexistent (Box 29.5).

Diagnostic Studies

To diagnose PBS/IC, diseases that cause similar symptoms must be ruled out (see Box 29.5). Urine culture and urinalysis are performed to test for bacteria and signs of infection. A cystoscopy with hydrodistension, performed under general anesthesia, is the standard diagnostic procedure for PBS/IC. The bladder is filled to capacity with water (commonly) or gas. This allows for examination of the epithelium with a small, telescopic fiber-optic camera, or scope that is inserted through the urethra to the bladder. Glomerulations (tiny hemorrhages that are the telltale sign of IC) are revealed only while the bladder is distended. These hemorrhages are present in 95% of IC cases (Graham & Chai, 2006; Hurst et al., 1996; Slobodov et al., 2004; van de Merwe et al., 2008).

Less frequently, epithelial ulcerations (Hunner's ulcers), lesions, and scars are found (Tomaszewski et al., 2001). Hunner's ulcers are indicative of PBS/IC, though hydrodistension is not needed to see them. A biopsy is performed to distinguish between ulcers and cancer and to evaluate the presence of mast cells, which are sometimes seen in abundance in PBS/IC-affected bladders. Some PBS/IC sufferers do not have epithelial glomerulations or ulcers. Cystoscopy may also reveal bladder stones, which can cause symptoms similar to PBS/IC.

Cystoscopy and hydrodistension are performed under anesthesia because distending the bladder of a PBS/IC sufferer is painful and otherwise causes urgent urination. Hydrodistension may also have therapeutic effects. Some patients repeat the procedure occasionally as treatment for PBS/IC because it may temporarily alleviate pain and pressure.

Cystoscopy

Cystoscopy is not mandatory and is performed at the discretion of the clinician. In the United States, it is usually reserved for patients with hematuria (gross or microscopic) or with symptoms that raise suspicion for other processes. As an example, synthetic mesh is frequently used for urologic and gynecologic surgery, and mesh erosion into the lower urinary tract has become an increasingly important cause of urinary symptoms. When a patient has a history of pelvic surgery that predates their symptoms, it is important to use cystoscopy to exclude the presence of foreign body in the lower urinary tract.

HYDRODISTENSION

Hydrodistension of the bladder is not required for diagnosis or treatment of PBS/IC, although strong opinions are voiced on both sides of this issue (Fall & Peeker, 2006; Ottem & Teichman, 2005). Patients are placed under anesthesia and the bladder is filled with water or saline until 70 cm of water pressure is reached, usually at a bladder volume that is far greater than the awake capacity of the patient (e.g., 1,000 mL). This bladder dilation is maintained for several minutes, and then the dilating fluid is released.

POTASSIUM SENSITIVITY TEST

The potassium sensitivity test (PST) has also been proposed by some researchers as useful for diagnosis of PBS/IC (Barber, 2007; Hohlbrugger & Riedl, 2001; Parsons, 2005a), but is not recommended for routine use because its results are nonspecific for PBS/IC (Hanno, 2005). During this test, 40 mL sterile water is instilled into the bladder, and note is made of any associated pain. The bladder is drained and then filled with a 40 mL of 0.4 M potassium chloride; a finding of increased pain during this second fill is considered indicative of bladder hypersensitivity and suggestive of PBS/IC.

SYMPTOM SCALES

Some centers use symptom scales to aid in diagnosis of PBS/IC; however, in practice, use of these scales adds little to the ability to make a diagnosis and thus use is not widespread. Symptom scales can be useful in the monitoring of clinical progress after diagnosis. Three such scales are the O'Leary–Sant IC symptom and problem index (American College of Obstetricians and Gynecologists, 2008; Propert et al., 2006), the Pelvic Pain and Urgency/Frequency (PUF) patient symptom scale (American College of Obstetricians and Gynecologists, 2008; Propert et al., 2006), and the University of Wisconsin Interstitial Cystitis Scale (Goin et al., 1998).

Treatment/Management

NONSPECIFIC THERAPIES

Common sense dictates that the following components are part of all treatment programs.

Psychosocial Support • Psychosocial support is an integral part of treatment of any chronic pain disorder. Patients may benefit from identification of a support person within the clinical practice whom they may contact as needed. They may benefit from pain support groups such as the Interstitial Cystitis Society (www.ichelp.org) or the Interstitial Cystitis Network (www.ic-network.com). Referral to a mental health clinician with expertise in support of patients with chronic illness may be helpful as well.

Pain Specialist • Referral to specialists in pain management should be considered if the full range of pain management options are not available within the practice.

Treatment of Comorbid Conditions • Depression is common in patients with chronic pain and may impede treatment success. Referral for mental health evaluation may be useful when there is any suspicion that depression is present.

Acute genitourinary disorders (e.g., UTI, vulvovaginitis) can exacerbate PBS/IC symptoms and need to be addressed promptly. Other disorders associated with visceral pain also require treatment because sensitization of any viscera probably results in increased bladder sensitivity. Thus, it is critically important to treat concomitant inflammatory bowel disease (Crohn's disease, ulcerative colitis, and diverticulitis), irritable bowel syndrome, dysmenorrhea and/or endometriosis. As PBS/IC patients often carry more than one of these diagnoses, treatment decisions can be complex, and collaboration with other medical professionals is usually necessary.

Avoidance of Activities Associated With Flares • Patients frequently note that some exercises or recreational activities, sexual activities, or body positions seem to worsen their bladder symptoms. Others note that some foods or beverages are troublesome. Common sense suggests that these factors be avoided until symptoms are resolved, at which time they may be reintroduced. Some practitioners strongly recommend the highly restrictive IC diet (DeLancey, 1994), but its benefit has never been studied, and in practice, most patients with food sensitivities are already aware of them and have already excluded them from their diet.

Behavioral Therapy • Behavioral therapy forms the cornerstone of all treatment packages. It includes avoidance of exacerbating activities, and also some form of a timed voiding reeducation protocol to expand functional bladder capacity. Such protocols are critical because frequent voiding leads to diminished functional bladder capacity (possibly because of shrinkage of smooth muscle, similar to diminished stomach capacity after fasting or after chronic intake of smaller amounts of food).

A typical bladder reeducation protocol involves teaching patients to "void by the clock" rather than voiding when they feel an urge to do so. For example, a patient who is currently voiding every half an hour is asked to void only on the hour during the daytime (drills are not typically continued through the night), whether they feel the need to void or not, and not to void more frequently than the prescribed interval. This voiding interval is continued for a full week, and if patients are successful at that voiding interval, it is increased. This might result in the prescription of a voiding interval of 90 minutes for the second week, of 2 hours for the third week, 2.5 hours for the fourth week, and 3 hours for the fifth week. Other similar bladder retraining therapies are widely used because they are inexpensive, without side effects, and universally available.

Specific Therapies

Because the exact cause of PBS/IC is poorly understood, there are several approaches to care that are based on various theories of the cause.

UROTHELIUM THERAPIES

Clinicians who favor the theory that urothelial abnormalities are responsible for symptoms often use therapies directed at the urothelium. These include the following.

Pentosan Polysulfate Sodium • Pentosan polysulfate sodium (PPS) is the only oral medication approved by the FDA for treatment of IC. The approved dose is 100 mg three times daily, although off-label treatment using 200 mg twice daily is clinically common (Erickson, Sheykhnazari, & Bhavanandan, 2006; Sant et al., 2003). PPS is a protein that is supposed to be filtered by the kidneys and appear in the urine so that it can reconstitute the deficient GAG layer over the urothelium. In fact, only a tiny proportion of the drug is absorbed by the gastrointestinal tract and excreted in the urine (Erickson et al., 2006). Urinary levels in patients who respond to treatment are not significantly different from the levels in nonresponders (Erickson et al., 2006; Sant et al., 2003).

A systematic review of randomized trials assessing pharmacologic treatments of PBS/IC found that PPS was more effective than placebo in overall improvement of patient-reported symptoms (pain, urgency, frequency) but the magnitude of effect was modest (Dimitrakov et al., 2007). There was considerable heterogeneity in the studies that addressed this question.

Intravesical Heparin and Lidocaine • Some clinicians recommend intravesical instillations of heparin and/or lidocaine, PPS, and sodium bicarbonate in various nonstandardized drug cocktails. No controlled studies of these therapies exist. As an example, use of a solution consisting of 40,000 U of heparin, 8 mL of 2% lidocaine, and 3 mL of 8.4% of sodium bicarbonate to reach a total fluid volume of 15 mL instilled into the bladder has been described as effective, with more than 80% of patients experiencing good remissions after 2 weeks of three treatments per week (Parsons, 2005b). Similar solutions have been recommended for use in patients with severe symptoms as a "rescue" intervention (Peeker, Haghsheno, Holmäng, & Fall, 2000; Perez-Marrero, Emerson, & Feltis, 1988). Patients can be taught to perform the instillations themselves at home.

Intravesical Dimethyl Sulfoxide • Dimethyl sulfoxide (DMSO) was approved by the FDA for use in IC in 1997 on the basis of data from one uncontrolled clinical trial. The action of DMSO is thought to be nonspecific, including anti-inflammatory, analgesic, smooth muscle relaxing, and mast cell inhibiting effects (Peeker, Haghsheno, Holmäng, & Fall, 2000; Perez-Marrero, Emerson, & Feltis, 1988). Treatment involves bladder catheterization with instillation of 50 mL DMSO weekly for 6 to 8 weeks, followed by 50 mL every 2 weeks for 3 to 12 months. Small randomized trials initially suggested benefit; however, adverse effects, including pain and significant exacerbation of symptoms, limited its use (Peeker, Haghsheno, Holmäng, & Fall, 2000; Perez-Marrero, Emerson, & Feltis, 1988). DMSO is currently less commonly used than in the past, because other, less painful treatments have become available.

Hydrodistension • Hydrodistension is usually used as a diagnostic aid for PBS/IC. It has also been used as a treatment because some patients report prolonged relief of symptoms after the procedure, possibly because of disruption of sensory nerves within the bladder wall. One uncontrolled study reported a positive effect in 35 of 50 patients (70%) who underwent 30 minutes of hydrodistension and another reported that hydrodistension followed by bladder training reduced flares related to menses and sexual intercourse in 80% of 361 patients (Dunn, Ramsden, Roberts, Smith, & Smith, 1977; Hsieh et al., 2008; Yamada, Murayama, & Andoh, 2003). Others have reported improvement in only 40% of patients (Dunn et al., 1977; Hsieh et al., 2008; Yamada et al., 2003).

When there is benefit, it is usually short-lived; many patients experience worsening of their symptoms after hydrodistension. Thus, many clinicians feel that the risk–benefit ratio of hydrodistension therapy is not appropriate for their patients. It may be appropriate to reserve use of repetitive therapeutic hydrodistension for patients who generally obtain significant and prolonged relief. Risks of hydrodistension include bleeding (from ruptured vessels) and, rarely, rupture of the bladder wall.

Intravesical Botulinum Toxin • The use of intravesical botulinum toxin for treatment of PBS/IC is controversial and is not approved by the FDA (Kuo & Chancellor, 2009). Investigation into this therapy is based on the ability of botulinum toxin to modulate sensory neurotransmission. Initial results regarding symptom relief with botulinum are promising; however, this therapy is also associated with chronic urinary retention. The need for catheterization would be particularly devastating for a patient with a painful bladder.

In the only randomized trial ($n = 67$) to evaluate this treatment, suburethral injection of botulinum toxin (100 or 200 U) followed by hydrodistension was compared with hydrodistension alone (Kuo & Chancellor, 2009). Successful treatment (based on multiple measures) was found in significantly more patients treated with botulinum toxin plus hydrodistension versus hydrodistension alone at 12-month (55% vs. 26%) and 24-month follow-up (30% and 17%). However, the rate of complications in the botulinum groups was concerning. Use of 200 U of botulinum toxin was decreased to 100 U after 1 year because of adverse reactions in 9 of 15 patients (e.g., urinary retention, severe dysuria) and these complications were found in more patients treated with 100 U botulinum than with hydrodistension alone (5 of 29 vs. 1 of 23; Kuo & Chancellor, 2009).

NEUROMODULATION THERAPIES

Proponents of the theory that PBS/IC represents a neurological hypersensitivity disorder tend to favor use of neuromodulation treatments. These include the following.

Amitriptyline • Medications used to treat other pain syndromes are commonly used for IC patients. Amitriptyline is commonly prescribed for relief of PBS/IC symptoms. In Germany, one trial randomly assigned 50 subjects with IC to amitriptyline or placebo (IC was defined according to NIDDK criteria; Wein et al., 2010). Subjects were treated for 4 months with a self-titration protocol that allowed them to escalate drug dosage by 25 mg increments weekly to a maximum of 100 mg. Amitriptyline use resulted in greater improvement in symptom scores than placebo. In addition, significantly more subjects taking amitriptyline rated their satisfaction with treatment as being "good" or "excellent" (63%) than those given placebo (4%). However, only 42% of patients in the amitriptyline group experienced more than a 30% decrease in symptom score, suggesting that benefits are modest. An open-label study of the long-term use of amitriptyline in 94 patients followed for a mean of 19 months reported similar results (van Ophoven & Hertle, 2005). Almost one half of patients rated satisfaction with treatment as "good" or "excellent" and designated themselves as being "moderately" or "markedly" improved. However, about one third dropped out of the study after a mean treatment period of 6 weeks, with nonresponse to treatment being the primary reason for dropout. Side effects of amitriptyline include sedation, dry mouth, and weight gain. A National Institutes of Health-sponsored randomized trial comparing behavioral therapy to amitriptyline-plus-behavioral therapy for treatment of PBS is ongoing (Richter, 2006).

Side effects of amitriptyline include anticholinergic effects, sedation, weight gain, orthostatic hypotension, and conduction abnormalities.

Gabapentin • In an uncontrolled study, 21 patients with refractory genitourinary pain were treated with gabapentin at a dose of 300 to 1,200 mg/d (Sasaki et al., 2001). About one half of the patients reported improvement in pain, including five of eight patients who had a diagnosis of IC. Anecdotal reports also suggest that pregabalin can be effective for pain relief in PBS/IC, but no formal studies support its use.

Electrical Stimulation Therapy • Several reports support treatment of PBS/IC symptoms with implanted sacral neuromodulation (e.g., InterStim® device, Medtronic Inc., Minneapolis, MN; Comiter, 2003; Peters & Konstandt, 2004; Peters, Feber, & Bennett, 2007; Zabihi, Mourtzinos, Maher, Raz, & Rodríguez, 2008). This device is FDA approved for treatment of urinary urgency and frequency, but not specifically for treatment of PBS/IC (Comiter, 2003; Peters, Feber, & Bennett, 2007; Peters & Konstandt, 2004; Zabihi, Mourtzinos, Maher, Raz, & Rodríguez, 2008). The device consists of an implanted lead that lies along a sacral nerve root (usually S3) and is attached to an implanted pulse generator. An uncontrolled study from a single center described 17 patients diagnosed with IC according to NIDDK criteria who received InterStim® implants and were followed for an average of 14 months (Nygaard et al., 2004). Mean daytime and nighttime voiding frequencies decreased from 17 and 9 to 4 and 1, respectively. Average pain rating decreased from 5.8/10 at baseline to 1.6/10 (Nygaard et al., 2004). Another case series documented "moderate" or "marked" improvement in pain in 20 of 21 IC patients (NIDDK criteria) during 1 year of follow-up (Nieminen et al., 2003).

InterStim® is a costly procedure; adverse events include surgical site infections and pain, and repeat operation for revisions at the lead or pulse generator site(s) is common. The sacral neuromodulation lead can be placed either along the sacral nerve root (most common) or to stimulate the pudendal nerve. A randomized crossover trial compared the efficacy of leads placed at these two sites in 22 patients with IC/PBS. The pudendal placement was chosen as the "better" lead in 77% of patients (Jelovsek et al., 2007).

Another study reported results after placement of bilateral neuromodulation leads to simultaneously stimulate bilateral sacral nerve roots S2 through S4 (Santaniello, Giannantoni, Cochetti, Zucchi, & Costantini, 2007). Among 30 patients, 77% responded initially to this therapy and 42% reported at least 50% improvement in symptoms at a minimum of 6-month follow-up. In this study, there was a 22% removal rate because of infection or malfunction (Comiter, 2003; Peters et al., 2007; Peters & Konstandt, 2004; Zabihi et al., 2008).

A less expensive and noninvasive alternative to sacral nerve stimulation is percutaneous posterior tibial nerve stimulation (Peters et al., 2010). One study reported guardedly positive results after tibial nerve stimulation was applied twice weekly in 18 patients with IC/PBS: eight (44%) experienced benefit from the treatment (Zhao, Bai, Zhou, Qi, & Du, 2008).

SOMATIC THERAPIES

Proponents of the theory that bladder symptoms are caused or maintained by somatic (body wall) abnormalities favor somatic therapies. At present, physical therapy is the only somatic therapy in routine use.

Physical Therapy • Treatment of the somatic abnormalities in PBS/IC patients is not within the scope of training of most physical therapists, even those who are skilled in treatment of UI. Resolution of the tender points, trigger points, connective tissue restrictions, and muscular abnormalities of the soft tissues requires specialized training in pelvic soft tissue manual manipulation and rehabilitation. The therapist may also suggest that manual therapy treatments be supplemented by heat or ice treatments.

The effectiveness of myofascial physical therapy for treatment of PBS/IC was illustrated by a randomized trial in which 50% of patients reported they were moderately or markedly improved after a course of targeted treatments, while only 7% of controls who received global massage therapy reported improvement (Burrows et al., 2004). The duration of this response after completion of therapy remains to be established. Several case series have also described symptom relief from manual physical therapies (Fitzgerald et al., 2009; Oyama et al., 2004; Weiss, 2001). As an example, one study reported that 70% of IC patients who were treated with manual physical therapy to the pelvic floor tissues for 12 to 15 visits experienced moderate to marked improvement (Fitzgerald et al., 2007). Another study of 21 women with IC and associated pelvic floor hypertonicity demonstrated decreased symptom scores after 5 weeks of pelvic floor massage (Richter et al., 2007). A second randomized trial of physical therapies for treatment of PBS/IC is currently ongoing (Richter, 2006).

MAST CELL THERAPY

Proponents of the theory that mast cells play a critical role in the development and/or maintenance of IC symptoms favor therapies directed at mast cells and allergic phenomena (Sant et al., 2003; Theoharides, Kempuraj, & Sant, 2001). These include the following.

Hydroxyzine and Cimetidine • Until recently, the antihistamine hydroxyzine was a mainstay of IC treatment, with an initial dosing of 10 mg in the evening (Keay, Zhang, Shoenfelt, & Chai, 2003; Sant et al., 2003; Theoharides, 1994), increasing to 50 to 100 mg daily as needed. However, a randomized controlled trial found hydroxyzine had no benefit over placebo (Keay et al., 2003; Sant, Kempuraj, Marchand, & Theoharides, 2007). Two small studies suggested benefit of treatment with cimetidine, an H2-receptor blocker, but clinical experience has not generally supported these smaller studies and cimetidine is not commonly used (Seshadri, Emerson, & Morales, 1994; Thilagarajah, Witherow, & Walker, 2001).

Montelukast • The presence of leukotriene D4 receptors in human detrusor myocytes and increased urinary leukotriene E4 in patients with IC and detrusor mastocytosis suggest that cysteinyl-containing leukotrienes may have a role as proinflammatory mediators in this disease (Reena, Kekre, & Kekre, 2007). One small study of 10 women with IC (NIDDK criteria) and detrusor mastocytosis received a single dose of montelukast daily for 3 months (Bouchelouche, Nordling, Hald, & Bouchelouche, 2001). After 1 month of montelukast treatment, there was a statistically significant decrease in 24-hour urinary frequency, nocturia, and pain which persisted during the 3 months of treatment. After 3 months, 24-hour urinary frequency decreased from 17.4 to 12 voids, nocturia decreased from 4.5 to 2.8 voids, and pain decreased from 46.8 to 19.6 mm on a visual analog scale. No side effects were observed during treatment. Further investigation of this modality is required.

Dimethyl Sulfoxide • See the Intravesical Dimethyl Sulfoxide section on page 552.

IMMUNOMODULATORY TREATMENTS

There is interest in exploring immunomodulatory treatments for PBS/IC.

Cyclosporine A • In one trial, 64 patients were randomized in a 1:1 ratio to 1.5 mg/kg cyclosporine A twice daily or 100 mg PPS three times daily for 6 months (Ustinova et al., 2006). Cyclosporine A was superior to PPS in all clinical outcome parameters measured: micturition frequency in 24 hours was significantly reduced (–6.7 ± 4.7 vs. –2.0 ± 5.1 times) and the clinical response rate (according to global response assessment) was significantly higher for cyclosporine than PPS (75% vs. 19%). Adverse effects of cyclosporine A include hair growth, gingival hyperplasia, paresthesias, abdominal pain, flushing, and muscle pain (Sairanen at al., 2005).

Bacillus Calmette–Guerin • Although intravesical instillation of bacillus Calmette–Guerin (BCG) triggers a variety of local immune responses and has an acceptable safety profile, it has not provided significantly greater relief of IC symptoms than placebo in randomized trials (Mayer et al., 2005; Teichman & Parsons, 2007).

GUIDED IMAGERY

One randomized study suggests benefit from the use of guided imagery for treatment of IC/PBS symptoms (Carrico, Peters, & Diokno, 2008; Teichman et al., 2007). For 8 weeks, twice daily for 25 minutes, a group of women either listened to a guided imagery recording or rested. Significantly more women responded to treatment in the guided imagery group (45% vs. 14%).

■ CYSTITIS

Acute cytitis refers to infection of the bladder, which is one component of the lower urinary tract system and includes the urethra.

Definition and Scope

Cystitis is inflammation (-itis) in the bladder (cyst-), usually caused by bacteria entering through the urethra. UTIs are a serious health problem affecting millions of people each year. Infections of the urinary tract are common—only respiratory infections occur more often. In 1997, UTIs accounted for about 8.3 million doctor visits (American College of Obstetricians and Gynecologists, 2008; Hooton, 2012; Nicolle et al., 2005).

Etiology

Women are especially prone to UTIs for reasons that are poorly understood. One woman in five develops a UTI during her lifetime. The most common bacteria causing uncomplicated UTI in women is *Escherichia coli*, followed by *Enterobacteriaceae*, *Proteus mirabilis*, *Klebsiella pneumoniae*, and *Staphylococcus saprophyticus*.

The key elements in the urinary system are the kidneys. The kidneys remove liquid waste from the blood in the form of urine, keep a stable balance of salts and other substances in the blood, and produce a hormone that aids the formation of RBCs. The ureters carry urine from the kidneys to the bladder. Urine is stored in the bladder and emptied through the urethra. The average adult passes about 1.5 quarts of urine each day. The amount of urine varies, depending on the fluids and foods a person consumes. The volume formed at night is about half that formed in the daytime.

Symptoms

Common symptoms reported in women with a UTI include a frequent urge to urinate and a painful, burning feeling in the area of the bladder or urethra during urination. Some will report malaise, myalgias, and urinary pain even when not urinating. Uncomfortable pressure above the pubic bone is common as is the complaint of passing only a small amount of urine despite a strong urge to urinate. The urine may look milky or cloudy, even reddish if blood is present. Pyelonephritis may be present in women with fever, flank pain, nausea, or vomiting.

Evaluation/Assessment

The history provides strong data in favor of a UTI. Physical examination may reveal suprapubic tenderness. Flank pain may be present in women with pyelonephritis.

Differential Diagnosis

Differential diagnoses that may be considered in women who present with symptoms suggestive of UTI include IC, pyelonephritis, and STDs.

Diagnostic Studies

Often an office dipped urine sample with positive leukocytes and positive nitrates confirms a UTI. If results are equivocal, or a women has a UTI within 1 month of a prior UTI, culture and sensitives are useful to identify the exact pathogen so that appropriate antibiotic therapy can be selected.

Treatment/Management

The mainstay of UTI treatment is antibiotic therapy. Antibiotics are selected based on the pathogenic bacteria. In the absence of a culture, antibiotic therapy is selected based on the most common bacterial causes of UTI and includes trimethoprim/sulfamethoxazole, fosfomycin, nitrofurantoin, cephalexin, and ciprofloxacin. Knowledge of resistant bacteria in the community is important as trimethoprim/sulfamethoxazole has become ineffective because of resistance in many communities.

In women with significant urinary tract pain on urination, use of phenazopyridine (Pyridium) can be helpful until the antibiotic has eradicated the causative bacteria. It is important to warn women that this medication will change the color of their urine to an orange red color.

Complementary medicine options such as cranberry and vitamin C are thought to be helpful by some patients; however, data supporting their use are lacking.

UTI prevention measures such as wiping front to back, urinating when the urge is present (not "holding it"), wearing cotton underwear, and hydrating well are also important.

Recurrent UTI

Recurrent UTIs are more common in women and are frequently defined as greater than or equal to two episodes in the last 6 months or greater than or equal to three episodes in the last 12 months (American College of Obstetricians and Gynecologists, 2008; Hooton, 2012; Nicolle et al., 2005). In a primary care setting, 53% of women above the age of 55 years and 36% of younger women report a UTI recurrence within 1 year. Recurrent UTI can be managed with low dose preventive antibiotic therapy after evaluation to ensure that no mechanical urinary system concerns are present (American College of Obstetricians and Gynecologists, 2008; Hooton, 2012; Nicolle et al., 2005).

▦ FUTURE DIRECTIONS

Treatment of urinary and pelvic floor problems in women has evolved tremendously over the past few decades. As science continues to identify new methods for therapy, resolution of these problems that negatively affect QOL for women will be simpler and less invasive, providing options for women that are not available today.

▦ REFERENCES

Abramov, Y., Gandhi, S., Goldberg, R. P., Botros, S. M., Kwon, C., & Sand, P. K. (2005). Site-specific rectocele repair compared with standard posterior colporrhaphy. *Obstetrics and Gynecology, 105*(2), 314–318.

Abrams, P., Cardozo, L., Fall, M., Griffiths, D., Rosier, P., Ulmsten, U.,...Wein, A.; Standardisation Sub-committee of the International Continence Society. (2002). The standardisation of terminology of lower urinary tract function: Report from the Standardisation Sub-committee of the International Continence Society. *Neurourology and Urodynamics, 21*(2), 167–178.

American College of Obstetricians and Gynecologists. (2008). ACOG Practice Bulletin No. 91: Treatment of urinary tract infections in non-pregnant women. *Obstetrics and Gynecology, 111*(3), 785–794.

Ashton-Miller, J. A., & DeLancey, J. O. (2007). Functional anatomy of the female pelvic floor. *Annals of the New York Academy of Sciences, 1101*, 266–296.

Barber, M. D. (2007). Questionnaires for women with pelvic floor disorders. *International Urogynecology Journal and Pelvic Floor Dysfunction, 18*(4), 461–465.

Barber, M. D., Amundsen, C. L., Paraiso, M. F., Weidner, A. C., Romero, A., & Walters, M. D. (2007). Quality of life after surgery for genital

prolapse in elderly women: Obliterative and reconstructive surgery. *International Urogynecology Journal and Pelvic Floor Dysfunction, 18*(7), 799–806.

Barber, M. D., Lambers, A., Visco, A. G., & Bump, R. C. (2000). Effect of patient position on clinical evaluation of pelvic organ prolapse. *Obstetrics and Gynecology, 96*(1), 18–22.

Barber, M. D., Walters, M. D., & Bump, R. C. (2005). Short forms of two condition-specific quality-of-life questionnaires for women with pelvic floor disorders (PFDI-20 and PFIQ-7). *American Journal of Obstetrics and Gynecology, 193*(1), 103–113.

Barber, M. D., Walters, M. D., & Cundiff, G. W.; PESSRI Trial Group. (2006). Responsiveness of the Pelvic Floor Distress Inventory (PFDI) and Pelvic Floor Impact Questionnaire (PFIQ) in women undergoing vaginal surgery and pessary treatment for pelvic organ prolapse. *American Journal of Obstetrics and Gynecology, 194*(5), 1492–1498.

Bernier, F., & Jenkins, P. (1997). The role of vaginal estrogen in the treatment of urogenital dysfunction in postmenopausal women. *Urologic Nursing, 17*(3), 92–95.

Blackwell, H. (2003). The role of the specialist nurse in pelvic floor dysfunction. *Hospital Medicine, 64*(6), 340–343.

Bogart, L. M., Berry, S. H., & Clemens, J. Q. (2007). Symptoms of interstitial cystitis, painful bladder syndrome and similar diseases in women: A systematic review. *The Journal of Urology, 177*(2), 450–456.

Bouchelouche, K., Nordling, J., Hald, T., & Bouchelouche, P. (2001). The cysteinyl leukotriene D4 receptor antagonist montelukast for the treatment of interstitial cystitis. *The Journal of Urology, 166*(5), 1734–1737.

Bruch, H. P., & Schwandner, O. (2004). [What is evidence based in the therapy of pelvic floor insufficiency?]. *Der Chirurg; Zeitschrift für alle Gebiete Der Operativen Medizen, 75*(9), 849.

Burrows, L. J., Meyn, L. A., Walters, M. D., & Weber, A. M. (2004). Pelvic symptoms in women with pelvic organ prolapse. *Obstetrics and Gynecology, 104*(5, Pt. 1), 982–988.

Carlström, K., Karlgren, E., Furuhjelm, M., & Ryd-Kjellén, E. (1982). Effects of intravaginal oestrogen treatment upon the vaginal absorption of conjugated equine oestrogens. *Maturitas, 4*(4), 277–283.

Carrico, D. J., Peters, K. M., & Diokno, A. C. (2008). Guided imagery for women with interstitial cystitis: Results of a prospective, randomized controlled pilot study. *Journal of Alternative and Complementary Medicine, 14*(1), 53–60.

Castelo-Branco, C., Cancelo, M. J., Villero, J., Nohales, F., & Juliá, M. D. (2005). Management of post-menopausal vaginal atrophy and atrophic vaginitis. *Maturitas, 52*(Suppl. 1), S46–S52.

Chiarelli, P., Brown, W., & McElduff, P. (1999). Leaking urine: Prevalence and associated factors in Australian women. *Neurourology and Urodynamics, 18*(6), 567–577.

Clemens, J. Q., Meenan, R. T., O'Keeffe Rosetti, M. C., Brown, S. O., Gao, S. Y., & Calhoun, E. A. (2005). Prevalence of interstitial cystitis symptoms in a managed care population. *The Journal of Urology, 174*(2), 576–580.

Clemens, J. Q., Meenan, R. T., Rosetti, M. C., Gao, S. Y., & Calhoun, E. A. (2005). Prevalence and incidence of interstitial cystitis in a managed care population. *The Journal of Urology, 173*(1), 98–102; discussion 102.

Close, C. E., Carr, M. C., Burns, M. W., Miller, J. L., Bavendam, T. G., Mayo, M. E., & Mitchell, M. E. (1996). Interstitial cystitis in children. *The Journal of Urology, 156*(2, Pt. 2), 860–862.

Comiter, C. V. (2003). Sacral neuromodulation for the symptomatic treatment of refractory interstitial cystitis: A prospective study. *The Journal of Urology, 169*(4), 1369–1373.

Committee on Practice Bulletins-Gynecology, American College of Obstetricians and Gynecologists. (2007). ACOG Practice Bulletin No. 79: Pelvic organ prolapse. *Obstetrics and Gynecology, 109*(2, Pt. 1), 461–473.

Cundiff, G. W., Amundsen, C. L., Bent, A. E., Coates, K. W., Schaffer, J. I., Strohbehn, K., & Handa, V. L. (2007). The PESSRI study: Symptom relief outcomes of a randomized crossover trial of the ring and Gellhorn pessaries. *American Journal of Obstetrics and Gynecology, 196*(4), 405.e1–405.e8.

Curhan, G. C., Speizer, F. E., Hunter, D. J., Curhan, S. G., & Stampfer, M. J. (1999). Epidemiology of interstitial cystitis: A population based study. *The Journal of urology, 161*(2), 549–552.

Daneshgari, F., Moore, C., Frinjari, H., & Babineau, D. (2006). Patient related risk factors for recurrent stress urinary incontinence surgery in women treated at a tertiary care center. *The Journal of Urology, 176*(4, Pt. 1), 1493–1499.

Dannecker, C., Wolf, V., Raab, R., Hepp, H., & Anthuber, C. (2005). EMG-biofeedback assisted pelvic floor muscle training is an effective therapy of stress urinary or mixed incontinence: A 7-year experience with 390 patients. *Archives of Gynecology and Obstetrics, 273*(2), 93–97.

Davis, K., & Kumar, D. (2005). Posterior pelvic floor compartment disorders. *Best Practice & Research. Clinical Obstetrics & Gynaecology, 19*(6), 941–958.

Davis, R., Jones, J. S., Barocas, D. A., Castle, E. P., Lang, E. K., Leveillee, R. J.,...Weitzel, W.; American Urological Association. (2012). Diagnosis, evaluation, and follow-up of asymptomatic microhematuria in adults: AUA Guideline. *Journal of Urology, 188*(Suppl. 6), 2473–2481.

de Tayrac, R., Deffieux, X., Gervaise, A., Chauveaud-Lambling, A., & Fernandez, H. (2006). Long-term anatomical and functional assessment of trans-vaginal cystocele repair using a tension-free polypropylene mesh. *International Urogynecology Journal and Pelvic Floor Dysfunction, 17*(5), 483–488.

Deger, R. B., Menzin, A. W., & Mikuta, J. J. (1993). The vaginal pessary: Past and present. *Postgraduate Obstetrics and Gynecology, 13*, 1–8.

DeLancey, J. O. (1994). The anatomy of the pelvic floor. *Current Opinion in Obstetrics & Gynecology, 6*(4), 313–316.

DeLancey, J. O., Morgan, D. M., Fenner, D. E., Kearney, R., Guire, K., Miller, J. M.,...Ashton-Miller, J. A. (2007). Comparison of levator ani muscle defects and function in women with and without pelvic organ prolapse. *Obstetrics and Gynecology, 109*(2, Pt. 1), 295–302.

Dezarnaulds, G., & Fraser, I. S. (2003). Vaginal ring delivery of hormone replacement therapy—A review. *Expert Opinion on Pharmacotherapy, 4*(2), 201–212.

Dietz, V., de Jong, J., Huisman, M., Schraffordt Koops, S., Heintz, P., & van der Vaart, H. (2007). The effectiveness of the sacrospinous hysteropexy for the primary treatment of uterovaginal prolapse. *International Urogynecology Journal and Pelvic Floor Dysfunction, 18*(11), 1271–1276.

Diez-Itza, I., Aizpitarte, I., & Becerro, A. (2007). Risk factors for the recurrence of pelvic organ prolapse after vaginal surgery: A review at 5 years after surgery. *International Urogynecology Journal and Pelvic Floor Dysfunction, 18*(11), 1317–1324.

Digesu, G. A., Chaliha, C., Salvatore, S., Hutchings, A., & Khullar, V. (2005). The relationship of vaginal prolapse severity to symptoms and quality of life. *BJOG: An International Journal of Obstetrics and Gynaecology, 112*(7), 971–976.

Digesu, G. A., Khullar, V., Cardozo, L., Robinson, D., & Salvatore, S. (2005). P-QOL: A validated questionnaire to assess the symptoms and quality of life of women with urogenital prolapse. *International Urogynecology Journal and Pelvic Floor Dysfunction, 16*(3), 176–181; discussion 181.

Dimitrakov, J., Kroenke, K., Steers, W. D., Berde, C., Zurakowski, D., Freeman, M. R., & Jackson, J. L. (2007). Pharmacologic management of painful bladder syndrome/interstitial cystitis: A systematic review. *Archives of Internal Medicine, 167*(18), 1922–1929.

Drutz, H. P., & Alarab, M. (2006). Pelvic organ prolapse: Demographics and future growth prospects. *International Urogynecology Journal and Pelvic Floor Dysfunction, 17*(Suppl. 1), S6–S9.

Dunn, M., Ramsden, P. D., Roberts, J. B., Smith, J. C., & Smith, P. J. (1977). Interstitial cystitis, treated by prolonged bladder distension. *British Journal of Urology, 49*(7), 641–645.

Erickson, D. R., Sheykhnazari, M., & Bhavanandan, V. P. (2006). Molecular size affects urine excretion of pentosan polysulfate. *The Journal of Urology, 175*(3, Pt. 1), 1143–1147.

Fall, M., & Peeker, R. (2006). What is the value of cystoscopy with hydrodistension for interstitial cystitis? *Urology, 68*(1), 236; author reply 236–236; author reply 237.

Fitzgerald, M. P., & Brubaker, L. (2002). Urinary incontinence symptom scores and urodynamic diagnoses. *Neurourology and Urodynamics, 21*(1), 30–35.

Fitzgerald, M. P., Anderson, R. U., Potts, J., Payne, C. K., Peters, K. M., Clemens, J. Q.,...Nyberg, L. M.; Urological Pelvic Pain Collaborative Research Network. (2009). Randomized multicenter feasibility trial of myofascial physical therapy for the treatment of urological chronic pelvic pain syndromes. *The Journal of Urology, 182*(2), 570–580.

Fitzgerald, M. P., Janz, N. K., Wren, P. A., Wei, J. T., Weber, A. M., Ghetti, C., & Cundiff, G. W.; Pelvic Floor Disorders Network. (2007). Prolapse severity, symptoms and impact on quality of life among women planning sacrocolpopexy. *International Journal of Gynaecology and Obstetrics, 98*(1), 24–28.

Ghibaudo, C., & Hocke, C. (2005). Is colpocleisis still indicated for the treatment of female genitourinary prolapse?. *Progrés en urologie: Journal de l'Association française d'urologie et de la Société française d'urologie, 15*(2), 272–276.

Ghielmetti, T., Kuhn, P., Dreher, E. F., & Kuhn, A. (2006). Gynaecological operations: Do they improve sexual life? *European Journal of Obstetrics, Gynecology, and Reproductive Biology, 129*(2), 104–110.

Gimbel, H., Zobbe, V., Andersen, B. M., Filtenborg, T., Gluud, C., & Tabor, A. (2003). Randomised controlled trial of total compared with subtotal hysterectomy with one-year follow up results. *BJOG: An International Journal of Obstetrics and Gynaecology, 110*(12), 1088–1098.

Glavind, K., & Kempf, L. (2005). Colpectomy or Le Fort colpocleisis—A good option in selected elderly patients. *International Urogynecology Journal and Pelvic Floor Dysfunction, 16*(1), 48–51; discussion 51.

Goin, J. E., Olaleye, D., Peters, K. M., Steinert, B., Habicht, K., & Wynant, G. (1998). Psychometric analysis of the University of Wisconsin Interstitial Cystitis Scale: Implications for use in randomized clinical trials. *The Journal of Urology, 159*(3), 1085–1090.

Goode, P. S., Burgio, K. L., Locher, J. L., Roth, D. L., Umlauf, M. G., Richter, H. E.,...Lloyd, L. K. (2003). Effect of behavioral training with or without pelvic floor electrical stimulation on stress incontinence in women: A randomized controlled trial. *Journal of the American Medical Association, 290*(3), 345–352.

Graham, E., & Chai, T. C. (2006). Dysfunction of bladder urothelium and bladder urothelial cells in interstitial cystitis. *Current Urology Reports, 7*(6), 440–446.

Guralnick, M. L., Kelly, H., Engelke, H., Koduri, S., & O'Connor, R. C. (2015). InTone: A novel pelvic floor rehabilitation device for urinary incontinence. *International Urogynecology Journal, 26*(1), 99–106.

Hagen, S., Stark, D., Glazener, C., Sinclair, L., & Ramsay, I. (2009). A randomized controlled trial of pelvic floor muscle training for stages I and II pelvic organ prolapse. *International Urogynecology Journal and Pelvic Floor Dysfunction, 20*(1), 45–51.

Hagen, S., Stark, D., Maher, C., & Adams, E. (2006). Conservative management of pelvic organ prolapse in women. *The Cochrane Database of Systematic Reviews, 2006*(4), CD003882.

Hall, S. A., Link, C. L., Pulliam, S. J., Hanno, P. M., Eggers, P. W., Kusek, J. W., & McKinlay, J. B. (2008). The relationship of common medical conditions and medication use with symptoms of painful bladder syndrome: Results from the Boston area community health survey. *The Journal of Urology, 180*(2), 593–598.

Hanno, P. (2005). Is the potassium sensitivity test a valid and useful test for the diagnosis of interstitial cystitis? Against. *International Urogynecology Journal and Pelvic Floor Dysfunction, 16*(6), 428–429.

Hanson, L. A., Schulz, J. A., Flood, C. G., Cooley, B., & Tam, F. (2006). Vaginal pessaries in managing women with pelvic organ prolapse and urinary incontinence: Patient characteristics and factors contributing to success. *International Urogynecology Journal and Pelvic Floor Dysfunction, 17*(2), 155–159.

Hilger, W. S., Poulson, M., & Norton, P. A. (2003). Long-term results of abdominal sacrocolpopexy. *American Journal of Obstetrics and Gynecology, 189*(6), 1606–1610; discussion 1610.

Hohlbrugger, G., & Riedl, C. R. (2001). Re: A new direct test of bladder permeability. *The Journal of Urology, 165*(3), 914–915.

Hooton, T. M. (2012). Clinical practice. Uncomplicated urinary tract infection. *New England Journal of Medicine, 366*(11), 1028–1037.

Hsieh, C. H., Chang, S. T., Hsieh, C. J., Hsu, C. S., Kuo, T. C., Chang, H. C., & Lin, Y. H. (2008). Treatment of interstitial cystitis with hydrodistention and bladder training. *International Urogynecology Journal and Pelvic Floor Dysfunction, 19*(10), 1379–1384.

Hsu, Y., Chen, L., Delancey, J. O., & Ashton-Miller, J. A. (2005). Vaginal thickness, cross-sectional area, and perimeter in women with and those without prolapse. *Obstetrics and Gynecology, 105*(5, Pt. 1), 1012–1017.

Hullfish, K. L., Bovbjerg, V. E., Gibson, J., & Steers, W. D. (2002). Patient-centered goals for pelvic floor dysfunction surgery: What is success, and is it achieved? *American Journal of Obstetrics and Gynecology, 187*(1), 88–92.

Hurst, R. E., Roy, J. B., Min, K. W., Veltri, R. W., Marley, G., Patton, K.,…Parsons, C. L. (1996). A deficit of chondroitin sulfate proteoglycans on the bladder uroepithelium in interstitial cystitis. *Urology, 48*(5), 817–821.

Interstitial Cystitis Association (ICA). Retrieved from http://www.ichelp .org/living-with-ic/icdiet/what-we-know-about-ic-diet

Jelovsek, J. E., & Barber, M. D. (2006). Women seeking treatment for advanced pelvic organ prolapse have decreased body image and quality of life. *American Journal of Obstetrics and Gynecology, 194*(5), 1455–1461.

Jelovsek, J. E., Maher, C., & Barber, M. D. (2007). Pelvic organ prolapse. *Lancet, 369*(9566), 1027–1038.

Jones, C. A., & Nyberg, L. (1997). Epidemiology of interstitial cystitis. *Urology, 49*(5A Suppl.), 2–9.

Kaaki, B., & Mahajan, S. T. (2007). Vesicovaginal fistula resulting from a well-cared-for pessary. *International Urogynecology Journal and Pelvic Floor Dysfunction, 18*(8), 971–973.

Kahn, M. A., Breitkopf, C. R., Valley, M. T., Woodman, P. J., O'Boyle, A. L., Bland, D. I., … Swift, S. E. (2005). Pelvic Organ Support Study (POSST) and bowel symptoms: Straining at stool is associated with perineal and anterior vaginal descent in a general gynecologic population. *American Journal of Obstetrics and Gynecology, 192*(5), 1516–1522.

Kammerer-Doak, D. (2009). Assessment of sexual function in women with pelvic floor dysfunction. *International Urogynecology Journal and Pelvic Floor Dysfunction, 20*(Suppl. 1), S45–S50.

Karram, M., Goldwasser, S., Kleeman, S., Steele, A., Vassallo, B., & Walsh, P. (2001). High uterosacral vaginal vault suspension with fascial reconstruction for vaginal repair of enterocele and vaginal vault prolapse. *American Journal of Obstetrics and Gynecology, 185*(6), 1339–1342; discussion 1342.

Keay, S., Zhang, C. O., Shoenfelt, J. L., & Chai, T. C. (2003). Decreased in vitro proliferation of bladder epithelial cells from patients with interstitial cystitis. *Urology, 61*(6), 1278–1284.

Kelly, C. E. (2003). Which questionnaires should be used in female urology practice? *Current Urology Reports, 4*(5), 375–380.

Kincade, J. E., Dougherty, M. C., Busby-Whitehead, J., Carlson, J. R., Nix, W. B., Kelsey, D. T.,…Rix, A. D. (2005). Self-monitoring and pelvic floor muscle exercises to treat urinary incontinence. *Urologic Nursing, 25*(5), 353–363.

Klauschie, J. L., Suozzi, B. A., O'Brien, M. M., & McBride, A. W. (2009). A comparison of laparoscopic and abdominal sacral colpopexy: Objective outcome and perioperative differences. *International Urogynecology Journal and Pelvic Floor Dysfunction, 20*(3), 273–279.

Koziol, J. A. (1994). Epidemiology of interstitial cystitis. *The Urologic Clinics of North America, 21*(1), 7–20.

Koziol, J. A., Clark, D. C., Gittes, R. F., & Tan, E. M. (1993). The natural history of interstitial cystitis: A survey of 374 patients. *The Journal of Urology, 149*(3), 465–469.

Kuo, H. C., & Chancellor, M. B. (2009). Comparison of intravesical botulinum toxin type A injections plus hydrodistention with hydrodistention alone for the treatment of refractory interstitial cystitis/painful bladder syndrome. *BJU International, 104*(5), 657–661.

Lagro-Janssen, A. L., Smits, A. J., & van Weel, C. (1994). Beneficial effect of exercise therapy in urinary incontinence in family practice depends largely on therapy compliance and motivation. *Nederlands Tijdschrift Voor Geneeskunde, 138*(25), 1273–1276.

Lamers, B. H., & van der Vaart, C. H. (2007). Medium-term efficacy of pelvic floor muscle training for female urinary incontinence in daily practice. *International Urogynecology Journal and Pelvic Floor Dysfunction, 18*(3), 301–307.

Lukacz, E. S., & Luber, K. M. (2002). Rectocele repair: When and how? *Current Urology Reports, 3*(5), 418–422.

MacLennan, A. H., Taylor, A. W., Wilson, D. H., & Wilson, D. (2000). The prevalence of pelvic floor disorders and their relationship to gender, age, parity and mode of delivery. *BJOG: An International Journal of Obstetrics and Gynaecology, 107*(12), 1460–1470.

Maher, C. F., Qatawneh, A. M., Dwyer, P. L., Carey, M. P., Cornish, A., & Schluter, P. J. (2004). Abdominal sacral colpopexy or vaginal sacrospinous colpopexy for vaginal vault prolapse: A prospective randomized study. *American Journal of Obstetrics and Gynecology, 190*(1), 20–26.

Maher, C., & Baessler, K. (2006). Surgical management of anterior vaginal wall prolapse: An evidence based literature review. *International Urogynecology Journal and Pelvic Floor Dysfunction, 17*(2), 195–201.

Maher, C., Baessler, K., Glazener, C., Adams, E., & Hagen, S. (2007). Surgical management of pelvic organ prolapse in women. *The Cochrane Database of Systematic Reviews, 2007*(3), CD004014.

Maito, J. M., Quam, Z. A., Craig, E., Danner, K. A., & Rogers, R. G. (2006). Predictors of successful pessary fitting and continued use in a nurse-midwifery pessary clinic. *Journal of Midwifery & Women's Health, 51*(2), 78–84.

Martin, P. L., Greaney, M. O., Burnier, A. M., Brooks, P. M., Yen, S. S., & Quigley, M. E. (1984). Estradiol, estrone, and gonadotropin levels after use of vaginal estradiol. *Obstetrics and Gynecology, 63*(4), 441–444.

Mayer, R., Propert, K. J., Peters, K. M., Payne, C. K., Zhang, Y., Burks, D.,…Foster, H. E.; Interstitial Cystitis Clinical Trials Group. (2005). A randomized controlled trial of intravesical bacillus calmette-guerin for treatment refractory interstitial cystitis. *The Journal of Urology, 173*(4), 1186–1191.

Misraï, V., Rouprêt, M., Seringe, E., Vaessen, C., Cour, F., Haertig, A.,…Chartier-Kastler, E. (2008). Long-term results of laparoscopic sacral colpopexy for high-grade cystoceles. *Progrés en urologie: Journal de l'Association française d'urologie et de la Société française d'urologie, 18*(13), 1068–1074.

Moen, M. D. (2004). Surgery for urogenital prolapse. *Revista de medicina de la Universidad de Navarra, 48*(4), 50–55.

Morse, A. N., O'Dell, K. K., Howard, A. E., Baker, S. P., Aronson, M. P., & Young, S. B. (2007). Midline anterior repair alone vs anterior repair plus vaginal paravaginal repair: A comparison of anatomic and quality of life outcomes. *International Urogynecology Journal and Pelvic Floor Dysfunction, 18*(3), 245–249.

Mouritsen, L. (2005). Classification and evaluation of prolapse. *Best Practice & Research. Clinical Obstetrics & Gynaecology, 19*(6), 895–911.

Mouritsen, L., & Larsen, J. P. (2003). Symptoms, bother and POPQ in women referred with pelvic organ prolapse. *International Urogynecology Journal and Pelvic Floor Dysfunction, 14*(2), 122–127.

Muir, T. W., Stepp, K. J., & Barber, M. D. (2003). Adoption of the pelvic organ prolapse quantification system in peer-reviewed literature. *American Journal of Obstetrics and Gynecology, 189*(6), 1632–1635; discussion 1635.

Naumann, G., & Kolbl, H. (2006). [Operative treatment of genital prolapse of the female: Pros and cons of mesh materials]. *Gynäkologisch-Geburtshilfliche Rundschau, 46*(3), 96–104.

Nazif, O., Teichman, J. M., & Gebhart, G. F. (2007). Neural upregulation in interstitial cystitis. *Urology, 69*(Suppl. 4), 24–33.

Nickel, J. C., Teichman, J. M., Gregoire, M., Clark, J., & Downey, J. (2005). Prevalence, diagnosis, characterization, and treatment of prostatitis, interstitial cystitis, and epididymitis in outpatient urological practice: The Canadian PIE Study. *Urology, 66*(5), 935–940.

Nicolle, L. E., Bradley, S., Colgan, R., Rice, J. C., Schaeffer, A., & Hooton, T. M.; Infectious Diseases Society of America; American Society of

Nephrology; American Geriatric Society. (2005). Infectious Diseases Society of America guidelines for the diagnosis and treatment of asymptomatic bacteriuria in adults. *Clinical Infectious Diseases,* 40(5), 643–654.

Nieminen, K., Huhtala, H., & Heinonen, P. K. (2003). Anatomic and functional assessment and risk factors of recurrent prolapse after vaginal sacrospinous fixation. *Acta Obstetricia et Gynecologica Scandinavica,* 82(5), 471–478.

North American Menopause Society. (2007). The role of local vaginal estrogen for treatment of vaginal atrophy in postmenopausal women: 2007 position statement of the North American Menopause Society. *Menopause, 14,* 355–369; quiz 370–371.

North, C. E., Hilton, P., Ali-Ross, N. S., & Smith, A. R. (2010). A 2-year observational study to determine the efficacy of a novel single incision sling procedure (Minitape) for female stress urinary incontinence. *BJOG: An International Journal of Obstetrics and Gynaecology,* 117(3), 356–360.

Nygaard, I. E., McCreery, R., Brubaker, L., Connolly, A., Cundiff, G., Weber, A. M., & Zyczynski, H.; Pelvic Floor Disorders Network. (2004). Abdominal sacrocolpopexy: A comprehensive review. *Obstetrics and Gynecology,* 104(4), 805–823.

Nygaard, I., Bradley, C., & Brandt, D.; Women's Health Initiative. (2004). Pelvic organ prolapse in older women: Prevalence and risk factors. *Obstetrics and Gynecology,* 104(3), 489–497.

O'Leary, M. P., Sant, G. R., Fowler, F. J., Whitmore, K. E., & Spolarich-Kroll, J. (1997). The interstitial cystitis symptom index and problem index. *Urology,* 49(5A Suppl.), 58–63.

Oravisto, K. J. (1975). Epidemiology of interstitial cystitis. *Annales chirurgiae et Gynaecologiae Fenniae,* 64(2), 75–77.

Ottem, D. P., & Teichman, J. M. (2005). What is the value of cystoscopy with hydrodistension for interstitial cystitis? *Urology,* 66(3), 494–499.

Oyama, I. A., Rejba, A., Lukban, J. C., Fletcher, E., Kellogg-Spadt, S., Holzberg, A. S., & Whitmore, K. E. (2004). Modified Thiele massage as therapeutic intervention for female patients with interstitial cystitis and high-tone pelvic floor dysfunction. *Urology,* 64(5), 862–865.

Paraiso, M. F., Barber, M. D., Muir, T. W., & Walters, M. D. (2006). Rectocele repair: A randomized trial of three surgical techniques including graft augmentation. *American Journal of Obstetrics and Gynecology,* 195(6), 1762–1771.

Parsons, C. L. (2005a). Argument for the use of the potassium sensitivity test in the diagnosis of interstitial cystitis. *International Urogynecology Journal and Pelvic Floor Dysfunction,* 16(6), 430–431.

Parsons, C. L. (2005b). Successful downregulation of bladder sensory nerves with combination of heparin and alkalinized lidocaine in patients with interstitial cystitis. *Urology,* 65(1), 45–48.

Parsons, C. L. (2007). The role of the urinary epithelium in the pathogenesis of interstitial cystitis/prostatitis/urethritis. *Urology,* 69(Suppl. 4), 9–16.

Parsons, C. L., Bullen, M., Kahn, B. S., Stanford, E. J., & Willems, J. J. (2001). Gynecologic presentation of interstitial cystitis as detected by intravesical potassium sensitivity. *Obstetrics and Gynecology,* 98(1), 127–132.

Parsons, C. L., Dell, J., Stanford, E. J., Bullen, M., Kahn, B. S., Waxell, T., & Koziol, J. A. (2002). Increased prevalence of interstitial cystitis: Previously unrecognized urologic and gynecologic cases identified using a new symptom questionnaire and intravesical potassium sensitivity. *Urology,* 60(4), 573–578.

Parsons, C. L., Greenberger, M., Gabal, L., Bidair, M., & Barme, G. (1998). The role of urinary potassium in the pathogenesis and diagnosis of interstitial cystitis. *The Journal of Urology,* 159(6), 1862–1866; discussion 1866.

Parsons, C. L., & Koprowski, P. F. (1991). Interstitial cystitis: Successful management by increasing urinary voiding intervals. *Urology,* 37(3), 207–212.

Parsons, J. K., Kurth, K., & Sant, G. R. (2007). Epidemiologic issues in interstitial cystitis. *Urology,* 69(Suppl. 4), 5–8.

Patel, M., O'Sullivan, D., & Tulikangas, P. K. (2009). A comparison of costs for abdominal, laparoscopic, and robot-assisted sacral colpopexy. *International Urogynecology Journal and Pelvic Floor Dysfunction,* 20(2), 223–228.

Peeker, R., Haghsheno, M. A., Holmäng, S., & Fall, M. (2000). Intravesical bacillus Calmette-Guerin and dimethyl sulfoxide for treatment of classic and nonulcer interstitial cystitis: A prospective, randomized double-blind study. *The Journal of Urology,* 164(6), 1912–1915; discussion 1915.

Perez-Marrero, R., Emerson, L. E., & Feltis, J. T. (1988). A controlled study of dimethyl sulfoxide in interstitial cystitis. *The Journal of Urology,* 140(1), 36–39.

Peters, K. M., & Konstandt, D. (2004). Sacral neuromodulation decreases narcotic requirements in refractory interstitial cystitis. *BJU International,* 93(6), 777–779.

Peters, K. M., Carrico, D. J., Perez-Marrero, R. A., Khan, A. U., Wooldridge, L. S., Davis, G. L., & Macdiarmid, S. A. (2010). Randomized trial of percutaneous tibial nerve stimulation versus Sham efficacy in the treatment of overactive bladder syndrome: Results from the SUmiT trial. *The Journal of Urology,* 183(4), 1438–1443.

Peters, K. M., Carrico, D. J., Wooldridge, L. S., Miller, C. J., & MacDiarmid, S. A. (2013). Percutaneous tibial nerve stimulation for the long-term treatment of overactive bladder: 3-year results of the STEP study. *The Journal of Urology,* 189(6), 2194–2201.

Peters, K. M., Feber, K. M., & Bennett, R. C. (2007). A prospective, single-blind, randomized crossover trial of sacral vs pudendal nerve stimulation for interstitial cystitis. *BJU International, 100*(4), 835–839.

Powers, K., Lazarou, G., Wang, A., LaCombe, J., Bensinger, G., Greston, W. M., & Mikhail, M. S. (2006). Pessary use in advanced pelvic organ prolapse. *International Urogynecology Journal and Pelvic Floor Dysfunction,* 17(2), 160–164.

Price, N., Jackson, S. R., Avery, K., Brookes, S. T., & Abrams, P. (2006). Development and psychometric evaluation of the ICIQ Vaginal Symptoms Questionnaire: The ICIQ-VS. *BJOG: An International Journal of Obstetrics and Gynaecology,* 113(6), 700–712.

Propert, K. J., Mayer, R. D., Wang, Y., Sant, G. R., Hanno, P. M., Peters, K. M., & Kusek, J. W.; Interstitial Cystitis Clinical Trials Group. (2006). Responsiveness of symptom scales for interstitial cystitis. *Urology,* 67(1), 55–59.

Reena, C., Kekre, A. N., & Kekre, N. (2007). Occult stress incontinence in women with pelvic organ prolapse. *International Journal of Gynaecology and Obstetrics,* 97(1), 31–34.

Richter, H. E. (2006). Cesarean delivery on maternal request versus planned vaginal delivery: Impact on development of pelvic organ prolapse. *Seminars in Perinatology,* 30(5), 272–275.

Richter, H. E., Nygaard, I., Burgio, K. L., Handa, V. L., Fitzgerald, M. P., Wren, P., ... Weber, A. M.; Pelvic Floor Disorders Network. (2007). Lower urinary tract symptoms, quality of life and pelvic organ prolapse: Irritative bladder and obstructive voiding symptoms in women planning to undergo abdominal sacrocolpopexy for advanced pelvic organ prolapse. *The Journal of Urology,* 178(3, Pt. 1), 965– 969; discussion 969.

Rortveit, G., Brown, J. S., Thom, D. H., Van Den Eeden, S. K., Creasman, J. M., & Subak, L. L. (2007). Symptomatic pelvic organ prolapse: Prevalence and risk factors in a population-based, racially diverse cohort. *Obstetrics and Gynecology,* 109(6), 1396–1403.

Rosenbaum, T. Y. (2007). Pelvic floor involvement in male and female sexual dysfunction and the role of pelvic floor rehabilitation in treatment: A literature review. *Journal of Sexual Medicine,* 4(1), 4–13.

Ross, J. W. (1996). Routine pelvic support procedures for laparoscopic vaginal hysterectomies. *Journal of the American Association of Gynecologic Laparoscopists,* 3(Suppl. 4), S43.

Sairanen, J., Tammela, T. L., Leppilahti, M., Multanen, M., Paananen, I., Lehtoranta, K., & Ruutu, M. (2005). Cyclosporine A and pentosan polysulfate sodium for the treatment of interstitial cystitis: A randomized comparative study. *The Journal of Urology,* 174(6), 2235–2238.

Salomon, L. J., Detchev, R., Barranger, E., Cortez, A., Callard, P., & Darai, E. (2004). Treatment of anterior vaginal wall prolapse with porcine skin collagen implant by the transobturator route: Preliminary results. *European Urology,* 45(2), 219–225.

Sampselle, C. M. (2003). Behavioral intervention: The first-line treatment for women with urinary incontinence. *Current Urology Reports,* 4(5), 356–361.

Sant, G. R., Kempuraj, D., Marchand, J. E., & Theoharides, T. C. (2007). The mast cell in interstitial cystitis: Role in pathophysiology and pathogenesis. *Urology,* 69(4 Suppl.), 34–40.

Sant, G. R., Propert, K. J., Hanno, P. M., Burks, D., Culkin, D., Diokno, A. C., ... Nyberg, L. M.; Interstitial Cystitis Clinical Trials Group. (2003). A pilot clinical trial of oral pentosan polysulfate and oral hydroxyzine in patients with interstitial cystitis. *The Journal of Urology, 170*(3), 810–815.

Santaniello, F., Giannantoni, A., Cochetti, G., Zucchi, A., & Costantini, E. (2007). Body mass index and lower urinary tract symptoms in women. *Archivio Italiano Di Urologia, Andrologia, 79*(1), 17–19.

Sasaki, K., Smith, C. P., Chuang, Y. C., Lee, J. Y., Kim, J. C., & Chancellor, M. B. (2001). Oral gabapentin (neurontin) treatment of refractory genitourinary tract pain. *Techniques in Urology, 7*(1), 47–49.

Schulz, J. A. (2001). Assessing and treating pelvic organ prolapse. *Ostomy/Wound Management, 47*(5), 54–59.

Segal, J. L., & Karram, M. M. (2002). Evaluation and management of rectoceles. *Current Opinion in Urology, 12*(4), 345–352.

Sergent, F., Sentilhes, L., Resch, B., Diguet, A., Verspyck, E., & Marpeau, L. (2007). [Prosthetic repair of genito-urinary prolapses by the transobturateur infracoccygeal hammock technique: medium-term results]. *Journal de gynécologie, obstétrique et biologie de la reproduction, 36*(5), 459–467.

Seshadri, P., Emerson, L., & Morales, A. (1994). Cimetidine in the treatment of interstitial cystitis. *Urology, 44*(4), 614–616.

Silva, W. A., Pauls, R. N., Segal, J. L., Rooney, C. M., Kleeman, S. D., & Karram, M. M. (2006). Uterosacral ligament vault suspension: Five-year outcomes. *Obstetrics and Gynecology, 108*(2), 255–263.

Slobodov, G., Feloney, M., Gran, C., Kyker, K. D., Hurst, R. E., & Culkin, D. J. (2004). Abnormal expression of molecular markers for bladder impermeability and differentiation in the urothelium of patients with interstitial cystitis. *The Journal of Urology, 171*(4), 1554–1558.

Suckling, J., Lethaby, A., & Kennedy, R. (2006). Local oestrogen for vaginal atrophy in postmenopausal women. *The Cochrane Database of Systematic Reviews, 2006*(4), CD001500.

Swift, S., Woodman, P., O'Boyle, A., Kahn, M., Valley, M., Bland, D., ... Schaffer, J. (2005). Pelvic Organ Support Study (POSST): The distribution, clinical definition, and epidemiologic condition of pelvic organ support defects. *American Journal of Obstetrics and Gynecology, 192*(3), 795–806.

Swift, S., Woodman, P., O'Boyle, A., Kahn, M., Valley, M., Bland, D., ... Schaffer, J. (2005). Pelvic Organ Support Study (POSST): The distribution, clinical definition, and epidemiologic condition of pelvic organ support defects. *American Journal of Obstetrics and Gynecology, 192*(3), 795–806.

Tegerstedt, G., Miedel, A., Maehle-Schmidt, M., Nyrén, O., & Hammarström, M. (2006). Obstetric risk factors for symptomatic prolapse: A population-based approach. *American Journal of Obstetrics and Gynecology, 194*(1), 75–81.

Teichman, J. M., & Parsons, C. L. (2007). Contemporary clinical presentation of interstitial cystitis. *Urology, 69*(Suppl. 4), 41–47.

Theoharides, T. C. (1994). Hydroxyzine in the treatment of interstitial cystitis. *The Urologic Clinics of North America, 21*(1), 113–119.

Theoharides, T. C., Kempuraj, D., & Sant, G. R. (2001). Mast cell involvement in interstitial cystitis: A review of human and experimental evidence. *Urology, 57*(6, Suppl. 1), 47–55.

Thilagarajah, R., Witherow, R. O., & Walker, M. M. (2001). Oral cimetidine gives effective symptom relief in painful bladder disease: A prospective, randomized, double-blind placebo-controlled trial. *BJU International, 87*(3), 207–212.

Tomaszewski, J. E., Landis, J. R., Russack, V., Williams, T. M., Wang, L. P., Hardy, C., ... Nyberg, L. M.; Interstitial Cystitis Database Study Group. (2001). Biopsy features are associated with primary symptoms in interstitial cystitis: Results from the interstitial cystitis database study. *Urology, 57*(6, Suppl. 1), 67–81.

Ustinova, E. E., Fraser, M. O., & Pezzone, M. A. (2006). Colonic irritation in the rat sensitizes urinary bladder afferents to mechanical and chemical stimuli: An afferent origin of pelvic organ cross-sensitization. *American Journal of Physiology. Renal Physiology, 290*(6), F1478–F1487.

van de Merwe, J. P., Nordling, J., Bouchelouche, P., Bouchelouche, K., Cervigni, M., Daha, L. K., ... Wyndaele, J. J. (2008). Diagnostic criteria, classification, and nomenclature for painful bladder syndrome/interstitial cystitis: An ESSIC proposal. *European Urology, 53*(1), 60–67.

van Ophoven, A., & Hertle, L. (2005). Long-term results of amitriptyline treatment for interstitial cystitis. *The Journal of Urology, 174*(5), 1837–1840.

Warren, J. W., Keay, S. K., Meyers, D., & Xu, J. (2001). Concordance of interstitial cystitis in monozygotic and dizygotic twin pairs. *Urology, 57*(6, Suppl. 1), 22–25.

Weber, A. M., & Richter, H. E. (2005). Pelvic organ prolapse. *Obstetrics and Gynecology, 106*(3), 615–634.

Weber, A. M., & Walters, M. D. (1997). Anterior vaginal prolapse: Review of anatomy and techniques of surgical repair. *Obstetrics and Gynecology, 89*(2), 311–318.

Weber, A. M., Abrams, P., Brubaker, L., Cundiff, G., Davis, G., Dmochowski, R. R., ... Weidner, A. C. (2001). The standardization of terminology for researchers in female pelvic floor disorders. *International Urogynecology Journal and Pelvic Floor Dysfunction, 12*(3), 178–186.

Weber, A. M., Walters, M. D., Schover, L. R., & Mitchinson, A. (1995). Vaginal anatomy and sexual function. *Obstetrics and Gynecology, 86*(6), 946–949.

Wein, A. J., Hanno, P. M., & Gillenwater, J. Y. (2010). Interstitial cystitis: An introduction to the problem. In P. M. Hanno, D. R. Staskin, R. J. Krane, & A. J. Wein (Eds.), *Interstitial Cystitis* (p. 25). London, UK: Springer Verlag London.

Weiss, J. M. (2001). Pelvic floor myofascial trigger points: Manual therapy for interstitial cystitis and the urgency-frequency syndrome. *The Journal of Urology, 166*(6), 2226–2231.

Wheeler, T. L., Richter, H. E., Burgio, K. L., Redden, D. T., Chen, C. C., Goode, P. S., & Varner, R. E. (2005). Regret, satisfaction, and symptom improvement: Analysis of the impact of partial colpocleisis for the management of severe pelvic organ prolapse. *American Journal of Obstetrics and Gynecology, 193*(6), 2067–2070.

Yamada, T., Murayama, T., & Andoh, M. (2003). Adjuvant hydrodistension under epidural anesthesia for interstitial cystitis. *International Journal of Urology, 10*(9), 463–468; discussion 469.

Zabihi, N., Mourtzinos, A., Maher, M. G., Raz, S., & Rodríguez, L. V. (2008). Short-term results of bilateral S2–S4 sacral neuromodulation for the treatment of refractory interstitial cystitis, painful bladder syndrome, and chronic pelvic pain. *International Urogynecology Journal and Pelvic Floor Dysfunction, 19*(4), 553–557.

Zhao, J., Bai, J., Zhou, Y., Qi, G., & Du, L. (2008). Posterior tibial nerve stimulation twice a week in patients with interstitial cystitis. *Urology, 71*(6), 1080–1084.

▪ ADDITIONAL READING

ACOG Committee on Practice Bulletins—Gynecology. (2007). ACOG Practice Bulletin No. 85: Pelvic organ prolapse. *Obstetrics and Gynecology, 110*(3), 717–729.

Barber, M. D., Brubaker, L., Burgio, K. L., Richter, H. E., Nygaard, I., Weidner, A. C., ... Meikle, S. F.; Eunice Kennedy Shriver National Institute of Child Health and Human Development Pelvic Floor Disorders Network. (2014). Comparison of 2 transvaginal surgical approaches and perioperative behavioral therapy for apical vaginal prolapse: The OPTIMAL randomized trial. *Journal of American Medical Association, 311*(10), 1023–1034.

Clemons, J. L., Aguilar, V. C., Tillinghast, T. A., Jackson, N. D., & Myers, D. L. (2004). Risk factors associated with an unsuccessful pessary fitting trial in women with pelvic organ prolapse. *American Journal of Obstetrics and Gynecology, 190*(2), 345–350.

Cundiff, G. W., Amundsen, C. L., Bent, A. E., Coates, K. W., Schaffer, J. I., Strohbehn, K., & Handa, V. L. (2007). The PESSRI study: Symptom relief outcomes of a randomized crossover trial of the ring and Gellhorn pessaries. *American Journal of Obstetrics and Gynecology, 196*(4), 405.e1–405.e8.

Diwadkar, G. B., Barber, M. D., Feiner, B., Maher, C., & Jelovsek, J. E. (2009). Complication and reoperation rates after apical vaginal prolapse surgical repair: A systematic review. *Obstetrics and Gynecology, 113*(2, Pt. 1), 367–373.

Gilchrist, A. S., Campbell, W., Steele, H., Brazell, H., Foote, J., & Swift, S. (2013). Outcomes of observation as therapy for pelvic organ prolapse: A study in the natural history of pelvic organ prolapse. *Neurourology and Urodynamics, 32*(4), 383–386.

Nygaard, I., Barber, M. D., Burgio, K. L., Kenton, K., Meikle, S., Schaffer, J.,…Brody, D. J.; Pelvic Floor Disorders Network. (2008). Prevalence of symptomatic pelvic floor disorders in US women. *Journal of the American Medical Association, 300*(11), 1311–1316.

Unger, C. A., Abbott, S., Evans, J. M., Jallad, K., Mishra, K., Karram, M. M.,…Barber, M. D. (2014). Outcomes following treatment for pelvic floor mesh complications. *International Urogynecology Journal, 25*(6), 745–749.

Wu, V., Farrell, S. A., Baskett, T. F., & Flowerdew, G. (1997). A simplified protocol for pessary management. *Obstetrics and Gynecology, 90*(6), 990–994.

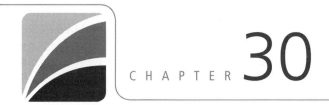

CHAPTER 30

Sexually Transmitted Diseases

Catherine Ingram Fogel

Sexual relations are a natural and healthy part of a woman's life and should be free of infection (Hatcher et al., 2011). However, sexually transmitted diseases (STDs) are a substantial health challenge in the United States (Centers for Disease Control and Prevention [CDC], 2015a) and preventing, diagnosing, and treating STDs has become even more challenging as an increasing number of persons are infected with more severe infections (CDC, 2015a; Hatcher et al., 2011). STDs are a variety of clinical syndromes and infections caused by pathogens that can be acquired and transmitted through sexual activity. This chapter covers STD infections and introduces STD sequelea as the most common health problems in the United States today.

■ DEFINITION AND SCOPE

The CDC estimates that nearly 20 million new STDs occur every year in the United States with half among young people aged 15 to 25 years old (CDC, 2015a). Furthermore, it is estimated that there are more than 110 million total STDs among women and men in the United States (Carcio & Secor, 2015). Rates of curable STDs in the United States are the highest among developed countries and are higher than the rates in some developing countries (CDC, 2015a). Individuals with an STD are often undiagnosed regardless of whether they are asymptomatic and are a huge risk for the spread of infection. At the current rate, at least one in four—and possibly as many as one in two—Americans will contract an STD during their lifetime (CDC, 2015a).

■ ETIOLOGY

STDs are a direct cause of tremendous human suffering, place heavy demands on health care services, and account for more than $16 billion in yearly health care costs (CDC, 2015a). The human costs are equally overwhelming. A diagnosis of cervical cancer or living with chronic pelvic pain can be devastating, and experiencing a preterm delivery or stillbirth can cause prolonged grief and suffering. Couples faced with a diagnosis of infertility because of STDs may require invasive diagnostic procedures and assisted reproductive technology such as in vitro fertilization.

■ RISK FACTORS

STDs are a group of contagious diseases. The risk of transmission is from person to person by close intimate contact (CDC, 2015a). The organisms causing STDs include a wide variety of microorganisms: bacteria, viruses, spirochetes, protozoans, and obligate intracellular organisms that infect the mucosal surfaces of the genitourinary tract as well as ectoparasites (organisms that live on the outside of the body such as lice) and the dozens of clinical syndromes that they cause (Table 30.1; CDC, 2015a). These terms have replaced the older designation, venereal disease, which primarily described gonorrhea and syphilis. Common STDs are listed in Table 30.1. The common STDs in women are chlamydia, human papillomavirus (HPV), gonorrhea, herpes simplex virus (HSV) type 2 (HSV-2), syphilis, hepatitis B virus (HBV), and HIV infection (CDC, 2015b).

In the past, public health efforts were aimed at the control of gonorrhea and syphilis; however, more recently, when it appeared that these diseases were controlled, the concern focused on other diseases, including chlamydia, HSV, HPV, and HIV. Unfortunately, this shifting of focus does not mean that gonorrhea and syphilis are no longer a concern, and, in recent years, increases in the number of primary, secondary, and congenital syphilis, chlamydia cases, gonorrhea cases, and drug-resistant strains of gonorrhea have become increasingly more common (CDC, 2015a). In the United States, STDs are among the most common infections and are a potential threat to an individual's immediate and long-term health and well-being (CDC, 2015a).

■ IMPACT OF STDs ON WOMEN

Although, historically, STDs were considered to be symptomatic illnesses usually afflicting men, women and their children have the most severe symptoms and sequelae of

TABLE 30.1	Characterized STDs in Women

Diseases characterized by genital ulcers

- Chancroid
- Genital herpes simplex virus infection
- Granuloma inguinale
- Lymphogranuloma
- Syphilis

Diseases characterized by urethritis and cervicitis

- Chlamydia
- Gonococcal infections
- Mucupurulent cervicitis

Diseases characterized by vaginal discharge

- Bacterial vaginosis
- Trichomoniasis
- Vulvovaginal candidiasis

Human papillomavirus infection

Vaccine-preventable STDs

- Hepatitis A
- Hepatitis B
- Hepatitis C

Ectoparasitic infections

- Pediculosis pubis
- Scabies

Human immunodeficiency virus

STDs, sexually transmitted diseases.
Adapted from Centers for Disease Control and Prevention (2015a).

these diseases. STDs have a greater and more long-lasting impact on the health of women than on the health of men. STDs in women and children are associated with multiple severe complications and death (Table 30.2).

Reproductive Health Concerns

Pelvic inflammatory disease (PID), a preventable complication of some STDs, such as chlamydia and gonorrhea, is a serious threat to women's reproductive capabilities. More than a million women every year experience an episode of PID (CDC, 2015a). Furthermore, at least 25% of women who have had PID experience long-term sequelae, including pelvic abscesses, chronic pelvic pain, dyspareunia, ectopic pregnancy because of partial tubal scarring and blockage, tubal infertility, increased need for reproductive tract surgery, and recurring PID (CDC, 2015a). Among women with PID, tubal scarring can cause infertility in 8% of women, ectopic scarring in 9%, and chronic pelvic pain in 18% (CDC, 2015a).

Women who have had PID are 6 to 10 times more likely to have an ectopic pregnancy compared with women who have not. Ectopic pregnancy occurs in about 2% of all pregnancies and is an important cause of pregnancy-related mortality (CDC, 2015a). Approximately 4% to 10% of all pregnancy-related deaths are attributed to ectopic pregnancy (UpToDate.com, 2016). Half of all women's

infertility is attributable to STDs (Brookmeyer, Hogben, & Kinsey, 2016). At least 15% of infertile U.S. women are infertile because of tubal damage caused by PID, and no more than half have been previously diagnosed with PID. Ectopic pregnancy also substantially increases the risk of tubal-factor infertility. In contrast, STDs rarely cause infertility in men.

Adverse Pregnancy Outcomes

STDs may cause acute complications for pregnant women and their offspring. Pregnant women may transmit the infection to their newborn, infant, or fetus through vertical transmission (through the placenta before delivery, during vaginal birth, or after birth through breastfeeding) or horizontal transmission (close physical or household contact). Some of the complications associated with an STD experienced by pregnant women can include spontaneous abortion, stillbirth, premature rupture of membranes, and preterm delivery. Vaginal and cervical STD infections during pregnancy can lead to inflammation of the placental or fetal membranes, resulting in maternal fever during or after delivery, wound and pelvic infections after cesarean section, and postpartum endometritis. Sexually transmitted pathogens that have serious consequences for women tend to have even more serious, potentially life-threatening health conditions in the fetus or newborn. Damage to the brain, spinal cord, eyes, and auditory nerves are of particular concern with STDs in the fetus and the infant. For example, severe, permanent central nervous system manifestations or fetal or neonatal death can occur with congenital syphilis. Currently, all transmission of HIV to infants in the United States is attributable to mother-to-infant transmission. Ophthalmia neonatorum can occur when infants of women with vaginal gonorrheal or chlamydial infections are infected during delivery and, if untreated, can result in corneal ulcers and blindness (CDC, 2015a).

Cancer-Related Consequences

HPV infections are highly prevalent in the United States, especially among young, sexually active women (CDC, 2015a). Furthermore, persistent infection with some types can cause cancer and genital warts. HPV types 16 and 18 account for approximately 70% of cervical cancer worldwide and HPV types 6 and 11 for 90% of genital warts (CDC, 2015a). Cervical cancer is the second most common cancer among women worldwide, and about 95% of cervical cancers are associated with 10 to 15 HPV subtypes. Furthermore, women with HPV infection of the cervix are 10 times more likely to develop invasive cervical cancer compared with women without HPV (Lowy, 2016). HIV infection may increase the risk that HPV infection will progress to cervical vaginal, vulvular, and anal cancers.

Increased HIV Risk

A synergistic relationship appears to exist between HIV and STDs (Duan et al., 2016). The inflammation or

TABLE 30.2	Consequences of STDs for Women and Children	
HEALTH CONSEQUENCES	**WOMEN**	**CHILDREN**
Cancers	Cervical cancer Vulva cancer Vaginal cancer Anal cancer Liver cancer T-cell leukemia Body cavity lymphoma	Liver cancer as adult
Reproductive health problems	Pelvic inflammatory disease Infertility Spontaneous abortion Tubal scarring	
Pregnancy-related problems	Ectopic pregnancy Preterm delivery Premature rupture of membranes Puerperal sepsis Postpartum infection	Stillbirth Neonatal death Prematurity Low birth weight Conjunctivitis Pneumonia Neonatal sepsis Hepatitis, cirrhosis Hepatitis B virus infection Neurologic damage Laryngeal papillomatosis Congenital abnormalities
Neurologic problems	Human T-lymphotropic virus-associated myelopathy (paralysis) Neurosyphilis	Cytomegalovirus-, herpes simplex virus-, and syphilis-associated neurologic problems
Other health consequences	Chronic liver disease Cirrhosis Disseminated gonococcal infection Septic arthritis Tertiary syphilis (cardiovascular and gumma)	Chronic liver disease Cirrhosis

Adapted from Center for Disease Control and Prevention (2015b).

disruption of genital mucosa that can occur with ulcerative and inflammatory STDs is a risk factor for contracting HIV during a sexual encounter (Duan et al., 2016). The increased risk for HIV acquisition in women with genital ulcer diseases and gonococcal and chlamydial cervicitis is estimated to be two- to fourfold (Duan et al., 2016).

Preventing, identifying, and managing STDs are essential components of women's health care. Advanced practice nurse practitioners play an essential role in promoting women's reproductive and sexual health by counseling women about STD risk, encouraging sexual and other risk-reduction measures, incorporating education regarding STD disease prevention in their nursing practice, and being current on management strategies. By doing so, advanced practice nurse practitioners can assist women in avoiding STDs and in living better with the sequelae and chronic infections of STDs.

■ TRANSMISSION OF STDs

The chance of contracting, transmitting, or suffering complications from HIV and STDs depends on multiple biological, behavioral, social, and relationship risk factors. However, most individuals are reluctant to discuss sexual health issues openly because of the biological and social factors associated with these infections. Microbiological, hormonal, and immunological factors influence individual susceptibility and transmission potential for STDs. These factors are partially influenced by a woman's sexual practices, substance use, and other health behaviors. Health behaviors, in turn, are influenced by socioeconomic factors and other social factors. In general, the prevalence of STDs tends to be higher in those who are unmarried, young (aged 15–35 years), and live in urban areas. A perceived shortage of available men that may lead to acceptance of partner concurrent sexual relationships, partner concurrency, and an inability to insist on partner condom use. Furthermore, intimate partner violence is associated with the lack of the use of sexual protection (Stults, Javdani, Greenbaum, Kapadia, & Halkitis, 2016; Wenzel et al., 2016).

Biological Factors

Biological factors place women at a greater risk than men for acquiring STDs and for suffering more severe health consequences associated with STDs (CDC, 2015a; Secor, 2015); for example, the risk of a woman contracting gonorrhea from a single act of intercourse is 60% to 90%, whereas the risk for a man is 20% to 30%. Furthermore, men are two to three times more likely to transmit HIV to women than the reverse. The vagina has a larger amount of genital mucous membranes exposed and has an environment more conducive for infections than does the penis. Moreover, the risk for trauma is greater during vaginal intercourse for women than for men. The cervix, particularly the squamocolumnar junction/transformation zone and endocervical columnar epithelial cells, are most susceptible to HIV; however, the virus can invade the vaginal epithelium as well.

More than 50% of bacterial and 90% of viral STDs are asymptomatic and are likely to be undetected in women. Additionally, when or if symptoms develop, they may be confused with those of other diseases not transmitted sexually. The frequency of asymptomatic and unrecognized infections results in delayed diagnosis and treatment, chronic untreated infections, and complications. Furthermore, it is more difficult to diagnose STDs in a woman because the anatomy of her genital tract makes clinical examination more difficult. For example, to diagnose gonorrhea in men, all that is needed is a urethral swab and Gram stain; in women, a speculum examination and specific cervical culture are necessary. Lesions that occur inside the vagina and in the cervix are not readily seen, and the normal vaginal environment (warm, moist, enriched medium) is ideal for infection.

Age and gender influence an individual's risk for an STD; specifically, young women (age 20–24 years) and female adolescents (15–19 years) are more susceptible than are their male counterparts (CDC, 2014). STDs tend to occur at a younger age in females than in males. Compared with women before menopause, female adolescents and young women are more susceptible to cervical infections, such as chlamydial infections and gonorrhea, and HIV because of the ectropion of the immature cervix and resulting larger exposed surface of cells unprotected by cervical mucus. The cells eventually recede into the inner cervix as women age. Postmenopausal women also are at increased risk because of thin vaginal and cervical mucosa. Furthermore, women who are pregnant have higher rates of cervical ectropion.

Other biological factors that may increase a woman's risk for acquiring, transmitting, or developing complications of certain STDs include vaginal douching, risky sexual practices, and use of hormonal contraceptives. Risk for contracting the infections that can lead to PID may be increased with vaginal douching, and risk for PID may increase with greater frequency of douching (Bui et al., 2016). Certain sexual practices, such as anal intercourse, sex during menses, and "dry sex" (inserted vaginal sex without sufficient lubrication) may predispose a woman to acquiring an STD. This may be because bleeding and tissue trauma can result from these practices and facilitate invasion by pathogens. Although normal vaginal flora may confer nonspecific immunity, both younger and postmenopausal women may be at a greater risk of acquiring HIV because of a thinner vaginal epithelium and resulting increased friability, thus providing direct access to the bloodstream.

Social Factors

Preventing the spread of STDs and HIV is difficult without addressing individual and community issues that have a tremendous influence on prevention, transmission, and treatment of these diseases. Societal factors such as poverty, lack of education, social inequity, and inadequate access to health care indirectly increase the prevalence of STDs and HIV in risk populations.

Persons with the highest rates of many STDs are often those with the poorest access to health care, and health insurance coverage influences if and where a woman obtains STD services and preventive services. Furthermore, even if a poor woman perceives herself to be at risk for an STD, she may not practice protective behaviors if survival is an overarching concern or if there are other risks that appear to be more threatening or imminent. The need to secure shelter, food, and clothing, safety for self and children, and money may override concerns about preventive health and thus prevent women from changing risky behaviors.

Social Interactions and Relationships

STDs are the only illnesses whose spread is directly caused by the human urge to share sexual intimacy and reproduce. Because intimate human contact is the common vehicle of transmission, sexual behavior in the context of relationships is a critical risk factor for preventing and acquiring STDs. The gender-power imbalance and cultural proscriptions sometimes associated with sexual relationships make it difficult for women to protect themselves from infection (Park, Nordstrom, Weber, & Irwin, 2016; Paterno & Jordan, 2012). Women may have less say over when and under what circumstances intercourse occurs. Young women are particularly at risk because they may have sex with older men and—because of the power difference in the relationship, feelings of low self-efficacy, and lack of self-confidence—may be unable to negotiate safer sex practices (Hewitt-Stubbs, Zimmer-Gembeck, Mastro, & Boislard, 2016; Parker et al., 2016). Lifestyles of premarital, intermarital, and extramarital sexual activity are common for many women; because of the secrecy and cultural proscriptions surrounding such activities, women often engage in them without preparation, leading to risk for themselves and their partners.

A woman may be dependent on an abusive male partner or a partner who places her at risk by his own risky behaviors (Hewitt-Stubbs et al., 2016; Paterno & Jordan, 2012). The risk of acquiring STDs or HIV infection is high among women who are physically and sexually abused. Past and current experiences with violence, particularly sexual abuse, erode women's sense of self-efficacy to exercise control over sexual behaviors, engender feelings of anxiety and depression, and increase the likelihood of risky sexual behaviors (Paterno & Jordan, 2012). Additionally, fear of physical harm and loss of economic support hamper women's efforts to enact protective practices. Furthermore, past and current abuse is strongly associated with substance abuse, which also increases the risk of contracting an STD.

A woman's risk of acquiring an STD is determined not only by her actions but by her partner's as well. Although prevention counseling customarily includes recommending that women identify the partner who is at high risk because of drugs and medical factors and also determine his sexual practices, this advice may be unrealistic or culturally inappropriate in many relationships. Women who engage in sexual activities with other women only may or may not be at risk for infection. Many women who identify themselves as lesbian have had intercourse with a man at one time by choice, by force, or by necessity. Their female partners may have had intercourse with a man. In addition, lesbians may use drugs and share needles.

Societal Norms

Cultural and religious attitudes regarding appropriate sexual behaviors affect risk at the individual and community levels. Relationships and sexual behavior are regulated by cultural norms that influence sexual expression in interpersonal relationships. Often, women are still socialized to please their partners and to place men's needs and desires first and may find it difficult to insist on safer sex behaviors. Traditional cultural values associated with passivity and subordination may diminish the ability of many women to adequately protect themselves.

Power imbalances in relationships are the product of and contributors to the maintenance of traditional gender roles that identify men as the initiators and decision makers of sexual activities and women as passive gatekeepers (Hewitt-Stubbs et al., 2016; Paterno & Jordan, 2012). As long as traditional gender norms define the roles for sexual relationships as men having the dominant role in sexual decision making, negotiating condom use by women will remain difficult. Additionally, cultural norms define talking about condoms as implying a lack of trust that runs counter to the traditional gender norm expectations for women. Women may not request condom use because of a need to establish and maintain intimacy with partners. Research has demonstrated that women at risk for HIV place significant importance on and investment in their heterosexual relationships, and these dynamics impact on the women's risk taking and risk management (Hewitt-Stubbs et al., 2016). Urging women to insist on condom use may be unrealistic, because traditional gender roles do not encourage women to talk about sex, initiate sexual practices, or control intimate encounters.

Recognition of Risk

Lack of a perception of risk is often given as a reason for not using sexual protective practices. Younger women may incur more STDs because they have less knowledge of reproductive health, less effective skills in communicating and negotiating with their partners about safer sex practices, and more barriers to access to health care services. Taking risks is a universal human element. In the throes of passion, people can make unwise sexual decisions. Furthermore, safer sex is not always perceived to be the most enjoyable sex.

Substance Use

Substance use (alcohol and drugs) is associated with increased risk of HIV and STDs (Welty et al., 2016), and STD rates are higher in areas where rates of substance abuse are high. Women drug users are at high risk for HIV and STD because of both drug-related and sexual transmission (Welty et al., 2016). For example, in many areas, cocaine and heroin use has paralleled trends in syphilis, gonorrhea, and HIV infection. There are several possible reasons for this association, including social factors, such as poverty and lack of educational and economic opportunities and individual factors such as risk taking and low self-efficacy. In addition to the risk from sharing needles, use of drugs and alcohol may contribute to the risk of HIV infection by undermining cognitive and social skills, thus making it more difficult to engage in HIV-protective actions. Furthermore, depression and other psychological problems and/or a history of sexual abuse are associated with substance abuse and thus contribute to risky behaviors (Braje, Eddy, & Hall, 2016). Being high and thus not able or willing to clean drug paraphernalia can be a pervasive barrier to protective practice. Moreover, drug use may take place in settings where persons participate in sexual activities while using drugs. Many cocaine users routinely engage in high-risk sexual behaviors that place them at high risk of HIV and other blood-borne STD infections (Cardozo et al., 2016). Finally, women who use drugs may be at a higher risk because of the practice of exchanging sex for drugs or money and high numbers of sexual partners and encounters (Cardozo et al., 2016).

Past and current physical, emotional, and sexual abuse characterize the lives of many, if not most, drug-using women (Imtiaz, Wells, & Macdonald, 2016). For women who have experienced violence, use of alcohol and drugs can become a coping mechanism by which they self-medicate to relieve feelings of anxiety, depression, guilt, fear, and anger stemming from the violence (Imtiaz et al., 2016). Women's drug use is strongly linked to relationship inequities and some men's ability to mandate women's sexual behavior. Sexual degradation of women has been described as an intimate part of crack cocaine use (Cardozo et al., 2016; Imtiaz et al., 2016).

Cultural and religious attitudes and beliefs also affect health care services. The loss of support for safer sex education programs in favor of an abstinence-only program does not protect adolescents. Teens who pledge to remain a virgin until marriage have the same, if not higher, rates of STDs than those who do not commit to abstinence. In response to these findings, a more pragmatic abstinence-plus or "ABC" message based on harm-reduction principles has been instituted. The message is "Abstinence, Be Faithful" for married couples or those in committed relationships, and "Use a Condom" for individuals who put themselves at risk for HIV infection.

■ SPECIAL POPULATIONS

Incarcerated Women

Incarcerated women experience STD/HIV infection at a rate 13 times greater than that of women in the general population (CDC, 2015a). This heightened risk is because of a unique confluence of factors, including histories of sex work, substance abuse, experienced violence, mental illness, concurrent partners, and infection with other STDs (Farel et al., 2013; Fogel et al., 2014). Additionally, before incarceration, many women have limited access to medical care. To date no comprehensive national guidelines have been developed regarding STDs and management for incarcerated persons; however, the multiple risk factors and high incidence of STDs in women prisoners demonstrated the need for STD screening and treatment in jails and prisons. Women 35 years and younger in juvenile and adult detention facilities have higher rates of chlamydia and gonorrhea than nonincarcerated females in the community (CDC, 2015a). Furthermore, syphilis rates are considerably higher in adult incarcerated women than in nonincarcerated females (CDC, 2015a). In short-term correctional facilities (jails and juvenile detention facilities), retention rates are short (often 48 hours) and as a result treatment completion may be less than optimal. Furthermore, the mobility of this population in and out of the community increases the risk for further infections.

The current CDC STD screening recommendation is that all women 35 and younger in correctional facilities be screened for chlamydia and gonorrhea and that universal syphilis screening be conducted on the basis of the local area and institutional prevalence of primary, secondary, and early latent syphilis (CDC, 2015a).

Women Who Have Sex With Women

Women who have sex with women (WSW) are a diverse group with variations in sexual identity, sexual behaviors, sexual practices, and risk behaviors (CDC, 2015a). Some WSW, particularly younger women and adolescents and women who have sex with both men and women may be at increased risk for STDs and HIV (CDC, 2015a). WSW have exposures to STDs such as trichomoniasis, gonorrhea, chlamydia, genital herpes, HPV, hepatitis C (HCV), syphilis, and HIV and should be screened for all of these diseases (Petti, 2015). HPV, which can be transmitted through skin-to-skin contact, is common in WSW and sexual transmission of HPV also occurs among female sex

partners (CDC, 2015a). Many women who identify as lesbians have experienced physical, emotional, and sexual violence and the health history should include assessment for these issues. Examples of specific questions to include in the health history are: Are you having sex with males, females, and/or both males and females? Do you participate in oral-to-vaginal contact with your partner(s)? Do you participate in finger-to-vaginal or anal contact with your partners(s)? Do you use sex toys (vibrators, strap-on penis, pelvic balls)? Do you share these with your partner(s)? and/or Do you participate in oral-to-anal contact with your partner(s)? Use of barrier protection with female partners (gloves during digital-genital sexual activities, condoms with sex toys, and latex or plastic barriers, e.g., dental dams) has been found to be infrequent (CDC, 2015a).

WSW are at risk for acquiring bacterial, viral, and protozoal STDs from their partners, both male and female, and should not be presumed to be at low or no risk for STDs based on sexual orientation. Effective screening requires that health care providers and their female patients have open and comprehensive discussion of sexual and behavioral risks that are beyond sexual identity. It is also essential that nurse practitioners understand their own comfort level in order to have open, candid discussion with women regarding their sexual practices and behaviors.

■ PREVENTION

Preventing infection (primary prevention) is the most effective way of reducing the adverse consequences of STDs for women, their partners, and society. With the advent of serious and potentially lethal STDs that are not readily cured or are incurable, primary prevention becomes critical. Prevention and control of STDs are based on five major strategies: (1) accurate risk assessment, education, and counseling of persons at risk on ways to avoid STDs through changes in sexual behaviors and use of recommended prevention services; (2) pre-exposure vaccination of persons at risk for vaccine-preventable STDs; (3) identification of asymptomatically infected person and persons with STDs; (4) effective diagnosis, treatment, counseling, and follow-up of infected persons; and (5) evaluation, treatment, and counseling of sex partners of persons who are infected with an STD (CDC, 2014). Prompt diagnosis and treatment of current infections (secondary prevention) also can prevent personal complications and transmission to others. Primary prevention of STDs begins with changing those behaviors that place persons at risk for infection. Moreover, treatment of infected individuals is a form of primary prevention of spread within the community in that it reduces the likelihood of transmission of STDs to sexual partners (CDC, 2014). Furthermore, the key to real progress in STD prevention is coordination of prevention programs for unintended pregnancy and HIV with those for other STDs, because all are the consequences of unprotected sexual activity. Risk factors for STDs and HIV are summarized in Box 30.1.

BOX 30.1   RISK FACTORS FOR STDs AND HIV

Women who are at an increased risk of contracting STDs and HIV include those:

- who have unprotected vaginal, anal, or oral intercourse
- who have multiple sex partners
- who use alcohol or illicit drugs during sexual activity
- with high-risk sex practices, including fisting, oral–anal contact, anal intercourse
- who share sex toys and douching equipment
- who share needles or other drug-use paraphernalia
- who have partners who are bisexual men who also have sex with other men
- with a previous history of a documented STD or HIV infection
- with partners who have a previous history of STDs or HIV
- involved in the exchange of sex for drugs or money
- who live in areas with a high STD/HIV incidence or prevalence
- at their initiation of sexual activity

STD, sexually transmitted disease.

Adapted from Centers for Disease Control and Prevention (2015a); Fogel (2006); Institute of Medicine (1997); Schmid (2001); Star (2004).

TABLE 30.3	Strategies for Reducing Personal Risk

- Avoiding all sexual contact (abstinence) with others is the only sure way to avoid contracting an STD
- Have sex with only one person who does not have sex with anyone else and who is free of STDs
- Always use a condom and use it correctly
- If you inject using needles, always use clean needles and other drug paraphernalia
- Prevent and treat all STDs to decrease your susceptibility to HIV infection and to decrease your infectiousness if you are HIV positive
- Delay starting to have sex as long as possible because the younger you are when you start having sex, the greater your risk for catching an STD
- Decrease the number of partners you have, because the risk of contracting an STD increases with the number of partners you have at one time and over your lifetime

If you are sexually active:

- Always use protection unless you are having sex with only one person who is also monogamous and who has no infection
- Have regular checkups for STDs even if you have no symptoms
- Always have a checkup when having sex with a new person
- Know the symptoms for STDs and see a health care provider if any suspicious symptoms develop, no matter how minor they are
- Do not have sex during your menstrual period because you are more susceptible to contracting an STD at that time
- Avoid anal intercourse, and use a condom if you have anal intercourse
- Do not douche unless prescribed by your health care provider because it removes some of the normal protective bacteria and increases the risk of getting some STDs

If you are diagnosed with having an STD:

- Be treated to decrease your risk of transmitting an STD to your partner
- Notify all recent sex partners, and urge them to get a checkup and be treated if necessary
- Follow all of your health care provider's recommendations
- Take all medications as prescribed
- Have a follow-up test if indicated
- Do not have sex during your treatment

STD, sexually transmitted disease.
Adapted from Fogel (2006).

Education

Educational efforts, both population-based and individual, that are gender and culture specific and are at an appropriate literacy level are important to STD control. Educational messages about specific infections, personal protective practices, and communication skills should be delivered in age-appropriate, culturally sensitive, appealing formats. Specific patient education messages are found in Table 30.3.

Unfortunately, mass educational efforts in the United States are limited largely to schools and the media. Furthermore, the culture-imposed secrecy surrounding sexual issues prevalent in the U.S. society results in a tremendous lack of information about STD prevention. To change risky behaviors, Americans need to become more comfortable discussing sexuality and sexual health issues between health care providers and patients, among sexual partners, and between parents and children. Comprehensive sexual health education provides information about STDs and HIV transmission, prevention, treatment and abstinence, and protective practice as well as training to build negotiation and communication skills. Although knowledge is essential in preventing STDs and HIV, it is not sufficient

to change behavior (Goldsberry, Moore, MacMillan, & Butler, 2016).

Individual Counseling

Since the advent of HIV and other incurable viral STDs, counseling individual women has become even more important. As incurable infections have emerged, the role of treatment with cure has lessened, and the need for risk-reduction counseling has increased. Woman-centered counseling to prevent acquisition or transmission of STDs should be a standard component of STD care regardless of where it is provided in the health care system. Counseling skills that are characterized by respect, compassion, and a nonjudgmental attitude toward all patients are essential to obtaining a complete sexual-risk history and counseling women effectively about prevention. Specific techniques that have been found to be effective in providing prevention counseling include using open-ended questions (e.g., "What has your experience with using condoms been like?"), using understandable language ("Have you ever had a sore or a scab on your private parts or lips?"), normalizing language ("Some of my patients tell me that it is hard to use a condom every time they have sex. How has it been for you?"), and reassuring the women that treatment will be provided regardless of consideration, such as ability to pay, language spoken, or lifestyle (CDC, 2014).

Assurances of confidentiality are equally important in providing effective risk-reduction counseling. Prevention messages should include descriptions of specific actions to be taken to avoid acquiring or transmitting STDs (e.g., refrain from sexual activity if you have STD-related symptoms, be vaccinated against HPV and hepatitis B) and should be tailored to the individual woman with attention given to her specific risk factors (CDC, 2015a).

Safer Sex Practices

Risk-free individual activities aimed at deterring infection include complete abstinence from sexual activities that transmit semen, blood, or other body fluids or that allow for skin-to-skin contact (Hatcher et al., 2011). Counseling that encourages abstinence from sexual intercourse is critical for women who are being treated for an STD, for women whose partner is being treated for an STD, and for persons wanting to avoid all possible consequences of sex (e.g., STDs, HIV, and unintended pregnancies). Alternatively, involvement in a mutually monogamous relationship with an uninfected partner also eliminates risk of contracting an STD. For women beginning a mutually monogamous relationship, screening for common STDs before beginning sex might decrease the risk for future transmission of asymptomatic STDs (CDC, 2015a). When neither of these options is realistic for a woman, however, the nurse practitioner must focus on other, more feasible measures.

An essential component of primary prevention is counseling women regarding safer sex practices, including knowledge of her partner, reduction of number of partners, low-risk sex, and avoiding the exchange of body fluids. No aspect of prevention is more important than knowing one's partner. Reducing the number of partners and avoiding partners who have had many previous sexual partners decreases a woman's chance of contracting an STD. Deciding not to have sexual contact with a casual acquaintance may be helpful too. Discussing each new partner's previous sexual history and exposure to STDs will augment other efforts to reduce risk. Women must be cautioned that, in any sexual encounter other than a mutually monogamous relationship, safer sex measures are always advisable, even when partners insist otherwise. Critically important is whether male partners resist wearing condoms. This is crucial when women are not sure about their partner's sexual history. Women should be cautioned against making decisions about a partner's sexual

and other behaviors based on appearances and unfounded assumptions such as:

- Single people have many partners and risky practices
- Older people have few partners and infrequent sexual encounters
- Sexually experienced people know how to practice safer sex
- Married people are heterosexual, low risk, and monogamous
- People who look healthy are disease free
- People with good jobs do not use drugs (Guest, 2006)

Women should be taught low-risk sexual practices and which sexual practices to avoid (Table 30.4). Sexual fantasizing is safe, as are caressing, hugging, body rubbing (frottage), and massage. Mutual masturbation is low risk as long as there is no contact with a partner's semen or vaginal secretions. All sexual activities when both partners are monogamous, trustworthy, and known by testing to be free of disease are safe.

When used correctly and consistently, male latex condoms are highly effective in preventing sexual transmission of HIV infection and can reduce the risk for other STDs (gonorrhea, chlamydia, and trichomonas; see Box 30.2). However, because they do not cover all exposed surfaces, they are more likely to be most effective in preventing infections that are transmitted by fluids from mucosal surfaces (gonorrhea, chlamydia, trichomonas, and HIV) than those transmitted by skin-to-skin contact (e.g., HSV, HPV, syphilis, chancroid). Furthermore, by limiting lower genital infections, condoms may also reduce the risk of PID (CDC, 2015a). Rates of latex condom breakage during sexual intercourse and withdrawal are low (about 2 condoms per 100 condoms used) in the United States (CDC, 2014). Nonlatex condoms (e.g., those made of polyurethane) can be substituted for persons with latex allergies (CDC, 2014) to prevent pregnancy. However, nonlatex condoms can have pores up to 1,500 nm in diameter, which is more than 10 times the diameter of HIV and more than 25 times the diameter of HBV. They also have higher rates of breakage and slippage than do latex condoms. The failures of condoms to protect women against STD transmission or unintended pregnancy are usually the result of inconsistent or incorrect use rather than from condom breakage.

Thus, counseling women about correct condom use is critical (see Boxes 30.3 and 30.4). Nurse practitioners can help to motivate clients to use condoms by first discussing the subject with them. This gives women an opportunity to discuss any concerns, misconceptions, or hesitations they may have about using condoms. The nurse practitioner may initiate a discussion of how to purchase and use condoms. Information to be discussed includes importance of using latex or plastic condoms rather than natural skin condoms. The nurse practitioner should remind women to use condoms with every sexual encounter, only use them once, use condoms with a current expiration date, and handle them carefully to avoid damaging them with fingernails, teeth, or other sharp objects. Condoms should be stored away from high heat. Contrary to popular myth, a recent study found no increase in breakage after carrying condoms in a wallet for a lengthy period of time (Hatcher et al., 201). Although

TABLE 30.4	Behavior and Levels of Risk		
SAFEST	**LOW RISK**	**POSSIBLE RISK**	**HIGH RISK**
Behavior Abstinence Self-masturbation Mutual monogamy (both partners monogamous and no high-risk activities) Hugging, touching, massaging[a] Dry kissing Mutual masturbation Drug abstinence **Prevention** Avoid all drug and sexual high-risk behaviors	**Behavior** Wet kissing Vaginal intercourse with condom Fellatio interruptus Urine contact with intact skin **Prevention** Avoid exposure to any potentially infected body fluids Consistently use latex or polyurethane condoms	**Behavior** Cunnilingus Fellatio Mutual masturbation with skin breaks Anal intercourse with condom **Prevention** Avoid anal intercourse Use dental dam, unlubricated male condom cut in half, female condom, or plastic wrap with cunnilingus Use latex gloves with masturbation	**Behavior** Unprotected anal intercourse Unprotected vaginal intercourse Unprotected oral–anal contact Vaginal intercourse after anal intercourse without a new condom Fisting Multiple sex partners Sharing sex toys, needles, or other drug paraphernalia, or douching equipment **Prevention** Avoid exposure to potentially infected body fluids Consistent condom use with vaginal and anal intercourse Avoid anal penetration If having anal penetration, use condom with intercourse, latex glove with hand penetration Avoid oral–anal contact Do not share sex toys, drug paraphernalia, or douche equipment Clean needles and drug paraphernalia with bleach and water before and after use

Note: [a]Assumes no breaks in the skin.
Adapted from Centers for Disease Control and Prevention (2015a); Fogel (1995, 2006).

BOX 30.2   SUGGESTIONS ON HOW TO USE A MALE CONDOM

Use new condoms every time you perform any vaginal, anal, and oral sex (try flavored).

- Open the package carefully to avoid damage
- Do not unroll before placing it on the penis
- Gently press out air at the tip before putting it on
- Put it on when the penis is erect
- Unroll to cover the entire erect penis
- If it tears or comes off in the vagina, stop immediately and withdraw; put on a new one before you continue
- After ejaculation and before the penis gets soft, withdraw the penis and the condom together
- Hold on to the rim as you withdraw so nothing spills
- Gently pull the condom off the penis
- Discard in waste containers
- Do not flush down the toilet
- Never reuse condoms

not ideal, women may choose to safely carry condoms in wallets, shoes, or inside a bra. Women can be taught the differences among condoms, price ranges, sizes, and where they can be purchased. This information can be found on the website of the American Social Health Association (www.ashastd.org) or in any drug store.

Laboratory studies have demonstrated that the female condom, a lubricated polyurethane sheath with a ring on each end that is inserted into the vagina, is an effective mechanical barrier to viruses, including HIV, and to semen (CDC, 2015a; see Box 30.5). Furthermore, clinical studies have documented its effectiveness in providing protection from recurrent trichomonas. If used consistently and correctly, the female condom should reduce the risk of contracting or transmitting an STD.

Selection of a contraceptive method has a direct impact on STD risk. Many women view condoms first, and perhaps only, as a method of contraception. Women who have another method of birth control, such as sterilization or hormonal contraceptives are less likely to use condoms when compared with other women. The effectiveness of contraceptive methods against STDs including HIV is summarized in Table 30.5. Women should be counseled that the contraceptive methods that are most protective against STDs usually are not the most effective pregnancy prevention methods. For example, condoms

BOX 30.3   QUESTIONS AND ANSWERS ABOUT USING MALE CONDOMS

■ **How many condoms will I need?**
You need to use a new condom every time you have sexual intercourse (however you have it). If you think you might have sex more than once, you should carry several with you. Never reuse the same condom—it will not work. Carry more condoms than you think you might need.

■ **Where should I keep my condoms?**
You need to keep condoms cool and dry (and in the dark), so keep them in the pocket of a jacket or in a bag. Do not keep them in the pocket of your jeans or the glove compartment of your car, because they will get too hot.

■ **What do I need to do before I have sex?**
Make sure the package the condom is sold in looks okay and check the expiration date. Carefully open the condom package at one corner. Do not attack it with your teeth or fingernails (this is the most common reason for a condom to be torn). You might tear a hole in the condom. The condom will be rolled up ready for use. Make sure you use it the right way around (so that the condom rolls down smoothly).

■ **What do I need to do before I have intercourse?**
You need to put the condom on when the penis is erect but before you have made any contact between the penis and any part of your partner's body.

■ **How do I put a male condom on?**
If your partner has not been circumcised, you will need to roll back his foreskin a bit before putting the condom on. Put the still rolled-up condom over the tip of the hard (erect) penis. If the condom does not have a reservoir (the blob at the end, which most condoms do have), you need to pinch half an inch at the end of it to make room for the semen (sperm) to collect. Pinch the air out of the condom tip between your finger and thumb of one hand, and unroll the condom over the penis with the other hand. Roll the condom all the way down to the base of the penis, and smooth out any air bubbles (air bubbles can cause a condom to break).

■ **How do I put extra lubrication on a condom?**
If you want or need to use some extra lubrication, put it on the outside of the condom before you use it. Only use a water-based lubricant, because an oil-based lubricant will dissolve the latex of the condom, making it useless.

■ **What if I cannot get the condom on?**
Most of the time (and when you have practiced a bit) condoms will roll down a penis very easily and smoothly. If it is getting stuck or is difficult to roll down, it probably means you are putting it on inside out. You will need to get this condom off by holding its rim. Throw this condom away and start again with a new one.

■ **When do I take the condom off?**
When your partner is wearing a condom, he needs to come out of you when his penis is still hard. To make sure that that no semen (sperm) is spilled, which will be at the end of the condom, you need to hold the condom against the base of the penis while it is removed. Have a look at the condom to look for tears or spills, and then pull the condom off.

■ **What do I do with the used condom?**
It is best to tie a knot in the used condom and then throw it in a bin (preferably wrapped in some tissue). Do not litter, and do not flush them down the toilet because they are not biodegradable and can be dangerous for marine life.

■ **What if I have not used it perfectly or have found a tear?**
No one is perfect and accidents happen. If you think the condom you have used might not have been used perfectly or you find a tear in it, do not panic. Try to get to a family planning clinic, your general practitioner, or a genitourinary medicine clinic soon (preferably within 24 hours) for emergency contraception. The earlier you start to take the emergency contraceptive pills, the more likely they are to prevent a pregnancy. If the condom has not worked properly, the sex you have had is unprotected, and you and your partner are both at risk of getting an infection. Get yourselves to a clinic and get checked out.

Adapted from Sexual Health Advice Center (2016).

are the most protective method against STDs and HIV but are not the most effective in preventing pregnancy. Use of dual protection to prevent pregnancy and STDs is critical for women. Because it is unclear how many women understand the need for dual protection, nurse practitioners can play an important role in counseling women in this regard and in the importance of other risk-reduction practices.

Until recently, women were counseled to use spermicides—specifically nonoxynol-9 (N-9)—with condoms for the prevention of HIV and other STDs. Research has found no significant reduction in the risk of HIV and STDs with the addition of N-9 spermicide to condom use. Furthermore, there is some evidence of harm disruption of genital or rectal epithelium, slightly higher rates of urogenital gonorrhea, and an increased risk for bacterial urinary tract infections in women who are nonoxynol-9 users (CDC, 2015a; Hatcher et al., 2011). At this time, no proven topical antiretroviral agents exist for the prevention of HIV (CDC, 2015a).

BOX 30.4   DOs AND DON'Ts OF CONDOM USE

- DO use only latex or polyurethane (plastic) condoms.
- DO keep condoms in a cool, dry place.
- DO put the condom on an erect (hard) penis before there is any contact with a partner's genitals.
- DO use plenty of water-based lubricant (like K-Y Jelly or Astroglide) with latex condoms. This reduces friction and helps prevent the condom from tearing.
- DO squeeze the air out of the tip of the condom when rolling it over the erect penis. This allows room for the semen (cum).
- DO hold the condom in place at the base of the penis before withdrawing (pulling out) after sex.
- DO throw the condom away after it has been used.

- DO NOT use out-of-date condoms. Check the expiration date carefully. Old condoms can be dry, brittle, or weakened, and can break easily.
- DO NOT unroll the condom before putting it on the erect penis.
- DO NOT leave condoms in hot places, such as your wallet or in your car.
- DO NOT use oil-based products, such as baby oil, cooking oil, hand lotion, or petroleum jelly (Vaseline), as lubricants with latex condoms. The oil quickly weakens latex and can cause condoms to break.
- DO NOT use your fingernails or teeth when opening a condom wrapper. It is very easy to tear the condom inside. If you do tear a condom while opening the wrapper, throw that condom away and get a new one.
- DO NOT reuse a condom. Always use a new condom for each kind of sex you have.

Source: Retrieved from www.ashastd.org

The exact risk of HIV transmission through ingestion of male or female sexual secretions is not known definitively; however, a few HIV cases have been linked to transmission through oral sex (CDC, 2015a). HBV and HCV can rarely be spread through saliva, and HSV type 1 (HSV-1) and HSV type 2 (HSV-2), syphilis, gonorrhea, and chlamydia can be spread through oral sex. Therefore, women should use barriers such as dental dams, male unlubricated condoms cut in half, or non-microwaveable saran wrap when engaging in cunnilingus or unlubricated condoms for fellatio.

With most of the condoms now available to women in the United States, active male cooperation is essential. A key issue in condom use as a preventative strategy is that, in sexual encounters, men must comply with a woman's suggestion or request that they use a condom. Moreover, condom usage must be renegotiated with every sexual contact, and women must address the issue of control of sexual decision making every time they request a male partner to use a condom. Women may fear that their partner will be offended if a condom is introduced. Some women may fear rejection and abandonment, conflict, potential violence, or loss of economic support if they suggest the use of condoms to prevent STD transmission. For many individuals, condoms are symbols of extra-relationship activity. Introduction of a condom into a long-term relationship where they have not been used previously threatens the trust assumed in most long-term relationships.

Many women do not anticipate or prepare for sexual activity in advance; embarrassment or discomfort in purchasing condoms may prevent some women from using them. Cultural barriers also may impede the use of condoms. Latino gender roles make it difficult for Latina women to suggest using condoms to a partner

(Morales-Alemán & Scarinci, 2016). Suggesting condom use implies that a woman is sexually active, that she is available for sex, and that she is seeking sex; these are messages that many women are uncomfortable conveying given the prevailing mores in the United States. In a society that may view a woman who carries a condom as overprepared, possibly oversexed, and willing to have sex with any man, expecting her to insist on the use of condoms in a sexual encounter is unrealistic. Finally, women should be counseled to watch out for situations that make it hard to talk about and practice safer sex. These include romantic times when condoms are not available and when alcohol or drugs make it impossible to make wise decisions about safer sex.

Certain sexual practices should be avoided to reduce one's risk of infection. Abstinence from any sexual activities that could result in exchange of infective body fluids will help decrease risk. Anal–genital intercourse, anal–oral contact, and anal–digital activity are high-risk sexual behaviors and should be avoided (Hatcher et al., 2011; CDC, 2015a). Sexual transmission occurs through direct skin or mucous membrane contact with infectious lesions or body fluids. Because mucosal linings are delicate and subject to considerable mechanical trauma during intercourse, small abrasions often may occur, facilitating entry of infectious agents into the bloodstream. The rectal epithelium is especially easy to traumatize with penetration. Sexual practices that increase the likelihood of tissue damage or bleeding such as fisting (inserting a fist into the rectum) should be avoided. Deep kissing when lips, gums, or other tissues are raw or broken also should be avoided (Hatcher et al., 2011). Because enteric infections are transmitted by oral–fecal contact, avoiding oral–anal, rimming (licking the anal area), and digital–anal activities

BOX 30.5   FEMALE CONDOMS

What Are Female Condoms?

Female condoms are made of very thin polyurethane. They are already lubricated to help you use them, but they do not have any spermicide (which is useful for people who are allergic to spermicide). Because they are made of a type of plastic, they can be used by people who are allergic to latex. They can also be used with oil-based lubricants and products (but be sure to not use oil-based lubricants with male condoms by mistake). Female condoms can provide protection from acquiring and transmitting an STD (CDC, 2015a).

Where Do They Go?

Female condoms are placed in a woman's vagina to line it and prevent sperm entering her cervix. It also helps protect her from infections that can be caught by having unprotected sex. (This will also protect her from most infections.) If used perfectly, they can be as effective as other contraceptives. If you use them with the birth control (or contraceptive) pill, they will be even more effective.

What Are the Advantages of Female Condoms?

- The woman is in control of her contraception
- Female condoms can protect against infections
- There are no side effects
- You do not have to remember to take a pill
- You can put a female condom in any time before sex

What Makes Them Less Effective?

- If the penis touches the vagina or area around it before a female condom is inserted
- If the condom splits
- If the female condom gets pushed too far into the vagina (the open end must stay outside the vagina during sex)
- If the penis enters the vagina outside the condom

How to Use Female Condoms

A new packet will have full instructions, including diagrams.

1. Check if it is new and check the use-by date.
2. You can put one in when you are lying down, squatting, or have one leg on a chair (like using a tampon, find the position that suits you best).
3. Take it out of the packet with care (fingernails and rings can tear polyurethane).
4. Hold the closed end of the condom and squeeze the inner ring (at the closed end) between your thumb and middle finger. If you keep your index finger on the inner ring too, it will help to keep it steady.
5. With your other hand, spread the outer and inner lips (labia), which are the folds of skin around your vagina. Push the squeezed ring into the vagina and as far up as you can (about a long-finger length). Now put your index finger or both your index and middle finger inside the open end of the condom, until you can feel the inner ring at the top. Push the inner ring at the top as far as you can into your vagina. (You will be able to feel the hard front of your pelvis—pubic bone—just in front of your fingers if you curve them forward a bit.)
6. The outer ring should be close against the outside of your vagina (vulva).
7. The female condom is loose fitting, so it is a good idea for the woman to help guide the penis into the ring. It will move about a bit during sex, but you will be protected from pregnancy and most infections as long as the penis stays inside the condom.

How to Remove Female Condoms

Take hold of the outer ring (the open end), and give it a twist to trap any semen inside it. Pull it out gently.

What to Do With Used Female Condoms

Never reuse a female condom. Wrap it up in a tissue and throw it in a trash bin. Do not put it in the toilet.

STD, sexually transmitted disease.

---

should reduce the likelihood of infection. Vaginal intercourse should never follow anal contact unless a condom has been used and then removed and replaced with a new condom.

Nurse practitioners can suggest strategies to enhance a woman's condom negotiation and communication skills. Suggesting that she talk with her partner about condom use at a time removed from sexual activity may make it easier to bring up the subject. Role-playing possible partner reactions with a woman and her alternative responses can be helpful. Asking a woman who appears particularly uncomfortable to rehearse how she might approach the topic is useful, particularly when a woman fears her partner may be resistant. The nurse practitioner might suggest her client begin by saying, "I need to talk with you about something that is important to both of us. It's hard for me and I feel embarrassed but I think we need to talk about safe sex." If women are able to sort out their feelings and

TABLE 30.5	Effectiveness of Contraceptives Against Sexually Transmitted Diseases	
	SEXUALLY TRANSMITTED DISEASE	
Contraceptive Method	**Bacterial**	**Viral (Including HIV)**
Condoms	Reduces risk; most protective in preventing infections transmitted by fluids	Protective
Sterilization	No protection	No protection
Vaginal spermicides with nonoxynol-9	Not effective in preventing cervical gonorrhea, chlamydia[a,d]	No protection, possibly increased risk[a,d]
Diaphragm, cervical cap	Modest protection against cervical infection (gonorrhea, chlamydia, trichomoniasis)	Questionable
Oral contraceptives	No known protection	Not protective; some studies suggest increased risk of HIV, others do not
Implantable/injectable contraceptives	Not protective	Not protective; some studies suggest increased risk of HIV[b]
Intrauterine device	Associated with pelvic inflammatory disease in first month after insertion[c]	No protection
Natural family planning	No protection	No protection

Notes: [a] Frequent use is associated with genital lesions, which may be associated with an increased risk of HIV transmission (Hatcher et al., 2011).
[b] Progestin-only contraceptives cause vaginal thinning, which may increase risk of HIV and may increase viral shedding if the woman has HIV (Hatcher et al., 2011).
[c] Likely to be caused by microbiological contamination at insertion (Hatcher et al., 2011).
[d] Efficacy in receptive anal intercourse is unknown.
Adapted from Centers for Disease Control and Prevention (2015a, pp. 1–94); Institute of Medicine (2015); Hatcher et al. (2011).

fears before talking with their partners, they may feel more comfortable and in control of the situation. Women can be reassured that it is natural to be uncomfortable and that the hardest part is getting started. Nurse practitioners should help their clients clarify what they will and will not do sexually because it is easier to discuss it if they are clear. Women can be reminded that their partner may need time to think about what they have said and that they must be paying attention to their partner's response. If the partner seems to be having difficulty with the discussion, a woman may slow down and wait a while. She can be reminded that if her partner resists safer sex, she may wish to reconsider the relationship. In addition, if a woman indicates fear for her safety if she suggests using a condom, the nurse practitioner must provide her with resources for prevention of violence and emphasize that her safety is paramount.

Women who have been diagnosed with an STD also need prevention counseling. Because of their behavior, both the woman and her partner need treatment for their infection and counseling to avoid reinfection. Key aspects to emphasize for women already infected include: (a) responding to disease suspicion by obtaining appropriate assessment promptly; (b) taking oral medications as directed; (c) returning for follow-up tests when applicable; (d) encouraging sex partners to obtain examination and treatment when indicated; (e) avoiding sexual exposure while infectious; (f) preventing future exposure by practicing protective practices; and (g) confidentiality.

■ SCREENING AND DETECTION

Symptoms

Prompt diagnosis and treatment are predicated on the assumption that any person who believes he or she may have contracted an STD, has symptoms of an STD, has had sexual relations with someone who has symptoms of an STD, or has a partner who has been diagnosed with an STD will seek care. Women must know how to recognize the major signs and symptoms of all STDs and obtain health care if they experience symptoms or have sexual contact with someone who had an STD. Nurse practitioners have the responsibility of educating their clients regarding the signs and symptoms of STDs. This may be done when a woman comes in for a well-woman examination, seeks contraception, obtains pre-conceptual care, or comes to her health care provider for prenatal care. Nurse practitioners also must ensure that clients know where and how to obtain care if they suspect they might have contracted an STD. Many local health departments have clinics specifically designed to treat STDs, and free treatment sometimes can be obtained at local emergency rooms. A critical first step to detecting STDs is for nurse practitioners to routinely and regularly obtain STD histories from their patients. To identify those at risk, specific questions should be asked during the collection of a health history.

Evaluation

Key aspects of obtaining a useful STD history include assurances of confidentiality and a nonjudgmental attitude. It is important that the history be conducted in a private room with the woman fully clothed. Be sure to begin with a rationale for why the questions are being asked, which assures the patient that you are not singling her out for some reason and also reinforces the importance of sexual health as a part of total health. When possible, use nonmedical terminology and be specific, for example, "How many partners have you had in the past month, past year?" Although it is advisable to collect a complete STD history, there may be times when this is not possible. If only a few minutes are available, ask something such as, "What are you doing to protect yourself from AIDS?" or "Thinking about AIDS and other sexual infections, what do you think is the riskiest thing you do?" From the answers to these questions, the clinician can get a sense of STD awareness and safer sex behaviors and can respond with at least one individualized, focused suggestion to add to knowledge and/or skill (Goldsberry et al., 2016). If it is possible to take a few more minutes, nurse practitioners can ask questions that elucidate a fuller history of infection, risk taking, and relationships in more detail. To obtain a comprehensive STD history, the questions in Tables 30.6 and 30.7 can be used to shape a risk assessment and STD history that is tailored to the cultural and social context of a patient's life and the prevalence of various STDs in a specific area.

Risk assessment depends on a woman's willingness to self-identify risk factors that may be seen as socially unacceptable or stigmatizing. It is possible that women may not reveal such risk factors directly to health care providers but will do so if they are asked to fill out a questionnaire using questions similar to those given in the sexual-risk history. Current recommendations (CDC, 2015a) are that all women from age of first sexual act until age 25 years should be screened at least yearly for STDs; after age 25 years, the timing of screening depends on risk factors present and whether the woman is pregnant. Furthermore, any woman who has been diagnosed with an STD should be screened for other STDs, because many of these infections (e.g., chlamydia, gonorrhea, syphilis, HBV) can be asymptomatic in women.

All pregnant women must be screened for gonorrhea, syphilis, chlamydia, and HBV. In addition, all pregnant women should be tested for HIV infection at the first prenatal visit, even if they have been previously tested (CDC, 2015a). Retesting in the third trimester (before 36 weeks)

is recommended for women at high risk for acquiring HIV infections including those who use illicit drugs, have a history of STDs during pregnancy, have multiple sex partners, or live in an area with high HIV prevalence (CDC, 2015a). A serological test for syphilis should be performed for pregnant women at the first prenatal visit and those at high risk for syphilis or who live in areas of high syphilis morbidity should be rescreened at approximately 28 weeks gestation and at delivery. Furthermore, neonates should not be discharged from the hospital unless the syphilis serological status of the mother has been obtained at least one time during pregnancy and preferably again at delivery. Any woman who delivers a stillborn infant should be tested for syphilis (CDC, 2015a). All pregnant women should be tested for HBV at the first prenatal visit even if they had previously been vaccinated or tested (CDC, 2015a). All pregnant women who are 25 years or older or at high risk of infection should be screened for chlamydia, gonorrhea, and HCV at the first prenatal visit.

Infected individuals should be asked to identify and notify all partners who might have been exposed. In addition, all persons infected with an STD must be thoroughly and appropriately treated. General procedures for reporting and treating STDs are discussed in the next section, and information specific to screening for individual STDs is presented in subsequent sections devoted to individual STDs.

■ CARING FOR A WOMAN WITH AN STD

Women may delay seeking care for STDs because they fear social stigma, have limited access to health care services, or may be asymptomatic or unaware that they have an infection. In this age of widespread and often sensational media publicity about STDs, being told she has any STD may be terrifying for a woman. She may not understand the difference between one infecting organism and another. Instead, she may hear a diagnosis of illness, possibly incurable. Symptoms such as increased vaginal discharge, malodor, and itching, associated with some STDs, may be perceived as dirty, and the woman may be embarrassed and concerned that she will offend those caring for her. When a woman is diagnosed with an STD, her reactions may range from acceptance to hurt, disbelief, anger, or concern. These reactions may vary with the expectations in the woman's subculture and personal experience.

Assessment

The diagnosis of an STD is based on an integration of relevant historical, physical, and laboratory data (see Tables 30.6, 30.7, and 30.8). A history that is accurate, comprehensive, and specific is essential for accurate diagnosis. Because many women are embarrassed or anxious, generally the history should be taken first, with the woman dressed. Information should be collected in a nonjudgmental manner, avoiding assumptions of sexual preference. All partners should be referred to as partners and not by gender. It is helpful to begin with open-ended questions that might

TABLE 30.6	Risk Screening

- ■ Are you sexually active? That is, have you engaged in sexual activities (had sex or intercourse) with anyone in the past 6 months? In the past year?
  - ● If no, have you engaged in sexual activities in the past?
  - ● If yes,
    - ○ Have your partners been men, women, or both?
    - ○ With how many different people? _____1 _____2–3 _____4–10 _____more than 10
    - ○ How many different people are you having sex with right now?
    - ○ Does your partner have any other partners that you know of?
    - ○ Have you ever had sex with someone who had been in jail or prison?
    - ○ Have you ever had sex with someone whom you were afraid put you at risk for HIV or other sexually transmitted diseases?
      - – Someone who had a positive AIDS test?
      - – Someone you think might have AIDS?
      - – Someone who uses illicit drugs? IV drugs?
      - – Someone who might have had sex with a sex worker?
      - – Someone who might have had sex with both men and women?
      - – Have you ever been told that you had a sexually transmitted infection?
        - _____ Never
        - _____ Chlamydia
        - _____ Gonorrhea
        - _____ Trichomonas
        - _____ Syphilis
        - _____ Other (list): _____
- ■ Have you ever been told that you had a pelvic infection or pelvic inflammatory disease?
- ■ Many women have sex when they have drunk too much alcohol or have been using drugs. Has this happened to you?
- ■ What kinds of drugs do you use?
  - _____ Opioids: Types _____ Route of administration _____ Frequency _____
  - _____ Stimulants: Types _____ Route of administration _____ Frequency _____
  - _____ Crack cocaine: Frequency _____ Have you had sex in a crack house? _____
  - _____ Alcohol: Types: _____ Frequency _____
- ■ Have you ever blacked out from alcohol or drugs, especially during sex?
- ■ Have you ever traded sex for drugs, money, food, housing, or anything else?
- ■ Do you ever have sex when you are high?
- ■ Can you tell me the kinds of sex that you have? This will help us figure out what your risks are.

Mouth on penis or vulva	protected _____	unprotected _____
Penis in vagina	protected _____	unprotected _____
Penis in the butt	protected _____	unprotected _____
Mouth on butt	protected _____	unprotected _____

For every sexually active woman, ask
- ● Are you worried about catching a sexually transmitted disease or HIV (the AIDS virus)?
- ● Do you do anything to prevent catching a disease?
- ● Have you had sex without a condom?
- ● When did you start using condoms?
- ● Have you performed oral sex on a man or woman without a barrier (dental dam, plastic wrap, condom)?

Adapted from Brown (2000); Carcio (1999); Fogel and Lauver (1990); Fogel and Woods (1995); Kurth (1998); MacLauren (1995); Star, Lommel, and Shannon (1995).

elicit information that otherwise would be missed; these can be followed with symptom-specific questions and relevant history. Specific areas to address include the reason why the woman has sought care and any symptoms she has noticed; a sexual history, including a description of the date and type of sexual activity; number of contacts; whether she has had contact with someone who recently had an STD; and potential sites of infection (mouth, cervix, urethra, and rectum). Pertinent medical history includes anything that will influence the management plan: history of drug allergies,

previously diagnosed chronic illnesses, and general health status. A menstrual history, including the date of the client's last menstrual period, must always be obtained so that pregnancy may be ruled out, because certain medications used to treat STDs are contraindicated in pregnancy. When indicated, an HIV-oriented systems review should be conducted (Chapter 31). Any positive answers regarding symptoms should be followed up to elicit information about onset, duration, and specific characteristics, such as color, amount, and consistency of discharge.

TABLE 30.7	Menstrual/Gynecologic History Questions to Assess Risk of STDs

Do you experience now or have you ever experienced:

- Frequent vaginal infections?
- Unusual vaginal discharge or odor?
- Vaginal itching, burning, sores, or warts?
- STDs? (Ask about individual diseases.)
- Abdominal pain?
- PID or infection of the uterus, tubes, or ovaries?
- Rape or violent intercourse?
- Physical, emotional, or sexual abuse?
- Abnormal Pap smear?
- Pain or bleeding with intercourse?
- Severe menstrual cramps occurring at the end of your period?
- Ectopic pregnancy?
- HIV testing?
- STD testing?
- Immunizations for the prevention of STDs?

PID, pelvic inflammatory disease; STDs, sexually transmitted diseases.

Unless the woman is reporting rape, a physical examination is not appropriate to diagnose STDs. If indicated, before the actual physical examination is performed, the nurse practitioner should discuss the examination with her client so that she is prepared for it. The physical examination begins with careful visualization of the external genitalia including the perineum. Erythema, edema, distortions, lesions or trauma from scratching, sexual activity, sports activity, or injury are noted. Palpation can locate areas of tenderness. The most common STDs can be diagnosed with a vaginal swab or urine screen. If rape is suspected a speculum exam and cultural are indicated. During the speculum examination, the vagina and cervix are inspected for edema, thinning, lesions, abnormal coloration, trauma, discharge, and bleeding. Thorough palpation of inguinal area and pelvic organs; milking of the urethra for discharge; and assessment of vaginal secretion odors are essential. Lesions should be evaluated and cultures obtained when appropriate. Because the speculum is usually not lubricated before insertion into the vagina as cultures of vaginal secretions may have to be obtained, insertion may be somewhat uncomfortable. Clients should be informed of this and reassured that every effort will be made to make the speculum examination as comfortable as possible. Appropriate laboratory studies will be suggested, in part, by the history and physical examination results. Because women are often infected with more than one STD simultaneously and many are asymptomatic, additional laboratory studies may be done, including a Pap smear, wet mounts, gonococcal culture, Venereal Disease Research Laboratory (VDRL) or rapid plasma reagent (RPR) for syphilis, and a hepatitis B panel (hepatitis B core antibody [HBcAb], hepatitis B surface antigen [HBsAg], hepatitis B surface antibody [HBsAb]). Cultures for HSV are obtained when indicated by history or physical examination. The woman should be offered HIV testing (Chapter 31). When indicated, a complete blood count,

sedimentation rate, urinalysis, or urine culture and sensitivity should be obtained. Further, if history or physical examination indicates, a pregnancy test should be performed.

Treatment

A woman with an STD will need support in seeking care at the earliest stage of symptoms. Counseling women about STDs is essential for (a) preventing new infections or reinfection; (b) increasing compliance with treatment and follow-up; (c) providing support during treatment; and (d) assisting patients in discussions with their partner(s). Clients must be made aware of the serious potential consequences of STDs and the behaviors that increase the likelihood of infection.

Box 30.6 outlines necessary client education for all STDs. The nurse practitioner must make sure that her client understands what disease she has, how it is transmitted, and why it must be treated. Clients should be given a brief description of the disease in language that they can understand. This description should include modes of transmission, incubation period, symptoms, infectious period, and potential complications. Effective treatment of STDs necessitates careful, thorough explanation of treatment regimen and follow-up procedures. Thorough, careful instructions about medications must be provided, both verbally and in writing. Side effects, benefits, and risks of the medication should be discussed. Unpleasant side effects or early relief of symptoms may discourage women from completing their medication course. Clients should be strongly urged to continue their medication until it is used up regardless of whether their symptoms diminish or disappear in a few days. Comfort measures that decrease symptoms such as pain, itching, or nausea should be suggested. Providing written information is a useful strategy, because this is a time of high anxiety for many clients and they may not be able to hear or remember what they were told. A number of booklets on STDs are already available, or the nurse practitioner may wish to develop literature that is specific to her practice setting and clients.

In general, women will be advised to refrain from intercourse until all treatment is finished and a re-culture, if appropriate, is done. After the infection is cured, women should be urged to continue using condoms to prevent recurring infections, especially if they have had one episode of PID or continue to have intercourse with new partners. Women may wish to avoid having sex with partners who have many other sexual partners. All women who have contracted an STD should be taught safer sex practices if this has not been done already. Follow-up appointments should be made as needed.

Addressing the psychosocial component of STDs is essential. It is never easy to tell a woman that she has an STD. Learning that one has an STD may be extremely upsetting, particularly if the STD is serious, has complications, or is incurable. Knowledge of an STD may unsettle a sexual relationship. Remember that a woman may be afraid or embarrassed to tell her partner, ask her partner to seek treatment, admit her sexual practices, or she may be concerned about confidentiality. The nurse practitioner may need to help the client deal with the effect of a diagnosis of

TABLE 30.8	History, Physical Examination, and Laboratory Test for STDs	
HISTORY	**PHYSICAL EXAMINATION**	**LABORATORY TESTS**

Current symptoms
Vaginal discharge: onset, color, odor, consistency, amount, constant versus intermittent, related to sexual contact, relationship to menses
Lesions or rashes anywhere on body
Genital itching, burning, swelling, rash, sores, or tears
Pain: location, intensity, any radiation, associated aggravating or alleviating factors, description
Abdominal or pelvic pain
Dysuria: internal versus external
Dyspareunia and/or postcoital bleeding
Symptoms of generalized infection (myalgia, arthralgia, malaise, fever)
Menstrual history
Last menstrual period
Sexual history
Sexual preference
Type and time of sexual activity
Frequency
Areas of contact
Partners: number, known partner history, history of new partner(s) in past month
Past history of similar problems: dates, times, follow-up, treatment response
History of:
    Previous infection or STD
    Chronic cervicitis
    Cervical surgery
    Abnormal Pap smear
    Unintended pregnancy
    Death in utero or stillbirth
    Preterm delivery or low-birth-weight delivery
    Allergies
    Adult health problems
    Diet, alcohol, cigarettes, drugs, use of sex toys, stimulants
    Contraceptive methods used
    Medications: recent antibiotics, use of vaginal medications (over-the-counter and prescription)
Frequency of douching, use of feminine sprays and deodorants, new toiletry products, perfumed toilet tissue
Change in laundry soaps, fabric softener, body soap
	Vital signs: blood pressure, pulse, respiration, temperature
	General examination of skin:
	Alopecia
	Rash on soles of feet, palms
	Condyloma lata
	Inguinal lymph nodes
	Abdominal examination rebound, bowel sounds, suprapubic tenderness, masses, organomegaly, enlarged bladder, costovertebral angle tenderness
	External genitalia examination (tenderness, enlargement, discharge, excoriations, erythema, lesions):
	Bartholin's glands, Skene's glands, sores, rash, genital warts, urethra
	Vaginal examination (speculum):
	Vaginal lesions, tears, discharge (color, odor, amount, odor)
	Cervix: friability, ectropion, cervical erosion, discharge from os, cervical tenderness, color
	Bimanual examination:
	Pain on cervical motion (positive Chandelier sign), fullness or pain in adnexa, tenderness of uterus, size of uterus
		As indicated by history or finding:
		Wet prep with KOH, normal saline
		KOH "whiff" test
		Gram stain
		Urinalysis or urine culture
		Vaginal swabs
		Gonorrhea culture
		Chlamydia culture
		Herpes culture
		Cervical culture
		pH with nitrazine testing
		HIV testing
		Serology test for syphillis
		Hepatitis B and hepatitis C testing
		Papanicolaou test
		Complete blood count

KOH, potassium hydroxide; STD, sexually transmitted disease.
Adapted from Carcio and Secor (2015a); Centers for Disease Control and Prevention (2015a); Hawkins, Roberto-Nichols, and Stanley-Haney (2008).

an STD on a committed relationship for the woman who is now faced with the necessity of dealing with uncertain monogamy. In other instances, the woman may be afraid that telling her partner may place her in danger of escalating abuse. This potential consequence must be discussed with each client.

For most STDs, sexual partners should be examined; thus, the infected woman is asked to identify and notify all partners who might have been exposed (partner notification). She may find this difficult to do. Empathizing with the client's feelings and suggesting specific ways of talking with partners will help decrease anxiety and assist in efforts to control infection. For example, the nurse practitioner might suggest that the woman say,

I care about you and I'm concerned about you. That's why I'm calling to tell you that I have a sexually transmitted disease. My clinician is _____ and she will be happy to talk with you if you would like (Fogel, 1995).

BOX 30.6 PATIENT STD PREVENTION EDUCATION

What Can You Do to Prevent STDs?

The only certain way to prevent STDs is to avoid sexual contact with others. If you choose to be sexually active, there are things you can do to decrease your risk of developing an STD:

- Have sex with only one person who does not have sex with anyone else and who has no infections.
- Always use a condom and use it correctly.
- Use clean needles if you inject any drugs.
- Prevent and control other STDs to decease your susceptibility to HIV infection and to reduce your infectiousness if you are HIV-infected.
- Wait to have sex for as long as possible. The younger you are when you start having sex for the first time, the more likely are to catch an STD. The risk of acquiring an STD also increases with the number of partners you have over a lifetime.

Anyone Who Is Sexually Active Should:

- Always use protection unless you are having sex with only one person who does not have sex with anyone else and who has no infections.

- Have regular checkups for STDs even if you have no symptoms and especially when having sex with a new partner.
- Learn the common symptoms of STDs. Seek health care immediately if any suspicious symptoms develop, even if they are mild.
- Avoid having sex during menstruation. HIV-infected women are probably more infectious, and HIV-uninfected women are probably more susceptible to becoming infected during that time.
- Avoid anal intercourse, but, if practiced, use a condom.
- Avoid douching because it removes some of the normal protective bacteria in the vagina and increases the risk of getting some STDs.

Anyone Diagnosed as Having an STD Should:

- Be treated to reduce the risk of transmitting an STD to another person.
- Notify all recent sex partners and urge them to get a checkup as soon as possible to decrease the risk of catching the infection again from them.
- Follow the health care provider's recommendations and complete the full course of medication prescribed. Have a follow-up test if this is necessary.
- Avoid sexual activity while being treated.

STDs, sexually transmitted diseases.

Offering literature and role-playing situations with the client may also be of assistance. It can be helpful to remind the client that, although this is an embarrassing situation, most persons would rather know than not know that they have been exposed. Health professionals who take time to counsel their clients on how to talk with their partner(s) can improve compliance and case finding. In situations when patient referral may not be effective or possible, health departments should be prepared to assist the woman either through contact referral or through provider referral. Contact referral is the process by which a woman agrees to notify her partners by a certain time. If her partners do not obtain medical evaluation and treatment within the given time period, then provider referral is implemented. Provider referral is the process by which partners named by identified patients are notified and counseled by health department providers.

Accurate identification and timely reporting of STDs are integral components of successful disease control efforts. All states require that gonorrhea, syphilis, and HIV/AIDS be reported to public health officials. Chlamydial infection is reportable in most states. The requirements for reporting other STDs differ from state to state. Nurse practitioners are legally responsible for reporting all cases of those diseases identified as reportable in the state in which they are employed and should make that sure they know what

the requirements are in the state in which they practice. The client must be informed when a case will be reported and told why. Failure to inform the client that the case will be reported is a serious breach of professional ethics. Confidentiality is a crucial issue for many clients. When an STD is reportable, women need to be told that they may be contacted by a health department representative. They should be assured that the information reported to and collected by health authorities is maintained in strictest confidence; in most jurisdictions, reports are protected by statute from subpoena. Every effort, within the limits of one's public health responsibilities, should be made to reassure clients.

The following sections outline the treatments for specific STDs following guidelines of the CDC. When available, they also delineate self-help measures and preventive strategies. Instructions specific to individual diseases are given in the appropriate sections.

■ CERVICITIS

Cervicitis is characterized by two major diagnostic signs: (1) a purulent or mucopurulent endocervical discharge seen in the endocervical canal or on a swab specimen and

(2) sustained endocervical bleeding easily induced by gentle passage of a cotton swab in the cervical opening (os). Either or both may be present. Additionally, cervicitis is frequently asymptomatic; however, some women complain of abnormal vaginal discharge and intermenstrual bleeding (e.g. after intercourse). When a cause of cervicitis is determined, it is typically chlamydia or gonorrhea. Additionally, cervicitis can also be seen in trichomoniasis and genital herpes (primary HCV-2) infections (CDC, 2015a). Because cervicitis may be a sign of upper genital tract infection, women with a new episode of cervicitis should be assessed for PID and tested for chlamydia and gonorrhea. Additionally, women with cervicitis should also be assessed for bacterial vaginosis (BV) and trichomoniasis and treated if indicated. Treatment as indicated is discussed in the following sections specific to each disease. Women should return for follow-up as indicated by treatment regimen selected. All sex partners in the past 60 days should be referred for evaluation, testing and treatment if chlamydia, gonorrhea, or trichomoniasis was identified or suspected in a woman with cervicitis (CDC, 2015a). In order to avoid reinfection, women and sex partners should not have intercourse until they have been adequately treated. Women with persistent or recurrent cervicitis despite having been treated should be reevaluated for possible reexposure or treatment failure to cervicitis or gonorrhea. If relapse and/or reinfection with an STD is ruled out, BV is not present, and sex partners have been treated, the effectiveness of subsequent antibiotic treatment is unknown.

Chlamydia Infection

Chlamydia trachomatis is the most frequently reported infectious disease in the United States and its prevalence is highest in persons aged 24 years or younger (CDC, 2015a). Severe sequelae can result from chlamydial infection in women including PID, ectopic pregnancy, and infertility. Acute salpingitis, a form of PID, is the most serious complication of chlamydial infections and is a major etiological factor in subsequent development of tubal-factor infertility, ectopic pregnancy, and chronic pelvic pain. Further, chlamydial infection of the cervix causes inflammation resulting in microscopic cervical ulcerations and thus may increase the risk of acquiring HIV infection. Chlamydia infection in pregnancy has been associated with premature rupture of the membranes, preterm birth, stillbirth, and low-birth-weight infants. Maternal chlamydial infectious morbidity includes increased risk of postabortion endometritis and salpingitis and postpartum endometritis. Chlamydial infection of neonates results from perinatal exposure to the mother's infected cervix. Initial infections involve the mucous membranes of the eye, oropharynx, urogenital tract, and rectum. Conjunctivitis usually develops 5 to 12 days after delivery in 20% to 50% of exposed infants. Chlamydia is also a common cause of subacute, afebrile pneumonia in infants aged 1 to 3 months of age (CDC, 2015a).

Chlamydia is more common among adolescents than in older women. Sexually active women younger than 20 years are two to three times more likely to become infected with chlamydia than women between 20 and 29 years; women older than 30 years of age have the lowest rate of infection (CDC, 2015a). Risky behaviors—including multiple partners and nonuse of barrier methods of birth control—increase a woman's risk of chlamydial infection. Lower socioeconomic status may be a risk factor, especially with respect to treatment-seeking behaviors.

ASSESSMENT AND DIAGNOSIS

Annual screening of all sexually active women 25 years and younger is recommended as is screening of older women at increased risk for infection, including those who have a new sex partner, multiple sex partners, a partner with concurrent partners, or a partner with an STD. A sexual-risk history should always be done and may indicate more frequent screening for some women. With attention to obtaining information regarding the presence of risk factors, the nurse practitioner should inquire about the presence of any symptoms. Although usually asymptomatic, some women may experience spotting or postcoital bleeding, mucoid or purulent cervical discharge, increased urinary frequency, or dysuria. Bleeding results from inflammation and erosion of the cervical columnar epithelium. Women who are taking oral contraceptives may also experience breakthrough bleeding. Occasionally, women report lower abdominal pain and dyspareunia.

All pregnant women should be routinely screened for chlamydia at the first prenatal visit (CDC, 2015a). Additionally, screening for chlamydia should be done in the third trimester (36 weeks) for women at increased risk. First-trimester screening might prevent the adverse effects of chlamydia during pregnancy; however, evidence for adverse effects in pregnancy is minimal, and, when screening is done only early during the first trimester, a longer period exists for acquiring infection before delivery (CDC, 2015a).

Recommended screening procedure for chlamydial infection in women is by testing first-catch urine or collecting swab specimens from the endocervix or vagina (CDC, 2015a). Nucleic acid amplification test (NAAT) of an endocervical sample (if a pelvic examination is acceptable) or a urine sample (if not acceptable). Endocervical NAAT is preferred because it provides the highest sensitivity of any screening test. Self-collected vaginal specimens are equivalent to those collected by a clinician and women find this screening procedure highly acceptable (CDC, 2015a).

Genital/pelvic examinations should be done on all women who have a positive urine test to identify complications such as PID. Endocervical (columnar) cells are required; cell scrapings provide better specimens, so the cervix should be swabbed with cotton or rayon swabs before collecting the specimen to remove mucus and discharge from the cervical os. Special culture media and proper handling of specimens are important, so the nurse practitioner should always know what is required at her individual practice site. Furthermore, chlamydial culture testing is not always available primarily because of expense. NAATs such as ligase chain reaction and polymerase chain reaction are the new gold standard, with sensitivity and specificity near 100%.

There is a high prevalence of reinfection in women who have had chlamydial infections in the preceding several months, usually from reinfection by a partner who was untreated. Because reinfection rates are high and the risk of complications increases with reinfection, nurse practitioners should advise all women, especially adolescents, with a chlamydial infection to be rescreened 3 to 4 months after treatment.

TREATMENT

Recommended treatments for chlamydial infections are azithromycin 1 g orally in a single dose or doxycycline 100 mg orally twice a day for 7 days. Alternative regimens include erythromycin base 500 mg orally four times a day for 7 days or erythromycin ethylsuccinate 800 mg orally four times a day for 7 days or levofloxacin 500 mg orally once daily for 7 days or ofloxacin 300 mg twice a day for 7 days (CDC, 2015a). Repeat culture is not necessary for women who complete treatment with doxcycline or azithromycin unless symptoms persist or reinfection is a possibility. A test of cure may be considered if the woman is treated with erythromycin.

Doxycycline and ofloxacin are contraindicated for pregnant women; however, clinical experience and research data suggest that azithromycin 1 g orally in a single dose is safe and effective (CDC, 2015a). It has fewer gastrointestinal side effects than erythromycin and has an equivalent cure rate. Alternative regimens include amoxicillin 500 mg orally three times a day or erythromycin base 500 mg orally four times a day for 7 days, erythromycin base 250 mg orally four times a day for 14 days, erythromycin ethylsuccinate 800 mg orally four times a day for 7 days, or erythromycin ethylsuccinate 400 mg orally four times a day for 14 days. Because of concern about chlamydia persisting following treatment with penicillin-class antibiotics, amoxicillin is now considered an alternative treatment for chlamydial infections in pregnant women (CDC, 2015a). Persons who have chlamydia infection and are also infected with HIV should be treated with the same regimen as those who are HIV negative. Because chlamydia is often asymptomatic, the patient should be cautioned to take all medication prescribed. All exposed sexual partners should be treated to avoid reinfection.

Gonorrhea

Gonorrhea is probably the oldest communicable disease in the United States and is the second most commonly reported communicable disease. Furthermore, many cases continue to be undiagnosed and unreported. Cases of gonorrhea in females has fluctuated throughout the 1980s, 1990s, and 2000s reaching a 40-year low in 2009. Gonorrhea rates in women are highest among young women and adolescents (CDC, 2014). Gonorrhea is caused by the aerobic, gram-negative diplococci *Neisseria gonorrhoeae*. Gonorrhea is almost exclusively transmitted by sexual activity, primarily genital-to-genital contact; however, it is also spread by oral-to-genital and anal-to-genital contact. Sites of infection in women are cervix, urethra, oropharynx, Skene's glands, and Bartholin's glands. Gonorrhea can be transmitted to the newborn in the form of ophthalmia neonatorum during

delivery by direct contact with gonococcal organisms in the cervix.

Age is an important risk factor associated with gonorrhea with the majority of those contracting gonorrhea aged 20 years and younger (CDC, 2016). In a single act of unprotected sex with an infected partner, a teenage woman has a 50% change of contracting gonorrhea. Other risk factors include early onset of sexual activity and multiple sexual partners. Traditionally, the reported incidence of gonococcal disease has been higher in non-Whites. Many of the apparent differences in infection rates can be explained by the disproportionate representation of African Americans among the nation's poor and among inner city dwellers. Rates of gonorrhea are higher in urban than rural areas, with even higher rates in inner cities.

Common sites of gonococcal infection in women are the endocervix (primary site), urethra, Skene's and Bartholin's glands, and rectum. The main complication of gonorrheal infections is PID and subsequent infertility; women also may have pelvic abscess or Bartholin's abscess. Gonococcal infections in pregnancy potentially affect both mother and infant. Women with cervical gonorrhea may develop salpingitis in the first trimester. Perinatal complications of gonococcal infection include spontaneous septic abortion, premature rupture of membranes, preterm delivery, chorioamnionitis, neonatal sepsis, intrauterine growth retardation, and maternal postpartum sepsis. Endometritis after elective abortion or chorionic villus sampling procedures may also occur. Amniotic infection syndrome manifested by the placental, fetal, and umbilical cord inflammation following premature rupture of the membranes may result from gonorrheal infections during pregnancy. Opthlamia neonatorum, the most common manifestation of neonatal gonococcal infections, is very contagious and, if untreated, may lead to blindness of the newborn.

Disseminated gonococcal infections (DGI) are a rare (0.5%–3%) complication of untreated gonorrhea. DGI occurs in two stages: The first stage is characterized by bacteremia with chills, fever, and skin lesions and is followed by stage two, during which the patient experiences acute septic arthritis with characteristic effusions, most commonly of the wrists, knees, and ankles (Star & Deal, 2004a). The most common clinical presentation of gonorrhea in pregnancy is DGI, and risk increases in the second and third trimester.

ASSESSMENT AND DIAGNOSIS

Up to 80% of women are asymptomatic; when symptoms are present, they are often less specific than the symptoms in men. Women may have a purulent, irritating endocervical discharge, but discharge is usually minimal or absent. Menstrual irregularities may be the presenting symptom, or women may complain of pain—chronic or acute severe pelvic or lower abdominal pain or longer, more painful menses. Unilateral labial pain and swelling may indicate Bartholin's glands infection, and periurethral pain and swelling may indicate inflamed Skene's glands. Infrequently, dysuria, vague abdominal pain, or low backache prompts a woman to seek care. Later symptoms may include fever (possibly high), nausea and vomiting, joint pain and swelling, or upper abdominal pain (liver involvement). Gonococcal rectal infection may occur in women following anal intercourse. Individuals with rectal gonorrhea may be completely asymptomatic or, conversely, experience severe symptoms with profuse purulent anal discharge, rectal pain, and blood in the stool. Rectal itching, fullness, pressure, and pain are also common symptoms, as is diarrhea. Gonococcal pharyngitis may appear to be viral pharyngitis; some individuals will have a red, swollen uvula and pustule vesicles on the soft palate and tonsils similar to strep infections. A diffuse vaginitis with vulvitis is the most common form of gonococcal infection in prepubertal girls. There may be few signs of infection, or vaginal discharge, dysuria, and swollen, reddened labia may be present.

Given that gonococcal infections are often asymptomatic, they cannot be diagnosed reliably by clinical signs and symptoms alone. Individuals may present with classic symptoms, with vague symptoms that may be attributed to a number of conditions, or with no symptoms at all. When symptoms are present, they typically are less specific than those seen in men. Specific microbiological diagnosis of infection with *N. gonorrhoeae* should be done in all women at risk for or suspected to have gonorrhea; a specific diagnosis can potentially reduce complications, reinfections, and transmission (CDC, 2015a). Cultures are considered as the gold standard for diagnosis of gonorrhea because of their ease of testing and the need to test for antibiotic resistance. Cultures should be obtained from the endocervix, rectum, and, when indicated, the pharynx. NAAT or nucleic acid hybrization of an endocervical swab specimen is superior to culture for detection in urogenital and nongenital anatomic sites (CDC, 2015a). Any woman suspected of having gonorrhea should have a chlamydial culture and serological test for syphilis if one has not been done in the past 2 months. A test for gonorrhea should be done at the first prenatal visit. A repeat culture should be obtained in the third trimester for women at risk or women living in an area in which the prevalence is high (CDC, 2015a).

Infants with gonococcal opthalmia should be hospitalized and assessed for signs of disseminated infection (sepsis, arthritis, meningitis). A single dose of ceftriaxone 25 to 50 mg/kg intravenous (IV) or intramuscular (IM) is adequate for gonococcal conjunctivitis (CDC, 2015a). Mothers of infants who have gonococcal infection and the mother's sex partners should be assessed and treated.

TREATMENT

Management of gonorrhea is straightforward, and the cure is usually rapid with appropriate antibiotic therapy (see Table 30.9). Single-dose efficacy is a major consideration in selecting an antibiotic regimen for women with gonorrhea. Another important consideration is the high percentage (45%) of women with coexisting chlamydial infections. Penicillin is no longer used to treat gonorrhea because of the high rate of penicillin-resistant strains of the organism. The CDC suggest concomitant treatment for chlamydia because coinfection is common. All women with gonorrhea and syphilis should be treated for syphilis according to CDC guidelines (see Ulcerative Genital Infection, Syphillis).

TABLE 30.9	Recommended Treatment Regimens for Gonococcal Infections	
NONPREGNANT WOMEN	**PREGNANT WOMEN**	
Ceftriaxone 250 mg IM in a single dose PLUS Azithromycin 1 g orally single dose If ceftriaxone is not available: Cefixime 400 mg orally in a single dose PLUS Azithromycin 1 g orally in a single dose	Ceftriaxone 250 mg IM once PLUS Azithromycin 1 g orally single dose If cephalosporin allergic, spectinomycin 2 g IM once (not available in the United States) Do not use quinolones or tetracyclines	

IM, intramuscular.
Adapted from Centers for Disease Control and Prevention (2015a).

All patients with gonorrhea should be offered confidential counseling and testing for HIV infection.

Gonorrhea is a highly communicable disease. Recent (past 30 days) sexual partners should be examined, cultured, and treated with appropriate regimens. Most treatment failures result from reinfection. Women need to be informed of this, as well as of the consequences of reinfection in terms of chronicity, complications, and potential infertility. Women are counseled to use condoms.

Gonorrhea is a reportable communicable disease. Health care providers are legally responsible for reporting all cases to the health authorities, usually the local health department in the client's county of residence. Women should be informed that the case will be reported, told why, and informed of the possibility of being contacted by a health department representative.

Treatment failure in uncomplicated gonorrhea in women who are treated with any of the recommended regimens is rare (less than 5%); therefore, follow-up culture (test of cure) is not essential. A more cost-effective approach is reexamination with culture 1 to 2 months after treatment. This approach will detect both treatment failures and reinfections. Patients also should be counseled to return if symptoms persist after treatment.

■ PELVIC INFLAMMATORY DISEASE

PID is a spectrum of inflammatory disorders of the upper female genital tract, including any combination of endometritis, salpingitis, tubo-ovarian abscess, and pelvic peritonitis. Multiple organisms have been found to cause PID, and most cases are associated with more than one organism. In the past, the most common causative agents were thought to be *N. gonorrhoeae* and *C. trachomatis*; however, recent studies suggest that PID infections are attributable to a wide variety of anaerobic and aerobic bacteria, such as *Streptococcus, E. coli, Gardnerella vaginalis* and cytomegalovirus (CMV; CDC, 2015a). Because PID may be caused by a wide variety of infectious agents and encompasses a wide variety of pathological processes, the infection can be acute, sub-acute, or chronic and has a wide range of symptoms. All women who are diagnosed with acute PID should be tested for HIV as well as gonorrhea and chlamydia using NAAT (CDC, 2015a).

Most PID results from an ascending spread of micro-organisms from the vagina and endocervix to the upper genital tract. This spread most frequently happens at the end of or just after menses following reception of an infectious agent. During the menstrual period, several factors facilitate the development of an infection: the os is slightly open; the cervical mucus barrier is absent; and menstrual blood is an excellent medium for growth. PID also may develop following an abortion, pelvic surgery, or delivery.

Each year, more than 1 million women in the United States have an episode of symptomatic PID (Sheperd, 2013) and there are nearly 18,000 hospitalizations. Teenagers have the highest risk for PID associated with their decreased immunity to infectious organisms and increased risk of gonorrhea and chlamydia (Sheperd, 2013). Young age at first intercourse, frequency of sexual intercourse, multiple sex partners, and a history of STDs also increase a woman's risk for PID. In addition, cigarette smoking and douching may increase a woman's risk for acute PID. Until recently, it was believed that the use of intrauterine devices (IUDs) increased a woman's risk for acquiring PID.

Major medical complications are associated with PID. Short-term consequences include acute pelvic pain, tubo-ovarian abscess, tubal scarring, and adhesions. Long-term complications include an increased risk (12%–16%) of infertility, ectopic pregnancy, chronic pelvic pain, dyspareunia, and recurrent episodes of PID (Sheperd, 2013). Because PID caused by chlamydia is more commonly asymptomatic, it more often results in tubal obstruction from delayed diagnosis or inadequate treatment.

Assessment and Diagnosis

Diagnosis of acute PID is difficult, because the symptoms of PID vary and almost all of the most common signs and symptoms could accompany other urinary, gastrointestinal, or reproductive tract problems. Symptoms may mimic other disease processes, such as ectopic pregnancy, endometriosis, and ovarian cyst with torsion, pelvic adhesions, inflammatory bowel disease, or acute appendicitis. Box 30.7 contains detailed information on diagnosing PID.

History taking must be comprehensive. A menstrual history is useful in establishing the relationship of onset of pain to menses and in identifying any variations from normal in the cycle. Other relevant history includes recent pelvic surgery, delivery, and dilation of the cervix, abortion, recent (within 1 month) IUD insertion, purulent vaginal discharge, irregular bleeding, and a longer, heavier menstrual period. A thorough sexual risk history should be obtained—including current or most recent sexual activity, number of partners, and method of contraception—and will assist in identifying possible increased risk for STD

> ## BOX 30.7   DIAGNOSING PID
>
> Empirical treatment of PID should be initiated for sexually active young women and others at risk of STDs if these minimum criteria are present and no other cause(s) for the illness can be found:
>
> - Uterine/adnexal tenderness, or
> - Cervical motion tenderness
>
> Additional criteria to support a diagnosis of PID include:
>
> - Oral temperature more than 101° F (more than 38.3° C)
> - Abnormal cervical or vaginal mucopurulent discharge
> - Presence of abundant white blood cells on saline microscopy of vaginal fluids
> - Elevated erythrocyte sedimentation rate
> - Elevated C-reactive protein
> - Laboratory documentation of cervical infection with *N. gonorrheae* or *C. trachomatis*
>
> The most specific criteria for diagnosing PID are:
>
> - Endometrial biopsy with histopathologic evidence of endometriosis
> - Transvaginal sonography or magnetic resonance imaging techniques showing thickened, fluid-filled tubes with or without free pelvic fluid or tubo-ovarian complex
> - Laparoscopic abnormalities consistent with PID
>
> PID, pelvic inflammatory disease; STD, sexually transmitted disease.
>
> Adapted from Centers for Disease Control and Prevention (2015a, p. 79).

---

exposure. Intestinal and bladder symptoms are important to review. Women may report various symptoms ranging from minimal pelvic discomfort to dull cramping and intermittent pain or severe, persistent, and incapacitating pain. Pelvic pain usually develops within 7 to 10 days of menses, remains constant, is bilateral, and is most severe in the lower quadrants. Pelvic discomfort is exacerbated by Valsalva maneuver, intercourse, or movement. Women with acute PID also may complain of intermenstrual bleeding. Symptoms of an STD in a woman's partner(s) also should be noted.

Vital signs are obtained, and a complete physical examination performed. A fever of 102°F or more is characteristic. Physical examination reveals adnexal tenderness, with or without rebound, and exquisite tenderness with cervical movement (chandelier sign). Pelvic tenderness is usually bilateral. There may or may not be a palpable adnexal swelling or thickening. Fever and peritonitis are more characteristic of gonococcal PID than of PID caused by other organisms, which are more likely to be "silent."

Subacute PID is far less dramatic, with a great variety in the severity and extent of symptoms. At times, symptoms are so mild and vague that the woman ignores them. Symptoms that suggest subacute PID are chronic lower abdominal pain, dyspareunia, menstrual irregularities, urinary discomfort, low-grade fever, low backache, and constipation. Abdominal examination usually reveals no rebound tenderness; there is slight adnexal tenderness with cervical movement, and cervical or urethral discharge, often purulent in nature, may be present.

Most women with PID have either mucopurulent cervical discharge or evidence of white blood cells (WBCs) on microscopic evaluation of saline preparation of vaginal fluids (i.e., wet prep). Essential laboratory studies are a complete blood count with differential, erythro-sedimentation rate (highest in chlamydial infections) and cervical cultures for gonorrhea and chlamydia. Laboratory data are useful only when considered in conjunction with history and physical examination findings.

Clinical diagnosis of PID is imprecise; nevertheless, most diagnoses of PID are clinical because laparoscopy and biopsy are too expensive and invasive to be practical screening tools. Because delay in diagnosis and treatment of PID is associated with severe sequelae, the CDC guidelines established new minimum criteria for beginning treatment. The CDC recommends a "low threshold for diagnosing PID" because of the risk of damage to reproductive health. The 2015 guidelines recommend empiric treatment of PID if one or both of two minimum criteria are present and if no other cause(s) of the illness can be identified: (1) uterine or adnexal tenderness or (2) cervical motion tenderness (CDC, 2015a). Furthermore, a diagnosis of PID must be considered in a woman with any pelvic tenderness and any sign of lower genital tract inflammation.

Treatment

Perhaps the most important nursing intervention for PID is prevention. Primary prevention would be education in avoiding acquisition of STIs, whereas secondary prevention involves preventing a lower genital tract infection from ascending to the upper genital tract. Instructing women in self-protective behaviors, such as practicing safer sex and using barrier methods, is critical. Also important is the detection of asymptomatic gonorrheal and chlamydial infections through routine screening of women with risky behaviors and/or specific risk factors such as age. Partner notification when an STD is diagnosed is essential to prevent reinfection.

In the past, most women with PID were hospitalized so that bed rest and parental therapy could be started. However, today approximately three-quarters of women with PID are not hospitalized (CDC, 2015a) because there are no available data that compare the efficacy of inpatient versus outpatient treatment. The decision of whether to hospitalize should be based on each woman's individual circumstances. To guide the nurse practitioner's decision regarding hospitalization, the following criteria have been offered by the CDC (2015a):

■ Surgical emergencies (e.g., appendicitis) cannot be excluded
■ Tubo-ovarian abscess
■ Pregnancy
■ No clinical response to oral antimicrobial therapy
■ Inability to follow or tolerate an outpatient oral regimen
■ Severe illness, nausea and vomiting, or high fever

There are no current data to suggest that adolescents would benefit from hospitalization for treatment; however, there is some evidence that women older than 35 years of age are likely to have a more complicated course and thus may benefit from hospitalization (CDC, 2015a). The guidelines recommend that pregnant women with PID be hospitalized and treated with antibiotics because of the high risk for preterm delivery, fetal wastage, and maternal morbidity (CDC, 2015a).

Although treatment regimens vary with the infecting organism, a broad-spectrum antibiotic is generally used. Several antimicrobial regimens have proved to be effective and no single therapeutic regimen of choice exists (see Table 30.10). Women with acute PID should be on bed rest in a semi-Fowler's position. Comfort measures include analgesics for pain and all other nursing measures applicable to a patient confined to bed. Minimal pelvic examinations should be done during the acute phase of the disease. During the recovery phase, the woman should restrict laboratory

TABLE 30.10	Treatment of Pelvic Inflammatory Disease	
	TREATMENT OF CHOICE	**ALTERNATIVES**
Parenteral regimen	Cefotetan 2 g IV every 12 hours plus doxycyline 100 mg IV or orally every 12 hours	Clindamycin 900 mg IV every 8 hours plus gentamycin loading dose IV or IM (2 mg/kg of body weight), followed by maintenance dose (1.5 mg/kg) every 8 hours; single daily dosing (3–5 mg/kg) may be substituted
Oral regimen	Doxycycline 100 mg orally every 12 hours	

IM, intramuscular.

studies after treatment and should include endocervical cultures for a test of cure.

Health education is central to effective management of PID. Nurse practitioners should explain to women about the nature of the disease and should encourage them to comply with all therapy and prevention recommendations, emphasizing the necessity of taking all medication, even if symptoms disappear. Any potential problems, such as lack of money for prescriptions or lack of transportation to return to the clinic for follow-up appointments that would prevent a woman from completing a course of treatment should be identified, and the importance of follow-up visits should be stressed. Women should be counseled to refrain from sexual intercourse until their treatment is completed. Contraceptive counseling should be provided. The nurse practitioner can suggest that the client select barrier methods, such as condoms, contraceptive sponge, or diaphragm. A woman with a history of PID should not use an IUD.

Women who suffer from PID may be acutely ill or may experience long-term discomfort. Either takes an emotional toll. Pain in itself is debilitating and is compounded by the infectious process. The potential or actual loss of reproductive capabilities can be devastating and can affect the patient's self-concept adversely. Part of the nurse practitioner's role is to help her client adjust her self-concept to fit into reality and to accept alterations in a way that promotes health. Because PID is so closely tied to sexuality, body image, and self-concept, women who are diagnosed with it will need supportive care. The woman's feelings need to be discussed and her partner(s) included when appropriate.

■ ULCERATIVE GENITAL INFECTION

Syphilis

Syphilis, one of the earliest described STDs, is a systemic disease caused by *Treponema pallidum*, a motile spirochete. The disease is characterized by periods of active symptoms and periods of symptomless latency. It can affect any tissue or organ in the body. Transmission is thought to be by entry in the subcutaneous tissue through microscopic abrasions that can occur during sexual intercourse. The disease can also be transmitted through kissing, biting, or oral–genital sex. A single sexual exposure to a person with active mucocutaneous syphilis has up to a 50% risk of acquiring the disease (CDC, 2015a). Transplacental transmission may occur at any time during pregnancy; the degree of risk is related to the quantity of spirochetes in the maternal bloodstream. Women with early syphilis are most likely to transmit the disease to their infants (CDC, 2015a).

There are an estimated 40,000 cases of primary and secondary syphilis in the United States each year. However, since 2001, primary and secondary syphilis rates have increased, particularly in women and men having sex with men (CDC, 2014). Syphilis rates are higher for heterosexual African American and Hispanic women than they are for White women. Much of the rise in cases seen is directly attributable to illicit drug use, particularly crack cocaine; the exchange of sex for drugs or money; reduction in the resources for syphilis control programs; and rising poverty rates. Rises in cases of congenital syphilis have paralleled these rates for women. In contrast to other bacterial STIs, which affect mostly teens and adults younger than 34 years of age, syphilis persists into the early 30s in both men and women.

Syphilis is a complex disease that can lead to serious systemic disease and even death when untreated. Infection manifests itself in distinct stages with different symptoms and clinical manifestations (see Table 30.11). Primary syphilis is characterized by a primary lesion, a chancre that often begins as a painless papule at the site of inoculation and then erodes to form a nontender, shallow, indurated, clean ulcer several millimeters to centimeters in size. The chancre is loaded with spirochetes and is most commonly found on the genitalia, although other sites include the cervix, perianal area, and mouth. Secondary syphilis is characterized by a widespread, symmetrical maculopapular rash on the palms and soles and generalized lymphadenopathy. The infected individual may experience fever, headache, and malaise. Condyloma lata (wart-like infectious lesions) may develop on the vulva, perineum, or anus. If the patient is untreated, she enters a latent phase that is asymptomatic for most individuals. If left untreated, about one third of the patients will develop tertiary syphilis. Cardiovascular (chest pain, cough), dermatological (multiple nodules or ulcers), skeletal (arthritis, myalgia, myositis), or neurological (headache, irritability, impaired balance, memory loss, tremor) symptoms can develop in this stage. Neurological complications are not limited to tertiary syphilis; rather, a variety of syndromes (e.g., meningitis, meningovascular syphilis, general paresis, and tabes dorsalis) may span all stages of the disease.

SCREENING AND DIAGNOSIS

Dark-field examination and direct fluorescent antibody tests of lesion exudates or tissue provide definitive diagnosis of early syphilis. Diagnosis is dependent on serology during latency and late infection. Any test for antibodies may not be reactive in the presence of active infection, because it takes time for the body's immune system to develop antibodies to any antigens. A presumptive diagnosis is possible with the use of two serological tests: nontreponemal and treponemal. Nontreponemal antibody tests such as the VDRL or RPR are used as screening tests; they are relatively inexpensive, sensitive, moderately nonspecific, and fast. False-positive results are not unusual with these tests, particularly when conditions such as acute infection, autoimmune disorders, malignancy, pregnancy, and drug addiction exist and after immunization or vaccination. A high titer (greater than 1:16) usually indicates active disease. A fourfold drop in the titer indicates a response to treatment. Treatment of primary syphilis usually causes a progressive decline to a negative VDRL within 2 years. In secondary, latent, or tertiary syphilis, low titers persist in about 50% of cases after 2 years. Rising titer (four times) indicates relapse, reinfection, or treatment failure. The treponemal tests, fluorescent treponemal antibody absorbed, and microhemagglutination

TABLE 30.11	Stages of Syphilis				
	PRIMARY	**SECONDARY**	**EARLY LATENT**	**LATE LATENT**	**TERTIARY**
Time after exposure	9–90 days	6 weeks to 6 months	3–12 months	More than 1 year	Years
Duration	Weeks	Weeks	Less than 2 years	More than years	Variable
Infectious	Yes	Yes	No	No	Yes
Clinical symptoms	Chancre Painless lympha-denopathy	Skin lesions; papular rash of soles and palms; patchy alopecia; condylomata; symptoms of systemic illness (fever, malaise, anorexia, weight loss, headache, myalgias)	No symptoms at this stage	No symptoms at this stage	Symptomatic central nervous system disease Cardiovascular syphilis Skin lesions (gumma) Progressive bone destruction
Laboratory changes	Dark-field serology[a] often negative or rising titers VDRL and FTA-ABS	Dark-field positive; peak antibody titers Seroconversion of FTA-ABS or MHA-TP positive CSF abnormal in up to 50% of women Proteinuria	CSF: Falling VDRL titers	CSF: Falling VDRL titers	CSF: VDRL positive or increased cells and protein, serum treponemal positive; nontreponemal positive or negative VDRL remains positive indefinitely with declining titer

[a]Dark field is only useful when examining moist lesions of primary syphilis.
CFS, cerebrospinal fluid; FTA-ABS, fluorescent treponemal antibody absorption test; MHA-TP, microhemagglutination assay for Treponema pallidum antibodies; VDRL, venereal disease research laboratory test.
Adapted from Augenbraum (2007); Barron (1998); Centers for Disease Control and Prevention (2006); Livengood (2001); Star (1999); Varney, Kriebs, and Gegor (2004).

assays for antibody to *T. pallidum* are used to confirm positive results. Test results in patients with early primary or incubating syphilis may be negative. Seroconversion usually takes place 6 to 8 weeks after exposure, so testing should be repeated in 1 to 2 months when a suspicious genital lesion exists. Treponemal antibody tests frequently stay positive for life regardless of treatment or disease activity; therefore, treatment is monitored by the titers of the VDRL or RPR. Sequential serologic tests should be obtained by using the same testing method (VDRL or RPR), preferably by the same laboratory.

Tests for concomitant STIs should be done, HIV testing offered, and, if indicated, wet preps carried out. All pregnant women should be screened for syphilis at the first prenatal visit and again in the late third trimester for high-risk patients. Some states also mandate screening of all patients in the third trimester and/or at delivery. No infant should be discharged from the hospital without the syphilis serological status of its mother having been determined at least once during pregnancy.

TREATMENT

Parenteral penicillin G is the preferred drug for treating patients with all stages of syphilis (see Table 30.12). It is the only proven therapy that has been widely used for patients with neurosyphilis, congenital syphilis, or syphilis during pregnancy. Intramuscular benzathine penicillin G

(2.4 million units IM once) is used to treat primary, secondary, and early latent syphilis. Women who have had syphilis for more than a year (late latent or tertiary stage) require weekly treatment of 2.4 million units of benzathine penicillin G for 3 weeks.

Although doxycycline, tetracycline, and erythromycin are alternative treatments for penicillin-allergic patients, both tetracycline and doxycycline are contraindicated in pregnancy and erythromycin is unlikely to cure a fetal infection. Therefore, pregnant women should, if necessary, receive skin testing and be treated with penicillin, or be desensitized (CDC, 2015a). Specific protocols for desensitization are recommended by the CDC (2015a). Some pregnant women treated for syphilis may experience a Jarisch–Herxheimer reaction. This is an acute febrile reaction to the toxins given off by treponemes when killed rapidly by treatment; the reaction occurs within 24 hours after treatment with penicillin and is characterized by fever up to 105° F, headache, myalgia, and arthralgia that lasts 4 to 12 hours (CDC, 2015a). Women treated in the second half of pregnancy who experience a Jarisch–Herxheimer reaction are at risk of preterm labor and delivery or fetal distress. They should be advised to contact their health care provider if they notice any change in fetal movement or experience cramping, contractions, or persistent low-back pain or pressure.

Monthly follow-up is mandatory so that retreatment may be given if needed. The nurse practitioner should emphasize the necessity of long-term serological testing even

TABLE 30.12	Treatment of Syphilis	
NONPREGNANT WOMEN OLDER THAN 18 YEARS OF AGE	**PREGNANT WOMEN**	**LACTATING WOMEN**
Primary, secondary, early latent disease: Benzathine penicillin G 2.4 million units IM single dose Late latent or unknown duration disease: Benzathine penicillin G 7.2 million units total, administered as three doses 2.4 million units IM each at 1-week intervals Penicillin allergy: Doxycycline 100 mg orally four times per day for 28 days *or* tetracycline 500 mg orally four times per day for 28 days[a]	Primary, secondary, early latent disease: Penicillin G 2.4 million units IM once Late latent or unknown duration disease: Benzathine penicillin G 7.2 million units total, administered as three doses 2.4 million units each at 1-week intervals No proven alternatives to penicillin in pregnancy. Pregnant women who have a history of allergy to penicillin should be desensitized and treated with penicillin.	Primary, secondary, early latent disease: Benzathine penicillin G 2.4 million units IM once

[a]Use only with close clinical follow-up.
IM, intramuscular.
Adapted from Centers for Disease Control and Prevention (2015a, pp. 36–39); Jacobs (2001).

in the absence of symptoms. The patient should be advised to practice sexual abstinence until treatment is completed, all evidence of primary and secondary syphilis is gone, and serologic evidence of a cure is demonstrated. Women should be told to notify all partners who may have been exposed. They should be informed that the disease is reportable. Preventative measures should be discussed.

Genital Herpes Simplex Virus Infection

Unknown until the middle of the 20th century, genital herpes is now one of the most common STDs in the United States, especially for women, who contract it far more often than men. Genital herpes is a chronic, lifelong incurable viral disease characterized by painful vesicular eruption of the skin and mucosa of the genitals. Two types of HSV can cause genital herpes: HSV-1 and HSV-2. HSV-2 is usually transmitted sexually and HSV-1 nonsexually. Although HSV-1 is more commonly associated with gingivostomatitis and oral labial ulcers (fever blisters) and HSV-2 with genital lesions, both types are not exclusively associated with the respective sites.

Although HSV infection is not a reportable disease, it is estimated that approximately 50 million persons in the United States are infected with HSV-2 and approximately half a million cases are diagnosed annually (CDC, 2015a). Most persons infected with HSV-2 have not had the condition diagnosed and as a result, most genital herpes infections are transmitted by persons who are unaware that they have the infection or are asymptomatic when the condition is diagnosed. Prevalence is higher in women with multiple sex partners. Most new cases occur in individuals between 15 and 34 years of age.

An initial herpetic infection (primary genital herpes) characteristically has both systemic and local symptoms and lasts about 3 weeks. Women generally have a more severe clinical course than do men. Flu-like symptoms with fever, malaise, and myalgia appear first about a week after exposure, peak within 4 days, and subside over the next week. Multiple genital lesions develop at the site of infection, usually the vulva; other common sites are the perianal area, vagina, and cervix. The lesions begin as small painful blisters or vesicles that become "unroofed," leaving ulcerated lesions. Individuals with primary herpes often develop bilateral tender inguinal lymphadenopathy, vulvar edema, vaginal discharge, and severe dysuria. Ulcerative lesions last 4 to 15 days before crusting over. New lesions may develop up to the 10th day of the course of the infection. Herpes simplex viral cervicitis also is common with initial HSV-2 infections; the cervix may appear normal or be friable, reddened, ulcerated, or necrotic. A heavy, watery to purulent vaginal discharge is common. Extra genital lesions may be present because of auto-inoculation. Urinary retention and dysuria may occur secondary to autonomic involvement of the sacral nerve root.

Women experiencing recurrent episodes of HSV infections commonly will have only local symptoms, which are usually less severe than those associated with the initial infection. Systemic symptoms are usually absent, although the characteristic prodromal genital tingling is common. Recurrent lesions are unilateral, less severe, and usually last 7 to 10 days without prolonged viral shedding. Lesions begin as vesicles and progress rapidly to ulcers. Very few women with recurrent disease have cervicitis.

Most mothers of newborns who acquire neonatal herpes do not have a history of clinically evident genital herpes (Pinninti & Kimberlin, 2013). Infection of the newborn is acquired by exposure to the virus in the maternal genital tract at the time of delivery. Neonates who develop HSV infection usually have severe disseminated or central nervous system infection resulting in mental retardation or death. Most mothers of infants who acquire neonatal herpes do not have a history of clinically evident genital herpes (CDC, 2015b). The risk for transmission to the neonate is high (30%–50%) among women who have an initial herpetic infection near time of delivery and low (less than 1%)

in women who have a history of recurrent herpes at or near term or who acquire genital herpes during the first half of pregnancy (CDC, 2015a).

SCREENING AND DIAGNOSIS

The risk profile for herpes is less clear-cut than in other STDs, and screening for asymptomatic women is not recommended. Diagnosis of genital herpes can be difficult because the typical painful, multiple vesicular and ulcerative lesions associated with HSV may be absent in many infected persons. Although a clinical diagnosis of genital herpes is both insensitive and nonspecific, a careful history provides much information when making a diagnosis of herpes. A history of exposure to an infected person is important, although infection from an asymptomatic individual is possible. A history of having viral symptoms, such as malaise, headache, fever, or myalgia, is suggestive. Local symptoms, such as vulvar pain, dysuria, itching or burning at the site of infection, and painful genital lesions that heal spontaneously also are suggestive of HSV infections. The nurse practitioner should ask about an earlier history of a primary infection, prodromal symptoms, vaginal discharge, dysuria, and dyspareunia.

During the physical examination, the nurse practitioner should assess for inguinal and generalized lymphadenopathy and elevated temperature. The entire vulvular, perineal, vaginal, and cervical areas should be carefully inspected for vesicles or ulcerated or crusted areas. A speculum examination may be very difficult for the patient because of the extreme tenderness associated with herpes infections.

Although a diagnosis of herpes infection may be suspected from the history and physical examination, it is confirmed by laboratory studies. Isolation of HSV in cell culture is the preferred virological test in women who have genital ulcers or other mucocutaneous lesions. Viral culture has a sensitivity of 70% to 80% (CDC, 2015a). Culture yield is best if the specimen is taken during the vesicular stage of the disease; however, the sensitivity of a culture declines rapidly as lesions begin to heal. In a primary infection, viral shedding is prolonged and the HSV is more easily isolated.

Because false-negative HSV cultures are common, especially with healing lesions or recurrent infection, type-specific serological tests are useful in confirming a clinical diagnosis. The HSV-specific glycoprotein G2 (HSV-2) assay is a point-of-care test that provides results for HSV-2 antibodies from capillary blood or serum during a clinical visit (CDC, 2015a). Sensitivity varies from 80% to 99%, and false-negative results can occur, especially in early stages of infection. Specificity of the assay is greater than 96%; false-positive results occur in patients with a low likelihood of HSV infection.

TREATMENT

Genital herpes is a chronic and recurring disease for which there is no known cure. Antiviral drugs do not eradicate the latent virus and do not affect subsequent risk, frequency, or severity of recurrence after administration. Systemic antiviral drugs partially control the symptoms and signs of HSV infections when used for the primary or recurrent episodes or when used as daily suppressive therapy. However, these drugs do not eradicate the infection nor alter subsequent risk, frequency, or reoccurrence after the drug is stopped. Three antiviral medications provide clinical benefit for genital herpes: acyclovir, valacyclovir, and famciclovir (CDC, 2015a). Treatment recommendations are given in Table 30.13.

Safety and efficacy have been shown clearly in persons taking acyclovir daily for up to 3 years. The safety of acyclovir, valacyclovir, and famciclovir therapy during pregnancy has not been definitively established. However, available data do not indicate an increased risk for major birth defects compared with the general population in women treated with acyclovir in the first trimester (Stone et al., 2004). The first clinical episode of genital herpes during pregnancy may be treated with oral acyclovir. In the presence of life-threatening maternal HSV infection, acyclovir IV is indicated (CDC, 2015a).

Women in their childbearing years should be counseled regarding the risk of herpes infection during pregnancy. They should be instructed to use condoms if there is any risk of contracting any STI from a sexual partner. If they are using acyclovir therapy, they should be counseled to use contraception because of the potential teratogenicity of acyclovir. Women currently breastfeeding should not use acyclovir.

Because neonatal HSV infection is such a devastating disease, prevention is critical. Current recommendations include carefully examining and questioning all women about symptoms at onset of labor (CDC, 2015a). Diagnosis of genital herpes in any pregnant women with active, visible lesions should be confirmed with culture. The results of viral cultures during pregnancy with or without visible herpetic lesions do not predict viral shedding at delivery, and therefore weekly surveillance cultures for HSV are not indicated for pregnant women who have a history of recurrent genital herpes (CDC, 2015a). All pregnant women should be asked whether they have a history of genital herpes. When a woman is admitted to the labor and delivery unit, she should be carefully questioned about the symptoms of genital herpes, including prodromal symptoms, and all women should be examined carefully for herpetic lesion. For women with no symptoms or signs of genital herpes or its prodromal at onset of labor, vaginal delivery is acceptable (CDC, 2015a). Cesarean delivery within 4 hours after labor begins or membranes rupture is recommended if visible lesions are present in order to prevent neonatal herpes. However, cesarean delivery does not completely eliminate the risk for HVS transmission to the infant. Any infant who is delivered through an infected vagina should be carefully observed and cultured and followed carefully by a specialist. Some experts recommend presumptive treatment with systemic acyclovir for infants who were exposed to HSV at delivery.

Cleaning lesions twice a day with saline will help prevent secondary infection. Bacterial infection must be treated with appropriate antibiotics. Measures that may increase comfort for women when lesions are active include warm sitz baths with baking soda; keeping lesions warm and dry by using a hair dryer on a cool setting or patting dry with soft towel; wearing cotton underwear and

TABLE 30.13	Treatment of Genital Herpes		
NONPREGNANT WOMEN OLDER THAN 18 YEARS OF AGE		**PREGNANT WOMEN**	**LACTATING WOMEN**
Primary infection: Acyclovir 400 mg orally three times per day for 7–10 days or Acyclovir 200 mg orally five times per day for 7–10 days or Valacyclovir 1 g orally twice a day for 7–10 days or Famciclovir 250 mg orally three times a day for 7–10 days Treatment may be extended if healing is incomplete after 10 days of therapy Recurrent infection: Acyclovir 400 mg orally three times per day for 5 days or Acyclovir 800 mg orally twice a day for 5 days or Acyclovir 800 mg orally three times per day for 2 days or Valacyclovir 500 mg orally twice a day for 3 days or Valacyclovir 1 g orally once a day for 5 days or Famciclovir 125 mg orally twice daily for 5 days or Famciclovir 1 gram orally twice a day for 1 day or Famciclovir 500 mg once, followed by 250 mg twice daily for 2 days Suppression therapy: Acyclovir 400 mg orally twice per day or Valacyclovir 500 mg orally twice a day or Valacyclovir 1 g orally once a day or Famciclovir 5 250 mg orally twice a day		Acyclovir 400 mg orally three times a day or Valacyclovir 500 mg orally twice a day Safety of systemic valacyclovir or famciclovir therapy has not been definitively established in pregnancy	Safety of systemic acyclovir, valacyclovir, or famciclovir therapy has not been established

Notes: Acyclovir, famciclovir and valacyclovir appear equally effective for episodic treatment of genital herpes, but famciclovir appears less effective for suppression of viral shedding.
Adapted from Centers for Disease Control and Prevention (2015a, pp. 28–29, 31–32).

loose clothing; using drying aids, such as hydrogen peroxide, Burrow's solution, and oatmeal baths; compresses of cold milk or Domeboro solution; applying cool, wet black tea bags to lesions; and applying compresses with an infusion of cloves or peppermint oil and clove oil to lesions (CDC, 2015s).

Oral analgesics such as aspirin or ibuprofen may be used to relieve pain and systemic symptoms associated with initial infections. Because the mucous membranes affected by herpes are very sensitive, any topical agents should be used with caution. Ointments containing cortisone should be avoided. Women should be informed that occlusive ointments may prolong the course of infections.

A diet rich in vitamins C, B-complex and B6, zinc, and calcium is thought to help prevent recurrences. Daily use of kelp powder (two capsules) and sunflower seed oil (one tablespoon) also have been recommended to decrease recurrences. The amino acid L-lysine has been used in doses of 750 to 1,000 mg daily while lesions are active and 500 mg during asymptomatic periods. It is thought that L-lysine has an inhibitory effect on the multiplication of the HSV (Fogel, 1995).

Counseling and education are critical components of the nursing care of women with herpes infections. Information regarding the etiology, signs and symptoms, sexual and perineal transmission, methods to prevent transmission, and treatment should be provided. The nurse practitioner should explain that each woman is unique in her response to herpes and emphasize the variability of symptoms. Women should be helped to understand when viral shedding and thus transmission to a partner is most likely, and that they should refrain from sexual contact from the onset of prodrome until complete healing of lesions. All persons with genital herpes should consistently use condoms with intercourse or oral–genital activity, and women should be encouraged to avoid intercourse when active lesions are present. Women can be encouraged to maintain close contact with their partners while avoiding contact with lesions. Women should be taught how to look for herpetic lesions using a mirror and a good light source and a wet cloth or finger covered with a finger cot to rub lightly over the labia. The nurse practitioner should ensure that patients understand that, when lesions are active, sharing intimate articles (e.g., washcloths, wet towels) that come into contact with the lesions should be avoided. Plain soap and water is all that is needed to clean hands that have come in contact with herpetic lesions; isolation is neither necessary nor appropriate.

The nurse practitioner should explain the role of precipitating factors in the reactivation of the latent virus and recurrent episodes. Stress, menstruation, trauma, febrile illnesses, chronic illness, and ultraviolet light have all been found to trigger genital herpes. Women may wish to keep a diary to identify which stressors seem to be associated with recurrent herpes attacks for them so that they can then avoid them when possible. Referral for stress reduction therapy, yoga, or meditation classes may be done when indicated. The role of exercise in reducing stress can be discussed. Avoiding excessive heat, sun, and hot baths and using a lubricant during sexual intercourse to reduce friction also may be helpful.

The emotional impact of contracting herpes is considerable. Media publicity regarding this disease can make receiving a diagnosis of genital herpes a devastating experience. No cure is available, and most women will experience recurrences. At diagnosis, many emotions may surface—helplessness, anger, denial, guilt, anxiety, shame, or inadequacy. Women need to be given the opportunity to discuss their feelings and help in learning to live with the disease. A woman can be encouraged to think of herself as a person who is not diseased but rather healthy and inconvenienced from time to time. Herpes can affect a woman's sexuality, her sexual practices, and her current and future relationships. She may need help in raising the issue with her partner or with future partners.

A common misconception that may cause anxiety for women is that HSV causes cancer. This myth should be dispelled because the role of HSV-2 in cervical cancer is at most that of a cofactor rather than a primary etiologic agent (CDC, 2015a).

Chancroid

Chancroid or soft chancre is a bacterial infection of the genitourinary tract caused by the gram-negative bacteria *Haemophilus ducreyi*. The prevalence of chancroid has declined in the United States and when infection does occur is usually associated with sporadic outbreaks. Worldwide, chancroid also appears to have declined, though infection still occurs in some regions of Africa and the Caribbean (CDC, 2015a). Because chancroid is a genital ulcer, it is a risk factor in the transmission and acquisition of HIV infection. The major way chancroid is acquired is through sexual contact; trauma or an abrasion is necessary for the organism to penetrate the skin. Chancroid is characterized by a rapidly growing ulcerated lesion formed on the external genitalia. The incubation period is usually 3 to 10 days but may be as long as 3 weeks.

Typically, the client presents with a history of a painful macule on the external genitalia, which rapidly changes to a pustule and then to an ulcerated lesion. Auto-inoculation of fingers or other sites occasionally occurs. The patient may develop enlarged unilateral or bilateral enlarged inguinal nodes known as buboe. After 1 to 2 weeks, the skin overlying the lymph node becomes erythematous, the center necrosis, and the node becomes ulcerated.

ASSESSMENT AND DIAGNOSIS

The combination of a painful genital lesion and tender suppurative inguinal adenopathy suggest the diagnosis of chancroid. A probable diagnosis can be made if all of the following criteria are met: presence of one or more painful genital ulcers; no evidence of syphilis or herpes genitalia infection is present; and the clinical presentation, appearance of genital ulcers, and regional lymphadenopathy are typical for chancroid (CDC, 2015a). Definitive diagnosis of chancroid is difficult because the organism can only be identified by culture on a special media that is not used routinely. A cotton or calcium alginate swab is used to obtain the specimen from the ulcer base after gentle removal of necrotic exudate with saline. Culture sensitivity is 80% or lower (CDC, 2006). Gonorrheal and chlamydia cultures should be obtained, and syphilis and HIV testing should be done at the time of diagnosis.

TREATMENT

The recommended treatment for chancroid includes azithromycin 1 g orally single dose or ceftriaxone 250 mg IM single dose or ciprofloxacin 500 mg orally twice a day for 3 days or erythromycin base 500 mg orally three times a day for 7 days (CDC, 2015a). HIV-infected persons may require retreatment after single-dose therapy. No adverse effects of chancroid on pregnancy outcome or on the fetus have been reported. Ciprofloxacin is contraindicated for pregnant and lactating women. Medications for use in pregnancy include ceftriaxone 250 mg IM single dose or erythromycin base 500 mg orally four times a day for 7 days.

Women should be instructed to have no sexual contact until all medication is taken and the importance of completing the entire course of medication must be stressed. Comfort measures the nurse practitioner can suggest are tepid sitz baths followed by drying carefully with a cool air hair dryer; avoiding tight, restricting clothes; and exposing the perineum to air flow as much as possible (e.g., wear a skirt without underpants when at home).

Patients should be reexamined 3 to 7 days after beginning therapy. If treatment is successful, there should be symptomatic improvement within 3 days of starting therapy and objectively within 7 days after therapy. If no clinical improvement is seen, the clinician should consider whether the diagnosis is correct; the patient is co-infected with another STD; the patient is infected with HIV; the treatment was not used as recommended; or the strain causing the infection is resistant to the prescribed antimicrobial (CDC, 2015a). It should be noted that it may take more than 2 weeks for complete healing of the ulcers to occur. All sexual partners who have had sexual contact within 10 days preceding the onset symptoms with a person diagnosed with chancroid should be evaluated regardless of whether symptoms are present.

DISEASES CHARACTERIZED BY VAGINAL DISCHARGE

Vaginal discharge and itching of the vulva and vagina are among the most common reasons a woman seeks help from a health care provider. Indeed, more women complain of vaginal discharge than any other gynecologic symptom. Vaginal discharge resulting from infection must be distinguished from normal secretions. Normal vaginal secretion or leukorrhea are clear to cloudy in appearance and may turn yellow after drying; the discharge is slightly slimy, non-irritating, and has a mild inoffensive odor. Normal vaginal secretions are acidic, with a pH range of 3.8 to 4.2. The amount of leukorrhea present differs with phases of the menstrual cycle, with greater amounts occurring at ovulation and just before menses. Leukorrhea also increases during pregnancy. Normal vaginal secretions contain lactobacilli and epithelial cells. Women who have adequate endogenous or exogenous estrogen will have vaginal secretions.

Vaginitis, an inflammation of the vagina characterized by an increased vaginal discharge containing numerous WBCs, occurs when the vaginal environment is disturbed, either by a microorganism (see Table 30.14) or by a disturbance that allows the pathogens that are found normally in the vagina to proliferate.

Factors that can disturb the vaginal environment include douches, vaginal medications, antibiotics, hormones, contraceptive preparations (oral and topical), stress, sexual intercourse, and changes in sexual partners (CDC, 2015a). Vulvo vaginitis or inflammation of the vulva and vagina may be caused by vaginal infection; copious amounts of leukorrhea, which can cause maceration of tissues; and chemical irritants, allergens, and foreign bodies, which may produce inflammatory reactions. BV, vulvovaginal candidiasis (VVC), and trichomoniasis are the most common causes of abnormal vaginal discharge.

Trichomoniasis

Trichomonas vaginalis vaginitis is the most prevalent nonviral STD, affecting an estimated 3.7 million persons (CDC, 2015a). Higher rates of infection are seen in Black women, women younger than 40 years of age, STD clinic patients, and incarcerated women. Trichomoniasis is caused by *T. vaginalis*, an anaerobic one-celled protozoan with characteristic flagellae. The organism lives in the vagina, urethra, and Bartholin's and Skene's glands in women, and in the urethra and prostate gland in men. It is readily transmitted during vaginal–penis intercourse. Although trichomoniasis may be asymptomatic, commonly women experience characteristically yellowish to greenish, frothy, mucopurulent, copious, malodorous discharge. Inflammation of the vulva, vagina, or both may be present, and the woman may complain of irritation and pruritis. Dysuria and dyspareunia are often present. Typically, the discharge worsens during and after menstruation. Often the cervix and vaginal walls will demonstrate the characteristic "strawberry spots" or tiny petechiae, and the cervix may bleed on contact. In severe infections, the vaginal walls, cervix, and occasionally the vulva may be acutely inflamed. Vaginal trichomoniasis is associated with two- to threefold increase in HIV acquisition. Preterm has been associated with adverse pregnancy outcomes, especially premature rupture of the membranes, preterm delivery, and other adverse pregnancy outcomes in pregnant women, including low birth weight. In women with HIV, trichomoniasis is associated with an increased risk for PID (Moodley, Wilkinson, Connolly, Moodley, & Sturm, 2002).

Trichomoniasis is the most common curable STD in the United States and worldwide and is the cause of up to 20% of all vaginitis with discharge occurring in approximately 3 million women annually (Hatcher, 2011).

ASSESSMENT AND DIAGNOSIS

In addition to obtaining a history of current symptoms, a careful sexual history including last intercourse and last sexual contact should be obtained, because trichomoniasis is an STI (see Table 30.15). Any history of similar symptoms in the past and treatment used should be noted. The nurse practitioner should determine whether her client's partner(s) was treated and whether she has had subsequent relations with new partners. Additional important information includes last menstrual period, method of birth control, if any, and other medications. The external genitalia should be observed for excoriation, erythema, edema, ulceration, and lesions. A speculum examination always is done, even though it may be very uncomfortable for the woman; relaxation techniques and breathing exercises may help the woman with the procedure. Any of the classic signs may be present on physical examination. The pH is elevated. The NAAT test is highly sensitive and can detect up to three to five times more *T. vaginalis* infections than wet-mount microscopy (CDC, 2015a); however, it is expensive and may not be widely available. Culture of a woman's vaginal secretions is another method of diagnosis with a sensitivity of 75% to 96% (CDC, 2015a). The most common method for diagnosing trichomoniasis is microscopic evaluation of wet prep of genital secretions; however, the sensitivity is low (51%–65%) in vaginal specimens. Although Pap smear results frequently include reports of trichomonads, sensitivity of the method is low because false negatives and false positives can frequently occur and it is not considered diagnostic. Because trichomoniasis is an STI, once the diagnosis is confirmed, gonorrhea and chlamydia cultures, and serology testing for syphilis if history indicates, should be carried out.

TREATMENT

Treatment reduces symptoms and signs of *T. vaginalis* infection and might reduce transmission. The recommended treatment for trichomoniasis (see Table 30.15) is metronidazole 2 g orally in a single dose (CDC, 2015a). Metronidazole (Flagyl) is an antiprotozoal and antibacterial agent. Complementary and alternative therapies for vaginitis are found in Table 30.16.

Until recently, metronidazole was contraindicated in the first trimester of pregnancy; however, multiple studies and meta-analyses have not demonstrated a consistent association between metronidazole use during pregnancy and teratogenic or mutagenic effects in offspring (CDC, 2015).

TABLE 30.14	Conditions Characterized by Vaginal Discharge			
	NORMAL DISCHARGE	**TRICHOMONIASIS**	**BACTERIAL VAGINOSIS**	**VULVOVAGINAL CANDIDIASIS**
STD	No	Yes	No	No
Vaginal pH	3.8–4.2	> 4.7	> 4.5	< 4.5 (usually normal)
Wet prep	Normal flora	With normal saline: delay results in drying and loss of characteristic shape of protozoan	With saline solution: positive for clue cells, decreased lactobacilli	With potassium hydroxide (KOH): pseudohyphae with yeast buds
Discharge	White/clear Thin/mucoid	Malodorous, copious, frothy or nonfrothy, thin or thick, white/yellow-green/gray	Thin, homogeneous, grayish-white, adherent, coats the vaginal walls	Thick white, curd-like; cottage cheese-like, adherent
Amine odor (KOH "whiff" test)	Normal body odor	Unpleasant smell may be present	Present (fishy)	None/yeasty, musty odor
Vulvular puritis	No	Soreness rather than itching, swelling, redness; burning and soreness of thighs and perineum	Mild if present at all	Yes, swelling, excoriation, redness
Genital ulceration	No	No	No	Skin may crack in severe cases
Pelvic pain	No	Yes, in severe cases; severe pelvic pain with tender inguinal lymph nodes	No	No
Dysuria	No	Yes	Occasionally	Severe cases
Dyspareunia	No	Yes	Occasionally	Occasionally
Main patient complaint	No	Excessive discharge, vulvar purities, dysuria, vaginal irritation, dyspareunia, postcoital bleeding	May be asymptomatic discharge, bad odor, possibly worse after intercourse; may report suprapubic pain	Itching/burning, discharge
Risk of pelvic inflammatory disease	No	May develop	Yes	No

Adapted from Carcio and Secor (2015b) and Centers for Disease Control and Prevention (2015a, pp. 69–78).

Symptomatic pregnant women should be treated with 2 g orally in a single dose. Treatment of pregnant women with asymptomatic trichomoniasis is not indicated, because data have not demonstrated that this strategy is effective in preventing preterm delivery (CDC, 2015a). Metronidazole is secreted in breast milk. Although several reported case series have found no evidence of adverse effects in infants exposed to metronidazole in breast milk, some nurse practitioners advise deferring breastfeeding for 12 to 24 hours after maternal treatment (CDC, 2015a).

Side effects of metronidazole are numerous, including sharp, unpleasant metallic taste in the mouth, furry tongue, central nervous system reactions, and urinary tract disturbances. When oral metronidazole is taken, the client is advised not to drink alcoholic beverages, or she will experience severe abdominal distress, nausea, vomiting, and

headache. Metronidazole can cause gastrointestinal symptoms regardless of whether alcohol is consumed and can also darken urine. The nurse practitioner should stress the importance of completing all medication even if symptoms disappear.

Although the male partner is usually asymptomatic, it is recommended that he receive treatment also, because he may harbor the trichomonads in the urethra or prostate. It is important that nurse practitioners discuss the importance of partner treatment with clients. If partners are not treated, it is likely that the infection will occur.

Women with trichomoniasis need to understand the sexual transmission of this disease. It is important that the client know that the organism may be present without symptoms being present, perhaps for several months, and that it is not

TABLE 30.15	Treatment of Vaginal Infections		
INFECTION	**NONPREGNANT WOMEN**	**PREGNANT WOMEN**	**LACTATING WOMEN**
Trichomoniasis	Metronidazole 2 g orally in single dose or Tinidazole 2 g orally in a single dose or Metronidazole 500 mg twice per day for 7 days	Metronidazole 2 g orally in single dose	Metronidazole 2 g orally in single dose Breast milk should be expressed and discarded during treatment. Resume breastfeeding 12–24 hours after completing treatment
Bacterial vaginosis	Metronidazole 500 mg orally twice per day for 7 days or Metronidazole gel 0.75%, one full applicator (5 g) intravaginally once per day for 5 days or clindamycin cream 2%, one full applicator (5 g) intravaginally at bedtime for 7 days Clindamycin 300 mg orally twice per day for 7 days or clindamycin ovules 100 g intravaginally once at bedtime for 3 days or Tinidazole 2 g orally daily for 2 days or Tinidazole 1 g orally daily for 5 days	Metronidazole 250 mg orally three times per day for 7 days or clindamycin 300 mg orally twice per day for 7 days before the 16th week of pregnancy	Metronidazole 2 g orally in a single dose Breast milk should be expressed and discarded during treatment. Resume breastfeeding 12–24 hours after completing treatment
Uncomplicated VVC	Butoconazole 2% cream 5 g intravaginally × 3 days or butoconazole 2% cream 5 g (sustained release) single intravaginal application or clotrimazole 1% cream 5 g intravaginally for 7–14 days[a] or clotrimazole 100 mg vaginal tablet for 7 days or clotrimazole 100 mg vaginal tablet, two tablets for 3 days or clotrimazole 500 mg vaginal tablet, one tablet in single application or miconazole 2% cream 5 g intravaginally for 7 days[a] or miconazole 100 mg vaginal suppository, one for 7 days[a] or miconazole 200 mg vaginal suppository, one for 3 days[a] or nystatin 100,000-unit vaginal tablet, one for 14 days or tioconazole 6.5% ointment 5 g intravaginally in a single application or terconazole 0.4% cream 5 g intravaginally for 7 days or terconazole 0.8% cream 5 g intravaginally for 3 days or terconazole 80 mg vaginal suppository, one for 3 days or fluconazole 150 mg oral tablet, 1 tablet single dose	Butoconazole 2% cream 5 g intravaginally for 3 days[a] or butoconazole 2% cream 5 g (sustained release) single intravaginal application or clotrimazole 1% cream 5 g intravaginally for 7–14 days[a] or clotrimazole 100 mg vaginal tablet for 7 days or miconazole 2% cream 5 g intravaginally for 7 days[a] or miconazole 100 mg vaginal suppository, one for 7 days[a]	Butoconazole 2% cream 5 g intravaginally for 3 days[a] or butoconazole 2% cream 5 g (sustained release) single intravaginal application or clotrimazole 1% cream 5 g intravaginally for 7 to 14 days[a] or clotrimazole 100 mg vaginal tablet for 7 days or miconazole 2% cream 5 g intravaginally for 7 days[a] or miconazole 100 mg vaginal suppository, one for 7 days[a]
Complicated VVC	*Recurrent VVC initial therapy* 7–14 days of topical therapy or 100, 150, or 200 mg dose of fluconazole every third day for a total of three doses (days 1, 4, and 7)	*Recurrent VVC initial therapy* 7 to 14 days of topical therapy	*Recurrent VVC initial therapy* 7–14 days of topical therapy or 100, 150, or 200 mg dose of fluconazole every third day for a total of three doses (days 1, 4, and 7)

(continued)

TABLE 30.15	Treatment of Vaginal Infections *(continued)*		
INFECTION	**NONPREGNANT WOMEN**	**PREGNANT WOMEN**	**LACTATING WOMEN**
	Maintenance therapy Clotrimazole 500 mg vaginal suppository weekly Ketoconazole 100 mg each day Fluconazole 100–150 mg dose weekly Itraconazole 400 mg once monthly or 100 mg daily *Severe VVC* 7–14 days of topical azole or fluconazole 150 mg in two sequential doses, second dose 72 hours after initial dose *Nonalbicans VVC* Optimal treatment is unknown. Nonfluconazole azole drug for 7–14 days is first-line therapy. For recurrent episodes, 600 mg boric acid in gelatin capsule vaginally once per day for 14 days	or 100, 150, or 200 mg dose of fluconazole every third day for a total of three doses (days 1, 4, and 7) *Maintenance therapy* 100, 150, or 200 mg dose of oral fluconazole weekly for 6 months	*Maintenance therapy* 100, 150, or 200 mg dose of oral fluconazole weekly for 6 months

aOver-the-counter preparations.
VVC, vulvovaginal candidiasis.

TABLE 30.16	Alternative Therapies for Vaginitis		
INTERVENTION	**DOSAGE**	**ADMINISTRATION**	**USE**
Vinegar (white)	1 T per pint water	Douche or local application	VVC
Acidophilus culture	1 to 2 T per quart water	Douche every 5 to 7 days or twice per day for 2 days or douche once or twice per week	VVC trichomoniasis, BV
Vitamin C	500 mg two to four times per day	Orally	VVC
Acidophilus tablet	40 million to 1 billion units (1 tablet) daily	Orally	VVC
Plain yogurt	1 T	Apply to labia or vagina hourly as needed	VVC
Chaparral	Steep 1 handful in 1 quart water for 30 minutes	Douche two to three times per week	Trichomoniasis
Chickweed	Steep 3 T in 1 quart water for 10 minutes, strain	Douche daily	Trichomoniasis
Goldenseal	1 tsp in 3 cups water, strain and cool	Douche	BV
Garlic clove	1 peeled clove wrapped in cloth dipped in olive oil	Overnight in vagina, change daily	BV
Boric acid powder	600 mg in gelatin capsule	Daily in vagina for 14 days	BV
Sassafras bark	Steep in warm water	Compress or insert into vagina	BV, VVC
Cold milk, cottage cheese, plain yogurt	No specific amount	Apply to affected area	Puritis
Gentian violet	Few drops in water, 0.25%–2%	Douche or local application	VVC

BV, bacterial vaginosis; VVC, vulvovaginal candidiasis.

possible to determine when she became infected. Women should be informed of the necessity for treating all sexual partners and helped with ways to raise the issue with her partner(s).

Bacterial Vaginosis

BV—formerly called nonspecific vaginitis, hemophilus vaginitis, or Gardnerella—is the most common type of vaginal discharge or malodor in childbearing women; however, up to 50% of women with BV are asymptomatic (CDC, 2015a). BV is a clinical syndrome in which normal H_2O_2-producing *Lactobacilli* are replaced with high concentrations of anaerobic bacteria (*Prevotella sp.* and *Mobiluncus sp.*) *Gardnerella vaginalis* and *Mycoplasm hominis*. With the proliferation of anaerobes, the level of vaginal amines is raised, and the normal acidic pH of the vagina is altered. Epithelial cells slough and numerous bacteria attach to their surfaces (clue cells). When the amines are volatilized, the characteristic fishy odor of BV occurs. The cause of the microbial alteration is not completely understood.

BV is a sexually associated condition associated with multiple sex partners, a new sex partner, douching, lack of condom use, and a lack of vaginal lactobacilli and is rarely found in women who have never been sexually active (CDC, 2015a).

BV infection is associated with miscarriage, chorioamnionitis, premature rupture of fetal membranes, preterm labor and delivery, postpartum or postabortion endometritis, and postpartum complications in the infant (CDC, 2015a). In addition, new evidence suggests that BV increases a woman's risk of acquiring STDs and HIV infection and of transmitting HIV infection (CDC, 2015a). Further, failure to treat BV infection before insertion of an IUD is associated with increased incidence of PID in the first month after insertion.

Women with BV may be asymptomatic or complain of a malodorous discharge. The fishy odor may be noticed by the woman or her partner after heterosexual intercourse as semen releases the vaginal amines. When present, the BV discharge is usually increased, thin and white or gray, or milky in appearance. Some women also may experience mild irritation, vulvar pruritus, postcoital spotting, irregular bleeding episodes, or vaginal burning after intercourse while others complain of urinary discomfort. Many women have no symptoms at all.

ASSESSMENT AND DIAGNOSIS

A careful history may help distinguish BV from other vaginal infections if the woman is symptomatic. Reports of fishy odor and increased thin vaginal discharge are most significant, and report of increased odor after intercourse is also suggestive of BV. Previous occurrence of similar symptoms, diagnosis, and treatment should be asked about because women may experience repeated episodes associated with repeated insults, such as antibiotic use, douching, or life stresses.

BV can be diagnosed by the use of clinical criteria or gram stain. A speculum examination is done to inspect the vaginal walls and cervix. A microscopic examination of vaginal secretions is always done. Both normal saline and 10% potassium hydroxide smears should be completed. Clinical criteria require three of the following symptoms or signs: homogenous, thin white discharge that smoothly coats the vaginal walls; clue cells on microscopic examination; and a fishy odor of vaginal discharge before or after addition of 10% potassium hydroxide (KOH; i.e., the whiff test; CDC, 2015a).

TREATMENT

Treatment is recommended for women with symptoms. The benefits of treatment for nonpregnant women are to relieve vaginal symptoms and signs of infection. Other potential benefits to treatment are reduction in risk of acquiring chlamydia, gonorrhea, HIV, and HSV-2. Treatment of BV with oral metronidazole (Flagyl) is most effective. Treatment guidelines are found in Table 30.15. The CDC 2015 guidelines recommend that regimens in pregnancy be limited to systemic therapy of longer duration rather than a single-dose or topical therapy. Intravaginal clindamycin cream is preferred in case of allergy or intolerance to metronidazole. Patients with a known allergy to oral metronidazole should not be given vaginal metronidazole gel (CDC, 2015a). Treatment of male sexual partners has not been beneficial in preventing recurrent BV infections (CDC, 2015a). A test for BV may be done early in the second trimester for symptomatic pregnant women who are at risk for preterm labor and whenever high-risk women report increased vaginal discharge or symptoms of preterm labor. The effectiveness of the treatment of BV in asymptomatic pregnant women who are at high risk for preterm delivery has been evaluated by several studies with mixed results (CDC, 2015a). Although metronidazole crosses the placenta, no evidence of teratogenicity or mutagenic effects in infants has been found (CDC, 2015a) and the data suggest that metronidazole therapy poses low risk in pregnancy. Metronidazole is secreted in breast milk in doses that are less than those used to treat infections in infants; however, some nurse practitioners advise deferring breastfeeding for 12 to 24 hours following maternal treatment with a single 2 g dose of metronidazole (CDC, 2015a).

■ HEPATITIS

Hepatitis is an acute, systemic viral infection that occurs as hepatitis A (HAV); hepatitis B (HBV); non-A; non-B, which includes HCV, hepatitis G (HGV or GBV-C), hepatitis E (HEV), and hepatitis D (HDV; see Table 30.17).

Hepatitis A

Hepatitis A, caused by infection with hepatitis A virus (HAV) is the most common form of hepatitis, is highly contagious, self-limiting, and does not result in chronic illness

TABLE 30.17	Viral Hepatitis			
TYPE	**TRANSMISSION**	**VACCINE**	**COMPLICATIONS**	
Hepatitis A virus (HAV)[a]	Person to person (fecal–oral) Contaminated water or food Sexual practices associated with oral–anal contact	Available	Fulminant hepatitis	
Hepatitis B virus (HBV)[a]	Blood or body fluids Sexually During delivery	Available	Fulminant hepatitis Cirrhosis Cancer Chronic liver disease Hepatitis B carriers	
Hepatitis C virus (HCV)	Via blood Transfusion-associated Sexual exposure	Not available	Chronic liver disease Cirrhosis Cancer	
Hepatitis D virus (HDV)	Via blood Only in presence of active hepatitis B	Not available	Chronic liver disease Fulminant hepatitis	
Hepatitis E virus (HEV)	Fecal–oral	Not available	High mortality in pregnant women	

[a]Women who have a laboratory-confirmed HAV or HBV diagnosis and women who have had a previous vaccination for either HAV or HBV are not candidates for concurrent vaccination. If a susceptible woman has never been vaccinated for either HAV or HBV, a combination vaccine (TWINRIX) may be given in a three-dose schedule.
Adapted from Centers for Disease Control and Prevention (2015a).

or chronic liver disease. HAV infection is primarily acquired through a fecal–oral route by ingestion of contaminated food—particularly milk, shellfish, or polluted water—or person-to-person contact. Women living in the western United States, Native Americans, Alaska Natives, and children and employees in day care centers are at high risk for contracting hepatitis A. Hepatitis A, like other enteric infections, can be transmitted during sexual activity. Many sexual practices facilitate fecal–oral transmission, and unapparent fecal contamination is common with sexual intercourse (CDC, 2015a). Some studies have associated more sexual partners, frequent oral–anal contact, and insertive anal intercourse with HAV infection (CDC, 2015a).

Unlike other persons with STDs, HAV-infected persons are infectious for only a brief period of time. HAV infection is a mild, self-limited disease characterized by flu-like symptoms with malaise, fatigue, anorexia, nausea, pruritus, fever, and upper right quadrant pain; usually, there are no chronic sequelae to infection.

DIAGNOSIS

Diagnosis is not done on clinical findings alone and requires serologic testing. The presence of the immunoglobulin M (IgM) antibody is diagnostic of acute HAV infection. The IgM antibody is detectable 5 to 10 days after exposure and can remain positive for up to 6 months. Because HAV infection is self-limited and does not result in chronic infection or chronic liver disease, treatment is usually supportive. Women who become dehydrated from nausea and vomiting or who have fulminating hepatitis A may need to be hospitalized. Medications that might cause liver damage or that are metabolized in the liver should be used with

caution. No specific diet or activity restrictions are necessary. Immunoglobulin (IG) or immune-specific globulin is indicated for any pregnant woman exposed to HAV to provide passive immunity through injected antibodies. Perinatal transmission of HAV has not been demonstrated. Two products are available for the prevention of hepatitis A: hepatitis A vaccine and immune globulin for IM administration. Inactivated hepatitis A vaccines are available in the United States for anyone older than 2 years. It is administered in a two-dose series and induces protective immunity in virtually all adults following the second dose. A combined hepatitis A and B vaccine is available for adults. Administered on a 0-, 1-, or 6-month schedule, its effectiveness is equal to the monovalent vaccine (CDC, 2006). All household contacts should receive IG. When administered before or within 2 weeks after exposure to HAV, IG is 85% effective in preventing HAV. Persons in the following groups who are likely to be treated in STD clinics should be offered the HAV vaccine: all women who have sex with men having sex with men; illegal drug users (both injecting and non-injecting drugs); and persons with chronic liver disease (CDC, 2015a).

Hepatitis B

HBV is a blood-borne pathogen transmitted by exposure to infectious blood or body fluids (e.g., semen, saliva). HBV is more infectious than HIV and hepatitis C (CDC, 2015a). The highest concentrations are in blood with lower concentrations found in other body fluids including wound exudates, semen, vaginal secretions, and saliva. Chronically infected persons can transmit the infection and are at 15% to 25% increased risk for premature death from cirrhosis or hepatocellular carcinoma (CDC, 2015a). Women who are infected with HBV can transmit the virus to their neonates during delivery; the risk of chronic infection in the infant is as high as 90% (CDC, 2015a). HBV infection is caused by a large DNA virus and is associated with three antigens and their antibodies. Screening for active or chronic disease or disease immunity is based on testing for these antigens and their antibodies.

Overall prevalence of HBV infection differs among racial/ethnic populations and is highest among persons who have emigrated from areas with a high endemicity of HBV infections, that is, Asia, Pacific Islands, Africa, and the Middle East (CDC, 2015a). Factors considered to place a woman at risk for HBV are those associated with STI risk in general (history of multiple sexual partners, multiple STIs, IV drug use), behaviors that are associated with blood contact (e.g., work or treatment in a dialysis unit, history of multiple blood transfusions, public safety workers exposed to blood in the work place, health care workers), and persons born in a country with a high incidence of HBV infection. Although HBV can be transmitted via blood transfusion, the incidence of such infections has decreased significantly because testing of blood for the presence of HBsAg became possible. Women who abuse drugs and share needles are at risk, as are women with a history of jail or prison experience and/or a history of needlestick injury, tattoos, or body piercing. Also at risk for HBV are day care workers who are exposed to body fluids and health care workers who are exposed to blood and needle sticks.

HBV infection is transmitted parentally and through intimate contact. Hepatitis B chronic infection affects 5% of the world population, with higher percentages found in tropical areas and Southeast Asia. Hepatitis B surface antigen has been found in blood, saliva, sweat, tears, vaginal secretions, and semen. Perinatal transmission does occur; however, the fetus is not at risk until it comes in contact with contaminated blood at delivery. HBV has also been transmitted by artificial insemination.

HBV infection is a disease of the liver and is asymptomatic in up to onethird of infected persons. In children and adults, the course of the infection can be fulminating and the outcome fatal. Symptoms of HBV infection are similar to those of HAV: arthralgias, arthritis, lassitude, anorexia, nausea, vomiting, headache, fever, and mild abdominal pain. Later, the patient may have clay-colored stools, dark urine, increased abdominal pain, and jaundice. Between 6% and 10% of adults with HBV have persistence of HBsAg and become chronically infected. Up to 25% of chronically infected individuals will die from primary hepatocellular carcinoma or cirrhosis of the liver.

ASSESSMENT AND DIAGNOSIS

All women at high risk for contracting hepatitis B should be vaccinated. Screening only high-risk individuals may not identify up to 50% of HBsAg-positive women; therefore, current CDC 2015 guidelines recommend screening for the presence of HBsAg in all women at their first prenatal visit and repeating screening in the third trimester of pregnancy for women with high-risk behaviors.

Components of the history to be obtained when hepatitis B is suspected include inquiry about the symptoms of the disease and risk factors outlined earlier. Women also should be asked about taste and smell peculiarities and intolerance of fatty foods and cigarettes. The nurse practitioner should ask about darkened urine and light-colored stools as well. Physical examination includes inspection of the skin for rashes, inspection of the skin and conjunctiva for jaundice, and palpation of the liver for enlargement and tenderness. Weight loss, fever, and general debilitation should be noted. If the HBsAg is positive, further laboratory studies may be ordered: anti-HBe, anti-HBc, SGOT, alkaline phosphatase, and liver panel. If the HBsAg is negative in early pregnancy and the woman could be in the "window phase" or if high-risk behaviors continue during pregnancy, a repeat HBsAg should be ordered in the third trimester. HIV testing should be done.

Interpretation of testing for hepatitis B is complex (see Table 30.18). Patients with acute hepatitis B generally have detectable serum HBsAg levels in the late incubation phase of the disease, 2 to 5 weeks before symptoms appear. Anti-HBs with a negative HBsAg test signals immunity. Anti-HBs with a positive antigen denotes a chronic state; during this time, the disease can be transmitted. During the recovery phase, the patient may continue to be infectious even though HBsAg cannot be detected. This is called the window phase and is identified by anti-HBc in the absence of anti-HBs. Women should be prepared for repeat testing because HBV screening tests may be used to monitor the progression of the disease.

TREATMENT

There is no specific treatment for hepatitis B. Recovery is usually spontaneous in 3 to 16 weeks. Usually pregnancies complicated by acute viral hepatitis are managed on an outpatient basis. Rest and a high-protein, low-fat diet are important. Women should be advised to increase their fluid intake and avoid medications that are metabolized in the liver, drugs, and alcohol. Women with a definite exposure to hepatitis B should be given hepatitis B immunoglobulin IM in a single dose as soon as possible, preferably within 24 hours after exposure (CDC, 2015a). HB vaccine is indicated for newborns of women who have tested positive for HBsAg or who are high risk with unknown status to stimulate the newborn's active immunity. The vaccine should be given as soon as possible after birth up to 7 days and again at 30 and 60 days. The CDC recommends routine vaccination of all newborns and vaccination of older children at high risk for HBV infection.

TABLE 30.18	Parameters of Hepatitis B Testing
HBsAg	Hepatitis B surface antigen
HBsAb	Hepatitis B surface antibody
IgM HBcAb	Hepatitis B core antibody (IgM class-recent infection)
IgG HBcAb	Hepatitis B core antibody (IgG class-past infection)
HBeAg	Hepatitis B e antigen
HBeAb	Hepatitis B e antibody

Ab, antibody; Ag, antigen; IgG, immunoglobulin G; IgM, immunoglobulin M.

All nonimmune women at high or moderate risk of hepatitis B should be informed of the existence of the hepatitis B vaccine. Vaccination is recommended for all individuals who have had multiple sex partners within the past 6 months. In addition, IV drug users, residents of correctional or long-term care facilities, persons seeking care for an STD, sex workers, women whose partners are IV drug users or are bisexual, and women whose occupation exposes them to high risk should be vaccinated. Vaccination is not associated with serious side effects and does not carry a risk for contracting HIV. The vaccine is given in a series of three (some authorities recommend four) doses over a 6-month period with the first two doses given within 1 month of each other. In adults, the vaccine should be given in the deltoid muscle, never in the gluteal or quadriceps muscle. The vaccination is not contraindicated during pregnancy.

Patient education includes explaining the meaning of hepatitis B infection, including transmission, state of infectivity, and sequelae. The nurse practitioner should also explain the need for immunoprophylaxis for household members and sexual contacts of women with acute or chronic infection. To decrease transmission of the virus, women with hepatitis B or who test positive for HBV should be advised to maintain a high level of personal hygiene: wash hands after using the toilet; carefully dispose of tampons, pads, and adhesive bandages in plastic bags; do not share razor blades, toothbrushes, needles, or manicure implements; have male partners use a condom if unvaccinated and without hepatitis B; avoid sharing saliva through kissing or sharing of silverware or dishes; wipe up blood spills immediately with soap and water. Women with hepatitis B should inform all health care providers of their chronic infective status; all HBsAg-positive pregnant women should be reported to the local and state health departments to ensure that they are entered into a case management system and appropriate prophylaxis is provided for their infants. In addition, household and sexual contacts of HBsAg-positive women should be vaccinated (CDC, 2015a). Newly delivered women should be reassured that breastfeeding is not contraindicated if their infants received prophylaxis at birth and are currently on the immunization schedule.

■ STDs DURING PREGNANCY

Perinatal outcomes can be affected by various STDs in that pregnant women may transmit the infection to their fetus, newborn, or infant through vertical transmission (via the placenta, during vaginal birth, or after birth through breastfeeding) or horizontal transmission (close physical or household contact). Some STDs (like syphilis) can cross the placenta and infect the fetus in utero. Other STDs (like gonorrhea, chlamydia, hepatitis B, and genital herpes) can be transmitted as the baby passes through the birth canal. The harmful effects of STDs may include stillbirth, low birth weight (less than 5 pounds), conjunctivitis, pneumonia, neonatal sepsis, neurological damage (such as brain damage or lack of coordination in body movements), blindness, deafness, acute hepatitis, meningitis, chronic liver disease, and cirrhosis. Some of these problems can be prevented if the woman is screened and treated for STDs during pregnancy.

Other problems can be treated if the infection is found in the newborn. A pregnant woman with an STD may have early onset of labor, premature rupture of the membranes, and uterine infection after delivery.

Treatment

STD treatment regimens may differ for pregnant women. Nurse practitioners should consult the most current CDC treatment guidelines and selected chapter references for further information about STDs in pregnancy.

■ FUTURE DIRECTIONS

STDs are among the most common health problems of women in the United States and around the world. Women experience a disproportionate amount of the burden associated with these illnesses, including complications of infertility, perinatal infections, poor pregnancy outcomes, chronic pelvic pain, genital tract neoplasms, and potential death. Additionally, these infections interfere with one's lifestyle and cause considerable distress, both emotional and physical. Nurse practitioners can help to ameliorate the misery, morbidity, and mortality associated with STDs and other common infections through accurate, safe, sensitive, and supportive care. Nurse practitioners should be aware that STD knowledge is constantly increasing and changing with new and improved prevention, diagnostic, and treatment modalities being developed and reported. All nurse practitioners have a responsibility to stay current with these developments through reviewing current journals, attending conferences, and being knowledgeable about recommendations and bulletins from the CDC. Furthermore, it is important that practitioners be aware of policies, recommendations, and guidelines of the state in which they practice, which also may change frequently.

■ REFERENCES

Augenbraun, M. (2007). Syphilis. In J. D. Klausner III & E. W. Hook (Eds.), *Current diagnosis and treatment of sexually transmitted diseases* (pp. 119–129). New York, NY: McGraw-Hill Medical.

Barron, M. L. (1998). *Nursing assessment of the pregnant woman: Antepartal screening and laboratory evaluation*. New York, NY: March of Dimes Birth Defects Foundation.

Braje, S. E., Eddy, J. M., & Hall, G. C. (2016). A comparison of two models of risky sexual behavior during late adolescence. *Archives of Sexual Behavior*, 45(1), 73–83.

Brookmeyer, K. A., Hogben, M., & Kinsey, J. (2016). The role of behavioral counseling in sexually transmitted disease prevention program settings. *Sexually Transmitted Diseases*, 43(2, Suppl. 1), S102–S112.

Brown, K. (2000). *Management guidelines for women's health nurse practitioners*. Philadelphia, PA: F. A. Davis.

Bui, T. C., Tran, L. T., Hor, L. B., Scheurer, M. E., Vidrine, D. J., & Markham, C. M. (2016). Intravaginal practices in female sex workers in Cambodia: A qualitative study. *Archives of Sexual Behavior*, 45(4), 935–943.

Carcio, H. A. (1999). *Advanced health assessment of women*. Philadelphia, PA: Lippincott Williams & Wilkins.

Carcio, H. A. & Secor, R. M. (2015a). *Advanced health assessment of women* (3rd ed.). Philadelphia, PA: Lippincott Williams & Wilkins.

Carcio, H. A. & Secor, R. M. (2015b). Vaginal microscopy. In *Advanced health assessment of women* (pp. 445–483). New York, NY: Springer Publishing.

Cardozo, T., Shmelkov, S. V., Carr, K., Rotrosen, J., Mateu-Gelabert, P., & Friedman, S. R. (2016). Cocaine and HIV infection. In *Biologics to treat substance use disorders* (pp. 75–103). Cham, Switzerland: Springer International Publishing.

Centers for Disease Control and Prevention (CDC). (2006). Sexually transmitted diseases treatment guidelines 2006. *Morbidity and Mortality Weekly Report, 55*(RR-11), 1–94.

Centers for Disease Control and Prevention (CDC). (2014). *STDs in adolescents and young adults.* Retrieved from www.cdc.gov/std/stats14/womenandinf.htm

Centers for Disease Control and Prevention (CDC). (2015a). Sexually transmitted diseases treatment guidelines, 2015. *Morbidity and Mortality Weekly Report, Recommendations and Reports, 64*(3), 2.

Centers for Disease Control and Prevention. (2015b). *STDs in women and children.* Retrieved from www.cdc.gov/std/stats14/womenandinf.htm

Duan, S., Ding, Y., Wu, Z., Rou, K., Yang, Y., Wang, J., Gao, M., Ye, R., Xiang, L., & He, N. (2016). The prevalence of HSV-2 infection in HIV-1 discordant couples. *Epidemiology and Infection, 144*(1), 97–105.

Farel, C., Parker, S. D., Muessig, K. E., Grodensky, C. A., Jones, C., Golin, C. E., . . . Wohl, D. A. (2013). Sexuality, sexual practices, and HIV risk among incarcerated African-American women in North Carolina. *Women's Health Issues, 26*(6), e357–e365.

Fogel, C. I. (1995). Sexually transmitted diseases. In N. F. Woods and C. I. Fogel (Eds.), *Women's health care* (pp. 571–609). Thousand Oaks, CA: Sage.

Fogel, C. I. (2006). Sexually transmitted infections. In K. D. Schuiling & F. K. Likis (Eds.), *Women's gynecological health* (pp. 421–469). Boston, MA: Jones & Bartlett.

Fogel, C. I., Gelaude, D. J., Carry, M., Herbst, J. H., Parker, S., Scheyette, A., & Neevel, A. (2014). Context of risk for HIV and sexually transmitted infections among incarcerated women in the south: Individual, interpersonal, and societal factors. *Women & Health, 54*(8), 694–711.

Fogel, C. I., & Lauver, D. (1990). *Sexual health promotion.* Philadelphia, PA: Saunders.

Fogel, C. I., & Woods, N. F. (Eds.). (1995). *Women's health care.* Thousand Oaks, CA: Sage.

Goldsberry, J., Moore, L., MacMillan, D., & Butler, S. (2016). Assessing the effects of a sexually transmitted disease educational intervention on fraternity and sorority members' knowledge and attitudes toward safe sex behaviors. *Journal of the American Association of Nurse Practitioners, 28*(4), 188–195.

Grosso, A. (2010). Social support as a predictor of HIV testing in at-risk populations: A research note. *Journal of Health and Human Services Administration, 33*(1), 53–62.

Guest, F. (2006). Patient-centered communication and STI care. In A. L. Nelson & J. Woodward (Eds.), *Sexually transmitted diseases* (pp. 279–294). Totowa, NJ: Humana Press.

Hatcher, R., Trussel, J., Nelson, A., Cates, W., Kowal, D., & Policar, M. (2004). *Contraceptive technology* (18th rev. ed.). New York, NY: Ardent Media.

Hatcher, R., Trussel, J., Nelson, A., Cates, W., Kowal, D., & Policar, M. (2011). *Contraceptive technology* (20th rev. ed.). New York, NY: Ardent Media.

Hawkins, J. E., Roberto-Nichols, D. M., & Stanley-Haney, J. L. (2008). *Sage protocols for nurse practitioners in gynecologic settings* (7th ed.). New York, NY: Tiresias Press.

Hewitt-Stubbs, G., Zimmer-Gembeck, M. J., Mastro, S., & Boislard, M. A. (2016). A longitudinal study of sexual entitlement and self-efficacy among young women and men: Gender differences and associations with age and sexual experience. *Behavioral Sciences (Basel, Switzerland), 6*(1), 4–18.

Imitiaz, S., Wells, S., & Macdonald, S. (2016). Sex differences among treatment clients with cocaine-related problems. *Journal of Substance Abuse, 21*(1), 22–28.

Institute of Medicine (IOM). (1997). *The hidden epidemic: Confronting sexually transmitted diseases.* Washington, DC: National Academies Press.

Institute of Medicine (IOM). (2015). *The hidden epidemic: Confronting sexually transmitted diseases.* Washington, DC: National Academies Press.

Jacobs, R. A. (2001). Infectious diseases: Spirochetal. In L. M. Tierney, S. J. McPhee, & M. A. Papadakis (Eds.), *Current medical diagnosis and treatment, 2001* (pp. 205–227). New York, NY: Lange Medical Books/McGraw-Hill.

Kurth, A. (1998). Promoting sexual health in the age of HIV/AIDS. *Journal of Nurse-Midwifery, 43*(3), 162–181.

Livengood, C. H. (2001). Syphilis. In S. Faro and D. E. Soper (Eds.), *Infectious diseases in women* (pp. 403–429). Philadelphia, PA: Saunders.

Lowy, D. R. (2016). HPV vaccination to prevent cervical cancer and other HPV-associated disease: From basic science to effective interventions. *The Journal of Clinical Investigation, 126*(1), 5–11.

MacLauren, A. (1995). Primary care for women: Comprehensive sexual health assessment. *Journal of Nurse-Midwifery, 40*, 104–119.

Moodley P., Wilkinson D., Connolly C., Moodley, J., & Sturm, A. W. (2002). *Trichomonas vaginalis* is associated with pelvic inflammatory disease in women infected with human immunodeficiency virus. *Clinical Infectious Disease, 34*, 519–522.

Morales-Alemán, M. M., & Scarinci, I. C. (2016). Correlates and predictors of sexual health among adolescent Latinas in the United States: A systematic review of the literature, 2004–2015. *Preventive Medicine, 87*, 183–193.

Park, J., Nordstrom, S. K., Weber, K. M., & Irwin, T. (2016). Reproductive coercion: Uncloaking an imbalance of social power. *American Journal of Obstetrics and Gynecology, 214*(1), 74–78.

Paterno, M. T., & Jordan, E. T. (2012). A review of factors associated with unprotected sex among adult women in the United States. *Journal of Obstetric, Gynecologic, and Neonatal Nursing, 41*(2), 258–274.

Petti, Y. M. (2015). Lesbian health (don't ask . . . won't tell: Lesbian women who have sex with women. In H. A. Carcio & R. M. Secor (Eds.), *Advanced Health Assessment of Women* (3rd ed., pp. 177–184). New York, NY: Springer Publishing.

Pinninti, S. G., & Kimberlin, D. W. (2013). Maternal and neonatal herpes simplex virus infections. *American Journal of Perinatology, 30*(2), 113–119.

Schmid, G. P. (2001). Epidemiology of sexually transmitted infections. In S. Faro and D. E. Soper (Eds.), *Infectious diseases in women* (pp. 395–402). Philadelphia, PA: Saunders.

Secor, M. R. (2015). Sexually transmitted infections. In H. A. Carcio & R. M. Secor (Eds.). *Advanced health assessment of women: Clinical skills and procedures* (3rd ed.). New York, NY: Springer Publishing.

Sexual Health Advice Center. (2016). *How to use a male condom.* Retrieved from http://www.addenbrookes.org.uk/serv/clin/shac/advice/contraception/types/mcondom.htm

Star, W. (1999). Syphilis. In W. L. Star, M. T. Shannon, L. L. Lommel, and Y. M. Gutierrez (Eds.), *Ambulatory obstetrics* (3rd ed., pp. 1031–1056). San Francisco, CA: UCSF Nursing Press.

Star, W. (2004). Sexually transmitted diseases. In W. L. Star, L. L. Lommel, and M. T. Shannon (Eds.), *Women's primary health care* (2nd ed., pp. 13–1–13–59). San Francisco, CA: UCSF Nursing Press.

Star, W., & Deal, M. (2004). Gonorrhea. In W. L. Starr, L. L. Lommel, & M. T. Shannon (Eds.), *Women's primary health care* (2nd ed., pp. 13–24). San Francisco, CA: UCSF Nursing Press.

Star, W. L., Lommel, L. L. & Shannon, M. T. (1995). *Women's health primary care: Protocols for practice.* Washington, DC: American Nurses Publishing.

Stone, K. M., Reiff-Eldridge, R. A., White, A. D., Cordero, J. F., Brown, Z., Alexander, E. R., & Andrews, E. B. (2004). Pregnancy outcomes following systemic prenatal acyclovir: Conclusions from the International Acyclovir Pregnancy Registry, 1984–1999. *Birth Defects Research Part A: Clinical and Molecular Teratology, 70*(4), 201–207.

Stults, C. B., Javdani, S., Greenbaum, C. A., Kapadia, F., & Halkitis, P. N. (2016). Intimate partner violence and sex among young men who have sex with men. *Journal of Adolescent Health, 58*(2), 215–222.

Varney, H., Kriebs, J. M., & Gegor, C. L. (2004). *Varney's midwifery* (4th ed.). Sudbury, MA: Jones & Bartlett.

Welty, L. J., Harrison, A. J., Abram, K. M., Olson, N. D., Aaby, D. A., McCoy, K. P., . . . Teplin, L. A. (2016). Health disparities in drug- and alcohol-use disorders: A 12-year longitudinal study of youths after detention. *American Journal of Public Health, 106*(5), 872–880.

Wenzel, S. L., Cederbaum, J. A., Song, A., Hsu, H. T., Craddock, J. B., Hantanachaikul, W., & Tucker, J. S. (2016). Pilot test of an adapted, evidence-based HIV sexual risk reduction intervention for homeless women. *Prevention Science: The Official Journal of the Society for Prevention Research, 17*(1), 112–121.

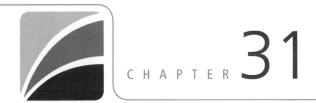
Women and HIV/AIDS

Catherine Ingram Fogel

In the summer of 1981, the Centers for Disease Control and Prevention (CDC, 1981) reported the occurrence of clusters of several rare illnesses—*Pneumocystis carinii* pneumonia (PCP), *Mycobacterium avium* intracellulare, cryptosporidiosis—and tumors (Kaposi's sarcoma, non-Hodgkin's lymphoma) in homosexual and bisexual men in California and New York. This was the beginning of the AIDS pandemic and represented a medical mystery that was solved with the identification of a single infectious agent destroying the immune system of infected persons: human immunodeficiency virus (HIV). Initially, HIV infection appeared to be associated with homosexual activities, but symptoms of the syndrome were identified in a woman within 2 months of the earliest reports of the disease in men. It soon became clear that heterosexual activity and direct blood contact could also transmit the virus. The first female AIDS case was reported to the CDC in July 1982, and, within the first year of the epidemic, women partners of infected hemophiliacs, female intravenous (IV) drug abusers, and women partners in heterosexual relationships were diagnosed with AIDS. Early misunderstanding of the nature of transmission of HIV led researchers and the medical community to grossly underestimate the numbers of women who were or would become infected with HIV.

■ DEFINITION AND SCOPE

The term *diagnosis of HIV infection* is defined as HIV infection regardless of stage of disease, referring to all persons with the diagnosis (CDC, 2015a). HIV infection and AIDS have spread rapidly throughout the world, affecting millions of persons and resulting in millions of deaths. From 2010 through 2014, the annual estimated number of all people living with HIV and the rate of diagnoses of HIV infections in the United States remained stable at 13.8%. In 2014, the highest rate for HIV was for persons aged 25 to 29 years. From 2005 to 2014, the number of new HIV diagnosis among African American women fell 42%. In 2014, an estimated 1,350 Hispanic/Latina women and 1,483 White women were diagnosed with HIV, compared with 5,128 African American women. Promising news is that

from 2010 through 2013, in the United States, a decrease in HIV deaths was noted.

■ SOCIAL CONTEXT

Deeply ingrained social and cultural forces that tend to devalue women, and particularly poor women of color, perpetuated the tendency for HIV and AIDS to be underdiagnosed in women, resulting in the delay of treatment. HIV infection was long considered to be a men's disease and, more specifically, a disease of homosexual men. However, most new HIV diagnoses in women are attributed to heterosexual sex (CDC, 2016).

Very few diseases in history have had the level of stigma that accompanies an HIV diagnosis. Many persons with HIV choose to keep their diagnosis a secret from family, friends, and coworkers. Although this means that they must hide clinic visits, medications, and HIV-related illnesses, they may feel this is preferable to experiencing the stigma that accompanies the diagnosis. Persons with HIV may face dissolution of important relationships when and if the diagnosis becomes known. Nurse practitioners can assist patients in identifying supportive others who can be helpful as the patient adapts to the diagnosis and antiretroviral therapy (ART) when initiated. Nurse practitioners should respect the patient's decisions about disclosure of the diagnosis (CDC, 2015a).

The woman may also want to make explicit her wishes regarding end-of-life care by establishing advance directives and entrusting a friend or family member with power of attorney in the event she becomes incapacitated. Nurse practitioners can be useful in explaining the meanings of various levels of advanced care and the implications of aggressive care in advanced HIV disease and AIDS. Young women with children may want more aggressive therapies and interventions than older women whose children are grown. This is a personal decision based on a variety of considerations, including spiritual and theological issues. Nurse practitioners must be careful not to make assumptions about what is desirable and appropriate for each woman.

Nurse practitioners can help patients reframe their understanding of HIV, particularly in terms of understanding it as a chronic disease that can be managed, rather than the "death sentence" it once was. When a woman learns of her HIV diagnosis, she may become seriously depressed, expecting to die soon and in much pain. Intervening early with these patients may prepare them to live with the disease, rather than simply waiting to die. Furthermore, many persons with HIV are recognized as long-term nonprogressors who, although infected with HIV, do not progress to AIDS even years after infection. Researchers have found psychological and behavioral factors that may play a role in the continuing viral suppression of nonprogressors. These factors include: (a) viewing HIV as a manageable illness; (b) taking care of their physical health; (c) staying connected with others in supportive relationships; (d) taking care of their emotional and mental health; and (e) nurturing their spiritual well-being. These means of adapting to the very serious diagnosis of HIV can assist the HIV-infected patient in regaining a sense of control and hope. Nurse practitioners are in a unique position to understand the multiplicity of factors and issues that face persons with HIV. Awareness of these factors can enhance nursing interventions to improve both physical and mental health and the long-term health outcomes for their HIV-positive patients.

At the beginning of the pandemic, researchers and scientists sought to identify the mechanism of infection and to seek a cure. In the ensuing two decades, scientists have identified the means of infection, although a cure remains elusive. However, in contrast to the early days of the epidemic, when HIV infection typically meant premature death from AIDS-related complications, a diagnosis of HIV infection now means a less-certain trajectory toward AIDS and death. With improved antiviral therapy, HIV infection in many persons has evolved into a treatable chronic infection.

In the course of their practice, most advanced practice nurse practitioners will likely have occasion to provide care for women infected with HIV. Although AIDS is a long-term sequela of unchecked viral replication and immune system damage with its attendant infections, the more salient effect of the HIV epidemic on advanced nursing practice is the management of patients chronically infected with this virus, not those who have developed AIDS. For many women, HIV is treated as a chronic condition, and it may never progress to AIDS. Therefore, this chapter addresses the issues more closely associated with management of HIV infection rather than AIDS.

Untreated HIV disease progresses relentlessly. In untreated patients, the time between HIV infection and the development of AIDS ranges from a few months to 17 years, with the median interval without treatment being 10 years (CDC, 2010). The rate of disease progression in an individual is determined by interactions between the host (the infected person), the virus, and the environment. The clinical goal is to minimize viral replication by determining the particular combination of antiretroviral therapies, health-related behaviors, and psychosocial support needed to sustain a woman's health, limit the number of acute illness episodes related to HIV, and prevent mother-to-child transmission.

■ EPIDEMIOLOGY OF HIV

Early in the epidemic, HIV infection and AIDS were diagnosed in relatively few women, although current knowledge suggests that many women were infected but were not diagnosed (CDC, 2007a; Thomas et al., 2015). The growing number of women living with HIV/AIDS is a dominant feature of the AIDS epidemic; approximately one of every four people living with HIV in the United States is a woman (AIDS info, 2015b). Additionally, an increasing number of women living with HIV/AIDS are older than 50 years. Although the increase can be explained in part by AIDS-delaying benefits of combination ART—thus women infected early in life are now being diagnosed with AIDS later in life—it may also be associated with women being infected later in life and being overlooked because of the assumption that older women are not as sexually active. Women who were married for 20 or more years and subsequently divorced have found themselves single again and have begun having sex (Kalibala, 2016; Milrod & Monto, 2016).

Women of color, particularly African American women, are disproportionately affected by HIV/AIDS. Of the total number of women diagnosed and living with HIV at the end of 2013, 63% were African American, 17% were White, and 15% were Hispanic/Latinas (AIDS info, 2015b). Although African American and Hispanic women represent less than one quarter of the U.S. population, 66% of new HIV infections occur in Black women, and almost 80% of women with AIDS in the United States are African American or Hispanic (CDC, 2015b). AIDS infection is the third leading cause of death for Black women aged 25 to 34 years; it is the sixth leading cause for women overall in this age group (CDC, 2016). Furthermore, the U.S. age-adjusted death rate of all Black women with HIV is roughly 15 times higher than that of the total number of HIV-infected women (CDC, 2015b).

In the United States, the HIV/AIDS epidemic is not evenly distributed throughout the states. Generally, HIV/AIDS cases are concentrated in urban areas with states containing major metropolitan areas reporting higher rates of HIV/AIDS (CDC, 2015d). The states with the highest number of women and girls estimated to be living with an HIV diagnosis are those in the Northeast and South including New York, Florida, Texas, California, New Jersey, Maryland, Pennsylvania, Georgia, North Carolina, and Illinois (CDC, 2013).

Women are more likely to be diagnosed at younger ages than men, with the majority (77%) of women with AIDS diagnosed between the ages of 25 and 44 years, indicating that many were infected at a young age. In 2010, almost 2,000 girls and young women aged 13 to 24 years were diagnosed with a new HIV/AIDS infection (CDC, 2016). The CDC recommends that each state and U.S. territory conduct HIV case surveillance in addition to ongoing AIDS case surveillance. Early in the epidemic, AIDS surveillance data were adequate to allow public health officials to understand and evaluate the impact of the illness and to make programmatic decisions regarding prevention efforts. However, the widespread use of effective ART has diminished the numbers of AIDS cases, even though the numbers of persons infected with HIV have increased. Therefore, it has become necessary for the CDC to recommend expanded HIV case surveillance to monitor the epidemic and shape policy, prevention, and care services in response to surveillance data.

This is particularly important for women with HIV, because women tend to be under-represented in AIDS surveillance data, as are ethnic minorities. HIV case surveillance is likely to reflect the epidemic in women earlier than AIDS data, which may be reported late in the disease after treatment failure or the onset of serious immunocompromised and health sequelae. The CDC has recommended HIV case surveillance rather than AIDS prevalence reports alone as it can provide a more realistic, useful estimate of the resources needed for patient care and services (Thomas et al., 2015).

■ NATURAL HISTORY AND HIV DISEASE PROGRESSION

The human immune system functions to protect the body from invasion by a variety of types of microbes and tumor cells. The immune system is comprised of two arms: humoral immunity, which is involved with antibody production, and cellular immunity, which is effected largely through cytotoxic T-cells. Central components of the cellular arm of the immune system are macrophages and CD4+ T-cells.

HIV is a retrovirus that specifically targets CD4+ T-cells, binding to the cell surface protein known as the CD4+ receptor. The virus affects the cells two ways: first, the absolute numbers of these cells are depleted; second, the function of the remaining cells is impaired, resulting in a gradual loss of immune function. Progressive depletion of CD4 cells in peripheral blood is the hallmark of advancing HIV disease (Hessol, Gandhi, & Greenblatt, 2005). Unimpeded, HIV can destroy up to 1 billion CD4 cells per day. In addition to its aggressive destruction, HIV is genetically highly variable, mutating with apparent ease.

Untreated HIV infection is a chronic illness that progresses relentlessly through several characteristic clinical stages. AIDS, the endpoint of HIV infection, results from severe immunologic damage, loss of effective immune response to specific opportunistic pathogens, and tumors. AIDS is diagnosed when one of these specific infections or cancers occurs or when CD4 cell levels are less than $200/mm^3$.

■ HIV STAGING AND PROGRESSION

HIV infection causes a wide range of symptoms and clinical conditions reflecting the level of immunologic injury and other predisposing factors. Certain conditions tend to occur at the same time and at specific CD4 cell counts. Staging systems for HIV disease facilitate clinical evaluation and therapeutic intervention, help to determine individual level of infirmary, and provide information with which to make diagnoses. The most widely used system for classifying HIV infection and AIDS in adults and adolescents in industrialized countries was developed by the CDC. When a patient has been diagnosed with HIV, clinicians need two important pieces of data in planning appropriate therapies and in estimating the patient's prognosis: (1) how far the disease has progressed already and (2) how fast the disease is progressing. The CD4+ count provides a clue as to how far the disease has progressed, whereas the viral load provides a clue as to the rate of progression. Clinically, these data are more relevant to direct appropriate care than are strict categories of illness in which individuals may or may not receive the best care tailored to their own particular state of illness or relative health. However, stages of HIV disease described in general terms are clinically relevant (Table 31.1).

Initially, women appeared to have a more rapid progression of illness than men and to present with different opportunistic infections. However, current data suggest that the incidence and distribution of HIV-related illnesses are similar in men and women with the exception of Kaposi's sarcoma, which is seen more often in men, and the gynecologic manifestations of HIV. In general, predictors of the rate of HIV disease progression and survival among women are the same as those in men. CD4 cell count depletion and higher HIV ribonucleic acid (RNA) level are strong predictors of a woman's progression and survival.

TABLE 31.1	Stages of HIV Infection
Acute infection	Virus establishes itself in the body; acute HIV syndrome (viral flu-like syndrome) occurs within 2–4 weeks of exposure to HIV. Characterized by fever, swollen glands, rash, muscle and joint aches and pains, and headaches. May last for several weeks. May become transiently immunocompromised. Takes 6–12 weeks for immune system to produce antibodies. Newly infected individual's blood may not test positive; however, individual may be highly contagious.
Clinical latency	Viral load stabilizes. Period of clinical latency with few or no symptoms; however, viral replication in lymphoid tissues continues. The individual is relatively symptom free but may have transient episodes of HIV-related infections. Women may be prone to aggressive cervical dysplasia. If on ART, clinical latency may last for several decades because the treatment helps keep the virus in check. For those not on ART, the clinical latency stage lasts an average of 10 years, although some may progress through this stage faster.
AIDS	CD4+ count < 200. Immune system is badly damaged and individual is vulnerable to opportunistic infections such as PCP. Individuals can respond to aggressive ART. CD4+ count < 50. Individual is severely ill with extensive organ involvement, aggressive neoplasia (Karposi's sarcoma), wasting disease syndromes, severe disseminated infections such as *M. tuberculosis* and extrapulmonary histoplasmosis. Death occurs with vascular collapse and organ failure.

ART, antiretroviral therapy; PCP, Pneumocystis carinii pneumonia.
Source: Centers for Disease Control and Prevention (2014).

■ TRANSMISSION

Virtually all cases of HIV are transmitted by three primary routes: sexual, parenteral (blood-borne), and perinatal. Rates of transmission from the infected host to the uninfected recipient vary by mode of transmission and specific circumstances of transmission (Hessol et al., 2005). Because HIV is a relatively large virus, has a short half-life in vitro, and only lives within primates, it is not transmitted through casual contact (i.e., hugging or shaking hands), surface contact (i.e., toilet seat), or from insect bites. Myths and misconceptions about HIV transmission are found in Table 31.2.

Sexual Activity

The most common mode of transmission involves depositing HIV on mucosal surfaces, especially genital mucosa (Landovitz et al., 2016). Sexual transmission of HIV occurs through male-to-female, female-to-male, male-to-male, and female-to-female sexual contact. Receptive anal and vaginal intercourse appears to have the greatest risk of infection; however, insertive anal or vaginal intercourse also is associated with HIV infection. The majority (72%) of HIV infections in women occur through unprotected heterosexual intercourse (AIDS info, 2015a). A much smaller percentage of HIV-infected women report having had sex with women; however, most of these had other risk factors, including injection drug use and sex with men who were infected or who had risk factors of infection (CDC, 2015b). In addition, a few cases of female-to-female HIV transmission have been reported, primarily through acts that may result in vaginal trauma such as sharing sex toys without condoms or digital play with fingers with cuts or sharp nails (CDC, 2015b; Thomas et al., 2015). Assuming that a woman is of very low risk for HIV because she has an expressed sexual preference for women overlooks the fact that many lesbians have a history of sexual intercourse with men or may have other risk factors for HIV infection (Para, Gee, & Davis, 2016).

Parental

HIV can reach a person's infectable cells via infected blood or blood products, most commonly through injection drug use, but also via razor blades or tattoo needles. In 2005, approximately 26% of cases of HIV/AIDS in women occurred through injection drug use (CDC, 2012, 2016).

HIV also can be transmitted from person to person through transfusion of blood or blood products; however, strict standards regarding testing of blood and blood products before administration have reduced the risk of exposure to HIV through this route. Once the presence of HIV was recognized in the blood supply in the early 1980s, very strict standards for donors regarding behavioral risk factors were set, and testing of donor blood was initiated. Since the institution of these standards, the risk of exposure to HIV through blood and blood product administration is negligible.

Vertical (Perinatal)

Perinatal transmission of HIV can occur in utero, during labor and delivery, or postpartum through breastfeeding. Transmission rates vary by maternal stage of disease, use of ART, duration of ruptured membranes, and breastfeeding (Thomas et al., 2015).

Occupational

Occupational transmission of HIV to nurse practitioners and other health care providers is extremely rare. Direct inoculation of HIV via needle-stick injury imposes a risk

TABLE 31.2	Myths and Facts About HIV Transmission
MYTH	**FACT**
HIV is transmitted through casual contact.	HIV is not transmitted through everyday, casual contact, including shaking hands and sharing eating utensils, even when living in close contact.
HIV is transmitted through insect bites.	There is no evidence of HIV transmission through bloodsucking or biting insects, including mosquitoes, flies, ticks, and fleas.
Donating or receiving blood is risky in the United States.	There are numerous safeguards to the U.S. blood supply, including only allowing persons with clean bills of health to donate, drawing blood with sterilized needles, and performing nine screening tests on all donated blood that ensure a safe blood supply.
Pets and other animals can carry HIV and transmit the virus to people.	Humans are the only animal that can harbor HIV. Some animals do carry similar viruses that can cause immune disease in their species; however, these cannot be transmitted to humans.
HIV can be transmitted through tears, sweat, and saliva.	Saliva, sweat, tears, and urine either carry no HIV or contain quantities too small to result in infection.

Sources: Derose et al. (2016), Mwamwenda (2016).

of infection of 0.3% (3 in 1,000) to the health care worker (Thomas et al., 2015). Casual contact with patients, even those known to be HIV positive, has not been determined to increase one's risk of acquiring HIV. Nurse practitioners can care for patients who are HIV positive with the knowledge that their risk of contracting HIV is limited to those contacts identified as being sources of transmission. Nurse practitioners need not be afraid to touch HIV-positive patients in the course of providing routine care. The use of standard precautions in caring for all patients minimizes the risk of exposure and infection by HIV and other serious illnesses (Table 31.3).

TABLE 31.3	Standard Precautions for HIV Prevention
Hand washing	1. Wash hands after touching blood, body fluids, secretions, excretions, and contaminated items, even if gloves are worn. Wash hands immediately after gloves are removed, between patient contacts, and when otherwise indicated to avoid transfer of microorganisms to other patients or environments. It may be necessary to wash hands between tasks and procedures on the same patient to prevent cross-contamination of different body sites. 2. Use a plain (nonantimicrobial) soap for routine hand washing. 3. Use an antimicrobial agent or a waterless antiseptic agent for specific circumstances (e.g., control of outbreaks or hyperendemic infections), as defined by the infection control program.
Gloves	Wear gloves (clean, nonsterile gloves are adequate) when touching blood, body fluids, secretions, excretions, and contaminated items. Put on clean gloves just before touching mucous membranes and nonintact skin. Change gloves between tasks and procedures on the same patient after contact with material that may contain a high concentration of microorganisms. Remove gloves promptly after use, before touching noncontaminated items and environmental surfaces, and before going to another patient, and wash hands immediately to avoid transfer of microorganisms to other patients or environments.
Mask, eye protection, face shield	Wear a mask and eye protection or a face shield to protect mucous membranes of the eyes, nose, and mouth during procedures and patient care activities that are likely to generate splashes or sprays of blood, body fluids, secretions, and excretions.
Gown	Wear a gown (a clean, nonsterile gown is adequate) to protect skin and to prevent soiling of clothing during procedures and patient care activities that are likely to generate splashes or sprays of blood, body fluids, secretions, or excretions. Select a gown that is appropriate for the activity and amount of fluid likely to be encountered. Remove a soiled gown as promptly as possible, and wash hands to avoid transfer of microorganisms to other patients or environments.
Patient care equipment	Handle used patient care equipment soiled with blood, body fluids, secretions, and excretions in a manner that prevents skin and mucous membrane exposures, contamination of clothing, and transfer of microorganisms to other patients and environments. Ensure that reusable equipment is not used for the care of another patient until it has been cleaned and reprocessed appropriately. Ensure that single-use items are discarded properly.
Environmental control	Ensure that the hospital has adequate procedures for the routine care, cleaning, and disinfection of environmental surfaces, beds, bedrails, bedside equipment, and other frequently touched surfaces, and ensure that these procedures are being followed.
Linens	Handle, transport, and process used linens soiled with blood, body fluids, secretions, and excretions in a manner that prevents skin and mucous membrane exposures and contamination of clothing and that avoids transfer of microorganisms to other patients and environments.
Occupational health and blood-borne pathogens	1. Take care to prevent injuries when using needles, scalpels, and other sharp instruments or devices; when handling sharp instruments after procedures; when cleaning used instruments; and when disposing of used needles. Never recap used needles or otherwise manipulate them using both hands or use any other technique that involves directing the point of a needle toward any part of the body; rather, use either a one-handed "scoop" technique or a mechanical device designed for holding the needle sheath. Do not remove used needles from disposable syringes by hand, and do not bend, break, or otherwise manipulate used needles by hand. Place used disposable syringes and needles, scalpel blades, and other sharp items in appropriate puncture-resistant containers, which are located as close as practical to the area in which the items were used, and place reusable syringes and needles in a puncture-resistant container for transport to the reprocessing area. 2. Use mouthpieces, resuscitation bags, or other ventilation devices as an alternative to mouth-to-mouth resuscitation methods in areas where the need for resuscitation is predictable.
Patient placement	Place a patient who contaminates the environment or who does not (or cannot be expected to) assist in maintaining appropriate hygiene or environmental control in a private room. If a private room is not available, consult with infection control professionals regarding patient placement or other alternatives.

Source: Centers for Disease Control and Prevention (2015c).

■ FACTORS FACILITATING TRANSMISSION

Transmission of HIV infection can be influenced by several factors, including characteristics of the infected host and the recipient, as well as the amount and infectivity of the virus itself.

Standard precautions synthesize the major features of blood and body fluid precautions (designed to reduce the risk of transmission of blood-borne pathogens) and body substance isolation (BSI; designed to reduce the risk of transmission of pathogens from moist body substances) and applies them to all patients receiving care in hospitals, regardless of their diagnosis or presumed infection status. Standard precautions apply to (a) blood; (b) all body fluids, secretions, and excretions except sweat, regardless of whether they contain visible blood; (c) nonintact skin; and (d) mucous membranes. Standard precautions are designed to reduce the risk of transmission of microorganisms from both recognized and unrecognized sources of infection in hospitals. Use standard precautions, or the equivalent, for the care of all patients.

Infectivity of the Host

There is an association between the amount of virus transmitted and the risk of HIV infection. Transmission is more likely to occur when viral replication is high during the initial stage of infection and in the advanced stages of HIV disease. Individuals with high blood viral loads are more likely to transmit HIV to their sexual partners, persons with whom they share drug paraphernalia, and their offspring. Furthermore, viral load has been found to be the chief predictor of heterosexual transmission risk of HIV-1 (Herbeck et al., 2016). Factors that decrease viral load, such as ART, may decease but not eliminate the risk of HIV transmission. Factors that increase the risk of exposure to blood, such as genital ulcer disease, sexual trauma, and menstruation of an HIV-infected woman during sexual contact, may increase transmission risk (Herbeck et al., 2016; Toren, Buskin, Dombrowski, Cassels, & Golden, 2016).

Factors that decrease viral load, including ART, may decrease but not eliminate the risk of transmission. Persons receiving ART have shown reduced HIV transmission rates to sexual partners, with studies demonstrating reduced HIV concentration in semen and vaginal secretion (Thomas et al., 2015).

Vasectomy in men does not significantly affect HIV concentration in seminal secretion (Rieg, 2006). Although circumcised men have a lower risk of acquiring HIV than do those who are uncircumcised, circumcision does not appear to decrease risk of transmission to a woman and may increase the risk if sexual activity is resumed before the circumcision wound is completely healed.

Susceptibility of Women

Women are biologically more vulnerable to HIV infection than men for several reasons. Sexual transmission of HIV is two to four times more efficient from male to female than from female to male (Thomas et al., 2015) because HIV in semen is in higher concentrations than in cervical and vaginal infections and because the vaginal area has a much larger mucosal area of exposure to HIV than does the penis. Certain characteristics of an uninfected woman may increase her likelihood of infection. Age and female anatomy are directly related to HIV transmission risk. Younger women have increased exposure of vaginal and cervical columnar epithelium, known to be a risk factor in the transmission of other sexually transmitted diseases (STDs). Pregnant women also have an increased exposure of columnar epithelium. This tissue is associated with endocervical inflammatory cells and can bleed more easily during intercourse. Normal vaginal flora may confer nonspecific immunity, and data suggest that women with bacterial vaginosis are at increased risk for HIV seroconversion (Thomas et al., 2015). Both younger and postmenopausal women may be at greater risk for acquiring HIV because of a thinner vaginal epithelium, resulting in increased friability and risk of trauma during intercourse, thus providing direct access to the bloodstream (AIDS info, 2015b; CDC, 2015c).

The integrity of the tissues of the female lower genital tract also influences HIV transmission risk. Trauma during intercourse, STD-related inflammation or cervicitis, cervical dysplasia, and an STD ulcer or chancre increase susceptibility to HIV infection. Any activity or condition that disrupts the tissues of the vagina may predispose a woman to infection with HIV. This includes the use of highly absorbent tampons, which are associated with vaginal desquamation with long-term use. Furthermore, higher rates of HIV transmission should be expected in sexual assault cases when trauma to the genital area occurs. Cases of domestic violence and sexual abuse also have been identified as important correlates of HIV in women (Chakraborty, 2016).

Sexual activity during menstruation may increase a woman's risk of acquiring HIV (CDC, 2016). Similarly, the disruption of tissues through receptive penile–anal intercourse provides a highly efficient means of HIV transmission. Some contraceptive methods (i.e., barrier methods) may decrease HIV transmission; however, others may afford no protection or increase the risk of transmission (AIDS info, 2015b). The effect of hormonal contraception on viral shedding is unclear, and these agents may interact with antibiotics and antiretrovirals (Phillips et al., 2015). Although some research findings suggest that oral contraceptive use increases the risk of cervical ectopy and thus the risk of infection, others do not find this to be the case after adjusting for behavioral risk factors (CDC, 2016). Use of the vaginal and rectal microbicide nonoxynol-9 provides no protection against HIV acquisition and may even increase susceptibility to infection because of mucosal barrier disruption, particularly with frequent use (Hatcher et al., 2011).

Douching, which can destroy the protective lactobacilli of the vagina, may increase a woman's susceptibility to bacterial vaginosis, STDs (gonorrhea, chlamydia, trichomonias), and HIV (Hatcher et al., 2011). Douching also dries out the vagina, traumatizes vaginal mucosa, and makes it more susceptible to tears. In addition, douching after sexual intercourse can push infectious agents further into the genital system, increasing the likelihood of infection. Douching is pointless and should be discouraged.

RISK FACTORS FOR HIV

Unlike many viruses that are easily transmitted through the air, water, food, and/or casual contact, HIV transmission usually requires risky behaviors. Common risky behaviors in women include vaginal, anal, and oral sex without a condom or vaginal barrier, concurrent partners, numerous lifetime partners, substance use or abuse, and a history of intimate partner violence. However, these behaviors do not occur in a vacuum, and biological, behavioral, psychological, demographic, and sociocultural factors all affect the likelihood and consequences of these behaviors (Thomas et al., 2015).

Cultural and religious attitudes and beliefs also affect health care services. The loss of support for safer sex education programs in favor of an abstinence-only model does not protect adolescents. Teens who pledge to remain a virgin until marriage have the same, if not higher, rates of STDs than those who do not commit to abstinence (Sathe, 2016). In response to these findings, a more pragmatic abstinence-plus or "ABC" message based on harm-reduction principles has been instituted. The message is Abstinence, Be Faithful for married couples or those in committed relationships, and use a Condom for individuals who are or put themselves at risk of HIV infection.

Biological Factors

Heterosexual transmission of HIV is 12 times more likely from men to women (Derose et al., 2016). A number of biological factors make HIV transmission easier or more difficult. These include the presence of STDs, tissue/ membrane vulnerability, viral load, and anatomical characteristics (see Susceptibility of Women section).

A person's biological sex (i.e., female, male) as well as the social roles associated with biological sex (gender) influence other risk factors of HIV/AIDS. For example, women are more likely to acquire HIV through heterosexual sexual activity than men because of their anatomy. Similar rates of exposure through heterosexual contact are seen in White (65%), Black (74%), and Hispanic (69%) women (Thomas et al., 2015). HIV can be transmitted through receptive oral sex with ejaculation. Any condition that interrupts the integrity of oral tissues, including periodontal disease, increases the risk of HIV transmission in this manner.

Demographic Characteristics

Demographic factors such as gender, ethnicity, and age shape HIV risk behaviors and influence social networks, making it more or less likely that an individual who engages in risky behaviors will associate with persons who are HIV positive.

In the United States, the majority of new AIDS cases, persons living with AIDS, and the majority of AIDS deaths are found among racial and ethnic minorities. Black/ African American and Hispanic/Latina women are disproportionately affected by HIV compared with women of other races/ethnicities (CDC, 2016). Furthermore, HIV-infected African Americans and Latinas are more likely than infected Whites to be uninsured, have less access to antiretroviral drugs, and lack access to health care (Thomas et al., 2015). Closely connected to ethnicity and race is socioeconomic status, one of the most powerful predictors of health and illness. Ethnicity may also be associated with certain contextual factors. Specific factors for African American women include the gender-ratio imbalance and historical and personal victimization.

Social Factors

Factors such as poverty, lack of education, social inequity, and inadequate access to health care indirectly increase the prevalence of HIV in at-risk populations. Persons with the highest rates of HIV are often those with the poorest access to health care, and health insurance coverage influences if and where a woman has access to care and whether she can afford antiretroviral medications. Furthermore, even if a poor woman perceives herself to be at risk of contracting HIV, she may not be able to practice protective behaviors if survival is an overarching concern or if there are other risks that appear to be more threatening or imminent. Survival concerns, such as secure shelter, food, safety for self and children, and money may override any concerns about protecting a woman's own health (Thomas et al., 2015).

Recognition of Risk

Beliefs and misconceptions about personal risk can increase an individual's risk of getting HIV infection. A woman who believes she has no risk factors for contacting an STD—including HIV—is unlikely to practice any risk-reducing behaviors. In addition, persons who believe they are not at risk of HIV infection are more apt to have risky behaviors. Younger women may be at higher risk because they have less knowledge of reproductive health, less skill in communicating and negotiating with their partners about risk-reduction practices, and more barriers to access to health care services. Taking risks is a universal human element. In the throes of passion, people can make unwise sexual decisions. Furthermore, safer sex is not always perceived to be the most enjoyable sex.

Personality Characteristics

Personality characteristics, such as low self-esteem, feelings of low self-efficacy, impulsivity, narcissism, tendency to take risks, and tendency to seek out new sensations are related to sexual risk behaviors. Furthermore, women with a sense of low self-efficacy and lack of self-confidence may be unable to negotiate safer sex practices. Coping strategies, such as high-risk sexual behaviors or drug and alcohol use to relieve or escape stress, can increase personal risk of HIV infection.

Social Interactions and Relationships

Because intimate human contact is a common vehicle of HIV transmission, sexual behavior in the context of relationships is a critical risk factor for preventing and acquiring HIV. Cultural and religious attitudes regarding appropriate sexual behaviors affect risk at the individual and community levels. Relationships and sexual behaviors are regulated by cultural norms that influence sexual expression in interpersonal relationships. Often women are still socialized to please their partners and to place men's needs and desires first; thus, they may find it difficult to insist on safer sex behaviors. Traditional cultural values associated with passivity and subordination may diminish the ability of many women to adequately protect themselves.

Power imbalances in relationships are the product of and contributors to the maintenance of traditional gender roles that identify men as the initiators of and decision makers about sexual activities and women as passive gatekeepers. As long as traditional gender norms define the roles for sexual relationships as men having the dominant role in sexual decision making, negotiating condom use by women will remain difficult. Additionally, cultural norms define talking about condoms as implying a lack of trust that runs counter to the traditional gender norm expectations for women (Maman, Campbell, Sweat, & Gielen, 2000). Women sometimes do not request condom use because of a need to establish and maintain intimacy with partners. Research has demonstrated that women at risk of HIV place significant importance on and investment in their heterosexual relationships and that these dynamics impact on the women's risk taking and risk management. Urging women to insist on condom use may be unrealistic, because traditional gender roles do not encourage women to talk about sex, initiate sexual practices, or control intimate encounters.

A woman who is dependent upon an abusive male partner or a partner who places her at risk by his own risky behaviors is at higher risk for contracting HIV than are women who are not dependent (Milrod, 2016; Chakraborty, 2016). The risk of acquiring HIV infection is high among women who are physically and sexually abused. Past and current experiences with violence—particularly sexual abuse—erode women's sense of self-efficacy to exercise control over sexual behaviors, engender feelings of anxiety and depression, and increase the likelihood of risky sexual behaviors (Chakraborty, 2016). Additionally, fear of physical harm and loss of economic support hamper women's efforts to enact protective practices. Furthermore, past and current abuse is strongly associated with substance abuse, which also increases the risk of contracting a sexually transmitted infection (STI).

The risk of acquiring an STI is determined not only by the woman's actions, but by her partner's as well. Although prevention counseling customarily includes recommending that women identify the partner who is at high risk

because of drugs and medical factors and also determine his sexual practices, this advice may be unrealistic and/or culturally inappropriate in many relationships. Women who engage in sexual activities with other women only may or may not be at risk of infection. Many women who identify themselves as lesbian have had intercourse with a man at one time by choice, by force, or by necessity or may have used drugs and shared drug paraphernalia such as needles.

Behavioral Risks

Any behavior that increases a woman's contact with bodily fluids of another person increases the likelihood of HIV transmission. During sexual activity, infected blood, semen, vaginal fluids, and anal fluids can enter the uninfected woman's body through cuts, tears, and lesions on the penis or labia and in or on the vagina or anus. Cuts and tears are more likely to occur during forced or rough sex, anal sex, dry sex, or when women are very young and their cervixes are not fully developed and thus more likely to rip or tear during sex (Sathe et al., 2016).

Substance Use

Drug and alcohol use is associated with increased risk of HIV (CDC, 2016). Sharing unclean drug paraphernalia—particularly needles and syringes—increases the risk of HIV transmission, particularly in areas where there is a high incidence of HIV infection among drug users. For example, in many areas, crack use parallels trends of HIV infection. Among several possible reasons for this association are social factors such as poverty and lack of educational and economic opportunities and individual factors such as risk taking and low self-efficacy. In addition to the risk from needle sharing, use of drugs and alcohol may contribute to the risk of HIV infection by undermining cognitive and social skills, thus making it more difficult to engage in HIV-protective actions. Furthermore, depression and other psychological problems and/or a history of sexual abuse are associated with substance abuse and thus contribute to risky behaviors. Being high and thus not able to clean drug paraphernalia can be a pervasive barrier to protective practice. Furthermore, drug use may take place in settings where persons participate in sexual activities while using drugs. Cocaine abusers have demonstrated higher levels of sexual risk behaviors than other addict populations. Finally, women who use drugs may be at higher risk because of the practice of exchanging sex for drugs or money and high numbers of sexual partners and encounters (Chakraborty et al., 2016; Klevens et al., 2016).

Past and current physical, emotional, and sexual abuse characterizes the lives of many, if not most, drug-using women (Chakraborty et al., 2016; Klevens et al., 2016). For women who have experienced violence, the use of alcohol and drugs can become a coping mechanism by which they self-medicate to relieve feelings of anxiety, depression, guilt, fear, and anger stemming from the violence. Women's drug use is strongly linked to relationship inequities and some men's ability to mandate women's sexual behavior. Sexual degradation of women is described as an intimate part of crack cocaine use.

PREVENTION

Primary prevention or preventing the transmission of HIV is the most effective way of reducing the adverse consequences of HIV/AIDS for women, their partners, and society. In addition, the diagnosis, counseling, and treatment of HIV/AIDS infection (secondary prevention) can prevent disease progression and complications for the individual and transmission to others. (Readers are referred to Chapter 30 for a discussion of primary prevention of STDs, including HIV.)

Pre-Exposure Prophylaxis for HIV Prevention

Given that some women may not have control over sexual health decisions, including primary prevention methods like condoms, there is a need for female-controlled methods. Although topical microbicides are an acceptable alternative, an efficacious product has not yet been found (Guest et al., 2010). When taken consistently for pre-exposure prophylaxis (PrEP), tenofovir–emtricitabine (Truvada) has been shown to reduce the risk of contracting HIV in 93% of high-risk individuals (CDC, 2016) and HIV-negative men and transgendered women who had sex with men (Grant et al., 2014). PrEP is recommended as one preventative option for adult heterosexually active men and women who are at substantial risk of contracting HIV. It is also recommended for adult injection drug users (IDU) at risk of HIV and heterosexually active women whose partners are known to have HIV. Currently, the efficacy and safety of PrEP for adolescents are insufficient. Before prescribing PrEP, acute and chronic infection with HIV must be excluded by patient history and HIV testing immediately. The only currently FDA-approved medication regimen for PrEP for heterosexual women and IDU is daily, continuing oral doses of TDF/FTC (Truvada). Additionally, women should have follow-up visits every 3 months to provide HIV testing, medication adherence counseling, behavioral risk-reduction support, and side-effect assessment. Additionally, women should be seen at 6 months and every 6 months thereafter to assess renal function and test for bacterial STDs (Smith et al., 2014).

There are significant secondary benefits associated with use of PrEP including frank discussion about sex and risk and increased attention to screening, prevention, and treatment of STDs (Grossman, 2015).

Types of HIV Tests

Beginning in 1985, HIV has been perhaps most associated with antibody testing, either for determination of serostatus or screening blood and tissue donations (Bennett, 2006).

TABLE 31.4	Indications for HIV Testing

- Physical symptoms consistent with HIV-related illness
- History of multiple sexual partners
- History of crack cocaine, cocaine, or methamphetamine use
- History of injection drug use
- History of sex with an HIV-positive person or one suspected to be HIV positive
- History of sex with an IV drug user
- History of a direct inoculation with HIV from an occupational exposure (e.g., operating room, emergency room)
- Social history that includes injection drug use or illicit drugs such as crack cocaine
- Pregnancy
- History of intimate partner violence
- Tattoos or body piercing

IV, intravenous.
Source: From basic information about HIV and AIDS, including information on the virus, its origins, symptoms, and testing. Retrieved from www.cdc.gov/hiv/default.html

HIV infection is diagnosed by serologic tests to detect antibodies against HIV-1 and HIV-2 and by virologic tests that detect HIV antigens or RNA. Available serological tests are highly sensitive and specific and can detect all known subtypes of HIV-1 (Thomas et al., 2015). Additionally, most can also detect HIV-2 and uncommon variants of HIV-1. Rapid HIV tests are available to allow clinicians to make a preliminary diagnosis of HIV infection in 30 minutes; however, they can produce negative results in recently infected individuals because they become reactive later than conventional laboratory-based serologic assays (Thomas et al., 2015). The specific recommendations for testing for HIV infection are found in Table 31.4.

The standard of practice for HIV diagnostic testing requires two tests on the same sample to be reactive for a person to be considered HIV positive. When an individual shows HIV antibodies on two or more serologic tests, an independent, highly specific supplemental test—commonly the HIV-1/HIV-2 antibody differentiation assay, Western blot test, or indirect immunofluorescent-antibody assay—is used (Thomas et al., 2015). The Western blot test is less sensitive than the enzyme-linked immunosorbent assay (ELISA) test, but rarely is there a false-positive result, and therefore it is used for confirming the ELISA test.

HIV Testing Guidelines

HIV testing is a serious matter with a number of social, ethical, and psychological implications, in addition to the obvious health care issues. Certain persons have histories or clinical indications that warrant HIV testing (Table 31.4). Counseling for risk factors will help health care providers determine the relative risk of a patient for HIV. Testing for HIV is recommended and should be offered to all women seeking evaluation for and treatment of STIs (Thomas et al., 2015).

The first guidelines for HIV testing were issued by the U.S. Public Health Service in 1987. In 1993, the CDC expanded the guidelines to include hospitalized patients and individuals receiving health care as outpatients in acute care settings. An important component of these guidelines was HIV counseling and testing as a priority prevention strategy for at-risk persons regardless of the health care setting. The CDC expanded current guidelines to recommended anonymous testing, which allowed persons to find out their status while minimizing their concern that their identities could be revealed.

The most recent recommendations for HIV testing in primary care settings were released in 2015 (Thomas et al., 2015). Specific recommendations include the following:

- HIV screening is recommended for all persons seeking evaluation or treatment for STDs. Testing should be done at the time of an STD diagnosis in populations at high risk of HIV infections.
- HIV testing must be voluntary and free from coercion. Persons should not be tested without their knowledge.
- Opt-out HIV screening (notifying the individual that the HIV test will be performed, unless she declines) is recommended in all health care settings.
- Specific signed consent for HIV testing should not be required. General informed consent for medical care is considered sufficient to encompass informed consent for HIV testing.
- Use of antigen/antibody combination tests are encouraged unless persons are unlikely to receive their results.
- Preliminary positive-screening tests for HIV infection must be followed with additional testing to definitively establish the diagnosis.
- Providers should be alert to the possibility of acute infection and perform antigen/antibody immunoassay or HIV RNA in conjunction with an antibody test.
- Persons suspected of recently acquired HIV infection should be immediately referred to an HIV clinical care provider.

Although a negative antibody test usually indicates that a person is not infected, these tests cannot exclude a recent infection. A patient with a negative test who is at very high risk of contracting the virus should be retested 3 to 6 months after the initial baseline test. A person with a specific exposure to HIV—for example, in an occupational setting or via unprotected sexual contact with a person known to have HIV—should be tested serially: first, at the time of the exposure to determine the baseline serologic status, and then at 3- and 6-month intervals until seroconversion is determined or the person remains seronegative for 1 year.

HIV Counseling

Researchers found that interactive client-centered counseling can reduce risk behaviors and the incidence of new STDs (Thomas et al., 2015) The impact of counseling and testing

is likely to be greatest for HIV-positive individuals, because the information gained could be used to avoid transmitting HIV to others (Thomas et al., 2015). Although prevention counseling is desirable for all persons at risk of HIV, it is recognized that counseling may not be feasible in all settings.

Although prevention counseling is no longer required as a part of the HIV screening programs in health care settings, it is strongly encouraged for all persons at high risk of HIV. It is also recommended that easily understood informational materials should be available in the languages of the persons using the health care services.

State laws vary regarding disclosure of a positive diagnosis for HIV to persons other than the patient, such as spouses or sexual contacts. Health care providers must be aware of the regulations governing their practice and should inform the patient of these regulations before testing, so that the patient can be fully informed as to the social and legal implications of a positive test. For many women, partner notification may make her vulnerable to abuse and violence in the event she is HIV positive.

Table 31.5 lists the issues that should be addressed in counseling a patient seeking HIV testing. All women seeking HIV testing should also be tested for hepatitis B. The posttest visit can be stressful for the patient, regardless of the results; therefore, test results should be disclosed as soon as possible in the visit, because the patient may be very anxious regarding the outcome. If the results are positive for HIV, the woman must be given time to accept the message and to react emotionally as needed. She must assimilate a lot of information at the time of this visit. Allowing her to express her feelings before discussing issues related to partner notification, treatments, and other issues may help her to take in some of the important information that must be conveyed at this time.

Seropositive patients must understand that, although they may exhibit no signs or symptoms of HIV disease, they are still infectious and will be for life. Basic information regarding minimizing transmission risk must be relayed to the patient at this time. A specific goal is to minimize the risk of transmission of the virus to others; therefore, the woman needs to understand immediately the implications of her HIV seropositivity in terms of transmission risk. Furthermore, advanced practice

TABLE 31.5	HIV-Test Counseling

- Explain the meaning and implications of negative and positive test results and the meaning of indeterminate results
- Discuss HIV risk reduction, including behaviors specific to the woman being tested
- Inform the woman of state-mandated reporting requirements
- If relevant, explain anonymous versus confidential testing
- Determine the woman's support system and coping and stress management strategies that may be enlisted based on test results
- Arrange for a return visit to discuss test results

Sources: Centers for Disease Control and Prevention (2001), Fogel and Black (2008a).

nurse practitioners must assess the newly diagnosed HIV-positive patient's need for further psychological and emotional supportive services.

TREATMENT PLANNING

A plan for treatment must be established. Often this requires a referral to an infectious disease health care setting that can provide expert care for the infection. Unless the patient is clearly immunocompromised and needs immediate treatment for an opportunistic infection, there is likely to be an interval between diagnosis and treatment decisions. This time can be used by the woman to begin to emotionally and psychologically integrate her diagnosis. She will need to make decisions regarding who must be told about her infection and begin to integrate behaviors that are required to minimize her risk of transmitting the virus to others.

The impact of HIV on future childbearing is an important consideration in counseling women with HIV. Many women are diagnosed with HIV during pregnancy. They must be given adequate information regarding vertical transmission and treatment during pregnancy in order to make informed decisions regarding their pregnancy. Many HIV-positive women are diagnosed during their childbearing years. Making the decision to become pregnant or to forego future childbearing should be made only when the woman is fully informed regarding HIV and pregnancy. The risk for perinatal transmission of HIV can be reduced with the use of antiretroviral treatment. Without treatment the risk of transmitting HIV to a neonate is approximately 30%, but can be reduced to less than 2% with antiretroviral treatment and obstetrical intervention, including cesarean section at 38 weeks gestation and not breastfeeding (Panel on Treatment of HIV-Infected Pregnant Women and Prevention of Perinatal Transmission, 2012). Pregnant women with HIV infection should be linked to care with an HIV care provider and be given appropriate prenatal and postpartum treatment and advice (Thomas et al., 2015). A women can choose to become pregnant with a relatively small risk of vertical transmission of the virus to the fetus; however, the possibility of a shortened life expectancy because of her HIV may shape a woman's decision to forego any further childbearing. This is an emotional and personal decision that will require ongoing support.

Unfortunately, many women are diagnosed later after infection than are men and may have more advanced HIV disease at the time of diagnosis. Furthermore, because HIV-positive women are more likely to be African American or Hispanic, they may have diminished economic resources and social support available to them. A comprehensive plan of care that takes into consideration the multiplicity of stressors that HIV-positive women experience has a greater chance at making a healthy impact on their lives.

A patient who is seronegative for HIV should receive counseling and education regarding behavior changes to reduce the risk of contracting HIV. The news that one is negative for HIV will be met with relief and an immediate reduction of anxiety. However, it is essential that all women who are tested for HIV based on risky behaviors be counseled regarding the need to be retested at 3 and 6 months given the delay in seroconversion after infection. Women who engage in very high-risk behaviors should be counseled to be tested serially. This is to prevent the ongoing assumption that the woman is seronegative for HIV, when in fact she may have been tested between the time of infection and the development of antibodies.

■ TREATMENT OF HIV/AIDS IN WOMEN

Women infected with HIV manifest a more heterogeneous viral population than do men, which may result in a more diverse immune response (Baril et al., 2016; CDC, 2016). Because women tend to progress to AIDS with viral loads that are significantly lower than men, decisions about beginning ART should be primarily based on CD4 counts rather than viral load (Baril et al., 2016; CDC, 2016).

Women with undiagnosed HIV often seek care for a gynecologic infection or condition. One of the most common symptoms of HIV infection in women is recurrent vaginal candidiasis. HIV-infected women are also more likely than uninfected women to have abnormal cervical cytology (40%), human papillomavirus infection (58%), more severe pelvic inflammatory disease, and bacterial vaginosis (Nyitray et al., 2016). In addition, HIV-infected women have higher incidences of toxoplasmosis, herpes, genital ulcerations, and esophageal candidiasis (CDC, 2016). The care of HIV-positive persons should be supervised by an expert in infectious disease (Thomas et al., 2015). Furthermore, current recommendations emphasize using laboratory monitoring of plasma levels of HIV-1 RNA (viral load) to direct practitioners in instituting, assessing, and changing ART.

Individuals with a new diagnosis of HIV infection should be informed about (a) the importance of promptly beginning medical care for their health and to reduce further transmission of HIV, and (b) the effectiveness of HIV treatments and what to expect when they begin health care of HIV infection (Thomas et al., 2015). All women newly diagnosed with HIV should undergo an extensive medical history review, physical examination, and laboratory evaluation. The medical history (Tables 31.6 and 31.7) should include inquiries related to sexual behaviors, STDs, and chronic illnesses unrelated to but affected by HIV and its treatments, such as heart disease and diabetes mellitus. The history also should include inquiries about illnesses and conditions associated with immunosuppression, such as tuberculosis, herpes zoster, and genitorectal herpes; acute and chronic skin disorders such as fungal infections and molluscum contagiosum; severe and repeated episodes of vaginal candidiasis; diarrhea associated with various fungi or bacteria; and frequent bouts of pneumonia and sinusitis (Thomas et al., 2015). The presence or frequency of these infections not typically found in persons with normal immunological status may help pinpoint the time of infection. In addition, women with HIV should be asked about their gynecologic and obstetrical history, including birth-control method and plans for future childbearing.

TABLE 31.6	Medical History for HIV-Positive Women
TOPIC	**SPECIFIC POINTS TO ADDRESS**
HIV diagnosis	When were you first tested? Why were you tested?
HIV treatment history	Pretherapy CD4 count, viral load Specific antiretroviral treatment history
STI and other infection history	Syphilis; gonorrhea; herpes simplex; pelvic inflammatory disease; anogenital warts; tuberculosis; hepatitis A, B, or C; prior vaccinations; history of chicken pox or shingles
Obstetrical and gynecologic history	Pregnancies and their resolution, menstrual disorders, anovulation, perimenopause, uterine fibroids or polyps, abnormal vaginal discharge, cancer, genital tract infections
Other medical diagnoses	Hypertension, type 2 diabetes mellitus, cardiovascular disease, premalignant or malignant conditions, thyroid disease
Sexual practices	Condoms use; other birth-control methods; number of current partners; sexual activity with men, women, or both; history of trading sex for drugs or money; history of anal sex
HIV-associated signs and symptoms	See Table 31.7; bacterial pneumonia, thrush, severe headache, midline substernal discomfort with swallowing, visual changes including flutters or visual field deficits
Mental health history	Past and current problems, evidence of depression (change in appetite, trouble sleeping, loss of interest in usual activities, anhedonia)
Family history	Age and health of children, including HIV tests if done; HIV in other family members; hypertension; type 2 diabetes; cardiovascular disease; malignancy
Medications	Prescription and over the counter; history of and attitude toward regular medication use; use of complementary and alternative therapies; drug allergies
Social history	Place of birth, where raised, who lived with, child care responsibilities, history of interpersonal violence, education and occupational history, travel history, substance use or abuse, illicit drug use
Sources of support	Who has the woman told of her diagnosis, and what were their reactions? Does she have friends and family members she can talk to? Does she have a job? Does she have health insurance?

STI, sexually transmitted infection.
Source: Department of Health and Human Services Panel on Antiretroviral Guidelines for Adults and Adolescents (2006).

The physical examination for patients with HIV should be very thorough (Table 31.8). Vital signs should be carefully monitored, especially temperature and weight. The wide-scale and subtle effects of HIV on various body systems requires careful examination, especially of the mouth, eyes, skin, lungs, heart, lymph nodes, abdomen, genitalia, rectum, and nervous system. HIV may cause subtle or obvious changes in each of these systems. Clinical abnormalities in these systems will give the practitioner evidence of the level of immune system compromise in the patient with HIV. In addition, certain laboratory tests (Table 31.9) should be included in the initial examination of the HIV-positive woman. In addition, all patients should be tested for tuberculosis initially and annually thereafter (AIDS info, 2016; Thomas et al., 2015).

General clinical findings in HIV-positive women are similar to those found in men, with the exception of a high frequency of reproductive tract disorders, including cervical dysplasia and refractory vaginal candidiasis (Thomas et al., 2015). Women with HIV should have an initial Pap smear to test for the presence of cervical dysplasia and at least yearly thereafter. Some women will require Pap smears more frequently based on initial findings and gynecological history. For women with cervical dysplasia, referral may be made for follow-up with a gynecologist for colposcopy and treatment.

The management of lower genital tract neoplasia represents a specific treatment issue in the care of women with HIV. Women with HIV are at risk of developing lower genital tract neoplasia, particularly as the HIV disease progresses and the woman becomes increasingly immunocompromised. Cervical intraepithelial neoplasia and invasive cervical cancer can be persistent and progressive and difficult to manage effectively in women with HIV. Women with these conditions should be referred to a gynecologist for management.

Appropriate vaccinations will be offered based on patient history and lab findings. Common vaccinations include yearly influenza immunizations, pneumonia immunizations, and the hepatitis A and hepatitis B series, as indicated.

TABLE 31.7	Signs and Symptoms of HIV
General observation	■ Extreme fatigue ■ Rapid weight loss ■ Anorexia ■ Frequent low-grade fevers and night sweats ■ Frequent yeast infections (in the mouth) ■ Vaginal yeast infections and other STDs
Skin	■ Rashes ■ Red, brown, or purplish blotches on/under skin or inside the mouth, nose, or eyelids ■ Generalized drying ■ Pruritus
Lymphatics	■ Localized or generalized lymph node involvement ■ Lymphadenopathy
Head, eyes, ears, nose, and throat	■ Headaches ■ Nasal discharge ■ Sinus congestion ■ Changes in visual acuity ■ Sore throat ■ Whitish or painful lesions of the oral mucosa
Cardiopulmonary	■ Cough ■ Shortness of breath
Gastrointestinal	■ Abdominal pain ■ Change in bowel habits ■ Persistent diarrhea
Musculoskeletal	■ Myalgias ■ Arthralgia
Neurological/ psychological	■ Depression ■ Personality change ■ Cognitive difficulties ■ Bowel or bladder dysfunction ■ Peripheral weakness ■ Parenthesis
Pain	■ Pain that is not musculoskeletal

STDs, sexually transmitted diseases.
Source: Department of Health and Human Services Panel on Antiretroviral Guidelines for Adults and Adolescents (2006).

TABLE 31.8	Physical Examination of Patients With HIV
General	■ Evidence of wasting ■ Fat distribution syndromes: buffalo hump, enlarged breasts, truncal obesity, subcutaneous fat loss in extremities, face, buttocks
Eyes	■ Purplish spots of Kaposi's sarcoma in conjunctiva ■ Petechiae ■ Hemorrhages caused by cytomegalovirus retinitis
Oropharynx	■ Thrush ■ Oral hairy leukoplakia ■ Purplish spots or plaques on mucosal surfaces
Lymph nodes	■ Nontender or minimally tender generalized adenopathy, which may indicate HIV infection or lymphoma
Lungs	■ Fine, dry "cellophane" rales, diagnostic for *Pneumocystis carinii* pneumonia
Hepatosplenomegaly	■ Sign of disseminated infection with *Mycobacterium avium* complex, tuberculosis, histoplasmosis, or lymphoma
Pelvic	■ External genitalia: sores or ulcers indicative of herpes simplex or syphilis ■ Condyloma acuminata ■ Abnormal vaginal discharge from vaginitis or cervicitis ■ Cervical motion and uterine and adnexal tenderness suggestive of pelvic inflammatory disease
Neurologic	■ Motor deficits ■ Peripheral neuropathy, including symmetrical distal sensory deficits, more often of feet ■ AIDS dementia complex: poor short-term memory, diminished concentration, sensorimotor retardation
Skin	■ Early manifestations: pruritic papular eruptions, bacterial folliculitis, scabies ■ Molluscum contagiosum ■ Shingles ■ Seborrheic dermatitis ■ Psoriasis ■ Kaposi's sarcoma

Source: Department of Health and Human Services Panel on Antiretroviral Guidelines for Adults and Adolescents (2006).

Based on the patient's history and physical and the laboratory findings, the health care team will devise a plan of follow-up care. Decisions related to the initiation of ART, chemoprophylaxis against opportunistic infections, and follow-up evaluation may be deferred until all test results are received if the patient appears to be generally healthy at the time of the initial examination. Patients who are obviously immunocompromised with signs and symptoms of AIDS-related illness or opportunistic infection at the time of initial evaluation may be treated presumptively, with further

refinements and changes in treatments possible at the time all laboratory data are reviewed.

Two specific lab values that shape treatment decisions in persons with HIV are the viral load (HIV-1 RNA) and the CD4+ count. With increasing emphasis in HIV care on maintaining viral load levels at an undetectable level, these

TABLE 31.9	Baseline HIV Lab Tests
Serology	■ Confirm HIV diagnosis ■ CD4 count, lymphocyte count ■ Viral load ■ Complete blood count, including white blood cell count differential ■ Chemistry panel, including liver and renal function ■ Lipid profile ■ Syphilis, toxoplasmosis, cytomegalovirus, varicella-zoster virus if no history of chicken pox or shingles ■ Hepatitis A, B, C
Cultures	■ Urinalysis ■ Pap smear ■ Chlamydia culture ■ Gonorrhea culture ■ Cervical human papillomavirus assay
Other	■ Chest x-ray ■ Purified protein derivative

Source: Department of Health and Human Services Panel on Antiretroviral Guidelines for Adults and Adolescents (2006).

TABLE 31.10	Benefits and Risks of ART
Benefits	■ Control of viral replication and reduction of viral load ■ Prevention of progressive immunosuppression by control of viral load ■ Delayed progression of clinical disease and progression to AIDS ■ Prolonged life ■ Decreased risk of resistant virus ■ Decreased risk of drug toxicity ■ Possible decreased risk of viral transmission
Risks	■ Reduction of quality of life from adverse drug effects, including headaches, occasional dizziness, and more serious ones such as swelling of the mouth and tongue or liver damage ■ Drug interactions with other HIV medicines and other medications ■ Limitations of future options for therapy if drug resistance develops in current agents ■ Potential for transmission of drug-resistant virus ■ Limitation of future drug choices because of the development of resistance ■ Potential long-term toxicity of therapy ■ Unknown duration of effectiveness of current therapies

ART, antiretroviral therapy.
Sources: AIDS info (2016), Department of Health and Human Services Panel on Antiretroviral Guidelines for Adults and Adolescents (2006), Fogel and Black (2008).

lab values are important in ascertaining appropriate ART and adherence to the medication regimen. The CD4 count is an important tool in assessing the overall status of the immune system. Also known as helper T-cells, CD4 cells signal other immune system cells to fight infection. Depletion of these cells is the hallmark of advancing HIV disease.

Antiretroviral Therapy

ART is the use of HIV medications to treat HIV infection. Effective ART involves using a combination of medications that slow viral replication. The goals of ART are (a) to improve the patient's quality of life; (b) to reduce HIV-related morbidity and mortality; (c) maximal, durable suppression of viral load; and (d) restoration and/or preservation of immunologic function (AIDS info, 2016). ART is likely to involve complex dosage schedules and uncomfortable side effects.

Specific characteristics of HIV infection have important implications for ART (AIDS info, 2016):

■ Between initial diagnosis and development of clinical disease, there is progressive immunosuppression evidenced by the decline in CD4 counts.
■ Viral replication is extremely rapid; the half-life of HIV in plasma is less than 48 hours and a turnover of up to 1 billion viruses per day.
■ HIV has a high capacity for genetic mutability, and thus resistance to ART can occur rapidly.

There is a rationale for beginning ART before symptom onset to prevent immunosuppression. Further therapy must be continuous to prevent viral replication. Benefits and risks exist in initiating ART in treatment-naïve, asymptomatic patients (see Table 31.10) that must be considered before the initiation of ART. The risks and benefits of treatment of asymptomatic patients must be weighed carefully on a case-by-case basis to determine the appropriate course for any particular patient. The decision to initiate treatment in an asymptomatic patient must balance several competing factors that influence risk and benefit.

Asymptomatic patients considering the initiation of ART must receive thorough education and counsel regarding this decision. Patients must be fully informed and willing to initiate therapy. Although this seems to be an obvious consideration in any therapeutic regimen, it is of particular importance in initiating ART. The patient must be reasonably likely to adhere to her regimen as prescribed, although no patient should automatically have ART withheld based on behaviors that some may assume are associated with a likelihood of nonadherence (CDC, 2016). Thorough patient education and counsel and ongoing follow-up counsel and support increase the likelihood of effective adherence to ART.

It is important that individuals infected with HIV start ART as soon as possible (AIDS info, 2016). Persons with the following conditions should start ART immediately: pregnancy, AIDS, HIV-related illnesses and coinfections, and early HIV infection (the first 6 months after infection). All patients who show signs of HIV disease progression should be offered ART. These signs can include thrush,

TABLE 31.11	AIDS-Defining Criteria

- CD4+ count below 200 cells/mm³
- Candidiasis, esophageal, tracheal, bronchi, or lungs
- Cervical cancer, invasive
- Coccidioidomycosis, disseminated or extrapulmonary
- Cryptococcosis, extrapulmonary
- Cryptosporidiosis with diarrhea for more than 1 month
- Cytomegalovirus of any organ other than liver, spleen, or lymph nodes
- HIV encephalopathy
- Herpes simplex infection: chronic ulcers of more than 1 month's duration; or bronchitis, pneumonitis, or esophagitis
- Histoplasmosis, disseminated or extrapulmonary
- Isosporiasis with diarrhea for more than 1 month
- Kaposi's sarcoma
- Lymphoma, Burkitt's, immunologic, primary central nervous system
- *Mycobacterium avium* complex or *Mycobacterium kansasii*, disseminated
- Mycobacterium, other or unidentified species, disseminated or extrapulmonary
- *Pneumocystis carinii* pneumonia
- Pneumonia, recurrent bacterial with more than two episodes in 12 months
- Progressive multifocal leukoencephalopathy
- Salmonella septicemia
- Toxoplasmosis of internal organ or brain
- Wasting syndrome caused by HIV

Source: Department of Health and Human Services Panel on Antiretroviral Guidelines for Adults and Adolescents (2006).

wasting, unexplained fever for more than 2 weeks, and symptoms of opportunistic infection. Any patient with AIDS-defining criteria (Table 31.11) should be offered ART. Patients who present with advanced HIV disease or AIDS can recover some degree of immune function after the initiation of ART. Patients with opportunistic infection must have it treated before or at the same time as the initiation of ART. Doing so, however, raises the issue of drug tolerance, interactions, and toxicities, in addition to the issues surrounding the complexities of scheduling multiple medications.

Specific ARTs

The development of effective ART represents one of the biggest scientific challenges in controlling and eventually eradicating HIV. A caveat is necessary before discussing ART in the treatment of HIV infection: The research and development of new therapies and the testing of different combinations of therapies can quickly change the state of the science. Advanced practice nurse practitioners are encouraged to use reliable sources (e.g., the CDC and the National Institutes of Health) available on the Internet for the most current recommendations and practices in HIV care.

Highly active antiretroviral therapy (HAART) consists of three or more antiretroviral agents used in combination

to try to decrease an individual's plasma viral load to an undetectable level. Issues to be considered when choosing an antiretroviral regimen include (a) the patient's daily routines and social support as they influence her ability to adhere to a particular regimen; (b) the side effects of the medications, including evaluation of the patient's other medical conditions that may increase the risk of certain adverse effects; and (c) any drug interactions with other medications the woman may be taking (Beal & Orrick, 2006a). Currently, four classes of antiretroviral medications are available: nucleoside reverse transcriptase inhibitors (NRTIs), non-nucleoside reverse transcriptase inhibitors (NNRTIs; e.g., efavirenz, delavirdine, and nevirapine), protease inhibitors (PIs; e.g., atazanavit, darunavir, nelfinar), and fusion inhibitors (enfuvirtide; AIDS info, 2016). NRTIs and NNRTIs work by disrupting the work of reverse transcriptase. Reverse transcriptase is an enzyme that changes the virus's chemical genetic message into a form that can be easily inserted inside the nucleus of an infected cell. This process occurs early in the viral replication cycle. Reverse transcriptase inhibitors interrupt the duplication of genetic material necessary for the virus to replicate. PIs are an important class of antiviral medications that are currently in the forefront of treatment options. Prescribed with reverse transcriptase inhibitors, they work inside infected cells late in the HIV-replication process. After HIV has infected a cell, it continues relentlessly to replicate itself. However, the newly produced genetic material, in the form of long chains of proteins and enzymes, is functional only after these long chains have been cut into shorter pieces by the HIV enzyme protease. By inhibiting the function of protease, PIs reduce the number of new infectious copies of HIV. Saquinavir, indinavir, and ritonavir are examples of PIs. Although ART medications have demonstrated a high level of effectiveness in reducing viral load in persons with HIV, they also have significant side effects that can adversely affect quality of life.

RTIs and PIs work together effectively to reduce the circulating viral load. With two different points of disruption of the replication cycle, concurrent use of these medications represents the best hope of managing HIV infection as a chronic illness. Regimens with the most experience in demonstrating serologic and immunologic efficacy are those composed of one NNRTI plus two NRTIs or one PI plus two NRTIs. The preferred NNRTI-based regimen (one NNRTI plus two NRTIs) is efavirenz (except during the first trimester of pregnancy or in women who are trying to conceive or who are not using effective, consistent contraception); the preferred alternative is nevirapine (Department of Health and Human Services [DHHS] Panel on Antiretoviral Guidelines for Adults and Adolescents, 2006).

Highly active ART is usually initiated in instances of failure of less potent ART, evidence of viral resistance, or in the case of serious immunocompromise requiring intense therapy and rapid viral reduction. HAART also may be initiated for treatment-naïve patients. Intense patient counseling to ensure maximal adherence to HAART is a crucial component of care for HIV-positive patients who are starting a HAART regimen in order to prevent early development of resistant virus and to maximize viral suppression.

Post-exposure prophylaxis (PEP) with ART is recommended for health care workers who have an occupational exposure to HIV through a needle-stick injury or cut with a contaminated object, contact of a mucous membrane or nonintact skin with potentially infectious material or body fluids, or prolonged exposure (several minutes or more) of intact skin to potentially infectious materials (Thomas et al., 2015). The basic regimen is used when there is an exposure with a recognized risk of HIV transmission. This regimen includes 28 days of zidovudine 600 mg daily in divided doses and lamivudine 150 mg twice a day. For HIV exposures that pose an increased risk of transmission, such as a larger volume of blood or exposure to blood with a high viral load, the basic PEP regimen is initiated, plus indinavir 800 mg every 8 hours or nelfinavir 750 mg three times a day.

Patients on ART may have other chronic conditions requiring medications and frequent monitoring of lab values. For any patient for whom ART is initiated, the interactions between HIV medications and other medications the patient takes regularly must be examined. Furthermore, scheduling of medications to minimize untoward interactions is a critical component of care for these patients.

Adherence to ART

Adherence to ART is crucial. The complexities of these regimens, however, can be very difficult to understand for some patients and very difficult to follow over time. A critical nursing challenge is to teach and counsel HIV-positive patients in adhering to the prescribed medication regimen. Failure to adhere to an ART protocol results in a rapid increase in viral load with concurrent immune system damage. The likelihood of developing AIDS is directly related to viral load. Simply, the presence of more virus means more immune system damage and a worsening ability to fend off aggressive opportunistic infections.

The development of ART-resistant strains of virus is a primary concern in treatment failure and represents a serious sequelea of nonadherence. Cross-resistance among treatment options limits the availability of effective therapy. Furthermore, the transmission of resistant strains complicates therapies for treatment-naïve patients, who may have few options available from the onset of the infection. Patients who fail to follow their ART regimen as prescribed face the risk of developing a resistant strain of virus. The danger of nonadherence is dual: First, an increased viral load with a resistant virus is an alarming clinical situation associated with a poor outcome for the patient. Second, additional treatments for opportunistic infections, with their concomitant side effects, will be necessary as symptoms of advancing disease manifest themselves.

Nurse practitioners have a distinct role in the preparation of patients as they begin ART. Effective nursing care must take into consideration the following issues related to the initiation of a treatment protocol that demands careful adherence:

■ *What is the patient's understanding of HIV?* Nurse practitioners in settings that see HIV patients regularly may take for granted that patients have a more thorough understanding of HIV than they really do. With much of the knowledge about HIV filtered through rumor, innuendo, and incomplete or misleading media reports, patients may be woefully lacking in substantive knowledge of their disease. Recent developments in ART have allowed the health care professional to understand HIV as a chronic and manageable disease; however, this understanding has not reached all segments of the general public. Emphasizing the chronic rather than fatal nature of the infection may help patients to reframe their understanding of the illness. Basic to the establishment of an effective nursing care plan is the thorough assessment of the patient's understanding of the disease, including its meaning to the patient.

■ *Can the patient understand how the medications are to be taken?* The patient may have a limited ability to understand the issues surrounding ART and adherence. It is incumbent on the nurse practitioner to ensure that the patient or the patient's caregiver understands the importance of taking the medications as ordered. The nurse practitioner may have to be creative in devising charts, journals, pill boxes, or other reminders for the patient and the caregiver to enhance the chances of successful adherence.

■ *What is the patient's daily schedule, and how does ART fit into the schedule?* The nurse practitioner must consider shift work, sleep–wake patterns, meal times, and family responsibilities in assisting the patient in establishing a medication schedule to which the patient can adhere. If is it clear that the patient is likely to fail in following a complex schedule of medications in the context of a busy and active life, the nurse should consult with the physician or nurse practitioner in identifying alternative medications that may be more suitable for the patient.

■ *Are there any social constraints on the patient related to taking ART?* ART represents the constant presence of HIV, an incurable infection that is fraught with social implications in addition to its health implications. Some persons find that the frequent reminder of the infection through taking ART is onerous and psychologically painful, lessening the likelihood of long-term adherence.

Many women keep their HIV infection a secret from their closest family members and friends. The presence of ART medications in the home increases the risk that someone will discover the patient's diagnosis. The patient must be counseled about that possibility and encouraged to think about the social implications if the HIV is discovered.

Beginning ART represents a small step in going public with the diagnosis. The patient must understand that the pharmacist filling the prescriptions will know the patient's diagnosis. The patient may prefer to have prescriptions filled in a place that is likely to offer more anonymity, such as a hospital pharmacy or a discount store pharmacy with a high volume of business. Finances may be an important consideration for the patient, who may have to seek outside sources of funds to enable the purchase of ART.

The goal for nurse practitioners is always the same: Patients will adhere to their ART schedules as evidenced by decreasing and ultimately nondetectable viral loads, maintaining that level for as long as possible. Simply handing a patient several prescriptions for expensive medications requiring complicated schedules and having a number of uncomfortable and potentially serious side effects is likely to result in treatment failure. Nurse practitioners are in a unique position to make a substantial positive impact on the lives of persons living with HIV by spending time in careful assessment, planning, intervening, and goal setting.

Prevention of Opportunistic Infections

In the 35 years since the identification of HIV/AIDS, great improvements have been made in the prevention of opportunistic infections that ravaged the earliest victims of the HIV pandemic. Increasingly, aggressive use of ART has helped in maintaining the immune systems of persons with HIV, reducing the need for routine chemoprophylaxis against opportunistic infections. Furthermore, infections such as PCP, toxoplasmosis, *Mycobacterium avium* complex disease, and other bacterial diseases have been effectively prevented in patients requiring chemoprophylaxis. A single daily dose of double-strength trimethoprim-sulfamethoxazole (Septra, Bactrim) has reduced the incidence of PCP, toxoplasmosis, and bacterial infections (Thomas et al., 2015). This is a particularly useful medication because it is effective, generally well tolerated, simple to take, and inexpensive. However, for those who are sensitive to or allergic to trimethoprim-sulfamethoxazole, dapsone is an effective alternative.

Persons with HIV should follow some specific, although not overly restrictive, guidelines regarding minimizing exposure to potential sources of opportunistic infection. For women who are likely to be managing the care of the home and children, understanding how to preserve and maintain her own health while fulfilling her household and parenting obligations is very important. Nurse practitioners should counsel women in basic good hygiene practices that can minimize the risk of many exposures. These practices include:

- Thorough hand washing with water and soap after toileting, after assisting children in toileting, and at intervals throughout the day. Paper towels in the bathroom provide a more sanitary means of drying hands than a hand towel that stays damp and may be used by others.
- Minimizing exposure to animal or human wastes by using disposable gloves. This includes wearing disposable gloves when doing yard work and when changing a baby's diaper.
- Drinking water only from sources known to be dependable and clean; avoiding ingestion of water from lakes, rivers, and recreational swimming pools.
- Avoiding contact with animals in specific circumstances:
  - pets younger than 6 months old (increased likelihood of exposure to parasites)
  - any animal with diarrhea
  - all reptiles: turtles, lizards, snakes, iguanas (risk of salmonella exposure)
  - situations that may expose the patient to bird droppings
- Treating cats with special care:
  - adopting cats that are more than 1 year old (risk of exposure to bacteria and parasites)
  - daily cleaning of litter box, preferably by a person without HIV
  - keeping the cat indoors, not allowing the cat to hunt
  - avoiding cat scratches or bites and washing scratches or bites thoroughly and immediately
  - controlling fleas on cats
- Avoiding raw or undercooked eggs, poultry, meat, or seafood, and preventing cross-contamination by using separate kitchen utensils and cutting boards when processing these foods. Cutting boards should be thoroughly scrubbed after each use. Careful kitchen and cooking practices can decrease greatly the risk of foodborne infection.

In addition, HIV-positive patients should be counseled to consult with a health care provider before traveling to developing countries that may result in exposure to opportunistic pathogens. The CDC website provides travelers with up-to-date information regarding endemic diseases and recommendations regarding vaccinations before travel.

Basic health practices, such as adequate sleep and rest, good nutrition, exercise, smoking cessation, and avoidance of stress should not be overlooked in counseling HIV-positive persons. Seven to eight hours of sleep a night is ideal for most adults. This amount may be difficult to achieve; however, nurse practitioners can assist the patient in developing a sleep schedule that allows adequate rest.

Principles of good nutrition apply to persons with HIV, and, in fact, are especially necessary to provide adequate vitamins, minerals, electrolytes, and protein. Persons with HIV who are significantly under- or overweight should be encouraged to improve their nutritional status through support groups, nutritional counseling, or other means of weight management. Persons with a high intake of alcohol should be counseled to decrease their intake, because alcohol does not have any significant nutritional value, can interfere with vitamin absorption, and contains excess calories. Furthermore, chronic alcohol abuse can exacerbate liver problems. It is important to note that excessive alcohol intake will impair one's ability to make good judgments regarding health and sexual behaviors and to adhere to the ART regimen.

Exercise improves muscle tone and cardiovascular health and reduces stress—all important factors in maintaining a state of health. HIV-positive persons should be encouraged to engage in some form of exercise on a regular basis. Nurse practitioners can assist the patient in identifying simple means of increasing activity, even if the patient is somewhat debilitated or reluctant to engage in regular workouts. Walking is a simple form of exercise that is within the abilities of most persons and can be incorporated into one's daily routine with little effort.

TABLE 31.12	Contraception for HIV-Infected Women	
METHOD	BENEFITS	DISADVANTAGES
Male condom	Protects against STIs and HIV; protects partner	Partner cooperation required
Female condom	Protects against STIs and HIV; protects partner	Partner cooperation helpful
Oral contraceptive	Effective when used consistently	Some HIV medications may reduce the effectiveness of hormonal contraceptives No HIV protection for partner No STI protection Risk of cervical ectopy Possible interaction with antibiotics and antiretrovirals
Depo-provera	Effective Limited compliance needed	No STI protection No HIV protection for partner
Intrauterine device	Effective	No HIV protection for partner No STI protection
Diaphragm	Effective Female controlled	Leave in 6–8 hours after ejaculation May increase risk of urinary tract infection
Patch	Avoids first-pass metabolism Easy to use	No STI protection No HIV protection for partner
Tubal ligation	One-time procedure Permanent	No STI protection No HIV protection for partner

STIs, sexually transmitted infections.
Sources: AIDS info (2016), Cotter, Potter, and Tessler (2006).

Patients should be encouraged and supported in their efforts to stop smoking. In addition to the well-documented negative effects of smoking on health, the propensity of HIV-positive persons to pulmonary infections makes smoking cessation imperative. Nurse practitioners should be cognizant of the difficulty of stopping smoking and support any efforts the patient makes to decrease the number of cigarettes per day. However, the nurse practitioner is also in an excellent position to help the patient find therapies, group support, and other means to stop smoking.

Stress reduction plays an important role in health maintenance. Nurse practitioners can assist patients in identifying changeable stressors and in developing strategies to decrease overall stress. Many persons with HIV have significant social stressors related to poverty and other sociocultural issues that may be difficult to ameliorate. Nurse practitioners can help these patients understand management of their HIV infection to lessen the effects of HIV on their lives. An important nursing intervention, then, is to help HIV patients understand the chronic, manageable aspects of the infection. Careful planning with patients in terms of making regular clinic visits, initiating and adhering to an ART regimen, and improving general health behaviors can be an effective means of reducing some of the HIV-related stresses for these patients.

■ SPECIAL POPULATIONS

HIV-Infected Women of Childbearing Age

Special considerations must be taken into account when managing HIV in women of childbearing age. Goals of their treatment include improving overall health and quality of life; minimizing disease progression; minimizing unwanted pregnancies; preventing heterosexual transmission; and avoiding prescribing medical treatments with teratogenic potential. Contraception and safer sex counseling are essential for HIV-positive women. The benefits and drawbacks of various contraceptives are found in Table 31.12. Barrier methods are necessary for HIV and STI prevention. The effect of hormonal contraceptives on viral shedding is not clear, and the bioavailability of ethinyl estradiol in hormonal contraceptives may be significantly reduced by some antiretroviral medications, including ritonavir, nelfinavir, or ritonavir-boosted lopinavir-nevirapine. Women using oral contraceptives methods, an intrauterine device, or tubal ligation should be counseled to use a barrier method as well to reduce the risk of contracting an STD or transmitting HIV or an STD to her partner. It is essential that advanced practice nurse practitioners be aware of the drug interactions between oral contraceptives and ART, because some of the interactions may compromise the effectiveness of either the contraceptive method by lowering oral contraceptive drug levels (e.g., nevirapine, nelfinavir, ritonavir) or lowering the effectiveness of the ART (amprenavir; AIDS info, 2016).

HIV in Pregnancy

Childbearing in women with HIV is a complex issue to be addressed carefully and thoroughly by clinicians working with this population. Reproduction is a major life activity, and refusing to help someone based solely on their HIV status is considered illegal discrimination. The American College of Obstetricians and Gynecologists (ACOG, 2010) stated that HIV-infected couples should not be denied assisted reproductive techniques based solely on their seropositive status (Fogel & Black, 2008b).

Preconception counseling for women known to have HIV is an important means of optimizing maternal health before pregnancy. Elements of preconception counseling for women with HIV should include appropriate contraceptive methods to reduce unintended pregnancy; safer sex practices; avoidance of alcohol, illicit drug use, and cigarette smoking; risk factors of perinatal transmission and effective strategies to reduce and prevent transmission; and potential effects of HIV on pregnancy and maternal health (Thomas et al., 2015). Elements to be considered in providing care to HIV-infected women considering pregnancy include avoiding antiretroviral agents with a potential for teratogenicity; attaining a stable, maximally suppressed HIV-1 RNA; evaluating the need for prophylaxis or preconception immunizations (influenza, pneumococcal, hepatitis B); optimizing nutritional status and folic acid supplementation; evaluating for opportunistic infections and initiating appropriate treatments or prophylactic regimens; screening for psychiatric and substance abuse disorders and domestic violence; standard genetic and reproductive health screening; and planning for pediatric and perinatal consultation (Thomas et al., 2015).

Protection of the health of the pregnant woman and the fetus is the primary therapeutic goal in all prenatal and perinatal care, and this goal is the same for all women regardless of their HIV status. For women with HIV, minimizing the risk of vertical transmission is an additional therapeutic goal. Without intervention, HIV is effectively transmitted from mother to child. Before antiretroviral prophylaxis use, vertical transmission rates ranged from 13% to 32% in industrialized countries. Transmission can occur at any time during a pregnancy; however, without any prevention measures, most transmission occurs during the intrapartum period (AIDS info, 2016). Factors affecting vertical transmission are found in Table 31.13. Perinatal transmission of HIV to the fetus has decreased significantly in the past decade because of the prophylactic administration of antiretroviral prophylaxis to pregnant women in the prenatal and perinatal periods. Health care providers should follow the same guidelines used for women who are not pregnant (AIDS info, 2016). During labor, women take HIV medicines to reduce the risk of mother-to-child transmission. The newborn infant then receives HIV medicines for the first 6 weeks of life, beginning at 8 to 12 hours after birth (AIDS info, 2016).

Use of ART during pregnancy involves two aims: (1) safeguarding maternal health and (2) reducing mother-to-child transmission. As with nonpregnant women, decisions regarding therapy initiation and selection should be based on standard clinical criteria (Table 31.9) applicable to all HIV-infected adults. Balancing potentially conflicting needs of mother and infant health may be challenging because data regarding the safety, efficacy, and pharmacokinetics of ART in pregnancy may limited, particularly with newer drugs. Women who are pregnant or considering pregnancy must be counseled regarding the potential short- and long-term risks and benefits associated with antiretroviral management strategies. Given zidovudine's proven efficacy and the availability of longer term safety

TABLE 31.13	Factors Affecting Vertical HIV Transmission		
DISEASE-RELATED FACTORS	**MATERNAL HEALTH AND SOCIAL FACTORS**	**OBSTETRICAL FACTORS**	**INFANT FACTORS**
Maternal HIV-1 RNA (plasma and genital tract) Maternal CD4+ count Viral genotype Viral resistance mutations	Clinical stage STDs during pregnancy Vitamin A deficiency Ongoing intrauterine device Tobacco use Multiple sexual partners during pregnancy	Duration of ruptured membranes Chorioamnionitis from use of invasive antenatal procedures Mode of delivery	Prematurity Breastfeeding

RNA, ribonucleic acid; STDs, sexually transmitted diseases.
Sources: Anderson (2005), Centers for Disease Control and Prevention (2015b), Squires (2007).

data on this medication, the *Perinatal HIV Guidelines* recommend that zidovudine ideally be used in pregnancy, either with or without additional antiretrovirals (AIDS info, 2016).

Before the widespread use of HAART, elective cesarean was routinely recommended as the preferred delivery method for HIV-infected women. Whether cesarean delivery continues to be the optimal method of delivery today, given that current transmission rates are very low and multiagent chemoprophylaxis is the norm, has not been established (Fogel & Black, 2008b). Fogel and Black, 2008b advise that women with HIV-1 RNA greater than 1,000 copies/mL in the third trimester should be counseled regarding the potential benefits of elective cesarean delivery.

Breastfeeding has been implicated in the transmission of HIV. The current recommendation is that HIV-positive mothers in the United States formula-feed their infants to avoid possible transmission of the virus (AIDS info, 2016). However, in developing countries, women may not have access to safe alternatives to breast milk for their infants.

Mothers face the difficult issue regarding guardianship of their children in the event of their death. Women with HIV are more likely to be poor and may have limited financial and social support. A single mother may have little or no contact with the father of her children, or he may be a poor candidate for parenting the children full-time. Making choices regarding her children's welfare may be difficult at best, and impossible if she has severely limited familial or social support. She may face the possibility that her children will be placed into foster care if she becomes very ill or dies. Nurse practitioners can assist HIV-infected mothers in expressing fear and grief over this possible, if not likely, scenario. Furthermore, nurse practitioners can assist the woman in seeking community services dedicated to managing the legal affairs of persons with HIV if those services are available. HIV case managers at the local level can also assist HIV-infected women in making decisions about the eventual care of their children. Women who address this issue early after their diagnosis may feel relieved that the issue of guardianship is resolved and formalized.

Incarcerated Women

Incarcerated women are 15 times more likely to be HIV infected than women in the general population because the behaviors for which they are incarcerated place them at higher risk (www.thebody.com, 2016). Among jail populations, African American women are over two times more likely to have a diagnosis of HIV as are White or Hispanic/Latina women (CDC, 2015a, 2015b). They are often substance abusers including injection drugs, have partners who are IDUs, have experienced intimate partner violence, or have been forced to have unprotected sex and/or trade sex for food or housing. Often they have few or no marketable job skills, have little or no access to HIV prevention

methods, and are afraid to ask their partners to use protection (www.body.com, 2016; Farrel et al., 2013; Fogel & Belyea, 1999; Fogel et al., 2014).

Prevention challenges include a lack of awareness about HIV and lack of resources for HIV testing and treatment in correctional facilities in their home counties. Although prisons are more likely to have HIV programs, most incarcerated individuals are detained in jails (Thomas et al., 2015). The majority of jail inmates are released within 72 hours and the rapid turnover in jail populations contributes to a lack of testing and connection with treatment. Additionally, inmate concerns regarding privacy and fear of stigma lead to a lack of disclosure of high-risk behaviors.

Transgender Women

Persons who are transgender identify as a gender that is not the same as the sex assigned to them at birth. Transgender women identify as women, but were born with male anatomy. The prevalence of HIV infection in transgender women is among the highest rates of HIV infection in the United States (Thomas et al., 2015; Mizuno, Fraiser, Huang, & Skarbiniski, 2015) and their odds of HIV infection compared with all adults of reproductive age is estimated as 27.7% (Herbst et al., 2008). Providers caring for transgendered women should have knowledge of their patients' current anatomy and patterns of sexual behavior before counseling them about STD/HIV prevention. Most transgendered women have not had genital affirmation surgery and may have a functional penis and therefore may have insertive oral, vaginal, or anal sex with men and women (CDC, 2015b).

■ SUMMARY

HIV/AIDS is associated with multifaceted dimensions of morbidity, mortality, and societal costs that are often disproportionately experienced by women and their infants. The need for prevention is critical, and nurse practitioners must assume a primary role in helping women decrease risky behaviors and increase protective practices.

■ FUTURE DIRECTIONS

To decrease the burden of HIV on women, screening and early detection are essential. Again, nurse practitioners are a first-line defense in providing these services. Finally, treatment of HIV can lessen the impact of the disease. Education and counseling are essential to ensure that women obtain the maximum benefit from treatment.

■ REFERENCES

AIDS info. (2015a). *HIV treatment: The basics.* Retrieved from https://aidsinfo.nih.gov/education-materials/fact-sheets/print/21/0/1

AIDS info. (2015b). *HIV and women.* Retrieved from https://aidsinfo.nih.gov/education-materials/fact-sheets/print/24/0/1

AIDS info. (2016). *Recommendations for use of antiretroviral drugs in pregnant HIV-1-infected women for maternal health and interventions to reduce perinatal HIV transmission in the United States.* Retrieved from https://aidsinfo.nih.gov/guidelines

American College of Obstetricians and Gynecologists (ACOG). (2001). *Human immunodeficiency virus. Ethics in obstetrics and gynecology.* Retrieved from http://www.acog.org

Anderson, J. R. (2005). *A guide to the clinical care of women with HIV.* Rockville, MD: U.S. Department of Health and Human Services, HIV/AIDS Bureau.

Baril, J. G., Angel, J. B., Gill, M. J., Gathe, J., Cahn, P., van Wyk, J., & Walmsley, S. (2016). Dual therapy treatment strategies for the management of patients infected with HIV: a systematic review of current evidence in ARV-naïve or ARV-experienced, virologically suppressed patients. *Plos One, 11*(2), e0148231.

Beal, J., & Orrick, J. J. (2006a). Antiretroviral therapy. In J. Beal & J. J. Orrick (Eds.), *HIV/AIDS primary care guide* (pp. 45–87). Norwalk, CT: Crown House.

Bennett, B. (2006). HIV testing. In J. Beal & J. J. Orrick (Eds.), *HIV/AIDS primary care guide* (pp. 9–16). Norwalk, CT: Crown House.

Centers for Disease Control and Prevention (CDC). (1981). Pneumocystis pneumonia—Los Angeles. *Morbidity and Mortality Weekly Report, 30,* 250–252.

Centers for Disease Control and Prevention (CDC). (2001). Revised guidelines for HIV counseling, testing, and referral: Technical expert panel review of CDC HIV counseling, testing, and referral guidelines. *Morbidity and Mortality Weekly Report, 50*(RR19), 1–58. Retrieved from www.cdc.gov/mmwr/preview/mmwrhtml/rr5019a1.htm

Centers for Disease Control and Prevention (CDC). (2007a). HIV/AIDS among women. Retrieved from http://www. cdc.gov/hiv

Centers for Disease Control and Prevention (CDC). (2007b). *HIV/AIDS Surveillance Report, 17,* 1–54.

Centers for Disease Control and Prevention (CDC). (2012). HIV transmission risk. Retrieved from http://www.cdc.gov/hiv/law/pdf/Hiv tranmsmision.pdf

Centers for Disease Control and Prevention (CDC). (2015a). *HIV among incarcerated populations.* Retrieved from www.cdc.gov/hiv/group/correctional.html

Centers for Disease Control and Prevention. (2015b). *Special populations.* Retrieved from www.cd.gov/std/tg2015/specialpops.htm

Centers for Disease Control and Prevention (CDC). (2015c). Universal precautions for the prevention of transmission of HIV and other blood borne infections. Retrieved from www.cdc.gov/niosh/yopics/bbp/html

Centers for Disease Control and Prevention (CDC). (2015d). HIV in the United States: At a glance. Retrieved from www.cdc.gov/hiv/statistics/overview/ataglance.html

Centers for Disease Control and Prevention (CDC). (2016). *HIV among women.* Retrieved from www.cdc.gov/hiv/group/gender/women/index.hyml

Chakraborty, H. (2016). Determinants of intimate partner violence among HIV-positive and HIV-negative women in India. *Journal of Intimate Partner Violence, 31*(3), 515–530.

Cotter, A., Potter, J. E., & Tessler, N. (2006). Management of HIV/AIDS in women. In J. Beal & J. J. Orrick (Eds.), *HIV/AIDS primary care guide* (pp. 533–546). Norwalk, CT: Crown House.

Derose, K. P., Griffin, B. A., Kanouse, D. E., Bogart, L. M., Williams, M. V., Haas, A. C.,...Oden, C. W. (2016). Effects of a pilot church-based intervention to reduce HIV stigma and promote HIV testing among African Americans and Latinos. *AIDS and Behavior, 20*(1), 1–14.

DHHS Panel on Antiretroviral Guidelines for Adults and Adolescents. (2006). *Guidelines for the use of antiretroviral agents in HIV-1 infected adults and adolescents.* Retrieved from http://www.AIDSinfo.nih.gov

Farrel, C. E., Parker, S. D., Muessig, K. E., Grodensky, C. A., Jones, C., Golin, C. E.,...Wohl, D. A. (2013). Sexuality, sexual practices, and HIV risk among incarcerated African-American women in North Carolina. *Women's Health Issues: Official Publication of the Jacobs Institute of Women's Health, 23*(6), e357–e364.

Fogel, C. I., & Belyea, M. (1999). The lives of incarcerated women: Violence, substance abuse, and at risk for HIV. *Journal of the Association of Nurses in AIDS Care, 10*(6), 66–74.

Fogel, C. I., & Black, B. (2008a). *Sexually transmitted infections, including HIV: Impact on women's reproductive health.* White Plains, NY: March of Dimes.

Fogel, C. I., & Black, B. (2008b). Women and HIV/AIDS. In C. I. Fogel & N. Fugate Woods (Eds.), *Women's health care in advanced practice nursing.* New York, NY: Springer Publishing.

Fogel, C. I., Gelaude, D. J., Carry, M., Herbst, J. H., Parker, S., Scheyette, A., & Neevel, A. (2014). Context of risk for HIV and sexually transmitted infections among incarcerated women in the south: Individual, interpersonal, and societal factors. *Women & Health, 54*(8), 694–711.

Grant, R. M., Anderson, P. L., McMahan, V., Liu, A., Amico, K. R., Mehrotra, M.,...Glidden, D., for the iPrEx study team (2014). Results of the iPrEx open-label extension (iPrEx OLE) in men and transgender women who have sex with men: PrEx uptake, sexual practices, and HIV incidence. Abstract. AIDS 2014 20th International AIDS Conference. Melbourne, Australia, July 20-25, 2014. Retrieved from http://pag.aids2014.org/Abstracts.aspx?SID=1106&AID=11143

Grossman, H. (2015). *The overlooked secondary benefits of PrEP.* Retrieved from www.thebodypro.com.content/7637

Guest, G., Shattuck, D., Johnson, L., Akumatey, B., Clarke, E. E., Chen, P. L., & Macqueen, K. M. (2010). Acceptability of PrEP for HIV prevention among women at high risk for HIV. *Journal of Women's Health (2002), 19*(4), 791–798.

Hatcher, R. A., Trussel, J., Nelson, A., Cates, W., Kowal, D., & Policar, M. (2011). *Contraceptive technology.* New York, NY: Springer Publishing.

Herbeck, J., Mittler, J., Gottlieb, G., Goodreau, S., Murphy, J., Cori, A., ...Fraser, C. (2016). *Evolution of HIV virulence in response to widespread scale up of antiretroviral therapy: A modeling study.* Retrieved from http://dx.doi.org.libproxy.lib.unc.edu

Herbst, J. H., Jacobs, E. D., Finlayson, T. J., McKleroy, V. S., Neumann, M. S., & Crepaz, N.; HIV/AIDS Prevention Research Synthesis Team. (2008). Estimating HIV prevalence and risk behaviors of transgender persons in the United States: A systematic review. *AIDS and Behavior, 12*(1), 1–17.

Hessol, N. A., Gandhi, M., & Greenblatt, R. M. (2005). Epidemiology and natural history of HIV infection in women. In J. R. Anderson (Ed.), *A guide to the clinical care of women with HIV* (pp. 1–34). Rockville, MD: Department of Health and Human Services, HIV/AIDS Bureau.

Jemmott, L. S., Jemmott, J. B., & O'Leary, A. (2007). Effects on sexual risk behavior and STD rate of brief HIV/STD prevention interventions for African American women in primary care settings. *American Journal of Public Health, 97*(6), 1034–1040.

Maman, S., Campbell, J., Sweat, M. D., & Gielen, A. C. (2000). The intersections of HIV and violence: Directions for future research and interventions. *Social Science & Medicine (1982), 50*(4), 459–478.

Mwamwenda, T. S. (2016). Myths and misconceptions about global HIV/AIDS: University students in Zimbabwe. *Transylvanian Review, 24*(6).

Panel on Treatment of HIV-Infected Pregnant Women and Prevention of Perinatal Transmission. (2012). Recommendations for use of antiretroviral drugs in pregnant HIV-1 infected women and maternal health and interventions to reduce perinatal HIV transmission in the United States (pp. 1–235). Retrieved from http://aidsinfo.nih.gov/contentfiles/IVguidelines/perinatalgl.pdf

Rieg, G. (2006). HIV infection and AIDS. In A. L. Nelson & J. Woodward (Eds.), *Sexually transmitted diseases* (pp. 99–125). Totowa, NJ: Humana Press.

Smith, D. K., Koenig, L. J., Martin, M., Mansergh, G., Heneine, W., Ethridge, S.,...PrEP Guidelines Writing Team Centers for Disease Control and Prevention. (2014). *Pre-exposure prophylaxis for the prevention of HIV infection in the United States – 2014. A clinical practice guideline* (pp. 1–67). Retrieved from https://www.cdc.gov/hiv/pdf/prepguidelines2014.pdf

Squires, K. E. (2007). Management of pregnancy in HIV-infected women. In E. P. Seekins, E. King, K. Obholtz, & S. McGuire (Eds.), *HIV/AIDS annual update 2007* (pp. 151–169). London, UK: Postgraduate Institute for Medicine and Clinical Care Options. Retrieved from http://www.clinicaloptions.com/ccohiv2007

Thomas R. Frieden, T. R., Jaffe, H. W., Cono, J., Richards, C. L., Iademarco, M. F., & Centers for Disease Control and Prevention. (2015). Sexually transmitted diseases treatment guidelines, 2015. *Morbidity and Mortality Weekly Report, 64*(3); 1–138. Retrieved from https://www.cdc.gov/std/tg2015/tg-2015-print.pdf

Toren, K. G., Buskin, S. E., Dombrowski, J. C., Cassels, S. L., & Golden, M. R. (2016). Time from diagnosis to viral load suppression: 2007–2013. *Sexually Transmitted Diseases, 43*(1), 34–40.

Wechsberg, W. M., Lam, W. K., Zule, W., Hall, G., Middlesteadt, R., & Edwards, J. (2003). Violence, homelessness, and HIV risk among crack-using African-American women. *Substance Use & Misuse, 38*(3–6), 669–700.

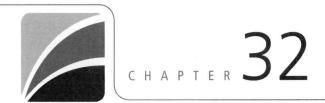

CHAPTER 32

Human Papillomavirus

Elizabeth A. Kostas-Polston • Versie Johnson-Mallard • Naomi Jay

■ CERVICAL HUMAN PAPILLOMAVIRUS–RELATED DISEASE

There was a time when our understanding of the human papillomavirus (HPV) was limited. The discovery of the Pap smear 60 years ago by Dr. George Papanicolaou, the subsequent discovery made by Dr. Harald zur Hausen regarding HPV as *the* necessary cause of cervical cancer, and the clinical evidence that we have learned as a result of our cervical cancer screening program—perhaps the most successful cancer screening model in America (National Cancer Institute [NCI], 2014)—have helped to make great strides in our understanding of the natural history of HPV, its association with sexual intimacy, and the role it plays in anogenital disease and cancer. Although HPV infection can lead to disease and cancer in primarily anogenital sites (e.g., cervix, vulva, vagina, anus, and penis), it has more recently been associated with head and neck (oropharyngeal) disease and cancer. This chapter focuses on the two anatomical sites where HPV infection wreaks the majority of its havoc in women; namely, the cervix and the anus.

Definition and Scope

According to the Centers for Disease Control and Prevention (CDC), HPV is the most common sexually transmitted infection (STI) in the United States (CDC, 2015a). It is estimated that there are currently 79 million individuals in the United States infected with HPV, and an additional 14 million who will become infected this year (CDC, 2015a). In fact, it is postulated that greater than 90% sexually active individuals will develop an HPV infection during their lifetime (CDC, 2015a; Chesson, Dunne, Hariri, & Markowitz, 2014). HPV-associated morbidity includes external genital warts (EGW) and cancer precursors. Cancer precursors may lead to HPV-associated cancer should an HPV infection persist. Only about 10% of all HPV infections persist.

Cost of HPV-Associated Disease

In 2012, Chesson et al. estimated the direct medical costs of preventing and treating HPV-associated disease and cancer for the purpose of quantifying economic burden and building a case for HPV vaccination (Chesson et al., 2012). The overall annual direct medical cost of preventing and treating HPV-associated disease was estimated to be about $8.0 billion. Of this, $6.6 billion was for routine cervical cancer screening and follow-up, $960 million for cancer treatment ($660 millon for cervical and $300 million for orpharyngeal [OP]), $300 million for treatment of EGWs, and $200 million for recurrent respiratory papilloma (RRP; Chesson et al., 2012).

Etiology

It is widely accepted that HPV infection is the cause of almost all cases of precancerous and cancerous lesions of the cervix. There are more than 150 types of HPV, of which approximately 30 infect the anogenital mucosa. These include low-risk or nononcogenic types that often cause benign changes and mild cellular abnormality, and high-risk or oncogenic types that have the potential to cause neoplasia and cancer. Although most HPV cases are subclinical, present no physical symptoms, and clear spontaneously within 2 years, others develop into benign papillomas or malignant cancers (Markowitz et al., 2014). HPV 16 and HPV 18 are particularly of interest, as 70% of HPV-associated cervical cancers are associated with at least one of the two strains (Uyar & Rader, 2014).

HPV infection is epidemic, but cancer is a rare occurrence; the infection is usually transient and clears as a result of a woman's immune response. Progression to cancer occurs when an HPV infection with a high-risk HPV type persists over time. Persistent infection is defined as the detection of the same HPV type, two or more times within a given interval of time.

The HPV type affects both the likelihood of persistence and the risk of progression to precancer. HPV type 16 persists longer than other types and also is especially carcinogenic, with a risk of cervical intraepithelial neoplasia (CIN)-3 of 40% at 5 years (Moscicki et al., 2006). High-risk HPV can cause neoplastic changes of other lower genital tract sites (e.g., vagina, vulva, anus, and penis) as well as nongenital sites (e.g., oral cavity, esophagus, and oropharynx). We still have much to learn about the impact of oncogenic HPV in the carcinogenesis of nongenital cancers.

HPV TYPES

The most common anogenital low-risk (nononcogenic) HPV types are 6 and 11 (which cause 90% of genital warts), and types 40, 42, 43, 44, 53, 54, 61, 72, 73, and 81. Most low-risk HPV infection clear spontaneously within the first year after infection, however may take up to 2 years to clear. High-risk (oncogenic) HPV types 16, 18, 31, 33, 35, 39, 45, 51, 52, 56, 58, 59, and 68 are associated with cervical neoplasia and cancer. HPV 16 is most commonly associated with high-grade CIN and invasive cancers. Although women infected with HPV 16 are at greater risk for developing high-grade cervical lesions, most HPV 16 infections will not develop into abnormal cellular changes. HPV type 18 is most commonly associated with cervical adenocarcinoma. This type of cervical cancer is more difficult to detect on cytology because it occurs in the upper portion of the endocervical canal. For the same reason, it is also more difficult to detect adenocarcinoma using colposcopy-directed biopsies.

Risk Factors

HPV is a skin cell virus and is transmitted through skin-to-skin contact. The number of sexual partners a woman has, as well as the number of partners that her sexual partner(s) have had, is directly related to the woman's risk of acquiring an HPV infection. However, given the HPV epidemic, we now understand that it is not a matter of who will acquire an HPV infection, but rather when. Immune status is also considered to be a risk factor. HPV infection is more likely to be detected in immunosuppressed women. Consistent condom use appears to reduce risk of cervical and vulvovaginal HPV infection. Furthermore, and as a result, there appears to be a higher rate of HPV infection clearance and evidence of the regression of cervical lesions (Hogenwoning et al., 2003; Manhart & Koutsky, 2002; Winer et al., 2006). It is important for health care providers to remember that there is no way to determine when or by whom a woman was infected with HPV.

Clinical Presentation

In most cases, HPV infection is transient and has no clinical manifestations or sequelae. In cases of condylomata acuminata (genital warts), lesions may be visible. However, it is important for health care providers to note that this may not always be the case. Condylomas develop as a result of HPV types 6 and 11, which are low risk or nononcogenic, and may appear as flat, fleshy, or exophitic; cauliflower-like in appearance; and/or pink or hyperpigmented lesions in either squamous epithelium and/or on mucous membranes.

Most often, HPV infection is detected through cervical cancer screening—specifically, because of an abnormal Pap smear or positive, high-risk HPV DNA test.

Evaluation and Assessment

Collecting a thorough medical and sexual health history is the first step in evaluating risk. Smoking and the use of immunosuppressive medications, for example, significantly increase the likelihood of HPV infection persistence. Inquiring as to whether a woman has a history of abnormal cervical cytology and treatment is also an important data gathering point. The health care provider must become proficient and comfortable when conducting a complete sexual history. Sexual health history questions are sensitive and may be perceived to be invasive by the woman. Health care provider sensitivity is needed.

Physical Examination

GENITAL LESIONS

Although usually benign, genital warts are highly infectious. As a result, infection with HPV 6 and/or 11 creates a significant amount of morbidity and health care costs related to treatment. Furthermore, a diagnosis of genital warts, especially in younger women, often carries with it psychological distress. Women with extensive disease are likely to have an alteration in the integrity of their immune system. This can be seen during times of pregnancy, where a woman's immune response is physiologically altered; if the HIV status of a woman changes; or if a woman begins smoking. Smoking carries a significant risk for persistent or recurrent HPV disease. Genital warts may be self-limiting and clear on their own, or may clear as a result of treatment. The development of new warts is not necessarily indicative of new infection or even reinfection, but rather may be caused by active disease which develops as a result of a persistent HPV infection.

Occasionally, genital warts may be cancerous. In order to avoid missing a rare diagnosis of verrucous carcinoma or squamous cell carcinoma, health care providers should biopsy all atypical lesions and send for histological evaluation. Missing such a diagnosis would be detrimental by leading to a delay in treatment, thereby leading to needless morbidity or even mortality.

Differential Diagnoses • Disease caused by HPV infection, unless an overt genital wart, does not usually cause visible changes that can readily be noted on inspection and physical examination. It is important to differentiate a woman's normal anatomy from HPV disease.

- Micropapilliferous and microfilamentous changes of the micropapillomatosis labialis
- Skin tags, hymenal remnants
- Raised pigmented red, dark, or white, or cauliflower-like lesions on the external genitalia
- Nevi
- Dermatoses (e.g., lichen sclerosus)
- Melanomas
- Molluscum contagiosum
- Verrucous carcinoma

CERVICAL CANCER

In 2016, 12,990 new cases of cervical cancer will be diagnosed among American women. Of these newly diagnosed cases, it is expected that 4,120 women will not survive (American Cancer Society [ACS], 2016a, 2016b). These statistics are most unfortunate as cervical cancer is a *preventable* and *curable* cancer! What is more, most of the women who will succumb to cervical cancer will have never have undergone cervical screening. In fact, in the United States, greater than 60% of cervical cancer cases occur in women in underserved populations (Scarinci, et al., 2010). Although most women with cervical cancer are asymptomatic, some women do experience bleeding with intercourse, or notice an unusual vaginal discharge and unpleasant odor.

Cervical Cancer Screening

The overall goal of cervical cancer screening is to prevent morbidity and mortality. This goal is accomplished by (a) identifying, treating, and surveilling high-grade cervical cancer precursors, thereby reducing a woman's risk of developing invasive cancer, and (b) avoiding unnecessary or overtreatment of benign and transient HPV infections and cancer precursor lesions that most likely will regress. Loop electrosurgical excision procedure (LEEP), one such method, has been associated with an untoward outcome of incompetent cervix during pregnancy (Saslow et al., 2012).

Diagnostic Tests

There are two screening tests available for use when screening for cervical cancer: cytology alone (conventional Pap smear or liquid-based Pap smear) and HPV DNA testing. There are three recommended screening modalities: cytology alone, HPV DNA testing alone, and finally cotesting using both cytology and HPV DNA testing.

CERVICAL CYTOLOGY

Cervical cytology consists of two collection methods: conventional Pap (exfoliated cells are smeared onto a slide and fixed with preservative) and liquid-based thin layer (exfoliated cells are collected using an endocervical brush and then transferred into a liquid preservative). Both methods are acceptable cervical screening methods. In fact, little difference has been found in the performance of the two methods when identifying high-grade disease (Davey et al., 2006). Most health care providers use liquid-based cytology as its sensitivity is greater when compared with conventional cytology. Liquid-based cytology is often most preferred as it allows for reflex HPV testing as well as gonorrhea and chlamydia testing. Regardless of method, a low-grade squamous intraepithelial lesion (LSIL) cytology triages many women into a low-risk category. An LSIL cytology result is typically translated to be an active HPV infection, of which most are self-limiting. In contrast, high-grade squamous intraepithelial lesion (HSIL) cytology identifies women who are at the greatest risk of developing an invasive cancer. Treatment of this cancer precursor is indicated to prevent transformation into invasive cancer.

HPV DNA TESTING

We have identified HPV as a necessary cause of cervical cancer. What is more, women infected with HPV types 16 and 18 have a tenfold increased risk of developing cervical cancer (Khan et al., 2005). HPV DNA testing uses advanced molecular biological methodologies for the detection of high-risk HPV. It is important that health care providers only use HPV DNA tests that are approved by the U.S. Food and Drug Administration (FDA).

COTESTING

Cotesting with cervical cytology and HPV DNA testing has been shown to increase sensitivity, thereby increasing early detection rates. An increased sensitivity translates into greater clinical confidence in the lengthening of screening intervals. In turn, lengthening screening intervals allows for transient HPV infection clearance and minimizes opportunites to overtreat.

Positive HPV DNA testing allows for risk stratification and identification in women who, for example, cytology alone was reported as normal. In these cases, a woman with a negative cytology result and a positive high-risk HPV result will require additional evaluation (e.g., colposcopy). When requesting an HPV DNA test, the health care provider may also request HPV genotyping (either at initial collection or after the HPV DNA test results are reported). Postive HPV 16 and 18 genotyping results help guide the health care provider in further stratifying a woman's risk of developing a cancer precursor and invasive cancer. A positive HPV DNA test or cytology result that is reported as CIN-1 identifies a woman who at that time is not at risk for cervical cancer.

For a more information regarding U.S. cervical cancer screening guidelines for average-risk women please go to www.cdc.gov/cancer/cervical/pdf/guidelines.pdf.

Treatment and Management

CONDYLOMATA ACUMINATA (GENITAL WARTS)

The primary purpose of treating genital warts is cosmetic in nature. Occasionally, genital warts may grow and spread and obstruct the birth canal. During pregnancy, when it is physiologically normal for the woman's immune system to be suppressed, shifts in hormone levels may cause preexisting genital warts to grow. In cases where genital warts grow and obstruct the birth canal, surgical removal and sometimes cesarean section may be indicated. In cases where genital warts are present during pregnancy, treatment should occur around 32 weeks gestation. This is the recommended period of gestation for treatment as there is a chance of recurrence. During pregnancy, genital warts may be treated with, for example, trichloroacetic acid, excision, and laser (see Table 32.1 for CDC treatment recommendations).

Treatment of genital warts includes both health care provider administered and patient self-administered therapies. When contemplating a treatment plan, health care providers should consider all of the following: genital wart size, number, location, morphology, woman's choice, health care provider experience, convenience, and adverse effects.

TABLE 32.1	Treatment Regimens for Genital Warts

RECOMMENDED REGIMENS FOR EXTERNAL GENITAL WARTS

Patient self-applied	*Podofilox* 0.5% solution or gel *Imiquimod* 5% cream *Sinecatechins* 15% ointment
Health care provider administered	*Cryotherapy* with liquid nitrogen or cryoprobe; repeat applications every 1–2 weeks *Podophyllin resin* 10%–25% in a compound tincture of benzoin *TCA* or *BCA* 80%–90% *Surgical removal* either by scissor excision, shave excision, curettage, or electrosurgery

ALTERNATIVE REGIMENS (MORE SIDE EFFECTS, LESS DATA ON EFFICACY)

Recommended regimen for cervical warts	For those with exophytic cervical warts, a biopsy evaluation to exclude high-grade SIL must be performed before treatment is initiated. Management of exophytic cervical warts should include consultation with a specialist.
Recommended regimens for vaginal warts	*Cryotherapy with liquid nitrogen.* The use of a cryoprobe in the vagina is not recommended because of the risk for vaginal perforation and fistula formation. *TCA or BCA 80%–90% applied to warts.* A small amount should be applied only to warts and allowed to dry, at which time a white frosting develops. If an excess amount of acid is applied, the treated area should be powdered with talc, sodium bicarbonate, or liquid soap preparations to remove unreacted acid. This treatment can be repeated weekly, if necessary.
Recommended regimens for urethral meatus warts	*Cryotherapy with liquid nitrogen.* *Podophyllin 10%–25% in compound tincture of benzoin.* The treatment area and adjacent normal skin must be dry before contact with podophyllin. This treatment can be repeated weekly, if necessary. The safety of podophyllin during pregnancy has not been established. Data are limited on the use of podofilox and imiquimod for treatment of distal meatal warts.
Recommended regimens for anal warts	*Cryotherapy with liquid nitrogen.* *TCA or BCA 80%–90% applied to warts.* A small amount should be applied only to warts and allowed to dry, at which time a white frosting develops. If an excess amount of acid is applied, the treated area should be powdered with talc, sodium bicarbonate, or liquid soap preparations to remove unreacted acid. This treatment can be repeated weekly, if necessary. *Surgical removal*

BCA, bichloroacetic acid; TCA, trichloroacetic acid.
Adapted from Centers for Disease Control and Prevention (2015b).

Treatment of CIN

There are two treatment modalities that are used to address CIN if it is determined that there is an increase and that the CIN will progress to cervical cancer. These modalities include ablative therapy and excisional therapy.

ABLATIVE THERAPY

This treatment modality includes the use of cryotherapy and laser vaporization. When performing cryotherapy or laser vaporization, it is important to note that no surgical specimen will be available for histologic testing. For this reason, many health care providers prefer using excisional therapies. Advantages of cryotherapy include that is is easy to perform in an outpatient setting, there is minimal health care provider training, it is inexpensive, and there are minimal long-term fertility issues. Significant cramping and a watery, malodorous vaginal drainage for up to 3 weeks are the most commonly reported disadvantages to cryotherapy. Laser vaporization is also readily performed in the outpatient

setting with minimal risk to the woman. The fact that health care providers must undergo special training and the cost of equipment are the common reasons why health care providers choose not to perform this procedure. Women tolerate laser vaporization well, and often receive some type of sedative before the procedure to help with any discomfort/pain and to minimize patient movement throughout. The biggest advantage of laser vaporization is the precision at which the tissue/area of concern is destroyed.

EXCISIONAL THERAPY

This therapy includes LEEP procedure and cold knife cone (CKC) biopsy. The result of these procedures is a tissue specimen, which is sent to pathology for histological evaluation and diagnosis. Women are most often treated with a local anesthesia during the procedures and with nonsteroidal anti-inflammatory medication for postprocedure cramping. Vaginal bleeding and discharge are common and may last for up to 2 weeks. Thermal artifacts are evident on the margins of a specimen, and care must be taken by both the health care provider and pathologist to ensure that the margins are clear; this is evidence that no high-grade lesions were missed during the procedure. In contemporary clinical practice, a CKC biopsy procedure is typically performed when there is evidence and concern for an increased possibility of invasive cancer. The biggest advantage of a CKC versus a LEEP procedure has to do with the fact that the biopsy specimen collected via CKC will not have undergone any thermal damage to the tissue margins. Because more tissue is collected during a CKC procedure, the woman is at greater risk for developing acute bleeding and long-term cervical stenosis and cervical insufficiency which may lead to, for example, premature delivery.

Current Approaches to Cervical Cancer Prevention

Current approaches to cervical cancer prevention include (a) vaccination, (b) cervical cancer screening, (c) follow-up evaluation using colposcopy and cervical biopsy, and (d) treatment for biopsy-confirmed high-grade cervical cancer precursors. Approaches (b) to (d) have previously been discussed. In the following section, we discuss HPV vaccination as a means of prevention.

HPV Vaccinations

In 2006, the FDA licensed an HPV quadrivalent vaccine to protect against HPV genotypes 6, 11, 16, and 18, which are responsible for 70% of cervical cancers and 80% of EGWs (Maktabi, Ludwig, Eick-Cost, Yerubandi, & Gaydos, 2013). Unfortunately, uptake of the vaccine in the United States has been less than hoped for. Decreasing persistent HPV infection rates, disease, and cancer burden will only be achieved if HPV-cancer prevention vaccine uptake increases through the implementation of interventions that are successful at improving vaccine uptake.

Widespread, HPV-cancer prevention vaccination will sharply reduce high-grade cervical, vaginal, vulvar, and anal dysplasia and cancer, and EGWs.

In the United States, there are three licensed, safe, and effective HPV-cancer prevention vaccines recommended by the CDC's Advisory Committee on Immunization Practices (ACIP; CDC, 2011) (Table 32.2). The ACIP recommends routine vaccination at age 11 to 12 and may begin as early as age 9 years. HPV vaccination is also recommended as catch-up for females aged 13 to 26 years and for males aged 13 to 21 years, for those who have not been previously vaccinated or who have not completed the three-dose vaccine series. Males aged 22 to 26 years may be vaccinated. Additionally, men who have sex with men (MSM) and immunocompromised individuals through age 26 years may be vaccinated (Ault, 2007).

In clinical trials, the quadrivalent and bivalent vaccines have shown prophylactic efficacy against EGWs (73% decrease in women younger than 26 years; Paavonen et al., 2007) and CIN 2/3 and adenocarcinoma in situ (AIS) associated with HPV 16 or HPV 18 and thus could be used for cervical cancer prevention (Donovan et al., 2011; Paavonen et al., 2007). In Australia and Canada, mandatory HPV-cancer prevention vaccination programs have been shown to significantly decrease HPV-related disease and cancer (Donovan et al., 2011) (Tables 32.3 and 32.4).

Poor HPV Vaccine Uptake and the Fight Against Cancer in America

In 2012, The President's Cancer Panel determined that low rates of adolescent HPV vaccine uptake were a threat to America's progress against cancer (The President's Cancer Panel, 2014). At that time, the CDC estimated that increasing current low vaccination rates up to 80% (a *Healthy People 2020* target) would prevent an additional 53,000 future cervical cancer cases in the United States in adolescent girls less than or equal to 12 years or younger, over the course of their lifetimes (CDC, 2013). Barriers to vaccine uptake were identified. They included (a) missed clinical opportunities, (b) misinformation, (c) mistrust, (d) lack of knowledge, (e) insufficient access and/or system gaps, and (f) cost concerns (The President's Cancer Panel, 2014). In an effort to address these barriers, the Panel recommended three critical goals that must be achieved to increase HPV vaccine uptake in the United States. The overall goal is completion of the full three-dose vaccine series by all vaccine-eligible

TABLE 32.2	U.S. Licensed HPV-Cancer Prevention Vaccines		
	QUADRIVALENT (GARDASIL®)	**BIVALENT (CERVARIX®)**	**9-VALENT (GARDASIL 9®)**
Manufacturer	Merck	GlaxoSmithKline	Merck
HPV genotypes	6, 11, 16, and 18	16 and 18	6, 11, 16, 18, 31, 33, 45, 52, and 58
Year licensed in the United States	2006 (females 9–26 years) 2009 (males 9–26 years)	2009 (females 15–25 years)	2015 (females 9–26 years) 2015 (males 9–15 years)
Schedule (months)	0, 1–2, 6 months	0, 1–2, 6 months	0, 1–2, 6 months
Cost/per dose[a]	$147.00/dose (×3 doses)	$128.75/dose (×3 doses)	$163.09/dose (×3 doses)

HPV, human papillomavirus.

[a]Adapted from http://www.cdc.gov/vaccines/programs/vfc/awardees/vaccine-management/price-list/#f5

TABLE 32.3	HPV 16/18-Related CIN 2/3 or AIS Efficacy Study Results for Quadrivalent Vaccine	
PRINCIPAL ENDPOINTS	**% EFFICACY**	**97.9% CI**
CIN 2/3 or AIS	99	93, 100
HPV 16-related CIN 2/3 or AIS	99	92, 100
HPV 18-related CIN 2/3 or AIS	100	78, 100
CIN 2	100	93, 100
CIN 3	98	89, 100
AIS	100	31, 100

AIS, adenocarcinoma in situ; CI, confidence interval; CIN, cervical intraepithelial neoplasia; HPV, human papillomavirus.
Adapted from Paavonen et al. (2007); Donovan et al. (2011).

TABLE 32.4	HPV 16/18-Related CIN2+ or AIS Efficacy Study Results for Bivalent Vaccine	
PRINCIPAL ENDPOINTS	**% EFFICACY**	**97.9% CI**
CIN 2/3 or AIS	90.4	53.4, 99.3
HPV 16-related CIN 2/3 or AIS	93.3	47.0, 99.9
HPV 18-related CIN 2/3 or AIS	83.3	−78.8, 99.9

AIS, adenocarcinoma in situ; CI, confidence interval; CIN, cervical intraepithelial neoplasia; HPV, human papillomavirus.
Adapted from Paavonen et al. (2007) and Donovan et al. (2011).

adolescents for whom the vaccine is not contraindicated. Critical goals include (a) reduce missed clinical opportunities to recommend and administer the vaccines; (b) increase parents', caregivers', and adolescents' acceptance of the vaccine; and (c) maximize access to HPV vaccination services (The President's Cancer Panel, 2014).

Missed Clinical Opportunities

It has been determined that the most important reason why the United States has not achieved the *Healthy People 2020* target of 80% vaccine uptake is missed clinical opportunities (Chaturvedi, Engels, Anderson, & Gillison, 2008). Often times, adolescents receive other recommended vaccines during visits with their health care providers, but not HPV vaccines. Health care providers should strongly encourage HPV vaccination whenever other vaccines are administered and health care organizations should use electronic health records and immunization info systems to avoid missed opportunities for HPV vaccination.

Knowledge, Attitudes, and Beliefs

Parental and caregiver knowledge, attitudes, and beliefs affect whether children receive any vaccine, including

HPV vaccines. Most parents believe that vaccines protect their children from potentially life-threatening diseases, but some refuse one or more recommended vaccines based on concerns, such as safety. The most important predictor of vaccination in the clinical setting is a strong recommendation from a health care provider. Failure of health care providers to strongly recommend HPV vaccines, as well as a lack of parental understanding of HPV vaccine safety and efficacy, has contributed to poor HPV vaccine uptake.

Maximizing Access to Vaccination Services

In an effort to maximize HPV vaccine uptake in the United States, settings other than traditional health care provider offices should be considered for vaccine administration. Schools and pharmacies are two examples of promising alternative settings.

Future Directions

The best approach to cervical cancer prevention is continued education, screening, and prevention. Thanks to improved technologies for biomedical analysis, how we screen women for cervical cancer is ever evolving. Vaccine development is also pushing the ticket for the many choices women have with regard to cancer-vaccine prevention. HPV vaccines are cancer-prevention vaccines. Health care providers must make it a priority to not allow women to be subjected to missed opportunities for HPV-cancer vaccine prevention.

The most commonly used HPV vaccine in the United States is the quadrivalent vaccine. This vaccine is indicated for prevention of cervical, vulvar, vaginal, and anal cancer as well as genital warts in women and penile and anal cancer and genital warts in men. Although many professional organizations have made the leap by recommending HPV vaccination for the prevention of HPV-related head and neck cancers, the science, and therefore the evidence, does not exist to support this as a clinical recommendation (it is not an FDA approved indication). There is still much to learn in regard to HPV and a lot of impact to make in the decreasing HPV morbidity and mortality.

■ ANAL HPV-RELATED DISEASE

Definition and Scope

In addition to the female genital tract, HPV is also associated with a spectrum of abnormal changes in the anal canal including infection with the virus, its associated lesions, LSIL and HSIL, and cancer. Anal cancer itself is rare. In 2015, there were an estimated 7,200 new cases in the United States (NCI, 2016) and an incidence rate of approximately 2.1 per 100,000 women and 1.5 per 100,000 men (Shiels, Kreimer, Coghill, Darragh, & Devesa, 2015). However, the incidence is increasing annually at a rate of 2.2% (ACS, 2016a, 2016b; NCI, 2016), and in women the incidence has doubled since the mid-1970s (Henley et al., 2015). There are identified populations considered at increased risk for anal cancer. The highest risk populations are HIV-seropositive men who have sex with men (MSM) with anal cancer rates estimated to be as high as 30/100,000 (Silverberg et al., 2012), surpassing the highest rates of cervical cancer for any other group. Women identified as high risk for anal cancer include women with a history of gynecologic HSIL and cancer and those who are immunocompromised. Current anal cancer rates in HIV-seropositive women are reported as high as 30 per 100,000 (Silverberg et al., 2012). There are elevated rates of anal cancer in other immune-suppressed populations as well. Increases in anogenital cancers of up to 100-fold were reported in the mid-1980s in solid organ transplant recipients (Blohmé & Brynger, 1985; Penn, 1986); this is believed to be because of the iatrogenic effect of immunosuppressive medications. More recent data also showed elevated incident rates of anal (11.6) as well as vulvar cancer (20.3) in a study analyzing data from the U.S. Transplant Cancer Match (Madeleine, Finch, Lynch, Goodman, & Engels, 2013). Similar data have been reported in studies analyzing transplant registries in Italy and Denmark (Busnach et al., 1993; Sunesen, Norgaard, Thorlacius-Ussing, & Laurberg, 2010). The risk increased after 2 years, with an average diagnosis of a cancer in the fourth or fifth year following transplant (Madeleine et al., 2013). Elevated risks for anal cancer are also found in patients on long-term steroid therapy for conditions such as systemic lupus erythematosus (Dreyer, Faurschou, Mogensen, & Jacobsen, 2011) and Crohn's disease (Sunesen et al., 2010). Finally, the association of gynecologic cancers with anal canal disease has been well documented. In an early study, nearly 13% of women with a history of vulvar cancer had anal cancer, and a total of 47.5% had HPV-associated lesions (Ogunbiyi et al., 1994). Elevated risks for anal cancer have been documented in women with a history of cervical, vaginal, or vulvar HSIL, and/or cancer (Chaturvedi et al., 2007: Jiménez, Paszat, Kupets, Wilton, & Tinmouth, 2009; Saleem et al., 2011).

Etiology

ANAL HPV AND SQUAMOUS INTRAEPITHELIAL LESION

Although anal cancer is rare, both HPV infection and HPV-associated anal lesions are common. The prevalence of HPV infection ranged from 4% to 22% among women in the general population compared with 23% to 36% in women with a history of gynecologic HPV-associated disease. In HIV-seropositive women, the prevalence was as high as 85% (Stier et al., 2015). The incidence is consistently higher in HIV-seropositive versus negative women; 76% of HIV-positive women were HPV positive as compared with 42% of HIV-negative women (Palefsky, Holly, Ralston, Da Costa, & Greenblatt, 2001).

RISK FACTORS

Risk factors include the presence of cervical HPV, CD4 less than 200 in HIV-positive women, smoking, and concurrent or a history of perianal and/or vulvar warts (Stier et al., 2015). A reported history of anal intercourse and higher number of lifetime sexual partners was associated with HPV prevalence in some but not all studies (Castro et al., 2012; Kojic et al., 2011). HPV persistence is a known risk factor for the development of cervical HSIL, although less studied in anal canal. The average clearance of anal HPV infection was reported at 5 months in one study (Goodman et al., 2008), and the majority of anal HPV had cleared by 3 years in another study (Moscicki et al., 2014). Persistence was associated with immunosuppression (Suardi et al., 2014) and recent anal sexual activity, as well as persistent cervical HPV infection (Moscicki et al., 2014).

The incidence of anal LSIL or HSIL has been measured by cytology, histology, or a composite of the two, by which the highest grade of disease was reported. Histology results usually are based on anoscopy or high-resolution anoscopy (HRA). HRA may only have been provided to subjects with abnormal cytology or a convenience sample subset of those that followed up with a referral for HRA following abnormal cytology. The literature reports any SIL, or may report LSIL and HSIL separately.

As a screening test, anal cytology, like cervical, is not a reliable indication of the grade of disease and its low sensitivity means many patients with disease will have false-negative results. Fortunately, this is not problematic in a slow-developing disease such as HPV-associated lesions, as repeated screening tests, over time, will eventually test positive. False-positive cytology is considered rare and therefore a positive cytology requires referral for higher level evaluation. For anal disease, like cervical, the gold standard is colposcopy-directed biopsy.

There are few studies that evaluated all subjects with HRA. In cohorts that were nonimmunocompromised, the incidence of anal SIL ranged from 4% to 20% and anal HSIL ranged from 2% to 9% (ElNaggar & Santoso, 2013; Heráclio et al., 2011; Jacyntho et al., 2011; Koppe et al., 2011; Likes, Santoso, & Wan, 2013; Santoso, Long, Crigge, Wan, & Haefner, 2010; Tatti et al., 2012). In comparison, a single study of 31 HIV-positive women all referred for HRA reported 52% SIL and 26% HSIL (Tatti et al., 2012). These data, however, may provide low estimates and reflect the overall inexperience of this relatively new practice. Health care providers with at least 10 years of HRA experience report anal HSIL in more than 40% of immunocompromised women, or in those women with a history of gynecologic HSIL or cancer (unpublished personal data). Unlike the cervical literature, longitudinal natural history studies are not yet available for anal disease. Finally, the heterogeneity of the data is difficult to synthesize and to statistically analyze, underscoring the need for continued research.

Symptoms

EXTERNAL GENITAL WARTS

Anal cancers and HSIL are more difficult and expensive to diagnose and treat, but overall they have a lower burden of disease as compared with anogenital warts, with estimates as high as 120 cases per 100,000 person-years in women. Although these data include all EGWs (Hoy, Singhal, Willey, & Insinga, 2009), anal warts are rarely reported separately. EGWs are found most frequently in younger women aged

20 to 24 years (Hoy et al., 2009). Although genital warts are benign, the diagnosis and treatment can have substantial economic as well as psychological impact on an individual.

Evaluation and Assessment

SQUAMOCOLUMNAR JUNCTION

The cervix has served as a hypothetical model for anal cancer screening because of biological similarities between the anus and the female genital tract. Both the cervix and anus have a squamocolumnar junction where squamous epithelium borders columnar epithelium, inducing a transformation zone in which normal metaplasia occurs. The dynamic process of metaplasia is conducive to the development of an abnormal transformation or dysplasia, and both LSIL and HSIL frequently occur here.

HPV STRAINS

The same strains of HPV affect the anus and genital tract, including the low-risk types associated with most LSIL and the high-risk types associated with most HSIL and cancers (Williams et al., 1994). The high-risk strain HPV 16 is found in a greater percentage of anal cancers (77%) than cervical (51%) (Steinau et al., 2013). Anal LSIL and HSIL lesions are morphologically similar to their respective cervical lesions, and HSIL is known to be the cancer precursor lesion in both sites (Berry et al., 2014). The natural history of cervical HSIL and cancer are better characterized because of decades of research. There are compelling data supporting a similar natural history development for anal cancer (Berry, Palefsky, & Welton, 2004; Kreuter et al., 2010; Watson, Smith, Whitehead, Sykes, & Frizelle, 2006). Screening programs for anal cancer, based on the cervical model, have been proposed and initiated in many communities. Natural history studies are underway to validate whether treating and managing anal HPV disease and cancer using the cervical cancer model is efficacious. We are anxiously awaiting the outcome of longitudinal trials such as the Study of the Prevention of Anal Cancer (SPANC) in Australia and the Anal Cancer HSIL Outcome Research (ANCHOR) trial in the United States.

ANAL CANCER SCREENING

The goal of anal cancer screening, like cervical cancer screening, is primarily to identify anal HSIL allowing for targeted treatment of these lesions, thereby preventing progression to cancer. In the general population, anal cancer is a rare cancer. However, there are special populations which are at higher risk; thus, health care providers focus their attention on these populations. Most anal cancer screening programs are targeting HIV-seropositive MSM. Additionally, elevated rates of anal cancer are found in specific populations of women, including those who are immunocompromised and those with a history of lower genital tract HSIL and cancers. Many health care providers include these women in anal cancer screening programs as well.

SCREENING TOOLS

Techniques for evaluation of the cervix have been adapted for anal canal disease. These include validation of anal cytology (Palefsky et al., 1997), HPV DNA testing (Palefsky et al., 2001), and HRA. HRA requires the use of a colposcope and colposcopic techniques for evaluation of the anal canal (Jay et al., 1997). The screening modality is dependent on available resources. HRA remains a relatively young field and there are few Centers of Excellence or trained health care providers across the United States. Therefore, *anal cytology should only be provided if there is a referral source for abnormal results*. If HRA is not available, consideration should be given to alternate options (see sections on DARE and cytology). The aim of anal cancer screening is to identify individuals with potential HSIL for evaluation with HRA, who can then be treated and followed with the overall goal of preventing progression to anal cancer. In high resource settings, screening would include anal cytology and digital anal rectal examination (DARE) with referral to HRA for abnormal findings, including ≥ atypical squamous cells of undetermined significance (ASC-US) cytology.

ANAL CYTOLOGY AND HISTOLOGY

Anal cytology and histology are classified with the same taxonomy as the cervix and genital tract, now unified using the newer Lower Anogenital Squamous Terminology (LAST) system (Darragh et al., 2013). The sensitivity of anal cytology ranges from 69% to 93% and specificity from 32% to 59%, similar to cervical cytology (Chiao, Giordano, Palefsky, Tyring, & El Serag, 2006). False-positive cytology results are rare, and the positive predictive value of abnormal cytology has been reported as 96% for the presence of any lesion in HIV-positive MSM (Cranston et al., 2007). Cytology results are not predictive of the level of dysplasia and will commonly underestimate the actual severity of disease. As much as 50% of ASC-US cytology will result in a finding of HSIL on HRA (Jay et al., 2012). This is true regardless of an individual's risk. Therefore, it has become common practice to refer any abnormal cytology for follow-up HRA (e.g., ≥ ASC-US) provided there are adequate referral resources.

TREATMENT AND MANAGEMENT ALGORITHMS

Algorithms for triage to colposcopy following abnormal cervical cytology, similar to those considered standard of care for cervical screening, are not yet established for anal canal disease. The newer triage protocols for cervical cytology including less frequent screening and incorporation of HPV DNA testing have not been validated for anal canal disease. In part, this is caused by the high prevalence of anal HSIL in populations considered at risk and therefore cannot be compared with cervical screening programs targeted at the general population of women. However, the essential principle that abnormal cytology results in referral for follow-up colposcopy, or in this case HRA, is the same. Different health care centers may establish different guidelines for triage to colposcopy and treatment until standards of care can be validated (Figure 32.1).

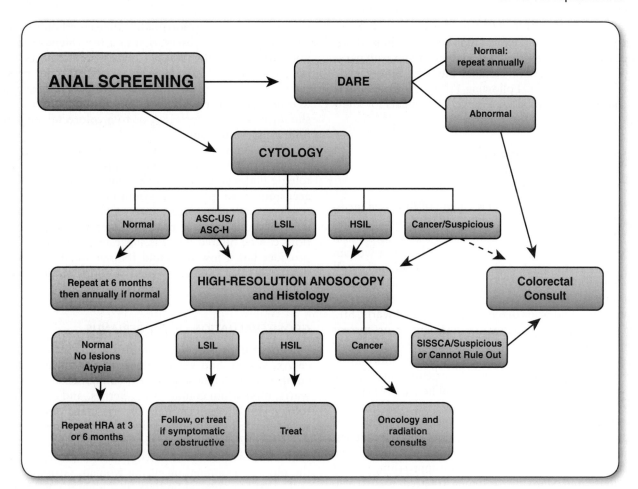

FIGURE 32.1

Anal screening triage chart.

ASC-US/ASC-H, atypical squamous cells of undetermined significance/atypical squamous cells, cannot rule out high-grade squamous intra-epithelial lesion; DARE, digital anal rectal examination; HRA, high-resolution anoscopy; HSIL, high-grade squamous intra-epithelial lesion; LSIL, low-grade squamous intraepithelial lesion.

Adapted from Donovan et al. (2011); Paavonen et al. (2007).

Although frequently incorporated into research studies, HPV testing is *not FDA approved* for the anal canal. Although yet to be determined, its utility may be similar to approved tests developed for the cervix, and eventually may help guide practice decisions. Occasionally, HPV testing is used, without clinical evidence, for its negative predictive value. For example, in women who have been treated for anal cancer, a negative HPV test might indicate the need for less frequent, follow-up HRA examinations.

HIGH-RESOLUTION ANOSCOPY

HRA, like cervical colposcopy, requires advanced training which can be obtained in courses provided by specialized professional organizations (e.g., the American Society for Colposcopy and Cervical Pathology [ASCCP]). However, all health care providers should have an understanding of abnormalities that require referral to a specialist providing HRA. These include abnormal clinical findings as well as abnormal cytology. Clinical findings that would prompt referral to an HRA-trained health care provider

include grossly evident perianal disease such as warts, lesion, erosions, atypical appearing hemorrhoids, and/or vulvar disease that extends to the perianus. In these cases, it is important to determine if intra-anal disease is present as well. The colposcopic evaluation (HRA) allows the trained health care provider to determine if microscopic lesions are present in addition to the macroscopic findings. Persistent symptoms such as bleeding, pain, and pressure, that cannot be explained by a clinical examination, may be better evaluated by HRA or, if unavailable, by a colorectal surgeon. Abnormal findings on the DARE should also prompt referral. These would include a mass, pain with palpation, and a hemorrhoid or wart that is hard or painful.

The HRA examination itself is a relatively short procedure generally lasting no longer than 15 to 20 minutes. The examination is usually well tolerated with only a feeling of minor discomfort caused by the pressure of the anoscope on the sphincter. The evaluation includes thorough examination of the anus and perianus using a small anoscope, which is inserted into the anus, and the application of acetic acid and Lugol's solutions applied to highlight potential lesions.

As most women referred for HRA have documented abnormal cytology, they should expect that biopsies will be done. Biopsies are not generally painful as there are no pain nerve endings in the anal canal. Perianal biopsies, however, do require local anesthesia. Following HRA, individuals may experience minor bleeding with bowel movements for a few days.

Evaluation and Assessment

MEDICAL AND SEXUAL HEALTH HISTORY

All women should be evaluated with an HPV-focused medical and sexual reproductive history of the entire genital tract. The woman's reported medical and sexual history will help the health care provider determine whether a woman (a) is considered high risk and should be offered anal cytology, (b) needs a DARE, and/or (c) requires referral for HRA. For the anus specifically, it is important to ascertain whether the woman has had prior diagnoses such as anal warts, SIL, and/or cancer, and/or whether she has a prior or current history/diagnosis of hemorrhoids, fissures, fistulas, and/or abscess. The health care provider should collect information on any treatment(s) and response(s) to treatment(s). While collecting a woman's medical and sexual health history, current symptoms such as bleeding, pain, irritation, and pruritus should be documented. Symptoms present with anal intercourse (voluntary or coerced), including frequency, duration, and if stable or worsening over time, should also be documented. A history of immunosuppression, steroid medications, and smoking or other tobacco use is also important to note, because they may play a role in persistent HPV disease, a necessary cause of anal cancer (Daling et al., 1992). Finally, inquiring as to whether there are new, severe, or persistent diarrhea, constipation, urgency, and/or any changes in bowel patterns or incontinence would be important to note in the woman's medical and sexual history. Health care providers should be aware that these questions are sensitive and women may be reluctant to discuss them.

WHAT TO LOOK FOR

The hallmarks of anal cancer include pain and bleeding. It is important to ascertain whether or not these symptoms are new, persistent, or worsening over time. Early or micro-invasive cancers may present with only minor symptoms or none at all, and may be an incidental finding during a hemorrhoidectomy. Vague symptoms such as minor pressure or a sudden change in bowel habits may indicate that a mass is developing. Once a cancer is established, the onset of symptoms may be sudden (e.g., bleeding with bowel movements) or subclinical (e.g., mistaken for a fissure or hemorrhoid).

DIGITAL ANAL RECTAL EXAMINATION

The most important service that can and should be provided by any health care provider is the DARE. The common story described by many anal cancer survivors is that despite complaining of discomfort and/or bleeding for months and sometimes years, no one looked or palpated, and they were told it was "just a hemorrhoid." All hemorrhoids should be evaluated by both observation and feel. Hemorrhoids are not hard (unless thrombosed, which also requires referral for treatment). It is important that health care providers remember that atypical presentation or persistent symptoms that do not resolve with common, short-term interventions should be referred for HRA or to a colorectal surgeon for follow-up evaluation.

Other findings that may require referral to a specialist include fissures, fistula openings, pruritus ani, and dermatologic findings. Unfortunately, women sometimes become accustomed to persistent symptoms that can be easily resolved with the correct intervention (which sometimes is beyond our scope of practice). Treatments and interventions can be offered but it is suggested that the health care provider has a low threshold for referral if symptoms do not resolve or improve within a short framework (e.g., 1 month).

GROSS EVALUATION OF THE PERIANUS

Health care providers are accustomed to evaluating the cervix, vagina, and vulva with gross visualization and are competent to diagnose and treat conditions such as genital warts, molluscum contagiosum, herpes, and simple dermatologic conditions. Persistent disease that does not resolve with standard treatment requires referral to the appropriate specialist. With the proper education and training, perianal evaluation with simple anoscopy can be incorporated into the physical examination of the woman. Gross evaluation will assess for atypical findings, including warts, changes in skin contour or color, redundant tissue or anal tags, hemorrhoids, fissures, ulcerations, denuded epithelium, or rashes. Visualized abnormalities should be queried for any accompanying symptoms such as pruritus, discomfort, or pain. If the patient has peripheral neuropathy or is on pain medication for other health care problems, she may have decreased anal sensation and may not report pain or discomfort. The health care provider should also assess for the extension of any abnormalities to or from the vulva and perineum or into the anal canal. Warts may seem typical in appearance but consideration should be given to providing a biopsy for histologic confirmation, especially if there are any atypical qualities such as fissuring, bleeding, or pigmentation changes. If a health care provider is uncertain, consultation with a specialist should be considered.

ANAL CYTOLOGY

Following the visual inspection, anal cytology can be performed and cells collected, if indicated. If a referral source for abnormal cytology is available, annual anal cytology can then be provided to women considered in high-risk groups (e.g., immunosuppression of any etiology, those with a history of gynecologic HSIL or cancer).

With minimal training, anal cytology specimens can be collected by any licensed health care provider. Patients should be instructed to avoid douching, using enemas, or inserting anything into their rectum a minimum of 24 hours before the exam. Fewer cells exfoliate from the anus and this will increase the yield of cells for cytological evaluation. Health care providers should monitor their results for adequacy; the unsatisfactory rate should be maintained at less than 3%. Applying additional pressure, longer contact with the anal walls (compared with the cervical specimen collection), and longer agitation of the swab in the collection medium will all help improve the satisfactory rate of anal cytology.

ANAL CYTOLOGY STEPS

1. The woman can be positioned in any position that provides adequate visualization of the anal opening (e.g., left or right lateral or lithotomy).
2. Using a synthetic swab (e.g., Dacron or polyester), moistened with tap water. Avoid use of the cytobrush, which is unnecessarily uncomfortable.
3. Insert the swab approximately 3 to 4 cm into the anus; this will ensure that cells are collected from the distal rectum to the anal verge. If initial resistance is encountered, change the position or angle of the swab and re-insert. It may be helpful if the patient retracts the upper buttock while lying in a lateral position.
4. Gently, but with pressure, rotate the swab in a slow circular motion. This will ensure sampling from all aspects of the anal canal. The swab should be in contact with the anal mucosa with more pressure and more time as compared with cervical cytology collection.
5. Women have shorter anal canals, and the anal squamocolumnar junction may be just within the verge; therefore, be certain to maintain pressure and continue rotating the swab even as the tip of the swab is nearly out of the canal.
6. Agitate the swab in the liquid medium for at least 30 seconds, or if using conventional slides preserve the exfoliated cells quickly to avoid air-dried artifacts.

Following the visualized assessment and cytology collection, the DARE should be performed. This should be done annually or more frequently if needed. The DARE emphasizes palpation of the anal walls rather than just the distal rectum (as with a digital rectal examination [DRE]). Abnormal thickening, hard masses, and bright red bleeding evidenced on exam should be referred for HRA or, if unavailable, to simple anoscopy.

DARE Instructions

1. Mix a small amount of 2% to 5% lidocaine gel or cream into K-Y Jelly. Use this mixture to lubricate the gloved finger.
2. Gently insert a gloved and lubricated finger slowly into the rectum.
3. Apply firm pressure on the external sphincter, allowing it to relax before advancing into the rectum.
4. Once inside the rectum, carefully palpate the entire circumference. Beginning in the distal rectum, feel the mucosa over the internal sphincter and the walls of the distal anal canal.
5. Palpate for warts, masses, ulcerations, fissures, and focal areas of discomfort or pain with palpation.
6. Complete the examination by performing a perianal sweep noting any thickening or areas of hardness,

particularly in relation to any redundant tags or hemorrhoids.
7. Correlate findings with a visual inspection of the perianus.

■ SUMMARY

Populations of women who are at risk of anal HPV-associated pathology have been identified and health care providers should have a heightened awareness, to include the anus and perianus for clinical evaluation. Prevention of anal cancer is the best "treatment strategy" for anal cancer and this requires using a screening model similar to cervical disease. In 2010, the FDA added prevention of anal intraepithelial neoplasia (AIN) and anal cancer in both men and women as an approved indication for the quadrivalent HPV vaccine. It is hoped that this will have an impact on the natural history of anal HSIL and cancer for future generations.

■ ACKNOWLEDGMENT

The authors thank Natalie Watt, Genevieve Banaag, and Olivia Sims, BSN Honor Students at the University of Florida, for their contribution to the preparation and writing of this chapter. Gator Nursing!

■ REFERENCES

American Cancer Society (ACS). (2016a). *Cancer facts & figures, 2016.* Atlanta, GA: American Cancer Society.

American Cancer Society (ACS). (2016b). *What are the key statistics about anal cancer?* Retrieved from http://www.cancer.org/cancer/analcancer/detailedguide/anal-cancer-what-is-key-statistics

Ault, K.A. (2007). Effect of prophylactic human papillomavirus L1 virus-like-particle vaccine on risk of cervical intraepithelial neoplasia grade 2, grade 3, and adenocarcinoma in situ: A combined analysis of four randomized clinical trials. *The Lancet 369*(9576), 1861–1868.

Berry, J. M., Jay, N., Cranston, R. D., Darragh, T. M., Holly, E. A., Welton, M. L., & Palefsky, J. M. (2014). Progression of anal high-grade squamous intraepithelial lesions to invasive anal cancer among HIV-infected men who have sex with men. *International Journal of Cancer, 134*(5), 1147–1155.

Berry, J. M., Palefsky, J. M., & Welton, M. L. (2004). Anal cancer and its precursors in HIV-positive patients: Perspectives and management. *Surgical Oncology Clinics of North America, 13*(2), 355–373.

Blohmé, I., & Brynger, H. (1985). Malignant disease in renal transplant patients. *Transplantation, 39*(1), 23–25.

Busnach, G., Civati, G., Brando, B., Broggi, M. L., Cecchini, G., Ragazzi, G,...Minetti, L. (1993). Viral and neoplastic changes of the lower genital tract in women with renal allografts. *Transplantation Proceedings, 25*(1, Pt. 2), 1389–1390.

Castro, F. A., Quint, W., Gonzalez, P., Katki, H. A., Herrero, R., van Doorn L. J.,...Kreimer, A. R.; Costa Rica Vaccine Trial Group. (2012). Prevalence of and risk factors for anal human papillomavirus infection among young healthy women in Costa Rica. *Journal of Infectious Diseases, 206*(7), 1103–1110.

Centers for Disease Control and Prevention (CDC). (2011). General recommendations on immunization: Recommendations of the Advisory Committee on Immunization Practices. *Morbidity and Mortality Weekly Report, 60*(RR-2).

Centers for Disease Control and Prevention (CDC). (2013). Human papillomavirus vaccination coverage among adolescent girls, 2007–2012, and postlicensure vaccine safety monitoring, 2006–2013—United States. *Morbidity and Mortality Weekly Report, 62*(29), 591–595.

Centers for Disease Control and Prevention (CDC). (2015a). *Genital HPV infection: Fact sheet.* Retrieved from http://www.cdc.gov/std/hpv/stdfact-hpv.htm

Centers for Disease Control and Prevention (CDC). (2015b). *2015 Sexually transmitted diseases guidelines.* Retrieved from http://www.cdc.gov/std/tg2015/warts.htm

Chaturvedi, A. K., Engels, E. A., Anderson, W. F., & Gillison, M. L. (2008). Incidence trends for human-papillomavirus-related and unrelated oral squamous cell carcinomas in the United States. *Journal of Clinical Oncology, 26*, 612–619.

Chaturvedi, A. K., Engels, E. A., Gilbert, E. S., Chen, B. E., Storm, H., Lynch, C. F.,...Travis, L. B. (2007). Second cancers among 104,760 survivors of cervical cancer: Evaluation of long-term risk. *Journal of the National Cancer Institute, 99*(21), 1634–1643.

Chesson, H. W., Dunne, E. F., Hariri, S., & Markowitz, L. E. (2014). The estimated lifetime probability of acquiring human papillomavirus in the United States. *Sexually Transmitted Diseases, 41*(11), 660–664.

Chesson, H. W., Ekwueme, D. U., Saraiya, M., Watson, M., Lowy, D. R., & Markowitz, L. E. (2012). Estimates of the annual direct medical costs of the prevention and treatment of disease associated with human papillomavirus in the United States. *Vaccine, 30*(42), 6016–6019.

Chiao, E. Y., Giordano, T. P., Palefsky, J. M., Tyring, S., & El Serag, H. (2006). Screening HIV-infected individuals for anal cancer precursor lesions: A systematic review. *Clinical Infectious Diseases, 43*(2), 223–233.

Cranston, R. D., Hart, S. D., Gornbein, J. A., Hirschowitz, S. L., Cortina, G., & Moe, A. A. (2007). The prevalence, and predictive value, of abnormal anal cytology to diagnose anal dysplasia in a population of HIV-positive men who have sex with men. *International Journal of STD & AIDS, 18*(2), 77–80.

Daling, J. R., Sherman, K. J., Hislop, T. G., Maden, C., Mandelson, M. T., Beckmann, A. M., & Weiss, N. S. (1992). Cigarette smoking and the risk of anogenital cancer. *American Journal of Epidemiology, 135*(2), 180–189.

Darragh, T. M., Colgan, T. J., Thomas, C. J., Heller, D. S., Henry, M. R., Luff, R. D.,...Wilbur, D. C.; Members of the LAST Project Work Groups. (2013). The Lower Anogenital Squamous Terminology Standardization project for HPV-associated lesions: Background and consensus recommendations from the College of American Pathologists and the American Society for Colposcopy and Cervical Pathology. *International Journal of Gynecological Pathology, 32*(1), 76–115.

Davey, E., Barratt, A., Irwig, L., Chan, S. F., Macaskill, P., Mannes, P., & Saville, A. M. (2006). Effect of study design and quality on unsatisfactory rates, cytology classifications, and accuracy in liquid-based versus conventional cervical cytology: A systematic review. *Lancet, 367*(9505), 122–132.

Donovan, B., Franklin, N., Guy, R., Grulich, A. E., Regan, D. G., Ali, H.,...Fairley, C. K. (2011). Quadrivalent human papillomavirus vaccination and trends in genital warts in Australia: Analysis of national sentinel surveillance data. *Lancet Infectious Diseases, 11*(1), 39–44.

Dreyer, L., Faurschou, M., Mogensen, M., & Jacobsen, S. (2011). High incidence of potentially virus-induced malignancies in systemic lupus erythematosus: A long-term followup study in a Danish cohort. *Arthritis and Rheumatism, 63*(10), 3032–3037.

ElNaggar, A. C., & Santoso, J. T. (2013). Risk factors for anal intraepithelial neoplasia in women with genital dysplasia. *Obstetrics and Gynecology, 122*(2, Pt. 1), 218–223.

Goodman, M. T., Shvetsov, Y. B., McDuffie, K., Wilkens, L. R., Zhu, X., Ning, L.,...Hernandez, B. Y. (2008). Acquisition of anal human papillomavirus (HPV) infection in women: The Hawaii HPV Cohort study. *Journal of Infectious Diseases, 197*(7), 957–966.

Henley, S. J., Singh, S. D., King, J., Wilson, R. J., O'Neil, M. E., & Ryerson, A. B. (2015). Invasive cancer incidence and survival—United States, 2012. *Morbidity and Mortality Weekly Report, 64*(49), 1353–1358.

Heráclio, S. d. e. A., Souza, A. S., Pinto, F. R., Amorim, M. M., Oliveira, M. d. e. L., & Souza, P. R. (2011). Agreement between methods for diagnosing HPV-induced anal lesions in women with cervical neoplasia. *Acta Cytologica, 55*(2), 218–224.

Hogenwoning, C. J. A., Bleeker, M. C. G., van den Brule, A. J. C., Voorhorst, F. J., Snijders, P. J., Berkhof, J.,...Meijer, C. J. (2003). Condom use promotes regression of cervical intraepithelial neoplasia and clearance of human papillomavirus: A randomized clinical trial. *International Journal of Cancer, 107*, 811–816.

Hoy, T., Singhal, P. K., Willey, V. J., & Insinga, R. P. (2009). Assessing incidence and economic burden of genital warts with data from a US commercially insured population. *Current Medical Research and Opinion, 25*(10), 2343–2351.

Jacyntho, C. M., Giraldo, P. C., Horta, A. A., Grandelle, R., Gonçalves, A. K., Fonseca, T., & Eleutério, J. (2011). Association between genital intraepithelial lesions and anal squamous intraepithelial lesions in HIV-negative women. *American Journal of Obstetrics and Gynecology, 205*(2), 115.e1–115.e5.

Jay, N., Berry, J. M., Hogeboom, C. J., Holly, E. A., Darragh, T. M., & Palefsky, J. M. (1997). Colposcopic appearance of anal squamous intraepithelial lesions: Relationship to histopathology. *Diseases of the Colon and Rectum, 40*(8), 919–928.

Jay, N., Berry, M., Park, I., Rubin, M., Darragh, T., & Palefsky, J. (2012). *ASCUS cytology is highly predictive of high-grade anal intraepithelial neoplasia (HGAIN) in at-risk populations.* 28th International Papillomavirus Conference. San Juan, Puerto Rico.

Jiménez, W., Paszat, L., Kupets, R., Wilton, A., & Tinmouth, J. (2009). Presumed previous human papillomavirus (HPV) related gynecological cancer in women diagnosed with anal cancer in the province of Ontario. *Gynecologic Oncology, 114*(3), 395–398.

Khan, M. J., Castle, P., Lorincz, A. T., Wacholder, S., Sherman, M., Scott, D. R.,...Schiffman, M. (2005). The elevated risk of cervical precancer and cancer in women with human papillomavirus (HPV) type 16 or 18 and the possible utility of type-specific HPV testing in clinical practice. *Journal of the National Cancer Institute, 97*(14), 1072–1079.

Kojic, E. M., Cu-Uvin, S., Conley, L., Bush, T., Onyekwuluje, J., Swan, D. C.,...Brooks, J. T. (2011). Human papillomavirus infection and cytologic abnormalities of the anus and cervix among HIV-infected women in the study to understand the natural history of HIV/AIDS in the era of effective therapy (the SUN study). *Sexually Transmitted Diseases, 38*(4), 253–259.

Koppe, D. C., Bandeira, C. B., Rosa, M. R., Cambruzzi, E., Meurer, L., & Fagundes, R. B. (2011). Prevalence of anal intraepithelial neoplasia in women with genital neoplasia. *Diseases of the Colon and Rectum, 54*(4), 442–445.

Kreuter, A., Potthoff, A., Brockmeyer, N. H., Gambichler, T., Swoboda, J., Stücker, M.,...Wieland U; German Competence Network HIV/AIDS. (2010). Anal carcinoma in human immunodeficiency virus-positive men: Results of a prospective study from Germany. *British Journal of Dermatology, 162*(6), 1269–1277.

Likes, W., Santoso, J. T., & Wan, J. (2013). A cross-sectional analysis of lower genital tract intraepithelial neoplasia in immune-compromised women with an abnormal Pap. *Archives of Gynecology and Obstetrics, 287*(4), 743–747.

Madeleine, M. M., Finch, J. L., Lynch, C. F., Goodman, M. T., & Engels, E. A. (2013). HPV-related cancers after solid organ transplantation in the United States. *American Journal of Transplantation, 13*(12), 3202–3209.

Maktabi, H., Ludwig, S. L., Eick-Cost, A., Yerubandi, U. D., & Gaydos, J. C. (2013). Incidence of genital warts among US service members before and after the introduction of the quadrivalent human papillomavirus vaccine. *Medical Surveillance Monthly Report, 20*(2), 17–20.

Manhart, L. E., & Koutsky, L. A. (2002). Do condoms prevent genital HPV infection, external genital HPV infection, external genital warts, or cervical neoplasia? A meta-analysis. *Sexually Transmitted Diseases, 29*, 725–735.

Markowitz, L. E., Dunne, E. F., Saraiya, M., Chesson, H. W., Curtis, C. R., Gee, J.,...Unger, E. R.; Centers for Disease Control and Prevention (CDC). (2014). Human papillomavirus vaccination: Recommendations of the Advisory Committee on Immunization Practices (ACIP). *Recommendations and Reports: Morbidity and Mortality Weekly Report, 63*(RR-05), 1–30.

Moscicki, A. B., Ma, Y., Farhat, S., Jay, J., Hanson, E., Benningfield, S.,...Shiboski, S. (2014). Natural history of anal human papillomavirus infection in heterosexual women and risks associated with persistence. *Clinical Infectious Diseases, 58*(6), 804–811.

Moscicki, A.-B., Schiffman, M., Kjaer, S., & Villa, L. L. (2006). Updating the natural history of HPV and anogenital cancer. *Vaccine, 24*(Suppl. 3), S3/42–S3/51.

National Cancer Institute (NCI). (2014). *A snapshot of cervical cancer.* Retrieved from http://www.cancer.gov/research/progress/snapshots/cervical

National Cancer Institute (NCI). (2016). *Surveillance, epidemiology, and end results program.* Retrieved from http://seer.cancer.gov/index.html

Ogunbiyi, O. A., Scholefield, J. H., Robertson, G., Smith, J. H., Sharp, F., & Rogers, K. (1994). Anal human papillomavirus infection and squamous neoplasia in patients with invasive vulvar cancer. *Obstetrics and Gynecology, 83*(2), 212–216.

Paavonen, J., Jenkins, D., Bosch, F. X., Naud, P., Salmeron, J., Wheeler, C. M.,…Dubin, G. (2007). Efficacy of a prophylactic adjuvanted bivalent L1 virus-like-particle vaccine against infection with human papillomavirus types 16 and 18 in young women: An interim analysis of a phase III double-blind, randomized controlled trial. *The Lancet, 369*(9580), 2161–2170.

Palefsky, J. M., Holly, E. A., Hogebbom, C. J., Berry, J. M., Jay, N., & Darragh, T. M. (1997). Anal cytology as a screening tool for anal squamous intraepithelial lesions. *Journal of Acquired Immune Deficiency Syndromes and Human Retrovirology, 14,* 415–422.

Palefsky, J. M., Holly, E. A., Ralston, M. L., Da Costa, M., & Greenblatt, R. M. (2001). Prevalence and risk factors for anal human papillomavirus infection in human immunodeficiency virus (HIV)-positive and high-risk HIV-negative women. *Journal of Infectious Diseases, 183*(3), 383–391.

Penn, I. (1986). Cancers of the anogenital region in renal transplant recipients. Analysis of 65 cases. *Cancer, 58*(3), 611–616.

The President's Cancer Panel. (2014). *Accelerating HPV vaccine uptake: Urgency for action to prevent cancer.* A report to the President of the United States from the President's Cancer Panel. Bethesda, MD: National Cancer Institute.

Saleem, A. M., Paulus, J. K., Shapter, A. P., Baxter, N. N., Roberts, P. L., & Ricciardi, R. (2011). Risk of anal cancer in a cohort with human papillomavirus-related gynecologic neoplasm. *Obstetrics and Gynecology, 117*(3), 643–649.

Santoso, J. T., Long, M., Crigger, M., Wan, J. Y., & Haefner, H. K. (2010). Anal intraepithelial neoplasia in women with genital intraepithelial neoplasia. *Obstetrics and Gynecology, 116*(3), 578–582.

Saslow, D., Solomon, D., Lawson, H. W., Killackey, M., Kulasingam, S. L., Cain, J.,…Myers, E. R.; ACS-ASCCP-ASCP Cervical Cancer Guideline Committee. (2012). American Cancer Society, American Society for Colposcopy and Cervical Pathology, and American Society for Clinical Pathology screening guidelines for the prevention and early detection of cervical cancer. *CA: Cancer Journal for Clinicians, 62,* 147–172.

Scarinci, I. C., Garcia, F., Kobetz, E., Partridge, E., Brandt, H., Bell, M., …Castle, P. (2010). Cervical cancer prevention: New tools and old barriers. *Cancer, 116,* 2531–2542.

Shiels, M. S., Kreimer, A. R., Coghill, A. E., Darragh, T. M., & Devesa, S. S. (2015). Anal cancer incidence in the United States, 1977–2011: Distinct patterns by histology and behavior. *Cancer Epidemiology, Biomarkers & Prevention, 24*(10), 1548–1556.

Silverberg, M. J., Lau, B., Justice, A. C., Engels, E., Gill, M. J., Goedert, J. J.,…Dubrow, R.; North American AIDS Cohort Collaboration on Research and Design (NA-ACCORD) of IeDEA. (2012). Risk of anal cancer in HIV-infected and HIV-uninfected individuals in North America. *Clinical Infectious Diseases, 54*(7), 1026–1034.

Steinau, M. U. E., Hernandez, B. Y., Goodman, M. T., Copeland, G., Hopenhayn, C., Cozen, W.,…Saraiya, M. (2013). Human papillomavirus prevalence in invasive anal cancers in the United States before vaccine introduction. *Journal of Lower Genital Tract Disease, 4,* 397–403.

Stier, E. A., Sebring, M. C., Mendez, A. E., Ba, F. S., Trimble, D. D., & Chiao, E. Y. (2015). Prevalence of anal human papillomavirus infection and anal HPV-related disorders in women: A systematic review. *American Journal of Obstetrics and Gynecology, 213*(3), 278–309.

Suardi, E., Bai, F., Comi, L., Pandolfo, A., Rovati, M., Barco, A., …Monforte, A. D. (2014). Factors associated with HPV-DNA clearance in a cohort of HIV-positive patients: Role of cART and gender. *Journal of the International AIDS Society, 17*(4, Suppl. 3), 19717.

Sunesen, K. G., Nørgaard, M., Thorlacius-Ussing, O., & Laurberg, S. (2010). Immunosuppressive disorders and risk of anal squamous cell carcinoma: A nationwide cohort study in Denmark, 1978–2005. *International Journal of Cancer, 127*(3), 675–684.

Tatti, S., Suzuki, V., Fleider, L., Maldonado, V., Caruso, R., & Tinnirello, M. d. e. L. (2012). Anal intraepithelial lesions in women with human papillomavirus-related disease. *Journal of Lower Genital Tract Disease, 16*(4), 454–459.

Uyar, D., & Rader, J. (2014). Genomics of cervical cancer and the role of human papillomavirus pathobiology. *Clinical Chemistry, 60*(1), 144–146.

Watson, A. J., Smith, B. B., Whitehead, M. R., Sykes, P. H., & Frizelle, F. A. (2006). Malignant progression of anal intra-epithelial neoplasia. *ANZ Journal of Surgery, 76*(8), 715–717.

Williams, A. B., Darragh, T. M., Vranizan, K., Ochia, C., Moss, A. R., & Palefsky, J. M. (1994). Anal and cervical human papillomavirus infection and risk of anal and cervical epithelial abnormalities in human immunodeficiency virus-infected women. *Obstetrics and Gynecology, 83*(2), 205–211.

Winer, R. L., Hughes, J. P., Feng, Q., O'Reilly, S., Kiviat, N. B., Holmes, K. K., & Koutsky L. A. (2006). Condom use and the risk of genital human papillomavirus infection in young women. *New England Journal Medicine, 354,* 2645–2654.

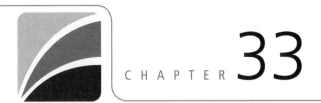

CHAPTER 33

Gynecologic Cancers

Barbara J. Silko • Leslie J. Heron

■ WOMEN'S EXPERIENCE WITH GYNECOLOGIC CANCER

Women's experience with cancer of the gynecologic tract can be life threatening and involves dramatic changes in their lives and lifestyles. There are multiple areas in which primary care providers can have a positive impact on the woman's experience with the prevention, diagnosis, treatment, and survivorship of a gynecologic malignancy. This chapter allows the reader to identify areas where primary providers of women's health care can have a major positive influence on women's knowledge of, and experience with, gynecologic cancer.

■ IMPORTANCE OF PRIMARY CARE RELATED TO GYNECOLOGIC CANCERS

In providing primary care to women, the advanced practice nurse is both educator and advocate. From prevention through diagnosis, treatment, and survivorship, both education and advocacy are essential for optimal outcomes of a potential gynecologic cancer.

Education

Primary prevention of gynecologic cancers begins with education. This may be the education of the patient about her anatomy, normal physiological function, and normal variations that are not a concern. It may also include education of the patient about prevention, screening, risk factors, and warning signs of cancer. Additionally, the advanced practice nurse may be involved in educating parents, schools, religious communities, cultural groups, health care organizations, and government bodies regarding the prevention needs of the patients in their care.

Education for the patient with a gynecologic cancer regarding the next steps in their care, including seeking specialist providers, the urgency of obtaining treatment, the expected diagnostic and treatment modalities that they may encounter, and even the need for routine health care during and after her cancer diagnosis is essential. This will assist the patient to have some sense of knowledge and control in an otherwise unfamiliar and fearful life situation.

Advocacy

The primary provider plays an important role as a patient advocate across the span of the disease spectrum from prevention through survivorship. Advocacy for health education, easy access to a broad range of women's health care services, the availability of affordable health care, and that all care be provided in a way that is respectful of the person continues to be the role of the advanced practice nurse.

False assumptions by health care providers regarding women's awareness of their bodies may limit the ability to effectively assess and examine a genital concern until it is past the point of primary treatment. Women and girls often lack adequate knowledge of their own body and its functioning. They may be unaware of what to anticipate with regard to normal age-related body changes, from puberty to menopause. If they are not sure what is "normal," they may be unable to identify normal versus abnormal states. Women's awareness of their bodies may be limited by individual, family, religious, societal, and cultural norms. Women's access to education about their bodies may be limited by financial, geographical, cultural, religious, and societal barriers. There may be limited access to books, education, health care providers, or types of health care services that are required. Personal history of physical, psychological, or sexual abuse may create fear and hesitation to seek care. Social stigma regarding the words used for female genitals, and an assumption that the use of these words is discouraged or shameful in general conversation, may also prevent girls and women from clearly speaking their concerns.

■ ACCESS TO, AND USE OF, WOMEN'S HEALTH SERVICES

Socioeconomic and Geographical Risk Factors

Women, as a population, are at greater socioeconomic risk, resulting in multiple disadvantages to accessing health care services (www.apa.org). Women's wages are routinely 66% to 77.3% of their male counterparts (www.apa.org). Women are more likely to be single parents and/or unpaid caregivers to family and community members in need. In 2013, the U.S. Census Bureau reported that there were about 15 million female heads of household, compared to 5 million male heads of household in the United States (U.S. Census Bureau, 2013). Working longer hours, or more than one job, to meet their economic needs places limits on the amount of time women have to access health care, especially during regular business hours. With limited childcare options, women may need to bring children into the examination room with them for health care visits. This may be a deterrent to seeking a women's health (pelvic) examination. Women heads of households are less likely to have disposable income to spend on health care, and are more likely to use those health care dollars for the care of their children rather than on themselves. Longer life expectancy for women compounds socioeconomic risk by limiting funds available for health care needs in old age.

In addition to socioeconomic issues, geography plays a role in access to health care. Women living in rural areas frequently commute long distances to access routine health care services. If there is a gynecologic concern requiring a specialist for diagnosis or treatment, the woman may need to travel as far as another state to obtain care. Up to 14.8 million women nationwide have difficulty with access to care centers that specialize in gynecologic cancers (Shalowitz, Vinograd, & Giuntoli, 2015). Limited access to gynecologic and oncologic specialized care may lead to delayed detection, misdiagnoses, incorrect chemotherapy or surgeries, incomplete treatment protocols, and limited follow-up after oncology treatment.

Social Stigma of Sexual Activity

Social stigma around sexual activity limits access to preventative and diagnostic gynecologic services. Parents may decline immunization against human papillomavirus (HPV) for their daughters due to worry of promoting promiscuity or denial that their child will eventually be sexually active and therefore will not be at risk of contracting HPV. Stigma that presenting to the clinic with any gynecologic concern might imply having been sexually active, and worry that symptoms might be related to a sexually transmitted disease (STD) may delay access to care for single and partnered women. A new onset of gynecologic symptoms may also imply sexual activity with multiple partners, or infidelity in a long-term relationship, leading to delayed evaluation of symptoms. There is lack of clarity regarding symptoms of STDs versus gynecologic cancers, time from exposure to symptom occurrence with HPV, low-risk versus high-risk HPV, and even with screening guidelines for gynecologic examinations and Pap testing (Lemieux, 2010).

Sexual Minorities

Lesbian, bisexual, and gender nonconforming women statistically present later for gynecologic concerns, including gynecologic cancers. Self-perception that routine gynecologic care is unnecessary if one is not seeking contraception, discomfort with the potential for discrimination by health care providers and staff, and decreased socioeconomic status all limit access to care (Carroll, 2015). There may be decreased sharing and trust in provider–patient interactions due to earlier visits with providers who are insensitive or uneducated around the needs of sexual minorities.

Many factors make this population of women at increased risk for gynecologic cancers. These include falsely assumed low risk for STD exposure, even though up to 90% of women who have sex with women report sex with a man at some point in their lifetime, and that there is a greater than 30% prevalence of HPV in women who have sex with women (Carroll, 2015). They are at increased risk of sexual victimization over their lifetime, yet may avoid both the medical and legal systems due to the fear of stigmatization. Gender nonconforming women may not feel engaged with their genitals and may not report if there are changes in tissues or menstrual patterns. There is also a correlation of increased risk for gynecologic cancers with increased body mass index (BMI), smoking, and alcohol intake, all which have been statistically associated with lesbian, bisexual, and transgendered populations (Carroll, 2015; Flemmer, Doutrich, Dekker, & Rondeau, 2012).

Religious and Cultural Factors

In many cultures and religions, women are discouraged from discussing gynecologic issues or being aware of their genitals. Information is passed down from one generation to the next, limiting new information regarding risks and symptoms of gynecologic cancers. There may be shame and a risk of being outcast for seeking knowledge outside of family or religious boundaries. Arranged marriages, marriage contracts, the importance placed on both virginity at marriage and on an ability to produce children all may impact women's patterns of seeking gynecologic care.

For non-English-speaking women, language barriers create yet another layer of risk for missed diagnosis of gynecologic conditions. Limited comfort with an unfamiliar or foreign medical system may delay access to care, and miscommunication may limit understanding of diagnosis, treatment, and referrals. The use of interpreters can assist in these situations, but is not always a complete solution. Patients may not feel comfortable speaking freely if the interpreter is a family member; a male; a part of, or not a part of their specific community or religion; or speaking a different dialect. These women frequently have compounded barriers, including lower socioeconomic status, transportation issues, limited knowledge of where or how to access care, and potentially, fear of accessing care due to undocumented residency.

Conclusion

Advanced practice nurses have a unique and vital opportunity to educate and advocate for the women in their care. Socioeconomic, sexual, religious, cultural, and other societal risk factors may limit trust of, and access to, gynecologic care. Knowledge and awareness of sociocultural risk factors will assist the primary care provider to effectively negotiate their patient interactions for gynecologic concerns.

■ DEFINITION AND SCOPE OF GYNECOLOGIC CANCERS

The risk for and incidence of gynecologic cancers is dependent on which of the gynecologic organs is affected. There are five major organs or sites for malignancy in the female genital tract: the vulva, vagina, cervix, uterus, and the ovary/fallopian tube/primary peritoneum. Each separate gynecologic organ cancer is diagnosed uniquely, and therefore the cancer treatment will vary by primary organ site. Women's experiences of the diagnosis and the treatment of their gynecologic cancer is likely to be related to the physical effects of the treatment as well as the emotional elements of having cancer of a female organ.

■ OCCURRENCE, DIAGNOSIS, AND TREATMENT OF THE CANCERS OF THE FEMALE GENITAL TRACT BY SITE

Vulvar Cancer

INCIDENCE/PREVALENCE

In the United States, vulvar cancer may affect up to 4,900 women per year (Elkas, Berek, Goff, Mundt, & Dizon, 2016) (see Table 33.1). The vulva refers to the external genital tissue that surrounds the clitoris, urethra, and vaginal opening (introitus), and extends from the midline of the clitoral hood, around the vaginal opening to the perirectal tissue. Often referred to as the labia majora and labia minora, the vulva serves to protect the structures of the urethra and introitus and is also capable of expanding and stretching significantly to allow for vaginal childbirth. The vulva is primarily a structure made of layers of skin and glandular tissue. The majority of vulvar cancers affect the epithelium or skin and therefore are treated similarly to other skin cancers of the body. The vulvar skin cells at risk for malignancy include squamous epithelial cells, basal

TABLE 33.1	Incidence of Gynecologic Cancers by Organ Site in the United States
Vulva	4,900 cases/yr
Vagina	4,070 cases/yr
Cervix	12,900 cases/yr
Uterus	54,870 cases/yr
Ovary	21,290 cases/yr

Adapted from Cancer.net, Cancer Facts and Figures (2015).

cells, and melanin cells. The majority of vulvar cancers are squamous cell carcinomas (Elkas et al., 2016). Squamous cell vulvar carcinomas may be related to underlying vulvar dystrophies, or more often may be related to HPV infection. Women may harbor or carry HPV for many years without a detectable lesion, though sometimes they may report that they had genital wart/lesions in the past. If the virus is present and active, and the woman's immune system or genital skin is compromised, it may be a trigger for the virus to become more virulent, causing cellular skin changes. More rare vulvar cancers include melanomas, basal cell carcinomas and glandular or adenocarcinomas, and sarcomas. Combined, these rarer vulvar cancers make up only approximately 10% of all vulvar cancers (Elkas et al., 2016).

SYMPTOMS

Symptoms of vulvar dysplasia, a precancerous lesion, can be a visible or a palpable lesion, or it can be an area of persistent itching, burning, or pain. The most common symptom is prolonged itching or pain in the vulva. Sometimes, a woman will report that she has noted a lump or bump that has persisted over time. Based on the somewhat vague symptoms and their location these lesions are frequently initially treated as a benign condition, such as a candidal infection or lichen sclerosus. However, if an irritating condition is related to either dysplasia or neoplasia, it will not get better with the treatment for either of those presumed benign etiologies. If a woman presents with persistent symptoms, which do not improve with topical over-the-counter or prescription treatments, the primary provider needs to perform a thorough examination of the vulvar skin, with a biopsy of any suspicious-looking areas. The skin may be erythematous, or whitish gray in appearance, and sometimes an ulcerative area is present. If there is a squamous invasive malignancy, the provider may note a nodular firm area at the site of the irritation, as this invasive carcinoma will infiltrate the lymphatic tissues, forming a mass, and will have potential to metastasize.

There are several rare types of vulvar cancers. Vulvar basal cell skin cancers resemble basal cell malignancies of other skin areas. They are typically pink, with raised edges, with a characteristic appearance of irritation, sometimes called a "rodent" lesion (Elkas et al., 2016). These lesions are usually well demarcated and do not invade deeply into the lymphatic tissue, and thus they do not typically metastasize. However, basal cell carcinomas may be associated with abnormal skin lesions in other areas of the body, and thus dermatology referral for a total body evaluation might be warranted. Other rare types of precancerous vulvar process affect glandular cells. These glandular dysplasias of the vulva are known as non-mammary Paget's lesions. These are noninvasive neoplasms, which become inflamed and roughened in appearance, and typically, women will report intense itching and irritation at the site of the lesion. The risk for recurrence is high in women with vulvar Paget's disease, and thus regular surveillance and follow-up are necessary (Fanning, Lambert, Hale, Morris, & Schuerch, 1999) with biopsy of any suspicious area. The Bartholin's gland in young women may become inflamed from an infectious process, but after age 40 years these glands rarely enlarge. Any woman older than 40 years presenting with an enlarged painful Bartholin's glandular process should undergo a thorough evaluation with biopsy to ensure that malignancy is ruled out.

Melanoma is the second most common malignancy affecting vulvar tissue (Elkas et al., 2016). As with melanomas in other parts of the body, vulvar melanomas are aggressive and must not be ignored. If a woman presents with a new or persistent skin discoloration that is dark blue or nearly black, this should be thoroughly evaluated and biopsied. Early diagnosis with biopsy and referral for surgical excision is the best chance for cure from any melanomatous lesion.

RISK FACTORS

Risk factors for vulvar cancers include, but are not limited to, old age, smoking history, HPV infection, immune system deficiency, and lichen sclerosus. Age is a risk factor, as about 85% of all vulvar cancers are diagnosed in women older than 50 years of age (Elkas et al., 2016). HPV-related skin changes of the vulva can be a risk factor for squamous cell vulvar cancer (Centers for Disease Control and Prevention [CDC], Division of Cancer Prevention and Control, 2013). The use of tobacco increases HPV-related premalignant changes of the vulva (Elkas et al., 2016). Women who have autoimmune disorders, HIV, or who are on any chronic immunosuppressive medications are at an increased risk for HPV-related vulvar disease (CDC, 2013). A benign chronic vulvar condition called lichen sclerosus may also increase a woman's risk for vulvar dysplasia or cancer (Cooper, Madnani, & Margesson, 2015). The various cell types of vulvar cancer may have different predisposing risk factors. Vulvar squamous epithelial cells are the most likely cells to be affected by either premalignancy or malignancy. The squamous cells of the vulva serve as the first line of defense and are thus often affected by skin irritants or viruses. A common potential threat to the vulvar tissue is HPV (WHO IARC, 2007). Multiple strains of HPV exist, and many are benign. However, there are several strains of HPV that are considered high risk and these have the potential to cause precancerous changes in the skin, which may lead to cancer if undetected and/or untreated (CDC, 2013) (Table 33.2). Skin-to-skin contact during sexual activity may expose a woman to HPV. HPV may be present but may go undetected, as often as there may be no visible or palpable lesion. Healthy intact tissue of the vulva is normally able to ward off the skin damaging effects of HPV, and women can be sexually active without any symptoms of HPV exposure. However, for some high-risk HPV types, it is harder for the body to resist infection with HPV, and genital lesions may arise. Vulvar squamous cell carcinomas are associated with strains 6, 11, 16, 18, and 33 (WHO IARC, 2007).

DIAGNOSIS AND TREATMENT

Diagnosis of vulvar cancer is dependent on pathological confirmation from a biopsy. The primary care provider can perform a punch biopsy of the suspicious area, or make referral to a gynecologic colleague for biopsy. The pathologist will make a diagnosis of the particular type of vulvar cancer. The patient should be referred to a gynecologic oncologist for further evaluation and planning for treatment.

Staging of vulvar cancer involves clinical examination and sometimes imaging (CT scans to detect enlarged lymph nodes) may be needed in planning for appropriate treatment (Table 33.3).

Treatment may include one or more modality, such as surgery alone, radiation alone, or surgery plus radiation and/or chemotherapy. Precancerous lesions are treated with surgical management, either CO_2 laser or surgical excision or a combination thereof. If there is no evidence of invasive disease and surgical margins are clear, a woman has an excellent prognosis for survival but will need close surveillance. Invasive vulvar cancers are treated with surgical excision with possible lymph-node dissection for staging and treatment. Survival rates from invasive vulvar cancers are based on the histological type of vulvar cancer and the stage of the disease at the time of diagnosis. Women with early-stage vulvar cancer have a very high likelihood of surviving to 5 years and beyond, whereas advanced-stage vulvar cancers that spread to distant nodes and/or organs have a higher risk of cancer recurrence. Women with a diagnosis of vulvar carcinoma will need close gynecologic surveillance for several years after treatment is completed.

TABLE 33.2	HPV Strains and Their Association With Gynecologic Organs
HIGH-RISK HPV STRAINS	**GYNECOLOGIC SITE THAT MAY BE AFFECTED**
16, 18, 31, 33, 35, 39, 45, 51, 52, 56, 58, 59, 66	Cervix
6, 11, 16, 18, 33	Vulva
16, 18	Vagina

HPV, human papillomavirus.
Adapted from WHO IARC (2007).

TABLE 33.3	Vulvar Cancer Stages
Stage I	Cancer confined to vulva; tumor is 2 cm or smaller
Stage II	Tumor is greater than 2 cm and remains confined to vulva
Stage III	Cancer spread to nearby tissue (anus, vagina, urethra) and/or lymph nodes of one side of body
Stage IV	Cancer has spread to both sides of body or to a distant part of the body

Adapted from Cancer.net, Cancer Facts and Figures (2015).

Vaginal Cancer

INCIDENCE/PREVALENCE

Vaginal cancer is the rarest of the gynecologic cancers. More than 4,000 women in the United States are diagnosed each year with vaginal cancer (Cancer.net, 2014b). The vagina refers to the canal or tube, which leads from the external vulvar tissue to the upper genital organs (cervix, uterus, ovaries, and fallopian tubes). Vaginal cancer can originate in the outermost layer of vaginal skin, called a squamous cell cancer, or the deeper glandular tissue, called adenocarcinoma. There are several rare types of vaginal cancer including melanoma (Frumovitz et al., 2010) and clear cell carcinoma, which may occur in women whose mothers took the drug diethylstilbestrol (DES) to prevent miscarriage (prescribed from 1940s up to the early 1970s; Verloop, Rookus, & van Leeuwen, 2000).

RISK FACTORS

Many risk factors associated with vaginal cancer exist. These risks include age greater than 60 years, HPV infection, history of precancerous lesions of the cervix or vagina, cigarette smoking, exposure to DES in utero, and altered immune system (Karem et al., 2015).

SYMPTOMS

Vaginal cancer may present as a symptom of an unusual discharge or discomfort in the pelvic or vaginal area. Frequently, women present with symptoms of irritation or burning inside the vagina. Women with vaginal cancer also commonly describe symptoms of pain and/or bleeding with intercourse. The vaginal mucosal skin may be discolored, abraded or ulcerated, and may be friable on examination.

DIAGNOSIS AND TREATMENT

As with vulvar cancers, the diagnosis of a vaginal cancer is made by examination and biopsy of the visibly or palpably abnormal vaginal tissue. Biopsy can be done in office with a punch or a Tischler instrument. Treatment of vaginal cancers is determined by the stage of the cancer (Table 33.4). Preinvasive, or early-stage vaginal cancer may be treated with laser surgery or surgical excision. Advanced-stage vaginal cancers may be treated with chemotherapy and/or radiation plus chemotherapy (Shah, Goff, Lowe, Peters, & Li, 2009).

TABLE 33.4	Vaginal Cancer Stages
Stage I	Tumor confined to the vaginal surface
Stage II	Tumor invades the wall of the vagina
Stage III	Cancer spreads to pelvic lymph nodes or pelvic wall
Stage IV	Cancer spreads to bladder, rectum, or beyond pelvis

Adapted from Cancer.net, Cancer Facts and Figures (2014b).

Cervical Cancer

INCIDENCE

Cervical cancers at one time were a common gynecologic cancer. Better screening has resulted in earlier detection of precancerous changes of the cervix, which has resulted in fewer diagnoses of invasive cervical cancer. Despite the decline in cervical cancer diagnosis, there are still approximately 12,900 women diagnosed with cervix cancer annually in the United States (Cancer.net, 2012). The cervix refers to the most external portion of the uterus; it is essentially the mouth of the uterine body. Only the outermost part of the cervix of the uterus is visible/palpable on clinical pelvic examination. The cervix contains both squamous and glandular cells, and cancer can affect either type of cell. The most external cells of the cervix are called the ectocervical cells, made up of squamous cells, and the most common cervix cancer is a squamous cell carcinoma. Glandular cells line the interior portion of the cervix, and these endocervical cells may develop an endocervical adenocarcinoma. Pap smears, which are a screening test for abnormal cells of the cervix, are ideally able to screen for both ectocervical and endocervical abnormalities. There are several rare cervix cancers, including neuroendocrine, small cell, and glassy cell carcinomas. These rare cancers are aggressive and usually very fast growing and prompt referral to gynecologic oncology is important.

SYMPTOMS

Symptoms of cervix cancer may or may not be present. Sometimes, cervix cancer is found when a woman has an abnormal Pap smear and the workup demonstrates cancer on pathology analysis. Other times the woman with cervix cancer will present for evaluation of new symptoms, such as pain or bleeding/spotting with intercourse. A woman may report abnormal menstrual pattern with intermenstrual bleeding or prolonged menstrual bleeding. Cervix cancer may be identified when a woman presents with a persistent foul-smelling vaginal discharge. Women with an advanced cervix cancer may also present with unexplained changes in bowel or bladder habits; unexplained pain in the pelvis, hips, back, or flank areas; or unilateral leg swelling and/or pain.

RISK FACTORS

Risk factors for cervix cancer are typically categorized according to the type of cervix cancer that is detected. Squamous cell carcinomas are the most common of all cervix cancers and these are highly associated with HPV infection, early coitarche, multiple sexual partners, cigarette smoking, and altered immune status. Cervical adenocarcinomas, which are the second most common of the cervix cancers, account for approximately 15% to 20% of all cervix cancers (Cancer.net, 2012). These glandular cell abnormalities are typically a more aggressive or faster growing abnormality. Risk factors for adenocarcinomas of the cervix include HPV infection and past birth control pill usage.

DIAGNOSIS AND TREATMENT

Guidelines for cervix screening have changed with advances in research on HPV. Primary and gynecologic care providers for women will want to consult with the published Pap smear guidelines to determine when to begin, and how often to obtain, screening Pap smears, and how to follow-up on the results (Lemieux, 2010; Limmer, LoBiondo-Wood, & Dains, 2014; Saslow et al., 2012) (Table 33.5). Abnormal or atypical Pap smears may be followed clinically, or may require a referral for a colposcopy, where the cervix can be evaluated under magnification to look for abnormal skin and vessel changes (American Congress of Obstetricians and Gynecologists [ACOG], 2012). The colposcopist will be able to provide a thorough evaluation of the cervical appearance and an opportunity for biopsy of any abnormal tissue. Precancerous cervical lesions can be effectively treated with noninvasive surgery, which can result in the prevention of cervix cancer. However, the woman treated for a precancerous lesion of the cervix requires a long-term close surveillance to ensure early detection of subsequent abnormal Pap results (Fields, 2013). According to the current guidelines, women with precancerous cervical changes will need to be examined every year for many years after the treatment is completed (ACOG, 2012; Feldman et al., 2015; Saslow et al., 2012).

Diagnosis of cervix cancer is based on the clinical findings of the pelvic examination and cervical biopsies. Neither Pap smears nor HPV testing are a diagnostic tool, although a Pap smear may detect an abnormality of the cervix, which in turn will lead to a more thorough investigation of the cervix, including HPV testing and/or a biopsy to determine if there is a high-risk HPV present or a precancerous or cancerous lesion of the cervix (Wright et al., 2011). If the biopsy confirms a cervix cancer, the stage of the cancer is based on the findings of the cervical lesion on pelvic examination (Table 33.6). Early-stage cervix cancers are confined to the cervix and are less than 4 cm in size. Advanced stages of cervical cancer are based on whether the tumor has spread to surrounding tissues, such as the vaginal walls, the rectum, or the bladder (Cancer.net, 2012).

Treatment of cervical cancer may involve surgery alone for an early-stage cancer. The surgery for a cervix cancer is a radical hysterectomy that includes surgery to remove the uterus and cervix, as well as the surrounding parametrial tissue of the vagina that could be at risk for a cancer spread. If the tumor is larger than 4 cm or if there is evidence of spread of the cancer beyond the cervix, the cancer will likely be treated with radiation therapy with or without radio-sensitizing chemotherapy. Sometimes, a patient with an advanced cervix cancer will have a surgical lymph node sampling in order to reduce the amount of tumor burden and/or to help in designing the radiation field for treatment. Cancer of the cervix that has spread beyond the pelvis will likely be treated with systemic chemotherapy.

Uterine Cancer

INCIDENCE

The most common of all gynecologic cancers is cancer of the uterus. The uterus, also called the womb, has a primary function to provide a place for a pregnancy to grow. The uterus is typically a small pear-shaped organ, but when it is supporting a pregnancy the uterus can enlarge to accommodate a full-term pregnancy and may occupy a large portion of the pelvis. The uterus is made up of the outer myometrium or muscle portion, and the inner endometrial or glandular lining of the uterus. Cancers of the uterus can affect either the endometrium or the myometrium. More than 54,000 women in the United States are diagnosed each year with uterine cancer (Cancer.net, 2014a). The endometrium, which comprises the inner lining or glandular portion of the uterus, is the area most often affected by cancer, and these endometrial adenocarcinomas account for more than 80% of all uterine cancers (Cancer.net, 2014a). A small percentage of endometrial cancers are a rare, serous carcinoma.

TABLE 33.5	Guidelines for Pap Smear Screening Among General Population
AGE GROUP	**RECOMMENDATION FOR SCREENING**
Women younger than 21 years	No Pap smear
Women 21–29 years	Screening with Pap cytology alone every 3 years
Women 30–65 years	Screening with cytology and HPV co-testing every 5 years
Women older than 65 years	No screening if no abnormal cytology (CIN 2+) in past 20 years
Posthysterectomy	No screening cytology if no past history of abnormal cytology (CIN 2+); if prior abnormal cytology (CIN 2 or 3 or cancer), will need long-term surveillance after hysterectomy

CIN, cervical intraepithelial neoplasia; HPV, human papillomavirus.
Adapted from Saslow et al. (2012).

TABLE 33.6	Cervical Cancer Stages
Stage I	Cancer has spread to the deep cervix lining but has not spread beyond the cervix
Stage II	Cancer has spread beyond the cervix to the vagina or adjacent tissue but still in the pelvis, no spread to lymph nodes
Stage III	Cancer has spread to the pelvic sidewall or distal or lowest part of the vagina
Stage IV	Cancer has invaded bladder or rectum, spread to distant parts of the body

Adapted from Cancer.net, Cancer Facts and Figures (2015a).

The second type of uterine cancer affects the myometrium, or outer muscle portion of the uterus, and they are referred to as sarcomas. Uterine sarcomas account for 2% to 4% of all uterine carcinomas (Cancer.net, 2014a).

SYMPTOMS

Women with endometrial cancer frequently present with postmenopausal spotting or bleeding. Perimenopausal or premenopausal women may report a sudden change in their menstrual cycle, such as very heavy or prolonged menstrual periods. Uterine cancer may also present as a feeling of pain, congestion, or pressure or cramping in the pelvis with or without bleeding.

RISK FACTORS

Risk factors for uterine cancer vary depending on where the uterine cancer originates. Several risk factors may increase the risk for endometrial carcinomas (Crosbie, Zwahlen, Kitchener, Egger, & Renehan, 2010). Women older than 60 years are at a higher risk of endometrial cancer than younger premenopausal women (Cancer.net, 2014a). Postmenopausal hormone therapy may increase a woman's risk for endometrial cancer (Grady, Gebretsadik, Kerlikowske, Ernster, & Petitti, 1995; Jaakkola, Lyytinen, Dyba, Ylikorkala, & Pukkala, 2011; Yuanyuan et al., 2014). Obesity is associated with endometrial cancer (Crosbie et al., 2010; Engel, 2014). A personal history of breast cancer and/or a family history of uterine or colon cancer may place a woman at an increased risk for uterine cancer (Lancaster, Powell, Chen, & Richardson, 2015). Stromal or myometrial tumors are rare and are not associated with particular risk factors.

DIAGNOSIS AND TREATMENT

Diagnosis of uterine cancer is made based on biopsy of the uterus either through an in-office endometrial biopsy or by intraoperative dilation and curettage (D&C) of the endometrial tissue. Once the biopsy has confirmed a neoplasm, which can range from preinvasive to invasive carcinoma, the woman should be referred to a gynecologic oncologist for evaluation and planning for treatment. Depending on the pathology and presenting symptoms, imaging—either a pelvic ultrasound or a CT scan of the chest/abdomen/pelvis—may be necessary to formulate a treatment plan.

Treatment for endometrial precancers and cancers almost always involves surgery. The type of surgery may depend on the level of abnormality diagnosed on the biopsy, and how much of the uterus and surrounding tissues are involved based on the imaging. Young women with precancers or low-grade neoplasms who are still interested in pursuing pregnancy may have the opportunity for conservative treatment. This conservative management may involve a therapeutic D&C to remove all of the abnormal endometrial tissue; then the woman is placed on hormonal management to reverse the process. She is monitored frequently and if the hyperplasia and/or atypia do not recur, she may be allowed to pursue a pregnancy. However, if the woman has completed childbearing when she is diagnosed with an endometrial neoplasm, she will likely be counseled to undergo hysterectomy for definitive

TABLE 33.7	Uterine Cancer Stages
Stage IA	Cancer confined to uterus lining, invading less than one half of lining-thickness
Stage IB	Cancer invades greater than one half lining-thickness, but is confined to the uterus
Stage II	Cancer has spread from uterus to cervix
Stage III	Cancer has spread from uterus to pelvis, such as lymph nodes
Stage IV	Cancer invades rectum or bladder, groin lymph nodes, or spreads from pelvis to distant part of body, such as lung

Adapted from Cancer.net, Cancer Facts and Figures (2014a).

management. If there is a true invasive endometrial cancer the treatment is surgical removal of the uterus (including the cervix) and the fallopian tubes/ovaries. The disease is staged based on the pathology results (Table 33.7). Early-stage low-grade neoplasms may be treated by surgery alone. Higher grade neoplasms or advanced-stage disease noted at the time of the initial workup will be treated with a full staging surgery, which would include complete hysterectomy, removal of the bilateral fallopian tube/ovaries, and dissection of the pelvic and para-aortic lymph nodes, followed by an adjuvant treatment, which may include chemotherapy, radiation, or a combination of chemotherapy plus radiation.

Cancers of the Ovary/Fallopian Tube/Primary Peritoneum

INCIDENCE/PREVALENCE

The ovaries are located in the pelvis on either side of the uterus. The fallopian tubes play a role in the transport of the eggs released from the ovaries to the uterus. The epithelial surface of the ovary, the inner epithelium of the fallopian tubes, and the lining of the pelvis are all made up of cells known as Müllerian cells. These cells arise from fetal gonadal stem cells (Dubeau, 2008). These Müllerian cells in any of the sites can develop epithelial carcinoma. The disease is identified based on where it originates, such as ovarian, fallopian tube, or primary peritoneal carcinoma. All of these carcinomas tend to behave similarly, and thus their treatment is similar. For simplicity, the term *ovarian cancer* will be used to refer to any of these cancers. Ovarian cancer affects 21,290 women in the United States annually (Cancer.net, 2015b) and 14,180 succumb to ovarian cancer per year. Epithelial ovarian cancers are the most common type of ovarian cancers, and these typically affect women older than 50 years of age (Cancer.net, 2015b). Another rare type of ovarian cancer, which is called a germ cell tumor, arises from within the ovarian egg or yolk sac. These tumors most often arise in young women aged less than 20 years (Billmire et al., 2004), and may be called a dermoid or teratoma. Germ cell tumors may be benign or malignant. Malignant germ cell tumors are diagnosed and treated with surgery alone or by a combination of surgery with chemotherapy.

SYMPTOMS

Ovarian cancer is most often detected after it has spread to an advanced stage (Andersen et al., 2008). The symptoms of ovarian cancer may be vague, as in pressure or discomfort or a sense of feeling full, or the symptoms may be more pronounced, such as significant pain or discomfort, bowel or bladder dysfunction, or even increased abdominal distention from a buildup of fluid in the pelvis. Occasionally, the symptoms of the neoplasm may be specific to one area, such as unilateral pelvic pain. Presenting symptoms of primary peritoneal tumors may be abnormal distention related to the accumulated pelvic fluid known as ascites (Urban, McIntosh, Andersen, & Karlan, 2003). Frequently, the woman with pelvic ascites describes symptoms of increased waist size, feeling full too fast (early satiety), and/or chronic sense of bloating (Slatnik & Duff, 2015). Primary and gynecologic providers are encouraged to discuss and assess any unusual pelvic symptoms and to work up persistent, unexplained symptoms for evaluation (Goff, Mandel, Melancon, & Muntz, 2004; Goff et al., 2012).

RISK FACTORS

Risk factors associated with ovarian cancer include age, obesity, family history, genetics, ethnicity, having a diagnosis of breast cancer, diagnosis of endometriosis, and never being pregnant (Cancer.net, 2015b; Lacey et al., 2006). Women with a strong family history of ovarian or breast cancer, or family history of cancer of the gastrointestinal (GI) tract (colorectal, stomach, pancreas, or liver) may wish to undergo genetic counseling and possible genetic testing (Pennington & Swisher, 2012). Risk factors for malignant ovarian germ cell tumors have not been clearly identified, though there is a higher risk among individuals with germ cell XY chromosomes combined with androgen insensitivity syndrome (Cancer.net, 2015b).

DIAGNOSIS AND TREATMENT

The majority of ovarian cancers are diagnosed when a woman presents with symptoms of an abnormal feeling in the pelvis. Due to vagueness of symptoms associated with ovarian cancer, the disease is often not detected until it is in its advanced stage, and thus it is often called "the silent killer" (Andersen et al., 2008). Early-stage ovarian cancers may be detected on a routine screening pelvic bimanual examination if there is nodularity or a firm mass on palpation. Women undergoing pelvic imaging for the workup of infertility may have an abnormality of their ovary and this may prompt referral to a gynecologic oncologist and result in an early-stage diagnosis. Pelvic ultrasound ordered to evaluate the adnexal structures may show a cystic or solid component within, or adjacent to, the ovary or fallopian tube. Women who are still ovulating may have ovarian follicular cysts with their cycle, and these may be enlarged and causing discomfort. Serial, short-interval follow-up ultrasounds and repeat CA-125 testing can be helpful in monitoring these ovarian cystic masses to ensure that these resolve with time. However, postmenopausal women, who no longer menstruate, should have small ovaries without cysts; thus, any cystic or solid mass in or near the ovary of an older woman should be evaluated by a gynecologic oncologist. A blood test of the tumor marker CA-125 may be obtained to determine if it is elevated in order to help in planning for management of a pelvic mass (Bast et al., 2005).

Treatment of ovarian cancers typically involves multiple modalities, including surgery and chemotherapy. Women will likely have a preoperative staging CT scan of the chest, abdomen, and pelvis to evaluate the pelvic structures, the lymph nodes of the pelvis and along the midline, and the omentum. If there is evidence of a significant amount of disease outside the pelvis at the time of the staging CT scan, the gynecologic oncologist may recommend initial treatment with three to four cycles of chemotherapy to reduce the disease volume and then take her to surgery to achieve optimal surgical results. Many women with ovarian cancer will undergo surgery first for debulking to reduce the burden of the tumor load to a very small residual volume, and then will receive chemotherapy to treat any remaining microscopic disease (Bristow et al., 2002). The success of placing the woman into remission after chemotherapy is positively influenced by the ability of the surgeon to reduce the disease to a volume of less than a centimeter at the completion of the surgery (Bristow et al., 2002). The staging is calculated based on where the disease is identified by the imaging as well as the pathology results of the surgery (Table 33.8). The patient and her gynecologic oncologist will set up a plan for treatment, which may include observation alone for stage I disease,

TABLE 33.8	Ovarian Cancer Stages
Stage IA	Cancer confined to one ovary or one fallopian tube
Stage IB	Cancer involves both ovaries or both fallopian tubes
Stage IC	Cancer of ovary or fallopian tube and pelvic washings are positive for malignant cells
Stage IIA	Cancer of ovary has spread to uterus or fallopian tube
Stage IIB	Cancer of ovary or fallopian tube has spread to rectum or bladder
Stage III	Cancer has spread to the pelvic organs, such as lymph nodes or omentum, or there are deposits of cancer on surface of bowel, spleen, or liver
Stage IV	Cancer invades spleen, liver, or is outside of the peritoneum to distant organ such as lungs

Adapted from Cancer.net Editorial Board (2013).

versus stage II to III and IV disease, which is treated with chemotherapy delivered either through an intravenous method or a combination of intravenous and intraperitoneal method (Cancer.net, 2015b).

■ PRIMARY CARE CONSIDERATIONS IN THE TREATMENT AND MANAGEMENT OF GYNECOLOGIC CANCERS

Screening and Diagnosis of Gynecologic Cancers

Nurses are trained in patient assessment from their first day of nursing school and continue to add to their skills with history taking, physical assessment, and patient care over years of patient interactions. With advanced practice training, nursing skills are both refined and expanded. Moving into the field of primary care allows the advanced practice nurse an opportunity to bring their expanded skill set to an ever changing population of patients with diverse and unexpected health care needs. Staying alert to key findings with each patient, from history to physical examination, will prevent missed diagnoses and build trust in the patient–provider relationship (Boxes 33.1 and 33.2).

Care of the Whole Person

Women facing gynecologic cancers continue to have responsibilities to their family, workplace, or school. Ask if there are family members or support people who should be invited in to medical visits. Offer assistance with Family Medical Leave Act (FMLA) paperwork or letters of support for reduced work hours or a leave of absence from school. Assisting patients with medical decision options that take their other responsibilities into consideration will go a long way to encouraging compliance with follow through on any plan of care.

Fertility Preservation

The suspicion of a gynecologic cancer leads rapidly to biopsy, diagnosis, and treatment. With every additional intervention, there is the possibility of disrupting fertility. Assessing the desire for future children is recommended for any patient of childbearing age, but becomes an essential assessment when there is the possibility of a gynecologic malignancy. Fertility preservation needs to be addressed before any treatment with the potential to affect fertility, including surgical biopsy, surgery, chemotherapy, and radiation exposure. Become familiar with the reproductive endocrinologists in your area and be ready to urgently refer a woman with a potential gynecologic cancer. Fertility preservation techniques may or may not be appropriate to initiate, but this decision needs to be made by the woman herself. Alternative

> **BOX 33.1   KEY COMPONENTS OF A SYMPTOM ANALYSIS: WHAT NOT TO MISS IN PRIMARY CARE**
>
> - Unexplained change in menstrual bleeding pattern
> - Any postmenopausal bleeding or spotting
> - Unusual vaginal discharge
> - Persistent vulvar/perineal discomfort or itching
> - Did not received HPV vaccine, or did not complete all three doses
> - History of abnormal Pap smears in the past
> - History of workup or surgery for abnormal Pap smears
> - Pain and/or bleeding with sexual activity
> - Family history of gynecologic, gastrointestinal, genitourinary cancers, or melanoma
> - Two office visits with persistent concern of abdominal or pelvic pain that has not resolved in more than 2 to 4 weeks, with or without treatment, warrants further assessment and workup, including pelvic examination, ultrasound of pelvis, and possible lab work

> **BOX 33.2   KEY COMPONENTS OF A GYNECOLOGIC PHYSICAL EXAMINATION: WHAT NOT TO MISS IN PRIMARY CARE**
>
> - Thoroughly palpate the abdomen and groin areas, noting any masses, firmness, or discomfort with examination
> - Evaluate any adenopathy of groin areas
> - Inspect external genital structures
> - Evaluate any skin lesions or discolorations with special attention to palpable thickened, nodular, or plaque-like lesions
> - Inspect vaginal tissues by gentle rotation of the speculum to allow for visualization of the superior and inferior vaginal tissue for any skin discoloration or ulcerations
> - Palpate for thickened or nodular areas on bimanual examination
> - Evaluate for size, shape, and density of pelvic organs

fertility options available post treatment will also be reviewed by the reproductive endocrinologist, allowing the woman to understand the full range of options available to her.

BOX 33.3 KEY DIAGNOSTIC STUDIES: WHAT NOT TO MISS IN PRIMARY CARE

- Pap smear
- HPV testing and typing
- Return, or referral, for colposcopy and biopsy if Pap result is abnormal
- Biopsy, or referral for biopsy, of any abnormal looking area of vulva or vagina
- Endometrial biopsy for abnormal bleeding pattern, including any postmenopausal spotting or bleeding
- If the cervix looks abnormal, obtain biopsy of abnormal tissue and an endocervical curettage; Pap is not diagnostic
- Ultrasound of the pelvis (transvaginal) to evaluate uterine endometrial stripe (thickness) or any endometrial lesions if there is abnormal bleeding pattern
- Ultrasound of the pelvis (transvaginal) if there is concern for persistent pelvic pain and/or palpable mass or "fullness" on examination

HPV, human papillomavirus.

TABLE 33.9	Vaccine Options for Gynecologic Cancer Prevention
HPV VACCINE	HPV STRAIN TARGETED
Cervarix	16, 18
Gardasil	6, 11, 16, 18
Gardasil 9	6, 11, 16, 18, 31, 33, 45, 52, 58

HPV, human papillomavirus.

Communication

It may be necessary to request medical records, laboratory results, and the treatment plan from the oncology team. Doing so will keep you informed regarding your patient's oncology care and will assist you in knowing if and when primary care assistance might be helpful. Symptom management, assistance with local referrals for counseling or family support services, and routine health care needs can be addressed by the primary care provider, even during active cancer treatment. Request records from the treatment providers themselves, to decrease the burden of care coordination on the patient.

■ PROMOTING PREVENTION OF GYNECOLOGIC CANCERS IN PRIMARY CARE

Role of the Advanced Practice Nurse

Advanced practice nurses, in their role as both educator and advocate, have an opportunity to assist patients in health promotion across their life span. Prevention of gynecologic cancers begins with role modeling body acceptance and providing a safe environment for women to address genital concerns.

Educating parents on timely administration and life saving potential of cancer preventing vaccines begins when the child is still in elementary school (Table 33.9). Encouraging girls from an early age to have a portion of their well-child examination independently in the room with their health care provider will set the expectation of their wellness visit being a safe opportunity to share information and concerns. Providing open and unbiased education regarding normal form and function of the genitals, sexuality, physical and psychological safety, and ways of avoiding STD set the stage for comfort and trust with health care providers. This trust will promote scheduling compliance for routine health screenings, willingness to ask questions, and comfort in seeking early consultation for genital concerns.

Risk Factors for Gynecologic Cancers

Some risk factors cannot be prevented. Genetic predisposition, in utero exposures to toxins and aging, for example, are out of our direct control. Educating women regarding these risks can assist them in seeking care without delay if they have a concern. Each area of the gynecologic tract has its own risks factors that can be prevented or attenuated (Cancer.gov). Advanced practice providers can advocate for lifestyle changes and educate regarding risk reduction.

VULVAR

Increased risk: Exposure to tobacco/nicotine; HPV exposure through unprotected sexual contact; repeated HPV exposure through multiple partners; history of autoimmune disorder; history of lichen sclerosus; long-term prednisone therapy; lack of HPV vaccination.

Decreased risk: No exposure to tobacco/nicotine; safer sex practices; timely vaccination with HPV vaccine (National Cancer Institute, 2015).

VAGINAL

Increased risk: DES exposure in utero; HPV exposure through unprotected sexual contact; repeated HPV exposure through multiple partners; lack of HPV vaccination; history of abnormal Pap cytology.

Decreased risk: Regular gynecologic surveillance; routine surveillance of abnormal Pap cytology; timely vaccination with HPV vaccine.

CERVICAL

Increased risk: Family history of pelvic cancers; DES exposure in utero; exposure to tobacco/nicotine; alcohol intake; HPV exposure through unprotected sexual contact; repeated HPV exposure through multiple partners; lack of HPV vaccination; history of abnormal Pap cytology; lack of surveillance for abnormal Pap cytology; exposure to other STD or sexual assault; cervical trauma; pelvic radiation; lack of HPV vaccine.

Decreased risk: No exposure to tobacco/nicotine; limited alcohol intake; safer sex practices; timely vaccination with HPV vaccine; regular surveillance with pelvic examination and Pap evaluation; routine surveillance for abnormal Pap cytology.

ENDOMETRIAL

Increased risk: Family history of pelvic and colorectal cancers; age older than 50 years; hyper-estrogen status, such as in obesity, polycystic ovary syndrome, nulliparity, unopposed estrogen replacement, and Tamoxifen use.

Decreased risk: Lower estrogen states generally decrease risk for endometrial cancer. Some of these include multiparity, late menarche, early menopause, oral contraceptive use, levonorgestrel-releasing intrauterine device (IUD), and combination estrogen and progesterone hormone replacement therapy.

OVARIAN

Increased risk: Between 30 and 50 years of age, there is a progressive increased risk for ovarian cancer, which slows after 50 years of age; obesity; nulliparity; fertility drugs without pregnancy; menopausal hormone replacement therapy; prolonged use of hormone replacement with sequential estrogen and progesterone; ovarian cysts; family history of breast, pelvic, and colorectal cancers.

Decreased risk: Oral contraceptives; tubal ligation; hysterectomy and salpingo-oophorectomy; regular surveillance with annual pelvic examinations.

■ GENETIC RISK FACTORS FOR GYNECOLOGIC CANCERS

Genetic Risk

Ovarian cancers were previously thought to be somewhat random in occurrence. With the advances made in unraveling the genetics of diseases, many ovarian cancers have been found to be associated with genetic traits identifiable in testing for specific genetic mutations. Genetic causes have been found for cervical, uterine, and endometrial cancers as well. Although there are many genetic traits and syndromes, there are three that are most frequently associated with gynecologic cancers: BRCA, Lynch syndrome, and Peutz–Jeghers syndrome (Table 33.10).

Genetic Counseling and Testing

Genetic counseling is a process to evaluate and understand a family's risk of an inherited medical condition. A genetic counselor is a health care professional with specialized

TABLE 33.10	Genetic Traits Associated With Gynecologic Cancers		
	BRCA 1 OR 2 MUTATION	LYNCH SYNDROME	PEUTZ–JEGHERS SYNDROME
Cervical			X
Uterine			X
Endometrial		X	
Ovarian/ fallopian	X	X	X
Primary peritoneal	X		

training in medical genetics and counseling (National Society of Genetic Counselors [NSGC], nsgc.org).

Women in your practice who should be encouraged to seek genetic counseling include those with a personal or family history of breast, ovarian, or uterine cancer at an early age, both breast and ovarian cancer diagnosed in the same person, or a family history of male breast cancer. Being of Ashkenazi Jewish descent has long been known as a risk factor for cancer, and there is some evidence that women of Hispanic and Caribbean heritage may be at increased risk as well (Cancer.gov). Women without these indications, but who have had a gynecologic cancer not fitting the risk profiles outlined earlier in this chapter may also benefit from genetic counseling.

Genetic counseling provides a venue for education and evaluation of risk. Genetic testing is not always appropriate once the assessment has taken place. Genetic testing is best done on the person who has had cancer. When that is not possible, testing can be done on other family members. With new knowledge regarding genetics, and seemingly ever expanding genetic testing possibilities, returning to a genetic counselor every 3 to 5 years is recommended for women with high-risk family histories but inconclusive findings or positive findings with unknown significance. There are many medical, ethical, and financial considerations involved in genetic counseling and testing, which are covered in Chapter 16.

■ SURVEILLANCE RECOMMENDATIONS FOR GYNECOLOGIC CANCERS

High-Risk Patient Surveillance

Women with a strong family history of cancer of the breast, uterus, or ovary should be referred for genetic counseling. The genetic counselor may recommend genetic testing, which includes evaluation for various genetic variants based on their specific family's cancer history. Women who carry a genetic variant that places them at a heightened risk for a specific cancer (such as breast or colon) may then be counseled to undergo high-risk surveillance for those cancers (Lebensohn, Kingham, Chun, & Kurian, 2011). Some women may have a strong family history of breast or gynecologic cancer but are found to be negative for genetic testing. If their family history is compelling, they may be advised to begin a regular high-risk surveillance pattern despite their negative test result. This will be recommended by their genetic counselor (Pruthi, Gostout, & Lindor, 2010).

If a woman is found to have an increased risk for breast, ovarian, or endometrial cancer, she may be counseled to consider chemoprevention, or to undergo risk-reducing surgery, including removal or ovaries and fallopian tubes, and hysterectomy (Finch et al., 2014; Lancaster et al., 2015). If a woman is interested in preserving her fertility options, she will be counseled to begin high-risk surveillance of her breasts and pelvic organs. High-risk gynecologic surveillance for these women will include being seen every 6 months for physical examinations, pelvic imaging, and blood work, as indicated by their genetic test result.

Women with Lynch syndrome are at increased risk for ovarian and/or endometrial cancer and will need to undergo yearly pelvic examination, pelvic ultrasound to evaluate the ovaries, uterus, and endometrial lining, and endometrial biopsy on an annual basis (Helder-Woolderink et al., 2013). Women found to be at increased risk for ovarian, fallopian tube, or primary peritoneal cancer will be counseled to undergo pelvic surveillance approximately every 6 months, including symptom screening, pelvic ultrasound, pelvic examination and screening blood tests for a tumor marker (Goff et al., 2012; Lacey et al., 2006). If a woman does not have access to a gynecologic oncology specialist, a primary care provider can provide high-risk surveillance in her local community. If surveillance detects an abnormality, the primary provider can then refer the patient to the gynecology oncology specialist in a timely manner.

Surveillance of the Cancer Survivor

Women who have been diagnosed and treated for a gynecologic malignancy will likely need close surveillance for several years after the completion of treatment. Many women will be followed by their gynecologic oncologist, but sometimes women may choose to be followed in their local community due to travel and cost issues, or because they have a trusting relationship with their primary provider. The primary care provider may see such women for surveillance as the sole provider or in conjunction with the gynecologic oncologist in an alternating fashion. Depending on their particular gynecologic diagnosis, the long-term follow-up may vary but will usually include examination, imaging, blood work, and possibly Pap smear surveillance.

Vulvar and Vaginal Cancer Posttreatment Surveillance

Women with vulvar and vaginal dysplasia (precancerous conditions) will require close surveillance for several years. Surveillance should include thorough examination of the vulva, vagina, and cervix every 3 months for the

first year after treatment, and then, as long as there is no recurrence, visits can be extended out to every 6 months for several years. Pap smears may be indicated yearly for evaluation of the lower genital tract, though this may vary based on whether the patient has undergone earlier hysterectomy and/or whether she has had an earlier abnormal Pap smear. The provider will need to follow the algorithm for abnormal Pap smear follow-up based on the most current ACOG guidelines for Pap surveillance. Women diagnosed with either stage I invasive vulvar or stage I invasive vaginal cancer are typically treated with surgery alone, and may be followed in their local community for surveillance. There are no clear guidelines for extended follow-up of these cancers. With extrapolation from the recommendations for the follow-up of cervical cancer, the suggestion is for vulvar and vaginal examination every 3 months for the first year and then every 6 months until they are 5 years from diagnosis (Salani et al., 2011). Women diagnosed with advanced-stage vulvar or vaginal cancer will likely undergo surgery and receive adjuvant treatment, including radiation and/or chemotherapy. The gynecologic oncology team will direct the long-term follow-up of these advanced cancers.

Cervical Cancer Posttreatment Surveillance

Cervical dysplasias (precancerous lesions) require long-term surveillance with pelvic examinations and Pap smears and/or HPV testing every 6 months for 1 to 2 years and then every year for many years according to the guidelines (ACOG, 2014; ASCCP, 2014; Huh et al., 2015). Women with early invasive cervix cancers that are stage I and treated with surgery alone will require pelvic examinations and Pap smears every 3 months for 1 year, then examinations with Pap smears every 6 months until they are 5 years from their surgery. If a woman is diagnosed with an advanced cervix cancer, which requires adjuvant treatment such as chemotherapy and/or radiation, she is considered at increased risk for recurrence and her gynecologic oncologist will likely follow her closely. If she elects to follow-up with her primary provider it will be important that the primary provider have a clear understanding of the oncologist's recommendations for follow-up.

Endometrial Cancer Posttreatment Surveillance

Women diagnosed with early-stage endometrial cancer are often treated with surgery alone and may be followed in their primary care setting. They will need to undergo thorough examination of the vagina and bimanual examination of the pelvis every 6 months for the first year and then will need to have yearly gynecologic examinations. No Pap smears are required after hysterectomy for endometrial cancer (Salani et al., 2011). Advanced-stage endometrial cancers will be treated with both surgery and adjuvant treatment, such as radiation and/or chemotherapy. Women with advanced endometrial cancer are likely to be followed by the gynecologic oncologist at least for the first several years after completion of treatment, until the risk of recurrence starts to decrease. The woman treated with radiation for endometrial cancer may experience complications from radiation treatment and the primary provider may need to refer her for follow-up with specialists in either urology or gastroenterology.

Ovarian Cancer Posttreatment Surveillance

Young women diagnosed with ovarian germ cell tumors will undergo surgery and may receive chemotherapy. They will be followed by their gynecologic oncologist during their highest risk for recurrence, the first 1 to 2 years post treatment. As their risk for recurrence decreases, they will likely be referred back to their primary care setting. Long-term surveillance for young women with history of germ cell tumor would include yearly pelvic examinations and blood work to test for tumor markers (Billmire et al., 2013).

Women diagnosed with stage I ovarian epithelial cancer have an excellent prognosis. Initially, they are likely to be followed by the gynecologic oncologist every 3 to 6 months for the first 2 years, and then they may be referred back to primary care for clinical examinations, blood work, and pelvic imaging (if they have a retained contralateral ovary). After 2 years, stage I ovarian cancer survivors are seen every 6 months until they are 5 years from their diagnosis. After 5 years of close surveillance they return to annual follow-up with yearly pelvic examinations and CA-125 testing (Salani et al., 2011). Women diagnosed with stages II, III, or IV epithelial cell ovarian cancers will be followed closely by their gynecologic oncologist after treatment, as there is a high risk for recurrence.

One important component of the posttreatment surveillance for all women diagnosed with ovarian cancer is to recommend genetic counseling and possible testing. Women diagnosed with ovarian cancer who are found to be genetic mutation carriers may be offered additional modalities of treatment and possible chemoprevention options, which may prolong their disease-free state (McLaughlin et al., 2013).

■ SYMPTOM MANAGEMENT DURING TREATMENT FOR GYNECOLOGIC CANCER

Managing Treatment-Related Symptoms

Most patients undergoing cancer treatment will be under the direct care of their oncology team and will have their treatment-related symptoms managed by their oncologist, radiation oncologist, or surgeon. In some cases, such as in more rural areas, patients may seek assistance from their primary care provider. It is always appropriate to request chart notes and treatment information from the oncology team for coordination of care. Reaching out to the oncology team for assistance with symptom management will assure that the patient is receiving the most appropriate treatment, that treatments will not interfere with oncology agents, and that therapies are not being duplicated. The primary

symptoms for patients undergoing active gynecologic cancer treatment are pain, nausea, hot flashes, radiation-related skin issues, and fatigue.

PAIN

Pain may be because of surgery or the cancer itself. Acute surgical pain needs to be addressed by the surgical provider. Cancer-related pain management often requires escalating doses of narcotic pain medicines and is not routinely managed in primary care. If the on-treatment cancer patient is seeking narcotic pain control from the primary care provider, communicating with the treatment team is the most appropriate action to initiate. Offering referrals for complementary therapies, such as massage, reflexology, acupuncture, reiki, meditation, and hypnosis can assist the patient with pain management and will not interfere with cancer treatments.

NAUSEA

Nausea and other GI symptoms may be due to chemotherapy, inflammation from radiation, or tumor burden. Medication management for nausea is best done by, or through consultation with, the oncology team. There is strong evidence to support the use of acupuncture for chemotherapy-related nausea, and acupressure, guided imagery, hypnosis, and music therapy can also be effective. Ginger has anti-nausea properties and can be used as a tea, chew, or in a powdered capsule form.

HOT FLASHES

Hot flashes, also called vasomotor symptoms, during gynecologic cancer treatment are caused by the disruption in estrogen production that occurs with surgery, chemotherapy, or radiation of the reproductive organs. Some women who have already gone through natural, age-related menopause report a recurrence of hot flashes with cancer treatment. Treatment with supplemental estrogen can be helpful, but should have approval from the oncology team as it may be contraindicated with some diagnoses or treatments. Supportive care with acupuncture, acupressure, and layered clothing, as well as stress reduction techniques, such as breathing exercises and meditation, are effective for many women.

RADIATION DERMATITIS

The most common radiation-related skin condition is radiation dermatitis. This may begin two or more weeks after the start of radiation therapy and may last 6 or more weeks after completion of treatment (Lacouture, 2012). Itching, pain, swelling, redness, dryness, and even blistering may occur. Encourage patients to use cool to lukewarm water and gentle soaps without fragrance for washing, to wear loose-fitting, light cotton clothing, and to avoid direct sun exposure. Topical corticosteroids, aloe, and fragrance-free moisturizers can be used over intact skin. Topical antibiotics may be used on open or peeling areas. Check with the radiation oncology team before using any antioxidant supplements, as these may protect cancer cells as well as healthy cells and thereby limit the therapeutic effect of radiation.

MUCOSITIS

Mucositis is another condition that can be caused by radiation and chemotherapy. Mucositis can affect the mucosa of the mouth, esophagus, genitals, intestines, and rectum. Soft, bland foods, cool or lukewarm beverages, and supportive care with pain-relieving mouthwashes may be helpful. Mucositis may be more severe, and there is increased risk of secondary infection, when radiation is combined with chemotherapy. Contact the oncology team for assistance if mucositis is severe, if eating or elimination is affected, or if there are symptoms of infection.

FATIGUE

Fatigue is the most common side effect reported by cancer patients and cancer survivors alike. Fatigue is multifactorial and may be caused by stress, depression, or cancer treatments, and may be related to an inflammatory reaction to the cancer itself (Cavallo, 2014). Cancer-related fatigue is treated symptomatically the way non-cancer-related fatigue is treated, but it does not rebound or reverse as easily. Rest, supportive nutrition and hydration, and stress reduction are essential for fatigue management. Daily exercise is to be encouraged, even if only slow walking, stretching, or gentle yoga is tolerated. Encouraging realistic time management allowing for balance of activity and rest may be the best recommendation for fatigue management during and after active cancer treatment.

■ SYMPTOM MANAGEMENT FOR SURVIVORS OF GYNECOLOGIC CANCER

Cancer Survivorship

The National Coalition for Cancer Survivorship (NCCS) has defined cancer survivorship as "the process of living with, through, and beyond cancer" (NCCS, 2014). By this definition, cancer survivorship begins at diagnosis and extends to the end of life. It includes people who continue to have treatment to either reduce risk of recurrence or to manage chronic disease, and is inclusive of family members or caregivers of the person diagnosed with cancer. In this section of the text, we focus on care of the person diagnosed with cancer after their acute treatment phase has been completed.

More people than ever before are surviving cancer. With advances in prevention, screening, detection, treatment, and research, cancer survivors numbered an estimated 15.5 million in the United States as of January 2016. That number is expected to increase to 20 million by 2026 (ACA, 2016; Miller et al., 2016), with approximately 8% of those being survivors of cervical, uterine, or ovarian cancers (Cancer.net, 2013).

In 2005, the Institute of Medicine published a report titled *From Cancer Patient to Cancer Survivor: Lost in Transition* (Hewitt, Greenfield, & Stovall, 2005). This report made several recommendations to assist patients and health care providers with the transition from active treatment to cancer survivorship. Slowly, in response to this report, survivorship services are being mandated, developed, and expanded in cancer centers across the United States. Documents called treatment summaries and survivorship care plans are being created with the intent of providing a summary of treatment as well as information on potential long-term and late effects of that treatment, risk surveillance, lifestyle recommendations, and resources for cancer survivors and their non-oncology health care providers.

Transition to a Shared Care Model

Although actively on cancer treatment, patients look to their oncology team for the majority of their care. The oncology team may see the patient on a weekly or even a daily basis, and may temporally assume management of chronic medical conditions. As treatment ends, many cancer survivors continue to consider their cancer specialists as their main care providers (Chubak et al., 2014). Even though the oncology provider will see the survivor back for surveillance and monitoring, even for many years after treatment, they do not provide primary care. Many cancer survivors do not comprehend the need to transition back to primary care, or the concept of shared care, at the end of cancer treatment. Patients lose trust in the ability of a primary care provider to manage the complexities of their care after a life-threatening diagnosis (Chubak et al., 2014). Over time, some patients will become lost to follow-up for any care, as they are released from the care of their oncologist but do not return to primary care. Cancer survivors are frequently not up to date on routine age-related health screenings, preventative interventions such as immunizations, or monitoring of chronic conditions, such as high blood pressure, due to this loss of connection to primary care during and after cancer treatment.

As primary care providers, advanced practice nurses have the opportunity to continue providing care to their patients during and after cancer treatment, promoting a shared care model with the oncology team. Advocating for communication with the oncology team throughout active treatment and after treatment with a treatment summary and survivorship care plan will build trust and confidence in this shared care model. By educating patients regarding the need to maintain a connection to primary care, and educating themselves regarding symptom management during and after treatment, advanced practice nurses will be ready to assist their patients as they transition from cancer patient to cancer survivor.

Physical Symptom Management

LONG-TERM AND LATE EFFECTS

Cancer treatments can cause acute, long-term, and late effects. Acute symptoms are generally addressed by the oncology team and resolve shortly after treatment ends (see

Managing Treatment-Related Symptoms discussed earlier). Long-term effects begin during the treatment phase and persist after treatment ends. Fatigue and peripheral neuropathy are classic long-term effects. Late effects may not be evident for years after treatment ends. Cardiomyopathy, osteoporosis, and secondary cancers are a few examples of known late effects. Some effects, such as peripheral neuropathy, may completely resolve over time, while others, such as infertility, will not. Some effects, such as cardiomyopathy and metabolic syndrome can be prevented or attenuated with lifestyle measures.

Long-term and late effects are dependent on the type of treatment, total dose or exposure, and targeted region of cancer therapy. Table 33.11 demonstrates common long-term and late effects from treatments used for gynecologic cancers.

Systematic Treatment of Symptoms

Treatment of reversible long-term and late effects begins with symptomatic and supportive care. Adequate rest, nutrition, hydration, and exercise are routinely the best measures for all body-system symptom management after cancer treatment. Primary care providers will need to assess for underlying issues that may interfere with a woman's ability to manage the long-term effects after cancer treatment. The primary provider will want to look for factors that affect her ability to acquire adequate sleep, such as anxiety; that affect her ability to maintain adequate nutrition and hydration, such as nausea; or that may affect her ability to exercise, such as pain or fatigue. Identifying and treating these underlying issues will help move her toward self management and a sense of control in her adjustment to the role of cancer survivor.

VISION/ORAL

Dry eyes can be treated with lubricating drops or artificial tears. Dry mouth is reduced by staying well hydrated, although this may not be fully effective. Gum recession and dental caries should be assessed and if indicated primary providers will want to encourage and promote routine dental care with a dental professional.

CARDIAC/RESPIRATORY

Cardiac and respiratory late effects are best managed with awareness and prevention. A progressive exercise program,

TABLE 33.11	Long-Term and Late Effects of Cancer Treatment by Body System		
AFFECTED AREA	**SURGERY**	**RADIATION**	**CHEMOTHERAPY**
Vision/eye			Dry eyes
Oral/teeth			Dry mouth, dental carries
Cardiac	Lower extremity edema and varicosities	Pelvic and leg lymphedema, atherosclerosis	Cardiomyopathy, congestive heart failure, hypertension, hyperlipidemia
Respiratory			Restriction, cough, fatigue with exertion
Gastrointestinal	Adhesions, bowel changes	Colitis, proctitis, chronic nausea	Colitis, irritable bowel syndrome, nausea, food intolerances
Hepatic		Altered function, secondary cancers	Altered liver function
Urological	Adhesions, incontinence, urgency, urinary frequency	Altered kidney function, urinary incontinence, urgency, urinary frequency, cystitis, secondary cancer	Altered kidney function, cystitis, hematuria, urinary tract infections
Pelvis	Infertility, adhesions, incontinence, lymphedema	Infertility, adhesions, incontinence, lymphedema, atrophic vaginitis, dyspareunia	Infertility, atrophic vaginitis, dyspareunia
Musculoskeletal	Incontinence, adhesions	Osteoporosis, adhesions, contractures, myalgia, arthralgia	Muscle wasting, myalgia, arthralgia
Skin	Adhesions	Adhesions, secondary cancer	Dry skin, urticaria
Endocrine	Infertility, menopause	Infertility, menopause, hypothyroid, fatigue	Metabolic syndrome, infertility, fatigue, menopause
Neurological	Pain, paresthesia	Pain, paresthesia, fatigue	Tinnitus, pain, peripheral neuropathy, fatigue, cognitive dysfunction

potentially guided by a physical therapist, and use of compression garments can prevent or stabilize lymphedema and assist with edema and varicosities. Exercise and a heart healthy diet can prevent hypertension, hyperlipidemia, and help delay or attenuate atherosclerosis, cardiomyopathy, and congestive heart failure. Exercise assists with respiratory restriction and symptoms of fatigue. Smoking cessation is essential, and prevention of respiratory illness with pneumonia and influenza vaccines is recommended. Careful cardiovascular and respiratory evaluation, to include lipid, blood pressure, and vascular evaluation, is encouraged with an annual well-physical examination.

GASTROINTESTINAL

GI symptoms caused by adhesions may be improved with massage and yoga. Constipation, loose stools, fecal incontinence, and colitis symptoms often respond to soluble fiber and probiotics. Dietary changes, stress reduction strategies, and acupuncture may also be successful in addressing these conditions. Referrals to specialists, such as a naturopath, nutritionist, physical therapist, massage therapist, and gastroenterologist can assist in the management of GI symptoms. If liver function tests remain abnormal at the end of cancer treatment, referral to gastroenterology is indicated. Urological symptoms of adhesions, pain, or incontinence may be reduced with pelvic floor physical therapy, core exercises, and massage therapy. Altered kidney function, hematuria, interstitial cystitis, and other conditions may require the assistance of a urology specialist.

PELVIC

Pelvic symptoms of incontinence and adhesions are well managed with assistance from massage and physical therapy. Atrophic vaginitis after treatment for gynecologic cancers can be managed with systemic estrogen replacement and/or vaginal estrogen. In some situations, systemic estrogen replacement may be contraindicated, but frequently vaginal estrogen may be allowed. Consult with the treating oncologist or a gynecologist if you are unsure if estrogen is contraindicated for your patient. Non-estrogen vaginal moisturizers are also available and these products can be used independently or in conjunction with estrogen products to assist with both function and comfort of vulvar and vaginal tissues. Dyspareunia related to hormone deficiency or radiation-induced vaginal atrophy can be managed with pelvic floor physical therapy, consistent use of a vaginal dilator well lubricated with a vaginal moisturizer or a water-based lubricant three or more times a week, and relaxation techniques. The addition of a small amount of viscous lidocaine may be added to water-based lubricants for use with the vaginal dilator as well. Counseling may be helpful if there is posttraumatic stress, persistent pelvic pain, body image, or sexuality concerns after gynecologic cancer treatments that are not resolving.

SKELETAL

Osteoporosis is a risk with both radiation exposure and reduction in estrogen production. Prevention with resistance exercise, adequate dietary and/or supplemental calcium, and supplemental vitamin D is advised. A bone density (dual-energy x-ray absorptiometry [DEXA]) examination and vitamin D level are recommended at the completion of cancer treatment to assess baseline risk status. Follow-up at least yearly with assessment of exercise participation, calcium, and vitamin D intake. Repeat assessment of vitamin D level and DEXA can be done every 1 to 5 years, depending on baseline study results. Myalgia, arthralgia, adhesions, and weakness can be addressed with physical therapy, massage, acupuncture, nutrition, and exercise.

INTEGUMENT

Dry skin, skin sensitivity, urticaria, and rash are common after cancer treatments. Routine use of fragrance-free moisturizes and gentle soaps are often enough to reduce symptoms. After radiation exposure, cancer survivors are at increased risk for various skin cancers in their radiation field. Sunscreen use and avoiding prolonged direct sun exposure is encouraged. Dermatological evaluation of the radiation field is recommended yearly and is needed for evaluation and treatment of other skin conditions after cancer treatments. Hair loss in the radiation field may persist for months or years after treatment.

ENDOCRINE

Endocrine changes with cancer treatments may be acute, such as with surgical menopause, or late, with changes in thyroid function or risk of metabolic syndrome. Symptomatic management of hot flashes, osteoporosis risk, and fatigue, as outlined earlier, assist with acute or long-term effects. Monitoring annually for hypothyroidism, hypertension, and hyperlipidemia are recommended over the lifetime of the cancer survivor.

INFERTILITY

Infertility is likely, but not consistently an outcome of radiation and/or chemotherapy exposure. Avoidance of pregnancy for one full year after cancer treatment is recommended, and contraception is advised if there is the potential for pregnancy in that time. A fertility evaluation, which includes ultrasound evaluation of the reproductive organs, laboratory evaluation of hormone levels, physical examination, and a consultation with a reproductive specialist is recommended if the survivor of gynecologic cancer is interested in childbearing. The support of a mental health counselor or support group may be helpful if there is a sense of grief around loss of fertility.

PAIN

Symptom management of post-cancer pain includes massage, physical therapy, acupuncture, acupressure, guided imagery, hypnosis, meditation, exercise, counseling, and distraction. Medications, such as anti-inflammatories, nonnarcotic pain relievers, muscle relaxants, antidepressants, anticonvulsants, and narcotic pain relievers may be appropriate for some patients. It is good to remember that this pain may be temporary or chronic, and treatments need to be monitored and re-assessed for appropriateness over time. Treatment of chronic post-cancer pain is not managed with escalating doses of narcotics the way cancer pain is treated, but with symptomatic and supportive care. Narcotics are used sparingly and in stable doses, as in a classic chronic pain model (Davies & D'Arcy, 2013, p. 294). Referral to a pain management specialist is recommended if assistance is needed for chronic pain management.

NEUROPATHY

Peripheral neuropathy naturally decreases over the first few years after cancer treatment, but may never fully resolve. Excellent supportive care assists in symptom reduction over time. Massage, acupuncture, nutritional support, and exercise are effective in the reduction of symptoms for many cancer survivors. Physical and occupational therapy may be needed if balance concerns create a fall risk for survivors with persistent lower extremity neuropathy.

COGNITIVE DYSFUNCTION

Cognitive dysfunction, often referred to as "chemo brain," is common in cancer survivors, but a specific cause has not been found. Cognitive dysfunction is related to the inflammatory response in the body to cancer, to cancer treatments, to stress, and to individual predisposition due to age, cognitive reserve, and genetics (Meadows, 2014). Reports of cognitive dysfunction range from mild, intermittent word finding concerns to complete memory blocks. Inability to organize and prioritize tasks may alter the ability to return to previous employment, and decreased short-term memory may severely alter the ability to learn new skills. As with other survivorship symptoms, supportive care and time generally improve cognitive function. Compensatory devices, such as keeping appointment reminders in a notebook or cell phone, mapping the route and list of errands to run, and having a routine for work-related tasks can be helpful. If cognitive dysfunction persists, or impacts performance and quality of life at work or home, referral for neuropsychological evaluation is indicated.

Psychological Symptom Management and Support

It is normal for the cancer survivor to have fear of cancer recurrence and a sense of living with uncertainty. Reassurance that this is normal, and reduces over time, may be all your patient needs to move forward. Encourage her to discuss her feelings of worry with family, friends, and support groups of other cancer survivors. If worry begins to interfere in functioning, or there are signs of posttraumatic stress disorder, referral for counseling is indicated. Depression, anxiety, posttraumatic stress disorder, insomnia, body image concerns, and relationship issues are all common after cancer treatment. These may be transient or persistent; they may be situational or global. Careful assessment of the cancer survivor at each visit will allow for early intervention and appropriate management. Supportive care

with support groups, counseling, and cognitive behavioral therapy may need to be augmented with medications for anxiety, depression, or insomnia. Exercise, yoga, meditation, hypnosis, acupuncture, and massage all have shown demonstrable impact on mental health for cancer survivors. Referral for a sleep medicine evaluation may be indicated if the cancer survivor reports persistent fatigue, insomnia, or disordered sleep–wake cycles after treatment.

SEXUAL HEALTH

The impact to intimacy and sexual health can be profound in the survivor of a gynecologic cancer. Relationship roles may have shifted during treatment to more of a caregiver–patient relationship than that of a sexual couple. Fear of pain, altered body image, and feeling that the genital area is no longer sensual or a source of pleasure is common after gynecologic cancer treatment. Encourage communication between partners, offer assistance with vaginal moisturizers, sexual lubricants, and hormone replacement as appropriate (see Symptom Management discussed earlier), and offer referrals for counseling as needed. For nonpartnered women, reentering the dating arena poses additional stressors with body image concerns, fear of rejection, and emotional vulnerability. Support groups can be helpful to address these issues. Providers certified by the American Association of Sexuality Educators, Counselors, and Therapists (aasect .org) can be especially helpful to address issues of intimacy and sexuality after cancer.

SPIRITUAL DISTRESS

Spiritual distress, including feelings of doubt, guilt, shame, hopelessness, and fear, in cancer survivors is well documented. Feeling in conflict with, or abandoned by, family, friends, or community is common. Questioning faith and trying to find meaning after cancer can lead to a sense of hopelessness and spiritual struggle. Many cancer survivors find that talking with a professional chaplain, a trusted religious or spiritual advisor, or a therapist about these issues is helpful. Being able to "give back," through volunteering or paid work with organizations providing assistance to various populations in need, is often therapeutic for management of spiritual distress.

Returning to work, inability to return to work, resuming routine activities of daily living, finding assistance with care needs, lack of control, and the financial burden of medical costs are all stressors related to cancer survivorship without easy solutions. Advanced-care planning discussions, including encouraging completion of documents, such as living wills and durable powers of attorney for health care, can assist cancer survivors to have a feeling of control over end-of-life issues. Assisting patients with referrals to community agencies, filling out FMLA or disability paperwork, and advocating for social services are all within the role of the advanced practice nurse in primary care.

Wellness and Lifestyle Management

Exercise, nutrition, hydration, sleep, stress management, and mental and spiritual wellness contribute to healthy cancer survivorship. Lifestyle management, including addressing substance use, relationship issues, and finding meaning promote healthy coping. Supportive care with routine health maintenance visits, surveillance for illness or cancer recurrence, and preventative health care services promote early detection and treatment for physical and mental health issues. Education and advocacy for healthy lifestyle management for the gynecologic cancer survivor is well within the scope of the advanced practice nurse in primary care.

END-OF-LIFE CONSIDERATIONS

Not all cancer patients become long-term cancer survivors. As noted at the beginning of this chapter, many women will present late for evaluation of pelvic symptoms, or will have limited warning symptoms and will present for care with late-stage or metastatic disease. The primary care provider frequently has a longstanding relationship with the patient and may be looked to for information and advice on end-of-life care. Advance knowledge regarding resources available in your community for end-of-life care will assist you in directing your patient with confidence to the appropriate resource.

Palliative care services are becoming more available, both in inpatient and outpatient settings. Palliative care providers can assist with management of symptoms such as pain, fatigue, and spiritual distress. Unlike hospice, palliative care may be pursued during active cancer treatment. Hospice becomes available to patients who are no longer seeking curative cancer treatments. A person does not need to be actively dying to qualify for hospice care, but does need to be estimated to have fewer than 6 months to live. Hospice, like palliative care, assists with symptom management—pain, fatigue, mobility issues, altered nutrition status—but not while under treatment with a curative intent. Patients, and health care providers, often believe that these services are only helpful at the very end of life. Both palliative care and hospice focus on function and quality of life, and can assist the patient and family with staying comfortable, functional, and in control of their symptoms for long periods of time. Knowing how, and when, to access and refer to these services in your community can make a dramatic difference in the quality of life for the cancer patient and her family members.

There may be significant distress for the woman, and her entire support network at the end of life (DellaRipa et al., 2015). She may be afraid to ask about resources for symptom management, end-of-life issues, funeral services, and may not have previously arranged to have a durable power of attorney for health care (DPAHC) decisions. She may not have had a safe place or opportunity to discuss her end-of-life wishes, distress, and fears. As an advanced practice nurse in primary care, you may be the one addressing these issues and providing support for the woman at the end of life, as well as for her family. Knowledge of referral sources for counselors, legal assistance, funeral services, and supportive care services in your community can be an essential skill set to have for these situations. Continuing to educate and advocate for your patient at the end of life brings full circle the role of the advanced practice nurse in primary care.

FUTURE DIRECTIONS

There are technological advances in the areas of genetic screening, genomics, molecular medicine, biomarkers, and biological agents in the news headlines. Vaccines for both cancer prevention and treatment are in development. Cancer survivorship is being recognized as a specific phase of cancer care, and there are more people surviving cancer than ever before. With an ever expanding number of primary care patients having cancer as part of their past medical history, cancer is rapidly becoming a chronic medical illness to be managed in the primary care setting.

REFERENCES

American Cancer Society. (2016). *Cancer treatment & survivorship: Facts & figures 2016–2017*. Atlanta, GA: American Cancer Society.

American Congress of Obstetricians and Gynecologists (ACOG). (2012). *New cervical cancer screening recommendations from the US Preventive Services Task Force and the American Cancer Society/American Society for Colposcopy and Cervical Pathology/American Society for Clinical Pathology*. Retrieved from https://www.acog.org/About_ACOG/Announcements/New_Cervical_Cancer Screening

American Psychological Association, Task Force on Socioeconomic Status. (2007). *Women and socioeconomic status*. Retrieved from http://www.apa.org/pi/ses/resources/publications/factsheet-women.aspx

Andersen, M. R., Goff, B. A., Lowe, K. A., Scholler, N., Bergan, L., Dresher, C. W.,...Urban, N. (2008). Combining a symptoms index with CA 125 to improve detection of ovarian cancer. *Cancer, 113*(3), 484–489.

ASCO Connection. (2014). *From patient to survivor: ASCO resources for survivorship continue to grow*. Retrieved from http://connection.asco.org/magazine-archives, http://read.uberflip.com/i/405796-november-2014

Bast, R. C., Badgwell, D., Lu, Z., Marquez, R., Rosen, D., Liu, J.,...Lu, K. (2005). New tumor markers: CA125 and beyond. *International Journal of Gynecological Cancer, 15*(Suppl. 3), 274–281.

Billmire, D. F., Cullen, J. W., Rescorla, F. J., Davis, M., Schlatter, M. G., Olson, T. A.,...Frazier, A. L. (2013). Surveillance after initial surgery for pediatric and adolescent girls with stage I ovarian germ cell tumors: Report from the children's oncology group. *Journal of Clinical Oncology, 32*(5), 465–470. doi:10.1200/JCO.2013.51.1006

Billmire, D., Vinocur, C., Rescorla, F., Cushing, B., London, W., Schlatter, M.,...Olson, T.; Children's Oncology Group (COG). (2004). Outcome and staging evaluation in malignant germ cell tumors of the ovary in children and adolescents: An intergroup study. *Journal of Pediatric Surgery, 39*(3), 424–429; discussion 424.

Bristow, R. E., Tomacruz, R. S., Armstrong, D. K., Trimble, E. L., & Montz, F. J. (2002). Survival effect of maximal cytoreductive surgery for advanced ovarian carcinoma during the platinum era: A meta-analysis. *Journal of Clinical Oncology, 20*(5), 1248–1259.

Cancer.gov. (2015). Retrieved from http://www.cancer.gov/types/breast/hp/breast-ovarian-genetics-pdq

Cancer.net. (2013). *About cancer survivorship*. Retrieved from http://www.cancer.net/survivorship/about-cancer-survivorship

Cancer.net. (2014a). *Uterine cancer: Overview approved by the Cancer.net editorial board 08/2014*. Retrieved from http://www.cancer.net/cancer-types/uterine-cancer/overview

Cancer.net. (2014b). *Vaginal cancer: Statistics approved by the Cancer.net editorial board, 04/2014*. Retrieved from http://www.cancer.net/cancer-types/vaginal-cancer/statistics

Cancer.net. (2015a). *Cervical cancer: Overview approved by the Cancer .net editorial board, 04/2012*. Retrieved from http://www.cancer.net/ cancer-types/cervical-cancer/overview

Cancer.net. (2015b). *Ovarian cancer: Overview approved by the Cancer .net editorial board, 04/2015*. Retrieved from http://www.cancer.net/ cancer-types/ovarian-cancer/overview

Cancer.net Editorial Board. (2013). Ovarian cancer: Stages and grades. Retrieved from http://www.cancer.net/cancer-types/ovarian-cancer/ stages-and-grades

Carroll, N. M. (2015). *Medical care of women who have sex with women*. Retrieved from http://www.uptodate.com/contents/medical -care-of-women-who-have-sex-with-women

Cavallo, J. (2014). Benefits of exercise for relieving fatigue in cancer survivors. *The ASCO Post, 5*(20). Retrieved from http:// www.ascopost.com/issues/december-15-2014/benefits-of-exercise -for-relieving-fatigue-in-cancer-survivors

Centers for Disease Control and Prevention (CDC), Division of Cancer Prevention and Control. (2013). *Basic information about HPV and cancer*. Division of Cancer Prevention and Control, Centers for Disease Control and Prevention. Retrieved from https://www.cdc.gov/ cancer/hpv/basic_info

Chubak, J., Aiello Bowles, E. J., Tuzzio, L., Ludman, E., Rutter, C. M., Reid, R. J., & Wagner, E. H. (2014). Perspectives of cancer survivors on the role of different healthcare providers in an integrated delivery system. *Journal of Cancer Survivorship: Research and Practice, 8*(2), 229–238.

Cooper, S. M., Madnani, N., & Margesson, L. (2015). Reduced risk of squamous cell carcinoma with adequate treatment of vulvar lichen sclerosus. *Journal of the American Medical Association Dermatology, 151*(10), 1059–1060.

Crosbie, E. J., Zwahlen, M., Kitchener, H. C., Egger, M., & Renehan, A. G. (2010). Body mass index, hormone replacement therapy, and endometrial cancer risk: A meta-analysis. *Cancer Epidemiology, Biomarkers & Prevention, 19*(12), 3119–3130.

DellaRipa, J., Conlon, A., Lyon, D. E., Ameringer, S. A., Lynch Kelly, D., & Menzies, V. (2015). Perceptions of distress in women with ovarian cancer. *Oncology Nursing Forum, 42*(3), 292–300.

Dubeau, L. (2008). The cell of origin of ovarian epithelial tumours. *The Lancet. Oncology, 9*(12), 1191–1197.

Elkas, J. C., Berek, J. S., Goff, B. A., Mundt, A. J., Dizon, D. S., & Falk, S. J. (2016). *Vulvar cancer: Clinical manifestations, diagnosis, and pathology*. UpToDate, Wolters Kluwer. Retrieved from http://www .uptodate.com/contents/vulvar-cancer-clinical-manifestationsdiagnosis andpathology?source=preview&search=vulvar+cancer&language=en US&anchor=H3&selectedTitle=3~76#H3

Engel, M. (2014). *Weighty matters: Another cancer linked to being heavy*. Retrieved from http://www.fhcrc.org/en/news/center-news/2014/03/ ovariancancerlinked

Fanning, J., Lambert, H. C., Hale, T. M., Morris, P. C., & Schuerch, C. (1999). Paget's disease of the vulva: Prevalence of associated vulvar adenocarcinoma, invasive Paget's disease, and recurrence after surgical excision. *American Journal of Obstetrics and Gynecology, 180*(1, Pt. 1), 24–27.

Feldman, S., Goodman, A., Peipert, J. F., Goff, B. A., Elmore, J. G., & Park, L. (2015). *Screening for cervical cancer*. UpToDate, Wolters Kluwer. Retrieved from http://www.uptpdate.com/contents/screening -for-cervical-cancer

Fields, M. M. (2013). New cervical cancer screening guidelines: Was the annual Pap too much of a good thing? *Journal of the Advanced Practitioner in Oncology, 4*(1), 59–64.

Finch, A. P. M., Lubinski, J., Moller, P., Singer, C. F., Karlan, B., Senter, L., …Narod, S. A. (2014). Impact of oopherectomy on cancer incidence and mortality in women with a BRCA1 or BRCA2 mutation. *Journal of Clinical Oncology, 32*(15), 1547–1553. doi:10.1200/JCO.2013.53.2820

Flemmer, D., Doutrich, D., Dekker, L., & Rondeau, D. (2012). Creating a safe and caring healthcare context for women who have sex with women. *Journal for Nurse Practitioner, 8*, 464–469. Retrieved from http://www.medscape.com/viewarticle/765550

Frumovitz, M., Etchepareborda, M., Sun, C. C., Soliman, P. T., Eifel, P. J., Levenback, C. F., & Ramirez, P. T. (2010). Primary malignant melanoma of the vagina. *Obstetrics and Gynecology, 116*(6), 1358–1365.

Goff, B. A., Lowe, K. A., Kane, J. C., Robertson, M. D., Gaul, M. A., & Andersen, M. R. (2012). Symptom triggered screening for ovarian cancer: A pilot study of feasibility and acceptability. *Gynecologic Oncology, 124*(2), 230–235.

Goff, B. A., Mandel, L. S., Melancon, C. H., & Muntz, H. G. (2004). Frequency of symptoms of ovarian cancer in women presenting to primary care clinics. *Journal of the American Medical Association, 291*(22), 2705–2712.

Grady, D., Gebretsadik, T., Kerlikowske, K., Ernster, V., & Petitti, D. (1995). Hormone replacement therapy and endometrial cancer risk: A meta-analysis. *Obstetrics and Gynecology, 85*(2), 304–313.

Helder-Woolderink, J. M., De Bock, G. H., Sijmons, R. H., Hollema, H., & Mourits, M. J. (2013). The additional value of endometrial sampling in the early detection of endometrial cancer in women with Lynch syndrome. *Gynecologic Oncology, 131*(2), 304–308.

Hewitt, M., Greenfield, S., & Stovall, E. (Eds.). (2005). *From cancer patient to cancer survivor: Lost in transition*. Committee on Cancer Survivorship: Improving care and quality of life, National Cancer Policy Board. Institute of Medicine and National Research Council of the National Academies. Retrieved from http://books.nap.edu/ openbook.php?record_id=11468

Huh, W. K., Ault, K. A., Chelmow, D., Davey, D. D., Goulart, R. A., Carcia, A. R. F.,…Einstein, M. H. (2015). Use of primary high risk human papillomavirus testing for cervical cancer screening: Initial clinical guidance. *Gynecologic Oncology, 136*(2), 178–182. Retrieved from http://dx.doi.org/10.1016/j.ygyno.2014.12.022

Jaakkola, S., Lyytinen, H. K., Dyba, T., Ylikorkala, O., & Pukkala, E. (2011). Endometrial cancer associated with various forms of postmenopausal hormone therapy: A case control study. *International Journal of Cancer, 128*(7), 1644–1651.

Karem, A., Berel, K. S., Lodd, E. A., Goff, B. A., Mundt, A. Z. J., & Dizon, D. S. (2015). Vaginal cancer. UpToDate, Wolters Kluwer. Retrieved from http://www.uptodate.com/contents/vaginal-cancer. 2015-8-31

Lacey, J. V., Greene, M. H., Buys, S. S., Reding, D., Riley, T. L., Berg, C. D., …Hartge, P. (2006). Ovarian cancer screening in women with a family history of breast or ovarian cancer. *Obstetrics and Gynecology, 108*(5), 1176–1184.

Lacouture, M. E. (2012). *Dr. Lacouture's skin care guide for people living with cancer*. Cold Spring Harbor, NY: Harborside Press.

Lancaster, J. M., Powell, C. B., Chen, L. M., & Richardson, D. L.; SGO Clinical Practice Committee. (2015). Society of Gynecologic Oncology statement on risk assessment for inherited gynecologic cancer predispositions. *Gynecologic Oncology, 136*(1), 3–7.

Lebensohn, A., Kingham, K. E., Chun, N. M., & Kurian, A. W. (2011). Hereditary cancer: Counseling women at risk. *Contemporary OB/ GYN, 56*(4), 30–38.

Lemieux, M. L. (2010). Primary screening for cervical cancer: Incorporating new guidelines and technologies into clinical practice. *Journal for Nurse Practitioners, 6*, 417–424.

Limmer, K., LoBiondo-Wood, G., & Dains, J. (2014). Predictors of cervical cancer screening adherence in the United States: A systematic review. *Journal of the Advanced Practitioner in Oncology, 5*(1), 31–41.

McLaughlin, J. R., Rosen, B., Moody, J., Pal, T., Fan, I., Shaw, P. A., …Narod, S. A. (2013). Long-term ovarian cancer survival associated with mutation in BRCA1 or BRCA2. *Journal of the National Cancer Institute, 105*(2), 141–148.

Meadows, M. E. (2014). *Cognitive function after cancer and cancer-related treatment*. UpToDate. Wolters Kluwer. Last updated August 6, 2014. Retrieved from www.uptodate.com

Miller, K. D., Siegel, R. L., Lin, C. C., Mariotto, A. B., Kramer, J. L., Rowland, J. H.,…Jemal, A. (2016), Cancer treatment and survivorship statistics, 2016. *CA: A Cancer Journal for Clinicians, 66*(4), 271–289. Retrieved from http://www.ncbi.nlm.nih.gov/pubmed/27253694. doi: 10.3322/caac.21349

National Cancer Institute. (2015). *Human papilloma virus (HPV) vaccines*. Retrieved from http://www.cancer.gov/about-cancer/ causes-prevention/risk/infectious-agents/hpv-vaccine-fact-sheet

National Coalition for Cancer Survivorship (NCCS). (2014). *Defining cancer survivorship*. Retrieved from http://www.canceradvocacy.org/ news/defining-cancer-survivorship

National Society of Genetic Counselors. (NSGC). (2015). *Your genetic health: Patient information. What is genetic counseling?* Retrieved from http://nsgc.org/p/cm/ld/fid=386

Pennington, K. P., & Swisher, E. M. (2012). Hereditary ovarian cancer: Beyond the usual suspects. *Gynecologic Oncology, 124*(2), 347–353.

Pruthi, S., Gostout, B. S., & Lindor, N. M. (2010). Identification and management of women with BRCA mutations or hereditary predisposition for breast and ovarian cancer. *Mayo Clinic Proceedings, 85*(12), 1111–1120.

Salani, R., Backes, F. J., Fung, M. F., Holschneider, C. H., Parker, L. P., Bristow, R. E., & Goff, B. A. (2011). Posttreatment surveillance and diagnosis of recurrence in women with gynecologic malignancies: Society of Gynecologic Oncologists recommendations. *American Journal of Obstetrics and Gynecology, 204*(6), 466–478.

Saslow, D., Solomon, D., Lawson, H. W., Killackey, M., Kulasingam, S., Cain, J., ... Myers, E. R. (2012). American Cancer Society, American Society for Colposcopy and Cervical Pathology, and American Society for Clinical Pathology Screening Guidelines for the Prevention and Early Detection of Cervical Cancer. *CA: A Cancer Journal for Clinicians, 62*(3), 147–172. doi.org/10.3322/caac.21139

Shah, C. A., Goff, B. A., Lowe, K., Peters, W. A., & Li, C. I. (2009). Factors affecting risk of mortality in women with vaginal cancer. *Obstetrics and Gynecology, 113*(5), 1038–1045.

Shalowitz, D. I., Vinograd, A. M., & Giuntoli, R. L. (2015). Geographic access to gynecologic cancer care in the United States. *Gynecologic Oncology, 138*(1), 115–120.

Slatnik, C. L., & Duff, E. (2015). Ovarian cancer: Ensuring early diagnosis. *The Nurse Practitioner, 40*(9), 47–54.

U.S. Census Bureau. (2013). America's Families and Living Arrangements: 2012. Retrieved from http://www.census.gov/prod/2013pubs/p20-570.pdf

Urban, N., McIntosh, M. W., Andersen, M., & Karlan, B. Y. (2003). Ovarian cancer screening. *Hematology/Oncology Clinics of North America, 17*(4), 989–1005, ix.

Verloop, J., Rookus, M. A., & van Leeuwen, F. E. (2000). Prevalence of gynecologic cancer in women exposed to diethylstilbestrol in utero. *New England Journal of Medicine, 342*(24), 1838–1839.

WHO International Agency for Research on Cancer. (2007). Human papillomaviruses. *IARC Monographs on the Evaluation of Carcinogenic Risks to Humans, 90.* Retrieved from https://monographs.iarc.fr/ENG/Monographs/vol90/mono90.pdf

Wright, T. C., Stoler, M. H., Sharma, A., Zhang, G., Behrens, C., & Wright, T. L.; ATHENA (Addressing THE Need for Advanced HPV Diagnostics) Study Group. (2011). Evaluation of HPV-16 and HPV-18 genotyping for the triage of women with high-risk HPV+ cytology-negative results. *American Journal of Clinical Pathology, 136*(4), 578–586.

Yuanyuan, Z., Liu, H., Yang, S., Zhang, J., Oian, L., Chen, X. (2014). Overweight, obesity and endometrial cancer risk: Results from a systematic review and meta-analysis. *International Journal of Biological Markers, 29*(1), e21–e299. Retrieved from http://www.pubfacts.com/detail/24170556/Overweight-obesity-and-endometrial-cancer-risk

■ BIBLIOGRAPHY

Anderson, G. L., Judd, H. L., Kaunitz, A. M., Barad, D. H., Beresford, S. A., Pettinger, M.,...Lopez, A. M.; Women's Health Initiative Investigators. (2003). Effects of estrogen plus progestin on gynecologic cancers and associated diagnostic procedures: The Women's Health Initiative randomized trial. *Journal of the American Medical Association, 290*(13), 1739–1748.

Andreyev, H. J., Davidson, S. E., Gillespie, C., Allum, W. H., & Swarbrick, E.; British Society of Gastroenterology; Association of Colo-Proctology of Great Britain and Ireland; Association of Upper Gastrointestinal Surgeons; Faculty of Clinical Oncology Section of the Royal College of Radiologists. (2012). Practice guidance on the management of acute and chronic gastrointestinal problems arising as a result of treatment for cancer. *Gut, 61*(2), 179–192.

ASCO Post. (2014). *Many insured patients alter their lifestyles and medical care to cope with cancer treatment costs.* 2014 Palliative Care in Oncology Symposium (Abstract 161). Retrieved from http://www.ascopost.com

Berek, J. S., Chalas, E., Edelson, M., Moore, D. H., Burke, W. M., Cliby, W. A., & Berchuck, A.; Society of Gynecologic Oncologists Clinical Practice Committee. (2010). Prophylactic and risk-reducing bilateral salpingo-oophorectomy: Recommendations based on risk of ovarian cancer. *Obstetrics and Gynecology, 116*(3), 733–743.

Bergner, D. (2015). The orthodox sex guru. *The New York Times,* January 22, 2015. Retrieved from http://www.nytimes.com/2015/01/25/magazine/the-orthodox-sex-guru.html?_r=0

Bober, S. L., Recklitis, C. J., Campbell, E. G., Park, E. R., Kutner, J. S., Najita, J. S., & Diller, L. (2009). Caring for cancer survivors: A survey of primary care physicians. *Cancer, 115*(Suppl. 18), 4409–4418.

Campagna, N. (2011). Hereditary breast and ovarian cancer syndrome. *Journal of Advanced Practical Oncology, 2,* 257–262.

Cassileth, B. (2014). *Survivorship: Living well during and after cancer.* Ann Arbor, MI: Spry Publishing.

Cavallo, J. (2013). Sexual health after cancer: Communicating with your patients. *The ASCO Post, 4*(6). Retrieved from http://www.ascopost.com/issues/april-15-2013/sexual-health-after-cancer-communicating-with-your-patients.aspx

Cooper, J. M., Loeb, S. J., & Smith, C. A. (2010). The primary care nurse practitioner and cancer survivorship care. *Journal of the American Academy of Nurse Practitioners, 22*(8), 394–402.

Dallal, C. M., Brinton, L. A., Bauer, D. C., Buist, D. S., Cauley, J. A., Hue, T. F.,...Lacey, J. V. Jr.; B-FIT Research Group. (2012). Obesity-related hormones and endometrial cancer among postmenopausal women: A nested case-control study within the B-FIT cohort. *Endocrine-Related Cancer, 20*(1), 151–160.

Davies, P. S., & D'Arcy, Y. (2013). *Compact clinical guide to cancer pain management: An evidence-based approach for nurses.* New York, NY: Springer Publishing.

Flamos, C., & Bracken, M. (2015). Utilization of the acronym ALBUMINS to screen gynecologic cancer survivors. *Journal for Nurse Practitioners, 11*(4), 430–435.

Gray, L. (2011). *Linking of mutations in 12 genes to ovarian cancers may lead to more effective prevention.* UW Health Science/UW Medicine. Retrieved from http://www.washington.edu/news/articles/linking-of-mutations

Hershman, D. L., Lacchetti, C., Dworkin, R. H., Smith, E. M. L., Bleeker, J., Cavaletti, G.,...Loprinzi, C.; American Society of Clinical Oncology. (2014). Prevention and management of chemotherapy-induced peripheral neuropathy in survivors of adult cancers: American Society of Clinical Oncology Clinical Practice Guideline. *Journal of Clinical Oncology, 32*(18), 1941–1967. Retrieved from http://jco.ascopubs.org/cgi/doi/10.1200/JCO.2013.54.0914

Hopenhayn, C., Christian, A., Christian, W. J., Watson, M., Unger, E. R., Lynch, C. F.,...Saraiya, M. (2014). Prevalence of human papillomavirus types in invasive cervical cancers from seven US cancer registries prior to vaccine introduction. *Journal of Lower Genital Tract Disease, 18*(2), 182–189.

Katz, A. J. (2007). *Breaking the silence on cancer and sexuality: A handbook for healthcare providers.* Pittsburgh, PA: Oncology Nursing Society.

Kloor, M., Voigt, A. Y., Schackert, H. K., Schirmacher, P., von Knebel Doeberitz, M., & Bläker, H. (2011). Analysis of EPCAM protein expression in diagnostics of Lynch syndrome. *Journal of Clinical Oncology, 29*(2), 223–227.

Lee, C. O., & Decker, G. M. (2012). *Cancer and complimentary medicine: Your guide to smart choices in symptom management.* Pittsburgh, PA: Oncology Nursing Society.

Loren, A. W., Mangu, P. B., Beck, L. N., Brennan, L., Magdalinski, A. J., Partridge, A. H.,...Oktay, K.; American Society of Clinical Oncology. (2013). Fertility preservation for patients with cancer: American Society of Clinical Oncology clinical practice guideline update. *Journal of Clinical Oncology, 31*(19), 2500–2510.

Manchio, J. V., & Sanders, B. M. (2013). Fecal incontinence: Help for patients who suffer silently. *Journal of Family Practice, 62*(11), 640–650.

Matei, D., Brown, J., & Frazier, L. (2013). Updates in the management of ovarian germ cell tumors. *American Society Clinical Oncology Education Book,* 210–216.

Medicalxpress. (2015). *Breast cancer survivors who experience pain during intercourse may benefit from lidocaine.* Retrieved from http://medicalxpress.com/print357274215.html

Morris, K. S., & Fruh, S. M. (2015). Reducing ethnic disparities in cancer care. *Clinical Advisor, 18*(3), 108–108.

Oeffinger, K. C., & Nekhlyudov, L. (2011). Optimizing health: Primary care. In M. Feuerstein & P. Ganz (Eds.), *Health services for cancer survivors* (pp. 189–203). New York, NY: Springer Publishing.

Rahn, D. D., Carberry, C., Sanses, T. V., Mamik, M. M., Ward, R. M., Meriwether, K. V.,...Murphy, M.; Society of Gynecologic Surgeons Systematic Review Group. (2014). Vaginal estrogen for genitourinary syndrome of menopause: A systematic review. *Obstetrics and Gynecology, 124*(6), 1147–1156.

Shulman, L. N., Jacobs, L. A., Greenfield, S., Jones, B., McCabe, M. S., Syrjala, K.,...Ganz, P. A. (2009). Cancer care and cancer survivorship care in the United States: Will we be able to care for these patients in the future? *Journal of Oncology Practice/American Society of Clinical Oncology, 5*(3), 119–123.

Soini, T., Hurskainen, R., Grénman, S., Mäenpää, J., Paavonen, J., & Pukkala, E. (2014). Cancer risk in women using the levonorgestrel-releasing intrauterine system in Finland. *Obstetrics and Gynecology, 124*(2, Pt. 1), 292–299.

Solheim, O., Kærn, J., Tropé, C. G., Rokkones, E., Dahl, A. A., Nesland, J. M., & Fosså, S. D. (2013). Malignant ovarian germ cell tumors: Presentation, survival and second cancer in a population based Norwegian cohort (1953–2009). *Gynecologic Oncology, 131*(2), 330–335.

Vadaparampil, S. T., & Quinn, G. P. (2013). Improving communication between oncologists and reproductive specialists to promote timely referral of patients with cancer. *Journal of Oncology Practice, 31*, 2500–2510.

Von Ah, D., Jansen, C. E., & Allen, D. H. (2014). Evidence-based interventions for cancer- and treatment-related cognitive impairment. *Clinical Journal of Oncology Nursing, 18*(Suppl.), 17–25.

Walsh, T., Casadei, S., Lee, M. K., Pennil, C. C., Nord, A. S., Thornton, A. M.,...Swisher, E. M. (2011). Mutations in 12 genes for inherited ovarian, fallopian tube, and peritoneal carcinoma identified by massively parallel sequencing. *Proceedings of the National Academy of Sciences of the United States of America, 108*(44), 18032–18037.

Weinstock, M. A. (1994). Malignant melanoma of the vulva and vagina in the United States: Patterns of incidence and population-based estimates of survival. *American Journal of Obstetrics and Gynecology, 171*(5), 1225–1230.

Whitney, R. L., Bell, J. F., Reed, S. C., Lash, R., Bold, R. J., Kim, K. K., ... Joseph, J. G. (2016). Predictors of financial difficulties and work modifications among cancer survivors in the United States. *Journal of Cancer Survivorship: Research and Practice, 10*(2), 241–250. http://doi.org/10.1007/s11764-015-0470-y

CHAPTER 34

Menopause

Ivy M. Alexander • Annette Jakubisin Konicki • Seja Jackson • Devangi Ladani • Jenna LoGiudice • Lauren Vo

Women experience several rites of passage throughout their life span; among these woman-specific passages are menarche, motherhood, and menopause. The stages of menopause are comprised of a progression of physical and psychological processes identified as perimenopause, menopause, and postmenopause. Premature menopause caused by surgical removal of ovaries, ovarian failures, or other etiologies and its impact on a woman's life is generally not addressed by either women or the medical profession. Attitudes toward menopause are culturally based; societies that value age and experience bestow "wise woman," elder or grandmother status as a revered achievement (Hall, Callister, Berry, & Matsumura, 2007, p. 110).

Negative attitudes are common in developed countries, which tend to put high value on youth, with descriptions of postmenopausal women as "irritable and cranky" and portrayal as sexless, useless, or crazy. In a study of Mexican and American college students, participants from both countries defined a postmenopausal woman as "old *and* irritable" (Marvan, Islas, Vela, Chrisler, & Warren, 2008, p. 678). Anthropologists studying menopause found that symptoms vary between cultures; in some cultures there are not even words for menopause-related symptoms such as "hot flashes" (HFs) or even menopause itself (Sievert, 2014). Some ethnic groups consider speaking of menopause a "private matter," saved for those of their own race and gender (Dillaway, Byrnes, Miller, & Rehan, 2008).

Male perceptions of menopause have rarely been explored; however, one study of British men found that sharing the responsibility for being in a relationship was common, including when the women partners were experiencing menopause. For many men "the impression here was of a joint endeavor where the woman's well-being was prioritized," but some men felt "helpless and redundant" and unable to be supportive (Liao, Lunn, & Baker, 2015, p. 173).

Western societies tend to medicalize menopause, concentrating on pharmaceuticals, including hormone replacement therapy (HRT), antidepressants, and other medications to relieve symptoms. "The introduction of the first synthetic replacement hormone in 1938 led to the construction of menopause as a 'hormone deficiency disease'" (Newhart, 2013, p. 366). As early as 1966, Wilson described menopause as "an estrogen deficiency" and touted HRT to provide youth, beauty, and sexuality for menopausal women (Wilson, Marino, & Wilson, 1966). Currently, there is less use of synthetic hormone therapy (HT) and an increased interest in biologically identical hormone therapy (BHRT), yet menopause remains a medicalized construct in Western society. A recent study investigated the use of BHRT and found that "the predominant complaint of women was that their symptoms were misunderstood, minimized, and even dismissed by their primary care physicians—which led them to anti-aging medicine as an 'alternative' solution" (Fishman, Flatt, & Settersten, 2015, p. 83). Although decreased estrogen may be the biological etiology and pharmaceuticals, synthetic or natural, are one way to address it, we know that menopause encompasses many more transformations for women.

For many women the transition to postmenopause is associated with changed perceptions of health, family, and social situations and presents an opportunity for women to reevaluate their lives and reaffirm their desire to improve and maintain their health (Alexander et al., 2003; Kaufert, Boggs, Ettinger, Woods, & Utian, 1998). The importance of health during and following the transition to postmenopause is receiving greater attention in part because of the increasing number of women living through and past menopause. The number of women becoming postmenopausal is expanding daily. Because of the increased life span, women today live a full one third of their lives after menopause. According to the 2010 U.S. Census, 23,768,592 women were between 50 and 74 years of age and in total 34,776,606 were between 50 and 100 years of age (U.S. Census Bureau, 2010, p. 2). Approximately 6,000 women become postmenopausal each day (North American Menopause Society [NAMS], 2014) and population experts project that more than 63 million women will be older than 50 years by the year 2020 (U.S. Census Bureau, 2012).

Women's adjustment to postmenopause incorporates both the response to the loss of fertility and perceived changes in appearance and health (Strauss, 2011). The heightened attention to health during and following menopause is also related to the changes in health risks that are associated with midlife. The natural alterations in a woman's hormonal milieu that accompany menopause and other natural aging processes increase her risk for heart disease, bone loss, diabetes, obesity, and various types of cancer. As estrogen and progesterone levels decline, women are likely to experience menopause-associated symptoms, often prompting them to seek health care. These consultations provide a unique opportunity to assist women in managing symptoms as well as to provide evaluation and education about other midlife health risks.

Harris (2008) suggests the use of a holistic model to optimize the care for women in this period of their lives. "Integrating into the whole also could mean an exploration of the community and the biosphere and how our sociocultural, socioeconomic, and sociopolitical contexts can support or inhibit our adult development process into more positive aging" (Harris, 2008, p. 977). She encourages learning from those who have already made the journey through menopause to optimize the opportunities to strengthen body, mind, and spirit during this transitional time.

■ DEFINITION AND SCOPE

Menopause is technically identified as a point in time following 12 consecutive months of amenorrhea occurring in response to normal physiologic changes in the hypothalamic–pituitary–ovarian (HPO) axis (Table 34.1; NAMS, 2014). These changes result in fewer follicles developing in the ovary during each menstrual cycle throughout the perimenopausal period, which encompasses the 2 to 10 years

preceding the final menstrual period and the 12 months of amenorrhea immediately before menopause. The follicles that develop during the perimenopausal period are less sensitive to follicle-stimulating hormone (FSH); in addition, ovarian production of estradiol, progesterone, and androgens declines. Therefore, the normal negative feedback system that causes hypothalamic production of gonadotropin-releasing hormone (GnRH) in response to elevated estrogen and progesterone levels is altered, allowing FSH and luteinizing hormone (LH) production by the anterior pituitary to continue. Over time, follicle production in the ovaries ceases, estrogen and progesterone hormone levels remain low, FSH and LH levels remain high, and menstruation ceases altogether. Although the term *postmenopausal* is commonly applied to any woman after menopause, the postmenopausal period technically refers to the first 5 years after menopause. Hormonal fluctuations are common during this period.

The average age for natural menopause is 51, with most women experiencing it between 48 and 55 years of age (NAMS, 2014). All women who live long enough will experience menopause. Predicting a woman's age for menopause is difficult. Gene mutation and statistical models have had minimal success in predicting the onset of menopause or risk of early menopause (Hefler et al., 2006; Huber, Grimm, Huber, et al., 2006). However, there is some correlation with the age when a woman's mother or older sisters experienced it (Bentzen et al., 2013; Cramer, Xu, & Harlow, 1995). There are substantial differences in age of menopause between geographical areas. Lifestyle (including alcohol use and street drugs), nutritional status, early life stress, smoking, environment, and HIV infection are among the factors that are being

TABLE 34.1	Terms and Definitions Used With Menopause
TERM/ABBREVIATION	**DEFINITION/COMMENT**
Perimenopause	Period preceding final menstrual period by 8–10 years, usually occurring between 48 and 55 years of age, associated with many symptoms of menopausal transition attributable to fluctuating hormone levels (see Box 34.1)
Menopause	Point in time occurring 12 consecutive months after natural cessation of menses; average age in North America is 51 years
Postmenopause	Period following menopause, commonly associated with symptoms attributable to waning estrogen and progesterone levels
HRT	Hormone replacement therapy; older term now replaced by preferred term, hormone therapy
HT	Hormone therapy; term encompasses ET, EPT, ETT, estrogen + bazedoxifene; preferred term for accurate communication; use urged by NAMS
MHT	Menopause hormone therapy
BHRT	Biologically identical hormone replacement therapy
ET	Estrogen therapy
EPT	Estrogen-progestogen therapy
ETT	Estrogen-testosterone therapy

NAMS, North American Menopause Society.
Adapted from North American Menopause Society (2014); Shifren and Gass (2014).

considered and explored in determining differences in the age of menopause, however, no distinct correlations have been identified as of yet other than cigarette smoking and nulliparity, which correlate with somewhat earlier menopause (Davis et al., 2015).

ETIOLOGY

Reduced levels of estrogen and progesterone are largely responsible for the menopause-related symptoms that women experience (NAMS, 2014). Alpha and beta estrogen receptors have been identified; these receptors have different affinities for the three different forms of endogenous estrogen. Both types of receptors are located throughout the body in the brain (cognitive and vasomotor centers), heart, skin, eyes, gastrointestinal tract, vascular system, urogenital tract, breast tissue, and bone. Similarly, progesterone receptors are located throughout the body in the pituitary, vasomotor, and hypothalamic areas in the brain; vascular tissues and heart; lung; pancreas; bones; and breast and reproductive organs. When the hormone levels fluctuate and decline, estrogen and progesterone receptors remain unbound, resulting in symptoms, such as vaginal dryness and HFs. As a result of the different affinities of receptors located throughout the body and among women, symptoms are individualized.

Although the perimenopausal transition sounds like a smooth process, it is anything but smooth for many women. Hormonal levels can fluctuate widely, causing abrupt changes that lead to many of the symptoms women experience. These fluctuating hormone levels explain in part why some women have wide variations of symptoms, being asymptomatic some days and manifesting severe symptoms on other days. Hormonal fluctuations are caused by multiple factors, including the reduced number of functioning ovarian follicles.

Interestingly, women continue to produce both estrogen and androgens after menopause (NAMS, 2014). Estrone (E1), the weakest estrogen, is the primary estrogen found in postmenopausal women. It is produced by adipose tissue conversion of androstenedione secreted by the adrenal glands (95%) and the ovaries and by estradiol metabolism (5%).

Following menopause the ovaries cease to produce functional follicles. However, the hilar and corticostromal cells of the ovarian stromal tissue are steroidogenic and continue to produce significant levels of both testosterone and androstenedione for several years. In postmenopausal women, circulating levels of androstenedione are about half those of their premenopausal counterparts. In contrast, circulating testosterone levels are relatively constant in pre- and postmenopausal women, partially attributable to the effects of high FSH levels, which stimulate ovarian stromal tissue to increase testosterone production. Dehydroepiandrosterone (DHEA), produced primarily in the adrenals, and DHEA-S, a sulfated metabolite of DHEA, levels are unaffected by menopause. Aromatization of DHEA, testosterone, and androgen to estrone and estradiol does increase with age. Overall, androgen metabolism is more heavily affected by the aging process than by the decline in ovarian function associated with menopause (NAMS, 2014).

In women, androgens are responsible for sexual sensation, libido, and motivation to pursue sexual activity, as well as for maintaining muscle and bone strength. Testosterone exists in both bound and unbound forms (NAMS, 2014). Circulating unbound or free levels of testosterone constitute approximately 2% of the total testosterone that exists in a woman's body. The rest of the circulating testosterone binds to either sex hormone binding globulin (SHGB) or albumin. Higher SHBG levels (as seen when oral estrogen therapy is used) can reduce free testosterone levels. Conversely, lower levels of SHBG (a condition that can occur with hypothyroidism and obesity) can increase free testosterone levels (NAMS, 2014). Although total testosterone levels are usually fairly constant in postmenopause, free levels might increase or decline slightly in some women. Women with higher free testosterone levels may have ovarian stromal hyperplasia with luteinization (NAMS, 2014).

Multiple factors besides natural aging can cause menopause (see Box 34.1; NAMS, 2014).

FACTORS AFFECTING THE TIMING OF MENOPAUSE

Multiple factors that may affect the age of menopause have been studied (e.g., age at menarche, height, body mass index [BMI], weight change, exercise participation, level of education, parity, breastfeeding, diet, alcohol consumption, and oral contraceptive use; Canavez, Werneck, Parente, Celeste, & Faerstein, 2013; Forman, Mangini, Thelus-Jean, & Hayward, 2011; Morris et al., 2012; Sapre & Thakur, 2014). Although there is no unequivocal evidence that any of these factors have a significant effect on the timing of menopause, smoking has emerged as having a fairly consistent correlation with earlier menopause by approximately 1.5 years (Butts et al., 2014; Sapre & Thakur, 2014). Similarly, changes in menstrual cycling (e.g., cycle length, amount of bleeding, and 60- or 90-day periods of amenorrhea) suggest a shorter length of time to the final menstrual period (Gracia, Sammel, Freeman, et al., 2005; Harlow et al., 2006). Heavy bleeding was associated with fibroids or obesity (Van Voorhis, Santoro, Harlow, Crawford, & Randolph, 2008). The data gathered by the U.S.-based Study of Women's Health Across the Nation (SWAN) suggest that several variables together may be useful in predicting the final menstrual period, such as age, irregular menstrual cycling, serum hormone levels, and smoking (Gold et al., 2013). Many studies (Butts et al., 2014; Chen et al., 2014; Lu, Liu, Recker, Deng, & Dvornyk, 2010; Spencer et al., 2013) examine the effect of genetics on onset of menopause, and more than 17 (He & Murabito, 2014) specific genetic markers are associated with earlier onset.

Ethnicity could also affect the timing of menopause. The Multiethnic Cohort Study (Henderson, Bernstein, Henderson, Kolonel, & Pike, 2008) revealed that Hispanic women, especially those born outside the United States, experienced significantly earlier menopause than White women. African American women experienced menopause

BOX 34.1   MENOPAUSE FROM CAUSES OTHER THAN NATURAL AGING

- *Primary ovarian insufficiency* (POI) or *premature ovarian failure* (POF) is transient or permanent loss of ovarian function in women younger than 40 years. It is usually associated with other health problems such as genetic anomalies, autoimmune disorders, or metabolic disturbances, as well as pelvic surgery, radiation, or chemotherapy. Further assessment is appropriate if a woman younger than 40 years of age misses three or more consecutive menstrual cycles.

- *Induced menopause* results from surgical removal of both ovaries (bilateral oophorectomy) or ablation of ovarian function from chemotherapy, medications, or radiation. Fertility and menstruation cease abruptly following surgical menopause and symptoms can be quite severe because of the sudden cessation of ovarian hormone production and subsequent abrupt drop in circulating estrogen levels. For women who experience induced menopause following ablative therapies, fertility and menstruation may continue for several months until they finally cease.

- *Premature menopause* occurs before the age of 40 years and frequently follows the same pattern as natural menopause including the permanent cessation of menstruation and fertility.

- *Early menopause* occurs in women between the age of 40 and 45 years and about 5% of women are affected.

- *Temporary menopause* can occur at any age if normal ovarian function is interrupted and then resumes. Temporary menopause can be medication induced, related to a disease process, or idiopathic.

Sources: North American Menopause Society (2014), Shifren and Gass (2014).

---

at the same age as White women, and Japanese women experienced significantly later menopause. Conversely, a longitudinal analysis as part of the SWAN study (Gold et al., 2013) found that racial and ethnic differences are no longer statistically significant once socioeconomic, lifestyle, and health variables are controlled. This supports the finding that social determinants of health are more strongly related to age at menopause than ethnicity or race alone. Body size may also play a role in the timing of menopause, possibly because adipose tissues store androstenedione and convert it to estrogen.

■ SYMPTOMS

Despite the negative press often associated with menopause, it is a normal life transition for most women. Hormonal fluctuations can cause symptoms that are distressing and that negatively affect a woman's overall quality of life (QOL; NAMS, 2014; Shifren & Gass, 2014). However, for some women, the transition is essentially silent. Approximately one third of women experience little or no menopause-related symptoms. Another one third may experience mild symptoms that are only bothersome on occasion. The final one third may have moderate to severe symptoms that can interfere with daily activities and sleep, leading to disruptions in work performance and causing moodiness or irritability.

Every woman presenting with symptoms suggestive of menopause is carefully assessed as there is a wide variation in the experience for individual women. Common symptoms are listed in Box 34.2.

The severity of the symptoms a woman experiences may vary. Generally, symptoms begin during the perimenopausal period and slowly increase in severity over time (Avis et al., 2001; NAMS, 2014). Irregular menses are common during the perimenopause and may include alterations in flow or cycle length, missed periods, and increased or newly developing premenstrual symptoms. The most common menopause-associated symptoms include HFs or flushes, sweats, and vaginal dryness. The frequency, severity, and incidence of HFs are highest for 5 to 7 years after menopause; however, many women continue to experience flashes for several more years (Kronenberg, 1990).

HFs are the single most common menopause-associated symptom among postmenopausal women, affecting about 75% of women (NAMS, 2014). Predictors of a woman experiencing HFs include cigarette smoking (quitting may mediate this somewhat; Smith, Flaws, & Gallicchio, 2015), increased abdominal adiposity, and a history of HFs in the woman's mother (Staropoli, Flaws, Bush, & Moulton, 1998; Thurston et al., 2008). Most women experience HFs as an intense heat sensation, beginning at the head and moving down the body or beginning at the feet and moving upward. Some women have a prodromal sensation. HFs cause a measurable increase in skin conductance and temperature and may or may not be accompanied by sweating. The heat sensation is followed by a decrease in core body temperature, often causing a chill, which can be exacerbated with sweating. Some women also experience flushing of the upper chest and face (hot flushes) and many experience night sweats (NAMS, 2014).

HFs are associated with a surge in the LH level. Because of a narrowing of the thermoneutral zone, small changes in core body temperature may precipitate HFs, sweating, or chills when the core body temperature rises above or falls below the thermoneutral thresholds (Freedman & Blacker, 2002).

Sleep problems are also common during the menopausal transition. Some sleep changes are related to aging: there is an overall reduced need for sleep (8 hours per night for

BOX 34.2   MENOPAUSE-RELATED SYMPTOMS

Acne
Anxiety/nervousness
Arthralgia
Asthenia
Cognitive changes
Cystitis, recurrent
Depression
Dizziness
Dry eyes
Dry skin and hair
Dyspareunia
Dysuria
Fatigue
Forgetfulness
Formication
Frequent urinary tract infection (UTI)
Genitourinary burning
Headache
Hirsutism/virilization
Hot flashes/flushes
Insomnia
Irregular menstrual bleeding
Irritability/mood disturbances

Mastalgia
Myalgia
Night sweats
Nocturia
Odor
Palpitations
Paresthesia
Periodontal inflammation
Poor concentration
Postcoital bleeding
Reduced libido
Skin dryness/atrophy
Sleep disturbances
Stress urinary incontinence[a]
Thinning hair/female pattern hair loss (FPHL)
Urinary frequency
Urinary urgency
Vaginal atrophy
Vaginal dryness
Vaginal/vulvar irritation
Vaginal/vulvar pruritus
Vaginal discharge
Vaginitis, recurrent

[a]Data are inconclusive.

Sources: Alexander et al. (2003), Alexander and Andrist (2005), North American Menopause Society (2014).

younger women, 5–7 hours for older women), more frequent periods of brief arousal, and less time spent in sleep stages III (early deep sleep) and IV (deep sleep and relaxation; Blackman, 2000). HFs and night sweats can further interrupt sleep (NAMS, 2014; Kronenberg, 1990). Sleep loss causes fatigue and has been associated with stress; headache; depression; poor work, home, or school functioning; diabetes; hypertension; emotional lability; irritability; and difficulty with reasoning, concentrating, and remembering (National Center on Sleep Disorder Research, 2011).

Cognition and memory problems are common. Although some research suggests these changes may not be related to menopause (Woods, Mitchell, & Adams, 2000), sleep interruptions and increased stress with resultant increased cortisol levels can interfere with cognition and memory. Additionally, studies have demonstrated the positive correlation between normal estrogen levels and improved memory, cognition, and cerebral blood flow (Hogervorst, De Jager, Budge, & Smith, 2004; Resnick, Maki, Golski, Kraut, & Zonderman, 1998; Shaywitz et al., 2003). Even with adequate sleep and relatively low levels of stress, some midlife women have difficulties with concentration and memory during menopausal transition; however, they return to baseline after menopause (NAMS, 2014).

Genitourinary syndrome of menopause (GSM) is a group of signs and symptoms associated with decrease in estrogen and other gonadal steroids, resulting in vulvovaginal atrophy (NAMS, 2014). Urogenital changes will affect all women during the transition and after menopause.

However, urogenital changes are not bothersome to all women. Atrophy of the vaginal epithelium causes vaginal dryness and dyspareunia, and can predispose women to urinary incontinence and recurrent urinary tract infections (UTIs). Menopausal women are vulnerable to infection because of micro-tears during intercourse and atropic genital tissues (NAMS, 2014). Falling estrogen levels also lead to urethral atrophy, which can further increase the likelihood of urinary incontinence (NAMS, 2014). Although midlife changes may predispose women to urinary incontinence, it is never normal and is evaluated and treated accordingly (see Chapter 29).

Other normal changes of aging can negatively affect sexual function (NAMS, 2014). As they age, women produce less vaginal secretions overall and need more time during sexual activity to achieve adequate vaginal lubrication. Vaginal dryness (Dennerstein, Dudley, Hopper, Guthrie, & Burger, 2000), atrophy, and superficial dyspareunia (Versi, Harvey, Cardozo, Brincat, & Studd, 2001) increase progressively as women approach menopause and after. Their vaginal elasticity, rugae, pigmentation, and superficial cell numbers all decline, leading to petechiae and even bleeding following minor trauma such as intercourse or other forms of sexual activity (NAMS, 2014). The risk for vaginal infection increases because of the increased vaginal pH resulting from reduced numbers of lactobacilli. Vulvar collagen and adipose tissues atrophy, further increasing the likelihood of dyspareunia. Libido may also decline. All of these changes, combined with possible relationship concerns, partner sexual difficulties, and/or reduced sexual activity may lead to reduced interest in sex (Dennerstein, Dudley, & Burger, 2001). Regardless of the causes of sexual dysfunction or dyspareunia, women often find the subject difficult to broach. Clinicians should ask about sexual satisfaction and function and remain open to the fact that sexual expression takes many forms (see Chapters 19 and 26).

Skin and hair changes are also frequently associated with menopause. As estrogen levels decrease, unbound estrogen receptors in the skin and normal changes of aging lead to a reduction in all of the following: number of collagen fibers, degree of elasticity, thickness of the skin, levels of glycosaminoglycans, and vascularity of the skin. Collagen loss of 30% occurs in the first 5 years postmenopause, with an average loss of 2.1% per year (Brincat et al., 1987). Skin dryness and hair changes, such as increased coarseness, thinning hair on the head, and increased body hair, especially at the nares or ear canals, are common.

Menopause-related symptoms may be affected by cultural or racial background. In the SWAN study, the number of psychosomatic symptoms (e.g., headache, moodiness, and palpitations) was highest among White and Hispanic women (Avis et al., 2001). However, the severity of vasomotor symptoms (e.g., sweats, HFs) was highest among Black women, followed by Hispanic, White, Chinese, and Japanese women, respectively (Gold et al., 2000). Vaginal dryness was more common among Black and Hispanic women. Hispanic women were more likely than White women to report urine leakage, heart racing or pounding, and forgetfulness. Sleeping difficulty was reported by White women more than any other group (Gold et al., 2000). In the Women's Health Initiative (WHI) trials, baseline data indicated the prevalence of urogenital symptoms (e.g., dryness, discharge, irritation, itching, and dysuria) was higher among Hispanic women (Pastore, Carter, Hulka, & Wells, 2004). The level of bother from some symptoms may also be higher among different ethnic groups. For example, Black women reported high bother from night sweats and sleep changes, vaginal and body odor, moodiness, "rage," weight gain, and irritability (Alexander et al., 2003). Asian women reported more problems with joint stiffness and pain, especially in the back, shoulders, and neck (Gold et al., 2000). The frequency, intensity, and bother from specific symptoms may be related to genetic, cultural, or environmental effects.

■ EVALUATION/ASSESSMENT

Evaluation of a woman presenting with symptoms suggestive of menopause includes a comprehensive personal and family history focusing on her unique experience of symptoms and symptom combinations, a complete physical examination, and selective diagnostic studies to determine the true cause of her symptoms.

History

Given the extensive list of possible differential diagnoses for the various symptom combinations associated with menopause, the approach to the history must be comprehensive. Symptoms suggestive of menopause may vary in duration and severity and many women will go through the transition to postmenopause without seeking health care (Martin & Manson, 2008). Health questionnaires are available to assist clinicians in reviewing the history of menopause-related symptoms such as the Greene Climacteric Scale (Greene, 1976) and the Menopause Health Questionnaire developed by the North American Menopause Society (NAMS, 2015a).

The history of presenting illness includes information on the presence and severity of symptoms associated with the menopause transition (Box 34.2). Further information on the onset, frequency, and severity of each of the symptoms and the menstrual cycle of the woman will inform the clinician on the progression in the transition to postmenopause.

The medication history includes review of any current or past use of hormonal contraceptives. Long-acting contraceptives may induce amenorrhea and limit the use of amenorrhea as an indicator of becoming postmenopausal. Both prescription and over-the-counter (OTC) treatments used for menopause-related symptoms are noted, including the duration of use, effect, any side effects experienced, and why they are no longer being used. Ask about any known allergies or sensitivities to hormonal contraceptives as it may influence treatment options (Goodman, Cobin, Ginzburg, Katz, & Woode, 2011).

The gynecologic history includes information on age of menarche, typical menses patterns during the reproductive years, and what is currently being experienced. Many women will report a progressively lengthened menstrual cycle (Nelson, 2008) as they get closer to menopause. All gynecologic-related problems and surgeries are reviewed and documented. Notations of the dates of the last cervical cytology test, self-breast examinations, and mammogram are listed.

The obstetrical history includes any pregnancy history including total number of pregnancies, full-term births, premature births, abortions, and living children. The age at the first pregnancy and any pregnancy-related complications are included. The sexual history is reviewed in a nonjudgmental manner facilitating an environment that encourages the woman to share any concerns or issues. Questions that address the five areas of sexual functions that change during the menopausal transition are (1) decline in sexual desire, (2) decreased sexual activity, (3) diminished sexual responsiveness, (4) dyspareunia, and (5) a partner with sexual function concerns.

The past medical history includes a review of any existing health problems, focusing on identifying established cardiovascular disease (CVD), previous cancers, obesity, or osteoporosis as these have implications for the woman becoming postmenopausal. Ask about induced menopause factors such as hysterectomy, chemotherapy, or radiation therapy (Goodman et al., 2011). The surgical history includes both gynecologic and other surgeries

Family history is reviewed and maternal age at onset of menopause is noted as there may be a correlation between mothers and daughters (Bentzen et al., 2013). The presence and age of onset is documented for family members with gynecologic or breast cancers, CVD, diabetes mellitus, or osteoporosis.

Social history includes behaviors and activities that may influence the woman's health and disease risk. Sleep patterns and concerns are documented as well as the current level of physical activity. Identify and note stressors and supports, recreational or illicit drug use, present or past tobacco use, alcohol consumption, occupation, and marital or relationship status as these may have implications for her health status, QOL, and ability to access care. Mood changes or mood disorders are reviewed keeping in mind that those having experienced hormone-related mood issues before menopause are more likely to experience mood-related issues during the menopause transition (Freeman, Sammel, Boorman, & Zhang, 2014). Other health-related behaviors (nutrition, stress management, caffeine intake, etc.) are also identified with a goal of identifying modifiable risk factors that may reduce the frequency and severity of menopause-related symptoms and improve overall health (Butts et al., 2012).

Physical Examination

The comprehensive physical examination is geared to identify health risks as well as other potential causes of symptoms. Include the vital signs of heart rate, blood pressure (BP), height, weight, BMI, waist circumference, and breast and pelvic examinations.

Significant bone loss occurs at the beginning of postmenopause and slows later (see Chapter 35). Documenting maximum adult height with current height will allow for assessment of bone loss; loss of height greater than 1.5 inches is suspect for vertebral compression fractures and thus osteoporosis (Nasto et al., 2012). Assessment of weight allows calculation of BMI stratifying the weight-associated health risk if the BMI is elevated. Waist circumference measurements of 35 inches or greater are indicative of central adiposity, which has been associated with the risk of coronary heart disease, hypertension, dyslipidemia, and type 2 diabetes mellitus in women (Weight-Control Information Network [WIN], 2014; see Chapters 43 and 44).

A clinical breast examination is a low-risk endeavor, though expert panels disagree on the value of the clinical breast examination in reducing breast cancer mortality (U.S. Preventive Services Task Force, 2009). The pelvic examination may reveal changes associated with decreasing estrogen levels: thinning hair distribution, thinning of the epithelium at the introitus and into the vagina, and bladder, rectal, or uterine descensus may be observed as evidence of decreased pelvic support (see Chapter 29). Women presenting with dyspareunia may be sensitive to gentle pressure distal to the hymen. The internal examination includes direct visualization of the cervix and cervical cytology and sexually transmitted infection (STI) screenings if appropriate. High levels of vaginal pH obtained from the vaginal sidewall suggest low estrogen levels. The internal reproductive organs are assessed during bimanual pelvic examination noting any pain, masses, size, and location of each. The benefit of a digital rectal examination is not clear given the current colonoscopy screening recommendations.

Differential Diagnoses

Several different health problems or the use of medication, drugs, or alcohol can mimic symptoms commonly associated with menopause and are considered in the differential (Table 34.2; NAMS, 2014).

TABLE 34.2	Sample Differential Diagnoses to Consider in Women Presenting With Menopause-Related Symptomatology
DIAGNOSIS	**SYMPTOMS SIMILAR TO PERIMENOPAUSE/MENOPAUSE**
Adenomyosis, endometriosis, fibroids, ovarian cysts, ovarian tumors, pregnancy, spontaneous abortion, uterine polyps	Menstrual changes, menorrhagia, worsening PMS
Anemia	Cognitive changes, fatigue
Anovulation, pregnancy	Amenorrhea, irregular bleeding
Arrhythmias	Fatigue, palpitations
Arthritis	Joint aches/pain
Depression	Anxiety, fatigue, insomnia, irritability, moodiness, sleep disturbances
Diabetes	Fatigue, HFs/heat intolerance, lack of energy
Hypertension	Headaches, HFs/heat intolerance
Hyperthyroidism	Heat intolerance, insomnia, irritability, nervousness, sleep disturbance
Hypothyroidism	Cognitive complaints, dry skin, fatigue, sleep disturbances, weight gain
Infections (fever, HIV, influenza, STIs, tuberculosis, viral illnesses)	Cystitis symptoms, dyspareunia, fatigue, vaginitis, vasomotor symptoms
Vulvar dystrophy	Dyspareunia, vaginal atrophy

HFs, hot flashes; PMS, premenstrual syndrome; STIs, sexually transmitted infections.
Adapted from Alexander and Andrist (2005); North American Menopause Society (2014); Shifren and Gass (2014).

■ DIAGNOSTIC STUDIES

The most accurate way to diagnose natural menopause is the clinical absence of a menstrual period for 12 consecutive months together with age and symptoms indicative of the menopausal transition (Box 34.2). Serum FSH testing is not recommended for determining perimenopausal or menopausal status. FSH levels are too variable and may unexpectedly return to normal, causing a rise in estrogen levels that may trigger the LH surge that prompts ovulation (NAMS, 2014). In women for whom the clinical picture is not clear, selected testing for conditions that commonly cause symptoms suggestive of menopause (Table 34.2) may be appropriate, such as thyroid stimulating hormone (TSH) levels and blood glucose or hemoglobin A1c.

■ TREATMENT/MANAGEMENT

Menopause management focuses on control of symptoms and reduction of health risks. Several approaches are used: self-management measures such as lifestyle changes, complementary and alternative medicine (CAM), HT, and nonhormonal prescription medications. It is important to inform the woman of the various symptom treatment options available and encourage active involvement in the decision-making process.

Often a woman at midlife has several diagnoses to contend with simultaneously, such as diabetes, hypertension, and perimenopause. Control of concomitant medical problems may also reduce a woman's menopausal symptoms to the point that they no longer affect her QOL.

Self-Management Measures

DIETARY CHANGES

Several food substances have been associated with increased frequency or severity of HFs: caffeine (cold and hot beverages, other substances that contain caffeine such as chocolate), sugar (especially refined sugars), alcohol, and spicy foods (Alexander et al., 2003; NAMS, 2014). Women are counseled to avoid or use these substances moderately to reduce or remove HF triggers.

Extra water ingestion is also recommended to replace the added insensible fluid lost through sweating. Drinking extra water, especially cold water, has been reported to reduce discomfort with sweating and HFs, as well as to minimize other symptoms such as dry skin (Alexander et al., 2003; NAMS, 2014). Water intake of at least 6 to 8 glasses each day is recommended. Women who experience nocturia are counseled to ingest most of their daily water in the morning to reduce nighttime wakening for urination. Only when bathroom access may be limited is moderate restriction of water intake warranted for women who experience urinary incontinence (NAMS, 2014).

VITAMINS AND SUPPLEMENTS

Some vitamins and supplements may reduce menopause-related symptoms and midlife health risks. Studies evaluating vitamin E for HF reduction have demonstrated conflicting results (Barton et al., 1998; Blatt, Weisbader, & Kupperman, 1953). Diets high in vitamin E and vitamin E supplements have been found to reduce the risk of developing Alzheimer's type dementia (Klatte, Scharre, Nagaraja, Davis, & Beversdorf, 2003; Onofrj et al., 2002). However, in two meta-analyses vitamin E not only was found to fail to protect against CVD, but it also was associated with increased mortality (Moyer & U.S. Preventive Services Task Force, 2014; Myung et al., 2013; Ye, Li, & Yuan, 2013). Beta-carotene and vitamin A were also associated with increased mortality (Bjelakovic, Nikolova, Gluud, Simonetti, & Gluud, 2007). Vitamin C and selenium did not affect mortality (Bjelakovic et al., 2007). Calcium and vitamin D have not been evaluated for mortality effects. They are critical for maintaining bone strength and preventing osteoporosis (National Osteoporosis Foundation, 2014) and thus are recommended for midlife women. High levels of homocysteine are associated with osteoporotic fracture, CVD, cerebrovascular accident, and Alzheimer's disease. A daily multivitamin with B complex is recommended because the B vitamins (folate, B_6, and B_{12}) are known to reduce homocysteine levels and the U.S. diet usually lacks sufficient fruits and vegetables, which are high in B complex vitamins (Fairfield & Fletcher, 2002; van Meurs et al., 2004). Omega-3 fatty acid supplements in a randomized trial showed no efficacy for vasomotor symptom management (Cohen et al., 2014); the omega-3 polyunsaturated fatty acids do have a powerful effect on reducing triglycerides level, which are associated with increased CVDs and are typically elevated in postmenopausal women. Unless (Dayspring, 2011) a specific iron deficiency is documented, use of iron supplementation and multivitamins with iron is not recommended. Excess iron has deleterious effects over time on the liver and cardiovascular system.

EXERCISE

Regular aerobic exercise is recommended for maintaining cardiovascular health, reducing the risk for osteoporosis and falls, and moderating glucose metabolism and weight gain. Regular aerobic exercise has also been shown to reduce the severity of menopause-related symptoms such as depression, forgetfulness, sleep disturbances (Afonso et al., 2012), and vasomotor symptoms (Daley, Stokes-Lampard, & MacArthur, 2011), and to improve QOL among postmenopausal women (NAMS, 2014; Reed et al., 2014). Additionally, lower levels of physical activity were associated with increased frequency of menopausal symptoms, particularly sleep disturbances, forgetfulness, soreness or stiffness, and heart racing or pounding (Gold et al., 2000). Emphasizing the benefits of regular exercise may serve as a motivator to continue or begin an exercise program. All women older than 50 years need to be evaluated before initiating a new exercise regimen to rule out any underlying CVD (see Chapter 14). Aerobic exercise for 1 hour per day is the goal. However, small amounts of exercise are also beneficial; therefore, beginning at even 10 or 20 minutes per day is a reasonable recommendation for a woman starting a new exercise program.

ENVIRONMENT AND CLOTHING CHANGES

The goal for clothing and environmental changes is to minimize core temperature changes to reduce vasomotor symptoms such as sweating or shivering. Wearing layered clothing that can be easily removed when room or air temperatures rise and using breathable fabrics, such as linen or cotton, help to reduce HF triggers (NAMS, 2014). Wearing high-neck or turtleneck shirts; tight clothing or clothing that does not allow for air circulation; extra layers, such as full-length stockings, girdles, or slips; and fabrics that do not absorb sweat, such as silk or polyester, are avoided. Wicking fabrics that dry quickly, such as those used by runners, can help to pull moisture away from the body when sweating does occur. There are pajamas designed specifically for women experiencing night sweats. Using these fabrics can reduce nighttime sleep disruptions attributable to night sweats.

Environmental adjustments can also reduce HF triggers. Circulating air with an open window or room fan, or both, and keeping the room temperature cool are beneficial, especially at night, because a woman's core temperature tends to rise under blankets and sheets while sleeping. Using sheets and blankets made of breathable fabrics to allow for air movement can reduce HF triggers at night. Similarly, using fabrics with imbedded Thermocules™ can be helpful. Based on space travel temperature regulation technologies, Thermocules are imbedded into fabrics used for mattresses, pillows, mattress pads, and sleepwear, and absorb excess body heat. Stored heat is released when the body cools, thus helping to maintain a steady temperature. Ingesting cold beverages or foods to reduce the core body temperature can also be beneficial (Alexander et al., 2003; NAMS, 2014).

VAGINAL LUBRICANTS AND MOISTURIZERS

Both water-based lubricants and moisturizers can help to reduce the discomfort and dyspareunia experienced as a result of vaginal atrophy. Water-based, nonhormonal lubricants such as Astroglide, K-Y Personal Lubricant, Moist Again, Lubrin, and Intimate Options Personal Lubricant Mousse are available OTC. Lubricants can be used for daily discomfort and are most beneficial for reducing vaginal dryness and thereby increasing comfort during sexual activity. More severe dryness that causes discomfort when walking or sitting is best managed using long-acting vaginal moisturizers such as K-Y Long-Lasting Vaginal Moisturizer and Replens. Compared with lubricants, moisturizers help to replenish and sustain fluids in the epithelial cells of the vaginal walls and provide longer lasting relief. Moisturizers can be especially beneficial for women who have daily discomfort; in addition, moisturizers are preferable because they support a normal vaginal pH and are therefore effective in reducing the likelihood of vaginitis (Nachtigall, 1994).

Oil-based products (e.g., petroleum jelly, baby oil) are not used on the vaginal epithelial tissue because they can be irritating and injure the tissue by causing cell clumping; also they are difficult to remove. Oil-based products can cause breakdown of diaphragms and condoms. An exception is vitamin E oil, which is nonirritating, does not interfere with condom or diaphragm function, and is safe for application directly to the vaginal walls. Other products that contain fragrances or oils, including toilet tissue, soaps, tampons, powders, or perfumes, are discouraged because they frequently cause irritation or vaginitis. Douching increases dryness and infection risks by removing normal vaginal flora and altering the vaginal pH (NAMS, 2014).

SLEEP AIDS

If HFs, night sweats, or other menopause-related symptoms are causing sleep disruption, then treating the symptoms will usually restore normal sleeping patterns. HT or non-hormonal medications can assist with HFs and night sweats. Less-severe HFs may be managed with lifestyle modifications. However, sleep disturbances are often related to other etiologies than menopause-related symptoms; in these cases, a more general approach is appropriate (see Chapter 15).

If stimulants are identified as potential problems then avoidance of alcohol, caffeine, and other stimulants can help to restore normal sleep patterns. Alcohol can have an initial sedative effect; however, it frequently causes sleep pattern disruptions after falling asleep such as rebound awakening and fragmented sleep (Landolt, Roth, Dijk, & Borbély, 1996). Because stimulant effects from caffeine can last more than 20 hours, complete elimination is recommended (Landolt, Werth, Borbély, & Dijk, 1995). To provide relief from common caffeine withdrawal side effects, such as headache, it is preferable to slowly reduce caffeine intake by substituting a caffeine-free beverage in increasing amounts over 1 month. Nicotine also increases sleep latency and causes reduced overall duration of sleep; thus smoking cessation is encouraged. Regular exercise and yoga (Afonso et al., 2012) can improve sleep quality and reduce sleep latency. Timing of exercise is critical, as exercising too close to bedtime can act as a stimulant and increase sleep latency (see Chapter 14).

In women with short duration of sleep, sleep-restriction therapy or sleep retraining can be helpful (Morin et al., 1999). Before initiation of a sleep-retraining program, the woman's current average number of sleep hours per night is determined. This time is subtracted from the desired morning rising time to identify when she will go to bed. After the woman has successfully (i.e., 95% of time) achieved this sleeping goal, the bedtime is moved back by 0.5 to 1 hour. This pattern is repeated gradually until she is sleeping the desired amount of time most nights. For the program to be successful, the woman must avoid *all* stimulants and sleep medications and must remain awake (no napping) except for the specified sleep hours. For example, if she is sleeping 4 hours at night and needs to rise at 6:30 a.m. for work, she is instructed to go to bed at 2:30 a.m. and rise at 6:30 a.m. each day. She continues with this pattern until she is sleeping the full 4 hours 95% of the time. When this goal is reached she changes her bedtime to 2:00 a.m. After she is sleeping the 4.5 hours for 95% of the time she changes her bedtime to 1:30 a.m. She continues with this pattern until she is sleeping the desired number of hours. Education also includes the normal amount of sleep that the woman needs (see Chapter 15).

Regardless of the underlying cause for sleep disruption, sleep hygiene is an important part of the management plan (Joffe, Massler, & Sharkey, 2010). Good sleep hygiene will reduce sleep latency and nocturnal wakening. Sleep hygiene practices cue the brain that it is time to sleep, prompting the brain's reticular activating system (RAS), which controls sleep–wake functions, to assume control. Just like children, adults sleep best when they follow a familiar and soothing routine before sleep. This is especially important for perimenopausal and postmenopausal women because sleep disruptions are so common. Bedtime routines that signal the mind for sleep might include grooming and relaxing activities. Activities that are stimulating are avoided just before bedtime, especially for those who have extended sleep latency. Reserving the bedroom for only sleep and sexual activity can further increase positive environmental triggers for sleep (see Chapter 15).

There are limited data on the nonprescriptive remedies of melatonin or sedative botanicals for the treatment of sleep disorders in menopausal women, but may be considered as options to improve sleep (Taavoni, Ekbatani, Kashaniyan, & Haghani, 2011) in addition to sleep hygiene practices.

SMOKING CESSATION

Smoking is linked to increased morbidity and mortality, particularly for CVD, cancer, bone loss, earlier age of menopause, and a higher prevalence of several menopause-related symptoms (Gold et al., 2000; NAMS, 2014). Several approaches can assist women with smoking cessation, the most important of which is clinician recommendation to stop smoking. Smoking cessation may mediate menopause-related HFs (Smith, Flaws, & Gallicchio, 2015) and reduce the risk of developing dementia (Williams, Plassman, Burke, Holsinger, & Benjamin, 2010).

TECHNIQUES FOR STRESS MANAGEMENT

Stress is an identified trigger for menopausal symptoms (Alexander et al., 2003). Stress is also linked to poor sleep and may cause moodiness or depression. At midlife, many women face multiple sources of stress, encompassing their work life, home life, relationships, and personal health (see Chapter 9).

Stress management techniques are tailored to the individual woman, because different women will find different activities relaxing. Some common activities that support relaxation include meditation, yoga, reading, spirituality or religion, regular exercise, massage, tai chi, a warm bath, deep or paced breathing, or seeking support from friends or family members. CAM therapies have been shown to provide sleep benefits in midlife women (Frame & Alexander, 2013). Biofeedback and progressive muscle relaxation have not been shown to change HFs significantly. Paced respiration had been associated with significantly reducing HFs (Freedman & Woodward, 1992; Irvin et al., 1996); however, in a recent randomized trial paced respirations was not found to be any better at reducing HF bother, interference, frequency, or severity (Sood et al., 2013). Some women report that effective management or avoidance of stress minimizes HF intensity and frequency (Alexander et al., 2003). Women can use deep breathing for relaxation and HF reduction by inhaling over a count of four, holding the breath over a count of seven, and exhaling slowly over a count of nine. Mindfulness-based stress reduction has shown some reduction in the intensity of HFs and bother, but was not statistically significant (Carmody et al., 2011), whereas both cognitive behavioral therapy (Hunter, 2014) and hypnosis (Elkins, Fisher, Johnson, Carpenter, & Keith, 2013) significantly reduced HF frequency and bother. Yoga has been shown to reduce vasomotor symptoms, joint pain, fatigue, and sleep disturbances, and increase QOL among postmenopausal breast cancer survivors (Reed et al., 2014).

ACTIVITIES FOR MEMORY FUNCTION ENHANCEMENT

Although some decline in mental function is normal with aging, many women experience more abrupt, bothersome cognitive changes that they associate with menopause. Most cognitive changes at midlife, such as difficulty remembering and concentrating, are related to poor sleep patterns or high stress levels. However, cognitive problems can also be associated with numerous medical problems. Thus, a comprehensive assessment is completed to identify the most likely cause of the cognitive changes before a treatment plan is determined.

Reasonable activities worth implementing that may help memory or potentially protect against dementia included remaining active both physically and mentally, increasing dietary intake of omega-3 fatty acids (Sydenham, Dangour, & Lim, 2012), keeping to no more than a moderate alcohol intake and not smoking (Williams et al., 2010). These activities, though not confirmed with rigorous studies, do have observational data for their implementation in the support of memory. Evidence does not support the use of HT for the improvement of cognitive function in postmenopausal woman (Henderson & Popat, 2011).

Establishing routines may help with memory; for example, store keys and accessories in the same location, note appointments and important events in a calendar, and keep an easily accessible list so that shopping needs and tasks can be monitored. Storing paper and pens at the bedside to note thoughts during the night can alleviate stress and may reduce nighttime awakenings. Attending to sleep hygiene and using relaxation methods can also improve memory. Keeping the mind actively engaged by participating in stimulating mental activities can also help retain cognitive function.

Complementary and Alternative Medicine

Use of CAM for menopause-related symptom management is increasing (Peng, Adams, Sibbritt, & Frawley, 2014). Because many patients do not report CAM use, it is critical that clinicians ask women about their use of these modalities. CAM therapies can provide reductions in vasomotor symptoms, assist with improving sleep, and reduce moodiness. (Frame & Alexander, 2013; NAMS, 2014; Peng et al., 2014).

ISOFLAVONES

Isoflavones are manufactured from plants that have both nonestrogenic and estrogenic properties. Isoflavones are found in foods, such as red clover and soy, and in commercially manufactured products and are converted to estrogenic compounds in the intestines. Because isoflavones have the ability to weakly bind with systemic estrogen receptors, particularly the beta receptors, they are frequently called phytoestrogens and have been studied extensively for managing HFs. Red clover and soy extracts also bind with progesterone and androgen receptors (Beck, Unterrieder, Krenn, Kubelka, & Jungbauer, 2003). A meta-analysis from 2012 found soy isoflavones to be significantly more effective in reducing the frequency and severity of HFs than placebo (Taku, Melby, Kronenberg, Kurzer, & Messina, 2012); no effect on vaginal dryness (Nikander et al., 2005) was identified. Results from other studies evaluating isoflavone efficacy on HF reduction have been contradictory. One meta-analysis identified efficacy for HFs with soy extract in 4 of 11 trials and no efficacy or mixed results with red clover in 6 trials (Nelson et al., 2006). Similarly, a Cochrane Review identified no efficacy in five trials of red clover extract, seven of nine trials of dietary soy, four of nine trials of soy extract, and six trials with other phytoestrogens (Lethaby et al., 2007). In a comparison of the most recent randomized, blinded, comparative clinical trials, the review found soy isoflavonids to be no more effective than a placebo (Chen, Lin, & Liu, 2015). Additionally, long-term use of soy phytoestrogens (5 years or longer) may increase the risk for endometrial hyperplasia (Unfer et al., 2004).

HERBAL PRODUCTS

Many herbal preparations are used for managing menopause-related symptoms (Table 34.3). Clinical studies evaluating the efficacy and safety of herbal remedies are increasing, especially for HFs. Study results have been inconclusive and contradictory for many products. Additionally, because herbal preparations are generally identified as dietary supplements, they are not held to the same U.S. Food and Drug Administration (FDA) regulations as are prescription medications or other OTC products, leading to concerns regarding purity and consistency. Product strength and use may also differ depending on the preparation (e.g., extract vs. tincture vs. poultice).

Many herbs are packaged in combination products or in Chinese herbal mixtures, sometimes making it difficult to determine the specific products that are being used. Women need to be asked specifically if they are using any of these products, because herbal products can interact with both other herbs and prescription medications.

BIOIDENTICAL OR "NATURAL" HORMONES

Many women request "natural" hormones for menopause-related symptom management. "Natural" hormones are mistakenly believed by many women to cause fewer side effects and to demonstrate higher safety than pharmaceutically manufactured hormones (Alexander, 2006). However, all commercially available hormones are manufactured. Furthermore, the term *natural* refers to substances with primary components derived from animal, plant, or mineral sources, which encompasses all pharmaceutically manufactured hormones as well. Many women also mistakenly believe that "natural" hormones are identical to the hormones produced in a woman's body (Alexander, 2006).

In contrast, "bioidentical" hormones are manufactured hormones that are chemically identical to those produced by a woman's body. Often, women who request "natural" hormones are actually interested in "bioidentical" products. Several bioidentical hormones (e.g., 17 estradiol, estriol, estrone, and micronized progesterone) are FDA-approved prescription products; others are available from compounding pharmacies.

Compounded estrogen products such as Bi-Est or Tri-Est can be prescribed. These topical creams are used for vasomotor and vaginal atrophy symptoms. Estriol vaginal cream can also be prescribed through a compounding pharmacy. Tri-Est (10% estradiol, 0.25 mg; 10% estrone, 0.25 mg; and 80% estriol, 2 mg) and Bi-Est (20% estradiol, 0.5 mg; and 80% estriol, 2 mg) are often advertised only identifying the estriol content of 80%, which is accurate. However, both Bi-Est and Tri-Est contain enough estradiol (0.25 to 0.5 mg) to also require use of progesterone for endometrial protection in women with an intact uterus (Gaudet, 2004). Advertisements by compounding companies were known to frequently infer that their products were safer than pharmaceutical grade hormones. The FDA took action against these companies to stop false advertisement claims for unsupported efficacy, safety, and superiority that are misleading to women and clinicians (FDA, 2008).

PROGESTERONE CREAM

OTC progesterone creams are available (e.g., Pro-Gest, PhytoGest, MenoBalance, and Endocreme). Progesterone content in these creams varies from less than 2 mg to greater than 700 mg per ounce. Progesterone creams can be prescribed through compounding pharmacies. These creams are considered dietary supplements. Thus, FDA regulations for prescription medications do not apply and concerns about concentration and purity are considered.

Although some women would like to use progesterone cream to avoid the potential systemic effects of oral progesterone, data do not support the use of progesterone creams for endometrial protection in women taking systemic estrogen therapy (ET). Transdermal progesterone cream does have some efficacy for reducing HFs (Leonetti, Longo, & Anasti, 1999) and may be a more frequently used option in the future.

ACUPUNCTURE

Acupuncture is a widely recognized modality for pain relief and relaxation. A meta-analysis of published acupuncture studies found a lack of convincing evidence to support the use of acupuncture for HF management (Lee, Shin, & Ernst, 2009). However, a more recent study showed an equal effect for vasomotor symptom control between acupuncture and venlafaxine (Walker et al., 2010). Despite these controversial findings, acupuncture is a safe, well-accepted form of

TABLE 34.3	Herbal Therapies for Menopause-Related Symptoms[a]		
PRODUCT	**USUAL DOSAGE[b]**	**PURPOSE IN MENOPAUSE**	**COMMENTS**
Black cohosh (*Cimicifuga racemosa*)	20 mg twice a day (proprietary standardized extract)	■ Vasomotor symptoms	■ Research evidence controversial; some data show beneficial effects close to that of estrogen for HF relief, and other data show no benefit ■ Safety for use greater than 6 months not established ■ Can potentiate antihypertensives ■ Multiple products and formulations available ■ Wide variations in product ingredients, purity, and extraction processes ■ Product labels frequently recommend much higher doses ■ Rare cases of hepatitis reported ■ Side effects rare, usually intestinal upset, dizziness, headache, hypotension, painful extremities; more common with higher doses
Chaste tree berry (*Vitex agnus-castus*)	Effective dose unknown; hard to find standardized extract	■ Menstrual irregularity	■ No data on relief of menopause-related symptoms ■ More popular in Europe than United States; approved in Germany for PMS, mastalgia, and menopause-related symptoms ■ Often found in combination products ■ Side effects rare, usually headache, intestinal upset
Dong quai (*Angelica sinensis*)	Two capsules two to three times a day; usually in combination products	■ Gynecologic conditions	■ Research found no benefit for menopause-related symptoms ■ Widely used in Asia ■ Used in Chinese herb combinations; Chinese *materia medica* cautions not to give alone ■ A "heating" herb, can cause red face, HFs, sweating, irritability, or insomnia ■ Contains coumarin derivatives, contraindicated in those taking warfarin ■ Can cause photosensitivity, hypotension, anticoagulation, and possibly has carcinogenicity properties
Evening primrose oil (*Oenothera biennis*)	3–4 g daily in divided doses	■ HFs ■ Mastalgia	■ No benefit for menopause-related symptoms ■ Potentiates risk for seizure if taken by person with seizure disorder or person taking phenothiazines and other medications that lower seizure threshold ■ Side effects include diarrhea and nausea
Ginkgo (*Ginkgo biloba*)	40–80 mg three times a day of standardized extract	■ Memory changes	■ Insufficient research on safety and efficacy ■ Memory changes often related to sleep disturbances; menopausal sleep disturbances frequently related to HFs, stress ■ Side effects include intestinal distress, hypotension; chronic use has been linked with subarachnoid hemorrhage, subdural hematoma, and increased bleeding times
Ginseng (*Panax ginseng*)	1–2 g of root daily in divided doses	■ General "tonic" ■ Improved mood, fatigue	■ Little to no benefit to menopausal symptoms; benefits well-being, general health, and depression ■ Heavily adulterated ■ Can cause uterine bleeding, mastalgia ■ Contraindicated in women with breast cancer and in women who are also taking monoamine oxidase inhibitors, stimulants, or anticoagulants; may potentiate digoxin and others (multiple drug interactions) ■ Side effects include rash, nervousness, insomnia, hypertension

(continued)

TABLE 34.3	Herbal Therapies for Menopause-Related Symptoms[a] *(continued)*		
PRODUCT	**USUAL DOSAGE[b]**	**PURPOSE IN MENOPAUSE**	**COMMENTS**
Kava (*Piper methysticum*)	150–300 mg of root extract daily in divided doses	■ Irritability ■ Insomnia	■ Little data available to support use ■ Banned in several countries because of hepatotoxicity; thus not recommended ■ Contraindicated with depression ■ Side effects include gastrointestinal discomfort, impaired reflexes and motor function, weight loss, hepatotoxicity, rash
Licorice root (*Glycyrrhiza glabra*)	5–15 mg of root equivalent daily in divided doses	■ Menopause-related symptoms	■ No data supporting relief of HFs ■ Found in many Chinese herb mixtures ■ High doses can lead to primary aldosteronism, cardiac arrhythmias, cardiac arrest ■ Contraindicated in presence of hepatic or renal disease, diabetes, hypertension, pregnancy, hypertonia, hypokalemia, or arrhythmia, or when taking diuretics
Passion flower (*Passiflora incarnata*)	3–10 g daily, divided doses	■ Sedative	■ Mixed results in sleep improvement ■ Menopausal sleep disturbances frequently related to HFs, stress
St. John's wort (*Hypericum perforatum*)	300 mg three times a day (standardized extract)	■ Vasomotor symptoms ■ Irritability ■ Depression	■ No data supporting vasomotor relief ■ Research findings support use for depression; there are no clinical trials for menopause ■ Often combined with black cohosh for menopause symptom treatment ■ Interferes with metabolism of many medications that are metabolized in liver; affects cytochrome P_{450} enzymes (e.g., estrogen, digoxin, theophylline); reduces INR levels; not to be used concomitantly with antidepressants, monoamine oxidase inhibitors, or immunosuppressants ■ Side effects include photosensitivity, rash, constipation, cramping, dry mouth, fatigue, dizziness, restlessness, insomnia
Valerian root (*Valeriana officinalis*)	300–600 mg of aqueous extract 0.5 to 1 hour before bed (insomnia); 150–300 mg every morning and 300–400 mg every evening aqueous extract (anxiety)	■ Sedative ■ Antianxiety	■ Research showed improvement in sleep and depression/mood scales ■ Used for insomnia in intermittent dosing, for anxiety with chronic dosing ■ Side effects include headache, uneasiness, excitability, arrhythmias, morning sedation, GI upset, cardiac function disorders (with long-term use)
Wild yam (*Dioscorea villosa*)	Unknown	■ Menopausal symptoms	■ Research showed no benefit to menopausal symptoms ■ Products claim that creams are converted to progesterone; however, human body cannot convert topical or ingested wild yam into progesterone ■ Wild yam is used as main ingredient in some products to manufacture progesterone in laboratory; these products have demonstrated some efficacy ■ Many preparations have been adulterated with undisclosed steroids that may cause potential harm and therefore are not recommended for use.

[a]See prescribing reference for full information on doses, side effects, contraindications, and cautions.
[b]Dosages vary and frequently differ according to form (e.g., drops, essential oil, liquid extract, standardized extract, tincture).
GI, gastrointestinal; HFs, hot flashes; INR, international normalized ratio; PMS, premenstrual syndrome.
Adapted from Peng, Adams, Sibbritt, and Frawley (2014); North American Menopause Society (2014).

CAM. The relaxation and any placebo effects obtained with this CAM modality may reduce HFs enough to provide benefit for some women; it is not recommended for the treatment of menopause-associated vasomotor symptoms at this time (NAMS, 2015).

Pharmacotherapeutics

HORMONE THERAPY

HT, consisting of ET, estrogen-progestogen therapy (EPT)/estrogen+bazedoxifene, or estrogen-testosterone therapy (ETT), remains the most effective strategy for managing moderate to severe vasomotor and vaginal symptoms associated with menopause (NAMS, 2014). HF severity is defined by the individual woman according to its effect on her QOL (NAMS, 2014).

Multiple different estrogen compounds are available (Table 34.4). Estrogens have differing dose equivalencies and target tissue responses. Preparations for estrogen include systemic (oral, patch, cream, gel, spray, vaginal ring) and local (vaginal cream, tablet, or ring) delivery systems. With the exception of the 0.5- and 0.1-mg versions of the vaginal Femring, local vaginal estrogen therapy has little effect on systemic estrogen levels and is not indicated for HFs. Rather, local therapy is used for managing symptoms of vaginal atrophy (NAMS, 2014). Estrogens are FDA approved for relief of moderate to severe vasomotor symptoms and vaginal atrophy.

In the postmenopausal woman with a uterus, either progesterone or bazedoxifene, a selective ER modulator (SERM), are used to protect the woman against developing endometrial hyperplasia or adenocarcinoma when ET is used (Table 34.4; NAMS, 2014). Progesterone is occasionally used alone for HF management in a woman who cannot take estrogen.

Several formulations of testosterone together with estrogen (ETT) are FDA approved for use in postmenopausal women when other forms of HT do not adequately control vasomotor symptoms (Table 34.4). A progestogen is needed for endometrial protection in women with an intact uterus. Although testosterone is not currently FDA approved for treating low libido in women, studies have demonstrated the effectiveness of a testosterone patch on libido in surgically and naturally postmenopausal women (Buster et al., 2005; Shifren et al., 2006). Transdermal testosterone has also been linked to improved well-being, mood, and sexual function in premenopausal women (Goldstat, Briganti, Tran, Wolfe, & Davis, 2003). Testosterone cream, patches, and gels manufactured for use in men and combination testosterone products are used off-label in women for this purpose (see Chapter 26; NAMS, 2014).

When a woman considers HT for menopause-related symptom management, all of the contraindications, side effects, and cautions (Table 34.5) are first carefully reviewed. Her personal and family histories are evaluated to identify possible risk factors or contraindications. The woman must be engaged in the decision and comfortable with use of HT. The known risks and benefits, as well as the unanswered scientific questions about HT, are openly discussed. Results from the Heart and Estrogen/Progestin Replacement Study (HERS; Grady et al., 2002; Hulley et al., 1998; Hulley et al.,

2002) and WHI (Anderson et al., 2004; Heiss et al., 2008; Rossouw et al., 2002; Shumaker et al., 2003) trials indicate that HT may increase risks for CVD, stroke, thromboembolism, breast cancer, and dementia (Alexander, 2012). The possibility that these risks are lower for women who are in or just past menopause or early in the postmenopausal period are also reviewed (Grodstein, Manson, & Stampfer, 2006; Hsia et al., 2006; Rossouw et al., 2007; Salpeter et al., 2004) The controversies that surround the relationship between HT and breast cancer and dementia are also discussed. Some studies demonstrate protective effects against dementia with HT (Bagger et al., 2005; Craig et al., 2008; Zandi et al., 2002) and others show increased risks (Shumaker et al., 2003). Breast cancer risk likely increases after 3 to 5 years of EPT use (Chlebowski et al., 2009; Li et al., 2008; NAMS, 2014; Rossouw et al., 2002) and may return to baseline after cessation (Chlebowski et al., 2009; Coombs, Taylor, Wilcken, & Boyages, 2005; Coombs, Taylor, Wilcken, Fiorica, & Boyages, 2005; Heiss et al., 2008). Additionally, recent epidemiologic data identifying fluctuating rates of breast cancer following the decline in HT use (Alexander, 2011; Clarke et al., 2006; Ravdin et al., 2007) and the reduced rates of mammography screenings (Breen et al., 2007; Meissner, Breen, Taubman, Vernon, & Graubard, 2007) are reviewed. Finally, it is important to discuss the possibility of mammographic changes while the woman is taking HT; for example, increased breast density may obscure detection of an early breast cancer lesion or mammogram abnormalities may lead to unnecessary biopsy (Chlebowski et al., 2008). There are no data identifying an increased risk of breast cancer with estrogen+bazedoxifene. NAMS notes that bazedoxifene may reduce the risk for breast cancer as bazedoxifene is a SERM (NAMS, 2014).

QOL benefits from HT are also considered. Many women have a decline in QOL with the transition to postmenopause (NAMS, 2014). If menopause-related symptoms are bothersome and negatively affecting a woman's QOL, then HT may be an appropriate option. In addition to relief of vasomotor symptoms and vaginal atrophy, HT is known to preserve skin thickness and reduce the appearance of wrinkles (Brincat, 2000); reduce sleep latency and insomnia and increase rapid eye movement (REM) sleep (Antonijevic, Stalla, & Steiger, 2000; Schiff, Regestein, Schinfeld, & Ryan, 1980); improve mood (Soares, Almeida, Joffe, & Cohen, 2001); improve sexual function (Cayan, Dilek, Pata, & Dilek, 2008); decrease colon cancer incidence; and maintain bone strength, reducing the possibility of osteoporotic fractures (Rossouw et al., 2002).

If a woman is an appropriate candidate for HT and elects to use it for symptom management, she is counseled about the possible regimen combinations and methods of delivery. ET is prescribed only to women who do not have an intact uterus. Testosterone may be added to either ET or EPT as needed, it cannot be added to estrogen+bazedoxifene. EPT can follow several different patterns. One option is the continuous combined (CC-EPT) method in which a progestogen is taken daily with estrogen, either in the same tablet or pill or as a separate oral medication such as with creams or gels. An alternative to this method is the pulsed regimen in which the woman takes estrogen every day and "pulses" the progestin dose by taking progestin for two consecutive days,

TABLE 34.4	Hormone Therapy Products[a]		
TYPE	**PRODUCT NAME (MANUFACTURER)**	**ACTIVE INGREDIENT**	**DOSAGE**
Estrogens, oral	Enjuvia	Conjugated estrogens B	0.3 mg, 0.45 mg, 0.625 mg, or 1.25 mg once daily
	Estrace; generics	Micronized estradiol	0.5 mg, 1 mg, or 2 mg once daily
	Menest	Esterified estrogens	0.3 mg, 0.625 mg, 1.25 mg, or 2.5 mg once daily
	Generic	Estropipate	0.75 mg, 1.5 mg, or 3.0 mg once daily
	Premarin	Conjugated estrogens (formerly conjugated equine estrogens)	0.3 mg, 0.45 mg, 0.625 mg, 0.9 mg, or 1.25 mg once daily
Estrogens, transdermal	Alora	Estradiol	0.025 mg, 0.05 mg, 0.075 mg, or 0.1 mg daily Change patch twice weekly Apply to lower abdomen or upper outer buttocks
	Climara; generic	Estradiol	0.025 mg, 0.0375 mg, 0.05 mg, 0.06 mg, 0.075 mg, or 0.1 mg daily Change patch weekly Apply to lower abdomen or upper outer buttocks
	Divigel	Estradiol	0.1% gel packet 0.25 mg/d, 0.5 mg/d, or 1.0 mg/d Apply one packet to thigh daily
	Elestrin	Estradiol	0.06% gel pump 0.87 g per pump of gel delivers 0.52 mg of estradiol daily Apply gel once daily to upper arm
	Generic	Estradiol	0.025 mg, 0.037 mg, 0.05, 0.075 mg, or 0.1 mg daily Change patch twice weekly Apply patch to buttocks, upper inner thigh, or upper arm
	Estrasorb cream	Estradiol	2.5% (4.35 mg/1.74 g/packet) emulsion 3.48 g to skin daily Two packets rubbed into thighs every morning for more than 3 minutes
	EstroGel	Estradiol	0.06% gel 1.25 g per pump of gel delivers 0.75 mg of estradiol daily Apply gel once daily to arm from shoulder to wrists
	Evamist	Estradiol	1.7% solution 90 mcg/L spray delivers 1.53 mg of estradiol daily Start with one spray daily; increase to two to three sprays as needed One spray once daily to forearm
	Menostar	Estradiol	0.014 mg daily Change patch weekly Apply to lower abdomen FDA approved for osteoporosis prevention; recent study also showed efficacy for HF relief
	Minivelle, Vivelle-Dot; generics	Estradiol	0.025 mg, 0.0375 mg, 0.05 mg, 0.075 mg, or 0.1 mg daily Change patch twice weekly

(continued)

TABLE 34.4	Hormone Therapy Products[a] *(continued)*		
TYPE	**PRODUCT NAME (MANUFACTURER)**	**ACTIVE INGREDIENT**	**DOSAGE**
Progestogens, oral	Aygestin	Norethindrone acetate	2.5 mg to 10 mg continuously or on set cycle schedule Used for woman with intact uterus taking estrogen
	Ortho Micronor; Nor-QD; generics	Norethindrone	0.35 mg Off-label use
	Prometrium	Micronized progesterone	200 mg at bedtime continuously or on set cycle schedule Used for woman with intact uterus taking estrogen Contains peanut oil
	Provera; generics	Medroxyprogesterone acetate (MPA)	2.5 mg, 5 mg, or 10 mg continuously or on set cycle schedule Used for woman with intact uterus taking estrogen
Combination estrogens + progestogens, oral	Activella	Estradiol + norethindrone acetate	0.5/0.1 mg or 1.0/0.5 mg once daily (continuous combined)
	Angeliq	Estradiol + drospirenone	1/0.5 mg once daily (continuous combined)
	FemHRT	Ethinyl estradiol + norethindrone acetate	2.5 mcg/0.5 mg or 5 mcg/1 mg once daily (continuous combined)
	Prefest	Estradiol 3 tabs then estradiol + norgestimate 3 tabs	1 mg × 3 days alternating with 1 mg/0.9 mg × 3 days, once daily sequentially
	Premphase	Conjugated estrogens (14 tabs), then conjugated estrogens + MPA (14 tabs)	0.625 mg, then 0.625 mg + 5 mg Once daily sequentially
	Prempro	Conjugated estrogens + MPA	0.3 mg + 1.5 mg once daily; 0.45 mg + 1.5 mg once daily; 0.625 mg + 2.5 mg once daily; or 0.625 mg + 5 mg once daily Taken daily (continuous combined)
Combination estrogens + progestogens, transdermal	Climara Pro	Estradiol + levonorgestrel	0.045 mg + 0.015 mg daily Change patch once weekly Apply to lower abdomen Continuous combined regimen
	CombiPatch	Estradiol + norethindrone acetate	0.05 mg/0.14 mg or 0.05 mg/0.25 mg daily Change patch twice weekly Apply to lower abdomen; rotate sites Use in rotation with estradiol patch to provide sequential progestogen, or daily as continuous combined regimen
Combination estrogens + bazedoxifene, oral	Duavee	Estrogens, conjugated + bazedoxifene	0.45 mg + 20 mg once daily
Combination estrogens + androgens, oral	Generics	Esterified estrogens + methyltestosterone	0.625 mg + 1.25 mg once daily Start with HS dose; if additional symptom relief needed, increase to 1.25 mg + 2.5 mg once daily

(continued)

TABLE 34.4	Hormone Therapy Products[a] *(continued)*		
TYPE	**PRODUCT NAME (MANUFACTURER)**	**ACTIVE INGREDIENT**	**DOSAGE**
Estrogens, vaginal creams	Estrace Vaginal	Micronized estradiol-17β	0.01% cream, 1 g = 0. mg of estradiol 2–4 g daily for 1–2 weeks; then taper as symptoms tolerate
	Premarin Vaginal	Conjugated estrogens (formerly conjugated equine estrogens)	0.625 g cream 1–2 g daily for 1–2 weeks; then taper to lowest effective dose
Estrogens, vaginal tablets	Vagifem	Estradiol hemihydrate	0.025 mg tab 1 tab daily for 2 weeks; then taper to lowest effective dose
Estrogens, vaginal rings	Estring	Micronized estradiol-17β	7.5 mcg delivered in 24 hours Replace vaginal ring every 3 months
	Femring	Estradiol acetate	0.05 mg delivered in 24 hours or 0.1 mg delivered in 24 hours Start with 0.05 mg/d ring Replace vaginal ring every 3 months Effective for both systemic vasomotor symptoms and local vulvovaginal symptoms
Progestogens, vaginal gel	Crinone	Progesterone	8% vaginal gel Off-label use
	Prochieve	Progesterone	4%, 8% vaginal gel Off-label use
IUS	Mirena	Levonorgestrel	52 mg IUD Ensure not pregnant Off-label use Provides local progesterone to prevent endometrial hyperplasia and cancer 5-year use

[a]See prescribing reference for full information on doses, side effects, contraindications, and cautions; use lowest effective dose for shortest time possible; progestogen is needed for any woman with an intact uterus who is using estrogen (oral, patch, cream, gel, systemic ring, and possibly for vaginal products) to prevent endometrial hyperplasia and cancer.
HF, hot flash; IUD, intrauterine device; IUS, intrauterine system.
Adapted from ePocrates; Alexander and Andrist (2005).

then estrogen only for 1 day, then both estrogen and progestin for 2 consecutive days in a repeating pattern. Both the CC-EPT and pulsed regimens will reduce or remove withdrawal bleeds over time. The pulsed regimen was developed to provide similar benefits as CC-EPT with fewer progestogen-related side effects. However, breakthrough bleeding is more common when the pulsed regimen is used. In the combined sequential (CS-EPT) method, estrogen is taken daily and the progestogen is added for 12 to 14 days of the month, often starting on the first day of the month. When this method is used, the woman will usually have a withdrawal bleed following completion of the progestogen. This sequence is repeated monthly. Some women prefer to take the progestogen only 3 or 4 months of the year. This will reduce the frequency of withdrawal bleeds and does reduce the risk of endometrial overgrowth and cancer; however, it is not as effective as the monthly dosing pattern. Breakthrough bleeding is common for all forms of EPT in the first several months following initiation of therapy. It will decrease over time and with the CC-EPT method bleeding often will cease completely. The cyclic regimen is another CS-EPT option, in which estrogen is taken alone on days 1 to 11 and together with the progestogen on days 12 to 21 of the month. This method is rarely used because of the frequency of rebound symptoms that occur during the withdrawal bleed period (days 22 to 28) when no hormones are taken. If rebound symptoms are not experienced, then tapering the HT is considered. Estrogen + bazedoxifene is administered in a continuous pattern of one combined tablet daily. Progestogen administered through an intrauterine system (e.g., Mirena; Mirena PI; labeling.bayerhealthcare.com/html/products/pi/Mirena_PI.pdf) can be considered for off-label endometrial protection in women who are taking ET and who prefer not to use or cannot tolerate oral progestogens.

TABLE 34.5	Common Hormone Therapy Side Effects and Management Strategies[a]
SIDE EFFECT	**MANAGEMENT STRATEGY**
Alopecia, extra hair growth	■ Consider changing estrogen ■ Consider changing progestogen ■ Consider reducing or discontinuing testosterone
Abdominal bloating, cramping, flatulence	■ Advise her to avoid grapefruit and grapefruit juice ■ Advise her to ingest 6–8 glasses of water daily ■ Change to low-dose transdermal estrogen ■ Consider adding a low-dose diuretic ■ Consider reducing progestogen dose, changing to alternate progestogen, or using micronized progesterone
Bleeding, spotting (vaginal)	■ Ensure that she is taking HT at same time each day ■ Educate her that breakthrough bleeding is common with continuous combined EPT during first few months of therapy ■ Consider changing to a different HT or reducing dose ■ If bleeding begins after the first few months of continuous combined EPT, evaluate using ultrasound and/or endometrial biopsy
Breast changes, tenderness	■ Advise her to reduce salt, peanuts, chocolate, and caffeine ingestion ■ Advise her to wear a supportive bra ■ Consider changing progestogen ■ Consider reducing or changing estrogen ■ Consider use of evening primrose oil
Chloasma/malasma	■ Ensure that she uses sunscreen daily ■ Advise her to wear wide-brimmed hat to shield face
Depression, mood changes	■ Ensure that sleep is adequate ■ Ensure that daily water intake is adequate ■ Assess for stress and stress management ■ Advise her to limit salt, alcohol, and caffeine consumption ■ Consider changing or reducing progestogen ■ Consider changing to a continuous combined EPT regimen
Dry eyes, intolerance of contact lenses	■ Advise her to avoid antihistamines ■ Advise her to avoid smoke ■ Advise her to maintain adequate water intake ■ Consider referral to discuss change in contact lenses ■ Recommend reduced wearing time for contact lenses ■ Recommend use of ophthalmic lubricating drops or rewetting drops for contact lens wearers
Elevated blood pressure	■ Advise her to avoid alcohol ■ Advise her to avoid and discontinue (if applicable) smoking ■ Advise her to exercise regularly and remain active ■ Advise her to limit salt intake ■ Advise her to lose weight if BMI is greater than 25 kg/m^2 ■ Advise her to maintain adequate water intake ■ Assess for stress and stress management ■ Ensure that antihypertensives are being taken correctly ■ Consider reducing, changing, or discontinuing estrogen ■ Consider reducing or discontinuing testosterone ■ Monitor blood pressure; if consistently elevated, consider discontinuing hormone therapy
Elevated blood glucose levels, glucose intolerance	■ Ensure that she is consistently following diet and exercising ■ Consider adjusting diabetes medication(s) ■ Consider reducing estrogen

(continued)

TABLE 34.5	Common Hormone Therapy Side Effects and Management Strategies[a] *(continued)*
SIDE EFFECT	**MANAGEMENT STRATEGY**
Fluid retention	■ Advise her to ingest 6–8 glasses of water daily; consider adding lemon for a natural diuretic effect ■ Advise her to exercise regularly ■ Consider adding a low-dose prescription diuretic or herbal diuretic ■ Consider changing to transdermal estrogen patch, gel, or cream ■ Consider reducing or changing progestogen
Gastrointestinal upset, nausea, vomiting	■ Advise her to take hormones with meals ■ Ensure that daily water intake is adequate ■ Consider changing or reducing estrogen ■ Consider changing or reducing progestogen ■ Consider changing to transdermal estrogen
Loss of libido	■ Consider adding testosterone (off-label use) ■ Assess sexual function, social factors, and relationship; make recommendations (see Chapters 19 and 29)
Headache or migraine aggravation	■ Advise her to limit salt, caffeine, and alcohol use ■ Assess for stress and stress management (see Chapters 12 and 40) ■ Ensure that daily water intake is adequate ■ Consider change to continuous combined EPT regimen to reduce hormone fluctuations ■ Consider change to transdermal estrogen ■ Consider decreasing estrogen and/or progestogen
Rash	■ Ensure that patch is applied over clean, dry area ■ Ensure that patch location is rotated ■ If urticaria develops, stop medication and assess for allergic response

[a]See prescribing reference for full information on side effects, cautions, and contraindications for estrogen, progestogens, and testosterone hormone therapy products.
EPT, estrogen-progestogen therapy; HT, hormone therapy.
Adapted from Alexander and Knight (2005); North American Menopause Society (2014); Shifren and Gass (2014).

Although progestogen therapy (PT) can be used alone for menopause symptom management, this is uncommon because EPT generally provides better symptom relief. For women who cannot take estrogen, PT using Megace (i.e., megestrol), a progestogen used for breast cancer treatment, or injectable medroxyprogesterone acetate (Depoprovera) might be considered (Loprinzi et al., 2006). However, other alternatives to HT may be equally effective and are also considered and discussed with the woman.

HT is available in multiple routes of delivery. Oral products are available as tablets, pills, coated tablets, and timed-release tablets. All orally ingested hormones are rapidly metabolized to estrone in the liver. Although maximum serum concentrations are achieved in approximately 6 hours and a steady state is present in about 1 week, it may take up to 6 weeks for symptom control to manifest because circulating hormones bind slowly to open hormone receptors.

Transdermal products are available as patches, spray, cream, and gel. The hepatic first-pass effect is largely avoided when transdermal administration is used. As a result, lower doses of hormones can be used and clotting risks may be reduced (Canonico et al., 2007). Otherwise, transdermal hormones generally carry the same risks and benefits as oral products (Canonico et al., 2007). Although often more costly than oral products, this route

of administration is ideal for women with a history of thrombosis, high triglyceride levels, hypertension, or other chronic diseases. Transdermal administration, especially with patches, tends to provide more constant hormone levels than oral administration.

Vaginal hormones are available as creams, tablets, and rings. As with the transdermal products, they largely avoid the hepatic first-pass effect; in addition, for women with underlying chronic disease or history of thrombosis, they are considered safer than oral methods. They carry the same overall risks and benefits as oral products. Most vaginal products work locally in the vagina and are the preferred treatment option for women with primary symptoms attributable to atrophic vaginitis. Very low doses, such as 10 mcg, can be effective (Bachmann, Lobo, Gut, Nachtigall, & Notelovitz, 2008). Femring does have systemic properties, is effective for both HFs and vaginal atrophy, and may require use of a progestogen.

Injectable hormones are available in formulations intended to provide relatively immediate or prolonged effects. Injectable hormones that provide relatively immediate effects are most often used for treating bleeding or protecting pregnancy. Some forms of contraception (see Chapter 21) and HT are also available in longer-acting injectable forms. The HT formulations rapidly provide steady serum levels and remain effective over a period of

CATEGORY	DRUG	DOSAGE[a]	COMMENT[a]	COMMON SIDE EFFECTS[a]	CONTRAINDICATIONS[a]
Anticonvulsants	Gabapentin (Neurontin)	Initial dose 300 mg/d Increase at 3- to 4-day intervals to 300 mg three times daily as needed	Avoid abrupt cessation Effective in two out of two trials	Ataxia, dizziness, fatigue, somnolence	No antacids within 2 hours of use Alcohol potentiates CNS depression
Antihypertensives	Clonidine	0.05–0.1 mg twice daily	Available as a patch Less effective than SSRIs/ SNRIs or gabapentin Avoid abrupt cessation	Agitation, arrhythmias, constipation, dizziness, drowsiness, dry mouth, hypotension, impotence, insomnia, myalgia, nausea, orthostatic hypotension, rash, urticaria, weakness	Antagonized by tricyclic antidepressants Potentiates CNS depressants
	Methyldopa and Bellergal		Not recommended because of toxicity		
Breast cancer agent (progestin)	Megestrol (Megace)	20 mg daily (divided doses)	May increase insulin requirements	Asthenia, chest pain, decreased libido, dyspepsia, edema, fever, hyperglycemia, hypertension, insomnia, intestinal disturbance, rash, urinary frequency, weight gain	Use with caution in women with diabetes or history of thromboembolic disease
SSRIs/SNRIs[b]	Fluoxetine (Prozac)	Start at 20 mg/d Titrate up as needed	Avoid abrupt cessation Monitor weight	Anorgasmia, asthenia, GI upset, reduced libido, somnolence, insomnia, sweating	Avoid concomitant use of MAO inhibitors or thioridazine
	Paroxetine (Brisdelle)	7.5mg/d	Only SSRI with FDA approval for treatment of HFs Avoid abrupt cessation	See fluoxetine	Use with caution with warfarin Avoid use with alcohol Use with caution in women with diabetes, diseases that affect metabolism, or heart disease
	Desvenlafaxine (Pristiq)	Start at 50 mg/d Titrate up to max dose of 400 mg/d as needed	Avoid abrupt cessation	See fluoxetine	
	Venlafaxine (Effexor XR)	Start at 37.5 mg/d Titrate up as needed	Avoid abrupt cessation	See fluoxetine	

[a]See prescribing reference for full information on doses, side effects, contraindications, and cautions; use of these products for vasomotor symptom relief is off-label; efficacy for HF management with these products is less than that with estrogen.

[b]Effective in four out of six trials in meta-analysis.

CNS, central nervous system; FDA, Food and Drug Administration; GI, gastrointestinal; MAO, monoamine oxidase; SNRI, serotonin-norepinephrine reuptake inhibitor; SSRI, selective serotonin reuptake inhibitor.

Adapted from Alexander and Andrist (2005); ePocrates; North American Menopause Society (2014, 2015b).

approximately 1 month. As with other methods of delivery, receptor binding and thus symptom control may take up to 6 weeks.

When initiating HT, NAMS recommends using a low dose of estrogen (e.g., 0.3-mg CEE or 0.25- to 0.5-mg estradiol patch). Some women will require higher doses to obtain symptom control. Efficacy is determined by monitoring symptoms and dose is titrated to the lowest possible effective dose for the woman.

Women may experience different side effects depending on the type of estrogen or progesterone they are taking. Trying different types to determine which products are most acceptable is appropriate and often necessary. Similarly, some women will determine that the delivery method initially selected is not agreeable and may need to be changed.

Clinicians provide women with anticipatory guidance regarding normal HT side effects and management strategies (Table 34.5). Many women attribute HT with weight gain; however, research provides evidence that HT does not increase body weight; instead, it assists in preventing the weight increase and abdominal adiposity associated with midlife (Espeland et al., 1997; Margolis et al., 2004). HT also helps to prevent diabetes, which affects more women as they age (Margolis et al., 2004). A follow-up appointment approximately 1 to 2 months after HT is initiated provides an opportunity to reevaluate symptoms, answer questions, and reiterate patient education. Dose adjustments can be made at this time if symptoms are not at an acceptable level.

The need for HT is reevaluated at least annually; if symptom control is still necessary, then HT may be continued for the shortest period possible. If symptoms are well controlled using a specific dose, then reducing the dose to determine if symptom control continues is appropriate. Some women have symptoms for a few years, whereas others continue with moderate to severe symptoms for many years (Kronenberg, 1990). The decision to discontinue HT is made collaboratively with the woman and based on her individual risks, needs, and QOL. The discussion on discontinuation of HT needs to include the newest findings from the 2015 study by Mikkola et al. showing increased risk of cardiac, stroke death in the first year after stopping hormone therapy in women aged 60 years or younger, but not in those older than 60 years (Mikkola et al., 2015).

NONHORMONE PRESCRIPTION MEDICATIONS

Although ET and EPT/estrogen + bazedoxifene are superior for vasomotor symptom management (NAMS, 2014; Nelson et al., 2006), women who are unwilling or unable to take hormones may seek alternative prescription options (Table 34.6). These may be added to lifestyle changes and/or some CAM therapies. Many of the studies evaluating efficacy of nonhormonal oral prescription medications for HF management were conducted with breast cancer survivors who were experiencing HFs. Clinicians need to consider whether the results apply to women who have not had breast cancer and also whether treatment options need to be tailored because some nonhormonal medications may interfere with breast cancer therapies (NAMS, 2015b).

Considerations for Special Populations

Because hormonal fluctuations and ovulation are possible, perimenopausal women can become pregnant. Three fourths (75%) of all 131 pregnancies among women older than 40 years of age are unintended (American Congress of Obstetricians and Gynecologists [ACOG], 2011). Thus, perimenopausal women with male partners who do not wish to conceive require a reliable method of birth control (see Chapter 21).

Women with premature or temporary menopause (see Box 34.1) have early loss of fertility and may experience more severe symptoms than those with natural menopause. They are at a higher risk for osteoporosis and CVD because of the comparatively earlier reduction in estrogen and progesterone levels and may also face significant health concerns related to underlying disease processes (NAMS, 2014). Likewise, menopause generally occurs earlier in women following hysterectomy, most likely attributable to the reduced circulation to the remaining ovaries following surgical interruption of the uterine blood supply, which also partially feeds the ovaries.

■ FUTURE DIRECTIONS

Much has been learned about managing menopause-related symptoms in midlife women over the past 2 decades. Landmark research studies have clarified risks and benefits of HT, nonhormonal therapy, and various CAMs for managing menopause-related symptoms, and the importance of maintaining a high QOL for midlife women has been underscored. Current research is evaluating various other methodologies, such as alternative hormones, different nonhormone and CAM therapies, and transdermal delivery options, to evaluate their effectiveness in mitigating vasomotor symptoms while retaining a strong safety profile for midlife women's overall health. These new therapies are likely to provide important relief for women in the future.

■ REFERENCES

Afonso, R. F., Hachul, H., Kozasa, E. H., Oliveira, D. d. e. S., Goto, V., Rodrigues, D.,...Leite, J. R. (2012). Yoga decreases insomnia in postmenopausal women: A randomized clinical trial. *Menopause, 19*(2), 186–193.

Alexander, I. M. (2006). Bioidentical hormones for menopause therapy: Separating the myths from the reality. *Women's Health Care, 5*(1), 7–17, 2006.

Alexander, I. M. (2011). Hormone therapy and incidence of breast cancer. *Climacteric, 14*, 299–300. Menopause Live, International Menopause Society Electronic Forum. Retrieved from www.imsociety.org [invited commentary].

Alexander, I. M. (2012). The history of hormone therapy use and recent controversy related to heart disease and breast cancer arising from prevention trial outcomes. *Journal of Midwifery & Women's Health, 57*(6), 547–557.

Alexander, I. M., Ruff, C., Rousseau, M. E., White, K., Motter, S., McKie, C., & Clark, P. (2003). Menopause symptoms and management strategies identified by black women [Abstract]. *Menopause, 10*(6), 601.

Alexander, I. M., & Andrist, L. (2005). Menopause. In F. Likis & K. Shuiling (Eds.), *Women's gynecologic health* (Chapter 11, pp. 249–289). Sudbury, MA: Jones & Bartlett.

Alexander, I. M., & Knight, K. A. (2005). *100 Questions and answers about menopause*. Sudbury, MA: Jones & Bartlett.

American Congress of Obstetricians and Gynecologists (ACOG). (2011). 2011 Women's Health Stats & Facts. Retrieved from https://www.acog.org/-/media/NewsRoom/MediaKit.pdf

Anderson, G. L., Limacher, M., Assaf, A. R., Bassford, T., Beresford, S. A., Black, H.,…Wassertheil-Smoller, S.; Women's Health Initiative Steering Committee. (2004). Effects of conjugated equine estrogen in postmenopausal women with hysterectomy: The Women's Health Initiative randomized controlled trial. *Journal of the American Medical Association*, 291(14), 1701–1712.

Antonijevic, I. A., Stalla, G. K., & Steiger, A. (2000). Modulation of the sleep electroencephalogram by estrogen replacement in postmenopausal women. *American Journal of Obstetrics and Gynecology*, 182(2), 277–282.

Avis, N. E., Stellato, R., Crawford, S., Bromberger, J., Ganz, P., Cain, V., & Kagawa-Singer, M. (2001). Is there a menopausal syndrome? Menopausal status and symptoms across racial/ethnic groups. *Social Science & Medicine (1982)*, 52(3), 345–356.

Bachmann, G., Lobo, R. A., Gut, R., Nachtigall, L., & Notelovitz, M. (2008). Efficacy of low-dose estradiol vaginal tablets in the treatment of atrophic vaginitis: A randomized controlled trial. *Obstetrics and Gynecology*, 111(1), 67–76.

Bagger, Y. Z., Tankó, L. B., Alexandersen, P., Qin, G., & Christiansen, C.; PERF Study Group. (2005). Early postmenopausal hormone therapy may prevent cognitive impairment later in life. *Menopause*, 12(1), 12–17.

Barton, D. L., Loprinzi, C. L., Quella, S. K., Sloan, J. A., Veeder, M. H., Egner, J. R.,…Novotny, P. (1998). Prospective evaluation of vitamin E for hot flashes in breast cancer survivors. *Journal of Clinical Oncology: Official Journal of the American Society of Clinical Oncology*, 16(2), 495–500.

Beck, V., Unterrieder, E., Krenn, L., Kubelka, W., & Jungbauer, A. (2003). Comparison of hormonal activity (estrogen, androgen and progestin) of standardized plant extracts for large scale use in hormone replacement therapy. *Journal of Steroid Biochemistry and Molecular Biology*, 84(2–3), 259–268.

Bentzen, J. G., Forman, J. L., Larsen, E. C., Pinborg, A., Johannsen, T. H., Schmidt, L.,…Nyboe Andersen, A. (2013). Maternal menopause as a predictor of anti-Mullerian hormone level and antral follicle count in daughters during reproductive age. *Human Reproduction*, 28(1), 247–255.

Bjelakovic, G., Nikolova, D., Gluud, L. L., Simonetti, R. G., & Gluud, C. (2007). Mortality in randomized trials of antioxidant supplements for primary and secondary prevention: Systematic review and meta-analysis. *Journal of the American Medical Association*, 297(8), 842–857.

Blackman, M. R. (2000). Age-related alterations in sleep quality and neuroendocrine function: Interrelationships and implications. *Journal of the American Medical Association*, 284(7), 879–881.

Blatt, M. H. G., Weisbader, H., & Kupperman, H. S. (1953). Vitamin E and the climacteric syndrome. *Archives of Internal Medicine, 91*, 792–796.

Breen, N., Cronin, K. A., Meissner, H. I., Taplin, S. H., Tangka, F. K., Tiro, J. A., & McNeel, T. S. (2007). Reported drop in mammography: Is this cause for concern? *Cancer, 109*(12), 2405–2409.

Brincat, M. P. (2000). Hormone replacement therapy and the skin: Beneficial effects: The case in favor of it. *Acta Obstetricia Et Gynecologica Scandinavica*, 79(4), 244–249.

Brincat, M., Kabalan, S., Studd, J. W., Moniz, C. F., de Trafford, J., & Montgomery, J. (1987). A study of the decrease of skin collagen content, skin thickness, and bone mass in the postmenopausal woman. *Obstetrics and Gynecology*, 70(6), 840–845.

Buster, J. E., Kingsberg, S. A., Aguirre, O., Brown, C., Breaux, J. G., Buch, A.,…Casson, P. (2005). Testosterone patch for low sexual desire in surgically menopausal women: A randomized trial. *Obstetrics and Gynecology*, 105(5, Pt. 1), 944–952.

Butts, S. F., Freeman, E. W., Sammel, M. D., Queen, K., Lin, H., & Rebbeck, T. R. (2012). Joint effects of smoking and gene variants involved in sex steroid metabolism on hot flashes in late reproductive-age women. *Journal of Clinical Endocrinology and Metabolism*, 97(6), E1032–E1042.

Butts, S. F., Sammel, M. D., Greer, C., Rebbeck, T. R., Boorman, D. W., & Freeman, E. W. (2014). Cigarettes, genetic background, and menopausal timing: The presence of single nucleotide polymorphisms in cytochrome P450 genes is associated with increased risk of natural menopause in European-American smokers. *Menopause*, 21(7), 694–701.

Canavez, F. S., Werneck, G. L., Parente, R. C., Celeste, R. K., & Faerstein, E. (2011). The association between educational level and age at the menopause: A systematic review. *Archives of Gynecology and Obstetrics*, 283(1), 83–90.

Canonico, M., Oger, E., Plu-Bureau, G., Conard, J., Meyer, G., Lévesque, H.,…Scarabin, P. Y.; Estrogen and Thromboembolism Risk (ESTHER) Study Group. (2007). Hormone therapy and venous thromboembolism among postmenopausal women: Impact of the route of estrogen administration and progestogens: The ESTHER study. *Circulation*, 115(7), 840–845.

Carmody, J. F., Crawford, S., Salmoirago-Blotcher, E., Leung, K., Churchill, L., & Olendzki, N. (2011). Mindfulness training for coping with hot flashes: Results of a randomized trial. *Menopause*, 18(6), 611–620.

Cayan, F., Dilek, U., Pata, O., & Dilek, S. (2008). Comparison of the effects of hormone therapy regimens, oral and vaginal estradiol, estradiol + drospirenone and tibolone, on sexual function in healthy postmenopausal women. *Journal of Sexual Medicine*, 5(1), 132–138.

Chen, C. T., Liu, C. T., Chen, G. K., Andrews, J. S., Arnold, A. M., Dreyfus, J.,…Rajkovic, A. (2014). Meta-analysis of loci associated with age at natural menopause in African-American women. *Human Molecular Genetics*, 23(12), 3327–3342.

Chen, M. N., Lin, C. C., & Liu, C. F. (2015). Efficacy of phytoestrogens for menopausal symptoms: A meta-analysis and systematic review. *Climacteric: The Journal of the International Menopause Society*, 18(3), 260–269.

Chlebowski, R. T., Anderson, G., Pettinger, M., Lane, D., Langer, R. D., Gilligan, M. A., … McTiernan, A.; Women's Health Initiative Investigators. (2008). Estrogen plus progestin and breast cancer detection by means of mammography and breast biopsy. *Archives of Internal Medicine*, 168(4), 370–377; quiz 345.

Chlebowski, R. T., Kuller, L. H., Prentice, R. L., Stefanick, M. L., Manson, J. E., Gass, M.,…Anderson, G.; WHI Investigators. (2009). Breast cancer after use of estrogen plus progestin in postmenopausal women. *New England Journal of Medicine*, 360(6), 573–587.

Clarke, C. A., Glaser, S. L., Uratsu, C. S., Selby, J. V., Kushi, L. H., & Herrinton, L. J. (2006). Recent declines in hormone therapy utilization and breast cancer incidence: Clinical and population-based evidence. *Journal of Clinical Oncology: Official Journal of the American Society of Clinical Oncology*, 24(33), e49–e50.

Cohen, L. S., Joffe, H., Guthrie, K. A., Ensrud, K. E., Freeman, M., Carpenter, J. S.,…Anderson, G. L. (2014). Efficacy of omega-3 for vasomotor symptoms treatment: A randomized controlled trial. *Menopause*, 21(4), 347–354.

Coombs, N. J., Taylor, R., Wilcken, N., & Boyages, J. (2005). Hormone replacement therapy and breast cancer: Estimate of risk. *British Medical Journal (Clinical Research Ed.)*, 331(7512), 347–349.

Coombs, N. J., Taylor, R., Wilcken, N., Fiorica, J., & Boyages, J. (2005). Hormone replacement therapy and breast cancer risk in California. *The Breast Journal*, 11(6), 410–415.

Craig, M. C., Fletcher, P. C., Daly, E. M., Picchioni, M. M., Brammer, M., Giampietro, V.,…Murphy, D. G. (2008). A study of visuospatial working memory pre- and post-gonadotropin hormone releasing hormone agonists (GnRHa) in young women. *Hormonal Behavior, June 54*(1), 47–59.

Cramer, D. W., Xu, H., & Harlow, B. L. (1995). Family history as a predictor of early menopause. *Fertility and Sterility*, 64(4), 740–745.

Daley, A., Stokes-Lampard, H., & Macarthur, C. (2011). Exercise for vasomotor menopausal symptoms. *The Cochrane Database of Systematic Reviews*, 2011(5), CD006108.

Davis, S. R., Lambrinoudaki, I., Lumsden, M., Mishra, G. D., Pal, L., Rees, M.,…Simoncini, T. (2015). Menopause. *Nature Reviews: Disease Primers*, 1, 1–19. Retrieved from http://dx.doi.org/10.1038/nrdp.2015.4

Dayspring, T. D. (2011). Understanding hypertriglyceridemia in women: Clinical impact and management with prescription omega-3-acid ethyl esters. *International Journal of Women's Health, 3,* 87–97.

Dennerstein, L., Dudley, E. C., Hopper, J. L., Guthrie, J. R., & Burger, H. G. (2000). A prospective population-based study of menopausal symptoms. *Obstetrics and Gynecology, 96*(3), 351–358.

Dennerstein, L., Dudley, E., & Burger, H. (2001). Are changes in sexual functioning during midlife due to aging or menopause? *Fertility and Sterility, 76*(3), 456–460.

Dillaway, H., Byrnes, M., Miller, S., & Rehan, S. (2008). Talking "among us": How women from different racial-ethnic groups define and discuss menopause. *Health Care for Women International, 29,* 766–781. Retrieved from http://dx.doi.org/10.1080/07399330802179247

Elkins, G. R., Fisher, W. I., Johnson, A. K., Carpenter, J. S., & Keith, T. Z. (2013). Clinical hypnosis in the treatment of postmenopausal hot flashes: A randomized controlled trial. *Menopause, 20*(3), 291–298.

ePocrates. *Computerized pharmacology and prescribing reference,* updated daily. Retrieved from at www.epocrates.com

Espeland, M. A., Stefanick, M. L., Kritz-Silverstein, D., Fineberg, S. E., Waclawiw, M. A., James, M. K., & Greendale, G. A. (1997). Effect of postmenopausal hormone therapy on body weight and waist and hip girths. Postmenopausal Estrogen-Progestin Interventions Study Investigators. *Journal of Clinical Endocrinology and Metabolism, 82*(5), 1549–1556.

Fairfield, K. M., & Fletcher, R. H. (2002). Vitamins for chronic disease prevention in adults: scientific review. *Journal of the American Medical Association, 287*(23), 3116–3126.

Fishman, J. R., Flatt, M. A., & Settersten, Jr., R. A. (2015). Bioidentical hormones, menopausal women, and the lure of the "natural" in U.S. anti-aging medicine. *Social Science & Medicine, 132,* 79–87. Retrieved from http://dx.doi.org/10.1016/j.socscimed.2015.02.27

Food and Drug Administration (FDA). (2008). *FDA takes action against compounded menopause hormone therapy drugs.* Retrieved from http://www.fda.gov/newsevents/newsroom/pressannouncements/2008/ucm116832.htm

Forman, M. R., Mangini, L. D., Thelus-Jean, R., & Hayward, M. D. (2013). Life-course origins of the ages at menarche and menopause. *Adolescent Health, Medicine and Therapeutics, 4,* 1–21. http://doi.org/10.2147/AHMT.S15946

Frame, K., & Alexander, I. M. (2013). Mind-body therapies for sleep disturbances in women at midlife. *Journal of Holistic Nursing, 31*(4), 276–284. doi:10.1177/0898010113493504

Freedman, R. R., & Blacker, C. M. (2002). Estrogen raises the sweating threshold in postmenopausal women with hot flashes. *Fertility and Sterility, 77*(3), 487–490.

Freedman, R. R., & Woodward, S. (1992). Behavioral treatment of menopausal hot flushes: Evaluation by ambulatory monitoring. *American Journal of Obstetrics and Gynecology, 167*(2), 436–439.

Freeman, E. W., Sammel, M. D., Boorman, D. W., & Zhang, R. (2014). Longitudinal pattern of depressive symptoms around natural menopause. *Journal of American Medical Association Psychiatry, 71*(1), 36–43.

Gaudet, T. W. (2004). CAM approaches to menopause management: Overview of the options. *Menopause Management: Women's Health Through Midlife & Beyond* 13(Suppl. 1), 48–50.

Gold, E. B., Crawford, S. L., Avis, N. E., Crandall, C. J., Matthews, K. A., Waetjen, L. E., & Harlow, S. D. (2013). Factors related to age at natural menopause: Longitudinal analyses from SWAN. *American Journal of Epidemiology, 178*(1), 70–83.

Gold, E. B., Sternfeld, B., Kelsey, J. L., Brown, C., Mouton, C., Reame, N., & Stellato, R. (2000). Relation of demographic and lifestyle factors to symptoms in a multi-racial/ethnic population of women 40–55 years of age. *American Journal of Epidemiology, 152*(5), 463–473.

Goldstat, R., Briganti, E., Tran, J., Wolfe, R., & Davis, S. R. (2003). Transdermal testosterone therapy improves well-being, mood, and sexual function in premenopausal women. *Menopause, 10*(5), 390–398.

Goodman, N. F., Cobin, R. H., Ginzburg, S. B., Katz, I. A., & Woode, D. E.; American Association of Clinical Endocrinologists. (2011). American Association of Clinical Endocrinologists medical guidelines for clinical practice for the diagnosis and treatment of menopause. *Endocrine Practice: Official Journal of the American College of Endocrinology and the American Association of Clinical Endocrinologists, 17*(Suppl. 6), 1–25.

Gracia, C. R., Sammel, M. D., Freeman, E. W., Lin, H., Langan, E., Kapoor, S. & Nelson, D. B. (2005). Defining menopause status: Creation of a new definition to identify the early changes of the menopausal transition, *Menopause, 12*(2), 128–135.

Grady, D., Herrington, D., Bittner, V., Blumenthal, R., Davidson, M., Hlatky, M.,…Wenger, N.; HERS Research Group. (2002). Cardiovascular disease outcomes during 6.8 years of hormone therapy: Heart and Estrogen/progestin Replacement Study follow-up (HERS II). *Journal of the American Medical Association, 288*(1), 49–57.

Greene, J. G. (1976). A factor analytic study of climacteric symptoms. *Journal of Psychosomatic Research, 20,* 425–430. Retrieved from http://www.sciencedirect.com/science/article/pii/0022399976900052

Grodstein, F., Manson, J. E., & Stampfer, M. J. (2006). Hormone therapy and coronary heart disease: The role of time since menopause and age at hormone initiation. *Journal of Women's Health (2002), 15*(1), 35–44.

Hall, L., Callister, L. C., Berry, J. A., & Matsumura, G. (2007, June). Meanings of menopause: Cultural influences on perception and management of menopause. *Journal of Holistic Nursing, 23*(2), 106–118. Retrieved from http://dx.doi.org/10.1177/0890010107299432

Harlow, S. D., Cain, K., Crawford, S., Dennerstein, L., Little, R., Mitchell, E. S., & Yosef, M. (2006). Evaluation of four proposed bleeding criteria for the onset of late menopausal transition. *Journal of Clinical Endocrinology and Metabolism, 91*(9), 3432–3438.

Harris, M. T. (2008). Aging women's journey toward wholeness: New visions and directions. *Health Care for Women International, 29,* 962–979. Retrieved from http://dx.doi.org/10.1080/07399330802269659

He, C., & Murabito, J. M. (2014). Genome-wide association studies of age at menarche and age at natural menopause. *Molecular and Cellular Endocrinology, 382*(1), 767–779.

Hefler, L. A., Grimm, C., Bentz, E. K., Reinthaller, A., Heinze, G., & Tempfer, C. B. (2006). A model for predicting age at menopause in white women. *Fertility and Sterility, 85*(2), 451–454.

Heiss, G., Wallace, R., Anderson, G. L., Aragaki, A., Beresford, S. A., Brzyski, R.,…Stefanick, M. L.; WHI Investigators. (2008). Health risks and benefits 3 years after stopping randomized treatment with estrogen and progestin. *Journal of the American Medical Association, 299*(9), 1036–1045.

Henderson, K. D., Bernstein, L., Henderson, B., Kolonel, L., & Pike, M. C. (2008). Predictors of the timing of natural menopause in the Multiethnic Cohort Study. *American Journal of Epidemiology, 167*(11), 1287–1294.

Henderson, V. W., & Popat, R. A. (2011). Effects of endogenous and exogenous estrogen exposures in midlife and late-life women on episodic memory and executive functions. *Neuroscience, 191,* 129–138.

Hogervorst, E., De Jager, C., Budge, M., & Smith, A. D. (2004). Serum levels of estradiol and testosterone and performance in different cognitive domains in healthy elderly men and women. *Psychoneuroendocrinology, 29*(3), 405–421.

Hsia, J., Langer, R. D., Manson, J. E., Kuller, L., Johnson, K. C., Hendrix, S. L.,…Prentice, R.; Women's Health Initiative Investigators. (2006). Conjugated equine estrogens and coronary heart disease: the Women's Health Initiative. *Archives of Internal Medicine, 166*(3), 357–365.

Huber, A., Grimm, C., Huber, J. C., Schneeberger, C., Leodolter, S., Reinthaller, A.,…Hefler, L. A. (2006). A common polymorphism within the steroid 5-alpha-reductase type 2 gene and timing of menopause in Caucasian women. *European Journal of Obstetrics, Gynecology, and Reproductive Biology, 125*(2), 221–225.

Hulley, S., Furberg, C., Barrett-Connor, E., Cauley, J., Grady, D., Haskell, W.,…Hunninghake, D.; HERS Research Group. (2002). Noncardiovascular disease outcomes during 6.8 years of hormone therapy: Heart and Estrogen/progestin Replacement Study follow-up (HERS II). *Journal of the American Medical Association, 288*(1), 58–66.

Hulley, S., Grady, D., Bush, T., Furberg, C., Herrington, D., Riggs, B., & Vittinghoff, E. (1998). Randomized trial of estrogen plus progestin for secondary prevention of coronary heart disease in postmenopausal women. Heart and Estrogen/progestin Replacement Study (HERS) Research Group. *Journal of the American Medical Association, 280*(7), 605–613.

Hunter, M. S. (2014). Beliefs about hot flashes drive treatment benefit. *Menopause, 21*(8), 909.

Irvin, J. H., Domar, A. D., Clark, C., Zuttermeister, P. C., & Friedman, R. (1996). The effects of relaxation response training on menopausal symptoms. *Journal of Psychosomatic Obstetrics and Gynaecology, 17*(4), 202–207.

Joffe, H., Massler, A., & Sharkey, K. M. (2010). Evaluation and management of sleep disturbance during the menopause transition. *Seminars in Reproductive Medicine, 28*(5), 404–421.

Kaufert, P., Boggs, P. P., Ettinger, B., Woods, N. F., & Utian, W. H. (1998). Women and menopause: Beliefs, attitudes, and behaviors. The North American Menopause Society 1997 Menopause Survey. *Menopause, 5*(4), 197–202.

Klatte, E. T., Scharre, D. W., Nagaraja, H. N., Davis, R. A., & Beversdorf, D. Q. (2003). Combination therapy of donepezil and vitamin E in Alzheimer disease. *Alzheimer Disease and Associated Disorders, 17*(2), 113–116.

Kronenberg, F. (1990). Hot flashes: Epidemiology and physiology. *Annals of the New York Academy of Sciences, 592*, 52–86; discussion 123.

Landolt, H. P., Werth, E., Borbély, A. A., & Dijk, D. J. (1995). Caffeine intake (200 mg) in the morning affects human sleep and EEG power spectra at night. *Brain Research, 675*(1–2), 67–74.

Landolt, H. P., Roth, C., Dijk, D. J., & Borbély, A. A. (1996). Late-afternoon ethanol intake affects nocturnal sleep and the sleep EEG in middle-aged men. *Journal of Clinical Psychopharmacology, 16*(6), 428–436.

Lee, M. S., Shin, B. C., & Ernst, E. (2009). Acupuncture for treating menopausal hot flushes: A systematic review. *Climacteric, 12*(1), 16–25.

Leonetti, H. B., Longo, S., & Anasti, J. N. (1999). Transdermal progesterone cream for vasomotor symptoms and postmenopausal bone loss. *Obstetrics and Gynecology, 94*(2), 225–228.

Lethaby, A. E., Brown, J., Marjoribanks, J., Kronenberg, F., Roberts, H., & Eden, J. (2007). Phytoestrogens for vasomotor menopausal symptoms, *The Cochrane Database of Systematic Reviews, 2007*(4), CD001395.

Li, C. I., Malone, K. E., Porter, P. L., Lawton, T. J., Voigt, L. F., Cushing-Haugen, K. L.,...Daling, J. R. (2008). Relationship between menopausal hormone therapy and risk of ductal, lobular, and ductal-lobular breast carcinomas. *Cancer Epidemiology, Biomarkers & Prevention: A Publication of the American Association for Cancer Research, Cosponsored by the American Society of Preventive Oncology, 17*(1), 43–50.

Liao, L., Lunn, S., & Baker, M. (2015). Midlife menopause: Male partners talking. *Sexual and Relationship Therapy, 30*(1), 167–180. Retrieved from http://dx.doi.org/10.1080/14681994.2014.893290

Loprinzi, C. L., Levitt, R., Barton, D., Sloan, J. A., Dakhil, S. R., Nikcevich, D. A.,...Kugler, J. W. (2006). Phase III comparison of depomedroxyprogesterone acetate to venlafaxine for managing hot flashes: North Central Cancer Treatment Group Trial N99C7. *Journal of Clinical Oncology, 24*(9), 1409–1414.

Lu, Y., Liu, P., Recker, R. R., Deng, H. W., & Dvornyk, V. (2010). TNFRSF11A and TNFSF11 are associated with age at menarche and natural menopause in white women. *Menopause, 17*(5), 1048–1054.

Margolis, K. L., Bonds, D. E., Rodabough, R. J., Tinker, L., Phillips, L. S., Allen, C.,...Howard, B. V.; Women's Health Initiative Investigators. (2004). Effect of oestrogen plus progestin on the incidence of diabetes in postmenopausal women: results from the Women's Health Initiative Hormone Trial. *Diabetologia, 47*(7), 1175–1187.

Martin, K. A., & Manson, J. E. (2008). Approach to the patient with menopausal symptoms. *Journal of Clinical Endocrinology and Metabolism, 93*(12), 4567–4575.

Marvan, M. L., Islas, M., Vela, L., Chrisler, J. C., & Warren, E. A. (2008). Stereotypes of women in different stages of their reproductive life: Data from Mexico and the United States. *Health Care for Women International, 29*, 673–687. Retrieved from http://dx.doi.org/10.1080/07399330802188982

Meissner, H. I., Breen, N., Taubman, M. L., Vernon, S. W., & Graubard, B. I. (2007). Which women aren't getting mammograms and why? *Cancer Causes & Control, 18*(1), 61–70.

Mikkola, T. S., Tuomikoski, P., Lyytinen, H., Korhonen, P., Hoti, F., Vattulainen, P.,...Ylikorkala, O. (2015). Increased cardiovascular mortality risk in women discontinuing postmenopausal hormone therapy. *Journal of Clinical Endocrinology and Metabolism, 100*(12), 4588–4594.

Morin, C. M., Hauri, P. J., Espie, C. A., Spielman, A. J., Buysse, D. J., & Bootzin, R. R. (1999). Nonpharmacologic treatment of chronic insomnia. An American academy of sleep medicine review. *Sleep, 22*(8), 1134–1156.

Morris, D. H., Jones, M. E., Schoemaker, M. J., McFadden, E., Ashworth, A., & Swerdlow, A. J. (2012). Body mass index, exercise, and other lifestyle factors in relation to age at natural menopause: Analyses from the breakthrough generations study. *American Journal of Epidemiology, 175*(10), 998–1005.

Moyer, V. A.; U.S. Preventive Services Task Force. (2014). Vitamin, mineral, and multivitamin supplements for the primary prevention of cardiovascular disease and cancer: U.S. Preventive Services Task Force recommendation statement. *Annals of Internal Medicine, 160*(8), 558–564.

Myung, S. K., Ju, W., Cho, B., Oh, S. W., Park, S. M., Koo, B. K., & Park, B. J.; Korean Meta-Analysis Study Group. (2013). Efficacy of vitamin and antioxidant supplements in prevention of cardiovascular disease: Systematic review and meta-analysis of randomised controlled trials. *British Medical Journal (Clinical research ed.), 346*, f10.

Nachtigall, L. E. (1994). Comparative study: Replens versus local estrogen in menopausal women. *Fertility and Sterility, 61*(1), 178–180.

Nasto, L. A., Fusco, A., Colangelo, D., Mormando, M., Di Giacomo, G., Rossi, B.,...Pola, E. (2012). Clinical predictors of vertebral osteoporotic fractures in post-menopausal women: A cross-sectional analysis. *European Review for Medical and Pharmacological Sciences, 16*(9), 1227–1234.

National Center on Sleep Disorder Research. (2011). *National institutes of health sleep disorders research plan*. Retrieved from http://www.nhlbi.nih.gov/files/docs/resources/sleep/201101011NationalSleepDisordersResearchPlanDHHSPublication11-7820.pdf

National Osteoporosis Foundation. (2014). *Clinician's guide to prevention and treatment of osteoporosis*. Washington, DC: National Osteoporosis Foundation.

Nelson, H. D. (2008). Menopause. *Lancet, 371*(9614), 760–770.

Nelson, H. D., Vesco, K. K., Haney, E., Fu, R., Nedrow, A., Miller, J.,...Humphrey, L. (2006). Nonhormonal therapies for menopausal hot flashes: Systematic review and meta-analysis, *Journal of the American Medical Association, 295*(17), 2057–2071.

Newhart, M. R. (2013). Menopause matters: The implications of menopause research for studies of midlife health. *Health Sociology Review, 22*(4), 365–376.

Nikander, E., Rutanen, E. M., Nieminen, P., Wahlström, T., Ylikorkala, O., & Tiitinen, A. (2005). Lack of effect of isoflavonoids on the vagina and endometrium in postmenopausal women. *Fertility and Sterility, 83*(1), 137–142.

Onofrj, M., Thomas, A., Luciano, A. L., Iacono, D., Di Rollo, A., D'Andreamatteo, G., & Di Iorio, A. (2002). Donepezil versus vitamin E in Alzheimer's disease: Part 2: Mild versus moderate-severe Alzheimer's disease. *Clinical Neuropharmacology, 25*(4), 207–215.

Pastore, L. M., Carter, R. A., Hulka, B. S., & Wells, E. (2004). Self-reported urogenital symptoms in postmenopausal women: Women's Health Initiative. *Maturitas, 49*(4), 292–303.

Peng, W., Adams, J., Sibbritt, D. W., & Frawley, J. E. (2014). Critical review of complementary and alternative medicine use in menopause: Focus on prevalence, motivation, decision-making, and communication. *Menopause, 21*(5), 536–548.

Ravdin, P. M., Cronin, K. A., Howlader, N., Berg, C. D., Chlebowski, R. T., Feuer, E. J.,...Berry, E. D. (2007). The decrease in breast-cancer incidence in 2003 in the United States. *New England Journal of Medicine, 356*(16), 1670–1674.

Reed, S. D., Guthrie, K. A., Newton, K. M., Anderson, G. L., Booth-LaForce, C., Caan, B.,...LaCroix, A. Z. (2014). Menopausal quality of life: RCT of yoga, exercise, and omega-3 supplements. *American Journal of Obstetrics and Gynecology, 210*(3), 244.e1–244.e11.

Resnick, S. M., Maki, P. M., Golski, S., Kraut, M. A., & Zonderman, A. B. (1998). Effects of estrogen replacement therapy on PET cerebral blood flow and neuropsychological performance. *Hormones and Behavior, 34*(2), 171–182.

Rossouw, J. E., Anderson, G. L., Prentice, R. L., LaCroix, A. Z., Kooperberg, C., Stefanick, M. L., Ockene, J.; Writing Group for the Women's Health Initiative Investigators. (2002). Risks and benefits of estrogen plus progestin in healthy postmenopausal women: Principal results from the Women's Health Initiative randomized controlled trial. *Journal of the American Medical Association, 288*(3), 321–333.

Rossouw, J. E., Prentice, R. L., Manson, J. E., Wu, L., Barad, D., Barnabei, V. M.,...Stefanick, M. L. (2007). Postmenopausal hormone therapy and risk of cardiovascular disease by age and years since menopause. *Journal of the American Medical Association, 297*(13), 1465–1477.

Salpeter, S. R., Walsh, J. M., Greyber, E., Ormiston, T. M., & Salpeter, E. E. (2004). Mortality associated with hormone replacement therapy in younger and older women: A meta-analysis. *Journal of General Internal Medicine, 19*(7), 791–804.

Sapre, S., & Thakur, R. (2014). Lifestyle and dietary factors determine age at natural menopause. *Journal of Mid-Life Health, 5*(1), 3–5.

Schiff, I., Regestein, Q., Schinfeld, J., & Ryan, K. J. (1980). Interactions of oestrogens and hours of sleep on cortisol, FSH, LH, and prolactin in hypogonadal women. *Maturitas, 2*(3), 179–183.

Shaywitz, S. E., Naftolin, F., Zelterman, D., Marchione, K. E., Holahan, J. M., Palter, S. F., & Shaywitz, B. A. (2003). Better oral reading and short-term memory in midlife, postmenopausal women taking estrogen. *Menopause, 10*(5), 420–426.

Shifren, J. L., Davis, S. R., Moreau, M., Waldbaum, A., Bouchard, C., DeRogatis, L.,...Kroll, R. (2006). Testosterone patch for the treatment of hypoactive sexual desire disorder in naturally menopausal women: Results from the INTIMATE NM1 Study. *Menopause, 13*(5), 770–779.

Shifren, J. L., & Gass, M. S. (2014). The North American Menopause Society recommendations for clinical care of midlife women. *Menopause, 21*(10), 1038–1062. doi:10.1097/GME.0000000000000319

Shumaker, S. A., Legault, C., Rapp, S. R., Thal, L., Wallace, R. B., Ockene, J. K., Wactawski-Wende, J.; WHIMS Investigators. (2003). Estrogen plus progestin and the incidence of dementia and mild cognitive impairment in postmenopausal women: the Women's Health Initiative Memory Study: A randomized controlled trial. *Journal of the American Medical Association, 289*(20), 2651–2662.

Sievert, L. L. (2014). Anthropology and the study of menopause: Evolutionary, developmental, and comparative perspectives. *Menopause: The Journal of the North American Menopause Society, 21*(10), 1151–1159. Retrieved from http://dx.doi.org/10.97/gme.0000000000000341

Smith, R. L., Flaws, J. A., & Gallicchio, L. (2015). Does quitting smoking decrease the risk of midlife hot flashes? A longitudinal analysis. *Maturitas, 82*(1), 123–127.

Soares, C. N., Almeida, O. P., Joffe, H., & Cohen, L. S. (2001). Efficacy of estradiol for the treatment of depressive disorders in perimenopausal women: A double-blind, randomized, placebo-controlled trial. *Archives of General Psychiatry, 58*(6), 529–534.

Sood, R., Sood, A., Wolf, S. L., Linquist, B. M., Liu, H., Sloan, J. A.,...Barton, D. L. (2013). Paced breathing compared with usual breathing for hot flashes. *Menopause, 20*(2), 179–184.

Spencer, K. L., Malinowski, J., Carty, C. L., Franceschini, N., Fernández-Rhodes, L., Young, A.,...Crawford, D. C. (2013). Genetic variation and reproductive timing: African American women from the Population Architecture using Genomics and Epidemiology (PAGE) Study. *PloS One, 8*(2), e55258.

Staropoli, C. A., Flaws, J. A., Bush, T. L., & Moulton, A. W. (1998). Predictors of menopausal hot flashes. *Journal of Women's Health/the Official Publication of the Society for the Advancement of Women's Health Research, 7*(9), 1149–1155.

Strauss, J. R. (2011). Contextual influences on women's health concerns and attitudes toward menopause. *Health & Social Work, 36*(2), 121–127.

Sydenham, E., Dangour, A. D., & Lim, W. S. (2012). Omega 3 fatty acid for the prevention of cognitive decline and dementia. *The Cochrane Database of Systematic Reviews, 2012*(6), CD005379.

Taavoni, S., Ekbatani, N., Kashaniyan, M., & Haghani, H. (2011). Effect of valerian on sleep quality in postmenopausal women: A randomized placebo-controlled clinical trial. *Menopause, 18*(9), 951–955.

Taku, K., Melby, M. K., Kronenberg, F., Kurzer, M. S., & Messina, M. (2012). Extracted or synthesized soybean isoflavones reduce menopausal hot flash frequency and severity: Systematic review and meta-analysis of randomized controlled trials. *Menopause, 19*(7), 776–790.

The North American Menopause Society (NAMS). (2014). *Menopause practice: A clinician's guide* (5th ed.). Mayfield Heights, OH: North American Menopause Society.

The North American Menopause Society (NAMS). (2015a). *Menopause health questionnaire*. Retrieved from http://www.menopause.org/publications/clinical-practice-materials/menopause-health-questionnaire

The North American Menopause Society (NAMS). (2015b). Non hormonal management of menopause-associated vasomotor symptoms: 2015 Position Statement of the North American menopause Society. *Menopause, 22*(11), 1155–1174. doi:10.1097/GME.0000000000000546

Thurston, R. C., Sowers, M. R., Sutton-Tyrrell, K., Everson-Rose, S. A., Lewis, T. T., Edmundowicz, D., & Matthews, K. A. (2008). Abdominal adiposity and hot flashes among midlife women, *Menopause, 15*(3), 429–434.

Unfer, V., Casini, M. L., Costabile, L., Mignosa, M., Gerli, S., & Di Renzo, G. C. (2004). Endometrial effects of long-term treatment with phytoestrogens: A randomized, double-blind, placebo-controlled study, *Fertility and Sterility, 82*(1), 145–148.

U.S. Census Bureau. (2010). *Age and sex composition: 2010* [2010 Census Briefs]. Retrieved from www.Census.gov/topics/population/age-and-sex.html

U.S. Census Bureau. (2012). Population division. *Projections of the population by selected age groups and sex for the United States: 2015 to 2060.* Retrieved from www.census.gov/population/projections/data/national/2012/summarytables.html

U.S. Preventive Services Task Force. (2009). Screening for breast cancer: U.S. Preventive Services Task Force recommendation statement. *Annual Internal Medicine, 151*(10), 716–726, W-236. Erratum in: *Annual Internal Medicine,* 2010, *152*(3), 199–200; *Annual Internal Medicine,* 2010, *152*(10), 688.

van Meurs, J. B., Dhonukshe-Rutten, R. A., Pluijm, S. M., van der Klift, M., de Jonge, R., Lindemans, J.,...Uitterlinden, A. G. (2004). Homocysteine levels and the risk of osteoporotic fracture. *New England Journal of Medicine, 350*(20), 2033–2041.

Van Voorhis, B. J., Santoro, N., Harlow, S., Crawford, S. L., & Randolph, J. (2008). The relationship of bleeding patterns to daily reproductive hormones in women approaching menopause. *Obstetrics and Gynecology, 112*(1), 101–108.

Versi, E., Harvey, M. A., Cardozo, L., Brincat, M., & Studd, J. W. (2001). Urogenital prolapse and atrophy at menopause: A prevalence study. *International Urogynecology Journal and Pelvic Floor Dysfunction, 12*(2), 107–110.

Walker, E. M., Rodriguez, A. I., Kohn, B., Ball, R. M., Pegg, J., Pocock, J. R.,...Levine, R. A. (2010). Acupuncture versus venlafaxine for the management of vasomotor symptoms in patients with hormone receptor-positive breast cancer: A randomized controlled trial. *Journal of Clinical Oncology: Official Journal of the American Society of Clinical Oncology, 28*(4), 634–640.

Weight-Control Information Network (WIN). (2014). *Understanding adult overweight and obesity.* National Institute of Diabetes and Digestive and Kidney Diseases website. Retrieved from http://win.niddk.nih.gov/publications/understanding.htm

Williams, J. W., Plassman, B. L., Burke, J., Holsinger, T., & Benjamin, S. (2010). *Preventing Alzheimer's disease and cognitive decline.* Evidence Report/Technology Assessment No. 193. AHRQ Publication No.

10-E005. Rockville, MD: Agency for Healthcare Research and Quality.

Wilson, R. A., Marino, E. R., & Wilson, T. A. (1966). Norethynodrel-mestranol (enovid) for prevention and treatment of the climacteric. *Journal of the American Geriatrics Society, 14*(10), 967–985.

Woods, N. F., Mitchell, E. S., & Adams, C. (2000). Memory functioning among midlife women: observations from the Seattle Midlife Women's Health Study. *Menopause, 7*(4), 257–265.

Ye, Y., Li, J., & Yuan, Z. (2013). Effect of antioxidant vitamin supplementation on cardiovascular outcomes: A meta-analysis of randomized controlled trials. *PloS One, 8*(2), e56803.

Zandi, P. P., Carlson, M. C., Plassman, B. L., Welsh-Bohmer, K. A., Mayer, L. S., Steffens, D. C., & Breitner, J. C.; Cache County Memory Study Investigators. (2002). Hormone replacement therapy and incidence of Alzheimer disease in older women: The Cache County Study. *Journal of the American Medical Association, 288*(17), 2123–2129.

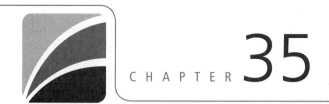

CHAPTER 35

Osteoporosis

Ivy M. Alexander • Danielle LaRosa • Emily Miesse • Matthew Witkovic

Osteoporosis (OP) is the most common bone disease in humans, representing a major public health problem (U.S. Department of Health and Human Services, 2004). Fracture attributable to OP is a significant health problem that women face, especially after menopause. As estrogen and progesterone levels fall, bone strength also declines. OP is a disorder of the skeletal system characterized by a reduction in bone strength and increased risk for fracture (U.S. Department of Health and Human Services, 2004). Osteopenia is similar to OP except that there is a lesser amount of bone lost. Two factors contribute to bone strength: bone mineral density (BMD) and bone quality. BMD refers to the thickness and volume of the bone. Bone quality refers to the bone architecture, mineralization, rate of turnover, and accumulated damage (Cosman et al., 2014; National Osteoporosis Foundation [NOF], 2014; U.S. Department of Health and Human Services, 2004). BMD is easily measured using densitometry testing such as the dual-energy x-ray absorptiometry (DEXA). Bone quality is more difficult to assess as simple measurement devices are not readily available.

Kyphosis causes a permanently stooped appearance, and may be recognized when a woman has a documented loss of height. Kyphosis also causes the rib cage to slump downward, eventually coming to rest on the ischial spines, thus minimizing thoracic and abdominal cavity space for organs. This restriction frequently leads to gastrointestinal problems, such as gastric reflux, anorexia, and constipation, and to respiratory disorders, such as shortness of breath. Self-image can also be negatively affected because of body changes and difficulty in finding clothing that fits properly over the kyphotic deformity.

Once the woman has an established diagnosis of OP or is at risk of the disease, other factors need to be considered by the clinician caring for these women. In a cross-sectional population-based study of persons aged 50 years or older using the Korea National Health and Nutrition Examination Survey, low socioeconomic status (SES) was associated with a greater need for health care, health outcomes, and health inequities (Kim, Lee, Shin, & Park, 2015). SES was also reported to affect health behavior and adherence to medication regimens. While primary prevention for OP can be managed, other factors, such as low SES, education, resources to promote recommended screenings, and

the money to pay for OP medications, need to be addressed with these women by their provider as part of the conversation in OP prevention, screening, and treatment (Kim et al., 2015).

■ DEFINITION

OP is defined by BMD at the hip or lumbar spine that is 2.5 or more standard deviations below the mean BMD of a young-adult reference population (Report of a WHO Study Group, 1994). OP is a risk factor for fracture, just as hypertension is a risk factor for stroke.

Primary OP occurs because of causes related to age, gender, and family history. It occurs with aging and accelerates in women at menopause. By age 60 years, half of the White women in the United States have low bone mass or OP (Watts et al., 2010). Low BMD at the femoral neck (T-score of –1.0 or below) is found in 21% of postmenopausal (PM) White women, 16% of PM Mexican American women, and 10% of PM African American women. More than 20% of PM women have prevalent vertebral fractures (Watts et al., 2010).

Secondary OP results from medical conditions or treatments that interfere with the attainment of peak bone mass and/or that may predispose to accelerated bone loss (Miazgowski, Kleerekoper, Felsenberg, Stěpán, & Szulc, 2012). Apart from the well-defined risk of secondary OP in patients requiring long-term corticosteroid therapy, an increasing list of dietary, lifestyle, endocrine, metabolic, and other causes of bone mass deterioration have been identified, such as smoking, sedentary lifestyle/low physical activity, Cushing's disease, diabetes, hyperthyroidism, and pregnancy (Cosman et al., 2014; Miazgowski et al., 2012).

OP affects approximately 10 million adults in the United States, and 43 million more have low bone mass (Cosman et al., 2014; U.S. Department of Health and Human Services, 2004). Women with OP, and especially low bone mass (which used to be called osteopenia), have an increased risk for fracture (Cosman et al., 2014; U.S. Department of Health and Human Services, 2004). OP is the most common bone disease, yet it is painless and often remains undiagnosed until a fracture occurs (Cosman et al., 2014; U.S. Department of Health and Human Services, 2004). Approximately 80% of the Americans affected with OP are women, most of them PM (Watts et al., 2010). At age 50, the lifetime risk of developing fractures is about 39% for White women. The U.S. surgeon general estimates that, by the year 2020, half of the adult U.S. population older than 50 years will be at risk of fractures related to OP (U.S. Department of Health and Human Services, 2004). By the year 2050, the number of people older than 65 years will increase from 32 million to 69 million, and more than 15 million people will live longer than 85 years of age (Watts et al., 2010). The incidence of hip and spine fractures increase with advancing age. Investigators estimate that incidences will increase from 2 to 3 million and associated costs will increase from $17 to $25 billion.

The real concerns associated with bone loss are related to fracture. In 2005, 2 million fractures were attributed to OP. Of these, 71% occurred in women; the direct cost was approximately $17 billion, 94% of which was attributable to fractures at nonvertebral sites (Watts et al., 2010). Many more women have osteoporotic fractures than new strokes, myocardial infarctions, or invasive breast cancer combined (Watts et al., 2010). Mortality risk increases by 10% to 25% in the year following a hip fracture (U.S. Department of Health and Human Services, 2004). The mortality during the first year after hip fracture is about 17% for women; more than half of hip fracture survivors will require skilled care away from their homes and many will have some degree of permanent disability (Watts et al., 2010). Among survivors, almost 50% are never able to live independently and approximately 25% require permanent nursing home care. Physical disability and inability to enjoy previous activities add to the burden of the disease by causing isolation and depression, factors that can increase risks for additional bone loss and falls through inactivity.

ETIOLOGY

Approximately 90% of bone mass is established by the age of 20 years, and adults achieve their peak bone mass around 30 to 35 years of age (U.S. Department of Health and Human Services, 2004). When peak bone mass is achieved, bone remodeling continues. Osteoclast cells secrete enzymes that digest bone and create microscopic holes, called resorption cavities, along the surface of the bone. Osteoblasts then migrate to the surface and secrete collagen to fill the resorption cavities with newly formed osteoid material. The osteoblasts are eventually replaced with lining cells, and the process repeats. Bone formation and remodeling are regulated by a number of endocrine and hormonal mechanisms. During childhood, when bone mass increases rapidly, the osteoblasts act independently and in response to growth hormones. However, in adulthood, osteoblasts act in response to osteoclast activity and functional load stress that is exerted on bone, such as the stress caused by physical exercise. Low bone mass and OP are caused when the normal processes of bone remodeling are unbalanced and

resorption rates exceed bone formation, resulting in reduced bone quality and strength (U.S. Department of Health and Human Services, 2004).

Primary OP is associated with aging and affects women more than men because of the rapid increase in bone loss that accompanies the decline in estrogen and progesterone levels during the menopausal transition (Management of osteoporosis in postmenopausal women, 2010; U.S. Department of Health and Human Services, 2004; Watts et al., 2010). The rate of bone turnover and bone loss accelerate during the 3- to 5-year span preceding and following menopause. During the menopausal transition a woman can have total bone loss of up to 10% (Watts et al., 2010). Age-related bone loss affects both men and women and begins in the sixth decade. It occurs at a slower rate, about 0.5% each year (Watts et al., 2010). Secondary OP is bone loss caused by other disease processes or medications (Box 35.1) that interfere with the normal process of bone formation; secondary OP can affect males or females at any age.

RISK FACTORS

Some risk factors for OP can be controlled; others cannot (Box 35.2). Risk factors for fracture and falls are distinct from those for bone loss (Box 35.3).

SYMPTOMS

OP itself is asymptomatic. The woman cannot tell that her bones are losing density until she loses one inch or more in height (usually due to silent vertebral fractures) or due to the pain associated with a fracture (Cosman et al., 2014).

EVALUATION/ASSESSMENT

Office assessment for OP includes a thorough history to identify personal and familial risk factors for bone loss; possible causes of secondary OP (Box 35.3) are also determined to identify any negative effects on bone health that can be eliminated or reduced (Cosman et al., 2014; U.S. Department of Health and Human Services, 2004; Watts et al., 2010).

History

Gathering information that will enable risk stratification and identification of potential secondary causes for OP is critical when taking a history. Medications used and health habits such as diet and exercise, smoking, and daily alcohol consumption are all important in understanding a woman's risk and determining nonpharmacologic treatments. Uncovering symptoms suggestive of systemic conditions that cause OP (e.g., hyperthyroidism) are also essential. Noting nonmodifiable risk factors such as age, ethnicity, history of fractures,

BOX 35.1 POSSIBLE CAUSES[a] OF SECONDARY OSTEOPOROSIS

Medications

Aluminum-containing antacids (e.g., Amphojel, Maalox, Mylanta)

Anticonvulsants (e.g., carbamazepine [Carbatrol, Tegretol], divalproex [Depakote], phenobarbital, phenytoin [Dilantin], valproate [Depacon])

Cholestyramine (e.g., Questran)

Chemotherapy/immunosuppressors (e.g., Methotrexate [Trexall])

Glucocorticosteroids (e.g., prednisone [Deltasone, Sterapred])

Gonadotropin-releasing hormone (GnRH)

Heparin

Lithium (e.g., Eskalith, Lithobid)

Medroxyprogesterone acetate injection (e.g., Depo-Provera)

Proton pump inhibitors (PPIs, e.g., rabeprazole [AcipHex], esomeprazole [Nexium], lansoprazole [Prevacid], omeprazole [Prilosec])

Selective serotonin reuptake inhibitors (SSRIs, e.g., paroxetine [Paxil], fluoxetine [Prozac], sertraline [Zoloft])

Thiazolidinediones (e.g., pioglitazone [Actos], rosiglitazone [Avandia])

Thyroid hormone (e.g., levothyroxine [Eltroxin, Levoxyl, Levathroid, Synthroid, Unithroid])

Warfarin (e.g., Coumadin)

Medical Conditions

Alcoholism

AIDS/HIV

Bone disorders (e.g., acromegaly, ankylosing spondylitis, osteogenesis imperfecta, posttransplant bone disease)

Chronic liver disease, cholestatic liver disease, primary biliary cirrhosis

Chronic renal failure, end-stage renal disease, renal tubular acidosis

Connective tissue diseases (e.g., lupus, multiple sclerosis, rheumatoid arthritis, sarcoidosis)

Depression

Eating disorders (e.g., anorexia nervosa, vitamin D deficiency, calcium deficiency)

Endocrine disorders (e.g., hypothyroidism, Cushing's syndrome, diabetes, hyperparathyroidism, hypophosphatasia, thyrotoxicosis)

Gastrointestinal disorders (e.g., celiac disease, malabsorption syndromes, gastrectomy, gastric bypass surgery, inflammatory bowel disease, pancreatic disease)

Genetic disorders (e.g., Gaucher's)

Hematologic disorders (e.g., hemochromatosis, hemophilia, leukemia, thalassemia)

Neuromuscular disorders (muscular dystrophy, paraplegia, quadriplegia, proximal myopathy)

Prolonged immobility

Respiratory disorders (e.g., cystic fibrosis, chronic obstructive pulmonary disease)

Seizure disorders (e.g., epilepsy)

[a]Representative list, not exhaustive.

Data from Miazgowski et al., (2012); National Osteoporosis Foundation (2014); U.S. Department of Health and Human Services (2004); Watts et al. (2010).

BOX 35.2 OSTEOPOROSIS RISK FACTORS

Potentially Modifiable Risk Factors

Amenorrhea (caused by eating disorder or excessive exercise)

Body weight less than 127 pounds, body mass index less than 21 kg/m²

Chronic diseases (Box 35.1)

Cigarette smoking (active or passive)

Frailty

Low estrogen level (e.g., menopause)

Medications (see Box 35.1)

Nulliparity

Poor nutrition (e.g., excessive vitamin A, excessive alcohol or caffeine intake, excessive soda intake, excessive sodium intake, inadequate calcium/vitamin D intake, protein deficiency)

Sedentary lifestyle

Nonmodifiable Risk Factors

Advanced age

Dementia

Delayed puberty

Endocrine disorders (Cushing's, thyrotoxicosis, diabetes mellitus)

Family history of OP

Female gender

First-degree relative with history of fracture

Fracture history (fracture at 40–45 years or older is associated with an increased risk for osteoporosis)

Genetic factors (variations in or absence of genes that regulate protein receptors or enzymes needed for bone development)

Race (Caucasian and Asian women at greatest risk, then Hispanic and African American)

Data from Cosman et al. (2014); U.S. Department of Health and Human Services (2004); Watts et al. (2010).

Adapted from Alexander and Andrist (2005).

BOX 35.3 RISK FACTORS FOR FALLS AND FRACTURE[a]

Evaluated in the WHO FRAX Algorithm

Age (especially greater than 65 years, fracture risk doubles with each 7–8 years after 50 years)

Current smoking

Femoral neck raw bone mineral density (BMD) in g/cm^2

Glucocorticoid use

Body mass index (BMI) (height and weight, BMI less than 21 kg/m^2)

Parent history of hip fracture (increases risk ~130%)

Personal prior fracture (risk for future fracture doubles)

Rheumatoid arthritis

Secondary OP

Gender (females at greater risk than males)

Ingestion of three or more units of alcohol per day

Selected Other Risk Factors

Weakness

History of falls, fainting, off balance

Poor vision

Neuropathy, especially lower extremities

Vertigo

Impaired mobility

Use of medications or substances that cause drowsiness, dizziness, lightheadedness, or imbalance; use of multiple medications

Neurologic disease

Frailty

Orthostatic hypotension

Low vitamin D levels

Sedentary lifestyle

Depression

[a]Risk factors have variable influences on fracture or fall risk. In the FRAX algorithm, all variables except age, height, weight, and gender are entered as yes/no. This limits the weighting of some variables that would carry a higher risk for fracture if values were entered on a continuum. For example, a woman with a history of two prior fractures and taking 30 mg of oral steroid daily is at greater risk than a woman with one prior fracture who is taking 5 mg of steroid daily. The FRAX does calculate fracture risk using all of the variables noted in the upper half of Box 35.3; therefore, the presence of multiple risks in one person is recognized.

BMD, bone mineral density; FRAX, fracture risk assessment; OP, osteoporosis.

Data from Cosman et al. (2014); U.S. Department of Health and Human Services (2004); World Health Organization (WHO, 2016).

and family history will help in determining if DEXA scanning is needed in women younger than 65 years of age. Using the fracture risk assessment (FRAX) algorithm scale will help quantify these risk factors (Cosman et al., 2014).

A comprehensive risk assessment for falls is completed in women with established OP, including hearing or vision impairments, neurologic status, and other medical problems or medications that may increase fall risk (Box 35.3).

Physical Examination

The physical examination includes assessment for physical risk factors, such as low body mass index (BMI) (less than 21 kg/m^2) or body weight (less than 127 pounds), kyphosis, tooth loss, or spinal tenderness; signs of low estrogen levels; signs of thyroid abnormalities; and clues to other secondary causes for OP. Height is measured accurately using a stadiometer, not taken via patient report. Reductions in height can be an important first clue for painless (or "silent") vertebral compression fractures (VCFs) (Cosman et al., 2014). Fall risk can also be assessed by observing gait when the patient is entering or leaving the room. If there is concern for falls, Romberg and orthostatic blood pressure readings can provide additional information.

VCFs can be painless; however, they are often associated with significant pain (Cosman et al., 2014; Watts et al., 2010). In women with OP, VCFs can be caused by normal activities of daily life, such as bending forward to pick up an item. The anterior edge of a vertebral bone crumbles in response to the increase in pressure exerted while bending forward, and changes into a wedge shape. Over time, having multiple wedge-shaped bones on top of one another, instead of the usual square cube shape, causes the spine to curve forward, causing kyphosis.

■ DIFFERENTIAL DIAGNOSES

The diagnosis of OP is based on DEXA results, physical exam findings, and laboratory results. A clinical diagnosis of OP is made when the patient has a low-trauma fracture of any type. A low-trauma fracture is a fracture sustained from relatively minor force, such as a fall from a standing height or less. Differentiating primary from secondary OP is important because some causes of secondary OP may be treatable and may rectify the bone loss. For example, some women with BMD test results that indicate OP may have disorders other than OP, such as osteomalacia or multiple myeloma that are treatable once identified. If serum calcium level is low, the cause needs to be identified and treated before an antiresorptive agent is administered, which may exacerbate the problem. If vitamin D levels are low, replacement is necessary.

OP can be missed in patients who sustain a low-trauma fracture. Recognition of OP is critical as medications and a multidisciplinary approach to management are most effective (Skorupski & Alexander, 2013).

■ DIAGNOSTIC STUDIES

DEXA is the gold standard for screening and diagnosing OP (Cosman et al., 2014; U.S. Department of Health and Human Services, 2004; Watts et al., 2010). DEXA testing can be done at the spine, wrist, or hip. However, central measures obtained at the hip and spine are used most often because they are most representative of the skeleton as a whole. Quantitative computed tomography (QCT) can also be used to evaluate central BMD. QCT is especially useful in evaluating women with osteoarthritis because it is less likely to detect osteophytes, which can falsely increase BMD measures identified with DEXA.

Other methods for evaluating bone density include peripheral DEXA, single-energy x-ray absorptiometry (SXA), peripheral QCT, radiographic absorptiometry (RA), quantitative ultrasound (QUS), and radiogrammetry. These methods are not used for diagnosis; they may be used when screenings are offered at health fairs. OP can also be incidentally identified on x-rays. However, it is apparent on x-rays only if there is bone loss of 30% to 40%; x-rays are not used to diagnose OP. When bone loss is identified with noncentral measures, the patient is referred for DEXA. See Box 35.4 for the NOF recommendations for DEXA screening.

BMD results by DEXA are reported as T-scores and Z-scores (Cosman et al., 2014; U.S. Department of Health and Human Services, 2004; Watts et al., 2010). The T-score indicates the number of standard deviations a woman's bone density is above or below that of a young adult, gender-matched norm. The WHO has determined classifications for various T-score results (Report of a WHO Study Group, 1994; Table 35.1). The Z-score indicates the number of standard deviations a woman's bone density is above or below the mean for an age- and gender-matched cohort. The Z-score is most often used for diagnosing bone loss in children or young adults, and is useful in identifying secondary OP. When the Z-score is low, it indicates either that her bone mass is lower than her age cohort due to secondary OP causes or that she did not achieve peak bone mass in young adulthood.

Before a diagnosis of OP is confirmed, even with DEXA results of –2.5 or below, diagnostic studies to identify suspected causes of secondary OP are needed (Cosman et al., 2014). Additionally, fasting serum calcium, serum 25-hydroxyvitamin D (25-OH D), and 24-hour urinary calcium levels are measured. Other helpful studies, which may be conducted for routine care independent of bone issues, include a complete blood count (CBC); creatinine level with calculated estimated glomerular filtration rate (eGFR); phosphorus, thyroid-stimulating hormone (TSH), and alkaline phosphatase levels; and measurement of hepatic enzymes. Other diagnostic studies may be indicated depending on the patient's presentation.

Serum or urinary by-products of bone turnover can be evaluated to determine rates of turnover (Cosman et al., 2014; U.S. Department of Health and Human Services, 2004). For example, N-teleopeptide crosslinks (NTx) are released into the blood with bone resorption and excreted by the kidneys in the urine. High levels of urinary NTx suggest higher levels of bone resorption. Osteoclastin is released into the bloodstream during bone formation. Higher levels of serum osteoclastin suggest higher levels of bone formation. Serum and urinary markers are not used to diagnose OP; instead, they may be useful for evaluating bone formation rates and thus bone quality (Cosman et al., 2014; U.S. Department of Health and Human Services, 2004). Standardized tests for these markers are not widely available. In the future, they may be more widely used to determine early response

---

BOX 35.4   NATIONAL OSTEOPOROSIS FOUNDATION RECOMMENDATIONS FOR DEXA SCREENING

■ All women 65 years old or older
■ Women younger than age 65 years who are PM or transitioning to postmenopause who have clinical risks[a] for OP
■ Individuals who sustain a fracture after age 50 years
■ Individuals who have a clinical condition or take medications that are associated with bone loss or decreased bone mass

DEXA, dual-energy x-ray absorptiometry.

[a]The U.S. Preventive Services Task Force identifies as woman as having "clinical risk" for bone loss/osteoporosis if her FRAX score (calculated without bone mineral density value) for a 10-year major osteoporotic fracture is 9.3% or higher (the calculated risk for a 65-year-old White woman without other risks; U.S. Preventive Services Task Force, 2011).

Data from Cosman et al. (2014).

TABLE 35.1	World Health Organization T-Score Classifications	
T-SCORE RESULT	**INTERPRETATION**
At or above –1.0	Normal
–1.0 to –2.5	Osteopenia
At or below –2.5	Osteoporosis
At or below –2.5 with low-trauma fracture(s)	Severe or established osteoporosis

Data from report of a WHO Study Group (1994).

to therapy rather than waiting 1 to 2 years for follow-up DEXA testing after medications have been initiated.

The FRAX, released by the WHO in 2008, uses data about 11 different risk factors as well as femoral neck bone density levels to provide added information to support clinical decision making for initiating medication therapy, especially among those with osteopenia (see Pharmacotherapeutics section) (WHO, 2016).

■ TREATMENT/MANAGEMENT

The goal of OP management begins early in life with the development of a high peak bone mass and the prevention of bone loss. Once bone loss has occurred, the goal continues with prevention of further bone loss as well as fracture prevention. Strategies for maximizing peak bone mass and bone loss prevention include changes in diet, use of supplements, and initiation of an exercise program. Fall prevention and use of pharmacotherapeutics are the mainstays of fracture prevention. Referral to a specialist is warranted when patients do not respond to pharmacotherapeutics or when comorbid disease makes management complicated.

Self-Management

DIET AND SUPPLEMENTS

OP prevention needs to start early in life by ingesting a diet rich in calcium, vitamin D, and minerals, which are necessary to achieve peak bone mass. Maintaining adequate intake of both calcium (Table 35.2) and vitamin D (600–1,000 U/d) remains necessary with aging and throughout postmenopause (Management of osteoporosis in postmenopausal women, 2010; U.S. Department of Health and Human Services, 2004; Ross et al., 2010; Watts et al., 2010).

Although ultraviolet sunlight exposure to bare skin can synthesize vitamin D, this is not the recommended modality to obtain adequate levels of vitamin D, both because of the increased risk for skin cancer and because of variables that interfere with a consistent amount of vitamin D production. Thus, supplementation or ingestion of vitamin D-fortified foods is recommended. Individuals with low serum 25-OH D levels (less than 32 ng/mL) require supplementation at higher rates. It may take up to 3 months for serum levels to achieve a steady state after a supplement is started. Calcium or calcium and vitamin D supplementation may reduce risks for all types of cancer (Lappe et al., 2007), including breast cancer (Lin et al., 2007), and inhibit weight gain during postmenopause (Caan et al., 2007).

Other dietary considerations include minimizing ingestion of soda and caffeinated beverages (Cosman et al., 2014; Miazgowski et al., 2012; Watts et al., 2010). The phosphorus in soda and the caffeine in other beverages may interfere with bone formation and remodeling processes if consumed in very high quantities. More important, for most people, is that frequent ingestion of these beverages can replace ingestion of calcium-rich milk, posing a greater harm to developing and maintaining bone strength. Adequate amounts of phosphorus are needed; however, phosphorus intake must

TABLE 35.2	Daily Calcium Recommendations for Females at Various Ages
AGE	DAILY CALCIUM RECOMMENDATION (MG)
Birth to 6 months	210
7–12 months	270
1–3 years	700
4–8 years	1,000
9–18 years	1,300
14–18 years and pregnant or lactating	1,300
19–50 years[a]	1,000
19–50 years and pregnant or lactating	1,000
≥ 51 years[a]	1,200–1,500
Postmenopausal[a]	1,200–1,500

[a]Postmenopausal women, regardless of age, are counseled to increase calcium intake to 1,200 to 1,500 mg daily.
Data from Ross et al. (2010); first published ahead of print November 29, 2010, as doi:10.1210/jc.2010-2704. National Academy of Sciences, Academy Press and U.S. Department of Health and Human Services (2004).

be balanced because either excessive or insufficient amounts can interfere with bone formation. Adequate citric acid, protein, and fiber are also needed for proper bone formation. Excessive protein or fiber intake can interfere with normal intestinal absorption of calcium. Moderate alcohol intake can improve bone strength; however, ingestion of more than three alcohol units per day (1 U = 12 oz. of beer, 4 to 5 oz. of wine, or 1 oz. of hard liquor) interferes with normal remodeling processes (Management of osteoporosis in postmenopausal women, 2010; U.S. Department of Health and Human Services, 2004; Watts et al., 2010).

Although supplementation with adequate amounts of calcium will increase bone density, it may not affect fracture risk (Jackson et al., 2006). Calcium from dietary sources is preferred over supplements; however, calcium intake from dietary sources is frequently below daily recommended levels and women with lactose intolerance may not tolerate the dairy products that are richest in calcium, making supplementation necessary (U.S. Department of Health and Human Services, 2004). Taking 1,000 mg of calcium supplement daily was not associated with increased risks for cardiovascular disease or stroke in the Nurses' Health Study (Paik et al., 2014). The recommended dietary allowances (RDAs) for calcium are based on elemental calcium—the amount of calcium that is actually absorbed from a food or supplement and used in the body. Most supplements now list elemental calcium levels on their labels; therefore, determining the amount of calcium that is absorbed is straightforward. Several different types of calcium supplements are available (Table 35.3).

TABLE 35.3	Calcium Supplements	
TYPE	**BRAND NAMES**	**COMMENTS**
Calcium carbonate	Calci-Fresh Gum, Caltrate, Os-Cal, Tums, Viactiv, others	■ Available in liquid, chewable tablet, and chewing gum forms ■ Needs to be taken with food; needs acidic environment for absorption ■ Not a good choice for women taking proton pump inhibitors because of lowered gastric acidity, even with meals ■ Often causes flatulence, constipation; can minimize these symptoms if taken in combination with magnesium ■ May contain lead if made from bone meal, dolamite, or oyster shell; concern mainly for children, pregnant or lactating women
Calcium citrate	Calci-Fresh Gum, Citrical	■ Available in liquid, tablet, and chewing gum forms ■ Can be taken with or without food; absorption not affected by acid level
Calcium phosphate tribasic	Posture, other fortified products	■ Can be taken with or without food; absorption not affected by acid level ■ Usual formulation added to calcium-fortified drinks
Calcium gluconate	Various	■ Less frequently used ■ Usually combined with calcium carbonate in vitamin or mineral supplement products
Calcium glubionate	Neo-glucagon syrup	■ Liquid form ■ Less frequently used

Data from U.S. Department of Health and Human Services (2004).

EXERCISE

Establishing an active lifestyle early in life and maintaining it throughout the older years is crucial to encourage normal bone formation and slow bone loss. The effects of exercise on bone are site specific because osteoblast activity increases locally in response to load stress caused by exercise (e.g., walking supports bone density in the hips, lower spine, and legs; hand weights benefit the arms and wrists; and overhead weights benefit the shoulders, upper arms, wrists, and upper spine) (U.S. Department of Health and Human Services, 2004). Both weight-bearing and resistance exercises are needed to create adequate load on bone tissue (U.S. Department of Health and Human Services, 2004). In addition to improving bone strength and providing overall fitness, exercise helps women maintain their balance, and thus reduces fall risk. Exercises that require forward bending are not recommended for women with established OP of the spine because of the risk of VCFs (U.S. Department of Health and Human Services, 2004). Activities that carry a high risk for falls are also discouraged in women with established OP. Encourage weight-bearing and resistance exercises, such as tai chi, walking, jogging, weight lifting, dancing, modified yoga (without forward bending), Pilates, swimming or water aerobics using resistive water weights, and bicycling against increasing resistance.

SMOKING CESSATION

Avoiding or quitting smoking to maximize peak bone formation and prevent bone loss is crucial (Cosman et al., 2014; U.S. Department of Health and Human Services, 2004; Watts et al., 2010). Nicotine in cigarettes interferes with hormonal functions that assist with balancing bone formation and can augment the negative effects that corticosteroids have on bone.

FALL PREVENTION

Fall prevention becomes more important in women with established bone loss who are at increased risk for fracture. A home assessment is done to determine and remedy the presence of loose rugs, exposed cords, or poor lighting that could increase the risk of falling, especially at night. Some patients can conduct this assessment and rectify problems themselves. In other instances, clinicians or family members need to intervene. Ingestion of sedating medications or substances are also avoided. For those with secondary OP, prevention through managing the underlying cause, changing medications, or reducing dosages can improve bone strength and reduce or reverse bone loss in addition to decreasing the risk of falls (Cosman et al., 2014; U.S. Department of Health and Human Services, 2004; Watts et al., 2010).

Complementary and Alternative Medicine

MASSAGE, RELAXATION THERAPIES, AND CHIROPRACTIC MANIPULATION

Massage may indirectly benefit bone strength because it can relax and assist in muscle flexibility, potentially increasing exercise tolerance. Chair massage is performed with caution because forward bending in women with established

OP potentially increases the risk of VCFs. Massage does not usually provide enough force to cause fracture with established OP and may provide relaxation that assists with pain reduction.

Other CAM modalities that enhance and encourage relaxation such as aromatherapy, yoga, and meditation may be helpful for pain management in women with OP fractures. Chiropractic manipulation techniques are modified by skilled chiropractors to avoid injury or fracture of weak bones. Some chiropractors do not perform manipulations on those with OP; instead, they counsel patients about dietary needs and safe exercise techniques.

BOTANICALS AND ACUPUNCTURE

Research evaluating the use of soy to improve bone density has provided conflicting results. Rimostil and genistein have both demonstrated increases in BMD (Clifton-Bligh, Baber, Fulcher, Nery, & Moreton, 2001; Marini et al., 2007). Epidemiologic studies have also suggested that women who consume high amounts of isoflavones found in soy products are at lower risk for OP (Adlercreutz & Mazur, 1997; Somekawa, Chiguchi, Ishibashi, & Aso, 2001). While a meta-analysis of randomized controlled trials found little overall support for the use of soy supplements to increase bone density (Liu et al., 2009), a systematic review found soy supplements to increase BMD (Wei, Liu, Chen, & Chen, 2012). Most soy products are available over the counter, such as Estroven®, Rimostil®, and Promensil®. Fosteum Rx® is available by prescription.

Treatment results for OP with acupuncture have been mixed. Acupuncture is more often used in combination with Chinese herbs for OP in the practice of traditional Chinese medicine (Guillaume, 1992). Herbs that might be used for OP management are intended to boost estrogen levels, such as cypress, black cohosh, sage, licorice, and ginseng (Decker & Myers, 2001). OsteoSine is a capsule containing minerals, vitamins, and a blend of *Cuscuta chinensis* herb ingredients, which contain flavonoids. Flavonoids are found in red wine and believed to contribute to reducing the risk of heart disease. NuLiv, the OsteoSine manufacturer, advertises the preparation for use in improving bone health; however, no published studies of large clinical trials are available at www.nulivlifestyle.com/index.html.

Pharmacotherapeutics

Several prescription medications are available for OP management. Prescription medications are recommended by the NOF and American Association of Clinical Endocrinologists (AACE) for PM women with T-score BMD values in the OP range (−2.5 or lesser) (Cosman et al., 2014; Watts et al., 2010). Most clinicians also agree that treatment is warranted if the T-score is −2.0 or less or if the woman has sustained a low-trauma fracture. The WHO developed the FRAX algorithm to identify 10-year fracture probabilities to assist in determining best practices for initiating medication therapy among patients with T-score BMDs in the osteopenic range (Cosman et al., 2014; WHO, 2016).

The FRAX algorithm is accessible online and applies only to patients who are naïve to OP pharmacotherapy. It is specific to country and in the United States is also categorized according to race/ethnicity. Ten-year fracture risk probability for hip fracture and any major osteoporotic fracture (e.g., forearm, hip, humerus, or vertebrae) is calculated on the basis of 11 risk factors for fracture (Box 35.5) and the femoral neck BMD (WHO, 2016). The calculated FRAX fracture probabilities are now printed on BMD DEXA results in the United States. The U.S. algorithm adapted to clinical scenarios provides the basis for the NOF clinical recommendations for initiating medication therapy for bone loss (Box 35.5) (Cosman et al., 2014; Dawson-Hughes et al., 2008; Tosteson et al., 2008; Watts et al., 2010; WHO, 2016). Another online fracture risk assessment tool, called QFracture, was released in 2009. It may have some improved discrimination over FRAX; however, it was based on data from England and Wales and is only applicable to these patient populations (Hippisley-Cox & Coupland, 2009).

Medication therapies that are currently U.S. Food and Drug Administration (FDA) approved for OP management in the United States include parathyroid hormone, estrogen agonist–antagonist, estrogen therapy (ET) or hormone therapy (HT), calcitonin, monoclonal antibody, and bisphosphonate agents (Table 35.4). There are two general categories among these medications. Antiresorptive agents compose the first category, and include estrogen and hormone therapies, bisphosphonates, estrogen agonist–antagonist (also known as selective estrogen receptor modulators [SERMs]), monoclonal antibody, and calcitonin. These medications inhibit osteoclast function, thus

---

BOX 35.5 NATIONAL OSTEOPOROSIS FOUNDATION RECOMMENDATIONS FOR INITIATING MEDICATION THERAPY FOR BONE LOSS

Medication therapy is recommended for postmenopausal women who present with the following:

BMD T-scores of the spine, total hip, or femoral neck of −2.5 or less (when causes of secondary osteoporosis have been ruled out)

Hip fracture(s) or clinical or incidental vertebral fracture(s)

T-scores of −1.0 to −2.5 at the femoral neck, total hip, or spine together with a calculated U.S.-adapted FRAX algorithm 10-year probability of hip fracture of greater than 3% or of any major osteoporotic fracture of greater than 20%

BMD, bone mineral density; FRAX, fracture risk assessment.
Data from Cosman et al. (2014).

TABLE 35.4	Prescription Options for Osteoporosis Management[a,b]	
MEDICATION	**FDA-APPROVED USE AND DOSE**	**CONSIDERATIONS**
Alendronate (Fosamax)	Prevention: 5 mg by mouth daily or 35 mg by mouth weekly Prevention and treatment: 10 mg by mouth daily or 70 mg by mouth weekly	■ Before any food ingestion, take oral doses in morning with 8-oz glass of plain water, remain upright, and ingest no food or drink for at least 30–60 minutes ■ Take oral doses 2 hour before antacids/calcium ■ Caution with oral forms if upper gastrointestinal disease present; clinical association with dysphagia, esophagitis, or ulceration ■ Beneficial effects may last for years after medication is discontinued ■ Fosamax plus D: combined bisphosphonate and vitamin D3 in a single tablet taken weekly ■ Actonel with calcium: blister pack for 28-day use; provides Actonel in one tablet taken on day 1 and calcium in other six tablets taken days 2–7; repeat sequence over 4 weeks ■ IV ibandronate and zoledronic acid are not associated with gastrointestinal side effects: no limitations on timing dose around food, water, calcium, or medication intake ■ Osteonecrosis of jaw (ONJ), exposed bone in mouth for > 3 months with nonhealing lesions, has been associated with high-dose IV bisphosphonate therapy among individuals with cancer-related bone disease (2–10%); cancer patients with dental problems, gum injury, oral bony abnormalities, or taking medications that interfere with healing; and, in very rare cases, healthy individuals with similar risk factors who are taking bisphosphonates for osteoporosis (incidence estimated at 0.001–0.002%). Consider stopping therapy for 2–3 months if invasive dental procedures are required and resume after healing is complete; encourage usual dental care (e.g., cleaning, fillings, crown work)
Alendronate + cholecalciferol (Fosamax Plus D)	Treatment: 70 mg plus 2,800 U of vitamin D3 or 70 mg plus 5,600 units of vitamin D3 in combined tablet by mouth weekly	
Risedronate (Actonel)	Prevention or treatment: 5 mg by mouth daily; 35 mg by mouth weekly; 75 mg by mouth 2 consecutive days each month; or 150 mg by mouth monthly	
Risedronate + calcium carbonate (Actonel with Calcium)	Prevention: 35 mg of risedronate day 1, 1,250 mg of calcium carbonate days 2 to 7	
Ibandronate (Boniva)	Prevention or treatment: 2.5 mg by mouth daily or 150 mg by mouth monthly Treatment: 3 mg IV every 3 months	
Zoledronic acid (Reclast)	Treatment: 5 mg IV yearly	
Calcitonin (Miacalcin, Fortical NS)	Treatment: 200 IU of intranasal spray daily (Miacalcin or Fortical NS) or 100 IU subcutaneously every other day (Miacalcin)	■ Usually administered as nasal spray ■ Alternate nares for nasal spray ■ Most often used for analgesic effect on acute pain resulting from vertebral compression fractures
Denosumab (Prolia)	60 mg subcutaneously every 6 months	■ Administered by a health care professional ■ Calcium and vitamin D needed ■ Contraindicated with hypocalcemia ■ May increase risk for infection ■ ONJ has been reported
Estrogen[b] (i.e., Alora, Climara, Estrace, Estraderm, Menest, Menostar, Premarin, Vivelle, Vivelle-Dot)	Prevention: doses and routes vary	■ Also effective in alleviating most symptoms related to menopause (even Menostar, which has a very low dose and was shown to effectively reduce severity and frequency of hot flashes in a 2007 study) ■ Available in several forms (e.g., pills, patch, ring, cream, gel) ■ Use for 2 to 3 years immediately following menopause; may provide some beneficial effects on bone health after discontinuation
Estrogen–progestin combination products[b] (i.e., Activella, Climara Pro, FemHRT, Prefest, Premphase, Prempro)	Prevention: doses and routes vary	
Genistein + citrated zinc bisglycinate + cholecalciferol (Fosteum Rx)	Prevention: 1 capsule twice daily (each capsule contains 27 mg of genistein, 20 mg of citrated zinc bisglycinate, 200 IU of cholecalciferol)	■ Medical food ■ Meets FDA standards for GRAS (generally recognized as safe) ■ Not recommended if taking hormone therapy, estrogen agonist–antagonists

(continued)

TABLE 35.4	Prescription Options for Osteoporosis Management[a,b] *(continued)*	
MEDICATION	**FDA-APPROVED USE AND DOSE**	**CONSIDERATIONS**
Raloxifene (Evista)	Prevention or treatment: 60 mg by mouth daily	■ May cause hot flashes ■ Not recommended if taking ET or EPT ■ Also approved for prevention of breast cancer in women at high risk for invasive breast cancer
Teriparatide (recombinant human PTH 1–34) (Forteo)	Treatment (high fracture risk): 20 mcg subcutaneously daily (a teriparatide patch for osteoporosis is under investigation)	■ Reserved for use after failure of first-line agents ■ Most effective when used sequentially following bisphosphonate

EPT, estrogen-progestogen therapy; ET, estrogen therapy; FDA, U.S. Food and Drug Administration.

[a]See prescribing reference for full information on doses, side effects, contraindications, and cautions. Combining therapies is uncommon and generally initiated only by an osteoporosis specialist because of potential side effects, including frozen bone syndrome—a condition in which bone turnover is suppressed to the point that bone quality declines despite increasing bone density, creating increased risk for fracture.

[b]Lowest effective dose is used; the FDA recommends considering non-estrogen osteoporotic agents when ET/EPT use is solely for the purpose of osteoporosis prevention.

Data from U.S. Department of Health and Human Services (2004); Cosman et al. (2014); Micromedex. Retrieved from www.thomsonhc.com/hcs/librarian; ePocrates. Retrieved from www.epocrates.com; Fosteum Prescribing Information. Retrieved from www.fosteum.com; Novartis Pharmaceuticals (2007). Reclast Prescribing Information, Novartis Pharmaceuticals (pdf); Roche Laboratories (2006, 2007); Boniva Injectable Prescribing Information, Roche Laboratories; Bachmann, Schaefers, Uddin, and Maggon (2016); Cosman et al. (2010); Prolia Prescribing Information (2010).

Adapted from Alexander and Andrist (2005).

reducing bone resorption and increasing bone density by allowing osteoblast activity to surpass osteoclast activity. Anabolic agents compose the second category. Currently, only one agent is U.S. FDA approved for use in this category—teriparatide (Forteo), which is a parathyroid hormone preparation. The mechanism of action of anabolic agents is to increase osteoblast activity and thereby stimulate formation of new bone. Additionally, one other prescription agent, a medical food, is available. Medical foods meet the FDA standard for GRAS, which means "generally regarded as safe." Fosteum meets this standard and includes a combination of genistein (an isoflavone that is purified from soy), vitamin D, and zinc. Studies evaluating Fosteum show that it does improve BMD; no data on fracture rates are available (Fosteum Prescribing Information).

Women who are treated for OP or low bone mass are monitored to evaluate the efficacy of their treatment. DEXA testing is done every 1 to 2 years until stability is achieved, and then the frequency of monitoring is reduced to every 3 years. In women with normal bone mass at baseline, repeat DEXA testing is done every 3 to 5 years, unless risk factors or history changes occur, prompting a need for earlier reevaluation (Cosman et al., 2014; U.S. Department of Health and Human Services, 2004; Watts et al., 2010).

Considerations for Special Populations

Temporary secondary bone loss can affect women receiving Depo-Provera injections for contraception and during pregnancy and lactation when calcium is leached from the bone. Bone mass usually reverts to prepregnancy and pre-Depo-Provera levels following birth, cessation of breast feeding, or discontinuation of Depo-Provera. A low-dose estrogen patch can be prescribed for women using Depo-Provera to preserve bone mass while taking the medication. Increasing calcium intake before pregnancy and maintenance of appropriate calcium intake during pregnancy and lactation are critical (U.S. Department of Health and Human Services, 2004).

■ FUTURE DIRECTIONS

Bone health is a critical issue for women across their lifetimes. Attending to building maximum bone mass during childhood and young adulthood will provide a strong foundation for fracture prevention with aging. Bone loss during midlife is managed for all women through diet, supplementation, and exercise. The FRAX algorithm can assist with determining who may benefit from pharmacologic therapy. Multiple pharmacotherapeutic options are available, making it realistic to tailor a medication plan for an individual woman. Future research is evaluating new delivery methods for existing pharmacotherapeutics as well as additional pharmacotherapeutic agents for bone health.

■ REFERENCES

Adlercreutz, H., & Mazur, W. (1997). Phyto-oestrogens and Western diseases. *Annals of Medicine, 29*(2), 95–120.

Alexander, I., & Andrist, L. (2005). Chapter 11: Menopause. In F. Likis & K. Shuiling (Eds.), *Women's gynecologic health*. Sudbury, MA: Jones & Bartlett.

Bachmann, G. A., Schaefers, M., Uddin, A., & Maggon, L. (2016). *Denosumab (Prolia, Amgen) FDA review and approval*. Retrieved from http://knol.google.com/k/denosumab-prolia-amgen-fda-review -approval

Caan, B., Neuhouser, M., Aragaki, A., Lewis, C. B., Jackson, R., LeBoff, M. S.,...LaCroix, A. (2007). Calcium plus vitamin D supplementation and the risk of postmenopausal weight gain. *Archives of Internal Medicine, 167*(9), 893–902.

Clifton-Bligh, P. B., Baber, R. J., Fulcher, G. R., Nery, M. L., & Moreton, T. (2001). The effect of isoflavones extracted from red clover (Rimostil) on lipid and bone metabolism. *Menopause, 8*(4), 259–265.

Cosman, F., de Beur, S. J., LeBoff, M. S., Lewiecki, E. M., Tanner, B., Randall, S., & Lindsay, R.; National Osteoporosis Foundation. (2014). *2014 Clinician's guide to prevention and treatment of osteoporosis.* Washington, DC: National Osteoporosis Foundation.

Cosman, F., Lane, N. E., Bolognese, M. A., Zanchetta, J. R., Garcia-Hernandez, P. A., Sees, K.,...Daddona, P. E. (2010). Effect of transdermal teriparatide administration on bone mineral density in postmenopausal women. *Journal of Clinical Endocrinology and Metabolism, 95*(1), 151–158.

Dawson-Hughes, B., Tosteson, A. N., Melton, L. J., Baim, S., Favus, M. J., Khosla, S., & Lindsay, R. L.; National Osteoporosis Foundation Guide Committee. (2008). Implications of absolute fracture risk assessment for osteoporosis practice guidelines in the USA. *Osteoporosis International, 19*(4), 449–458.

Decker, G. M., & Myers, J. (2001). Commonly used herbs: Implications for clinical practice. *Clinical Journal of Oncology Nursing, 5*(2), 13p.

ePocrates. *Computerized pharmacology and prescribing reference* (updated daily). Retrieved from www.epocrates.com

Fosteum Prescribing Information. Retrieved from http://www.fosteum .com/pi.pdf

Guillaume, G. (1992). Postmenopausal osteoporosis and Chinese medicine. *American Journal of Acupuncture, 20*, 105–111.

Hippisley-Cox, J., & Coupland, C. (2009). Predicting risk of osteoporotic fracture in men and women in England and Wales: Prospective derivation and validation of QFractureScores. *British Medical Journal, 339*, b4229.

Jackson, R. D., LaCroix, A. Z., Gass, M., Wallace, R. B., Robbins, J., Lewis, C. E.,...Barad, D.; Women's Health Initiative Investigators. (2006). Calcium plus vitamin D supplementation and the risk of fractures. *New England Journal of Medicine, 354*(7), 669–683.

Kim, J., Lee, J., Shin, J., & Park, B. (2015). Socioeconomic disparities in osteoporosis prevalence: Different results in the overall Korean adult population and single-person households. *Journal of Preventive Medicine and Public Health, 48*, 84–93.

Lappe, J. M., Travers-Gustafson, D., Davies, K. M., Recker, R. R., & Heaney, R. P. (2007). Vitamin D and calcium supplementation reduces cancer risk: Results of a randomized trial. *American Journal of Clinical Nutrition, 85*(6), 1586–1591.

Lin, J., Manson, J. E., Lee, I. M., Cook, N. R., Buring, J. E., & Zhang, S. M. (2007). Intakes of calcium and vitamin D and breast cancer risk in women. *Archives of Internal Medicine, 167*(10), 1050–1059.

Liu, J., Ho, S. C., Su, Y. X., Chen, W. Q., Zhang, C. X., & Chen, Y. M. (2009). Effect of long-term intervention of soy isoflavones on bone mineral density in women: A meta-analysis of randomized controlled trials. *Bone, 44*(5), 948–953.

Marini, H., Minutoli, L., Polito, F., Bitto, A., Altavilla, D., Atteritano, M.,...Squadrito, F. (2007). Effects of the phytoestrogen genistein on bone metabolism in osteopenic postmenopausal women: A randomized trial. *Annals of Internal Medicine, 146*(12), 839–847.

Miazgowski, T., Kleerekoper, M., Felsenberg, D., Stěpán, J. J., & Szulc, P. (2012). Secondary osteoporosis: Endocrine and metabolic causes of bone mass deterioration. *Journal of Osteoporosis, 2012,* 907214. doi:10.1155/2012/907214

Micromedex. Retrieved from www.thomsonhc.com/hcs/librarian

Novartis Pharmaceuticals. (2007). *Reclast prescribing information.* Novartis Pharmaceuticals (pdf).

Paik, J. M., Curhan, G. C., Sun, Q., Rexrode, K. M., Manson, J. E., Rimm, E. B., & Taylor, E. N. (2014). Calcium supplement intake and risk of cardiovascular disease in women. *Osteoporosis International, 25*(8), 2047–2056. doi:10.1007/s00198-014-2732-3

Prolia Prescribing Information. (2010). Retrieved from http://pi.amgen .com/united_states/prolia/prolia_pi.pdf

Report of a WHO Study Group. (1994). Assessment of fracture risk and its application to screening for postmenopausal osteoporosis. Geneva, Switzerland: World Health Organization (WHO Technical Report Series, No. 843).

Roche Laboratories. (2006). *Boniva tablet prescribing information.* Retrieved from www.rocheusa.com/products/Boniva/PI.pdf

Roche Laboratories. (2007). *Boniva injectable prescribing information.* Retrieved from www.rocheusa.com/products/Boniva/Injection_PI.pdf

Ross, A. C., Manson, J. E., Abrams, S. A., Aloia, J. F., Brannon, P. M., Clinton, S. K.,...Shapses, S. A. (2010). The 2011 report on dietary reference intakes for calcium and vitamin D from the Institute of Medicine: What clinicians need to know. *Journal of Clinical Endocrinology and Metabolism, 96*(1), 53–58. doi:10.1210/jc.2010-2704.

Skorupski, N., & Alexander, I. M. (2013). Multidisciplinary osteoporosis management of post low-trauma hip fracture patients. *Journal of the American Academy of Nurse Practitioners, 25*(1), 3–10.

Somekawa, Y., Chiguchi, M., Ishibashi, T., & Aso, T. (2001). Soy intake related to menopausal symptoms, serum lipids, and bone mineral density in postmenopausal Japanese women. *Obstetrics and Gynecology, 97*(1), 109–115.

Tosteson, A. N., Melton, L. J., Dawson-Hughes, B., Baim, S., Favus, M. J., Khosla, S., & Lindsay, R. L.; National Osteoporosis Foundation Guide Committee. (2008). Cost-effective osteoporosis treatment thresholds: The United States perspective. *Osteoporosis International, 19*(4), 437–447.

U.S. Department of Health and Human Services. (2004). *Bone health and osteoporosis: A report of the surgeon general.* Rockville, MD: U.S. Department of Health and Human Services, Office of the Surgeon General.

U.S. Preventive Services Task Force. (2011). Screening for osteoporosis: U.S. preventive services task force recommendation statement. *Annals of Internal Medicine, 154*(5), 356–364.

Watts, N. B., Bilezikian, J. P., Camacho, P. M., Greenspan, S. L., Harris, S. T., Hodgson, S. F.,...Petak, S. M.; AACE Osteoporosis Task Force. (2010). American Association of Clinical Endocrinologists Medical Guidelines for Clinical Practice for the diagnosis and treatment of postmenopausal osteoporosis. *Endocrine Practice, 16*(Suppl. 3), 1–37. Retrieved from https://www.aace.com/files/osteo-guidelines-2010.pdf

Wei, P., Liu, M., Chen, Y., & Chen, D.-C. (2012). Systematic review of soy isoflavone supplements on osteoporosis in women. *Asian Pacific Journal of Tropical Medicine, 5*(3), 243–248.

World Health Organization (WHO). (2016). *WHO FRAX technical report.* World Health Organization. Retrieved from www.shef.ac.uk/ FRAX

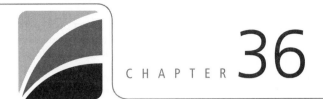

CHAPTER 36

The Challenge of Unintended Pregnancies

Katherine Simmonds • Lisa Stern

Since well before the advent of modern contraceptives, women and couples have employed various techniques and technologies to prevent pregnancy or to increase the chances of conception (Schneider & Schneider, 1995). For many, deciding when to become pregnant is crucial for their sense of personal well-being (Frost & Lindberg, 2013). Researchers and clinicians commonly classify pregnancies as "intended" or "unintended" depending on whether the woman (or, occasionally, the couple) was seeking pregnancy. The terms "unplanned" or sometimes "accidental" pregnancy are also used in the scientific literature. In recent years, a robust debate has emerged regarding the validity of this dichotomous approach for categorizing pregnancies. In this chapter—though we use the terminology of intent to describe epidemiologic trends—we acknowledge that this concept is flawed, and perhaps only useful at the population level, if at all. This tension is discussed here. However, because clinical care takes place between clinicians and individuals, this chapter focuses primarily on interventions at this level.

DEFINITIONS AND EPIDEMIOLOGY

Demography and public health define unintended pregnancy as "a pregnancy that is mistimed, unplanned, or unwanted at the time of conception" (Centers for Disease Control and Prevention [CDC], 2013b). Within this framework, if a woman did not want to become pregnant at the time she did or at any time in the future, the pregnancy is considered "unwanted." If she wanted to become pregnant at some point in the future but *not* at the time she did, it is classified as "mistimed."

Large-scale population surveys like the National Survey of Family Growth (NSFG) and the Pregnancy Risk Assessment Monitoring System (PRAMS) are the most commonly cited sources of data on unintended pregnancy in the United States. According to the most recent NSFG, just more than half of the 6.6 million pregnancies that occur annually in the United States are unintended, divided

between 20% unwanted and 31% mistimed. For women aged 15 to 44 years, the unintended pregnancy rate is 54 per 1,000 women (Finer & Zolna, 2014). Given this rate, more than half of U.S. women will experience an unintended pregnancy by age 45 years (Jones & Kavanaugh, 2011). The stated goal for *Healthy People 2020* is to increase the proportion of all pregnancies that are intended to 56% (U.S. Department of Health and Human Services [DHHS], 2010). Globally, 40% of the 85 million pregnancies that occur each year are unintended (Singh, Sedgh, & Hussain, 2010). Many public health experts have called for the improvement of family planning services as a critical component for achieving the United Nations' Millennium Development Goal of reducing maternal mortality (Nanda, Switlick, & Lule, 2005).

Disparities in Unintended Pregnancy

Unintended pregnancy rates have been found to vary by select geographic, personal, and population characteristics. Nationwide, states in the South and Southwest and those that are densely populated tend to have the highest rates: Delaware (62%), Hawaii, and New York (61% each) currently have the highest overall rates, while the lowest is in New Hampshire (32%). Economic factors and rates of insurance coverage have been offered as partial explanations for these variations (Kost, 2015).

At the population level, various demographic and socioeconomic factors are associated with unintended pregnancy. Unmarried women—particularly those who live with a partner—are more likely than married women to experience an unintended pregnancy. Low-income women, Black women, Hispanic women, those without a high school degree, and those aged 18 to 24 years are also more likely to experience unintended pregnancies (Finer & Zolna, 2014). Youth living in poverty and homeless women are also at high risk (Brooks-Gunn, Duncan, & Aber, 1997; Gelberg et al., 2008). Unintended pregnancy has also been found to occur frequently among women in violent relationships (Pallitto et al., 2013).

Broad social determinants of health, including poverty and racial inequality underlie disparities in unintended pregnancy rates. Encouraging women to plan for pregnancy is an inadequate strategy for overcoming the impact of these structural forces on general health outcomes, including those related to reproduction. Social and reproductive justice can provide a framework for providers of clinical care to better understand and promote the health of women and families in general, and within which to contextualize unintended pregnancy. Nursing scholars have called for a public health approach to unintended pregnancy that broadens the focus beyond the individual patient encounter promoting access to high-quality, evidence-based sexuality education and broad preventive health services that help women and families attain healthy pregnancy outcomes and time pregnancies as desired (Taylor, Levi, & Simmonds, 2010). For those who do become pregnant, high-quality, accessible obstetric and abortion services are also essential.

Clinicians and public health experts can play an important role in advocating for public policies that increase access to health care and health education, enhance women's economic power, and decrease racism and other forms of oppression. Although this chapter—intended for a clinical audience—focuses primarily on clinical interventions at the individual level, to succeed in reducing unintended pregnancy and improving maternal and child health outcomes, structural barriers to reproductive health care must be dismantled and health equity must be more broadly promoted (Bridges, 2011; List, 2011).

Outcomes and Clinical Implications of Unintended Pregnancy

Between 2001 and 2008, there was a slight increase (from 48% to 51%) in the proportion of pregnancies that was reported as unintended. In 2008 (the latest year for which data are available), excluding miscarriages, 40% of unintended pregnancies in the United States ended in abortion, and 60% in live births, reflecting a continuing downward trend in abortion rates since its peak in the 1980s (Finer & Zolna, 2014). Globally, 50% of unintended pregnancies end in abortion, 13% in miscarriage, and 38% in birth (Singh et al., 2010). Of pregnancies that end in live births, children may be raised by biological parents, adoptive parents, or within kinship networks. Although difficult to obtain precise numbers, approximately 20,000 domestic-born infants are placed for adoption annually in the United States (Carney, n.d.). Clinicians must be prepared to provide unbiased information, decision support, and referrals about each of these options to any woman who presents with an initial positive pregnancy test (Dobkin, Perrucci, & Dehlendorf, 2013). General information and resources as well as principles and specific techniques for fulfilling this clinical role are discussed subsequently.

Studies of the relationship of pregnancy intent and maternal and child health outcomes have yielded mixed results, especially when important variables such as income and age are controlled (Logan, Holcombe, Manlove, & Ryan, 2007). One recent study that considered the extent of both mistiming and desire found that intent positively affected whether women recognized a pregnancy early, entered prenatal care during the first trimester, and breast fed (Kost & Lindberg, 2015). Babies born of pregnancies that were classified as unwanted were also found more likely to be low birth weight. Early access to prenatal care is encouraged for all women to promote health pregnancy, yet women who experience an unintended pregnancy may be less likely to access early prenatal care (Braveman et al., 2003).

ISSUES IN THE MEASUREMENT OF UNINTENDED PREGNANCY

The intent of a pregnancy or birth is a complex and highly subjective concept. In order to enhance the validity and stability of the measurement of pregnancy intent, typically researchers do not directly ask whether a pregnancy was intended or unintended but rather pose a series of related questions (Klerman, 2000). In the NSFG, for instance, women are asked with regard to each pregnancy they have had whether they wanted to have a baby at the time they conceived; further questions are then based on this initial response (Guzzo & Hayford, 2013). It is important to note that this approach to the measurement of pregnancy intention is retrospective: participants are asked about their desire to become pregnant *before* conception, however, many are responding months or even years after that conception occurred. This leads to potential recall bias, threatening the validity of the findings (Joyce, Kaestner, & Korenman, 2002). Additionally, there is substantial evidence that women's views on intent may change over time, even within the course of a pregnancy (Poole, Flowers, Goldenberg, Cliver, & McNeal, 2000). One study that analyzed data from the National Longitudinal Survey of Adolescent Health found that 22% of women changed reports of birth intent for the same pregnancy among waves of the survey (Guzzo & Hayford, 2013).

Recently, there has been renewed interest in exploring men's role in pregnancy decision-making. Although the initial survey on which the NSFG is based (known as the Indianapolis Survey) attempted to capture pregnancy intent by querying couples, most subsequent studies have only engaged female participants. However, in light of the fact that most unplanned pregnancies occur as a result of heterosexual intercourse, more sexual health researchers have sought to understand men's attitudes toward pregnancy and their relationship to outcomes (Higgins, Popkin, & Santelli, 2012; Kågesten, Bajos, Bohet, & Moreau, 2015). However, researchers have critiqued the quality of existing surveys of male fertility intention and behavior (Joyner et al., 2012).

Though public health has long regarded unintended pregnancy as a problem, recent research suggests that some women may not view pregnancy planning as a priority, meaningful, or feasible, as the dominant public health approach assumes. Rather, many women express a feeling of ambivalence about pregnancy or regard it as something that "just happens" (Borrero et al., 2015; Higgins et al., 2012). Although some suggest that this argues for more widespread preconception planning, it also calls the assumptions underlying the framework of "intention" or "planning" into question. Regardless of an individual woman's personal stance on pregnancy intention or planning, clinicians have an ethical responsibility to uphold and promote fully autonomous reproductive decision making that includes high-quality comprehensive reproductive health services as part of a full spectrum of empowered women's health care. This is consistent with the client-centered approach to quality family planning care promulgated by the Centers for Disease Control and Prevention (CDC) and U.S. Office of Population Affairs (Gavin et al., 2014).

■ ASSESSMENT

For clinicians who provide care to women of reproductive age, assessment for a possible or confirmed pregnancy that is mistimed or unwanted will vary depending on a woman's particular situation and the point in the pregnancy at which she presents for care. Baker (1995) describes three distinct but related types of patient encounters that a clinician may be involved in: pregnancy testing, pregnancy options counseling, and abortion counseling. In the first instance, a woman may present already suspecting she is pregnant but seeking confirmation, or, less commonly, unaware she is pregnant until the clinician suggests the possibility. In either case, the clinician proceeds with a pregnancy test, physical examination (if indicated), and delivery of test results (discussed as follows). If this assessment leads to a pregnancy diagnosis, then the second type of encounter—pregnancy options counseling—may ensue. In other cases, a woman may present for care already certain she is pregnant. Although a pregnancy test may still be warranted or desired, the main purpose of the visit is to receive counseling and information about options. Suggested steps are discussed in the Pregnancy Options Counseling section. Finally, with the last type of encounter described by Baker, some women present to the health system already with a confirmed pregnancy and having made the decision about how to resolve a pregnancy. In such cases, the clinical visit may simply be to initiate desired services (abortion or prenatal care), or to obtain a referral. Abortion counseling is provided when a woman knows that she is pregnant and has decided to terminate the pregnancy, but is seeking support and information specifically about this option. This type of counseling is discussed further in the section on abortion.

History

As with all patient encounters, when assessing a woman who may be or is certain that she is pregnant, obtaining a relevant history is the first step. Beginning the visit with open-ended questions to determine why she has come in often yields important information about the possible pregnancy, as well as her feelings about it. The possibility of pregnancy should be considered if a reproductive age woman reports symptoms associated with early pregnancy, such as nausea, breast tenderness, fatigue, irregular vaginal bleeding, and/or amenorrhea. In some clinical encounters, a woman's presenting complaint may have nothing to do with pregnancy,

but the possibility emerges during a review of systems, or routine evaluation for another issue (e.g., before ordering x-rays or as part of a preoperative examination).

If a woman indicates she suspects or already knows she is pregnant, eliciting additional information can yield important historical data that informs clinical assessment and management. For example, recent unprotected intercourse may have prompted the visit and a pregnancy test may be premature (if it is less than 7–10 days since fertilization occurred). If a woman is not currently seeking pregnancy and it is less than 5 days since she had unprotected intercourse, the clinician should offer emergency contraception (see Chapter 22). If intercourse took place between 4 and 5 days earlier, ulipristal acetate (Ella) or—if she is interested in and eligible for long-acting reversible contraception—a Copper-T intrauterine device (IUD; Paragard) should be included in these offerings because of their greater efficacy after 72 hours as compared to levonorgestrel-containing methods (Plan B One-Step, Take Action, Next Choice One-Dose, My Way, or other generic forms).

If a woman reports she has had a positive pregnancy test, the clinician should determine if she has already made a decision about whether to continue or end the pregnancy, or whether she wants or needs additional information or counseling. If she indicates she has decided and is sure about the decision, the clinician can proceed with making a plan for her to obtain desired services. If, on the other hand, a woman is unsure of her decision or is lacking information, pregnancy options counseling and education may be the next step. Before proceeding with pregnancy testing or options counseling, the clinician should verify the date of the patient's last menstrual period (LMP) and whether it was normal (i.e., usual amount of flow, duration, etc.) in order to establish the estimated gestational age (EGA) of the pregnancy. If the LMP is unknown or unsure, a pelvic examination and/or ultrasound can establish the gestational age. Reports of any spotting, bleeding, pain, or other early pregnancy warning signs also warrant further evaluation (see Chapter 22 for further discussion). In addition, screening women for intimate partner violence and reproductive coercion should be routine when assessing a woman for a possible or confirmed pregnancy.

Physical Examination and Diagnosis

If history indicates that pregnancy is possible, and a pregnancy test has not already been performed, a qualitative, immunometric urine test for human chorionic gonadotropin (hCG) should be performed. Based on a woman's history and presentation, a clinician may also decide to perform a physical examination, including a pelvic examination. The presence of probable signs of pregnancy, including Chadwick's (bluish hue of the vagina and cervix), Goodell's (softening of the cervix), and Hegar's (softening of the uterine isthmus), as well as enlargement of the uterus can contribute to the diagnosis of pregnancy; however, these may not be present in early pregnancy or may be too subtle for a clinician to detect. Physical examination findings should be correlated with pregnancy test results and EGA; any discrepancy among these data needs to be further investigated, including by reviewing the menstrual and gynecologic history to confirm accuracy of the reported LMP. If a discrepancy persists, a quantitative hCG and/or transvaginal ultrasound may be warranted (see Chapter 22).

■ MANAGEMENT

Delivering Pregnancy Test Results

Once pregnancy has been ruled out or confirmed, the clinician should inform the woman using neutral language, such as "The result of your test is positive, which means you are pregnant." If the pregnancy test is negative, possible reasons for this result should be explained, including that it may be too early for the test to be positive or that the woman is actually not pregnant. If a review of the menstrual and sexual history reveals that it could be too early for a positive result, the woman can be instructed to repeat the test in 1 to 2 weeks. When performed correctly, 98% of women will have a positive test result within 7 days after implantation (Fjerstad & Stewart, 2011). With immunometric tests, the type used in most clinical settings, a false negative result is possible, though extremely rare. These rare false negatives are associated with elevated lipids, high immunoglobulin levels and low serum protein associated with severe kidney disease. If the clinician doubts the accuracy of a negative result, a quantitative beta subunit radioimmunoassay can be ordered (Fjerstad & Stewart, 2011).

Following a negative pregnancy test, if a woman does not want to become pregnant, the clinician should initiate a discussion about contraceptive options, encompassing a review of which method(s) she has been using, what has or has not worked for her in the past, and what her desires are for future pregnancies. Together, the clinician and woman can establish a contraceptive plan that includes follow-up before the close of the visit.

If the pregnancy test is positive or pregnancy is otherwise confirmed, verifying the gestational age and relaying this information to the woman is important as it may be a factor in her decision about how to proceed and may shape what options are available to her. The following section focuses on providing pregnancy options counseling.

Pregnancy Options Counseling

After confirming pregnancy or delivering a positive pregnancy test result, a clinician must determine whether a woman wants or needs additional information and support about what options are available to her. Though every patient encounter should be tailored for a particular individual, four general steps have been suggested for delivering options counseling (Simmonds & Likis, 2011): (1) explore how the patient feels about the pregnancy, which may include assessing baseline knowledge and providing education about each option; (2) help to identify support systems and assess for risks; (3) assist with decision making; and (4) provide desired service, or referral. Each of these four steps will now be discussed further.

EXPLORE FEELINGS

Pregnancy may precipitate an abrupt change in a woman's life, relationship(s), living arrangements, financial stability, or self-concept. Baker (1995) suggests that for some, pregnancy may represent a crisis as it can cause a variety of uncomfortable emotions or physical symptoms that interfere with the ability to function. Awareness of these possibilities can help a clinician to deliver nonjudgmental, patient-centered care.

Asking open-ended questions such as "How do you feel about the pregnancy (or pregnancy test result)?" at the start of a visit can establish a climate in which a woman feels comfortable to share her concerns and experience. Finding out if she has thought or already made up her mind about the outcome of the pregnancy allows the clinician to assess the woman's decision-making process, as well as her level of understanding about available options. Some women will report that they have already made a decision, while others may not yet know how they will proceed, or may not feel comfortable expressing their thoughts about this to the clinician. A nondirective statement that expresses support for a woman's decision—no matter what it is—can help establish an environment where a woman feels comfortable expressing her emotions and asking questions. For example, the clinician can say, "I want to be sure that you know what all of your options are, and I will help you get good care no matter what you decide to do about the pregnancy." Ascertaining whether a woman understands what all of her options are is important. This need may be greater for women from certain vulnerable populations (such as adolescents), or those considering abortion or adoption, which may be more stigmatized options than continuing a pregnancy and parenting for some women. (See the section Considerations for Special Populations that follows.)

If a pregnancy has just been diagnosed or confirmed, some women may need time to accept this news. Creating space—both psychologic and chronologic—that allows a woman to reflect and emote before discussing her options or making specific plans is optimal. Some women may prefer to do this outside of the clinical setting, in which case a follow-up plan should be established. Follow-up may consist of a telephone call or return visit when further counseling and education can be delivered, or simply confirmation that the woman has made a decision and knows how to arrange the next step of her care. Social and economic barriers that could interfere with follow-up, such as adolescents who do not plan to tell their parent or guardian that they are pregnant or a woman with insecure housing, should be taken into consideration when establishing the follow-up plan.

If a clinician determines that a woman is ready and wants to discuss her options, counseling and education should be delivered. In order to provide quality care, clinicians must stay informed about locally available resources for childrearing, adoption, and abortion. Assessing a woman's baseline knowledge and perceptions about each option can be accomplished by asking a question such as "Tell me what have you heard about adoption/abortion?" or "Do you have any questions about what it would be like to be a parent/place a child for adoption/have an abortion?" Strategies and tools for assisting women with making a decision are discussed next.

IDENTIFY SUPPORT SYSTEMS AND ASSESS FOR RISK

In addition to discussing feelings about being pregnant and, if warranted, providing education about options, the clinician should inquire about support systems and determine if a woman is at risk for violence or other personal harm that could be further exacerbated by the revelation of her pregnancy. Asking if she has told others that she is or might be pregnant allows the clinician to assess social network relationships and identify individuals who might be in need of more support, including additional follow-up or a referral for social/mental health services.

All women should be screened for risk of violence, abuse, or coercion as a routine component of a pregnancy options counseling visit. For some, a pregnancy may be a result of reproductive coercion, and/or coercion may be an important factor in decision making as partners, parents, or other influential people in her social network may exert excessive pressure or control regarding the outcome of a pregnancy. These situations can be ethically and legally complex in clinical practice. Resources to assist with identifying and managing such cases are available for clinicians (Chamberlain & Levenson, 2013). If coercion is or seems to be a factor in a woman's pregnancy decision making, additional counseling and follow-up are warranted.

ASSIST WITH DECISION MAKING

Many women who know or strongly suspect that they are pregnant may have already decided how they will proceed before presenting for clinical care; others may seek information or decision support from a health care provider before making their final decision. For a woman who has not made a decision yet, contextualizing her decision in relation to the current gestational age of the pregnancy is an important component of pregnancy options counseling. Women should be made aware that both early entry into prenatal care and early abortion are advised as they are associated with better health outcomes. Furthermore, the clinician may need to inform women that at advanced gestational ages abortion may be logistically difficult to obtain or illegal, and that this option may not be possible if decision making is delayed.

For women who are unsure about whether to continue a pregnancy or have an abortion, tools to assist with decision making may be helpful. A number of resources have been created for this purpose. These can be used during a clinical visit or recommended for use after the clinic visit, including with a partner or another trusted individual. Another suggested strategy to support decision making that can be used during a time-limited pregnancy options counseling session is to have a woman make a list of the pros and cons of each option. The Ottowa Personal Decision Guide is an evidence-supported, theory-based tool that has been designed to help patients with making health or social decisions (O'Connor, Jacobsen, & Stacey, 2015). Though there are no published studies on its use among women facing a pregnancy decision, it may be helpful in pregnancy options counseling. The Reproductive Health Access Project has also developed a model for providing options counseling to women who are ambivalent about pregnancy that includes counseling points and suggested exercises (www.reproductiveaccess.org/resource/pregnancy-options-counseling-model).

PROVIDE DESIRED SERVICE OR REFER TO APPROPRIATE PROVIDER

Establishing a plan for a woman to obtain desired prenatal care or abortion services is the final step in a pregnancy options counseling visit. If a woman is not ready to make a decision before the end of the visit, a follow-up plan should be established that takes into account the current EGA and encourages initiation of desired services in a timely manner.

Depending on certification, state-level advanced practice registered nurse (APRN) scope-of-practice regulations, and clinical protocols, a clinician may be the provider of desired services (prenatal care and/or abortion), or may need to refer a woman to another provider or facility. If a woman is considering adoption, referral to a social worker or an agency that can provide accurate information and supportive counseling is recommended. Resources on adoption are listed in the Resources section in the online ancillary accompanying this text.

With appropriate education and certification, many primary care clinicians are able to provide routine prenatal care. Determining whether a woman wants and is eligible to receive prenatal care from a particular type of clinician (e.g., nurse-midwife, obstetrician) depends on her insurance or available public assistance programs, as well as personal preference and whether these services are available in the area. Exploring these issues as part of establishing a prenatal care plan is essential for upholding patient autonomy and promoting patient satisfaction. Nurse practitioners', nurse midwives', and physician assistants' ability to provide abortion services varies from state to state.

Clinicians who do not or cannot provide the pregnancy-related service(s) a woman is seeking must refer her to another provider or site. By developing relationships with individual providers and/or referral sites, clinicians can gain a deeper understanding of the setting and quality of care delivered, which can be helpful to women, especially with regard to allaying anxiety in the face of a break in continuity of care. With abortion in particular, community perceptions of a site, based on reality or myth, or the presence of anti-abortion protesters may influence a woman's experience when going for an appointment (Kimport, Cockrill, & Weitz, 2012). In some communities, "full-spectrum" or "abortion doula" programs have been established to provide women undergoing abortions with support.

Once a plan for care is made, the pregnancy options counseling encounter is over. Unless a clinician will be providing the desired prenatal or abortion care, a woman may not return until she comes for a follow-up or to resume routine primary care; therefore, as with other referrals, if requested services will be obtained in a different facility, assistance with making an appointment, verifying that the woman was able to successfully access these services in a timely manner, and following up to determine if she was satisfied with the services are a responsibility of the clinician or clinical care team.

SPECIAL CONSIDERATIONS WHEN PROVIDING OPTIONS COUNSELING

Clinicians may experience conflicts between their personal feelings and professional responsibilities when providing care to a woman who has recently discovered that she is pregnant or is deciding whether to continue or terminate a pregnancy. Regardless of personal beliefs, health professionals are bound by professional Codes of Ethics, such as the American Nurses Association Code of Ethics for Nursing With Interpretive Statements (ANA, 2015) to uphold patient rights to autonomy and deliver care that is respectful and nonjudgmental. Although health professionals may refuse to provide care that violates their personal beliefs, if a patient faces a life-threatening situation, or is otherwise at risk of not receiving needed care, conscientious objection cannot be invoked. Conversely, Harris (2012) suggests that some clinicians may choose to invert this concept of conscience instead, using it to assert their *willingness* to provide certain types of care, such as abortion.

Before providing options counseling, ideally all clinicians should engage in a process of values clarification, reflecting on their personal beliefs regarding parenting, adoption, abortion, and related reproductive health issues, and how these may influence their interactions with patients. Tools and workshops designed to assist health care providers in exploring these personal and professional intersections have been developed. If personal values threaten or interfere with the delivery of unbiased, nondirective counseling or referrals, care should be transferred to another provider. Every effort should be made to minimize delays and limit the burden to women in obtaining alternative care.

■ ABORTION

Induced abortion—or the practice of terminating a pregnancy before viability—has been practiced throughout history and across different cultures. Extensive historical and anthropological evidence indicates that abortion has been practiced for thousands of years through a variety of means, and that it is a "universal phenomenon" across all human societies. Sociologist Carole Joffe asserts that when and wherever abortion has been forbidden, women have continued to seek it, and a culture of illegal provision has proliferated (Joffe, 2009).

Until about 1880, abortion was legal in the United States. After that time, most states banned it, except to save the life of the mother. In 1973, following the Supreme Court ruling on the case of *Roe vs. Wade*, the decision to terminate a pregnancy in its early stages, or before viability, became a legal right again for women in the United States. Before that ruling, many women still had abortions (estimates range from 200,000 to 1.2 million per year), including through legal channels in some cases, but more often by self-induction, underground, or "back alley" providers. As a result, many women died from sepsis, hemorrhage, or other complications due to poorly performed abortions. In 1930, 18% of maternal deaths in the United States were attributed to induced abortion. By 1965, the absolute number of deaths due to abortion had dropped considerably (to less than 200 per year), largely as a result of the discovery of antibiotics in the 1940s; however, this number still represented 17% of all maternal deaths for the year (Gold, 2003). In terms of global health, in countries where abortion is still illegal or highly restricted, unsafe abortion rates remain high. In 2008, worldwide some 47,000 deaths, or 13% of all maternal deaths, were attributed to unsafe abortion (World Health Organization [WHO], 2011).

As of this writing, abortion remains legal in the United States, but legislation at both the state and federal level has profoundly restricted its availability in many parts of the country. These policies include mandatory waiting periods, parental consent laws, and strict regulation of providers and sites where abortions are performed. An exhaustive discussion of abortion-related legislation is beyond the scope of this chapter, but it is essential for clinicians to stay apprised of both state and national abortion laws and regulations in order to provide accurate information to women about their legal rights and assist them with obtaining services.

In addition to legal restrictions, other factors can profoundly influence whether a woman is able to obtain an abortion. These include provider availability, geographic location, transportation, and economic resources. From 1982 until early 2000, there was a general decline in both the number of facilities and providers offering abortion in the United States. Although this trend plateaued between 2008 and 2011, more recently declines in the number of providers and facilities (4% and 1%, respectively) have again been observed (Jones & Jerman, 2014). In 2011, 89% of U.S. counties in which 38% of U.S. women reside had no abortion service (Jones & Jerman, 2014). For some, the distance to an abortion provider can be an insurmountable obstacle; when coupled with the time required for the visit itself—including any waiting period mandated by the state—this can present an excessively burdensome situation, especially for women with limited resources.

In addition to provider availability, other economic factors can determine whether a woman is able to obtain an abortion or not. In 2011 and 2012, the average cost for an aspiration abortion with local anesthesia at 10 weeks gestation in a nonhospital setting in the United States was $480; for an early medication abortion it was $504; and at 20 weeks gestation it was $1,350 (Jerman & Jones, 2014). In 2008, more than half of women paid out of pocket for their abortion. Although many of those (63%) had private insurance, either their insurance plan did not cover abortion, they were not aware that it covered abortion, their deductible was higher than the cost of the abortion, or they opted not to use it (Jones, Finer, & Singh, 2010). In recent years, state and federal trends toward greater restrictions on insurance coverage of abortion have caused even more women to use personal resources to pay for abortions. For some, this has led to significant delays in obtaining services (Guttmacher Institute, 2015; Roberts, Gould, Kimport, Weitz, & Foster, 2014). Because of the Hyde Amendment, which prohibits the use of federal funds for abortion except in cases of life endangerment, rape, or incest, women who are eligible for Medicaid also experience challenges with abortion coverage. Currently, only 17 states allow use of state Medicaid funds for abortion, while women who reside in the other 33 states and District of Columbia must pay out of pocket (Guttmacher Institute, 2015). In some sites, income eligible women may be able to access free care to pay for an abortion. However, because many women need financial support—for all of the aforementioned reasons—to be able to obtain an abortion, independent abortion funds have been established to help them pay for this service and related costs, such as transportation and lodging.

In addition, other factors, including lack of information, intimidation by protesters, stigma, and violence toward those working in abortion service have been identified as barriers to abortion. As a result of these obstacles, for many women obtaining an abortion can be difficult. Clinicians can play a vital role in recognizing and helping patients navigate these challenges, and where legally possible, alleviating the provider shortage by delivering abortion care in their clinical practice. Special considerations for APRNs regarding the provision of abortion are discussed further as follows.

Incidence

Since its peak in 1981, the abortion rate in the United States has been steadily declining. In 2011 (the most recent data available), 1.06 million abortions took place in the United States representing a rate of 16.9/1,000 women aged 15 to 44 years (Jones & Jerman, 2014). By the age of 45 years, approximately three out of every 10 women in the United States will have an abortion, making it one of the most common medical procedures in the country (Jones & Kavanaugh, 2011). According to the most current CDC surveillance data, 91% of abortions in the United States occurred before the end of the first trimester, the majority (64.5%) before 8 weeks gestation. Less than 2% took place after 21 weeks gestation. Fourteen percent of the women who had abortions were teenagers, and 33% were between 20 and 24 years old (Pazol, Creanga, Burley, & Jamieson, 2014). Most women who have abortions were never married (Jones et al., 2010).

Women from all economic levels, races, ethnicities, and religions have abortions; however, researchers have noted disparities in rates. These disparities reflect similar trends in unintended pregnancy (discussed previously), though with some subtle variations by subgroups. For example, Black women are more likely to end a pregnancy through abortion than White or Hispanic women, whereas poor and low-income women and those with lower educational achievement have been found to be less likely to resolve an unintended pregnancy through abortion than those who are more affluent and have higher levels of education. However,

because of the overarching disparities in unintended pregnancy rates, both abortion and unintended births rates are the highest among poor women in this country (Finer & Zolna, 2014). These variations in abortion rates should be interpreted with awareness of the larger sociocultural context in which women live, work, engage in sexual activity, use contraception, and make decisions about whether and when to have children (Dehlendorf, Harris, & Weitz, 2013).

Studies of why women decide to have abortions have identified multiple, diverse, interrelated factors. Among the most common reasons are finances, timing, partner issues, and responsibilities to others, including children (Biggs, Gould, & Foster, 2013). Approximately, 61% of women who terminate a pregnancy have already had at least one child (Jones et al., 2010). Other reported reasons for terminating a pregnancy include the disruption that having a baby would cause with current commitments, such as school or work, and feeling unready to parent (Finer, Frohwirth, Dauphinee, Singh, & Moore, 2005).

■ ASSESSMENT AND MANAGEMENT

When providing care to a woman who is seeking an abortion, the clinician's role includes providing information about which methods are options for her based on the gestational age of the pregnancy, her medical history, and availability of services in the area. In addition, as part of the abortion care team, the APRN's role may include offering decision-making support, screening for coercion, and providing the type of abortion selected. If a clinician cannot or chooses not to provide abortions, he or she must refer women to an alternative provider or site, optimally of known, high quality. Care coordination, which includes helping women make appointments, secure financial resources, arrange child care and/or transportation, and successfully navigate other logistic challenges, is another responsibility of clinicians providing abortion-related care. Follow-up to ensure that a woman was able to obtain services and is not experiencing complications is also the responsibility of the clinician and the abortion care team. Postabortion care is discussed further later in this chapter. The aim of this section is to provide a general overview of abortion methods to help clinicians with providing accurate, unbiased patient education and counseling. For those who decide to provide abortion care that extends beyond counseling and education, additional training is required.

Abortion Methods

Because most abortions in the United States take place during the first trimester (Pazol et al., 2014), this section focuses primarily on methods commonly used for early terminations; methods used after the first trimester are discussed only briefly.

There are two general approaches to early abortion. Aspiration abortion (also referred to as "surgical" abortion or "suction curettage") is the most common method. Medication abortion (also referred to as "medical" or sometimes "chemical" abortion) has become more widespread in the United States since the Food and Drug Administration (FDA) approval of mifepristone in 2000. Between 2002 and 2011, early medication abortions (less than or equal to 8 weeks gestation) increased more than 200% (from 5.3% to 18.3% of all abortions; Pazol et al., 2014).

Early abortions are most often performed or initiated in ambulatory settings, which is both safe and cost effective. In sites where both medication and aspiration abortion are offered, efforts are often made to keep costs roughly equivalent. In rare cases, a woman may have a complicating medical condition that requires the abortion to be performed in a hospital setting, which increases total cost.

ASPIRATION ABORTION

Aspiration abortion involves removal of a pregnancy by applying suction to the uterine cavity. Sharp curettage is an adjunct to this technique that was common in the past, but is no longer recommended as evidence has mounted against its safety and patient acceptability (International Federation of Gynecology and Obstetrics, 2011; WHO, 2012). A typical visit for an outpatient aspiration abortion begins with a review of the woman's medical and social history, laboratory tests (urine pregnancy test as indicated, hemoglobin, Rh factor), and counseling that includes a discussion of the procedure and obtaining informed consent. This is followed by a focused physical examination including pelvic, and if indicated by history or physical examination, screening for vaginitis, sexually transmitted infections, and/or cervical cancer. In some settings, ultrasound is routinely performed as part of the preoperative work up to confirm intrauterine pregnancy and gestational age, and rule out uterine anomalies, twin pregnancies, or other potentially complicating conditions. After all of these preliminary steps are completed, and if no contraindications have been detected, the abortion procedure can be initiated.

The first step in an aspiration abortion procedure involves dilating the cervix. This can be achieved in one of several ways, including by inserting a series of progressively larger dilators into the cervical opening (os) immediately before the application of suction, or by administering vaginal or oral misoprostol (a prostaglandin analogue) several hours earlier. Another technique (more commonly used in later abortions) involves placing osmotic dilators into the os a few hours to a day before the procedure, which slowly dilate the cervix.

After the cervix has been adequately dilated, the provider introduces a plastic cannula into the uterine cavity. The cannula is attached to an electric or manual vacuum aspirator that creates suction, causing the endometrial lining in which the pregnancy, or "products of conception" (POC), is embedded to separate from the uterine wall. Typically, the POC is examined before the woman is discharged from the facility to ensure that the pregnancy has been successfully and completely removed. Some facilities may also send the POC off-site for pathology evaluation, though this is not considered necessary (Paul, Lackie, Mitchell, Rogers, & Fox, 2002). This entire procedure—from dilation through uterine evacuation—is generally complete within several minutes.

Pain during abortion can be alleviated through a number of pharmacologic and nonpharmacologic interventions. Local anesthesia in the form of a paracervical block is considered a standard of care worldwide (Renner, Jensen, Nichols, & Edelman, 2010; WHO, 2012). Most settings in the United States offer additional options for relief of pain and anxiety, ranging from minimal to deep sedation, administered by mouth or parenterally. General anesthesia is available in some sites, but because it introduces both greater risk and cost, is not advised for most women undergoing first trimester abortion (Kapp, Whyte, Tang, Jackson, & Brahmi, 2013). In addition, nonpharmacologic strategies suggested to reduce pain during the procedure include respectful staff, a clean environment, ensuring confidentiality, and verbal support (Ipas, 2016). In some places, abortion or "full-spectrum" doulas are available to support women undergoing abortion.

Aspiration abortion has low rates of morbidity and mortality, making it among the safest of medical procedures (Raymond & Grimes, 2012). Complications following aspiration abortion can include infection, incomplete abortion or retained tissue, hemorrhage, continuing pregnancy, cervical laceration or uterine perforation, hematometra, and pain. An estimated 1.3% to 4.4% of women experience complications (Weitz et al., 2013), with less than 0.25% serious enough to warrant hospitalization (Upadhyay et al., 2015). Because of refinements in technique, improved prevention and management of complications, and trends toward earlier termination, the risk of death associated with abortion is less than 0.7 per 100,000 abortions overall (Raymond, Grossman, Weaver, Toti, & Winikoff, 2014), or approximately 14 times lower than the risk associated with childbirth (Raymond & Grimes, 2012). Risk of death with first trimester abortion is lower than the overall risk, which supports the recommendation for terminations to be carried out early in pregnancy when possible. The most common causes of death following aspiration abortion are infection (27%), hemorrhage (24%), embolism (17%), and adverse reaction to anesthesia (16%) (Bartlett et al., 2004).

Strategies to reduce infection risk include prescribing post-procedure prophylactic antibiotics and instructing women to avoid douching and intercourse in the weeks following the procedure (Grimes & Creinin, 2004; Stubblefield, Carr-Ellis, & Borgatta, 2004). Evidence to support recommendations against tub bathing, swimming, and the use of tampons are lacking; however, it is still frequently advised. To prevent uterine atony and potential hemorrhage, some providers give patients methergine for home administration, however, evidence to support this practice is also lacking. Hematometra, retained tissue, and continuing pregnancy are less frequent complications that may necessitate repeat uterine aspiration.

In addition to promoting understanding of potential complications, relaying accurate information about the long-term safety profile of abortion is an important duty of the clinician when providing abortion counseling. There is no evidence that first trimester abortion increases the risks of infertility, ectopic pregnancy, spontaneous abortion, birth defects, or preterm or low-birth-weight delivery with future pregnancies (Boonstra, Gold, Richards, & Finer, 2006). Following extensive reviews, both the National Cancer Institute (NCI) and American College of Obstetricians and Gynecologists (ACOG) have concluded that there is not a link between abortion and breast cancer (ACOG, 2009; NCI, 2003), nor has abortion been linked to any other type of cancer. Among women with unplanned pregnancies, those who have abortions have been found to have no greater risk of subsequent mental health problems than those who carry the pregnancy to term (Major et al., 2008).

Generally, most women are eligible for uterine aspiration for pregnancy termination. Certain conditions, such as cervical stenosis, uterine anomalies, or morbid obesity can make performing an aspiration abortion challenging, and may necessitate a more experienced provider. Other medical conditions, such as asthma, hypertension, and coagulopathies may also require special preparations for the service to be delivered safely. In rare cases, such as severe cardiac disease, an abortion may need to be performed in a hospital rather than in an outpatient setting. However, because of the greater risks associated with pregnancy and childbirth compared to abortion, there are essentially no absolute contraindications to aspiration abortion other than lack of patient consent.

Following aspiration abortion, patients are typically monitored for 30 to 90 minutes to ensure that they are clinically stable before discharge. During this time, after care and warning signs are usually reviewed (Box 36.1) and RhoGAM is administered to those who are Rh negative (if it was not already given earlier in the visit). Women are given information about who to contact in case of emergency, and are encouraged to follow-up for a routine evaluation 2 to 3 weeks after the procedure, either at the site where the abortion was performed or with their primary care provider. Though many abortion providers recommend routine follow-up, evidence that it is beneficial is limited (Kapp et al., 2012). Nevertheless, clinicians need to be prepared to provide routine post-abortion care, as well as assess for complications following aspiration abortion, which will be discussed further in the section on post-abortion care in the following.

MEDICATION ABORTION

Medication abortion is the term used to describe administration of pharmaceutical agents to intentionally disrupt a pregnancy. Although this definition technically encompasses methods used for later pregnancy terminations, such as labor induction, only the use of medications for abortions in early pregnancy are discussed in this section. Later pregnancy termination methods are discussed in another section in this chapter.

In the United States, the most common method of medication abortion involves the use of mifepristone (also called Mifeprex, RU-486, or "the abortion pill") in combination with misoprostol (Creinin & Grossman, 2014). Methotrexate (also administered in combination with

---

BOX 36.1 POST-ABORTION WARNING SIGNS AND SELF-CARE INSTRUCTIONS

Following an abortion, all patients should be given 24-hour contact information about who to contact in case of emergency and instructions about warning signs.

Warning Signs

- Temperature greater than or equal to 100.4°F
- Chills
- Foul-smelling discharge
- Persistent/increasing abdominal pain
- Bleeding: saturating more than one pad an hour for 2 hours, or twice as much as a heavy period

Other Self-Care Instructions

- Rest immediately after the abortion, and for up to 24 hours if possible.
- Avoid strenuous exercise or heavy lifting for at least a week, or at least until comfortable doing so.
- Avoid use of alcohol or drugs that could interfere with noticing complications.
- Abstain from intercourse for at least 1 week. Use contraception as soon as resuming intercourse to avoid pregnancy.
- Change pads/tampons frequently.
- Do not douche.
- Take all prescribed medications as directed.
- Take ibuprofen (400–800 mg every 4–8 hours) or acetaminophen (up to 1,000 mg) every 4 hours for pain as needed. Heating pads/hot water bottles and massage can also help to relieve pain.
- Pregnancy symptoms should resolve within a week after the abortion. If they do not, contact the provider. Do not perform a pregnancy test, as it may be positive even if no longer pregnant.

Adapted from McIntosh, Stewart, and Teplin (2009).

---

misoprostol) and misoprostol only are alternative pharmacologic approaches that have also been found to be effective for inducing early abortion; however, compared to mifepristone, these regimens are somewhat less effective and less acceptable to women overall (Creinin & Grossman, 2014; Wiebe, Dunn, Guilbert, Jacot, & Lugtig, 2002). As a result, mifepristone is currently the most widely used method for medication abortion in the United States, and therefore is the main focus of this section.

Mifepristone is an "anti-progestin" that blocks the activation of receptors by endogenous progesterone. When given to a woman in early pregnancy this causes the endometrial lining in which the pregnancy sac is embedded to separate from the underlying decidua. This endometrial and pregnancy tissue is eventually expelled from the uterus, a process that is accelerated through the administration of misoprostol, a prostaglandin that promotes uterine contractions. The efficacy of this form of medication abortion is 95% to 98% for pregnancies of less than 63 days gestation (9 weeks; Gatter, Cleland, & Nucatola, 2015). After this gestational age, efficacy decreases, however, it has been shown to be comparably effective for up to 70 days gestation (Winikoff et al., 2012). Medication abortions that deploy methotrexate, a folic acid antagonist, in combination with misoprostol have been found to have similar rates of success as mifepristone–misoprostol regimens. Misoprostol (alone) has also been under investigation as a method for inducing abortion; however, to date, none of the misoprostol-only regimens studied has been found to be as effective as the other combination regimens (Kulier et al., 2011). Use of misoprostol without medical supervision to self-induce abortion is a well-known phenomenon in parts of the world where abortion is illegal or highly restricted, and has also been observed in the United States, particularly within immigrant communities (Grossman et al., 2010; Rosing & Archbald, 2000).

No matter which regimen is selected, it is important for a woman considering medication abortion to understand that it is a process that involves several steps. As with a typical visit for an aspiration abortion, the first step (or visit) for a medication abortion includes reviewing a woman's medical and social history, providing appropriate counseling, including obtaining informed consent, and performing laboratory testing. Because medication abortion is most effective for terminating pregnancies in the first trimester (Creinin & Grossman, 2014), confirmation of gestational age is critical. In the United States, transvaginal ultrasound is commonly performed to confirm gestational age, as well as to rule out ectopic pregnancy, uterine anomalies, or other relevant obstetric or gynecologic conditions. However, menstrual history and uterine sizing by physical examination are acceptable, evidence-based approaches for confirming gestational age (Bracken et al., 2011). Following pre-abortion evaluation, if no contraindications are detected (Box 36.2), the primary abortifacient (mifepristone, methotrexate, or misoprostol) is administered on site. Because mifepristone is currently the most common type of medication abortion in the United States, only this method will be discussed further in this chapter.

Although the FDA-approved regimen for medication abortion advises a 600 mg dose of mifepristone, doses as little as 200 mg have been found to be equally efficacious and more cost effective, and, therefore, have become standard in the United States. Many providers have adopted other evidence-based practices that differ from the FDA-approved regimen as well; some of these are highlighted in Table 36.1.

The next step of a medication abortion involves use of misoprostol. In the United States, at-home misoprostol administration is a standard, evidence-based practice. Timing of administration has been studied extensively, and a number of approaches have been found to be equivalent in terms of efficacy (Creinin & Grossman, 2014). Evidence supports self-administration of vaginal misoprostol immediately or up to several days after mifepristone is taken. With

---

BOX 36.2   CONTRAINDICATIONS FOR USE OF MIFEPRISTONE–MISOPROSTOL MEDICATION ABORTION

- Hemorrhagic disorder, or concurrent anticoagulant therapy
- Chronic adrenal failure
- Concurrent long-term systemic corticosteroid therapy
- Confirmed or suspected ectopic pregnancy or undiagnosed adnexal mass
- Inherited porphyrias
- IUD in place (must remove before treatment)
- History of allergy to mifepristone, misoprostol, or other prostaglandins
- Gestation *beyond limits* (depending on the protocol followed)
- Inability to give informed consent and comply with treatment requirements

In addition, women electing medication abortion must have access to a telephone and transportation to a medical facility equipped to provide emergency treatment for incomplete abortion, blood transfusions, and emergency resuscitation (Creinin & Grossman, 2014).

Data on the effects of mifepristone and misoprostol on infants who are breastfeeding are limited; however, pumping and discarding milk for several days is an option some providers offer breastfeeding women seeking a medication abortion. Evaluation of women with other severe medical conditions (i.e., liver disease, cardiac disease, uncontrolled seizure disorders) must be done on an individual basis to determine the safest method of pregnancy termination for their particular case (Creinin & Grossman, 2014).

IUD, intrauterine device.

---

buccal or oral misoprostol administration, waiting 24 to 36 hours after mifepristone is standard (Reproductive Health Access Project, 2014).

At this time, the recommended route of administration for misoprostol is a dynamic area of practice. Although the FDA protocol advises oral administration, vaginal administration has been shown to be more effective and causes less nausea and diarrhea (Creinin & Grossman, 2014). As a result, evidence-based protocols for vaginal administration of misoprostol have been widely adopted. However, the death of six women from atypical infections following medication abortions in the United States precipitated changes in practice related to route of misoprostol administration (Dempsey, 2012). Though no clear causal relationship has been found between the medications, route of administration, and these fatal infections (Creinin & Grossman, 2014), in an attempt to decrease risk, many clinicians now instruct women to administer misoprostol buccally or orally, rather than vaginally.

TABLE 36.1	Comparison of FDA-Approved Versus Evidence-Based Mifepristone Regimens	
	FDA-APPROVED REGIMEN	**EVIDENCE-BASED REGIMEN**
Dose of mifepristone	600 mg	200 mg
Dose and route of misoprostol administration	400 mcg oral	800 mcg vaginal or buccal; or 800 mcg oral, given in two divided doses
Site of misoprostol administration	In office/clinic	At home
Timing of misoprostol administration	48 hours	Varies: Between 6 and 72 hours with vaginal administration; 24 and 72 with buccal
Gestational age limit for use	49 days	< 63 days
Follow-up visit	Day 14	4 to 14 days after mifepristone administration for vaginal and buccal misoprostol; 7 days and again at 14 days if incomplete for oral regimens

FDA, Food and Drug Administration.
Adapted from Creinin and Grossman (2014); http://www.reproductiveaccess.org/wp-content/uploads/2014/12/mifepristone_protocol.pdf

Regardless of the specific protocol used, most women begin to bleed between 1 and 3 hours following the administration of misoprostol (Creinin, Schwartz, Pymar, & Fink, 2001). For the majority, bleeding peaks after 4 to 6 hours, coinciding with expulsion of the pregnancy from the uterus. After that, bleeding usually slows but continues, with a mean duration of 14 to 17 days and a range of 1 to 69 days (Schaff et al., 1999). Typically, bleeding is heaviest during the first day after misoprostol use. It is considered excessive if the patient soaks more than two thick sanitary pads for two consecutive hours at any point during the abortion process (Grimes & Creinin, 2004). Women who do not experience bleeding may be offered an additional dose of misoprostol, or undergo uterine aspiration to complete the abortion (Reeves, Kudva, & Creinin, 2008).

Cramping is normal and should be expected with medication abortion. Intensity ranges widely; for most women, cramps tend to be strongest when bleeding is heaviest. Pain can be relieved with oral pharmaceutical agents, including nonsteroidal anti-inflammatory drugs (NSAIDs) or narcotics if necessary (Creinin & Grossman, 2014), as well as nonpharmacologic methods, such as heating pads/hot water bottles and relaxation techniques.

In addition to bleeding and cramping, nausea, vomiting, and diarrhea are common with misoprostol use; vaginal administration may reduce these side effects (Kulier et al., 2011). To lessen nausea, some providers routinely prescribe an antiemetic for prophylactic use before administration of misoprostol.

As part of self-care during and after a medication abortion, women are instructed to monitor their bleeding and pain, watch for signs of infection (fever, foul odor), and report any abnormalities (Box 36.1). Contraceptive counseling, education, and provision are also a standard component of the first (or second) medication abortion visit. As with aspiration abortion, return to fertility following medication abortion is rapid. For this reason, women are encouraged to initiate contraception immediately. Hormonal methods can be started immediately after the mifepristone has been taken, and IUDs can be inserted at a follow-up visit as soon as the gestational sac has been expelled (CDC, 2010; Ipas, 2007; see Table 36.2).

Risks and Complications • Risks and complications associated with medication abortion are similar to those of aspiration abortion, absent those that result from uterine instrumentation (cervical laceration, uterine perforation) and anesthesia. As discussed earlier, although a very small number of atypical, fatal infections have been reported following medication abortion, less severe uterine infections are a possible, though uncommon (less than 1%) complication (Shannon, Brothers, Philip, & Winikoff, 2004).

In addition to risk of infection, excessive bleeding is another possible complication of medication abortion. Acute hemorrhage or prolonged excessive bleeding can both lead to decreases in hemoglobin severe enough to warrant treatment, including uterine evacuation or rarely, transfusion. Death due to hemorrhage following medication abortion has not been reported in the United States. Because of the risk of bleeding, women with severe anemia are generally not eligible for medication abortion.

Persistent pregnancy is another complication with medication abortion, though this occurs in fewer than 1% of gestations of less than 63 days (Creinin & Grossman, 2014). Management of such cases may be expectant (watchful waiting up to several more weeks), or involve repeat administration of misoprostol or uterine evacuation. As a routine component of pre-abortion counseling, all women who elect medication abortion are informed about the possibility of a failed or incomplete abortion, and—because of the potential teratogenicity of misoprostol—are required to consent for uterine evacuation if the medication is not successful.

Follow-Up After Medication Abortion • After completing the first two steps of a medication abortion as described earlier, women are instructed to contact the provider in case of any signs or symptoms of complications, and to return for routine follow-up between several days and 2 weeks after the use of mifepristone. Ultrasound is often performed at the follow-up visit to confirm completion of the abortion, though it may also be confirmed by clinical examination and/or the use of quantitative hCG testing (Creinin & Grossman, 2014). Studies have also investigated the use of

TABLE 36.2	Initiating Contraception Following Abortion		
METHOD	WHEN TO INITIATE AFTER ASPIRATION ABORTION	WHEN TO INITIATE AFTER MEDICATION ABORTION	COMMENTS
Condoms (external or internal), spermicide, sponge	With resumption of intercourse	With resumption of intercourse	
Diaphragm, cervical cap	With resumption of intercourse	With resumption of intercourse	New users: do not fit until cervical changes from pregnancy have resolved (~2 weeks after abortion); Continuing users: checking for correct fit at the follow-up visit is advised Diaphragm and cap should not be used for 6 weeks following a second trimester abortion (Kaunitz, 2015)
Oral contraceptives, vaginal ring (Nuvaring), patch	Immediately or up to 7 days later (OCs), or any time if reasonably certain not pregnant	Immediately, or at time of confirmation of abortion completion (follow-up visit), or any time if reasonably certain not pregnant	
Injectable depot medroxyprogesterone acetate (Depo-provera)	Immediately or any time if reasonably certain not pregnant	Immediately, at the time of confirmation of abortion completion (follow-up visit), or any time if reasonably certain not pregnant	Can be administered before discharge following aspiration abortion or at return visit after medication abortion Abstain/back up if not within 7 days
Copper IUD (Paragard)	Immediately and up to 7 days; or any time if reasonably certain not pregnant	Little research on immediate insertion after medication abortion; clinical guidelines recommend within 14 days of mifepristone use if abortion confirmed (Planned Parenthood Federation of America, 2003); or any time if reasonably certain not pregnant (CDC, 2013a)	If not placed at time of abortion, abstain/back up for 7 days after insertion Evidence of slight increase in risk of expulsion following 2nd trimester abortion (Steenland, Tepper, Curtis, & Kapp, 2011)
Levonorgestrel intrauterine system (Mirena, Skyla, Liletta)	Immediately and up to 7 days; or any time if reasonably certain not pregnant	Little research on immediate insertion after medication abortion; clinical guidelines recommend within 14 days of mifepristone use if abortion confirmed (Planned Parenthood Federation of America, 2003); or any time if reasonably certain not pregnant (CDC, 2013a)	If not placed at time of abortion, abstain/back up for 7 days after insertion
Implant (Nexplanon)	Immediately and up to 7 days; or any time if reasonably certain not pregnant	At time of confirmation of abortion completion (follow-up visit), or any time if reasonably certain not pregnant	If not placed at time of abortion, abstain/back up for 7 days after insertion
Sterilization	Immediately, if abortion is uncomplicated		Laparascopic methods are recommended (Kaunitz, 2015) Complications that warrant postponement of sterilization include cervical tear/uterine perforation, hematometra, and hemorrhage

IUD, intrauterine device; OCs, oral contraceptives.
Based on Centers for Disease Control and Prevention (2013a, 2013b); Kapp, Whyte, Tang, Jackson, and Brahmi (2011).

urine pregnancy tests and self-administered questionnaires for assessing completion of medication abortion (Jackson, Dayananda, Fortin, Fitzmaurice, & Goldberg, 2012).

Early Abortion Counseling: Aspiration Versus Medication

In practice, clinicians may encounter women who have decided to terminate an early pregnancy but are unaware or unsure of what their options are. Some women may hold beliefs about abortion based on inaccurate information relayed by friends, family members, or media sources. As with pregnancy options counseling, the clinician's role in abortion counseling is to provide an overview of available methods, correct misinformation, support decision making, and ultimately provide the desired service or, alternatively, an appropriate referral. For women who are eligible for both medication or aspiration abortion, counseling may include comparing the two approaches, providing information about where each can be obtained, and supporting selection of a method (Box 36.3). The Reproductive Health Access Project has created a fact sheet (available in English and Spanish) comparing these two early abortion options that may be a useful patient decision aid when providing abortion education and counseling.

BOX 36.3   COMPARISON OF ASPIRATION AND MEDICATION ABORTION

MEDICATION ABORTION	ASPIRATION ABORTION
Some contraindications, including gestational age limit (7–10 weeks)	Rare contraindications
Usually avoids invasive procedure	Invasive procedure
Abortion takes place over period of several days; at least two visits to provider generally required	Requires only one visit to complete abortion; follow-up visit recommended
Involves heavy bleeding, may persist for several weeks	Bleeding after procedure generally light
Woman may feel she has more control	Abortion provider has more control
Most of abortion experience occurs at home (may offer greater privacy)	Takes place in clinic, office, or hospital setting (may be less private)

Adapted from Breitbart (2000); see also Reproductive Health Access Project.

Later Abortion

Currently in the United States, there are two general approaches to abortion after the first trimester, or that take place after 14 to 16 weeks gestation: dilation and evacuation (D&E) and labor induction. A brief overview of these methods is provided in this section.

Regardless of method, abortions after the first trimester have low rates of complications and mortality, however, risk of mortality increases exponentially with advancing gestational age and consequently, gestational age at the time of an abortion has been found to be the largest risk factor for abortion-related death (Bartlett et al., 2004). Although there has been a general trend toward earlier pregnancy termination in the United States (Pazol et al., 2014), women continue to seek abortions after the first trimester due to a number of both individual and structural causes, including logistical factors, such as difficulty finding a provider, being referred to a different clinic, and problems with child care; emotional factors, such as difficulty deciding and fear of having an abortion; late discovery of pregnancy; and financial barriers (Drey et al., 2006). Poor women have been found to be twice as likely to experience delays in having an abortion due to difficulties with making arrangements (Finer, Frohwirth, Dauphinee, Singh, & Moore, 2006).

DILATION AND EVACUATION

D&E is the most common method used for abortions after the first trimester in the United States (Pazol et al., 2014). Studies have shown that compared to labor induction, D&E is both safer and better for the psychological health of women (Grimes, 2008). However, D&E is a procedure that requires advanced clinical skills, and in many parts of the country no such providers are available (Jerman & Jones, 2014). As a result, women seeking later abortions may have to undergo labor induction, travel long distances to reach an experienced D&E provider, or continue an unwanted pregnancy.

As with aspiration abortion, D&E is accomplished by dilating the cervix and applying suction to the uterine cavity to remove the endometrial lining and POC. In later gestations (beyond 15–16 weeks), forceps may also be used. D&Es require greater cervical dilation than procedures performed at earlier gestations; this process is often carried out through the use of osmotic dilators (discussed in the previous section on aspiration abortion). Alternatively or in addition, prostaglandins may be given to achieve the degree of dilation needed while minimizing trauma to the cervix. Although mechanical dilation can be used, risks of hemorrhage, cervical, or unsuccessful uterine evacuation increase with this approach.

D&Es can be performed in an outpatient setting, but are more likely than first trimester abortions to be performed in a hospital. Regardless of setting, preoperative assessment and counseling are carried out and informed consent is obtained before the procedure. Clinical standards in the United States include universal ultrasound after 14 weeks EGA to ensure accurate pregnancy dating, which allows for appropriate cervical dilation as well as compliance with laws pertaining to gestational age limits and abortion (National Abortion Federation [NAF], 2015). In addition to a paracervical block, pain relief options may include light sedation, or if desired, general anesthesia. Although D&E is similar to aspiration abortion, it is a more time-consuming and difficult procedure to perform, and as previously discussed, risks of serious morbidity and mortality increase with gestational age. The causes of serious complications and death following D&E are the same as with terminations performed earlier in pregnancy.

Postoperative care following D&E is generally the same as with earlier terminations. Immediately after the procedure, women are monitored for complications and provided with education about self-care, signs and symptoms of complications, who to contact in case of emergency, and contraception. A routine follow-up visit is generally advised several weeks after completion of the procedure.

ABORTION BY LABOR INDUCTION

The administration of systemic and/or locally applied medications, herbs, or other agents to provoke uterine contractions and eventual expulsion of a fetus is referred to as labor induction abortion, or sometimes medical induction abortion. Various forms of this practice have been documented across different cultures throughout history, and as far back as 1,500 BCE in Egyptian medical writings (Potts & Campbell, 2009). Before the refinement of aspiration abortion, labor induction was the most common method for inducing abortion; however, in recent years D&E has become the primary method for terminating later pregnancies in the United States (Pazol et al., 2014). As discussed previously, this shift in practice can be attributed to the lower rates of maternal mortality and better psychological outcomes associated with D&E (Grimes, 2008).

Women seeking later abortions do not always have the option of electing D&E because of lack of access to a skilled provider (Turok et al., 2008). In addition, at times medical or psychological considerations may drive the decision to use labor induction abortion instead of D&E. For example, labor induction may be selected because it is believed to facilitate parental grieving, however, several studies, including a 2005 study of women who terminated pregnancies because of a fetal anomaly, did not find any significant difference in resolution of grief symptoms between those who elected D&E and those who chose labor induction (Burgoine et al., 2005). The authors suggest that with "adequate information and support, patients will be able to select the method of termination that best meets their needs for well-being and convenience, as well as the long-term resolution of their loss" (Burgoine et al., 2005, p. 1932). Thus, clinicians can play an important role in assisting and supporting women in the selection and referral process with regard to later terminations.

Complications associated with labor induction are similar to those associated with aspiration procedures, including hemorrhage, infection, and retained pregnancy tissue. In addition, this method carries additional risks of uterine rupture and retained placenta. Although it is well established that D&E is safer than labor induction for pregnancy terminations after the first trimester, data indicate that both methods have low mortality and complication rates overall, and lower mortality rates than continuing pregnancy to term (Pazol et al., 2014; Turok et al., 2008).

■ APRNs AS ABORTION PROVIDERS

A number of studies have demonstrated that with appropriate training, nonphysician clinicians can be safe, competent providers of early abortion care (Weitz et al., 2013). Recognizing this capacity to provide quality early abortion care, as well as the potential of advanced practice nurses and physician assistants to increase women's access to abortion, a number of professional organizations, including the American Academy of Physician Assistants, American College of Nurse Midwives, ACOG, American Medical Women's Medical Association, American Public Health Association, NAF, National Association of Nurse Practitioners in Women's Health, and Physicians for Reproductive Choice and Health have issued statements in support of this role for advanced practice nurses (Committee on Health Care for Underserved Women, 2014; Taylor, Safriet, Dempsey, Kruse, & Jackson, 2009).

To determine whether a nurse clinician can legally provide abortions in a specific state, both regulations regarding APRN practice and abortion laws must be considered. Currently in the United States, four states allow nonphysician clinicians to provide both medication and aspiration abortion; nine states only permit provision of medication abortion. The remaining 37 states either expressly prohibit nonphysician clinicians from providing abortion, or have extant physician-only laws or other legal barriers to APRNs abortion provision (ANSIRH, 2015). APRNs interested in providing abortion as part of their practice are advised to seek professional support, including from state or national organizations familiar with this issue, gather information about current, relevant state laws and regulations, and seek appropriate training. A guide ("The APC Toolkit") has been created to assist clinicians with all aspects of this process (Taylor et al., 2009).

Personal beliefs and considerations may also influence a clinician's decision about whether to provide abortions. Resources have been designed to help health professionals clarify their personal values about abortion in the context of their professional roles and responsibilities. Regardless of personal beliefs, ensuring access to abortion services is a professional responsibility of all clinicians. As discussed in the section on options counseling, clinicians are bound by ethical codes to respect patients' rights and autonomy, including women seeking abortion. Although health professionals may refuse to participate in the provision of abortion, their personal beliefs should never prevent access to or present an undue burden for women seeking an abortion. Referral to another provider or facility should not lead to untimely delays or a lessening in the quality of care provided.

■ POST-ABORTION CARE

Primary care clinicians may be expected to provide routine follow-up care, as well as manage complications that women may experience following an abortion. This section provides an overview of current recommendations and guidelines for both of these aspects of post-abortion care.

As previously discussed, when abortions are performed safely, the risk of complications is very low (Upadhyay et al., 2015). As a result, the need for routine follow-up after aspiration abortion has been challenged (Grossman, Ellertson, Grimes & Walker, 2004; Kapp et al., 2012). On the other hand, though the Society for Family Planning (SFP) and ACOG state that "in-clinic evaluation" after medication abortion is "important... but not always necessary" (Creinin & Grossman, 2014, p. 158), the standard of care in many sites continues to be to advise women to return to the abortion provider for confirmation of successful termination of pregnancy. For this reason, this section focuses primarily on the role of primary care clinicians in providing follow-up after aspiration or D&E abortion procedures.

Follow-Up After Aspiration Abortion

Although standard practice has been to recommend a routine follow-up visit 2 to 3 weeks after an aspiration abortion, Grossman et al. (2004) assert that there is limited evidence to support this practice. The authors noted that routine follow-up visits did not typically reveal complications that women could not be taught to identify themselves, and that the recommended timing for routine follow-up is not well-suited for detecting the most severe potential complications associated with abortion (infection and ectopic pregnancy). Furthermore, they argue that the costs of these visits to women and the health care system are considerable. Their clinical recommendations included advising follow-up appointments only for women in need of other routine reproductive or general health care, while others could simply be given instruction on self-monitoring and reporting complications and possibly receive routine follow-up by phone. Nevertheless, many abortion providers continue to recommend routine follow-up, either at the site where a woman had her abortion or with her primary care provider.

Routine Post-Abortion Assessment and Management

Although only about half of all women present for routine follow-up care after an aspiration abortion (Grossman et al., 2004), for those who do, clinicians have the opportunity to assess physical and emotional well-being, provide contraceptive counseling and management, and address other identified reproductive or general health needs. At the start of the visit, the clinician should review the abortion experience with the woman by asking her how she has been feeling since the procedure and whether she experienced any complications during or since that time. Some women may bring a procedure or pathology report from the abortion provider, or the clinician may be able to obtain a copy of the medical record from the abortion visit; this can be helpful for verifying that pregnancy tissue was successfully removed and was normal. The clinician should ask about bleeding patterns, pain, signs and symptoms of infection or continuing pregnancy, and emotional state since the procedure. Although the American Psychological Association (APA) has refuted the claim that abortion leads to mental health problems (Major et al., 2009) and the predominant emotion women report following abortion is relief (Rocca, Kimport, Gould, & Foster, 2013), some may experience grief, sadness, or depression. Offering support, and—for any who need it—a referral for counseling, is an important aspect of the post-abortion visit.

POST-ABORTION CONTRACEPTION

Establishing an acceptable contraceptive method is an important component of post-abortion care. Because a woman may ovulate as early as 8 days after an abortion (mean: 21–29 days; Schreiber, Sober, Ratcliffe, & Creinin, 2011; Stoddard & Eisenberg, 2011), contraceptive counseling, selection, and provision at the time of the procedure is advised. Most types of contraception can be initiated immediately after an abortion is complete; evidence shows that same day initiation of IUDs, implants, and injectables is an effective strategy for decreasing subsequent abortions and births among women in the year following an abortion (Langston, Joslin-Roher, & Westhoff, 2014). When providing routine abortion follow-up care, clinicians should assess contraceptive acceptability, side effects, and adherence, and establish a patient-centered management plan that takes these factors into account. Additional education, counseling, provision of supplies, and follow-up should be part of the plan. If warranted, initiation of an alternative or additional contraceptive method should also be made if the woman expresses a preference for this (Table 36.2).

If a woman did not start or resume the use of a method after her abortion, finding out her reasons is essential for developing a contraceptive plan to effectively address her needs and preferences. Also, if a woman has resumed sexual activity, the clinician must determine whether she is at risk for a repeat pregnancy. Emergency contraception can be taken at any time after an abortion if it is indicated.

POST-ABORTION PHYSICAL EXAMINATION AND DIAGNOSTICS

In addition to vital signs, a clinician may perform a physical examination including speculum and bimanual examination to assess for signs of infection (purulent discharge, soft, tender uterus, fever), excessive bleeding, ongoing pregnancy, or retained POC (bleeding, uterus not well involuted) as part of a routine post-abortion visit. Screening for sexually transmitted infections, vaginitis, and cervical dysplasia may also be clinically warranted. Routine performance of a pregnancy test is generally not advised in women who report resolution of pregnancy symptoms, as it may be positive for up to 4 to 8 weeks after an abortion due to lingering hCG and the high sensitivity of pregnancy tests (Cappiello, Beal, & Simmonds, 2011).

Given the low rate of complications, in most cases post-abortion assessments are normal. The visit can be concluded by arranging with the woman to obtain care for any additional health concerns identified during the visit or for routine follow-up according to recommended screening guidelines.

Assessment and Management of Post-Abortion Complications

Occasionally, a woman may present to a primary care clinician with concerns or complications following an aspiration or medication abortion. In such cases, referring the woman back to the provider or setting where the abortion was performed is recommended. However, if this is not feasible or desirable, a primary care clinician may be able to manage the case independently, or in consultation with the abortion provider or other qualified health care provider. A brief review of possible complications and general information about management of complications is provided as follows.

BLEEDING

Following aspiration abortion, women experience a wide range of bleeding patterns, from none to moderate amounts for a week or longer. Before discharge, they are instructed to contact the abortion provider, or seek emergency care if bleeding is excessive at any point after the procedure. Although difficult to quantify, suggestions for determining if bleeding is excessive include saturating a sanitary pad in less than an hour for two consecutive hours, or bleeding twice as much as with normal menstrual flow. Passing clots is also normal after an abortion; however, if the amount is greater than a cup in 2 hours, it may be excessive (McIntosh, Stewart, & Teplin, 2009).

Women may contact their primary care clinician with concerns about bleeding, and in-person assessment may be warranted to ensure that the amount is not excessive. In addition to a pelvic examination, checking for signs of orthostatic hypotension and hemoglobin or hematocrit are appropriate ways to evaluate hematologic stability. Management depends on the degree of blood loss and may include iron supplementation, intravenous therapy, or rarely, transfusion.

In addition to excessive bleeding, women may report persistent bleeding after an abortion. The clinician must determine whether this is normal or if it could be due to an infection, ongoing pregnancy (including ectopic), retained POC, or some other cause unrelated to the abortion, such as cervical pathology. Women who engage in strenuous activity soon after an abortion may experience persistent bleeding. In general, avoiding rigorous physical activity for 1 to 2 weeks following the procedure is advised; however, there is little evidence to support this recommendation. Women who initiate a hormonal method of contraception following abortion may also experience persistent bleeding or

spotting. Ruling out other possible causes of bleeding (mentioned earlier) can support the diagnosis of vaginal bleeding due to exogenous hormone use.

Women who report no bleeding and increasing pain or cramps following aspiration abortion may be experiencing hematometra. This uncommon complication is caused when a blood clot or multiple clots accumulate in the uterus, preventing blood flow through the cervix. Typically, hematometra occurs immediately or within hours after the procedure, and therefore, is not likely to arise after a woman has left the facility where the abortion was performed. Management usually involves re-evacuation of the uterus (Yonke & Leeman, 2013).

Menses typically resumes 4 to 6 weeks after an abortion. Failure to menstruate can indicate a repeat pregnancy or rarely, Asherman's syndrome, a complication of instrumentation of the uterus in which cervical stenosis or intrauterine adhesions lead to amenorrhea. If repeat or continued pregnancy have been ruled out, post-abortion amenorrhea requires referral to a gynecologist; hysteroscopy may be indicated.

INFECTION

As previously discussed, in the United States many providers routinely prescribe prophylactic antibiotics to prevent infection following abortion. However, in spite of this practice, there is still a small risk of post-abortal infection (less than 1%; Achilles, Reeves & Society of Family Planning, 2011). Women who call or present with reports of fever greater than 100.4, chills, severe or persistent pelvic pain, body aches, or general malaise should be evaluated for this complication. Typically, signs and symptoms of infection emerge within 48 to 96 hours after the procedure. On examination, pelvic tenderness is likely and an elevated white blood cell count is expected. Screening for sexually transmitted infections should be performed, and broad-spectrum antibiotics administered promptly to prevent serious sequelae, such as infertility, chronic pelvic pain, and sepsis. Treatment can be oral, but if the woman fails to respond within 48 to 72 hours, parenteral therapy should be initiated.

Reported cases of post-abortal infection associated with *Clostridium sordellii* (discussed in the previous section on medication abortion) differed from more typical infections in that the women were often afebrile, and—though they complained of intense pelvic pain—did not have uterine tenderness on examination. They also presented with tachycardia, hypotension, elevated white blood cell count (with left shift), hemoconcentration, and generally felt sicker than clinical findings would indicate. Though extremely rare, because of the high fatality rate associated with these atypical infections, any woman who has had a recent medication abortion and reports signs or symptoms suggestive of infection should be referred to an emergency setting for immediate evaluation and treatment (Creinin & Grossman, 2014).

ONGOING PREGNANCY

Following aspiration abortion, very occasionally a woman may report persistent pregnancy symptoms when she presents for routine follow-up. However, though pregnancy symptoms usually resolve within a week after an abortion, hCG may be detectable for up to 8 weeks. For this reason, patients should be instructed not to perform a home pregnancy test following an abortion, as the test may be positive even though the woman is no longer pregnant. Those who report persistent pregnancy symptoms (e.g., nausea, breast tenderness) should be assessed for continued pregnancy. Though it occurs in less than 1% of procedures (Lichtenberg & Grimes, 2009), ongoing pregnancy (or "failed abortion") can be attributed to a number of factors including that the pregnancy was not successfully disrupted because it was very small or was outside of the uterus (ectopic), the woman had a uterine anomaly that interfered with removal, there was more than one gestation (twin, multiples, or heterotopic, in which one pregnancy is in the uterus and another is outside of the uterus), or the provider was inexperienced. In most settings the uterine aspirate is reviewed after the procedure to verify the presence of pregnancy tissue to identify women at risk of these complications. If ectopic pregnancy is suspected, a plan for close follow-up is established and the woman is given special instruction about related warning signs. For any woman who presents for routine or emergency care, if ongoing pregnancy (including ectopic) is suspected, serial quantitative hCGs and/or ultrasound are warranted. Ideally, she should be referred back to the abortion provider, or if this is not possible, the abortion provider should be consulted. Ultimately management depends on the clinical diagnosis. If an ongoing pregnancy is detected and verified as intrauterine following attempted aspiration abortion, a woman may opt to repeat the abortion or continue the pregnancy. Ectopic pregnancy following abortion is managed according to current standards of clinical care. As previously discussed, because of the teratogenic effects associated with misoprostol, women with ongoing pregnancies following medication abortion are required to undergo uterine evacuation to complete the abortion.

One of the most common complications following abortion is retained tissue in the uterus (0.29%–1.96% in first trimester; 0.4%–2.7% in second trimester). Women with retained tissue may experience lower abdominal pain or cramps and persistent bleeding including expulsion of clots. They may present before the recommended routine follow-up visit with these complaints or wait for their scheduled visit to report these symptoms. Accompanying infection is not common, unless large amounts of tissue are present. On examination, the uterus may feel somewhat enlarged and soft. Ultrasound will often reveal heterogeneous material in the uterine cavity that is indistinguishable from blood clots. If the amount of tissue present is small and the woman prefers to avoid a repeat uterine aspiration, it may be postponed to allow time for the tissue to pass on its own. However, if bleeding is heavy or a large amount of tissue is present in the uterus, evacuation may be warranted. When there is evidence of retained POC following medication abortion, expectant management may be acceptable if the woman is not bleeding excessively or does not have signs of infection. However, in such cases, referring the woman back to the abortion provider is advised.

CONSIDERATIONS FOR SPECIAL POPULATIONS

Providing pregnancy options counseling to some women may require special knowledge or present particular challenges for some clinicians. Adolescents, immigrants, and women with mental disabilities are among those who may warrant specialized knowledge and efforts on the part of the clinician to ensure that the dignity-, autonomy-, and pregnancy-related needs and wishes of these individuals are adequately and appropriately addressed.

Adolescents

In most states, adolescents are legally entitled to receive confidential sexual and reproductive health (SRH) services, including family planning, sexually transmitted infection testing and treatment, and prenatal care, however, specific laws vary. With regard to abortion, minors must secure the consent of at least one parent or guardian or obtain a judicial waiver to this requirement in most states. Before providing SRH care to a minor, clinicians need to become familiar with relevant laws and policies in the state where they are practicing. For more and up-to-date information about legislation related to minors' reproductive health care, including abortion.

Personal values may subtly or overtly influence the SRH care a clinician provides to adolescents. In order to deliver quality care that respects emerging adults' rights to autonomy, clinicians are advised to engage in a process of self-reflection to clarify how their attitudes about adolescents' sexual behaviors, pregnancies, parenting, and abortion intersect with their professional responsibility of delivering care that is ethically sound. Sexually active adolescents and pregnant teenagers have the same right to health care that is free of judgment, unbiased, and nondirectional as adults.

Immigrant Women

Women who immigrate to the United States may not be aware of what their legal reproductive rights are in the United States. In addition, some may not know about state-based public assistance programs that provide coverage for pregnancy-related care or support to families (such as the Women, Infants, and Children nutritional supplementation program or childcare assistance programs). For some immigrant women, abortion may be illegal in their country of origin, with punishment, including incarceration for attempting an abortion. Dependence on male partners, limited language abilities, and/or fear of deportation may be factors that prevent some non-United States born women from accessing services, or from being fully aware of all of their pregnancy options. Clinicians who provide care to immigrant women are advised to stay up to date regarding the status of health-related assistance programs, including SRH services, as well as programs that support families.

Women With Mental Disabilities

Providing pregnancy options counseling and appropriate referrals for women with mental illness or disability can be challenging. Ethical dilemmas that arise in providing health care to women in this subpopulation have been extensively debated and described in the literature. Reproductive rights are a particularly sensitive topic, especially in light of the extensive history of abuse that women with mental disabilities have been subjected to. Exhaustive discussion of these issues is beyond the scope of this chapter, however, it is important for clinicians who provide pregnancy options counseling and related services to have an understanding of the legal safeguards that have been put in place to protect women with mental disabilities from future abuse, as well as ethical guidelines that inform practice. In general, when providing options counseling or referrals for women with mental illness, consultation with the patient's psychiatrist or therapist is advised. For women with cognitive impairment, the ACOG recommends "obtaining the assistance of individuals trained in communicating with mentally disabled individuals...these may include special educators, psychologists, nurses, attorneys familiar with disability law, and physicians accustomed to working with mentally disabled patients" when obtaining informed consent for sterilization procedures (ACOG, 2007, p. 219). This guidance is also relevant for clinicians caring for women with mental disabilities who are making decisions about pregnancy and abortion.

■ SUMMARY

Clinicians who provide care to women of reproductive age need to be prepared to provide pregnancy testing, options counseling, and direct services for continuing or terminating a pregnancy, or referrals to providers who are qualified to deliver these services. In addition, routine follow-up care of women who have had abortions and managing or referring those with complications is within the scope of practice of primary care clinicians. Ensuring that the care provided is accurate, compassionate, and nonjudgmental is paramount and requires clinicians to engage in a process of continuing education and self-reflection. Women deserve no less.

■ REFERENCES

Achilles, S. L., & Reeves, M. F.; Society of Family Planning. (2011). Prevention of infection after induced abortion: Release date October 2010: SFP guideline 20102. *Contraception, 83*(4), 295–309.

American College of Obstetricians and Gynecologists (ACOG). (2007). Sterilization of women, including those with mental disabilities. ACOG Committee Opinion No. 371. *Obstetrics and Gynecology, 110*, 217–220.

American College of Obstetricians and Gynecologists (ACOG). (2009). Committee on gynecologic practice. ACOG Committee Opinion. No. 434: Induced Abortion and Breast Cancer Risk. *Obstetrics and Gynecology, 113*, 1417–1418.

American Nurses Association (ANA). (2015). *Code of ethics with interpretive statements.* Silver Spring, MD: Nursebooks.org.

Advancing New Standards in Reproductive Health (ANSIRH). (2015). *Landscape of health professional regulation of abortion provision in the U.S.* Retrieved from http://www.ansirh.org/research/pci/access.php

Baker, A. (1995). *Abortion and options counseling: A comprehensive reference.* Granite City, IL: Hope Clinic for Women.

Bartlett, L. A., Berg, C. J., Shulman, H. B., Zane, S. B., Green, C. A., Whitehead, S., & Atrash, H. K. (2004). Risk factors for legal induced abortion-related mortality in the United States. *Obstetrics and Gynecology, 103*(4), 729–737.

Biggs, M. A., Gould, H., & Foster, D. G. (2013). Understanding why women seek abortions in the U.S. *BMC Women's Health, 13*, 29.

Boonstra, H., Gold, R., Richards, C., & Finer, L. (2006). *Abortion in women's lives.* New York, NY: Guttmacher Institute.

Borrero, S., Nikolajski, C., Steinberg, J. R., Freedman, L., Akers, A. Y., Ibrahim, S., & Schwarz, E. B. (2015). "It just happens": A qualitative study exploring low-income women's perspectives on pregnancy intention and planning. *Contraception, 91*(2), 150–156.

Bracken, H., Clark, W., Lichtenberg, E. S., Schweikert, S. M., Tanenhaus, J., Barajas, A.,...Winikoff, B. (2011). Alternatives to routine ultrasound for eligibility assessment prior to early termination of pregnancy with mifepristone-misoprostol. *British Journal of Obstetrics and Gynaecology, 118*(1), 17–23.

Braveman, P., Marchi, K., Sarnoff, R., Egerter, S., Rittenhouse, D., & Salganicoff, A. (2003). *Promoting access to prenatal care: Lesson from the California experience.* Retrieved from http://www.cdph.ca.gov/data/surveys/MIHA/MIHAPublications/MO-MIHA-PromotingAccessToPrenatalCare.pdf

Breitbart, V. (2000). Counseling for medical abortion. *American Journal of Obstetrics and Gynecology, 183*(Suppl. 2), S26–S33.

Bridges, E. (2011). *Unintended pregnancy among young people in the United States: Dismantling structural barriers to prevention.* Retrieved from http://www.advocatesforyouth.org/storage/advfy/documents/unintended%20pregnancy_5.pdf

Brooks-Gunn, J., Duncan, G. J., & Aber, J. L. (1997). *Neighborhood poverty. Context and consequences for children* (Vol. 1). New York, NY: Russell Sage Foundation.

Burgoine, G. A., Van Kirk, S. D., Romm, J., Edelman, A. B., Jacobson, S. L., & Jensen, J. T. (2005). Comparison of perinatal grief after dilation and evacuation or labor induction in second trimester terminations for fetal anomalies. *American Journal of Obstetrics and Gynecology, 192*(6), 1928–1932.

Cappiello, J. D., Beal, M. W., & Simmonds, K. E. (2011). Clinical issues in post-abortion care. *The Nurse Practitioner, 36*(5), 35–40.

Carney, E. N. (n.d.). *The truth about domestic adoption.* Retrieved from https://www.adoptivefamilies.com/talking-about-adoption/domestic-adoption-myths-and-truths

Centers for Disease Control and Prevention (CDC). (2006). Recommendations to improve preconception health and health care—United States. *Morbidity and Mortality Weekly Report Recommendations and Reports, 55*(RR-06), 1–23.

Centers for Disease Control and Prevention (CDC). (2010). Medical eligibility criteria for contraceptive use, 2010. *Morbidity and Mortality Weekly Report, 59*(RRO4), 1–6.

Centers for Disease Control and Prevention (CDC). (2013a). U.S. selected practice recommendations for contraceptive use, 2013: Adapted from the World Health Organization selected practice recommendations for contraceptive use, 2nd edition. Recommendations and Reports: Morbidity and Mortality Weekly Report. Recommendations and Reports/Centers for Disease Control, 62(RR-05), 1–60.

Centers for Disease Control and Prevention (CDC). (2013b). Unintended pregnancy prevention. Retrieved from http://www.cdc.gov/reproductivehealth/unintendedpregnancy

Chamberlain, L., & Levenson, R. (2013). *Addressing intimate partner violence, reproductive and sexual coercion: A guide for obstetric, gynecologic and reproductive health care settings* (3rd ed.). Washington, DC: American College of Obstetricians and Gynecologists; San Francisco, CA: Futures Without Violence. Retrieved from http://www.acog.org/About_ACOG/ACOG_Departments/Health_Care_for_Underserved_Women/~/media/Departments/Violence%20Against%20Women/Reproguidelines.pdf

Committee on Health Care for Underserved Women. (2014). ACOG Committee opinion no. 612: Abortion training and education. *Obstetrics and Gynecology, 124*(5), 1055–1059.

Creinin, M. D., Schwartz, J. L., Pymar, H. C., & Fink, W. (2001). Efficacy of mifepristone followed on the same day by misoprostol for early termination of pregnancy: Report of a randomised trial. *British Journal of Obstetrics and Gynaecology, 108*(5), 469–473.

Creinin, M., & Grossman, D. (2014). Medical management of first-trimester abortion. *Contraception, 89*(3), 148–161.

Dehlendorf, C., Harris, L. H., & Weitz, T. A. (2013). Disparities in abortion rates: A public health approach. *American Journal of Public Health, 103*(10), 1772–1779.

Dempsey, A. (2012). Serious infection associated with induced abortion in the United States. *Clinical Obstetrics and Gynecology, 55*(4), 888–892.

Dobkin, L. M., Perrucci, A. C., & Dehlendorf, C. (2013). Pregnancy options counseling for adolescents: Overcoming barriers to care and preserving preference. *Current Problems in Pediatric and Adolescent Health Care, 43*(4), 96–102.

Drey, E. A., Foster, D. G., Jackson, R. A., Lee, S. J., Cardenas, L. H., & Darney, P. D. (2006). Risk factors associated with presenting for abortion in the second trimester. *Obstetrics and Gynecology, 107*(1), 128–135.

Finer, L. B., Frohwirth, L. F., Dauphinee, L. A., Singh, S., & Moore, A. M. (2005). Reasons U.S. women have abortions: Quantitative and qualitative perspectives. *Perspectives on Sexual and Reproductive Health, 37*(3), 110–118.

Finer, L. B., Frohwirth, L. F., Dauphinee, L. A., Singh, S., & Moore, A. M. (2006). Timing of steps and reasons for delays in obtaining abortions in the United States. *Contraception, 74*(4), 334–344.

Finer, L. B., & Zolna, M. (2014). Shifts in intended and unintended pregnancies in the United States, 2001–2008. *American Journal of Public Health, 104*(S1), S44–S48.

Fjerstad, M., & Stewart, F. (2011). Pregnancy testing and management of early pregnancy. In R. Hatcher, J. Trussell, A. L. Nelson, W. Cates, Jr., D. Kowal, & M. S. Policar (Eds.), *Contraceptive technology* (20th revised edition). New York, NY: Ardent Media.

Frost, J. J., & Lindberg, L. D. (2013). Reasons for using contraception: Perspectives of US women seeking care at specialized family planning clinics. *Contraception, 87*(4), 465–472.

Gatter, M., Cleland, K., & Nucatola, D. L. (2015). Efficacy and safety of medical abortion using mifepristone and buccal misoprostol through 63 days. *Contraception, 91*(4), 269–273. Retrieved from doi:http://dx.doi.org/10.1016/j.contraception.2015.01.005

Gavin, L., Moskosky, S., Carter, M., Curtis, K., Glass, E., Godfrey, E.,…Zapata, L.; Centers for Disease Control and Prevention (CDC). (2014). Providing quality family planning services: Recommendations of CDC and the U.S. Office of Population Affairs. *Recommendations and Reports: Morbidity and Mortality Weekly Report. Recommendations and Reports/Centers for Disease Control, 63*(RR-04), 1–54.

Gelberg, L., Lu, M. C., Leake, B. D., Andersen, R. M., Morgenstern, H., & Nyamathi, A. M. (2008). Homeless women: Who is really at risk for unintended pregnancy? *Maternal and Child Health Journal, 12*(1), 52–60.

Gold, R. B. (2003). Lessons from before Roe: Will past be prologue? *Guttmacher Report on Public Policy, 6*(1), 8–11.

Grimes, D. A. (2008). The choice of second trimester abortion method: Evolution, evidence and ethics. *Reproductive Health Matters, 16* (Suppl. 31), 183–188.

Grimes, D. A., & Creinin, M. D. (2004). Induced abortion: An overview for internists. *Annals of Internal Medicine, 140*(8), 620–626.

Grossman, D., Ellertson, C., Grimes, D. A., & Walker, D. (2004). Routine follow-up visits after first-trimester induced abortion. *Obstetrics and Gynecology, 103*(4), 738–745.

Grossman, D., Holt, K., Peña, M., Lara, D., Veatch, M., Córdova, D.,…Blanchard, K. (2010). Self-induction of abortion among women in the United States. *Reproductive Health Matters, 18*(36), 136–146.

Guttmacher Institute. (2015). *State funding of abortion under Medicaid, state policies in brief.* Retrieved from http://www.guttmacher.org/statecenter/spibs/spib_SFAM.pdf.

Guzzo, K. B., & Hayford, S. R. (2013). *Revisiting retrospective reporting of birth intendedness.* Paper Presented at the Annual Meeting of the Population Association Meeting of America, New Orleans, LA.

Harris, L. H. (2012). Recognizing conscience in abortion provision. *New England Journal of Medicine, 367*(11), 981–983.

Higgins, J. A., Popkin, R. A., & Santelli, J. S. (2012). Pregnancy ambivalence and contraceptive use among young adults in the United States. *Perspectives on Sexual and Reproductive Health, 44*(4), 236–243.

International Federation of Gynecology and Obstetrics. (2011). *Consensus statement on uterine evacuation: Uterine evacuation: Use vacuum aspiration or medications, not sharp curettage.* London, UK: FIGO.

Ipas. (2007). *Starting contraception after first trimester medication abortion.* Retrieved from http://www.ipas.org/~/media/Files/Ipas%20Publications/MAFactsheet1.ashx

Ipas. (2016). *Clinical updates in reproductive health.* In A. Mark (Ed.). Chapel Hill, NC: Ipas. Retrieved from file:///C:/Users/ima00001/Downloads/CURHE16.pdf

Jackson, A. V., Dayananda, I., Fortin, J. M., Fitzmaurice, G., & Goldberg, A. B. (2012). Can women accurately assess the outcome of medical abortion based on symptoms alone? *Contraception, 85*(2), 192–197.

Jerman, J., & Jones, R. K. (2014). Secondary measures of access to abortion services in the United States, 2011 and 2012: Gestational age limits, cost, and harassment. *Women's Health Issues, 24*(4), e419–e424.

Joffe, C. (2009). Abortion and medicine: A sociopolitical history. In M. Paul, E. Lichtenberg, L. Borgatta, D. A. Grimes, P. G. Stubblefield, & M. D. Creinin (Eds.), *Management of unintended and abnormal pregnancy: Comprehensive abortion care.* Chichester, UK: Wiley Blackwell.

Jones, R., Finer, L., & Singh, S. (2010). *Characteristics of U.S. abortion patients, 2008.* New York, NY: Guttmacher Institute.

Jones, R. K., & Jerman, J. (2014). Abortion incidence and service availability in the United States, 2011. *Perspectives on Sexual and Reproductive Health, 46*(1), 3–14.

Jones, R. K., & Kavanaugh, M. L. (2011). Changes in abortion rates between 2000 and 2008 and lifetime incidence of abortion. *Obstetrics and Gynecology, 117*(6), 1358–1366.

Joyce, T., Kaestner, R., & Korenman, S. (2002). On the validity of retrospective assessments of pregnancy intention. *Demography, 39*(1), 199–213.

Joyner, K., Peters, H. E., Hynes, K., Sikora, A., Taber, J. R., & Rendall, M. S. (2012). The quality of male fertility data in major U.S. surveys. *Demography, 49*(1), 101–124.

Kågesten, A., Bajos, N., Bohet, A., & Moreau, C. (2015). Male experiences of unintended pregnancy: Characteristics and prevalence. *Human Reproduction, 30*(1), 186–196.

Kapp, N., Whyte, P., Tang, J., Jackson, E., & Brahmi, D. (2013). A review of evidence for safe abortion care. *Contraception, 88*(3), 350–363.

Kaunitz, A. (2015). *Postpartum and postabortion contraception.* In K. Eckler (Ed.), *UpToDate.* Retrieved from http://www.uptodate.com/home

Kimport, K., Cockrill, K., & Weitz, T. A. (2012). Analyzing the impacts of abortion clinic structures and processes: A qualitative analysis of women's negative experience of abortion clinics. *Contraception, 85*(2), 204–210.

Klerman, L. K. (2000). The intendedness of pregnancy: A concept in transition. *Maternal and Child Health Journal, 4*(3), 155–162.

Kost, K. (2015). *Unintended pregnancy rates at the state level: Estimates for 2010 and trends since 2002.* Retrieved from http://www.guttmacher.org/pubs/StateUP10.pdf

Kost, K., & Lindberg, L. (2015). Pregnancy intentions, maternal behaviors, and infant health: investigating relationships with new measures and propensity score analysis. *Demography, 52*(1), 83–111.

Kulier, R., Kapp, N., Gülmezoglu, A., Hofmeyr, G., Cheng, L., & Campana, A. (2011). Medical methods for first trimester abortion. *The Cochrane Database of Systematic Review, 2011*(11), CD002855. doi:10.1002/14651858.CD002855.pub4

Langston, A. M., Joslin-Roher, S. L., & Westhoff, C. L. (2014). Immediate postabortion access to IUDs, implants and DMPA reduces repeat pregnancy within 1 year in a New York City practice. *Contraception, 89*(2), 103–108.

Lichtenberg, E., & Grimes, D. (2009). Surgical complications: Prevention and management. In M. Paul, E. Lichtenberg, & L. Borgatta, D. A. Grimes, P. G. Stubblefield, & M. D. Creinin (Eds.), *Management of unintended and abnormal pregnancy: Comprehensive abortion care.* Chichester, UK: Wiley Blackwell.

List, J. M. (2011). Beyond charity-social justice and health care. *The Virtual Mentor, 13*(8), 565–568.

Logan, C., Holcombe, E., Manlove, J., & Ryan, S. (2007). *The consequences of unintended childbearing* [White paper]. Washington, DC: Child Trends.

Major, B., Appelbaum, M., Beckman, L., Dutton, M. A., Russo, N. F., & West, C. (2009). Abortion and mental health: Evaluating the evidence. *The American Psychologist, 64*(9), 863–890.

Major, B., Appelbaum, M., Beckman, L., Dutton, M., Russo, N. F., & West, C. (2008). *Report of the task force on mental health and abortion.* Washington, DC: American Psychological Association Task Force on Mental Health and Abortion. Retrieved from http://www .apa.org/pi/wpo/mental-health-abortion-report.pdf

McIntosh, K., Stewart, G., & Teplin, D. (2009). Routine aftercare and contraception. In M. Paul, E. Lichtenberg, & L. Borgatta, D. A. Grimes, P. G. Stubblefield, & M. D. Creinin (Eds.), *Management of unintended and abnormal pregnancy: Comprehensive abortion care.* Chichester, UK: Wiley Blackwell.

Nanda, G., Switlick, K., & Lule, E. (2005). *Accelerating progress towards achieving the MDG to improve maternal health: A collection of promising approaches* [Discussion paper]. Washington, DC: The International Bank for Reconstruction and Development/The World Bank.

National Abortion Federation (NAF). (2015). *Clinical policy guidelines.* Washington, DC: National Abortion Federation.

National Cancer Institute. (2003). Summary report: Early reproductive events and breast cancer workshop. Retrieved from www.cancer.gov/ cancertopics/causes/ere/workshop-report

O'Connor, Stacey, & Jacobsen. (2015). *Ottawa personal decision guide.* Ottawa Hospital Research Institute & University of Ottawa, Canada. Retrieved from https://decisionaid.ohri.ca/docs/das/OPDG.pdf

Pallitto, C. C., Garcia-Moreno, C., Jansen, H. A. F. M., Heise, L., Ellsberg, M., & Watts, C. (2013). Intimate partner violence, abortion, and unintended pregnancy: Results from the WHO Multi-country Study on Women's Health and Domestic Violence. *International Journal of Gynecology and Obstetrics, 120*(1), 3–9.

Paul, M., Lackie, E., Mitchell, C., Rogers, A., & Fox, M. (2002). Is pathology examination useful after early surgical abortion? *Obstetrics and Gynecology, 99*(4), 567–571. doi:10.1016/ S0029-7844(01)01782-3

Pazol, K., Creanga, A., Burley, K., & Jamieson, D. (2014). Abortion surveillance—United States, 2011. *Morbidity and Mortality Weekly Report, 63*(SS11), 1–41.

Planned Parenthood Federation of America. (2003). *Medical abortion.* New York, NY: Planned Parenthood Federation of America.

Poole, V., Flowers, J., Goldenberg, R., Cliver, S., & McNeal, S. (2000). Changes in intendedness during pregnancy in a high-risk multiparous population. *Maternal and Child Health Journal, 4*(3), 179–182.

Potts, M., & Campbell, M. (2009). History of contraception. *The Global Library of Women's Medicine.* doi:10.3843/GLOWM.10376

Raymond, E., & Grimes, D. (2012). The comparative safety of legal induced abortion and childbirth in the United States. *Obstetrics and Gynecology, 119*(2, Pt. 1), 215–219.

Raymond, E., Grossman, D., Weaver, M., Toti, S., & Winikoff, B. (2014). Mortality of induced abortion, other outpatient surgical procedures and common activities in the United States. *Contraception, 90*(5), 476–479. doi:10.1016/j.contraception.2014.07.012

Reeves, M., Kudva, A., & Creinin, M. (2008). Medical abortion outcomes after a second dose of misoprostol for persistent gestational sac. *Contraception, 78*, 332–335.

Renner, R. M., Jensen, J. T., Nichols, M. D., & Edelman, A. B. (2010). Pain control in first-trimester surgical abortion: A systematic review of randomized controlled trials. *Contraception, 81*, 372–388.

Reproductive Health Access Project. (2014). *Mifepristone/misoprostol abortion protocol.* Retrieved from http://www.reproductiveaccess.org/ wp-content/uploads/2014/12/mifepristone_protocol.pdf

Roberts, S., Gould, H., Kimport, K., Weitz, T., & Foster, D. (2014). Out-of-pocket costs and insurance coverage for abortion in the United States. *Womens Health Issues, 24*(2), E211–E218. doi:10.1016/j .whi.2014.01.003

Rocca, C., Kimport, K., Gould, H., & Foster, D. (2013). Women's emotions one week after receiving or being denied an abortion in the United States. *Perspectives on Sexual and Reproductive Health, 45*(3), 122–131. doi:10.1363/4512213

Rosing, M. A., & Archbald, C. D. (2000). The knowledge, acceptability, and use of misoprostol for self-induced medical abortion in an urban U.S. population. *Journal of the American Medical Women's Association (1972), 55*(Suppl. 3), 183–185.

Schaff, E. A., Eisinger, S. H., Stadalius, L. S., Franks, P., Gore, B. Z., & Poppema, S. (1999). Low-dose mifepristone 200 mg and vaginal misoprostol for abortion. *Contraception, 59*(1), 1–6.

Schneider, P., & Schneider, J. (1995). Coitus interruptus and family respectability in Catholic Europe: A Sicilian case study. In F. D. Ginsburg & R. Rapp (Eds.), *Conceiving the new world order: The global politics of reproduction* (pp. 177–194). Berkeley and Los Angeles, CA: University of California Press.

Schreiber, C. A., Sober, S., Ratcliffe, S., & Creinin, M. D. (2011). Ovulation resumption after medical abortion with mifepristone and misoprostol. *Contraception, 84*(3), 230–233.

Shannon, C., Brothers, L. P., Philip, N. M., & Winikoff, B. (2004). Infection after medical abortion: A review of the literature. *Contraception, 70*(3), 183–190.

Simmonds, K., & Likis, F. E. (2011). Caring for women with unintended pregnancies. *Journal of Obstetric, Gynecologic, and Neonatal Nursing, 40*(6), 794–807.

Singh, S., Sedgh, G., & Hussain, R. (2010). Unintended pregnancy: Worldwide levels, trends, and outcomes. *Studies in Family Planning, 41*(4), 241–250.

Steenland, M. W., Tepper, N. K., Curtis, K. M., & Kapp, N. (2011). Intrauterine contraceptive insertion postabortion: A systematic review. *Contraception, 84*(5), 447–464.

Stoddard, A., & Eisenberg, D. L. (2011). Controversies in family planning: Timing of ovulation after abortion and the conundrum of postabortion intrauterine device insertion. *Contraception, 84*(2), 119–121.

Stubblefield, P. G., Carr-Ellis, S., & Borgatta, L. (2004). Methods for induced abortion. *Obstetrics and Gynecology, 104*(1), 174–185.

Taylor, D., Levi, A., & Simmonds, K.; Board of the Society of Family Planning. (2010). Reframing unintended pregnancy prevention: A public health model. *Contraception, 81*(5), 363–366.

Taylor, D., Safriet, B., Dempsey, G., Kruse, B., & Jackson, C. (2009). *Providing abortion care: A professional toolkit for nurse-midwives, nurse practitioners, and physician assistants.* San Francisco, CA: Regents of the University of California, University of California-San Francisco.

Turok, D. K., Gurtcheff, S. E., Esplin, M. S., Shah, M., Simonsen, S. E., Trauscht-Van Horn, J., & Silver, R. M. (2008). Second trimester termination of pregnancy: A review by site and procedure type. *Contraception, 77*(3), 155–161.

U.S. Department of Health and Human Services (DHHS). (2010). *Healthy People 2020.* Retrieved from http://www.healthypeople.gov/2020/ topics-objectives/topic/family-planning/objectives

Upadhyay, U. D., Desai, S., Zlidar, V., Weitz, T. A., Grossman, D., Anderson, P., & Taylor, D. (2015). Incidence of emergency department visits and complications after abortion. *Obstetrics and Gynecology, 125*(1), 175–183.

Weitz, T. A., Taylor, D., Desai, S., Upadhyay, U. D., Waldman, J., Battistelli, M. F., & Drey, E. A. (2013). Safety of aspiration abortion performed by nurse practitioners, certified nurse midwives, and physician assistants under a California legal waiver. *American Journal of Public Health, 103*(3), 454–461.

Wiebe, E., Dunn, S., Guilbert, E., Jacot, F., & Lugtig, L. (2002). Comparison of abortions induced by methotrexate or mifepristone followed by misoprostol. *Obstetrics and Gynecology, 99*(5, Pt. 1), 813–819.

Winikoff, B., Dzuba, I. G., Chong, E., Goldberg, A. B., Lichtenberg, E. S., Ball, C.,…Swica, Y. (2012). Extending outpatient medical abortion services through 70 days of gestational age. *Obstetrics and Gynecology, 120*(5), 1070–1076.

World Health Organization (WHO). (2011). *Unsafe abortion: Global and regional estimates of the incidence of unsafe abortion and associated mortality in 2008* (6th ed.). Geneva, Switzerland: World Health Organization.

World Health Organization (WHO). (2012). *Safe abortion: Technical and policy guidance for health systems* (2nd ed.). Geneva, Switzerland: World Health Organization.

Yonke, N., & Leeman, L. M. (2013). First-trimester surgical abortion technique. *Obstetrics and Gynecology Clinics of North America, 40*(4), 647–670.

CHAPTER 37

Infertility

Rachel Oldani Bender • Elizabeth A. Kostas-Polston

Infertility is rapidly becoming a routine evaluation often performed by the advanced practice nurse practitioner. As such, having a solid foundation and resources to turn to will be invaluable in practice. The purpose of this chapter is to give an overview of fertility evaluation and treatments, as well as the many ethical and psychological dilemmas that may be encountered when caring for the patient and her family. Infertility should be treated systematically and care should be standardized throughout all practices. The American Society for Reproductive Medicine (ASRM) serves as an invaluable resource for health care providers and provides invaluable information on reproductive, evidence-based practice guidelines.

■ DEFINITION AND SCOPE

Infertility is a couple's condition and is defined by the inability to achieve pregnancy after 12 months or more of regular, unprotected, and well-timed intercourse in women younger than 35 years, and after 6 months beyond the age of 35 years (ASRM, 2004/2008). A woman is considered to have primary infertility if she has never achieved pregnancy after regular, unprotected, and well-timed intercourse as discussed previously (ASRM, 2012a). Secondary infertility is defined as a woman who has not been able to conceive after having a prior pregnancy or who has recurrent pregnancy loss. *Fecundability* is defined as a woman's likelihood of achieving pregnancy within one menstrual cycle (ASRM, 2012a). By age 24, a woman reaches her maximum fertility potential with declining rates beginning at age 35. Today, the average age at which many women deliver their first child in the United States has increased. Between 1990 and the early 2000s, the first-time birth rate for women aged 35 to 45 years old was 53% (Martin et al., 2007).

Infertility is not specifically a female issue; thus, both sexual partners should be evaluated simultaneously for factors impairing infertility, if possible. It is important to remember that recognition, evaluation, and treatment of infertility is highly stressful for most couples.

Prevalence

The National Survey of Family Growth (NSFG) study included interviews of 12,279 women ages 15 to 44 years to estimate the prevalence of infertility in the United States. Infertility was determined if a woman reported continuous cohabitation during the previous 12 months or more and intercourse each month with no use of contraception and had not become pregnant (Chandra et al., 2013). In 2002, 2% of women of childbearing age desired infertility counseling and an additional 10% received infertility management. The 2013 data showed that 64% of nulliparous married women with infertility desired to have a child, and 53% of parous, married, infertile women desired to have another child (Chandra et al., 2013).

■ ETIOLOGY

Approximately one third of infertility is caused by male factors, one third by female factors, and one third by a combination of factors in both partners. Overall, 20% of infertility cases are unexplained (ASRM, 2008). A woman has a 20% chance of becoming pregnant in each month or menstrual cycle. Over 1 year, the cumulative pregnancy rate is 85% (ASRM, 2012a). According to the National Center for Health Statistics of the Centers for Disease Control and Prevention (CDC), in the United States, married women aged 15 to 44 years who have difficulty getting pregnant or carrying a baby to term has increased from 21.2% (2006–2010) to 24.2% (2011–2013; CDC, 2015b). Fertility peaks from the late teenage years through the late 20s, and then declines thereafter. A woman's risk for miscarriage increases beginning age 30 years (ASRM, 2008). Approximately one in every five women in the United States now has her first child after age 35 years and fertility problems affect one third of these women (ASRM, 2012a). Earlier evaluation and treatment after 6 months of unprotected intercourse may be justified based on medical history and physical findings for older women as recommended by ASRM (2008).

RISK FACTORS

According the CDC, ASRM, American Fertility Association, and Resolve, an organization to support men and women on their journey of infertility, many of the risk factors for both male and female infertility are the same (CDC, 2015a). The strongest evidence supports smoking, alcohol, and weight as modifiable risk factors. Couples trying to conceive should be counseled to stop smoking, consuming alcohol, and to maintain a healthy weight (ASRM, 2012f; CDC, 2015a). Being overweight or underweight with a body mass index (BMI) of 25 kg/m² or greater, or of 20 kg/m² or less, can lead to hormone imbalances and ovulatory dysfunction (CDC, 2015a). At-risk women include those with eating disorders (e.g., anorexia nervosa, bulimia) and women on a very low-calorie or restrictive diet. Strict vegetarians also may experience infertility problems because of a lack of important nutrients such as vitamin B₁₂, zinc, iron, and folic acid. Marathon runners, dancers, and others who exercise very intensely are also more prone to menstrual irregularities and infertility. As previously mentioned, fertility declines with age, so women in their late 30s are about 30% less fertile than those in their early 20s. Furthermore, as a woman ages, there is a decrease in ovarian reserve, quality of oocyte, and irregularity of ovulation, thus increasing the risk of pregnancy loss. It is important to consider that more and more women are choosing to delay childbearing because of many factors (e.g., education, career). Other risk factors for infertility include chronic diseases, such as diabetes, hyper or hypothyroidism, lupus, arthritis, hypertension, or asthma, all of which increase in prevalence as a woman ages (CDC, 2015a).

Some 2.86 million cases of chlamydia and 820,000 cases of gonorrhea occur annually in the United States (CDC, 2015c). Some sexually transmitted infections (STIs) can be asymptomatic and are transmitted more easily to women. STIs can lead to pelvic inflammatory disease (PID) in women and epididymitis in men and are responsible for much of the tubal occlusion in women and men; chlamydia is the most prevalent organism responsible (CDC, 2015c). Complications are more common in women including subsequent scarring, miscarriage, adhesions, blocked tubes, and ectopic pregnancy (CDC, 2015c).

Approximately 10% to 15% of infertility cases are unexplained (ASRM, 2008). Risk factors that may be attributable to the unexplained cases include exposure to toxic substances and/or hazards on the job (e.g., lead, cadmium, mercury, ethylene oxide, vinyl chloride, radioactivity, x-rays). Cigarette or marijuana smoke and heavy alcohol consumption can contribute to infertility (CDC, ASRM, & Society for Assisted Reproductive Technology [SART], 2015). For men, exposure of the genitals to elevated temperatures such as hot baths, whirlpools, steam rooms, and bicycle riding are also factors that can lead to infertility issues. Also, men with a history of hernia repair, undescended testicles, prostatitis or genital infection(s), and/or mumps after puberty are at risk (CDC, ASRM, & SART, 2015).

EVALUATION/ASSESSMENT

Completion of a thorough history and physical examination is an important, first-step process that will be used by the health care provider to determine appropriate plan for a patient's infertility workup and diagnostic testing. The ASRM website offers the most current guidelines regarding optimal evaluation of the infertile female and of the infertile male (www.asrm.org/?vs=1).

Female Assessment

MEDICAL AND SURGICAL HISTORY

A thorough family, medical, surgical, and reproductive health history must be obtained from the couple to include a complete review of systems (ROS) with documentation of any allergies. If applicable, proven fertility in one partner with all details should be obtained. Duration of infertility, previous evaluation and treatment(s), and menstrual cycle history (including cycle length and characteristics) should be discussed. Previous history of STIs, history of PID, abnormal cervical cytology and histology, and all treatment(s) should be noted. Furthermore, the health care provider should be sure to rule out, either by history or testing, thyroid dysfunction, galactorrhea, hirsutism, pelvic and/or abdominal pain, dysmenorrhea, and dyspareunia (ASRM, 2015b, 2015c). A comprehensive medical history is helpful to identify any systemic conditions. Calculation of BMI and history of significant weight gain or loss can reveal underlying eating disorders. Exercise levels should be assessed as excessive amounts impact ovulation. If underlying medical problems are identified, evaluation and treatment are recommended to ensure management of infertility, conception, and pregnancy would not pose a threat to the mother's health (ASRM, 2015f).

Again, it is important not to label one partner with fertility issues. Instead, it is important that the health care provider objectively complete the history, physical examination, and diagnostic tests, as necessary, for both partners. The history should be obtained with the couple together as well as apart, as there may be confidential issues related to past relationships that are unknown in the current relationship.

SOCIAL HISTORY

A history of tobacco, alcohol, and drug use should be obtained. Occupational history is necessary to identify risk factors and exposure to known carcinogens/toxins (past or present). Absence because of work-related travel or military deployments should be discussed as they relate to availability of the partner in infertility management.

GYNECOLOGIC HISTORY

Gynecologic history should begin with a description of the menstrual cycle. This includes age at menarche, cycle length, duration and amount of menstrual flow, and history of dysmenorrhea. Any periods of amenorrhea, spotting, or irregular bleeding are important to document. A history of irregular cycles, defined as less than 24 days or greater than 35 days, is the basis for further evaluation of ovulatory dysfunction (ASRM, 2015b, 2015c).

Questions regarding types and use of contraceptives and as well as discontinuation of methods are necessary in assessing expectations for return to fertility. History of any past pregnancies, mode of delivery, and/or abortions (spontaneous or therapeutic) with outcomes or complications should be obtained (ASRM, 2015b, 2015c). A sexual history that includes number of partners, STIs, and frequency of coitus, as well as the correlation of intercourse with the time of ovulation, is essential. Any previous infertility treatments should be recorded. Previous history of pelvic and abdominal surgeries and cervical procedures such as loop electrosurgical excision procedure (LEEP) and cold knife cone (CKC) biopsy are also important to note (ASRM, 2015a, 2015d). Finally, a complete physical and pelvic examination should be performed.

FAMILY HISTORY

Significant family history that should be obtained includes history of infertility, premature ovarian failure, recurrent pregnancy loss, endometriosis, thyroid disease, cancer, and endocrine or genetic problems (ASRM, 2015b, 2015c).

PHYSICAL EXAMINATION

Physical examination should be focused on assessing signs for potential causes of infertility (Box 37.1). The health care provider should calculate body mass index and distribution of fat, as extremes are associated with decreased fertility (ASRM, 2015f). Disproportional abdominal fat can be correlated to increased insulin resistance and may lead to a diagnosis of polycystic ovarian syndrome (PCOS; ASRM, 2014c, 2015f). Body shape and development or underdevelopment of secondary sex characteristics should be noted to rule in or out hypogonadotropic hypogonadism or Turner's syndrome. Presence of thyroid abnormalities, galactorrhea, hirsutism, acne, or male-pattern baldness can suggest endocrinopathies such as hyper-/hypothyroidism, hyperprolactinemia, PCOS, or adrenal disorder. Pelvic examination should include evaluation of the adnexa and posterior cul-de-sac for masses or tenderness, possibly suggesting PID or endometriosis. The vagina and cervix should be inspected for normality to rule out mullerian anomaly, infection, or cervical factors. The uterus should be palpated for enlargement, nodularity, irregularity, and lack of mobility suggesting a uterine anomaly, leiomyoma, endometriosis, and pelvic adhesion disease (ASRM, 2012c, 2015b).

DIAGNOSTIC STUDIES

The order of testing is related to the history and physical examination and is specific to the body process(es) that may be causing infertility. Testing usually progresses from the least to the most invasive. Preconception evaluation may be done at this time as it can be used for diagnostic and

---

BOX 37.1   FEMALE CAUSES OF INFERTILITY

- Endocrine
- Ovulatory
  - Follicle stimulating hormone/luteinizing hormone
  - Polycystic ovarian syndrome
  - Luteal phase defect
  - Premature ovarian failure
  - Thyroid
  - Pituitary
- Anatomic
  - Tubal
  - Endometriosis
  - Cervical
  - Uterine
- Genetic
  - Sheehan syndrome
  - Kallman syndrome
  - Turner syndrome
  - Hypothalamic hypogonadism
- Immunologic
  - Antibodies
- Unexplained

---

therapeutic counseling. Preconception evaluation includes blood type and Rh, rubella status, cystic fibrosis screening, chlamydia and gonorrhea screening, and Pap smear collection. Diagnostic testing can be divided into three categories: (1) semen analysis (to be discussed in male section), (2) ovulatory function and reserve, and (3) tubal patency (ASRM, 2012c, 2015b, 2015c).

Assessment of Ovulatory Function • Ovulatory disorders account for approximately 40% of all infertility in women (Mosher, 1991). The occurrence of regular monthly menstrual cycles is a good indicator of ovulation, with 95% to 98% being ovulatory cycles. Irregular cycles (less than 21 days or greater than 35 days) are generally not ovulatory cycles. Laboratory assessment of ovulation should be preformed in women who do not have grossly abnormal menstrual cycles (ASRM, 2015b). A mid-luteal phase progesterone level will establish ovulation approximately 1 week before the expected menses. A progesterone level greater than 3 ng/mL is consistent with ovulation (Luciano et al., 1990). Ovulation predictor kits (OPK) are another reliable method to monitor the level of luteinizing hormone (LH), which begins to rise before ovulation. Kits are dependent on monoclonal antibodies to LH. OPKs are useful in improving the timing of intercourse, as they predict ovulation prospectively compared with basal body temperature charts, which do so retrospectively (McGovern et al., 2004). Ovulation most commonly occurs 12 to 24 hours following a random urine sample positive test result (McGovern et al., 2004). Daily ultrasounds to follow the development and eventually the disappearance of a follicle (most accurate method of documenting ovulation) and endometrial biopsy (which show secretory changes of the endometrium) are too expensive or invasive to use for routine diagnostic assessment of ovulation. Patients requiring this level of diagnostic testing should be referred to a reproductive endocrinologist (RE; ASRM, 2015b, 2015a).

Assessment of Ovarian Reserve •

Decreased ovarian reserve refers to decreased oocyte quality, quantity, or reproductive potential. Many screening tests are utilized; however, there is *no single test* that is highly reliable for predicting pregnancy potential. Ovarian reserve can be assessed by measuring follicle stimulating hormone (FSH) and estradiol (E_2) on cycle day 2 or 3. FSH values greater than 10 to 20 international units (IU) suggest decreased reserve and deceased fertility potential, while FSH values less than 20 IU are predictive of a decrease in reproductive potential (ASRM, 2015b).

In 2004, Tarun, Soules, and Collins conducted a meta-analysis comparing basal FSH and the clomiphene citrate challenge test (CCCT) as predictors for ovarian reserve. Basal FSH testing requires a single serum measurement on cycle day 2, 3, or 4. Tarun et al. (2004) found that basal FSH and the CCCT were similar in predicting the ability of a woman to achieve a clinical pregnancy, with the normal result being of limited value. However, they found that an abnormal result virtually confirmed that pregnancy will not occur without treatment (Tarun et al., 2004). These tests are indicated in women suspected of having premature ovarian failure or early menopause. Clomiphene citrate 50 to 100 mg is given on days 5 to 9 of the menstrual cycle with a basal FSH obtained on days 3 and 10. The FSH response to clomiphene reflects ovarian follicular inhibin capability. If the FSH is elevated on either day, the test is abnormal, a significant predictor for infertility (Tarun et al., 2004). The CCCT is more costly than a single, basal FSH level and associated with greater inconvenience and potential side effects. Present-day use of CCCT has decreased as serum antral follicular count (AFC) and anti-Müllerian hormone (AMH) are easier and highly predictive of ovarian response (ASRM, 2015b). Both AMH and AFC have been shown to be markers for ovarian reserve.

Antral follicle counts are the sum total of antral follicles of both ovaries measured via transvaginal ultrasound on days 2 and 4 of a normal menstrual cycle (Hsu et al., 2011). Antral follicles are defined as follicles measuring 2 mm to 10 mm in diameter. A low AFC (4–10) suggests poor ovarian reserve. AFC is a good predictor of ovarian reserve and response, but is a poor predictor of oocyte quality, the ability to conceive with in vitro fertilization (IVF), or pregnancy outcome (Hsu et al., 2011).

AMH is expressed by the small (less than 8 mm) preantral and early antral follicles (Dewailly et al., 2014). AMH level shows the size of the primordial follicle pool, and as such, may be the best biochemical marker of ovarian function. In adult women, AMH gradually declines as the primordial pool declines and is indictable at menopause (Hsu et al., 2011). AMH may play an especially important role in special patients, such as cancer patients, and in those who have had ovarian injury either from radiation

or surgery. AMH is used in IVF to determine the number of oocytes to be retrieved after stimulation or determine hyperstimulation (Dewailly et al., 2014). AMH levels are dependent on the laboratory; it is important that the health care provider should reference their own laboratory's reference range.

Assessment of Uterine Cavity and Tubal Patency •

After the determination of ovulation and semen analyses have been completed, more invasive testing can be started. Assessment of tubal patency can be done through hysterosalpingography, ultrasound, sonohystogram, hysteroscopy, and laparoscopy. The hysterosalpingogram (HSG) demonstrates tubal patency and uterine cavity abnormalities. The most common reason for occlusion of the tubes is PID (Coppus et al., 2007). Other uterine abnormalities that can be implicated in infertility include septa, polyps, and submucosal myomata. The ideal timing for an HSG is approximately 2 to 3 days after the cessation of menstrual flow, in the mid-follicular phase of the cycle (Wass et al., 2014). HSG should be scheduled before an intrauterine insemination (IUI) or ovulation induction for those women with unexplained infertility (ASRM, 2012d). HSG is performed under fluoroscopy usually by a physician and/or radiologist. Mild analgesic or prostaglandin synthesis inhibitor may be administered orally 30 to 40 minutes before the HSG to minimize cramping pain and discomfort (ASRM, 2015b). HSG is contraindicated in the presence of tenderness palpated on bimanual examination (ASRM, 2015b).

The diagnostic value of HSG has been clearly established; however, its value as a therapeutic modality in infertility is controversial (ASRM, 2015b). HSG can be used to diagnose proximal or distal tubal occlusion, salpingitis isthmica nodosa, and rule in or out tubal structure abnormality (ASRM, 2015b). Studies have demonstrated that the performance of an HSG enhances fertility in subsequent months (ASRM, 2012c, 2015b; Panchal & Nagori, 2014). HSG may increase fertility by opening the tubes from the mechanical lavage of the dye, dislodging any mucus plugs, and breaking down peritoneal adhesions. It may also stimulate the cilia within the lumen of the tubes (ASRM, 2012c, 2015b; Panchal & Nagori, 2014).

Vaginal ultrasonography may be used as part of an evaluation to detect any uterine or ovarian abnormalities (ASRM, 2012c, 2015b). If the HSG or vaginal ultrasound is abnormal or suspicious, a sonohysterogram should be completed, as it is more sensitive for identifying intrauterine pathology such as polyps and intrauterine fibroids (ASRM, 2015b). Sonohysterography involves the injection of saline into the uterine cavity followed by careful ultrasound examination of the uterus. Sonohysterography is often used concomitantly with HSG to differentiate between fibroids that are submucous versus fibroids that have an intramural component (ASRM, 2015b).

For abnormalities requiring direct visualization of the uterine cavity, hysteroscopy can be performed (Panshy et al., 2006). The procedure involves placing a small hysteroscope through the internal os into the uterine cavity and filling the cavity with warm Ringer's lactate solution (Panshy et al., 2006). The procedure can be performed either under local anesthesia with paracervical block and sedation or under light general anesthesia. An operative hysteroscope is commonly used to exclude and treat polyps, fibroids, and uterine septa (Panshy et al., 2006). The treatment of Asherman's syndrome (intrauterine adhesions) is frequently performed by either hysteroscopy or by hysteroscopy combined with laparoscopy (National Organization for Rare Disorders [NORD], 2005). Asherman's syndrome is a rare, acquired gynecologic disorder characterized by changes in menstrual pattern. These changes are most often a result of surgical scraping of tissue from the uterine wall (such as with dilatation and curettage [D&C]) and infections of the endometrium (such as PID; NORD, 2005).

Unexplained Infertility

Peritoneal factors, endometriosis, and/or adnexal adhesions must be considered when all other diagnosis have been ruled out. As the health care provider begins to rule in and rule out diagnoses based on the patient's history, physical examination, and diagnostic evaluation, this information, in itself, is not sufficient for diagnosis (ASRM, 2015b). For example, in the most severe stages of endometriosis (stages 3 and 4), ultrasonography may be able to identify an endometrioma, but again, is not diagnostic (Bulletti et al., 2010). Direct visualization is required to make a diagnosis of endometriosis or adnexal adhesion during laparoscopy (Bulletti et al., 2010; Hsu, Khachikyan, & Stratton, 2010). However, mild endometriosis (stages 1 and 2) has minimal impact on fertility. Most women who have significant adnexal adhesions or stage 3 and 4 endometriosis will have risk factors such as pelvic pain, previous pelvic infection or surgery, or an abnormal HSG (Bulletti et al., 2010). Laparoscopy is indicated for these select individuals where treatment of disease may provide benefit to potential fertility and is not used routinely for evaluation of infertility (ASRM, 2015b). There is no evidence to support superior results related to the treatment of endometriosis (Bulletti et al., 2010). For cases of failed laparoscopic treatment and/or failed medical treatment, assisted reproductive technology (ART), technology used to achieve pregnancy (e.g., fertility medication, artificial insemination, IVF), is appropriate as the next step to enable fertility (ASRM, 2015a).

Unexplained infertility (UI) is a *definition of exclusion* made in the presence of a normal assessment of ovulation, evaluation of uterotubal function, and semen analysis. The incidence of UI is about 30% in infertile couples (Nardo & Chouliaras, 2015). Treatment consists of ovulation induction on clomiphene citrate or FSH combined with IUI or ART. If treatment fails, gamete intrafallopian transfer (GIFT), IVF, and/or IVF with intracytoplasmic sperm injection (ICSI) may be considered (Guzick et al., 1998).

Male Assessment

HISTORY

The medical history in the male is focused on identifying systemic conditions that could impact fertility (Box 37.2;

BOX 37.2 MALE CAUSES OF INFERTILITY

- Low sperm count
- Low sperm motility
- Anatomic
  - Obstruction of the tract
- Immunologic
  - Sperm antibodies
- Ejaculatory disorders
- Genetic
- Toxins
- Idiopathic

ASRM, 2015c). Important considerations include age at puberty; history of undescended testicles; erectile dysfunction; significant illness with high fever; mumps-related orchitis; radiography of groin; trauma to groin; and/or infections such as epididymitis, prostatitis, urinary tract infections, and penile discharge (ASRM, 2015c). Diabetes mellitus may also cause impotence and retrograde ejaculation. Medications used to treat hypertension can also cause impotence, as well as those used for treatment of peptic ulcer disease, ulcerative colitis, Crohn's disease, and cystic fibrosis, which can alter semen quality (ASRM, 2015c). Surgical history is also important. It is important to note procedures such as hernia repair, testicular surgery, pelvic surgery, varicocele repair, and vasectomy and/or vasectomy reversal. Family history would be remarkable for endocrine or genetic conditions. Referral to an urologist is recommended if further evaluation at any time is warranted (ASRM, 2015c).

PHYSICAL ASSESSMENT

Evaluation of the male for infertility begins with the semen analysis (ASRM, 2015c; Cooper et al., 2010). Semen analysis is performed as a first step in the assessment of the infertile couple. It is an easy, noninvasive test to perform, and abstinence for 2 to 3 days before collection is optimum.

Semen can be collected by means of masturbation into a specimen container or via intercourse with the use of a special semen collection condom that is chemical free so as not to interfere with sperm viability (ASRM, 2015c; Cooper et al., 2010). The specimen should be taken to the laboratory with within 1 hour of ejaculation for semen analysis. Sperm volume, concentration, motility, morphology, pH, and cellularity are reported. Sperm parameters that have been suggested to predict male fertility include a sperm count of 48 million/mL, sperm motility greater than 63%, and sperm morphology greater than 12% normal set by strict criteria for evaluation (ASRM, 2015c; Cooper et al., 2010; World Health Organization [WHO], 2010). Of importance to the health care provider is evidence that suggests that some men with an *optimal* semen analysis may be infertile, whereas those with a suboptimal analysis may be fertile. Hence, semen analysis alone has not proven to be powerful discriminator when evaluating male infertility (ASRM, 2015c; Cooper et al., 2010; Guzick et al., 2001; WHO, 2010). Patients with semen analyses that do not fall within laboratory reference ranges should be referred to a urologist for further testing, including endocrine evaluation, postejaculatory urinalysis, ultrasonography (e.g., transrectal, scrotal), and specialized clinical tests on semen and sperm (e.g., quantification of leukocytes, antisperm antibodies, sperm viability, and deoxyribonucleic acid [DNA] fragmentation tests; ASRM, 2015c; Cooper et al., 2010). Genetic screening may also be warranted and may include (a) testing for cystic fibrosis gene mutations, (b) karyotypic chromosomal abnormalities (e.g., Klinefelter syndrome, inversion, and balanced translocations), (c) Y-chromosome microdeletions, and (d) chromosome aneuploidy (ASRM, 2015c; Cooper et al., 2010; Guzick et al., 2001).

Management of Infertile Couples

The treatment and management of infertile couples begins with health promoting behaviors. Health care providers should counsel couples about the avoidance of modifiable, negative health behaviors (ACOG, 2005/2015).

HEALTH BEHAVIORS

Smoking • Both active and passive smoking reduce female and male fertility (ASRM, 2012f). Chemicals in cigarettes accelerate egg loss and decreases reproductive function by interfering with the ability of ovarian cells to make estrogen. This leads to an increase in susceptibility of the oocytes to genetic abnormalities (ASRM, 2012f). Men who smoke have been shown to have lower sperm counts and sperm motility with increased abnormalities in sperm shape and function (ASRM, 2012a, 2012f). Smoking is also associated with an increased risk of spontaneous abortion, and is thought to be linked to an increased risk for ectopic pregnancy. In all cases, health care providers should recommend smoking cessation as it may improve fertility and success rates with infertility treatments (ASRM, 2012f).

Advanced Maternal Age • Couples should be counseled to attempt pregnancy before the maternal age of 35 years. Studies have shown that both the number and quality of oocytes decrease, and the incidence of genetic abnormalities and spontaneous pregnancy loss increases in women older than 35 years (ASRM, 2012a, 2015b; Chandra et al., 2013; Mosher & Pratt, 1991). Women should take a supplement of 0.4 mg of folic acid every day. Megadose supplements of vitamins are not advised; recommended daily allowances should not exceed 100% (ACOG, 2014; CDC, 1992).

Body Weight • Regular exercise and a well-balanced diet should be encouraged (ACOG, 2013/2015; CDC, 2014).

Overweight and underweight both have effects on a woman's ability to conceive by causing hormone imbalances and ovulatory dysfunction (ACOG, 2013/2015; CDC, 2014). Obesity is defined as a BMI of 30 or above and is often associated with three physical alterations that physiologically interfere with ovulation and thus fertility: (1) increased peripheral aromatization of androgens to estrogens, (2) decreased levels of sex hormone binding globulin resulting in increased levels of free estradiol and testosterone, and (3) increased insulin levels that can stimulate ovarian stromal tissue producing androgens (ACOG, 2013/2015, 2014; CDC, 2014). Fertility issues with low body weight or obesity include (a) irregular or infrequent menstrual cycles, (b) increased risk of infertility, (c) increased risk during fertility surgical procedures, (d) increased risk of miscarriage, and (e) decreased success with fertility treatments (ACOG, 2013/2015, 2014; CDC, 2014). In obese patients, a weight loss of 5% to 10% may improve ovulation and pregnancy rates. In underweight patients (10%–15% below recommended weight), abnormal menstrual function and ovulatory dysfunction may occur (ASRM, 2015b). Referral is appropriate for women with a BMI that is less than 19 or underweight.

Stress • Couples who are being treated for infertility experience stress (ASRM, 2014e). Although stress has not been proven to cause infertility, it can affect the autonomic nervous, endocrine, and immune systems; change hormone levels; and interfere with ovulation (ASRM, 2014e; Homan et al., 2007). With each passing menstrual cycle, it is important for the health care provider to address stress in couples hoping for a pregnancy. This is important because there is some evidence that increased stress level negatively affects, for example, the outcome of fertility treatment, and also a couple's decision to discontinue fertility treatments (Brandes et al., 2009).

Alcohol and Caffeine • Although it is well known that no amount of alcohol is safe at any given time during pregnancy, there are limited studies regarding the impact of alcohol on fertility. Similarly, there is no consistent evidence supporting a negative effect of routine caffeine consumption on fertility (CDC, 2012; Chang et al., 2006; Homan et al., 2007). Even so, it has been postulated that any alcohol and caffeine effects on fertility are probably dose dependent (ACOG, 2014). Women actively trying to conceive and those who are pregnant should avoid drinking any amount and/or type of alcohol. It is recommended that all pregnant women limit their caffeine consumption to no more than 200 mg each day (equivalent to one 12-ounce cup of coffee; March of Dimes, 2015).

Ovulation Disorders

WHO CLASSIFICATION

WHO classifies ovulation disorders into three categories. WHO Class 1, *hypogonadotropic hypogonadal anovulation*, occurs in approximately 5% to 10% of infertile couples.

Low or low-normal FSH levels and low estradiol levels are caused by decreased hypothalamic secretion of or pituitary response to gonadotropin releasing hormone (GnRH; WHO Technical Report Series, 1992). Hypothalamic amenorrhea, caused from an excessively low BMI or extreme exercise, is an example of a WHO Class 1 ovulation disorder.

WHO Class 2, *normogonadotropic normoestrogenic anovulation*, is the most common type of ovulation disorder; it occurs in approximately 75% to 80% of infertile couples. With this ovulatory disorder, normal amounts of gonadotropins are secreted; however, FSH levels during the follicular phase are low (WHO Technical Report Series, 1992). PCOS is an example of a WHO Class 2 ovulation disorder.

WHO Class 3, *hypergonadotropic hypoestrogenic anovulation*, is estimated to occur in approximately 5% to 10% of couples experiencing infertility. In women with WHO Class 3 ovulatory disorder, there is an absence of follicular development because of premature ovarian failure or gonadal dysgenesis (WHO Technical Report Series, 1992).

POLYCYSTIC OVARIAN SYNDROME

PCOS can oftentimes be treated with behavioral changes (ASRM, 2014c). Weight loss, improved nutrition, and exercise are the recommended first-line therapy. Insulin-sensitizing agents help to improve the body's response to insulin, thereby working to restore normal insulin levels. Metformin (Glucophage), an antihyperglycemic, reduces insulin and androgen levels. According to the ASRM, both clomiphene citrate or letrozole are recommended as first-line treatment, followed by injectable gonadotropins (ASRM, 2014c, 2014b).

■ TREATMENT AND MANAGEMENT

Treatment of Oligomenorrhea or Anovulation

Oligomenorrhea and anovulation can lead to infertility. Oligomenorrhea is defined as light or infrequent menstruation, whereas anovulation is the failure of the ovary to release ova over a period (ASRM, 2008/2014). There are three categories of medications used to treat oligomenorrhea and anovulation. These medications are targeted for the purpose of inducing ovulation.

CLOMIPHENE CITRATE (CLOMID)

Clomiphene citrate (Clomid) is an oral medication and is a selective estrogen receptor modulator (SERM) with both estrogen antagonist and agonist properties, thus increasing gonadotropin release. Clomiphene citrate is indicated only for the treatment of WHO Class 2 ovulation disorders (Legro et al., 2014). Treatment typically begins on cycle day 5 and continues through day 9, with FDA-approved dosages ranging from 50 to 150 mg/d (Legro et al., 2014). Approximately 50% of women will ovulate on 50 mg of clomiphene citrate (ASRM, 2012e).

For those women who remain anovulatory, the dosage can be increased is subsequent cycles, up to 100 mg daily, for five days (ASRM, 2012e). The maximum dose is typically 200 mg daily, for 5 days (ASRM, 2012e). If a woman remains anovulatory and does not achieve pregnancy after three or four ovulatory cycles, she should be referred to a reproductive endocrinologist (RE) specialist (ASRM, 2012e).

Monitoring ovulation activity can be performed with (a) self-monitoring for urinary LH surge, and/or (b) serial ultrasound. Common side effects of clomiphene citrate include vasomotor flushes and abdominal discomfort. Less common side effects include breast tenderness, nausea, vomiting, nervousness, insomnia, and visual symptoms (ASRM, 2012e). Symptoms do not usually appear to be dose dependent. The patient should be informed that a fairly common side effect of clomiphene citrate therapy is the antiestrogenic effect on the uterus and cervix. This effect can result in a decrease in the quantity and quality of cervical mucus, as well as a thinning of the endometrium (ASRM, 2012e).

Clomiphene therapy is encouraging with an 80% success rate in inducing ovulation and an overall pregnancy rate of 30% of pregnancies occurring in the first three ovulatory cycles. Less than 10% of all gestations will be multiple, and those are predominantly twins (ASRM, 2012f). Pregnancies resulting from clomiphene therapy are not associated with increased risk of congenital abnormalities; risks are the same as for the general population. Current nationwide studies have shown no association between ovarian stimulation and an increased risk of endometrial or colorectal cancer (ASRM, 2014c).

AROMATASE INHIBITORS

Aromatase inhibitors (AIs) are most widely used for the treatment of breast cancer and prevention of reoccurrence. In regard to infertility, AIs have been proven to be effective when treating women with WHO Class 2 ovulatory disorders (those women who have failed to respond to clomiphene or those who have a thin endometrium; ASRM, 2012e). AIs block the action of aromatase, the cytochrome P450 enzyme that is responsible for the conversion of androstenedione and testosterone into estrone and estradiol, respectively (ASRM, 2012e). Administration of AIs in the early follicular phase prevents the normal negative feedback from estradiol on the hypothalamopituitary axis, resulting in an increased secretion of pituitary gonadotropins, predominantly FSH (Legro et al., 2014). AIs are usually administered orally in doses between 2.5 and 5 mg/d, between cycle days 3 and 7 (ASRM, 2012e).

AIs are usually well tolerated, although there are reported side effects. The most frequently reported side effects include hot flashes, nausea and vomiting, and leg cramps (ASRM, 2012e). There are advantages to using AIs instead of clomiphene for induction of ovulation. When using AIs, there is a reduced number of follicles produced, thus decreasing the risk for multiples during gestation. Furthermore, AIs have a shorter half-life (50 hours versus days), resulting in less antiestrogenic effect on the endometrium and cervical mucus (Legro et al., 2014). Studies have shown that pregnancy rates may be higher, and with fewer miscarriages, with AI use as compared with clomiphene citrate (Legro et al., 2014). AIs have been proven to equally safe when compared with clomiphene citrate (ASRM, 2012e).

GONADOTROPINS

Gonadotropins are used to induce follicular development and ovulation for anovulatory women, and also used in women undergoing ART. The treatment and management of gonadotropin therapy extends beyond the scope of the primary care health care provider's clinic and laboratory; it requires highly specialized laboratory and radiology services be available on site and on a daily basis. Gonadotropin preparations include agents with recombinant FSH or human menopausal gonadotropins containing FSH combined with LH. There are few studies that have evaluated the effectiveness of gonadotropin therapy (ASRM, 2012e). Many different protocols and combinations of drugs exist for ovulation induction during the follicular phase for recruitment of ovarian follicles (gonadotropin regimens are beyond the scope of this chapter). The success rate of gonadotropin therapy is influenced by the age and cause(s) of a woman's infertility (ASRM, 2012e). Approximately 20% to 60% of infertile women become pregnant after ovulation induction with gonadotropin therapy (ASRM, 2012e).

GnRH Analogs • GnRH agonists work by binding to pituitary GnRH receptors, resulting in an initial increase in both FSH and LH secretion (commonly known as the *flare effect*; ASRM, 2012e). Continued binding of the agonist results in a down regulation of GnRh receptors, with subsequent suppression of pituitary gonadotropin release, thereby preventing an endogenous LH surge (ASRM, 2012e). GnRh antagonists work by competitively binding to GnRh receptors in the anterior pituitary gland. These synthetic drugs are also utilized to prevent spontaneous LH surges and ovulation. Studies have shown a higher pregnancy rate in cycles utilizing GnRH (ASRM, 2012e). Another advantage of GnRh antagonists is that fewer injections are required and stimulation cycles are shorter. However, both GnRh agonists and antagonists are equally effective in preventing spontaneous LH surges. Although slightly more expensive, GnRh antagonists may also be associated with a lower risk of ovarian hyperstimulation (ASRM, 2012e).

Human Chorionic Gonadotropin • Human chorionic gonadotropin (hCG) stimulates the LH surge that causes ovulation at mid-cycle (ASRM, 2012e). The alpha subunit of hCG is identical to that of LH. Additionally, there are similarities between the beta chains (ASRM, 2012e). Ovulation occurs between 32 and 38 hours after hCG administration. Health care providers should note that a pregnancy test will be falsely positive if taken 10 days or less post-hCG administration (ASRM, 2012e).

Infertility Treatment Procedures

INTRAUTERINE INSEMINATION

IUI is theoretically grounded in the belief that the likelihood of fertilization is increased when a large number of sperm are placed high in the reproductive tract. The procedure involves the placement of motile, concentrated sperm directly into the uterine cavity (ASRM, 2012d). In order for IUI to be performed, a woman's cycle must be ovulatory, there must be at least one patent fallopian tube, an adequate number of sperm must be available at hand, and there can be no suspicion or evidence of cervical, uterine, or pelvic infection (ASRM, 2012d). IUI is generally well tolerated; however, it may be associated with cramping. IUI has been shown to improve the pregnancy rate when used in conjunction with clomiphene and gonadotropins (ASRM, 2012e).

Proper sperm collection is critical when preforming IUI. The specimen should be collected the morning of the IUI, after abstaining from ejaculation for 2 to 3 days. On ejaculation, the specimen should be collected in a sterile container. The sperm is then washed for the purpose of separating the ejaculate from the prostaglandins and seminal fluid. This procedure concentrates the amount of motile sperm by removing cellular debris (ASRM, 2012d).

Donor Insemination • Donor insemination (DI) can be used for women with a partner who has any of the following: (a) azospermia, (b) low sperm count, (c) issues with sperm motility or abnormal morphology, (d) absence of testes and/or vas deferens, (e) presence of antisperm antibodies, and/or (f) previous vasectomy (Guzick et al., 2001; WHO, 2010). Couples may choose to use DI when (a) there is a personal or family history of genetic disease or birth defect, (b) an individual is serodiscordant for sexually transmitted viruses (Sauer et al., 2009), (c) when the patient is a woman without a male partner (ASRM, 2012b), and/or (d) when an individual has hemolytic disease. Donors are blood typed and screened for STIs, cytomegalovirus, Tay-Sachs, thalassemia, and sickle cell. Donor matching is performed to ensure compatibility in donor and female patient characteristics. Over time, DI has become less common because of the success of both IVF and ICSI (ASRM, 2012d). Rates of miscarriage and birth defects for donor sperm are comparable to those of spontaneous conceptions (ASRM, 2012d).

ASSISTED REPRODUCTIVE TECHNOLOGIES

ART is a complex procedure that is usually conducted by an RE specialist (ASRM, 2015a). This section is a brief overview of the procedure and is presented through the lens of patient counseling. As such, a discussion on the technique/procedure and follow-up is limited. Assisted reproductive technologies consists of a conglomerate of all techniques involved with the direct retrieval of oocytes from the ovary. These technologies have expanded exponentially over the past 10 years. They include (a) GIFT, (b) zygote intrafallopian transfer (ZIFT), (c) IVF, and (d) ICSI. Advanced techniques used to harvest sperm for ART procedures include testicular sperm extraction (TESE) and microsurgical epididymal sperm aspiration (MESA; ASRM, 2015a).

The average percentage of ART cycles leading to live births was 37.4% for women younger than 35 years, 31.1% for women aged 35 to 37 years, and 20.6% for women aged 37 to 40 years (CDC, ASRM, SART, 2015; Luke et al., 2012; Sunderam et al., 2015).

OOCYTE RETRIEVAL

Ovarian stimulation is monitored by serial measurements of serum estradiol and ultrasound imaging of ovarian follicles. Transvaginal ultrasound-guided follicle aspiration is universally used for oocyte retrieval. Oocyte retrieval is approximately a 30-minute procedure and is performed approximately 34 hours to 36 hours after hCG (trigger) administration (ASRM, 2013b). Although bleeding and/or infection are noted complications, they are uncommon (ASRM, 2013b, 2014b).

PRESERVATION OF EMBRYOS

As multiple follicles are aspirated during retrieval, much discussion has occurred over the preservation of embryos. Specific guidelines have been established to address concerns of numbers of embryos to implant and how to preserve embryos that are not used (ASRM, 2013a, 2013b, 2013c). The ASRM recommends that (a) no more than three embryos be transferred in women younger than 35 years, (b) no more than four transferred in women aged 35 to 40 years, and (c) no more than five embryos be transferred in patients older than 40 years (ASRM, 2013a). If more than three embryos implant inside the uterus, multifetal reduction can be performed to reduce the number of implantations (ASRM, 2013a). Extra embryos can be cryopreserved for use at a later stage. Approximately two thirds of embryos survive after freezing and thawing, and the transfer of cryopreserved embryos significantly increases the success rate from single oocyte retrieval (ASRM, 2013a).

GAMETE INTRAFALLOPIAN TRANSFER

GIFT is a modified version of IVF. This procedure is indicated for couples without fallopian tube pathology and a normal sperm count. GIFT is a basic form of ART, whereby oocytes are obtained from the ovaries and sperm are washed and placed directly into the fallopian tubes laparoscopically, via the use of a transfer catheter (ASRM, 2015a). Individuals may choose GIFT over IVF (e.g., for religious beliefs) as it relies on the body's natural processes to produce pregnancy (ASRM, 2015a).

ZYGOTE INTRAFALLOPIAN TRANSFER

ZIFT is a variation of GIFT in which fertilization occurs in vitro, after egg retrieval, from the ovaries. Ejaculated or surgically retrieved sperm are prepared by washing, centrifuging, and then fertilizing using a swim-up technique (ASRM, 2015a). Approximately 50,000 sperm are placed around each oocyte, allowing fertilization to occur naturally (ASRM, 2015a). The fertilized egg, a zygote, is transferred to the fallopian tubes laparoscopically. ZIFT procedures constitute only approximately 1% of total ART (ASRM, 2015a).

IN VITRO FERTILIZATION

IVF accounts for more than 99% of ART procedures (ASRM, 2013b). IVF was introduced in the United States in 1981. Between 1985 and 2007, more than 500,000 babies were born in the United States as a result of ART procedures (IVF, GIFT, ZIFT, and combination procedures; ASRM, 2013b). By 2011, 36% of all fresh nondonor ART cycles resulted in pregnancy and 29% results in a live birth (Sunderam et al., 2015). Because of advances in ART, in the general population, a single IVF cycle now has a higher fecundability (29%) compared with a natural conception cycle (27.7%; Luke et al., 2012). The average cost of an IVF cycle in the United States is $12,000; medications run an additional $3,000 to $5,000 (Sunderam et al., 2015). Indications for IVF include: (a) male factor infertility, (b) tubal endometrial factor infertility, (c) failed conservative therapy, (d) multifactorial infertility, (e) advanced maternal age and/or declining ovarian reserve, (f) ovarian failure (donor eggs needed), (g) uterine factor (surrogacy), (h) genetic abnormalities, and/or (i) a history of recurrent miscarriage (ASRM, 2013a, 2015a).

PREIMPLANTATION GENETIC DIAGNOSIS

Preimplantation genetic diagnosis (PGD) is a reproductive technology used with an IVF cycle. Specifically, the procedure involves removing a cell from an IVF embryo for genetic testing before transferring the embryo to the uterus. PGD can also be used for prenatal aneuploidy screening and the diagnosis of chromosomal abnormalities (e.g. translocations, inversions; ASRM, 2014d; Genetics & IVF Institute, n.d.). For example, in the case where one of the parents is a known translocation carrier, testing by PGD is helping to reduce the risk of spontaneous abortion. The use of PGD for sex selection, for nonmedical reasons, is an ethical dilemma and is not recommended by ASRM (Ethics Committee, 2015).

Oocyte Donation

Using donated oocytes can be a highly effective infertility treatment for women (a) who are older than 35 years, (b) have experienced premature ovarian failure, (c) are younger and have failed to achieve a pregnancy with IVF using their own oocytes, and/or (d) with poor-quality oocytes (ASRM, 2013c). The use of donated oocytes through IVF has achieved pregnancy rates of approximately 55% (ASRM, 2013c; CDC, 2015a; Ethics Committee, 2013c). Donors are carefully selected and, ideally, are younger than 28 years of age. There are clear criteria for physical and psychological screening and record keeping for all gamete donors. These criteria are available at www.asrm.org/uploadedFiles/ASRM_Content/News_and_Publications/Practice_Guidelines/Guidelines_and_Minimum_Standards/2008_Guidelines_for_gamete (1).pdf (ASRM, 2013c).

Fertilization is typically accomplished with the recipient's husband's sperm and the resultant embryo(s) placed into the recipient. The endometrium of the recipient is prepared for implantation with medications and monitoring of the endometrium is undertaken by ultrasound to ensure that the endometrial stripe is greater than 6 mm in thickness (ASRM, 2013c). Typically only one or two embryos are placed, with extra embryos being cryopreserved for future use (ASRM, 2013b). There are many ethical concerns about gamete donation and compensation (Ethics Committee, 2007). The ASRM created an excellent document, *Recommendations for gamete and embryo donation: a committee opinion* (ASRM, 2013c), which addresses compensation, informed consent, and many other ethical issues regarding oocyte donation (www.asrm.org).

Technologies for Men

Sperm aspiration techniques are used to obtain viable sperm from men with no sperm (azospermia), sperm without motility, or dead sperm (Guzick et al., 2001). Azospermia occurs because of a blockage in the male reproductive tract with sperm trapped in the epididymis (obstructive), or as the result of impaired or nonexistent sperm production (nonobstructive; ASRM, 2015c). ICSI must be used for conception after sperm are collected. The following paragraphs include a discussion about the three sperm-harvesting techniques used to obtain sperm from men with obstructive azospermia.

MICROSURGICAL EPIDIDYMAL SPERM ASPIRATION

MESA can be used for men with a congenital absence of the vas deferens or for those men who have had a vasectomy. MESA is a relatively safe procedure with minimal complications when performed by a specialist in microsurgery (ASRM, 2015c).

TESTICULAR SPERM EXTRACTION

TESE involves removal of testicular tissue to retrieve sperm from within the seminiferous tubules. This is the recommended method for sperm retrieval in men with nonobstructive azospermia and an alternative option for men with obstructive azospermia (ASRM, 2015c, 2015a). As with other sperm-harvesting techniques, sperm can be frozen and stored for later use (ASRM, 2015c, 2015a).

INTRACYTOPLASMIC SPERM INJECTION

In cases of severe male factor infertility, ICSI is a technique that is frequently used for sperm harvesting. A single mature sperm is isolated, and by means of a microneedle (using a micromanipulator), the single sperm is injected directly into the oocyte, allowing fertilization to occur (ASRM, 2015c, 2015a). As a result of ICSI, fertilization occurs in approximately 50% to 80% of oocytes (ASRM, 2015c, 2015a).

Integrative Medicine

There is little found in the literature supporting the use of integrative methods for treating infertility, although this is an area in need of more research. One study demonstrated that acupuncture on the day of embryo transfer might increase pregnancy rates; however, the study involved a small sample size (Cheong et al., 2008). Another study identified that the most common strategies used in one clinic to address infertility included religious intervention, changes in sexual practices, and diet (Schaffir et al., 2009). The authors also reported that younger patients, irrespective of education, parity, and/or duration of infertility, were more willing to consider and use alternative methods/interventions (Schaffir et al., 2009).

Psychological Aspects of Infertility

The psychological aspects of infertility cannot be minimized. The inability to conceive and carry a child to term is often viewed as the first failure in a couple's life experience. This experience often leads to stress, grief, depression, a sense of loss, a sense of failure, and disappointment, with anger toward or resentment of the spouse. Resolve is an infertility support group with many local chapters that offers support for couples experiencing infertility.

Furthermore, the need for assistance in conception and carrying a child to term takes away from the privacy and intimacy of the act of procreation, instead moving it into a public and technologically oriented arena. This is not how most people believe creating a family should occur. Very private moments become mechanized, and time becomes scrutinized and graded by health care providers. Therapeutic communication techniques are a necessity.

It is useful for the health care provider to use screening tools for depression and resources for patients. These include recognition of and management of stressors, coping with holidays, families, other people's expectations, and creating alternate plans to avoid situations that could provoke discomfort. Health care providers need to assess for stress, which can be done through a list of questions (Domar et al., 2015).

1. Do you feel uncomfortable being around pregnant women and or children/babies?
2. Do you find that you try to avoid situations where there may be pregnant women and/or small children/babies?
3. Is your sexual relationship very satisfying, satisfying, or dissatisfying? If dissatisfying, do you feel that your infertility has led to a negative impact on your sex life?
4. Do you only make love during the fertile times of your cycle?
5. Do you feel that you and your partner mostly agree about how to proceed with infertility treatment?
6. Do you feel that your partner is sympathetic and supportive of you?
7. How is your mood? How have you been feeling? Are you able to enjoy your usual activities?

8. Are you worried? Do you have difficulty concentrating or sleeping? Are you restless?
9. Has your appetite changed?

Patients need to be given permission to cry, be angry, mourn, and grieve. They need to be provided with a safe place to vent. It is useful to identify several therapists who are experienced with the infertility process and make appropriate referrals. The health care provider must recognize there are different styles of coping between partners, and one fix does not work for each partner or all couples. Finally, holidays and special occasions such as Mother's Day, Father's Day, birthdays, and holidays can all increase a couple's stressors.

Ethical Issues Related to Reproductive Technologies

As the scope of assisted reproductive technologies continues to expand, there are an increasing number of medical, social, moral, and ethical dilemmas that arise. Clinical treatment strategies should ensure a stepwise progression from conservative to invasive therapies to avoid excessive treatments and costs. Furthermore, to offer fertility treatments when the prognosis is poor is a dilemma. It is imperative that health care providers provide full disclosure before the initiation of all treatments regarding the success rates of each option in that particular center (Ethics Committee, 2012a).

Using family members as gamete donors and/or surrogates is also becoming a more frequent occurrence. In all cases, counseling for all parties, including the partners of donors and surrogates, is strongly encouraged (Ethics Committee, 2012b). Although it is now acceptable to use family members as donors or surrogates, consanguineous gamete donations from first-degree relatives is unacceptable and not medically advised (Ethics Committee, 2012b). Should offspring be informed of the facts of their conception by gamete donation, and if so, how much information about donors should be revealed (Ethics Committee, 2013b)? Both counseling and informed consent about disclosure are essential for the donor and recipients, and parties should agree in advance on how and when ART programs and sperm banks will release donor information to the recipients. Although disclosure to offspring regarding the use of donor gametes is encouraged, it is ultimately the choice of recipient parents (Ethics Committee, 2013b).

Another medical, social, moral, and ethical dilemma is whether to donate spare embryos for embryonic stem cell research (Ethics Committee, 2013a). This question has elicited diverse and conflicting perspectives since the advent of IVF. The ASRM Ethics Committee (2013b) regards embryo research as ethically acceptable if it is likely to provide significant new knowledge that will benefit human health and if it is conducted in ways that render the embryo with the utmost respect. Another unresolved issue relates to financial incentives to recruit gamete donors (Ethics Committee, 2007). Although financial remuneration has been well established for male donors, compensation for oocyte donors is more challenging. The question of what constitutes fair compensation to oocyte donors remains unresolved. Should these donors be compensated for their time and/or loss of work, or should additional compensation be offered to them as an incentive? ASRM recommends either no compensation, or, if compensation is warranted, it should not be in excess of $5,000 (Ethics Committee, 2007). Sex selection with PGD for family balancing is another unresolved and controversial issue (Ethical Committee, 2015). Most fertility clinics do not offer PGD for sex selection in the absence of screening for sex-linked diseases (Ethics Committee, 2015).

In the cases of gamete donation, there are issues about the health history of the donor and their availability should certain unforeseen conditions arise (Ethics Committee, 2013b). Should the child be told of his or her heritage? If not, why not? If so, how? These and many other medical, social, moral, and ethical dilemmas are yet to be determined.

Considerations for Special Populations

CANCER SURVIVORS

Another issue that is becoming more prevalent is fertility preservation and reproduction in cancer patients (ASRM, 2015d). The improvement in cancer treatment has enabled many younger individuals with cancer to survive. Furthermore, many women aged 20 to 49 diagnosed with cancer have excellent (5–10 year) survival rates (ASRM, 2015d). Unfortunately, successful treatment in younger patients may lead to reduced fertility; this varies and is dependent on the age at diagnosis as well as the type of cancer and treatment. If damage to reproductive organs as a result of treatment is unavoidable, cryopreservation of gametes, embryos, and/or gonadal tissue may help address later fertility. Techniques for freezing oocytes and ovarian tissue should be considered. It is imperative that patients whose gametes, embryos, and/or tissues are cryopreserved and stored give very specific directions for future disposition (ASRM, 2015d). Another issue to consider is whether the offspring of these patients are at an increased risk of congenital abnormalities, chromosomal defects, or cancer as a result of any cancer treatment/s or effects of ART. To date, studies that have examined pregnancy outcomes in cancer survivors have found no significant increase in congenital malformations or cancer in the resulting offspring (ASRM, 2015d). Infertility after cancer certainly can increase the likelihood of stress, loss, and anger (ASRM, 2015d).

HUMAN IMMUNODEFICIENCY VIRUS

Over the past three decades, a prevalent issue has surfaced regarding the use of infertility treatment in patients who are HIV positive (Ethics Committee, 2010). In 1994, the Ethics Committee of the ASRM published guidelines concerning patients with HIV who require reproductive assistance (2010). Since then, the understanding and treatment of HIV-infected individuals and laboratory techniques for the preparation of virus-free sperm for reproductive assistance have changed substantially (Ethics Committee, 2010). Today, HIV infection is now recognized as a chronic disease and women are able to achieve a healthy pregnancy.

Previously, ethical issues were also raised by knowingly risking the birth of a child with HIV. More recently, the risk has been greatly reduced with antiretrovirals that are taken by the pregnant woman before and throughout her pregnancy (Ethics Committee, 2010). Additionally, the risk of transmitting HIV to health care professionals as a result of accidental exposure from a patient's blood or contamination with body fluids at birth continues to be a concern. It is important for health care providers to consider HIV-positive patients seeking fertility evaluation, treatment, and management as disabled, and therefore protected under the Americans with Disabilities Act (Ethics Committee, 2010). IVF with ICSI has resulted in 170 live births with no instances of HIV transmission to mother or child (Sauer, 2009).

OTHER STIs

The CDC (2015c) and ASRM have published guidelines for treating patients with most STIs.

LESBIAN WOMEN

A significant number of women choose to have children through donor insemination or in vitro fertilization with donor sperm after identifying themselves as lesbian, bisexual, or single (ASRM, 2012b). Many of the needs of these patients who have access to ART will be similar to those of heterosexual women. There is no persuasive evidence of harm to children or support for restricting access to ART on the basis of marital status or sexual orientation (ASRM, 2012b). The ASRM advises that programs should treat all requests for ART equally without regard to sexual orientation (ASRM, 2012b).

ADOPTION

If all available options have been attempted and pregnancy has not occurred, referral to area agencies to facilitate adoption should be offered (ASRM, 2014a). International adoption is another opportunity available to infertile couples, although financial costs are more substantial. Adoption is not an option for all couples, however, there are many resources available at Resolve support groups (ASRM, 2014a).

■ SUMMARY

The goal of the health care provider is to (a) conduct a complete medical investigation, (b) treat abnormalities, (c) educate a couple as to their treatment choices, and (d) refer to support services in the case of adoption. Advances in the treatment of infertility are occurring rapidly and it is challenging for the primary care health care provider to be aware of the most advanced and appropriate treatment regimens for patients with fertility issues. The ASRM Practice Committee has established evidence-based guidelines to assist health care providers with best clinical practices recommendations (ASRM, 2015a, 2015c). Finally, the

psychological impact on couples facing infertility should not be minimized; myths and misconceptions should be dispelled.

■ REFERENCES

American College of Obstetricians and Gynecologists (ACOG). (2005/2015). *The importance of preconception care in the continuum of women's health care.* Number 313. Retrieved from https://www.acog.org/-/media/Committee-Opinions/Committee-on-Gynecologic-Practice/co313.pdf?dmc=1&ts=20160118T0849387653

American College of Obstetricians and Gynecologists (ACOG). (2013/2015). Obesity in pregnancy. Committee Opinion No. 548. *Obstetrics & Gynecology, 126*(6), 1321–1322.

American College of Obstetricians and Gynecologists (ACOG). (2014). Preconception and interconception care. In *Guidelines for women's health care: A resource manual* (4th ed., pp. 381–398). Washington, DC: American College of Obstetricians and Gynecologists.

American Society for Reproductive Medicine (ASRM). (2004/2008). *Definition of infertility and recurrent pregnancy loss; committee opinion.* Birmingham, AL: Fertility and Sterility. Retrieved from http://dx.doi.org/10.1016/j.fertnstert.2012.09.023

American Society for Reproductive Medicine (ASRM). (2008). *Recommendations for reducing the risk of viral transmission during fertility treatment with the use of autologous gametes: A committee opinion.* Retrieved from http://www.asrm.org/uploadedFiles/ASRM_Content/News_and_Publications/Practice_Guidelines/Guidelines_and_Minimum_Standards/Guidelines_for_reducing(1).pdf

American Society for Reproductive Medicine (ASRM). (2012a). *Age and fertility.* Retrieved from http://www.asrm.org/uploadedFiles/ASRM_Content/Resources/Patient_Resources/Fact_Sheets_and_Info_Booklets/agefertility.pdf

American Society for Reproductive Medicine (ASRM). (2012b). *Counseling issues regarding gay men and lesbians seeking assisted reproductive technologies.* Retrieved from https://www.asrm.org/uploadedFiles/ASRM_Content/Resources/Patient_Resources/Fact_Sheets_and_Info_Booklets/Counseling%20issues%20for%20gay%20men%20and%20lesbians%20FINAL%204-23-12.pdf

American Society for Reproductive Medicine (ASRM). (2012c). *Diagnostic testing for female infertility.* Retrieved from https://www.asrm.org/FACTSHEET_Diagnostic_Testing_for_Female_Infertility

American Society for Reproductive Medicine (ASRM). (2012d). *Intrauterine insemination.* Retrieved from http://www.asrm.org/uploadedFiles/ASRM_Content/Resources/Patient_Resources/Fact_Sheets_and_Info_Booklets/IUI_3-19-12_FINAL.pdf

American Society for Reproductive Medicine (ASRM). (2012e). *Medications for inducing ovulation: A guide for patients.* Retrieved from http://www.asrm.org/BOOKLET_Medications_for_Inducing_Ovulation

American Society for Reproductive Medicine (ASRM). (2012f). *Smoking and infertility: A committee opinion.* Retrieved from http://www.asrm.org/uploadedFiles/ASRM_Content/News_and_Publications/Practice_Guidelines/Educational_Bulletins/Smoking_and_infertility(1).pdf

American Society for Reproductive Medicine (ASRM). (2013a). *Criteria for number of embryos to transfer: A committee opinion.* Retrieved from http://www.asrm.org/uploadedFiles/ASRM_Content/News_and_Publications/Practice_Guidelines/Guidelines_and_Minimum_Standards/Guidelines_on_number_of_embryos(1).pdf

American Society for Reproductive Medicine (ASRM). (2013b). *Mature oocyte cryopreservation: A guideline.* Retrieved from http://www.asrm.org/uploadedFiles/ASRM_Content/News_and_Publications/Practice_Guidelines/Committee_Opinions/Ovarian_tissue_and_oocyte(1).pdf

American Society for Reproductive Medicine (ASRM). (2013c). *Recommendations for gamete and embryo donation: A committee opinion.* Retrieved from http://www.asrm.org/uploadedFiles/ASRM_Content/News_and_Publications/Practice_Guidelines/Guidelines_and_Minimum_Standards/2008_Guidelines_for_gamete(1).pdf

American Society for Reproductive Medicine (ASRM). (2014a). *Adoption: Where to start and what to think about.* Retrieved from http://www.asrm.org/FACTSHEET_Adoption

American Society for Reproductive Medicine (ASRM). (2014b). *Ovarian stimulation for IVF does not increase the risk for endometrium or colorectal cancer: Nationwide Cohort Study.* Retrieved from http://www.asrm.org/Ovarian_Stimulation_for_IVF_Does_Not_Increase_Risk_of_Endometrial_or_Colorectal_Cancer_Results_from_a_Nationwide_Cohort_Study

American Society for Reproductive Medicine (ASRM). (2014c). *Polycystic ovarian syndrome.* Retrieved from http://www.asrm.org/uploaded-Files/ASRM_Content/Resources/Patient_Resources/Fact_Sheets_and_Info_Booklets/PCOS.pdf

American Society for Reproductive Medicine (ASRM). (2014d). *Preimplantation genetic testing.* Retrieved from http://www.asrm.org/FACTSHEET_Preimplantation_genetic_testing

American Society for Reproductive Medicine (ASRM). (2014e). *Stress and infertility.* Retrieved from http://www.asrm.org/uploadedFiles/ASRM_Content/Resources/Patient_Resources/Fact_Sheets_and_Info_Booklets/Stress-Fact.pdf

American Society for Reproductive Medicine (ASRM). (2015a). *Assisted reproductive technology: A guide for patients.* Retrieved from http://www.asrm.org/uploadedFiles/ASRM_Content/Resources/Patient_Resources/Fact_Sheets_and_Info_Booklets/ART.pdf

American Society for Reproductive Medicine (ASRM). (2015b). *Diagnostic evaluation of the female patient: A committee opinion.* Retrieved from http://www.asrm.org/uploadedFiles/ASRM_Content/News_and_Publications/Practice_Guidelines/Committee_Opinions/Diagnostic_eval_infertile_female_inpress-noprint.pdf

American Society for Reproductive Medicine (ASRM). (2015c). *Diagnostic evaluation of the infertile male: A committee opinion.* Retrieved from http://www.asrm.org/uploadedFiles/ASRM_Content/News_and_Publications/Practice_Guidelines/Committee_Opinions/optimal_evaluation_of_the_infertile_male(1).pdf

American Society for Reproductive Medicine (ASRM). (2015d). *Female cancer, cryopreservation, and fertility.* Retrieved from https://www.asrm.org/uploadedFiles/ASRM_Content/Resources/Patient_Resources/Fact_Sheets_and_Info_Booklets/Female_Cancers_Cryopreservation_and_Fertility_7-25-11.pdf

American Society for Reproductive Medicine (ASRM). (2015f). *Obesity and reproduction: A committee opinion.* Retrieved from http://www.asrm.org/uploadedFiles/ASRM_Content/News_and_Publications/Practice_Guidelines/Committee_Opinions/Obesity_and_reproduction-noprint.pdf

Brandes, M., van der Steen, J. O., Bokdam, S. B., Hamilton, C. J., de Bruin, J. P., Nelen, W. L., & Kremer, J. A. (2009). When and why do subfertile couples discontinue their fertility care? A longitudinal cohort study in a secondary care subfertility population. *Human Reproduction, 24*(12), 3127–3135.

Bulletti, C., Coccia, M. E., Battistoni, S., & Borini, A. (2010). Endometriosis and infertility. *Journal of Assisted Reproduction and Genetics, 27*(8), 441–447.

Centers for Disease Control and Prevention (CDC). (1992). *Recommendations for the use of folic acid to reduce the number of cases of spina bifida and other neural tube defects.* Retrieved from http://www.cdc.gov/mmwr/preview/mmwrhtml/00019479.htm

Centers for Disease Control and Prevention (CDC). (2012). Alcohol use and binge drinking among women of childbearing age—United States, 2006–2010. *Morbidity and Mortality Weekly Report, 61*(28), 534–538.

Centers for Disease Control and Prevention (CDC). (2014). *Women's health: Overweight and obesity.* Retrieved from http://www.cdc.gov/women/az/overweight.htm

Centers for Disease Control and Prevention (CDC). (2015a). *Infertility FAQs: What is infertility?* Retrieved from http://www.cdc.gov/reproductivehealth/Infertility/index.htm

Centers for Disease Control and Prevention (CDC). (2015b). *Key statistics from the National Survey of Family Growth.* Retrieved from http://www.cdc.gov/nchs/nsfg/key_statistics.htm

Centers for Disease Control and Prevention (CDC). (2015c). *STDs and infertility.* Retrieved from http://www.cdc.gov/std/infertility/default.htm

Centers for Disease Control and Prevention (CDC), American Society for Reproductive Medicine (ASRM), & Society for Assisted Reproductive Technology (SART). (2015). *2013 Assisted reproductive technology fertility clinic success rates report.* Atlanta, GA: U.S. Department of Health and Human Services.

Chandra, A., Copen, C. E., & Stephen, E. H. (2013). Infertility and impaired fecundability in the United States, 1982–2010: Data from the National Survey of Family Growth. *National Health Statistics Report, 14*(67), 1–18.

Chang, G., McNamara, T. K., Haimovici, F., & Hornstein, M. D. (2006). Problem drinking in women evaluated for infertility. *American Journal of Addiction, 15*(2), 174–179.

Cheong, Y. C., Hung, Y. N. G., & Ledger, W. L. (2008). Acupuncture and assisted conception. *The Cochrane Database of Systematic Reviews.* doi:10.1002/14651858.CD006920.pub2

Cooper, T. G., Noonan, E., von Eckardstein, S., Auger, J., Baker, H. W., Behre, H. M., ... Vogelsong, K. M. (2010). World Health Organization reference values for human semen characteristics. *Human Reproduction Update, 16*, 231–245.

Coppus, S. F., Opmeer, B. C., Logan, S., van der Veen, F., Bhattacharya, S., & Mol, B. W. (2007). The predictive value of medical history taking and chlamydia IgG ELISA antibody testing (CAT) in the selection of subfertile women for diagnostic laparoscopy: A clinical prediction model approach. *Human Reproduction Update, 22*, 1353–1358.

Dewailly, D., Andersen, C. Y., Balen, A., Broekmans, F., Dilaver, N., Fanchin, R., ... Anderson, R. A. (2014). The physiology and clinical utility of anti-Mullerian hormone in women. *Human Reproduction Update, 20*, 370.

Domar, A. D., Gross, J., Rooney, K., & Boivin, J. (2015). Exploratory randomized trial on the effect of a brief psychological intervention on emotions, quality of life, discontinuation, and pregnancy rates in in vitro fertilization patients. *Fertility and Sterility, 104*(2), 440.

Ethics Committee of the American Society for Reproductive Medicine. (2007). *Financial compensation for oocyte donors.* Retrieved from http://www.asrm.org/uploadedFiles/ASRM_Content/News_and_Publications/Ethics_Committee_Reports_and_Statements/financial_incentives.pdf

Ethics Committee of the American Society for Reproductive Medicine. (2010). *Human immunodeficiency virus and infertility treatments: A committee opinion.* Retrieved from http://www.asrm.org/uploadedFiles/ASRM_Content/News_and_Publications/Ethics_Committee_Reports_and_Statements/hivethics.pdf

Ethics Committee of the American Society for Reproductive Medicine. (2012a). *Fertility treatment when the prognosis is poor or futile: A committee opinion.* Retrieved from http://www.asrm.org/uploadedFiles/ASRM_Content/News_and_Publications/Ethics_Committee_Reports_and_Statements/futility.pdf

Ethics Committee of the American Society for Reproductive Medicine. (2012b). *Using family members as gamete donors or surrogates.* Retrieved from http://www.asrm.org/uploadedFiles/ASRM_Content/News_and_Publications/Ethics_Committee_Reports_and_Statements/family_members.pdf

Ethics Committee of the American Society for Reproductive Medicine. (2013a). *Donating embryos for human embryonic stem cell (hESC) research: A committee opinion.* Retrieved from http://www.asrm.org/uploadedFiles/ASRM_Content/News_and_Publications/Ethics_Committee_Reports_and_Statements/donatingspare.pdf

Ethics Committee of the American Society for Reproductive Medicine. (2013b). *Informing offspring of their conception by gamete or embryo donation: a committee opinion.* Retrieved from http://www.asrm.org/uploadedFiles/ASRM_Content/News_and_Publications/Ethics_Committee_Reports_and_Statements/informing_offspring_donation.pdf

Ethics Committee of the American Society for Reproductive Medicine. (2013c). *Oocyte or embryo donation to women of advanced age: A committee opinion.* Retrieved from http://www.asrm.org/uploadedFiles/ASRM_Content/News_and_Publications/Ethics_Committee_Reports_and_Statements/postmeno.pdf

Ethics Committee of the American Society for Reproductive Medicine. (2015). *Use of reproductive technology for sex selection for nonmedical reasons.* Retrieved from https://www.asrm.org/uploadedFiles/ASRM_Content/News_and_Publications/Ethics_Committee_Reports_and_Statements/Recc_practices_mgmt_embryology_andrology_endocrinology_labs2014-members.pdf

Genetics & IVF Institute (n.d.). *Genetic services: What is PGD?* Retrieved from http://www.givf.com/geneticservices/whatispgd.shtml

Guzick, D. S., Sullivan, M. W., Adamson, G. D., Cedars, M. I., Falk, R. J., Peterson, E. P., & Steinkampf, M. P. (1998). Efficacy of treatment for unexplained infertility. *Fertility and Sterility, 70*, 207–213.

Guzick, D. S., Overstreet, J. W., Factor-Litvak, P., Brazil, C. K., Nakajima, S. T., Coutifaris, C., & Vogel, D. L.; National Cooperative Reproductive Medicine Network. (2001). Sperm morphology, motility, and concentration in fertile and infertile men. *New England Journal of Medicine, 345*(19), 1388–1393.

Homan, G. F., Davies, M., & Norman, R. (2007). The impact of lifestyle factors on reproductive performance in the general population and those undergoing infertility treatment: A review. *Human Reproduction Update, 13*(3), 209–223.

Hsu, A., Khachikyan, I., & Stratton, P. (2010). Invasive and non-invasive methods for the diagnosis of endometriosis. *Clinical Obstetrics & Gynecology, 53*(2), 413–419.

Hsu, A., Arny, M., Knee, A. B., Bell, C., Cook, E., Novak. A. L., & Grow, D. R. (2011). Antral follicle count in clinical practice: Analyzing clinical relevance. *Fertility and Sterility, 95*, 474.

Legro, R. S., Bryzyski, R. G., Diamond, M. P., Coutifaris, C., Schlaff, W. D., Casson, P.,.... Zhang, H.; NICHD Reproductive Medicine Network. (2014). Letrozole versus clomiphene for infertility in the polycystic ovarian syndrome. *New England Journal of Medicine, 371*, 119.

Luke, B., Brown, M. B., Wantman, E., Lederman, A., Gibbons, W., Schattman, G. L.,...Stern, J. E. (2012). Cumulative birth rates with linked assisted reproductive technology cycles. *New England Journal of Medicine, 366*, 2483.

March of Dimes. (2015). *Caffeine in pregnancy.* Retrieved from http://www.marchofdimes.org/pregnancy/caffeine-in-pregnancy.aspx

Martin, J. A., Hamilton, B. E., Sutton, P. D., Ventura, S. J., Menacker, F., Kirmeyer, S., & Munson, M. L. (2007). Births: Final data for 2005. *National Vital Statistics Reports, 56*(6). Hyattsville, MD: National Center for Health Statistics.

McGovern, P. G., Myers, E. R., Silva, S., Coutifaris, C., Carson, S. A., Legro, R. S.,...Diamond, M. P.; NICHD National Cooperative Reproductive Medicine Network. (2004). Absence of secretory endometrium after false-positive home urine luteinizing hormone testing. *Fertility and Sterility, 82*, 1273–1277.

Mosher, W. D., & Pratt, W. F. (1991). Fecundity and infertility in the United States: Incidence and trends. *Fertility and Sterility, 56*(2), 192–193.

Nardo, L. G., & Chouliaras, S. (2015). Definitions and epidemiology of unexplained female infertility. In *Unexplained fertility: Pathophysiology, evaluation, & treatment* (pp. 21–25). New York, NY: Springer Publishing.

National Organization for Rare Disorders (NORD). (2005). *Asherman's syndrome.* Retrieved from http://rarediseases.org/rare-diseases/ashermans-syndrome

Panchal, S., & Nagori, C. (2014). Imaging techniques for assessment of tubal status. *Journal of Human Reproductive Sciences, 7*(1), 2–12.

Panshy, M., Feingold, M., Sagi, R., Herman, A., Schneider, D., & Halperin, R. (2006). Diagnostic hysteroscopy as a primary tool in a basic infertility workup. *Journal of the Society of Laparoendoscopic Surgeons, 10*(2), 231–235.

Sauer, M. V., Wang, J. G., Douglas, N. C., Nakhuda, G. S., Vardhana, P., Jovanovic, V., & Guarnaccia, M. M. (2009). Providing fertility care to men seropositive for human immuno-deficiency virus: Reviewing 10 years of experience and 420 consecutive cycles of in vitro fertilization and intracytoplasmic sperm injection. *Fertility and Sterility, 91*(6), 2455–2460.

Schaffir, J., McGee, A., & Kennard, E. (2009). Use of nonmedical treatments by infertility patients. *Journal of Reproductive Medicine, 54*(7), 415–420.

Sunderam, S., Kissin, D. M., Crawford, S. B., Folger, S. G., Jamieson, D. J., Warner, L., & Barfield, W. D. (2015). Assisted reproductive technology surveillance—United States, 2013. *Morbidity and Mortality Weekly Report: Surveillance Summaries MMWR Surveillance Summary, 64*(11), 1–25.

Tarun, J., Soules, M. R., & Collins, J. A. (2004). Comparison of basal follicle-stimulating hormone versus the clomiphene citrate challenge test for ovarian reserve screening. *Fertility and Sterility, 82*(1), 180–185.

Wass, J., Owen, K., & Turner, H. (2014). Reproductive endocrinology. In J. Wass & K. Owen (Eds.), *Oxford handbook of endocrinology and diabetes* (3rd ed.). Oxford, UK: Oxford University Press.

World Health Organization (WHO) Technical Report Series. (1992). *Recent advances in medically assisted conception: Report of a WHO Scientific Group.* No. 820, 1–111.

World Health Organization (WHO). (2010). *WHO laboratory manual for the examination and processing of human semen* (5th ed.). Retrieved from http://apps.who.int/iris/bitstream/10665/44261/1/9789241547789

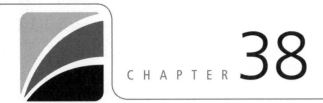

CHAPTER 38

High-Risk Childbearing

Marianne T. Stone-Godena

ADVANCED MATERNAL AGE

Human beings are capable of bearing children in their early to mid-teens (sometimes younger). In ancient times, women married and birthed young and often died as a result. When a woman's average life span was less than 40 years, women who gave birth in their 30s were relatively rare and referred to as older, elderly, or senile gravidas during pregnancy. This state of being of an "elderly parturient" was first defined in 1958 by the Council of International Federations of Obstetrics (FIGO) as "one aged 35 years or more at the first delivery" (Kirz, Dorchester, & Freeman, 1985). Beginning the latter quarter of the 20th century in developed nations, women began delaying childbearing. Focusing on a career, getting advanced education, establishing financial stability, marrying later, having second families, greater access to birth control, and favorable economic conditions have solidified this trend (Dulitzki et al., 1998). In the United States, the median age at first birth went from 21.3 years in 1969 to 24.4 years in 1994. When stratified by years of education, the difference was more dramatic. In 1969, only 10% of U.S. college graduates giving birth for the first time were older than 30 years compared with 45% of first births to college graduates occurring after the age of 30 years in women in 1994 (Heck, Schoendorf, Ventura, & Kiely, 1997). The first section of this chapter describes the incidence, prevalence, and risk factors associated with childbearing and advanced maternal age. The second section presents common causes and possible contributory factors to complications of pregnancy during advanced years. This content is meant to assist with anticipatory guidance to providing safe competent care to this population of women. Evidence-based diagnostic studies and suggested management plans based on current national protocol/guidelines are also presented. This chapter concludes with an important national issue affecting women: intimate partner violence (IPV).

Definition and Scope

With the advent of assisted reproductive technologies including the use of donor eggs, births to women more than 40 years of age are relatively common with an increase of 70% in 10 years (Heffner, 2004). According to U.S. 2015 birth certificate data, 10.6 births per 1,000 women in 2014 were to women between ages 40 and 44 years, and 677 births were reported in women beyond 45 years of age in 2013 (Hamilton, Martin, Osterman, Curtin, & Matthews, 2015; Heffner, 2004). The oldest spontaneously conceived pregnancy resulting in a viable fetus was in a woman 57 years of age, while pregnancies conceived through assisted reproductive technology (ART) have been successful in women as old as 66 years of age (Salihu, Shumpert, Slay, Kirby, & Alexander, 2003). Although the numbers of births to women older than 35 years have increased, advanced maternal age (AMA) continues to be defined as age greater than 35 years at delivery and very AMA as pregnancy after age 45 years.

Etiology

Pregnancy loss from all etiologies is greater among women older than 35 years (Lagrew, Morgan, Nakamoto, & Lagrew, 1996; Nybo Andersen, Wohlfahrt, Christens, Olsen, & Melbye, 2000). The risk of early, spontaneous abortion (SAB) increases largely due to aneuploidy, though there is also an increase in euploid (normal complement of chromosomes) losses. The baseline risk for pregnancy loss at age 20 to 29 years is 10% to 15%. The risk of loss doubles by age 35 years and, by age 45 years, this risk rises to 90% for women pregnant with their own eggs (Nybo Andersen et al., 2000). Although the exact cause of pregnancy loss in AMA is unknown, there is research to support the hypothesis that elevated gonadotropin levels occurring with decreased ovarian function may induce chromosomal abnormalities (Lagrew et al., 1996).

Other anomalies with or without loss are noted with increased frequency in women older than 35 years. In a series of 2,000 in vitro fertilization (IVF) pregnancies, which reached a point of fetal cardiac activity, the incidence of SAB was 13% at age 35 years and 22% at age 40 years demonstrating processes other than aneuploidy at play. In another study of more than 100,000 SABs, stillborns, and liveborn infants, the risk of cardiac defects was four times

TABLE 38.1	Pregnancy Loss by Maternal Age at Conception		
MATERNAL AGE (YEARS)	SPONTANEOUS ABORTIONS (%)	ECTOPIC PREGNANCY (%)	STILLBIRTHS/1,000
< 20	13.3	2.0	5.0
20–24	11.1	1.5	4.2
25–29	11.9	1.6	4.0
30–34	15.0	2.8	4.4
35–39	24.6	4.0	5.0
40–44	51.0	5.8	6.7
> 45	93.4	7.0	8.2

Adapted from Nybo Andersen, Wohlfahrt, Christens, Olsen, and Melbye (2000).

greater at age 40 compared to age 25 (McIntosh, Olshan, & Baird, 1995; Nybo Andersen et al., 2000).

As a woman ages, multiple partners, endometriosis, and pelvic adhesions can all contribute to an increased risk for tubal pathology and interference with the orderly progress of the fertilized ovum in the tube. Two studies demonstrated a four to eight times greater risk of ectopic pregnancy in women older than 35 years compared with younger women (McIntosh et al., 1995; Storeide, Veholmen, Eide, Bergsjø, & Sandvei, 1997) (Table 38.1). In addition to the obvious risk to the pregnancy, ectopic pregnancy can result in significant maternal morbidity and mortality.

The number of multiple pregnancies (twins, triplets, quadruplets, and higher) in the random population remained relatively stable until the 1970s. Since then, with delayed childbearing and advances in reproductive technologies (ovarian hyperstimulation, oocyte retrieval, and embryo transfer), the prevalence of dizygotic (DZ) multiple births has risen in all the developed nations despite the overall decline in fertility after the age of 35 (Figure 38.1) (Martin et al., 2002; Russell, Petrini, Damus, Mattison, & Schwarz, 2003).

Spontaneous DZ multiple pregnancy increases as ovaries age and is compounded with increased parity (previous numbers of births). A woman of 40 years having her fourth child is four times more likely to have a multifetal gestation than a woman of 20 years having her first child (Figure 38.2). The rise in multiples comes at a public health care price. Fetal mortality in multiples is four times greater than in singletons and neonatal mortality is six times greater (Prapas et al., 2006). The increased mortality is due to prematurity, diabetes, growth restriction, and preeclampsia (PEC). The greatest increase in multifetal gestations is among women of AMA. Their infants are at greater risk for a very low birth weight than infants born to younger women (Petrou et al., 2003) (Figure 38.3).

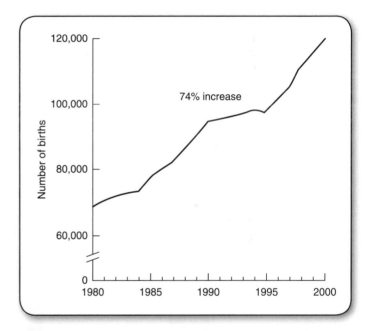

FIGURE 38.1

Rise in multifetal gestations from assisted reproductive technology.

From Martin et al. (2002).

■ MEDICAL DISORDERS

Comorbid conditions, while strongly associated with AMA, rarely have a clear-cut cause and effect relationship. Hypertension is the most frequently encountered health problem in pregnancy in women of all ages (Abu-Heija, Jallad, & Abukteish, 2000).

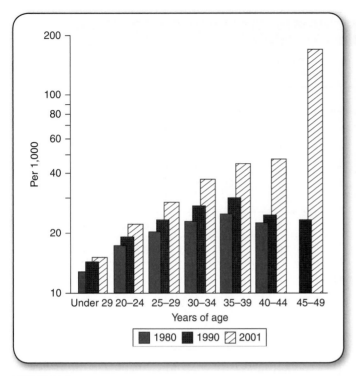

FIGURE 38.2

Age-related incidence of dizygotic twin gestations.

From Martin et al. (2002).

Preeclampsia

Preeclampsia (PEC) is a disease in pregnancy of hypertension with proteinuria and/or multiple organ edema. PEC occurs primarily in primiparous women at the extremes of their childbearing years. It is the presence of preexisting hypertension that increases the probability that PEC will develop in multiparous women as well as nulligravidas (Sibai, 1996). The incidence of PEC more than quadruples between 25 years of age at 3% to 4% to 17% of women older than 35 years and up to 35% of women older than 50 years (Bobrowski & Bottoms, 1995). The risks of hypertension include maternal morbidity and mortality from stroke (Hoyert, Danel, & Tully, 2000; van Katwijk & Peeters 1998).

Gestational Diabetes

Gestational diabetes is more common in women of advancing age; all women older than 35 years of age should be screened with a 50-g load of glucose between 24 and 28 weeks of pregnancy and earlier if they have any personal or family historical factors increasing the risk. During pregnancy, human placental lactogen, secreted by the placenta, acts on insulin receptor sites binding them, raising

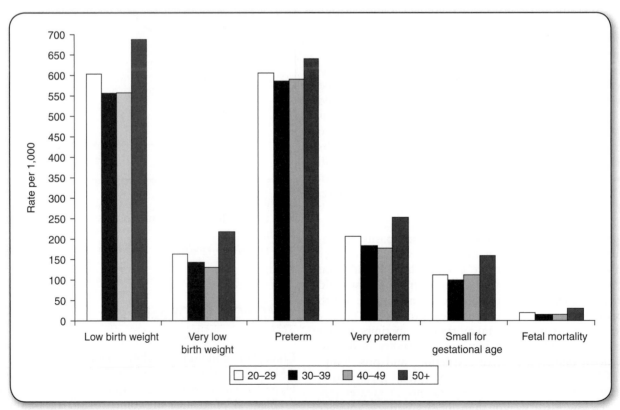

FIGURE 38.3

Gestational age, birth weight, and mortality among multiples by maternal age.

Adapted from Salihu, Shumpert, Slay, Kirby, and Alexander (2003).

circulating levels of maternal glucose. Prepregnant maternal weight and weight at term are noted to increase with age. Glucose impairment increases at all ages with increasing weight. Pancreatic B cell function and insulin sensitivity fall with age; the incidence of gestational and overt diabetes increases. The combination of age, obesity, and pregnancy increases the likelihood of overt and gestational diabetes from 3% of the random obstetric population to 12% of women older than 40 years and 20% of women older than 50 years. The complications of diabetes in pregnancy include an increased risk for congenital anomalies, PEC, induction of labor, fetal macrosomia, and cesarean delivery (Michlin et al., 2003; Roach, Hin, Tam, Ng, & Rogers, 2000). See Chapter 44 for more details on diabetes in pregnancy.

Uterine Leiomyomata

Uterine leiomyomata, often known as fibroids, are found with increasing frequency in women in their 30s and 40s. Uterine leiomyomata are independently associated with placental abruption, dysfunctional labor, fetal malpresentation, and cesarean delivery.

The baseline incidence of breech (buttocks first) presentation is 3% to 4% at term. One study reported an incidence of 11% of fetuses in the breech presentation at term in women 45 years of age. It may be a function of uterine leiomyomata, laxity of the abdominal wall, or laxity of the muscles of the pelvis (Williams, Lieberman, Mittendorf, Monson, & Schoenbaum, 1991).

Risk Factors

Women in the latter third of their reproductive lives can bear children safely; however, preexisting comorbidities and complications during pregnancy and delivery are inherent, especially after the age of 50 years (Table 38.2)

(Heffner, 2004). The deleterious effects of childbearing at the outer edge of fertility are compounded by the influence of ethnicity and socioeconomics. African American women in all age groups have an increased incidence of perinatal morbidity and mortality and this incidence rises more rapidly with age than in Caucasian women (Salihu et al., 2003). A prudent clinician is aware of these risks and plans care accordingly.

The risks of complications of pregnancy associated with AMA fall loosely into two categories: those attributed to declining ovarian function, which manifest in early pregnancy, and complications of medical disorders whose incidence rises with age and which tend to occur in late pregnancy.

Symptoms

Ovarian dysfunction is a common symptom occurring with AMA. A woman is born with all the eggs she will ever have. Over time, these eggs diminish in quantity and ability to divide properly with chromosomes failing to pass evenly to separate cells during the final stage of division after fertilization. This failure to pass evenly is known as nondisjunction. It results in aneuploidy, which is a deviation from the normal number of chromosomes. The incidence of nondisjunction and aneuploidy in embryos begins to rise at approximately 35 years of age, rising sharply at 40 years of age (Lagrew et al., 1996; Snijders, Sebire, & Nicolaides, 1995). Aneuploidy may present as monosomy, when one of a pair of chromosomes is missing. More commonly, nondisjunction results in a trisomy, which is an additional chromosome of a particular type, as in Down syndrome (Trisomy 21), Edward syndrome (Trisomy 18), and Patau syndrome (Trisomy 13). There may be aneuploidy of the sex chromosomes as well leading to Klinefelter's syndrome (47 XXY) and triple X syndrome (46 XXX). One study on preimplantation genetic diagnosis (PGD) looked at 1,029 conception cycles in women older than 37 years using florescence in

TABLE 38.2	Average Age-Related Risk for Most Common Aneuploidies in Live Births			
AGE (YEARS)	ALL TRISOMIES	TRISOMY 21	TRISOMY 18	TRISOMY 13
< 22	1:526	1:1,667	1:17,000	1:33,000
25	1:476	1:1,250	1:14,000	1:25,000
29	1:417	1:1,000	1:11,000	1:20,000
34	1:238	1:485	1:7100	1:14,000
36	1:156	1:289	1:2,400	1:4,800
39	1:83	1:136	1:1,505	1:3,500
44	1:26	1:38	1:700	1:1,600
49	1:8	1:11	1:300	1:800

Adapted from Snijders, Sebire, and Nicolaides (1995).

situ hybridization techniques (FISH) and found that 50% of them were abnormal for Trisomy 21, 18, 13, and the sex aneuploidies but an additional 12% were aneuploid for less common trisomies of 1, 16, and 22, for an overall trisomy rate of 62% (Gianaroli, Magli, & Ferraretti, 2005). Rates of aneuploidy are calculated per live birth, but fetuses with trisomies have a higher miscarriage or early stillborn rate, meaning the incidence of a given trisomy is higher if calculated earlier in pregnancy.

The risk for aneuploidy does not increase with advancing paternal age as sperm are made fresh shortly before being disbursed. There is evidence to suggest that in children of fathers of advanced age there is an increased risk of spontaneous mutations in autosomal dominant disorders such as achondroplasia, Marfan's syndrome, Apert's syndrome, and neurofibromatosis as well as some X lined disorders including hemophilia A and Duchenne muscular dystrophy. The risk of the individual diseases is small, so the risk is presented as a pooled risk for all the disorders (McIntosh et al., 1995). The risk occurs across ethnic and socioeconomic lines.

Evaluation/Assessment

Women of AMA have a higher preterm birth rate, with a significant number occurring before 32 weeks (Jolly, Sebire, Harris, Robinson, & Regan, 2000). Pugliese et al. found an 18% preterm birth rate in women older than 40 years of age compared with 12% in the control group of younger women (Hui, Muggli, & Halliday, 2016). Infants of older women are also at risk of being small for gestational age. According to the 2013 U.S. fetal and neonatal mortality statistics, fetal mortality in infants of mothers older than 35 years continued to rise though the rates declined in women between 20 and 34 years of age (MacDorman & Gregory, 2015). Several prospective population-based studies have confirmed an increased risk for preterm birth even when adjusted for confounding variables, such as smoking, preexisting disease, multifetal pregnancies, and parity.

Controlling for abruption and hypertension, the incidence of intrauterine growth restriction (IUGR) and stillbirth is higher in women older than 35 years than in younger women (Abu-Heija et al., 2000; Humphrey, Griffin, Senz, Shaffer, & Caughey, 2016; Jolly et al., 2000; Lagrew et al., 1996). The incidence of unexplained stillbirth increases after 37 weeks gestation. In an 8-year retrospective cohort analysis, stillbirth occurred at twice the rate in women older than 35 years compared with their younger counterparts (Miller, 2005). This risk for unexplained fetal death is substantially higher in African American women. Across all age groups, the risk for adverse perinatal outcomes in African Americans is twice the rate for Caucasians. This disproportion increases more rapidly in older, poor Black women (MacDorman & Gregory, 2015).

Cesarean delivery nationwide for women younger than 30 years of age is 25% to 30% compared with a 40% to 52% surgical delivery rate in women 35 to 45 years and an 80% cesarean rate in women beyond age 50 years (Abu-Heija et al., 2000; Jolly et al., 2000; Lagrew et al., 1996).

Some reasons include increased rates of placental abruption and placenta previa, malpresentations, fetal intolerance of labor, maternal request, clinician intolerance of labor, and multiple gestations. However, a disproportionate number is performed for dystocia compared with a similar cohort of younger women (Dulitzki et al., 1998; Miller, 2005; Williams, Lieberman, Mittendorf, Monson, & Schoenbaum, 1991). Deteriorating myometrial function may be a contributing factor. Popov, Ganchev, and Bakurdzhiev (1990) observed that with advancing age in primiparous women there was a progressive thickening of the muscular layer of myometrial arteries due to fibrosis, which may ultimately lead to reduced uterine contractility.

A number of studies have demonstrated that the incidence of cerebral palsy (CP) in infants has a bimodal pattern with peaks in mothers younger than 20 years and older than 35 years. As with other risks associated with age, there is no clear evidence that age per se is the culprit. As an example, the same groups of women at risk for an infant with CP are at risk for prematurity, PEC, and fetal growth restriction. Although the risks of maternal mortality in industrialized nations are small, nine of 100,000 births of women between 20 and 24 years of age, the risk triples between 35 and 39 years and is five times higher in women older than 40 years (Hoyert et al., 2000).

Assessment is a critical component to anticipatory guidance and decision making. Findings of diagnostic testing are essential to maternal future planning since AMA is associated with an increased risk for some adverse outcomes. With careful assessment, planning, monitoring, and appropriately timed interventions, morbidity and mortality can be reduced.

Diagnostic Studies

Older women are at increased risk or chromosomal abnormalities. Therefore, prenatal genetic diagnostic studies, counseling, and testing of women should be offered. Counseling before diagnostic studies should include a definition of chromosomes, aneuploidy, and nondisjunction. The most common trisomy, Trisomy 21 (Down syndrome) is a result of having three copies of chromosome 21. The syndrome is associated with mild to moderate mental retardation, congenital heart disease, and other chronic health problems. There are often external physical characteristics associated with Down syndrome including low-set ears, eyes with epicanthal folds, and protuberant tongue. A second trimester fetal survey ultrasound may reveal choroids plexus cysts, disturbances in the heart outflow tract (calcium deposits which appear as bright spots in the left ventricle), shortened humerus or femur, and growth restriction (Gross & Bombard, 1998). There is no correlation between the severity of physical signs and the degree of mental retardation. Trisomy 13 (Patau syndrome) and Trisomy 18 (Edward syndrome) are also caused by the presence of three copies of a chromosome. Both of these syndromes have more severe health issues than Down syndrome and are usually fatal prenatally or within the first year of life.

Chromosomal abnormalities 47 XXY (Klinefelter's syndrome) and 47 XXX (Triplo X) are caused by the presence of an extra X chromosome. Klinefelter's is associated with phenotypical males with androgen deficiency and mild mental retardation.

Treatment/Management

PRECONCEPTION COUNSELING

Preconception counseling may reduce the risk of comorbidities, such as smoking, obesity, uncontrolled diabetes, or hypertension. The recommended daily allowance (RDA) for pregnant women is 800 mcg of folic acid and 1,200 mg of calcium. In the absence of lactose intolerance, it is possible to consume adequate calcium with dairy products. For those with intolerance, calcium-fortified juices or foods may be substituted. Many women benefit from calcium supplementation to approach the RDA. The volume of greens necessary to consume 800 mcg of folic acid daily is quite large. Most women need folic acid supplementation. Organically grown grains and produce are the best sources of vitamins, minerals, and nutrients. The use of herbs is controversial. They are not regulated by the Food and Drug Administration and may vary widely in quality. Many women purchase herbs without input from a provider, but providers should be aware of those herbs that have been shown to have untoward effects on pregnancy and those that are generally considered safe.

Management also consists of a detailed description of prenatal diagnostic options, including invasive and noninvasive testing. Amniocentesis and chorionic villus sampling are diagnostic tests. Chorionic villus sampling involves taking a sample of placental tissue between 10 and 12 weeks gestation. As the placenta is of the same embryonic origin of the fetus, the chromosomes are the same. Amniocentesis involves passing a needle through the maternal abdomen and withdrawing fetal cells from the amniotic fluid after 15 weeks gestation (Gross & Bombard, 1998). The loss of a normal pregnancy as a result of an invasive procedure is approximately 1/200 to 300 pregnancies (Gross & Bombard, 1998). As age 35 years is the point at which the risk of one is equivalent to the risk of the other, it has become the standard time for offering a diagnostic procedure based on age alone; thus, with increasing numbers of women bearing children after age 35 years, the use of invasive prenatal testing has risen, though exact numbers are unknown. Some women do not want invasive testing. A study in California found women of African American or Hispanic descent were more likely to decline testing than Caucasians or women of Asian descent (Baker, Teklehaimanot, Hassan, & Guze, 2004; Halliday, Lumley, & Watson, 1995). In Australia, where prenatal diagnostic testing is available to women for free, one author found a substantial number of women chose not to use the option. Of the women younger than 39 years of age, 43% declined testing. Even in older women (greater than 40) 29% of the women declined testing.

Although only invasive testing is diagnostic, there is noninvasive screening available allowing the woman to decide based on more information than age whether she desires invasive testing. For women receiving care in the first trimester, maternal serum testing with nuchal translucency evaluation to adjust the age-related risk can be offered. Women in the second trimester can be offered a blood screening test for Down syndrome, Trisomy 18 and 13, and open neural tube defects. This "quad screen" test is done between 15 and 22 weeks gestational age and provides an indirect measurement of four hormones secreted in pregnancy: alpha-fetoprotein, human chorionic gonadotropin (hCG), estriol, and inhibin. With the quad screen, 70% of children with Down syndrome will be detected in women older than 35 years and 60% of children with trisomy 13 will be diagnosed. A second trimester fetal survey may identify stigmata (structural abnormalities; Figure 38.4), some of which are associated with chromosomal abnormalities. Women may choose to combine a fetal anatomic survey with the quad screen before making a decision about a diagnostic amniocentesis. Prenatal genetics and chromosomal abnormalities are addressed in Chapters 16, 22, and 23.

Nonstress Test

Based on the observations of increased risk of stillbirth to women older than 35 years, the American College of Obstetricians and Gynecologists (ACOG) recommends fetal surveillance in the form of nonstress testing or biophysical profiles. Using data from McGill University, weekly antepartum testing from 37 weeks with labor induction between 39 and 40 weeks seems to be associated with the lowest risk for adverse outcomes (Humphrey et al., 2006). This increased surveillance has resulted in increased intervention, but there is no consensus the practice has reduced the incidence of stillbirth.

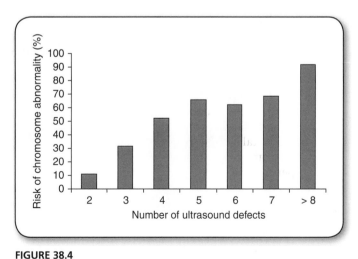

FIGURE 38.4

Risk of chromosomal abnormalities based on number of ultrasound defects.

Adapted from Gross and Bombard (1998).

■ MULTIPLE PREGNANCY

The overwhelming majority of human pregnancies are singleton. Because multiples are rare, in primitive cultures, they were imbued with special powers. Some cultures revered multiples while others feared and killed them (Devereux, 1941). Multiple pregnancies occur through one of two mechanisms. Monozygotic (MZ) or identical twins occur when one fertilized egg splits within the first 2 weeks after conception. DZ twinning is a result of multiple eggs being fertilized. MZ twins originating from one ovum share genetic make-up. They may each have their own sac and placenta (amnion and chorion) and are known as diamnionic/dichorionic (Figure 38.5). The placentas can be separate or they may fuse if the splitting of the ovum occurs within the first 2 days after fertilization.

Definition and Scope

Diamnionic/monochorionic twins account for 70% of MZ twins. This di/mono state occurs when splitting happens 3 to 8 days after fertilization, resulting in a shared chorion but separate amnions. The rarest time for splitting is 9 to 12 days after fertilization as only 1% of twins share the amnion and the chorion, that is, monoamnionic/monochorionic. When twins share chorion, they share vasculature which puts the twins at risk of twin–twin transfusion, a situation in which one fetus grows excessively large (the recipient) often with excessive amniotic fluid, while the other languishes with diminished fluid (the donor). (See the section on abnormalities in amniotic fluid regulation). The ovum splitting more than 12 days after fertilization results in conjoined twins, which are always mono/mono (Cunningham et al., 1997). The precise mechanism of splitting of MZ twins is unknown. The incidence of MZ twins is 1/81 pregnancies worldwide (Zach, 2006).

DZ twins share genetic material in the same way siblings born of different pregnancies would. Levels of follicle-stimulating hormone appear to correlate with DZ twinning. This correlation has been noted in women who have born multiple sets of twins and has been compared in Nigeria where in one tribe the incidence of spontaneous twins is 45 of 1,000 births and in Japan where the frequency of DZ twins is low.

Risk Factors

Spontaneous twinning varies with ethnicity, age, and the use of fertility drugs. Drugs used to induce ovulation are associated with hyperstimulation of the ovary and a release of multiple eggs which when fertilized can result in triplets and higher order multiples. These multiples can be MZ, DZ, or trizygotic.

Evaluation/Assessment

MZ and DZ twins should be assessed for cord entanglement, congenital anomalies, and discordant birth weights. Whenever overcrowding occurs in the uterus, the woman should be assessed for signs and symptoms of preterm birth. Additionally, the more fetuses competing for nutrition, the more likely the placenta will be unable to keep up the supply and the more likely one or more fetuses will experience decreased growth rate. Discordance in weight of more than 20% has been associated with fetal and neonatal mortality (Hartley, Hitti, & Emanuel, 2002). Maternal hypertension and PEC further stress the placenta. A larger placental mass produces more human placental lactogen and places the mother at greater risk of gestational diabetes. The demands of two fetuses almost guarantee maternal anemia unless the mother uses iron supplementation. Over distension of the uterus predisposes to antepartum and postpartum hemorrhage (PPH), preterm delivery, abnormal presentation, and cesarean delivery. Growth restriction with low birth weight

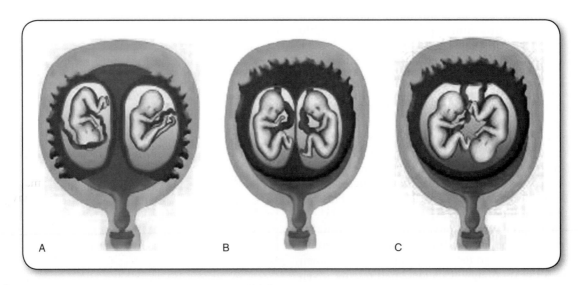

FIGURE 38.5

Types of placentation: (A) diamnionic, dichorionic; (B) diamnionic, monochorionic; and (C) monoamnionic, monoamnionic.

Reprinted with permission from Terrence Zachary (2007). Available at: http://www.emedicine.com/ped/topic2599.htm

and prematurity contribute significantly to the perinatal mortality rate and morbidity among multiples. Twins have a perinatal mortality rate five to seven times greater than singletons, and triplets are more than 20 times as likely to die in the first month of life. Preterm birth is associated with anatomic and physiologic immaturity, including hypothermia, respiratory difficulties, hypoglycemia, necrotizing enterocolitis (NEC), infection, intraventricular hemorrhage, and iatrogenic complications like retinopathy (Henderson, Hockley, Petrou, Goldacre, & Davidson, 2004). Second twins have a higher perinatal mortality when delivered vaginally. Death due to perinatal hypoxia is 1:350 twin births. This raises the issue of mode of delivery. Many believe all multiples should be delivered operatively. However, at least one study demonstrated that CP in twins is greater than in singleton births regardless of mode of birth (Pharoah, 2001).

Diagnostic Studies

Diagnosis of spontaneously occurring multiples used to be made based on clinical information: uterine size greater than expected, fetal parts in all quadrants, and palpation of two fetal heads. With the advent of ultrasonography most multiple pregnancies are diagnosed early in pregnancy allowing appropriate time for evaluation, education, discharge planning, and gathering of resources.

Treatment/Management

DZ twins and MZ twins may be collaboratively managed by a nurse-practitioner or nurse-midwife as long as the fetuses have individual amnions and chorions and remain growth concordant. The medical plan of care may be determined by the obstetrician but mothers of multiples can benefit from psychosocial support. One study recently reported increased maternal depression, anxiety, and negative impact on quality of life of women bearing multiples.

Women bearing multiples need to increase their caloric intake by about 600 kcal/day to meet the need of two growing fetuses and they need additional iron supplementation. The maternal center of gravity changes earlier in pregnancy than with a singleton, the incidence of peripheral edema is higher, and the added weight increases lower back pain. Although all of these are common concerns in pregnancy, they may limit activity earlier in pregnancy than with a singleton and lead to isolation. Multiple gestations are associated with more nausea and vomiting, heartburn, and sleep disturbances than single gestations. Because of the risk for prematurity, women carrying multiples will usually begin fetal assessment by 30 weeks and if they have other children, this additional testing may present transportation or babysitting challenges. Once the babies are born, the mother will need support with lactation and the peculiar challenges of nursing more than one infant.

■ GESTATIONAL TROPHOBLASTIC DISEASE

Currently, there is disagreement regarding histology but for convenience, the nonmolar forms of gestational trophoblastic disease (GTD) are grouped together in this chapter. Hydatidiform moles can be complete (CHM) or partial (PHM). In 2000, the International Federation of Obstetricians and Gynecologists (FIGO) reduced the classification to molar pregnancy and postmolar gestational trophoblastic neoplasia (GTN) (FIGO Oncology Committee, 2000). In 2004, the ACOG applied the terms molar pregnancy and malignant GTD (Committee on Practice Bulletins-Gynecology, ACOG, 2004). The supposition in 1983 was that each GTD is histologically distinct (Novak & Sheah, 1954).

Definition and Scope

In 1983, the WHO defined GTD as a spectrum of disorders arising from the trophoblastic epithelium of placental tissue marked by excessive quantities of the beta subunit of beta-hCG (World Health Organization [WHO], 1983). They comprise 80% of GTD and are the most treatable forms. Invasive mole, choriocarcinoma, placental site trophoblastic tumors (PSTTs), and miscellaneous or unclassified trophoblastic tumors complete the list generally referred to as GTN or malignant trophoblastic disease. (Scully, Bonfiglio, Kurman, & Silverberg, 1994). All GTN, though relatively rare, have the potential to metastasize and can be fatal if untreated.

The incidence of GTD varies due to the difference in diagnostic criteria nationally and internationally. In the United States, reported incidence is about 110 to 120 per 100,000 pregnancies. A normal pregnancy begins when a sperm fertilizes an egg and half of the chromosomes from each parent are contributed to the newly developing products of conception. Approximately 10% of CHMs arise from an anuclear egg, which is fertilized by two sperms (Lawler, Fisher, & Dent, 1991). These pregnancies may be 46 XX or 46 XY but with no maternal contribution to the genes. There is no fetal tissue in a complete mole and the tissue ultimately destined to be placental tissue develops abnormally as a vacuolar mass consisting of diffuse, enlarged villi (hydropic) and hyperplastic trophoblasts, which have a grape-like resemblance. Trophoblasts are epithelial cells that form the outermost layer of the blastocyst (a very early embryonic structure) and are responsible for the production of beta-hCG. The disorder in the trophoblasts with a molar pregnancy results in excessive production of beta-hCG (Dawood, Saxena, & Landesman, 1977). While trophoblasts invade the maternal decidua, there is no placental tissue to receive blood flow. The blood flow from the maternal system flows into the uterus and becomes apparent as painless vaginal bleeding, one of the hallmarks of a molar pregnancy. The bleeding may be massive, though most commonly is minimal to moderate but may persist for months.

A PHM may has an embryo (dead or alive) and is usually triploid 69 XXX or 69 XXY, rarely 69 XYY (Table 38.3). It arises from an ovum with a 23 X haploid set of maternal chromosomes (Philipp, Grillenberger, Separovic, Philipp, & Kalousek, 2004). The egg is fertilized by two sperms. It results in a zygote with duplication of the paternal haploids plus the single set of maternal haploids. While a twin may exist with a molar pregnancy, the incidence of

TABLE 38.3	Characteristics of Complete and Partial Molar Pregnancies	
CHARACTERISTIC	**COMPLETE MOLE**	**PARTIAL MOLE**
Chromosomes	46 XX or 46 XY	Mostly 69 XXX or 69 XXY
Fetus	Absent	Often present, often nonviable
Hydropic villi	Diffuse, often severe	Focal, variable
Postmolar malignancy	6%–32%	< 5%
Uterine size	50% larger than dates	May be small for dates
Theca lutein cysts	25%	Rare

Adapted from Committee on Practice Bulletins-Gynecology, American College of Obstetricians and Gynecologists (2004).

chromosomal anomalies and fetal loss is high with the twin. PHM is characterized by less bleeding, often presenting as a missed abortion (Berkowitz, Goldstein, & Bernstein, 1991). The level of beta-hCG while elevated is usually not as dramatic as seen with a CHM, often less than 100,000 mIU/mL. Only rarely does PHM progress to invasive disease.

Etiology

Most molar pregnancies are of androgenetic origin, consisting primarily of two paternal haploid complements (Wolf & Lage, 1995). A complete (classic) mole (CHM) is almost exclusively (greater than 99%) paternal in chromosomal origin and 85% to 90% of the time is 46 XX. Ninety-nine percent of the time, a CHM pregnancy arises from a sperm entering an egg that has no nucleus (anuclear). Since there is nothing within the egg to contribute chromosomes (no maternal haploid sets), the sperm contributes two morphologically identical haploid sets (23X) of paternal chromosomes.

Risk Factors

Maternal age and past history are consistent risk factors for GTD. Women younger than 20 years of age, particularly those younger than 16 years, and women older than 35 years and especially older than 40 years are at greatest risk (Buckley, 1996). This association is not as strong with PHM (Sebire et al., 2002). The geographic, ethnic, and age differences in distribution have not been fully explained. Some proposed theories for variation of rates are diets low in protein, carotene, and folic acid, as well as trends in ages of childbearing with the highest risk being at times of general instability of ovarian tissue early and late in the reproductive span (Berkowitz, Im, Bernstein, & Goldstein, 1998; Semer & Macfee, 1995).

The second most consistent predictive risk factor for GTD is a previous history of GTD. A woman with a history of one prior GTD event has a 10 times greater risk of having a second event than a woman in the random population (Lorigan, Sharma, Bright, Coleman, & Hancock, 2000). A previous diagnosis of GTD carries a low risk of about 1% in subsequent pregnancies. This risk increases to about 25% with more than one prior GTD. Choriocarcinoma can arise after any pregnancy, but the risk is highest after a molar pregnancy. A review of 3,000 GTD pregnancies demonstrated choriocarcinoma in only 0.1% (Seckl et al., 2000). CHMs have a 25% incidence of progression to invasive disease. A more aggressive form of molar pregnancy known as invasive mole, invasive trophoblastic disease (ITD), or chorioadenoma destruens occurs in about 20% of CHM pregnancies and 0.5% of PHM pregnancies. The villi in ITD grow through to the muscular layer of the uterus, often presenting with profuse bleeding and abdominal pain. Developing months after the original benign mole, 15% of these tumors limit invasion to the uterus and another 5% metastasize to other organs (Lurain, 2002). The incidence of choriocarcinoma after a normal pregnancy is 1:16,000. Both choriocarcinoma and ITD can produce metastases, sometimes invading pulmonary tissue with resultant pulmonary embolus.

Symptoms

BLEEDING

When bleeding is noted early and continues, the source of bleeding as well as the amount needs to be differentiated. Up to 50% of normal pregnancies may be accompanied by some bleeding. There are multiple etiologies during each trimester. One study found 58% of women with a CHM presented with vaginal bleeding as the only sign (Gemer, Segal, Kopmar, & Sassoon, 2000). Another study found that between 84% and 97% of molar pregnancies were accompanied by bleeding (Soto-Wright, Bernstein, Goldstein, & Berkowitz, 1995).

UTERINE SIZE

Uterine size greater than dates was the only symptom identified associated with molar pregnancy 15% of the time in a small study done in Germany (Gemer et al., 2000). When a uterus is larger than expected for dates, complete hydatidiform mole (CHM), partial hydatidiform mole (PHM), ITD, and choriocarcinoma must be distinguished from multiple pregnancy, uterine myomas (benign tumors of the muscle), or polyhydramnios (excessive amniotic fluid). Even without an embryo, the uterus enlarges from the proliferation of the mole and from intrauterine bleeding.

NAUSEA AND VOMITING

When the amount is excessive or persists beyond the first trimester other explanations for the nausea must be sought. Nausea and vomiting accompany approximately 50% of normal pregnancies. But excessive vomiting is often noted in direct proportion to the levels of beta-hCG or to uterine size (Soper, Clarke-Pearson, & Hammond, 1988).

HYPERTHYROIDISM

Hyperthyroidism is noted to accompany approximately 3% to 7% of molar pregnancies. As with nausea, there is a strong correlation between symptoms and levels of beta-hCG. hCG has a weak thyroid-stimulating effect (Mann, Schneider, & Hoermann, 1986). Unlike patients with Graves' disease, women with molar hyperthyroidism may be asymptomatic. If they are symptomatic, women may experience flushing, tremors, unexpected weight loss, heat intolerance, and tachycardia. Rarely do they experience exopthalmus (Yamazaki et al., 1995).

A complaint of pain in the region of the adnexa should prompt the clinician to rule out torsion, ectopic pregnancy, large physiologic cysts, or theca lutein cysts, which occur in up to 40% of women with GTD (Hancock & Tidy, 2002).

HYPERTENSION

Chronic hypertension may first be noted in a normally progressing pregnancy. Hypertension with proteinuria and edema early in pregnancy is a rare occurrence but historically has occurred with measurable frequency. In one study comparing symptoms of molar pregnancy before and since the advent of ultrasonography, pregnancies later in the study were identified earlier in the pregnancy and the incidence of PEC was greatly reduced, from 27% to 1% (Kirk, Papageorghiou, Condous, Bottomley, & Bourne, 2007).

Disseminated intravascular coagulation (DIC) may occur as a complication of a molar pregnancy with PEC, without evidence of PEC or during treatment for the disease (Schorge, Goldstein, Bernstein, & Berkowitz, 2000).

A woman developing shortness of breath, cough, tachycardia, or cyanosis without documentation of fetal viability could be experiencing thromboplastic emboli, which occur in 2% to 3% of molar pregnancies and are immediately life threatening.

Evaluation/Assessment

A woman who presents with elevated beta-hCG, hyperemesis, tachycardia, flushing, tremor, or thyroid enlargement should have her thyroid function assessed. After 12 weeks of pregnancy, beta-hCG values of greater than 100,000 mIU/mL are usually associated with molar pregnancies though may be reached in multiple gestations. A beta-hCG in this range warrants an ultrasound. A complete blood count (CBC) with platelets is helpful when bleeding is excessive and anemia is suspected, to exclude an infectious process and to rule out thrombocytopenia. Choriocarcinoma commonly presents as unexplained vaginal bleeding 6 weeks to 1 year after a pregnancy. Bleeding may be mild or hemorrhagic. On physical examination, the uterus may be enlarged with bilateral ovarian cysts. Metastases most commonly present as respiratory, urinary, cerebral, or hepatic symptoms.

Diagnostic Studies

Ultrasonography done transvaginally in early pregnancy or abdominally in later pregnancy may be diagnostic of CHM (Kirk et al., 2007). With PHM the ultrasound results must be assessed in the context of symptoms and beta-hCG values. Because of the risk of metastases to the lungs, a plain chest film is indicated when a molar pregnancy has been confirmed. Morphologically, choriocarcinoma and ITD appear the same. Diagnosis is made histologically. ITD has villi present and can regress spontaneously (Wolf & Lage, 1995).

Choriocarcinoma has no villi and will not regress without treatment, growing rapidly and causing death within months. The precise mechanism of the evolution from a benign disease to a neoplastic one is not known.

PSTTs are a result of invasion of the placental bed and myometrium by trophoblasts; these rare tumors originate weeks to years after a normal pregnancy. A PSTT is often malignant and unlike other trophoblastic tumors may have minimal beta-hCG. These tumors may be resistant to chemotherapy (Altieri, Franceschi, Ferlay, Smith, & La Vecchia, 2003).

Molar pregnancies are diagnosed in increased numbers on both extremes of childbearing, younger than 20 years and older than 40 years. Women of African descent in all geographic locations experience molar pregnancies at an increased rate. In some Asian countries, the diagnosis is estimated as high as 1:120 pregnancies (Song & Wu, 1986). The diagnosis of choriocarcinoma appears to mirror the geographic prevalence of molar pregnancies though inconsistency in histological confirmation of clinical diagnoses is often missing in epidemiologic studies (Altieri et al., 2003).

Treatment/Management

The first step in management is to confirm the diagnosis. On diagnosis, referral is made to an obstetrician-gynecologist or a gynecologic oncologist for surgical intervention. The uterus will be emptied of the mole by a surgical procedure called dilatation and curettage (D&C). Suction curettage removes the bulk of the mass (Song, Wu, Wang, Yang, & Dong, 1988). Sharp curettage is then performed ensuring all material obtained is sent for pathological and histological evaluation. As excessive bleeding is characteristic of a molar pregnancy, an intravenous infusion of oxytocin will accompany the procedure to promote uterine contractility and decrease postoperative bleeding. If the woman is Rhesus factor (Rh) negative she will receive a full dose of Rh immune globulin. A CT scan of the abdomen and pelvis, chest film, or MRI of the head may be used to determine whether there is any spread of molar tissue to other organs. Liver and kidney functions and clotting studies may be evaluated especially if there has been evidence of PEC (Committee on Practice Bulletins-Gynecology, ACOG, 2004). If there is no invasion, in PHM with a viable twin the pregnancy may be allowed to continue (Garner, Lipson, Bernstein, Goldstein, & Berkowitz, 2002). At the time of surgery if there is no evidence of invasive disease, levels of beta-hCG will be drawn weekly until no beta-hCG is detected in three specimens, then monthly for 6 months, then bimonthly until a year has passed from the procedure. Serial beta-hCG levels are drawn because although the incidence of invasive disease is low, it can still occur months after evacuation of the uterus.

Periodic pelvic examinations to rule out uterine enlargement and ovarian cysts may be indicated and a chest film may be repeated. If there is invasive disease, whether it is an invasive mole or choriocarcinoma, the woman will also receive antineoplastic treatment usually in the form of methotrexate (MTX); or, if there are metastases, a combination of therapeutic agents will be used (Song, Wu, Wang, Yang, & Dong, 1988).

Once the pregnancy has been terminated, care may be collaborative between the primary clinician and the consulting physician. The consulting physician will monitor the follow-up plan but the primary clinician will perform the follow-up physical examinations, monitor the frequent hCG levels, interpret the results for the woman, and provide her with education including planning for future pregnancies. Women are advised to delay conception to ensure clearance of all beta-hCG from the molar pregnancy for 12 months. The beta-hCG level usually returns to nonpregnant levels within 3 months after a CHM and 2 months after a PHM. Should beta-hCG levels indicate the presence of GTN, care of the woman is referred to the consulting physician.

In industrialized nations, most women with molar pregnancies can preserve their reproductive capacity with early, aggressive treatment. Even invasive tumors can be treated with surgery and medication, though invasive tumors may require a hysterectomy and therefore a loss of fertility.

Traditionally, molar pregnancies were diagnosed in second trimester when the woman developed protracted vaginal bleeding beginning between the sixth and 16th weeks of pregnancy, experienced a severe, persistent form of hyperemesis, uterine size greater than expected by the date of the pregnancy, fatigue from the chronic blood loss, early-onset PEC, and/or absence of fetal heart tones and passage of grape-like tissue vaginally. Up to 20% of women presented with persistent pelvic pain and were noted to have enlarged ovaries from theca lutein cysts, which form in response to the high circulating levels of beta-hCG. With the utilization of serum beta-hCG levels and ultrasonography, molar pregnancies are now more likely to be diagnosed first trimester, often before the development of symptoms. Ultrasonography and beta-hCG levels are important adjuncts to clinical judgment, but no substitute. One series of more than 1,000 women referred for GTD found that ultrasound was correct for diagnosis of GTD of any type only about half the time (Fowler, Lindsay, Seckl, & Sebire, 2006). A CHM is easier to identify as there is no embryo, no amniotic fluid, and a heterogeneous mass of grape-like clusters visualized as a "snow storm pattern" in the area of the placenta (Kirk et al., 2007). A PHM will demonstrate more of a Swiss cheese effect than a snowstorm because the villi are not as hydropic. Either a gestational sac without an embryo or an embryo usually without cardiac activity may also be seen. If there is cardiac activity, the fetus is often growth restricted. Amniotic fluid, if present, is diminished. Because the picture with PHM is less clear, it was confused with an incomplete abortion more than 50% of the time in one series (Benson et al., 2000). hCG levels in a CHM can run to the hundreds of thousands and with

TABLE 38.4	B-hCG Criteria for Postmolar Gestational Trophoblastic Disease
1. hCG level plateau of four values ± 10% over 3 weeks duration, days 1, 7, 14, 21	
2. hCG level increase of > 10% of 3 values over 2 weeks duration, days 1, 7, 14	
3. Persistent, detectable hCG > 6 months after molar evacuation	

hCG, human chorionic gonadotropin.
Adapted from Committee on Practice Bulletins-Gynecology, American College of Obstetricians and Gynecologists (2004).

choriocarcinoma can reach millions, though a PHM may have only nominally elevated beta-hCG levels (Table 38.4).

Pharmacotherapeutics

Women are encouraged to use a highly effective form of birth control to ensure no conception for 12 months. The use of combination hormonal contraceptives is controversial. Two studies found an increased risk for molar pregnancy amongst women using oral contraceptives, before conception as well as post evacuation (Curry et al., 1989; Parazzini et al., 2002). One randomized trial found no increased risk for GTD with the use of low-dose combined oral contraceptives (Stone, Dent, Kardana, & Bagshawe, 1976).

The ACOG expert panel has determined that oral contraceptives are a safe and effective method for use after molar pregnancy unless other medical contraindications are noted (Committee on Practice Bulletins-Gynecology, ACOG, 2004). Recurrence in a woman with more than one previous molar pregnancy is 25% (Sebire et al., 2003). The clinician can reassure the woman that the pregnancy rate after treatment with MTX is 80%, the same as the random population (Song, Wu, Wang, Yang, & Dong, 1988). After all subsequent pregnancies, beta-hCG levels will be followed for up to 1 year.

Complementary/Alternative Treatments

Although no complementary treatments are in the literature for the treatment of molar pregnancies, emphasis on nutrition including folic acid supplementation is always a good basis for supporting the immune system. The association between certain nutritional deficits and molar pregnancy also supports the need for foods high in carotene, protein, and folate. Because of the risk of a subsequent molar pregnancy and because a woman may have anxiety approaching a subsequent pregnancy, an early pelvic ultrasound in a subsequent pregnancy and serial beta-hCG levels should be performed until a fetus with cardiac activity is confirmed and molar pregnancy is excluded.

The sensitive clinician will remember that while this was an abnormal pregnancy, the woman may have been as attached as if it were a normally developing pregnancy. Care should be taken in discussion, acknowledging the loss of the pregnancy and potential feelings of despair regarding one's reproductive "fitness." Referral should be made for care of women beyond the scope of the primary clinician. There are websites for support of pregnancy loss and grief counselors listed in the phone directory.

■ ABNORMALITIES IN AMNIOTIC FLUID REGULATION

During pregnancy, the fetus is bathed in amniotic fluid, which cushions the baby and umbilical cord from trauma, allows it to move its extremities, contributes to the development of the gastrointestinal (GI) tract, provides nutrients, and allows it to practice expanding its lungs by swallowing the fluid. In addition, the fluid is important because it has some bacteriostatic qualities (Brace, 1997).

Definition and Scope of Problem

Amniotic fluid is minimal in early pregnancy (about 1 oz. during the first trimester). Mid trimester, the fetus begins to secrete pulmonary fluid, to produce urine, and to swallow the fluid, which increases in production with advancing gestation. Peaking at about a liter between 34 and 36 weeks, the fluid declines slightly at term to 700 to 800 mL (Brace, 1997).

Mechanisms producing pathophysiologic changes in amniotic fluid are not clearly understood but they are known to be the result of a problem with movement of the fluid through the fetus and the amniotic sac (Rabinowitz, Peters, Vyas, Campbell, & Nicolaides, 1989). It has been estimated that the exchange rate is in excess of 3,000 mL/hr; thus, any significant, persistent alteration in the amniotic fluid level can have a negative impact on the developing fetus. During the second trimester, amniotic fluid that is secreted by the fetal lungs and kidneys is absorbed primarily through the permeable fetal skin. As the keratin layer develops, the dominant mode of amniotic fluid clearance in the last half of pregnancy is through fetal swallowing and urination with some fluid clearing across the fetal surface of the placenta (Wang, Kallichanda, Song, Ramirez, & Ross, 2001).

Historically, alterations in amniotic fluid regulation were associated with poor perinatal outcomes. However, defining the alteration was subjective, sometimes being made postpartum. Even with the advent of ultrasound defining alteration is a source of much debate.

Polyhydraminios

Polyhydramnios, also known as hydramnios, means too much fluid. Polyhydramnios occurs from either increased amniotic fluid production or decreased absorption complicating pregnancies. Findings consistent for polyhydramninous include:

■ A maximum vertical pocket (MVP) of fluid greater than 8 cm (Magann et al., 2003)

■ An amniotic fluid index (AFI) of greater than 25 (Manning, 1995)
■ Amniotic fluid greater than 95th percentile for a given gestational age (Phelan, Smith, Broussard, & Small, 1987)

Etiology

Idiopathic is a diagnosis of exclusion, when all other sources have been ruled out. When polyhydramnios is severe, a cause is identified close to 90% of the time. Severe polyhydramnios is associated with fetal anomalies (Yeast, 2006). When polyhydramnios is in the mild to moderate range, a cause is identified only about one third of the time (Magann et al., 1997). Risks of polyhydramnios include preterm delivery (about 26% of the time), premature rupture of the membranes, abruptio placentae, cord prolapse, malpresentation with resultant cesarean section, and PPH. Perinatal mortality rates are influenced by the presence of anomalies (87%), prematurity 10% to 30%, and idiopathic nature (13%).

Multiple pregnancies can have the unusual circumstance of simultaneous polyhydramnios (too much amniotic fluid) in one fetus and oligohydramnios in another. In twin–twin transfusion, the donor twin may be growth restricted with oligohydramnios while the recipient twin grows excessively large and has polyhydramnios (Magann et al., 2003).

Amniotic fluid production may be increased in diabetes, with certain congenital anomalies such as anencephaly, some infections such as syphilis or viral hepatitis, or maternal substance abuse. Decreased absorption can occur with GI blockage, with neurological abnormalities with high output cardiac failure (hydrops), or from idiopathic causes (Storeide et al., 1997).

Evaluation/Assessment

Women with polyhydramnios are frequently assessed for signs and symptoms of preterm delivery, premature rupture of the membranes, abruptio placentae, cord prolapse, malpresentation, and PPH.

Treatment/Management

Polyhydramnios is usually treated expectantly unless it is severe enough to compromise maternal pulmonary or cardiac function. A woman with severe, early-onset polyhydramnios should have her care transferred to a maternal–fetal specialist. While there are no randomized controlled trials comparing treatment regimens, nonsteroidal agents are used for their inhibitory effect on fetal urine production. Due to concerns over fetal ductus arteriosus closure, indomethacin or other nonsteroidal agent should only be administered in a high-risk unit where fetal ductus flow can be monitored ultrasonographically. Because of the risk for preterm birth, steroids may be administered if diagnosis is before 34 weeks (Piantelli et al., 2004). Therapeutic amniocentesis is sometimes performed as a palliative measure for maternal comfort (Yeast, 2006).

Oligohydraminios

Oligohydramnios from the Greek means little amniotic fluid, and is variously defined as:

- An absolute value of less than 500 mL of amniotic fluid between 32 and 36 weeks of pregnancy (Brace, 1997)
- A MVP of fluid less than 2 cm (Magann et al., 2003)
- An AFI of less than 5 cm (Manning, 1995)
- Amniotic fluid at less than 5th percentile for a given gestational age (Phelan et al., 1987)

Oligohydramnios that occurs in 4% to 5% of all pregnancies may be acute or chronic. The etiology may be renal, postrenal, or nonrenal in origin. The most common cause of oligohydramnios at term is nonrenal from loss of fluid with rupture of the amniotic membranes (ROM). Although most often an acute event at term, ROM can cause chronic oligohydramnios when occurring remote from term. Postterm oligohydramnios is hypothesized by some to be from placental insufficiency, with decreased perfusion to the fetal kidneys leading to decreased fetal urine production. This has not been confirmed histologically. Up to 12% of postdate pregnancies are accompanied by oligohydramnios (Manning, 1995; Phelan et al., 1987).

Etiology

Very early occurring oligohydramnios (first trimester or early second trimester) is largely caused by fetal renal malformations including agenesis occurring in about 1:4,000 births, polycystic or dysplastic kidneys, or ureteral atresia (Dubbins, Kurtz, Wapner, & Goldberg, 1981). Oligohydramnios may result from decreased urine production or blockage of urine passage. The risk of preterm oligohydramnios varies from 0.5% to 8% (Manning, 1995; Phelan et al., 1987). After 24 weeks, prerenal etiologies of oligohydramnios are most common. Viral diseases, PEC, autoimmune diseases such as lupus erythematosus, smoking, or substance abuse can all result in placental insufficiency. Placental insufficiency leads to growth restriction. Growth-restricted fetuses are hypoxemic and shift blood to the heart, the brain, and the adrenal glands as the most critical organs and away from the kidneys. The redistribution of blood flow results in decreased renal perfusion leading to decreased fetal urinary output (Yoshimura, Masuzaki, Gotoh, & Ishimaru, 1997). Any condition that can affect maternal urinary output can also affect fetal urinary output, such as diabetes and maternal dehydration (Piepert & Donnenfield, 1991). A rarer cause of oligohydramnios is from the use of ACE inhibitors or indomethacin in pregnancy (Kirshon, Moise, Mari, & Willis, 1991). Morbidity and mortality in late onset are lower with a perinatal survival rate of about 85% (Yeast, 2006). Adverse outcomes are influenced by the severity of the fluid deficit and the degree of prematurity at birth, presence of fetal growth restriction, and presence of confounding

variables, such as uteroplacental insufficiency, meconium aspiration, abnormal fetal positioning, and umbilical cord compression (Piepert & Donnenfield, 1991).

Evaluation/Assessment

Oligohydramnios after amniocentesis is a possibility. Leakage of amniotic fluid is a known complication of amniocentesis but the membranes usually seal over and the oligohydramnios corrects itself (Abboud et al., 2000). If oligohydramnios develops after 24 weeks, it is commonly associated with fetal IUGR. Amniotic fluid production may be increased in diabetes, with certain congenital anomalies such as anencephaly, some infections such as syphilis or viral hepatitis, or maternal substance abuse. Decreased absorption can occur with GI blockage, with neurological abnormalities with high output cardiac failure (hydrops), or from idiopathic causes (Yeast, 2006).

Oligohydramnios is commonly associated with decreased placental perfusion; high intra-amniotic fluid pressure can impair uteroplacental perfusion as well causing fetal hypoxemia and acidemia. The earlier in pregnancy the oligohydramnios occurs, the more profound the impact on the fetus. When oligohydramnios is noted before 24 weeks, the fetus will often have hypoplastic lungs or limb defects including clubbing dislocation. It may also have what is known as a Potter's face: flat nose, recessed chin, and low-set ears. The mortality rate in infants developing oligohydramnios second trimester is as high as 90% (Shipp, Bromley, Pauker, Frigoletto, & Benacerraf, 1996). The possibility of oligohydramnios increases past 41 weeks and because the AFI has been shown to be subject to technical variability it is contested whether noting it as an isolated finding in low-risk pregnancies represents a complication or variation of normal (Alchalabi, Obeidat, Jallad, & Khader, 2006; Magann et al., 1997; Ott, 2004). Shime and his group found a 79% false-positive rate and a 0.4% false-negative rate when oligohydramnios was diagnosed after term by ultrasound. This means the majority of fetuses were not hypoxic and experienced healthy outcomes, supporting a description of isolated postterm oligohydramnios as idiopathic (Shime et al., 1984). If oligohydramnios is confirmed, there is no evidence of growth restriction, and there is no evidence of fetal renal problems, a sterile speculum examination can be performed to assess for rupture of the membranes. If this test reveals no evidence or rupture, indigo carmine (a blue dye) might be injected into the uterus transabdominally, with visualization vaginally for leakage of blue fluid (Piepert & Donnenfield, 1991).

Diagnostic Studies

Diagnosis of alterations in amniotic fluid is made ultrasonographically, either coincidentally or when performed for a clinical indication. Diminished fluid may be suspected clinically based on lag in fundal growth, fetal parts easily palpable abdominally, or maternal report of diminished fetal movement. Excessive fluid may be suspected clinically when the fundal height greatly exceeds expectations for gestational age, the mother experiences abdominal discomfort with shortness of breath, or there is difficulty identifying fetal parts. Fluid may be estimated qualitatively by abdominal palpation or subjective assessment of pockets of fluid on ultrasound.

Ultrasound will usually identify or rule out renal issues such as agenesis, dysplastic or cystic kidneys, and ureteral atresia (Magann et al., 2004). Fetal growth parameters as well as the amount of fluid and its distribution are determined. Fluid is measured quantitatively by one of two methods. The first method was developed by Phelan and associates as a predictor for the success of external cephalic version of breeches (Phelan et al., 1987). It is considered the standard method for diagnosing oligohydramnios, though several studies have disputed the accuracy of Phelan's findings especially in the upper and lower levels of amniotic fluid (Magann et al., 2004). Fluid is measured in four quarters of the maternal abdomen with the umbilicus as the central point. The largest vertical pocket of fluid identified is measured in each quadrant and an AFI is obtained by summing the four pockets. The second method measures the depth of the single MVP. This method may be more reliable in twin pregnancies and pregnancies in early gestation (Manning, 1995).

Treatment/Management

Treatment for oligohydramnios is gestational age dependent. There is no effective long-term treatment. Because of the risks of chronic oligohydramnios, once a diagnosis is made, care of the woman is made in consultation with a maternal–fetal specialist and the role of the nurse-midwife or nurse-practitioner is supportive and educational. Preterm, expectation management is usually the treatment of choice. The woman is encouraged to be on bed rest and consume large quantities of fluid. Studies have shown ingestion of 2 L of fluid is associated with an increase in amniotic fluid of 30% within several hours (Hofmeyr & Gulmezoglu, 2006). Periodic amniotic fluid monitoring and fetal status monitoring are performed until the fetus is at least 34 weeks unless fetal status appears to be deteriorating. The frequency of assessment is determined by the presence of growth restriction, the severity of the oligohydramnios, and the rapidity of the decline in fluid. Beyond 40 weeks gestation AFI has been correlated with fetal tolerance of labor and is used as a measurement of fetal surveillance. When the AFI is less than 5 cm, induction is usually the treatment of choice when the cervix is favorable. Studies have not demonstrated an improvement in perinatal outcome with induction, so fetal surveillance may be performed while the cervix is ripening (Ek, Andersson, Johansson, & Kublicas, 2005). Given AFI can be influenced by pressure of the ultrasound transducer, angle placed against the maternal abdomen, presence of the umbilical cord, and other factors, some authors have suggested that, in the face of an isolated finding of oligohydramnios at term with an unripe cervix, the risks of intervention must be weighed against the risks of inaction. Some authors suggest it is prudent to hydrate the mother orally or intravenously and repeat the AFI (Ek, Andersson, Johansson, & Kublicas, 2005; Hofmeyr & Gulmezoglu, 2006; Leeman & Almond, 2005).

First and early second trimester oligohydramnios is most commonly associated with genetic and congenital anomalies and has a very high mortality rate, so counseling should include signs and symptoms of miscarriage and genetic counseling. If the infant is diagnosed with renal agenesis, the family will need grief counseling as the mortality rate is 100%. Milder forms of renal cysts or dysplasia may be associated with low normal kidney function or might be associated with long-term renal failure (Dubbins et al., 1981). Second trimester oligohydramnios prognosis depends on etiology and presence of pulmonary hypoplasia.

Grief counseling is important if a life-threatening congenital anomaly is seen ultrasonographically. The risks of prematurity should be discussed with early-onset polyhydramnios. If diabetes is present, maintaining euglycemia is emphasized. An abdominal support band may provide symptomatic relief.

There is virtually no research on the use of complementary therapy in the treatment of oligohydramnios but there is one case study report of successful induction of labor with acute oligohydramnios at term using homeopathic Caulophyllum thalictroides (Kistin & Newman, 2007).

■ POSTTRANSPLANT PREGNANCY

This section details some of the factors common amongst posttransplant pregnancies regardless of the type of graft. Posttransplant, the woman has ongoing care from the specialist that performed the transplant but she might receive her primary or gynecologic care from a nurse practitioner or nurse-midwife. This person may be the one who provides preconceptional care and may be the person who diagnoses a pregnancy.

Definition and Scope

The U.S. National Transplantation Pregnancy Register (NTPR) was established in 1991. They have followed 1,400 graft recipients through 2,200 pregnancies (Armenti et al., 2003). Transplant registries exist in most developed countries or in blocs of countries such as Western Europe. Although registries remain the largest source of data regarding transplants, registration is voluntary and the data collected across registries are not consistent (Davison & Redman, 1997).

In 1963, the *New England Journal of Medicine* reported the case of the first woman successfully carrying a posttransplant pregnancy in 1958 (Murray, Reid, Harrison, & Merrill, 1963). Since that time, more than 14,000 successful posttransplant pregnancies have been documented worldwide, with most of them being renal transplants (Atallah et al., 2015).

Etiology

We will not address cause of renal disease in this chapter. Successful pregnancies occur after solid organ transplant.

Contraceptive precautions should be taken to ensure the graft is well accepted before pregnancy. In general, hormonal contraception is not contraindicated. The woman should be encouraged to stay current on her immunizations to decrease the risk of infections during pregnancy.

Risk Factors

Posttransplantation pregnancy is considered to be of high risk and should not be undertaken without counseling regarding risks and benefits (Davison & Bailey, 2003). Even with its high-risk status, most women who become pregnant posttransplant elect to continue their pregnancies as evidenced by the therapeutic abortion rate reported at equivalent to the random population. Before transplant, most women in renal, pancreatic, or heart failure have almost no chance of maintaining a pregnancy; after transplant, the overall successful pregnancy rate is 20% (Table 38.5) (Handelsman & Dong, 1993). Patients with cystic fibrosis who receive a pancreas transplant may still have difficulty achieving a pregnancy because of the presence of thick cervical mucus (McKay & Josephson, 2006).

The incidence of SABs demonstrates no increase over expected baseline based on maternal age at conception. Ninety-four percent of posttransplant pregnancies surviving first trimester have viable outcomes (Branch et al., 1998). The most common transplants with successful pregnancies subsequent are renal; the least common are combined heart–lung transplants.

Treatment/Management

Pregnancy is not recommended within the first 1 to 2 years after organ graft, as medications are at their highest level during this time and the risk of organ rejection is greatest (Armenti et al., 2003; Atallah et al., 2005; McKay & Josephson, 2006). As part of preventative care, during this time, women with transplants should be carefully screened

TABLE 38.5	Numbers of Successful Pregnancies Posttransplant by Type of Graft
ORGAN	NUMBER OF PREGNANCIES AS OF 2003
Kidney	> 1,000
Liver	187
Pancreas–kidney	56
Heart	54
Lung	15
Kidney–liver	6
Heart–lung	3

Adapted from Armenti et al. (2003).

for infections such as herpes simplex virus (HSV), cytomegalovirus (CMV), toxoplasmosis, pneumococcus, influenza, and hepatitis B (Armenti et al., 2003). Other principles of counseling and screening any reproductive-age woman could apply: The woman should strive toward a healthy weight and nutritional counseling should focus on sources of iron, folic acid, calcium, and low-mercury sources of omega-3 fatty acids. Folic acid supplementation should be initiated and risk avoidance encouraged. In preconception counseling to a posttransplant patient it is important to remember, in addition to the risks from the graft, the regular anatomical and physiological changes of the pregnancy. These women will need to structure their lives to allow for extra nutritional support, more fluids, and more rest. If they have other children, they will need to make plans early in pregnancy for care of the other children in the event of an unexpected hospitalization. While cesarean section should be performed for obstetric indications, not because of the graft, the cesarean section rate is about 50%, so the woman should include that in her plans.

Once a woman with a graft has a pregnancy diagnosed, her care should be with a high-risk service in a tertiary care center since the rate of prematurity and the need for critical care services are high. Her care is best coordinated between her graft specialist, transplant center, and a maternal–fetal specialist. The greatest risks across graft types include prematurity and fetal growth restriction, infection, hypertension, and PEC. Lesser risks include graft rejection and the risk of the immunesuppressives to the fetus.

The major goals of coordinated care are "to optimize maternal health including graft function, to maintain a normal metabolic environment (i.e., maintaining normoglycemia), minimize complications associated with preterm birth, detect and manage hypertensive complications especially PEC (which occurs in as much as 20% of transplant recipients) and to ensure adequate fetal growth" (Davison & Bailey, 2003).

Risk of graft rejection is increased when there is minimal time between graft and pregnancy. In presence of "adequate stable graft function" most pregnancies do well. In some women, the first pregnancy after graft has been successful but subsequent pregnancies resulted in more maternal complications including graft rejection (Table 38.6) (Branch et al., 1998). In renal transplants, if prepregnancy renal function was normal no increased risk of graft rejection has been noted. Conversely, in pregnancies conceived while the serum creatinine was 2.5 mg/dL or higher, women were three times more likely to experience graft rejection compared with women whose serum creatinine was less than 1.5 mg/dL at conception (Atallah et al., 2015).

Pharmacotherapeutics

Risks of immunosuppressive drugs to the fetus vary. It is beyond the scope of this chapter to have an in-depth discussion of various immunosuppressives but general principles are reviewed. The pharmacokinetics and fetal effects during pregnancy are not well understood. The longest experience in the United States has been with prednisone, azathioprine (AZA), cyclosporine (CsA), and tacrolimus. Prednisone is a

TABLE 38.6	Percentage of Complication by Type of Graft				
	HYPERTENSION (%)	PREECLAMPSIA (%)	INFECTION (%)	PRETERM DELIVERY (%)	LOW BIRTH WEIGHT (%)
Kidney	60–70	30	30	> 50	50
Liver	35	23	27	36	34
Pancreas–kidney	75	35	55	78	64
Heart	46	10	11	32	32
Lung	53	13	20	68	63

Adapted from Armenti et al. (2003).

category B drug and in low to moderate doses has not been demonstrated to have any negative effects on pregnancy or the fetus. In high doses, the drug may be associated with low birth weight. Tacrolimus, CsA, and AZA are category C drugs with which there is sufficient experience for it to be considered safe in pregnancy (Armenti, Moritz, Cardonick, & Davison, 2002). Other drugs used include sirolimus (SRL) and mycophenolate mofetil (MMF). MMF has been demonstrated to have teratogenicity in animals and there are two case reports of structural abnormalities recorded in the National Pregnancy Transplantation Registry (NPTR). Immunosuppressive drug levels are monitored at least monthly. The goal is the lowest level of drug that maintains the integrity of the graft.

Hypoglycemic medications to manage diabetes in pregnancy do not seem to be increased after transplant. Even pancreas and pancreas/kidney grafts have demonstrated an ability to maintain euglycemia in pregnancy but have the same risks of other grafts (Armenti et al., 2003).

Antihypertensive medications to manage hypertension and PEC in pregnancy are common with all postgraft pregnancies, occurring in up to one third of women, and are managed aggressively (Davison & Redman, 1997). There is little agreement on ideal antihypertensive agents or management strategies but early use of antihypertensives appears to prevent maternal hypertensive crisis.

Preterm delivery occurs in between 45% and 60% of postgraft pregnancies. Contributing factors include severe PEC and severe growth restriction. Despite the pelvic location, transplanted kidneys do not seem to have a negative impact on pregnancy (Davison & Redman, 1997).

Anticipate management of certain infection in pregnancy such as urinary tract infections (UTIs), HSV, CMV, toxoplasmosis (toxo), and hepatitis B. Frequent (at least monthly) urine monitoring should be done. The UTI rate is about 40% and many of the immunosuppressives at high doses can cause renal insufficiency (McKay & Josephson, 2006).

Growth restriction is carefully monitored and managed by standard surveillance techniques. Up to half of infants born to posttransplant mothers will have low birth weights. It is unclear whether this is a function of the increased rate of hypertension, the effect of the drugs, or other unidentified factors.

Breastfeeding is not currently recommended on immunosuppressives as the drugs have been found in breast milk

(American Academy of Pediatrics Committee on Drugs, 1994); however, the NTPR has followed several children whose postgraft mothers breastfed between 6 weeks and 18 months with no current untoward effects having been noted (Armenti et al., 2003). The amount of drug in the milk was measured at a subtherapeutic level. What requires further study is the effect of immunosuppressives on infant T cell formation.

■ HEMOLYSIS, ELEVATED LIVER ENZYMES, AND LOW PLATELETS

A complication of pregnancy involving coagulation defects and microthrombi was first described in 1892 (Barton & Sibai, 2004). In 1982, Dr Louis Weinstein first coined the acronym HELLP for this syndrome consisting of *h*emolysis, *e*levated *l*iver enzymes, and *l*ow *p*latelets (thrombocytopenia) (Weinstein, 1982).

Definition and Scope

Considered by some to be a severe form of PEC, by others to be a mild form of DIC, the precise pathogenesis of all three entities is unknown. They may be separate diseases with some common pathways or they may be extreme variations of one another (Barton, & Sibai, 2004). A leading investigator of HELLP, Dr. Baha Sibai, estimates the incidence of HELLP at 1 in 1,000 pregnancies in the general population (Table 38.7). He further estimates that approximately 10% to 20% of women with severe PEC or eclampsia develop HELLP but up to 20% of women with HELLP are diagnosed without the PEC criteria of proteinuria and hypertension. This lack of association with PEC seems to be especially true with postpartum onset of HELLP (Sibai et al., 1993). The timing of HELLP is slightly different from PEC in that PEC is relatively rare second trimester and postpartum.

The incidence of HELLP rises with advancing gestation, peaking in late third trimester. The peak occurrence of HELLP is mid-third trimester. Approximately 30% of the time, HELLP is not noted until the postpartum period, most commonly within the first 48 hours after birth, but occasionally up to 7

TABLE 38.7	Epidemiology of HELLP Versus Preeclampsia	
FACTOR	**HELLP**	**PREECLAMPSIA**
Incidence	0.2%–0.6% all pregnancies	5%–7% all pregnancies
Parity	Multiparous	Nulliparous
Age	> 25 years	< 20 and > 40 years
Ethnicity	More Caucasian	More African American
Genetics	Family history	Family history
Incidence postpartum onset	30%	5%
Predisposing comorbidities	Previous history Antiphospholipid antibody syndrome	Diabetes Multiple gestation Chronic hypertension Antiphospholipid antibody syndrome
Occurrence rates of HELLP in subsequent pregnancies	17%–29%	20% if severe preeclampsia
Occurrence of preeclampsia in subsequent pregnancies	43%–50%	2.5%–10%

HELLP, hemolysis, elevated liver enzymes, and low platelets.
Adapted from Sullivan et al. (1994).

days after birth (Table 38.8) (Barton & Sibai, 2004; Sibai et al., 1993). PEC has been diagnosed as late as 6 weeks postpartum but the overall incidence of postpartum onset PEC is 5%.

Etiology

Like PEC, HELLP is a disease of endothelial dysfunction and vasospasm. Whether the endothelial dysfunction is the cause or effect of vasospasm is not known. What is known is this dysfunction untreated results in microangiopathic hemolysis, destruction of red blood cells (RBCs) from narrowing or obstruction of small vessels which can be observed on a peripheral smear as schistocytes, spherocytes, and other abnormally shaped RBCs. Microangiopathic hemolysis is also associated with an elevated indirect bilirubin, decreased haptoglobin, and elevated lactic acid dehydrogenase levels. The damage occurs chiefly in the liver and kidneys, though the heart, lungs, and brain may also be affected. Sibai's group found the degree of cellular damage could not be directly correlated with the lab abnormalities or the clinical picture (Sibai, 1990). As the elevated liver enzymes portion of the acronym HELLP implies, some degree of liver damage is inherent in the disease. The liver enzyme abnormalities are not specific to HELLP, and other diseases, especially acute fatty liver of pregnancy, must be excluded. Liver enzyme abnormalities are generally higher with HELLP and jaundice occurs much later in HELLP (Padden, 1999).

Risk Factors

It is estimated about half of the women with HELLP have a risk of renal involvement and up to 20% experience acute renal failure with DIC. Coagulopathy, if present, is a late sign of HELLP syndrome, though some authors speculate all

TABLE 38.8	Timing of HELLP and Preeclampsia by Week of Gestation	
WEEKS AT ONSET	**HELLP (%)**	**PREECLAMPSIA (%)**
< 20	3	< 1
24–27	11	5
27–36	50	10 at < 34 weeks
36+	15	78.5
Postpartum	30	5.4

HELLP, hemolysis, elevated liver enzymes, and low platelets.
Adapted from Sibai et al. (1993).

patients with HELLP have an underlying coagulopathy that remains subclinical because the woman is delivered before becoming fulminant or because laboratory tests have not been fully explored. Most women will have normal coagulation studies (Padden, 1999). In pregnancy onset HELLP, once the fetus is delivered, even severe renal involvement typically resolves (Weinstein, 1982). However, HELLP syndrome with postpartum onset is associated with greater risk for pulmonary edema and renal failure (Sibai et al., 1993).

Symptoms

Women with high blood pressure and proteinuria may or may not have symptoms preceding the signs, which give them a diagnosis of PEC. When PEC is diagnosed first, clinicians are more alert for complications and HELLP syndrome may be more readily recognized. In some women, HELLP symptoms occur without hypertension and the condition is initially misdiagnosed. Patients with HELLP often present with general malaise of a few days duration. GI disturbances in the form of epigastric pain and nausea and vomiting are common. Some women experience a headache as well (Table 38.9). This combination of symptoms may be interpreted initially as flu or other illness or in the case of postpartum onset might be attributable to exaggerated postpartum sensations.

One study reported an average of 8 days between onset of symptoms and diagnosis in patients with HELLP (Schroder & Heyl, 1985).

Evaluation/Assessment

Physical assessment often provides less information than patient history. The liver may be enlarged or tender to palpation. A liver capsule hematoma may cause pain referred to the shoulder. If preceded by PEC, central edema of the face, abdomen, and sacrum may be noted and deep tendon reflexes may be brisk. A ruptured liver capsule can cause rapid abdominal distension and shock. Rarely, less than 5% of the time, jaundice is evident (Wolf, 1996). As HELLP has overlapping symptoms with many other diseases, diagnosis is often based on timing of symptoms and history and less often based on laboratory studies (see Box 38.1).

Diagnostic Studies

Diagnosis is supported by laboratory testing.

1. Liver test abnormalities cannot predict the clinical severity of the disease, complications, or recovery; they support the diagnosis. The transaminases aspartate aminotransferase (AST) or alanine aminotransferase (ALT) will be moderately elevated and lactic acid dehydrogenase will be markedly elevated. Elevated liver enzymes are thought to result from obstruction of the hepatic blood flow by fibrin deposits, leading to periportal necrosis (Wolf, 1996).

2. The most sensitive marker for HELLP is the platelet count, which is markedly to severely depressed (Magann et al., 1994).
3. Hemoglobin and hematocrit may be in the normal range but abnormal cells will be noted on the peripheral smear.
4. A mildly elevated indirect bilirubin may be noted.
5. D-Dimer may be positive in the presence of an abnormally high level of fibrin degradation products. It indicates significant clot (thrombus) formation and breakdown in the body, but it does not tell the location or cause. In women with PEC this test is predictive of who will develop HELLP. The D-dimer will be positive before coagulation studies change (Neiger, Trofatter, & Trofatter, 1995).
6. Prothrombin time and partial thromboplastin time are usually normal (Table 38.10).

Treatment/Management

HELLP syndrome is most appropriately managed by a physician, preferably in a tertiary care center. Deterioration in maternal or fetal status can occur rapidly. The fetus is assessed and the mother stabilized, then transported to the hospital. There is no place for home management of HELLP syndrome. The woman is maintained on left lateral bed rest with intravenous hydration, careful monitoring of blood pressure and fluid balance, preferably in a tertiary care center. While a diagnosis is being established and if conservative management is appropriate, laboratory markers should be followed. Classification of severity of HELLP syndrome that is based on laboratory markers may be useful in directing management.

There are two commonly employed classification systems used in managing HELLP syndrome The first system developed by Sibai's group in Tennessee quantifies the number of abnormalities, with partial HELLP having only one or two abnormalities and full HELLP having all three: hemolysis, elevated liver enzymes, and low platelets (Mol et al., 2016). The treatment of choice for full HELLP is to expedite birth within 48 hours of diagnosis, even if the fetus

TABLE 38.9	Presenting Symptoms of HELLP by Frequency
SYMPTOM	**PERCENTAGE**
General malaise	90
RUQ or epigastric pain	65–90
Headache	31
Nausea, vomiting	30
Bleeding	9
Visual disturbances	5
Shoulder pain	5

HELLP, hemolysis, elevated liver enzymes, and low platelets; RUQ, right upper quadrant.
Adapted from Sibai (1990); Wolf (1996).

BOX 38.1   DIFFERENTIAL DIAGNOSIS AND HELLP SYNDROME

Acute fatty liver of pregnancy (AFLP)
Idiopathic thrombocytopenia purpura (ITP)
Thrombotic thrombocytopenia purpura (TTP)
Viral hepatitis
Gastroenteritis
Pancreatitis
Gall bladder disease
Pyelonephritis
Hemolytic uremic syndrome
Systemic lupus erythematosus (SLE)
Kidney stones
Peptic ulcer

TABLE 38.10	Laboratory Values With HELLP Syndrome		
LABORATORY TEST	**NORMAL VALUE IN PREGNANCY**	**MEDIAN VALUE WITH HELLP**	**RANGE**
Platelets	150,000–450,000/mm³	<60,000/mm³	6,000–150,000/ mm³
Peripheral smear	RBCs with normal configuration	Schistocytes (Helmut cells) Target cells	—
Aminotransferases ALT AST	<35 U/L <25 U/L	200 U/L 249 U/L	70–6,000 U/L
Lactic acid dehydrogenase	250–450 U/mL	853 U/mL	600–23,000 U/mL
Hemoglobin and hematocrit	11.0–14 g/dL 33%–42%	Usually within normal limits	Depression in relationship to RBC destruction
D-Dimer	Negative	Positive if preeclampsia also present	—
Bilirubin	0.3–1.0 mg/dL	1.5 mg/dL	0.5–25.5 mg/dL

ALT, alanine transaminase; AST, aspartate transaminase; HELLP, hemolysis, elevated liver enzymes and low platelets; RBC, red blood cells.
Adapted from Barton and Sibai (2004).

is premature. Maternal liver function can decline rapidly and the risk for DIC is high. If there are only one to two manifestations, conservative management may be appropriate to get the pregnancy to 34 weeks gestation. One study suggested that conservative management for up to 15 days between 28 and 32 weeks was not associated with increased perinatal or maternal morbidity if the woman is normotensive and does not have right upper quadrant pain (Audibert, Friedman, Frangieh, & Sibai, 1996).

The second classification system developed by Martin and colleagues in Mississippi is based on the platelet count. Class I is the most severe with platelets less than 50,000/mm³. Class II is a nadir of 50,000 to 100,000 platelets per mm³ and Class III is 100,000 to 150,000 per mm³. Those women in Class III may be candidates for conservative management if remote from term (Martin et al., 1997).

Pharmacotherapeutics

Although ACOG practice guidelines on HELLP do not currently endorse the routine use of steroids for HELLP, for women in whom administration of glucosteroids is being employed to decrease the consequences of prematurity, the steroids show promise of reducing maternal complications as well as fetal. Three small studies employed corticosteroids in the form of dexamethasone 10 mg: IM two doses 12 hours apart immediately postpartum followed by 5 mg at 24 hours and 36 hours in the treatment of HELLP syndrome. This treatment was associated with improvement in laboratory functions (increased platelets, decreased lactic acid dehydrogenase and alanine aminotransferase) and improvement in maternal urinary output. These improvements were associated with a quicker recovery (Magann et al., 1994; Martin et al., 1997, 2003; Vigil de Garcia & Garcia de Caceres, 1997). Because of the association with

severe PEC, patients with HELLP often receive seizure prophylaxis in the form of magnesium sulfate (Waisman, Mayorga, Cámera, Vignolo, & Martinotti, 1988). See Chapter 45 for details on hypertension management.

If a diastolic blood pressure of less than 100 is unable to be maintained, antihypertensive therapy in the form of Apresoline, labetalol, or nifedipine will be initiated. Apresoline is typically administered with a 5 mg initial dose intravenously followed every 15 to 20 minutes by another 2.5 to 5 mg until the blood pressure is in the target range. When nifedipine and magnesium sulfate are used concurrently, there is a risk of potentiation of effect (Waisman et al., 1988).

PPH is a common sequela of HELLP. However, prophylactic blood transfusion is usually not necessary if vaginal birth is anticipated, unless the platelets fall below 25,000/mm³. Transfusion does not reduce the risk of PPH or accelerate the rate of platelet recovery. Vaginal delivery is not contraindicated. Cesarean section should be performed for the same indications as for all women. For patients undergoing cesarean section, transfusion is considered when platelets decline below 50,000/mm³. More than half of patients with HELLP will receive some form of blood product, most often postpartum. Administered postpartally, plasmapheresis appears to increase platelet count and facilitate normalization of LDH (Barton & Sibai, 1996).

Pain relief options can generally be decided by the patient in conjunction with her obstetric and anesthesia providers. If platelets are greater than 100,000 per mm³, with no evidence of coagulopathy, epidural may be appropriate. Intravenous narcotics, local anesthetics, or general anesthesia can be used if epidural is considered unsafe (Portis, Jacobs, Skerman, & Skerman, 1997).

If the disease is not treated early, up to 25% of women develop serious complications including PPH. A small number of women die (1.1%) (Sibai et al., 1993). Risk for developing HELLP in subsequent pregnancies is high, 19% to 27% (Sullivan et al., 1994). These women also have an almost 50% risk of developing PEC in subsequent pregnancies (Chames, Haddad, Barton, Livingston, & Sibai, 2003). Morbidity rates among babies born to mothers with HELLP syndrome vary (10%–60%), influenced by comorbidities such as prematurity and IUGR. Hypoglycemia may be profound and hypotension may be present (Barton & Sibai, 2004).

Women with HELLP should be screened for antiphospholipid antibodies (APLA). There are no known preventative measures for HELLP, though calcium and aspirin supplementation have been studied. The woman may have permanent liver damage, which may require a transplant or can be fatal. When counseling the woman for future pregnancy, it is important to strike a balance between conveying the risk for future pregnancies with a sense of optimism. The woman should be encouraged early in the pregnancy to make plans for who will watch her older child(ren) should she become ill again; if she works, she might advise her employer she is at risk for preterm delivery. Discuss mode of delivery, for example, if she had a cesarean section the first time, discuss whether she absolutely has to have one in future pregnancies (van Pampus, Wolf, Mayruhu, Treffers, & Bleker, 2001). At her first prenatal visit, she should have baseline liver functions drawn with the routine lab work of pregnancy.

Complementary/Alternative Medicine

Although no CAM method has been demonstrated useful in the acute treatment of HELLP, root vegetables and their leaves have historically been thought to be liver purifiers. Dandelion, beets, and carrots, both the vegetable and the root, may be consumed as a vegetable or steeped as a tonic. They are high in vitamins and potassium and may serve as a natural diuretic. They are safe for consumption between and during pregnancy.

■ ISOIMMUNIZATION

RBCs are covered with a variety of proteins called antigens. The antigens are divided into groups. One of the best known groups is the Rh. There are three alleles (variations) in the Rh factor group: Cc, D, and Ee. The D allele of the Rh factor, the most clinically relevant, is found on the RBC membranes in most people. Those with this antigen are called Rh positive. Those without this antigen are known as Rh negative. If the fetus has a different Rh factor from the mother, any mixing of fetal and maternal blood can stimulate an immune reaction from the mother.

Definition and Scope

Fetal blood cell production begins within a few weeks of conception (Manogura & Weiner, 2006). When a fetus of an Rh negative mother is carrying antigens of the CDE (RH)

system and the mother has no antibodies, she can become sensitized or alloimmunized to her fetus and produce immunoglobulin G (IgG) anti D antibodies that readily cross the placenta, bind to fetal RBCs, and are ultimately destroyed by the fetal spleen. The initial antibody response to the D antigen can take up to 6 months, so immunization during a first pregnancy is uncommon. However, if untreated, about 20% of women will become sensitized at the time of birth.

Etiology

Subsequent pregnancy of an Rh-positive fetus will result in a rapid secondary immunological response in days, not months. The spleen rapidly destroys RBCs, which affects fetal organs, interferes with placental perfusion, and can result in hydrops fetalis. This process is known as hemolytic disease of the newborn (HDN) or hemolytic disease of the fetus.

Symptoms

Infants born with HDN demonstrate:

- Pallor
- Jaundice that begins within 24 hours after delivery
- Unexplained bruising or petechiae
- Tissue swelling (edema)
- Respiratory distress
- Seizures
- Lack of normal movement
- Poor reflex response

Evaluation/Assessment

Prenatal determination of maternal blood type, Rh status, and antibody screening is a standard of care in most industrialized nations at the initial prenatal visit. If antibodies are present they are measured as a titer. A titer of greater than 1:4 is considered sensitized. Although the majority of alloimmunization occurs in response to the D Rh, there are other non-Rh groups that can be associated with HDN.

Treatment/Management

The groups Kell, Kidd, and MNS account for a small percentage of HDN and the treatment is very similar, but there is no current preventative strategy. ABO incompatibility is also a source of hemolysis but is rarely severe and when present with RH incompatibility reduces the risk of immunization to about 5% (Manogura & Weiner, 2006).

For the unsensitized woman, obtain the blood type and Rh of the father of the baby if available. If it is unknown or Rh positive, the woman should receive Rh-immune globulin at various points in the pregnancy. If there is no bleeding during pregnancy, a 300-mcg dose of RhIgG at 27 to 28 weeks is adequate to cover up to 15 mL of fetal RBCs, which may mix with maternal blood for the next 12 weeks. If there is first trimester bleeding, a smaller dose of RhIgG may be administered. If there is bleeding, or risk of bleeding, as from an amniocentesis or abdominal trauma, the full 300mcg dose should be administered. After birth, the newborn blood type will be available and if it is Rh +, Du+, the woman should receive another dose of RhIgG within 72 hours of birth (ACOG, 2006).

A sensitized woman during her initial sensitized pregnancy should have the blood type and Rh of the father if not already known and the father is available. An antibody titer will be obtained on the mother during the first prenatal visit. If the titer is less than 1:16, the woman may be followed collaboratively between the APRN and a collaborating physician. Titers will be repeated every 2 to 4 weeks depending on gestation and levels of dilution (ACOG, 2006).

If the titer on the initial prenatal visit is greater than 1:16, the woman's care will be per physician management and will include periodic assessment of amniotic bilirubin levels. As RBCs are being destroyed by the fetal spleen, the red cell pigment is released and can be detected as bilirubin in the maternal amniotic fluid. If an antibody titer is greater than 1:16, fetal blood typing may eliminate the need for more invasive testing. Fetal blood type can be obtained through a process called percutaneous umbilical blood sampling (PUBS) where a small amount of blood is taken directly from the fetal umbilical cord under ultrasonographic guidance. If the fetal blood type is determined to be Rh negative, no further evaluation is necessary. If the fetus is Rh positive and the maternal antibody titer is greater than 1:16, the fetal bilirubin can be followed by periodic PUBS procedures, or more commonly, the bilirubin will be measured indirectly by spectrophotometric analysis of the amniotic fluid obtained during amniocentesis. If the titer surpasses 1:32 for the first time after 27 to 28 weeks, usually the fetus can grow safely to term with the periodic amniotic fluid analyses and concomitant ultrasonographic evaluation of the fetus for hydrops. Hydrops fetalis is a condition of severe edema in fetal tissue. As RBCs are destroyed in the fetus, anemia develops and subsequently hypoproteinuria. Hypoproteinuria causes a drop in the colloidal osmotic pressure and blood is pushed from the vasculature into the tissue. Organs including the heart, liver, and spleen are unable to compensate. The heart experiences high output failure; fluid collects in the heart, lungs, and abdomen (ascites). The changes are seen ultrasonographically as an enlarged heart, liver, and spleen. The placenta becomes thickened. Edema is even observed subcutaneously in the fetal scalp (Socol, 1998).

In large medical centers, fetuses can be followed with Doppler flow ultrasonography, which is useful as a noninvasive measure of fetal disease. The blood flow in the middle cerebral artery is visualized. The expected peak systolic flow is calculated. This functions as a surrogate for cardiac function (Mari et al., 2000).

Subsequent sensitized pregnancies are followed similarly but with surveillance beginning earlier and occurring more often based on the changes during the previous affected pregnancy. Changes in the bilirubin concentration of the amniotic fluid are plotted on a graph called a Liley curve with certain values being associated with no to minimal disease (zone 1), higher numbers with moderate disease, and highest numbers (above med zone 2 to 3) indicating severe disease and the need for immediate intervention in the form of fetal transfusion or delivery.

■ RECURRENT PREGNANCY LOSS

Miscarriage or SAB is more than simply loss of a gestation. It is loss of a potential family member, which is an emotionally charged experience. It may evoke feelings of reproductive failure, loss of femininity or masculinity, and general decline in self-worth.

Definition and Scope

The natural occurrence rate of spontaneous pregnancy loss is unknown. The baseline for a single pregnancy loss of a clinically recognized pregnancy is estimated at one in five pregnancies in women during their peak reproductive lives (ages 20–34 years). In the very young and the older reproductive groups, the incidence of a single loss is higher. One study involving monthly immunoassays for pregnancy hormones reported an overall loss rate including pregnancies not detected clinically in excess of one in two pregnancies. Three or more consecutive pregnancy losses of a confirmed pregnancy before the 20th week of gestation are generally considered recurrent pregnancy loss (RPL). Some clinicians define RPL as two or more consecutive losses or three or more with interspersed viable pregnancies (Ansari & Kirkpatrick, 1998).

While a single pregnancy loss is a common phenomenon, it may be overwhelming to a couple. It may be difficult for them to believe it does not statistically increase the likelihood of a second loss. After two miscarriages, the loss rate rises to one in three pregnancies and after three miscarriages the rate is one in two pregnancies. Having a viable pregnancy drops the recurrence rate back to one in three. Using the criterion of three or more losses the incidence of RPL is 1% of the childbearing population, and using the criterion of two or more the incidence is 2% (Salat-Baroux, 1988).

RPL can be primary or secondary. Primary RPL indicates a woman has never carried a pregnancy to viability. Secondary RPL implies one or more pregnancies have been carried beyond 20 weeks. Few level 1 studies exist on the etiology and management of RPL. Reported rates of causes vary with the study and since loss is probably multifactorial, assigned percentages may overlap. General categories of etiology for RPL include genetic, anatomic, immunologic, endocrine, thrombophilic, and other.

Etiology

Chromosomal abnormalities in the fetus are a common cause of pregnancy loss first trimester and account for 30% of losses second trimester but are not usually associated with RPL.

Genetic factors in the parents in the form of a major chromosomal rearrangement account for 3% to 5% of RPL. The majority of these rearrangements are translocations, where genetic material breaks off of one part of a chromosome and fuses with another part in such a way the rearranged chromosome still contains the same genetic material (Franssen et al., 2005).

Structural defects associated with congenital weakness of the muscle fibers have been associated with underdevelopment of the cervix from maternal DES exposure in utero. Before 1971, some women were given the drug diethylstilbesterol (DES) in the mistaken notion that it could reduce the incidence of miscarriage. After the discovery of clear cell carcinoma in female children whose mothers had received DES in pregnancy, the drug was withdrawn from the market; children born from 1972 onward should not have been exposed. However, with the increase in pregnancies in women more than 35 years, the influence of DES will be felt for another 15 years and is still a public health issue. About 25% to 50% of the women exposed to DES in utero have an abnormality of the upper third of the vagina inducing inadequate development of the cervix and abnormalities in the size and shape of the uterine cavity (Herbst, Kurman, & Scully, 1972). The risks do not decrease even when the cervix appears normal or the woman has born a term child before.

Mullerian duct structure abnormality accounts for most congenital uterine anomalies, affecting between 1/200 and 1/600 women. Depending on the timing of the abnormality embryologically, the woman may have a bicornuate uterus, which often receives and carries a pregnancy to term, or in the most severe form will have a unicornuate uterus, which carries an extremely high risk of mid-trimester loss (Pui, 2004). A woman with a unicornuate uterus often will have other anatomical abnormalities including short cervix and kidney defects. If a woman does carry a fetus to viability, the pregnancy is still at risk for preterm birth, abnormal presentation, cervical insufficiency (CI), and fetal growth restriction (Raga et al., 1997). A septate uterus has the poorest pregnancy outcome of the Mullerian duct abnormalities. The length of the septum affects the incidence of pregnancy loss. A septum is easily correctible with surgery. One report indicates the RPL rate declines from 80% to 10% to 15% after surgery to remove a uterine septum (Proctor & Haney, 2003).

Cervical muscle fibers may be damaged by trauma such as birth or mechanical dilatation during a second trimester termination or forcible dilatation during a D&C. The treatment of cervical intraepithelial neoplasis (CIN) has become safer in recent years with replacement of the cone biopsy with a LEEP or laser ablation, but there are still reproductive women who have had a conization of their cervix. Cervical lacerations have even been noted after vaginal and cesarean births and are probably associated with prolonged pushing (Smith & Kirsop, 1991).

One indirect cause of cervical shortening may be uterine overdistention with multiples and polyhydramnios (Goldenberg et al., 1996; Many, Lazebnik, & Hill, 1996). Multiple pregnancies and those conceived with ovulation induction by menotropins have been demonstrated to have a higher circulating level of the hormone relaxin (Haning et al., 1996). Relaxin causes connective tissue reorganization, which is beneficial in relaxing pelvic architecture but may result in cervical shortening.

Endocrine disorders probably account for the largest percentage of RPL. A luteal phase defect possibly accounts for about 5% of RPL (Daya, 1996). Luteal phase defect is the term applied to the second half of a woman's menstrual cycle when there is inadequate protestational effect on the endometrium from a disruption in corpus luteum formation. The role of progesterone in pregnancy is well documented. Progesterone is produced by the corpus luteum cyst on the ovary after ovulation. Supported by luteinizing hormone (LH) from the pituitary after conception, the corpus luteum supports a pregnancy for the first 7 weeks and then gradually diminishes its progesterone production as the placenta develops and hCG dominates.

Assumptions have been made that a shortened luteal phase results in insufficient progesterone to support a pregnancy. As the methods for diagnosing luteal phase defects and the effects of progesterone supplementation have not been consistently demonstrated in the literature, the role of a luteal defect in infertility is unclear (Arredondo & Noble, 2006).

During pregnancy, a woman carries her fetus without rejection. The process by which this happens is unknown and therefore the process by which an autoimmune response results in pregnancy loss is also unknown. Autoimmune disorders account for approximately 5% to 15% of RPL. An autoimmune condition is where the body attacks its own organs (Martin et al., 2002). Phospholipids make up a portion of cell walls including the cells of the placenta. Anything which interferes with phospholipid synthesis (antiphospholipid) will disrupt placental function. The most widely studied of the APLA are lupus anticoagulant and anticardiolipin antibody (ACL). Women with these autoimmune antibodies are at increased risk of fetal loss in any trimester from placental thrombosis or growth restriction (Empson, Lassere, Craig, & Scott, 2002).

Two other autoimmune associations with RPL include a biological false positive on syphilis screening and the presence of antithyroid antibodies (Abramson & Stagnaro-Green, 2001; Stagnaro-Green & Glinoer, 2004). The mechanism for these reactions is felt to be one of general autoimmune disruption rather than disruption at the level of a single organ. Alloimmune disorders as a cause of pregnancy loss are still largely theoretical and often assigned as a cause of RPL only as a diagnosis of exclusion.

Uncontrolled diabetes is associated with a higher than normal risk for congenital anomalies and pregnancy loss. The mechanism is felt to be partly immunologic and partly from maternal vascular disease (Greene et al., 1989). Other chronic maternal illnesses like renal failure and severe cardiac disease are associated with a high degree of infertility, both inability to conceive and early pregnancy loss. The mechanisms are felt to be the same as for diabetes.

Normal prolactin levels are felt to be important in maintaining pregnancy. Hyperprolactinemia has been associated with a higher rate of miscarriage and possibly accounts for 15% to 60% of early pregnancy loss (Hirahara et al., 1998).

Polycystic ovary syndrome (PCOS) accounts for a significant portion of early pregnancy losses (20%–40%). High levels of LH and testosterone may affect ovulation, endometrial development, and alterations in the prostaglandin/cytokine balance. Insulin resistance is known to play a role but the precise mechanism is not known (Glueck, Wang, Goldenberg, & Sieve-Smith, 2002).

During pregnancy, development of the placental bed requires alterations of various clotting factors. Thrombosis impairs spiral arteriole development. Inherited thrombophilias including factor V Leiden, prothrombin gene mutation, and deficiencies in protein S and C or antithrombin can all contribute to thrombosis. Although fetal wastage from thrombosis is well documented, the effect of these disorders on early pregnancy has not been consistently demonstrated (Barbieri, 2001; Kutteh & Triplett, 2006; Sotiriadis, Makrigiannakis, Stefos, Paraskevaidis, & Kalantaridou, 2007).

Environmental teratogens such as anesthetic gases, lead, and mercury are known to account for 10% of congenital anomalies and probably account for a small percentage of RPL. Smoking, ethyl alcohol (EtOH), and illicit substances are rare causes and probably dose dependent (Summers, 1994).

Radiation and teratogenic medications are associated with individual pregnancy loss but have not been demonstrated to be associated with RPL (Gopalkrishnan et al., 2000).

Miscellaneous causes of infertility include obesity, hypothesized to be partly from insulin resistance and untreated celiac disease. Even when subclinical, celiac disease is associated with menstrual irregularity and miscarriage.

The male factor accounts for 40% of infertility and some studies have found an increase in miscarriage amongst women whose partners have poor sperm quality (ACOG, 2002).

Anecdotally, many infectious agents have been associated with RPL. A recent review of the literature failed to show any association between a specific infectious agent and RPL.

There has been no evident to link moderate exercise and exposure to electromagnetic fields to RPL (Rai, Backos, Baxter, Chilcott, & Regan, 2000).

Risk Factors

Many factors can be associated with RPL. Uterine myomas and intrauterine polyps are thought to interfere with implantation. Leiomyomas are benign muscular tumors, which may develop in the endometrial cavity.

Polyps are an organized overgrowth of the endometrium occurring in response to estrogen. The role of the myoma or polyp on pregnancy loss depends on the size, number, and position of the masses. There is little literature regarding the treatment of myomas or polyps in pregnancy. Some recommend removal before a pregnancy as large myomas or polyps may disrupt the endometrium and prevent a pregnancy from implanting (Pérez-Medina et al., 2005). Risks of surgical removal should be weighed against the benefits in planning a pregnancy. Any surgery that disrupts the lining of the uterus places the uterus at risk of scar formation. Asherman syndrome is an especially damaging form of scar formation in which bands of tissue called synechiae form throughout the uterine cavity in the face of a hypoestrogenic state. Asherman syndrome accounts for a relatively small percentage of RPL. The incidence has declined with the decrease in the use of inappropriate D&C procedures, but can still occur with uterine surgery, as a result of some infections and as a result of radium implants (Christiansen et al., 2005).

CI, sometimes called cervical incompetence, is the most common cause of mid-trimester fetal loss, accounting for 2% of all pregnancy losses and 25% of second trimester losses. CI is probably not one disorder but an end result of multiple biophysical and structural factors (Iams et al., 1995). The most distal portion of the uterus is the cervix, which is composed of smooth muscle and extracellular tissue matrix held together with collagen, elastin, and fibronectin (Leppert, 1995). The muscle content is in a gradient with the highest portion of the muscle at the internal os and the lowest at the external os (Rorie & Newton, 1967). The elastic, muscular internal os supports the weight of the pregnancy. In a normal pregnancy, the cervical components remain in a stable mix until shortly before labor when point collagen bundles begin to decrease and extracellular matrix begins to rearrange, a process known as effacement (Leppert, 1995). Before these changes, the cervix is digitally and visually appreciated as a structure about 3 to 4 cm long with the consistency of the cartilage at the tip of the nose. As the matrix dissociates, the cervix shortens and the texture becomes more the consistency of the human lips (Rorie & Newton, 1967). How this change occurs is not fully understood, so where and how it goes awry is also not understood.

Evaluation/Assessment

Women presenting with CI exhibit premature, progressive dilatation of the cervix without painful contractions and occurring before fetal viability, often resulting in a previable birth. If dilatation begins mid-trimester, progress may be slow and result in a severely premature infant.

Diagnostic Studies

Diagnosis may be made by manual cervical assessment of transvaginal ultrasonography (TVUS). Because the lower uterine segment and the cervix are poorly differentiated before 20 weeks, there is little interobserver reliability in measurement of the cervix manually or ultrasonographically. After 20 weeks there is more consistency in measurements on TVUS. The normal cervical length is 3 to 4 cm and a cervical length less than 2 cm was found to have a 50% preterm delivery risk in one study (Christiansen et al., 2005). Other studies have looked at the response of the internal os to pressure on top of the uterus or the Valsalva maneuver. This funneling is associated with a diagnosis of CI (Iams et al., 1995).

A comprehensive workup for a diagnosis of RPL is best performed by a specialist in the field of infertility. Portions of the work up which can be performed by a nurse practitioner or nurse midwife include detailed history, lifestyle modifications to correct environmental risks, counseling regarding weight loss and glucose control, and treatment of any vaginal infections.

A medical surgical history for RPL includes:

- Any maternal disease including diabetes, lupus, thyroid disease, deep vein thrombosis
- History of abdominal or pelvic trauma including instrumentation
- Exposure to environmental teratogens, including tobacco, alcohol, illicit drugs, anesthetic gases, lead, radiation or mercury
- Current medications including herbs

Obstetric and gynecologic history includes:

- Description of menstrual cycles
- Description of timing in pregnancy of any losses
- Was fetal cardiac activity detected?
- Was there cytogenetic analysis?
- Is there a history of gestations ending progressively earlier in pregnancy?

A family history includes:

- History of birth defects or chromosomal abnormalities in family
- Question consanguinity

A general full physical examination includes:

- Attention to hirsutism, acanthosus nigracans Galactorrhea
- Reproductive organ abnormalities

Diagnostic studies can be very expensive and often need special timing within the menstrual cycle; specialty testing is most appropriately performed by an infertility expert. Those tests done by the nurse practitioner include common tests for health such as

- Sexually transmitted disease screening and Pap smear screening
- Thyroid-stimulating hormone, blood glucose or insulin levels, CBC including platelets

Tests performed by a specialist may include:

- Karyotyping for translocations and mosaicism (Scott, 2003)

Sonohysteroscopy is performed to assess uterine cavity shape and cervical abnormalities, particularly Müllerian duct abnormalities and diagnosis of Asherman syndrome. When the dye is injected into the uterus, the adhesions appear as thick, muscular bands or as defects in the wall. The adhesions can be removed hysteroscopically but there is some risk of further adhesion formation. The pregnancy rate after adhesion removal is 60% to 80% but risk of placenta accreta and preterm labor/birth is high.

Immunology workup will include ACL IgG and IgM, anti-lupus coagulant (done twice, 6–8 weeks apart), factor V Leiden, and protein S and C. Endocrine workup may include day 3 follicle-stimulating hormone (FSH) and estradiol.

Antithyroid peroxidase antibodies (TPO) presence is associated with a miscarriage rate five times greater than random population. Often, women have no clinical evidence of thyroid disease.

Endometrial biopsy is considered by some to be the gold standard for determining a luteal phase defect. Other authors feel that results of an endometrial biopsy have no predictive value for whether a pregnancy will be supported.

Treatment/Management

Surgical repair may be done of any uterine wall defects, synechiae may be lysed, and septums removed. Counseling includes informing the woman that after a completed workup only 50% of the time will there be an identified cause for her recurrent loss. Although not identifying the cause is frustrating for the couple and the provider, the good news is that even when the cause is not identified most women with RPL have a 70% chance of having a viable pregnancy.

Once pregnancy has been achieved, the woman's care is most appropriately provided by maternal–fetal medicine specialists. Treatment often includes the use of baby aspirin, steroids, and heparin or immune globulin therapy for immune problems (Gross & Bombard, 1998; Halliday, Lumley, & Watson, 1995). Metformin may be initiated before conception and continued through pregnancy. It effectively decreases insulin resistance (Michlin et al., 2000). Progesterone may be used if a luteal phase defect has been identified (Oates-Whitehead, Haas, & Carrier, 2003). A woman with a shortened cervix may have a cerclage, which is a stitch in the upper cervix to provide support normally provided by the cervix. This stitch is usually done as a "rescue" procedure when shortening is detected during pregnancy (Final Report of the Medical Research Council/Royal College of Obstetricians and Gynaecologists Multicentre Randomised Trial of Cervical Cerclage, 1993). In one large, randomized study in England, the birthrate before 33 weeks was reduced by half with women who had a therapeutic cerclage placed. The rates of infection and premature rupture of the membranes were higher, leading the authors to conclude that cerclage should be confined to those women in whom the benefits outweigh the risks (ACOG Practice Bulletin, 2014; Drakeley, Roberts, & Alfirevic, 2003).

RPL and its evaluation are emotionally imbued experiences for a couple and may lead to unproven therapies and mental distress. Caring, empathy, and interpreting tests and interventions for the couple can assist them in choosing appropriate therapies.

■ IPV IN PREGNANCY

IPV in the form of battering is the most common cause of injury to women, crossing race, ethnic, and socioeconomic lines. Serious injuries with resultant health costs, lost days of work, and family breakdown make abuse a public health issue (Breiding, Basile, Smith, Black, & Mahendra, 2015).

Definition and Scope

IPV is misuse of power by dominating or coercive behaviors perpetrated against someone who is physically, economically, or mentally less powerful. Abuse is not just a personal problem. While violence is gender blind, more than 95% of the IPV occurs between a man and a woman. About one third of female homicide victims are murdered by their current or ex-partner, usually a male (Breiding et al., 2015).

Homicide during pregnancy is the second leading cause of death by injury.

It is estimated that in the United States, 5 million women each year are physically or sexually abused by their current or former partner (Tjaden & Thoennes, 2000). The incidence of violence against pregnant women has been reported between 23% and 40%, higher than all other complications of pregnancy (Gazmararian et al., 1996). Up to 40% of those women experienced the battering from that partner first during the pregnancy and of those women, 60% reported more than one episode of violence during pregnancy (McFarlane, Campbell, Sharps, & Watson, 2002). One study addressing patient identification versus provider identification found IPV occurs in up to 25% of pregnant women but providers detect only 4% to 10% of cases (Guth & Pachter, 2000). While IPV crosses demographics, certain populations are more vulnerable. Teens have higher incidences of most complications of pregnancy and IPV is no exception.

Etiology

Physical insult on a pregnant woman is magnified because of the physiologic changes of pregnancy. Some of trauma seen during pregnancy can be accounted for by orthostatic hypotension, pelvic and abdominal wall laxity, pain, and the awkwardness of movement caused by alteration of the center of gravity and a protuberant abdomen (Esposito, Gens, Smith, Scorpio, & Buchman, 1991). Trauma in pregnancy is estimated at 6% to 7%, with blunt trauma being most common (Eyler & Cohen, 1999). Blunt trauma occurs most often due to motor vehicle accidents. The incidence of minor trauma, especially falls, increases as pregnancy progresses. However, falls and accidents may also be how the victim of IPV tries to cover her abuse. When a pregnant patient suffers trauma, maternal survival does not guarantee fetal survival. Fetal death rates in pregnant trauma victims exceed maternal death rates three to ninefold (Table 38.11) (Hedin & Janson,

TABLE 38.11	Health Risks of Intimate Partner Violence	
	DIRECT	**INDIRECT**
Obstetric	Miscarriage	Poor maternal weight gain
	Preterm labor/birth	Sexually transmitted diseases including HIV
	Low-birth-weight babies	Fetal infection
	Abruption/hemorrhage	Chronic stress
	Stillbirth	
Medical	Contusions	Chronic pelvic pain
	Lacerations	Chronic back pain
	Fractures	Temporomandibular joint pain
	Abdominal organ rupture	GI disorders: irritable bowel syndrome, constipation, diarrhea
	Concussions	Arthritis
	Orifice injury: mouth, anus, vagina	Chronic urinary or kidney infections
	Blood loss/anemia	Headaches
	Disfigurement	Traumatic arthritis
	Unwanted pregnancy	
	Maternal death	
Psychological	Depression	Low self-esteem
	Anxiety	Sleep disturbances
	Fear	Drug/EtOH/tobacco abuse
	Suicidal ideation	Sexual dysfunction
	Homicidal ideation	

EtOH, ethyl alcohol.
Adapted from Eyler and Cohen (1999); Breiding et al. (2015).

2000). Even with minor trauma, the fetal death rate is estimated at 1% to 5% (Agnoli & Deutchman, 1993).

Risk Factor

Pregnancy is a time when battering tends to increase by abusive partners. IPV crosses all socioeconomic statues, race, ethnic, sex, and gender lines. However, African American women seem to be particularly vulnerable with rates of seven times that of non-Hispanic Caucasians (Chang, Berg, Saltzman, & Herndon, 2005; Jacoby, Gorenflo, Black, Wunderlich, & Eyler, 1999; Tjaden & Thoennes, 2000). During pregnancy when IPV does not result in death, it still poses health risks to the woman and her fetus. Complications can be acute or chronic, physical, and emotional.

Evaluation/Assessment

Any report of a fall needs to be investigated for its association with interpersonal violence. Each prenatal site should develop a program for assessing the safety of pregnant women and other vulnerable members of the family (Poole et al., 1996). ACOG recommends screening women minimally at the initial prenatal visit and at least every trimester during pregnancy (Clark et al., 2000). With the stresses of new parenting, there is often an escalation in IPV, so postpartum encounters should also include screening (ACOG, 1999). There is research to demonstrate the value of screening for IPV, but no study has shown any one tool improves outcomes (Stewart, 1994). Some authors recommend screening only women who demonstrate signs or symptoms of IPV, others recommend screening be universal (Feldhaus et al., 1997; Nelson, Nygren, McInerney, & Klein, 2004). When screening is universal, it is easier to ask hard questions about abuse, to reassure the woman her answers will only be used to protect her safety and to remain current on available resources (McFarlane, Parker, Soeken, & Bullock, 1992). Regardless of screening method, to be effective screening should be done in private. If the partner never allows the woman to be alone, the provider or a staff member must separate the woman from her partner to give an appropriate space to assess the woman's safety. If the only safe place is the bathroom, the provider or staff may follow the woman under the pretense of teaching her how to collect a clean catch urine specimen.

Screening for IPV

There are a number of screening tools published with validated results (Brown, Lent, Schmidt, & Sas, 2000; Coker, Pope, Smith, Sanderson, & Hussey, 2001; Feldhaus et al., 1997; Fogarty, Burge, & McCord, 2002; Sherin, Sinacore, Li, Zitter, & Shakil, 1998; Wasson et al., 2000). Table 38.12 includes various questions that may be included.

The partner violence screen (PVS) consists of direct, closed-ended questions that can be answered with "yes" or "no." This screen has been used for more than 20 years and has been assessed as detecting 65% to 71% of women with a history of IPV (Table 38.13) (Feldhaus et al., 1997). The first question "Have you been hit, kicked, punched or

TABLE 38.12	IPV Screening Questions
Does anyone with whom you have a relationship physically hurt you or make you feel afraid?	
Is there someone who makes you feel bad in other ways like shaming or name calling?	
Have you been in a previous relationship in which you were hurt, threatened, or made to have unwanted sex, including your family of origin?	
Is there someone with whom you have a relationship who threatens or hurts your children?	
Does anyone with whom you have a current relationship force you to have unwanted sex or make you do things sexually that you don't like or find uncomfortable?	
Has your partner ever refused to wear condoms when you wanted them?	
Are there guns in your house or anywhere you spend a lot of time?	
Does anyone with whom you have a relationship have alcohol or substance problems?	
How does that person behave when drinking or using drugs?	
What happens when you get in an argument with your partner or others with whom you have a relationship?	
Has anyone with whom you have a relationship ever stolen or destroyed your things?	
Does anyone try to stop you from seeing friends, leaving the house, going to school or work?	

IPV, intimate partner violence.
Adapted from Flitcraft and Hadley (1992).

otherwise physically hurt by someone in the last year?" correlates with the results of all three questions and is used by many as a very brief screen. The Woman Abuse Screening Tool (WAST) has been refined from seven questions to two and asks about IPV indirectly (Brown, Lent, Schmidt, & Sas, 2000). This tool is reported to identify 92% of victims of IPV (Flitcraft & Hadley, 1992). A patient-centered (PC) approach has been validated as a tool for screening in a population in which the women have demonstrated verbal or nonverbal cues to IPV. The study found the PC approach to be preferred most and the direct PVS method to be least effective (McCord-Duncan, Floyd, Kemp, Bailey, & Lang, 2006). The PC approach consists of open-ended questions based on verbal or nonverbal clues offered by the woman during an interview. This tool, though more time intense to administer, focuses on a woman's "ideas, concerns, expectations and personal experience regarding their problem" (Stewart et al., 1995). Because the study has not been independently confirmed, this screening tool is not recommended over any other. A screening tool should never substitute for careful observation. Providers and staff need to be trained to recognize the signs and symptoms of IPV.

TABLE 38.13	Alert Indicators for IPV
Late prenatal care or erratic care	
Multiple trips to the emergency room with episodes of falls or accidents	
Multiple trips to the emergency room for children with episodes of falls or accidents	
Bruising or injuries in unusual places	
Bruising or injuries in various stages of healing	
Injuries more severe than expected from explanation	
Keeping extremities covered at all times	
Wearing sunglasses indoors	
Inability to make eye contact or always looking at partner	
Appearing withdrawn or agitated	
Admission for suicidal gestures or drug or alcohol abuse	
Chronic, unexplained, often changing somatic complaints	
Woman or her partner demonstrating abusive behavior to her children	
Woman or her partner who appear under the influence of substances	
A partner who never lets the woman come to her prenatal appointments alone	
A partner who always speaks for the woman	
A partner who threatens the woman, her children, or staff	
A woman who is not allowed to answer the telephone at home	

IPV, intimate partner violence.
Adapted from McFarlane, Parker, Soeken, and Bullock (1992); Stewart (1994).

If staff or provider suspect IPV based on injuries or behaviors and the woman denies it, having resource materials in waiting rooms and restrooms allows patients to gather information without confrontation. The provider may also supply resources or phone numbers with the suggestion the information might be helpful for a friend. Screening of teens is particularly important, because they have higher rates of prenatal injuries from motor vehicle crashes and domestic violence. With teens being cautious, the perpetrator may be a parent or older sibling. Teens like to be accompanied during their visits, but the same rules of privacy apply to teens as well as adults (Jacoby et al., 1999).

Differential Diagnosis

In establishing a differential diagnosis the following must be considered: child abuse, drug, EtOH abuse, depression, suicidal ideation, psychosis (self or partner), and risk for homicide.

No specific diagnostic testing is available; testing is based on injuries.

Treatment/Management

For very complicated reasons, many women choose not to leave their abuser (Bacchus, Mezey, & Bewley, 2006). Continuing to offer support and resources will allow the woman to know the provider cares. For a woman who acknowledges situations of IPV, the provider should assess for her personal safety and inquire specifically about guns. Since IPV often extends to other vulnerable members of a family, the provider should inquire about the safety of any children in the home or any elders. Each state has regulations regarding reporting of elder and child abuse or endangerment. Each provider should know the rules of her or his state (ACOG, 2012).

All discussions of IPV must be documented as well as evidence of physical abuse and any management plans or implementations (Table 38.14). If the office has access to a camera, pictures are supportive documents. If a camera is not available, injuries should be drawn on a body diagram. When documenting, in addition to the standard date and time, define time since the violence in weeks, days, hours, or minutes. It is difficult to assess triggers to violence or the extent to which violence can escalate, so the woman should be assisted in identifying supports and in developing an escape plan and given information on legal supports. If the woman needs to call resources, the provider should find a safe place for her in the office and either place a phone call, then hand the phone to the woman or at least provide her with privacy to initiate calls (McCord-Duncan et al., 2006). The provider should assess whether it is safe to take home written materials or receive phone calls, then develop a follow-up plan. If the provider has access to a social worker, involving the social worker is appropriate. If there is no social worker available, the provider or staff may need to call police if the perpetrator is in the office.

The woman needs to be educated about the cycle of abuse. The cycle begins with a tension-building period. The controller begins to argue. He or she looks for stressors, like job dissatisfaction, money issues, or even the way the woman dresses. The controller escalates controls, imposing limits on the partner, perhaps imposing minor degrees of physical insult. The partner tries to accommodate but rage builds in the controller anyway. The acute violence period or abuse stage is often triggered by a trivial event. Once the assault starts no behavior on the part of the woman will stem the rage. The violence spins out of control. The controller usually picks the fight; but, occasionally, a woman will bait the controller because she knows the assault is coming and she wants it over. A honeymoon phase follows. The controller will give gifts, apologize for previous behaviors, and beg for forgiveness. Both parties will want to believe it will never happen again. The cycle will then begin again with the violence becoming more frequent and escalating in intensity until it becomes lethal (Walker, 1979).

IPV management plans are only as effective as the setting in which they are context. Community resources include social service, law enforcement, shelters, counselors, and the criminal justice system.

TABLE 38.14	Management Plan for Women in At-Risk Relationships
Be aware of signs and symptoms of intimate partner violence	
Provide universal screening	
Maintain confidentiality	
Take any report seriously	
Suspend judgment	
Affirm for the woman you can provide help	
Perform a thorough examination looking for inappropriate bruising or lacerations	
Document findings, make photos if possible	
Assess potential for homicide or suicide	
Provide support and referral	
Be aware of state mandated reporting laws	
Provide follow-up	

With the statistics on IPV it is easy to become pessimistic and might be convenient to assume that it is an issue which crosses all cultures. It is true there are many cultures in which the problem is even greater than the United States. There are however, cultures in which interpersonal violence is rare. These cultures demonstrate common characteristics: strong sanction against violence with support for the victims, flexible gender roles, and equality of resources and decision making between sexes.

■ FUTURE DIRECTIONS

Women are living longer and delaying childbirth beyond 35 years of age. With the advancement of genetic testing, assisted reproductive technology at advanced maternal age (ART AMA) is a reality of the future. Practice, research, and reproductive policies will be challenged to keep up with the science. Prolonged fertility will impact the definition of family and is stacked with pros and cons. Age is not the single risk to pregnancy outcome but is complicated by smoking, higher BMI, and chronic health conditions. Age cannot be controlled but health conditions are modifiable.

■ REFERENCES

Abboud, P., Zejli, A., Mansour, G., Monnoyer, Y., Houareau, L. G., Bart, H., & Bock, S. (2000). Amniotic fluid leakage and premature rupture of membranes after amniocentesis. A review of the literature. *Journal de Gynécologie, Obstétrique Et Biologie De La Reproduction, 29*(8), 741–745.

Abramson, J., & Stagnaro-Green, A. (2001). Thyroid antibodies and fetal loss: An evolving story. *Thyroid: Official Journal of the American Thyroid Association, 11*(1), 57–63.

Abu-Heija, A. T., Jallad, M. F., & Abukteish, F. (2000). Maternal and perinatal outcome of pregnancies after the age of 45. *The Journal of Obstetrics and Gynaecology Research, 26*(1), 27–30.

ACOG Practice Bulletin. (2014). Cerclage for the management of cervical insufficiency. *Obstetrics and Gynecology, 123*, 372–329.

Agnoli, F. L., & Deutchman, M. E. (1993). Trauma in pregnancy. *The Journal of Family Practice, 37*(6), 588–592.

Alchalabi, H. A., Obeidat, B. R., Jallad, M. F., & Khader, Y. S. (2006). Induction of labor and perinatal outcome: The impact of the amniotic fluid index. *European Journal of Obstetrics, Gynecology, and Reproductive Biology, 129*(2), 124–127.

Altieri, A., Franceschi, S., Ferlay, J., Smith, J., & La Vecchia, C. (2003). Epidemiology and aetiology of gestational trophoblastic diseases. *The Lancet. Oncology, 4*(11), 670–678.

American Academy of Pediatrics Committee on Drugs. (1994). Transfer of drugs and other chemicals into breast milk. *Pediatrics, 93*, 137–150.

American College of Obstetricians and Gynecologists (ACOG). (2002). ACOG practice bulletin. Management of recurrent pregnancy loss. Number 24, February 2001. (Replaces Technical Bulletin Number 212, September 1995). American College of Obstetricians and Gynecologists. *International Journal of Gynaecology and Obstetrics, 78*(2), 179–190.

American College of Obstetricians and Gynecologists (ACOG). (2006). Management of isoimmunization in pregnancy. *ACOG Technical Bulletin 75, 108*(2), 457–464.

American College of Obstetricians and Gynecologists (ACOG). (2012). Intimate partner violence. *ACOG Committee Opinion, 119* (2, Pt. 1), 412–417. doi:10.1097/AOG.0b013e318249ff74

Ansari, A. H., & Kirkpatrick, B. (1998). Recurrent pregnancy loss. An update. *Journal of Reproductive Medicine, 43*(9), 806–814.

Armenti, V. T., Moritz, M. J., Cardonick, E. H., & Davison, J. M. (2002). Immunosuppression in pregnancy: Choices for infant and maternal health. *Drugs, 62*(16), 2361–2375.

Armenti, V. T., Radomski, J. S., Moritz, M. J., Gaughan, W. J., McGrory, C. H., & Coscia, L. A. (2003). Report from the National Transplantation Pregnancy Registry (NTPR): Outcomes of pregnancy after transplantation. *Clinical Transplantation*, 131–141.

Arredondo, F., & Noble, L. S. (2006). Endocrinology of recurrent pregnancy loss. *Seminars in Reproductive Medicine, 24*(1), 33–39.

Atallah, D., El Kassis, N., Salameh, C., Safi, J., Bejjani, L., Lutfallah, F., Ghaaname, W., & Moukarzel, M. (2015). Pregnancy and renal transplantation. *Le Journal Médical Libanais. The Lebanese Medical Journal, 63*(3), 131–137.

Audibert, F., Friedman, S. A., Frangieh, A. Y., & Sibai, B. M. (1996). Clinical utility of strict diagnostic criteria for the HELLP (hemolysis, elevated liver enzymes, and low platelets) syndrome. *American Journal of Obstetrics and Gynecology, 175*(2), 460–464.

Bacchus, L., Mezey, G., & Bewley, S. (2006). A qualitative exploration of the nature of domestic violence in pregnancy. *Violence Against Women, 12*(6), 588–604.

Baker, D., Teklehaimanot, S., Hassan, R., & Guze, C. (2004). A look at a Hispanic and African American population in an urban prenatal diagnostic center: Referral reasons, amniocentesis acceptance, and abnormalities detected. *Genetics in Medicine, 6*(4), 211–218.

Barbieri, R. L. (2001). The initial fertility consultation: Recommendations concerning cigarette smoking, body mass index, and alcohol and caffeine consumption. *American Journal of Obstetrics and Gynecology, 185*(5), 1168–1173.

Barton, J. R., & Sibai, B. M. (1996). Hepatic imaging in HELLP syndrome (hemolysis, elevated liver enzymes, and low platelet count). *American Journal of Obstetrics and Gynecology, 174*(6), 1820–1825; discussion 1825.

Barton, J. R., & Sibai, B. M. (2004). Diagnosis and management of hemolysis, elevated liver enzymes, and low platelets syndrome. *Clinics in Perinatology, 31*(4), 807–33, vii.

Benson, C. B., Genest, D. R., Bernstein, M. R., Soto-Wright, V., Goldstein, D. P., & Berkowitz, R. S. (2000). Sonographic appearance of first trimester complete hydatidiform moles. *Ultrasound in Obstetrics & Gynecology, 16*(2), 188–191.

Berkowitz, R. S., Goldstein, D. P., & Bernstein, M. R. (1991). Advances in management of partial molar pregnancy. *Contemporary Obstetrics and Gynecology, 36*, 33–44.

Berkowitz, R. S., Im, S. S., Bernstein, M. R., & Goldstein, D. P. (1998). Gestational trophoblastic disease. Subsequent pregnancy outcome, including repeat molar pregnancy. *Journal of Reproductive Medicine, 43*(1), 81–86.

Bobrowski, R. A., & Bottoms, S. F. (1995). Underappreciated risks of the elderly multipara. *American Journal of Obstetrics and Gynecology, 172*(6), 1764–1767; discussion 1767.

Brace, R. A. (1997). Physiology of amniotic fluid volume regulation. *Clinical Obstetrics and Gynecology, 40*(2), 280–289.

Branch, K. R., Wagoner, L. E., McGrory, C. H., Mannion, J. D., Radomski, J. S., Moritz, M. J., … Armenti, V. T. (1998). Risks of subsequent pregnancies on mother and newborn in female heart transplant recipients. *Journal of Heart and Lung Transplantation, 17*(7), 698–702.

Breiding, M. J., Basile, K. C., Smith, S. G., Black, M. C., & Mahendra, R. R. (2015). *Intimate partner violence surveillance: Uniform definitions and recommended data elements, version 2.0.* Atlanta, GA: National Center for Injury Prevention and Control, Centers for Disease Control and Prevention.

Brown, J. B., Lent, B., Schmidt, G., & Sas, G. (2000). Application of the Woman Abuse Screening Tool (WAST) and WAST-short in the family practice setting. *Journal of Family Practice, 49*(10), 896–903.

Buckley, J. D. (1996). Choriocarcinoma. In D. Schottenfeld & J. F. Fraumeni (Eds.), *Cancer epidomology and prevention* (2nd ed.). Philadelphia, PA: Oxford University Press.

Centers for Disease Control and Prevention. (2003). *Intimate partner violence against women in the United States* (pp. 1–53). Atlanta, GA: Department of Health and Human Services.

Chames, M. C., Haddad, B., Barton, J. R., Livingston, J. C., & Sibai, B. M. (2003). Subsequent pregnancy outcome in women with a history of HELLP syndrome at < or = 28 weeks of gestation. *American Journal of Obstetrics and Gynecology, 188*(6), 1504–1507; discussion 1507.

Chang, J., Berg, C. J., Saltzman, L. E., & Herndon, J. (2005). Homicide: A leading cause of injury deaths among pregnant and postpartum women in the United States, 1991–1999. *American Journal of Public Health, 95*(3), 471–477.

Christiansen, O. B., Nybo Andersen, A. M., Bosch, E., Daya, S., Delves, P. J., Hviid, T. V., … van der Ven, K. (2005). Evidence-based investigations and treatments of recurrent pregnancy loss. *Fertility and Sterility, 83*(4), 821–839.

Clark, K. A., Martin, S. L., Petersen, R., Cloutier, S., Covington, D., Buescher, P., & Beck-Warden, M. (2000). Who gets screened during pregnancy for partner violence? *Archives of Family Medicine, 9*(10), 1093–1099.

Coker, A. L., Pope, B. O., Smith, P. H., Sanderson, M., & Hussey, J. R. (2001). Assessment of clinical partner violence screening tools. *Journal of the American Medical Women's Association (1972), 56*(1), 19–23.

Committee on Practice Bulletins-Gynecology, American College of Obstetricians and Gynecologists (ACOG). (2004). ACOG Practice Bulletin #53. Diagnosis and treatment of gestational trophoblastic disease. *Obstetrics and Gynecology, 103*(6), 1365–1377.

Cunningham, F. G., MacDonald, P. C., Gant, N. F., Leveno, K. J., Gilstrap, L. C., Hankins, G. D. V., & Clark, S. L. (1997). *Williams obstetrics* (20th ed.). Stamford, CT: Appleton and Lange.

Curry, S. L., Schlaerth, J. B., Kohorn, E. I., Boyce, J. B., Gore, H., Twiggs, L. B., & Blessing, J. A. (1989). Hormonal contraception and trophoblastic sequelae after hydatidiform mole (a Gynecologic Oncology Group Study). *American Journal of Obstetrics and Gynecology, 160*(4), 805–809; discussion 809.

Davison, J. M., & Bailey, D. J. (2003). Pregnancy following renal transplantation. *The Journal of Obstetrics and Gynaecology Research, 29*(4), 227–233.

Davison, J. M., & Redman, C. W. (1997). Pregnancy post-transplant: The establishment of a UK registry. *British Journal of Obstetrics and Gynaecology, 104*(10), 1106–1107.

Dawood, M. Y., Saxena, B. B., & Landesman, R. (1977). Human chorionic gonadotropin and its subunits in hydatidiform mole and choriocarcinoma. *Obstetrics and Gynecology, 50*(2), 172–181.

Daya, S. (1996). Evaluation and management of recurrent spontaneous abortion. *Current Opinion in Obstetrics & Gynecology, 8*(3), 188–192.

Devereux, G. (1941). Mohave beliefs concerning twins. *American Anthropologist, 43*(4), 573–592.

Drakeley, A. J., Roberts, D., & Alfirevic, Z. (2003). Cervical cerclage for prevention of preterm delivery: Meta-analysis of randomized trials. *Obstetrics and Gynecology, 102*(3), 621–627.

Dubbins, P. A., Kurtz, A. B., Wapner, R. J., & Goldberg, B. B. (1981). Renal agenesis: Spectrum in utero findings. *Journal of Clinical Ultrasound, 9*(4), 189–193.

Dulitzki, M., Soriano, D., Schiff, E., Chetrit, A., Mashiach, S., & Seidman, D. S. (1998). Effect of very advanced maternal age on pregnancy outcome and rate of cesarean delivery. *Obstetrics and Gynecology, 92*(6), 935–939.

Ek, S., Andersson, A., Johansson, A., & Kublicas, M. (2005). Oligohydramnios in uncomplicated pregnancies beyond 40 completed weeks. A prospective, randomised, pilot study on maternal and neonatal outcomes. *Fetal Diagnosis and Therapy, 20*(3), 182–185.

Empson, M., Lassere, M., Craig, J. C., & Scott, J. R. (2002). Recurrent pregnancy loss with antiphospholipid antibody: A systematic review of therapeutic trials. *Obstetrics and Gynecology, 99*(1), 135–144.

Esposito, T. J., Gens, D. R., Smith, L. G., Scorpio, R., & Buchman, T. (1991). Trauma during pregnancy. A review of 79 cases. *Archives of Surgery (1960), 126*(9), 1073–1078.

Eyler, A. E., & Cohen, M. (1999). Case studies in partner violence. *American Family Physician, 60*(9), 2569–2576.

Feldhaus, K. M., Koziol-McLain, J., Amsbury, H. L., Norton, I. M., Lowenstein, S. R., & Abbott, J. T. (1997). Accuracy of 3 brief screening questions for detecting partner violence in the emergency department. *Journal of the American Medical Association, 277*(17), 1357–1361.

FIGO Oncology Committee. (2000). FIGO staging for gestational trophoblastic neoplasia 2000. FIGO Oncology Committee. *International Journal of Gynaecology and Obstetrics, 77*(3), 285–287.

Final Report of the Medical Research Council/Royal College of Obstetricians and Gynaecologists Multicentre Randomised Trial of Cervical Cerclage. (1993). MRC/RCOG Working Party on Cervical Cerclage. *British Journal of Obstetrics and Gynaecology, 100*, 516.

Flitcraft, A. H., & Hadley, S. M. (1992). AMA diagnosis and treatment guidelines on domestic violence. In C. Warshaw, A. Flitcraft, S. Haldey, S. McLeer, & M. B. Hendricks-Mathews (Eds.), *Diagnostic and treatment guidelines on domestic violence.* Chicago, IL: American Medical Association.

Fogarty, C. T., Burge, S., & McCord, E. C. (2002). Communicating with patients about intimate partner violence: Screening and interviewing approaches. *Family Medicine, 34*(5), 369–375.

Fowler, D. J., Lindsay, I., Seckl, M. J., & Sebire, N. J. (2006). Routine pre-evacuation ultrasound diagnosis of hydatidiform mole: Experience of more than 1000 cases from a regional referral center. *Ultrasound in Obstetrics & Gynecology, 27*(1), 56–60.

Franssen, M. T., Korevaar, J. C., Leschot, N. J., Bossuyt, P. M., Knegt, A. C., Gerssen-Schoorl, K. B., … Goddijn, M. (2005). Selective chromosome analysis in couples with two or more miscarriages: Case-control study. *British Medical Journal (Clinical Research Ed.), 331*(7509), 137–141.

Garner, E. I., Lipson, E., Bernstein, M. R., Goldstein, D. P., & Berkowitz, R. S. (2002). Subsequent pregnancy experience in patients with molar pregnancy and gestational trophoblastic tumor. *Journal of Reproductive Medicine, 47*(5), 380–386.

Gazmararian, J. A., Lazorick, S., Spitz, A. M., Ballard, T. J., Saltzman, L. E., & Marks, J. S. (1996). Prevalence of violence against pregnant women. *Journal of the American Medical Association, 275*(24), 1915–1920.

Gemer, O., Segal, S., Kopmar, A., & Sassoon, E. (2000). The current clinical presentation of complete molar pregnancy. *Archives of Gynecology and Obstetrics, 264*(1), 33–34.

Gianaroli, L., Magli, M. C., & Ferraretti, A. P. (2005). Sperm and blastomere aneuploidy detection in reproductive genetics and medicine. *Journal of Histochemistry and Cytochemistry, 53*(3), 261–267.

Glueck, C. J., Wang, P., Goldenberg, N., & Sieve-Smith, L. (2002). Pregnancy outcomes among women with polycystic ovary syndrome treated with metformin. *Human Reproduction, 17*(11), 2858–2864.

Goldenberg, R. L., Iams, J. D., Miodovnik, M., Van Dorsten, J. P., Thurnau, G., Bottoms, S., … McNellis, D. (1996). The preterm prediction study: Risk factors in twin gestations. National Institute of Child

Health and Human Development Maternal-Fetal Medicine Units Network. *American Journal of Obstetrics and Gynecology, 175*(4, Pt. 1), 1047–1053.

Gopalkrishnan, K., Padwal, V., Meherji, P. K., Gokral, J. S., Shah, R., & Juneja, H. S. (2000). Poor quality of sperm as it affects repeated early pregnancy loss. *Archives of Andrology, 45*(2), 111–117.

Greene, M. F., Hare, J. W., Cloherty, J. P., Benacerraf, B. R., & Soeldner, J. S. (1989). First-trimester hemoglobin A1 and risk for major malformation and spontaneous abortion in diabetic pregnancy. *Teratology, 39*(3), 225–231.

Gross, S. J., & Bombard, A. T. (1998). Screening for the aneuploid fetus. *Obstetrics & Gynecology Clinics of North America, 87*, 948–952.

Guth, A. A., & Pachter, L. (2000). Domestic violence and the trauma surgeon. *American Journal of Surgery, 179*(2), 134–140.

Halliday, J., Lumley, J., & Watson, L. (1995). Comparison of women who do and do not have amniocentesis or chorionic villus sampling. *Lancet, 345*(8951), 704–709.

Hamilton, B. E., Martin, J. A., Osterman, M. J., Curtin, S. C., & Matthews, T. J. (2015). Births: Final Data for 2014. *National Vital Statistics Reports, 64*(12), 1–64.

Hancock, B. W., & Tidy, J. A. (2002). Current management of molar pregnancy. *Journal of Reproductive Medicine, 47*(5), 347–354.

Handelsman, D. J., & Dong, Q. (1993). Hypothalamo-pituitary gonadal axis in chronic renal failure. *Endocrinology and Metabolism Clinics of North America, 22*(1), 145–161.

Haning, R. V., Canick, J. A., Goldsmith, L. T., Shahinian, K. A., Erinakes, N. J., & Weiss, G. (1996). The effect of ovulation induction on the concentration of maternal serum relaxin in twin pregnancies. *American Journal of Obstetrics and Gynecology, 174*(1, Pt. 1), 227–232.

Hartley, R. S., Hitti, J., & Emanuel, I. (2002). Size-discordant twin pairs have higher perinatal mortality rates than nondiscordant pairs. *American Journal of Obstetrics and Gynecology, 187*(5), 1173–1178.

Heck, K. E., Schoendorf, K. C., Ventura, S. J., & Kiely, J. L. (1997). Delayed childbearing by education level in the United States, 1969–1994. *Maternal and Child Health Journal, 1*(2), 81–88.

Hedin, L. W., & Janson, P. O. (2000). Domestic violence during pregnancy. The prevalence of physical injuries, substance use, abortions and miscarriages. *Acta Obstetricia Et Gynecologica Scandinavica, 79*(8), 625–630.

Heffner, L. J. (2004). Advanced maternal age—How old is too old? *New England Journal of Medicine, 351*(19), 1927–1929.

Henderson, J., Hockley, C., Petrou, S., Goldacre, M., & Davidson, L. (2004). Economic implications of multiple births: Inpatient hospital costs in the first 5 years of life. *Archives of Disease in Childhood. Fetal and Neonatal Edition, 89*(6), F542–F545.

Herbst, A. L., Kurman, R. J., & Scully, R. E. (1972). Vaginal and cervical abnormalities after exposure to stilbestrol in utero. *Obstetrics and Gynecology, 40*(3), 287–298.

Hirahara, F., Andoh, N., Sawai, K., Hirabuki, T., Uemura, T., & Minaguchi, H. (1998). Hyperprolactinemic recurrent miscarriage and results of randomized bromocriptine treatment trials. *Fertility and Sterility, 70*(2), 246–252.

Hofmeyr, G. J., & Gülmezoglu, A. M. (2006). Maternal hydration for increasing amniotic fluid in oligohydramnios and normal amniotic fluid volume. *The Cochrane Database of Systematic Reviews, 2006,* CD00011134.

Hofmeyr, G. J., Gülmezoglu, A. M., Novikova, N. (2002). Maternal hydration for increasing amniotic fluid volume in oligohydramnios and normal amniotic fluid volume. *The Cochrane Database of Systematic Reviews 2002,* Issue 1. Art. No.: CD000134. doi: 10.1002/14651858 .CD000134

Hoyert, D. L., Danel, I., & Tully, P. (2000). Maternal mortality, United States and Canada, 1982–1997. *Birth, 27*(1), 4–11.

Hui, L., Muggli, E. E., & Halliday, J. L. (2016). Population-based trends in prenatal screening and diagnosis for aneuploidy: A retrospective analysis of 38 years of state-wide data. *BJOG: An International Journal of Obstetrics and Gynaecology, 123*(1), 90–97.

Humphrey, W. M., Griffin, E. E., Senz, K. L., Shaffer, B. L., & Caughey, A. B. (2016). Routine amniocentesis versus serum screening for detection of aneuploidy in women of advanced maternal age. *American Journal of Obstetrics & Gynecology, 214*(1, Suppl. S82).

Iams, J. D., Johnson, F. F., Sonek, J., Sachs, L., Gebauer, C., & Samuels, P. (1995). Cervical competence as a continuum: A study of ultrasonographic cervical length and obstetric performance. *American Journal of Obstetrics and Gynecology, 172*(4, Pt. 1), 1097–1103; discussion 1104.

Jacoby, M., Gorenflo, D., Black, E., Wunderlich, C., & Eyler, A. E. (1999). Rapid repeat pregnancy and experiences of interpersonal violence among low-income adolescents. *American Journal of Preventive Medicine, 16*(4), 318–321.

Jolly, M., Sebire, N., Harris, J., Robinson, S., & Regan, L. (2000). The risks associated with pregnancy in women aged 35 years or older. *Human Reproduction, 15*(11), 2433–2437.

Kirk, E., Papageorghiou, A. T., Condous, G., Bottomley, C., & Bourne, T. (2007). The accuracy of first trimester ultrasound in the diagnosis of hydatidiform mole. *Ultrasound in Obstetrics & Gynecology, 29*(1), 70–75.

Kirshon, B., Moise, K. J., Mari, G., & Willis, R. (1991). Long-term indomethacin therapy decreases fetal urine output and results in oligohydramnios. *American Journal of Perinatology, 8*(2), 86–88.

Kirz, D. S., Dorchester, W., & Freeman, R. K. (1985). Advanced maternal age: The mature gravida. *American Journal of Obstetrics and Gynecology, 152*(1), 7–12.

Kistin, S. J., & Newman, A. D. (2007). Induction of labor with homeopathy: A case report. *Journal of Midwifery & Women's Health, 52*(3), 303–307.

Kutteh, W. H., & Triplett, D. A. (2006). Thrombophilias and recurrent pregnancy loss. *Seminars in Reproductive Medicine, 24*(1), 54–66.

Lagrew, D. C., Morgan, M. A., Nakamoto, K., & Lagrew, N. (1996). Advanced maternal age: Perinatal outcome when controlling for physician selection. *Journal of Perinatology, 16*(4), 256–260.

Lawler, S. D., Fisher, R. A., & Dent, J. (1991). A prospective genetic study of complete and partial hydatidiform moles. *American Journal of Obstetrics and Gynecology, 164*(5, Pt 1), 1270–1277.

Leeman, L., & Almond, D. (2005). Isolated oligohydramnios at term: Is induction indicated? *Journal of Family Practice, 54*(1), 25–32.

Leppert, P. C. (1995). Anatomy and physiology of cervical ripening. *Clinical Obstetrics and Gynecology, 38*(2), 267–279.

Lorigan, P. C., Sharma, S., Bright, N., Coleman, R. E., & Hancock, B. W. (2000). Characteristics of women with recurrent molar pregnancies. *Gynecologic Oncology, 27*, 678.

Lurain, J. R. (2002). Advances in management of high-risk gestational trophoblastic tumors. *Journal of Reproductive Medicine, 47*(6), 451–459.

MacDorman, M. F., & Gregory, C. W. (2015). Fetal and perinatal mortality: United States, 2013. *National Vital Statistics Reports, 64*(8), 1–24.

Magann, E. F., Chauhan, S. P., Doherty, D. A., Barrilleaux, P. S., Martin, J. N., & Morrison, J. C. (2003). Predictability of intrapartum and neonatal outcomes with the amniotic fluid volume distribution: A reassessment using the amniotic fluid index, single deepest pocket, and a dye-determined amniotic fluid volume. *American Journal of Obstetrics and Gynecology, 188*(6), 1523–1527; discussion 1527.

Magann, E. F., Doherty, D. A., Chauhan, S. P., Busch, F. W., Mecacci, F., & Morrison, J. C. (2004). How well do the amniotic fluid index and single deepest pocket indices (below the 3rd and 5th and above the 95th and 97th percentiles) predict oligohydramnios and hydramnios? *American Journal of Obstetrics and Gynecology, 190*(1), 164–169.

Magann, E. F., Perry, K. G., Chauhan, S. P., Anfanger, P. J., Whitworth, N. S., & Morrison, J. C. (1997). The accuracy of ultrasound evaluation of amniotic fluid volume in singleton pregnancies: The effect of operator experience and ultrasound interpretative technique. *Journal of Clinical Ultrasound, 25*(5), 249–253.

Magann, E. F., Perry, K. G., Meydrech, E. F., Harris, R. L., Chauhan, S. P., & Martin, J. N. (1994). Postpartum corticosteroids: Accelerated recovery from the syndrome of hemolysis, elevated liver enzymes, and low platelets (HELLP). *American Journal of Obstetrics and Gynecology, 171*(4), 1154–1158.

Mann, K., Schneider, N., & Hoermann, R. (1986). Thyrotropic activity of acidic isoelectric variants of human chorionic gonadotropin from trophoblastic tumors. *Endocrinology, 118*(4), 1558–1566.

Manning, F. A. (1995). Dynamic ultrasound-based fetal assessment: The fetal biophysical profile score. *Clinical Obstetrics and Gynecology, 38*(1), 26–44.

Manogura, A., & Weiner, C. (2006). Maternal alloimmunization and fetal hemolytic disease. In E. A. Reece & J. Hobbins (Eds.), *Clinical obstetrics: The fetus and mother* (3rd ed., Chapter 49). New York, NY: Wiley-Blackwell.

Many, A., Lazebnik, N., & Hill, L. M. (1996). The underlying cause of polyhydramnios determines prematurity. *Prenatal Diagnosis, 16*(1), 55–57.

Mari, G., Deter, R. L., Carpenter, R. L., Rahman, F., Zimmerman, R., Moise, K. J.,...Blackwell, S. C. (2000). Noninvasive diagnosis by Doppler ultrasonography of fetal anemia due to maternal red-cell alloimmunization. Collaborative Group for Doppler Assessment of the Blood Velocity in Anemic Fetuses. *New England Journal of Medicine, 342*(1), 9–14.

Martin, J. A., Hamilton, B. E., Ventura, S. J., Menacker, F., Park, M. M., & Sutton, P. D. (2002). Births: Final data for 2001. *National Vital Statistics Reports, 51*(2), 1–102.

Martin, J. N., Perry, K. G., Blake, P. G., May, W. A., Moore, A., & Robinette, L. (1997). Better maternal outcomes are achieved with dexamethasone therapy for postpartum HELLP (hemolysis, elevated liver enzymes, and thrombocytopenia) syndrome. *American Journal of Obstetrics and Gynecology, 177*(5), 1011–1017.

Martin, J. N., Thigpen, B. D., Rose, C. H., Cushman, J., Moore, A., & May, W. L. (2003). Maternal benefit of high-dose intravenous corticosteroid therapy for HELLP syndrome. *American Journal of Obstetrics and Gynecology, 189*(3), 830–834.

McCord-Duncan, E. C., Floyd, M., Kemp, E. C., Bailey, B., & Lang, F. (2006). Detecting potential intimate partner violence: Which approach do women want? *Family Medicine, 38*(6), 416–422.

McFarlane, J., Campbell, J. C., Sharps, P., & Watson, K. (2002). Abuse during pregnancy and femicide: Urgent implications for women's health. *Obstetrics and Gynecology, 100*(1), 27–36.

McFarlane, J., Parker, B., Soeken, K., & Bullock, L. (1992). Assessing for abuse during pregnancy. Severity and frequency of injuries and associated entry into prenatal care. *Journal of the American Medical Association, 267*(23), 3176–3178.

McIntosh, G. C., Olshan, A. F., & Baird, P. A. (1995). Paternal age and the risk of birth defects in offspring. *Epidemiology, 6*(3), 282–288.

McKay, D. B., & Josephson, M. A. (2006). Pregnancy in recipients of solid organs–effects on mother and child. *New England Journal of Medicine, 354*(12), 1281–1293.

Michlin, R., Oettinger, M., Odeh, M., Khoury, S., Ophir, E., Barak, M.,...Strulov, A. (2000). Maternal obesity and pregnancy outcome. *The Israel Medical Association Journal, 2*(1), 10–13.

Miller, D. A. (2005). Is advanced maternal age an independent risk factor for uteroplacental insufficiency? *American Journal of Obstetrics and Gynecology, 192*(6), 1974–1980; discussion 1980.

Mol, B. W., Roberts, C. T., Thangaratinam, S., Magee, L. A., de Groot, C. J., & Hofmeyr, G. J. (2016). Pre-eclampsia. *Lancet, 387*(10022), 999–1011.

Murray, J. E., Reid, D. E., Harrison, J. H., & Merrill, J. P. (1963). Successful pregnancies after human renal transplantation. *New England Journal of Medicine, 269*, 341–343.

Neiger, R., Trofatter, M. O., & Trofatter, K. F. (1995). D-dimer test for early detection of HELLP syndrome. *Southern Medical Journal, 88*(4), 416–419.

Nelson, H. D., Nygren, P., McInerney, Y., & Klein, J.; U. S. Preventive Services Task Force. (2004). Screening women and elderly adults for family and intimate partner violence: A review of the evidence for the U.S. Preventive Services Task Force. *Annals of Internal Medicine, 140*(5), 387–396.

Novak, E., & Sheah, C. S. (1954). Choriocarcinoma of the uterus. *American Journal of Obstetrics and Gynecology, 67*, 933.

Nybo Andersen, A. M., Wohlfahrt, J., Christens, P., Olsen, J., & Melbye, M. (2000). Maternal age and fetal loss: Population based register linkage study. *British Medical Journal (Clinical Research Ed.), 320*(7251), 1708–1712.

Oates-Whitehead, R. M., Haas, D. M., & Carrier, J. A. (2003). Progesterone for preventing miscarriage. *The Cochrane Database of Systematic Reviews, 2003*(4), CD003511.

Ott, W. J. (2004). Re-evaluation of the relationship between amniotic fluid volume and perinatal outcome. *American Journal of Obstetrics and Gynecology, 192*, 1803–1809.

Padden, M. O. (1999). HELLP syndrome: Recognition and perinatal management. *American Family Physician, 60*(3), 829–36, 839.

Parazzini, F., Cipriani, S., Mangili, G., Garavaglia, E., Guarnerio, P., Ricci, E.,...La Vecchia, C. (2002). Oral contraceptives and risk of gestational trophoblastic disease. *Contraception, 65*(6), 425–427.

Pérez-Medina, T., Bajo-Arenas, J., Salazar, F., Redondo, T., Sanfrutos, L., Alvarez, P., & Engels, V. (2005). Endometrial polyps and their implication in the pregnancy rates of patients undergoing intrauterine insemination: A prospective, randomized study. *Human Reproduction, 20*(6), 1632–1635.

Petrou, S., Mehta, Z., Hockley, C., Cook-Mozaffari, P., Henderson, J., & Goldacre, M. (2003). The impact of preterm birth on hospital inpatient admissions and costs during the first 5 years of life. *Pediatrics, 112*(6, Pt. 1), 1290–1297.

Pharoah, P. O. (2001). Twins and cerebral palsy. *Acta Paediatrica (1992). Supplement, 90*(436), 6–10.

Phelan, J. P., Smith, C. V., Broussard, P., & Small, M. (1987). Amniotic fluid volume assessment with the four-quadrant technique at 36–42 weeks' gestation. *Journal of Reproductive Medicine, 32*(7), 540–542.

Philipp, T., Grillenberger, K., Separovic, E. R., Philipp, K., & Kalousek, D. K. (2004). Effects of triploidy on early human development. *Prenatal Diagnosis, 24*(4), 276–281.

Piantelli, G., Bedocchi, L., Cavicchioni, O., Verrotti, C., Cavallotti, D., Fieni, S., & Gramellini, D. (2004). Amnioreduction for treatment of severe polyhydramnios. *Acta Bio-Medica: Atenei Parmensis, 75*(Suppl. 1), 56–58.

Piepert, J. F., & Donnenfield, A. E. (1991). Oligohydramnios: A review. *Obstetrical and Gynecological Survey, 46*, 325–339.

Poole, G. V., Martin, J. N., Perry, K. G., Griswold, J. A., Lambert, C. J., & Rhodes, R. S. (1996). Trauma in pregnancy: The role of interpersonal violence. *American Journal of Obstetrics and Gynecology, 174*(6), 1873–1877; discussion 1877.

Popov, I., Ganchev, S., & Bakurdzhiev, G. (1990). The morphological findings in the myometrial arteries and in the placenta with reference to the age of primaparae. *Akusherstvo i Ginekologiia, 29*(4), 20–23.

Portis, R., Jacobs, M. A., Skerman, J. H., & Skerman, E. B. (1997). HELLP syndrome (hemolysis, elevated liver enzymes, and low platelets) pathophysiology and anesthetic considerations. *American Association of Nurse Anesthetists, 65*(1), 37–47.

Prapas, N., Kalogiannidis, I., Prapas, I., Xiromeritis, P., Karagiannidis, A., & Makedos, G. (2006). Twin gestation in older women: Antepartum, intrapartum complications, and perinatal outcomes. *Archives of Gynecology and Obstetrics, 273*(5), 293–297.

Proctor, J. A., & Haney, A. F. (2003). Recurrent first trimester pregnancy loss is associated with uterine septum but not with bicornuate uterus. *Fertility and Sterility, 80*(5), 1212–1215.

Pui, M. H. (2004). Imaging diagnosis of congenital uterine malformation. *Computerized Medical Imaging and Graphics, 28*(7), 425–433.

Rabinowitz, R., Peters, M. T., Vyas, S., Campbell, S., & Nicolaides, K. H. (1989). Measurement of fetal urine production in normal pregnancy by real-time ultrasonography. *American Journal of Obstetrics and Gynecology, 161*(5), 1264–1266.

Raga, F., Bauset, C., Remohi, J., Bonilla-Musoles, F., Simón, C., & Pellicer, A. (1997). Reproductive impact of congenital Müllerian anomalies. *Human Reproduction, 12*(10), 2277–2281.

Rai, R., Backos, M., Baxter, N., Chilcott, I., & Regan, L. (2000). Recurrent miscarriage: An aspirin a day. *Human Reproduction, 15*(10), 2220–2223.

Roach, V. J., Hin, L. Y., Tam, W. H., Ng, K. B., & Rogers, M. S. (2000). The incidence of pregnancy-induced hypertension among patients with carbohydrate intolerance. *Hypertension in Pregnancy, 19*(2), 183–189.

Rorie, D. K., & Newton, M. (1967). Histologic and chemical studies of the smooth muscle in the human cervix and uterus. *American Journal of Obstetrics and Gynecology, 99*(4), 466–469.

Russell, R. B., Petrini, J. R., Damus, K., Mattison, D. R., & Schwarz, R. H. (2003). The changing epidemiology of multiple births in the United States. *Obstetrics and Gynecology, 101*(1), 129–135.

Salat-Baroux, J. (1988). Recurrent spontaneous abortions. *Reproduction, Nutrition, Développement, 28*(6B), 1555–1568.

Salihu, H. M., Shumpert, M. N., Slay, M., Kirby, R. S., & Alexander, G. R. (2003). Childbearing beyond maternal age 50 and fetal outcomes in the United States. *Obstetrics and Gynecology, 102*(5, Pt. 1), 1006–1014.

Schorge, J. O., Goldstein, D. P., Bernstein, M. R., & Berkowitz, R. S. (2000). Recent advances in gestational trophoblastic disease. *The Journal of Reproductive Medicine, 45*(9), 692–700.

Schroder, W., & Heyl, W. (1985). HELLP syndrome Weinstein L, pre-eclampsia/eclampsia with hemolysis, elevated liver enzymes and thrombocytopenia. *Obstetrics and Gynecology, 66,* 657–660.

Scott, J. R. (2003). Immunotherapy for recurrent miscarriage. *The Cochrane Database of Systematic Reviews, 2003*(1), CD000112. doi: 10.1002/14651858.CD000112. Retrieved from http://onlinelibrary.wiley.com/doi/10.1002/14651858.CD000112/full

Scully, R. E., Bonfiglio, T. A., Kurman, R. J., & Silverberg, S. G. (1994). *Histological typing of female genital tract tumors. WHO international histological classification of tumors* (2nd ed.). New York, NY: Springer Verlag.

Sebire, N. J., Fisher, R. A., Foskett, M., Rees, H., Seckl, M. J., & Newlands, E. S. (2003). Risk of recurrent hydatidiform mole and subsequent pregnancy outcome following complete or partial hydatidiform molar pregnancy. *BJOG: An International Journal of Obstetrics and Gynaecology, 110*(1), 22–26.

Sebire, N. J., Foskett, M., Fisher, R. A., Rees, H., Seckl, M., & Newlands, E. (2002). Risk of partial and complete hydatidiform molar pregnancy in relation to maternal age. *BJOG: An international Journal of Obstetrics and Gynaecology, 109*(1), 99–102.

Seckl, M. J., Fisher, R. A., Salerno, G., Rees, H., Paradinas, F. J., Foskett, M., & Newlands, E. S. (2000). Choriocarcinoma and partial hydatidiform moles. *Lancet, 356*(9223), 36–39.

Semer, D. A., & Macfee, M. S. (1995). Gestational trophoblastic disease: Epidemiology. *Seminars in Oncology, 22*(2), 109–112.

Sherin, K. M., Sinacore, J. M., Li, X. Q., Zitter, R. E., & Shakil, A. (1998). HITS: A short domestic violence screening tool for use in a family practice setting. *Family Medicine, 30*(7), 508–512.

Shime, J., Gare, D. J., Andrews, J., Bertrand, M., Salgado, J., & Whillans, G. (1984). Prolonged pregnancy: Surveillance of the fetus and the neonate and the course of labor and delivery. *American Journal of Obstetrics and Gynecology, 148*(5), 547–552.

Shipp, T. D., Bromley, B., Pauker, S., Frigoletto, F. D., & Benacerraf, B. R. (1996). Outcome of singleton pregnancies with severe oligohydramnios in the second and third trimesters. *Ultrasound in Obstetrics & Gynecology, 7*(2), 108–113.

Sibai, B. M. (1990). The HELLP syndrome (hemolysis, elevated liver enzymes, and low platelets): Much ado about nothing? *American Journal of Obstetrics and Gynecology, 162*(2), 311–316.

Sibai, B. M. (1996). Hypertension in pregnancy. In N. Gleicher, L. Buttino, U. Elkayam, M. Evans, R. Galbraith, S. Gail, & B. Sibal (Eds.), *Obstetrics: Normal and problem pregnancies* (3rd ed., pp. 935–996). New York, NY: Churchill Livingstone.

Sibai, B. M., Ramadan, M. K., Usta, I., Salama, M., Mercer, B. M., & Friedman, S. A. (1993). Maternal morbidity and mortality in 442 pregnancies with hemolysis, elevated liver enzymes, and low platelets (HELLP syndrome). *American Journal of Obstetrics and Gynecology, 169*(4), 1000–1006.

Smith, D. H., & Kirsop, R. (1991). Cervical incompetence occurring after caesarean section: A case report. *Asia-Oceania Journal of Obstetrics and Gynaecology, 17*(3), 225–226.

Snijders, R. J., Sebire, N. J., & Nicolaides, K. H. (1995). Maternal age and gestational age-specific risk for chromosomal defects. *Fetal Diagnosis and Therapy, 10*(6), 356–367.

Socol, M. (1998). Management of blood group isoimmunization. In M. M. Kaplan, D. A. Meier, N. Gleicher, & L. Buttino (Eds.), *Principles and practice of medical therapy in pregnancy.* New York, NY: Appleton and Lange.

Song, H. Z., & Wu, P. C. (1986). Incidence of hydatidiform mole in China. *International Journal of Epidemiology, 15*(3), 429–430.

Song, H. Z., Wu, P. C., Wang, Y. E., Yang, X. Y., & Dong, S. Y. (1988). Pregnancy outcomes after successful chemotherapy for choriocarcinoma and invasive mole: Long-term follow-up. *American Journal of Obstetrics and Gynecology, 158*(3, Pt. 1), 538–545.

Soper, J. T., Clarke-Pearson, D., & Hammond, C. B. (1988). Metastatic gestational trophoblastic disease: Prognostic factors in previously untreated patients. *Obstetrics and Gynecology, 71*(3, Pt. 1), 338–343.

Sotiriadis, A., Makrigiannakis, A., Stefos, T., Paraskevaidis, E., & Kalantaridou, S. N. (2007). Fibrinolytic defects and recurrent miscarriage: A systematic review and meta-analysis. *Obstetrics and Gynecology, 109*(5), 1146–1155.

Soto-Wright, V., Bernstein, M., Goldstein, D. P., & Berkowitz, R. S. (1995). The changing clinical presentation of complete molar pregnancy. *Obstetrics and Gynecology, 86*(5), 775–779.

Stagnaro-Green, A., & Glinoer, D. (2004). Thyroid autoimmunity and the risk of miscarriage. *Best Practice & Research. Clinical Endocrinology & Metabolism, 18*(2), 167–181.

Stewart, D. E. (1994). Incidence of postpartum abuse in women with a history of abuse during pregnancy. *Canadian Medical Association Journal, 151*(11), 1601–1604.

Stewart, M., Brown, J. B., Weston, W. W., McWhinney, L., McWilliam, C. L., & Freeman, T. R. (1995). *Patient centered medicine transforming the clinical method.* Thousand Oaks, CA: Sage.

Stone, M., Dent, J., Kardana, A., & Bagshawe, K. D. (1976). Relationship of oral contraception to development of trophoblastic tumour after evacuation of a hydatidiform mole. *British Journal of Obstetrics and Gynaecology, 83*(12), 913–916.

Storeide, O., Veholmen, M., Eide, M., Bergsjø, P., & Sandvei, R. (1997). The incidence of ectopic pregnancy in Hordaland County, Norway 1976–1993. *Acta Obstetricia Et Gynecologica Scandinavica, 76*(4), 345–349.

Sullivan, C. A., Magann, E. F., Perry, K. G., Roberts, W. E., Blake, P. G., & Martin, J. N. (1994). The recurrence risk of the syndrome of hemolysis, elevated liver enzymes, and low platelets (HELLP) in subsequent gestations. *American Journal of Obstetrics and Gynecology, 171*(4), 940–943.

Summers, P. R. (1994). Microbiology relevant to recurrent miscarriage. *Clinical Obstetrics and Gynecology, 37*(3), 722–729.

Tjaden, P., & Thoennes, N. (2000). *Extent, nature and consequences of intimate partner violence, finding from the national violence against women survey.* Washington, DC: National Institute for Justice, publication 2000; #19167.

van Katwijk, C., & Peeters, L. L. (1998). Clinical aspects of pregnancy after the age of 35 years: A review of the literature. *Human Reproduction Update, 4*(2), 185–194.

van Pampus, M. G., Wolf, H., Mayruhu, G., Treffers, P. E., & Bleker, O. P. (2001). Long-term follow-up in patients with a history of HELLP syndrome. *Hypertension in Pregnancy, 20*(1), 15–23.

Vigil de Garcia, P., & Garcia de Caceres, E. (1997). Dexamethasone in the postpartum treatment of HELLP syndrome. *Journal of Obstetrics and Gynaecology, 59,* 217–221.

Waisman, G. D., Mayorga, L. M., Cámera, M. I., Vignolo, C. A., & Martinotti, A. (1988). Magnesium plus nifedipine: Potentiation of hypotensive effect in preeclampsia? *American Journal of Obstetrics and Gynecology, 159*(2), 308–309.

Walker, L. (1979). *The battered woman.* New York, NY: Harper & Row.

Wang, S., Kallichanda, N., Song, W., Ramirez, B. A., & Ross, M. G. (2001). Expression of aquaporin-8 in human placenta and chorioamniotic membranes: Evidence of molecular mechanism for intramembranous amniotic fluid resorption. *American Journal of Obstetrics and Gynecology, 185*(5), 1226–1231.

Wasson, J. H., Jette, A. M., Anderson, J., Johnson, D. J., Nelson, E. C., & Kilo, C. M. (2000). Routine, single-item screening to identify abusive relationships in women. *Journal of Family Practice, 49*(11), 1017–1022.

Weinstein, L. (1982). Syndrome of hemolysis, elevated liver enzymes, and low platelet count: A severe consequence of hypertension in pregnancy. *American Journal of Obstetrics and Gynecology, 142*(2), 159–167.

Williams, M. A., Lieberman, E., Mittendorf, R., Monson, R. R., & Schoenbaum, S. C. (1991). Risk factors for abruptio placentae. *American Journal of Epidemiology, 134*(9), 965–972.

Wolf, J. L. (1996). Liver disease in pregnancy. *The Medical Clinics of North America, 80*(5), 1167–1187.

Wolf, N. G., & Lage, J. M. (1995). Genetic analysis of gestational trophoblastic disease: A review. *Seminars in Oncology, 22*(2), 113–120.

World Health Organization (WHO). (1983). *Gestational trophoblastic diseases: Report of a WHO Scientific Group.* WHO Technical Report Series No, 692, 16–18.

Yamazaki, K., Sato, K., Shizume, K., Kanaji, Y., Ito, Y., Obara, T., …Nishimura, R. (1995). Potent thyrotropic activity of human chorionic gonadotropin variants in terms of 125I incorporation and de novo synthesized thyroid hormone release in human thyroid follicles. *The Journal of Clinical Endocrinology and Metabolism, 80*(2), 473–479.

Yeast, J. (2006). Polyhydramnios: Etiology, diagnosis and treatment. *Neo Reviews, 7*, e300–e304.

Yoshimura, S., Masuzaki, H., Gotoh, H., & Ishimaru, T. (1997). Fetal redistribution of blood flow and amniotic fluid volume in growth-retarded fetuses. *Early Human Development, 47*(3), 297–304.

Zach, T. (2006). *Multiple births: eMedicine.* Retrieved from http://www.emedicine.com/ped/topic2599.htm

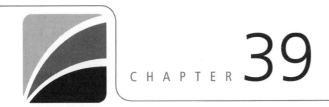

CHAPTER 39

Intrapartum and Postpartum Care

Heather Dawn Reynolds • Allison McCarson • Lilyan Kay • Meredith Goff

No matter how much a mother-to-be and her health care provider(s) prepare and plan, birth is a spontaneous, unpredictable event. Furthermore, the care provided to a woman during the intrapartum and postpartum periods has the potential to affect a woman for the rest of her life. This chapter focuses on the care rendered to a woman during the life-altering event known as childbirth.

■ INTRAPARTUM CARE

The intrapartum period is the period of care received during labor and delivery or childbirth. Specifically, the intrapartum period begins with the onset of labor and ends at the completion of the third stage of labor.

Labor and Delivery

LABOR

The antenatal, intrapartum, and postpartum health care provider's knowledge of the normal physiological changes that occur during labor, delivery, and postpartum is essential when managing the care of a woman during childbirth. Intrapartum providers in hospitals are most often certified nurse-midwives (CNMs), certified nurse anesthetists (CNAs), and medical doctors (MDs) with a certification in obstetrics. The role of the women's health nurse practitioner (WHNP) as an intrapartum health care provider mostly occurs in triage units, education, and sometimes involves the management of labor but not delivery (in most states). However, all health care providers must be familiar with the assessment and management of labor and possible delivery of the antenatal client in an emergency situation. The cause of labor is not implicit; diagnosis of labor is based on clinical judgment and has no clear-cut, explicit, agreeable starting point and can be problematic if assigned prematurely (Cheyne, Dowding, & Hundley, 2006). If a woman is admitted before active labor, she is at risk for inappropriate medical intervention. If the health care provider fails to diagnose labor, the woman is at risk for a medically unattended birth.

The initiation of human parturition is affected by a course of speculated causes involving changes in the maternal uterus and probably fetoplacental hormonal stimulation. Labor is the presence of uterine contractions of adequate intensity, frequency, and duration to convey consistent, progressive effacement and/or dilation of the cervix. Labor is usually divided into three phases. The first phase of labor, known as the latent phase, is when uterine contractions are becoming coordinated and lasts until onset of the active phase. Once cervical dilation is 5 cm in multiparous and 6 cm in primiparous women the laboring woman is usually entering the active phase, which is illustrated by organized, strong contractions and the most rapid changes in cervical dilation as plotted against time (King & Pinger, 2014). The active phase of labor includes both an increased rate of cervical dilation and, ultimately, descent of the presenting fetal part.

On the contrary, Braxton Hicks contractions are weak, irregular contractions, and can occur for weeks before the onset of actual labor, resulting in no progressive cervical change. The transformation of the uterus from calm to active contraction remains a conundrum. Some shared theories include fetal maturation, cervical ripening, and stretching of the uterus. Other theories deserve further explanation, such as a shift in estrogen and progesterone level and uterine sensitivity to oxytocin and inflammatory process.

Physiology of Labor

ESTROGEN AND PROGESTERONE SHIFT

Estrogen and progesterone, as well as several other hormones, play an important role in maintaining pregnancy. During pregnancy, these hormones increase sevenfold as compared to a nonpregnant woman. Elevated estrogen levels in pregnancy have significant effects on the maternal cardiovascular system, liver protein synthesis, and on the uterus itself. These effects include an increase in various aspects, such as binding proteins and clotting factors, uterine blood flow and sodium retention, and a decrease in vascular resistance. Estrogen stimulates uterine growth, increases the blood supply to the uterine vessels, and increases uterine contractions near term. It also aids in the development of the glands and ducts in the breasts in preparation for lactation. These are all necessary in the maternal adaptation to pregnancy and can have a profound effect on pregnancy. During the last 6 weeks of pregnancy, there is a rapid increase in estrogen levels, causing a change in the ratio between estrogen and progesterone before the onset of labor.

Progesterone synthesis, initially occurring in the corpus luteum, takes place in the placenta following the seventh week of pregnancy. Progesterone induces changes in the endometrium that are required for implantation; these levels must be maintained for the pregnancy to progress. This hormone acts to relax the smooth muscles of the uterus, preventing spontaneous abortion; however, withdrawal of progesterone in early pregnancy results in spontaneous abortion. Progesterone also plays a role in changes that occur in immune function during pregnancy to prevent rejection of the fetus or placenta as foreign antigens (Chan et al., 2002; Druckmann & Druckmann, 2005). A drop in the ratio between progesterone and estrogen has been thought to signal the onset of labor. Progesterone withdrawal, the most frequently recognized model of labor initiation, is thought to interrupt the myometrium or the smooth core tranquil state, resulting in uterine contractions (Chan et al., 2002; Druckmann & Druckmann, 2005).

OXYTOCIN

Oxytocin, a cyclic nonapeptide (a peptide made up of nine amino acids) biochemically similar to vasopressin, is synthesized as a large precursor peptide in the paraventricular and supraoptic nuclei of the hypothalamus. This precursor peptide, which undergoes cleavage during its transport to the posterior pituitary, is stored in association with another protein, neurophysin, in granules in the nerve terminals located in the posterior pituitary (Chan et al., 2002; Druckmann & Druckmann, 2005). In response to peripheral stimuli from the cervix and vagina, the neurophysin–oxytocin complex is released from the storage granules into the plasma in a pulsatile fashion. Once in the plasma, the oxytocin–neurophysin complex dissociates and oxytocin becomes a free molecule, able to bind to its receptors in myometrial, endometrial, and amnion cells.

The role of oxytocin in the regulation of uterine myometrial contractility is well documented. Myometrial oxytocin receptor sites increase by almost 200% during pregnancy, reaching their peak in early labor. This rise in oxytocin receptivity and stimulation of prostaglandin release in the uterus are thought to mediate contractions, which transform the uterus from quiescent to active contractions (Chan et al., 2002; Druckmann & Druckmann, 2005). It is known that the frequency of oxytocin cyclic pulses increase during spontaneous labor, reaching maximal frequency during the second and third stages of labor. This increased oxytocin production is probably necessary for the expulsive efforts needed for the birth of the baby and placenta (Chan et al., 2002; Druckmann & Druckmann, 2005). However, uterine contraction pressures and cervical dilation do not correlate with peripheral plasma oxytocin levels, so it remains unclear what role oxytocin plays in the initiation of parturition.

INFLAMMATORY PROCESS

It has been suggested that a major proportion of genes (e.g., interleukin-8 [IL-8], manganese superoxide dismutase, and metalloproteinase-9) upregulated during labor is associated with inflammatory-immune pathways of the lower segment of the myometrium (Chan et al., 2002). Another theory purports a mild proinflammatory state with increased IL-6 levels and may prime neonatal neutrophils to maximize their antibacterial potential (Chan et al., 2002). Labor at term or early onset could potentially boost neutrophil numbers by delaying apoptosis without excessive neutrophil activation or tissue damage.

As noted, many aspects of labor are not clearly understood. However, the regulation of uterine activity by progesterone, estrogen, and oxytocin appear to hold a role in parturition. The first stage of labor ends with full dilation of the cervix. This phase is initiated with regular contractions resulting in progressive effacement and dilation of the cervix. However, just as the mechanism for the initiation of labor is not yet determined, the precise onset of labor is not readily discernible. A major challenge is presented when a woman's self-diagnosis of labor does not coincide with clinical diagnosis and time of admission to hospital (Gross, Hecker, Matterne, Guenter, & Keirse, 2006).

Assessment

SIGNS OF LABOR

Standard signs of labor are painful contractions resulting in cervical dilatation of at least 5 cm, which progressively changes; an increase in bloody show; and spontaneous rupture of membranes. Women and health care providers struggle with identifying the *right time* to make the transition to the health care facility with complete accuracy (Gross et al., 2006). Teaching women when to transition from home to hospital includes instructions about the timing, frequency, duration, and strength of contractions and status of the amniotic bag of water.

Women are encouraged to report to their health care provider the following signs of labor: regular uterine contractions that increase in frequency, discomfort, and duration; spontaneous rupture of membranes; and/or bloody show. These preliminary signs may or may not lead to cervical change. Women who wait too long to seek medical assistance increase their risk for an unattended birth at home or birth en route to the health care facility. On the other hand, premature admission to the labor and delivery unit may result in an increased risk of maternal/fetal infection, obstetrical intervention, and/or cesarean delivery (Gross et al., 2006). A critical point of assessment for the health care provider is to be open to the varied types of unique experiences women may be having and actively listening to their concerns (Slade, Escott, Henderson, & Fraser, 2003). The clinician can accomplish this by explaining to women the range of normal while also adding that there is not one *right way* to identify labor or to define it (Slade et al., 2003).

Any woman reporting leaking of vaginal fluids or suspicion for rupture of membranes should be encouraged to seek medical care to rule out or confirm the suspicion of ruptured membranes. Home testing kits such as AmniScreen™ are available for consumer use; however, results need to be interpreted cautiously and confirmed by a health care provider. False readings can occur if fewer than 12 hours have passed since sexual intercourse or vaginal douching. Additionally, AmniScreen should not be used if there is vaginal bleeding or spotting. Regardless of results, a health care provider should be consulted if a woman experiences unexplained wetness, vaginal bleeding or spotting, or suspicion of vaginal infection.

The function of labor contractions is to dilate the cervix and move the fetus through the birth canal. Progress of labor can be plotted using graphs with an expectation of 1 cm/hour dilation for nulliparous women (1–2 cm/hr for multiparous), which is considered as normal labor progression (Cesario, 2004; Friedman, 1978).

The strength of contractions varies with the stage of labor, state of the cervix, exogenous oxytocin administration, and pain medication. The strength of contraction is assessed by observation of the mother, palpation of the fundus, external tocodynamometry, and internal pressure transducer.

When the evaluation of contractions is difficult due to various factors (e.g., body habitus) or when the response to oxytocin is unclear, intrauterine pressure catheters may be beneficial. The intrauterine pressure of the uterus during a contraction is reported in Montevideo units (MVUs); MVUs are calculated by multiplying the average peak of contraction in millimeters of mercury (mmHg) by the number of contraction in a 10-minute window or period. The use of MVUs for evaluation of contraction strength varies by institutional protocol and may not be used in all areas of the United States. Caution must be taken when using intrauterine pressure monitoring as a substitute for one-on-one nursing care during labor.

Health care providers who manage labor are concerned with fetal size, lie, presentation, attitude, position, station, and pelvis. The fetal head attempts to accommodate the birth canal through a process known as the cardinal movements of labor. These movements are engagement, descent, flexion, internal rotation, extension, external rotation, and expulsion. Engagement is the arrival of a fetal presenting part below the pelvic inlet, at or below the ischial spines, and is determined by palpation of the fetal head in relation to the ischial spines. Descent is the downward passage of the presenting part through the pelvis. Ideally, the fetus is in a cephalic presentation, with a completely flexed fetal head descending through the pelvis. The presenting part rotates anteriorly or posteriorly as it passes through the pelvis, resulting in the widest axis of the fetal head lining up with the widest axis of the pelvis. Once the head is in line with the pelvis, it descends to the level of the introitus and extension occurs. The fetal head is delivered and the fetal torso rotates as the body of the fetus is delivered (expulsion). Cardinal movements are described as passive actions synchronized with contractions and maternal pushing.

Stages of Labor

The indication of the first stage of active labor is generally signified with regular uterine contractions with cervical dilation of 5 to 6 cm or greater; this is also commonly the accepted criteria for admission to a labor and delivery unit in many institutions. The onset of active versus latent labor is usually arbitrarily assigned based on subjective reports. Being decisive as to when a woman is in true labor can be challenging even for the most experienced health care provider. A goal for the health care provider is to avoid the temptation to admit a patient in the latent phase of labor in order to relieve her pain or soothe her fear. A mutual understanding of the diagnosis of labor can be exasperating for both the patient and health care provider.

STAGE ONE

Stage one of labor consists of three phases: latent, active, and transition. This stage of labor is marked by psychological and physical changes; it consists of distention of the lower uterine segment and ending with full dilation of the cervix. Anxiety and fear of personal injury and fetal injury are the most commonly verbalized psychological concerns and vary from female to female. A woman experiencing excessive anxiety produces increased catecholamine secretions, which make her brain perceive physical pain that is out of proportion to the physiological stimulus. Physical change is the consequence of mechanical stretching of cervical tissue and pressure on adjacent structures surrounding the vagina and distention of the pelvic floor as the fetus descends into the pelvis. The physical changes associated with the first stage of labor can last 12 to 14 hours as the cervix thins and dilates.

Latent Phase • During the latent phase, a woman or her support person may call the office or hospital to report regular, somewhat uncomfortable contractions, which may be described as lower back pain. This phase of labor is usually marked by slow, progressive change. Contractions usually increase in frequency, duration, and intensity of discomfort. The woman may note an increase in bloody show as well as experience a spontaneous rupture of her amniotic membranes.

The most frequently asked question directed at the health care provider during the latent phase is, when should I go to the hospital? The health care provider should instruct the woman to seek medical care when her contractions are 3 to 5 minutes apart; when her contractions become progressively stronger, longer, and more uncomfortable (e.g., can't walk or talk through contractions); or immediately if her amniotic membranes rupture. During this phase, anticipatory guidance regarding labor and pain management options becomes more important to the woman. Education is most effective, with the inclusion of family along with the laboring woman. The family member or support person is encouraged to provide emotional support to the laboring woman. The use of complementary therapies (e.g., back rubs, baths, meditation) may assist with discomfort during this phase.

Active Phase • As the woman's cervical dilation progresses from 5 to 6 to 8 cm (the active phase of labor), she will report more intense discomfort (King & Pinger, 2014). The fetus continues to descend into the pelvis, contributing to the woman's increased discomfort, which oftentimes results in a request for greater pain management—such as an epidural.

Admission is ensured with the onset of painful, regular uterine contractions resulting in progressive cervical effacement and/or dilatation. Full evaluation of the laboring patient includes fetal presentation, position, uterine contraction pattern and strength, fetal heart rate (FHR) pattern, and evaluation of the woman's prenatal record.

Transition • Transition (8–10 cm of cervical dilation) is the period where the woman experiences the strongest, most frequent contractions, commonly marked by a transition to high anxiety and fear of losing control (even in the previously calm, cooperative patient). The laboring woman may exhibit nausea with vomiting, shivering, and shaking; all of which are normal during labor.

STAGE TWO

The second stage of labor begins with full cervical dilatation (10 cm) and ends with the delivery of the infant. This stage varies from a few minutes to a few hours. The mean length is 19 minutes for a multiparous woman and 54 minutes for a nulliparous woman. A fetus with a large presenting diameter may increase the mean duration of stage two. If the second stage exceeds 3 hours without an epidural or 4 hours with an epidural in a nulliparous woman, she is considered to be in a prolonged second stage. In a multiparous woman, the second stage is considered prolonged if labor exceeds 2 hours without an epidural, or 3 hours with an epidural (Kopas, 2014; Spong, Berghella, Wenstrom, Mercer, & Saade,, 2012).

A woman in this stage may report rectal pressure and an involuntary urge to bear down with contractions. The health care provider may note an increase in bloody show and rapid fetal descent as the laboring woman responds to the urge to push.

STAGE THREE

Time from delivery of the infant to separation and expulsion of the placenta is the third stage of labor. Following delivery of the fetus, the upper segment of the uterus retracts rapidly. Separation of the placenta then occurs due to the shrinking of the site and the area of attachment. The placenta is forced down into the lower uterine segment and as the abdominal muscles and diaphragm contract, the placenta is then expelled through the vagina. The mechanism of action behind this separation is a decrease in placental site, a decrease in intrauterine pressure, formation of a line of cleavage in the decidua, and formation of a retroplacental clot. Bleeding from the newly uncovered implantation site continues until the placenta is expelled. The placenta can be expelled through either the Schultze mechanism or the Duncan mechanism.

The Schultze mechanism is used when the placenta separates from the central area to the margins with inversion, causing the fetal side to present first. With the Duncan mechanism, the placenta separates from the margins to the center and the maternal side is presented first. Placental separation is marked by the lengthening of the umbilical cord, a gush of fluid from the vagina, and a globular shape of the fundus. After the expulsion of the placenta, the maternal and fetal surfaces, as well as the umbilical cord, should be inspected for intactness and abnormalities. The placenta usually weighs about one seventh of the neonatal weight. The fetal surface is shiny and the maternal surface consists of cotyledons (each cotyledon consists of a main stem of chorionic villus). The normal appearance of the umbilical cord consists of three vessels (two arteries and one vein) and measures 50 to 60 cm in length. The cord should be inserted far from the margin on the fetal surface of the placenta and should have a coiled pattern.

If the placenta does not separate spontaneously or copious bleeding occurs, an abnormal implantation must be considered. Such an abnormal invasion of the placental villi to the uterine wall can be a life-threatening condition (Wiedaseck & Monchek, 2014). Placenta accreta occurs when the placental villi abnormally adhere to the myometrium, with partial or complete absence of the decidua basalis. Placenta increta occurs when the placental villi embed deeply into the muscular walls of the uterus. Placenta percreta occurs when the placenta penetrates through the entire uterine wall and attaches to the bladder or other organs. This diagnosis may require advanced medical intervention or surgery and can lead to the necessity of a peripartum hysterectomy.

A previous cesarean delivery is associated with more significant risk for placenta accreta, placenta previa, uterine rupture, injury to internal organs during surgery, excessive blood loss, need for hysterectomy, and maternal death. Uterine scarring secondary to previous cesarean delivery may lead to abnormal trophoblast invasion and subsequent placenta accreta (Hundley, 2002). Approximately 50% of pregnancies complicated by placenta accreta are in women who have had a previous cesarean section; the risk increasing with each subsequent cesarean delivery, reaching a rate of more than 60% in women with greater than three cesarean deliveries (Hundley, 2002).

Management of Labor

STAGE ONE

If not already ruptured, an amniotomy may be performed to assess the amount and color of amniotic fluid as well as the fetal presentation. Maintaining adequate uterine contractions, monitoring for cervical progression of 1 to 2 cm/hr, evaluation of fetal descent, as well as monitoring maternal and fetal well-being is the focus of this stage of labor (Box 39.1). If spontaneous contractions fail to effect progressive cervical dilation or descent of the fetus, artificial stimulation of uterine contractions with oxytocin augmentation should be considered. Measures such as massage, controlled breathing, baths, and previously established epidurals can be used to facilitate comfort and relaxation during this phase of labor (Impey, Hobson, & O'Herlihy, 2000; Slade et al., 2003).

STAGE TWO

During stage two, the health care provider focuses on fetal descent and well-being. If an unexpected birth occurs outside of the hospital, the health care provider needs to be prepared with an emergency delivery kit and appropriate supplies (Box 39.2).

BOX 39.1   SUMMARY OF ACOG RECOMMENDATIONS FOR LABOR MANAGEMENT

- Counsel patients that walking during labor does not enhance or improve progress in labor nor is it harmful.
- It is beneficial for women and their newborns to have continuous support during labor.
- Although active management of labor may shorten labor in nulliparous women, it has not consistently been shown to reduce the rate of cesarean delivery.
- Amniotomy may be used to enhance progress in active labor but may increase the risk of maternal fever.
- Intrauterine pressure catheters may be helpful in the management of dystocia (slow, abnormal progression of labor) in selected patients, such as those who are obese.
- Women with twin gestations may undergo augmentation of labor.

ACOG, American College of Obstetricians and Gynecologists.
Data from ACOG (2009).

BOX 39.2   EMERGENCY DELIVERY KIT

Delivery Supplies

Towels, sheets, and blankets
Sterile gloves
Sterile scissors
Pitocin (oxytocin)
Intravenous infusion start kit (optional)
Bulb syringe
Cord clamps
Kelly clamps
Methylergonovine (Methergine)
1,000 mL lactated ringers (optional)

Data from Cheyne, Dowding, and Hundley (2006).

Before any invasive management interventions during the second stage, the health care provider should consider reassessment of the maternal pelvis, cervix, expulsive forces, and the fetus for size, position, and presentation. Maternal position for pushing and birth have shifted with the transition to hospital birth and increased assisted vaginal delivery with forceps. In recent decades, after the shift of childbirth to the hospital, the lithotomy position has become the norm for the second stage of labor. Evidence suggests that the lithotomy or a supine position increases the risk for FHR abnormalities and fewer spontaneous vaginal deliveries. The upright position, either sitting or squatting, is optimal for fetal descent with a lateral or hands–knees position for decreased lacerations during birth (Kopas, 2014). Evidence strongly supports delayed pushing or laboring down, when a woman is fully dilated without the urge to push. Although there is no consensus on absolute maximum time, pushing can be delayed for up to 2 hours or until the woman has a strong urge to push or the fetal head is visualized at the introitus. When bearing down efforts are not reflexive or spontaneous, coaching may be needed. Directed pushing, or coaching, should be considered an intervention; it is the most common management of the second stage of labor. Directed pushing methods are conducted with the woman in a lithotomy position while holding her breath and pushing for 10 seconds. Spontaneous pushing has been found to be safer for both mom and fetus, but if guidance is needed, encourage the laboring woman to push instinctively with three to four focused pushes of less than 6 seconds with each contraction. There are a variety of ways to encourage a woman to push; however, the paramount method is what works best for her.

If the woman has not attended childbirth classes or does not have a coach, she should be encouraged to do what comes naturally and to follow her body's urge (Bloom, Casey, Schaffer, McIntire, & Leveno, 2006). Women may choose to squat, stand, kneel, or sit on the toilet. The woman may also use a squatting bar or birthing ball. Other than in the Western culture, women rarely choose to push lying in bed.

STAGE THREE

Management of the third stage of labor includes clamping of the umbilical cord, delivery of the placenta, and evaluation of the maternal status to include close assessment for postpartum hemorrhage (PPH). There have been many documented studies that show the benefits of delayed umbilical cord clamping, including increasing neonatal iron stores and preventing anemia in both full-term and preterm infants (American College of Obstetricians and Gynecologists [ACOG], 2012; Arca, Botet, Palacio, & Carbonell-Estrany, 2010). Conversely, the possibility of an increased incidence of hyperbilirubinemia and polycythemia in the infant and the possible increased risk for PPH in the mother continues to be debated; therefore, this practice is not a standard of care in the United States (ACOG, 2012; Cesario, 2004).

As in most cases at least three contractions are necessary to separate the placenta, and it is important to wait at least 10 minutes before initiating any intervention to assist with placenta delivery. Failure to wait the 10 minutes greatly increases the risk of uterine inversion, a condition in which the uterus turns inside out often protruding from the cervix and occasionally, even the vagina. These obstetrical emergencies can lead to PPH, shock, and even maternal death.

If the placenta does not separate and deliver spontaneously, active management of the third stage of labor is initiated to help prevent PPH due to uterine atony. This active management of the third stage includes the administration of oxytocin immediately following fetal delivery, gentle cord traction, and uterine massage (Magann & Lanneau, 2005).

Several maneuvers can be used to deliver the placenta and should be considered if the placenta has not separated after 20 to 30 minutes. The Brandt–Andrews maneuver is used frequently to assist with the delivery of the placenta. The abdominal hand secures the uterine fundus to prevent inversion and downward traction is exerted on the umbilical cord with the other hand. Another method is the Crede maneuver, by which the cord is fixed with the lower hand and the uterine fundus is secured while traction is exerted upward using the abdominal hand.

After the placenta delivers, putting the infant to breast or giving a dose of Pitocin (oxytocin) may decrease the risk of hemorrhage. Retained products of conception will contribute to continued uterine bleeding, in which case manual uterine exploration should be considered to remove any retained products of conception. Synthetic oxytocin should be given intramuscularly (IM) or intravenously (IV) as a continuous infusion, not as a bolus, as rapid IV dosing has been linked to maternal cardiovascular collapse (Magann & Lanneau, 2005). If IV access is not available, and oxytocin is given IM, this route will take 3 to 5 minutes to stimulate contraction of the uterus.

The average blood loss during a vaginal delivery is 500 mL. A loss of more than 500 mL during a vaginal delivery is defined as PPH, though an even lower blood loss in a woman with anemia can result in hemodynamic instability. Further, a loss of more than 1,000 mL for a primary cesarean or 1,500 mL for a repeat cesarean also constitutes PPH. PPH is usually a subjective diagnosis. This is problematic as, in many instances, the amount of bleeding is underestimated due to the fact that blood is mixed with amniotic fluid and is often absorbed in linens and towels used during labor and delivery (Magann & Lanneau, 2005). After the delivery of the placenta, assessment should also include a thorough evaluation of the labia, perineum, cervix, and vagina for lacerations.

Obstetric Interventions

The most frequent obstetric interventions performed to manage labor are induction or augmentation of labor with oxytocin, amniotomy, episiotomy, and cesarean section. As previously mentioned, oxytocin is used to stimulate labor and to differentiate functional uterine disorders from dystocia, which are frequently caused by four abnormalities (Fraser, Marcoux, Moutquin, & Christen, 1993):

- Expulsive forces (e.g., contractions)
- Conditions, position, or development of the fetus (e.g., large for gestational age, malpresentation)
- Maternal bony pelvis (e.g., cephalopelvic disproportion [CPD])
- Other factors such as soft tissue dystocia

AMNIOTOMY

An amniotomy is frequently performed to induce or augment labor. A reduction in labor duration of 1 to 2 hours has been associated with performing an amniotomy after cervical effacement and dilatation has occurred (Fraser et al., 1993). Amniotomy may increase progress of active labor and reduce the need for oxytocin augmentation but may increase the risk of chorioamnionitis as well as a woman's pain during contractions. Once cervical dilatation has reached 5 cm, amniotomy usually has little effect on labor progression.

OXYTOCIN

Oxytocin is a medication used for induction and augmentation of human labor. The goal of oxytocin use is to strengthen uterine contractions, effecting cervical change and fetal descent, while simultaneously avoiding uterine tachysystole and fetal compromise. The role oxytocin plays in the initiation of labor is unclear; however, its role in establishing labor is better understood. In addition, the contractile response of the uterine myometrium to oxytocin is to some extent predictable; the higher concentration of receptors to the uterine fundus increases the response of synthetic oxytocin.

Oxytocin protocols vary according to institutional policy. A fairly consistent starting dose of oxytocin (low dose) is 1 mU/min. At term (pregnancy), 1 to 2 mU is the amount of oxytocin needed to stimulate oxytocin receptor sites, increasing the dosage by 1 mU/min every 30 minutes until regular uterine contractions or a maximal dose is reached. The health care provider or practicing institution prescribes the maximum dose; the most common maximum dose is 20 mU/min (Patka, Lodolce, & Johnston, 2005). More and more, laboring patients are usually not restricted to staying in bed during a Pitocin infusion. Issues regarding whether to be bedridden or not during Pitocin administration have been centered around a laboring woman's increased risk for uterine tachysystole (historically monitored with continuous fetal monitoring). With the advent of ambulatory fetal monitoring capability, many institutions now allow a laboring woman to freely move about during Pitocin administration.

RISK FACTORS

Tachysystole is a major potential risk of oxytocin and is defined as more than five contractions in 10 minutes, averaged over a 30-minute window (Robinson & Nelson, 2008). Tachysystole may occur without corresponding FHR abnormalities. However, the fetus is monitored closely for signs of fetal distress, which could be a direct result of tachysystole, resulting in decreased oxygenation to the fetus.

The risk for uterine rupture increases with tachysystole and is particularly increased if the woman has an earlier history of uterine surgery. Other risks associated with exogenous oxytocin use include maternal water intoxication, hypotension, and with prolonged use (such as with a long and difficult labor induction), postpartum uterine atony and subsequent hemorrhage. Water intoxication, though relatively rare, should be considered the differential diagnosis of laboring patients with acute changes in mental status or seizures (Ophir, Solt, Odeh, & Bornstein, 2007).

In the presence of tachysystole, immediate discontinuation of the oxytocin infusion, increasing IV fluids, positioning the mother in a lateral position, and offering oxygen at 10 L/min via facemask usually result in a quick termination of tachysystole and potential fetal distress

(Robinson & Nelson, 2008). However, if the problem persists, the maintenance IV fluids should be increased and a subcutaneous dose of terbutaline can be given. Terbutaline is a beta-adrenergic receptor agonist that causes relaxation of the smooth muscle of the uterus and therefore can be useful as a tocolytic. However, terbutaline is not without side effects, including jitteriness, increased heart rate, tremors, headaches, dizziness and very rarely, increased blood sugar and seizures (Smith & Merrill, 2006). If tachysystole is prolonged and results in ominous signs of fetal distress, a prompt cesarean section is often indicated.

OPERATIVE VAGINAL INTERVENTIONS

Operative obstetric vaginal delivery interventions include episiotomy, vacuum extraction, and obstetric forcep-assisted deliveries. Operative vaginal delivery procedures are only appropriate after complete dilation. They may be indicated to minimize valsalva maneuvers in light of maternal cardiac compromise, prevent severe perineal trauma, and minimize risk of traumatic delivery for the fetus. Potential maternal risks associated with the use of these techniques includes soft tissue damage, PPH, thromboembolic events, puerperal infections, and wound infections. Potential risks to the neonate include bruising, lacerations, cephalohematoma, retinal hemorrhage, and brachial plexus palsy.

EPISIOTOMY

Episiotomy is a constituent of operative vaginal delivery (forceps and vacuum) with the goal of avoidance of perineal trauma, such as anal sphincter injury, perineal pain, fecal incontinence, urgency, and/or sexual dysfunction (Box 39.3) (Hudelist et al., 2005; Macleod & Murphy, 2008). Mediolateral episiotomy is associated with fewer anal sphincter lacerations than midline episiotomy. Midline (also known as median) episiotomy increases perineal laceration length as well as incidence for sphincter disruption. Midline episiotomy over mediolateral episiotomy preference varies according to the station and position of the presenting part in addition to the experience of the health care provider (Macleod & Murphy, 2008). Mediolateral episiotomies are associated with higher blood loss than midline and some studies have demonstrated higher pain scores in women. The choice of whether or not to perform an episiotomy when using forceps or vacuum is made by the health care provider (Hudelist et al., 2005).

Fetal Monitoring

Electronic fetal monitoring (EFM) was made available in the United States around the 1960s. Fetal compromise has been associated with changes in the baseline FHR, repetitive decelerations, and prolonged decreased variability of the FHR noted during fetal monitoring. EFM was projected to improve perinatal outcome, possibly associated with fetal acidosis. However, false-positive results have led to increased

---

> ### BOX 39.3   WOMEN AT RISK OF EPISIOTOMY
>
> Nulliparous
> Prolonged second stage of labor
> Terminal bradycardia
> Fetal malpresentation at full dilation
> Macrosomia
> Epidural
> History of severe laceration
> Shoulder dystocia
> Nondistending vaginal introitus
> Cardiac conditions
>
> Data from Hastings-Tolsma, Vincent, Emeis, and Francisco (2007).

---

surgical intervention without the expected decline in neonatal morbidity and mortality. Combining visual assessment of FHR tracing with automated analysis of the fetal EKG has been shown to reduce false-positive results (Gonsalves, Rocha, Ayres-de-Campos, & Bernardes, 2006). A fetal EKG examination, when supplemented with standard EFM analysis, has been shown to detect, within a term, pregnancy labor, lowered rates of both fetal metabolic acidosis, and operative delivery for fetal distress. Intrapartum fetal assessment can be performed using intermittent or continuous fetal monitoring.

Intermittent monitoring (IA) is accomplished with the use of a handheld Doppler—an external transducer or, in low-resource settings, a fetoscope held against the maternal abdomen. Continuous monitoring can be accomplished using an external transducer, held in place by an elastic belt on the woman's gravid abdomen or an internal monitor applied as an electrode attachment to the fetal scalp. The internal monitor requires the cervix to be dilated and amniotic membrane to be ruptured. The decision as to the method of fetal monitoring may vary among stage of labor, institution, and health care provider. Interpretation of fetal monitoring patterns includes notation of baseline rate and variability, presence or absence of accelerations, presence of periodic or episodic decelerations in reference to contractions, depth of deceleration, length of deceleration, and trends in patterns, including frequency and duration of contractions.

ASSESSMENT

EFM can be classified as reassuring, non-reassuring, or ominous. Non-reassuring patterns are classified as fetal tachycardia, bradycardia, prolonged decelerations, and late decelerations. The timing of the patterns (baseline, periodic, or episodic) is also of importance. Periodic patterns are associated with uterine contractions, whereas episodic patterns are not associated with uterine contractions.

Prolonged fetal compromise will result in ominous patterns, requiring immediate delivery and possible neonatal resuscitation. Ominous patterns are recurrent, late, or prolonged variable decelerations, or substantial bradycardia with absent FHR variability.

EFM should be used as a screening tool for fetal distress. The reporting or recording of fetal monitoring patterns must be inclusive of baseline rate and variability, presence or absence of accelerations, periodic or episodic decelerations, and trends and patterns, and should include frequency and duration of contractions to adequately evaluate fetal well-being and tolerance of labor. It is important that gestational age be considered in the explanation of the pattern. Note that a lack of agreement in visual interpretation of FHR patterns, definition, and nomenclature exists. Fetal monitoring is a procedure performed in 99% of labors occurring in a hospital; however, evidence does not support that fetal monitoring can detect acid-base metabolic changes that reflect fetal well-being during labor (Hadar et al., 2001). There is no complete agreement concerning guidelines for clinical management of, or interpretation of, non-reassuring FHR patterns using EFM. This lack of agreement may delay or prevent clinical intervention for interpretation of fetal monitoring.

■ COMPLICATIONS IN LABOR

Pain Management

Coping with labor pain represents both a physiological and psychological challenge to the woman (Cyna, McAuliffe, & Andrew, 2004; Smith, Collins, Cyna, & Crowther, 2006). Uterine contraction, dilation of the cervix, and stretching of the pelvic floor are the contributing factors to labor pain. Women may fear that their inability to control themselves during labor may cause harm to their unborn child. Also, if a woman chooses to use pain medication, an additional fear may include the concern for harm to herself. The uncertainty of labor (including the length of time that pain will be experienced, as well as the uncertainty of how stronger contractions will get) can lead to increased anxiety in the laboring woman as well as the inability to control her response to pain as labor progresses.

The health care provider aims to reduce the amount of pain a laboring woman experiences during childbirth by informing her of interventions available to her, including parenteral medications, epidural, and nondrug interventions (e.g., the use of a doula or other support person to coach relaxation and breathing techniques, imagery, acupressure, therapeutic touch, biofeedback, and hypnosis).

Complementary therapies are gaining interest. In 2006, approximately 36% of health care providers recommended some form of complementary alternative therapies (Zwelling, Johnson, & Allen, 2006). The use of complementary alternative therapies is increasing due to overwhelming support by, for example, professional organizations, such as state boards of nursing.

Complementary and Alternative Therapies

Complementary and alternative medicine (CAM), a group of diverse medical and health care systems, practices, and products that are not considered part of conventional medicine, is recognized by the National Institutes of Health, specifically by the National Center for CAM (Table 39.1). Published research supports CAM therapies as safe and effective. In labor and delivery, complementary and alternative therapies, such as the use of doulas, Lamaze techniques, and guided imagery have been shown to reduce the use of pharmaceuticals and epidurals (Cyna et al., 2004).

DOULAS

Ideally, a woman in labor receives one-on-one professional nursing support and care. In reality, the amount of labor support provided is directly related to the availability of staff and the acuity of the patient. Charting, monitoring, medication distribution, high numbers of patients, and low numbers of staff may leave very little time to provide emotional, spiritual, and physical care to the laboring woman. Therefore, women should be educated during prenatal care about other options for support, such as a doula or other support person.

Traditionally, doulas are women assisting women and their partners during active labor and immediately postpartum, providing continuous comfort measures. These paraprofessionals assist women and their partners to carry out their labor plan. The assistance is accomplished by facilitating communication among the woman, her partner, and the health care provider. Doulas have no medical or clinical care responsibilities. A doula is not a nurse, but a person skilled to provide emotional, spiritual, and physical support

TABLE 39.1	Five Domains of CAM
TYPE	**EXAMPLE**
Alternative medical systems	Homeopathic, naturopathic, Chinese medicine, and ayurveda medicine
Mind–body medicine	Support groups, biofeedback, Lamaze, cognitive behavioral therapy, meditation, prayer, mental healing, art, music and dance therapies
Biological-based therapies	Herbs, foods, vitamins
Manipulative and body-based therapies	Chiropractic or osteopathic manipulation, massage
Energy therapies	Biofeedback (qigong, reiki, healing touch) Bioelectromagnetic (pulsed fields, magnetic fields, alternating current, or direct current fields)

CAM, complementary and alternative medicine.
Data from Smith, Collins, Cyna, and Crowther (2006).

during labor and delivery—not clinical or medical care. These skilled persons are not friends, family, or relatives, but rather birth assistants. Doulas usually charge a set price for agreed on services, although some doulas do volunteer their services to certain populations. Doulas are trained and apply national standards set forth by their professional organization, Doulas of North America International (Kane Low, Moffat, & Brennan, 2006; Papagni & Buckner, 2006). Standards include knowledge related to the physiology of labor, the stages of labor, comfort measures, and breastfeeding techniques (Kane Low et al., 2006; Papagni & Buckner, 2006). Doulas use imagery, massage, and acupressure to minimize fear and anxiety for the laboring woman. Health care providers should inform pregnant women, during their routine prenatal care, that doulas are an option and may be included in their birth plan. Access to doula services is, however, limited by geographic location, ability to pay, and type of insurance. Continuous support by a doula has resulted in reduced cesarean section rates, decreased oxytocin augmentation, and shortened duration of labor (Kane Low et al., 2006; Papagni & Buckner, 2006).

PREPARED CHILDBIRTH CLASSES

Another form of CAM is active involvement in prepared childbirth classes. Various types of childbirth classes are available, such as the Bradley Method, hypnobirthing, birthing from within, and the most common, Lamaze International. Lamaze is a childbirth education program focused on teaching women to trust their ability to give birth with minimal medical interventions (Hotelling, 2006; Zwelling et al., 2006). Women are encouraged to use self-help measures, such as breathing and relaxation techniques. Lamaze International teaches pregnant women six practice strategies that they believe promote normal birth: labor begins on its own, freedom of movement throughout labor, continuous labor support, no routine interventions, non-supine (e.g., upright or side-lying) positions for birth, and no separation of mother and baby with unlimited opportunity for breastfeeding (Hotelling, Amis, Green, & Sakala, 2004; Lothian, Amis, Crenshaw, & Goer, 2004). The health care provider should be aware that women who have taken classes may present with a birthing plan requesting no restrictions on eating and drinking during labor, the avoidance of IV fluids, and no continuous EFM unless absolutely medically necessary (Hotelling et al., 2004; Lothian et al., 2004). The requests of the laboring woman may challenge the medical model and may have to be worked on an individual basis.

GUIDED IMAGERY

Guided imagery is a cognitive activity that embraces the notion that the mind is linked to a physiologic process of decreased awareness of pain (Brown, Douglas, & Flood, 2001). The thought is to engage a laboring woman's mind with breathing and deep relaxation techniques so that the awareness of the pain from the contraction is reduced. Relaxation increases pain tolerance by reducing feelings of anxiety. Catecholamine response decreases as the laboring woman becomes less anxious, resulting in an increased uterine blood flow and decreased muscle tension. Pain tolerance increases even more when the laboring woman's thoughts are guided to pleasant experiences with an end point in relaxation.

HYPNOSIS

Hypnosis is a psychological intervention that reduces awareness of external stimuli and increases response to suggestions (Cyna et al., 2004; Smith et al., 2006). Suggestions can be in the form of verbal and nonverbal communication that results in noticeable spontaneous changes in perception, mood, or behavior. The therapeutic communication of medical hypnosis is directed at the laboring woman's subconscious (Cyna et al., 2006; Smith et al., 2006). Women can be taught self-hypnosis, which can be used in labor as an adjunct to facilitate and enhance other analgesics for the purpose of reducing labor pain. Evidence suggests that hypnosis in childbirth allows the laboring woman to reduce her need for pharmacological analgesia, resulting in increased chance of having a spontaneous vaginal birth (Cyna et al., 2006).

ACUPRESSURE AND THERAPEUTIC TOUCH/MASSAGE

Acupressure is the application of finger pressure or deep massage to the traditional acupuncture points on the hands, feet, and ears or energy flow lines to reduce labor pain (Brown et al., 2001). Therapeutic touch/massage is an effective therapy to manage labor pain and to lower anxiety and agitation. There are three main goals of therapeutic touch: (1) reduction of pain and anxiety, (2) initiation of relaxation, and (3) stimulation of healing process (Fischer & Johnson, 1999).

Therapeutic touch/massage therapy can be taught quickly and effectively at the bedside to a friend, family member, or significant other. Laboring women who receive therapeutic touch/massage have been shown to have shorter labors and less postpartum depression (Brown et al., 2001). However, not every woman desires to be touched during contractions, therefore techniques must be individualized for each woman.

Applying hot compresses to the abdomen, groin, or perineum or ice packs to the lower back, anus, or perineum are also effective alternative and adjunct measures to massage (Brown et al., 2001). Aromatherapy oils and/or lotions are often used in conjunction with massage. Popular essential oils for use in labor include lavender or jasmine, mixed with a carrier oil or lotion. Peppermint oil can be used to decrease nausea and vomiting (Zwelling et al., 2006). A few drops of an essential oil (ginger or lemongrass) to hydrotherapy baths can also promote relaxation. At the time of publication of this textbook, no national nursing standards were available regarding the use of aromatherapy. Hence, guidelines for use of oils in late pregnancy and labor need to be followed according to the policy of institutions.

HYDROTHERAPY

Another technique frequently used in the first stage of labor is hydrotherapy (laboring in water). To accommodate a laboring patient's request for hydrotherapy, some hospitals have added oversized showers and jetted tubs to their labor units. Although literature to support hydrotherapy is limited, researchers agree that hydrotherapy does not cause harm to the mother or fetus. Hydrotherapy appears to assist with decreasing pain and anxiety in the first stage of labor, resulting in the decreased need of labor augmentation, decreased pain, and increased labor satisfaction (Cluett, Pickering, Getliffe, & St George Saunders, 2004). The goal of managing labor pain without causing harm to the mother or her fetus can be met by using complementary and alternative pain control methods.

Epidural Analgesia

Another intervention for controlling labor and surgical pain is epidural analgesia. Epidurals have been shown to be effective and safe and are the most commonly used method of pain control in the United States. Small doses of epidural or spinal opioids alone or combined with low doses of local anesthetics have been shown to not affect the well-being of the neonate at birth (Capogna & Camorcia, 2004). The process consists of medications, such as ropivacaine and levobupivacaine, with the addition of an opioid administered through a catheter into the epidural space. During and after the placement of an epidural, the laboring woman must be monitored closely for hypotension and fetal bradycardia, both of which are commonly associated with an epidural. These complications can be resolved by maternal position change and hydration. Epidural analgesia is also associated with maternal fever, post-epidural headache, decreased sensation for pushing, inability to ambulate, potential need for urinary catheterization, and narcotic use in labor (Cluett et al., 2004).

Perineal Trauma

Perineal trauma, or genital tract injury, occurs in more than 65% of all vaginal births (Christianson, Bovbjerg, McDavitt, & Hullfish, 2003). Most perineal trauma is less than or equal to a second degree laceration. Factors contributing to an increased risk of perineal lacerations include squatting position during birth in primiparous women, disruption of spontaneous bearing down efforts, epidural use, pudendal anesthesia, and oxytocin use (Hastings-Tolsma, Vincent, Emeis, & Francisco, 2007). Other contributing risk factors include poor maternal nutrition, untreated vaginal infections, and uncontrolled expulsion of the fetus. The occurrence of third- or fourth-degree tears are relatively rare, but are potential complications of vaginal delivery. Fourth degree tears occur more often with operative episiotomies, and carry long-term risk of fecal incontinence, fecal urgency, and/or sexual dysfunction.

Lacerations may occur with or without an episiotomy. Some interventions used during labor and birth that are known to minimize the risk of perineal trauma include pushing in the lateral position, upright, and on hands and knees; delivery of the fetal head between contractions; warm compresses; and flexion/counter pressure to slow birth of the fetal head. Prenatal perineal massage with sweet almond oil, evening primrose oil, or other vegetable-based oil for 5 to 10 minutes daily from 34 weeks until delivery (particularly in nulliparous women) is a protective perineal intervention that can promote elasticity of the perineum (Eason, Labrecque, Wells, & Feldman, 2000; Hastings-Tolsma et al., 2007).

MANAGEMENT

Attention should be focused on signs of infection and hemorrhoids during the first few hours to days postdelivery. Monitor the patient at least every 4 hours for elevated temperature (which could indicate infection of the genitourinary tract). Careful and close inspection of the perineum for the development of a hematoma should also be done every 4 hours postdelivery. Ice applied to the perineum the first 12 hours after a vaginal delivery will help to discourage the development of edema or a hematoma and provides comfort. The episiotomy site should be free of heat, drainage, or redness. The acronym REEDA can be used as a reminder that the site should be assessed for redness (R), edema (E), ecchymosis (E), discharge (D), and approximation (A). Sutures, used for homeostasis and to approximate tissue, may or may not be visible or palpable.

Assess the postpartum woman's pain level and encourage her to empty her bladder. Encourage warm or cool sitz baths and benzocaine spray to promote comfort and healing. If hemorrhoids are present, offer Tucks® pads (infused with witch hazel) and stool softeners and instruct the patient to increase her fluid and fiber intake. Stool softeners may also be helpful the first few weeks following delivery, in the case of a third- or fourth-degree laceration. Kegel exercises should be encouraged to strengthen perineal tone once soreness has decreased and healing of the perineum has occurred.

Cesarean Section

Cesarean delivery is the most common surgical procedure in women in the United States. It accounted for 32.7% of all births in the United States in 2013 (Martin, Hamilton, & Osterman, 2014). Cesarean section carries a risk of major abdominal surgery, infection, pelvic structure injury, and potential for blood transfusion. An increase in elective cesarean delivery has stimulated debate in the medical community. In a committee opinion published in April of 2013, the ACOG did not recommend elective cesarean delivery. Instead, ACOG supports a planned vaginal delivery in the absence of maternal or fetal indications for a cesarean section (ACOG, 2013). ACOG has offered recommendations to assist with counseling and decision making, should the health care provider and pregnant woman, together, decide on elective cesarean (ACOG, 2013). This recommendation became necessary because elective or unnecessary cesarean deliveries have been performed in the absence of documented maternal and/or neonatal medical risk factors (Kabir et al., 2004). It has been suggested that women elect cesarean to reduce a personal perceived risk of maternal pelvic organ prolapse, urinary and fecal incontinence, and the avoidance of anxiety and the pain of labor. Furthermore, health care providers have reported that, at times, they have elected cesarean delivery due to the convenience of a scheduled delivery, as a means to decrease the risk of stillbirth, and to deal with FHR abnormalities and breech presentation (Armson, 2007).

Cesarean delivery can be a life-saving intervention for the fetus when the pregnancy is complicated by HIV, active herpes, fetal malpresentation, macrosomia, multiple gestation, fetal structural abnormalities, cord prolapse, placental abruption, and fetal distress as noted via fetal heart monitoring. In emergent situations, such as fetal distress, ACOG has recommended abdominal incision within 30 minutes of the decision to undertake emergency cesarean. Even so, the time from decision to incision exceeds 30 minutes in one third to one half of pregnant women experiencing cesarean sections for non-reassuring fetal heart tracing. There remains a need for improvement from decision to incision (Chauhan et al., 2003).

LABOR DYSTOCIA

Labor dystocia is an idiom used to suggest abnormal labor caused by ineffective expulsive forces of the uterus (power); the position, size, or presentation of the fetus (passenger); and the maternal pelvis or soft tissues (passage). A leading cause of operative vaginal and cesarean delivery and any accompanying complications has been attributed to labor dystocia (ACOG, 2003). Any combination of these factors may result in mechanical interferences with the passage of the fetus through the birth canal. The International Classification of Diseases (ICD) coding for labor dystocia includes the diagnoses of failure to progress (FTP), arrest of dilation, arrest of descent, and CPD.

A lack of correspondence between the size of the maternal pelvis and the fetal head that results in arrest of fetal descent is termed dystocia secondary to CPD (Althaus et al., 2006). However, the clinical diagnosis of dystocia cannot be made until the completion of the latent phase of labor and the initiation of active labor (an increase rate of cervical dilatation and descent of fetus), to include an adequate trial of labor. Clinical diagnosis of dystocia as defined by ACOG's 2003 Practice Bulletin includes the protraction (slower than normal) or arrest (complete cessation of progress) of labor over time (Ressel, 2004). This definition allows for a less restrictive consideration for diagnosis. Many maternal and fetal characteristics may play a role in labor dystocia (see Box 39.4). Other factors labeled as *potentially contributing* to a diagnosis of labor dystocia include hospital admission before active labor has been established (< 5–6 cm dilated), induction of labor, use of epidural analgesia, and lack of labor support (King & Pinger, 2014; Lowe, 2007).

For a diagnosis of labor dystocia, the provider should assess and document:

■ Frequency of contractions if less than three contractions per 10 minutes
■ Quantification of uterine activity less than 25 mmHg above baseline using an intrauterine pressure catheter
■ Four hours of contraction patterns less than 200 MVUs resulting in insignificant cervical change

---

BOX 39.4   FACTORS CONTRIBUTING TO LABOR DYSTOCIA

Maternal Factors

Nulliparous women
Age older than 35 years
Height less than 5 feet
Pregnancy weight gain more than 35 lbs
Emotional distress and fear

Fetal Factors

Fetal weight more than 4,000 g
Occipitoposterior position
Breech presentation
Infection/sepsis
Fetal station above zero with active labor

Data from Lowe (2007).

Additionally, assessment of maternal cervix, pelvis, fetal position, station, and well-being should be performed before labor augmentation. Failed augmentation is the inability to achieve cervical dilatation of 4 cm and 90% effacement or at least 5 cm (regardless of effacement) after a minimum of 12 to 18 hours of membrane rupture and oxytocin administration (Lin & Rouse, 2006).

HYPOTONIC LABOR

Dysfunctional labor can be the result of abnormal uterine activity. This can be categorized as hypotonic or hypertonic labor. Hypotonic labor is present when contractions are occurring with normal frequency, but the peak pressure is too low to achieve cervical dilation or descent of the fetus. Although effective contractions can vary in strength from woman to woman, MVUs less than 200 is generally the considered criterion for a diagnosis of hypotonic labor. This type of labor dysfunction usually occurs during the active phase of labor when contractions have been previously established, but then diminish in frequency and strength.

Management • Interventions that can be used for hypotonic labor include rest, ambulation, artificial rupture of membranes, and if no improvement is evident in 1 to 2 hours, labor augmentation with oxytocin.

HYPERTONIC LABOR

Hypertonic labor is characterized by either a high uterine resting tone or by frequent, uncoordinated contractions. This is sometimes referred to as uterine irritability. The contractions will often be perceived by the laboring woman as very strong, yet will not cause dilation of the cervix. It is important to rule out placental abruption and chorioamnionitis when this type of labor pattern is encountered as this irritability can be a direct result of these issues. Hypertonic labor typically occurs during the latent phase of labor and can be associated with precipitous labor.

Management • This dysfunctional labor pattern can be managed with oxytocin administration in an attempt to establish a more regular, adequate contraction pattern. In contrast to this intervention, analgesia and/or sedation may be used in an effort to cause relaxation of the uterus and then subsequently a new trial of labor can be initiated.

PRECIPITOUS LABOR

Precipitous labor is defined as labor that progresses from start to delivery of an infant in less than 3 hours. Precipitous labor should not be confused with precipitous delivery, which can occur after a labor of any length, and can occur in or out of the hospital or birth center, when a trained assistant is not present for the delivery. Complications that can occur as a result of precipitous labor and delivery include uterine rupture, cervical lacerations, severe perineal lacerations, and hematomas of the vagina or vulva.

MALPRESENTATION/MALPOSITION

The most common fetal presentation is the vertex of the fetal head. Malpresentations are all presentations of the fetus, other than vertex, and can include complete breech, frank breech, footling or double footling breech, or transverse lie. Although complete or frank breech presentations can sometimes be delivered vaginally, it is up to the discretion of the health care provider who will take into consideration pelvimetry, absence of macrosomia, and a flexed fetal head.

By contrast, fetal malpositions are abnormal presentations of the vertex fetal head (in reference to the occiput) relative to the maternal pelvis. This includes most commonly the occiput posterior (OP) position. Spontaneous rotation of the fetal head occurs in approximately 90% of cases during the labor process (Simkin, Ancheta, & Myers, 2005). If this rotation does not occur, arrested labor can result as the head does not rotate and descend further into the pelvis. Furthermore, delivery in these cases may be complicated by perineal tears or extension of an episiotomy. Other malpositions that must be addressed are brow presentation, face presentation, chin anterior or posterior presentation, and compound presentation. Each of these presentations are managed differently depending on the individual circumstances (Simkin et al., 2005).

Management • One of the most commonly used interventions to encourage the rotation of the fetus from the OP position is to help the laboring woman get into an open knee–chest position, with her head resting on the bed and her hips flexed to greater than 90°. This position tilts the pelvis forward with the inlet lower than the outlet. This allows gravity to encourage the unengaged fetal head to move out of the pelvis and to reposition more favorably toward the occiput anterior position (Simkin et al., 2005).

The knee–chest position may also offer relief to women who are experiencing back labor secondary to laboring with a fetus in the OP position.

BREECH PRESENTATION

Planned cesarean section has been shown to be the safest form of delivery for an infant in a persistent breech presentation. However, cesarean sections are not without risk for mother and baby. Decision aids such as booklets or audio-CDs have been found to be an effective, useful, and acceptable adjunct to standard counseling about management options for breech presentation (Nassar, Roberts, Raynes-Greenow, Barratt, & Peat, 2007; Tiran, 2004). During the last weeks of prenatal visits, when breech presentation is persistent, this information has been shown to be effective in helping a pregnant woman make an informed decision regarding her delivery options (Tiran, 2004).

Management • Research findings reflect that pregnant women who reviewed decision aids reported feeling significantly more informed and experienced less uncertainty (Nassar et al., 2007). If the pregnant woman wishes to avoid cesarean section when the fetus is in breech, there are several nonsurgical options that may be useful. An external cephalic version can be attempted to turn the fetus to a vertex position so vaginal delivery can be attempted. This is generally done with the aid of ultrasound and tocolytics in order to relax the uterine smooth muscle so the fetus can be manipulated by placing manual pressure on the abdomen to guide the fetus into a vertex position. In addition to this method, there are various alternative techniques that can be used to encourage breech fetuses to spontaneously turn to a vertex position. These methods include pelvic tilt, light, music, the Webster technique, moxibustion, acupressure, homeopathics such as *Pulsatilla*, and herbs such as Bach's Bougainvillea Essence (Tiran, 2004).

Twin Gestation

In the United States, twin (and multiples) gestation has increased in part due to assisted reproductive technology. Although the incidence of twinning has increased, risks associated with twin pregnancy (including during labor and birth) remain greater than with a singleton pregnancy.

RISK FACTORS

A significant risk seen with a multiple pregnancy is preterm birth. The average duration of pregnancy in twins is 35.3 weeks. The choice of augmentation, induction, vaginal delivery, or cesarean section is influenced heavily by ultrasonographic confirmation of fetal position and size—ideally on the day of delivery.

ASSESSMENT

In almost 50% of twin pregnancies, both infants are vertex. Most experts agree that in an otherwise uncomplicated twin pregnancy, a trial of labor and vaginal delivery in vertex/

vertex twins is not contraindicated. Twin pregnancies in which the presenting twin is not vertex (approximately 20% of twin gestations) are considered safer if delivered by cesarean. It is important to note that consensus regarding mode of delivery for the 30% of twin deliveries that are vertex/breech presentation has not been agreed on by experts (Cruikshank, 2007).

MANAGEMENT

ACOG makes no recommendation regarding the route of delivery of twins, suggesting that delivery be determined by position, ease of FHR monitoring, and maternal and fetal size. Ultimately, more than 60% of all twin births have been delivered by cesarean (Gherman et al., 2006). Due to uterine overdistension and increased incidence of anemia in twin gestations, there is a greater risk for atony and PPH (Cruikshank, 2007). High-dose, IV oxytocin infusion should be considered, as well as methylergonovine and prostaglandin analogues (such as hemabate and misoprostol), and should be readily available for administration in cases of continuous, immediate postpartum bleeding.

Shoulder Dystocia

Shoulder dystocia, a component of labor dystocia, can have serious consequences and cause major concern and even fear among health care providers. The incidence of shoulder dystocia is frequently unpredictable and has been linked with PPH and neonatal death (Gherman et al., 2006). Shoulder dystocia occurs infrequently and represents a size discrepancy between the fetal shoulders and the pelvic inlet, resulting in the failure of delivery of the fetal shoulder (usually the anterior shoulder). The risk for shoulder dystocia increases when truncal rotation does not occur.

RISK FACTORS

Shoulder dystocia is largely unpredictable with about half occurring in fetuses of average gestational size. There are associated factors, the most prominent of which is higher birth weight. Fetal weight greater than 5,000 g in pregnant women without diabetes and greater than 4,500 g in pregnant women with diabetes is a common denominator connecting maternal and fetal risk for shoulder dystocia (Athukorala, Crowther, & Willson, 2007). Infants of diabetic mothers experience shoulder dystocia at an increased rate over nondiabetic women because of the distribution of the fetal weight. Higher birth weight (fetal macrosomia and large for gestational age) is common among infants of diabetic mothers. Women with gestational diabetes are classified as at risk for shoulder dystocia, operative vaginal delivery, and fetal macrosomia (Athukorala et al., 2007).

MANAGEMENT

Up to 42% of shoulder dystocia is reported to be correctable using the McRoberts maneuver as an initial step for the disimpaction of the shoulder during a vaginal delivery. This maneuver is performed by sharply flexing the maternal thighs onto the abdomen. It results in a straightening of the maternal sacrum relative to the lumbar spine, consequently increasing the mean angle of inclination between the symphysis pubis and sacral promontory (Gherman et al., 2006).

Calling for pediatric support is important during shoulder dystocia, an emergency in which fetal hypoxia-acidosis is common (Crofts et al., 2006; Kovavisarach, 2006). Although shoulder dystocia is not a soft tissue issue, an episiotomy may allow the fetal rotational maneuvers to be performed and create more room for attempted delivery of the posterior arm. Suprapubic pressure is usually given before or with the McRoberts maneuver. Pressure is directed posterior in an attempt to force the anterior shoulder under the symphysis pubis. Other maneuvers include:

- Woods' corkscrew: Abduct the posterior shoulder by exerting pressure onto the anterior surfaces of the posterior shoulder.
- Rubin's maneuver: Pressure is applied to the posterior surface of the most accessible part of the fetal shoulder to effect shoulder adduction.
- All fours maneuver (also known as the Gaskin maneuver): Have the woman roll from her existing position onto her hands and knees. The downward force of gravity or favorable change in pelvic diameters produced by this technique may allow disimpaction of the fetal shoulder (Kovavisarach, 2006).
- To deliver the posterior fetal arm, pressures should be applied at the antecubital fossa in order to flex the fetal forearm. The arm is subsequently swept out over the infant's chest and delivered over the perineum. Rotation of the fetal trunk to bring the posterior arm anterior is sometimes required. Grasping and pulling directly on the fetal arm, as well as application of pressure onto the mid-humeral shaft, should be avoided because bone fracture may occur.
- The Zavanelli maneuver is reserved when all attempts at correction of the shoulder dystocia have failed. The goal of the maneuver is to replace the fetus into the pelvis, relieving the impaction while preparing for cesarean delivery. This maneuver is accomplished by the reversal of the cardinal movements of labor with manual replacement of the fetal vertex into the vagina. There are significant maternal and neonatal complications inherent in this procedure.
- Fundal pressure is not a maneuver believed to alleviate shoulder dystocia and is discouraged as practice in the United States. This technique has been associated with an increased risk of Erb's palsy and thoracic spinal cord injury in the neonate. Fundal pressure may further impact the anterior shoulder behind the symphysis pubis (Gherman et al., 2006).

A contemporary approach to preparing personnel for a shoulder dystocia is simulation training. As with cardiopulmonary resuscitation, shoulder dystocia simulation drills provide repeated practice and acquisition of the aforementioned techniques improving clinical performance of these maneuvers and reducing the incidence of medical negligence (Maslovitz, Barkai, Lessing, Ziv, & Many, 2007).

ACOG recommends a cesarean delivery be considered for an estimated birth weight of greater than 5,000 g, as a prevention to avoid shoulder dystocia. The decision to perform a cesarean delivery for labor dystocia should be made based on clinical assessment of the woman, the fetus, and the skills of a trained obstetrician (ACOG, 2003; Crofts et al., 2006).

Nuchal Cord

Nuchal cord, a common fetal complication, can be associated with an increased risk of variable decelerations, acidemia, meconium-stained amniotic fluid, and emergency cesarean section. The degree of tightness of the umbilical cord around the fetal neck has been found to correlate to the degree of fetal distress. A moderately tight cord around the fetal neck may impair cephalic venous blood flow and a very tight nuchal cord may compromise the umbilical circulation and produce systemic hypoxia, hypercapnia, acidemia, and ultimately fetal death.

Meconium-stained amniotic fluid is another common occurrence seen in infants with nuchal cord. Meconium passed by the fetus in labor is often interpreted as a sign of fetal distress or compromise. The risk of fetal compromise is greater when meconium accompanies a nuchal cord. Conversely, the presence of clear amniotic fluid can be an unreliable sign of fetal well-being (Greenwood et al., 2003).

■ CONSIDERATIONS FOR SPECIAL POPULATIONS

Teen Intrapartum Care

Young maternal age carries with it much pregnancy risk. Being a pregnant young teen has been linked to low birth weight, preterm labor, fetal growth restriction, and infant mortality (Wilson, Alio, Kirby, & Salihu, 2008). Pregnant teens have a higher prevalence of anemia, eclampsia, and preeclampsia than pregnant women between the ages of 20 and 34 years. The risk of intrapartum stillbirth among teens less than 15 years of age has also been found to be about three times that of older adolescents (Wilson et al., 2008). Therefore, intrapartum fetal surveillance and supportive labor care are important contributions to a positive labor and delivery outcome for the younger teen.

Regardless of the outcome of the pregnancy, teens are at greater risk for repeat pregnancies and sexually transmitted infections than their older counterparts. Safer sex and reproductive education should be a priority with teens during the immediate postpartum period and before discharge from a health care facility. Parenting skills and support system should be assessed and referrals made when necessary.

Pregnant Athletes

Most professional athletes continue to work out during their pregnancy. Current data show that athletic women are likely to have term, average-sized infants and may even have an enhanced labor and delivery experience due to their physical fitness (Duncombe et al., 2006). Due to their rigorous regimen and their focus on a healthy lifestyle, these women may prefer CAM methods of managing labor pain. Many times, these women seek medical advice to identify any potential risk to themselves or their unborn fetus in reference to continued vigorous exercise during pregnancy and any potential effects at delivery. The ACOG (2015) committee opinion on exercise during pregnancy and during the postpartum periods recommends that the average woman can perform moderate exercise for 30 minutes a day, 7 days a week, and that recreational and competitive athletes can remain active during pregnancy but should modify their usual exercise routines as indicated by their health care provider. Women should be instructed not to initiate a vigorous exercise program during the first trimester of pregnancy and limit themselves to moderate exercise a few times a week with medical supervision (Duncombe et al., 2006).

Summary

The health care provider's knowledge of antenatal, intrapartum, and postpartum physiology is essential in managing the care of a woman and her unborn child. Health care providers who manage labor are concerned with two patients and the safety of both during the course of labor and delivery. Recognizing aberrancies in the normal physiology and pathophysiology of labor and birth and developing an alternative plan of care is critical to ensure the safety and well-being of the laboring woman and her neonate.

■ POSTPARTUM CARE

The postpartum period begins immediately at birth and extends for up to 12 weeks. This period is a time of taking in and great change. What is more, it is also a time of great vulnerability: the mother's health and recovery; the need to acquaint herself with her infant's needs; if she elects, the need to establish lactation; figuring out where the husband or partner fit in; and the list goes on. Health care providers play an integral role in supporting the newly delivered mom and her family to take in all of these changes, which impact the family from delivery and beyond.

During the postpartum period, which is also known as the puerperium, women and their families adapt physically, psychologically, and socially to the changes that have taken place following birth. Commonly, this transition is defined as lasting from 6 to 12 weeks, and it is described as a return to the normal, nonpregnant state (Gabbe, Niebyl, & Simpson, 2007). However, the implication that all will be as it once was is misleading. In immeasurable ways, the new mother and those around her are forever changed.

The postpartum period begins after the delivery of the placenta, with the first hour being referred to as the fourth stage of labor. Although seemingly anticlimactic, it is a crucial juncture calling for vigilance on the part of caregivers. During this first hour, the new mother and her infant are monitored closely for a number of physiologic risks, including maternal PPH or respiratory distress in the newborn. During this time, caregivers need to address the mother's comfort needs in addition to assisting her and her family with bonding with the newborn.

The first 24 hours after birth is referred to as the immediate postpartum period, whereas the second day through the first week is called the early postpartum period. The term late postpartum period refers to the second through sixth weeks. Although some sources claim that these designations are arbitrary, it is worth noting that a number of disparate cultures practice postpartum rituals that entail 40-day periods of seclusion for new mothers and babies (Hundt et al., 2000; Kim-Godwin, 2000) (see Box 39.5).

Social upheavals of the late 19th and 20th centuries profoundly changed family life, including women's experiences of birth and child rearing. The feminist movement, the evolution of family structure, and women's roles have coincided with changes to the health care system as a result of managed care, thus bringing about major shifts in the delivery of maternal child health care. Shortened length of hospital stay, the changed configuration of care for mothers and babies during and after birth, legislation related to breastfeeding in the workplace, welfare reform, and shifting immigration patterns are examples of social and political issues that significantly impact maternal child health outcomes. Health care providers need to be aware of these issues to plan and implement effective maternity care.

Physical Changes of the Postpartum Period

BREASTS

By the end of pregnancy, each breast has gained nearly 1 pound in weight as a result of increased fat, myoepithelial cells, connective tissue, electrolytes, water retention, and the hypertrophy of blood vessels. Blood flow to the breasts has nearly doubled, which is necessary to perfuse the enlarged, lobular structures of the alveolar milk ducts. Colostrum may be secreted at varying times during pregnancy up until the first 2 to 3 days postpartum, and this is followed by

transitional and then full milk. Before mature milk comes in, the growth of blood vessels, lymphatics, alveoli, and the further enlargement of the lobules may cause a painful hardening of the breasts known as engorgement. This condition is less likely to occur if the mother is able to breastfeed early and often. The transition to mature milk may be accompanied by low-grade fever; however, significant temperature elevation (e.g., greater than 38°C or 100.4°F) warrants further assessment to identify symptoms (e.g., erythema of one breast, systemic myalgias) that may suggest mastitis (Berens, 2009).

After the delivery of the placenta, the hormones estrogen and progesterone diminish, while prolactin is secreted by the anterior pituitary gland; this in turn stimulates the breasts to secrete colostrum. In response to the stimulus of the infant's suckling, the mother's posterior pituitary gland secretes oxytocin, which stimulates the contractile tissue around the milk ducts and the alveoli, a process known as the letdown reflex. Oxytocin also continues to stimulate uterine contractions preventing PPH (Lee, 2007). Thus, breastfeeding serves an important physiologic function for the mother as well as the baby, particularly during the period immediately following delivery.

UTERUS

Immediately after delivery, the uterus decreases to about half of the size that it was before labor (e.g., the size that it was at ~20 weeks gestation) and weighs about 2 pounds. The uterine fundus is palpable at or just below the level of the umbilicus, although the exact location may vary with factors such as the woman's habitus and the baby's size. For each postpartum day after delivery, the fundus normally descends approximately one fingerbreadth below the umbilicus. By the end of the first week, the uterus reduces in size to a weight of approximately 1 pound. The fundus is palpable just above the pubic symphysis, which is approximately the size that it was at 12 weeks' gestation. The fundus is usually not palpable after 10 days postpartum.

Strong coordinated contractions of the uterus are necessary for involution to occur. The primiparous uterus tends to remain contracted, whereas multiparous experience contractions at intervals; these cause *after pains*, which tend to escalate in severity with higher parity and which are stimulated by breastfeeding. After pains may last for 2 to 3 days, and they can be relieved with the application of heat to the lower abdomen. Nonsteroidal anti-inflammatory drugs (NSAIDs) may be taken safely if necessary, or narcotic analgesics may be given in the event of cesarean section delivery.

The sudden decompression and diminished size of the uterus after the baby's birth causes the placenta to shear off and deliver. When this occurs, the uterine muscle, the placental site, and the adjacent arterial muscle walls all contract vigorously to ensure hemostasis and to prevent hemorrhage.

CERVIX

Pregnancy- and birth-induced changes to the cervix, including hypervascularity, any lacerations that may have occurred during the birth, and ecchymosis, have normally resolved by 6 weeks, while edema and hyperplasia of the

---

BOX 39.5   CULTURES THAT PRACTICE 40 DAYS OF POSTPARTUM SECLUSION

Non-Western cultures in which the 40th day has cultural significance include the following:

  Palestinian Bedouin
  Jordanian
  Lebanese
  Egyptian
  Ancient Hebraic (according to Leviticus 12)
  Indian
  Mexican American

Data from Hundt et al. (2000); Kim-Godwin (2003).

cervical glands may last for up to 3 months. Because small amounts of lateral tearing to the cervix commonly occur during delivery, at the completion of involution the parous cervical os is changed appearing as a horizontal slit rather than the characteristically small, round opening of the nulliparous cervical os.

Profound changes also take place within the cervix at the cellular level. Ahdoot et al. (1998) found that 50% of women diagnosed with high-grade cervical dysplasia prenatally had markedly improved condition after vaginal delivery. Although these findings have been replicated by some investigators (Strinić, Buković, Karelović, Bojić, & Stipić, 2002), others have failed to find a significant association between pregnancy and improved cervical cytology (Kaneshiro, Acoba, Holzman, Wachi, & Carney, 2005).

LOCHIA

The vaginal discharge following birth, which is called lochia rubra, contains blood and epithelial cells as well as the superficial layer of the deciduas (e.g., the lining of the uterus). This red, menses-like flow diminishes in quantity after several hours and lasts for 2 to 3 days. As the blood diminishes in proportion to the serous component, the discharge becomes reddish brown and is called lochia serosa; this continues for 3 to 6 weeks. Normally the woman needs to change her pad two to three times per day during this stage. From the tenth day on, the discharge may become yellowish white in color as a result of an increase in leukocytes; at this point it is called lochia alba. Meanwhile, between the 10th day and the 8th week, a new endometrial lining is generated from the decidua basalis (e.g., the deep layer of the uterine lining).

PLACENTAL INVOLUTION

As the process of uterine involution progresses, the placental site undergoes its own involution process. As the outer layer of the decidua is shed with the lochia, the surrounding margins draw downward and the endometrium is regenerated from the decidua basalis underneath. This process is normally complete by the sixth week postpartum.

VAGINA AND PERINEUM

The distended vaginal wall, which has been stretched and smoothed out during the birth process, returns to its rugated and contracted state by the third week postpartum, although it does not go back to its previous size. The extent to which the voluntary muscles of the pelvic floor regain their tone will depend on a variety of factors: parity, nutritional status, the size of the baby, the type of delivery, and the degree to which the mother has exercised her pelvic floor muscles (e.g., performed Kegel exercises). Changes to the appearance of the vaginal introitus result from tears of the hymenal tags that occur during delivery; these form remnants known as carunculae myrtiformes.

Severe stretching or laceration of the vagina or perineum can lead to relaxation and decreased pelvic support, the prolapse of the pelvic organs, and, eventually, problems with incontinence. The management of the perineum at the time of delivery has consequences for the integrity of the pelvic floor musculature postpartum. In the past, prophylactic episiotomy has been widely believed to preserve pelvic muscle function and to prevent perineal laceration. However, episiotomy has actually been found to be associated with more perineal pain, trauma, and long-term complications, and is no longer common practice (Hartmann et al., 2005). A comparative study of women who had episiotomies, women with an intact perineum, women with first-degree lacerations, and women with second- and third-degree lacerations after delivery, found that those in the episiotomy group had the poorest perineal muscle endurance postpartum, and they were also the only group whose muscle endurance decreased postpartum from what it had been antepartally (Fleming, Newton, & Roberts, 2003). Antenatal perineal massage performed one to two times per week beginning at 35 weeks' gestation is an evidence-based intervention that has been demonstrated to prevent birth-related trauma to the perineum, including episiotomy (Beckmann & Garrett, 2006).

Assessment • The thorough assessment of the perineum can be ensured by using the acronym REEDA, which will help the clinician to remember to look for redness, ecchymosis, edema, discharge, and wound approximation. This systematic assessment will reveal problems such as infection, hematoma, dehiscence of repair, excessive bleeding, and hemorrhage (Kindberg, Stehouwer, Hvidman, & Henrikson, 2008).

Management • Management includes the application of ice packs for 20-minute periods for the initial 24 hours. Thereafter, either warm or cold sitz baths may be recommended. A randomized trial demonstrated no difference in REEDA score with the use of heat or cold on the perineum during the first 24 hours postpartum (Hill, 2006). However, cold sitz baths are more effective in reducing edema and hematoma formation and provide more effective pain relief by causing local vasoconstriction and decreasing nerve conduction and muscle spasm (Gabbe et al., 2007; Ramler & Roberts, 1986). Nevertheless, cold treatments may not be acceptable in some cultures that hold the belief that the loss of blood during birth creates a cold state in the body, which would necessitate the provision of warmth to the postpartum woman. Belief in the need to balance hot and cold in the body, which is known as the humoral theory, is prevalent in Asia, Africa, Latin America, and the Middle East (Kim-Goodwin, 2003).

Pharmacotherapeutics • Ibuprofen is effective orally or rectally, and it is safe during lactation. A Cochrane Review of rectal analgesia for pain from perineal trauma after delivery points out that 50% of the medication bypasses the liver and thus results in faster and more effective pain relief than oral medication. This meta-analysis identified rectal analgesia with NSAIDs as an effective means of analgesia postpartum (Hedayati, Parsons, & Crowther, 2003). In the event of a fourth-degree laceration necessitating repair of the rectal sphincter, suppositories are not given. Oral NSAIDs are appropriate and stool softeners and avoidance of constipation or straining of any kind is important.

HORMONES

Ovarian Function • Ovarian function is suppressed in lactating women and it typically returns around 6 months postpartum. Estrogen and progesterone levels are diminished, while prolactin levels rise in response to the stimulus of breastfeeding, thus increasing the secretion of milk. Therefore, giving supplemental bottles may sabotage the breastfeeding effort, because this reduces the prolactin secretion needed to ensure an adequate milk supply. Thus, the reason for giving up on breastfeeding (e.g., "I don't have enough milk") becomes a self-fulfilling prophecy if caregivers or well-meaning family members attempt to help the breastfeeding mother rest during the initial postpartum days by giving her baby a bottle.

The postpartum suppression of ovulation is determined to a large extent by the frequency and duration of breastfeeding and whether there is exclusive breastfeeding or supplementary feeding with formula, which diminishes the amenorrheic properties of lactation (Kennedy & Visness, 1992). Maternal nutritional status has also been shown to significantly affect the resumption of ovulation postpartum. Women with a lower body mass index (BMI) have been shown to consistently remain amenorrheic longer after birth, regardless of breastfeeding behavior, child nutritional status, and child age, suggesting that maternal nutritional status has an effect that is independent of breastfeeding behavior (Peng, Hight-Laukaran, Peterson, & Perez-Escamilla, 1998).

The hypoestrogenic state of the puerperium is extended in lactating women. The elevation in prolactin leads to a decreased libido and the thinning and dryness of the vaginal mucosa; this, in addition to healing vaginal and perineal trauma, may contribute to frequent complaints of dyspareunia and sexual dysfunction postpartum (Henderson & MacDonald, 2004).

POSTPARTUM THYROIDITIS

The thyroid gland, which increases in size and function during pregnancy, returns to its normal size by 12 weeks postpartum. Thyroid hormones normally return to prepregnant levels by 4 weeks postpartum. Postpartum hypothyroidism is a relatively common condition that is also known as postpartum thyroiditis or postpartum thyroid dysfunction (PPTD), and may or may not be associated with autoimmune antibodies. It is estimated to occur in 7% to 11.3% of women during the first year after childbirth, and it involves symptoms of fatigue, depression, palpitations, and irritability (Abalovich et al., 2007; Golden, Robinson, & Saldanha, 2009). Serum thyroid-stimulating hormone with antithyroid peroxidase antibodies are checked in women with these symptoms postpartum. Risk factors for PPTD include type 1 diabetes, previous thyroid problems, and a family history of thyroid disease or autoimmune disease. About 30% of these women go on to develop hypothyroidism (Mestman, 2002).

MUSCULOSKELETAL AND DERMATOLOGIC CHANGES

Striae Gravidarum • The distention of the pregnant abdomen causes the rupture of the elastic fibers in the skin and stretches the broad and round ligaments. These anatomic changes may result in a soft and flaccid abdomen and striae gravidarum, which are purple or dark-brown lines (depending on the woman's skin color) that may appear on the abdomen, breasts, and buttocks. These will eventually fade; however, they will not disappear completely. Two herbal creams have been shown to have some beneficial effect in minimizing striae. One cream contained the active ingredients vitamin E, essential fatty acids, panthenol, hyaluronic acid, elastin, and menthol. The second cream contained tocopherol, collagen-elastin hydrolysates, and centella asiatica. The active ingredients in both creams can be difficult to obtain (Young & Jewell, 1996). Although a Cochrane Review reported no adverse effects from these interventions, other researchers have noted that no studies have addressed the safety of these herbs or the many others that are commonly used during pregnancy (Ernst, 2002; Tunzi & Gray, 2007).

Diastasis Recti • The separation of the abdominal muscles may persist following delivery, which results in a condition called diastasis recti. This can be described by the number of fingerbreadths that the health care provider can fit between the abdominal muscles as the supine woman reaches her arms forward and lifts her head, neck, and shoulders; this number diminishes over time as the muscles come back together. Recovery is helped with the use of abdomen-strengthening exercises, such as leg lifts and curl-ups, which may begin as soon as the woman is able to after 6 weeks postpartum.

HAIR

During pregnancy, scalp hair generally thickens as a result of a decrease in the progression of hair growth from the anagen phase (e.g., the "growing" stage) to the telogen phase (e.g., the "resting" stage; Elling & Powell, 1997; Wong, 1996). This telogen phase persists during 1 to 5 months postpartum. During the postpartum period, the loss of scalp hair beyond this 1- to 5-month period is fairly common and is called telogen effluvium. Telogen effluvium usually ends within 15 months postpartum; however, the scalp hair may never regain its prepregnancy thickness (Winton & Lewis, 1982).

BONE DENSITY

Following delivery and lactation there is a temporary decrease in bone mineralization (Karlsson, Ahlborg, & Karlsson, 2005). Lactating women require the additional intake of calcium, although calcium needs are met with the reabsorption of maternal skeletal calcium and a decrease in the excretion of calcium by the kidneys. Lactating women are likely to experience a decrease in bone density, losing as much as 7% of their bone mass by 9 months of continued breastfeeding (Laskey & Prentice, 1999). However, this demineralization is reversible after weaning has occurred (Karlsson et al., 2005).

WEIGHT LOSS

With delivery comes the much-anticipated shedding of pounds as a result of the birth of the baby and the placenta and also because of amniotic fluid and blood loss, normally resulting in a loss of 10 to 13 pounds at the time of birth (Gabbe et al., 2007). Further diuresis normally accounts for an additional 4 to 7 pounds lost during the first week postpartum. Although 28% of women return to their prepregnant weight by 6 weeks postpartum, most remain about 3 pounds heavier than before pregnancy, and have increased waist-to-hip ratios. Multiparous women tend to retain more weight than primiparous women. Women who gain more than 35 pounds during their pregnancy remain an average 11 pounds heavier than their prepregnant weight (Gabbe et al., 2007).

CARDIOVASCULAR SYSTEM

There is increased risk of venous thromboembolism (VTE) during pregnancy as well as during the postpartum period. The three conditions that predispose women to VTE are referred to as Virchow's triad. They include increased occurrence of vascular endothelial injury, a hypercoagulable state, and venous stasis (Burrows, Meyn, & Weber, 2004; Greer, 1999). VTE occurs twice as frequently during the postpartum period as it does during pregnancy (Nisenblat et al., 2006; Simpson, Lawrence, Nightingale, & Farmer, 2003). There is vascular injury at the placental site during labor, delivery, and the postpartum period that contributes to vascular endothelial injury. Throughout pregnancy, there is a progressive increase in clotting factors I, II, VII, VIII, IX, and X; this, in combination with an increased number of fibrinogen and platelets and a decrease in fibrinolytic activity and free protein S, contribute to the hypercoagulable state of pregnancy that persists during the postpartum period (Beck, Froman, & Bernal, 2005; Marik & Plante, 2008). Women with inherited thrombophilic disorders, such as factor V Leiden and prothrombin gene mutations, may be at increased risk for VTE during pregnancy (Gerhardt et al., 2000; Tsu, 2004). Pulmonary embolism (PE) is more likely to occur during the postpartum period than the antepartum period, although deep vein thrombosis (DVT) occurs more frequently during the antepartum period (Ahmed, Jayawarna, & Jude, 2006; Beck et al., 2005; Heit et al., 2005). Another population-based study found that the VTE event of DVT in the postpartum population occurred four times more frequently than in the antenatal population (Greer, 1999). The incident of VTE was increased fourfold among women who delivered via cesarean section as compared with women who delivered vaginally.

Although the plasma volume increases by about 1,200 mL by the third trimester, it diminishes by about 1,000 mL as a result of blood loss immediately after delivery. By the third day postpartum, it has again increased by 900 to 1,200 mL as a result of the shift of extracellular fluid into the vascular space. Normally, a rise in systolic and diastolic blood pressure of about 5% occurs during the first 4 days postpartum (Henderson & MacDonald, 2004). After delivery, there is a sudden increase in venous return, because the newly emptied uterus no longer impedes blood flow from the extremities. This results in an abrupt rise in cardiac output, which causes bradycardia. Cardiac output returns to its prelabor value 1 hour after delivery and to its prepregnancy levels between 2 and 4 weeks after delivery (Gabbe et al., 2007).

KIDNEYS AND URINARY TRACT

The normal pregnancy-induced increase in renal plasma flow begins to fall during the third trimester; however, it takes 1 to 2 years to return to prepregnancy levels. Both the increased glomerular filtration rate (GFR) and the consequent rise in creatinine clearance rates that occur during pregnancy return to normal by 8 weeks postpartum. In response, blood urea nitrogen (BUN) also resumes its prepregnant level by 1-week postpartum (Gabbe et al., 2007). Urinary tract infection (UTI), is discussed further in the UTI and Pyelonephritis section.

METABOLISM, FLUIDS, AND ELECTROLYTES

In addition to the substantial blood and fluid loss that are sustained during labor and delivery, an additional 3.5 L of fluid are lost during the first 6 weeks postpartum. Although the total amount of sodium diminishes, its serum concentration increases as the loss of fluid surpasses it, and plasma potassium also rises. This results in a net increase of serum cations and anions and thus an increased plasma osmolality and a decreased serum chloride level as the serum bicarbonate level increases.

By the second postpartum day, fatty acids return to their normal concentration in the blood, whereas cholesterol and triglycerides take 6 to 7 weeks to return to their prepregnant levels. Both fasting and postprandial blood glucose levels decline after birth, dropping to their lowest levels on the second and third days postpartum and then increasing back up to prepregnant levels. This has important implications for the interpretation of blood sugar tests and insulin requirements during the first week postpartum.

Postpartum Complications

The incidence of postpartum complications is related to the mode of delivery: there are fewer complications associated with vaginal birth than with cesarean section delivery (Burrows et al., 2004). Cesarean section delivery is associated with an increased risk for infection, hemorrhage, VTE, anesthetic complications, and a longer and more painful recovery (Greer, 1999; Liu et al., 2007). After cesarean section delivery, maternal and neonatal complications exist for future pregnancies as well (Beck et al., 2005; Galyean, Lagrew, Bush, & Kurtzman, 2009).

ASSESSMENT AND MANAGEMENT AFTER CESAREAN SECTION

Postoperative care after cesarean section delivery is similar to that of other abdominal surgeries; however, it also encompasses the myriad needs that are common to all women who have just given birth (Hundt et al., 2000). For some women, a cesarean section delivery represents the loss of a hoped-for birth experience or even a personal failure as a woman. It is important to allow the mother to have time to talk about her birth experience soon afterward and then again several weeks postpartum.

Physical care is directed at detecting, preventing, and treating potential complications, which include hemorrhage, infection, thrombosis, pneumonia, and complications of anesthesia. Early ambulation and fluid intake may help to prevent some of the more common complications.

POSTDURAL PUNCTURE HEADACHE

Postdural puncture headaches, which are also known as spinal headaches, may occur after spinal anesthesia or after epidurals that have inadvertently become spinals. Spinal fluid leaks from the dural space through the puncture site and into the extradural space, which causes a headache that immediately improves when the woman is supine. An epidural blood patch with the woman's own blood is the most effective treatment; it provides immediate relief for most women (Ahmed et al., 2006; Reamy, 2009).

POSTPARTUM HEMORRHAGE

Excessive postpartum blood loss is the greatest cause of maternal mortality worldwide, responsible for up to 150,000 deaths per year. It is estimated that one woman dies every 4 minutes from postpartum hemorrhage (PPH), most often as a result of primary or early PPH, which occurs within the first 24 hours after birth (ACOG, 2006a). The estimation of postpartum blood loss is notoriously inaccurate and definitions of PPH vary. A commonly accepted definition is more than 500 mL during the first 24 hours after a vaginal birth and more than 1,000 mL after a cesarean section delivery. Perhaps a more useful definition that is based on less subjective data is excessive bleeding that makes the woman symptomatic or that results in signs of hypovolemia (Devine, 2009; Lowdermilk, Perry, & Bobak, 2000).

PPH occurs when there is a malfunction of one of the processes that control bleeding after birth, commonly called the "4 Ts": tone, tissue, trauma, and thrombin. The most common of these is tone, or uterine atony, which accounts for 75% to 85% of the cases of early PPH. Risks for atony include the over distention of the uterus caused by macrosomia, multiple gestation, fibroids, or polyhydramnios; uterine muscle fatigue caused by prolonged, rapid, or augmented labor; uterine infection; or a full bladder interfering with the ability of the uterine muscles to contract (Lowdermilk et al., 2000; Tsu, 2004). Tissue refers to retained fragments of placental tissue or membranes that may result in hemorrhage and may necessitate uterine exploration and removal of the retained tissue. Retained placenta occurs when there is abnormal placental adherence to the uterine wall, which occurs with placenta accreta and placenta percreta. These conditions are more likely to occur in pregnancies after cesarean section delivery as a result of the abnormal development of the placenta, which takes place over the site of the cesarean section scar. PPH caused by trauma is most commonly a result of genital tract laceration after a vaginal birth or the extension of a uterine incision during cesarean section delivery; infrequent causes include uterine rupture or inversion. The least frequent cause of hemorrhage is abnormalities of coagulation (e.g., thrombin), which may preexist or be acquired during pregnancy (see Box 39.6).

BOX 39.6   RISKS FOR AND ASSOCIATED FACTORS OF POSTPARTUM HEMORRHAGE

Uterine atony
Overdistended uterus
- Macrosomia
- Multiple gestation
- Polyhydramnios
- Fibroids
- Blood clots
- Prolonged labor
- Labor induction
Grand multiparity
Medications
- Magnesium sulfate
- Anesthesia
- Tocolytics
Pathology
- Pregnancy-induced hypertension
- Infection
- Prolonged rupture of membranes
- Internal monitoring
- Cesarean section delivery
Lacerations (perineal, cervical, or vaginal)
Macrosomia
Operative delivery (i.e., forceps, vacuum, or cesarean section delivery)
Precipitous delivery
Retained placenta
History of cesarean section delivery
- Abnormal adherence of placenta
- Placenta accreta
Placenta percreta
History of retained placenta
Hematoma (may have signs of shock without visible blood loss)
Traumatic delivery

Data from Dunn (2005) and Katz (2007).

Interventions to prevent or decrease the incidence of PPH have received international attention; the most effective of these is active management of the third stage of labor. Recommended by international obstetric and midwifery organizations, active management of the third stage consists of the administration of uterotonics immediately before or within 1 minute of the birth of the baby, controlled cord traction to deliver the placenta, and the massage of the uterine fundus immediately after the delivery of the placenta (Cunningham & Williams, 2005; Fahy, 2009). During the immediate postpartum period, attention is focused on detecting, preventing, and managing uterine atony. After delivery, the uterine fundus should be firm, midline, and approximately reaching the level of the umbilicus. As noted previously, it may be slightly higher or lower, depending on the size of the baby, the habitus of the mother, and the number of hours postpartum. The lochia should not be in excess of a normal menses; soaking through one or more large peri pads per hour is abnormal. If the fundus is deviated to the side or if the bladder itself is palpable, the woman is either helped to void or is catheterized. The uterus is then reassessed and the fundus firmly massaged while the uterus is stabilized with the other hand above the symphysis. Fundal massage usually causes the atonic uterus to contract, which results in a noticeable decrease in the amount of vaginal bleeding (Hofmeyr, Abdul-Aleem, & Abdul-Aleem, 2008; Mousa & Alfirevic, 2007). If bleeding continues after fundal massage, other sources of bleeding need to be considered. The perineum, vagina, and cervix are examined for lacerations. If no lacerations are found, retained fragments of placenta or membrane should be considered. Coagulation disorders are the least common cause, and most are known before the onset of labor (Anderson & Etches, 2007; Miller, Lester, & Hensleigh, 2004).

In cases of uterine atony, if active management of the third stage of labor has not been performed or if excessive bleeding persists after fundal massage, uterotonics are indicated. Oxytocin is the uterotonic of choice both for the active management of the third stage and as the first-line treatment of PPH. It can be given IV or IM, has a rapid onset of action, and has few side effects. It causes rhythmic uterine contractions, which constrict the spiral arteries in the myometrium, thereby decreasing blood flow. If excessive bleeding persists after oxytocin administration, additional medications are given. Methergine, which is an ergot alkaloid, is the usual second-line choice. It is given IM, which causes a sustained contraction of the uterine muscle; however, it is contraindicated in women with elevated blood pressure. If bleeding continues to be excessive, prostaglandins are given (Tsu, 2004). These uterotonics require skill for administration, and some also require refrigeration, which can present important limitations when caring for women in developing countries. Recently, there has been an effort to identify uterotonics that may be more appropriate for areas of the world in which access to skilled birth attendants capable of giving injections may be limited. Misoprostol is an inexpensive and stable prostaglandin analogue that is administered in tablet form. It may be given orally, rectally, or sublingually, and has been found to be effective for decreasing postpartum blood loss, although it has more side effects than the more commonly used uterotonics. Side effects that are commonly associated with prostaglandin use (e.g., fever, chills, nausea, vomiting, diarrhea, pain from uterine contractions) appear to be dose related (Blum, Alfirevic, Walraven, Weeks, & Winikoff, 2007; Geller, Adams, Kelly, Kodkany, & Derman, 2006; Hofmeyr et al., 2009; Vivio & Williams, 2004).

LATE PPH

Although most hemorrhages take place within the first 24 hours after birth (and most of these occur within the first 4 hours), "late" PPH can also occur. Late or secondary

PPH is defined as excessive bleeding that occurs more than 24 hours and up to 6 weeks postpartum; it most typically begins 1 to 2 weeks after delivery. Common causes are infection, retained products of conception, and subinvolution of the uterus, which occurs when there is a failure of the uterine muscle, the placental site, or the adjacent arterial muscle walls to contract adequately to ensure hemostasis. When assessing the quality and quantity of bleeding in women days or weeks after delivery, it is important to remember that a lesser yet steady amount of bleeding may appear deceptively insignificant relative to the more extensive bleeding that occurs at the time of birth; however, if this type of bleeding continues over time, it will result in significant blood loss. Diagnosis and management may include transvaginal ultrasound and curettage, if necessary; broad-spectrum antibiotics; and uterotonics (Dunn, 2005; Lausman, Ellis, Beecroft, Simons, & Shapiro, 2008).

LACERATIONS

If uterotonics and fundal massage successfully firm the uterus and bleeding still continues, the most likely cause is laceration of the vagina or cervix. A laceration of the perineum, peri urethra, or labia would likely be visualized and repaired by the health care provider at the time of delivery; however, a deep sulcus (vaginal) or cervical laceration may be missed. Identifying lacerations requires careful inspection with adequate visualization and pain control for the woman. This can be difficult if the laceration is deep and if the field is obscured by bleeding. It is crucial to summon expert help without delay, because severe blood loss can occur rapidly and is controllable only by the repair of the laceration with adequate anesthesia or analgesia.

HEMATOMA

On rare occasions, trauma to the soft tissue during delivery may cause lacerations to blood vessels in which significant invisible blood loss occurs and results in a hematoma. Most of these lacerations occur after an operative vaginal delivery with forceps or vacuum or after an episiotomy. The symptoms of hematoma of the vulva or, less commonly, of the vagina are pain, swelling, bruising, a palpable mass, and signs of shock (if blood loss is great enough). Vulvar hematomas will eventually become visible as they increase in size; however, vaginal hematomas may not be visible. If hemodynamically stable, the woman with a vulvar or vaginal hematoma may be followed with observation, ice packs, and analgesia for symptomatic relief, and a Foley catheter, if necessary. If hemodynamically unstable, the hematoma may need to be excised, drained, and packed with a drain left in, depending on the size of the hematoma. Retroperitoneal hematoma is a rare yet serious complication of cesarean section delivery that must be surgically repaired (Miller et al., 2004).

POSTPARTUM FEVER

The accepted definition of postpartum febrile morbidity is an oral temperature of 38°C (100.4°F) or more on any two of the first 10 days postpartum (exclusive of the first 24 hours). A temperature elevation of up to 38°C (100.4°F) during the first 24 hours after delivery or of up to 39°C (102.2°F) for 24 hours after the mother's milk comes in may be a normal finding. Maternal fever after the first 24 hours postpartum or fever that is unrelated to breast engorgement are most often the result of infection and require further evaluation to identify the source.

ENDOMETRITIS

Postpartum endometritis occurs after 1% to 3% of vaginal births and is up to 10 times more frequent after a cesarean birth. It is caused by the contamination of the uterine lining by vaginal organisms, which may include group A or B streptococci, *Chlamydia trachomatis*, *Neisseria gonorrhoeae*, *Mycoplasma hominis*, or *Ureaplasma urealyticum*, the prevalence of which vary depending on the population and the institution in which the delivery takes place. Postpartum endometritis may be a continuation of amnionitis that began during labor. A long labor, prolonged rupture of the membranes, multiple vaginal examinations, invasive monitoring, and forceps or vacuum extraction are all risks factors for this condition (Faro, 2005; French & Smaill, 2004).

In the past, puerperal fever was commonly spread by obstetricians and medical students who neglected to wash their hands between pelvic examinations or after handling cadavers. Ignaz Semmelweis, a 19th-century Hungarian physician, after studying the puerperal fever rate in two clinics, observed that in the clinic attended by midwives, as well as women who were unattended at birth, were more likely to survive and had lower rates of fevers than women who were delivered by doctors or medical students. Semmelweis deduced that hand washing by health care providers would improve the chances of a woman's survival. This discovery became the basis for infection control in all areas of health care. Even today, proper hand hygiene is emphasized as an important tool for the prevention of postpartum infection (French & Smaill, 2004; Maharaj & Teach, 2007).

The clinical diagnosis of postpartum endometritis is based on the presence of fever and uterine tenderness. Other signs include abdominal tenderness, foul-smelling lochia, and leukocytosis. Symptoms most frequently occur within 48 hours of delivery; a later onset of symptoms may present as a late PPH caused by the subinvolution of the uterus (Faro, 2005). A combination of gentamicin and clindamycin is the gold standard for the initial treatment of postpartum endometritis to cover the broad range of possible causative organisms. If this regimen is ineffective for resolving fever and other symptoms within 3 days, further workup is warranted to assess for the adequacy of antibiotic levels, the presence of resistant organisms, or another etiology of maternal fever. Further treatment is critical, because the progression of the infection can lead to life-threatening complications, such as peritonitis, sepsis, and abscess (Faro, 2005).

UTI AND PYELONEPHRITIS

A number of factors contribute to the development of UTIs during the postpartum period: decreased bladder tone that leads to urinary stasis, incomplete emptying of the bladder, the introduction of bacteria with pelvic examinations and catheterizations, and the prevalence of asymptomatic bacteriuria in pregnancy. *Escherichia coli* is the causative bacteria in 80% to 90% of cases. If left untreated, pyelonephritis may develop into a more serious infection that is characterized by fever, chills, flank pain, nausea, vomiting, and costovertebral angle tenderness (French & Smaill, 2004). UTI and pyelonephritis are treated with the use of appropriate antibiotic therapy. Some women with pyelonephritis require IV support for fluid management as a result of the associated nausea and vomiting.

MASTITIS

Postpartum mastitis is the inflammation of the breast associated with lactation characterized by fever and flu-like symptoms, pain that is most often unilateral, erythema, warmth, and possibly a streaked appearance to the breast. More commonly seen in primiparous women, it is associated with milk stasis, improper feeding, and cracked nipples, which allow for the entry of bacteria. This is differentiated from the generalized engorgement and temperature elevation that sometimes occurs with the onset of mature milk production around the third or fourth day postpartum. Treatment consists of bed rest, increased intake of fluids, the application of warm compresses, and the emptying of the breast either by the suckling of the infant or a breast pump. Antibiotics may lead to the faster resolution of symptoms (Barbosa-Cesnik, Schwartz, & Foxman, 2003; Jahanfar, Ng, & Teng, 2009).

POSTPARTUM WOUND INFECTION

Infection of an episiotomy or perineal laceration after a vaginal delivery is suspected in postpartum women who complain of perineal pain, swelling, and erythema. If the infection appears superficial, it may be treated with sitz baths and analgesia. Deeper infections may require surgical exploration and drainage and can then be allowed to heal by secondary intention. Wound infection is more commonly seen after a cesarean section delivery and occurs in up to 16% of women. Risk factors include obesity, length of surgery, amount of blood loss, and presence of chorioamnionitis. The risk is significantly decreased by the administration of perioperative antibiotics; additional antibiotics may need to be given postoperatively to those women who do develop a wound infection (French & Smaill, 2004).

VENOUS THROMBOEMBOLISM

Pregnancy and the postpartum period are hypercoagulable states, thereby increasing the risk for DVT and PE. This is most likely a protective mechanism that evolved to decrease women's risk of excessive bleeding after childbirth. Cesarean section delivery, obesity, increased parity, and advanced maternal age further increase this risk, with cesarean section delivery being associated with up to 75% of all fatal thromboembolic events. DVT is characterized by a unilateral redness (most often the left leg), tenderness, swelling of the calf or thigh, and a positive Homans' sign.

If DVT is suspected, compression ultrasonography is indicated to confirm the diagnosis. Because levels of D-dimer increase during pregnancy, this is less useful as a diagnostic test (Marik & Plante, 2008; Whitty & Dombrowski, 2002). Women with undiagnosed DVT have an increased risk of PE; therefore, prompt diagnosis and treatment are critical. Classic signs and symptoms include leg swelling, tachycardia, tachypnea, and dyspnea. Immediate medical attention is required (Whitty & Dombrowski, 2002). Early ambulation and the use of compression stockings during the postpartum period may decrease risk. After the condition is diagnosed, management consists of anticoagulation and referral may be appropriate (Marik & Plante, 2008; Whitty & Dombrowski, 2002).

PERIPARTUM CARDIOMYOPATHY

Postpartum hemodynamic stresses make this an extremely high-risk time for women with preexisting heart disease. In addition, postpartum or peripartum cardiomyopathy (PPCM) is a rare form of congestive heart failure that affects 1 in 3,000 to 1 in 15,000 women, with a mortality rate of 25% to 50% (Brown & Bertolet, 1998). PPCM is the onset of left ventricular dysfunction (e.g., an ejection fraction of less than 45%) during the last month of pregnancy or within 5 months of delivery in an otherwise previously healthy woman. PPCM cannot be explained by other etiologies, and its cause is still not completely understood (Pearson et al., 2000). However, most experts suggest that a myocarditis secondary to an autoimmune process is at the root of PPCM (Melvin, Richardson, Olsen, Daly, & Jackson, 1982; Oakley, 2005; Task Force on the Management of Cardiovascular Diseases During Pregnancy of the European Society of Cardiology, 2003). Many cases go undiagnosed or are misdiagnosed (Oakley, 2005). Heart failure (HF) is a common presenting feature of PPCM. However, the signs and symptoms of HF (e.g., shortness of breath, edema in the lower extremities) are also often experienced by healthy women during the final month of pregnancy. Postpartum women who present with marked fluid retention may be misdiagnosed as having had excessive IV fluids administered during delivery (Task Force on the Management of Cardiovascular Diseases During Pregnancy of the European Society of Cardiology, 2003). Women with PPCM also present with chest pain or a new onset of arrhythmia (Oakley, 2005). For women who present with symptoms before delivery, delivery is planned as soon as possible (Pearson et al., 2000; Task Force on the Management of Cardiovascular Diseases During Pregnancy of the European Society of Cardiology, 2003). Many of the standard pharmacologic therapies for HF (e.g., loop diuretics, spironolactone, angiotensin-converting enzyme [ACE] inhibitors, and angiotensin II receptor blockers [ARBs]) are contraindicated in pregnant women. Standard medical therapy is started for postpartum women (Oakley, 2005; Task Force on the Management of Cardiovascular Diseases During Pregnancy of the European Society of Cardiology, 2003). The prognosis is dependent on improvement in left ventricular function. If ventricular function normalizes, it is expected to do so within 6 months. Medical therapy is continued for at least 1 year after the return of normal left ventricular function (Oakley, 2005).

Psychosocial Issues

Even the arrival of the most hoped-for infant creates a stressful period of disequilibrium within the family while its members adjust to their new roles. On the basis of her observations of postpartum mothers during the 1960s, Rubin developed her classic theory on the nature of the new mother's evolving psyche. During the somewhat narcissistic *taking in* phase that immediately follows birth, the postpartum mother is primarily concerned with her own physical needs. This is followed by *taking hold*, when she gradually transfers her attentions onto her infant, and then the *letting go* phase occurs. During letting go, the woman finally becomes comfortable in her new role as mother (Davidson, London, & Ladewig, 2007). Since the late 20th century, this paradigm has been challenged by nurse researchers, who have applied social science's tests of validity and found the theory to be lacking (Ament, 1990; Martell, 1996). Rubin's work laid an important foundation during a time when the transition to new motherhood was poorly understood. Current social and cultural norms have shifted since Rubin's work, and the birth experience in America has been transformed. Women may no longer have the chance to take in before it is time to briefly take hold and then let go. Thus, although these experiences may no longer be distinct phases, the theory sheds important light on the transitions and emotions that new mothers experience.

POSTPARTUM PSYCHIATRIC DISORDERS

Public awareness of the prevalence and importance of postpartum emotional disorders has grown during recent years, primarily because of high-profile cases in the media, some of which have involved celebrities or resulted in catastrophic outcomes. A direct result of this attention has been the passage of both state and federal legislation to support research and mandate education for health care providers about postpartum depression. Nevertheless, postpartum psychiatric problems often remain undetected. Postpartum psychiatric disorders are commonly divided into three categories.

Baby Blues • These are the transient labile emotions that women frequently undergo during the first few weeks postpartum. This condition is considered benign and self-limiting, and is experienced by approximately 80% of all women after they have given birth (Payne, 2007).

Postpartum Depression • This is a more serious condition that affects approximately 10% to 20% of postpartum women and that occurs around 4 to 6 weeks postpartum (Campbell & Cohn, 1991; U.S. Department of Health and Human Services [USDHHS], 2005). It is characterized by the signs and symptoms of major depression. The woman may experience changes in eating habits, psychomotor agitation or retardation, insomnia or hypersomnia, feelings of worthlessness or guilt, or decreased concentration, and she may express or exhibit suicidal ideation (Beck, 2006; Pearlstein, Howard, Salisbury, & Zlotnick, 2009).

Postpartum Psychosis • This condition is related to severe depression and is characterized by delusions. Postpartum psychosis occurs in about one in 1,000 births (Brockington, 2004). It is more likely to occur among women with bipolar disease, particularly those with a family history of postpartum psychosis. Although the condition is relatively rare, postpartum psychosis is an extremely dangerous condition with a high risk of infanticide and suicide and of recurrence with future pregnancies. This condition requires immediate emergency hospitalization (Haessler & Rosenthal, 2007).

Anxiety disorders may actually be more common than depression postpartum. Preexisting panic or anxiety may be exacerbated or new-onset anxiety may be provoked, particularly if a woman is isolated and feels overwhelmed by the responsibilities of motherhood (Brockington, 2004).

POSTPARTUM DEPRESSION

It is crucial that women and their families be made aware of the signs of postpartum depression as they can

---

BOX 39.7 ANTENATAL RISKS FOR POSTPARTUM DEPRESSION

Lack of social support
Low self-esteem
Life stressors, including child care stress
Fatigue
Prenatal depression
Prenatal anxiety
Poor marital relationship
History of depression
Difficult infant temperament
"Baby blues"
Low socioeconomic status (e.g., financial problems with housing or income)
Single marital status
Unplanned or unwanted pregnancy
Age younger than 20 years
Medically indigent
Comes from a family of six or more children
Separated from one or both parents during childhood or adolescence
Received poor parental support and attention during childhood
Had limited parental support during adulthood
Has poor relationship with husband or boyfriend
Is dissatisfied with the amount of education
Shows evidence of past or present emotional problems

Data from Beck (2008); Hanretty and Miller (2003, p. 341); Katz (2007).

---

mimic the normal transient mood changes that follow delivery (e.g., baby blues) or the normal signs of postpartum fatigue. Postpartum depression has profound consequences for the children of affected mothers; their social and psychologic development are jeopardized as a result of their mother's diminished ability to interact or provide needed stimulation. Particularly in developing countries, a mother's postpartum depression is likely to lead to the malnutrition and poor health of her children. Antenatal risks for postpartum depression are identified in Box 39.7.

ETIOLOGY AND IMPORTANT FACTORS OF POSTPARTUM DEPRESSION

Hormones and Stress Response • Levels of adrenocorticotropic hormone (ACTH) and corticotropin-releasing hormone (CRH) have been found to be increased among postpartum women who are depressed, thus indicating an altered stress response (Jolley, Elmore, Barnard, & Carr, 2007). There is evidence that the hormones of breastfeeding have a protective effect against stress (Groer, Davis, & Hemphill, 2002); therefore, promoting breastfeeding antenatally is an important strategy for preventing postpartum depression, particularly with women who are at risk for postpartum depression.

Transcultural Factors • Although cross-cultural studies have found that postpartum depression occurs in disparate cultures throughout the world, it varies widely in prevalence and with regard to its associated risk factors. Some risks are common across cultures, such as poverty, a history of depression, a history of multiple miscarriages, and an unemployed or absent father of the baby. However, in parts of the world in which sons are valued over daughters (e.g., Turkey, India), the incidence of postpartum depression is higher among women who have daughters. Although the incidence of postpartum depression in Western societies has been estimated to be between 8% and 20%, the worldwide incidence is anywhere from close to 0% to as high as 60%. In societies in which stoicism is valued and mental illness is stigmatized, women may be disinclined to disclose feelings of depression. In cultures in which female family members are there to take care of the baby's siblings and household tasks, where women are given the support they need during the postpartum period, the rates of depression are significantly lower. Even when the condition exists, its roots are not perceived to be based in the biologic medical model, and thus the concept of its diagnosis and treatment as a disease may be incongruous with local customs (Halbreich & Karkun, 2006).

Considering the risk factors that are common to cultures throughout the world, it is clear that postpartum depression is a socially mitigated phenomenon. Poverty, single parenthood, and bearing a daughter in a place and time when it is considered a shameful misfortune are not biologically based phenomena. Even so, the puerperium is a time during which susceptible individuals experience a uniquely stressful situation that is potentiated by particular coexisting factors.

Assessment • Although women traditionally are not seen by their obstetric health care provider until 6 weeks after delivery, provisions are made for follow-up within the first 2 weeks postpartum. Women need to be aware of how to easily obtain help in the meantime. Home visits by nurses or doulas are known to be helpful to the new mother. These visits are also cost effective in that they reduce the number of newborn hospital readmissions (Paul, Phillips, Widome, & Hollenbeak, 2004).

The 2-week postpartum visit provides the opportunity to make a number of critical assessments; however, the onset of postpartum depression typically occurs between 4 to 6 weeks postpartum. Therefore, a second visit around 6 weeks is needed to screen for the condition again. Administering the Edinburgh Postpartum Depression Scale (EPDS), which is a well-validated 10-question instrument, is one method of screening women for depression during their postpartum visits. Women with a positive screen (e.g., a score greater than or equal to 12 on the EPDS) are evaluated for immediate safety and then referred with an appropriate level of urgency to psychiatric clinicians for diagnosis and treatment (Cox & Holden, 2015). If emergent care is not necessary, the woman is given information about crisis intervention resources should the need arise before her appointment date. She is also screened for other possible causes of depression, such as hypothyroidism. A thorough discussion of the issue of sleep deprivation is crucial, because it may be related to depression both as a contributing factor and as an effect. Pregnant women and their families are made aware of the signs of postpartum depression and given crisis referral information, which is reinforced before discharge from the hospital. Concrete plans for help at home and support after discharge are ensured for women who are at risk for postpartum depression.

Several days after discharge, all women should receive a screening phone call from a nurse or a health care provider during which they are asked open-ended questions about how they are doing, how breastfeeding is going (if they are breastfeeding), and their feelings about their birth experience.

COMPLEMENTARY AND ALTERNATIVE MEDICINE

Some evidence-based interventions have been shown to positively affect postpartum depression. Depressed mothers who were taught infant massage were found to have improved moods and more positive interactions with their infants, and their infants fell asleep faster and slept for longer periods. A number of other parent training and coaching programs have also been shown to have significant effects on maternal mental health outcomes by reducing anxiety and stress as well as depression (Weier & Beal, 2004).

PHARMACOTHERAPEUTICS

Antidepressant medications such as selective serotonin reuptake inhibitors (SSRIs) are commonly prescribed. The Cochrane Collaboration cautions that not enough is known about the efficacy of SSRIs for postpartum depression or about their effects on the breastfeeding infant. Researchers concluded that the risk of these drugs to breastfeeding infants probably does not outweigh their benefits in most cases (Howard, Hoffbrand, Henshaw, Boath, & Bradley, 2005). Although safety risks are a moot point for women who are not breastfeeding, the question of efficacy in postpartum depression remains. Thus, the management of these women by health care providers with psychiatric expertise is critical.

Changes in Low-Risk Obstetric Care

THE DECLINE OF THE DELIVERY ROOM AND THE NEWBORN NURSERY

Birth and postpartum care have evolved from the sterile operating room type of delivery involving a recovery room to birth rooms and postpartum care floors. In most instances, the mother–infant dyad is together in the same room and cared for by the same nurse throughout labor, delivery, and the immediate postpartum period through discharge. The newborn nursery is used for assessing newborns and for caring for infants whose mothers require special postpartum care themselves.

EARLY HOSPITAL DISCHARGE

The length of hospital stay for the delivery of an infant has also shifted. Mothers are discharged very quickly after delivery. In fact, hospital stays were so short that the Newborns' and Mothers' Health Protection Act was passed in 1996 to mandate at least 48 hours of guaranteed hospitalization after childbirth for normal vaginal deliveries, and a 96-hour stay for women after cesarean section delivery (Knutson, 1996). The American Academy of Pediatrics (AAP) clearly states that discharge should be determined by the health care provider and based on individual evaluation of each mother–infant dyad as opposed to being decided by third-party payers (AAP, 2004).

There has been no discernible impact on infant mortality since the legislation was passed; however, there have been significantly fewer readmissions during the first year of life for infection. The application of the act's protections has not been universal. Those populations who are more likely to experience infant mortality, are, unfortunately, still experiencing earlier hospital discharge after delivery. Thus, the full effects of the legislation on infant mortality remain unknown (Datar & Sood, 2006).

THE FAMILY MEDICAL LEAVE ACT

Unlike other countries in the industrialized world, leave from work after delivery is not protected by legislation in the United States. The only possible legislative protection is found in the federal Family and Medical Leave Act (FMLA). However, the application of this protection is very limited and it often leaves low-income families outside of its protection. Families who do fall under its protection are often forced to choose between caring for an ill family member or receiving paychecks to sustain family life (Association of Women's Health and Neonatal Nurses [AWHONN], n.d.). The AWHONN calls for expansion of the act's coverage so that, at a minimum, families who cannot afford the required 12 weeks without pay are able to have some basic protections.

Medical Concerns Before Hospital Discharge

The mother is offered a rubella vaccine before discharge if she is found to be nonimmune during her prenatal care. If she is Rh negative, the results of the RhoGAM workup are evaluated, and the mother is given Rh immunoglobulin (e.g., RhoGAM®) within 72 hours of delivery if the baby is Rh positive to prevent Rh isoimmunization. During the winter season, the flu vaccine is also offered. None of these preventive measures are contraindicated for breastfeeding mothers.

Rest and Recovery After Delivery

Fatigue is an expectation during the puerperium, and factors such as multiple gestation and complicated, high-risk, or operative deliveries may cause even greater fatigue. Many women and their families are neither prepared for the level of exhaustion that they experience nor the length of time that it lasts. Interventions include breastfeeding while side lying rather than sitting, which has been shown to be effective for reducing postpartum fatigue (Troy, 2003). After delivery, the new mother is counseled to sleep when the baby sleeps and wake with the baby for feedings. She is encouraged to arrange for help at home with household chores and other children for the first several weeks so that she has time to recover physically and to bond with the baby. Family and friends are asked to help with household chores rather than infant care. Health care providers have the authority to write work releases for 6 weeks postpartum, which is considered the standard period of recovery for an uncomplicated delivery. Women who are recovering normally may gradually increase their activity levels, both inside and outside of the home, as tolerated. Exercise is effective for preventing depression of any kind, including postpartum depression.

Sexuality

Women and their partners are counseled so they are prepared for the normal changes related to sexuality that occur during the months and sometimes years after delivery that are caused by a number of factors. Dyspareunia may occur as a result of perineal trauma suffered during birth, particularly if lacerations, episiotomy, forceps, or vacuum extraction were involved. It may also occur as a result of the changes in hormone levels postdelivery, especially those that are associated with breastfeeding. Diminished estrogen levels in relation to progesterone and decreased levels of androgens result in less lubrication, thinning of the vaginal mucosa, and diminished libido. Additionally, exhaustion and emotional lability come with being the parent of a newborn. For some breastfeeding women and their partners, it is difficult to accept the breasts as a mode of nourishing a child, while in another setting they are sexual organs. Rest, support, vaginal lubricants, taking things slowly, open communication, and a considerate partner are essential. A vaginal estrogen cream can be prescribed if over-the-counter lubricants are insufficient for treatment of atrophic vaginal tissue, which may occur during lactation (Gabbe et al., 2007). Desire discrepancy between partners around the birth of a child, as well as the new mother's understandable preoccupation with her baby, have been major challenges in relationships throughout the ages.

Contraception

Counseling the postpartum woman about contraceptive options takes into account religious, cultural, and personal beliefs as well as the desired method of infant feeding and any medical contraindications. For breastfeeding women, counseling addresses those methods that are known to have the least effect on breastfeeding, such as barrier methods, intrauterine devices (IUDs), surgical sterilization, and hormonal methods. A recent systematic review suggested that existing trials are insufficient to establish what effect hormonal contraception may have on the quality or quantity of breast milk (Truitt et al., 2003).

Women who are not breastfeeding may ovulate as early as day 25 postpartum; however, hypercoagulability of the postpartum period extends to 2 to 3 weeks after birth, thereby increasing the risk of VTE (ACOG, 2006b). Those women who desire combination oral contraceptives are advised to not start taking the pills until 6 weeks after birth. Progesterone-only methods may be started earlier, with various progesterone only methods offered before the woman is discharged from the hospital. For women who desire long-term contraception, the IUD may be a good option whether the mother is breastfeeding or not. This type of device is inserted either immediately postpartum, or, more typically, at the 6-week postpartum visit. Although it is possible to insert the IUD after the placenta has been delivered, this presents a greater risk for the expulsion of the device. Thus, insertion is usually delayed until 6 weeks postpartum, as are diaphragm or cervical cap fittings, if one of these methods is chosen. For exclusively breastfeeding women with amenorrhea, the lactational amenorrhea method (LAM) of birth control may be the woman's method of choice for birth control. LAM has a failure rate of less than 2% (Association of Reproductive Health Professionals [ARHP], 2003).

Diet

Dietary concerns of recently delivered mothers frequently center around their desire to lose weight. This needs to be balanced with nutritional needs, particularly if they are breastfeeding, in which case they are counseled to consume at least 1,800 calories per day. An adequate intake of nutrients, particularly fluids; calories from a balance of protein, vegetable, and fruit sources; fats; vitamins; and minerals are essential for establishing an adequate milk supply, the replacement of fluids and blood, and wound healing after delivery. The woman is counseled to eat foods that are rich in protein, iron, and calcium, and to continue to take prenatal vitamins and an iron supplement if she has been anemic or has experienced a large blood loss. Iron-deficiency anemia can contribute to the fatigue of the postpartum period, thus increasing the challenges of recovery, breastfeeding, and newborn care; this makes the intake of iron-rich foods especially important. Fiber intake is also important to prevent constipation, which can be quite painful if the woman has had a perineal repair. She must be followed closely if she has had a fourth-degree repair, with referral for any difficulty with bowel movements.

Exercise

There are no absolute contraindications to exercise after a normal vaginal delivery; healthy women can gradually resume prepregnancy exercise routines as they regain strength. A woman may start with head raises for abdominal muscles, Kegel exercises, and walking. Heavy lifting and aggressive exercise are discouraged until much later because excessive exercise during the earlier postpartum period may increase the risk for hemorrhage. Activity is modified in the event of cesarean section delivery; stress on the abdomen needs to be avoided until clearance is obtained from the health care provider. Maternal weight loss has not been shown to interfere with the weight gain of breastfeeding infants, with the caveat that the mother's fluid and nutritional intake is adequate to compensate for calories and fluid lost during exercise so that she produces a sufficient amount of milk. A review of diet and exercise for postpartum weight loss found that diet alone as well as diet plus exercise led to postpartum weight loss without compromising breastfeeding; exercise alone did not lead to weight loss (Amorim-Adegboye, Linne, & Lourenco, 2007).

Newborn Care

New mothers' early postpartum educational priorities range from the need to know things as basic as bathing and diaper changing to feeding, sleeping, and normal development. A multiparous woman is assessed for basic knowledge as well as her awareness of changes in infant or self-care that may have taken place since the birth of her last child. The health care provider assesses the woman's level of knowledge and support available from her family as well as the new mother's readiness and ability to take in information. Open-ended interviewing techniques are used to assess knowledge and needs rather than questions that can be answered with simple yes-or-no responses. It is also important to consider what has transpired during labor and delivery, because women who have experienced prolonged or difficult labors or operative deliveries are likely to take longer to bond with their infants and to experience more difficulty doing so.

Recent research suggests that parents play an important role in the development of the newborn's physical, cognitive, emotional, and social growth. The four key factors that have been identified as integral to this development are healthy attachment, responsive care, protection from harm, and breastfeeding (Bryanton & Beck, 2010).

An excellent method for teaching and assessing parents' knowledge, beliefs, and practices regarding infant care and for observing parents' interactions with their infants is to include them when performing the newborn examination. Adolescent parents in particular will benefit from this experience, because they can be taught the basics of baby care. The ability of the baby to actively interact with the environment, the infant's sleep–wake cycles, and the newborn's individual temperament should be discussed in concrete terms (Davidson et al., 2007).

SAFETY

Sleep Safety • Infant sleep practices are influenced by ethnic, social, economic, and other factors, including the method of infant feeding. There is a strong relationship between breastfeeding and bed sharing. Women who choose to bed share with their infants need to be informed about safe sleep practices. These include placing the baby on a firm, flat surface (e.g., no waterbeds or couches) in the supine position, with the bedding tucked in tightly (e.g., no pillows, stuffed animals, quilts, duvets, or comforters). There should be no spaces in which the infant's head could become trapped (e.g., between the bed and a headboard or a wall). Placing the baby on a firm mattress on the floor away from a wall or using a co-sleeper may be a safe alternative. Having an infant sleep in the same room as her or his parents appears to be protective against sudden infant death syndrome (SIDS; Academy of Breastfeeding Medicine, 2008) (Box 39.8).

Newborns need to be kept warm; however, it is equally important that parents not overdress their infants. In particular, heavy blankets and soft or furry bedding (e.g., lambskin) are hazardous and have been associated with an increased risk of SIDS. It is therefore essential that health care providers assess whether new parents have adequate heating or cooling available in their homes upon discharge. If they do not, the health care provider should arrange for social services to evaluate the home situation before discharging newly delivered mothers and infants. New families are also provided with safe sleep instructions.

Car Safety • All infants are discharged from the hospital in federally approved, rear-facing infant car seats that are correctly installed in the back seat. Therefore, staff need to know how to install them and be allowed enough time to teach parents appropriate techniques before discharge.

Social Support: Home Visits

Knowledge of community resources or the ability to refer to social service agencies is essential for health care providers

BOX 39.8   SAFE SLEEPING INSTRUCTIONS

Always put a baby to sleep on his or her back, and make sure that other caretakers always do this as well

If sleeping separately, put the baby on a firm mattress in his or her own crib or bassinet, close to parents or caregivers

If co-sleeping, follow specific safety recommendations[a]

Do not place pillows or blanket rolls in the crib

Do not smoke in a house with a baby

Breastfeeding reduces a baby's risk of sudden infant death syndrome

Pacifiers have been associated with decreased rates of sudden infant death syndrome; if breastfeeding, offer a pacifier after the first month, when breastfeeding has been well established

[a]The Association of Women's Health and Neonatal Nurses recommends separate sleeping, and the American Academy of Pediatrics Task Force states that co-sleeping may be hazardous in certain circumstances (e.g., with smokers or those who use alcohol or drugs) and recommends safety precautions for breastfeeding mothers who choose to co-sleep with their infants. These include placing the infant in a supine sleeping position, avoiding soft surfaces and loose bedding, moving the bed away from the wall and other furniture to avoid entrapment, and keeping anyone other than parents from sharing the bed.

Data from the Task Force on Sudden Infant Death Syndrome (2005); Association of Women's Health and Neonatal Nurses: Education and practice resource: AWHONN summarizes the American Academy of Pediatrics revised sudden infant death syndrome (SIDS) prevention recommendations and highlights issues raised (2005).

BOX 39.9   POSTPARTUM DISCHARGE INSTRUCTIONS

Follow-Up Appointments

1. Maternal: routinely in 4 to 6 weeks; may be sooner as needed for physical or psychosocial assessment
2. Infant: routinely in 2 weeks; may be sooner as needed for physical assessment or laboratory tests

Activity

1. Rest for first 2 to 4 weeks
2. Ask visitors and relatives to help with other children, household chores, and errands

Sudden Infant Death Syndrome Prevention

1. Pacifier use should not be stopped suddenly during the first 26 weeks of life
2. Safe sleep environment: the crib should meet safety regulations, and no pillows, soft bedding, or toys should be used
3. Bed sharing increases risk with a parent who smokes, drinks, or takes certain drugs or medications

Maternal Danger Signs

1. Sudden or persistent blood loss
2. Faintness or dizziness
3. Fever, chills, abdominal pain, and foul-smelling lochia
4. Headaches and visual disturbances
5. Red or painful area of the leg or breast
6. Persistent or severe feelings of depression

Infant Danger Signs

1. Jaundice (worsening or new onset) or pale stools
2. Diarrhea or constipation
3. Lack of wet diapers
4. Excessive or inconsolable crying
5. Fever of more than or equal to 38°C

Data from Demott et al. (2006).

who work with postpartum families. Postpartum home visiting programs that make use of nurses and paraprofessionals have demonstrated significant positive effects on a number of maternal–child health outcomes. The rate of hospital readmissions of infants for jaundice and dehydration was reduced by one such program, and indicators of positive family and mental health outcomes among mother–child dyads were still present at 2-year follow-up assessments in another. These included the mother's sense of mastery, improved mother–child interactions, increased child spacing, and improved child development (Meyer, Arnold, & Pascali-Bonaro, 2001).

Discharge Instructions

Discharge teaching includes verbal and written instructions about the following (Box 39.9):

- Follow-up appointments for mother and baby
- Danger signs, including a fever of more than 38°C (100.4°F); painful urination; lochia that has become

heavier than a period (lochia is usually lighter after cesarean section delivery); a reddened or tender area of the breast accompanied by flu-like symptoms; thigh or calf pain with redness and tenderness; separation of the wound or redness or oozing at the wound site;

and abdominal pain that increases in severity or that is unrelieved by prescribed pain medication

■ Seeking care for continuing severe depression or the woman's inability to care for herself or the baby; seeking help if she has thoughts of harming herself or the baby

Care is taken to ensure that there are functional systems in place for help after hours and for families that may require the services of a language interpreter.

■ SUMMARY

The postpartum mother has many concerns to address, including her own health, bonding with and nurturing her baby, and caring for other family members. She is carefully assessed and supported in meeting her extra-nutritional requirements as well as in her need to obtain restorative rest. Rest is important for her to properly recover from labor and delivery and also to facilitate the demanding physiologic processes of involution, lochia discharge, breastfeeding, and caring for her newborn. She is monitored for postpartum complications and provided with extensive education for recognizing problems in addition to having a thorough understanding of how to care for both herself and her newborn.

■ REFERENCES

Abalovich, M., Amino, N., Barbour, L. A., Cobin, R. H., De Groot, L. J., Glinoer, D., ... Stagnaro-Green, A. (2007). Management of thyroid dysfunction during pregnancy and postpartum: An Endocrine Society Clinical Practice Guideline. *Journal of Clinical Endocrinology and Metabolism, 92*(Suppl. 8), S1–47.

Academy of Breastfeeding Medicine. (2008). Protocol Committee: ABM clinical protocol #6: guideline on co-sleeping and breastfeeding. *Breastfeeding Medicine, 3*(1), 38–42.

Ahdoot, D., Van Nostrand, K. M., Nguyen, N. J., Tewari, D. S., Kurasaki, T., DiSaia, P. J., & Rose, G. S. (1998). The effect of route of delivery on regression of abnormal cervical cytologic findings in the postpartum period. *American Journal of Obstetrics and Gynecology, 178*(6), 1116–1120.

Ahmed, S. V., Jayawarna, C., & Jude, E. (2006). Post lumbar puncture headache: Diagnosis and management. *Postgraduate Medical Journal, 82*(973), 713–716.

Althaus, J. E., Petersen, S., Driggers, R., Cootauco, A., Bienstock, J. L., & Blakemore, K. J. (2006). Cephalopelvic disproportion is associated with an altered uterine contraction shape in the active phase of labor. *American Journal of Obstetrics and Gynecology, 195*(3), 739–742.

Ament, L. A. (1990). Maternal tasks of the puerperium reidentified. *Journal of Obstetric, Gynecologic, and Neonatal Nursing, 19*(4), 330–335.

American Academy of Pediatrics (AAP). (2004). American Academy of Pediatrics Committee on Fetus and Newborn: Policy statement: Hospital stay for healthy term newborns. *Pediatrics, 113*(5), 1434–1436.

American College of Obstetricians and Gynecologists (ACOG). (2003). Practice Bulletin No. 49, December 2003: Dystocia and augmentation of labor. *Obstetrics and Gynecology, 102*(6), 1445–1454.

American College of Obstetricians and Gynecologists (ACOG). (2006a). Practice Bulletin No. 76, Post Partum Hemorrhage: Clinical management guidelines. *Obstetrics and Gynecology, 108*(4), 1039–1047.

American College of Obstetricians and Gynecologists (ACOG). (2006b). Committee on Practice Bulletins—Gynecology: Practice Bulletin No. 73: Use of hormonal contraception in women with coexisting medical conditions. *Obstetrics and Gynecology, 107*(6), 1453–1472.

American College of Obstetricians and Gynecologists (ACOG). (2009). Practice bulletin no. 107: Induction of labor. *Obstetrics and Gynecology, 114*(2, Pt. 1), 386–397.

American College of Obstetricians and Gynecologists (ACOG). (2012). Timing of umbilical cord clamping after birth. Committee Opinion No. 543. *Obstetrics and Gynecology, 120*(6), 1522–1526.

American College of Obstetricians and Gynecologists (ACOG). (2013). Cesarean delivery on maternal request. Committee Opinion No. 559. *Obstetrics and Gynecology, 121*, 904–907.

American College of Obstetricians and Gynecologists (ACOG). (2015). Physical activity and exercise during pregnancy and the postpartum period. Committee Opinion No. 650. *Obstetrics and Gynecology, 126*, e135–e142.

Amorim-Adegboye, A. R., Linne, Y. M., & Lourenco, P. M. C. (2007). Diet or exercise, or both, for weight reduction in women after childbirth. *The Cochrane Database of Systematic Reviews, 2007*(3), CD005627. doi:10.1002/14651858.CD005627.pub2

Anderson, J. M., & Etches, D. (2007). Prevention and management of postpartum hemorrhage. *American Family Physician, 75*(6), 875–882.

Arca, G., Botet, F., Palacio, M., & Carbonell-Estrany, X. (2010). Timing of umbilical cord clamping: New thoughts on an old discussion. *Journal of Maternal-Fetal & Neonatal Medicine, 23*(11), 1274–1285.

Armson, B. A. (2007). Is planned cesarean childbirth a safe alternative? *Canadian Medical Association Journal, 176*(4), 475–476.

Association of Reproductive Health Professionals (ARHP). (2003). *Postpartum counseling: A quick reference guide for clinicians, 2003.* Retrieved from http://www.arhp.org/publications-and-resources/quick-reference-guide-for-clinicians/postpartum-counseling

Association of Women's Health and Neonatal Nurses (AWHONN). (n.d.). *FMLA position policy statement: Enhanced family medical leave protections.*

Athukorala, C., Crowther, C. A., & Willson, K.; Australian Carbohydrate Intolerance Study in Pregnant Women (ACHOIS) Trial Group. (2007). Women with gestational diabetes mellitus in the ACHOIS trial: Risk factors for shoulder dystocia. *The Australian & New Zealand Journal of Obstetrics & Gynaecology, 47*(1), 37–41.

Barbosa-Cesnik, C., Schwartz, K., & Foxman, B. (2003). Lactation mastitis. *Journal of the American Medical Association, 289*(13), 1609–1612.

Beck, C. T. (2006). Postpartum depression: It isn't just the blues. *American Journal of Nursing, 106*(5), 40–50; quiz 50.

Beck, C. T. (2008). State of the science on postpartum depression: What nurse researchers have contributed, part 1. *American Journal of Maternal Child Nursing, 33*(2), 121–126.

Beck, C. T., Froman, R. D., & Bernal, H. (2005). Acculturation level and postpartum depression in Hispanic mothers. *American Journal of Maternal Child Nursing, 30*(5), 299–304.

Beckmann, M. M., & Garrett, A. J. (2006). Antenatal perineal massage for reducing perineal trauma. *The Cochrane Database of Systematic Reviews, 2006*(1), CD005123.

Berens, P. (2009). The Academy of Breastfeeding Medicine (ABM) clinical protocol #20: Engorgement. *Breastfeed Medicine, 4*(2), 111–113. doi:10.1089/bfm.2009.9997

Bloom, S. L., Casey, B. M., Schaffer, J. I., McIntire, D. D., & Leveno, K. J. (2006). A randomized trial of coached versus uncoached maternal pushing during the second stage of labor. *American Journal of Obstetrics and Gynecology, 194*(1), 10–13.

Blum, J., Alfirevic, Z., Walraven, G., Weeks, A., & Winikoff, B. (2007). Treatment of postpartum hemorrhage with misoprostol. *International Journal of Gynaecology and Obstetrics, 99*(Suppl. 2), S202–S205.

Brockington, I. (2004). Postpartum psychiatric disorders. *Lancet, 363*(9405), 303–310.

Brown, C. S., & Bertolet, B. D. (1998). Peripartum cardiomyopathy: A comprehensive review. *American Journal of Obstetrics and Gynecology, 178*(2), 409–414.

Brown, S. T., Douglas, C., & Flood, L. P. (2001). Women's evaluation of intrapartum nonpharmacological pain relief methods used during labor. *Journal of Perinatal Education, 10*(3), 1–8.

Bryanton, J., & Beck, C. T. (2010). Postnatal parental education for optimizing infant general health and parent-infant relationships. *The Cochrane Database of Systematic Reviews, 2010*(1), CD004068. doi:10.1002/14651858.CD004068.pub3

Burrows, L. J., Meyn, L. A., & Weber, A. M. (2004). Maternal morbidity associated with vaginal versus cesarean delivery. *Obstetrics and Gynecology, 103*(5, Pt. 1), 907–912.

Campbell, S. B., & Cohn, J. F. (1991). Prevalence and correlates of postpartum depression in first-time mothers. *Journal of Abnormal Psychology, 100*(4), 594–599.

Capogna, G., & Camorcia, M. (2004). Epidural analgesia for childbirth: Effects of newer techniques on neonatal outcome. *Paediatric Drugs, 6*(6), 375–386.

Cesario, S. K. (2004). Reevaluation of Friedman's Labor Curve: A pilot study. *Journal of Obstetric, Gynecologic, and Neonatal Nursing, 33*(6), 713–722.

Chan, E. C., Fraser, S., Yin, S., Yeo, G., Kwek, K., Fairclough, R. J., & Smith, R. (2002). Human myometrial genes are differentially expressed in labor: A suppression subtractive hybridization study. *Journal of Clinical Endocrinology and Metabolism, 87*(6), 2435–2441.

Chauhan, S. P., Magann, E. F., Scott, J. R., Scardo, J. A., Hendrix, N. W., & Martin, J. N. (2003). Cesarean delivery for fetal distress: Rate and risk factors. *Obstetrical & Gynecological Survey, 58*(5), 337–350.

Cheyne, H., Dowding, D. W., & Hundley, V. (2006). Making the diagnosis of labour: Midwives' diagnostic judgement and management decisions. *Journal of Advanced Nursing, 53*(6), 625–635.

Christianson, L. M., Bovbjerg, V. E., McDavitt, E. C., & Hullfish, K. L. (2003). Risk factors for perineal injury during delivery. *American Journal of Obstetrics and Gynecology, 189*(1), 255–260.

Cluett, E. R., Pickering, R. M., Getliffe, K., & St George Saunders, N. J. (2004). Randomised controlled trial of labouring in water compared with standard of augmentation for management of dystocia in first stage of labour. *British Medical Journal (Clinical Research ed.), 328*(7435), 314.

Cox, J., & Holden, J. (2015). *Perinatal mental health: A guide to the Edinburgh Postnatal Depression Scale (EPDS).* Retrieved from www.netLibrary.com/urlapi.asp?action=summary&v=1&bookid=87488

Crofts, J. F., Bartlett, C., Ellis, D., Hunt, L. P., Fox, R., & Draycott, T. J. (2006). Training for shoulder dystocia: A trial of simulation using low-fidelity and high-fidelity mannequins. *Obstetrics and Gynecology, 108*(6), 1477–1485.

Cruikshank, D. P. (2007). Intrapartum management of twin gestations. *Obstetrics and Gynecology, 109*(5), 1167–1176.

Cunningham, F. G., & Williams, J. W. (2005). Obstetrical hemorrhage. In F. G. Cunningham & J. W. Williams (Eds.), *Williams obstetrics* (22nd ed.). New York, NY: McGraw-Hill Professional.

Cyna, A. M., Andrew, M. I., Robinson, J. S., Crowther, C. A., Baghurst, P., Turnbull, D.,...Whittle, C. (2006). Hypnosis antenatal training for childbirth: A randomised controlled trial. *BJOG, 120*(10), 1248–1259.

Cyna, A. M., McAuliffe, G. L., & Andrew, M. I. (2004). Hypnosis for pain relief in labour and childbirth: A systematic review. *British Journal of Anaesthesia, 93*(4), 505–511.

Datar, A., & Sood, N. (2006). Impact of postpartum hospital-stay legislation on newborn length of stay, readmission, and mortality in California. *Pediatrics, 118*(1), 63–72.

Davidson, M. R., London, M. L., & Ladewig, P. A. W. (2007). Postpartal family adjustment and nursing assessment. In M. R. Davidson, M. L. London, & P. A. W. Ladewig (Eds.), *Olds' maternal-newborn nursing & women's health across the lifespan* (8th ed.). Harlow, NJ: Prentice Hall.

Demott, K., Bick, D., Norman, R., Ritchie, G., Turnbull, N., Adams, C.,...Taylor, C. (2006). *Clinical guidelines and evidence review for post natal care: Routine post natal care of recently delivered women and their babies.* London, England: National Collaborating Centre for Primary Care and Royal College of General Practitioners.

Devine, P. (2009). Obstetric hemorrhage. *Seminars in Perinatology, 33*(2), 76–81.

Druckmann, R., & Druckmann, M. A. (2005). Progesterone and the immunology of pregnancy. *The Journal of Steroid Biochemistry and Molecular Biology, 97*(5), 389–396.

Duncombe, D., Skouteris, H., Wertheim, E. H., Kelly, L., Fraser, V., & Paxton, S. J. (2006). Vigorous exercise and birth outcomes in a sample of recreational exercisers: A prospective study across pregnancy. *The Australian & New Zealand Journal of Obstetrics & Gynaecology, 46*(4), 288–292.

Dunn, P. M. (2005). Ignac Semmelweis (1818–1865) of Budapest and the prevention of puerperal fever. *Archives of Disease in Childhood. Fetal and Neonatal Edition, 90*(4), F345–F348.

Eason, E., Labrecque, M., Wells, G., & Feldman, P. (2000). Preventing perineal trauma during childbirth: A systematic review. *Obstetrics and Gynecology, 95*(3), 464–471.

Elling, S. V., & Powell, F. C. (1997). Physiological changes in the skin during pregnancy, *Clinical Dermatology, 15*(1), 35–43.

Ernst, E. (2002). Herbal medicinal products during pregnancy: Are they safe? *BJOG: An International Journal of Obstetrics and Gynaecology, 109,* 227–235.

Fahy, K. (2009). Third stage of labor care for women at low risk of postpartum hemorrhage. *Journal of Midwifery Womens Health, 54*(5), 380–386.

Faro, S. (2005). Postpartum endometritis. *Clinical Perinatology, 32*(3), 803–814.

Fischer, S., & Johnson, P. G. (1999). Therapeutic touch. A viable link to midwifery practice. *Journal of Nurse Midwifery, 44*(3), 300–309.

Fleming, N., Newton, E. R., & Roberts, J. (2003). Changes in postpartum perineal muscle function in women with and without episiotomies. *Journal of Midwifery Womens Health, 48*(1), 53–59.

Fraser, W. D., Marcoux, S., Moutquin, J. M., & Christen, A. (1993). Effect of early amniotomy on the risk of dystocia in nulliparous women. The Canadian Early Amniotomy Study Group. *New England Journal of Medicine, 328*(16), 1145–1149.

French, L., & Smaill, F. M. (2004). Antibiotic regimens for endometritis after delivery. *The Cochrane Database of Systematic Reviews, 2004*(4), CD001067. doi:10.1002/14651858.CD001067.pub2

Friedman, E. A. (1978). *Labor: Clinical evaluation and management* (2nd ed.). Norwalk, CT: Appleton-Century-Crofts.

Gabbe, S. G., Niebyl, J. R., & Simpson, J. L. (2007). *Obstetrics: Normal and problem pregnancies* (5th ed.). New York, NY: Churchill Livingstone.

Galyean, A. M., Lagrew, D. C., Bush, M. C., & Kurtzman, J. T. (2009). Previous cesarean section and the risk of postpartum maternal complications and adverse neonatal outcomes in future pregnancies. *Journal of Perinatology, 29,* 726–730.

Geller, S. E., Adams, M. G., Kelly, P. G., Kodkany, B. S., & Derman, R. J. (2006). Postpartum hemorrhage in resource-poor settings. *International Journal of Gynecology & Obstetrics, 92,* 202–211.

Gerhardt, A., Scharf, R. E., Beckmann, M. W., Struve, S., Bender, H. G., Pillny, M.,...Zotz, R. B. (2000). Prothrombin and factor V mutations in women with a history of thrombosis during pregnancy and the puerperium. *New England Journal of Medicine, 342*(6), 374–380.

Gherman, R. B., Chauhan, S., Ouzounian, J. G., Lerner, H., Gonik, B., & Goodwin, T. M. (2006). Shoulder dystocia: The unpreventable obstetric emergency with empiric management guidelines. *American Journal of Obstetrics and Gynecology, 195*(3), 657–672.

Golden, S. H., Robinson, K. A., & Saldanha, I. (2009). Clinical review: Prevalence and incidence of endocrine and metabolic disorders in the United States: A comprehensive review. *Journal of Clinical Endocrinology and Metabolism, 94*(6), 1853–1878.

Gonsalves, H., Rocha, A. P., Ayres-de-Campos, D., & Bernardes, J. (2006). Internal versus external intrapartum fetal heart rate monitoring: The effect on linear and nonlinear parameters. *Physiological Measurement, 27*(3), 307–319.

Greenwood, C., Lalchandani, S., MacQuillan, K., Sheil, O., Murphy, J., & Impey, L. (2003). Meconium passed in labor: How reassuring is clear amniotic fluid? *Obstetrics and Gynecology, 102*(1), 89–93.

Greer, I. A. (1999). Thrombosis in pregnancy: Maternal and fetal issues. *Lancet, 353*(9160), 1258–1265.

Groer, M. W., Davis, M. W., & Hemphill, J. (2002). Postpartum stress: Current concepts and the possible protective role of breastfeeding.

Journal of Obstetric, Gynecologic, and Neonatal Nursing, 31(4), 411–417.

Gross, M. M., Hecker, H., Matterne, A., Guenter, H. H., & Keirse, M. J. (2006). Does the way that women experience the onset of labour influence the duration of labour? *British Journal of Obstetrics and Gynaecology, 113*(3), 289–294.

Hadar, A., Sheiner, E., Hallak, M., Katz, M., Mazor, M., & Shoham-Vardi, I. (2001). Abnormal fetal heart rate tracing patterns during the first stage of labor: Effect on perinatal outcome. *American Journal of Obstetrics and Gynecology, 185*(4), 863–868.

Haessler, A., & Rosenthal, M. B. (2007). Chapter 61: Psychiatric disorders of pregnancy and puerperium. In A. H. DeCherney & L. Nathan (Eds.), *Current diagnosis and treatment obstetrics and gynecology.* New York, NY: McGraw-Hill.

Halbreich, U., & Karkun, S. (2006). Cross-cultural and social diversity of prevalence of postpartum depression and depressive symptoms. *Journal of Affective Disorders, 91*(2–3), 97–111.

Hanretty, K. P., & Miller, A. W. F. (2003). *Obstetrics illustrated* (6th ed., p. 341). Edinburgh, Scotland and New York, NY: Churchill Livingstone.

Hartmann, K., Viswanathan, M., Palmieri, R., Gartlehner, G., Thorp, J. Jr., & Lohr, K. N. (2005). Outcomes of routine episiotomy: A systematic review. *Journal of the American Medical Association, 293*(17), 2141–2148.

Hastings-Tolsma M., Vincent D., Emeis C., & Francisco T. (2007). Getting through birth in one piece: Protecting the perineum. *American Journal of Maternal Child Nursing, 32*(3), 158–164.

Hedayati, H., Parsons, J., & Crowther, C. A. (2003). Rectal analgesia for pain from perineal trauma following childbirth. *The Cochrane Database of Systematic Reviews, 2003*(3), CD003931.

Heit, J. A., Kobbervig, C. E., James, A. H., Petterson, T. M., Bailey, K. R., & Melton, L. J., III. (2005). Trends in the incidence of venous thrombosis during pregnancy or postpartum: A 30-year population-based study. *Annals of Internal Medicine, 143*(10), 697–706.

Henderson, C., & MacDonald, S. (2004). *Maye's midwifery: A textbook for midwives* (13th ed.). New York, NY: Bailliere Tindall.

Hill, P. D. (2006). Effects of heat and cold on the perineum after episiotomy/laceration. *Journal of Obstetric, Gynecologic, and Neonatal Nursing, 18*(2), 124–129.

Hofmeyr, G. J., Abdul-Aleem, H., & Abdul-Aleem, M. A. (2008). Uterine massage for preventing postpartum hemorrhage. *The Cochrane Database of Systematic Reviews, 2008*(3), CD006431. doi:10.1002/14651858.CD006431.pub2

Hofmeyr, G. J., Gülmezoglu, A. M., Novikova, N., Linder, V., Ferreira, S., & Piaggio, G. (2009). Misoprostol to prevent and treat postpartum haemorrhage: A systematic review and meta-analysis of maternal deaths and dose-related effects. *Bulletin of the World Health Organization, 87*(9), 666–677.

Hotelling, B. A. (2006). Using the official Lamaze guide in childbirth education classes. *Journal of Perinatal Education, 15*(3), 47–49.

Hotelling, B., Amis, D., Green, J., & Sakala, C. (2004). Continuous labor support. *Journal of Perinatal Education, 13*(2), 16–22.

Howard, L. M., Hoffbrand, S., Henshaw, C., Boath, L., & Bradley, E. (2005). Antidepressant prevention of postnatal depression. *The Cochrane Database of Systematic Reviews, 2005*(2), CD004363.

Hudelist, G., Gelle'n, J., Singer, C., Ruecklinger, E., Czerwenka, K., Kandolf, O., & Keckstein, J. (2005). Factors predicting severe perineal trauma during childbirth: Role of forceps delivery routinely combined with mediolateral episiotomy. *American Journal of Obstetrics and Gynecology, 192*(3), 875–881.

Hundley, A. F. (2002). Managing placenta accreta. *OBG Management, 14*(8), 18–33

Hundt, G. L., Beckerleg, S., Kassem, F., Abu Jafar, A. M., Belmaker, I., Abu Saad, K., & Shoham-Vardi, I. (2000). Women's health custom made: Building on the 40 days postpartum for Arab women. *Health Care for Women International, 21*(6), 529–542.

Impey, L., Hobson, J., & O'Herlihy, C. (2000). Graphic analysis of actively managed labor: Prospective computation of labor progress in 500 consecutive nulliparous women in spontaneous labor at term. *American Journal of Obstetrics and Gynecology, 183*(2), 438–443.

Jahanfar, S., Ng, C. J., & Teng, C. L. (2009). Antibiotics for mastitis in breastfeeding women. *The Cochrane Database of Systematic Reviews, 2009*(1), CD005458. doi:10.1002/14651858.CD005458.pub2

Jolley, S. N., Elmore, S., Barnard, K. E., & Carr, D. B. (2007). Dysregulation of the hypothalamic-pituitary-adrenal axis in postpartum depression. *Biological Research for Nursing, 8*(3), 210–222.

Kabir, A. A., Steinmann, W. C., Myers, L., Khan, M. M., Herrera, E. A., Yu, S., & Jooma, N. (2004). Unnecessary cesarean delivery in Louisiana: An analysis of birth certificate data. *American Journal of Obstetrics and Gynecology, 190*(1), 10–19; discussion 13A.

Kane Low, L., Moffat, A., & Brennan, P. (2006). Doulas as community health workers: Lessons learned from a volunteer program. *Journal of Perinatal Education, 15*(3), 25–33.

Kaneshiro, B. E., Acoba, J. D., Holzman, J., Wachi, K., & Carney, M. E. (2005). Effect of delivery route on natural history of cervical dysplasia. *American Journal of Obstetrics and Gynecology, 192*(5), 1452–1454.

Karlsson, M. K., Ahlborg, H. G., & Karlsson, C. (2005). Female reproductive history and the skeleton: A review. *BJOG: An International Journal of Obstetrics and Gynaecology, 112*(7), 851–856.

Katz, V. L. (2007). Postpartum care. In S. G. Gabbe, J. R. Niebyl, & J. L. Simpson (Eds.), *Obstetrics: Normal and problem pregnancies* (5th ed.). New York, NY: Churchill Livingstone.

Kennedy, K. I., & Visness, C. M. (1992). Contraceptive efficacy of lactational amenorrhoea, *Lancet, 339*(8787), 227–230.

Kim-Godwin, Y. S. (2003). Postpartum beliefs and practices among non-Western cultures. *American Journal of Maternal Child Nursing, 28*(2), 74–78.

Kindberg, S., Stehouwer, M., Hvidman, L., & Henrikson, T. B. (2008). Postpartum perineal repair performed by midwives: A randomized trial comparing two suture technique leaving the skin unsutured. *BJOG: An International Journal of Obstetrics and Gynaecology, 115*(4), 472–479.

King, T. L., & Pinger, W. (2014). Evidence-based practice for intrapartum care: The pearls of midwifery. *Journal of Midwifery & Women's Health, 59*, 572–585.

Knutson, L. L. (1996). *Clinton asks Congress to require improved childbirth coverage.* Washington, DC: Associated Press, Dateline Washington.

Kopas, M. L. (2014). A review of evidence-based practices for management of the second stage of labor. *Journal of Midwifery & Women's Health, 59*, 264–276.

Kovavisarach, E. (2006). The "all-fours" maneuver for the management of shoulder dystocia. *International Journal of Gynecology & Obstetrics, 95*(2), 153–154.

Laskey, M. A., & Prentice, A. (1999). Bone mineral changes during and after lactation. *Obstetrics and Gynecology, 94*(4), 608–615.

Lausman, A., Ellis, C., Beecroft, J., Simons, M., & Shapiro, J. L. (2008). A rare etiology of delayed postpartum hemorrhage. *Journal of Obstetrics and Gynaecology Canada, 30*(3), 239–243.

Lee, N. (2007). Postpartum hemorrhage. *American Journal of Nursing, 107*(4), 15.

Lin, M. G., & Rouse, D. J. (2006). What is a failed labor induction? *Clinical Obstetrics and Gynecology, 49*(3), 585–593.

Liu, S., Liston, R. M., Joseph, K. S., Heaman, M., Sauve, R., & Kramer, M. S.; Maternal Health Study Group of the Canadian Perinatal Surveillance System. (2007). Maternal mortality and severe morbidity associated with low-risk planned cesarean delivery versus planned vaginal delivery at term. *Canadian Medical Association Journal, 176*(4), 455–460.

Lothian, J., Amis, D., Crenshaw, J., & Goer, H. (2004). No routine interventions. *Journal of Perinatal Education, 13*(2), 23–29.

Lowdermilk, D. L., Perry, S. E., & Bobak, I. M. (2000). *Maternity & women's health care* (7th ed.). St. Louis, MO: Mosby.

Lowe, N. K. (2007). A review of factors associated with dystocia and cesarean section in nulliparous women. *Journal of Midwifery & Women's Health, 52*(3), 216–228.

Macleod, M., & Murphy, D. J. (2008). Operative vaginal delivery and the use of episiotomy—A survey of practice in the United Kingdom and Ireland. *European Journal of Obstetrics and Gynecology and Reproductive Biology, 136*(2), 178–183.

Magann, E. F., & Lanneau, G. S. (2005). Third stage of labor. *Obstetrics & Gynecology Clinics of North America, 32*(2), 323–332, x–xi.

Maharaj, D., & Teach, D. T. (2007). Puerperal pyrexia: A review. Part II. *Obstetrical & Gynecological Survey, 62*(6), 400–406.

Marik, P. E., & Plante, L. A. (2008). Venous thromboembolitic disease and pregnancy. *New England Journal of Medicine, 359*(19), 2025–2033.

Martell, L. K. (1996). Is Rubin's "taking-in" and "taking-hold" a useful paradigm? *Health Care Women International, 17*(1), 1–13.

Martin, J. A., Hamilton B. E., & Osterman, M. J. K. (2014). *Births in the United States, 2013. NCHS data brief, no 175.* Hyattsville, MD: National Center for Health Statistics.

Maslovitz, S., Barkai, G., Lessing, J. B., Ziv, A., & Many, A. (2007). Recurrent obstetric management mistakes identified by simulation. *Obstetrics and Gynecology, 109*(6), 1295–1300.

Melvin, K. R., Richardson, P. J., Olsen, E. G., Daly, K., & Jackson, G. (1982). Peripartum cardiomyopathy due to myocarditis. *New England Journal of Medicine, 307*, 731–734.

Mestman, J. H. (2002). Endocrine diseases in pregnancy. In S. G. Gabbe, J. R. Niebyl, & J. L. Simpson (Eds.), *Obstetrics: Normal and problem pregnancies* (4th ed.). New York, NY: Churchill Livingstone.

Meyer, B. A., Arnold, J. A., & Pascali-Bonaro, D. (2001). Social support by doulas during labor and the early postpartum period. *Hospital Physician, 37*(9), 57–65.

Miller, S., Lester, F., & Hensleigh, P. (2004). Prevention and treatment of postpartum hemorrhage: New advances for low-resource settings. *Journal of Midwifery & Women's Health, 49*(4), 283–292.

Mousa, H. A., & Alfirevic, Z. (2007). Treatment for primary postpartum hemorrhage. *The Cochrane Database of Systematic Reviews, 24*(1), CD003249.

Nassar, N., Roberts, C. L., Raynes-Greenow, C. H., Barratt, A., & Peat, B. (2007). Evaluation of a decision aid for women with breech presentation at term: A randomised controlled trial [ISRCTN14570598]. *BJOG: An International Journal of Obstetrics and Gynaecology, 114*(3), 325–333.

Nisenblat, V., Barak, S., Griness, O. B., Degani, S., Ohel, G., & Gonen, R. (2006). Maternal complications associated with multiple cesarean deliveries. *Obstetrics and Gynecology, 108*(1), 21–26.

Oakley, C. (2005). Peripartum cardiomyopathy. In N. K. Wenger & P. Collins (Eds.), *Women and heart disease* (2nd ed., pp. 341–349). London, UK: Taylor & Francis.

Ophir, E., Solt, I., Odeh, M., & Bornstein, J. (2007). Water intoxication- a dangerous condition in labor and delivery rooms. *Obstetrical & Gynecological Survey, 62*(11), 731–738.

Papagni, K., & Buckner, E. (2006). Doula support and attitudes of intrapartum nurses: A qualitative study from the patient's perspective. *Journal of Perinatal Education, 15*(1), 11–18.

Patka, J. H., Lodolce, A. E., & Johnston, A. K. (2005). High- versus low-dose oxytocin for augmentation or induction of labor. *Annals of Pharmacotherapy, 39*(1), 95–101.

Paul, I. M., Phillips, T. A., Widome, M. D., & Hollenbeak, C. S. (2004). Cost-effectiveness of postnatal home nursing visits for prevention of hospital care for jaundice and dehydration. *Pediatrics, 114*(4), 1015–1022.

Payne, J. L. (2007). Antidepressant use in the postpartum period: Practical considerations. *The American Journal of Psychiatry, 164*, 1329–1332.

Pearlstein, T., Howard, M., Salisbury, A., & Zlotnick, C. (2009). Postpartum depression. *American Journal of Obstetrics and Gynecology, 200*(4), 357–364.

Pearson, G. D., Veille, J. C., Rahimtoola, S., Hsia, J., Oakley, C. M., Hosenpud, J. D.,...Baughman, K. L. (2000). Peripartum cardiomyopathy: National Heart, Lung, and Blood Institute and Office of Rare Diseases (National Institutes of Health) workshop recommendations and review. *Journal of the American Medical Association, 283*(9), 1219–1220.

Peng, Y. K., Hight-Laukaran, V., Peterson, A. E., & Perez-Escamilla, R. (1998). Maternal nutritional status is inversely associated with lactational amenorrhea in sub-Saharan Africa: Results from demographic and health surveys II and III. *Journal of Nutrition, 128*(10), 1672–1680.

Ramler, D., & Roberts, J. (1986). A comparison of cold and warm sitz baths for relief of postpartum perineal pain. *Journal of Obstetric, Gynecologic, & Neonatal Nursing, 15*(6), 471–474.

Reamy, B. (2009). Post-epidural headache: How late can it occur? *Journal of the American Board of Family Medicine, 22*(2), 202–205.

Ressel, G. W. (2004). ACOG releases report on dystocia and augmentation of labor. *American Family Physician, 69*(5), 1290–1292.

Robinson, B., & Nelson, L. (2008). A review of the proceedings from the 2008 NICHD Workshop on Standardized Nomenclature for Cardiotocography: Update on definitions, interpretative systems with management strategies, and research priorities in relation to intrapartum electronic fetal monitoring. *Reviews in Obstetrics & Gynecology, 1*(4), 186–192.

Simkin P., Ancheta, R., & Myers, S. (2005). *The labor progress handbook.* Oxford, UK: Blackwell.

Simpson, E. L., Lawrence, R. A., Nightingale, A. L., & Farmer, R. D. (2003). Venous thromboembolism in pregnancy and the puerperium: Incidence and additional risk factors from a London perinatal database. *BJOG: An International Journal of Obstetrics and Gynaecology, 108*(1), 56–60.

Slade, H., Escott, P., Henderson, D., & Fraser, R. B. (2003). Selected coping strategies in labor: An investigation of women's experiences. *Birth, 30*(3), 189–194.

Smith, C. A., Collins, C. T., Cyna, A. M., & Crowther, C. A. (2006). Complementary and alternative therapies for pain management in labour. *The Cochrane Database of Systematic Reviews, 2006*(4), CD003521.

Smith, J. G., & Merrill, D. C. (2006). Oxytocin for induction of labor. *Clinical Obstetrics and Gynecology, 49*(3), 594–608.

Spong, C. Y., Berghella, V., Wenstrom, K. D., Mercer, B. M., & Saade, G. R. (2012). Preventing the first cesarean delivery: Summary of a joint Eunice Kennedy Shriver National Institute of Child Health and Human Development, Society for Maternal-Fetal Medicine, and American College of Obstetricians and Gynecologists Workshop. *Obstetrics Gynecology, 120*(5), 1181–1193.

Strinić, T., Buković, D., Karelović, D., Bojić, L., & Stipić, I. (2002). The effect of delivery on regression of abnormal cervical cytologic findings. *Collegium Antropologicum, 26*(2), 577–582.

Task Force on Sudden Infant Death Syndrome. (2005). The changing concept of sudden infant death syndrome: Diagnostic coding shifts, controversies regarding the sleeping environment, and new variables to consider in reducing risk. *Pediatrics, 116*(5), 1245–1255.

Task Force on the Management of Cardiovascular Diseases During Pregnancy of the European Society of Cardiology. (2003). Expert consensus document on management of cardiovascular diseases during pregnancy. *European Heart Journal, 24*(8), 761–781.

Tiran, D. (2004). Breech presentation: Increasing maternal choice. *Complementary Therapies in Nursing and Midwifery, 10*(4), 233–238.

Troy, N. W. (2003). Is the significance of postpartum fatigue being overlooked in the lives of women? *American Journal of Maternal Child Nursing, 28*(4), 252–259.

Truitt, S. T., Fraser, A. B., Gallo, M. F., Lopez, L. M., Grimes, D. A., & Schulz, K. F. (2003). Combined hormonal versus nonhormonal versus progestin-only contraception in lactation. *The Cochrane Database of Systematic Reviews, 2003*(2), CD003988. doi:10.1002/14651858. CD003988

Tsu, V. D. (2004). New and underused technologies to reduce maternal mortality. *Lancet, 363*(9402), 75–76.

Tunzi, M., & Gray, G. R. (2007). Common skin conditions during pregnancy. *American Family Physician, 75*(2), 211–218.

U.S. Department of Health and Human Services (USDHHS). (2005). Health resources and services administration. *Women's health USA 2005.* Retrieved from mchb.hrsa.gov/whusa_05/pages/0429pd.htm

Vivio, D., & Williams, D. (2004). Active management of the third stage of labor: Why is it controversial? *Journal of Midwifery & Women's Health, 49*(1), 2–3.

Weier, K. M., & Beal, M. W. (2004). Complementary therapies as adjuncts in the treatment of postpartum depression. *Journal of Midwifery & Women's Health, 49*(2), 96–104.

Whitty, J. E., & Dombrowski, M. P. (2002). Respiratory diseases in pregnancy. In S. G. Gabbe, J. R. Niebyl, & J. L. Simpson (Eds.), *Obstetrics: Normal and problem pregnancies* (4th ed.). New York, NY: Churchill Livingstone.

Wiedaseck, S., & Monchek, R. (2014). Placental and cord insertion pathologies: Screening, diagnosis, and management. *Journal of Midwifery & Women's Health, 59*, 328–335.

Wilson, R. E., Alio, A. P., Kirby, R. S., & Salihu, H. M. (2008). Young maternal age and risk of intrapartum stillbirth. *Archives of Gynecology and Obstetrics, 278*(3), 231–236.

Winton, G. B., & Lewis, C. W. (1982). Dermatosis of pregnancy. *Journal of the American Academy of Dermatology, 6*(6), 977–998.

Wong, R. C. (1996). Physiologic skin changes in pregnancy. In M. Harahap & R. C. Wallach (Eds.), *Skin changes and diseases in pregnancy* (p. 37). New York, NY: Marcel Dekker.

Young, G. L., & Jewell, D. (1996). Creams for preventing stretch marks in pregnancy. *The Cochrane Database of Systematic Reviews, 1996*(2), CD000066.

Zwelling, E., Johnson, K., & Allen, J. (2006). How to implement complementary therapies for laboring women. *American Journal of Maternal Child Nursing, 31*(6), 364–370; quiz 371–362.

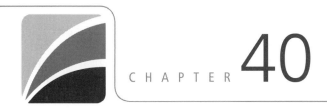

CHAPTER 40

Mental Health Challenges

Deborah Antai-Otong

The prevalence of psychiatric disorders in women seen in primary care settings is high, especially anxiety, major depression, substance use, and eating disorders. Approximately 20% to 30% of all women experience at least one psychiatric disorder during a given year (Kessler et al., 2005). Even more concerning is the exceptionally higher rate of psychiatric disorders in women of childbearing age (Kessler et al., 2005).

Complex biological and psychosocial factors contribute to psychiatric disorders in women. Female gender is a powerful constitutional determinant of mental health that interacts with individual characteristics, including age, race, reproductive cycle, developmental stage, personality traits, self-worth, and strengths. The concurrence of hormonal and reproductive events and biological factors in women's lives increase the risk for mood and anxiety disorders during various reproductive events, such as postpartum and perimenopausal depression (Chen, Su, Li, Chen, & Bai, 2013; DiFlorio et al., 2013; Soares, 2014). Social influences, which include environmental and sociocultural factors, life events, history of abuse, family dynamics, socioeconomic and educational status, and access to equitable and gender-centered health care, are equally linked to women's well-being and mental health (WHO, 2014). Situations in which women lack autonomy, independent income, decision-making power, and locus of control make managing stressful situations difficult and increase vulnerability to psychiatric conditions.

■ MENTAL HEALTH DISORDERS

Definition and Scope

Women are twice as likely as men to experience depressive and anxiety disorders, particularly posttraumatic stress disorder (PTSD; Kessler et al., 2006; Polusny et al., 2014; Sher, Oquendo, Burke, Cooper, & Mann, 2013; Wosu, Gelaye, & Williams, 2015). A disproportionate number of women experience trauma. Precipitating events associated with mental health problems include rape, deployment and combat-related stressors, other sexual assaults, intimate partner violence (IPV), history of childhood physical and/or sexual abuse, or being threatened with a weapon.

Common consequences associated with violence against women include development of depression, PTSD, anxiety and/or substance-use disorders during pregnancy and postpartum, as well as negative effects on children and adolescents exposed to environmental violence (Cohen, Field, Campbell, & Hien, 2013; Kessler et al., 2006; Vatnar & Bjørkly, 2011). In addition, suicide risk and gastrointestinal (GI) conditions are commonly associated with psychosocial stressors in women. For example, women exposed to psychological IPV were more likely to suffer from PTSD than controls (Vatnar & Bjørkly, 2011).

The prevalence of eating disorders varies with sampling and evaluation methodology. According to the lifetime estimates from the *Diagnostic and Statistical Manual of Mental Disorders*, fifth edition (*DSM-5*; American Psychiatric Association [APA], 2013), individuals diagnosed with anorexia nervosa, bulimia nervosa, and binge eating disorder are 0.8%, 2.3%, 3.5%, respectively, women (Smink, van Hoeken, Oldehinkel, & Hoek, 2014). Disordered eating or eating disorders are more common in older adolescents and young women and uncommon in men.

A common myth about eating disorders is that they are limited to middle and upper-middle-class White women. Although some studies suffering from population selection bias limitation support this myth, other studies indicate that the incidence of eating disorders are similar in women across ethnic and racial groups and that culturally sensitive interventions must be implemented to reduce the risk of eating disorders among vulnerable populations (Stojek & Fischer, 2013). Disordered eating is highly co-occurring with other psychiatric disorders such as anxiety, mood, substance use, and personality disorders. The mortality rate in this population has not improved during the past decade (Mendolicchio, Maggio, Fortunato, & Ragione, 2014). Thus, inquiring about symptoms of disordered eating in women of all races and ethnicities is necessary to ensure accurate diagnosis and appropriate management to reduce morbidity and mortality.

Access to timely and appropriate health care also challenges women with mental health problems. It is widely documented that many patients with a mental health problem receive mental health care from a primary care clinician rather than a mental health clinician. Growing concerns about the complexity of mental health care and provision of integrated mental health services in primary care practice remains a challenge because of the importance of timely monitoring and, in some cases, the need to collaborate with mental health clinicians. Primary care clinicians must bridge the gap and work with mental health and physical health services to develop collaborative approaches for managing mental health problems for women. Regardless of where a woman enters the health care system, clinicians must recognize and value the unique biological and psychosocial makeup that increases her risk for mental health problems and need for gender-specific interventions.

Etiology and Risk Factors

Mental health is influenced by one's capacity to cope with the daily stress of living, establish and maintain meaningful relationships, tolerate frustration and anxiety, and contribute to society. The stress-diathesis theory suggests that psychosocial, neurobiological, genetic, cultural, economic, and environmental as well as personality traits together modulate stressful events and vulnerability to psychiatric disorders (Oquendo et al., 2014). Furthermore, researchers submit alterations in neurobiological processes, particularly the hypothalamic–pituitary–adrenal (HPA) axis, demonstrate a significant role in the diathesis of suicide (Oquendo et al., 2014). These complex factors play principal roles in the development of psychiatric disorders and have implications for treatment considerations. Reproductive events mediated by psychosocial stressors and complex underpinnings predispose women to psychiatric disorders.

GENETIC VULNERABILITY

Major depression, anxiety, substance use, and eating disorders appear to be more heritable in women than men, and are associated with interactions between biological, genetic, hormonal, and psychosocial factors (Karg, Burmeister, Shedden, & Sen, 2011). Family and twin studies correlate genetic vulnerability to psychiatric disorders, seemingly particularly higher in women with personality disorders (e.g., borderline personality disorder) and a history of childhood trauma or trauma exposure (Karg et al., 2011; Salmela-Aro et al., 2014; Van der Auwera et al., 2014). Genetics also predispose women to early-onset, coexistent psychiatric conditions, including alcohol misuse, panic disorder (PD) and lifetime overall anxiety disorders, and recurrence of major depression (Karg et al., 2011; Schuch, Roest, Nolen, Penninx, & de Jonge, 2014). Explanations for genetic risk factors associated with psychiatric conditions involve alterations in serotonin transporter (5-HTT), less functional s-allele transporters, and tryptophan depletion (Karg et al., 2011; Moreno et al., 2010).

The extent to which genetic and environmental factors contribute to stress-induced mental health problems may also be based in the context of environmental risk factors (Karg et al., 2011). Given women's sensitivity and vulnerability to psychosocial stressors and higher incidence of early childhood and other trauma exposure, the diathesis-stress model suggests that anxiety and mood disorders are mediated by genetic and neurobiological vulnerability as well as psychosocial stressors. The diathesis-stress model can guide therapeutic interventions, such as pharmacological interventions that target both genetic and biological underpinnings (serotonin receptors sites) to reduce symptoms and strengthen coping skills.

BIOCHEMICAL

Alterations in complex brain regions and neurocircuitry pathways contribute to variability in thought processing, behavior, and mood—hallmark features of mood and anxiety disorders. Serotonin and its metabolite, cerebrospinal 5-hydroxylindoleacetic acid (5-HIAA), and tryptophan depletion are widely accepted as biologic markers of major depressive disorders. Lower cerebrospinal fluid (CSF) serotonin levels are implicated in women with severe major depression (Moreno et al., 2010). Neurotransmitters are target sites for antidepressant medications, particularly those that enhance serotonergic levels and norepinephrine. Increased CSF 5-HIAA levels have also been found in women with co-occurring major depression and PD and implicate increased serotonin release and greater serotonin metabolism and/or decreased 5-HIAA clearance. Co-occurring psychiatric conditions, such as borderline personality disorder (BPD), PTSD, and major depression, are associated with serious psychiatric disorders, increased disability and mortality, and poor treatment outcomes (Miller et al., 2013).

NEUROIMAGING ABNORMALITIES

Findings from neuroimaging studies involving psychiatric disorders point to alterations in three brain regions: the medial prefrontal cortex, amygdala, and hippocampus. For instance, in PTSD, dysregulation of the amygdala and prefrontal cortex appear to contribute to the exaggerated physiological responses to stimuli such as startle response, hypervigilance, avoidant behaviors, and increased heart rate and blood pressure (Shin et al., 2011). Similar findings were discovered in women with BPD, who often suffer from childhood trauma and PTSD (Frewen et al., 2011). Data from these studies also demonstrated abnormalities in the frontal-amygdala circuitry, namely hypometabolism and decreased volume (Jacob et al., 2013). Alterations in the medial prefrontal cortex are associated with poor impulse control, emotional instability, maladaptive coping behaviors, and suicide and self-injurious behaviors—core features of BPD and individuals with eating disorders. Selective serotonin reuptake inhibitor (SSRI) antidepressants are effective in treating major depression and aggressive impulsive behaviors, which are commonly found in women with BPD. The efficacy of these agents is their stabilizing effect of prefrontal cortex metabolism on impulsive behaviors commonly found in individuals with BPD and PTSD (Jacob et al., 2013).

NEUROENDOCRINE

Alterations in the HPA axis are often linked to medical and psychiatric conditions. Depression and anxiety disorder have long been linked to abnormalities in the HPA axis (McHugh et al., 2014; Petrowski, Wintermann,

Schaarschmidt, Bornstein, & Kirschbaum, 2013). Recent findings using combined dexamethasone (DEX) and corticotrophin-releasing hormone (CRF) demonstrated marked dysregulation in the HPA axis in persons with unipolar and bipolar depression (Sher et al., 2013). These data confirmed earlier findings implicating the role of neuroendocrine factors in the genesis of depression and other psychiatric conditions.

Prolonged stress reaction is also implicated in mood and anxiety disorders. Prolonged stress produces alterations in hippocampal function and structure in animal models, an effect mediated primarily by increased glucocorticoids and limited neurogenesis. These findings are consistent with magnetic resonance imaging (MRI) studies of individuals with PTSD who had reduced hippocampal volume and deficits in memory and cognition (Mahar, Bambico, Mechawar, & Nobrega, 2014). Antidepressants play a key role in the modulation of serotonin transmission by mediating stress-regulating processes in those with PTSD and major depression (Mahar et al., 2014). These agents enhance neurogenesis and neuroprotection, increase hippocampal volume, and improve cognitive and memory function.

REPRODUCTIVE EVENTS

The reproductive cycle has been implicated in the pathogenesis of psychiatric disorders in women and is associated with dysregulation of ovarian steroids. Estrogen is widely distributed to receptors in the brain and believed to modulate dopamine, norepinephrine, and acetylcholine neurotransmitters involved in mood and cognition. Hyperactivity of the HPA in women is linked to depression and believed to play a regulatory role in sex hormones. Greater emphasis has centered on the serotonin-estrogen connection in the modulation of mood and cognition, although the significance of this relationship is unclear. Estrogen's unique relationship with serotonin has spurred robust interest, mainly because serotonin is well studied, clearly connected with regulation of mood, and a primary target for pharmacologic treatment of unipolar depression (Bethea et al., 2011).

Premenstrual dysphoric disorder (PMDD) is a good example of the interrelationship among estrogen–serotonin, neuroendocrine, and the genesis of mood disorders. Although the precise cause of PMDD continues to be studied, most evidence suggests dysregulation in neuroendocrine, hormonal, or serotoninergic neurocircuitry. Abnormal serotonergic transmission and the efficacy of SSRIs further strengthen the premise of this neurotransmitter in the pathogenesis and treatment of mood and anxiety disorders (Marjoribanks, Brown, O'Brien, & Wyatt, 2013; McHugh et al., 2014).

ENVIRONMENTAL AND ADVERSE LIFE STRESSORS

Stressful life events increase vulnerability to mood and anxiety disorders (Karg et al., 2011). However, some women who experience life stressors do not develop mood and anxiety disorders. Emerging models posit that the effect of adverse life events is modulated by her repertoire of coping skills, quality of support systems, and personality style.

Heightened levels of perfectionism, low self-esteem, and perceived ineffectiveness are common traits in women with eating disorders and concomitant mood disorders. In addition, family and twin study results implicate genetic vulnerability in women contributing to adverse life events and susceptibility to psychiatric illness (Karg et al., 2011).

Psychosocial stressors contribute to depressive and anxiety disorders in women, and the nature of stress itself is a significant risk factor for mental health problems. Women often face significant stressors such as the demands of single parenthood, childrearing, and caring for aged parents. Lack of close and meaningful relationships, low self-esteem, low confidence, interpersonal violence, and marital discord further overburden women's coping skills. Psychosocial stressors and adverse life events must be thoroughly evaluated to determine their effects on current complaints, experience, adaptation, level of danger to self and others, functionality, and quality of life.

CULTURAL INFLUENCES

Emerging evidence demonstrates that women from various cultural and ethnic backgrounds experience discrimination, insensitivity, lack of knowledge about their religious and cultural practices, and poor access to mental health care. Collectively these issues interfere with the clinician–patient relationship, provision of quality emotional support, and culturally and linguistically sensitive mental health care (Du Mont et al., 2012; Lacey, McPherson, Samuel, Powell Sears, & Head, 2013). Implications from these findings emphasize the importance of respecting a woman's uniqueness and establishing therapeutic relationships that ensure her active participation in treatment and decision making based on her strengths, wishes, needs, and cultural and spiritual preferences.

Evaluation/Assessment

HISTORY AND SYMPTOMS

Women with psychiatric conditions typically seek help from their primary care clinicians with complaints of somatic problems such as fatigue or sleep disturbances. In these situations, it is imperative to ask about reasons for seeking treatment at this time, what has resolved somatic complaints in the past, and identify recent stressors. Clinicians must understand the basic concepts of diagnosing and treating women who present with mental health problems. The diagnosis of psychiatric disorders is determined by the quality of the interview, the level of clinical expertise with psychiatric evaluation, patient history, and patient motivation to change.

A successful comprehensive interview is built on establishing a therapeutic relationship in which the clinician displays empathy, genuine interest, respect, and competence (Box 40.1; Antai-Otong, 2008). An extensive chronology of mood changes, if any, during hormonal events, such as menstrual cycles, pregnancy, postpartum, and menopause, must be obtained. Systematic data collection and synthesis of a number of topics is important (Box 40.2).

PHYSICAL EXAMINATION

Women with psychiatric symptoms must receive a diagnostic evaluation to develop a differential diagnosis of a psychiatric and/or medical disorder. Routine data from vital signs, neurological evaluation, signs of abuse or self-injurious behaviors (e.g., bruises, rashes, cuts, and punctures), functional status, and nutritional status provide relevant information needed to make a differential diagnosis. Symptoms of eating disorders often manifest as serious medical conditions that require immediate management and stabilization. Throughout both the history and physical examination, the clinician observes her carefully to complete a mental status examination (MSE) and identify any signs of dysfunction (Table 40.1).

Differential Diagnoses

Psychiatric rating scales provide useful screening tools to both identify psychiatric conditions and monitor her response to treatment. They can be specific or comprehensive and measure internal experiences, such as depression, and external observable behaviors. Rating scales quantify her mental status, behavior, and relationships with others and society. Data collected from these tools provide baseline information and provides an objective strategy to monitor treatment efficacy. Because of the time involved in using various structured tools, most mental health clinicians and primary care clinicians may opt to use diagnostic criteria listed in the *DSM-5* (APA, 2013). The *DSM-5* is a nonaxial classification system that is based on diagnostic assessment based on *International Classification of Diseases* (ICD)-9 and ICD-10 diagnoses (formerly Axes I, II, and

---

BOX 40.1   KEY COMPONENTS OF A SUCCESSFUL COMPREHENSIVE INTERVIEW

Assuring adequate time to perform a psychiatric and physical evaluation

Eliciting the client's symptoms, experience, and level of distress

Consulting or collaborating with a mental health professional when appropriate

Developing a client-centered treatment plan, based on client preferences, wishes, gender, culture, and ethnicity

Source: Antai-Otong (2009).

BOX 40.2   DATA COLLECTED IN A SYSTEMATIC COMPREHENSIVE PSYCHIATRIC HISTORY

Reasons for seeking treatment
- Chief complaint—use her own words, that is, "I am depressed and can't sleep"
- Duration of symptoms and her goals or need to address psychiatric symptoms

Current stressors or significant changes the past 6 to 12 months

Strengths; quality of support system (marital status, significant other); interests, preferences, and values pertaining to health care

Sociocultural needs; spiritual and religious beliefs

Attitude concerning weight, shape, and eating, and associated psychiatric symptoms

History of current symptoms and chronology of remissions and exacerbation
- Description and severity of current symptoms—sleep disturbances, altered mood and anxiety states, hallucinations, delusions, cognitive deficits

Chronology of psychiatric history/treatment, including exposure to antipsychotic agents, medication side effects, response; most recent periods of stability and episodes when symptoms produced severe distress and impaired function

Family history of psychiatric problems, including eating disorders

Current medications, including OTC drugs, vitamins, herbs, or complementary therapies

Allergies or serious or distressful adverse drug reactions

Present and past general medical history and responses to previous treatment

Significant personal history—coping styles

Recent/past hospitalizations, surgeries

Current health status, last physical examination, diet

Trauma exposure—rape, military, natural disaster, witness to violence

Inquire and assess for emotional and physical signs of IPV

Legal history—past and present charges, arrests, incarceration, parole or probation, DUI charges

History of abuse and/or violence

Substance abuse/dependence history (illicit, licit), treatment, dual diagnosis (concurrent psychiatric and substance-use disorder)

Review of systems; focused medical history

Functional, occupational, psychosocial status

Relevant military history (e.g., combat, noncombat; military sexual trauma); discharge status

DUI, driving under the influence; IPV, intimate partner violence; OTC, over the counter.

Source: Antai-Otong (2008).

TABLE 40.1	Mental Status Function Examination: Key Points to Note During the History and Physical Examination
ASSESSMENT CATEGORY	**EVALUATION POINTS**
General	■ Appearance—hygiene, grooming, appropriateness of attire (e.g., wears warm clothing during cold weather) ■ Approximate age—based on general appearance ■ Level of distress ■ Responses to questions ■ Facial expression, posture, and gait ■ Attentiveness to details and understanding of the interview ■ Eye contact—consider cultural and ethnicity influences ■ Overt behavior and psychomotor activity—restlessness, pacing, irritability ■ Attitude—cooperative, distant, uncooperative, distrustful, or suspicious ■ Mode of arrival—alone, with significant other, friend
Mood and affect	■ Mood—internal and subjective pervasive or sustained emotion ■ Affect—present emotional responsiveness; note range, intensity, and stability ■ Blunted—severely decreased feeling tone ■ Restricted—minimal intensity of feeling tone ■ Flat—absence of emotional feeling tone ■ Appropriate versus mood incongruence—whether mood appropriately reflects what is being discussed
Speech	■ Quality ■ Fluency ■ Articulation ■ Accent ■ Rate—rapid during the manic phase of bipolar disorder, anxiety ■ Spontaneity—may be reduced in woman who is in shock from recent trauma exposure, depression ■ Pressured—normally found in bipolar disorder, manic episode ■ Rambling—may occur during psychosis or mania ■ Hesitant—often occurs during depression or psychosis ■ Mumbled—may occur with psychosis, paranoia, or suspiciousness ■ Loud—may indicate hearing disturbances or indicate anger or agitation
Perceptual and sensory function	■ Hallucinations—based on internal stimuli ■ Illusions—based on misinterpretation of external stimuli, such as a shadow for a person ■ Circumstances of hallucinations or illusions (i.e., stress, falling asleep) ■ Content of hallucinations or delusions
Thought processes (thought organization and flow of ideas)	■ Loose associations (unrelated, disconnected)—associated with psychosis ■ Flight of ideas (rapid thinking-connected and related)—usually indicates mania or psychosis ■ Racing thoughts, tangentiality, and circumstantiality—commonly found in bipolar disorder I, manic episode
Thought content	■ Delusions—false beliefs, which are not shared by a person's culture and cannot be substantiated with rational explanations. They are *very real* to the patient. Types of delusions include persecutory, grandiose, somatic, and jealousy. ■ Preoccupations ■ Obsessions ■ Paranoia ■ Phobias ■ Suicidal/homicidal ideations ■ Ideas of reference
Sensorium and cognition	A systematic evaluation of cognitive function, including: ■ Level of consciousness ■ Orientation ■ Attention ■ Concentration ■ Memory
Insight	■ Understanding of illness and motivation to adhere to treatment recommendations
Impulsivity	■ Degree and appropriateness in which client is able to control impulses
Judgment	■ Degree and appropriateness of decision making, assessed by asking "what if" questions

Source: Antai-Otong (2008, 2009).

III). ICD-10 diagnoses have yet to be published, but they will be linked to relevant conditions in the taxonomy (APA, 2013). This section includes mental health diagnosis and relevant medical conditions (APA, 2013). Axis IV (formerly psychosocial stressors) has been replaced with a WHO Disability Assessment Schedule (WHODAS) score, whereas Axis V (formerly referred to as global level of functioning [GAF]) has been deleted from *DSM-5*. The WHODAS classification evolves from the International Classification of Functioning, Disability and Health (ICF) for use in vast medical and health care settings (APA, 2013).

1. Diagnostic assessment psychiatric disorder, relevant medical condition; relevant specifier(s)
2. WHODAS score

Psychiatric emergency refers to a severe disturbance of mood, thought, or behavior that requires immediate medical and psychiatric attention. Specific presentations and management for common psychiatric problems are presented in the following separate sections.

Diagnostic Studies

The following diagnostic and laboratory studies are frequently needed: serum chemistry profile; liver and renal function panels; serum electrolytes; urinalysis; complete blood count (CBC); platelet count; erythrocyte sedimentation rate (ESR); thiamine, vitamin B_{12}, and folate levels; vitamin assay (in those with signs of eating disorders); fasting glucose, thyroid panel; comprehensive metabolic profile; pregnancy test for women of childbearing age, even if she reports using contraception; blood and urine cultures; toxicology screens; and electrocardiogram (EKG).

Treatment/Management

Treating psychiatric disorders in primary care requires evidence-based practice and use of best practices guidelines. Collaboration with a mental health clinician offers expertise, decision support, and additional resources to manage the mental health care of women. For example, although women suffering from major depression are commonly treated in primary care settings, the concurrent risk of suicide and other life-threatening behaviors must always be evaluated and managed. Failing to recognize worsening symptoms or assess suicide risk during brief primary care appointments may have dire consequences. The collaborative model provides greater resources (e.g., education about mental health) and decision support and improves clinical outcomes for women with mental health problems (Thota et al., 2012). Most psychiatric disorders require both pharmacological and psychotherapeutic interventions. The decision to initiate psychotropic medications in the primary care setting must include consideration of severity of illness and associated level of functioning, history of response, safety of medication (lethality in overdose), side effects (short term and long term), medication interactions, coexisting disorders, cost (affordability), patient preferences, and reproductive events including pregnancy and lactation.

More severe psychiatric disorders, such as acute or exacerbation of psychiatric conditions (e.g., schizophrenia, PTSD, generalized anxiety disorder [GAD], bipolar-manic episode, drug-induced psychosis, or acute suicidal ideations and behaviors), are best treated by a psychiatric clinician. Psychiatric emergencies are best treated in emergency settings to ensure staff and patient safety. Thus, in emergency presentations—such as those requiring immediate psychiatric and medical interventions or those where the patient complains of physical distress and mood or anxiety disorders—referral by primary care clinicians to an emergency facility is appropriate.

■ ANXIETY DISORDERS

Definition and Scope

Anxiety disorders affect an estimated 18% or 40 million Americans each year and occur in women twice as often as in men (Kessler et al., 2005). Anxiety disorders tend to run in families and often go unrecognized and under treated in primary care (Kessler, Petukhova, Sampson, Zaslavsky, & Wittchen, 2012). According to the National Comorbidity Replication Survey, the lifetime prevalence of anxiety disorders is 28.8%, mood disorders is 20.8%, and substance abuse is 14.6% (Kessler et al., 2005). The median age of onset for anxiety disorders is 11 years (Kessler et al., 2005). Findings from the National Comorbidity Replication Survey (Cougle, Keough, Riccardi, & Sachs-Ericsson, 2009) demonstrated that social anxiety, PTSD, GAD, and PD were predictors of suicidal ideation. Further analyses of these data indicated that women with all four anxiety disorders had a greater risk of suicidal ideation or suicide attempts when compared with men, whose risks increased with PTSD and PD (Cougle et al., 2009). Anxiety disorders are pervasive, disabling, and generally coexist with mood and other psychiatric disorders. Women tend to present with co-occurring mood and personality disorders, variables that adversely impact treatment outcomes.

Etiology

Anxiety disorders are caused by a multitude of factors as described above. Additional specific factors are specified in the following sections addressing specific diagnoses.

Treatment/Management

Documented poor treatment outcomes in primary care settings relate to the numerous physical complaints that dominate a woman's concerns and obscure complaints of anxiety-related symptoms; her beliefs, knowledge, and attitudes toward mental health services; realities of time constraints and competing demands placed on primary care clinicians to quickly assess, treat, and monitor treatment response; and clinician's lack of knowledge about current psychiatric treatment guidelines (Kessler et al., 2012). Even those who are accurately diagnosed with anxiety disorders in primary care settings have gaps in the continuum of care they receive as evidenced by poor adherence to medication, inadequate follow-up and monitoring, and rare exposure to effective evidence-based psychotherapies, such as cognitive behavioral therapy (CBT; Beck et al., 1985). Growing evidence indicates the effectiveness of CBT in the treatment of postpartum depression (PPD). In a recent study of women diagnosed with *DSM-IV* criteria, PPD (*n* = 45) researchers concluded that monotherapy CBT demonstrated superior outcomes after 12 weeks when compared with monotherapy SSRI (e.g., sertraline) and combined CBT and SSRI. Implications from these findings offer additional choices for women suffering from PPD (Milgrom et al., 2015).

SELF-MANAGEMENT MEASURES

Women can be taught stress management (e.g., journaling), relaxation techniques (e.g., muscle relaxation exercises), and deep-breathing exercises to aid in their management of anxiety.

COMPLEMENTARY AND ALTERNATIVE MEDICINE

Referral to a mental health clinician is imperative and provides a woman with access to various psychotherapeutic interventions such as pharmacotherapy and CBT. CBT is an empirically based, time-limited psychotherapy approach that has demonstrated effectiveness in the treatment of vast psychiatric and substance-use disorders, including depression and anxiety disorders. This structured approach centers on the interface among thoughts (cognitions), emotions (feelings), and behaviors. The success of this approach is often enhanced by a holistic and interdisciplinary approach that involves the nurse psychotherapist, patient, and primary care provider. Through various structured activities, such as homework assignments, the patient actively develops adaptive problem-solving and coping behaviors. Homework assignments can help her challenge anxiety-provoking thoughts and feelings and substitute these for realistic and positive thoughts and adaptive coping behaviors. Typically, there are weekly sessions for 6 to 12 weeks, although longer treatment demonstrates greater improvement.

PHARMACOTHERAPEUTICS

Because of the biological nature of anxiety and mood disorders, some clients may not benefit from the sole treatment of CBT and require pharmacological interventions depending on the severity and debilitation associated with their illness. Specific agents used in various types of anxiety disorders are delineated in the following sections.

Considerations for Special Populations

PREGNANCY AND ANXIETY DISORDERS

Anxiety disorders presenting during pregnancy can have deleterious effects on both mother and fetus. Evidence implicates pregnancy as one of the most stressful and emotional periods in a woman's life. Biological factors associated with increased estrogen and progesterone levels, coupled with psychosocial stress and anxiety about her personal health and those of the developing fetus and associated lifestyle risks increase the possibility of anxiety, mood disorders, and exacerbating preexisting psychiatric conditions.

Early screening for anxiety disorders during pregnancy and the postpartum period are critical to identifying women at risk and initiating appropriate interventions to reduce harm to the mother and child (Milgrom et al., 2015). The aim of treatment during pregnancy and the postpartum period is to employ interventions to minimize toxic exposure to the woman and the child. The high co-occurrence of major depression with GAD and panic attacks warrant concern and further evaluation. Left untreated, anxiety disorders increase the risk of harm to the developing child including premature preterm birth, low birth weight, and attention deficits (Mortazavi, Chaman, Mousavi, Khosravi, & Ajami, 2013). The high incidence of anxiety disorders during pregnancy and potential long-term effects on the mother, infant, and family makes it critical to discuss holistic and empirically based treatment options. Empirically based treatment options include antidepressants, CBTs, and relaxation techniques (Goodman, Chenausky, & Freeman, 2014).

Panic Disorder

ETIOLOGY

PD, one of the most debilitating and costly anxiety disorders, is associated with high co-occurrence with depression, physical symptom burden, functional impairment, suicide risk, and increased use of health care services. Women are twice as likely as men to present with PD with or without agoraphobia. Symptoms occur suddenly "out of the blue"; are repeated with no warning; and can result in alcohol or substance abuse, depression, and social and occupational impairment (APA, 2013). Women are more likely than men to present with multiple somatic complaints.

EVALUATION/ASSESSMENT AND SYMPTOMS

PD can present with and without agoraphobia (APA, 2013). Clinical features of PD generate substantial distress and fearfulness, which are often mistaken for medical conditions, such as "having a heart attack" or fears of "going crazy," mainly because of autonomic arousal and heightened anxiety level. Women with PD often present in emergency departments complaining of chest pain, dizziness, heart palpitations, diaphoresis, and intense anxiety. Agoraphobia refers to anxiety about being in open places or situations in which escape is embarrassing or difficult (e.g., standing in line or crowds or traveling over a bridge). Anxiety-provoking situations are usually avoided or tolerated. In the latter situation, she experiences intense anxiety and distress or chooses to be accompanied by a friend or family member. First symptoms of PD are rare during childhood, but usually occur during adolescence or early adulthood and often follow a chronic and remitting course (APA, 2013).

Normally panic attacks emerge rapidly, reach a peak within 10 minutes of increasingly worse intensity, and generate feelings of doom and gloom. Normal duration is 20 to 30 minutes, and rarely 1 hour. Attacks tend to occur two to three times a week. Clinicians must inquire if the panic attack was expected (generated by a stressful situation) or unexpected. Unexpected panic attacks are classic symptoms of PD. A question about the focus on anxiety or fear is equally significant in distinguishing PD from other anxiety disorders. A lack of focus is also common in PD. MSE during the attack reveals difficulty speaking, memory deficits, and stammering. Loss of control and sense of helplessness often generate depression during the attack. Symptoms abate quickly or gradually with a sense of exasperation.

DIFFERENTIAL DIAGNOSES

The first concern is to rule out potentially life-threatening medical illness such as a heart attack or endocrine disorders (e.g., hyperthyroidism, drug intoxication, or withdrawal). Diagnosis of PD using *DSM-5* criteria (Box 40.3; APA, 2013) can be complicated because of physical symptoms that are manifested and obscured co-occurring psychiatric disorders.

TREATMENT/MANAGEMENT

Clinical findings from the physical examination are critical in treating PD along with reassuring her that she is not dying or "going crazy." Presenting data from the physical examinations, such as a normal EKG and standard diagnostic laboratory studies, provides objective data concerning her symptoms.

Once a definitive diagnosis of PD is confirmed, treatment options are discussed to develop a plan of care that considers gender factors, preferences, and cultural considerations. In general, two approaches to treatment are available: pharmacotherapy and psychotherapeutic. Effective treatment outcomes are associated with combined therapies.

Complementary and Alternative Medicine • Women with PD should be referred to a qualified mental health clinician for psychotherapy, such as CBT, to address distorted cognitions that generate anxiety. Relaxation and deep-breathing exercises are also useful in controlling the physiological response to anxiety-provoking situations.

Pharmacotherapeutics • Primary care clinicians may prescribe pharmacotherapeutics to manage the biological basis of anxiety disorders in collaboration with a mental health clinician that provides psychotherapy.

Acute Management • Benzodiazepines offer rapid, limited relief to women with acute panic attacks by reducing the frequency and intensity of an attack (Sadock, Sadock, & Sussman, 2014). Benzodiazepines are contraindicated in women with a history of substance-use disorder. Although benzodiazepines were the mainstay treatment of anxiety disorders and have been extensively studied, concerns about potential for dependence, cognitive impairment, and abuse, particularly with long-term use, challenge clinicians to use

---

BOX 40.3   PANIC DISORDER

Diagnostic Criteria   300.01 (F41.0)

A. Recurrent unexpected panic attacks. A panic attack is an abrupt surge of intense fear or intense discomfort that reaches a peak within minutes, and during which time four (or more) of the following symptoms occur:

Note: The abrupt surge can occur from a calm state or an anxious state.

1. Palpitations, pounding heart, or accelerated heart rate
2. Sweating
3. Trembling or shaking
4. Sensations of shortness of breath or smothering
5. Feelings of choking
6. Chest pain or discomfort
7. Nausea or abdominal distress
8. Feeling dizzy, unsteady, light-headed, or faint
9. Chills or heat sensations
10. Paresthesias (numbness or tingling sensations)
11. Derealization (feelings of unreality) or depersonalization (being detached from one-self)
12. Fear of losing control or "going crazy"
13. Fear of dying

Note: Culture-specific symptoms (e.g., tinnitus, neck soreness, headache, uncontrollable screaming

or crying) may be seen. Such symptoms should not count as one of the four required symptoms.

B. At least one of the attacks has been followed by 1 month (or more) of one or both of the following:
   1. Persistent concern or worry about additional panic attacks or their consequences (e.g., losing control, having a heart attack, "going crazy").
   2. A significant maladaptive change in behavior related to the attacks (e.g., behavior designed to avoid having panic attacks, such as avoidance of exercise or unfamiliar situations).

C. The disturbance is not attributable to the physiological effects of a substance (e.g., a drug of abuse, a medication) or another medical condition (e.g., hyperthyroidism, cardiopulmonary disorders).

D. The disturbance is not better explained by another mental disorder (e.g., the panic attacks do not occur only in response to feared social situations, as in social anxiety disorder; in response to circumscribed phobic objects or situations, as in specific phobia; in response to obsessions, as in obsessive-compulsive disorder; in response to reminders of traumatic events, as in posttraumatic stress disorder; or in response to separation from attachment figures, as in separation anxiety disorder).

Reprinted with permission from the *Diagnostic and Statistical Manual of Mental Disorders,* Fifth Edition (Copyright © 2013). American Psychiatric Association. All Rights Reserved.

these medications sparingly and carefully monitor for signs of dependence. Alprazolam, a common high-potency benzodiazepine used to treat PD, has been linked to a discontinuation syndrome after regular dosing of only 6 to 8 weeks' duration. Slowly tapering these agents, particularly after chronic use, reduces discontinuation syndrome. Suggestions for tapering depend on the patient, duration of treatment, and medication potency and half-life. For instance, alprazolam must be decreased by 0.5 mg/week; faster tapering increases the risk of seizures and delirium (Sadock et al., 2014). Agents with a long half-life (e.g., clonazepam) have a propensity to cause impaired daytime sleepiness or "hangover"; however, they require less frequent dosing and may be more useful in acute and maintenance treatment. Shorter half-life agents (e.g., alprazolam) carry a higher risk of withdrawal and rebound between doses and require frequent dosing. Apart from the potential for dependence and abuse, additional side effects are few such as sedation, fatigue, and confusion. Side effects are usually managed with dose adjustment. As confusion and disorientation are especially common in older adults, these agents should be used cautiously in this age group.

Some patients find it comforting to carry a dose or two with them in the event they have an attack. The association and conditioning of ending the attack with a benzodiazepine is often helpful in allaying anxiety. It also offers control over an anxiety-related situation and their physiological responses, and thus empowers them to self-manage their condition.

Antidepressants: Maintenance Treatment • Antidepressants have demonstrated efficacy in the treatment of panic attacks and mitigating anticipatory and avoidance behaviors, which are core symptoms of PD. They are also effective for treating coexisting major depression. SSRIs (Table 40.2) are generally well tolerated and should be considered first-line treatment for PD (Sadock et al., 2014). Therapeutic effects have been observed in 1 to 2 weeks. Initially, these agents may increase anxiety. SSRIs must not be taken within 14 days of other antidepressant agents, such as monoamine oxidase inhibitors (MAOIs) and hypericum perforatum (St. John's wort), because of serious drug interactions. Careful patient education about desired and adverse effects along with the time required to reduce anxiety is imperative.

In addition to SSRIs, selective norepinephrine reuptake inhibitors (SNRIs) and dual-acting antidepressants, such as venlafaxine (regular or extended release), should also be considered for maintenance treatment. Venlafaxine is a potent inhibitor of both serotonin and norepinephrine and a weak inhibitor of dopamine. These medications are safe, well tolerated, and effective for preventing relapse in outpatients with PD and in treating major depression (Andrisano, Chiesa, & Serretti, 2013). SSRIs have proven efficacy in treating women with PD and/or co-occurring major depressive illness (Popovic, Vieta, Fornaro, & Perugi, 2015). Of these agents, paroxetine and paroxetine controlled release (CR) are particularly effective (Cameron, Habert, Anand, & Furtado, 2014).

Starting doses of antidepressants should be low and gradually titrated up until efficacy is achieved (Table 40.3). The starting dose of medications used to treat PD is usually one-half the starting dose used to treat depression. Age-related changes and medical conditions should also be considered when deciding the initial dose. Normally, 4 to 6 weeks are

TABLE 40.2	Common Major Side Effects Associated With SSRIs
SYSTEM	POTENTIAL EFFECTS
CNS	■ Headaches (most common), activation of mania or hypomania, hyperkinesia, aggressive reactions ■ Insomnia ■ Anxiety, nervousness, dizziness ■ Fatigue, sedation ■ Fine tremor ■ Akathisia (primarily with fluoxetine) ■ Nocturnal bruxism ■ Concentration disturbances, lightheadedness
GI	■ Nausea (most common), vomiting ■ Diarrhea (especially sertraline; normally abates after 10–14 days, reduced by food) ■ Weight gain
Cardiovascular	■ Palpitations ■ Hot flashes
Endocrine/metabolic	■ Induced syndrome of inappropriate secretion of antidiuretic hormone (SIADH) ■ Elevated prolactin levels
Genitourinary	■ Sexual dysfunction ■ Decreased libido ■ Orgasmic disturbances
Respiratory	■ Rhinitis ■ Cough ■ URI
Musculoskeletal	■ Asthenia ■ Myalgia
Miscellaneous	■ Fever ■ Fatigue ■ Taste disturbances

CNS, central nervous system; GI, gastrointestinal; SSRIs, selective serotonin reuptake inhibitors; URI, upper respiratory infection.
Adapted from American Psychiatric Association (2013); Gelenberg et al. (2010); National Institutes of Mental Health (2009, 2011); Sadock, Sadock, and Sussman (2014).

necessary to achieve a therapeutic response and she should continue taking the medication for at least 12 months (Cameron et al., 2014; National Institutes of Mental Health, 2011; Sadock et al., 2014). Follow-up and close monitoring are important to evaluate for response, side effects, and suicide risk and any needed medication adjustment.

SSRIs and SNRIs cannot be discontinued abruptly as this may precipitate a withdrawal syndrome. The syndrome is primarily associated with paroxetine and SSRIs with short half-lives and patients must be warned not to stop the medication abruptly. Hallmark features of this syndrome include dizziness, especially with head motion, dry mouth, rebound anxiety, sleep disturbances, headaches, and cognitive disturbances. It is time-limited and symptoms abate spontaneously in 3 weeks. This syndrome is associated with daily dosing of

TABLE 40.3	Suggested Dosing for Antidepressants Used to Treat Panic Disorder	
ANTIDEPRESSANT	**STARTING DOSE PER DAY**	**MAINTENANCE DOSE PER DAY**
Fluoxetine	5–10 mg	20 mg
Paroxetine	5–10 mg	20–40 mg
Paroxetine CR	12.5 mg	25 mg
Citalopram	10 mg	20–40 mg
Escitalopram	5 mg	10–20 mg
Sertraline	12.5–25 mg	50–200 mg
Nefazodone	100–200 mg BID	300–600 mg
Bupropion-SR-IR XR	150 mg 100 mg BID 150 mg	450 mg 300 mg (divided 150 mg) 450 mg
Venlafaxine	37.5 mg	75 mg once daily
Desvenlafaxine	50 mg	50–400 mg
Duloxetine	40–60 mg	60 mg
Levomilnacipran	40 mg	Up to 120 mg
Vortioxetine	10 mg	20 mg
Vilazodone	10 mg	20–40 mg
Mirtazapine	15 mg	15–45 mg

BID, twice a day.
Adapted from American Psychiatric Association (2013); Gelenberg et al. (2010); National Institutes of Health (2009, 2011); Sadock, Sadock, and Sussman (2014).

at least 6 weeks (Sadock et al., 2014). When discontinued, it should be gradually tapered over a 2- to 3-week period (Sadock et al., 2014). Long-acting SSRIs, such as fluoxetine, are less likely to precipitate this syndrome.

Adrenergic Receptor Antagonists (Alpha-Adrenergic Blockers) • The off-label use of adrenergic receptor antagonists for anxiety disorders continues to be explored. Preliminary findings from agents used to treat acute and chronic symptoms of stress-related anxiety support the efficacy of these agents in reducing physiological aspects of anxiety, sleep disturbances, nightmares, and memory consolidation, particularly with PTSD (Raskind et al., 2013; Writer, Meyer, & Schillerstrom, 2014). The course and chronicity of trauma-related anxiety or PD may be lessened using these agents (Hudson, Whiteside, Lorenz, & Wargo, 2012).

Propranolol and other beta blockers suppress acute biological symptoms of panic attacks such as racing heart, palpitations, and sweating. Major side effects associated with these agents include reduced blood pressure, bradycardia, drowsiness, and depression. They should be avoided in patients with a history of asthma or congestive heart failure.

CONSIDERATIONS FOR SPECIAL POPULATIONS

Benzodiazepines should not be prescribed during pregnancy as they freely cross the placenta, accumulate in fetal circulation, and have teratogenic properties (e.g., cleft palate). They are present in breast milk at sufficient levels to produce adverse effects in the newborn. The precise effects on the newborn continue to be researched; however, they are metabolized slowly in the newborn and can accumulate.

Generalized Anxiety Disorder

SCOPE AND ETIOLOGY

GAD is among the most common psychiatric conditions, affecting 8% to 10% of the general population, and is more prevalent in women than in men (APA, 2013; Haller, Cramer, Lauche, Gass, & Dobos, 2014). The 12-month prevalence of GAD varies from 2% to 9% and even higher in primary care settings (Kessler et al., 2012). An estimated 8% of all primary care visits are patients with GAD of whom a large percentage experience co-occurring major depression (Kessler et al., 2008; Ohaeri & Awadalla, 2012). Similar to other anxiety disorders, GAD usually begins in childhood and continues throughout adulthood. It is highly heritable and often coexists with other anxiety and mood disorders. Major depression is the most common co-occurring psychiatric condition in women with GAD (Kessler et al., 2005). PD has been found in 25% of those with GAD because of overlapping symptoms (Kessler et al., 2005). Twin studies suggest a shared genetic vulnerability to anxiety disorders, including GAD and major depression (Oathes, Hilt, & Nitschke, 2015).

EVALUATION/ASSESSMENT

Women with GAD typically complain of excessive worrying about everyday life, muscle tension, headaches, and exaggerated attentiveness. Clinically, they exhibit free-floating anxiety, unfocused anxiety, and are overly anxious. Cognitive vigilance often manifests as irritability and agitation. Similar to other anxiety disorders, symptoms are chronic, disabling, and involve extensive health care utilization, particularly in primary care settings. Chief complaints are usually somatic: headaches, GI disturbances, and sleep disturbances (Antai-Otong, 2009).

DIFFERENTIAL DIAGNOSES

Differential diagnosis is based on findings from physical and psychiatric evaluation, including the mental status examination and diagnostic physical workup. Because of the high prevalence of co-occurrence, depression, other anxiety disorders, and substance-use disorders must be ruled out. The

DSM-5 criteria include all of the following major symptoms of GAD (APA, 2013):

- Excessive worrying that occurs more days than not for at least 6 months, major focus on everyday issues, such as children, work, and home
- Difficulty controlling the worry
- Anxiety is associated with three of more of the following:
  - Restlessness, on edge, keyed up
  - Iirritability
  - Easily fatigued
  - Difficulty concentrating
  - Muscle tension
  - Sleep disturbances—difficulty falling or staying asleep or nonrestorative sleep
- Does not meet criteria for other anxiety disorders
- Symptoms significantly interfere with usual activities
- Symptoms are not associated with an underlying medical condition or substance induced

TREATMENT/MANAGEMENT

Early diagnosis, appropriate treatment, collaboration with mental health clinicians, and adherence to treatment offer hope to women suffering from GAD. In the case of coexisting major depression, treatment involves antidepressants and anxiolytic agents such as buspirone. When there is evidence of active or past alcohol or other substance-use disorders, she must be referred for evaluation and treatment for chemical dependency and subsequently treated for GAD and concomitant psychiatric disorders.

Pharmacotherapeutics • SSRI and novel antidepressant medications (e.g., venlafaxine, venlafaxine CR, mirtazapine, and buspirone) have demonstrated efficacy in the treatment of GAD (Alaka et al., 2014). Treatment considerations for women presenting with GAD are similar to those used to manage PD. Venlafaxine is also effective in treating comorbid major depression and social anxiety disorder (SAD), formerly known as social phobia. Dosing for venlafaxine or venlafaxine CR is titrated up gradually based on reduction of target symptoms of muscle tension, sleep disturbances, restlessness, agitation, and concentration disturbances (Sadock et al., 2014). Side effects associated with venlafaxine are similar to the central nervous system (CNS), GI, and sexual side effects caused by SSRIs (Table 40.1). Excessive diaphoresis and elevated blood pressure may also occur.

Buspirone has anxiolytic and mild serotonergic properties and has proven efficacy in the treatment of GAD and concomitant major depression (Bandelow et al., 2013). Its low potential for tolerance, abuse, or dependency makes it an excellent option for patients in which tolerance and addiction are concerns (Sadock et al., 2014). Buspirone also produces minimal cognitive deficits and can be used in those with a history of substance-related disorders. Major disadvantages include the length of time to produce anxiolytic effects (i.e., 2–4 weeks) and the need for regular use to reduce anxiety (versus as needed use with benzodiazepines). Common side effects associated with buspirone include headaches, dizziness,

lightheadedness, nervousness, and GI disturbances. Because this agent affects dopamine receptors, there is a risk of extrapyramidal side effects, especially when combined with antipsychotic agents. Hypomania and mania have been observed, primarily in older adults who do not meet criteria for bipolar disorder. Safety in pregnancy or lactation is not established.

Social Anxiety Disorder

DEFINITION, SCOPE, AND ETIOLOGY

The lifetime prevalence of SAD is about 12.1% (Kessler et al., 2005). Social phobia is an anxiety disorder characterized by extreme fear and phobic avoidance of social and performance situations and associated with reduced quality of life (APA, 2013). It may be associated with PD and GAD. More than 50% of people with SAD have coexisting major depression (Kessler et al., 2005). This potentially disabling anxiety disorder occurs equally in men and in women and affects about 15 million American adults (Kessler et al., 2005).

EVALUATION/ASSESSMENT AND SYMPTOMS

In general, women with SAD express fear and sensitivity to criticism from others associated with social or performance situations, resulting in distress and functional impairment (APA, 2013). Women with SAD tend to experience anxiety when presented with the phobic stimulus.

DIFFERENTIAL DIAGNOSES

Co-occurring psychiatric conditions, such as PD, GAD, and major depression, may make if difficult to distinguish symptoms from SAD. A comprehensive physical and psychiatric evaluation is needed to rule out underlying medical conditions. *DSM-5* criteria for SAD are as follows (APA, 2013):

- Persistent and exaggerated fear of social situations in which the person is exposed to possible scrutiny by others
- Exposure to feared social situations evokes intense anxiety
- The person recognizes the fear is unreasonable or excessive
- The person avoids the feared social situations or endures them with significant distress and anxiety
- Avoidance of social situations interferes significantly with the person's social, occupational, academic, and interpersonal relationships
- Symptoms persist for at least 6 months
- Symptoms are not related to underlying general medical conditions or substance-use disorders

TREATMENT/MANAGEMENT

Coexisting anxiety disorders and major depression increase the risk of suicide (Cougle et al., 2009). Throughout treatment it is imperative to monitor the woman's response, evaluate her sense of helplessness and hopelessness, and collaborate with a mental health clinician to ensure access to psychotherapeutic interventions such as CBT. CBT empowers women to understand the basis of their fears and challenge distorted thoughts that contribute to depression, anxiety, and reduced functionality and quality of life.

Pharmacotherapeutics • It is widely documented that SSRIs, SNRIs, and other novel antidepressants are effective in managing SAD or social phobia. Mirtazapine is effective in treating SAD because it enhances serotonergic function distinct from reuptake inhibition by disinhibiting the norepinephrine activation, thus ultimately increasing serotonergic transmission (Sadock et al., 2014). These properties allow mirtazapine to allay anxiety and sleep disturbances and increase appetite. It is also a potent histamine-1 (H_1) receptor blocker.

Major side effects associated with mirtazapine include somnolence, dry mouth, weight gain, and constipation. It may also increase liver enzyme levels and produce reversible blood dyscrasias (i.e., agranulocytosis) requiring a baseline CBC with differential at baseline and for monitoring. Because of this side effect, this medication is not used during pregnancy or lactation.

Obsessive-Compulsive Disorder

DEFINITION, SCOPE, AND ETIOLOGY

The prevalence of obsessive-compulsive disorder (OCD) is approximately 1.6% (APA, 2013). Although the treatment of this complex anxiety disorder should occur in mental health settings, it is important for the primary care clinician to recognize its prevalence and major symptoms in order to make a provisional diagnosis and refer. This anxiety disorder affects women and men equally and is highly heritable. Depression commonly coexists with OCD and heightens the risk of poor outcomes, suicide, and substance abuse. OCD tends to have a sudden onset following a stressful event, such as a pregnancy, sexual assault, or significant loss.

EVALUATION/ASSESSMENT AND DIFFERENTIAL DIAGNOSES

Characteristically, the patient recognizes that her behaviors are unreasonable, but she has difficulty controlling impulses or ritualistic behaviors to allay anxiety generated by obsessions. Patients with OCD often seek treatment for physical problems and, because of embarrassment and secrecy about irrational behaviors and thoughts, they seldom mention them during encounters with primary care clinicians. Diagnosis is seldom made until 5 or 10 years after onset, making it difficult to treat this chronic condition. Questions about ritualistic or compulsive behaviors must be asked. *DSM-5* clinical features of OCD include obsession(s), compulsion(s), or both (APA, 2013):

- *Obsessions*—recurrent persistent thoughts, impulses, or images that produce anxiety and distress
- *Compulsions*—repetitive behaviors or mental acts performed in response to obsessions

And each of the following (APA, 2013):

- The person recognizes that the compulsions or obsessions are unreasonable
- Obsessions or compulsions disrupt the person's normal activities, cause significant distress, or take a great deal of time
- Compulsions or obsessions exceed the focus of any other Axis I disorder the person may have
- Symptoms cannot arise from an underlying medical condition or be induced by substances

TREATMENT/MANAGEMENT

Major challenges for primary care clinicians are the patient's reluctance to adhere to medications and resistance to accepting a referral to a mental health clinician for psychotherapy to address underlying issues associated with OCD symptoms and behaviors (Cuijpers et al., 2014). Collaboration with a mental health clinician is imperative.

Pharmacotherapeutics • Antidepressants used to treat other anxiety conditions extend to OCD. The first-line approach is to start with an SSRI or clomipramine, a tricyclic antidepressant. Clomipramine is the first drug approved by the Food and Drug Administration (FDA) for treatment of OCD. Studies indicate that using combination exposure therapy and clomipramine may be superior to monotherapy with clomipramine (Cuijpers et al., 2014). Improvement is seen in 2 to 4 weeks, but symptoms may continue to abate over 4 to 5 months. Primary side effects of clomipramine include dry mouth, sedation, seizures, significant weight gain, and cardiac arrhythmias. Before prescribing clomipramine, routine screening for seizures and cardiovascular disease is necessary because of its cardiotoxic properties and seizure risk (Krebs, Waszczuk, Zavos, Bolton, & Eley, 2015; Sadock et al., 2014).

Fluvoxamine, an SSRI, is also approved for OCD (Seibell & Hollander, 2014). The side-effect profile is the same as other SSRIs (Table 40.1) except it has numerous drug–drug interactions. Higher doses need to be divided for bid dosing (Sadock et al., 2014).

Posttraumatic Stress Disorder

SCOPE, ETIOLOGY, AND RISK FACTORS

PTSD affects about 7.7 million American adults; however, it can occur at any age (APA, 2013; Mitchell, Mazzeo, Schlesinger, Brewerton, & Smith, 2012). Women are twice as likely to develop PTSD as men because of the increased lifespan likelihood of being a survivor of violence (APA, 2013). Women are 4.9 times as likely to experience violence before the age of 25 years as men and are more likely to report a coexisting major depression and anxiety disorder (Street, Gradus, Giasson, Vogt, & Resick, 2013). In addition, the growing number of women deployed during the Iraq and Afghanistan wars exposes them to additional stressors (e.g., sexual harassment) and the risk of PTSD. Although PTSD is not an inevitable consequence of trauma exposure, 10%

of women who experience trauma develop this psychiatric disorder (APA, 2013). Women diagnosed with PTSD usually have experienced or witnessed an overwhelming, life-threatening traumatic event that generates fear, anxiety, horror, disbelief, and self-blame (Chung & Breslau, 2008). Trauma exposure is most likely to occur among survivors of rape, childhood trauma, military warfare and confinement, physical assault, IPV, or threats of harm (APA, 2013).

EVALUATION/ASSESSMENT

The *DSM-5* (APA, 2013) definition of PTSD has undergone considerable changes. Primary changes include the removal of emotional reactions to trauma exposure as part of Criterion A. Manifestations of PTSD symptoms vary among individuals. Depending on the nature of the trauma and when it occurred (acute versus chronic symptoms), it is imperative to accept and believe the woman's perception of the event, avoid pressing for details to avoid retraumatization, express genuine concern, and use a nonjudgmental approach. Support and safety are principal interventions following acute trauma exposure. Inquire about recent stressors and be mindful of the difficulty she may have in sharing the experience. Fears of not being believed or understood are common barriers to sharing a painful emotional experience. Clinicians must be able to distinguish normal stress reactions from PTSD. Health education about normal stress reactions is critical to "normalizing" her feelings, thoughts, and behaviors.

Most women with PTSD present immediately following the attack for injury evaluation or later with somatic complaints such as fatigue and sleep problems. She may express difficulty going out at night because of concerns about personal safety. Her mental status examination may reveal hyper vigilance and that she is easily startled; however, findings are individual and depend on the acuteness and nature of the event and availability of quality support. Based on her mental status examination, it is vitally important to evaluate and understand the nature of her distress and precipitating stressors.

A woman with a history of trauma-related anxiety, such as military sexual trauma and/or rape trauma syndrome, may appear calm or distraught or in a "state of shock" (e.g., dissociation) and have difficulty believing what happened to her and/or providing details about the event. She must have time to respond to questions. For women presenting later with somatic symptoms, asking about a history of trauma may be the first indication she has suffered an unresolved traumatic event.

Routine screening for IPV or other trauma exposure events, especially in women of childbearing age, is recommended by some professional organizations. Clinicians must be cognizant of state laws governing how to report IPV and work with local agencies to ensure patient and family safety.

DIFFERENTIAL DIAGNOSES

A comprehensive psychiatric evaluation, physical examination, and diagnostic studies provide the basis for determining what differential diagnoses to consider. *DSM-5* criteria for PTSD include all of the following (APA, 2013):

- Exposure to an overwhelming traumatic or stressful event that threatens life/personal integrity or causes intense fear, horror, or helplessness
- The traumatic event is persistently reexperienced in one or more of the following:
  - Nightmares or distressing dreams of the event
  - Autonomic arousal when exposed to trauma reenactment
  - Intrusive-repeated reliving the event; flashbacks, intense emotional distress when exposed to trauma reenactment
  - Physical or psychological distress to cues/reminders of the event
- Persistent avoidance of the stimuli linked to the traumatic event (not present before the event) as evidenced by three or more of the following related to the trauma:
  - Inability to remember important aspects of the event
  - Avoiding people, places, and objects
  - Inability to recall important aspects of the trauma
  - Feelings of detachment or distance from others
  - Reduced interest in activities
  - Avoiding thoughts and reminders of the event
  - Foreshortened perspective of own future, no self-view for future
- Persistent symptoms of arousal such as:
  - Decreased sleep
  - Increased anger outbursts, agitation
  - Hyperarousal
  - Hypervigilance
  - Exaggerated startled response
- Duration of symptoms lasts more than 4 weeks
- Causes marked distress or impairment in functional abilities

TREATMENT/MANAGEMENT

Treatment considerations for PTSD must be individualized and target underlying symptoms and behaviors. Patients must be offered referral to a mental health clinician and encouraged to participate in psychotherapeutic approaches, including CBT and relaxation techniques, and maintain continuity with their clinicians.

Complementary and Alternative Medicine • Trauma-related symptoms can be ameliorated using several interventions: supportive counseling; CBT from a mental health clinician; education about normal stress reactions; learning and using simple stress-reduction exercises, such as deep breathing, sleep hygiene, and muscle relaxation; and participation in support groups to normalize reactions and receive ongoing support.

Pharmacotherapeutics • First-line treatment of PTSD is with SSRIs and novel antidepressants (Stein et al., 2013). Maintenance treatment of PTSD with SSRIs improves the psychiatric and clinical outcome of patients with the disorder and prevents relapse and symptom exacerbation (Jeffreys, Capehart, & Friedman, 2012).

Adrenergic-antagonist agents, such as propranolol, reveal promising results in the treatment of physiological and hyperarousal features of PTSD (Arnsten, Raskind, Taylor, & Connor, 2015; Hudson et al., 2012) and in preventing presynaptic norepinephrine receptors and reducing cortisol-mediated memories. They may also prevent consolidation of traumatic memories and fear conditioning 2 to 3 months posttrauma (Arnsten et al., 2015). Emerging evidence further indicates the efficacy of novel medications such as CRH receptor antagonists in the treatment of PTSD (Dunlop et al., 2014). Medications used in the treatment of PTSD are largely determined by coexisting psychiatric, substance use, and medical conditions and personal preferences.

CONSIDERATIONS FOR SPECIAL POPULATIONS

Exposure to trauma in pregnancy poses a unique danger to mother and child and is associated with a disproportionately high rate of PTSD. IPV remains a leading cause of death and is the second most common injury-related death during pregnancy (Samandari, Martin, & Schiro, 2010). Assaults during pregnancy generally occur in the abdomen and to the unborn child (Chu, Goodwin, & D'Angelo, 2010). High-risk factors associated with IPV and murder during pregnancy are being younger than age 20 years and receiving late or no prenatal care (Chu et al., 2010). Consequences of IPV during pregnancy include risk of depression, suicide, and substance-related disorders (Chung & Breslau, 2008; Devries et al., 2013).

A history of violence is common before the pregnancy and increased frequency during pregnancy. It is imperative to inquire or assess for IPV at all primary care visits. Besides pregnancy, women of childbearing age are at the greatest risk of trauma exposure, accounting for a lifetime range of 3.6% to 12.6% (Chu et al., 2010; Devries et al., 2013; Jackson et al., 2015).

■ MOOD DISORDERS ACROSS THE LIFE SPAN

Similar to most anxiety disorders, women are at a substantially higher risk for developing mood disorders than men. Some women may be more emotionally and physically sensitive during reproductive cycles and thus more vulnerable to mood disorders. Reasons for this disparity are poorly understood; however, fluctuating changes in female hormone levels across the life span may have a direct or indirect influence on mood. Clinicians should routinely screen women for mood disorders and collaborate with mental health clinicians to implement evidence-based treatment when appropriate to promote optimal functioning, reduce suicide risk, and improve quality of life.

Major Depressive Disorder

SCOPE AND ETIOLOGY

Lifetime prevalence of major depression in women (21.3%) is twice as common as in men (12.7%; Kessler et al., 2005).

This ratio has been documented worldwide and among diverse ethnic groups. One possible explanation is mood changes that correlate with reproductive and cyclic hormonal changes. Although cyclic hormonal changes are more noticeable during the childbearing years, they also occur during peri- and postmenopause (Soares, 2014).

It is interesting to note that despite the high prevalence of mood and anxiety disorders in women, until a decade ago or so, the inclusion of women of reproductive ages was limited or prohibited during early clinical trials. Although most epidemiological studies include a propronderance of women, there is a lack of consistent data that distinguishes gender-related interactions. Gender differences may play a vital role in the clinical manifestations of depression, namely its course, chronicity, and co-occurring psychiatric disorders (APA, 2013). Recent data indicate these earlier assertions were inconsistently found in women. However, treatment considerations that include psychopharmacology and psychotherapeutic approaches must be person-centered and based on the woman's needs, informed decision making, developmental stage, and presenting symptoms.

EVALUATION/ASSESSMENT

A comprehensive medical and psychiatric examination is necessary to differentiate major depression from medical and other psychiatric conditions. Queries and evaluation of mood changes that parallel hormonal changes, such as menstruation, pregnancy, postpartum, and peri- and postmenopause, provide invaluable data concerning treatment and management.

DIFFERENTIAL DIAGNOSES

Of particular importance is ruling out conditions such as hypothyroidism and certain cancers, such as pancreatic, that may manifest as depression, to ensure an accurate diagnosis and appropriate treatment. Co-occurring anxiety disorders complicate treatment and are associated with poor treatment outcomes and chronicity. *DSM-5* diagnostic criteria for major depression include persistent symptoms for at least 2 weeks, a change from prior functioning, include *either* a depressed mood *or* loss of interest in things that were once pleasurable *and* five of the following (APA, 2013):

- Depressed or sad mood
- Substantial loss of interest in things once considered important and pleasurable or anhedonia
- Significant appetite and weight disturbances—increased appetite results in weight gain and the reverse with poor appetite
- Sleep disturbances—difficulty staying asleep, waking up feeling tired, or increased sleep
- Fatigue
- Cognitive disturbances—difficulty concentrating, forgetfulness
- Feelings of worthlessness or excessive guilt
- Psychomotor agitation or retardation
- Thoughts of death or suicide

TREATMENT/MANAGEMENT

Pharmacological interventions are first-line treatment for women who present in primary care settings with unipolar and bipolar major depression. Referral for CBT is also needed.

Complementary and Alternative Medicine • CBT has proven efficacy as a sole or adjunct to medication treatment depending on severity of biological symptoms (e.g., psychomotor retardation, sleep disturbances). Regular exercise and stress management activities are also useful in coping with depression. Over-the-counter herbal preparations are available (e.g., St. John's wort, SAMe), but most have side effects that interfere with the efficacy of safety of prescribed antidepressants. Queries about herbal preparations must be a part of the initial history and physical and include health teachings about serious drug–drug and potentially fatal interactions, such as St. John's wort and SSRIs (e.g., serotonin syndrome)

Pharmacotherapeutics • Gender differences in responsivity and tolerability to SSRIs and tricyclic antidepressant medications have been identified. Earlier researchers asserted that women are more likely to have a greater response to SSRIs than tricyclic antidepressants than men because of gender-related neurobiological differences (e.g., estrogen; Young et al., 2009).

Premenstrual Dysphoric Disorder

SCOPE AND ETIOLOGY

PMDD is a distinct mood disorder that affects 3% to 8% of women of childbearing age (APA, 2013; Rapkin & Lewis, 2013; Yonkers, Vigod, & Ross, 2011). Mood disturbances emerge during the luteal phase of the menstrual cycle and cease shortly after the beginning of menses. Principal differences between major depressive episode and PMDD are its cyclic symptomatology and functional impairment. Although the precise cause of PMDD continues to be questioned, converging evidence links PMDD to an abnormal cyclic response to estrogen and progesterone and a heightened awareness of physical sensations and internal changes during this period (Rapkin & Lewis, 2013; Yonkers et al., 2011). Increased incidence of subsequent depression during pregnancy, postpartum, and perimenopause also parallel PMDD with dysregulation of neuroendrocrine processes including cortisol and hormonal levels and GABAergic and serotonergic neurocircuitry (Rapkin & Lewis, 2013; Yonkers et al., 2011).

EVALUATION/ASSESSMENT

Similar to other atypical depressive episodes, women with PMDD complain of a depressed mood, tension, anxiety, agitation, increased appetite, and sleep and concentration disturbances during the luteal phase of their menstrual cycle—core symptoms of PMDD. Headaches, muscle pain, bloating, and fatigue are also common.

DIFFERENTIAL DIAGNOSES

A definite diagnosis can be made when at least five core major depressive symptoms occur a week before menses and diminish several days after menses that produce global functional impairment similar to major depression for at least two cycles (APA, 2013).

TREATMENT/MANAGEMENT

Early treatment initiation offers relief for women suffering from PMDD and reduces the risk of future depressive episodes during pregnancy, postpartum, and perimenopause.

Pharmacotherapeutics • Increasingly, SSRIs have become the mainstay treatment of PMDD and may be used during the luteal phase or limited to duration of symptoms. However, SNRIs and clomipramine have also proven efficacy in the treatment of PMDD (Rapkin & Lewis, 2013; Yonkers et al., 2011).

Symptoms of PMDD respond to serotonin reuptake inhibitors when treatment is limited to 14 days of the menstrual cycle. Women with more severe PMDD may respond better to luteal-phase dosing than symptom-onset dosing (Cunningham, Yonkers, O'Brien, & Eriksson, 2009; Rapkin & Lewis, 2013). Although antidepressants are an integral part of treatment, there is mounting evidence that indicates a holistic approach that includes dietary considerations, complementary therapies, CBTs, and exercise, which may reduce symptoms and improve the quality of life in women with PMDD.

Bipolar Disorders I and II

SCOPE AND ETIOLOGY

Bipolar disorder affects 0.5% to 1.5% of individuals in the United States (APA, 2013). Typically, the onset of bipolar disorders in females occurs during adolescence and the early 20s, placing them at greater risk of episodes during reproductive years (APA, 2013). The initial episode is more likely to be depressive in women compared with manic in men. Women are also more likely than men to have the rapid-cycling form of the illness and to display depressive characteristics (APA, 2013). Bipolar disorder presents special challenges to women of reproductive age as well as to their families and clinicians. Problems include lower fertility rates, strong genetic loading, and potential fetal teratogenic risks, as well as high risks of illness recurrence if treatment is discontinued abruptly (Altshuler et al., 2010; Epstein, Moore, & Bobo, 2015). Bipolar disorders are highly prevalent with other psychiatric disorders such as substance-use disorder and personality disorders.

EVALUATION/ASSESSMENT

When evaluating women with major depressive symptoms, it is imperative to inquire about a past history of increased energy, decreased need for sleep, increased irritability, and engaging in pleasurable activities with a high risk of negative outcomes. This is important because an affirmative answer (Antai-Otong, 2009) may indicate either a manic or hypomanic episode that may or may not have been treated. Additional questions to elicit symptoms and to differentiate from major depression are listed in the following section as well as a comprehensive psychiatric and medical evaluation.

DIFFERENTIAL DIAGNOSES

This discussion is limited to manic and depressive episodes because of the difficulty in differentiating among rapid cycling, mixed type, and hypomania bipolar disorders. Women exhibiting bipolar disorder symptoms should be referred to a mental health clinician for diagnosis. *DSM-5* diagnostic criteria for major depression are noted above. *DSM-5* diagnostic criteria for manic and hypomanic episodes include each of the following, respectively (APA, 2013):

- Distinct period of abnormally and persistently elevated, expansive, or irritable mood, lasting at least 4 or more days for hypomanic and 1 week or more for manic
- Type I: at least one manic episode
- Type II: at least one hypomanic episode

Manic Episode
- During the period of mood disturbances *three or more* of the following occur:
  - Overblown self-esteem
  - Reduced need for sleep
  - Racing thoughts
  - Talkativeness; circumstantial, tangential, and pressured speech
  - Increased involvement with pleasurable activities, especially that can cause harm (e.g., shopping sprees)
  - Heightened goal-directed activity or agitation
  - Easily distracted by unimportant external stimuli

Hypomanic Episode
- During the period of mood disturbances, *three or more* of the symptoms listed with a manic episode occur and are:
  - Less severe than manic episode
  - Observable by others
  - Normally not severe enough to cause marked impairment in social or occupational performance or necessitate hospitalization
- Mood disturbance significant enough to impair usual function, risk of violence to self and others, or psychotic characteristics
- Symptoms are severe enough to cause marked global impairment or necessitate hospitalization to prevent harm to self or others or there are psychotic features
- Symptoms are not caused by other medical illness or substances

TREATMENT/MANAGEMENT

Bipolar disorders are serious, chronic disorders that require referral for management by an interdisciplinary mental health team. High suicide risk is common in bipolar disorders and requires close follow-up. One qualitative investigative study indicated the rate as high as 19% based on social factors and stigma (Owen, Gooding, Dempsey, & Jones, 2015). Treatment adherence is difficult in women with this disorder, making it difficult to reduce morbidity and mortality.

Pharmacotherapeutics

Manic Episode. Management of bipolar disorder is determined by the clinical presentation. A manic episode may present a psychiatric emergency requiring immediate pharmacological intervention. Early recognition and referral to psychiatric emergency services is critical to the safety of both the woman and the staff. Depending on the severity and nature of symptoms, haloperidol and lorazepam are administered intramuscularly to manage agitation, delusions, hallucinations, paranoia, and intense anxiety. Hospitalization is indicated to stabilize symptoms initially using atypical antipsychotic medications, such as quetiapine, lurasidone, and quetiapine XR (Carlborg, Thuresson, Fentoft, & Bodegard, 2015; McIntyre, Cha, Kim, & Mansur, 2013); monotherapy olanzapine; or lanzapine/fluoxetine and mood stabilizers, such as valproic acid, lithium, carbamazepine, or lamitrogine (McIntyre et al., 2013). Typically, mood stabilizers and lithium require 10 to 14 days to reach therapeutic serum levels. Because of serious side effects unique to each agent, specifically teratogenic side effects (Carlborg et al., 2015), baseline laboratory studies, including a pregnancy test, are vital to ensure safe treatment for women.

Bipolar Depression (Depressed Episode). Bipolar depression is often misdiagnosed as unipolar depression and treated with monotherapy antidepressants. The distinction between unipolar depression and bipolar depression is that the former is synonymous to major depression without a history of manic or hypomanic episodes. Initial symptoms of bipolar depression manifest as switching to a manic episode with monotherapy antidepressants and failure to respond to treatment. Quality of life in terms of duration and recurrence is significantly worse in women who suffer bipolar depression than bipolar-manic episodes. There is a paucity of research available for treatment of bipolar depression. Even more perplexing is a lack of data that monotherapy antidepressants are effective mood stabilizers in the treatment of bipolar depression. Ongoing controversy that indicates these agents need to be avoided to reduce the risk of mood-switching prevails. First-line considerations must include conventional mood stabilizers, such as lithium and valproic acid, and newer agents, including lamotrigine, and atypical antipsychotics. Atypical antipsychotic agents continue to demonstrate efficacy in treating both bipolar-manic and depressive episodes (McIntyre et al., 2013).

CONSIDERATIONS FOR SPECIAL POPULATIONS

Bipolar Disorder and Pregnancy • Management of bipolar illness in pregnancy is most difficult when the pregnancy is unplanned. Women with bipolar disorder are at high risk of symptom exacerbation during the immediate postpartum period and a recurrent episode after delivery (Epstein et al.,

2015). Among women with bipolar disorder who decide to discontinue therapy during the postpartum period, the estimated risk of relapse is substantially higher than for nonpregnant, nonpuerperal women. Relapse occurs rapidly with acute symptoms emerging a few weeks after delivery (Epstein et al., 2015).

General guidelines for the treatment of bipolar disorder from the APA (2013) were discussed earlier; however, serious concerns arise when these guidelines are applied in the treatment of pregnant and postpartum women (APA, 2013). The decision to treat depression during pregnancy has to be guided by considerations of risks associated with untreated depression along with potential adverse effects on fetal exposure to specific medications. No antidepressants are approved for use during pregnancy and all psychotropic medications cross the placenta and enter fetal circulation. Clinicians must carefully review all sources regarding medication side effects and adverse drug reactions in pregnant women, including the FDA category labeling, to determine risks and benefits of taking mood stabilizers, lithium, and other antimanic agents during pregnancy. Careful education of pregnant women and their significant others is needed.

Pregnancy and Mood Disorder • Despite the notion that pregnancy is a positive experience, many women experience tremendous stress and mood changes during this stage of life. Many are fearful of caring for a newborn and coping with the transition into motherhood. Pregnancy, similar to other reproductive events, actually heightens the risk of emotional stress, risk of mental health problems, and new onset or relapse of depression (Csaszar, Melichercikova, & Dubovicky, 2014). The occurrence of depression in pregnant women is estimated to be 13% to 20% (Csaszar et al., 2014). Women who have a history of depression during the nonpregnant period are at risk of relapse during pregnancy, even those currently euthymic (Csaszar et al., 2014). Hormonal changes, significant stressors, and discontinuation of antidepressant medications increase the risk of depression during pregnancy. Other risk factors include past history of major depression, inadequate social support, discontinuation or reduction of antidepressant medication, marital discord, and uncertainty about pregnancy (Csaszar et al., 2014).

Treatment/Management

Pharmacotherapeutics. Antidepressant medication should be considered during pregnancy if depressive symptoms are moderate to severe, or if withdrawal of maintenance medication is likely to result in recurrent depression. The potential benefits of using antidepressant medications in a pregnant or breastfeeding woman should be balanced against the potential risks to the newborn. Because of the risk of neonatal withdrawal syndrome, SSRIs should be used at the lowest effective dose during the third trimester of pregnancy and should be tapered before delivery (Weisskopf et al., 2015).

The primary goal of mental health treatment during pregnancy is full remission of depression to mitigate risk to mother and child during this period and the postpartum period. Early screening in women who are planning to get pregnant and those who are pregnant must be a priority to address the needs of women who are asymptomatic and symptomatic to educate them about treatment options, including risk-benefits, and managing their illness during and after pregnancy.

Pharmacological considerations for women with mood disorders during pregnancy necessitate an assessment and discussion with the client and significant others of the risks and benefits of treatment for both mother and child. Although there is growing consensus among researchers concerning the risk–benefit of antidepressant use during pregnancy in women with severe depression, others caution the overstated analysis of data implicating the safety of antidepressants during gestation (Toohey, 2012; Yonkers, Blackwell, Glover, & Forray, 2014). Risks associated with pharmacological treatment should be compared with the risks of not treating depression, which may include poor mother–infant bonding, infanticide, lifelong social and developmental delays and adjustment, suicide, poor maternal and fetal nutrition, and adverse neonatal obstetric outcome and the continuation of depression into the postpartum period (Toohey, 2012). As discussed earlier, poor medication management of psychiatric disorders during pregnancy and the postpartum period can have tragic consequences. Prevailing data indicate that most SSRIs are not major teratogens, except paroxetine (e.g., cardiac defects), but the ultimate treatment decision lies with the mother, spouse, and/or significant others. Before prescribing these agents, the risk of harm to the developing fetus versus benefits to the mother must be resolved case by case and requires careful discussion with the woman and her partner/spouse as part of the informed-consent process.

Agitation is a common cofeature of depression or mania and substance-use disorders, which manifests as abnormal and excessive verbal or physical aggression, intense anxiety and arousal, restlessness and agitation, and marked negative impact on global functioning. Data from several studies indicated that benzodiazepines and haloperidol are the most commonly used drugs for agitation during psychiatric emergencies. However, data failed to demonstrate efficacy in the treatment of agitation and combativeness specifically during pregnancy, but noted that the advent of atypical antipsychotics with or without benzodiazepines are comparable with haloperidol and benzodiazepines (MacDonald et al., 2012). In the absence of evidence-based practice guidelines and demonstrated effective or safe treatment of agitation in women, primary care clinicians must learn and employ verbal de-escalation and other means of security to manage these volatile situations.

Postpartum Depression

SCOPE AND ETIOLOGY

The incidence of PPD is relatively common and similar to rates of major depressive disorder in nonpregnant women, affecting 7% to 14% of women within 6 months of delivery (Yonkers et al., 2008). Moreover, 50% to 80% will experience the "blues" lasting 4 to 10 days (Yonkers et al., 2008). Risks associated with PPD include a prior history of major depression or PPD, current stressors, such as transitioning into motherhood, and socioeconomic issues. Untreated PPD can have acute and long-term deleterious effects on the overall social, physiological, and psychological well-being of the mother, newborn, and the entire family.

RISK FACTORS

Risk factors for PPD include (El-Hachem et al., 2014):

- Family or personal history of mood disorders (including PPD)
- Severe PMDD
- Psychosocial stressors, such as marital discord, financial problems, and so forth
- Limited or poor social support
- Mood instability during adolescence that caused severe distress
- Emotional reactivity to oral contraceptives leading to discontinuation
- Sadness, irritability, and mood disturbances during pregnancy
- Feelings of inadequacy as parent
- Sleep, appetite, and concentration disturbances

SYMPTOMS

Women with PPD often complain of fatigue, unexplained crying spells, irritability, sleep disturbances, anger, feelings of loss, and mild mood swings. Despite the high prevalence of PPD, many cases go unrecognized and untreated (Yonkers et al., 2008). Normally, most women experience PPD after the first 2 weeks postpartum; for some it occurs sooner (Yonkers et al., 2008). Symptoms usually begin during the third trimester. The incidence of PDD varies among cultures and ethnicities. Women with strong and quality social support and help with child care, meal preparation, feeding, and bathing tend to have a lower incidence of PDD (El-Hachem et al., 2014).

EVALUATION/ASSESSMENT

Symptoms and evaluation of PPD are similar to those for major depression. Postpartum "blues" are characterized by fluctuating mood, crying spells, irritability, anxiety, and sleep and appetite disturbances several weeks after delivery. Persistent symptoms that worsen during this period must be evaluated to distinguish a frank mood disorder from "postpartum blues." The Edinburgh Postnatal Depression Scale, a 10-item questionnaire, is a useful screening tool (Cox, Holden, & Sagovsky, 1987) that can be used during the early postpartum period. Women with PPD complain of mood, appetite, concentration, and sleep disturbances. Sleep problems involve difficulty sleeping even when the infant is asleep. A large number of women with PPD experience distressful and obsessional thoughts about harming their infants—although they are rarely acted on in the presence of nonpsychotic depression. Severe PPD concomitant with suicidal ideations heightens the risk of infanticide—not because of hatred of the infant, rather because of fears of abandonment with suicide (Nau, McNiel, & Binder, 2012). A history of PPD is associated with high prevalence and

recurrence with subsequent pregnancies. Queries about previous PPD are critical for prevention and management of this highly recurrent condition (Cox et al., 1987).

DIFFERENTIAL DIAGNOSES

A comprehensive physical and psychiatric evaluation helps distinguish PPD from other mood disorders, including postpartum blues and postpartum psychosis (see the following section). When symptoms of postpartum blues persist more than several weeks, she must be evaluated for PPD. PPD is diagnosed when symptoms of major depression emerge within 4 weeks of delivery using *DSM-5* criteria, which includes each of the following (APA, 2013):

- Either depressed mood or lack of interest or pleasure plus at least four additional symptoms, including:
  - Marked weight loss
  - Activity disruptions—overactive or slowed actions
  - Frequent sense of worthlessness or unwarranted guilt
  - Sleep disturbances
  - Concentration disturbances, indecisiveness
  - Daily fatigue or lack of energy
  - Suicidal ideations, thoughts of death
- Symptoms are not consistent with mixed depression
- Symptoms cause significant disruption in function and/or distress
- Symptoms are not caused by other medical illness or substances
- Symptoms are not caused by bereavement

TREATMENT/MANAGEMENT

Early screening of PPD and prompt initiation of pharmacological interventions are critical to symptom management to mitigate short- and long-term adverse consequences including functional deficits and newborn neglect that may negatively influence both mother–child bonding and the infant's mental and physical development (Toohey, 2012).

Complementary and Alternative Medicine • Health education and reassurance coupled with assuring home support for infant and self-care are usually adequate interventions for postpartum blues. These interventions are geared toward decreasing the likelihood of full-blown PPD, improving infant safety, and optimizing health for the mother–infant dyad.

Pharmacotherapeutics • No antidepressant or mood stabilizer has been endorsed as safe during lactation. When choosing an antidepressant or mood stabilizers, clinicians must consider the patient's previous response to medication, evidence-based data on efficacy, monotherapy, and flexible dosing.

First-line treatment for nonpsychotic PPD is based on the underlying psychiatric diagnosis. Unipolar PPD should be treated the same as any major depressive episode. Mainstay treatment for bipolar PPD should be the same as for bipolar I and II depression, and follow what was used for her most recent episode (see earlier discussed section).

Postpartum Psychosis

DEFINITION AND SCOPE

Postpartum psychosis is a rare disorder that is considered a psychiatric emergency. Care for women with postpartum psychosis extends beyond the scope of primary care clinicians. The role for clinicians in general obstetrical, gynecologic, and primary care is accurate recognition of the major symptoms and prompt referral to psychiatric emergency services for evaluation and treatment. Psychosis is the most severe of the PPD symptoms.

SYMPTOMS

Psychosis can occur 2 to 3 days postpartum; most women exhibit symptoms within the first 2 weeks postpartum. Psychosis may present as part of a continuum of major depression, bipolar disorder, or recurrent illness mood disorder. Delusions, hallucinations, depressed or elated mood, cognitive disturbances, and disorganized behavior and agitation are core symptoms of PPD with psychotic features.

TREATMENT/MANAGEMENT

Postpartum psychosis is often treated by using the same approach as with bipolar-manic psychosis (i.e., atypical antipsychotic medications, antimanic agents) and requires acute inpatient hospitalization. Untreated postpartum psychosis can have tragic consequences, including infanticide and suicide. Postpartum psychosis is recurrent and substantially worsens the risk of acting on homicidal thoughts toward the infant. When suspected, postpartum psychosis must be quickly evaluated and treated to reduce these potential outcomes.

Depression in Peri- and Postmenopause

ETIOLOGY

Although the role of estrogen deficiency and hormonal variance has been associated with depression during menopausal transition, it remains unclear if there is an increased vulnerability to depression during this developmental stage. Findings from several community and clinic-based studies indicate that perimenopausal women reported more depressive complaints than either premenopausal or menopausal women, implicating biological changes during this transitional stage as a risk for depression (Soares, 2014). Vasomotor symptoms, vaginal dryness, decreased libido, night sweats, and irritability, especially severe symptoms, frequently cause insomnia and depression in women around menopause. Left unresolved or inadequately treated, these symptoms often diminish functional status, quality of life, and overall health, and become the basis for seeking medical attention.

EVALUATION/ASSESSMENT

Apart from routine diagnostic studies and physical and mental status evaluations, a history of symptoms and chief complaints guide the primary care provider in distinguishing symptoms unique to perimenopausal and menopausal depression. A thorough history of mood changes during reproductive events across the life span must also be integrated in the diagnostic process.

DIFFERENTIAL DIAGNOSES

Differential diagnoses to consider in peri- and postmenopausal women that exhibit signs of depression are the same as for major depression (see earlier discussion).

Treatment/Management • Mounting data support that monotherapy with SSRIs and SNRIs mitigate depressive symptoms, reduce baseline vasomotor symptoms, and improve quality of sleep, functional status, and quality of life in perimenopausal women (Ensrud et al., 2012). These agents are well tolerated and have a relatively safe side-effect profile. The precise mechanisms of their actions are unknown, although vasomotor symptoms are linked to dysregulation of serotonin and norepinephrine (Tella & Gallagher, 2014). When prescribing short-term use of SSRIs and SNRIs to treat vasomotor symptoms, it is practical to start with a low dose (e.g., 10–20 mg escitalopram; 50–100 mg desvenlafaxine) and titrate based on response. When using for major depression, it is imperative to follow the APA (Gelenberg et al., 2010) practice guidelines to determine if continuation and maintenance treatment (e.g., 6–12 months) are indicated. Treatment must be periodically reassessed as vasomotor symptoms, a potential precursor to depression, are often time-limited and may subside without any intervention (see Chapter 34).

■ PSYCHOTIC DISORDERS

Schizophrenia

ETIOLOGY AND RISK FACTORS

Schizophrenia has genetic, neuroanatomical, neuroendocrine, and environmental underpinnings. Multiple factors are characteristic as the disorder has many subtypes with varying symptoms (APA, 2013; Jones, Chandra, Dazzan, & Howard, 2014). Typical symptoms of schizophrenia encompass cognitive, emotional, psychosocial, and behavioral deficits. Collectively, these symptoms result in a lack of insight about the importance of treatment to manage symptoms. The prevalence of schizophrenia in women and men is similar; however, women are more likely to have mood symptoms than men. As mentioned, under normal and healthy circumstances, pregnancy is a very stressful experience. It is particularly stressful and often overwhelming to women with coexisting psychiatric conditions, such as depression, bipolar disorder, and schizophrenia (Jones et al., 2014).

EVALUATION/ASSESSMENT

Women and men with schizophrenia present with hallucinations, delusions, agitation, and disorganized thoughts and behaviors. A comprehensive physical and psychiatric evaluation is needed to determine the underlying etiology.

DIFFERENTIAL DIAGNOSES

Acute psychosis must be differentiated from medical and other psychiatric conditions, substance intoxication, and withdrawal.

TREATMENT/MANAGEMENT

Acute psychosis is a psychiatric emergency requiring an immediate referral to the emergency department or psychiatric triage unit. Acute exacerbation of psychosis has been previously discussed and includes management of hallucinations, delusions, agitation, disorganized thinking, and risk of danger to self or others. Mainstay treatment for acute management involves administration of intramuscular (IM) antipsychotic agents such as haloperidol, and a benzodiazepine such as lorazepam. Patients are closely monitored for desired effect and side effects to ensure safe and effective symptom management. Explanations must occur before, during, and after medication administration to reduce anxiety and fear and ameliorate psychosis. Because of the complexity of schizophrenia, the importance of medications and a comprehensive treatment plan that includes psychotherapeutic interventions, and the high co-occurrence of psychiatric disorders, such as depression, substance use, and anxiety disorders, women with schizophrenia are managed by a mental health clinician and interdisciplinary team. Core elements of the interdisciplinary model include integrated symptom management, medication adherence, health education, and foster hope and empowerment to optimize and attain positive treatment outcomes.

■ EATING DISORDERS

Eating disorders are severe, debilitating, and chronic conditions associated with co-occurring psychiatric conditions and medical complications. Eating disorders carry the highest mortality rate of all psychiatric disorders, with high suicidality and deaths from physiologic causes (APA, 2013). An estimated 2% to 4% of young adult females meet criteria for an eating disorder (APA, 2013). The peak age at onset is between 16 and 20 years of age, during which time women are leaving home and are faced with enormous psychosocial stressors (Eddy et al., 2015). Eating disorders, especially anorexia nervosa, are psychiatric disorders depicted by an excessive fear of weight gain or persistent weight-avoidance behaviors. Collectively, these biological markers are associated with appetite regulatory hormones in women, which are highly heritable and familial. The incidence of eating disorders is similar among women from various cultures and ethnicities (Eddy et al., 2015). Demands for autonomy and social or sexual functioning may contribute to perception of eating, shape, and competence. The two major eating disorders include anorexia nervosa and bulimia nervosa.

Anorexia Nervosa

ETIOLOGY

Anorexia nervosa is one of the most serious and potentially fatal of the eating disorders (Pisetsky, Thornton, Lichtenstein, Pedersen, & Bulik, 2013). It is characterized by distorted body image and self-imposed nutritional limitations that result in serious malnutrition. Attitudes and behaviors in women with eating disorders have costly psychological and physiological consequences. Low self-esteem and confidence, disgust, and shame are common themes for women with eating disorders. Anorexia is classified as restricted type or binge eating/purging type.

EVALUATION/ASSESSMENT

A comprehensive physical and psychiatric evaluation, including appropriate diagnostic studies and vital signs, is performed to make a diagnosis and rule out co-occurring psychiatric and/or medical conditions. This process is complicated by her denial of symptoms, lack of insight into her illness, ritualistic behaviors, and resistance to treatment. Clinical findings often include low blood pressure, orthostatic hypotension, hypothermia, dependent edema, dental caries or erosion of enamel, and noticeable weight loss (Yager et al., 2012). Women with eating disorders often have a passion for preparing meals for others, while continuously restricting their own food intake. Binge eating tends to occur in secret, normally at night along with self-induced vomiting. Binge eating is associated with co-occurring substance-use disorder and borderline personality disorder. Denial is profound and withstands confrontation from others. Laxative and diuretic abuse and excessive exercising are used to maintain low body weight. Bizarre eating rituals are common such as cutting food into small pieces and spending enormous time rearranging it before eating. Medical attention tends to be sought when severe weight loss becomes obvious. A history of primary amenorrhea, hair loss, dry and brittle hair, fatigue, cold intolerance, and bruising and muscle weakness are common physical findings in women with eating disorders, especially anorexia nervosa. In suspected cases of eating disorders, queries about purging, dental integrity, and amenorrhea provide additional data to make a diagnosis (APA, 2013; Yager et al., 2012).

DIFFERENTIAL DIAGNOSES

Early recognition and treatment of eating disorders may mitigate morbidity and mortality. *DSM-5* diagnostic criteria for anorexia nervosa (APA, 2013) include each of the following:

- Refusal to maintain body weight at or above minimal body weight for age and height (e.g., body weight less than 85% of that expected)
- Marked fear of gaining weight and becoming obese, although underweight
- Distortion in a way body weight is experienced—self devaluation, negative self-image
- Amenorrhea—defined as the absence of menses three consecutive months (reproductive years)

- Restricted type: No regular purging or binge eating.
- Binge eating/purging type: Regular purging or binge eating has occurred during current episode.

DIAGNOSTIC STUDIES

Based on the answers and physical findings concerning eating disorders, additional diagnostic studies may be indicated such as a comprehensive metabolic profile, bone density, and referral for a dental examination.

MANAGEMENT

Referral for psychiatric treatment is needed. Hospitalization is indicated for nutritional and medical stabilization, dehydration, and electrolyte imbalance. Common physical findings in women with anorexia who require hospitalization include abnormal vital signs, specifically marked orthostatic hypotension with bradycardia; abnormal EKG; abnormal electrolytes, including hypokalemia; abnormal renal and liver function tests; inability to maintain normal body temperature; signs of malnourishment, such as generalized weakness, palpitations, shortness of breath, chest pain, cold extremities, and concentration and GI disturbances. These physiological disturbances jeopardize health, and in severe cases, result in death. Parameters used to determine choice of treatment include current weight, rate of weight loss, cardiac function, metabolic status, suicidality, degree of denial, and impact on health (Yager et al., 2012).

Women who are 20% below expected weight are referred for inpatient programs and those who are 30% below expected weight require psychiatric inpatient treatment for 2 to 6 months (Yager et al., 2012). A comprehensive approach that includes CBT, family and individual therapies, nutritional counseling, and rehabilitation are recommended. Pharmacological interventions have not demonstrated efficacy in the treatment of anorexia nervosa.

Bulimia Nervosa

SCOPE AND ETIOLOGY

Bulimia nervosa is more prevalent than anorexia nervosa. Characteristics of bulimia include episodic, uncontrolled, compulsive, and rapid ingestion of large quantities of food within a short duration (binge eating) followed by self-induced vomiting, misuse of laxatives and fasting, and excessive exercise to reduce weight gain (APA, 2013). Similar to anorexia nervosa, the onset is from 16 to 18 years of age and there is a higher male–female ratio of 1:10 (APA, 2013; Swanson, Crow, Le Grange, Swendsen, & Merikangas, 2011). Again similar to anorexia nervosa, bulimia nervosa also has a chronic and recurring course and is associated with medical complications, such as electrolyte imbalance, dental caries, suicidality, and metabolic acidosis.

EVALUATION/ASSESSMENT

As with anorexia nervosa, assessment includes a thorough and comprehensive physical and psychiatric evaluation to identify coexisting medical and/or psychiatric conditions.

Attitude about weight gain and food often provides the first clue of an eating disorder.

DIFFERENTIAL DIAGNOSES

Differentiating between eating disorders and other possible medical and/or psychiatric causes is needed. *DSM-5* diagnostic criteria for bulimia nervosa (APA, 2013) include each of the following:

- Recurrent episodes of binge eating, which includes *both* consuming a larger than normal quantity of food in a short period of time *and* feeling no control over eating during the event
- Recurring episodes of inappropriate compensatory behavior to reduce weight gain
- Binge eating and compensatory behaviors to reduce weight gain occur at least two times a week on average for 3 months or more
- Self-perception and evaluation is excessively affected by body weight and shape
- The disturbance is not limited to episodes of anorexia nervosa

TREATMENT/MANAGEMENT

Women with bulimia nervosa require referral to a psychiatric clinician for management. Hospitalization is limited to medical and psychiatric stabilization, similar to anorexia nervosa. A comprehensive treatment plan to address underlying issues associated with an eating disorder is recommended. Psychotherapeutic interventions include psychotherapy, nutritional rehabilitation and counseling, and health education. Dissimilar to anorexia nervosa, pharmacological interventions, such as mood stabilizers, antianxiety agents, SNRIs, and antipsychotic drugs, have proven efficacy in the treatment of bulimia nervosa.

■ SUBSTANCE-USE DISORDERS

Scope and Etiology

The co-occurrence between specific mood and anxiety disorders and specific drug-use disorders is pervasive in the U.S. population. Substance-use disorders are associated with increased morbidity, high risk of HIV or hepatitis infection, incarceration, and poor treatment outcomes. An epidemiologic study of gender differences in psychiatric disorders and co-occurring substance-related disorders initially found a higher incidence in women than men. However, when these data were adjusted for sociodemographics and coexisting psychiatric disorders, they found few gender differences associated with substance-use disorders (Goldstein, Dawson, Chou, & Grant, 2012).

The high prevalence of depression in women also increases the incidence of women presenting with coexisting depression and substance-use disorder. Research findings (Villena & Chesla, 2010) suggest substantial barriers to women with psychiatric disorders and co-occurring substance-use disorders. Major barriers include lack of knowledge concerning how to access health care services, childcare issues, and a lack of support and encouragement to seek mental health services.

EVALUATION/ASSESSMENT AND DIAGNOSTIC STUDIES

Evaluating psychiatric complaints in women with coexisting substance-use disorders is challenging as substance use can mimic or complicate diagnosis of psychiatric symptoms. When these disorders occur simultaneously, patients may have difficulty maintaining abstinence, have a higher risk of suicide, and use substantial medical and psychiatric services. Women seeking help in primary care may initially present with physical complaints that require an extensive evaluation. Women metabolize alcohol differently than men. Women are more likely to suffer earlier onset of medical complications associated with alcoholism and other drug use and to acquire sexually transmitted infection (STI). Diagnostic studies provide evidence of these changes, especially disease that is associated with chronic drug use (Antai-Otong, 2006). Inquiring about active and past alcohol and other drug use is critical to identifying substance-use disorders. Observing for signs of intoxication or withdrawal along with ordering drug screens and liver function tests can assist in making a diagnosis.

DIFFERENTIAL DIAGNOSES

Differentiating between organic medical disease and sequelae of alcohol or other substance use is essential for appropriate management of both the medical problems and the substance-abuse disorder. *DSM-5* diagnostic criteria for substance-related disorders (APA, 2013) are listed next.

Dependence

- Maladaptive substance-use pattern resulting in marked impairment or distress as demonstrated by three of more of the following, occurring during a given 12-month period:
  - Tolerance
  - Withdrawal
  - Larger amounts of substance use than intended
  - Persistent desire or unsuccessful effort to reduce use or control use
  - Increased substance-seeking behaviors
  - Global functional impairment (e.g., social, interpersonal, occupational)
  - Use is continued despite negative consequences

Abuse

- A maladaptive substance-use pattern resulting in significant impairment or distress as demonstrated by one or more of the following, occurring during a given 12-month period:
  - Recurrent use resulting in functional impairment
  - Use when it is physically hazardous such as driving or operating equipment
  - Repeated legal problems because of substance use
  - Continued use despite negative consequences
- Use does not meet criteria for substance dependence

MANAGEMENT

A referral to a mental health clinician for management of co-occurring psychiatric and substance-use disorders is critical to successful treatment outcomes. A gender-specific approach that addresses the needs of women is required as they use drugs for different reasons than men. Gender-specific treatment requires an integration of biological, psychosocial, and spiritual needs that impact individual substance use. It must also focus on the woman's experiences, relationships, and overall health. Women presenting with substance-use disorders tend to experience guilt, shame, and anxiety about substance use and exhibit low self-esteem and self-worth along with greater depression than their male counterparts. Treatment approaches must focus on their strengths, uniqueness, and personal needs rather than confrontation, which is highly used with men with substance-use disorders. In addition, treatment is guided by the specific active or past substance, patterns of abuse, quality of psychosocial support, current psychiatric symptoms, patient preferences and motivation for seeking treatment, and data from the medical and psychiatric evaluation. Health education about dangers of drug use during pregnancy must be an integral part of treatment planning.

Considerations for Special Populations

SUBSTANCE-USE DISORDERS AND INCARCERATED WOMEN

Despite the high prevalence of dual diagnoses in incarcerated women, symptoms are often unrecognized and untreated. The care of incarcerated women with co-occurring psychiatric and substance-use problems must include a gender-specific approach that includes assessing mood and substance-abuse problems; recognizing history of abuse, injury, or childhood trauma, and limited treatment choices; and determining if she has children and who is caring for them (Nargiso, Kuo, Zlotnick, & Johnson, 2014; Johnson, 2014). In addition, it is important to have pharmacological interventions to treat specific psychiatric disorders, abstinence from substances, and psychotherapeutic interventions, including relational and interpersonal psychotherapy, peer support, personal safety, parenting classes, and life skills to engage healthy relationships and facilitate transition into the community. Pharmacological and psychotherapeutic interventions and support of women with psychiatric and substance-use disorders can be effective (Nargiso, Kuo, Zlotnick, & Johnson, 2014).

■ FUTURE DIRECTIONS

The prevalence of mental health problems among women challenges primary care clinicians to recognize these problems. Women have unique presentations and needs and mental health problems often parallel reproductive events and are complicated by hormonal changes. As more and more women seek psychiatric help in primary care practices, it is imperative for clinicians to recognize the distinct risk factors among women associated with psychiatric disorders and initiate individualized treatment and referral to mental health services. More research is needed to address the needs of childbearing women during menses, pregnancy, and the postpartum period, as well as the unique needs of women during peri- and postmenopause.

■ REFERENCES

Alaka, K. J., Noble, W., Montejo, A., Dueñas, H., Munshi, A., Strawn, J. R.,... Ball, S. (2014). Efficacy and safety of duloxetine in the treatment of older adult patients with generalized anxiety disorder: A randomized, double-blind, placebo-controlled trial. *International Journal of Geriatric Psychiatry, 29*(9), 978–986.

Altshuler, L. L., Kupka, R. W., Hellemann, G., Frye, M. A., Sugar, C. A., McElroy, S. L.,... Suppes, T. (2010). Gender and depressive symptoms in 711 patients with bipolar disorder evaluated prospectively in the Stanley Foundation Bipolar Treatment Outcome Network. *American Journal of Psychiatry, 167*(6), 708–715.

American Psychiatric Association (APA). (2013). *Diagnostic and statistical manual of mental disorders (DSM-5*; 5th ed.). Washington, DC: Author.

Andrisano, C., Chiesa, A., & Serretti, A. (2013). Newer antidepressants and panic disorder: A meta-analysis. *International Clinical Psychopharmacology, 28*(1), 33–45.

Antai-Otong, D. (2006). Women and alcoholism: Gender-related medical complications: Treatment considerations. *Journal of Addictions Nursing, 17,* 33–42.

Antai-Otong, D. (2008). *Psychiatric nursing: Biological and behavioral concept* (2nd ed.). Clifton Park, NY: Thomson Delmar Learning.

Antai-Otong, D. (2009). *Psychiatric emergencies: Managing and assessing people in crisis* (2nd ed.). Eau Claire, WI: Professional Educational Systems.

Arnsten, A. F., Raskind, M. A., Taylor, F. B., & Connor, D. F. (2015). The effects of stress exposure on prefrontal cortex: Translating basic research into successful treatments for post-traumatic stress disorder. *Neurobiology of Stress, 1,* 89–99.

Bandelow, B., Boerner J, R., Kasper, S., Linden, M., Wittchen, H. U., & Möller, H. J. (2013). The diagnosis and treatment of generalized anxiety disorder. *Deutsches Ärzteblatt International, 110*(17), 300–309; quiz 310.

Beck, A. T., Emery, G., & Greenberg, R. (1985). *Anxiety disorders and phobias: A cognitive perspective.* New York, NY: Basic Books.

Bethea, C. L., Lima, F. B., Centeno, M. L., Weissheimer, K. V., Senashova, O., Reddy, A. P., & Cameron, J. L. (2011). Effects of citalopram on serotonin and CRF systems in the midbrain of primates with differences in stress sensitivity. *Journal of Chemical Neuroanatomy, 41*(4), 200–218.

Cameron, C., Habert, J., Anand, L., & Furtado, M. (2014). Optimizing the management of depression: Primary care experience. *Psychiatry Research, 220*(Suppl. 1), S45–S57.

Carlborg, A., Thuresson, M., Fentoft, L., & Bodegard, J. (2015). Characteristics of bipolar disorder patients treated with immediate- and extended-release quetiapine in a real clinical setting: A longitudinal, cohort study of 1761 patients. *Therapeutic Advances in Psychopharmacology, 5,* 13–21.

Chen, M. H., Su, T. P., Li, C. T., Chen, T. J., & Bai, Y. M. (2013). Symptomatic menopausal transition increases the risk of new-onset depressive disorder in later life: A nationwide prospective cohort study in Taiwan. *PLoS One, 152,* 334–339.

Chu, S. Y., Goodwin, M. M., & D'Angelo, D. V. (2010). Physical violence against U.S. women around the time of pregnancy, 2004–2007. *American Journal of Preventive Medicine, 38*(3), 317–322.

Chung, H., & Breslau, N. (2008). The latent structure of post-traumatic stress disorder: Tests of invariance by gender and trauma type. *Psychological Medicine, 38*(4), 563–573.

Cohen, L. R., Field, C., Campbell, A. N., & Hien, D. A. (2013). Intimate partner violence outcomes in women with PTSD and substance use: A secondary analysis of NIDA Clinical Trials Network "Women and Trauma" Multi-site Study. *Addictive Behaviors, 38*(7), 2325–2332.

Cougle, J. R., Keough, M. E., Riccardi, C. J., & Sachs-Ericsson, N. (2009). Anxiety disorders and suicidality in the National Comorbidity Survey-Replication. *Journal of Psychiatric Research, 43*(9), 825–829.

Cox, J. L., Holden, J. M., & Sagovsky, R. (1987). Detection of postnatal depression. Development of the 10-item Edinburgh Postnatal Depression Scale. *The British Journal of Psychiatry: The Journal of Mental Science, 150,* 782–786.

Csaszar, E., Melichercikova, K., & Dubovicky, M. (2014). Neuroendocrine and behavioral consequences of untreated and treated depression in pregnancy and lactation. *Neuro Endocrinology Letters, 35*(Suppl. 2), 169–174.

Cuijpers, P., Sijbrandij, M., Koole, S. L., Andersson, G., Beekman, A. T., & Reynolds, C. F. (2014). Adding psychotherapy to antidepressant medication in depression and anxiety disorders: A meta-analysis. *World Psychiatry: Official Journal of the World Psychiatric Association, 13*(1), 56–67.

Cunningham, J., Yonkers, K. A., O'Brien, S., & Eriksson, E. (2009). Update on research and treatment of premenstrual dysphoric disorder. *Harvard Review of Psychiatry, 17*(2), 120–137.

Devries, K. M., Mak, J. Y., Bacchus, L. J., Child, J. C., Falder, G., Petzold, M.,... Watts, C. H. (2013). Intimate partner violence and incident depressive symptoms and suicide attempts: A systematic review of longitudinal studies. *PLoS Medicine, 10*(5), e1001439.

Di Florio, A., Forty, L., Gordon-Smith, K., Heron, J., Jones, L., Craddock, N., & Jones, I. (2013). Perinatal episodes across the mood disorder spectrum. *JAMA Psychiatry, 70*(2), 168–175.

Du Mont, J., Hyman, I., O'Brien, K., White, M. E., Odette, F., & Tyyskä, V. (2012). Factors associated with intimate partner violence by a former partner by immigration status and length of residence in Canada. *Annals of Epidemiology, 22*(11), 772–777.

Dunlop, B. W., Rothbaum, B. O., Binder, E. B., Duncan, E., Harvey, P. D., Jovanovic, T.,... Mayberg, H. S. (2014). Evaluation of a corticotropin releasing hormone type 1 receptor antagonist in women with post-traumatic stress disorder: Study protocol for a randomized controlled trial. *Trials, 15,* 240.

Eddy, K. T., Lawson, E. A., Meade, C., Meenaghan, E., Horton, S. E., Misra, M.,... Miller, K. K. (2015). Appetite regulatory hormones in women with anorexia nervosa: Binge-eating/purging versus restricting type. *Journal of Clinical Psychiatry, 76*(1), 19–24.

El-Hachem, C., Rohayem, J., Bou Khalil, R., Richa, S., Kesrouani, A., Gemayel, R.,... Attieh, E. (2014). Early identification of women at risk of postpartum depression using the Edinburgh Postnatal Depression Scale (EPDS) in a sample of Lebanese women. *BMC Psychiatry, 14,* 242.

Ensrud, K. E., Joffe, H., Guthrie, K. A., Larson, J. C., Reed, S. D., Newton, K. M.,... Freeman, E. W. (2012). Effect of escitalopram on insomnia symptoms and subjective sleep quality in healthy perimenopausal and postmenopausal women with hot flashes: A randomized controlled trial. *Menopause, 19*(8), 848–855.

Epstein, R. A., Moore, K. M., & Bobo, W. V. (2015). Treatment of bipolar disorders during pregnancy: Maternal and fetal safety and challenges. *Drug, Healthcare and Patient Safety, 7,* 7–29.

Frewen, P. A., Dozois, D. J., Neufeld, R. W., Densmore, M., Stevens, T. K., & Lanius, R. A. (2011). Neuroimaging social emotional processing in women: fMRI study of script-driven imagery. *Social Cognitive and Affective Neuroscience, 6*(3), 375–392.

Gelenberg, A. J., Freeman, M. P., Markowitz, J. C., Rosenbaum, J. F., Thase, M. E., Trivedi, M. H., & Van Rhoads, R. S. (2010). *Practice guideline for the treatment of patients with major depressive disorder* (3rd ed.). Washington, DC: American Psychiatric Association.

Goldstein, R. B., Dawson, D. A., Chou, S. P., & Grant, B. F. (2012). Sex differences in prevalence and comorbidity of alcohol and drug use disorders: Results from wave 2 of the National Epidemiologic Survey on Alcohol and Related Conditions. *Journal of Studies on Alcohol and Drugs, 73*(6), 938–950.

Goodman, J. H., Chenausky, K. L., & Freeman, M. P. (2014). Anxiety disorders during pregnancy: A systematic review. *Journal of Clinical Psychiatry, 75*(10), e1153–e1184.

Haller, H., Cramer, H., Lauche, R., Gass, F., & Dobos, G. J. (2014). The prevalence and burden of subthreshold generalized anxiety disorder: A systematic review. *BMC Psychiatry, 14,* 128.

Hudson, S. M., Whiteside, T. E., Lorenz, R. A., & Wargo, K. A. (2012). Prazosin for the treatment of nightmares related to posttraumatic stress disorder: A review of the literature. *The Primary Care Companion for CNS Disorders*, 14(2). doi:10.4088/PCC.11r01222

Jackson, C. L., Ciciolla, L., Crnic, K. A., Luecken, L. J., Gonzales, N. A., & Coonrod, D. V. (2015). Intimate partner violence before and during pregnancy: Related demographic and psychosocial factors and postpartum depressive symptoms among Mexican American women. *Journal of Interpersonal Violence*, 30(4), 659–679.

Jacob, G. A., Zvonik, K., Kamphausen, S., Sebastian, A., Maier, S., Philipsen, A., ... Tüscher, O. (2013). Emotional modulation of motor response inhibition in women with borderline personality disorder: An fMRI study. *Journal of Psychiatry & Neuroscience*, 38(3), 164–172.

Jeffreys, M., Capehart, B., & Friedman, M. J. (2012). Pharmacotherapy for posttraumatic stress disorder: Review with clinical applications. *Journal of Rehabilitation Research and Development*, 49(5), 703–715.

Johnson, J. E. (2014). Integrating psychotherapy research with public health and public policy goals for incarcerated women and other vulnerable populations. *Psychotherapy Research: Journal of the Society for Psychotherapy Research*, 24(2), 229–239.

Jones, I., Chandra, P. S., Dazzan, P., & Howard, L. M. (2014). Bipolar disorder, affective psychosis and schizophrenia in pregnancy and the post-partum period. *Lancet*, 384(9956), 1789–1799.

Karg, K., Burmeister, M., Shedden, K., & Sen, S. (2011). The serotonin transporter promoter variant (5-HTTLPR), stress, and depression meta-analysis revisited: Evidence of genetic moderation. *Archives of General Psychiatry*, 68(5), 444–454.

Kessler, R. C., Berglund, P., Demler, O., Jin, R., Merikangas, K. R., & Walters, E. E. (2005). Lifetime prevalence and age-of-onset distributions of *DSM-IV* disorders in the National Comorbidity Survey Replication. *Archives of General Psychiatry*, 62(6), 593–602.

Kessler, R. C., Chiu, W. T., Jin, R., Ruscio, A. M., Shear, K., & Walters, E. E. (2006). The epidemiology of panic attacks, panic disorder, and agoraphobia in the National Comorbidity Survey Replication. *Archives of General Psychiatry*, 63(4), 415–424.

Kessler, R. C., Gruber, M., Hettema, J. M., Hwang, I., Sampson, N., & Yonkers, K. A. (2008). Co-morbid major depression and generalized anxiety disorders in the National Comorbidity Survey follow-up. *Psychological Medicine*, 38(3), 365–374.

Kessler, R. C., Petukhova, M., Sampson, N. A., Zaslavsky, A. M., & Wittchen, H. U. (2012). Twelve-month and lifetime prevalence and lifetime morbid risk of anxiety and mood disorders in the United States. *International Journal of Methods in Psychiatric Research*, 21(3), 169–184.

Krebs, G., Waszczuk, M. A., Zavos, H. M., Bolton, D., & Eley, T. C. (2015). Genetic and environmental influences on obsessive-compulsive behaviour across development: A longitudinal twin study. *Psychological Medicine*, 12, 1–11.

Lacey, K. K., McPherson, M. D., Samuel, P. S., Powell Sears, K., & Head, D. (2013). The impact of different types of intimate partner violence on the mental and physical health of women in different ethnic groups. *Journal of Interpersonal Violence*, 28(2), 359–385.

MacDonald, K., Wilson, M., Minassian, A., Vilke, G. M., Becker, O., Tallian, K., ... Feifel, D. (2012). A naturalistic study of intramuscular haloperidol versus intramuscular olanzapine for the management of acute agitation. *Journal of Clinical Psychopharmacology*, 32(3), 317–322.

Mahar, I., Bambico, F. R., Mechawar, N., & Nobrega, J. N. (2014). Stress, serotonin, and hippocampal neurogenesis in relation to depression and antidepressant effects. *Neuroscience and Biobehavioral Reviews*, 38, 173–192.

Marjoribanks, J., Brown, J., O'Brien, P. M., & Wyatt, K. (2013). Selective serotonin reuptake inhibitors for premenstrual syndrome. *The Cochrane Database of Systematic Reviews*, 2013(6), CD001396.

McHugh, R. K., Hu, M. C., Campbell, A. N., Hilario, E. Y., Weiss, R. D., & Hien, D. A. (2014). Changes in sleep disruption in the treatment of co-occurring posttraumatic stress disorder and substance use disorders. *Journal of Traumatic Stress*, 27(1), 82–89.

McIntyre, R. S., Cha, D. S., Kim, R. D., & Mansur, R. B. (2013). A review of FDA-approved treatment options in bipolar depression. *CNS Spectrums*, 18(Suppl. 1), 4–20; quiz 21.

Mendolicchio, L., Maggio, G., Fortunato, F., & Ragione, L. D. (2014). Update on eating disorders: Epidemiology, mortality and comorbidity. *Psychiatria Danubina*, 26(Suppl. 1), 85–88.

Milgrom, J., Gemmill, A. W., Ericksen, J., Burrows, G., Buist, A., & Reece, J. (2015). Treatment of postnatal depression with cognitive behavioural therapy, sertraline and combination therapy: A randomised controlled trial. *The Australian and New Zealand Journal of Psychiatry*, 49(3), 236–245.

Miller, J. M., Hesselgrave, N., Ogden, R. T., Zanderigo, F., Oquendo, M. A., Mann, J. J., & Parsey, R. V. (2013). Brain serotonin 1A receptor binding as a predictor of treatment outcome in major depressive disorder. *Biological Psychiatry*, 74(10), 760–767.

Mitchell, K. S., Mazzeo, S. E., Schlesinger, M. R., Brewerton, T. D., & Smith, B. N. (2012). Comorbidity of partial and subthreshold PTSD among men and women with eating disorders in the National Comorbidity Survey-Replication study. *International Journal of Eating Disorders*, 45(3), 307–315.

Moreno, F. A., Parkinson, D., Palmer, C., Castro, W. L., Misiaszek, J., El Khoury, A., ... Delgado, P. L. (2010). CSF neurochemicals during tryptophan depletion in individuals with remitted depression and healthy controls. *European Neuropsychopharmacology: The Journal of the European College of Neuropsychopharmacology*, 20(1), 18–24.

Mortazavi, F., Chaman, R., Mousavi, S. A., Khosravi, A., & Ajami, M. E. (2013). Maternal psychological state during the transition to motherhood: A longitudinal study. *Asia-Pacific Psychiatry: Official Journal of the Pacific Rim College of Psychiatrists*, 5(2), E49–E57.

Nargiso, J. E., Kuo, C. C., Zlotnick, C., & Johnson, J. E. (2014). Social support network characteristics of incarcerated women with co-occurring major depressive and substance use disorders. *Journal of Psychoactive Drugs*, 46(2), 93–105.

National Institutes of Mental Health. (2011). *Depression*. NIH Publication No. 11–3561 Revised. Bethesda, MD: U.S. Department of Health & Human Services.

National Institutes of Mental Health. (2009). *Women and depression*. NIH Publication No. 09 4779: Bethesda, MD: U.S. Department of Health & Human Services.

Nau, M. L., McNiel, D. E., & Binder, R. L. (2012). Postpartum psychosis and the courts. *Journal of the American Academy of Psychiatry and the Law*, 40(3), 318–325.

Oathes, D. J., Hilt, L. M., & Nitschke, J. B. (2015). Affective neural responses modulated by serotonin transporter genotype in clinical anxiety and depression. *PloS one*, 10(2), e0115820.

Ohaeri, J. U., & Awadalla, A. W. (2012). Characteristics of subjects with comorbidity of symptoms of generalized anxiety and major depressive disorders and the corresponding threshold and subthreshold conditions in an Arab general population sample. *Medical Science Monitor: International Medical Journal of Experimental and Clinical Research*, 18(3), CR160–CR173.

Oquendo, M. A., Sullivan, G. M., Sudol, K., Baca-Garcia, E., Stanley, B. H., Sublette, M. E., & Mann, J. J. (2014). Toward a biosignature for suicide. *American Journal of Psychiatry*, 171(12), 1259–1277.

Owen, R., Gooding, P., Dempsey, R., & Jones, S. (2015). A qualitative investigation into the relationships between social factors and suicidal thoughts and acts experienced by people with a bipolar disorder diagnosis. *Journal of Affective Disorders*, 176, 133–140.

Petrowski, K., Wintermann, G. B., Schaarschmidt, M., Bornstein, S. R., & Kirschbaum, C. (2013). Blunted salivary and plasma cortisol response in patients with panic disorder under psychosocial stress. *International Journal of Psychophysiology: Official Journal of the International Organization of Psychophysiology*, 88(1), 35–39.

Pisetsky, E. M., Thornton, L. M., Lichtenstein, P., Pedersen, N. L., & Bulik, C. M. (2013). Suicide attempts in women with eating disorders. *Journal of Abnormal Psychology*, 122(4), 1042–1056.

Polusny, M. A., Kumpula, M. J., Meis, L. A., Erbes, C. R., Arbisi, P. A., Murdoch, M., ... Johnson, A. K. (2014). Gender differences in the effects of deployment-related stressors and pre-deployment risk factors on the development of PTSD symptoms in National Guard Soldiers deployed to Iraq and Afghanistan. *Journal of Psychiatric Research*, 49, 1–9.

Popovic, D., Vieta, E., Fornaro, M., & Perugi, G. (2015). Cognitive tolerability following successful long term treatment of major depression and anxiety disorders with SSRI antidepressants. *Journal of Affective Disorders*, 173, 211–215.

Rapkin, A. J., & Lewis, E. I. (2013). Treatment of premenstrual dysphoric disorder. *Women's Health*, 9(6), 537–556.

Raskind, M. A., Peterson, K., Williams, T., Hoff, D. J., Hart, K., Holmes, H.,...Peskind, E. R. (2013). A trial of prazosin for combat trauma PTSD with nightmares in active-duty soldiers returned from Iraq and Afghanistan. *American Journal of Psychiatry*, 170(9), 1003–1010.

Sadock, B. J., Sadock, V. A., & Sussman, N. (2014). *Kaplan & Sadock's pocket handbook of psychiatric drug treatment* (6th ed.). Philadelphia, PA: Lippincott Williams & Wilkins.

Salmela-Aro, K., Read, S., Vuoksimaa, E., Korhonen, T., Dick, D. M., Kaprio, J., & Rose, R. J. (2014). Depressive symptoms and career-related goal appraisals: genetic and environmental correlations and interactions. *Twin Research and Human Genetics: The Official Journal of the International Society for Twin Studies*, 17(4), 236–243.

Samandari, G., Martin, S. L., & Schiro, S. (2010). Homicide among pregnant and postpartum women in the United States: A review of the literature. *Trauma, Violence & Abuse*, 11(1), 42–54.

Schuch, J. J., Roest, A. M., Nolen, W. A., Penninx, B. W., & de Jonge, P. (2014). Gender differences in major depressive disorder: Results from the Netherlands Study of Depression and Anxiety. *Journal of Affective Disorders*, 156, 156–163.

Seibell, P. J., & Hollander, E. (2014). Management of obsessive-compulsive disorder. *Prime Reports*, 6, 68.

Sher, L., Oquendo, M. A., Burke, A. K., Cooper, T. B., & Mann, J. J. (2013). Combined dexamethasone suppression-corticotrophin-releasing hormone stimulation test in medication-free major depression and healthy volunteers. *Journal of Affective Disorders*, 151(3), 1108–1112.

Shin, L. M., Bush, G., Milad, M. R., Lasko, N. B., Brohawn, K. H., Hughes, K. C.,...Pitman, R. K. (2011). Exaggerated activation of dorsal anterior cingulate cortex during cognitive interference: A monozygotic twin study of posttraumatic stress disorder. *American Journal of Psychiatry*, 168(9), 979–985.

Smink, F. R., van Hoeken, D., Oldehinkel, A. J., & Hoek, H. W. (2014). Prevalence and severity of *DSM-5* eating disorders in a community cohort of adolescents. *International Journal of Eating Disorders*, 47(6), 610–619.

Soares, C. N. (2014). Mood disorders in midlife women: Understanding the critical window and its clinical implications. *Menopause*, 21(2), 198–206.

Stein, D. J., Rothbaum, B. O., Baldwin, D. S., Szumski, A., Pedersen, R., & Davidson, J. R. (2013). A factor analysis of posttraumatic stress disorder symptoms using data pooled from two venlafaxine extended-release clinical trials. *Brain and Behavior*, 3(6), 738–746.

Stojek, M. M., & Fischer, S. (2013). Thinness expectancies and restraint in Black and White college women: A prospective study. *Eating Behaviors*, 14(3), 269–273.

Street, A. E., Gradus, J. L., Giasson, H. L., Vogt, D., & Resick, P. A. (2013). Gender differences among veterans deployed in support of the wars in Afghanistan and Iraq. *Journal of General Internal Medicine*, 28(Suppl. 2), S556–S562.

Swanson, S. A., Crow, S. J., Le Grange, D., Swendsen, J., & Merikangas, K. R. (2011). Prevalence and correlates of eating disorders in adolescents. Results from the national comorbidity survey replication adolescent supplement. *Archives of General Psychiatry*, 68(7), 714–723.

Tella, S. H., & Gallagher, J. C. (2014). Efficacy of desvenlafaxine succinate for menopausal hot flashes. *Expert Opinion on Pharmacotherapy*, 15(16), 2407–2418.

Thota, A. B., Sipe, T. A., Byard, G. J., Zometa, C. S., Hahn, R. A., McKnight-Eily, L. R.,...Williams, S. P.; Community Preventive Services Task Force. (2012). Collaborative care to improve the management of depressive disorders: A community guide systematic review and meta-analysis. *American Journal of Preventive Medicine*, 42(5), 525–538.

Toohey, J. (2012). Depression during pregnancy and postpartum. *Clinical Obstetrics and Gynecology*, 55(3), 788–797.

Van der Auwera, S., Janowitz, D., Schulz, A., Homuth, G., Nauck, M., Völzke, H.,...Grabe, H. J. (2014). Interaction among childhood trauma and functional polymorphisms in the serotonin pathway moderate the risk of depressive disorders. *European Archives of Psychiatry and Clinical Neuroscience*, 264(Suppl. 1), S45–S54.

Vatnar, S. K., & Bjørkly, S. (2011). Victim of and witness to violence: An interactional perspective on mothers' perceptions of children exposed to intimate partner violence. *Violence and Victims*, 26(6), 830–852.

Villena, A. L., & Chesla, C. A. (2010). Challenges and struggles: Lived experiences of individuals with co-occurring disorders. *Archives of Psychiatric Nursing*, 24(2), 76–88.

Weisskopf, E., Fischer, C. J., Bickle Graz, M., Morisod Harari, M., Tolsa, J. F., Claris, O.,...Panchaud, A. (2015). Risk-benefit balance assessment of SSRI antidepressant use during pregnancy and lactation based on best available evidence. *Expert Opinion on Drug Safety*, 14(3), 413–427.

World Health Organization (WHO). (2014). *Violence against women: Fact sheet*. Retrieved from http://www.who.int/mediacentre/factsheets/fs239/en

Wosu, A. C., Gelaye, B., & Williams, M. A. (2015). Childhood sexual abuse and posttraumatic stress disorder among pregnant and postpartum women: Review of the literature. *Archives of Women's Mental Health*, 18(1), 61–72.

Writer, B. W., Meyer, E. G., & Schillerstrom, J. E. (2014). Prazosin for military combat-related PTSD nightmares: A critical review. *Journal of Neuropsychiatry and Clinical Neurosciences*, 26(1), 24–33.

Yager, J., Devlin, M. J., Halmi, K. A., Herzog, D. B., Mitchell III, J. E., Powers, P., & Zerbe, K. J. (2012). *Guideline watch (2012): Practice guideline for the treatment of patients with eating disorders* (3rd ed.). Washington, DC: American Psychiatric Association.

Yonkers, K. A., Blackwell, K. A., Glover, J., & Forray, A. (2014). Antidepressant use in pregnant and postpartum women. *Annual Review of Clinical Psychology*, 10, 369–392.

Yonkers, K. A., Lin, H., Howell, H. B., Heath, A. C., & Cohen, L. S. (2008). Pharmacologic treatment of postpartum women with new-onset major depressive disorder: A randomized controlled trial with paroxetine. *Journal of Clinical Psychiatry*, 69(4), 659–665.

Yonkers, K. A., Vigod, S., & Ross, L. E. (2011). Diagnosis, pathophysiology, and management of mood disorders in pregnant and postpartum women. *Obstetrics and Gynecology*, 117(4), 961–977.

Young, E. A., Kornstein, S. G., Marcus, S. M., Harvey, A. T., Warden, D., Wisniewski, S. R.,...Rush, A. J. (2009). Sex differences in response to citalopram: A STAR*D report. *Journal of Psychiatric Research*, 43(5), 503–511.

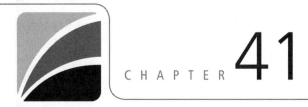

CHAPTER 41

Substance Abuse and Women

Susan Caverly

Substance use affects the health of women, their children, and their families, often in profound ways, while also affecting workplace productivity and societal resources. Primary care providers see women more frequently than they do their male counterparts. The 2012 rate for physician office visits by women age 18 ro 64 years old exceeded that of male counterparts by 57% (Ashman, Hing, & Talwalkar, 2012). Despite their more frequent use of primary care, women are not routinely evaluated for a substance-use disorder. Of the 17.3 million Americans aged 12 years and older who met criteria for alcohol abuse or dependence in 2013, only 6.3% had received treatment, whereas 90.6% neither received nor perceived a need for treatment. Primary care providers are in an important position for engaging at-risk and substance-using women and identifying needs for intervention. Primary care represents a critical area in which tremendous health opportunity can be realized through providers' awareness, empathy, use of open-ended questions, reflective listening, and understanding of the process and the treatment of addictive disorders.

In 1990 an Institute of Medicine (IOM) report concluded that the early detection and treatment of at-risk drinkers is as important as the identification and treatment of persons who are alcohol dependent. To meet the challenge of early detection and treatment, *Healthy People 2010* recommended a 75% increase in the number of primary health care providers who screen for substance-abuse problems (U.S. Department of Health and Human Services [USDHHS], 2000). The Substance Abuse and Mental Health Services Administration (SAMHSA) has advocated the integration of primary care, mental health, and substance-use treatment for decades, and the most recent IOM report, *Psychosocial Interventions for Mental and Substance Use Disorders: A Framework for Establishing Evidence-Based Standards* (2015), highlights the need for identifying, developing, and implementing practices with an evidence base for treating substance-use disorders.

In an update of the working definition of *recovery*, the SAMHSA (2012) identified "health, home, purpose, and community" as major dimensions in recovery while emphasizing that recovery emerges from hope; is person-driven; occurs via many pathways; is supported by peers and allies, as well as by relationships and social networks; is culturally based and influenced; is supported by addressing trauma;

involves individual, family, and community strengths and responsibility; and is based on respect (del Vecchio, 2012). The SAMHSA perspective provides a strong and holistic foundation for incorporating substance-use care in the primary care setting and is very closely aligned with current health care initiatives.

This chapter addresses the scope of the problem of substance use among women and its etiology, risk, and protective factors; diagnostic criteria; symptoms; evaluation process and screening for differential diagnoses; use of diagnostic studies; treatment and management, including risk reduction; and future directions. Additional resources, including web-based ones, will be recommended. As the field of substance use and care is evolving rapidly, the focus of this chapter is to provide a foundation for integrating new data and methods of care into practice as they become available.

■ DEFINITION AND SCOPE

The definition of *substance use* has changed with increasing understanding of how it is experienced as well as how it is caused. Revisions of the *Diagnostic and Statistical Manual of Mental Disorders* (5th ed.; *DSM-5*; American Psychiatric Association [APA], 2013) no longer include use of the diagnostic labels *substance abuse* and *substance dependence*. Instead, substance-use disorders are described as mild, moderate, or severe depending on criteria for severity met by an individual (see Box 41.1 for symptoms associated with substance-use disorders). "Substance use disorders occur when recurrent use of drugs and/or alcohol causes impairment (clinical or functional), exemplified by health problems, disability, and failure to meet major responsibilities at work, school, or home." The *DSM-5* guides the diagnosis of substance-use disorder, requiring that it be based on evidence of impaired control, social impairment, risky use, and pharmacological criteria (www.samhsa.gov/disorders/substance-use).

The most common substance-use disorders in the United States include alcohol-use disorder (AUD), tobacco-use disorder, cannabis-use disorder, stimulant-use disorder, hallucinogen-use disorder, and opioid-use disorder

BOX 41.1 COMMON SUBSTANCE-USE DISORDERS IN THE UNITED STATES

Alcohol-Use Disorder (AUD): A diagnosis of AUD requires that certain diagnostic criteria are met, including problems controlling intake of alcohol, continued use of alcohol despite problems resulting from drinking, development of a tolerance, drinking that leads to risky situations, or the development of withdrawal symptoms. *Moderate drinking* is defined as up to one drink per day for women and up to two drinks per day for men; *binge drinking,* five or more alcoholic drinks on the same occasion on at least 1 day in the past 30 days. (Four drinks for women and five drinks for men over a 2-hour period produces blood alcohol concentrations greater than 0.08 g/dL.)

Tobacco-Use Disorder: Symptoms of tobacco-use disorder include consumption of larger quantities of tobacco over a longer period than intended; unsuccessful efforts to quit or reduce tobacco intake; use of an inordinate amount of time acquiring or using tobacco products; cravings for tobacco; failure to attend to responsibilities because of tobacco use; continued use despite adverse social or interpersonal consequences; forfeiture of social, occupational, or recreational activities in favor of tobacco use; use in hazardous situations; and continued use despite awareness of physical or psychological problems directly attributed to tobacco use.

Cannabis-Use Disorder: Symptoms of cannabis-use disorder include disruptions in functioning, development of tolerance, cravings for cannabis, and development of

withdrawal symptoms, such as inability to sleep, restlessness, nervousness, anger, or depression within a week of ceasing heavy use.

Stimulant-Use Disorder: Symptoms of this disorder include craving for stimulants, failure to control use when tempted, continued use despite interference with major obligations or social functioning, use of larger amounts over time, development of tolerance, use of a great deal of time obtaining and using stimulants, and withdrawal symptoms occurring after stopping or reducing use, including fatigue, vivid and unpleasant dreams, sleep problems, increased appetite, or irregular problems in controlling movement.

Hallucinogen-Use Disorder: Symptoms of hallucinogen-use disorder include craving for hallucinogens, failure to control use when attempted, continued use despite interference with major obligations or social functioning, use of larger amounts over time, use in risky situations such as driving, development of tolerance, and use of a great deal of time obtaining and using hallucinogens.

Opioid-Use Disorder: Symptoms of opioid-use disorders include strong desire for opioids, inability to control or reduce use, continued use despite interference with major obligations or social functioning, use of larger amounts over time, development of tolerance, use of a great deal of time obtaining and using opioids, and withdrawal symptoms occurring after stopping or reducing use, such a s negative mood, nausea or vomiting, muscle aches, diarrhea, fever, and insomnia.

Definitions abstracted from www.samhsa.gov/disorders/substance-use

---

(www.samhsa.gov/disorders/substance-use). These are described in Box 41.1 and in later sections of this chapter.

■ INCIDENCE AND PREVALENCE

The use of new diagnoses that reduce stigma introduces a new lexicon into the field of substance use. Although the introduction of new *DSM-5* diagnoses addresses the disadvantages of stigmatizing diagnoses, it creates challenges when comparing the rates of particular diagnoses over time.

Although clinicians and women themselves may search for clearer definitions of substance use and substance-use disorders, there are multiple sources of definitions. Societal changes in the U.S. views of cannabis use have complicated identification of substance use, as reflected in lay literature replete with the putative benefits of cannabis as a safe herbal remedy. There is evidence showing that a lower perception of risk is associated with a greater likelihood of participation in an activity; hence, society may be redefining substance use as the use of cannabis increases. The National Survey on Drug Use and Health (SAMHSA, 2013c) revealed that an estimated 4.2 million people 12

and older met criteria for a substance-use disorder based on marijuana use (SAMHSA, 2013c).

Substance-use statistics are dynamic and complex to interpret. Changing patterns of substance use for one substance may result in changes in the use patterns for others. For example, as rates of use of cannabis increase, alcohol use may diminish. Substance-use statistical reports may reflect either current use (use within the prior month) and/or any past use. Thus reporting practices can be confusing. Also, as new data accumulate, the *DSM-5* criteria will be in place, making it somewhat challenging to compare data prior to 2016 in which differentiations between substance abuse and substance dependence were made. Another complexity of substance-use statistics is the reality that trends in use vary, challenging practitioners to maintain current knowledge. For example, the capacity of routine toxicology screens to detect new designer drugs and synthetic cannabinoids has not been adequate, as the chemical constituencies of these substances are purposefully altered to evade detection, making diagnosis of acute presentations imprecise.

The National Survey on Drug Use and Health (SAMHSA, 2013c) revealed that the current use of all illicit substances was lower among women (7.3%) than men (11.5%) for respondents 12 years and older. Among those 12 to 17 years old, only 8% of females reported current use of illicit substances compared with 9.6% of males. However, the nonmedical use of psychotherapeutic (prescription) medications has remained consistently higher among females aged 12 to 17 years old. This did diminish from 4.4% to 2.4% between 2002 and 2013 (males in same cohort reduced prescription drug use from 3.7% to 2.0% in the same time). This highlights the importance of the current shifts in prescribing practices that have begun to limit the generous dispensing of controlled substances (SAMHSA, 2013c). The CDC WONDER database shows that although death by overdose has remained lower for women than for men, from 2001 to 2014, death by overdose of opioid pain relievers has risen 3.4-fold; death by overdose of heroin, sixfold; and death by overdose of benzodiazepines, fivefold among all adults. In 2013, it was estimated that 4.6 million women older than 18 years had misused prescription drugs in the previous year (SAMHSA, 2013a) and that a woman was seen at a hospital emergency room every 3 minutes as a result of the misuse of prescription pain medication (CDC, 2013a). With regard to alcohol, 43.7% of women reported current and regular alcohol consumption in 2012 (Blackwell, Lucas, & Clarke, 2014), and in 2013, 4.6% of women met criteria for alcohol abuse or dependence (SAMHSA, 2013a).

Tobacco smoking has been reported to still be the greatest single cause of preventable deaths in the United States, and it is estimated that 16.8% (40.0 million) of American adults smoked tobacco in 2014 (CDC, 2014, 2015). Women who smoke tobacco have a 12 times greater risk of death associated with bronchitis and emphysema; a 12 times greater risk of death related to tracheal, lung, or bronchial cancer; and for middle-aged women, a five times greater risk of death resulting from coronary heart disease than women who do not smoke (CDC, 2014). There is a trend toward reduced tobacco use, with 16% of women identified as currently smoking tobacco, and 66% reported no history of smoking (Blackwell, Lucas, & Clarke, 2014). However, 2010 CDC data showed that 34% of women with a mental health condition smoked, and overall 48% of individuals who both suffer a mental illness and live in poverty smoke compared with 33% of those living above the poverty level (CDC, 2013b). Perinatal tobacco use was highest before pregnancy, with a 23.2% prevalence, dropping to 10.7% during pregnancy, and remaining low at 15.9% after delivery (CDC, 2013c). Nonetheless, between 2005 and 2009, 1,015 infant deaths per year were estimated to be attributable to tobacco smoking (CDC, 2014), and the estimated risk of stillbirth is two to three times greater in women who smoke tobacco or marijuana, take prescription pain relievers, or use illegal drugs during pregnancy (Tobacco, drug use in pregnancy, 2013). Combined 2012 and 2013 SAMHSA data show that use of illicit substances was more likely among younger pregnant women than among their older counterparts. The group reporting the highest percentage of use included pregnant women aged 15 to 17 years (14.6%). Comparatively, 8.6% of pregnant women aged 18 to 25 years and 3.2% of those aged 26 to 44 years reported current illicit substance use (SAMHSA, 2014). The relatively high prevalence of illicit substance use among adolescents who are pregnant serves to elevate their already high age-associated pregnancy risk.

Co-occurring mental health and substance-use disorders are common. In 2014, 5.7% of women met criteria for either alcohol- or illicit substance-use disorders compared with 8.4% of their male counterparts (SAMHSA, 2014). Although 1.8% of all adult women met criteria for a substance dependence or abuse diagnosis in the past year, 5.2% of women with a mental health diagnosis also met criteria for a co-occurring substance-use disorder. Among individuals whose mental illness was considered to be severe, 13.8% of women and 18.2% of men met criteria for a co-occurring disorder. It is clear that individuals who experience a psychiatric disorder have higher probability of also meeting criteria for a substance-use disorder.

In addition to co-occurring mental health problems, other factors increase the risk for substance use by women. In 2005, SAMHSA reported that women aged 18 to 49 years who were married had lower rates of substance use than women who were separated, divorced, or never married. In this same age group, women not living with children (12.9%) were nearly twice as likely to meet criteria for substance abuse or dependence compared with women living with children (5.5%) (SAMHSA, 2005a). Demographic data related to race/ethnicity and substance use are complicated. Patterns of alcohol use, the impact of this use, and access to treatment are somewhat more clear for alcohol than for other substances; however, when socioeconomic, legal system involvement, and geographic factors are taken into account, the racial/ethnic differences may be attenuated (Cook & Alegria, 2011; Smith et al., 2006). Certainly, the consequences of severe substance use in the context of geography, education, socioeconomic factors, legal system involvement, and resource accessibility serve to reinforce and to amplify the impact of the racial disparities that do exist. Also, ethnicity and culture are associated with specific challenges as well as resilience among individuals, and these specificities contribute to treatment response. Outcomes cannot help but be improved when practitioners are attuned to the needs, preferences, holistic resources, and beliefs or biases of the person they are striving to help, and they actively seek to accommodate these in the treatment provided.

In summary, younger women; women who are compromised by factors such as abuse, homelessness, poverty, lack of education, criminal justice involvement, and mental illness; and older woman who experience social isolation may be those most at risk for a substance-use disorder. Statistics do not account for the full spectrum of epigenomic risk factors known and not yet determined to exist. Practitioners need to remain mindful of the myriad risk factors for substance-use disorders that occur across patient populations and standardize a model to reduce biased selection into treatment, thereby ensuring that women are given access to respectful screening and/or evaluation for substance use.

ETIOLOGY OF SUBSTANCE-USE DISORDERS

Substance-use and other addictive disorders are complex biopsychosocial disorders, and the factors related to substance use among women of all ages and ethnicities are multifaceted. Increasingly, it is clear that the biology of women places those who use substances more at risk for substance-use disorders and also more at risk for negative physical and psychiatric effects of substances (www.drugabuse .gov/publications/drugfacts/substance-use-in-women). This has been linked to the hormonal differences, including the impact of progesterone on certain neuroreceptors, something particularly evident in regard to nicotine receptor upregulation (National Institute on Drug Abuse [NIDA], 2013). In addition smaller body weight and lower fluid volume are thought to contribute to increased risk.

Generally, the areas of the brain that are thought to be most involved with the development and maintenance of substance-use disorders are the ventral tegmental area (VTA), the nucleus accumbens (NAc), and the amygdala. Within these brain areas, multiple neurotransmitter receptor systems, including the gamma-aminobutyric acid (GABA), opioid, dopaminergic, serotonergic, endocannabinoid, nicotinic cholinergic, and N-methyl-Dasparatate (NMDA) glutamate systems, are implicated in substance-use disorders. A pattern of binge/intoxication, withdrawal/ negative affect, and preoccupation/anticipation has been described by Koob (2015). Rewarding neurotransmitter activity (dopamine in particular) has been found to increase during the intoxication phase of this cycle and to decrease during the withdrawal phase, whereas stress-related neurotransmitter activity, including dynorphin, corticotropin-releasing factor, and norepinephrine activity, is increased during withdrawal. Substances such as opioids and cannabis act as mimics for transmitters that are endogenous in the brain, whereas other substances, including stimulants, act by triggering the release of excess amounts of neurotransmitters into the neural synapses (Galanter, Kleber, & Grady, 2015).

The craving state is associated with other brain regions including the amygdala and the orbitofrontal and prefrontal cortices, and can be triggered by either cuing or internal distress. The term *salience* refers to the triggers that elicit increased attention or behavior-associated use of a particular substance. The plasticity of the neural network is affected through a variety of pathways creating changes that may be long lasting. At times this may be referred to as a *state of postacute withdrawal,* a phase during which the impact of salience and the experience of craving continue after sustained abstinence. Individuals may experience a response to salient cuing without full awareness, resulting in confusion as relapse occurs without their knowledge of when they decided to use. This distortion of the decision-making process represents a significant challenge to the maintenance of sobriety.

The nexus of genetics and environment is critical in the development of substance-use disorders. Studies to identify genetic polymorphisms and risk genes for individual substance categories are underway but are not yet clinically useful. A family history of substance-use disorders is a key element of the psychosocial history necessary to adequately evaluate and understand the substance-use risk for each individual. A positive family history yields both the potential for genetic predisposition to misuse substances and the increased probability of early exposure to substances, leading to enhanced opportunity for use at a young age. The environmental element may convey a normalization of substance overuse and a reduction in risk perspective related to substance use, thereby increasing the likelihood for early adoption of substance-using behavior. Evidence suggests that the earlier an individual initiates substance use, the greater the chance for developing a use disorder and the more the risk for negative consequences (Winters & Arria, 2011).

Risk Factors

Risk factors are attributes of individuals or environments that increase the chances of developing a substance-use disorder and contribute to a greater severity or a longer duration of the disorder (Wheaton, 1985). Protective factors decrease the risk of disorders by reducing exposure to risk factors, disrupting important processes involved in the development of the disorder, and interacting with the risk factor to reduce its effects (Wheaton, 1985). Three major types of risk and protective factors are biological, psychological, and social/environmental.

Biological risk factors include age, sex, ethnicity, genetic transmission, family history, personality disorders, and psychiatric disorders. Of these, genetic transmission, family history of disorders, and personal history of psychiatric disorders play a prominent role in the initiation and continuation of substance use (Hawkins, Catalano, & Miller, 1992; SAMHSA, 2005a).

Psychological risk factors for substance use include personality, belief systems, and coping styles (i.e., sensation seeking and appraisal of substances as having no consequences, minor consequences, or positive benefits). In addition, low self-esteem, lack of resistance skills, prior experimentation, and negative life events such as child abuse, trauma, and deaths of significant others represent significant risk factors (Pentz, 1994). Young women who have experienced sexual assault are at increased risk for substance use: Kilpatrick, Resnick, Saunders, & Best (1998) found that 29% of sexual assaults of women occurred by age 11 years, and 32% occurred between ages 11 and 17 years. The risk of lifetime alcohol dependence increased as a function of the number of lifetime assaults experienced. For 50% of the 638 assault victims who participated in the study, the first consumption of alcohol occurred within a year of the assault. Older women who do not reduce drinking as they age may have other risk factors predicting late-life drinking problems, such as friends' approval of alcohol use, avoidance coping strategies, deaths of significant others, depression, and isolation (Moos, Schutte, Brennan, & Moos, 2004).

Social environmental risk factors include parental substance misuse, exposure to poor parenting practices, negative peer bonding, poor interpersonal relationships, lack of social support, negative educational experiences, easy access to substances, the changing of social and gender norms, economic and social incentives for drug trafficking, and exposure to drinking environments (Pentz, Bonnie, & Shopland, 1996). A major risk factor for heterosexual women is their relationships with men who use substances (Henderson & Boyd, 1997), whereas for lesbian women, going to gay bars and clubs is a major influence (Hughes & Wilsnack, 1997).

Women who have sex with other women are predicted to have a higher use of injection drugs and a higher prevalence of sexually transmitted diseases (Bell, Ompad, & Sherman, 2004) and may be at heightened risk for consequences of drinking (McCabe, Hughes, & Boyd, 2004).

The initiation of substance use may involve all three types of risk factors: biological, psychological, and social/environmental. An early age of onset is one of the most important predictors of movement from smoking and alcohol use to illegal drug use. A frequently mentioned concern in the literature is the narrowing of the gap between boys' and girls' ages of initiation of substance use (Cyr & McGarry, 2002; Greenfield, Manwani, & Nargiso, 2003). Among high school senior girls, crack cocaine users began smoking cigarettes at 10.6 years of age compared with 13.5 years for those who remained exclusively cigarette smokers (Kandel & Yamaguchi, 1993). A second predictor of movement to illegal use is the substance itself. Tobacco and alcohol use among women are important "gateway" substances; that is, they lead to the use of drugs that are costly and obtained illegally (SAMHSA, 2002).

Findings suggest that gender differences for both the initiation and the heavy use of substances are associated with different perceptions of life problems and the drugs' effects on the individual. Liu and Kaplan (1996) showed that young women used substances primarily because of personal problems, such as arguments with significant others, anger directed toward someone, and "self-medication" of feelings of worthlessness and inadequacy.

Protective Factors

Protective factors decrease the risk of disorders by reducing exposure to risk factors, disrupting processes involved in the development of the disorder, and interacting with risk factors to reduce their effects (IOM, 1990). Differences in gender roles may be protective factors that prevent women from using substances at the same rates as men. For example, there are social sanctions against women's substance use, and women tend to be more nurturing, less aggressive, and less sensation seeking than men (Nolen-Hoeksema, 2004).

Events along the life course, such as pregnancy, may be protective factors. A longitudinal study of 100 pregnant women addicted to heroin found that pregnancy led to cessation of drug use. The women had concerns about the development of their unborn babies and concerns regarding losing custody of their children (Nolen-Hoeksema, 2004).

Linking Known Risk Factors With Prevention Programs

Outcome studies of prevention programs show reductions in substance use, that is, *prevention works* (Eggert, Thompson, Herting, Nicholas, & Dicker, 1994; Holder, 1999; Kumpfer, 1998; Pentz, 1994). Changing situational and environmental factors show *how programs work*.

The IOM (1994) identified three levels of prevention for alcohol, tobacco, and other drugs: universal, selective, and indicated. Universal prevention programs are "targeted to the general public or a whole population group that has not been identified on the basis of individual risk; i.e., the intervention is desirable for everyone in that group" (p. 24). Public education via the mass media and other sources can focus on the risks and consequences of the use of alcohol, tobacco, and other drugs, including risks to pregnant and childbearing women, such as smoking, which contributes to low-birth-weight infants and secondhand smoke damage in children.

Selective prevention programs counteract risk factors and promote individual, social, and environmental protective factors. The hallmark of selective prevention programs is not the type of intervention, but who receives the intervention (i.e., high-risk groups; Kumpfer, 1998). For example, a school-based intervention for 12-year-old girls demonstrated a faster increase over time on social assertiveness and a slower increase in initiation to substances (Lillehoj, Trudeau, Spoth, & Wickrama, 2004). Kumpfer (1998) initiated a "strengthening families" program that provides parent training, children's skill training, and family skills training to families who are at risk because of drug-abusing parents.

Indicated prevention programs target those already manifesting known precursors of substance use and who are in need of help. Eggert et al. (1994) designed a school-based prevention program that targeted negative peer bonding (i.e., encouraging involvement with peers who are successful in school rather than those who are skipping school).

Diagnostic Criteria

The implementation of the *DSM-5* (APA, 2013) as the nosology for diagnosing mental health and substance use disorders in 2015, has required practitioners to transition from use of the diagnoses substance abuse and substance dependence to the more inclusive category of substance use disorders. Substance use disorders are then categorized as mild, moderate, or severe, depending on the number of criteria that are met. One intended consequence of this change is to move away from stigmatizing language that has created a barrier to treatment access for many. This shift in language holds opportunity for substance-use disorders to begin to be viewed by patients and providers alike as a health concern in need of care. This transition likely requires rethinking on the part of health care providers, as more individuals may meet criteria for a disorder. The diagnosis of substance abuse has been problematic, as it was considered by many to not merit serious intervention, and its differentiation from substance dependence has been resolved by designating the spectrum of use disorders. Another change has been the extension of the time to reach criteria for early remission. In the past, early remission required only a 1-month period of sobriety, whereas now the substance-free interval must be 3 months. Sustained remission requires an interval of 12 months without any symptoms beyond craving, which does not prevent the designation of remission. The specification of a controlled environment, although important for understanding the process of abstinence, does not preclude the designation of remission.

The *DSM-5* includes 10 classes of drugs (alcohol, caffeine, cannabis, hallucinogens [with phencyclidine and arylcyclohexylamines separately considered, and other hallucinogens], inhalants, opioids, sedative/hypnotic/anxiolytics, stimulants [amphetamine, cocaine, and other], tobacco, and other or unknown substances). Individual substances may vary in regard to criteria. Although there is no use disorder specified for caffeine, the *DSM-5* (APA, 2013) includes intoxication, withdrawal, other caffeine-induced disorders, and unspecified caffeine-related disorder. Several substance-related diagnoses are listed for each substance category. Substance-use disorder, for most substances, requires, at minimum, two of 11 diagnostic symptoms to have occurred within a 12-month period. The presence of two or three symptoms is noted to be a mild-use disorder; four or five, a moderate-use disorder; and six or more, a severe-use disorder. Tolerance and withdrawal are no longer required for an individual to meet the criteria for even a severe substance-use disorder. This is a significant change from the prior *DSM* and one that takes into account a newer understanding of the disorders. When medication is taken as prescribed, the individual does not receive a substance-use disorder diagnosis even in the presence of tolerance or withdrawal.

The key criteria for substance-use disorders include:

- The substance is taken in larger amounts or over a longer period of time than was intended
- There has been a persistent desire or unsuccessful attempts to cut down or control use
- A great deal of time is spent in activities necessary to obtain, use, or recover from the substance
- There is a craving or strong desire or urge to use the substance
- Recurrent use results in failure to fulfill major role obligations at work, school, or home
- Continued use occurs, despite having persistent or recurrent social or interpersonal problems caused or exacerbated by the substance effects
- Important social, occupational, or recreational activities are given up or reduced because of the substance use.
- Recurrent substance use occurs in situations in which it is physically hazardous
- Substance use is continued despite knowledge of persistent or recurrent physical or psychological problems likely caused or exacerbated by the substance
- Tolerance
- Withdrawal

The diagnostic process takes place over time. Although practitioners are pressed to establish a diagnosis after an initial interview, by their very nature these diagnoses are provisional. Moreover, accurate diagnosis is often not possible after a single encounter, especially for individuals for whom substance use is problematic.

Symptoms

The *DSM-5* criteria provide helpful descriptions of symptoms associated with each category of substances (see Box 41.1 for examples). Generally, there is a variety of emotional, behavioral, and physical symptoms and clinical presentations that warrant a more specific assessment for substance use. Impulsivity and uncharacteristic changes in performance of age- and role-appropriate behaviors may be associated with substance use. These include school or work absenteeism or diminished performance in those settings; financial irresponsibility; diminished self-care; frequent, poorly explained accidents or injuries; missed appointments; involvement with agencies such as Child Protective Services or courts; evidence of physical or emotional hyperarousal or hypo-arousal; sleep dysregulation; and/or specific evidence of changes such as pupil size and reactivity, or abrupt changes in mental state characterized by emotional lability, cognitive clouding, psychosis or hypervigilance, and/or racing thoughts. Physical problems associated with liver or pancreatic illness, infection, skin erosions or lesions, dental erosion or extensive tooth pain, nasal excoriation, and sexually transmitted diseases warrant careful assessment for a substance-use disorder.

It is not uncommon for individuals engaged in substance use to experience symptoms of anxiety, depression, or a first episode of psychosis, with or without a prior episode of mental health treatment. Often, these individuals fail to respond as anticipated to interventions and historically may have been prescribed a variety of medications that were deemed ineffective or to have had untoward effects. At times the person who has a substance-use disorder presents with specific medication requests and compelling reasons why other medications are not acceptable options.

Women who have substance-use disorders may report significant past or current trauma (possibly presenting with frequent accident-related injuries). They may struggle to bond with their children, and the children may have symptoms of failure to thrive or behavior that is disruptive and unresponsive to parenting recommendations.

■ EVALUATION AND ASSESSMENT

Substance-use disorders among women may go unnoticed for several reasons. Women are reluctant to report use or misuse, particularly illicit drug use (Manwell, Fleming, Johnson, & Barry, 1998), and are more likely to seek health care for a substance-induced health problem rather than seeking treatment for substance abuse per se. For this reason, at-risk women drinkers are detected only about 10% of the time. Despite significant increases in substance abuse education over the past several decades, some health care providers have reported that they lack the assessment skills needed to work with this population; others have negative attitudes toward persons who misuse substances and hold a belief that individuals do not change substance-use behavior; and still other clinicians wish to avoid involvement in situations that may entangle them legally to report incidents such as child abuse (SAMHSA, 1997). A national sample of physicians considered a diagnosis of substance abuse only 1% of the time when presented with a vignette describing early symptoms of substance abuse among older women (Center for Substance Abuse, 1998). A recent review of the literature indicated that very little has changed in this regard.

Whether an artifact of true or perceived time constraints, knowledge or skill deficits, sociologic bias or stigma, and the reality that in years past there were no gender-specific treatments available, health care providers do not regularly assess female patients for substance use. Integrating substance-use assessment into routine and urgent health care encounters requires primary care providers to develop the necessary skill set, an understanding of the disorder, the knowledge of treatment alternatives, and self-reflection regarding personal biases and stigmatizing language or behavior. A supportive, patient-centered approach more likely engages women who are using substances and allows them adequate comfort to reveal the struggles they are experiencing.

History

Inclusion of substance-use questions in the health history requires specific questions in order to ascertain what substances have been used, the age at which the substances were first used, and the last episode of use. Context for the use, such as level of functioning before use and life events that occurred just before use or concurrent with initiation or exacerbation of use, help clarify the diagnosis and suggest treatment strategies. Often, asking specifically about the frequency and quantity of use for any substances used more than five times can focus the assessment. It is important to inquire about response to the use of each targeted substance, as well as the triggers for use after intervals of abstinence: This helps not only with understanding the substance use, but also with identifying potential co-occurring psychiatric diagnoses. Relapse is sometimes related to changes in hormone levels: Therefore asking about menstrual cycles and postpartum experiences in association with other triggers can be helpful. Asking about the person's own concerns regarding substance use, the benefits they perceive the substance provides, and explication of the negative impacts that substances may have had in their lives help the practitioner to formulate a functional analysis. As with any other disorder, it is important to ensure that women of childbearing age are asked if they are pregnant or planning to become pregnant. When feasible, the use of standardized assessment tools is recommended, as discussed later in this chapter.

Many individuals have prior experiences with substance-use treatment. When this is the case, it is important to document both inpatient and outpatient treatment experiences, treatment completed or not completed, any past pharmacologic therapy for addiction, the person's perception of what had been helpful or problematic about the intervention or the program, and the length of sustained sobriety after each treatment encounter. This information is helpful for conceptualizing an individualized treatment approach and parsing intervention options.

Health history is most useful when it incorporates the following elements:

- Full psychosocial history (including resilience factors as well as risks, family relationships, peer relationships and influences, school experiences, work success, and stability)
- History of mental health symptoms and if applicable past interventions (including the person's assessment of benefit or detrimental impact of treatment)
- Developmental history (including fetal exposure to substances, birth challenges, and milestones)
- Family history of blood relatives who have experienced mental health and or substance-use symptoms, clarifying the treatments they may have undertaken and the results

Physical Examination

A routine physical examination usually includes the following systems likely to be affected by substance use. Attentiveness to abnormalities, especially in the areas noted, can help identify the possibility of a substance-use disorder and informs the practitioner as to the extent of physical compromise sustained from the substance use. The examples provided, while not an exhaustive listing, include many physical findings commonly occurring in consort with substance use. If a specific substance is suspected, it can also be useful to consult a reference that describes physical presentation common to that substance.

- Neurologic assessment targeting coordination, falls, head trauma, seizure history, papillary reactivity and presentation, reflexes, gait, and temperature regulation
- Mental status assessment for orientation and alertness; memory and cognition; thought processing; and speech rate, pressure, and coherency
- Ear, nose, throat, and mouth assessment for dental health or damage, mucosal excoriation or erosion, and bleeding
- Integument assessment for evidence of needle tracks, skin picking, gooseflesh, abscess, cellulitis, or excoriation
- Respiratory assessment for evidence of infection, airway reactivity, and chronic pulmonary disease
- Cardiac assessment of heart rate and blood pressure and evidence of dependent edema and vascular insufficiency
- Gastrointestinal assessment of the liver, pancreas, stomach, and intestines, with emphasis on pain, hemorrhage, and inflammation
- Genitourinary assessment for evidence of pregnancy, trauma, infection, and renal impairment
- Musculoskeletal assessment for the presence of injuries resulting from substance use or possibly associated with chronic pain and therefore representing a barrier to sobriety

Laboratory Testing

Toxicology testing is not a common practice in primary care; yet it holds potential for reducing the time frame required to rule out substance use and differentially diagnose presenting problems. The American Society of Addiction Medicine (ASAM) recommends that drug testing become more regularly used in general practice settings, given the high prevalence of substance-use disorders among medical patients (ASAM, 2013, p. 64). The rationale for drug testing is supported by a Quest Diagnostics study in which 40% of samples were positive only for medications prescribed, 25% were negative for both prescribed and illicit substances, 15% were negative for prescribed medications yet positive for other medications or substances, and 20% were positive for both prescribed and other substances. (Quest Diagnostics, 2013).

Routine toxicology screening for women who are pregnant is supported by evidence that women who test positive and who are referred for an early intervention program have pregnancy outcomes consistent with women who screened negative for substances. Women who test positive for substances and do not receive treatment experienced a risk ratio for negative outcomes two to 16 times higher than those who were treated (Goler, Armstrong, Taillac, & Osejo, 2008).

A number of laboratory tests can be used to gain a greater understanding of substance use. Those specific for the assessment of current or recent substance use include the toxicology screen and the ethyl glucuronide (EtG) test. The standard toxicology evaluation has been performed using observed urine specimens. These samples can provide point-of-service, immediate-read results. However, when quantitative levels are desired the test must be sent to a toxicology laboratory for analysis. Saliva swabs may be utilized to access data comparable with that of a urine drug screen, depending on the specific laboratory performing the tests. Saliva swabs are not currently available for use as a point-of-care toxicology screening test. It can be uncomfortable for both practitioners and patients to request a urine drug screening unless it is a routine practice, and urine samples that not observed are easily adulterated. Newer oral drug screening swabs are very useful because observed collection is easy to achieve: Patients often find this sample less intrusive or offensive, oral screens do not require a person to urinate (less restricted by "shy bladder" issues), and the results have validity. Note that oral levels of substances are not directly associated with urine levels, making it a challenge to compare the results from different collection methods. Blood samples are most useful in emergency settings, where it is essential to know the current level of substance in order to intervene appropriately. Sweat patches, nail clippings, and hair samples are also utilized for toxicology testing, but their usefulness in the clinical setting is limited because of challenges in quantification and/or the length of time that a substance may be retained in the sample.

It is notable that individual labs use different methods of analysis and establish independent levels of detection. Therefore when interpreting toxicology results it is essential to have obtained information from the lab regarding detection limits as well as the other substances (including prescription medications) that may lead to false-positive or false-negative results. The laboratory is able to provide information regarding the detection window for specific substances and sample type. Often labs offer standard screens; however, these may or may not contain a particular substance. Most labs offer the option to order a screen and/or a confirmatory test for a specific substance, even if it is not included in a standard screen. Examples of drugs that are not commonly included in toxicology screens include dextromethorphan (DXM), Ecstasy, phencyclidine, and synthetic cannabinoids such as Spice or K2. Standard tests discover opioid substances such as heroin and morphine-based drugs but may not detect oxycodone, buprenorphine (Suboxone), or methadone.

When working with women for whom substance use is suspected, it is important to note that the CDC recommends that women younger than 25 years who are sexually active be screened for chlamydia and that there be universal testing for gonorrhea and chlamydia among incarcerated adolescent and adult females up to the age of 35 years because of the potential for health impacts. It is also important to consider a pregnancy test for women of childbearing age (CDC, 2010).

Laboratory studies to consider ordering when substance-use disorders are being evaluated are those that assess for infection and liver, pancreas, renal, and immune system compromise:

- CBC with differential and platelet
- Aspartate aminotransferase (AST)
- Alanine aminotransferase (ALT)
- Serum gamma-glutamyltransferase (SGGT)
- Hepatitis B and C screens
- HIV screen
- Amylase
- Blood urea nitrogen (BUN), creatinine, electrolytes
- Toxicology, including for EtG
- Electrocardiogram
- Sexually transmitted diseases
- Pregnancy

The physiological impact of AUD on the liver may be associated with abnormalities in laboratory results. Alkaline phosphatase, bilirubin, prothrombin time, ammonia, glucose, triglycerides, and AST/ALT ratio may be elevated. Mild macrocytic anemia may be present; phosphate, magnesium, and potassium levels may be low; and white blood cells may evidence abnormalities. Although an elevated SGGT will not be specific for excessive alcohol use, it can serve as both a screening tool and a means of monitoring use for individuals currently in treatment.

Differential Diagnosis

The symptoms related to the misuse of substances often co-occur with those of mental illness and commonly mimic psychiatric symptoms. This represents a challenge to practitioners to carefully evaluate for the possibility of a mental health diagnosis whenever considering the diagnosis of a substance-use disorder. In particular, mood disorders are often misdiagnosed when individuals are not adequately assessed for substance use. It is critical to develop a timeline of symptom occurrence and comparatively a timeline of substance use. A toxicology screen can be of particular help in the differential diagnosis of an acute-onset psychiatric disorder; however, if the symptoms have been present for more than a few days, it is possible that the substance levels in the blood, urine, or saliva have diminished such that a drug screen will be negative. For this reason, any diagnosis must be made utilizing the available history, taking into account not only symptoms and test results, but also context for the symptom presentation. At times, it is also necessary to nonjudgmentally consider the potential for the secondary gain associated with the presentation of specific symptoms.

Substances that are stimulating in nature (including nicotine and caffeine) may cause hyperarousal, sleep interruption or restriction, cardiac stimulation with elevated heart rate and blood pressure, hypersexuality, and appetite suppression or weight loss. When the stimulant is chronically used or when it is depleted, exhaustion and depression can present. Emotional lability may vary from euphoric or mixed-state hypomania, anxiety, agitation, and confusion to psychosis. The use of stimulants may trigger a first episode of mood disorder or psychosis that may not resolve with sobriety. The dilation of pupils, bruxism, and skin picking may aid in the differential diagnosis.

Substances that are central nervous system depressants create symptoms of physiological and mental sedation. Speech may be slurred, gait and coordination may be impaired (lots of dropping of belongings, bumps, and bruises), and complaints of constipation may be reported. An EKG may find changes in the QTC interval, and blood pressure and heart rate may be lowered during intoxication and elevated during withdrawal. When the substance is withdrawn, there can be a risk of seizure (depending on the substance), gastrointestinal distress, temperature dysregulation, insomnia, emotional agitation, or anxiety. Pupillary constriction during the intoxication phase may be helpful in the differential diagnosis. In overdose or in combination with other depressant substances, respiratory depression can lead to coma or death.

Hallucinogenic or dissociative substances, including over-the-counter substances such as DXM, may present with either stimulant- or depressant-like effects, depending on the specific substance. These substances have the potential to cause mental distortions that mimic psychosis. Anabolic steroid use often presents with symptoms similar to those of excessive testosterone (enhanced muscle mass, acne, hypertension, and in women, masculinization). Impulsivity and mood dysregulation with rage episodes may lead to the diagnosis of intermittent explosive disorder or physical disorders such as pheochromocytoma.

When substance use is diminished or discontinued, psychiatric symptoms may present for the first time or exacerbate. This is especially the case when the individual has experienced trauma and the symptoms of posttraumatic stress disorder have been suppressed by substance use. Patients with mood disorders, anxiety disorders, and in particular, obsessive compulsive disorder often become more acutely in need of psychiatric intervention with the onset of sobriety. Conversely, when these disorders are left untreated or unrecognized, patients' capacity to achieve or maintain sobriety is jeopardized. It is essential that both the psychiatric and the substance-use disorders are adequately managed in order for stability to be achieved. Therefore when established and patient accepted care is not helpful, it is necessary to reevaluate for additional psychiatric or substance-use disorders that have not been previously identified.

Screening

The goal of substance abuse screening is to identify individuals who have begun to develop problems or are at high risk for problems, as well as to accurately determine whether or not there is a problem (IOM, 1994). Good screening tools possess understandable directions, are quick to administer, and demonstrate sensitivity (accuracy in problem identification) and specificity (ruling out those not affected; IOM, 1994). It is important that the tools used for screening include an adequate number of questions regarding substance use and that these questions are framed in an open, nonjudgmental manner that encourages truthful response.

Assessment Instruments

There is one in-depth assessment tool designed specifically for women: the female version of the Addiction Severity Index (ASI-F; Brown, Frank, & Friedman, 1997). The ASI-F is based on the Addiction Severity Index (McLellan et al., 1992), which is considered the gold standard of addiction assessment. The ASI-F is very similar to the ASI except that it has a section pertaining to women's issues, albeit mostly reproductive. The ASI-F, like the ASI, is comprehensive. Items include medical, psychiatric, employment, and legal status; family and social relationships; family history of alcohol and other drug use; and current and past history of alcohol and other drug use. The assessment must be conducted in person the first time it is administered. Phone interviews can be conducted thereafter. The person being assessed responds verbally to items. At the end of each section, the clinician administering the ASI-F records what are referred to as *clinician confidence ratings*; that is, the clinician provides an opinion of the client's understanding of the questions in the section being completed and assesses the client's degree of distortion to each response. The ASI has an extensive history of psychometric development.

Screening Instruments for Varied Population Groups

A number of screening tools might be used for screening for specific substances, general substance use, and symptoms of withdrawal. These are described in Box 41.2.

Note that at each step in the decision trees for substance abuse (screening, assessment, brief intervention, treatment, family interview or intervention, follow-up, and relapse prevention), MI, and efforts to promote engagement are critical aspects of the interaction that contribute to successful outcome. Also note that the steps include ongoing assessment,

BOX 41.2   SCREENING TOOLS FOR SUBSTANCE-USE DISORDERS

The Alcohol Use Disorders Identification Test (AUDIT; Babor, de la Fuente, Saunders, & Grant, 1992) is a 10-item scale that can be self-administered or used in an interview. It requires 2 minutes for administration and 1 minute for scoring. A user's manual is available, and the tool has been translated into several non-English languages.

The Drug Abuse Screening Test (DAST; available from the Center for Addiction and Mental Health) is a 20-item instrument that can be self-administered or used as a structured interview and has been used for screening as well as determination of the level of treatment and goal planning. It has been validated with individuals who use psychoactive substances. The administration requires 5 minutes and yields a quantitative index score based on yes/no responses.

The Problem-Oriented Screening Instrument for Teenagers (POSIT; Gruenewald & Klitzner, 1991)

consists of 139 items with 10 subscales. It has a yes/no format and requires 20 minutes to administer. This scale has been determined to have adequate established validity and reliability.

The TWEAK, a phonetic acronym for five questions—tolerance, worried, eye-opener, amnesia, and cut down (Russell, 1994)—may be useful in assessing women who are pregnant. The items are drawn from the cut down, annoyed, guilty, and eye-opener (CAGE) questionnaire, which is considered more appropriate for use in assessing chronic alcohol users. Although the TWEAK has promising face validity and is useful at the clinical level, it has not been subjected to reliability testing.

The Michigan Alcoholism Screening Test—Geriatric Version (MAST-G) is a 24-item test (Blow et al., 1992) recommended for use in older adults.

For additional screening tools, the National Institute of Alcohol Abuse and Alcoholism (NIAAA) and the National Institute of Drug Abuse (NIDA) websites provide options for both brief and in-depth screening instruments and cite the literature supporting their use.

---

for factors that complicate the disorder or the treatment such as homelessness, health compromise, or mental illness, and integrate approaches for these disorders in further assessments or treatments.

■ TREATMENT MANAGEMENT

The 2015 IOM report framework for developing and strengthening the evidence base for psychosocial interventions in practice included as a priority that the consumer be central to the process and inform care providers as an agent in their own care. The report also made a point of developing a structure for evaluating the effectiveness of interventions and identifying the elements that are commonly packaged in standardized or manualized psychosocial interventions, rather than developing a listing of evidence-based practices (EBPs). The committee also recognized that accounting for context, different stakeholders (specified here are only consumers and providers) have access to a differentiated range of abilities to influence the implementation of interventions and improvement of outcomes. Consumers contribute through "meaningful participation in governance, in organizational leadership positions, and as board members." Providers contribute through "quality measurement and reporting such as tracking outcomes for practices and for populations served" (IOM, 2015, p. 40).

Recommendations for the treatment or management of substance-use disorders or co-occurring mental health and

substance-use disorders are commonly made after evaluation and diagnosis are completed but without having first engaged the individual and without factoring in their readiness for treatment, personal preferences, or needs. The consideration of treatment needs must include individual "fit" in order to promote the possibility of successful outcome. Likewise, the goals for treatment must reflect the goals of the person the practitioner is striving to help rather than those of the care team or family. Readiness for change is often assessed using the Transtheoretical, or Stages of Change, model first developed by Prochaska and DiClemente, which describes stages of precontemplation, contemplation, preparation, action, and maintenance. For engagement to occur, the practitioner needs to find ways of meeting the individual where they are and of matching communication and treatment recommendations to the individual's preparation for change (Prochaska, DiClemente, & Norcross, 1992).

Motivational Interviewing

MI represents one of the best practices for promoting engagement and helping move individuals toward the direction of healthy change. It is a purposeful model of communication that serves to activate a person's own motivation and resources for change. It is nondirective, yet mindfully directional (Miller & Rollnick, 2013). The spirit of MI conveys partnership and acceptance; it supports autonomy, affirms strength, and is evocative; and it does not strive to provide a remedy that may not have

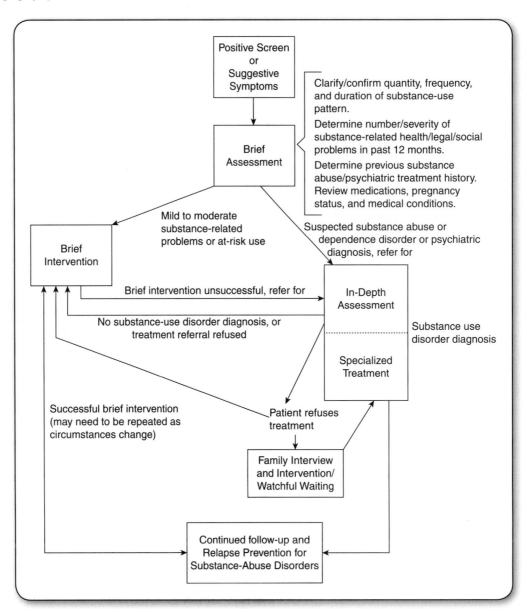

FIGURE 41.1

A decision tree for substance abuse assessment, diagnosis, and treatment for primary care clinicians.

Derived from National Institute on Alcohol Abuse and Alcoholism (1993).

been requested. Rather than convincing or coercing the individual to comply with treatment recommendations, the communication and the context of the relationship promote the explication of participants' desire and goals for health. The use of MI has been found to be especially effective in work with individuals who have substance-use disorders. The practitioner truly learns about the context and the goals of the patient, thereby allowing ultimate recommendations to be a good match for that individual. An added incentive for primary care providers to learn and utilize MI in routine practice is the diffusion of conflict with patients and the increased probability that agreed-upon follow-up or homework will take place (Miller,

Forcehimes, & Zweben, 2011; Miller & Rollnick, 2002; Miller & Rollnick, 2013; Miller, Zweben, DiClemente & Rychtarik, 1999).

Screening, Brief Intervention, and Referral to Treatment

The screening, brief intervention, and referral to treatment (SBIRT) process is grounded in MI and has been shown to be an effective means for identifying individuals who engage in substance misuse and for determining the severity of the disorder. SBIRT incorporates MI to provide brief intervention and to make referrals to treatment as indicated and accepted. This practice was initially implemented in the emergency care setting but is a natural fit for use in the primary care setting (SAMHSA, 2013b).

Level of Care

The ASAM provides an algorithm for recommending placement in outpatient (once-a-week treatment), intensive outpatient (three-times-a-week treatment, including group as well as individual therapy), or inpatient treatment. The criteria reflect the severity of the substance use, as well as the social context of the individual. As with any guideline, the ASAM placement criteria are not proscriptive and do not replace clinical judgment. Riggs found that one session per week of individual therapy (cognitive behavioral therapy [CBT] and motivational enhancement therapy [MET]) was equally effective for adolescents regardless of what level of care might have been recommended on the basis of the ASAM placement criteria (Riggs et al., 2007; Riggs, Caverly, & Grappone, 2013).

For women and adolescent girls, the circumstances of substance use often demand the selection of treatment level be tailored to fit individual need. For example, a woman in an untenable living situation fraught with opportunity or pressure to use substances may require an inpatient episode of care to stabilize in a supportive environment. Other women, who fear the loss of hard-to-replace jobs or have no one to care for their children, may find outpatient treatment to be most beneficial. Some women will need a short inpatient treatment episode for medically supervised substance discontinuation. Women who are pregnant or postpartum may also have medical complications best served in an inpatient setting. However, individuals who are extremely anxious may find the ordeal of the inpatient setting impossible to tolerate. Women who are in the military or who have careers that would be severely limited by employer knowledge of their substance use may need both support and help to find adequate treatment that will not create more circumstantial problems. When barriers to seeking care are perceived to be too great to overcome, women will be less likely to engage in treatment. However, when it is possible to match care to patient need and capacity, thereby removing unnecessary stress, it allows the person to focus on participating in getting healthier rather than surviving an ordeal or awaiting the next crisis.

Psychotherapeutic Interventions

Although the IOM has opted not to develop a list of approved evidence-based therapies for treating substance-use disorders, the National Registry of Evidence-Based Programs and Practices (NREPP) does provide such a list, and NIDA has identified CBT, contingency management (CM), MET, and family therapy as having particular benefit in the treatment of substance-use disorders. Many of the EBPs listed on the NREPP site are amalgamations of these psychotherapeutic interventions.

One element consistent among the EBPs is that the therapeutic intervention is applied with fidelity to a protocol, and there is a manual that provides structure to the intervention. Many of the EBPs explicitly indicate the number of sessions or weeks of therapy to be provided and for which outcomes have been determined. In substance-use treatment as usual, a key measurement has often been retention in treatment rather than a specific treatment goal our outcome. Certainly, for psychotherapeutic interventions, it is widely held that the more "doses" of treatment provided, the greater the possibility of improved outcome; retention in treatment does allow more opportunity for doses of therapy to be received, but it does not indicate treatment benefit or change associated with treatment.

Project Match was funded by the NIAAA in 1990 as a multisite clinical trial to explore treatment effectiveness. This project compared the outcomes of 12-step facilitation therapy, CBT, and MET. Each therapy was structured to be provided for 12 weeks by a therapist using a standardized protocol. The intention was to evaluate whether patient characteristics intersected with treatment outcomes differentially for the three therapies. The results showed that patient characteristics were related to different outcomes, depending upon the therapy provided. For example, although the 12-step group is commonly not considered an EBP, individuals who were without an abstinence social-support system benefitted most from this group. Those presenting with the greatest oppositionality and anger did best in the MET; individuals with co-occurring mental health disorders and those with less severe alcohol use benefitted from CBT, whereas those with more severe AUDs benefitted more from the 12-step facilitation group (Project Match Research Group, 1998). Women in Sobriety and Smart Recovery may represent alternatives to Alcoholics Anonymous or Narcotics Anonymous for women. In particular, Women in Sobriety represents an environment focusing on the needs and experiences of women (Miller et al., 2011).

Cognitive Behavioral Therapy

CBT is grounded in becoming aware of one's own automatic, possibly irrational thoughts and underlying assumptions that precede dysregulated emotional response and may result in behavior that is problematic, such as substance use. It is a skills-based learning therapy focused on developing replacement thoughts and a pattern of increased self-efficacy, but this does not diminish the importance of empathy and connection in the therapeutic relationship. CBT utilizes homework to practice skills and explores the role of beliefs, thoughts and behaviors using tools such as functional analysis. CBT can be especially helpful for individuals who need to reframe traumatic experiences, manage anxiety or depressive symptoms, manage mood volatility and impulsiveness, and tolerate the discomfort of abstaining from substances and instead experience feelings. For women who have substance-use disorders, CBT can often be of tremendous value in enhancing self-worth and reinforcing capability while becoming free of substance use. It is well studied with models for use in substance use and a myriad of mental health disorders. Seeking Safety is a manualized CBT therapy designed to treat co-occurring posttraumatic stress disorder and substance use. It has been found to be of particular benefit for women and girls who have experienced trauma and are engaged in substance use (Najavitis, 2002).

Contingency Management

CM is based on behavioral reinforcement theory. Nancy Petry developed a model for CM in which fishbowl draws are used in research studies as well as in the clinical setting and in drug courts to reward positive behaviors. Maintaining sobriety as evidenced by negative urine drug screens, completion of a CBT homework assignment, attendance at therapy sessions, or participation in a prosocial activity is rewarded by an opportunity to draw from the fishbowl. Often there is a perception that the use of CM represents bribery; however, the evidence is that it is a powerful tool found to have positive outcomes when used as an element of substance-use treatment. Programs using CM may enlist participants to help determine what prizes might be made available. Whether the participant wins or not, the conveyance of affirmation for having earned the fishbowl draw represents a reinforcement (Godley, Godley, Wright, Funk, & Petry, 2008; Stitzer, Petry, & Peirce, 2010).

Motivational Enhancement Therapy

MET is therapy consistent with MI and SBIRT, as previously described. The emphasis is on guiding the individual toward positive health decisions that are grounded in their own goals and personal strengths (Miller, Zweben, DiClemente, & Rychtarik, 1999).

Family Therapy

A number of family therapy approaches have been developed for use with families of young people who have behavioral disorders and substance use. Functional Family Therapy and Multi-Systemic Family Therapy are among the most widely implemented, often among youth involved with the juvenile justice system. In these models, the work is designed to assist families in managing the communication and the environment in a way that diminishes conflict and reduces oppositional behaviors as well as substance use. When these therapies are funded through the juvenile justice system, the reduction of what is known as criminogenic behavior and recidivism are the key outcomes measured (Schaeffer & Borduin, 2005; Sexton & Alexander, 2000).

■ PSYCHOPHARMACOLOGICAL INTERVENTIONS

The questions of when and what medication to prescribe for a woman known to have a substance-use disorder is always difficult. There is a very short list of medications that have indications for substance-use treatment and a much longer list of medications that are used off label to treat symptoms associated with substance withdrawal and/or the emotional symptoms that may be caused by a co-occurring psychiatric disorder or an artifact of the substance use. Certainly, when a psychiatric disorder is evident, it is appropriate to treat that disorder. Although in the past individuals experiencing co-occurring disorders were often required to defer treatment of psychiatric disorders pending a sustained interval of sobriety, this is not currently a standard of care. For women, decision making about prescribing medication is further complicated by known pregnancy, the possibility of unplanned pregnancy, and lactation. The prescribing decision must often be based in a risk–benefit analysis: whether treating the substance-use disorder specifically using an opioid antagonist, partial agonist/antagonist, or full agonist or determining whether to provide medication to stabilize symptoms of mood, anxiety, or psychotic disorders. Often this is a very individualized clinical decision, rather than a blanket approach to treatment. There is always a potential for unintended consequences whether prescribing a medication to a pregnant or nursing woman. The decision not to treat is also a treatment decision that has clinical consequences. Whenever possible, the decisions regarding a pharmacological intervention will be most effective when arrived at in collaboration with the person seeking care. Communicating treatment recommendations and the limits of the treatment in a mutually respectful manner while acknowledging the woman's goals and strengths, without succumbing to demands that may be contrary to best practice or clinical judgment, is critical to maintaining a healthy and safe relationship that permits future care to be accessible.

The first step toward any pharmacologic treatment decision is to be clear as to the diagnosis (whether the symptoms are related to substance use or a co-occurring disorder), the goal (for any intervention but especially for a pharmacologic therapy), the plan for care, and most important, the plan for assessing response and potentially discontinuing medication not found helpful. The next step is a risk–benefit assessment considering factors such as general health status, risks associated with potential QTC interval changes, drug–drug interactions (e.g., promethazine [Phenergan] is unsafe with methadone or other opioid medications), the self-harm or safety status of the individual, the risk of the medication being diverted or not safely stored, the prospect of adherence to the recommended dosing regimen, and the potential for benefit.

Prescriptions that offer high potential for abuse or which have a known street value should be avoided whenever possible, whether or not it is clear that the patient has a substance-use problem. When individuals are engaged in a methadone or buprenorphine (Suboxone) program, there are specific SAMHSA regulations specifying the management of these medications. Before providing a prescription or dispensing a take-home dose, it is necessary to assess whether the environment is stable enough for medication to be safely stored and administered. Safe storage is of particular importance when women have children in the home.

When methadone is dispensed, take-home doses must be placed in a locked box before being taken from the provider agency dispensary.

Once determined that medication is indicated and a prescription is the best clinical action, there remain some challenges. Substance-use disorders vary over time with regard to preferred substance, severity of use or cravings, and symptoms manifested in association with the substance. It can be difficult to know whether an apparent medication response is due to the medication prescribed or to a change in illicit substance use. This can lead to repetitive changes in prescribed medications before an adequate trial has been accomplished. Prescription medications can and do interact with over-the-counter medications, herbal remedies, and illicit substances that the practitioner may not be aware the patient is using. Adherence to prescription regimens is universally difficult and far more so for individuals who are accustomed to self-prescribing. A conversation about the challenges of medication adherence prior to providing the first prescription can help both the practitioner and the patient to be mindful of this possibility and adds a layer of transparency that may result in greater sharing of information. It is also common for prescription medications to unmask disorders that had not been evident before the initiation of a medication or to cause an exacerbation of reported symptoms; this may be more likely the case if the medication is not taken as prescribed.

■ FOOD AND DRUG ADMINISTRATION–APPROVED MEDICATIONS FOR TREATING SUBSTANCE-USE DISORDERS

Although numerous compounds are under development for the detoxification, antagonism, vaccination, craving reduction, and restoration of homeostasis, there is a very short list of currently approved medications. These are in the categories of sensitizing, antagonist, partial agonist, agonist, and replacement agents. The descriptions that follow are not intended as a full prescribing guide, but rather as a brief overview with a focus on use in pregnancy. Kranzler Ciraulo, and Zindel (2014) provide extensive information in the *Clinical Manual of Addiction Psychophramacology*, and the NIDA or ASAM websites are valuable resources. The Department of Veterans Affairs guidelines (U.S. Department of Veterans Affairs, 2015) highlight acamprosate, disulfiram, naltrexone oral or extended release, and the anticonvulsant topiramate as having strong evidence for, and the anticonvulsant gabapentin as having weak evidence, for the treatment of AUDs. Pharmacological treatments for opioid-use disorders with strong evidence include buprenorphine/naltrexone (or buprenorphine without naltrexone for the treatment of women who are pregnant), methadone, and extended-release injectable naltrexone. There is weak evidence cited for gradual-taper sedative–hypnotics using original benzodiazepine, a longer-acting benzodiazepine, or phenobarbital. There is no recommendation for the pharmacological treatment of cannabis-use disorders or stimulant-use disorders (www.healthquality.va.gov/guidelines/MH/sud/).

Alcohol

Disulfiram was approved in 1948 as an alcohol-sensitizing agent that inhibits the intermediate metabolism of alcohol, causing an elevation in serum acetaldehyde when alcohol is consumed. A cascade of physically uncomfortable symptoms known as the *disulfiram–ethanol reaction* arises, characterized by flushing, lowered blood pressure, elevated heart rate, nausea, vomiting, blurred vision, dizziness, or confusion. In some instances, psychotic symptoms may arise in susceptible individuals prescribed high doses. Common doses are 250 to 500 mg/d. A number of cautions exist, and safety in pregnancy or lactation is not clear.

Acamprosate was approved in 2004 as an agent that affects glutamate and GABA neurotransmitter systems to reduce alcohol cravings, although it is not entirely clear how it accomplishes this. The dosing of this medication has been challenging, as it is intended to be taken three times a day. Acamprosate is listed as pregnancy category C, so the manufacturer recommends cautious use among lactating women, as there are no clear data on the excretion of acamprosate in human milk.

Naltrexone (ReVia oral formulation as well as depot Vivitrol) was approved in 1984 as an opioid antagonist, blocking opioid receptors and thereby reducing the reward experienced in response to the use of alcohol. Vivitrol is the monthly injectable version of this medication. Both have been found to reduce cravings as well as use of alcohol. Naltrexone is pregnancy category C, and both it and 6-beta-naltrexol are excreted into human milk, with unknown effects on the nursing infant (Product Information, ReVia [naltrexone]).

Opioids

Methadone was approved in the 1960s as a long-acting opioid agonist medication that blocks opioid receptors, thereby preventing intoxication from short-acting opioids and/or withdrawal symptoms. Methadone is approved as an opioid substitution therapy only when provided through programs regulated by SAMHSA and the Drug Enforcement Agency (DEA). Nurse practitioners are now among the licensed professionals with the authority to initiate therapy (methadone induction) in settings that are directed by a physician. Methadone is pregnancy category C, yet it is considered the gold standard as an intervention for opioid-dependent pregnant women. Although methadone is present in breast milk, it is not uncommon for women to nurse while on methadone, although, to prevent infant opioid withdrawal, it is important for the infant to be weaned rather than to stop nursing abruptly. The management of care for pregnant women on methadone requires a team approach, and this team should include midwives or obstetric and pediatric practitioners, as well as chemical dependency professionals and social service providers. Doses may be given twice a day, and the dose requires adjustment over the course of the pregnancy and postpartum interval. The pregnant woman on methadone is a full participant in decisions regarding dosing and lactation after delivery and so must be given adequate information to make informed decisions and to follow recommendations for healthy infant outcomes. The inclusion of partners in this education and support process is highly recommended. Infants require monitoring for excessive sedation or for symptoms of withdrawal after birth and when nursing (U.S. National Library of Medicine, n.d.).

Buprenorphine was approved in 2002 as a partial mu-opioid agonist and kappa-opioid antagonist and was approved for the treatment of opioid dependence in 2002 in the United States. It is pregnancy category C and is available in the form of Subutex (buprenorphine) as well as Suboxone (buprenorphine/naloxone). Both are available as sublingual tablets or sublingual dissolving strips. Suboxone was developed to reduce the potential for overdose resulting from the injection of buprenorphine, and the naloxone is not absorbed unless injected. The Maternal Opioid Treatment: Human Experimental Research project (Jones, et al., 2012) found buprenorphine to have similar outcomes for mothers and infants as did methadone but with fewer neonatal abstinence symptoms. It is generally recommended that pregnant women be given buprenorphine rather than the combination of buprenorphine/naloxone to avoid potential toxicity associated with the naloxone. Buprenorphine is highly regulated but can be prescribed in office-based practices by medical practitioners who have completed mandatory training. Individuals who are treated with buprenorphine usually fill prescriptions at a local pharmacy. There are some settings in which dosing is more closely monitored, and daily dosing may be provided (Hendree et al., 2010; SAMHSA, 2004, 2005).

Naltrexone (oral and depot) is an opioid antagonist, blocking opioid receptors. Vivitrol is the monthly injectable version of this medication. Naltrexone is pregnancy category C, and both it and 6-beta-naltrexol are excreted into human milk, with unknown effects on the nursing infant. Methadone and buprenorphine are better established as safe treatments for pregnant and nursing women. It is important to educate individuals who achieve sobriety on naltrexone that if they do resume the use of opioid substances, they will have a lower tolerance and will be at risk of overdose if they resume their prior level of use immediately. This is somewhat different from individuals who have stabilized on an opioid agonist or on partial agonist medication. Still, for nonpregnant individuals who are early in the course of opioid-use disorder, naltrexone may be the most ethical first-trial medication, as it does not hold potential for escalating opioid use (Product Information, ReVia [naltrexone]).

Naloxone is an opioid antagonist that is administered by intravascular or intranasal methods to reverse opioid overdose. It has been available for medical use in emergency settings for years but was approved by the Food and Drug Administration (FDA) in November 2015 for use as a nasal spray for opioid overdoses. Naloxone is pregnancy category C. It rapidly crosses the placenta and is recommended only for use during pregnancy or in infants when it is essential and the only option for care. SAMHSA guidelines for the use of naloxone for first responders is available online or as a printed resource (SAMHSA, 2013a).

Nicotine

Nicotine replacement therapy (NRT) has been approved by the FDA in a variety of forms. Safety data during pregnancy are limited. Nicotine and NRT are classified as pregnancy category D and are not currently recommended for pregnant women. The American College of Obstetricians and Gynecologists (ACOG) recommends caution when considering the treatment of pregnant women with NRT and indicates it is something to consider only after other options and when the woman has clear intention of quitting the use of tobacco. Generally, there is inadequate data supporting the routine use of NRT in pregnant and nursing women (American College of Obstetricians and Gynecologists [ACOG], 2010).

Bupropion was FDA approved as Zyban for smoking cessation in 1997. It is a dopaminergic antidepressant that is classified as pregnancy category C. ACOG has indicated that although there is no known fetal or adverse pregnancy risk, there is insufficient evidence to evaluate safety in pregnancy and lactation (ACOG, 2010).

Varenicline is a nicotine partial agonist approved for smoking cessation in 2006. It is classified as pregnancy category C and is excreted in human milk. ACOG has indicated that there is inadequate information to ascertain safety during pregnancy and lactation (ACOG, 2010; Product Information, Chantix [varenicline]).

■ FUTURE DIRECTIONS

Women who experience substance-use disorders continue to be a somewhat hidden population, regardless of other characteristics. Stigmatizing language and potential threats of job loss or loss of child custody, coupled with limited resource allocation, serve to encourage women to hide substance use. Greater emphasis must be placed on preparing health care providers to be knowledgeable about and comfortable in assessing women for substance use. Efforts to change stigmatizing language used by health care providers represents a meaningful step. Additional efforts include:

- Advocate for the development of a variety of gender-specific treatment modalities and ensure that they become available in an affordable, geographically distributed manner to enhance the possibility that women will access treatment. Child-friendly settings that offer family programs and daycare if needed diminish barriers women experience in seeking help for substance use.
- Strive to increase funding to address epigenomics and grow the understanding of gender differences in the development of substance-use disorders.
- Prioritize the evaluation of women who have co-occurring mental health or substance-use disorders, and when these are present, have a capacity for providing of integrated care at the most accessible location.
- Focus on women veterans, determining the most acceptable and successful interventions by evaluating

the outcomes of current programs and asking women what they need that is not currently available to them.

- Incorporate evidence-based strategies in the development of any innovative models of care, evaluating outcomes in a prospective manner and comparing them to care as usual.
- Take action to press the pharmacology industry to gather the information that is lacking with regard to the safety of pharmacologic therapies for use in adolescent girls, women, and pregnant and lactating women.

■ REFERENCES

American College of Obstetricians and Gynecologists. (2010). Smoking cessation during pregnancy. Committee Opinion No. 471. American College of Obstetricians and Gynecologists. *Obstetrics and Gynecology, 116*, 1241–1244.

American Psychiatric Association. (2013). *Diagnostic and statistical manual of mental disorders* (5th ed.). Arlington, VA: American Psychiatric Publishing.

American Society of Addiction Medicine (ASAM). (2013). *Drug testing: A white paper of the American Society of Addiction Medicine (ASAM).* Chevy Chase, MD: Author. Retrieved from http://www.asam.org/docs/default-source/public-policy-statements/drug-testing-a-white-paper-by-asam.pdf

Ashman, J. J., Hing, E., & Talwalkar, A. (2012). *Variation in physician office visit rates by patient characteristics and state, 2012.* NCHS data brief, no 212. Hyattsville, MD: National Center for Health Statistics.

Babor, T. F., de la Fuente, J. R., Saunders, J., & Grant, M. (1992). *AUDIT: The alcohol use disorders identification test: Guidelines for use in primary health care.* Geneva, Switzerland: World Health Organization.

Bell, A. V., Ompad, D., & Sherman, S. (2004). Sexual and drug-risk behaviors among women who have sex with women. *American Journal of Public Health, 96*(6), 1066–1072.

Blackwell, D. L., Lucas, J. W., & Clarke, T. C. (2014). Summary health statistics for U.S. adults: National Health Interview Survey, 2012. National Center for Health Statistics. *Vital Health Statistics, 10*(260), 83.

Blow, F. C., Brower, K. J., Schulengerg, J. E., Demo-Dananberg, L. M., Young, J. P., & Beresford, T. P. (1992). The Michigan Alcoholism Screening Test—Geriatric Version (MAST-G): A new elderly specific screening instrument. *Alcoholism: Clinical and Experimental Research, 16*, 372.

Brown, E., Frank, D., & Friedman, A. (1997). *Supplementary administration manual for the expanded female version of the Addiction Severity Index (ASI) instrument, The ASI-F.* DHSH Publication No. SMA 96–8056. Rockville, MD: Center for Substance Abuse Treatment, Office of Evaluation, Scientific Analysis and Synthesis.

Center for Substance Abuse. (1998). *Under the rug: Substance abuse and the mature woman.* New York, NY: Columbia University Press.

Centers for Disease Control and Prevention (CDC). (2010). *2010 STD treatment guidelines.* Retrieved from http://www.cdc.gov/std/treatment/2010/qanda/screening.htm

Centers for Disease Control and Prevention (CDC). (2013a). *Vital signs: Prescription painkiller overdoses: A growing epidemic, especially among women.* Retrieved from www.cdc.gov/vitalsigns/prescriptionpainkilleroverdoses/index.html

Centers for Disease Control and Prevention (CDC). (2013b). Vital signs: Current cigarette smoking among adults aged ≥ 18 years with mental illness—United States, 2009–2011. *Morbidity and Mortality Weekly Report, 62*(05), 81–87.

Centers for Disease Control and Prevention (CDC). (2013c). Trends in smoking before, during, and after pregnancy—Pregnancy risk assessment monitoring system, United States, 40 sites, 2000–2010. *Morbidity and Mortality Weekly Report, 62*(SS06), 1–19.

Centers for Disease Control and Prevention (CDC). (2014). *The health consequences of smoking—50 years of progress: A report of the Surgeon General.* Atlanta, GA: U.S. Department of Health and Human Services (USDHHS), Centers for Disease Control and Prevention, National Center for Chronic Disease Prevention and Health Promotion, Office on Smoking and Health.

Centers for Disease Control and Prevention (CDC). (2015). Current cigarette smoking among adults—United States, 2005–2014. *Morbidity and Mortality Weekly Report, 64*(44), 1233–1240.

Center for Substance Abuse Treatment. (2004). *Clinical Guidelines for the use of buprenorphine in the treatment of opioid addiction: Treatment improvement protocol (TIP) series 40.* DHHS Publication No. (SMA) 04-3939. Rockville, MD: Substance Abuse and Mental Health Services Administration.

Center for Substance Abuse Treatment. (2005). *Medication-assisted treatment for opioid addiction in opioid treatment programs: Treatment improvement protocol (TIP) series 43.* HHS Publication No. (SMA) 12-4214. Rockville, MD: Substance Abuse and Mental Health Services Administration.

Cook, B. L., & Alegria, M. (2011). Racial-ethnic disparities in substance abuse treatment: The role of criminal history and socioeconomic status. *Psychiatric Services, 62*, 1273–1281.

Cyr, M. G., & McGarry, K. A. (2002). Alcohol use disorders in women. Screening methods and approaches to treatment. *Postgraduate Medicine, 112*, 31–32, 39–40, 43–47.

del Vecchio, P. (2012). SAMHSA's working definition of recovery updated. *Substance Abuse and Mental Health Services Administration (SAMHSA).* Retrieved from http://blog.samhsa.gov/2012/03/23/definition-of-recovery-updated

Eggert, L. L., Thompson, E. A., Herting, J. R., Nicholas, L. J., & Dicker, B. G. (1994). Preventing adolescent drug abuse and high school dropout through an intensive school-based social network development program. *American Journal of Health Promotion, 8*(3), 202–215.

Galanter, M., Kleber, H. D., & Brady, K. T. (2015). *Textbook of substance abuse treatment* (5th ed.). Arlington, VA: American Psychiatric Publishing.

Godley, S. H., Godley, M. D., Wright, K. L., Funk, R. R., & Petry, N. M. (2008). Contingent reinforcement of personal goal activities for adolescents with substance use disorders during post-residential continuing care. *American Journal on Addictions, 17*(4), 278–286.

Goler, N. C., Armstrong, M. A., Taillac, C. J., & Osejo, V. M. (2008). Substance abuse treatment linked with prenatal visits improves perinatal outcomes: A new standard. *Journal of Perinatology, 28*(9), 597.

Greenfield, S. F., Manwani, S. G., & Nargiso, J. E. (2003). Epidemiology of substance use disorders in women. *Obstetrics and Gynecology Clinics of North America, 30*(3), 413–446.

Gruenewald, P. J., & Klitzner, M. (1991). Results of a preliminary POSIT analyses. In E. Radhert (Ed.), *Adolescent assessment/referral system manual* (DHHS Pub. No. [ADM] 91–1735). Rockville, MD: National Institute on Drug Abuse.

Hawkins, J. D., Catalano, R. F., & Miller, J. Y. (1992). Risk and protective factors for alcohol and other drug problems in adolescence and early adulthood: Implications for substance abuse prevention. *Psychological Bulletin, 112*(1), 64–105.

Henderson, D., & Boyd, C. (1997). All my buddies was male: Relationship issues of addicted women. *Journal of Obstetric, Gynecologic, and Neonatal Nursing, 26*(4), 469–476.

Hendree, E. J., Kaltenbach, K., Heil, S. H., Stine, S. M., Coyle, M. G., Arria, A. M.,...Fischer, G. (2010). Neonatal abstinence syndrome after methadone or buprenorphine exposure. *New England Journal of Medicine, 363*, 2320–2331.

Holder, H. D. (1999). Prevention aimed at the environment. In B. S. McCrady and E. E. Epstein (Eds.), *Addictions: A comprehensive guidebook* (pp. 573–594). New York, NY: Oxford University Press.

Hughes, T. L., & Wilsnack, S. C. (1997). Use of alcohol among lesbians: Research and clinical implications. *American Journal of Orthopsychiatry, 67*(1), 20–36.

Institute of Medicine (IOM). (1990). *Broadening the base of treatment for alcohol problems.* Washington, DC: National Academies Press.

Institute of Medicine (IOM). (1994). *Reducing risks for mental disorders: Frontiers for preventive intervention research.* Washington, DC: National Academies Press.

Institute of Medicine (IOM). (2015). *Psychosocial interventions for mental and substance use disorders: A framework for establishing evidence-based standards.* Washington, DC: National Academies Press.

Jones, H. E., Fischer, G., Heil, S. H., Kaltenbach, K., Martin, P. R., Coyle, M. G.,...Arria, A. M. (2012). Maternal opioid treatment: Human experimental research (MOTHER)—approach, issues and lessons learned. *Addiction, 107*(S1), 28–35.

Kandel, D. B., & Yamaguchi, K. (1993). From beer to crack. *American Journal of Public Health, 83*, 851–855.

Kilpatrick, D. G., Resnick, H. S., Saunders, B. E., & Best, C. L. (1998). Victimization, posttraumatic stress disorder, and substance use and abuse among women. In C. L. Wetherington & A. B. Roman (Eds.), *Drug addiction research and the health of women,* 285–307. Rockville, MD: National Institue on Drug Abuse.

Koob, G. F. (2015). Neurobiology of addiction. In M. D. Galanter, H. D. Kleber, and K. T. Brady (Eds.), *Textbook of substance abuse treatment,* DSM-5 Edition (pp. 3–24). Washington, DC: American Psychiatric Publishing.

Kranzler, H. R., Ciraulo, D. A., & Zindel, L. R. (2014). *Clinical manual of addiction psychopharmacology* (2nd ed.). Washington, DC: American Psychiatric Publishing.

Kumpfer, K. L. (1998). Selective prevention interventions: The strengthening families program. In R. S. Ashery, E. B. Robertson, & K. L. Kumpfer (Eds.), *Drug abuse prevention through family interventions.* NIDA Research Monograph #177 (pp. 160–297). Rockville, MD: National Institute on Drug Abuse.

Lillehoj, C. J., Trudeau, L., Spoth, R., & Wickrama, K. A. (2004). Internalizing, social competence, and substance initiation: Influence of gender moderation and a preventive intervention. *Substance Use and Misuse, 39*(6), 963–991.

Liu, X., & Kaplan, H. (1996). Gender-related differences in circumstances surrounding initiation and escalation of alcohol and other substance use/abuse. *Deviant Behavior: An Interdisciplinary Journal, 17,* 71–106.

Manwell, L. B., Fleming, M. F., Johnson, K., & Barry, K. L. (1998). Tobacco, alcohol, and drug use in a primary care sample: 90-day prevalence and associated factors. *Journal of Addictive Diseases, 17,* 67–81.

McCabe, S. E., Hughes, T. L., & Boyd, C. J. (2004). Substance use and misuse: Are bisexual women at greater risk? *Journal of Psychoactive Drugs, 36*(2), 217–225.

McLellan, A. T., Kushner, H., Metzger, D., Peters, R., Smith, I., Grissom, G.,...Argeriou, M. (1992). The fifth addition of the Addiction Severity Index. *Journal of Substance Abuse Treatment, 9,* 199–213.

Miller, W. R., Forcehimes, A. A., & Zweben, A. (2011). Treating addiction: A guide for professionals (pp. 124–126). New York, NY: Guilford Press.

Miller, W. R., & Rollnick, S. (2002). *Motivational interviewing: Preparing people for change* (2nd ed.). New York, NY: Guilford Press.

Miller, W. R., & Rollnick, S. (2013). *Motivational interviewing, helping people change* (3rd ed.). New York, NY: Guilford Press.

Miller, W. R., Zweben, A., DiClemente, C. C., & Rychtarik, R. G. (1999). *Motivational enhancement therapy manual: A clinical research guide for therapists treating individuals with alcohol abuse and dependence.* Rockville, MD: National Institute on Alcohol Abuse and Alcoholism.

Moos, R. H., Schutte, K., Brennan, P., & Moos, B. S. (2004). Ten year patterns of alcohol consumption and drinking problems among older women. *Addiction, 99*(7), 829–838.

Najavitis, L. M. (2002). *Seeking safety: A treatment manual for PTSD and substance abuse.* New York, NY: Guilford Press.

National Institute on Alcohol Abuse and Alcoholism (NIAAA). (1993). *Assessing alcohol problems. A guide for clinicians and researchers.* NIAAA Treatment Handbook Series #4. Rockville, MD: Author.

National Institute of Health (NIH). (2013, December 11). *Tobacco, drug use in pregnancy can double risk of stillbirth. NIH network study documents: Elevated risk associated with marijuana, other substances* [News release]. Retrieved from www.nichd.nih.gov/news/releases/Pages/121113-stillbirth-drug-use.aspx

National Institute on Drug Abuse (NIDA). (2013). *Receptor may underlie gender differences in response to smoking cessation.* Retrieved from https://www.drugabuse.gov/news-events/nida-notes/2013/05/receptor-may-underlie-gender-differences-in-response-to-smoking-cessation-therapy

Nolen-Hoeksema, S. (2004). Gender differences in risk factors and consequences for alcohol use and problems. *Clinical Psychology Review, 24*(8), 981–1010.

Pentz, M. A. (1994). Adaptive evaluation strategies for estimating effects of community-based drug abuse prevention programs. *Journal of Community Psychology, 22*(1), 26–51.

Pentz, M. A., Bonnie, R. J., & Shopland, D. S. (1996). Integrating supply and demand reduction strategies for drug abuse prevention. *American Behavioral Scientist, 39*(7), 897–910.

Prochaska, J. O., DiClemente, C. C., & Norcross, J. C. (1992). In search of how people change: Applications to addictive behaviors. *American Psychologist, 47,* 1102–1114.

Product Information. *Chantix (varenicline).* New York, NY: Pfizer U.S. Pharmaceuticals Group.

Product Information. *ReVia (naltrexone).* Wilmington, DE: DuPont Pharmaceuticals.

Project Match Research Group. (1998). Matching alcohol treatment to client heterogeneity: Treatment main effects and matching effects on within treatment drinking. *Journal of Mental Health, 7*(6), 589–602.

Quest Diagnostics. (2013). *Health trends: Prescriptive drug monitoring report 2013.* Retrieved from http://www.questdiagnostics.com/dms/Documents/healthtrends/2013_health_trends_prescription_drug_misuse.pdf

Riggs, P, D., Mikulich-Gilbertson, S. K., Davies, R. D., Lohman, M., Klein, C., & Stover, S. K. (2007). A randomized controlled trial of fluoxetine and cognitive behavioral therapy in adolescents with major depressive disorder, behavior problems and substance use disorders. *Archives of Pediatrics and Adolescent Medicine, 161*(11), 1026–1034.

Riggs, P., Caverly, S., & Grappone, G. (2013). *Research to Practice: Real world implementation of integrated treatment for co-occurring psychiatric and substance use disorders.* Joint Meeting on Adolescent Treatment Effectiveness, Baltimore, MA.

Russell, M. (1994). New assessment tools for drinking in pregnancy: T-ACE, TWEAK, and others. *Alcohol, Health, and Research World, 18*(1), 55–61.

Schaeffer, C. M., & Borduin, C. M. (2005). Long-term follow-up to a randomized clinical trial of multisystemic therapy with serious and violent juvenile offenders. *Journal of Consulting and Clinical Psychology, 73*(3), 445–453.

Sexton, T. L., & Alexander, J. F. (2000). Functional family therapy. *Juvenile Justice Bulletin.* Retrieved from https://www.ncjrs.gov/pdffiles1/ojjdp/184743.pdf

Smith, S. M., Stinson, F. S., Dawson, D. A., Goldstein, R., Huang, B., & Grant, B. F. (2006). Race/ethnic differences in the prevalence and co-occurrence of substance use disorders and independent mood and anxiety disorders: Results from the national Epidemiologic Survey on Alcohol and Related Conditions. *Psychological Medicine, 7,* 987–998.

Stitzer, M. L., Petry, N. M., & Peirce, J. (2010). Motivational incentives in the National Drug Abuse Treatment Clinical Trials Network. *Journal of Substance Abuse Treatment, 38*(Suppl. 1), 561–569.

Substance Abuse and Mental Health Services Administration (SAMHSA), Office of Applied Studies. (1997). *A guide to substance abuse services for primary care clinicians.* Rockville, MD: Author.

Substance Abuse and Mental Health Services Administration (SAMHSA), Office of Applied Studies. (2002). *National household survey on drug abuse: Population estimates 2000.* Rockville, MD: Author.

Substance Abuse and Mental Health Services Administration (SAMHSA), Office of Applied Studies. (2005a). *The DASIS report for 2000.* Rockville, MD: Author.

Substance Abuse and Mental Health Services Administration (SAMHSA), Office of Applied Studies. (2005b). *The National Survey on Drug Abuse and Health for 2003.* Rockville, MD: Author.

Substance Abuse and Mental Health Services Administration (SAMHSA). (2012). *SAMHSA's Working Definition of Recovery: 10 Guiding Principles of Recovery.* Publication ID: PEP12-RECDEF. Rockville, MD: Author.

Substance Abuse and Mental Health Services Administration (SAMHSA). (2013a). *Opioid overdose prevention toolkit.* HHS Publication No. (SMA) 13–4742. Rockville, MD: Author.

Substance Abuse and Mental Health Services Administration (SAMHSA). (2013b). *Systems-level implementation of screening, brief intervention, and referral to treatment.* Technical Assistance Publication (TAP) Series 33. HHS Publication No. (SMA)13–4741. Rockville, MD: Author.

Substance Abuse and Mental Health Services Administration (SAMSHA). (2013c). *Results from the 2012 National Survey on Drug Use and*

Health: Summary of National Findings, NSDUH Series H-46. HHS Publication No. (SMA) 13-4795. Rockville, MD: Author.

Substance Abuse and Mental Health Services Administration (SAMHSA). (2014). *Results from the 2013 National Survey on Drug Use and Health: Summary of National Findings*. HHS Publication No. (SMA) 14–4863. NSDUH Series H-48. Rockville, MD: Author.

U.S. Department of Health and Human Services (USDHHS). (2000). *Healthy People 2010: With understanding and improving health and objectives for improving health* (2nd ed., 2 vols.). Washington, DC: U.S. Government Printing Office.

U.S. Department of Veterans Affairs. (2015). *Management of substance use disorders*. Retrieved from http://www.healthquality.va.gov/guidelines/MH/sud

U.S. National Library of Medicine. (n.d.). *Toxnet*. Toxicology Data Network. Retrieved from http://toxnet.nlm.nih.gov/cgi-bin/sis/htmlgen?LACT"

Wheaton, B. (1985). Models for the stress-buffering functions of coping resources. *Journal of Health and Social Behavior, 26*, 352–365.

Winters, K. C., & Arria, A. (2011). Adolescent brain development and drugs. *The Prevention Researcher, 18*(2), 21–24.

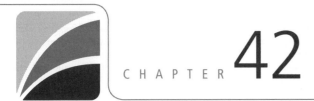
Gender-Based Violence and Women's Health

Angela Frederick Amar

Gender-based violence, also known as *violence against women*, is a public health and societal concern. It denotes violence inflicted on women because of their subordinate status in society. It includes any act or threat by men or male-dominated institutions that inflicts harm on a woman or girl because of gender. Gender-based violence includes physical, sexual, and psychological violence such as domestic or intimate partner violence (IPV) and sexual abuse, including rape and sexual abuse of children by family members. Additional examples are sexual slavery and trafficking; traditional practices harmful to women, such as honor killings, burning or acid throwing, female genital mutilation, dowry-related violence; violence in armed conflict; and sexual harassment and intimidation at work (World Health Organization [WHO], 2010). Gender violence occurs in both the "public" or general community and in "private," or family, spheres. In most cultures, traditional beliefs, norms, and social institutions legitimize and therefore perpetuate violence against women. The state perpetuates violence through policies or the actions of agents of the state, such as the police, military, or immigration authorities. Gender-based violence happens in all societies, across all social classes.

Gender-based violence is a major cause of injury that leads many survivors to seek care in the emergency departments of hospitals and clinics. However, long-term physical and mental health consequences cause survivors to seek health care in primary care, prenatal and postnatal areas, labor and delivery areas, pediatricians' offices, mental health services, and other areas within most hospitals and clinics (Laughon, Amar, Sheridan, & Anderson, 2010). Each of these encounters provides nurses and other health care providers with opportunities to identify and intervene for gender-based violence and health-related consequences (Sharps et al., 2001).

The purpose of this chapter is to orient the women's health nurse to IPV and sexual violence and their related behaviors such as stalking and strangulation. Limited aspects of perpetration, although not a focus of this chapter, are included to increase nurse's awareness. Information is provided to assist the women's health nurse in the identification and assessment of gender-based violence. Current evidence-based nursing responses and interventions are presented, as are resources useful to nurses and to survivors of IPV and sexual violence and their families, friends, and other sources of social support. Because this book is geared toward women's health nurses, we refer primarily to the experiences of women as it relates to IPV and sexual violence. Within the field, the term *victim* is used to connote victimization, and some feel that *survivor* should not be used until the process of healing is complete. However, in our society, the term *victim* is also identified with weakness. Others feel that the process of healing starts immediately and that living through a traumatic event confers survivor status. In this chapter, the term *survivor* is used in place of the term *victim*.

■ DEFINITION AND SCOPE (INCIDENCE/PREVALENCE)

IPV and sexual violence are both forms of gender-based violence that fall under the category of interpersonal violence. Both occur in the context of a social relationship that more often includes known perpetrators rather than strangers. IPV is a pattern of assaultive and coercive behaviors that adults or adolescents use against their intimate partners. Intimate partnerships include current or former dating, married, or cohabiting relationships of heterosexuals, lesbian women, or gay men. Both men and women are identified as victims/survivors and perpetrators of IPV (Groves, Augustyn, Lee, & Sawirds, 2002). However, women are often overrepresented in survivor status, and males are more likely to be identified as perpetrators (Archer, 2000; Breiding et al., 2014). Worldwide, 35% of women have experienced either physical and/or sexual IPV or nonpartner sexual violence (WHO, 2013a). A substantial proportion of U.S. female and male adults have experienced some form of sexual violence, stalking, or IPV during their lifetimes. Centers for Disease Control and Prevention (CDC) data suggest that 23.6% of women and 11.5% of men reported experiencing physical or sexual IPV in their lifetimes. Severe physical violence is experienced by 22.3% of women and 12% of men (Breiding et al., 2015).

IPV, also referred to as *domestic violence*, can take many forms. Physical IPV is inflicting physical pain or bodily harm against a partner. For example, physical IPV behaviors include hitting, punching, kicking, choking, pushing, burning, and throwing things. Emotional abuse involves inflicting mental anguish and includes threatening, humiliating, intimidating, and degrading behaviors. It also includes coercive behaviors, such as jealousy and withholding financial support, that are used to maintain control. Sexual IPV is any form of sexual contact or exposure without consent or forced sexual activity. Most survivors experience multiple forms of violent behaviors in their relationships.

Sexual Violence

Sexual violence includes all sexual acts that occur against one's wishes. It includes anal, vaginal, and oral sexual activities and intercourse. Sexual violence includes a range of behaviors from rape to a range of unwanted sexual behaviors with or without contact (Black et al., 2011). Rape involves some form of sexual penetration of the survivor; sexual assault is a broader category that includes any type of unwanted or nonconsensual sexual activity. An estimated 19.3% of women and 1.7% of men have been raped, and 43.9% of women and 23.4% of men have experienced other forms of sexual violence during their lifetimes. Among female rape survivors, 78.7% were raped before age 25 and 40% before age 18 years (Breiding et al., 2015). Adolescents and young adults are at highest risk of sexual victimization (Black et al., 2011). Although both men and women are victimized, survivors are more often women, and aggressors are more often male (Black et al., 2011; Breiding et al., 2015).

Rape is the most underreported crime to law enforcement (Rennison, 2002). Estimates of rape in general and victimization surveys are higher than actual crime reports from law enforcement. Societal stigma about sex, victim blaming, and the fact that most rapes are perpetrated by someone known to the survivor are all factors that make reporting to the police difficult (Sable, Danis, Mauzy, & Gallagher, 2006). Furthermore, survivors are concerned that they will not be believed or will be blamed (Amar, 2008). In fact, secondary victimization is often reported through experiences with health care providers and especially in the criminal justice system (Campbell, Wasco, Ahrens, Sefl, & Barnes, 2001). Men are particularly vulnerable to the stigma of sexual assault, especially because of the societal belief that it cannot happen to men, which could account for the lower reporting. Finally, the traumatic nature of experiencing violence could create a response involving high levels of psychological distress that may inhibit immediate reporting (Fisher, Daigle, Cullen, & Turner, 2003).

Stalking

Stalking is intimidation and psychological terror that often escalates into violence and has serious health consequences for its survivors (National Center for Victims of Crime, 2007).

Stalking behavior is "the willful, malicious, and repeated following or harassing of another person that threatens his or her safety" (Kamphuis & Emmelkamp, 2001, p. 795). Stalking can escalate to physical violence and is often a part of IPV (Fisher, Cullen, & Turner, 2000; Kohn, Flood, Chase, & McMahon, 2000). Furthermore, the intrusive and persistent nature of stalking can cause individuals to fear for their safety.

The National Violence Against Women Survey (NVAWS) indicated that 8% of women in the United States were stalked at some point in their lives, which, when compared with other types of violence, means that women are three times more likely to be stalked than raped and two times more likely to be physically assaulted than stalked (Tjaden & Thoennes, 1998). Furthermore, approximately 1,006,970 women and 370,990 men are stalked annually; 8% of women and 2% of men in the United States have been stalked at some time in their lives. The NVAWS revealed that the primary targets and 52% of survivors of violence were adults between 18 and 29 years of age. Although young adults are more likely to experience stalking, the behavior appears among all socioeconomic levels, often in highly educated survivors (Pathe & Mullen, 1997; Sheridan, Blaauw, & Davies, 2003).

Reproductive Coercion

Reproductive coercion is a newer identified form of IPV. It includes male partners' attempts to control pregnancy. Tactics include promoting pregnancy in their female partners through verbal pressure and threats; direct interference with contraception (birth control sabotage); and threats and coercion related to pregnancy continuation or termination (control of pregnancy outcomes; Miller et al., 2014). Abusive male partners have been found to actively promote pregnancy via behaviors such as verbal pressure to become pregnant, condom manipulation, threats, or actual violence in response to condom requests and direct acts of birth control sabotage (e.g., removing a vaginal ring, throwing out birth control pills, and blocking women from seeking access to contraception; Miller, Jordan, Levenson, & Silverman, 2010). In addition, once a female partner is pregnant, abusive male partners may initiate behaviors to control the outcomes of pregnancy, including violent acts, attempts to induce miscarriage, and coercion to either continue or terminate the pregnancy. It is suspected that reproductive coercion provides the link between IPV and unintended pregnancy. WHO's Multi-country Study on Women's Health and Domestic Violence provides compelling evidence that IPV is a strong and consistent risk factor for unintended pregnancy (Pallitto et al., 2013).

Etiology

The cycle of violence is a common explanation of the dynamics of IPV relationships; usually men are depicted as abusers and women as survivors. However, it can apply to both genders. The relationship usually begins without violence. The abuser presents as loving and caring. Tension builds gradually and eventually erupts in a violent episode. During the violent episode, the abuser is unpredictable and the survivor feels helpless. After the violent episode, the abuser is contrite and attentive and tries to make amends. The couple returns to the first stage, a honeymoon period. The survivor feels uncertain while trying to reconcile the loving partner of the first and last stages with the abusive person of the middle stage. Soon, however, the tension builds to an eruption, and the same cycle repeats (Walker, 2009). This cycle of violence helps explain the dynamics of the relationships and each partner's behavior. Most outsiders see only the violence and have difficulty understanding and responding to the relationship. This framework, depicted in Figure 42.1, is a useful aid in understanding the dynamics of an abusive relationship.

Societal factors also affect conceptualizations of gender-based violence. Myths about violence and victims/survivors prevail. Many of these myths blame survivors for their victimization. Discussions of sexual assault focus on what she was wearing, why she was there, and why she did not fight harder. We focus on why women stay in abusive relationships and ask why she does not leave rather than ask why he hits. These perceptions place the onus for preventing acts of interpersonal violence on the survivor rather than on the perpetrator. There is a large mismatch between the public perception of sexual assault and sexual assault offenders and the reality of sexual assault. The general public thinks of sexual

assault as a very violent act, often involving extreme force or a weapon, between people who do not know each other and occurring in a public place. Most sexual assaults are committed by someone known to the survivor; force is not always used, and the locations are usually private (Black et al., 2011; Fisher, Cullen, & Turner, 2000). Furthermore, as a society, we place family and intimate and sexual relationships in a private zone that makes witnesses reluctant to intervene and prevents conversations regarding violence. This makes it difficult for those affected to recognize the problem and to seek help.

The gender-based violence movement provides a new context in which to examine and understand the phenomenon of violence against women. It shifts the focus from women as victims to gender and the unequal power relationships between women and men created and maintained by gender stereotypes as the basic underlying cause of violence against women. Institutions within society often lend support for violence through historical interpretations, various customs, and social mores. A historical patriarchal structure lends support to societal factors such as gender roles and equality, normalization of violence, and objectification of women. Traditional gender role beliefs that support patriarchy and male dominance are associated with violence against

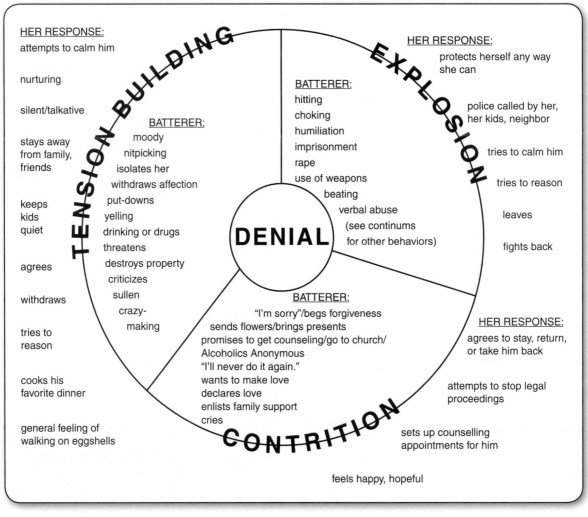

FIGURE 42.1
Cycle of violence.

women (Sokoloff & Dupont, 2005). It must be noted that not all men have violence-accepting attitudes or engage in violence against women. The term is not meant to suggest that all men are violent. Rather, it describes a context that normalizes violence and inequality with the institutions and structure of society.

One powerful societal institution used to support violence and to make it difficult to end violent relationships is organized religion. For example, the Bible is used to support husbands as in charge and wives as submissive. Popular media portrays violence and control as signs of a loving relationship that normalizes violence and makes it difficult for survivors to come forward. Misogynistic media that portray women as sexual objects negatively affect perceptions of gender equality. The objectification of women and their bodies is common. For example, women's bodies are used in advertisements for guns, alcohol, cars, and so on. Violence against women occurs in many countries in the world; however, the prevalence and severity of violence is higher in rural compared with industrialized areas (Moreno-Garcia, Jansen, Ellsberg, Heise, & Watts, 2009). The cause of gender-based violence is complex and multifactorial. Causes exist at the individual, familial, institutional, and societal level. Identification of causes helps identify solutions. The involvement of multiple entities is necessary to make change.

Risk Factors

Understanding risk factors is important so that a behavior can be prevented. A consistent risk factor that predicts future violence is past violence. Individuals who experienced one form of violence are more likely to experience subsequent violence (Classen, Palesh, & Aggarwal, 2005; Gagne, Lavoie, & Hebert, 2005; Halpern, Oslak, Martin, & Kupper, 2001; Smith, White, & Holland, 2003). Individuals who experienced child abuse are more vulnerable to experiencing sexual assault and physical partner violence than children who were not abused (Basile & Smith, 2011).

Findings from WHO's Multi-country Study on Women's Health and Domestic Violence identified secondary education, high socioeconomic status (SES), and formal marriage as factors that offer protection from IPV. Alcohol abuse, cohabitation, young age, attitudes supportive of violence, outside sexual partners, and experience with or perpetration of other forms of violence in adulthood are factors that increased the risk for IPV. The strength of the association increases when the woman and her partner share the risk factor (Abramsky et al., 2011). Jewkes (2002) also adds poverty, relationships full of conflict, and heavy alcohol consumption as risk factors of IPV. A woman's risk of being killed by an intimate partner is increased by the perpetrator's access to a gun or previous threat with a weapon, the perpetrator's stepchild in the household, and estrangement (Campbell et al., 2003). Furthermore, levels of social adversity are directly related to the experience of abuse, with women who report higher levels of adversity also reporting victimization (Bowen, Heron, Waylen, & Wolke, 2005).

Similarly, James, Brody, and Hamilton (2013) found that abuse before pregnancy and lower education level were strong predictors of abuse during pregnancy. An association exists between abuse while pregnant and unintentional pregnancy, lower SES, and single marital status. A longitudinal study of women during pregnancy and for 6 weeks after birth found that partner alcohol misuse was a risk factor for women's IPV victimization during pregnancy and that stress may increase the risk for IPV (Hellmuth, 2013). However, a longitudinal study of women during and after pregnancy found that pregnancy appeared to be protective against IPV (Bowen, Heron, Waylen, & Wolke, 2005). For example, the abusive partner may discontinue violence while his partner is pregnant.

Reasons posited for why abusers are violent include violence in the family of origin, alcohol and drug use, and mental illness or character defects. Thus far, these hypotheses have not been conclusively proven (Edleson, Eisikovits, & Guttmann, 1985). A meta-analytic review identified increased anger and hostility as more common with abusers than with nonabusers (Norlander & Eckhardt, 2005). Risk factors for identifying perpetrators of partner homicide include previous IPV, childhood survivors of abuse, drug and alcohol abuse, sexual jealousy, threat of separation, stalking behavior, and personality disorder (Aldridge & Browne, 2003).

Factors that increase the risk of sexual assault are women who are Native American, are African American, are single, have a low socioeconomic background, have emotional or mental difficulties, have a prior history of sexual violence, and report alcohol use (Söchting, Fairbrother, & Koch, 2004). The study of rapists has yielded four major typologies: power reassurance, power assertive, angry retaliatory, and anger excitation. The power reassurance rapist is also referred to as the *gentleman rapist*. He is the least violent and most common offender. He uses the assault to bolster his masculinity and self-esteem. The power assertive rapist is motivated by an ability to dominate another person. This rapist is sexually selfish and is not concerned about the survivor's emotional or physical well-being. The angry retaliatory rapist uses rape to punish women and express rage. These rapes are usually brutal and violent. The anger excitation rapist is a sadist who gets sexual gratification from inducing torture and suffering (Groth & Burgess, 1977; Hazelwood, 2009). These typologies are useful for nurses who care for offenders to understand their motivation.

▥ HEALTH CONSEQUENCES OF IPV

Violence against women is a significant public health issue costing society more than $4.1 billion in health care and mental health services for survivors (National Center for Injury Prevention and Control, 2003). Injuries are common in IPV and sexual assault. The U.S. health care community treats millions of intimate partner physical assaults and rapes annually, often unknown to the health care worker. Of the estimated 4.8 million intimate partner rapes and physical assaults perpetrated against women annually, approximately 2 million result in an injury to the survivor, and 552,192 result in some type of medical treatment for the survivor. Of the estimated 2.9 million intimate partner physical assaults perpetrated against men annually, 581,391 will result in an injury to the survivor, and 124,999 will result in some type of medical treatment for the survivor (Tjaden & Thoennes, 2000, 2006). Injury occurs in 36% of women who are raped, and in 41.5% of women and 19.9% of men who are physically assaulted by an intimate partner. Of those injured, most do not receive medical care.

The most common injuries received are minor, such as scratches, bruises, and welts. Common locations for genital injuries include tears or abrasions of the posterior fourchette, abrasion or bruising of the labia minora and fossa navicularis, and ecchymosis or tears of the hymen (Linden, 2011). A prospective study on sexual assault survivors presenting at an emergency department found that general body and genital trauma occurred in most cases (Riggs, Houry, Long, Markovchick, & Feldhaus, 2000). Finally, defensive injuries, such as lacerations, abrasions, and bruises, may be observed on the hands and the extensor surfaces of the arms and medial thighs.

Physical Health Consequences

The health consequences of experiencing physical, sexual, or psychological IPV can be found in every system of the body. A review by Campbell et al. (2002) reports that partner violence is associated with headache and back pain, vaginal infection and other gynecologic symptoms, and digestive problems. Common complaints of battered women include headaches, insomnia, choking sensations, hyperventilation, gastrointestinal symptoms, and chest, back, and pelvic pain (Campbell et al., 2002). Many of the symptoms commonly seen are stress related. Other conditions are the result of the impact of IPV on the cardiovascular, gastrointestinal, endocrine, and immune systems through chronic stress or other mechanisms. Examples of health conditions associated with IPV include asthma, bladder and kidney infections, circulatory conditions, cardiovascular disease, fibromyalgia, irritable bowel syndrome, chronic pain syndromes, central nervous system disorders, gastrointestinal disorders, joint disease, migraines, and headaches (Black, 2011; Campbell et al., 2002). Sexual assault is associated with a similar plethora of physical and mental health symptoms.

Strangulation is one of the most lethal forms of violence used against intimate partners. Asphyxia can induce loss of consciousness within about 10 seconds and death within 4 or 5 minutes. A person who was strangled can have substantial physical (dizziness, nausea, sore throat, voice changes, throat and neck injuries, breathing problems, ringing in ears, vision changes), neurological (eyelid droop, facial droop, left or right side weakness, loss of sensation, loss of memory, paralysis), and psychological (posttraumatic stress disorder [PTSD], depression, insomnia) concerns (Sheridan & Nash, 2007). Strangulation is also a strong risk factor of homicide and an important factor to assess (Campbell, 2002).

Reproductive Health Consequences

Gynecologic problems are the most consistent, longest lasting, and largest physical health differences between women who experienced violence and those who did not. Women with abuse histories are more likely to report gynecologic problems, including abdominal pain, urinary problems, decreased sexual desire, and genital irritation (Campbell, Woods, Chouaf, & Parker, 2000). Differential symptoms and conditions include sexually transmitted infections (STIs), vaginal bleeding or infection, fibroids, decreased sexual desire, genital irritation, pain on intercourse, chronic pelvic pain, and urinary tract infections (Campbell, 2002). Sexual assault and rape are also associated with symptoms of vaginal itching, vaginal discharge, pain or discomfort, and fear of STIs and pregnancy.

Women who are abused during pregnancy are more likely to experience all forms of violence report injury and are particularly likely to experience more severe forms of violence (Brownridge et al., 2011). Maternal exposure to IPV during pregnancy is associated with significantly increased risk of low birth weight and preterm birth (Shah & Shah, 2010). IPV coexisting with pregnancy is associated with late entry into prenatal care, low-birth-weight babies, premature labor, fetal trauma, and unhealthy maternal behavior (Jasinski, 2004; Shah & Shah, 2010). Adverse pregnancy outcomes, such as abortion, increased abortion rate, delayed prenatal care, fetal death, low birth weight, and preterm labor and delivery, are associated with IPV (Black, 2011). IPV is a strong risk factor for unintended pregnancy and abortion (Pallitto et al., 2013). Therefore reducing IPV can significantly reduce risks to maternal and reproductive health. Sexual violence during pregnancy is significantly associated with increased reporting of pregnancy-related physical symptoms (Lukasse, Henriksen, Vangen, & Schei, 2012).

■ HEALTH CARE USAGE AND PERCEPTIONS OF HEALTH

IPV and sexual violence have profound effects on the health of survivors that often translate to being heavy users of health care services. In a retrospective review of women who reported IPV in their lifetime, health care utilization was higher for all categories of service compared with women without IPV. Health care utilization decreased over time after the cessation of IPV; however, it was still 20% higher 5 years after the women's abuse ceased compared with women without IPV histories. Additionally, the adjusted annual total health care costs were higher for women with a history of IPV compared with other women (Rivara et al., 2007). Increased health care costs range from 1.4 to 4 times higher for women who have been exposed to IPV compared with other women (Bonomi et al., 2009; Fishman, Bonomi, Anderson, Reid, & Rivara, 2010; Rivara et al., 2007).

In contrast, survivors of forced sex were less likely to have seen a physician in the past 12 months for routine checkup and had lower health care utilization than women who had not been sexually assaulted (Kapur & Windish, 2011; Surís, Lind, Kashner, Borman, & Petty, 2004). However, rape creates additional costs to society. These include the direct costs of other services, including specialized nurse examiner programs in emergency rooms, mental health services, criminal justice response, social services, and substance abuse–treatment programs, as well as indirect costs such as estimates in dollars of the value of reduced quality of life for survivors (Basile & Smith, 2011).

Mental Health

The experience of trauma triggers intense emotions and disintegrating effects on the mind. The main findings of a recent systematic review suggest an association between IPV and depression, PTSD, and anxiety; the severity of mental health symptoms increases with the severity and extent of IPV exposure (Lagdon, Armour, & Stringer, 2014). Depression is the most common mental health symptom in response to violence. Anxiety is also a common consequence that often complicates the depression and continues for years after the traumatic experience. Lowered self-esteem often stems from self-blame. Self-blame is influenced by society's victim-blaming regarding sexual violence. Guilt and shame work to complicate the experience of depression. Substance use often starts as a way to self-medicate the pain of victimization (Kilpatrick, Acierno, Resnick, Saunders, & Best, 1997; Kilpatrick et al., 2003; Turchik & Hassija, 2014). Research on adolescents suggests an association of dating violence and substance abuse, unhealthy weight control, suicidality, depression, PTSD, general psychological distress, and low self-esteem (Amar & Gennaro, 2005; Coffey, Leitenberg, Henning, Bennett, & Jankowski, 1996; Silverman, Raj, Mucci, & Hathaway, 2001).

Depression

The experience of violent victimization can bring about fear, uncertainty, vulnerability, and helplessness. Depression is a common psychological response to gender-based violence. Depressive symptoms include irritable or sad mood; lack of interest in or pleasure from most activities; significant changes in weight and/or appetite, activity, and sleep patterns; loss of energy and concentration; excessive feelings of guilt or worthlessness; and suicidality (American Psychiatric Association, 2013). The loss of energy, interest, and concentration may cause problems academically, socially, or professionally. Depression can result in suicidal ideation and suicide attempts. In women, IPV is associated with incident depressive symptoms and suicide attempts, and depressive symptoms with incident IPV. In men, few studies have been conducted, but evidence suggests that IPV is associated with incident depressive symptoms (Devries et al., 2013). A meta-analytic review found that women who were exposed to partner violence had greater risk of experiencing depressive symptoms and being diagnosed with a depressive disorder (Beydoun, Beydoun, Kaufman, Lo, & Zonderman, 2012). Women with a history of sexual assault had a number of sleep difficulties, increased risk of depression, and overall poorer subjective well-being than their nonassaulted counterparts (Kendall-Tackett, Cong, & Hale, 2013).

Posttraumatic Stress Disorder

PTSD may be an acute or chronic response to physical or sexual violence. To be diagnosed with PTSD an individual must have experienced, witnessed, or been confronted with a traumatic event and have characteristic resulting symptoms, usually within the subsequent 3 months. Resulting symptoms include (a) persistent reexperiencing of the event, (b) persistent avoidance of stimuli associated with the trauma, and (c) symptoms of increased arousal (American Psychiatric Association, 2013). Persistent reexperiencing of a traumatic event creates an intrusion to daily functioning. Survivors may experience flashbacks, nightmares, or other reenacting experiences. Avoidance behaviors are efforts to avoid feelings, thoughts, activities, places, and people associated with the traumatic event. Numbing behaviors, such as difficulty expressing feelings, lack of interest in pleasurable activities, or isolation from others, are another way to avoid the traumatic event. The restrictions may interfere with normal life functioning.

Other survivors may have symptoms of increased arousal. Hyperarousal symptoms include being extremely watchful of the environment, insomnia, and anger and rage. Individuals with increased arousal symptoms are constantly alert and on guard for signs of danger or trauma. Exposure to severe and uncontrollable stressors desensitizes a person to trauma; that is, the person is so used to being on edge that they may react to milder stressors with a major stress response. Intrusions, avoidance, and hyperarousal symptoms may persist for a long time after the attack and usually disrupt the individuals' interpersonal, social, or occupational function.

Many people who experience traumatic events do not develop PTSD. Lifetime prevalence estimates suggest that about 8% of the general population have PTSD, with women being twice as likely as men to have PTSD at some point during their lifetimes (Kessler, Sonnega, Bromet, Hughes, & Nelson, 1995). Symptoms of PTSD often occur within 3 months of the stressor.

Acute stress disorder (ASD) is an immediate response to a traumatic event. ASD usually occurs within 1 month after the traumatic event. Individuals with ASD may experience dissociative symptoms, persistent reexperiencing of the event, marked avoidance, and marked arousal (American Psychiatric Association, 2013). Dissociative symptoms may occur during and after the trauma. They include numbing, detachment, reduced awareness of surroundings, depersonalization (feeling of lost identity), derealization (false perception that the environment is changed), and amnesia for important aspects of the trauma (American Psychiatric Association, 2013). These cognitive symptoms, during and after the trauma, provide an escape from the traumatic event by altering one's state of consciousness. The dissociative symptoms are not necessary for a diagnosis of PTSD. For a diagnosis of ASD, the symptoms must cause significant distress or impair functioning. Most people recover from ASD within a month; however, it is a significant predictor of PTSD (Brewin, Andrews, Rose, & Kirk, 1999). If the symptoms are unresolved, then the diagnosis is changed to PTSD. The symptom profile of ASD is similar to that of

PTSD. The main difference is that ASD has a shorter time of symptoms onset than PTSD.

Interpersonal Difficulties

Interpersonal responses to violence include problems with intimacy. Violence with a known offender can lead to feelings of betrayal and difficulty trusting others (Amar & Alexy, 2005). Forced sex can lead to feelings of repulsion and lack of pleasure (Turchik & Hassija, 2014). Alternately, forced sex has been associated with sexual risk taking such as promiscuity and unprotected sex (Deliramich & Gray, 2008; Johnson & Johnson, 2013; Turchik & Hassija, 2014). Social readjustment to the workplace seems to be the most difficult social impact of rape, and one study found productivity to suffer for up to 8 months after rape. Rape may be associated with deterioration of intimate relationships, which is often related to sexual problems or may stem from damage to beliefs such as those about the trustworthiness of others. Rape can also have a negative effect on the friends, family, and intimate partners of survivors, which further strains relationships (Basile & Smith, 2011).

■ EVALUATION/ASSESSMENT

Assessment Findings, Techniques, and Documentation

In clinical practice, nurses routinely encounter survivors of gender-based violence. Providers should ask patients of all ages about current and past experiences of violence at every visit (Amar, Laughon, Sharps, & Campbell, 2013). Routine inquiry promotes and increases early identification of gender-based violence. Survivors may seek health care because of injuries; however, inquiries about violence should occur at every visit, regardless of the absence or presence of abuse indicators (Groves, Augustyn, Lee, & Sawirds, 2002). The nurse should suspect abuse when the health visit is for ongoing emotional issues, drug or alcohol misuse, repeated sexually transmitted diseases, unexplained chronic pain, or repeated health consultations with no clear diagnosis (WHO, 2013b). Screening can occur at annual visits, new patient visits, visits for new presenting complaints, prenatal and postnatal visits, and pediatric well- and sick-child visits (Amar, Laughon, Sharps, & Campbell, 2013; Falsetti, 2007). The interview should be conducted in private, and patients should be informed of any reporting requirements or limits to confidentiality. Patients are asked about current and lifetime exposure to IPV, including physical, emotional, and sexual abuse and sexual assault.

Building Rapport

The nurse must build rapport while assessing for violence. Verbal and nonverbal communication is a key component. It is important for the nurse to be direct, honest, and professional while using language that the patient understands. Table 42.1 provides communication tips. Technical medical terms might be misinterpreted. For example, the nurse asks the survivor about choking rather than strangulation. Furthermore, individuals may answer affirmatively that they have experienced violent behaviors yet not identify themselves as abused, battered, or raped. Sample questions include, "Has your partner ever hit, shoved, or otherwise physically hurt you? Is your partner very jealous or controlling? Has your partner made you have sex when you didn't want to?" These questions are direct, gender neutral, and useful for identifying IPV (Rhodes & Levinson, 2003).

Verbal communication is important; however, nonverbal communication is equally important to assess. Behavioral clues from the survivor can be indicative of exposure to violence. For example, if a person cowers or flinches in response to touch, the nurse should suspect violence. Aspects of one's appearance can be used to conceal injuries. For example, hair in the face or makeup could be used to conceal bruises. Multiple injuries in various stages of healing should also raise suspicion and prompt the nurse to assess further. Another potential indicator of abuse is a mismatch between the injury and the story of how it happened (WHO, n.d.; e.g., being told that multiple injuries to the chest and face resulted from a fall).

Safety Concerns

Because of the dynamics of abuse and concern for safety, it is important to interview the patient alone, separate from their partner (Falsetti, 2007). Interviews with an abusive partner present can result in the partner dominating the interview and the survivor being too fearful of retaliation to disclose. One large urban hospital evaluated the use of a computerized screening protocol for patients during the

TABLE 42.1	Communication Tips	
DO	**DON'T**
Separate partners	Try to prove abuse by accusations or demands
Conduct the interview in private	Display horror, shock, anger, or disapproval
Be direct, honest, and professional	Place blame or make judgments
Use language the patient understands and ask about behaviors	Probe or press for answers that patient is not willing to give
Be understanding and attentive	Try to "prove" abuse using accusations or demands
Listen actively	Display horror, shock, anger, or disapproval

wait for services in the emergency department. Compared with face-to-face interview, screening for IPV using the computerized tool had a higher detection rate of IPV (Trautman, McCarthy, Miller, Campbell, & Kelen, 2007). Once a patient discloses violence, safety should be determined. Questions to assess immediate safety include:

- Are you in immediate danger?
- Do you have somewhere safe to go?
- Are you afraid your life is in danger?
- Has the violence gotten worse or scarier?
- Has your partner ever threatened to kill you, the children, or himself or herself

On receiving affirmative answers, the nurse should follow up with direct questions to determine the risk of danger. Safety assessments should be repeated at every follow-up visit (Groves, Augustyn, Lee, & Sawirds, 2002).

Screening Tools

Several tools have been developed and tested for use in identifying gender-based violence in a variety of settings. Screening tools are available and clearly described on the Futures without Violence website (www.futureswithoutviolence.org). The Abuse Assessment Screen (AAS) is a quick, easy-to-use measure that is effective in identifying IPV (Laughon, Renker, Glass, & Parker, 2008). This widely used questionnaire contains four questions on a range of violent behaviors, one of which asks about abuse during pregnancy. Male and female body maps are available to document injuries. In addition to assessing for past-year IPV, it assesses for sexual violence from any person and asks about fear, which could include current stalking threats.

For women who screen positive for IPV, the danger assessment (DA) can help the provider to determine the woman's risk of being killed by IPV (Campbell, Webster, & Glass, 2009). The provider needs to know the risk of homicide to determine the urgency and types of referrals to make. There are four levels of danger: variable risk, increased danger, severe danger, and extreme danger. High DA scores are associated with a greater risk of lethal violence. However, low scores do not mean that there is no risk. Rather, low scores are indicative of unknown risk. The nurse and survivor should review the findings together. It is important that survivors be aware of and appreciate the lethal risk of their partner's behavior. Significant factors to consider in determining the patient's safety are any increases in frequency and severity of the violence, threats of homicide or suicide, presence of firearms or weapons in the home, increased drug or alcohol use, and attempts or separation from or plans to leave the partner (Campbell, Webster, & Glass, 2009). Subsequent discussion with the woman should center on identifying resources and strategies for safety. If the woman is ready, discussions can also address leaving the partner or ending the relationship. The nurse respects the woman's choice and works with her to support her wishes and keep her safe.

Clinical red flags for reproductive coercion include inconsistent or no contraception use, frequent requests for emergency contraception, and frequent visits for pregnancy and STI testing (Miller et al., 2010). If reproductive coercion is suspected, the nurse should assess the women's pregnancy intention and ask direct questions regarding her partner's behavior. Assessing for other acts of violence is indicated for developing a comprehensive plan of action.

WHO recommends that providers should listen, inquire, validate, enhance safety, and support; the letters in the word *LIVES* can help providers remember (WHO, n.d.). Listening is important for communicating positive regard, understanding, and attentiveness. The nurse inquires as necessary to determine and respond to emotional, physical, social, and practical needs. Inquiring does not mean probing and making the women recount details and unnecessarily relive the trauma. Rather, the nurse gathers only the information needed to plan care. Validation shows the survivor that the nurse understands and believes what is being said. Enhancing safety is done by discussing a plan to prevent harm in future violence, and support is provided by giving referrals to services, information, and support (WHO, 2013b). Building rapport and a therapeutic relationship are the cornerstones that enable the nurse to work with the survivor to meet health and psychosocial needs.

Documentation

It is important to document the patient encounter. Documentation should include the patient's statements regarding the abuse, chief complaint, relevant history, results of physical examination, diagnostic procedures, and results of assessment, intervention, and referrals (Groves, Augustyn, Lee, & Sawirds, 2002).

◼ TREATMENT/MANAGEMENT

Focused Interventions

Routine screening must be followed by focused intervention. Patients who present for treatment after IPV episodes should receive immediate attention and care to treat their physical injuries. Once the medical or physical needs are attended to, the nurse can attend to safety and self-esteem needs. Abuse can erode the survivor's sense of self, and therefore the nurse is intentional in attempts to boost self-esteem. For example, the nurse can remind the survivor that it is not her fault. A critical area for assessment is determining the survivor's level of safety and planning strategies to maintain safety (Amar, Laughon, Sharps, & Campbell, 2013). Assessing and planning for safety is an ongoing process rather than a one-time event. Each visit represents an opportunity to reevaluate safety and to determine any immediate risk of harm. If it is not safe for a survivor to return home, the nurse should discuss options such as safe housing choices in domestic violence shelters or with friends and family. It is also useful to talk about legal resources such as the police and protective orders. Referrals to social workers can be helpful in identifying community resources. In addition, nurses can contact the local hotline to learn of community resources. If the survivor does not wish to leave the relationship, the nurse respects her wishes and does not try to coerce her to leave. Rather, the nurse should help her think about her safety at home. A discussion of an escape plan to be used for rapid escape in a crisis is essential. Questions such as "If you need to leave your home in a hurry, where would you go?" can be helpful.

Safety plans are used to help a survivor plan to leave the abusive partner. These plans are important because leaving an abusive partner increases the risk of being killed by the partner (Campbell, 2004). The nurse would make sure that the survivor understands that the increased risk of injury necessitates careful planning before leaving an abusive relationship. All patients in violent relationships should be engaged in a discussion of options and creation of a safety plan. Together, the nurse and survivor might consider options of places and people she can go to for help. For example, the survivor might keep spare keys, clothes, money, and important papers in a safe place with easy access after leaving. The nurse could provide referrals, phone numbers, and websites for external services and information (Dienemann, Campbell, Wiederhorn, Laughon, & Jordan, 2003). Although face-to-face interviews can be effective in planning for safety, the use of a computerized aid can improve the safety decision-making process related to IPV (Glass, Eden, Bloom, & Perrin, 2009).

Most women eventually leave a partner; however, some women make multiple attempts before they successfully leave (Campbell, 2001). Leaving is a process, and survivors need time to prepare emotionally for the ending of the relationship. Some women are not interested in leaving the partner; they only want the abuse to stop. It is important that the nurse respects the woman's choices and not assume she will leave. The nurse can ask direct questions to determine the woman's needs and perception of most useful forms of help. Providing information on domestic violence and resources with each visit helps prepare the woman. It is also important to be careful with handouts. Pamphlets and handouts related to IPV can alert the partner to the disclosure and prompt retaliatory violence and increased controlling behavior. A phone number on a prescription pad can be safe, effective, and nonthreatening.

Referrals

Experiencing violence creates multiple issues that require a multidisciplinary approach. Often, nurses work with social services and the criminal justice system to ensure that survivors' needs are met. Referrals to advocacy and counseling are beneficial. These services can link survivors with resources and have documented results in decreasing re-abuse and increasing quality of life (Wathen & MacMillan, 2003). Referrals are an important mechanism for connecting the survivor with resources for health, safety, and social support (WHO, 2013b). Examples include crisis lines, shelters, support groups, legal aid, and mental health programs. From a legal perspective, good documentation of injuries using body maps, photographs, and descriptions help with a court case. Referral to community resources includes notification of law enforcement and hospital social workers, as well as the provision of numbers to the domestic violence hotline,

IPV shelter, and IPV legal advocate (Glass, Dearwater, & Campbell, 2001).

Nursing Care of Sexual Assault Survivors

When a sexual assault survivor reports to the emergency department, they are evaluated for any injuries or physical problems. Injuries are treated. Once the survivor has been cleared as medically stable, the sexual assault nurse examiner (SANE), sexual assault response team (SART), or other trained professional responds and is involved in collecting forensic evidence, documenting assessment findings, and connecting the survivor to resources and support (Linden, 2011). The gathering of forensic evidence is a critical element of postrape care for women who want to pursue legal action. Using a special kit, the health care worker collects, documents, and turns over to law enforcement the evidence for processing and legal action. The survivor is offered testing and prophylactic treatment for STIs and pregnancy. There is also a legal obligation to provide court testimony if the case goes to trial. The SANE is specifically trained to respond in a supportive and sensitive manner to individuals who have experienced trauma. The nurses who provide these services have undergone specialized training in the collection of forensic evidence, assessment and treatment of STDs and HIV, crisis intervention, and rape trauma syndrome (Basile & Smith, 2011; Campbell, Patterson, & Lichty, 2005).

Crisis strategies, such as building rapport, encouraging verbalization of feelings, supporting existing coping strategies, helping mobilize social support systems, and providing referrals to resources, are used. It is important for all nurses to be aware of the available community resources. These include local and national hotlines, state coalitions, rape crisis centers and web-based resources. The resources are designed primarily to support survivors. However, providers may call to get advice on ways to approach the survivor, resources available in the community, and management strategies.

Prevention/Intervention

An overarching consideration is the inclusion of trauma informed care (TIC), which is a primary framework that emphasizes the effects of trauma and guides the entire organization and behavior of individuals in the system (Hopper, Bassuk, & Olivet, 2010). TIC services are those in which service delivery is influenced by an understanding of the impact of interpersonal violence and victimization on an individual's life and development. All staff of an organization, from the receptionist to direct care workers to the board of directors, must understand the influence of violence and trauma so that every interaction is consistent with the recovery process and reduces the possibility of retraumatization. Integrated services include core areas of outreach and engagement, screening and assessment, resource coordination and advocacy, crisis intervention, mental health and substance abuse services, trauma-specific services, parenting support, and health care.

Strategies for promoting a TIC system begin with education and training at all levels of the organization. Training helps the staff recognize that many of the problematic behaviors seen by survivors result from the trauma, often as means of coping with the abuse. This understanding shifts the focus from "What's wrong with you?" to "What happened to you?" The goal is to create a safe environment that minimizes the possibility of retraumatization. For example, when performing routine health assessments, the nurse recognizes the potential to trigger feelings of loss of control over one's body and provides detailed information on what will occur during the procedure. A TIC system is structured and organized to accommodate the vulnerabilities of trauma survivors and promotes service delivery in a manner that avoids inadvertent retraumatization and facilitates patient participation in treatment (Jennings, 2004). Incorporating knowledge about trauma in all aspects of service delivery ensures that treatment minimizes revictimization while facilitating recovery and empowerment.

Interventions used for IPV take a psychoeducational approach coupled with referrals. Most programs teach women about the cycle of violence and safety-promoting behaviors. Referrals are provided for local community-based IPV services, as well as other agencies for additional services. However, a systematic review of interventions targeting IPV showed that most programs focus on empowerment, safety, and community referrals and demonstrate patient-level benefits (Bair-Merritt et al., 2014). Limited success is demonstrated from programs targeting women in decreasing partner violence and also from programs targeting gender-based violence during pregnancy. A systematic review found that home visitation programs and multifaceted counseling interventions show promising effects for decreasing physical, sexual, and psychological violence and IPV during pregnancy (Van Parys, Verhamme, Temmerman, & Verstraelen, 2014). However, O'Reilly, Beale, and Gillies (2010) found limited evidence for effective interventions that reduced the amount of violence experienced by women but did find that recurring screening increased the identification of violence. In addition, a Cochrane Review also found insufficient evidence to assess the effectiveness of interventions for domestic violence on pregnancy outcomes (Jahanfar, Janssen, Howard, & Dowswell, 2013). Limited research demonstrates evidence-based strategies for reproductive coercion. However, Miller et al. (2011) report that an intervention with a trained family planning specialist decreased pregnancy coercion.

Another intervention strategy is to target men who abuse. Court-mandated batterer intervention programs are the most commonly used option. Most programs use the Duluth model, which focuses on power and control (Paymar & Pence, 1993). Group therapy, psychoeducation, and a profeminist approach are common elements of most programs (Price & Rosenbaum, 2009). Evidence supporting the effectiveness of batterer intervention programs is small from the perpetrator perspective and nonexistent when survivor perspective is considered (Feder & Wilson, 2005). Problems with these programs include the lack of non–English-language programs and a one-size-fits-all approach (Price & Rosenbaum, 2009). Other research has shown benefits to including substance abuse treatment as part of batterer intervention (Stover, Meadows, & Kaufman, 2009). The court-mandated approach, while appropriate, does not ensure that perpetrators are emotionally committed to the effort required to make and sustain behavioral change.

Gender-based violence is violence directed at girls and women because of their gender. IPV and sexual assault are two forms of gender-based violence that have significant health consequences for affected girls and women. Gender-based violence is an important public health and societal issue that requires major effort to eradicate. Because IPV and sexual violence affects the psychological and physical health of survivors, both increase the likelihood of contact with nurses in varied areas of health care. Nurses' understanding of the societal norms and attitudes regarding violence and the dynamics of abuse is crucial for providing the needed care. Nurses should screen for violence and its related consequences and provide counseling and referrals to survivors of gender-based violence.

■ REFERENCES

Abramsky, T., Watts, C. H., Garcia-Moreno, C., Devries, K., Kiss, L., Ellsberg, M.,…Heise, L. (2011). What factors are associated with recent intimate partner violence? Findings from the WHO multi-country study on women's health and domestic violence. *BMC Public Health, 11*(1), 109.

Aldridge, M. L., & Browne, K. D. (2003). Perpetrators of spousal homicide: A review. *Trauma, Violence, & Abuse, 4*(3), 265–276.

Amar, A., Laughon, K., Sharps, P., & Campbell, J. (2013). Screening and counseling for violence against women in primary care settings. *Nursing Outlook, 61*(3), 187–191.

Amar, A. F. (2008). African American college women's perceptions of resources and barriers when reporting forced sex. *Journal of the Black Nurses Association, 19*(2), 34–40.

Amar, A. F., & Alexy, E. M. (2005). "Dissed" by dating violence. *Perspectives in Psychiatric Care, 41*(4), 162–171.

Amar, A. F., & Gennaro, S. (2005). Dating violence in college women: Associated physical injury, healthcare usage, and mental health symptoms. *Nursing Research, 54*(4), 235–242.

American Psychiatric Association. (2013). *Diagnostic and statistical manual of mental disorders* (5th ed.). Arlington, VA: American Psychiatric Publishing.

Archer, J. (2000). Sex differences in aggression between heterosexual partners: A meta-analytic review. *Psychological Bulletin, 126*(5), 651–680.

Bair-Merritt, M. H., Lewis-O'Connor, A., Goel, S., Amato, P., Ismailji, T., Jelley, M.,…Cronholm, P. (2014). Primary care–based interventions for intimate partner violence: A systematic review. *American Journal of Preventive Medicine, 46*(2), 188–194.

Basile, K. C., & Smith, S. G. (2011). Sexual violence victimization of women: Prevalence, characteristics, and the role of public health and prevention. *American Journal of Lifestyle Medicine, 5*, 407–417.

Beydoun, H. A., Beydoun, M. A., Kaufman, J. S., Lo, B., & Zonderman, A. B. (2012). Intimate partner violence against adult women and its association with major depressive disorder, depressive symptoms and postpartum depression: A systematic review and meta-analysis. *Social Science and Medicine, 75*(6), 959–975.

Black, M. C. (2011). Intimate partner violence and adverse health consequences: Implications for clinicians. *American Journal of Lifestyle Medicine, 5*, 428–439.

Black, M. C., Basile, K. C., Walters, M. L., Merrick, M. T., Chen, J., & Stevens, M. R. (2011). *The National Intimate Partner and Sexual Violence Survey (NISVS)*. Atlanta, GA: National Center for Injury Prevention and Control, Centers for Disease Control and Prevention.

Bonomi, A. E., Anderson, M. L., Reid, R. J., Rivara, F. P., Carrell, D., & Thompson, R. S. (2009). Medical and psychosocial diagnoses in women with a history of intimate partner violence. *Archives of Internal Medicine, 169*(18), 1692–1697.

Bowen, E., Heron, J., Waylen, A., & Wolke, D. (2005). Domestic violence risk during and after pregnancy: Findings from a British longitudinal study. *BJOG: An International Journal of Obstetrics & Gynaecology, 112*(8), 1083–1089.

Breiding, M. J., Smith, S. G., Basile, K. C., Walters, M. L., Chen, J., & Merrick, M. T. (2014). Prevalence and characteristics of sexual violence, stalking, and intimate partner violence victimization—National intimate partner and sexual violence survey, United States, 2011. *Morbidity and Mortality Weekly Report. Surveillance Summaries, 63*(8), 1–18.

Breiding, M. J., Smith, S. G., Basile, K. C., Walters, M. L., Chen, J., & Merrick, M. T. (2015). Prevalence and characteristics of sexual violence, stalking, and intimate partner violence victimization—National intimate partner and sexual violence survey, United States, 2011. *American Journal of Public Health, 105*(4), e11.

Brewin, C. R., Andrews, B., Rose, S., & Kirk, M. (1999). Acute stress disorder and posttraumatic stress disorder in victims of violent crime. *American Journal of Psychiatry, 156*(3), 360–366.

Brownridge, D. A., Taillieu, T. L., Tyler, K. A., Tiwari, A., Chan, K. L., & Santos, S. C. (2011). Pregnancy and intimate partner violence: Risk factors, severity, and health effects. *Violence Against Women, 17*(7), 858–881.

Campbell, J., Dienemann, J., Kub, J., Schollenberger, J., O'Campo, P., Gielen, A. C., & Wynne, C. (2002). Intimate partner violence and physical health consequences. *Archives of Internal Medicine, 162*(10), 1157–1163.

Campbell, J. C. (2001). Safety planning based on lethality assessment for partners of batterers in intervention programs. *Journal of Aggression, Maltreatment & Trauma, 5*(2), 129–143.

Campbell, J. C. (2002). Health consequences of intimate partner violence. *The Lancet, 359*, 1331–1336.

Campbell, J. C. (2004). Helping women understand their risk in situations of intimate partner violence. *Journal of Interpersonal Violence, 19*(12), 1464–1477.

Campbell, J. C., Webster, D., Koziol-McLain, J., Block, C., Campbell, D., Curry, M.,…Sachs, C. (2003). Risk factors for femicide in abusive relationships: Results from a multisite case control study. *American Journal of Public Health, 93*(7), 1089–1097.

Campbell, J. C., Webster, D. W., & Glass, N. (2009). The danger assessment validation of a lethality risk assessment instrument for intimate partner femicide. *Journal of Interpersonal Violence, 24*(4), 653–674.

Campbell, J. C., Woods, A. B., Chouaf, K. L., & Parker, B. (2000). Reproductive health consequences of intimate partner violence: A nursing review. *Clinical Nursing Research, 9*(3), 217–237.

Campbell, R., Patterson, D., & Lichty, L. F. (2005). The effectiveness of sexual assault nurse examiner (SANE) programs: A review of psychological, medical, legal, and community outcomes. *Trauma, Violence, & Abuse, 6*(4), 313–329.

Campbell, R., Wasco, S. M., Ahrens, C. E., Sefl, T., & Barnes, H. E. (2001). Preventing the "second rape" rape survivors' experiences with community service providers. *Journal of Interpersonal Violence, 16*(12), 1239–1259.

Classen, C. C., Palesh, O. G., & Aggarwal, R. (2005). Sexual revictimization: A review of the empirical literature. *Trauma Violence Abuse, 6*(2), 102–129. doi:10.1177/1524838005275087

Coffey, P., Leitenberg, H., Henning, K., Bennett, R. T., & Jankowski, M. K. (1996). Dating violence: The association between methods of coping and women's psychological adjustment. *Violence & Victims, 11*(3), 227–238.

Deliramich, A. N., & Gray, M. J. (2008). Changes in women's sexual behavior following sexual assault. *Behavior Modification, 32*(5), 611–621.

Devries, K. M., Mak, J. Y., Bacchus, L. J., Child, J. C., Falder, G., Petzold, M.,…Watts, C. H. (2013). Intimate partner violence and incident depressive symptoms and suicide attempts: A systematic review of longitudinal studies. *PLoS Medicine, 10*(5), e1001439. doi:10.1371/journal.pmed.1001439

Dienemann, J., Campbell, J., Wiederhorn, N., Laughon, K., & Jordan, E. (2003). A critical pathway for intimate partner violence across the continuum of care. *Journal of Obstetric, Gynecologic, and Neonatal Nursing, 32*(5), 594–603.

Edleson, J. L., Eisikovits, Z., & Guttmann, E. (1985). Men who batter women: A critical review of the evidence. *Journal of Family Issues, 6*(2), 229–247.

Falsetti, S. A. (2007). Screening and responding to family and intimate partner violence in the primary care setting. *Primary Care: Clinics in Office Practice, 34*(3), 641–657.

Feder, L., & Wilson, D. B. (2005). A meta-analytic review of court-mandated batterer intervention programs: Can courts affect abusers' behavior? *Journal of Experimental Criminology, 1*(2), 239–262.

Fisher, B. S., Cullen, F. T., & Turner, M. G. (2000). *The sexual victimization of college women.* Washington, DC: National Institute of Justice.

Fisher, B. S., Daigle, L. E., Cullen, F. T., & Turner, M. G. (2003). Reporting sexual victimization to the police and others: Results from a national-level study of college women. *Criminal Justice and Behavior, 30*, 6–38.

Fishman, P. A., Bonomi, A. E., Anderson, M. L., Reid, R. J., & Rivara, F. P. (2010). Changes in health care costs over time following the cessation of intimate partner violence. *Journal of General Internal Medicine, 25*(9), 920–925.

Gagne, M. H., Lavoie, F., & Hebert, M. (2005). Victimization during childhood and revictimization in dating relationships in adolescent girls. *Child Abuse and Neglect, 29*(10), 1155–1172.

Glass, N., Dearwater, S., & Campbell, J. (2001). Intimate partner violence screening and intervention: Data from eleven Pennsylvania and Californina community hospital emergency departments. *Journal of Emergency Nursing, 27*(2), 141–149.

Glass, N., Eden, K. B., Bloom, T., & Perrin, N. (2009). Computerized aid improves safety decision process for survivors of intimate partner violence. *Journal of Interpersonal Violence, 25*(11), 1947–1964.

Groth, A. N., & Burgess, A. W. (1977). Rape: A sexual deviation. *American Journal of Orthopsychiatry, 47*(3), 400.

Groves, B. M., Augustyn, M., Lee, D., & Sawirds, P. (2002). *Identifying and responding to domestic violence: Consensus recommendations for child and adolescent health.* San Francisco, CA: Family Violence Prevention Fund.

Halpern, C. T., Oslak, S. G., Young, M. L., Martin, S. L., & Kupper, L. L. (2001). Partner violence among adolescents in opposite-sex romantic relationships: Findings from the National Longitudinal Study of Adolescent Health. *American Journal of Public Health, 91*(10), 1679–1685.

Hazelwood, R. R. (2009). Analyzing the rape and profiling the offender. In R. R. Hazelwood & A. W. Burgess (Eds.), *Practical aspects of rape investigation: A multidisciplinary approach* (4th ed., pp. 97–122). Boca Raton, FL: CRC Press.

Hellmuth, J. C. (2013). Risk factors for intimate partner violence during pregnancy and postpartum. *Archives of Women's Mental Health, 16*(1), 19–27.

Hopper, E. K., Bassuk, E. L., & Olivet, J. (2010). Shelter from the storm: Trauma-informed care in homelessness services settings. *The Open Health Services and Policy Journal, 3*(2), 80–100.

Jahanfar, S., Janssen, P. A., Howard, L. M., & Dowswell, T. (2013). Interventions for preventing or reducing domestic violence against pregnant women. *The Cochrane Database of Systematic Reviews,* (2), CD009414.

James, L., Brody, D., & Hamilton, Z. (2013). Risk factors for domestic violence during pregnancy: A meta-analytic review. *Violence and Victims, 28*(3), 359–380.

Jasinski, J. L. (2004). Pregnancy and domestic violence: A review of the literature. *Trauma, Violence, & Abuse, 5*(1), 47–64.

Jennings, A. (2004). *Models for developing trauma-informed behavioral health systems and trauma-specific services.* Alexandria, VA: National Association of State Mental Health Program Directors, National Technical Assistance Center for State Mental Health Planning.

Jewkes, R. (2002). Intimate partner violence: Causes and prevention. *The Lancet, 359*(9315), 1423–1429.

Johnson, N. L., & Johnson, D. M. (2013). Factors influencing the relationship between sexual trauma and risky sexual behavior in college students. *Journal of Interpersonal Violence, 28*(11), 2315–2331.

Kamphuis, J. H., & Emmelkamp, P. M. (2001). Traumatic distress among support-seeking female victims of stalking. *American Journal of Psychiatry, 158*(5), 795–798.

Kapur, N. A., & Windish, D. M. (2011). Health care utilization and unhealthy behaviors among victims of sexual assault in Connecticut: Results from a population-based sample. *Journal of General Internal Medicine, 26*(5), 524–530.

Kendall-Tackett, K., Cong, Z., & Hale, T. W. (2013). Depression, sleep quality, and maternal well-being in postpartum women with a history of sexual assault: A comparison of breastfeeding, mixed-feeding, and formula-feeding mothers. *Breastfeeding Medicine, 8*(1), 16–22.

Kessler, R. C., Sonnega, A., Bromet, E., Hughes, M., & Nelson, C. B. (1995). Posttraumatic stress disorder in the National Comorbidity Survey. *Archives of General Psychiatry, 52*(12), 1048–1060.

Kilpatrick, D. G., Acierno, R., Resnick, H. S., Saunders, B. E., & Best, C. L. (1997). A 2-year longitudinal analysis of the relationships between violent assault and substance use in women. *Journal of Consulting and Clinical Psychology, 65*(5), 834–847.

Kilpatrick, D. G., Ruggiero, K. J., Acierno, R., Saunders, B. E., Resnick, H. S., & Best, C. L. (2003). Violence and risk of PTSD, major depression, substance abuse/dependence, and comorbidity: Results from the National Survey of Adolescents. *Journal of Consulting and Clinical Psychology, 71*(4), 692–700.

Kohn, M., Flood, H., Chase, J., & McMahon, P. M. (2000). Prevalence and health consequences of stalking—Louisiana, 1998–1999. *Morbidity and Mortality Weekly Report, 49*(29), 653–655.

Lagdon, S., Armour, C., & Stringer, M. (2014). Adult experience of mental health outcomes as a result of intimate partner violence victimisation: A systematic review. *European Journal of Psychotraumatology, 5*, 24794.

Laughon, K., Amar, A. F., Sheridan, D. J., & Anderson, S. (2010). Legal and forensic nursing responses to family violence. In J. Humphreys & J. C. Campbell (Eds.), *Family violence and nursing practice* (2nd ed., pp. 367–380). New York, NY: Springer Publishing.

Laughon, K., Renker, P., Glass, N., & Parker, B. (2008). Revision of the Abuse Assessment Screen to address nonlethal strangulation. *Journal of Obstetric, Gynecologic, and Neonatal Nursing, 37*(4), 502–507.

Linden, J. A. (2011). Care of the adult patient after sexual assault. *New England Journal of Medicine, 365*(9), 834–841.

Lukasse, M., Henriksen, L., Vangen, S., & Schei, B. (2012). Sexual violence and pregnancy-related physical symptoms. *BMC Pregnancy and Childbirth, 12*(1), 83.

Miller, E., Decker, M. R., McCauley, H. L., Tancredi, D. J., Levenson, R. R., Waldman, J.,…Silverman, J. G. (2011). A family planning clinic partner violence intervention to reduce risk associated with reproductive coercion. *Contraception, 83*(3), 274–280.

Miller, E., Jordan, B., Levenson, R., & Silverman, J. G. (2010). Reproductive coercion: Connecting the dots between partner violence and unintended pregnancy. *Contraception, 81*(6), 457.

Miller, E., McCauley, H. L., Tancredi, D. J., Decker, M. R., Anderson, H., & Silverman, J. G. (2014). Recent reproductive coercion and unintended pregnancy among female family planning clients. *Contraception, 89*(2), 122–128.

Moreno-Garcia, C., Jansen, H. A. F. M., Ellsberg, M., Heise, L., & Watts, C. (2009). *WHO Multi-Country Study on Women's Health and Domestic Violence Against Women.* Geneva, Switzerland: World Health Organization.

National Center for Injury Prevention and Control. (2003). *Costs of intimate partner violence against women in the United States.* Atlanta, GA: Centers for Disease Control and Prevention.

National Center for Victims of Crime. (2007). Retrieved from www.nsvcc.org

Norlander, B., & Eckhardt, C. (2005). Anger, hostility, and male perpetrators of intimate partner violence: A meta-analytic review. *Clinical Psychology Review, 25*(2), 119–152.

O'Reilly, R., Beale, B., & Gillies, D. (2010). Screening and intervention for domestic violence during pregnancy care: A systematic review. *Trauma, Violence, & Abuse, 41*, 128–133.

Pallitto, C. C., García-Moreno, C., Jansen, H. A., Heise, L., Ellsberg, M., & Watts, C. (2013). Intimate partner violence, abortion, and unintended pregnancy: Results from the WHO Multi-country Study on Women's Health and Domestic Violence. *International Journal of Gynecology & Obstetrics, 120*(1), 3–9.

Pathe, M. T., & Mullen, P. E. (1997). The impact of stalkers on their victims. *British Journal of Psychiatry, 170*, 12–17.

Paymar, M., & Pence, E. (1993). *Education groups for men who batter: The Duluth Model.* New York, NY: Springer Publishing.

Price, B. J., & Rosenbaum, A. (2009). Batterer intervention programs: A report from the field *Violence and Victims, 24*(6), 757–770.

Rennison, C. M. (2002). Rape and sexual assault: Reporting to police and seeking medical attention, 1992–2000. Washington, DC: Bureau of Justice Statistics.

Rhodes, K. V., & Levinson, W. (2003). Interventions for intimate partner violence against women: Clinical applications. *Journal of the American Medical Association, 289*(5), 601–605.

Riggs, N., Houry, D., Long, G., Markovchick, V., & Feldhaus, K. M. (2000). Analysis of 1,076 cases of sexual assault. *Annals of Emergency Medicine, 35*(4), 358–362.

Rivara, F. P., Anderson, M. L., Fishman, P., Bonomi, A. E., Reid, R. J., Carrell, D., & Thompson, R. S. (2007). Healthcare utilization and costs for women with a history of intimate partner violence. *American Journal of Preventive Medicine, 32*(2), 89–96.

Sable, M. R., Danis, F., Mauzy, D. L., & Gallagher, S. K. (2006). Barriers to reporting sexual assault for women and men: perspectives of college students. *Journal of American College Health, 55*(3), 157–162.

Shah, P. S., & Shah, J. (2010). Maternal exposure to domestic violence and pregnancy and birth outcomes: A systematic review and meta-analyses. *Journal of Women's Health, 19*(11), 2017–2031.

Sharps, P. W., Koziol-McLain, J., Campbell, J., McFarlane, J., Sachs, C., & Xu, X. (2001). Health care providers' missed opportunities for preventing femicide. *Preventive Medicine, 33*(5), 373–380.

Sheridan, D. J., & Nash, K. R. (2007). Acute injury patterns of intimate partner violence victims. *Trauma, Violence, & Abuse, 8*(3), 281–289.

Sheridan, L. P., Blaauw, E., & Davies, G. M. (2003). Stalking: Knowns and unknowns. *Trauma, Violence, & Abuse, 4*(2), 148–162.

Silverman, J. G., Raj, A., Mucci, L. A., & Hathaway, J. E. (2001). Dating violence against adolescent girls and associated substance use, unhealthy weight control, sexual risk behavior, pregnancy, and suicidality. *Journal of the American Medical Association, 286*(5), 572–579.

Smith, P. H., White, J. W., & Holland, L. J. (2003). A longitudinal perspective on dating violence among adolescent and college-age women. *American Journal of Public Health, 93*(7), 1104–1109.

Söchting, I., Fairbrother, N., & Koch, W. J. (2004). Sexual assault of women: Prevention efforts and risk factors. *Violence Against Women, 10*(1), 73–93.

Sokoloff, N. J., & Dupont, I. (2005). Domestic violence at the intersections of race, class, and gender challenges and contributions to understanding violence against marginalized women in diverse communities. *Violence Against Women, 11*(1), 38–64.

Stover, C. S., Meadows, A. L., & Kaufman, J. (2009). Interventions for intimate partner violence: Review and implications for evidence-based practice. *Professional Psychology: Research and Practice, 40*(3), 223–233.

Surís, A., Lind, L., Kashner, T. M., Borman, P. D., & Petty, F. (2004). Sexual assault in women veterans: An examination of PTSD risk, health care utilization, and cost of care. *Psychosomatic Medicine, 66*(5), 749–756.

Tjaden, P., & Thoennes, N. (1998). Stalking in America: Findings from the National Violence Against Women Survey. Washington, DC: U.S. Department of Justice.

Tjaden, P., & Thoennes, N. (2000). *Extent, nature, and consequences of intimate partner violence.* Washington, DC: National Institute of Justice and the Centers for Disease Control and Prevention.

Tjaden, P., & Thoennes, N. (2006). *Extent, nature, and consequences of rape victimization: Findings from the National Violence Against Women Survey.* Washington, DC: National Institute of Justice.

Trautman, D. E., McCarthy, M. L., Miller, N., Campbell, J. C., & Kelen, G. D. (2007). Intimate partner violence and emergency department screening: Computerized screening versus usual care. *Annals of Emergency Medicine, 49*(4), 526–534.

Turchik, J. A., & Hassija, C. M. (2014). Female sexual victimization among college students: Assault severity, health risk behaviors, and sexual functioning. *Journal of Interpersonal Violence, 29*(13), 2439–2457.

Van Parys, A., Verhamme, A., Temmerman, M., & Verstraelen, H. (2014). *Intimate partner violence and pregnancy: A systematic review of interventions.* Retrieved from http://dx.org/10.1371/journal.pone.0085084

Walker, L. E. (2009). *The battered woman syndrome.* New York, NY: Springer Publishing.

Wathen, C. N., & MacMillan, H. L. (2003). Interventions for violence against women: Scientific review. *Journal of the American Medical Association, 289*(5), 589–600.

World Health Organization (WHO). (2010). Injuries and violence: The facts. Geneva, Switzerland: Author.

World Health Organization (WHO). (2013a). *Global and regional estimates of violence against women: prevalence and health effects of intimate partner violence and non-partner sexual violence.* Geneva, Switzerland: Author.

World Health Organization (WHO). (2013b). *Responding to intimate partner violence and sexual violence against women: WHO clinical and policy guidelines.* Geneva, Switzerland: Author.

World Health Organization (WHO). (n.d.). *Health care for women subjected to intimate partner violence or sexual violence: A clinical handbook.* Geneva, Switzerland: Author.

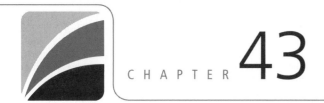

CHAPTER 43

Cardiovascular Disease in Women

Tina M. Chasse Mulinski • Karin V. Nyström • Catherine G. Winkler

All women face the threat of developing cardiovascular disease (CVD) regardless of race or ethnicity. CVD remains the leading cause of death in both men and women in the United States and is the leading global cause of death; 17.3 million people die each year from CVD (Mozaffarian et al., 2015). More specifically, heart disease is the number 1 cause of death in women, taking more lives than all forms of cancer combined. Regrettably, more than one in three women has some form of CVD, although the extent of disease risk varies among individuals based on demographic as well as biopsychosocial factors (Mozaffarian et al., 2015).

Furthermore, CVD is associated with significant health and financial burden; the estimated direct and indirect cost was $320.1 billion in 2011. Included in these expenses are cardiovascular operations and procedures, the number of which increased 28% from 2000 to 2010, totaling approximately 7.6 million annually (Mozaffarian et al., 2015).

In the United States, about 43 million women are living with some form of CVD or the aftereffects of stroke, and the population at risk is considerably larger (Mozaffarian et al., 2015). Likewise, more women than men die each year of CVD. In 2011, CVD was the cause of death for 398,035 women, which represents 51% of all deaths from CVD. Additionally, CVD is a major concern in minority populations, with half of all African Americans having some form of CVD, which represents 48% of women. Similarly, stroke affects 55,000 more women than men each year. This is in part because the average life expectancy for women is longer than that for men and the highest rates for stroke are in the oldest age groups. In 2011, women accounted for nearly 60% of stroke deaths nationwide (Mozaffarian et al., 2015).

Although there are a significant number of women with known CVD, many women remain poorly informed or uninformed about their cardiovascular risk, leading to missed opportunities to prevent or minimize the effects of a major cardiac event. Despite an increase in awareness of heart disease as the leading cause of death in women over the past 15 years, only 56% of women recognized it as a major health threat (Mosca et al., 2013). Among women in higher risk groups, specifically racial/ethnic minorities, this lack of awareness was more profound, with only 36% of Black and 34% of Hispanic females aware of the significance of CVD in women (Mosca et al., 2013).

In 2011, CVD caused about one death per minute among females. This represents around the same number of deaths in women from cancer, chronic lower respiratory disease, and diabetes combined. Although the number of men and women who die from CVD has decreased over the past 10 years by 30.8% (Mozaffarian et al., 2015), the decline is less notable for women. There has been a trend in reduced CVD death rates for women aged 35 to 44 years over the past 40 years. However, recently, there has been an increase in death rates in this group, likely because of the growing obesity epidemic (Ford et al., 2007). Advances in clinical care, implementation of evidence-based therapies for CVD, and modification of risk factors, as well as preventive strategies and increased public awareness, are major contributors to the overall decline in CVD. Nevertheless, more progress is needed to increase awareness on the part of both providers and patients, specifically, that heart disease is not exclusive to men. Despite widespread access to CVD prevention, health care providers continue to underestimate the cardiovascular risk in women.

The American Heart Association (AHA) has set a 2020 impact goal to improve cardiovascular health for all Americans by 20% while also reducing deaths from CVD and stroke by 20%. The goal statement describes "cardiovascular health" as the absence of disease and the presence of seven key health factors and behaviors, which include controlling blood pressure, cholesterol, and blood glucose and encouraging a healthy diet, weight, physical activity and a no-smoking status, all of which need to be monitored over time (Lloyd-Jones et al., 2010). Advanced practice nurses (APNs) have a unique opportunity to support the 2020 impact goal through screening and prevention, ensuring timely access to care, providing treatment, monitoring outcomes, educating patients, and advocating changes in care approaches for women to mitigate risk and better manage CVD.

■ DEFINITION AND SCOPE OF CVD

CVD includes many conditions that can affect the heart and coronary arteries as well as the blood vessels throughout the body, including the brain (cerebrovascular disease), kidneys (renal vascular disease), and extremities (peripheral vascular disease). Structural heart disease affects cardiac muscle and valves and can lead to other conditions of vascular dysfunction, such as hypertension (HTN) and conduction defects causing arrhythmias. In this chapter, the emphasis is on atherosclerosis, a type of arteriosclerosis in which there is thickening and hardening of the arteries and often a build-up of plaque, which is formed from fat, cholesterol, calcium, and other substances found in the blood. Together, these two processes cause narrowing and blockage of vessels, limiting the flow of oxygen-rich blood to the body and leading to ischemic changes and infarction or tissue death.

The Framingham Heart Study (FHS) was initiated in 1948 by the U.S. Public Health Service to assess the epidemiology and risk factors for CVD. From the data obtained in this longitudinal study, investigators were able to generate risk factors or general patterns that would suggest a likelihood of developing heart diseases (Lewandowski & Gracey, 2014). This work led to improved screening techniques and to many of the cardiovascular guidelines used today. More recent publications from the Framingham Study, which saw the evolution of heart disease in the overall population, noted the differences between men and women in prevalence, incidence, prognosis, and risk factors. Although CVD was historically considered a "man's disease," it is now understood to be the leading cause of death in women. Women lag behind men by 10 to 12 years in CVD incidence (Mozaffarian et al., 2015). The lifetime risk at age 50 years of developing CVD is approximately 51.1% in men and 39.2% in women, which nears a comparable risk between the genders with aging (Lloyd-Jones, Haykowsky, Swartz, Douglas, & Mackey, 2007; Novella, Dantas, Segarra, Medina, & Hermenegildo, 2012).

Although there has been progress in understanding the significance of CVD in women, women continue to be underrepresented in studies that form the basis of clinical standards of care. Gender differences in pathobiology, clinical symptoms, medication management, risk identification and prevention, treatment, and prognosis are still not fully understood. Only 30% of CVD clinical trials report sex-specific results despite the U.S. Food and Drug Administration (FDA) regulations and the National Institutes of Health (NIH) recommendations of increased inclusion of women in clinical trials (Kim & Menon, 2009). Enrollment of women in clinical trials did increase from 9% in 1970 to 41% in 2006, but the representation remains overall lower compared with men (Melloni et al., 2010). Although the research on women and CVD had been slow in the past, efforts to combat this major public health issue has been significant in recent years. The Women's Health Initiative, a large, multisite, randomized controlled trial focused on women, has provided important data informing CVD care for women over the past 10 years (Rossouw et al., 2002).

■ CARDIOVASCULAR RISK FACTORS

Recognizing the high burden of CVD among women, the AHA, the American College of Cardiology (ACC), and other organizations sponsored an expert panel to develop guidelines for CVD prevention in women that were published in 2004 and updated in 2007 and 2011 (Mosca et al., 2011). Of note, the new 2011 guidelines underwent an important modification from "evidence-based" to "effectiveness-based" recommendations. This change acknowledged the benefits and risks observed in clinical practice or the "effectiveness" of preventive therapies, which is different from efficacy or "evidence" of benefits observed in clinical research alone (Mosca et al., 2011). Figure 43.1 depicts the flow diagram for the evaluation of CVD risk in women.

Cardiovascular risk factors can be categorized as fixed/nonmodifiable (e.g., age, gender, and a family history of heart disease or genetics) or modifiable (e.g., dyslipidemia, tobacco use, HTN, diabetes, obesity, sedentary lifestyle, and a cluster of interrelated metabolic causes). Less well-understood modifiable risk factors, such as serum biomarkers and specific clinical conditions, continue to emerge and appear to be more prevalent among women. Clinical conditions include depression and other psychosocial risk factors, as well as autoimmune diseases such as lupus erythematous, rheumatoid arthritis (Salmon & Roman, 2008), and psoriasis (Neimann et al., 2006). More research is needed to understand the relationship of these clinical conditions with CVD, with the goal to direct interventions aimed at improving outcomes and adherence to therapy.

Classification of CVD in women is now based on the 2011 guidelines, with modifications that incorporate the new concept of "ideal cardiovascular health" as the baseline and two more categories listed as "at risk," defined as one or more major risk factor, and "high risk," or one or more high-risk states (Mosca et al., 2011). The new classification table includes the Framingham CVD risk profile, as before, and includes evolving factors that are unique to women and may be associated with the development of CVD (Table 43.1).

Nonmodifiable Risk Factors

AGE AND GENDER

The prevalence of heart disease in women rises sharply after menopause (Novella et al., 2012). Part of this increase is attributed to decreased endogenous estrogen (Novella et al., 2012). Other age-associated risk factors may also play a role. The onset of CVD at an older age is associated with a higher incidence of comorbid conditions, additional cardiovascular risk factors, and other disease states, including collagen vascular diseases or autoimmune problems, as noted earlier (Gopalakrishnan, Ragland, & Tak, 2009).

FAMILY HISTORY/GENETICS

A family history of premature CVD has been defined as the onset of CVD in a first-degree relative before the age of 55 years for men and 65 years for women (Mulders et al., 2011). These age cut points were selected based on the recommendations of the National Cholesterol Education Program Expert Panel (NCEP, 2002) Third Adult Treatment Panel (ATP-III) and Seventh Joint National Committee (JNC) on Prevention, Detection, Evaluation, and Treatment of High Blood Pressure (JNC 7; Chobanian et al., 2003).

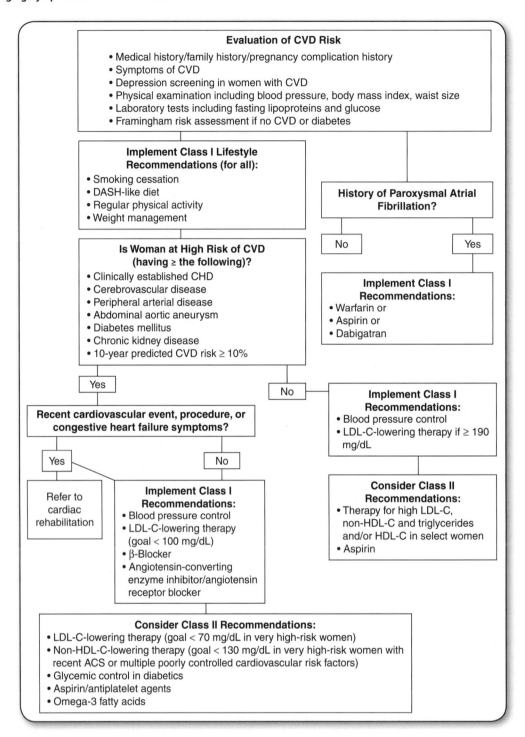

FIGURE 43.1

Evaluation of CVD risk.

CHD, coronary heart disease; CVD, cardiovascular disease; DASH, Dietary Approaches to Stop Hypertension; HDL, high-density lipoprotein; HDL-C, high-density lipoprotein cholesterol LDL, low-density lipoprotein; LDL-C, low-density lipoprotein cholesterol.
Source: Mosca et al. (2011).

Furthermore, a paternal history of premature heart attack has been shown to approximately double the risk of a heart attack in men and increase the risk in women by approximately 70% (Lloyd-Jones et al., 2004; Sesso et al., 2001). Premature CVD can also factor into some modifiable risk factors, including dyslipidemia, HTN, and diabetes. Therefore, it is difficult to assess exactly what percentage of CVD is directly related to the family history versus modifiable risk factors.

Genetic markers are still under investigation and have not been shown to add to cardiovascular risk predictions beyond the current models that include family history (Holmes, Harrison, Talmud, Hingorani, & Humphries, 2011). They have not been used yet to improve the prediction of subclinical atherosclerosis beyond the traditional risk factors (Hernesniemi et al., 2012). An association has been demonstrated between genetic markers and coronary artery calcification (Thanassoulis et al., 2012).

TABLE 43.1	Cardiovascular Disease Risk Classification for Women
RISK STATUS	**CRITERIA**

Ideal cardio-vascular health (women who meet all criteria)	Total cholesterol < 200 mg/dL (without treatment)
	Blood pressure < 120/< 80 mmHg (without treatment)
	Fasting blood sugar < 100 mg/dL (without treatment)
	Body mass index < 25 kg/m^2
	Smoking abstinence
	Goal physical activity for adults > 20 years old:
	   Moderate intensity ≥ 150 minutes/week
	   Vigorous intensity > 75 minutes/week
	   or, combination of 1 and 2
	DASH-like, healthy diet

At risk (women with ≥ 1 major risk factor[s])	Advanced subclinical atherosclerosis (e.g., carotid plaque, thickened intima-media thickness, coronary calcifications)
	Blood pressure ≥ 120/ ≥ 80 mm Hg
	Dyslipidemia, treated
	High density lipoprotein cholesterol < 50 mg/dL
	History of cardiovascular disease in a first-degree relative:
	   Women < 65 years of age
	   Men < 55 years of age
	Hypertension, treated
	Inactivity
	Metabolic syndrome
	Obesity (especially central adiposity)
	Poor diet
	Poor treadmill test exercise capacity and/or abnormal heart rate recovery after ceasing exercise
	Prior preeclampsia, gestational diabetes, or pregnancy-induced hypertension
	Smokes cigarettes
	Autoimmune collagen-vascular disease, systemic (e.g., rheumatoid arthritis or lupus)
	Total cholesterol ≥ 200 mg/dL

High risk (women with ≥ 1 high-risk states)	10-year predicted cardiovascular disease risk ≥ 10% Abdominal aortic aneurysm Cerebrovascular disease, clinically manifest Chronic or end-stage kidney disease Coronary heart disease, clinically manifest Diabetes mellitus Peripheral arterial disease, clinically manifest

Adapted from Mosca et al. (2011; Table 2, p. 34).

Modifiable Risk Factors

LACK OF AWARENESS OF SIGNIFICANT CARDIOVASCULAR RISK AND DELAYED TREATMENT

An often overlooked problem is women's underestimation of CVD risk factors and poor access to or use of health education materials. Targeted education that highlights the importance of knowledge about CVD in women, especially in racial/ethnic minorities, should be regularly updated and presented in a culturally sensitive format. Strategies for decreasing CVD have been developed to educate the public on traditional risk factors such as HTN, dyslipidemia, and smoking. Broader risk factor reduction has been recommended that includes cardiometabolic risk and metabolic syndrome in women (elevated fasting blood glucose, high-density lipoprotein cholesterol [HDL-C], and triglycerides, along with a waist size greater than 35 inches). Opportunities exist for increasing knowledge and awareness of CVD as the leading cause of death, including further education on the symptoms of myocardial infarction (MI; often different in women than in men) and the most appropriate response to a CVD emergency (Giardina et al., 2011).

Women, unaware of their own cardiovascular risk, often defer making an emergency 911 call. Delays in care can result in extensions of myocardial damage and poorer clinical outcomes. In a study of 5,887 individuals with suspected cardiac symptoms, women were 50% more likely than men to receive delayed treatment (Concannon et al., 2009). Although the reason for the delay was not specifically studied, research suggests that symptom presentation in women is different, is often more diffuse than in men, and therefore may not be readily recognized as a cardiac event by the patient and the emergency medical service (EMS) staff. Clearly, the lack of appreciation by many women for the need of emergency care for CVD and the lack of recognition of CVD symptoms by clinicians is a threat to women's mortality and morbidity and should be addressed through ongoing public education.

NONADHERENCE TO MEDICAL THERAPIES

Nonadherence to medical therapies, including taking prescribed medications, can be considered a risk factor for CVD. There are many patient, clinician, and system barriers that limit adherence to clinical treatments, ranging from lack of knowledge by the patient to lack of sufficient time with the primary care provider during routine clinic visits. In a meta-analysis of more than 100 medical adherence studies, women were as likely to be nonadherent to medical therapies as men (DiMatteo, 2004). Nonadherence to medications has been documented in more than 60% of cardiovascular patients (Kravitz et al., 1993) and continues to be problematic because of the expenses and complexities associated with managing health. In fact, self-reported adherence to cardiovascular medications in patients who have coronary artery disease (CAD) is less than 40% for the combination of aspirin, beta blocker, and lipid-lowering agent in both isolated and long-term follow-up surveys (Newby et al., 2006). Moreover, the highest risk of nonadherence occurs during the immediate discharge period; 24% of patients with acute MI do not fill their medications within 7 days of discharge (Jackevicius, Ping, & Tu, 2008). Almost one in four patients is partially or completely nonadherent in filling prescriptions after discharge (Jackevicius, Ping, & Tu, 2008). This is because many patients have difficulty adjusting their lifestyle if it is warranted, as well as adding new medications that increase expenses and complicate daily schedules.

Nonadherence to medical therapies is multifactorial and can be categorized as issues with communication, motivation, and socioeconomics (Baroletti & Dell'Orfano, 2010). Some specific causes of medication nonadherence are fragmentation of the health care system, problems with accessing information, complexity of some medication regimens, poor communication between the clinician and patient, low functional/health care literacy of the patient, concerns about costs by the patient, and unintentional behaviors such as forgetting to take the medication. Health care providers should use multiple approaches to improve their patients' short- and long-term medication adherence (Baroletti & Dell'Orfano, 2010). Identifying methods to improve compliance begins with assessing why patients are not taking their medications. In some cases it may help to change to a less expensive medication, offer samples, change to medications that require less-frequent dosing, recommend systems for reminders (e.g., smartphone chime or pill organizers), or provide additional education to the patient and/or a support person on the regimen on the importance of the medication.

Clinicians have been documented to make recommendations less often for preventative therapy in women (Mosca et al., 2005). This was thought to be a result of the lower perceived threat, despite the similar calculated risk for women and men. Educational interventions for clinicians and patients are needed in order to improve the quality of CVD preventive care, ensure adoption of CVD prevention guidelines, and lower CVD morbidity and mortality. CVD must be considered in all patients such that clinicians provide strategies for comprehensive health promotion and disease prevention and make both an early diagnosis and aggressive intervention plan when warranted.

SMOKING

Tobacco use continues to be the leading preventable risk factor for CVD development in women. Over the past half century, the risk of death from cigarette smoking continued to rise among women, with an overall increase from all causes to include lung cancer, chronic obstructive pulmonary disease (COPD), stroke, and CVD; the risk is now nearly identical in men and women, compared with those who do not smoke (Huxley & Woodward, 2011). Smoking has been associated with half of all coronary events in women. Among adult women, those who smoke include white women (19%), American Indian/Alaskan Native women (17%), African American women (15%), Hispanic women (7%), and Asian women (5%). There were approximately 6,300 new cigarette smokers every day based on an estimate in 2012 (Mozaffarian et al., 2015). Cigarette smoke affects not only smokers. Secondhand smoke can cause chronic respiratory conditions, cancer, and heart disease. Approximately 34,000 nonsmokers die from heart disease each year as a result of exposure to environmental tobacco smoke (U.S. Department of Health and Human Services, 2014).

Electronic cigarette products are another potential concern with respect to cardiovascular health. Since e-cigarettes are a relatively new product, data are still limited. E-cigarettes are changing quickly, and newer products could be safer; however, many e-cigarettes deliver larger dosages of nicotine and other by-products that are more detrimental to health than those of conventional cigarettes (Grana, Benowitz, & Glantz, 2014). Patterns of use need to be considered since e-cigarettes are often marketed as a smoking-cessation aid. However, many individuals use both e-cigarettes and conventional cigarettes, with no proven cessation benefits. Thus there may not be a lower disease burden with e-cigarrete use, since dose delivery is inconsistent, use patterns vary, and nicotine addiction remains a public health problem.

Marijuana use has been associated with threefold greater mortality after acute MI; the risk increased with more frequent use (Mukamal, Maclure, Muller, & Mittleman, 2008). Since marijuana use appears to be increasing among middle-aged and older adults and use is being legalized in some states, this finding may have importance in the future. Although marijuana use does not appear to be associated with mortality among the general population, it may carry particular risks for vulnerable populations with established CVD (Mukamal et al., 2008).

For women older than 35 years, the absolute risks associated with oral contraceptive (OCP) use and smoking are greater because of the steeply rising incidence of arterial diseases (Farley, Meirik, Chang, & Poulter, 1999). However, newer generation OCP formulations have no increased MI risk for current users to date, although there is an increased risk of venous thromboembolism (Shufelt & Bairey Merz, 2009). More cardiovascular data on the latest generation of contraceptive hormone formulations, including those that contain newer progestins that lower blood pressure and have nonoral routes (transdermal and vaginal), will need to be followed in the context of other cardiovascular risk factors, including smoking. More important, smoking cessation dramatically reduces mortality from all major smoking-related diseases, and it is never too late to quit.

OBESITY

Over 159 million U.S. adults (approximately 69%) are overweight or obese (Mozaffarian et al., 2015). According to the AHA's 2015 Women and CVD Update, an estimated 64.7% of women aged 20 years or above are overweight or obese, with 61.2% being non-Hispanic Whites; 81.9%, non-Hispanic Blacks; and 76.3%, Hispanic (Mozaffarian et al., 2015). Obesity is an independent risk factor for CVD and is associated with significant mortality and morbidity and health care costs. Furthermore, many comorbid conditions and CVD risk factors associated with obesity, including diabetes, CAD, sleep apnea, some cancers, HTN, low HDL-C, elevated triglycerides, and elevated levels of inflammatory markers; these make it imperative to treat obesity, which in and of itself has become a chronic disease. Even modest weigh gain during the adult years is highly related to an increased risk factor burden. The rise in the obesity rate is a significant contributor to the growing epidemic of type 2 diabetes. It is important that clinicians address risk reducing interventions to prevent and treat obesity with patients early and often.

DIABETES AND HYPERGLYCEMIA

Approximately 21.1 million American adults have a diagnosis of diabetes, and 10.6 million are women (Mozaffarian et al., 2015). In addition, an estimated 3.0 million women have undiagnosed diabetes. Of the 80.8 million Americans with prediabetes, about 34.3 million are women.

Diabetes is an even more potent risk factor for CVD among women, conferring a twofold to fourfold increase in women compared with a onefold to twofold increase in men (Calles-Escadon, Garcia-Rubi, Mirza, & Mortenson, 1999). The diagnosis of diabetes in a woman eliminates the usual 10-year gap seen between the sexes in the onset of CVD (Calles-Escadon et al., 1999). The American Diabetes Association (ADA, 2015) has set aggressive treatment goals for diabetic patients with regard to cardiovascular risk factors such as dyslipidemia and HTN. The 2015 ADA guidelines for the diagnosis and classification of diabetes recognized women with impaired fasting glucose levels (i.e., 100–125 mg/dL) and impaired glucose tolerance (i.e., 2-hour postglucose load of 140–199 mg/dL) as having "prediabetes"; these women are at the highest risk for developing diabetes, and these clinical entities are strongly associated with metabolic syndrome. In addition to the strong association of diabetes and CVD, patients with impaired fasting glucose levels are also at increased risk for CVD. Mechanisms that increase blood glucose levels and raise the CVD risk in women include endothelial dysfunction, the promotion of atheroma, and thrombus formation as a result of platelet overactivity and hypercoagulability (Bell, 1995). Women with diabetes require intensive cardiovascular screening. This is also the case with women who develop gestational diabetes and preeclampsia, who are further prone to develop subsequent diabetes along with adverse CVD profiles (Wenger, 1999). Diabetes mellitus is a concern for many reasons, especially its association with an increased overall risk of MI and stroke (Preis et al., 2009).

METABOLIC SYNDROME

Metabolic syndrome is a combination of conditions, which include HTN, elevated blood glucose, abnormal lipid levels, and an increased waist size, that together contribute to CVD and stroke in both men and women. Metabolic syndrome has been defined using the ATP-III guidelines (National Heart, Lung, and Blood Institute, National Cholesterol Education Program, 2002) and World Health Organization (WHO; Alberti & Zimmet, 1998) criteria separately and continues to evolve as more is known about the condition. The metabolic syndrome defined by ATP-III guidelines consists of three or more of the following: fasting plasma glucose of at least 110 mg/dL, serum triglycerides of at least 150 mg/dL, serum HDL-C of less than 40 mg/dL, BP of at least 130/85 mmHg or on BP medication, or waist girth of greater than 102 cm. The modified definition of the WHO criteria consists of hyperinsulinemia (the upper fourth of the fasting insulin level among nondiabetic subjects) or hyperglycemia (fasting glucose of at least 110 mg/dL) in addition to at least two of the following: waist girth of at least 94 cm, dyslipidemia (triglycerides of at least 150 mg/dL or HDL-C of less than 40 mg/dL), or BP of at least 140/90 mmHg or taking BP medication. This condition is estimated to be present in 47 million Americans, with a similar prevalence in men (24%) and women (23%). However, the gender equality is lost when comparing within ethnic groups. Although there were fewer White women with metabolic syndrome than White men, there are 57% more African American women with the metabolic syndrome than African American men and 26% more Mexican American women than Mexican American men (Ford, Giles, & Dietz, 2002). In addition, the National Health and Nutrition Examination Survey (NHANES) data demonstrated an age-adjusted increase in metabolic syndrome of 23.5% in women (P = .021) and only 2.2% among men (P = .831) from 1988–1994 to 1999–2000 (Ford et al., 2007). Over time, there likely will be more women with metabolic syndrome than men.

Metabolic syndrome is important to recognize because all patients with this condition are at risk for the development of diabetes and additional CVD. Women also have the specific circumstances of pregnancy, OCP use, menopause, and conditions such as polycystic ovary syndrome and preeclampsia that need to be factored into their clinical care because these factors increase the risk of weight gain and metabolic syndrome. In contrast, lactation or nursing decreased the incidence of metabolic syndrome by 22% (95% CI [1–39%]) among women who breastfed for more than 1 month compared with women who did not breastfeed or breastfed for less than 1 month (Cohen, Pieper, Brown, & Bastian, 2006). As it is with obesity, it is important to have a discussion early with patients to prevent and/or limit the progression of the condition through a proper diet and exercise plan.

PHYSICAL INACTIVITY

In 2013, in adults 18 years of age and older, inactivity was higher among women than among men (32.3% vs 28.6%, age adjusted; National Center for Health Statistics [NCHS], 2013). Only about 17.0% of women compared with 24.9% of men met the 2008 federal Physical Activity Guidelines for Americans in 2012 (Mozaffarian et al., 2015). This is an alarming statistic for both men and women and a concern, since physical inactivity is responsible for 12.2% of the global burden for MI after controlling for the CVD risk factors such as smoking, HTN, obesity, lipid profile, psychosocial causes, and diabetes (Yusef et al., 2004). The AHA 2020 Impact Goal for ideal cardiovascular health recommends 150 minutes of minimal/moderate activity/week, 75 minutes of vigorous activity/week, or 150 minutes of moderate and vigorous activity/week (NCHS, 2013).

PSYCHOSOCIAL FACTORS INCLUDING EMOTIONAL STRESS

Although the classic risk factors for CVD are similar among men and women, differences do appear to exist in certain conditions that may contribute to CVD. Conditions known to contribute to CVD that are more prevalent among women include depression and psychosocial factors such as anxiety and inadequate social and economic resources. These conditions and circumstances require effective interventions to manage issues of knowledge deficits and lack of adherence to medical recommendations. Accordingly, screening for depression has been added to the effectiveness-based guidelines for the prevention of CVD in women (Mosca et al., 2011). There is a growing recognition of the importance of emotional stress as a risk factor for heart disease. Women have higher levels of psychological risk factors that potentially contribute to heart disease through atherosclerosis development, with an earlier onset or more negative outcomes when there is existing disease. In particular, younger women (no older than 50 years) compared with age-matched men had twice (52% vs. 25%) the rate of mental stress-induced myocardial ischemia (Vaccarino et al., 2014). The investigators from the INTERHEART study suggested that acute MI was strongly associated with combined exposure to psychosocial stressors such as depression, major life events, and perceived stress at home or work (Yusef et al., 2004). Depressive symptoms were associated with increased risk of death, especially in young women with suspected or established CVD (Shah et al., 2014). Stress-induced Takotsubo cardiomyopathy is a condition that is unique to women; it occurs after menopause when there has been exposure to sudden, unexpected emotional or physical stress (Akashi, Goldstein, Barbaro, & Ueyama, 2008). This condition results in hospitalization and treatment by a cardiologist.

AUTOIMMUNE AND INFLAMMATORY CONDITIONS/CHRONIC ILLNESSES

In addition to the recognition that some psychosocial factors may contribute to CVD in women is the realization that certain autoimmune and inflammatory diseases, also more prevalent in women, may add to CVD development. Autoimmune diseases affect approximately 8% of the population, 78% of whom are women (Fairweather & Rose, 2004).

People with lupus have a significantly increased risk of premature coronary heart disease (CHD) or atherosclerosis, stroke, and other cardiovascular-related conditions than those without lupus (Manzi et al., 1997). Several other systemic autoimmune conditions, including rheumatoid arthritis, antiphospholipid syndrome, and primary Sjögren's syndrome, are also associated with atherosclerosis. Systemic inflammation associated with autoimmune diseases or the inflammatory components of the immune response are thought to accelerate the atherosclerotic process (López-Pedrera et al., 2011). Previous infection has also been linked to atherosclerosis (Fairweather & Rose, 2004). Further study will help to clarify this relationship; the link between autoimmune diseases and CVD, whether direct or indirect, seems to be related to inflammation and to damaging effect on the vasculature.

Emerging—Migraines, Low Vitamin Levels, Sleep Duration, Therapies to Treat Breast Cancer

Migraine is a common chronic disorder that affects women four times more often than men (Lipton & Bigal, 2005). People who have a migraine with aura have a twofold increased risk of ischemic stroke (Schürks et al., 2009). Data suggest a higher risk among women, with an increase in the risk associated with people who were younger than 45 years old, smoked, and with women who used OCPs. An overall association between migraine and MI or death from CVD was not found. Migraine physiology continues to be studied to better understand the etiology; nonetheless, the condition is thought to be related to vascular mechanisms such as endothelial dysfunction and hypercoagulability,

which are the same processes involved in the development of CVD (Tietjen, 2007).

Vitamin D deficiency may be associated with incident CVD. Further clinical and experimental studies are still warranted to determine whether correction of vitamin D deficiency could contribute to the prevention of CVD. Vitamin D receptors have a wide tissue network that includes vascular smooth muscle, endothelium, and cardiomyocytes; although the mechanism is unclear, there may be some relationship with low levels of vitamin D and CVD (Wang et al., 2010).

Short, self-reported sleep duration has also been associated with an increased risk of CVD in women, regardless of age, smoking status, obesity, HTN, diabetes mellitus, and other cardiovascular risk factors (Ayas et al., 2003). Further studies are needed to better understand the pathological changes underlying this association and to determine whether the cause of the sleep deprivation (insomnia vs. lifestyle choices) affects CVD development (Ayas et al., 2003).

Another risk factor for CVD primarily in women is the treatment used for breast cancer. Advancements in breast cancer treatment have led to improved survival, along with an unintended elevated risk of CVD, specifically ischemic heart disease. It remains unknown if the elevated risk result entirely from the specific therapies or from the disease itself, which is also associated with some of the same risk factors as ischemic heart disease (Gulati, Shaw, & Bairey Merz, 2012).

Novel Cardiac Risk Factors

Despite all that is known about the "traditional" risk factors for CVD, many individuals have few or none of these risk factors and still experience cardiovascular events. In fact, 50% of patients who experience an MI have normal lipid levels, and an estimated 20% have no traditional risk factors (Khot et al., 2003). These unsettling statistics have prompted a search for additional risk factors that contribute to the development of CVD. Homocysteine, lipoprotein(a) [LP(a)], and C-reactive protein (CRP) are three emerging risk factors that are believed to contribute to CVD.

HOMOCYSTEINE

Elevated plasma total homocysteine has been suggested as a possible modifiable risk factor for CVD and stroke, as well as other vascular conditions. Homocysteine, a sulfur-containing amino acid, has been linked to the development of atherosclerosis (Greenland, Smith, & Grundy, 2001). It promotes endothelial dysfunction and cell injury, enhances thromboxane A_2 and platelet aggregation, and has procoagulant effects (Harjari, 1999). The lack of controlled clinical intervention trials that demonstrate improved outcomes with the treatment of elevated homocysteine levels in women with CVD has kept this possible risk factor from being recommended as part of routine screening.

LIPOPROTEIN(A)

Lp(a) is produced in the liver and competes with plasminogen for binding sites, thereby inhibiting fibrinolysis (Scanu, Lawn, & Berg, 1991). Lp(a) has also been shown to increase cholesterol invasion into the arterial wall, enhance foam-cell formation, generate free radicals in monocytes, and promote smooth muscle cell proliferation (Loscalzo, Weinfeld, Fless, & Scanu, 1990); are all factors in the process of atherosclerosis. Up to 20% of individuals with premature CVD have elevated Lp(a) levels. The routine screening of Lp(a) in all persons at increased cardiovascular risk is not recommended; however, checking Lp(a) in women with premature CVD that is not explained by traditional risk factors is recommended (Shai et al., 2005). The treatment of elevated Lp(a) levels is still somewhat controversial because the specific effects on CVD from lowering Lp(a) levels are unknown (Suk Danik, Rifai, Buring, & Ridker, 2006).

C-REACTIVE PROTEIN

CRP is a nonspecific marker of acute inflammation that may play a role in the inflammatory process (Rifai & Ridker, 2001). CRP has been established as an independent risk factor for CVD and stroke (Ridker, Hennekens, Buring, & Rifai, 2000; Ridker, Rifai, Rose, Buring, & Cook, 2002). High-sensitivity CRP (hs-CRP) for the quantification of cardiovascular risk in women has been found to be a much better predictor of CVD risk than some traditional markers, such as the total cholesterol–to–HDL-C ratio (Ridker et al., 2002). In 2003, the AHA and the Centers for Disease Control and Prevention (CDC) issued a joint recommendation for the use of hs-CRP in clinical practice. In addition, obtaining the hs-CRP level is recommended for most individuals with intermediate risk as determined by their FHS score (10%–20% risk of MI during the next 10–20 years), because a high hs-CRP level in an intermediate-risk patient may guide the clinician to treat known traditional risk factors more aggressively (Pearson et al., 2003).

■ DIAGNOSTIC STUDIES

Resting EKG

Although the resting EKG is a routine component of many physical examinations, the sensitivity of resting abnormalities for the prediction of CVD events is overall rather low (Ashley, Raxwal, & Froelicher, 2001). Thus many women who experience their first cardiac event have a normal baseline EKG (Pignone, Fowler-Brown, Pletcher, & Tice, 2003). The resting EKG can also be helpful for stratifying risk in women who have HTN because the presence of left ventricular hypertrophy (LVH) identified by EKG increases the risk of sudden cardiac death (Kannel & Abbott, 1986).

Exercise EKG: Stress Testing

Historically, exercise stress testing in women has been thought to have a decreased diagnostic accuracy because of a lower prevalence of CAD in women; however, most early studies evaluating stress testing as a diagnostic tool were performed in almost exclusively male cohorts (Kohli & Gulati, 2010).

Since there are gender differences in assessing CVD and a high mortality resulting from CVD in women, it is critically important to identify disease as early as possible to interrupt the trajectory. However, it is very difficult to identify CVD in women. The presence of CVD in young women is low, with women tending to present with symptoms and CVD at older ages compared with men. Additionally, women may present with more diffuse symptoms. They also have a lower prevalence of obstructive coronary disease, making diagnostic testing designed to detect focal areas of coronary stenosis less sensitive and less specific in this population (Shaw et al., 2006).

Stress testing is useful for diagnostic as well as prognostic information. Exercise capacity is a stress-test measure that has been found to be a potent predictor of all-cause mortality (Gulati et al., 2003). The metabolic equivalent of a task (MET) is a multiple of the resting rate of oxygen consumption. One MET represents the oxygen consumption of a seated individual at rest (Pate et al., 1991). In 2005, the AHA and the ACC published a joint position statement regarding the role of noninvasive testing in women; it recommends separating women into low, intermediate, and high pretest risk categories on the basis of cardiovascular risk factors with the use of a tool such as the FHS scores (Mieres et al., 2005). In addition, assessing the likelihood that the symptoms are cardiac in nature is also important. Women can present with more atypical symptoms than men. The U.S. Preventive Services Task Force (USPTF) recommends using available risk-factor screening tools (e.g., the FHS score) and consider screening for CVD in those at intermediate risk for CVD, who could be reclassified as being high risk after additional testing and subsequently treated more aggressively with regard to risk-factor modification (Pignone et al., 2003).

In low- and intermediate-risk women who are having symptoms suggestive of typical or atypical angina, EKG stress testing with the use of a treadmill protocol is indicated as long as the woman has a normal baseline EKG and is capable of maximal exercise (Mieres et al., 2005). It is generally accepted that if a woman can achieve five METs, exercise stress testing can be undertaken. Many household tasks (e.g., vacuuming, washing floors) are equivalent to approximately four to five METs. If the woman cannot adequately exercise for any reason, pharmacological stress testing with an imaging modality is more appropriate.

Stress Testing With Imaging Modalities

The cardiac imaging modalities that are most widely studied and available are stress testing with nuclear imaging and stress echocardiography. Gated myocardial perfusion single-photon emission computed tomography (SPECT) is the most commonly performed stress test. SPECT provides information about perfusion defects (e.g., ischemia) as well as about global and regional left ventricular function and left ventricular volumes (Klocke et al., 2003).

The American Society of Nuclear Cardiology (ASNC) Task Force on Women and Heart Disease (Mieres, et al., 2003) recommends stress testing with nuclear imaging for women with an intermediate to high pretest likelihood of CVD (Mieres et al., 2005). Stress testing with cardiac imaging is indicated for high- and intermediate-risk women who have symptoms of CVD, diabetes, and a baseline abnormal EKG (Mieres et al., 2005). For women with symptoms who cannot exercise at a level of at least five METs, pharmacologic stress testing is indicated (Mieres et al., 2005). Stress echocardiography, like nuclear myocardial perfusion imaging, is indicated for women who are at intermediate and high risk of CVD who have symptoms suggestive of myocardial ischemia (Mieres et al., 2005). Stress echocardiography can also provide useful information regarding left ventricular function, systolic and diastolic dysfunction, and valvular heart disease (Mieres et al., 2005).

Computed Tomography

CT of the coronary vasculature detects and quantifies the amount of calcium in the coronary arteries and signifies the presence of atherosclerotic disease. The effect of calcium scoring on clinical outcomes has yet to be determined. Thus the USPSTF does not advocate CT in the routine screening of low-risk women (Pignone et al., 2003). However, the ACC/AHA guidelines suggest that the greatest potential for use of calcium scoring with CT could be as a screening tool for risk stratification in asymptomatic women at intermediate risk according to their FHS scores when added to traditional risk-factor scoring (Mieres et al., 2005). Furthermore, in a study by Lakowski et al. (2007) women classified as low risk based on the Framingham risk score (FRS) with prevalent coronary artery calcium (CAC) had a higher risk for future CVD compared with low-risk women without detectable CAC. Additionally, low-risk women with advanced CAC had especially high relative and absolute risks for CVD events. Therefore there is a need to continually review the indications for diagnostic studies and the associated benefits for assessment of CVD risks in middle-aged and older women.

Cardiovascular MRI

Cardiac MRI (CMRI) allows for the visualization of coronary arteries, determination of flow within the coronary arteries, evaluation of myocardial perfusion (similar to SPECT), assessment of wall motion during stress, and identification of infarcted myocardium. CMR angiography is also a promising imaging modality. CMRI may be especially useful in women without obstructive CAD who instead have microvascular coronary dysfunction (MCD), since magnetic resonance perfusion imaging, together with ejection fraction (EF), has been found to predict prognosis (Shufelt et al., 2013).

Carotid Intimal Medial Thickness

Carotid intimal medial thickness (IMT) has been well studied as a marker for CVD in women; it detects subclinical atherosclerosis in the carotid artery with the use of carotid ultrasonography. Many clinical studies, including the large Cardiovascular Health Study, demonstrated a relationship between IMT and cardiovascular events (Mieres et al., 2005; O'Leary et al., 1999). Carotid IMT is safe and noninvasive, does not use ionizing radiation, and is widely available. There had been a lack of accepted technical standards for IMT testing, and lack of outcome data prevent this test from being recommended for all women (Mieres et al., 2005); however, newer methodologies using multiple viewing angles have improved the sensitivity of this diagnostic test (Casella et al., 2008).

Coronary Angiography and Cardiac Catheterization

In the event of a positive stress test, many women are referred for coronary angiography and cardiac catheterization. Women who present with acute coronary syndromes (ACSs) may also undergo cardiac catheterization. The term *angiography* refers to the visualization of the arteries with the use of contrast medium. Cardiac catheterization encompasses coronary angiography and the assessment of left ventricular function; it can also include hemodynamic measurements and the assessment of valvular regurgitation and stenosis. Women have been shown to have a higher rate of normal cardiac catheterizations than men (Rosengren & Hasdai, 2005). Gender bias with regard to women and cardiac care in general, and to coronary angiography and cardiac catheterization specifically, has been researched and debated during the past two decades (Rosengren & Hasdai, 2005). Golden, Chang, and Hollander (2013) reported that women who presented to the emergency department with symptoms of ACS reported lower rates of referral for cardiovascular testing, as well as lower rates of counseling regarding cardiac causes of their chest pain. These findings suggest that sex differences in cardiovascular testing may be partly explained by the discussions between women and their clinicians.

■ CVD DIAGNOSES

Hypertension

DEFINITION AND SCOPE

HTN is both a diagnosis and a well-known, major risk factor for cardiovascular, cerebrovascular, and renal disease. Of the 80 million Americans who have high blood pressure, more than half are women. Within the African American and Mexican American communities, the prevalence of HTN in women is among the highest in the world (Mozaffarian et al., 2015). In patients older than the age of 75 years, the prevalence of HTN is nearly double that of patients aged 45 to 55 years, with about 84% of elderly women having a blood pressure higher than 140/90 mmHg. HTN is one of the leading causes of heart failure (HF) in women, particularly with the development of diastolic dysfunction. African American women older than 75 years have the highest prevalence at 75% (Mozaffarian et al., 2015). Despite efforts to increase community awareness of this risk factor for heart disease and stroke, more than 65% of Americans are either unaware that they have HTN or are insufficiently treated (Burt et al., 1995; Hajjar & Kotchen, 2003).

The lifetime risk of HTN is 90% in women who were normotensive at 55 to 65 years, as found by the FHS (Vasan et al., 2002). When women develop HTN, they are older, are postmenopausal, and have a higher propensity for isolated systolic HTN compared with men. Moreover, postmenopausal women with HTN have a propensity for CAD. It is thought that at this point in the lifespan, women are estrogen deficient and therefore have increased peripheral resistance and impaired endothelial function. HTN, however, is not limited to older women; 5% to 10% of all pregnancies are complicated by HTN (American College of Obstetricians and Gynecologists, 1996). Identifying and treating elevated blood pressure in women would dramatically change the health and longevity of women both pre- and postpartum.

Women are more likely to know that they have HTN and are more likely to be treated than men; the higher treatment rates are thought to be due to more frequent physician contact visits (Hajjar & Kotchen, 2003). However, data from NHANES indicate that though women have increased rates of treatment for HTN, they are less likely to achieve blood pressure control (Gu, Burt, Paulose-Ram, & Dillon, 2008). Women have lower systolic blood pressure than men until age 60 years. After age 60, women have higher systolic blood pressure than men. The highest incidence of HTN is in elderly African American women, in whom the prevalence of HTN is greater than 75% after 75 years of age. Though postmenopausal women are twice as likely to have HTN than premenopausal women, the results of research on hormone replacement therapy (HRT) as a treatment for HTN have not been consistent, and therefore hormone therapy is not indicated for the treatment of HTN (Mosca et al., 2007; Oparil, 2006).

Though most HTN (90%–95%) in the United States is essential HTN, renal artery stenosis resulting from fibromuscular dysplasia and vasculitis are more common in women than in men. HTN has been noted in users of OCPs. The Nurses' Health Study found that OCP users had significantly increased risk of HTN compared with nonusers, though the absolute risk was small. Return of blood pressure to pretreatment levels was noted within 3 months of discontinuing the OCPs. HTN in these women seemed to be related to the progesterone rather than the estrogen potency of the OCP (Pemu & Ofili, 2008). High blood pressure during pregnancy is a major concern for the sequelae of both maternal and fetal morbidity and mortality. HTN and pregnancy are discussed in detail in Chapter 38.

EVALUATION/ASSESSMENT

The National High Blood Pressure Education Program Coordinating Committee in collaboration with the National Heart Lung and Blood Institute issued the JNC 8. The purpose was to provide an evidence-based approach to the management of HTN in adults. The panel set a goal for blood pressure of less than 150/90 in persons aged 60 years or older and less than 140/90 in persons aged 30 to 59 years.

The same goals or thresholds are recommended for those persons with diabetes or nondiabetic kidney disease as the general population younger than 60 years of age. The JNC 8 guidelines provide a treatment algorithm to assist health care practitioners in a comprehensive treatment approach when caring for those with HTN (James et al., 2013).

TREATMENT/MANAGEMENT

Guidelines for the treatment of HTN are the same for men and women (see Figure 43.2), and the efficacy of pharmacological agents is similar for both genders.

Lifestyle Modifications • Rather than detailing comprehensive lifestyle modifications, which are a cornerstone for the treatment of HTN, JNC 8 endorses the 2013 AHA/ACC Guideline on Lifestyle Management to Reduce Cardiovascular Risk (Eckel et al., 2013). These guidelines encompass recommendations for lifestyle modifications to achieve optimal cardiovascular health, specifically for persons with HTN and hyperlipidemia. Dietary recommendations emphasize the intake of vegetables, fruits, whole grains, low-fat dairy products, poultry, fish, legumes, and nontropical oil and nuts (see Chapter 13). Limited intake of sweets, sugar-sweetened beverages, and red meats is advised. Limiting sodium intake to no more than 2,400 mg/day remains the current recommendation (Eckel et al., 2013).

Though weight management is detailed in a separate guideline, weight loss can be a powerful nonpharmacological treatment for HTN management. The loss of as few as 10 pounds can result in improved blood pressure control. Physical activity is an important part of HTN management as well as overall cardiovascular health. The 2013 Lifestyle Management guidelines advise adults to engage in moderate to vigorous aerobic physical activity at least three to four sessions per week for 40 minutes per session (Eckel et al., 2013).

Smoking cessation should be encouraged as a part of overall cardiovascular risk reduction, as discussed earlier.

Pharmacotherapeutics • The JNC 8 panel recommends that in the general non-Black population, the initial pharmacological treatment of HTN should include a thiazide-type diuretic, calcium-channel blocker, angiotensin-converting enzyme (ACE) inhibitor or angiotensin receptor blocker (ARB). The results of major trials showed consistent reduction in cardiovascular events and mortality with these agents. Moreover, evidence from these trials supports that actual blood pressure control, rather than a specific agent used to achieve that control, is the most relevant consideration for this recommendation. Beta blockers and alpha-blockers were not recommended as initial (first-line) therapy after a review of randomized controlled trials. However, these agents may be used as add-on agents to achieve optimal control, recognizing that many people require multiple agents. In the Black population, JNC 8 advises the use of thiazide-type diuretics or calcium-channel blockers as first-line agents over the use of ACE inhibitors, based on the ALLHAT trial, which indicated better outcomes in Black patients treated with these agents (James et al., 2013).

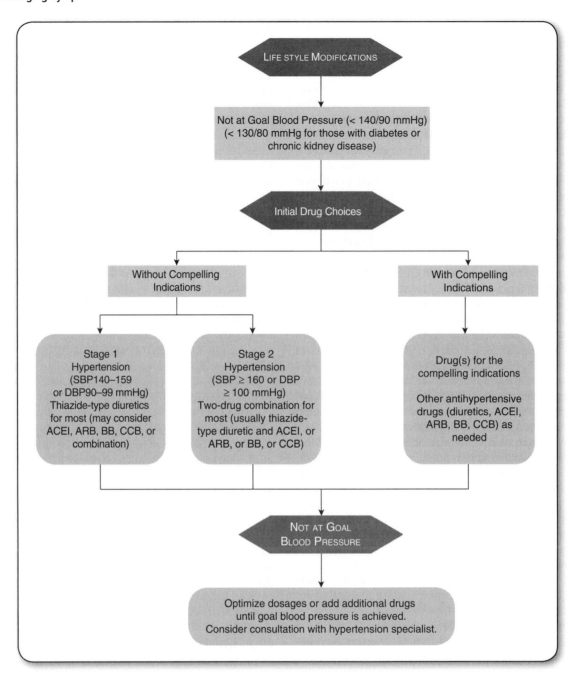

FIGURE 43.2

Algorithm for the treatment of hypertension.

ACEI, angiotensin converting enzyme inhibitor; ARB, angiotensin receptor blocker; BB, beta blocker; CCB, calcium channel blocker; DBP, diastolic blood pressure; SBP, systolic blood pressure.

Reproduced from www.nhlbi.nih.gov/guidelines/hypertension/jnc7full.pdf

JNC 8 also stresses the importance of attaining and maintaining blood pressure control by increasing the titration of the initial drug chosen or adding a second drug after 1 month of treatment. Additional agents can be added in the same manner to achieve blood pressure goals. However, the use of ACE inhibitors with an ARB in the same patient is not recommended. Referral to a HTN specialist is recommended if adding a third agent fails to achieve blood pressure control (James et al., 2013). Some caveats have

been noted regarding pharmacological treatment of HTN in women. The Treatment of Mild Hypertension Study (TOMHS) found that women reported twice as many side effects to common hypertensive medications compared with men. For instance, diuretics were more likely to cause hyponatremia and hypokalemia (August & Oparil, 1999). In addition, ACE inhibitors were three times more likely to cause cough (Os et al., 1994). Calcium-channel blockers were more likely to result in lower-extremity edema in women compared with men (August & Oparil, 1999; Pemu & Ofili, 2008). Though these factors do not preclude use of these agents in women, practitioners should be aware of the potential side effects.

Dyslipidemia

ETIOLOGY AND RISK FACTORS

Dyslipidemia results from excessive production of lipoproteins, defective removal of lipoproteins, or both. Drugs such as OCPs, hormones, corticosteroids, beta blockers, diuretics, and alcohol can all cause and contribute to dyslipidemia. Moreover, factors such as obesity and a high-fat diet and conditions such as diabetes, hypothyroidism, Addison's disease, and Cushing's disease can cause secondary dyslipidemia. Pregnancy can cause transient dyslipidemia but lipid levels return to normal within 6 to 8 weeks after birth (Gotto & Pownall, 1999). Women who breastfed their infants had lower low-density lipoprotein cholesterol (LDL-C) and insulin levels than those who did not breastfeed (Gunderson et al., 2007). The long-term implications of the lower LDL-C levels in these women are not known (Gunderson et al., 2007).

Disorders of lipoprotein metabolism are well-established risk factors for CHD in both sexes. In general, LDL-C levels are lower and HDL-C levels are higher in women compared with men, until menopause. After menopause, LDL-C levels climb, so that by age 70 years, women have higher LDL-C levels than men. Although HDL-C levels in women decline during menopause, they still remain overall higher than those of men (Duvall, 2003).

TREATMENT/MANAGEMENT

Guidelines for Dyslipidemia • Many clinical trials have demonstrated lower cardiac event rates with medical treatment of dyslipidemia. Women were underrepresented in earlier landmark clinical trials involving lipid-lowering drugs. However, one clinical study that included women in large numbers was the Heart Protection Study (HPS). The HPS enrolled 5,082 women and 15,454 men with known vascular disease. The investigators found a 24% reduction in major vascular events at 5 years, independent of gender, in participants taking simvastatin (HPS Collaborative Group, 2002). More recently, the Justification for the Use of Statin in Prevention: An Intervention Trial Evaluating Rosuvastatin (JUPITER) included 6,801 women with elevated hs-CRP levels (higher than 2 mg/L) and LDL-C levels lower than 130 mg/dL treated with rosuvastatin and showed a significant reduction in atherosclerotic CVD (ASCVD) events compared with placebo (Mora et al., 2010). Current treatment guidelines do not differentiate between men and women; target goals for lipid profiles are the same (Stone et al., 2014).

Historically, the National Heart, Lung and Blood Institute (NHLBI), National Cholesterol Education Program (NCEP) developed guidelines for the treatment of dyslipidemia (NHLBI, 2001). The guidelines for the treatment of blood cholesterol to reduce ASCVD in adults were revised in 2013 by the AHA and ACC, in collaboration with the NHLBI (Stone et al. 2014). With these guidelines, the focus of primary prevention shifted to evaluating absolute risk rather than treating to a specific cholesterol number. Individuals with established ASCVD are recommended for high-dose statin therapy (Stone et al., 2014). These guidelines recommend using a new Pooled Cohort Equation to estimate 10-year risk for ASCVD in White and Black men and women without known ASCVD (Stone et al., 2014). This risk calculator is available at http://www.cvriskcalculator.com and as an application for smartphones and tablets.

The risk calculator uses the cardiovascular risk factors of gender, age, race, total cholesterol, HDL-C, systolic blood pressure (mmHg), treatment of HTN, diabetes, and smoking to calculate a 10-year risk of developing ASCVD in individuals aged 20 to 79 years. The application also calculates a lifetime risk score in persons aged 20 to 59 years of age. In general, individuals with a 10-year ASCVD risk of less than 5% are not considered to benefit from pharmacological management of hyperlipidemia. However, for these individuals, clinicians may consider additional factors in deciding treatment options, including family history of premature CHD, LDL-C greater than 160 mg/dL, hs-CRP levels greater than 2 mg/dL, a high CAC by cardiac computed tomography angiogram (CTA), and evidence of peripheral arterial disease by the ankle–brachial index (Stone et al., 2014). Treatment of lipids in the guidelines is centered on the use of 3-hydroxy-3-methylglutaryl-coenzyme (HMG-CoA) reductase inhibitors, also known as *statins*. The presence of diabetes increases the risk substantially; at least moderate-intensity statin therapy is recommended for all adults aged 40 to 75 years with diabetes. Moderate-intensity statin therapy is recommended for individuals aged 40 to 75 years without diabetes whose lifetime risk is 5% to 7.5% and for those with a 10-year risk of greater than 7.5% (Stone et al., 2014).

The 2013 guidelines were met with some controversy, particularly related to a lack of specific LDL-C targets. In addition, the guidelines increased the overall number of primary prevention patients eligible for statin therapy. However, recent research has since validated the use of the guidelines. The first study compared the 2013 guidelines with the old NCEP guidelines. Using a CAC CT score in asymptomatic patients aged 35 years and older, the 2013 guideline was found to be more accurate at matching statin eligibility with the presence and extent of subclinical atherosclerosis as measured by CAC scores. The study's authors conclude that the 2013 guidelines are more accurate and efficient than the previous guidelines (Pursnani, Massaro, D'Agostino, O'Donnell, & Hoffmann, 2015). Other research using a microsimulation model predicted ASCVD events using data from NHANES, large clinical trials, and meta-analysis for statin benefits and treatment. The analysis demonstrated the cost-effectiveness of 10-year risk thresholds for initiating statin therapy for primary prevention (Pandya, Sy, Cho, Weinstein, & Gaziano, 2015).

Pharmacotherapeutics • The first-line drug therapy for dyslipidemia is primarily with HMG-CoA reductase inhibitors, otherwise known as *statins*, which lower total cholesterol and LDL-C. Statins currently available are simvastatin, lovastatin, fluvastatin, atorvastatin, rosuvastatin, pravastatin, and pitavastatin. They vary in dosage and potency. Statins are the only lipid-lowering drugs that produce plaque stabilization and lower LDL-C. Patients with active liver disease or women who are pregnant or may become pregnant are not candidates for statins (Ballantyne, O'Keefe, & Gotto, 2005).

Myopathy is a potential side effect of all statins, though the risk of myopathy is less than 1% in most individuals studied in large research trials. However, an incidence of approximately 5% has been observed (Pasternak et al., 2002). The risks of myositis or myopathy increases with high-intensity statin therapy and with concurrent use of medications such as niacin, verapamil, amiodarone, macrolide antibiotics, azole antifungals, fibric acid derivatives (especially gemfibrozil) and HIV protease inhibitors (Ballantyne et al., 2005; Meagher, 2004). In patients who have complaints of muscle aches, a creatine kinase (CK) level should be checked. However, routine monitoring of CK levels in patients without myositis symptoms is not recommended (Gotto & Pownall, 1999). As stated earlier, statins are contraindicated in women who are pregnant or may become pregnant, thus limiting their use in women of childbearing age. Though the incidence of statin myopathy is overall low in clinical trials, the authors concluded that there was a paucity of sex- and age-specific research in the area of statin-induced myotoxicity (Bhardwaj, Slevarajah, & Schneider., 2013).

Another approach to lower LDL-C is the use of bile acid sequestrants such as colesevelam, cholestyramine, colestipol, and colestimide, which bind bile acids in the intestinal lumen and interrupt enteropathic circulation of bile acids, thereby decreasing fecal excretion of acidic steroids. They are well suited as an "add-on" agent with a statin, and can be used in patients with statin intolerance or liver disease, as they act only in the gastrointestinal system and have no systemic effects. They are also are a good option for women of childbearing age for this same reason. There are no studies showing reduced cardiovascular events in women using these agents, though they were found to be modestly effective in men (Gotto & Pownall, 1999).

Fibric acid derivatives, also known as *fibrates*, act in the liver to increase lipoprotein lipase activity, increase bile acid secretion, and decrease triglyceride synthesis. Fibrates are used mainly to lower triglycerides. They also can increase HDL-C. Fenofibrate has been shown to decrease LDL-C mildly. A fibrate can be added to statin therapy to treat combined hyperlipidemias in many patients. There are limited outcome data regarding the use of fibrates in women, as most available outcome studies enrolled only men. However, treating women with a fibrate has shown some benefit (Diabetes Atherosclerosis Intervention Study Investigators, 2001; Mosca, 2005).

Niacin, a water-soluble B vitamin, is another option for the treatment of dyslipidemia, especially elevated triglycerides and low HDL-C. The main side effect with niacin is flushing, which can be minimized with taking aspirin ½ to 1 hour before the drug, as well as by taking the medication at night. Niacin should also be taken with food to increase its absorption and lessen the side effect of flushing (Gotto & Pownall, 1999). Women have been shown to achieve greater LDL-C lowering with niacin than did men. In addition, a

trend toward greater triglyceride lowering in women has been reported (Brown et al., 2001; Goldberg, 1998).

The cholesterol absorption inhibitor ezetimibe is approved for the treatment of hyperlipidemia. It lowers LDL-C modestly, has mild triglyceride-lowering capabilities, and works equally well in men and women (Ballantyne et al., 2005). Ezetimibe has a low incidence of side effects and only rarely causes an increase in liver transaminases. Clinical outcome studies with use of ezetimibe for the treatment of high LDL-C have been mixed. The ENHANCE trial investigated the effects of ezetimibe in combination with simvastatin versus simvastatin alone on carotid IMT in patients with heterozygous familial hyperlipidemia (Kastelein et al., 2008). Despite significant decreases in LDL-C in the ezetimibe–simvastatin group compared with the simvastatin group, the combination failed to demonstrate carotid IMT regression (Kastelein et al., 2008). However, the 2014 IMPROVE-IT study demonstrated improved outcomes in ACS patients treated with the combination ezetimibe–simvastatin over 7 years versus simvastatin alone. Individuals treated with ezetimibe had statistically significant fewer CHD-related deaths, MIs, and urgent coronary revascularizations (Cannon et al., 1994). The study validates the hypothesis that lowering LDL-C levels to below that of recommended targets in high-risk patients has benefit (Cannon et al., 1994). Ezetimibe is a reasonable therapy in patients who cannot tolerate a statin or are not at goal on high-dose statin alone (Drazen, Jarcho, Morrissey, & Curfman, 2008; Jackevicius, Tu, Ko, & Krumholtz, 2008; Kastelein et al., 2008).

Nonpharmacologic Management • Treatment of dyslipidemia requires a multifaceted approach, which includes diet modification and exercise. The AHA/ACC 2013 guideline notes state that adherence to a heart-healthy diet, regular exercise habits, maintenance of healthy weight, and avoidance of tobacco products remain crucial components of ASCVD risk reduction (Stone et al., 2014). The guideline endorses the 2013 AHA/ACC guideline on Lifestyle Management to Reduce Cardiovascular Risk for lifestyle modifications (Eckel et al., 2014). Consuming a diet that emphasizes the intake of vegetables, fruit, and whole grains and includes low-fat dairy products, poultry, fish, legumes, nontropical vegetable oils, and nuts is recommended. Limiting the intake of sweets, sugar-sweetened beverages, and red meats is advised. Additional recommendations are to aim for a dietary pattern that achieves 5% to 6% of calories from saturated fat, reduces the percentage of calories from saturated fat, and reduces the percentage of calories from trans-fat (Eckel et al., 2014).

Dietary plans such as the AHA diet, the U.S. Department of Agriculture (USDA) Food Pattern, or the Dietary Approaches to Stop Hypertension (DASH) diet are specifically recommended by the 2013 Lifestyle guideline. The U.S. Department of Health and Human Services 2010 Dietary Guidelines for Americans also recommend these diets (USDA, 2010).

Physical activity has modest effects on lowering LDL-C (3–6 mg/dL) and non–HDL-C (6–9 mg/dL) (Eckel et al., 2014). No consistent benefit of aerobic exercise alone has been demonstrated on either HDL-C or triglycerides (Eckel et al., 2014). The 2013 guideline committee recommended that adults engage in three to four sessions of moderate-to-vigorous-intensity exercise per week, lasting 40 minutes per session, to assist in lowering LDL-C and non–HDL-C (Eckel et al., 2014).

Complementary and Alternative Medicine Therapies • Omega-3 fish oil has been shown to be modestly effective in lowering triglycerides (20%–40%) and increasing HDL-C (5%–10%; Gotto & Pownall, 1999). Fish oil can be a useful add-on therapy in the treatment of dyslipidemia. Unfortunately, because of a significant "first pass" effect by the liver, the dose of fish oil needs to be quite high to achieve benefits. A minimum of 4,000 to 6,000 mg (four to six capsules, in divided doses, with meals) is needed to affect lipids positively. However, newer formulations are "odorless" and "tasteless," making it more palatable to take, and fish oil is very safe in combination with other medications (Gotto & Pownall, 1999).

Another option for the treatment of dyslipidemia, specifically LDL-C lowering, is use of a plant stanol. Plant stanols are naturally occurring substances found in some vegetables and the pulp of wood; they act as cholesterol inhibitors in the intestines. Plant stanols have been shown to reduce LDL-C cholesterol 8% to 16% and have been found to be effective in women (Gylling, Radhakrishnan, & Miettinen, 1997; Miettinen, Puska, Gylling, Vanhanen, & Vartianen, 1995). They are safe and well tolerated. Plant stanols are found in some commercially available margarine spreads and salad dressings and are also now available in tablet or capsule form over the counter. The recommended daily dose is 2 g in divided doses, with meals (Gylling et al., 1997; Miettinen et al., 1995).

Atherosclerotic Disease

ETIOLOGY

CVD and its root cause, atherosclerosis, are systemic disorders. As early as the 1960s, clinical experience, laboratory studies, and necropsy studies supported the concept that patients with disease in one vascular bed were likely to have disease in other vascular beds (Young, Gofman, Tandy, & Waters, 1960). More recent studies have confirmed that patients who had peripheral vascular disease were more likely to have CAD and/or cerebrovascular disease than those who did not (Johnson et al., 2004). The pathogenesis of this chronic and progressive illness that leads to atherosclerotic plaque formation and cardiac events is multifactorial and explained by several mechanisms, leading clinicians to direct preventive strategies, acute treatments, and secondary interventions to prevent or delay future events.

Atherosclerosis is a disorder of the vessel wall that involves complex relationships among hemodynamic and environmental factors, inflammatory pathways, thrombotic mechanisms, lipid metabolism, and various compositional elements of the vessel wall (Libby & Therous, 2005). Because plaque formation initially spares the vessel lumen, coronary angiography often underestimates the true burden of atheroma in the arterial wall. Risk factors associated with the development of atherosclerosis play key roles in the popular "response-to-injury" hypothesis.

The NHLBI-sponsored Women's Ischemic Syndrome Evaluation (WISE) 1999 study contributed numerous data that have improved the understanding of some unique differences among vasculopathies in women with heart disease (Johnson et al., 2004). Differences in both vascular structure and function and the unique circumstances of pregnancy and menopause predispose women to greater risk and more severe disease at a later age than men.

DIFFERENTIAL DIAGNOSES

Angina Pectoris (Chronic Stable Angina)
Etiology, Definition, Scope, and Diagnostic Studies. The term *chronic stable angina* or *stable ischemic heart disease* refers to angina symptoms that occur with exertion or psychological stress. The symptoms are relieved within 2 to 3 minutes of rest or with nitrates (i.e., sublingual nitroglycerin). In these individuals, coronary ischemia is caused by a mismatch between oxygen supply and demand in the presence of a fixed and stable coronary plaque. The presentation in women is often different than that in men. In men, heart disease more often occurs as a result of blockages in their coronary arteries, referred to as *obstructive CAD*, whereas women more frequently develop heart disease within the smaller arteries. This is referred to as *microvascular disease* (MVD) and occurs particularly in younger women in the 45- to 65-year time frame, although the process can occur at any time in women's lives if they have lower-than-normal estrogen levels. Women exhibit a greater symptom burden, more functional disability, and a higher prevalence of no obstructive CAD compared with men when evaluated for signs and symptoms of myocardial ischemia (Gulati, Shaw, & Bairey Merz et al., 2012).

MCD, defined as limited coronary flow reserve (CFR) and/or coronary endothelial dysfunction, is the predominant mechanism of ischemia in women with persistent chest pain, no obstructive CAD, and ischemia evidenced by stress testing. MCD is associated with a 2.5% yearly major adverse event rate of death, nonfatal MI, nonfatal stroke, and congestive HF (Kothawade & Bairey Merz, 2011). Although tests such as the adenosine stress CMRI can be useful noninvasive methods for predicting ischemia, the standard test to diagnose MCD is an invasive coronary reactivity testing (CRT; Kothawade & Bairey Merz, 2011). Early identification of MCD by CRT may be helpful in determining prognosis and the best approach for optimal medical therapy.

Evaluation/Assessment
HISTORY AND SYMPTOMS. Obtaining a complete history is the first step when evaluating the woman with chest pain. Typical angina is often described as pressure or tightness; common adjectives used to describe angina include *squeezing, vice-like,* and *heavy.* The condition can also mimic indigestion. Angina is rarely sharp or stabbing in nature, and it does not change in character with deep inspiration or movement. The duration of pain is often 10 to 20 minutes; it is neither brief nor fleeting nor is it constant (e.g., longer than 1 hour; Fraker & Fihn, writing on behalf of the 2002 Chronic Stable Angina Writing Committee, 2007). Women are more likely than men to present with stable angina as their first manifestation of CVD, whereas

men more often present with infarction (Lerner & Kannel, 1986). Although the AHA defines *angina* as chest, jaw, shoulder, back, or arm discomfort brought on by physical or emotional stress (Fraker & Fihn, 2007), it is important to recognize that this definition of *typical angina* was derived from studies done almost exclusively with male participants (Douglas & Ginsburg, 1996). Clinicians must be vigilant to the fact that women present more often with atypical symptoms (Jackson, 2005; Redberg & Shaw, 2003). Women have less exertional symptoms and instead, more chest discomfort that occurs at rest or during sleep. Moreover, women experience other nonspecific symptoms of fatigue, nausea, and shortness of breath (Jackson, 2005).

Women are also less likely to describe their chest discomfort as substernal and crushing; rather, their symptoms are more often described as burning or squeezing or as a feeling of upper abdominal fullness (Jackson, 2005). As women age, there is a change in symptoms, and older women are more likely to present with a "typical" pattern of angina than younger women. In addition, the more "typical" the pattern of angina, the more likely the diagnosis is CVD (Jackson, 2005). However, in a cluster analysis of women's prodromal and acute MI (McSweeney, Cleves, Zhaom, Lefler, & Yang, 2010), interesting symptom patterns emerged. During the prodromal phase, chest pain/discomfort was often lacking, and instead women experienced the same "early warning" symptoms of unusual fatigue, sleep disturbances, shortness of breath, change in thinking/remembering, heart racing, frequent indigestion, and anxiety. There is a high recurrence rate of the prodromal symptom cluster occurring in the acute phase of illness in those admitted with ACS (McSweeney et al., 2010). Other implications for practice included the following findings: (a) Older, White women without a history of diabetes or smoking were less likely to experience a cluster of prodromal symptoms but instead were likely to experience a single symptom, which was profound fatigue; and (b) Black women younger than 50 years with multiple risk factors compared with other women were more likely to experience a cluster of symptoms composed of many distressing prodromal symptoms, and Black women who smoked, were younger, were obese, and were diabetic and had a history of CVD reported the largest cluster of acute MI symptoms (McSweeney et al., 2010). These data demonstrate the importance of a careful history to determine if the woman is experiencing a cluster of prodromal MI symptoms, which may help with a diagnosis of CVD to facilitate early treatment and a better clinical outcome.

PHYSICAL EXAMINATION AND DIAGNOSTIC STUDIES. The physical examination of women with angina is often benign. However, it may provide clues regarding the presence of cardiovascular risk factors or other vascular disease. During an episode of chest pain, a transient gallop or murmur of mitral regurgitation (MR) can be auscultated. Likewise, although the resting EKG of a woman with angina who is pain free is often normal, EKG changes may or may not be observed when the woman is having angina symptoms (Fraker & Fihn, 2007).

DIFFERENTIAL DIAGNOSES AND TREATMENT/ MANAGEMENT. The medical management of stable angina is usually coordinated by a specialist, and it includes the aggressive control of cardiac risk factors, especially dyslipidemia, HTN, diabetes, obesity, and smoking. There are four types of medications used for the treatment of stable angina: nitrates, beta blockers or calcium-channel blockers if beta blockers cannot be used, ACE inhibitors or ARBs, and ranolazine. Lipid management should be considered in addition to good control of the patient's blood pressure. Aspirin had been recommended for the prevention of CVD in women younger than 65 years of age but is no longer recommended to prevent MI, like it is in men, although it does provide stroke benefit per the Women's Health Study (Ridker et al., 2005). Last, exercise is beneficial for reducing the morbidity associated with chronic stable angina and for improving quality of life (Fihn et al., 2012), as well as reducing other risk factors as they apply to the specific patient. The management of refractory angina with coronary artery bypass graft (CABG) surgery and percutaneous coronary intervention (PCI) as they relate to women are presented in the following sections.

Cardiac Syndrome X • The presence of typical angina symptoms and evidence of myocardial ischemia as determined by cardiac stress testing (yet with smooth coronary arteries as shown by coronary angiography) is known as *cardiac syndrome X* (Kaski, 2006). Suggested mechanisms for cardiac syndrome X include microvascular endothelial dysfunction with abnormal vasodilator reserve, estrogen deficiency, abnormal pain perception, and insulin resistance. Recent advances in technology have shed more light on this phenomenon. As cardiac syndrome X is found primarily among perimenopausal and postmenopausal women, a relationship between cardiac syndrome X and estrogen deficiency has been established (Kaski, 2006). Women with cardiac syndrome X have been found to have higher levels of anxiety and depression as well as fewer social supports than age-matched controls (Kaski, 2006). However, the psychological abnormalities seen among women with cardiac syndrome X may be secondary to the disease process and its symptoms and compounded by inadequate reassurance and education by the clinician (Kaski, 2006). It is prudent to conclude that chest pain symptoms are psychological in etiology only after exploring the possibility of CVD or other physiologic causes.

Scope. As many as 20% or more of patients diagnosed with angina and undergoing cardiac catheterization are said to have cardiac syndrome X, and they are predominantly women (Kaski, 2006). Women with cardiac syndrome X have been a perplexing group to manage because there are few randomized controlled studies available to help guide evaluation and treatment (Kaski, 2006).

The NHBLI's WISE study is the largest study of women with CVD to date (Johnson et al., 2004). In this study, nearly 60% of the 1,000 women referred for cardiac catheterization after an abnormal stress test did not have obstructive (flow-limiting) coronary lesions. Although women had lower angiographic disease burden and better left ventricular systolic function as determined by angiography, they had more symptoms and greater disability (Johnson et al., 2004). In addition, compared with age- and race-matched controls, women enrolled in the WISE study had higher cardiovascular event rates and mortality rates despite nonobstructive or angiographically normal coronary arteries (Kaski, 2006). Nearly 50% of women with normal coronary arteries in the WISE study had angiographic evidence of MCD as defined by reduced coronary flow velocity when injected with the vasodilator adenosine (Reis et al., 2001). These women had more cardiac events than women with normal microvascular vasodilator response. Moreover, MCD could not be predicted by traditional risk factors for heart disease (Reis et al., 2001). Patients with MCD have a 2.5% annual adverse cardiac event rate, which includes MI, congestive HF, stroke, and sudden cardiac death (Bugiardini & Bairey Merz, 2005). Data from the NHLBI-sponsored WISE study has shown that women with no obstructive CAD and evidence of myocardial ischemia have a poorer prognosis compared with women without obstructive CAD or myocardial ischemia (Johnson et al., 2004). Microvascular CAD is prevalent in women with signs and symptoms of ischemia and no obstructive CAD. The long-term prognosis is not benign, as previously thought, with new findings suggesting that these women are at increased risk for cardiac events. More research is needed to advance the understanding of MCD pathophysiology to guide diagnosis and therapy.

Evaluation/Assessment and Treatment/Management. The treatment of women with cardiac syndrome X or "nonobstructive" CAD is challenging. Nitrates, beta blockers, and calcium-channel blockers are useful for women with documented ischemia or abnormal myocardial perfusion imaging (Kaski, 2006). In small clinical trials, imipramine (Tofranil) (Cannon et al., 1994) and aminophylline (Somophylline) (Morris, 2005) have been found to be effective for decreasing chest pain symptoms. Although hormone therapy has been shown to be effective for the treatment of cardiac syndrome X (Orshal & Khalil, 2004), it carries significant cardiovascular risk as well. Currently, chest pain that is thought to be a result of cardiac syndrome X can be treated with nitrates and with the control of CVD risk factors (Fraker & Fihn, 2007; Kaski, 2006). The treatment of MCD can be challenging because of a current lack of uniform diagnostic criteria and multiple variables contributing to the pathophysiology. The goals of treatment are to control symptoms and improve quality of life, to reduce the incidence of hospitalization and repeated invasive testing, and to improve survival (Kothawade & Bairey Merz, 2011).

Acute Coronary Syndromes

Etiology. Approximately 70% to 80% of cases result from an unstable coronary plaque that fissures or ruptures and causes acute thrombosis (Morris, 2005). Further details of the process were presented in a review of vulnerable plaques (Finn, Nakano, Narula, Kolodgie, & Virmani, 2010) of more than 800 cases of sudden coronary death; at autopsy, 55% to 60% of subjects had underlying plaque rupture as the etiology, whereas 30% to 35% had erosion and 2% to 7% had thrombi attributed to calcified nodules.

ST-elevation MI (STEMI) is caused by the acute and complete closure of a coronary artery, which results in myocardial necrosis and cell death; non-STEMI (NSTEMI) and unstable angina (UA) are caused by subtotal coronary occlusion, which results in varying amounts of myocardial damage.

Definition and Scope. ACSs include UA, non–Q-wave MI (also known as *NSTEMI*), and Q-wave MI (also known as *STEMI*). It is now understood that these conditions are not distinct, separate entities; rather, they exist on a continuum.

Acute MI is less likely to be the first presenting event in women, especially in younger women. In fact, women are less likely to have an acute MI at any age. However, differences between men and women regarding morbidity and mortality decrease with advancing age (Lerner & Kannel, 1986). Autopsy studies reveal that plaque erosion is more common among women, particularly younger women, whereas plaque rupture is more common among men (Burke, Kolodgi, Farb, & Virmani, 2003). This may explain why men experience greater prehospital acute MI mortality rates and why women have greater in-hospital mortality rates (Bairey Merz, Shaw, & Reis, 2006).

Women generally present later during the course of MI because there is a delay in symptom recognition (Heer et al., 2002). One potential reason for the delay in treatment and poorer outcomes is that women are more likely to experience a prodromal cluster of nonchest pain symptoms than men, which adds to the difficulty of securing a correct diagnosis (McSweeney et al., 2010). Most deaths from acute MI occur outside of the hospital, with more men succumbing to sudden cardiac death than women; this may explain the disparity in mortality rates seen later in the course of the condition for women (Bairey Merz et al., 2006).

Evaluation/Assessment. ACS and MI often have atypical presentations in women (Chen, Woods, & Puntillo, 2005; Patel, Rosengren, & Ekman, 2004). Fewer than 30% of women reported having chest pain prior to their MIs and 43% reported no chest pain at any phase of MI (McSweeney et al., 2003). In contrast, others report that most (90%) women with acute MI experience some form of chest pain or discomfort during the acute event. Even in women, the more "typical" the symptoms are, the greater the chance of ACS (Milner, Funk, Arnold, & Vaccarino, 2002). Nonetheless, women are more likely than men to have associated symptoms of nausea, shortness of breath, cold sweats, palpitations, and dizziness (Chen et al., 2005; Milner et al., 2002; Patel et al., 2004) as well as sleep disturbances, weakness in the arms, and indigestion (McSweeney et al., 2003). These prodromal symptoms occurred up to 2 weeks before the MI and persisted until the acute event occurred (McSweeney et al., 2003).

Treatment/Management. Restoring coronary blood flow is the primary goal for a woman with STEMI (Kern, 2005), as it is with all patients per the 2013 American College of Cardiology Foundation (ACCF) and AHA Guideline for the Management of STEMI (O'Gara et al., 2013). For women with UA and NSTEMI, preventing further thrombosis and maintaining and improving existing coronary flow are the primary goals (Morris, 2005; Jneid et al., 2012).

In general, an early invasive approach (i.e., cardiac catheterization and potential revascularization) is indicated for women with refractory angina, hemodynamic instability, unstable serial EKGs, or positive cardiac biomarkers (specifically troponin). In the absence of the aforementioned criteria, an initial conservative (noninvasive) approach is appropriate. The preferences of the woman and the clinician are considered, as are any comorbid conditions. Current research does not support an invasive strategy in women with low-risk features, such as atypical chest pain in the absence of positive biomarkers, no EKG changes, and few cardiac risk factors (Dolor et al., 2012; Salisbury et al., 2014).

THROMBOLYTICS FOR STEMI. Reperfusion therapy with thrombolytics benefits both genders and is indicated for women with chest pain symptoms of less than 12 hours' duration with ST elevation or new left bundle branch block (O'Gara et al., 2013). Women exhibit a higher incidence of cerebral bleeding complications related to thrombolytic therapy, which may affect decisions to forego this therapy for women (Heer et al., 2002). Although findings of bleeding complications are controversial, factors such as an age of more than 65 years, a low body weight (i.e., less than 70 kg), and HTN on admission all increase the risk of bleeding and are more prevalent among women (Rosengren & Hasdai, 2005).

PCI FOR STEMI. In medical centers with appropriate resources immediately available, primary PCI (i.e., angioplasty with stenting) is preferred over intravenous thrombolytic therapy for the treatment of STEMI, and it is superior for decreasing mortality rates among both sexes (O'Gara et al., 2013). In medical centers with PCI available, the standard of care is to expedite the process so that the time from medical contact to balloon or stent implantation is 90 minutes or less (O'Gara et al., 2013). PCIs now have significantly lower complication rates and improved long-term patency rates (O'Gara et al., 2013). The use of drug-eluting stents (DESs) coated with either sirolimus (Rapamune) or paclitaxel (Abraxane) to ensure artery patency are commonplace as invasive cardiology technology continues to advance (Lansky et al., 2005). These first-generation DESs were used to minimize the restenosis process that had occurred with bare-metal stents. Some of these early DESs did reduce restenosis but were limited by suboptimal polymer biocompatibility, delayed stent endothelialization leading to late (more than 30 days) and very late thrombosis (more than 12 months) formation, and local drug toxicity (Abizaid & Costa, 2010; Agarwal, Shawl, Raman, & Binbrek, 2008). Newer DESs with biodegradable polymers and nonpolymeric DESs, as well as immunosuppressive and antiproliferative drugs added to the structure, are under study to prevent restenosis and decrease inflammation. Since then, cases of late (more than 30 days postimplantation) and very late (more than 12 months postimplantation) stent thrombosis (ST) have appeared with increasing frequency.

Both bare-metal stents and the newer DESs have been shown to be equally effective for men and for women (Anderson et al., 2012). The decision to use a bare-metal stent or a DES is based on patient profile. A bare-metal stent should not be used sin patients who have a high bleeding risk, who have an inability to tolerate 1 year of dual antiplatelet therapy (DAPT), or who may have an invasive or surgical procedure within 1 year of stent placement (O'Gara et al., 2013). Of particular importance to women is that stents appear to have favorable short-term and long-term results in smaller vessels as well as in larger vessels. Today, women remain at higher risk of in-hospital mortality and other complications. In contrast, long-term outcomes are similar or better in women and men. The use of a DES is associated with a similar benefit in both men and women (Anderson et al., 2012). Perhaps some of the higher complication rates, such as the increased in-hospital mortality rates among women in recent stent and DES studies, can be explained by the higher risk profile of women. After adjustments are made for clinical factors such as older age, small body surface area, and comorbidities, the difference in mortality rates between men and women are negated (Jacobs, 2003). Notably, in the more recent studies, the differences between men and women (adjusted) in in-hospital mortality has almost disappeared, even in large-scale registries, which are less likely to be underpowered, since 25% to 30% of patients are women (Lansky et al., 2005). However, the incidence of bleeding and vascular complications after the procedure continues to be significantly higher in women than in men and again might be related to the clinical differences noted earlier. In general, both women and men in recent studies have, compared with earlier studies, more complex anatomy and concomitant disease. Still, adjusted mortality after PCI has decreased, especially in women. Last, the reasons for a reduction in gender differences in mortality are uncertain, but it is likely that greater awareness of issues specific to women (periprocedural HF resulting from hypertensive heart disease) and improved technology, including smaller and more flexible stents (allowing access to smaller coronary vessels), have resulted in improvements (Jacobs, 2009).

PHARMACOTHERAPEUTICS. During the initial stages of ACS with or without PCI, aspirin has been the mainstay therapy. Women derive as much benefit as men do from aspirin therapy with ACS or MI (Antithrombotic Trialists Collaboration, 2002). Aspirin is recommended indefinitely for all women with CVD, particularly after revascularization procedures, unless a true allergy exists (Lansky et al., 2005). Clopidogrel is recommended for ACS in the acute phase and for 1 year after STEMI and NSTEMI, and it was found to be similarly beneficial for both sexes (Anderson et al., 2007; Mehta et al., 2001). Although unfractionated heparin anticoagulation has been a mainstay of the pharmacologic management of ACS and MI for more than a decade and is known to reduce mortality (Amsterdam et al., 2014; O'Gara et al., 2013) low-molecular-weight heparin (enoxaparin) has been found to be equally effective or better for the treatment of AMI. Enoxaparin is now preferable to heparin as an anticoagulant for acute MI unless the patient has renal failure (O'Gara et al., 2013).

Other treatment options for the patient with UA, NSTEMI, or STEMI include beta blockers, nitrates, ACE inhibitors, and calcium-channel blockers. Beta blockers prevent recurrent MI and ischemia and are effective antianginals and antihypertensive agents. They are contraindicated for women with bronchospasm, hypotension, or advanced atrioventricular-node block. The long-term use of ACE inhibitors helps with the prevention of recurrent ischemic events and the reduction of mortality, especially among women with left ventricular dysfunction. For women who are allergic to ACE inhibitors, ARBs are indicated (Krumholz et al., 2008). In addition to beta blockers and ACE inhibitors, the Task Force on Performance Measures also reiterated the importance of the evaluation and treatment of risk factors during the inpatient care of the post-MI patient, especially checking lipid levels and providing smoking-cessation advice and counseling (Krumholz et al., 2008).

CABG SURGERY. The decision to treat women with PCI or CABG surgery is complex. In general, multivessel disease and left main CAD are indications for a surgical approach (Hillis et al., 2011). Fewer women are referred for CABG and PCI, with women making up only 33% of patients who have had PCI. In the past, mortality rates for both PCI and CABG were higher in women (Lundberg & King, 2012). Some of the reasons for these results have been because women had presented at an older age and had more comorbidities such as HTN, diabetes mellitus, and LV dysfunction. Additionally, women have a smaller stature, lesser body surface area, and blood vessels with less multivessel disease and less obstructive CAD. Some have also thought that there still has been an underrecognition of heart disease in women and an underutilization of the guidelines. However, recent registries and studies have shown that women have mortality rates similar to men after correcting for age and comorbidities (Lundberg & King, 2012), and according to the 2011 ACCF/AHA guidelines women may have better long-term outcomes than men. Also reported was that women have higher rates of periprocedural morbidity and mortality. Women who have stable angina, NSTEMI, and STEMI have improved results with revascularization compared with the results from historical studies. Accordingly, women should be managed the same as their male counterparts, except for women with low-risk UA/NSTEMI.

The differences between genders may be improved through durable revascularization procedures and close postoperative care that is specific to women (Guru, Fremes, Austin, Blackstone, & Tu., 2006). It was noted in the literature that more studies are needed to be certain that the differences between the genders in outcomes has in fact, narrowed. Even so, there may be some factors that continue to contribute to the postoperative differences in men and women because after CABG surgery, women have a more difficult recovery period compared with men, which has not been explained by the severity of illness, the presurgery health status, or other patient characteristics (Vaccarino et al., 2014).

Of note, among patients with prior CABG surgery, there were no significant differences in death rates according to gender, and hence the "gender gap" was altered among prior CABG patients, per findings by Al-Aqeedi, Al Suwaidi, Singh, and Al Binalis (2012). Nevertheless, the authors noted that women with prior CABG need to be more represented in studies to better understand the findings (Al-Aqeedi et al., 2012).

CARDIAC REHABILITATION. Cardiac rehabilitation programs incorporate monitored exercise with extensive risk-factor modification, including smoking-cessation, lipid, and nutrition counseling; weight control; and disease management (Leon et al., 2005). Programs are designed to optimize the patient's physical and psychological well-being with the goals of improving cardiac fitness, preventing disease progression, and reducing cardiac mortality. Cardiac rehabilitation programs have also been shown to improve psychological functioning and health-related quality of life (HRQOL) (Oldridge et al., 1991). Candidates for cardiac rehabilitation traditionally include patients with MI or CABG, chronic stable angina, or chronic HF and those who have undergone PCI or cardiac transplant. Cardiac rehabilitation participation is associated with increased survival rates among patients who are more than 70 years old, independent of older age and comorbidities (Córtes & Arthur, 2006). Although cardiac referral programs are critically important in terms of recovery for all patients, participation rates are extremely low. Of eligible patients, only 14% to 35% of heart attack survivors and 1% of patients after CABG surgery participate in a cardiac rehabilitation program (Suaya et al., 2007).

One of the first steps to improving women's participation in cardiac rehabilitation programs is the promotion of greater clinician awareness of the benefits of cardiac rehabilitation. This is especially important because clinician referral has been cited as one of the important determinants of participation in a formalized cardiac rehabilitation program (Thompson et al., 2003). Low patient referral rate, especially of women, older adults, and ethnic minorities, is a challenge (Leon et al., 2005). Regrettably, women and minorities are vulnerable groups who are significantly more likely to die within 5 years after a first MI compared with White male patients, so they might benefit from early participation in cardiac rehabilitation (Mozaffarian et al., 2015).

After a first cardiac event, women report increased psychological distress and lower self-efficacy and self-esteem. Additionally older age, lower exercise levels, and reduced functional capacity or comorbid conditions, such as osteoporosis and urinary incontinence, were barriers to physical activities for women with heart disease (Bjarnason-Wehrens, Grande, Loewel, Völler, & Mittag, 2007). Women were significantly more likely to withdraw from cardiac rehabilitation than men because of greater medical problems, specifically musculoskeletal and multiple medical reasons (Marzolini, Brooks, & Oh, 2008). Lack of interest and work obligations were greater barriers for men, and transportation and family obligations more often affected women. Furthermore, gender alone was not the main reason for withdrawal; rather other factors common for women included less social support, obesity, lower fitness levels, smaller proportion of CABG referral, depression, and decreased use of preventative cardiac medications (Marzolini et al., 2008). There was a 23% increase in the odds of not completing the program for a 1 MET decrease in fitness level (Marzolini et al., 2008). Strategies that may help with encouraging participation by women would be to expand home-based services, assist with the provision of transportation to community-based programs where there are more sites that have modified hours and session times to meet family and work schedules, and add internet-based technologies that promote physical activity and lifestyle changes to reduce cardiovascular risk factors (Balady et al., 2011). Last, lack of insurance coverage has been a problem in the past for some; however, with health care reform, an essential benefit package has begun to improve access to cardiac rehabilitation for low-income and underinsured populations (Balady et al., 2011).

Heart Failure

DEFINITION, SCOPE, AND ETIOLOGY

HF is a complex syndrome that involves cardiac pump dysfunction (either systolic or diastolic) in combination with cardiac remodeling and the interaction of various hormonal and cytokine systems along with alterations in renal function, as well as activation of the rennin–angiotensin–aldosterone and sympathetic nervous systems that ultimately results in circulatory insufficiency (Koelling, Chen, Lubwama, L'Italien, & Eagle, 2004). HF can result from a structural or functional impairment of ventricular filling or ejection of blood (Yancy et al., 2013). The cardinal signs of HF are dyspnea and fatigue, which may limit exercise tolerance, and fluid retention, which may lead to pulmonary and/or splanchnic congestion and/or peripheral edema. Certain patients have exercise intolerance but little evidence of fluid retention, whereas others have edema, dyspnea, or fatigue. Per the AHA guidelines, as some patients do not have signs or symptoms of volume overload, the term *heart failure* is preferred over *congestive heart failure* (Yancy et al., 2013). It is important to keep in mind that there is no single diagnostic test for HF because it is largely a clinical diagnosis based on a careful history and physical examination (Yancy et al., 2013). Etiologies include CVD, HTN, valvular heart disease, and various cardiomyopathies (Koelling et al., 2004), as well as diabetes, arrhythmias, and congenital heart defects (Yancy et al., 2013). In an analysis of data from the Cardiovascular Health Study, in which patients presented for catheter ablation of premature ventricular contractions (PVCs), the data suggested that PVCs could be an "epiphenomenon," or a marker for future HF (Dukes et al., 2015). More specifically, a higher frequency of PVCs was associated with a decrease in left ventricular function, an increase in incident HF, and an increase in mortality (Dukes et al., 2015).

Women with HF are more likely to have preserved left ventricular systolic function with diastolic dysfunction (an inability of the heart muscle to relax normally), and they are typically older than their male counterparts (Givertz, Colucci, & Braunwald, 2005). Although age itself is a risk factor for diastolic HF, age-adjusted rates for diastolic HF are still higher among women. Although women present with diastolic HF or although this condition is often a precursor to systolic HF or an impaired ability to pump blood, HTN and diabetes play a greater role in the development of HF in women, whereas CVD remains the most common risk factor for men (Levy et al., 2002). In contrast to the view given by clinical trials primarily focusing on men with left ventricular systolic dysfunction linked to CVD, as opposed to the equally common form of HF associated with preserved systolic function typically found in hypertensive men and women, there were more female HF cases overall (51%)

(Stewart, Ekman, Ekman, Odén, & Rosengren, 2010). However, when women do have an MI, they are more likely to also have HF (Givertz et al., 2005). LVH is more frequent and more pronounced among women despite women having similar blood-pressure values as men (Barnard, 2005). In addition, in the FHS, the prevalence of LVH was greater among obese women with HTN than among normotensive obese women (Barnard, 2005).

More than 5.1 million people in the United States are estimated to have HF, with 650,000 new cases diagnosed each year (Yancy et al., 2013). About 3 million women have HF with approximately 455,000 new cases diagnosed each year. Further, in 2011, there were 33,700 deaths among women from HF, or 57.8% of all HF deaths (Mozaffarian et al., 2015). HF is the most common hospital diagnosis among patients who are more than 65 years old, with the overall rate of HF admissions representing 32% of all hospitalizations (Hall, Levant, & DeFrances, 2012) and 25% of all-cause readmission within 1 month (Krumholtz et al., 2009).

HF is an increasing financial burden to the health care system, with the cost of care in the United States exceeding $30 billion annually, over half of the costs associated with hospitalization. In 2010, HF hospitalization rates for males and females were similar (32.5 and 33.0 per 10,000 population respectively), and for those aged 65 years and over who were hospitalized for HF, there was a significant increase in the proportion of patients discharged to long-term care institutions but a significant decrease in the proportion who died in the hospital (Hall et al., 2012). An interesting trend occurred in the United States over the past several years: The number of primary HF hospitalizations decreased as the number of secondary HF admissions increased. This translates into patients with HF experiencing over 3 million secondary hospitalizations annually, often related to comorbid conditions. The common diagnoses for secondary HF hospitalizations included pulmonary disease, renal failure, and infections (Blecker, Paul, Taksler, Ogedegbe, & Katz, 2013). The work involved to decrease primary HF admissions has successfully reduced hospitalizations, lengths of stay, and readmissions; however, work needs to be done to identify patients admitted with the secondary diagnosis of HF who have primary noncardiac admitting diagnoses; these patients then need aggressive, concurrently treatment of the HF to reduce this large, growing burden on the health care system.

EVALUATION/ASSESSMENT

The diagnosis of HF is made clinically and is based on one or more clinical symptoms of volume overload, including elevated jugular venous pressure, hepatojugular reflux, lung crackles, and lower-extremity edema (Table 43.2) (Bristow & Lowes, 2005). Patients are classified based on functional capacity. The New York Heart Association (NYHA) classification system relates symptoms to everyday activities and to the woman's quality of life (Young & Mills, 2001). This system categorizes the severity of congestive HF by functional classes that depend on the degree of effort required to elicit symptoms. Class I patients have no limitation of physical activity: Ordinary activities do not produce symptoms of

TABLE 43.2	Signs to Evaluate in Patients With Heart Failure
CARDIAC ABNORMALITY SIGN	
Elevated cardiac filling pressures and fluid overload, elevated jugular venous pressure	
S3 gallop	
Rales	
Hepatojugular reflux	
Ascites	
Edema	
Cardiac enlargement, laterally displaced or prominent apical impulse	
Murmurs that suggest valvular dysfunction	

Adapted from Lindenfeld et al. (2010).

angina, dyspnea, or undue fatigue. Class II patients have a slight limitation of physical activity: Ordinary activities do produce cardiac symptoms. Class III patients have a marked limitation of physical activity: Although these patients are comfortable at rest, less-than-ordinary activities do produce cardiac symptoms. Those in Class IV have severe, persistent symptoms with any physical activity, and they can also have symptoms while at rest.

DIAGNOSTIC STUDIES

Diagnostic testing initially consists of a chest radiograph, which often shows increased intravascular markings, frank pulmonary edema, or pleural effusions; cardiomegaly is a common finding as well. The EKG often reveals LVH. It is not unusual to see tachycardia, rapid atrial fibrillation (AF), or ischemic EKG changes, as well as evidence of atrioventricular and intraventricular conduction blocks and changes in voltage (Madias, 2006).

Over the past few years, the measurement of B-type natriuretic peptide (BNP) levels has been used as a reliable indicator of HF and its severity. Currently, the Heart Failure Society of America (HFSA) recommends BNP testing for women who are suspected of having HF when the diagnosis is not certain (Lindenfeld et al., 2010). The AHA and ACC guidelines likewise indicate that elevated BNP levels may support a suspected diagnosis of HF (Lindenfeld et al., 2010). BNP levels are interpreted together with physical examination findings and other diagnostic testing to make the diagnosis of HF (Lindenfeld et al., 2010; Yancy et al., 2013).

DIFFERENTIAL DIAGNOSES

Systolic Versus Diastolic HF • A transthoracic echocardiogram (TTE) has become an integral part of the evaluation of the woman with HF. It is helpful for making the diagnosis

of diastolic HF by identifying LVH, which is the leading cause of diastolic HF (Jessup et al., 2009; Vasan & Levy, 2000). It provides important clues regarding the etiology of HF (i.e., ischemic, hypertensive, or the result of valvular disease, regurgitation, pericardial effusion, cardiomyopathy, cardiac amyloidosis, or a combination). Results of the TTE also help guide management because the test provides a measurement of the EF (Yancy et al., 2013). In a healthy adult, a normal EF is 55% to 75% (Shekelle et al., 2003). An EF of 40% to 49% is considered to be mild impairment; 31% to 39% is moderate impairment, and 30% or less is considered severe impairment of the left ventricular systolic function. Left ventricular systolic dysfunction is not synonymous with HF; many patients with left ventricular systolic dysfunction do not exhibit signs of HF, although they are at high risk for it (Yancy et al., 2013).

HF is often separated into two diagnostic categories, depending on left ventricular systolic function. Systolic HF involves left ventricular systolic dysfunction or an EF of less than 45%. The diagnosis of diastolic HF is made when left ventricular systolic function is normal or only slightly reduced but more than 45%. In the 2006 and 2013 ACCF/AHA Guideline for the Management of Heart Failure, new terms were introduced: HF-reduced EF (HFrEF), defined as the clinical diagnosis of systolic HF and an EF equal to or less than 40%, and HF with a preserved EF (HFpEF), defined as diastolic HF with an EF in the range of 40% to 50% or at an intermediate level (Yancy et al., 2013).

TREATMENT/MANAGEMENT

HF treatment has been revolutionized during the past 2 decades with the advent of new classes of medications and new indications for older medications. In addition, devices such as implantable defibrillators and biventricular pacemakers have been shown to improve morbidity and mortality rates among women with systolic HF (Agabiti-Rosei & Muiesan, 2002). Wilcox et al. (2014), in an analysis of data from the registry to Improve the Use of Evidence-Based Heart Failure Therapies in the Outpatient Setting (IMPROVE HF), found that cardiac resynchronization therapy (CRT) and internal cardiac defibrillator (ICD) therapy were equally effective in men and women with HF.

Self-Management Measures • Patient education is a critical component of HF self-management. HF can be difficult to understand, and it requires complicated lifestyle and medication regimens for management. Deviating from the diet or medication plan can have disastrous consequences (Bristow & Lowes, 2005). Many clinics have implemented disease-management programs for women with HF, and these have been shown to decrease frequent hospitalizations (Chan, Heidenreich, Weinstein, & Fonarow, 2008; Sanghavi et al., 2014). APN-run programs can be a cost-effective alternative to the traditional management of these women to improve health outcomes (Lowery et al., 2012; Stauffer et al., 2014).

Outpatient Emergency Department • In some parts of the United States, emergency departments have areas established exclusively to treat patients with HF who are volume overloaded with an intravenous diuretic or to assign the patient to observation for a few hours without admission. If patients in either program respond to treatment, they return home with continued outpatient management. Furthermore, in some extended-care facilities, patients with HF who require intravenous care may now receive the medication in place without transfer to the hospital. Home-care services can also assist with the monitoring of these women and with helping them to adhere to diet and medication regimens. Accordingly, home-monitoring programs appear to be the most effective in promoting long-term outcome benefit when they reinforce patient education toward medication adherence and patient self-efficacy (Konstam, 2012). Gandhi and Pinney (2014) in a review article have also found that a combination of biomarkers, monitoring devices, and disease-management programs together may work best for improving care for all patients with HF.

Pharmacotherapeutics

Left Ventricular Dysfunction. Treatment guidelines for the management of the patient with HF are outlined in the 2013 ACCF/AHA Guideline for the Management of Heart Failure (Yancey et al., 2013) and the European Society of Cardiology (ESC) guidelines for the diagnosis and treatment of acute and chronic HF (McMurray et al., 2012).

Diuretics to control the symptoms of volume overload are used in the smallest dose possible. Although they are useful for symptom management, diuretics have not been proven to reduce mortality. Loop diuretics (e.g., furosemide [Lasix], and torsemide [Demadox]) are the most frequently used (Yancy et al., 2013).

ACE inhibitors have been proven to decrease morbidity and mortality rates and to improve quality of life in patients with left ventricular systolic dysfunction and congestive HF, although women may derive less benefit than men (Pina & Daoud, 2005; Shekelle et al., 2003). Whether this is related to smaller numbers of women enrolled in these studies is not certain.

ARBs are indicated when women are intolerant to ACE inhibitors. For women who cannot take an ACE inhibitor or an ARB (e.g., women with renal disease), the combination of hydralazine and a nitrate is an acceptable alternative (Lindenfeld et al., 2010; Yancy et al., 2013).

Beta blockers, which were formerly absolutely contraindicated for women with HF, have become one of the cornerstone therapies (Lindenfeld et al., 2010; Yancy et al., 2013). Because beta blockers were a later addition to the treatment of congestive HF, women have not been adequately studied (Wenger, 2002). Beta blockers are equally effective for reducing morbidity and mortality rates in both women and men (CIBIS-II Investigators and Committees, 1999; Ghali, Pina, Gottlieb, Deedwania, & Wikstrand, 2002; Packer et al., 2001). This includes metoprolol (extended release, Toprol XL) and bisoprolol (Cardicor), which are both cardioselective agents, and carvedilol (Corgard), which is a noncardioselective beta blocker with alpha-blocking properties. Moreover, these drugs are effective for the treatment of both ischemic and nonischemic forms of congestive HF (Yancy et al. 2013).

For women who remain symptomatic despite the use of beta blockers and ACE inhibitors or ARB therapy, adding a combination of hydralazine (Unipres) and isosorbide dinitrate (Isordil) can be considered. This combination has been shown to reduce mortality among Blacks but not among Whites (Yancy et al., 2013). It is recommended as a part of standard therapy for Blacks (Yancy et al., 2013).

Digoxin (Lanoxin), which is one of the oldest pharmacological agents available, is currently indicated only for women with systolic dysfunction who are still symptomatic despite conventional therapies (Lindenfeld et al., 2010; Yancy et al., 2013). One important caveat with digoxin use in women is the higher risk of digoxin toxicity at low doses. The HFSA guidelines of 2013 recommend digoxin levels of less than 1.0 ng/mL (Yancy et al., 2013). Digoxin can also help with the management of heart rate in women with AF (Lindenfeld et al. 2010; Yancy et al., 2013).

Aldosterone blockers, such as spironalactone (Aldactone) and the newer eplerenone (Inspra), have been found to improve mortality rates among women with Class III and IV HF. This is primarily a result of these drugs' neurohormonal blockage effects and not because of their diuretic effects (Yancy et al., 2013).

Diastolic Dysfunction. Effective treatments for diastolic HF, the predominant presentation in women, remains understudied (Wenger, 2012). The management of diastolic HF is largely empiric. As with systolic HF, diuretics are used to control symptoms of fluid overload (Yancy et al., 2013). However, managing fluid balance with diastolic HF can be more challenging. Patients with diastolic HF are more dependent on preload to maintain cardiac output as a result of the stiffened left ventricle (Barnard, 2005). Current ACC and AHA guidelines regarding diastolic HF recommend the treatment of any underlying causative conditions (e.g., HTN). The 2010 HFSA guidelines are more specific regarding diastolic dysfunction, which the organization classifies as "Heart Failure with preserved left ventricular dysfunction" (Lindenfeld et al., 2010, p. 496).

Beta blockers are important for the treatment of diastolic dysfunction to control HTN and tachycardia, thereby increasing diastolic left ventricular filling time. Furthermore, measures to restore and maintain the sinus rhythm among women with AF who are symptomatic despite rate control can also be considered (Yancy et al., 2013).

ACE inhibitors and ARBs have been shown to reduce myocardial fibrosis and LVH; however, they have not been studied exclusively in the presence of diastolic HF. Even so, patients with diastolic dysfunction (as with systolic dysfunction) appear to have activation of the renin–angiotensin–aldosterone system, which makes these medications logical choices for the treatment of HF that results from diastolic dysfunction (Yancy et al., 2013).

Device Therapy for HF • Mortality rates among patients with HF and severely impaired left ventricular systolic function (≤ 30%) are high (Yancy et al., 2013). Regrettably, HF represents a sentinel prognostic event in patients with a high risk for readmission (50% in 6 months) and a high 1-year mortality rate of 30% (Giamouzis et al., 2011; Kociol et al., 2010). Death is attributable to arrhythmia, MI, progressive HF, pulmonary or systemic emboli, electrolyte disturbances, and other vascular events (Lindenfeld et al., 2010). The risk of sudden cardiac death is decreased with appropriate pharmacologic therapy, as described previously. However, certain women may benefit from the implantation of an ICD. The 2012 ACC/AHA guidelines for device therapy recommend the implantation of an ICD in patients with an EF of 35% or less who are NYHA class II or III or patients with an EF of less than 30% who are NYHA class I and in whom survival is anticipated for 1 year or more (Tracy et al., 2012). These devices are not recommended or appropriate for the end-stage (class D) woman with progressive and irreversible HF symptoms or with a limited life expectancy as a result of other disease states; such devices are unlikely to affect the overall prognosis of these women (Tracy et al., 2012; Yancy et al., 2013).

Another treatment option for the patient with HF, reduced left ventricular function, and widened QRS complex is CRT. Biventricular pacing improves hemodynamic measurements such as cardiac index and systemic vascular resistance (Blanc et al., 1997). Furthermore, medication therapy using ACE inhibitors, ARBs, and beta blockers along with CRT can slow and even partially reverse left ventricular remodeling (Lindenfeld et al., 2010). In addition, research has shown decreases in rehospitalization rates and increases in functional capacity and HRQOL scores (Lindenfeld et al., 2010). In fact, the only therapies shown to improve HRQOL are CRT and certain disease-management and educational approaches (Harrison et al., 2002; Inglis et al., 2010; Johansson, Dahlstrom, & Brostrom, 2006; McAlister, Stewart, Ferrua, & McMurray, 2004). Self-care and exercise may also improve HRQOL, but the results of studies evaluating these interventions are mixed (Chien, Lee, Wu, Chen, & Wu, 2008; Ditewig, Blok, Havers, & van Veenendaal, 2010; Karapolat et al., 2009). Recent data also noted improved survival rates among these patients (Bristow et al., 2004). Wilcox et al. (2014) found that the use of guideline-directed CRT and ICD therapy was associated with substantially reduced 24-month mortality in eligible men and women with HF and reduced EF. Device therapies should be offered to all patients.

Critical to the decision making for device implantation is the woman's overall prognosis and her functional capacity at baseline. Women with HF have been found to have poorer HRQOL than men (Heo, Moser, & Widener, 2007; Lesman-Leegte et al., 2009). In addition, many women need a great deal of psychological support because the implantation of such a device can be unnerving, impeding patient recovery and return to daily life—now with an ICD. Cultivation of social-support networks can cushion the impact of stress through support and online chat groups.

Arrhythmias

Aging is associated with many changes in the cardiovascular system that include decreased compliance of blood vessels, mild concentric LVH, increased atrial contraction contribution to left ventricular filling, and a higher incidence of many cardiac arrhythmias and conduction disorders (Chow, Marine, & Fleg, 2012). Some alterations in cardiac rhythm do not produce symptoms, whereas others cause hemodynamic changes requiring treatment. The prognostic significance of any conduction abnormality or rhythm disturbance is dependent primarily on the presence and severity of any accompanying cardiac disease (Chow et al., 2012).

ETIOLOGY

Early research regarding the pharmacological management of arrhythmias included few, if any, women. Newer treatments have been studied in women: Radiofrequency catheter ablation and implantable defibrillators have been found to be equally effective for both men and women. There is evidence that the conduction system of the female heart has important differences compared with that of the male heart (Hongo & Scheinman, 2005). The resting heart rate of a woman is three to five times higher than that of an age-matched man (Lui et al., 1989), thought to be the result of a short sinus node recovery time in women (Connolly et al., 2009). The average resting heart rate of a woman is increased during the menstrual phase compared with the follicular and luteal phases in premenopausal women (Taneja, Mahnert, Passman, Goldberger, & Kadish, 2001). Women have a longer rate-corrected QT interval than men. This difference occurs after males enter puberty: Androgen surges result in a shortening of the rate-corrected QT interval. The gender differences in the QT interval disappear after about the age of 50 years (Burke et al., 1997). Therefore there may be more complexity in diagnosing and treating arrhythmias in women over the life cycle. Last, women may also respond differently to treatments for arrhythmias, especially pharmacological management (Hongo & Scheinman, 2005).

DIFFERENTIAL DIAGNOSES

Supraventricular Arrhythmias

Definition and Etiology. The term *supraventricular arrhythmia (SVA)* encompasses rhythms that originate from the SA node (e.g., paroxysmal atrial tachycardia), from the atrial tissue (e.g., atrial flutter), and from the atrioventricular junction (e.g., supraventricular tachycardia [SVT]); it also includes accessory pathway–mediated tachycardias.

Symptoms. Women with SVA in addition to AF and ventricular arrhythmias can present with a variety of symptoms, including palpitations, heart racing, heart flutters, chest discomfort, lightheadedness, dizziness, presyncope, and fatigue. However, frank syncope is uncommon with SVA, occurring in only about 15% of patients (Blomström-Lundqvist et al., 2003).

Differential Diagnoses and Diagnostic Studies. A TTE may be used to evaluate structural heart disease, including valvular heart disease that will increase the risk of arrhythmias. Twenty-four-hour Holter monitoring is helpful for evaluating the woman with frequent symptoms. An event recorder or loop recorder is indicated for less-frequent symptoms. Exercise testing can be helpful if the symptoms are brought on by stress or exercise. Laboratory examination of the woman with palpitations and a suspected arrhythmia includes electrolyte, magnesium, and thyroid function tests. A complete blood count may be indicated if anemia or infection is suspected because both conditions may precipitate tachyarrhythmias (Blomström-Lundqvist et al., 2003).

Additionally, findings from these studies help the clinician to differentiate between SVA and ventricular tachycardia.

Treatment/Management. For women who have no evidence of pre-excitation on the 12-lead EKG, who have normal left ventricular function, and who tolerate the arrhythmia well, no specific therapy may be required, especially if the episodes are infrequent. Precipitating factors should be reviewed during the initial assessment, and if there is a history of excessive intake of alcohol, caffeine, or nicotine; use of recreational drugs; or hyperthyroidism, these factors should be discussed and eliminated (Blomström-Lundqvist et al., 2003). Treatment with pharmacological agents (e.g., beta blockers, calcium-channel blockers) is necessary if the episodes are frequent or not well tolerated. Digoxin (Lanoxin) is less effective for the prevention of SVA. For women with SVT and no evidence of structural heart disease, propafenone (Rythmol), and flecainide (Tambocor) are effective for the prevention of recurrence, and they may be prescribed by cardiologists who specialize in arrhythmia management (Blomström-Lundqvist et al., 2003). Radiofrequency catheter ablation has also been very successful for the treatment of SVA (especially SVT) in individuals who do not tolerate or who desire long-term drug therapy (Blomström-Lundqvist et al., 2003; Scheinman & Huang, 2003). Catheter ablation with SVT is 96% effective; complication rates are minimal, with a reported 1% rate of heart block necessitating permanent pacemaker implantation. Nevertheless, it is important to note that tamponade during AF ablation procedures, although very rare, can occur, with women having an approximately twofold higher risk for developing this complication (Michowitz et al., 2014). The risk of tamponade among women decreases in high-volume centers, so this should be considered when referring a patient. Additionally, the decision of whether or not to undergo ablation is highly individualized and often depends on the woman's tolerance to and the effectiveness of pharmacological therapy.

Atrial Flutter
Etiology, Symptoms, and Evaluation/Assessment. Women with atrial flutter can present with symptoms similar to those of SVT, and the diagnostic workup is identical (Blomström-Lundqvist et al., 2003). However, these women often have more comorbidities and are more likely to have symptoms of fatigue, shortness of breath, and chest discomfort, as well as palpitations. HF and pulmonary disease are commonly seen among these women, who are typically older than women with SVT (Scheinman & Huang, 2003).

Treatment/Management. Guidelines regarding the pharmacological management of atrial flutter are often combined with those of AF. Beta blockers and nondihydropyridine calcium-channel blockers can be used for initial rate control. However, the most common side effect is hypotension. Amiodarone (Pacerone) can also be considered (Blomström-Lundqvist et al., 2003; Miller & Zipes, 2005).

Although the stroke risk with atrial flutter is less than that seen with AF, anticoagulation with vitamin K antagonists is recommended unless contraindicated, as it is for women who are at increased risk for thromboembolism; this includes women with valvular heart disease, HTN, and

previous embolic history. Pharmacological or electrical cardioversion can be undertaken if the arrhythmia is clearly less than 48 hours old or if a transesophageal echocardiogram is negative for thrombus; other women need to have anticoagulation therapy to an international normalized ratio (INR) of 2.0 to 3.0 for at least 2 to 3 weeks before attempted cardioversion (pharmacological or electrical) by a specialist (Blomström-Lundqvist et al., 2003).

Atrial Fibrillation
Definition and Scope, Etiology. AF is a common arrhythmia that increases with age, affecting between 2.7 and 6.1 million people in the United States and accounting for 467,000 hospitalizations each year (January et al., 2014). AF and HF have become cardiovascular epidemics over the past 10 years (Anter, Jessup, & Callans, 2009; January et al., 2014). Patients with AF are hospitalized twice as often as those without AF and are three times more likely to have multiple admissions. It is estimated that caring for patients with AF adds $26 billion to U.S. health care expenses (January et al., 2014). The increase in hospitalizations for AF occur for many reasons, including aging of the population, the rising prevalence of chronic heart disease, and more frequent diagnosis as a result of increased monitoring and awareness of the condition by practitioners and patients. The prevalence is higher among men than women (Feinburg Blackshear, Laupacis, Kronmal, & Hart, 1995); however, because the incidence of AF increases overwhelmingly with aging and because there are more women in the population older than 75 years, the total number of women and men with AF in this age group is equal (Humphries et al., 2001). Women are more symptomatic than men, possibly because of faster heart rates and smaller body size, and unfortunately, have experienced more problems when the heart rate is controlled (Hector et al., 2010).

AF incidence and prevalence are increasing because of the growing number of older people in the U.S population, although the estimates of the rate of expected growth have varied widely. The incidence of AF is projected to double from 2010 to 2030, and the prevalence is expected to increase from 5.2 million cases in 2010 to 12.1 million in 2030 (Colilla et al., 2013).

AF can occur in the presence or absence of heart disease. However, as with atrial flutter, individuals with AF often have HTN, valvular heart disease, and/or CVD. AF is associated with an increased risk of stroke, HF, and all-cause mortality, especially among women (Stewart, Hart, Hole, & McMurray, 2002). Furthermore, perioperative AF is associated with an increased long-term risk of ischemic stroke, especially after noncardiac surgery (Gialdini et al., 2014). The prognosis of those with AF is most benign among individuals who are younger than 60 years with no known heart disease; these patients are often referred to as having *lone AF*. Most individuals move out of this category over time as they age and develop other heart diseases and HTN (Alpert et al., 2014).

Evaluation/Assessment and Diagnostic Studies. Women who present with AF can have the same symptoms as previously mentioned for women with SVA. The initial diagnostic workup is similar as well. The hemodynamic consequences of AF include the loss of "atrial kick," which can add up to 30% of cardiac output; this loss is particularly important to those with reduced heart function. In addition, the tachycardia itself can lead to a cardiomyopathy (Fuster et al., 2006).

Treatment/Management. The first goal of AF management is rate control with either a beta blocker or a calcium-channel blocker. As with the other tachyarrhythmias, if hemodynamic instability exists, referral for electrical cardioversion is the preferred management strategy. As long as the patient is hemodynamically stable, the rate may be controlled with beta blockers, nondihydropyridine calcium-channel blockers, or amiodarone (Pacerone). Digoxin can also be used to slow the ventricular rate in AF; however, it is rarely useful as monotherapy. Digoxin (Lanoxin) is not effective for controlling increased heart rate during times of exertion or exercise (Fuster et al., 2006).

Rate versus rhythm control is a difficult choice that most often requires referral to a cardiologist or an electrophysiology specialist. Most concerning with the diagnosis of AF is the risk of ischemic stroke, which averages 5% per year among patients with nonvalvular AF. Rates of ischemic stroke are two to seven times higher among women with AF than among those without AF (Cabin, Clubb, Hall, Perlmutter & Feinstein, 1990; Wolf, Abbott, & Kannel, 1991), and the risk for embolic stroke is higher among women (Cabin et al., 1990).

Some investigators have demonstrated a worse outcome and a higher rate of recurrence after cardioversion. Hector et al. (2010), who conducted a review of the literature, found that mortality was higher for women with AF than for men with AF and that women with AF have a higher risk of stroke compared with men. They also discovered through a review of the evidence that women, when taking sotalol or dofetilide, have an increased risk for torsades de pointes and a higher risk for bradyarrhythmias when taking antiarrhythmics. Catheter ablation for AF is beneficial for both men and women, although women may have higher procedural bleeding complications. Still, women tend to be referred for ablation less often and later than men. AF affects the current risks and the long-term prognosis of women differently than of men. An analysis from the Euro Heart Survey on Atial Fibrillation found that women with AF have more than double the thromboembolism risk of men with AF (Lip et al., 2010). In addition, a Swedish study found that the rate of ischemic stroke in AF patients younger than 65 years was 47% higher in women than men (Friberg, Benson, Rosenqvist, & Lip, 2012). Last, women overall have a significantly higher risk of AF-related stroke than men and are more likely to live with stroke-related disability, which in turn leads to a significantly lower quality of life (Volgman, Manankil, Mookherjee, & Trohman, 2009). The diagnosis, symptoms, and treatments of AF can differ for women too. A potential deadly difference in women 20 to 79 years old is that the risk of stroke is 4.6-fold greater in women than in men (Schnohr, Lange, Scharling, & Jensen, 2006). In addition, mortality for women with AF is up to 2.5 times greater than that for men (Michelena, Powell, Brady, Friedman, & Ezekowitz, 2010).

The decision to place patients with AF on anticoagulation therapy is based on a number of factors. The choice of agent to use is dependent on balancing the risk of stroke or thromboembolic event with the risk of bleeding. Current guidelines recommend using the CHA_2DS_2-VASc score to determine the appropriateness of anticoagulation (January et al., 2014). It is a 10-point scale found to be a clinical predictor for estimating stroke risk in patients with nonrheumatic AF (Lip et al., 2010; see Table 43.3). Individuals scoring two or greater on the CHA_2DS_2-VASc are considered at high risk for thromboembolic events and should have anticoagulation therapy, unless contraindicated (January et al., 2014). Those scoring less than two (zero or one) are candidates for aspirin therapy with either 81 or 325 mg (January et al., 2014).

For many years, the standard of therapy for anticoagulation was vitamin K antagonists, namely, warfarin (Fuster et al., 2006). Warfarin therapy has been demonstrated to be superior to aspirin therapy (Fuster et al., 2006), alone or in combination with clopidogrel, for stroke prevention (Connolly et al., 2009). The risk of intracranial hemorrhage (ICH) with the use of warfarin occurred in individuals with an INR greater than 4.0. The advantages of warfarin include its ability to be quickly reversed by parenteral vitamin K or fresh frozen plasma (Mookadam, Shamoun, & Mookadam, 2015). However, there are many disadvantages to warfarin therapy. INR monitoring is critical to the success of balancing this medication's anticoagulant effect with the risk for bleeding. It can take 5 days or longer for some individuals to reach the recommended therapeutic INR of 2.0 to 3.0. Warfarin's significant food and drug interactions affect the INR, and therefore guidelines recommend monitoring at least every 30 days (Mookadam et al., 2015). These factors discourage providers from prescribing anticoagulation and patients accepting their recommendations (Hohnloser, 2011). Warfarin therapy is highly unpredictable (Macedo et al., 2015). A population-based data analysis of 140,078 patients with AF in their first year of warfarin therapy in the United Kingdom found that only 44% had optimal INRs more than 70% of the time (Macedo et al., 2015).

The search for more predictable anticoagulation has led to the development of non–vitamin K anticoagulants

TABLE 43.3	CHA_2DS_2-VASc	POSSIBLE POINTS
C	Congestive heart failure	+ 1
H	Hypertension	+ 1
A	Age (older than 75 years)	+ 2
D	Diabetes mellitus	+ 1
S	Prior stroke or transient ischemic attack or thromboembolic event	+ 2
V	Vascular disease of any kind	+ 1
Sc	Sex category (female sex)	+ 1

Source: From Lip, Nieuwlaat, Pisters, Lane, and Crijns (2010).

(NOACs). The four available agents are all indicated for use in patients with nonvalvular AF and cannot be used in patients with prosthetic heart valves. These agents have the advantage of fixed dosing and do not require blood test monitoring. In addition, they do not have dietary precautions, as they are not vitamin K antagonists. Most require adjustment for renal dysfunction (Mookadam et al., 2015).

Dabigatran is an oral direct thrombin inhibitor prescribed twice daily. It is superior to warfarin in the prevention of the primary outcomes of stroke or systemic embolism (Connolly et al., 2009). A lower dose is approved for use in patients with renal dysfunction, but it should be avoided in patients with severe renal dysfunction (Mookadam et al., 2015). A risk of major bleeding was found, similar to warfarin, in the analysis of all patients, and in subgroup analysis the risk of intracranial bleeding was lower in patients older than 75 years (Connolly et al., 2009). The main concern with direct thrombin inhibitors is the lack of a direct antidote. However, the FDA is currently reviewing the drug idarucizumab as an antidote to dabigatran, which showed good effect in the reversal of the anticoagulant effects of dabigatran in patients needing urgent surgery (Pollack et al., 2015).

Rivaroxaban, apixaban, and the newest approved edoxaban are Factor Xa inhibitors approved for use in patients with nonvavular AF. All of the Factor Xa agents are fixed dose agents that do not require blood testing of anticoagulation levels. Rivaroxaban is a direct Factor Xa inhibitor approved in 2011. It is administered once daily and requires dose adjustment in patients with renal dysfunction. The ROCKET-AF trial demonstrated the noninferiority of rivaroxaban compared with warfarin in the prevention of stroke and embolism in patients with nonvalvular AF; rivaroxaban had no significant differences in rates of major bleeding and less risk of intracranial and fatal bleeding when compared with warfarin (Patel et al., 2011).

Apixaban is a direct Factor Xa inhibitor that was approved for use in 2012. It is administered twice daily. The ARISTOTLE study compared apixaban to warfarin in patients with AF. Apixaban was found to be superior to warfarin ($P = .01$), and rates for major bleeding were found to be less than with warfarin therapy (Granger et al., 2011). Moreover, apixaban therapy reduced rates of all-cause mortality (Granger et al., 2011). Apixaban is approved in 2.5- and 5-mg doses. The 2.5-mg dose is recommended for patients with two of three of the following factors: age more than 80 years, body weight less than 60 kg, or serum creatinine higher than 1.5 mg/dL (Granger et al., 2011).

Edoxaban is a direct Factor Xa inhibitor approved for use in 2015 for anticoagulation in AF. It is a once-daily medication and has a dose adjustment with renal impairment. The ENGAGE-AF TIMI 48 trial studied edoxaban versus warfarin in the prevention of thromboembolic events in patients with nonvalvular AF (Giugliano et al., 2013). Edoxaban was found to be equal to warfarin in the prevention of stroke and embolism. There were lower rates of fatal bleeding and intracranial bleeding. However, significantly higher rates of gastrointestinal bleeding were noted (Giugliano et al., 2013).

The decision to withhold or stop anticoagulation therapy in women who are at high risk for bleeding can be difficult.

The decision to initiate anticoagulation is individualized and discussed with the woman and her family as well as with all members of the health care team. Strategies to limit bleeding risk when prescribing anticoagulation have been studied. The European Society of Cardiology guidelines for the treatment of AF include utilization of a scoring system to assess patients at high risk for bleeding, called the HAS-BLED score (Lane & Lip, 2012). At the very least, patients at high bleeding risk require more frequent monitoring and follow-up (Mookadam et al., 2015).

Sinus Tachycardia

Definition and Scope. In many instances, women with symptoms of palpitations or heart racing will have a sinus tachycardia. Approximately 90% of patients with inappropriate sinus tachycardia are women. Interestingly, many are health care professionals (Blomström-Lundqvist et al., 2003; Krahn, Yee, Klein, & Morillo, 1995).

Evaluation/Assessment. In the case of sinus tachycardia, it is most appropriate to find and treat the underlying disorder. Before medication is prescribed, a history is obtained to check for possible precipitating factors, such as excessive caffeine, alcohol, nicotine intake, recreational drugs, or hyperthyroidism. The condition, such as hyperthyroidism, is treated or the precipitating agents eliminated first before proceeding to medical management.

Treatment/Management. A beta blocker is indicated for symptom management in many instances, especially in the case of hyperthyroidism. If a beta blocker is contraindicated or not tolerated, a nondihydropyridine calcium-channel blocker (e.g., diltiazem [Cardizem] or verapamil [Calan]) can be considered. Close monitoring is required because less rate-controlling medication is needed when the underlying condition has been successfully treated; often the medication can be tapered off completely (Blomström-Lundqvist et al., 2003).

Ventricular Arrhythmias • The presentation of ventricular arrhythmias ranges from single PVCs of little or no hemodynamic significance to life-threatening ventricular tachycardia or ventricular fibrillation. These arrhythmias can occur in women with and without heart disease or cardiac disorders.

Differential Diagnoses and Treatment/Management. The primary goal for managing life-threatening ventricular arrhythmias is the prevention of sudden cardiac death. Referral to an arrhythmia specialist is appropriate. Management is based on the etiology of the arrhythmia. Possible treatments are medications, ablation, implantable cardioverter device (ICD) placement, and sometimes a short-term intervention involving a wearable defibrillator in the form of a vest.

Long QT syndrome is a rare disorder that is more common in women than in men. Women who have it are more likely to faint or die from the disorder during menstruation or shortly after delivery. It is often goes undiagnosed, although 90% of these patients have experienced the condition by age 40 years. The problem arises from the ion channels in the heart muscle causing conduction defects, which predispose patients to torsades de pointes, which then can proceed to syncope and sudden cardiac death. A prolonged QT can be caused by some medications as well as hypokalemia and other nutritional and endocrine disorders. Long QT syndrome should be suspected in patients who have recurrent syncope during exertion and those with family histories of sudden, unexpected death (Meyer et al., 2003). A thorough history is key to protecting patients at risk.

Arrhythmias and Pregnancy • Fortunately, most arrhythmias during pregnancy are benign. In addition, most arrhythmias in the pregnant woman arise in the setting of a structurally normal heart and are therefore tolerated well (Shotan, Ostrzega, Mehra, Johnson, & Elkayam, 1997). In women with a history of arrhythmia, ectopy may increase. Premature atrial contractions and PVCs are relatively common during pregnancy and generally do not require pharmacological management. Often the heart rate increases by 25% in women who are pregnant; therefore sinus tachycardia, especially in the third trimester is common. Ectopic beats and nonsustained arrhythmia are found in more than 50% of pregnant women assessed for palpitations, whereas sustained tachycardias are uncommon in 2 to 3/1,000 (Blomström-Lundqvist et al., 2003; Shotan et al., 1997). The avoidance of triggers such as caffeine and emotional stress can be helpful.

SVT episodes may increase during pregnancy. Women with frequent SVT who are contemplating becoming pregnant may want to consider ablation therapy before conception to avoid medications while pregnant (Oakley et al. 2003). All antiarrhythmic medications cross the placenta, and pharmacokinetics can be altered during pregnancy, thereby necessitating more frequent monitoring of drug levels (Oakley et al., 2003). Therapeutic drug levels can be affected by an increase in intravascular volume requiring an increase in loading dose, a reduction of plasma proteins contributing to lower drug concentrations, increased renal blood flow with an increase in the clearance of drugs, increased hepatic metabolism of drug resulting from progesterone also increasing clearance, and changes in gastric absorption of medication, making serum drug concentrations variable (Perez-Silva & Merino, 2011).

For women who develop SVT during pregnancy, vagal maneuvers are attempted first to break the arrhythmia (Oakley et al., 2003). If these are not effective, adenosine is the drug of choice for terminating a sustained SVT (Elkayam & Goodwin, 1994; Hongo & Scheinman, 2005; Leffler & Johnson, 1992; Perez-Silva & Merino, 2011). If the condition is recurrent and suppression is necessary, cardioselective beta blockers (e.g., metoprolol) are recommended. However, atenolol is a pregnancy category D agent because it has been implicated in research studies as causing fetal growth retardation (Lip, Beevers, Churchill, Shaffer, & Beevers, 1997). Some experts recommend avoiding beta blockers altogether during the first trimester, if possible; however, others contend that beta blockers are acceptable during pregnancy (Hongo & Scheinman, 2005). Sotalol is more likely to cause fetal bradycardia

because it more readily crosses the placenta (Oakley et al., 2003). Nondihydropyridine calcium-channel blockers are not considered first-line therapy because verapamil has been shown in case reports to cause maternal and fetal bradycardia (Oakley et al., 2003). Although digoxin is not as effective, it has been found to be safe during pregnancy. Flecainide and propafenone have been safely used during pregnancy for the treatment of refractory SVT (Cox & Gardner, 1993). Ablation with the use of echocardiography-guided catheters has also been performed safely during pregnancy (Curry & Quintana, 1970; Perez-Silva & Merino, 2011).

AF is relatively rare during pregnancy, and it will most often present in women with known valvular or congenital heart disease (e.g., mitral stenosis [MS]) (Ogburn, Schmidt, Linman, & Cefalo, 1992). It can also occur in women with hypertrophic cardiomyopathy (Fuster et al., 2006). Unfortunately, many of these women may be previously undiagnosed, and the increased intravascular volume of pregnancy triggers a symptomatic arrhythmia. Occasionally, hyperthyroidism or hypothyroidism can also trigger AF during pregnancy (Shoob, Croft, Ayala, & Mensah, 2006). Digoxin, beta blockers, and calcium-channel blockers are all appropriate for the rate control of AF during pregnancy (Fuster et al., 2006; Oakley et al., 2003). Most women do not require anticoagulation during pregnancy unless they are at high risk for a thromboembolic event (e.g., women with valvular heart disease) (Fuster et al., 2006).

Warfarin crosses the placenta and has been implicated in fetal hemorrhage and death; therefore it is contraindicated during pregnancy. Low-molecular-weight heparin is the anticoagulant of choice in pregnancy (Fuster et al., 2006). Bradycardia that requires permanent pacemaker implantation is also uncommon during pregnancy; however, uterine compression of the inferior vena cava can rarely cause reflex bradycardia (Oakley et al., 2003). In addition, congenital heart block can become symptomatic during pregnancy. Permanent pacemaker implantation is safe during pregnancy if abdominal lead shielding is used (Oakley et al., 2003).

Ventricular tachycardia is much less common during pregnancy; however, it can present in women with congenital long QT interval syndrome or valvular heart disease. If ventricular tachycardia presents during the last 6 weeks of pregnancy or after birth, postpartum cardiomyopathy is ruled out. Because ventricular tachycardia during pregnancy can be exacerbated by increased catecholamines, beta blockers are used as first-line therapy. Amiodarone is used much less often because it has been shown to cause fetal thyroid problems, growth retardation, and premature birth (Cox & Gardner, 1993; Oakley et al., 2003).

Any hemodynamically unstable rhythm can seriously compromise blood flow to the fetus and is considered a medical emergency. Electrical cardioversion can be used to convert any hemodynamically unstable tachyarrhythmia. Very little electrical energy reaches the fetus, and it is advisable to convert the rhythm quickly rather than to risk decreased blood flow to the fetus (Curry & Quintana, 1970; Ogburn, Schmidt, Linman, & Cefalo, 1992; Zipes et al., 2006).

Valvular Heart Disease

DEFINITION AND SCOPE

In industrialized countries, the prevalence of valvular heart disease is estimated at 2.5%. Because of the increase in degenerative etiologies, the prevalence of valve disease increases after the age of 65 years, especially with aortic stenosis (AS) and MR, which is responsible for three of four cases of valve disease (Iung & Vahanian, 2014). Valvular heart disease has contributed to increasing cardiac mortality and morbidity rates in the United States for the last 2 decades (Shoob et al., 2006). Despite these trends, there have been advances in noninvasive cardiac monitoring, minimally invasive surgical techniques, and appropriate timing of surgical interventions, along with sophisticated prosthetic valves; these have improved the overall prognosis for acute and chronic valvular disorders. The etiology and pathophysiological consequences, evaluation, treatment, and continual care of women with valvular heart disease and consequent cardiac dysfunction necessitate a methodic approach to the efficient and practical use of a wide choice of diagnostic procedures, medical and surgical interventions, and long-term follow-up.

ETIOLOGY

The four heart valves normally regulate unidirectional blood flow through the heart's atria and ventricles and into the systemic circulation. Their structural and functional characteristics allow for efficient cardiac muscle contractility and relaxation and for optimal cardiac perfusion (Guyton & Hall, 2006).

Valvular diseases and the resultant changes in normal circulatory physiology are caused by either a forward flow through a narrow or irregular orifice (stenosis) or a regurgitant flow through an incompetent valve (insufficiency). Each of these structural abnormalities leads to hemodynamic changes that directly affect myocardial structure and function as well as coronary blood flow. With the widespread use of echocardiography to both diagnose and plot the trajectory of valve dysfunction, the guidelines for the management of specific valvular lesions have incorporated noninvasive and surgical interventions for patients with acute and chronic valve disease.

EVALUATION/ASSESSMENT

In general, patients with valve disease may present with a heart murmur, symptoms, or incidental findings of valvular abnormalities on chest imaging or noninvasive testing. Regardless, all patients with known or suspected valve disease should undergo an initial history and physical examination.

Cardiac auscultation as a screening method for valvular disease is an essential aspect of the cardiac evaluation. Murmurs are classified according to location, intensity, pitch, radiation, and duration on the basis of the timing of events during the cardiac cycle (Shipton & Wahba, 2001). Specific details of cardiac auscultation–associated physical examination findings that aid in the diagnosis of valvular dysfunction are provided in the ACC/AHA 2014 practice guidelines for the management of patients with valvular heart disease.

DIAGNOSTIC STUDIES

A chest x-ray study and EKG, as well as a TTE with two-dimensional imaging and Doppler, are performed to secure a diagnosis (Nishimura et al., 2014). There is a classification system to note the progression of valvular disease with four stages (A–D), similar to that of the HF guidelines (see earlier section). The stages range from A (at risk) through B (progressive), C (asymptomatic severe), and D (symptomatic severe). These stages are based on valve anatomy, valve hemodynamics, the hemodynamic consequences, and symptoms (Nishimura et al., 2014).

DIFFERENTIAL DIAGNOSES

Mitral Valve Prolapse

Definition, Scope, and Etiology. The term *mitral valve prolapse (MVP)* refers to the displacement of abnormally thickened redundant mitral valve leaflets that extend into the left atrium during systole and that may or may not be associated with MR. Other associated features of this syndrome may include left atrial dilatation, left ventricular enlargement, consequent SVA, and abnormalities that involve other valves as well.

It is estimated that 1% to 3% of the U.S. population is afflicted with MVP (Bonow et al., 2006), although the true prevalence is difficult to determine. MVP may have a much lower prevalence than previously estimated, and the prevalence may be similar among different ethnic groups (Theal et al., 2004). From a population perspective, the prevalence of serious cardiovascular complications associated with MVP is low. It is more commonly diagnosed in women than in men and is thought to be associated with either familial (e.g., Marfan syndrome or other connective-tissue diseases) or acquired disorders (e.g., CAD). The health trajectory of a patient with MVP is variable, ranging from a benign hemodynamic state and a normal life expectancy to severe comorbid complications and the need for surgical intervention.

Evaluation/Assessment. Although a formal diagnosis is made with the use of echocardiography, a routine physical examination reveals an abnormal auscultatory sound that prompts further workup. The salient auscultatory characteristic of MVP is a high-pitched midsystolic "click" that is best heard at or medial to the apex of the heart. A subsequent late-systolic crescendo murmur indicates mild MR. Changes in the patient's body position, which affects ventricular blood volume, can alter auscultatory findings: Standing to decrease the end-diastolic volume causes an earlier click during systole, whereas squatting to increase ventricular volume causes a delay in the click.

Diagnostic Studies. Noninvasive two-dimensional Doppler echocardiography provides the most specific and quantitative information to help define the degree of valve abnormality. For symptomatic women, transthoracic echocardiography is performed to help with the determination of the need for cardiac catheterization; transesophageal echocardiography is performed when surgical repair is being considered (Bonow et al., 2006; Nishimura et al., 2014).

Treatment/Management. The ACC and AHA guidelines have approached the evaluation and management of women with MVP on the basis of the presence or absence of symptoms, although some indications overlap (Bonow et al., 2006; Nishimura et al., 2014).

Monitoring and Surgical Management. Most women with MVP have a benign course. However, potential associated complications include embolic events, infective endocarditis, and MR that eventually requires surgery. Symptomatic women who develop severe MR require valve repair or replacement to prevent complications such as HF, cerebrovascular events, arrhythmias, and death (Bonow et al., 2006). Mitral valve repair is preferred whenever possible over replacement (Nishimura et al., 2014).

Mitral Regurgitation

Etiology. MR is usually classified as a chronic condition with a gradual worsening of the valve lesion as a result of MVP, CVD, or collagen vascular disease or as an acute and severe condition caused by ruptured papillary muscle, ruptured chordae tendineae, or infective endocarditis that requires immediate surgical intervention (Bonow et al., 2006; Nishimura et al., 2014). One of the initial hemodynamic changes that takes place with MR is an increase in the end-diastolic volume. An incompetent mitral valve allows for increased blood flow (and subsequent increased pressure) into the left atrium, which reduces afterload (thus decreasing the end-systolic volume). In a more chronic state, the heart compensates for changes in pressure and volume by increasing in size and becoming hypertrophied. A reduction in cardiac output with severe MR can result in pulmonary congestion, shock, and death (Chirillo, Salvador, & Cavallini, 2006).

Evaluation/Assessment and Diagnostic Studies. For the purpose of designing a treatment algorithm, the progression of MR can be categorized into three stages: (a) the asymptomatic patient with hemodynamically significant regurgitation, (b) the asymptomatic patient with decreased left ventricular function, and (c) the symptomatic patient with decreased left ventricular function (Carabello & Crawford, 1997; Nishimura et al., 2014). For women with chronic MR, cardiac enlargement with displacement of the left ventricular apical impulse can be appreciated during the physical examination. A holosystolic murmur can be auscultated and may also be accompanied by an S_3 or early diastolic flow rumble with or without the presence of HF. Transthoracic echocardiography provides a baseline evaluation of the severity of the MR.

Treatment/Management. Medical therapy is limited, although vasodilating agents such as nitroprusside are used to reduce afterload. For women who develop symptoms

in the presence of acute and severe MR, surgery is recommended, particularly if left ventricular function is preserved. Surgical options include mitral valve repair, mitral valve replacement with the preservation of the valve apparatus, and mitral valve replacement with the removal of the valve apparatus (Bonow et al., 2006; Nishimura et al., 2014). Valve repair is preferred over valve replacement to avoid the need for chronic anticoagulation. The European Heart Survey showed that women with severe MR were referred for surgery at a more advanced clinical state than men were; also, MV repair was performed less often in women and conferred a higher mortality rate than it did in men (Carabello & Crawford, 1997).

Mitral Stenosis

Etiology. MS generally traces back to a case of rheumatic fever. It is typically latent for an average of 20 years before symptoms appear, and it is the most common valvular disease discovered during pregnancy (Elkayam & Bitar, 2005). A funnel-shaped structure develops from both chordae and commissural fusions, and in conjunction with a thickening and calcification of the leaflets, it produces a narrowed orifice between the left atrium and the left ventricle. Other potential complications associated with MS are AF and embolization as a result of an increase in left atrial pressure and enlargement. MS affects women four times as often as men in developing countries. However, with the decline in the incidence of rheumatic fever in the United States and Europe, the ratio of women to men who present with MS is 2:1 (Bonow et al., 2006). Patients are generally 60 years old or older when they present with symptoms, and more than one third of patients who require surgical repair are more than 65 years old (Shoob et al., 2006).

Symptoms, Evaluation/Assessment, and Diagnostic Studies. Women may present early during the course of MS with fatigue, dyspnea, orthopnea, new-onset AF, pulmonary edema, or an embolic event (e.g., stroke). Symptomatic women with MS require evaluation of the extent of their valve disease, as well as an assessment of their NYHA functional class status. The ACC/AHA guidelines categorize MS severity as mild, moderate, or severe on the basis of hemodynamic data and symptom history (Nishimura et al., 2014). Patient history, physical examination, and noninvasive studies, including chest radiography, EKG, and echocardiography, facilitate the diagnosis. During the cardiac examination, the characteristic "opening snap" during early diastole, a low-pitched rumbling diastolic murmur, and an accentuated S_1 are indicative of MS. Findings with worsening valve disease include signs of right ventricular overload, such as distended neck veins, a right ventricular heave, ascites, and peripheral edema. On chest radiography, left atrial enlargement may be noted. Both the pulmonary arterial and venous circulations may be distorted, and there may be evidence of interstitial edema that is consistent with congestion. Echocardiography is the most sensitive and specific noninvasive test used to assess the degree of restricted opening of the mitral valve leaflets; leaflet mobility, flexibility, thickness, and calcification; and suitability of valvotomy (Bonow et al., 2006; Nishimura et al., 2014). Because women with

MS can remain clinically stable for years, there is generally no need for further immediate testing if the documented valve area is greater than 1.5 cm^2 and the mean gradient is less than 5 mmHg.

Treatment/Management. Medical therapy cannot correct mechanical obstruction of the mitral valve. Women who develop more severe MS can remain free of symptoms if they are educated to limit strenuous physical activity. Women are counseled to seek immediate evaluation if a sudden increase in shortness of breath occurs. Disease progression is monitored with an annual history and physical examination, EKG, and chest radiography. Surgical intervention generally correlates with clinical symptoms or with evidence of pulmonary HTN or ventricular dysfunction (Bonow et al., 2006; Nishimura et al., 2014).

Recommendations for the treatment of conditions associated with MS (e.g., AF) include anticoagulation, heart rate control, and chemical or electrical cardioversion. Long-term anticoagulation is warranted to prevent systemic embolic events. Without surgical intervention, mitral valve disease results in an 85% mortality rate at 20 years after symptom onset (Bonow et al., 2006).

Aortic Stenosis

Definition, Scope, and Etiology. Nonrheumatic AS has been described as a calcific disease in which there is an accumulation of lipids, smooth muscle cells, collagen inflammatory cells, and platelet adherence that produces plaque-laden areas along the leaflets and valve cusps; this imitates the atherosclerotic process that accompanies CAD (Carabello & Crawford, 1997). This generally idiopathic process results in the obstruction of blood flow through a narrowed orifice. Fewer women present with AS as a result of exposure to rheumatic fever. AS is the most common valvular lesion in the United States, affecting approximately 25% of individuals who are more than 65 years old, and it is associated with cardiovascular risk factors such as HTN, diabetes mellitus, gender, smoking, and dyslipidemia (Bonow et al., 2006). Furthermore, investigators pooled together databases and calculated an estimated prevalence of 12.4% for AS and 3.4% for severe AS as the burden of disease among the elderly. Using these calculations, approximately 290,000 elderly patients with severe AS are potential candidates for transcatheter aortic valve replacement (TAVR; Osnabrugge et al., 2013).

Evaluation/Assessment and Diagnostic Studies. During the cardiac examination, the most common sign of AS is a late-systolic ejection murmur heard in the aortic area. The murmur can frequently be heard radiating to the neck. The murmur can mimic MR in that it may also be auscultated over the apex; it may also be associated with a thrill. As the AS worsens, pulsus parvus et tardus may be elicited; when this occurs, the carotid upstrokes diminish in amplitude and are delayed during the cardiac cycle, and the clinician may also detect a paradoxically split S$_2$ as a result of delayed ventricular emptying. The development of symptoms such as angina, HF, or syncope indicates a poor short-term prognosis with a high risk for sudden death within 2 to 3 years. Two-dimensional Doppler echocardiography is used to confirm the diagnosis.

Treatment/Management. Although the progression rate of AS is slow, the individual rate of progression to hemodynamic consequences varies, thus necessitating the close monitoring of both symptomatic and asymptomatic women by a specialist. No medical therapy has been shown to effectively treat AS. Lipid-lowering therapy may slow the progression of the mechanisms associated with atherosclerosis; however, because symptoms can quickly progress, surgical intervention is considered if diagnostic testing reveals moderate to severe AS (Bonow et al., 2006; Nishimura et al., 2014).

Aortic Regurgitation

Etiology. Aortic regurgitation (AR) is caused by disease that involves at least one of the aortic leaflets (e.g., infective endocarditis, rheumatic fever) or the aortic root (e.g., collagen vascular disease, annuloaortic ectasia). Acute AR, which is usually a complication of an invasive procedure, aortic dissection, or chest trauma, is a rare and life-threatening event. Chronic AR is more prevalent and imposes a cardiac trajectory with an initial compensatory increase in left ventricular mass, a low EF, and subsequent HF symptoms. The prevalence of AR increases with age and is detected more often in men than in women (Carabello & Crawford, 1997).

Evaluation/Assessment. Multiple examination findings suggest regurgitant flow and increased systolic stroke volume. The classic murmur is a high-frequency decrescendo diastolic murmur heard at the left sternal border. An S$_3$ is sometimes noted, and S$_2$ may be absent altogether. With severe AR, women may present with bounding carotid pulses, head bobbing (i.e., de Musset's sign), a pulsating uvula (i.e., Miller's sign), and pistol-shot sounds heard over a compressed femoral artery (i.e., Traube's sign).

Treatment/Management. Referral to a specialist is appropriate for women with AR to manage resultant HF or to provide surgical intervention. The guidelines recommend (Class I) that the management of patients with severe heart valve disease is best achieved by a heart valve team composed minimally of a cardiologist and a cardiac surgeon but potentially including cardiologists, structural valve interventionalists, cardiovascular imaging specialists, cardiovascular surgeons, anesthesiologists, and nurses, all of whom have expertise in the management and outcome of patients with severe heart valve disease. Often, heart valve centers of excellence have a valve clinic with a valve team. The guidelines recommend (Class IIa) that consultation with or referral to a heart valve center of excellence is reasonable for asymptomatic patients with severe valve disease. Surgical risk is evaluated through the Society of Thoracic Surgeons (STS), where surgeons predict the risk of mortality by assessing the patients' fragility (e.g., Katz Index of Independence in Activities of Daily Living; Bach, 2014).

Infective Endocarditis

Prevention. The ACC/AHA 2008 guideline update regarding valvular heart disease revised the recommendations for infective endocarditis prophylaxis (Wilson et al., 2007). Infective endocarditis is less likely to be caused by a procedure than by random exposure to bacteria, such as when brushing teeth, chewing gum, or other oral hygiene procedures, and it was also found that prophylactic antibiotic treatment prevents only a very small number of cases of infective endocarditis. Thus prophylactic antibiotics are reserved for women who are at the highest risk of an adverse outcome from acquiring infective endocarditis (Wilson et al., 2007). The 2014 AHA/ACC Guideline for the Management of Patients With Valvular Heart Disease by Nishimura et al. (2014) recommend the same approach to care.

Considerations for Special Populations • The normal physiological changes related to a woman's cardiovascular system during pregnancy become more critical in the setting of valvular disease. There is a 50% increase in blood volume and a consequent 25% increase in cardiac output that influences valvular function such that stenotic valve murmurs are accentuated and regurgitant murmurs may be come nearly inaudible. Ideally, the management of women with known valvular lesions begins before conception. The 2006 ACC/AHA Guidelines for the Management of Patients with Valvular Heart Disease provide recommendations such as anticoagulation therapies, exercise restrictions, and prophylaxis endocarditis treatment for each specific valve condition (Bonow et al., 2006).

Cardiomyopathy

DEFINITION, SCOPE, AND ETIOLOGY

The AHA classified cardiomyopathies as primary (i.e., genetic, mixed, or acquired) or secondary (e.g., infiltrative, toxic, or inflammatory). The four major types are dilated cardiomyopathy, hypertrophic cardiomyopathy, restrictive cardiomyopathy, and arrhythmogenic right ventricular cardiomyopathy (Maron et al., 2006).

Dilated cardiomyopathy, the most common form and affects 5 in 100,000 adults and 0.57 in 100,000 children. It is the third leading cause of HF in the United States after CAD and HTN (Wexler, Elton, Pleister, & Feldman, 2009). The causes of cardiomyopathies are varied. Dilated cardiomyopathy in adults is most commonly caused by CAD (ischemic cardiomyopathy) and HTN, although viral myocarditis, valvular disease, and genetic predisposition may also play a role (Wexler et al., 2009).

Peripartum cardiomyopathy (PPCM) is an uncommon disorder associated with pregnancy; the heart dilates and weakens, leading to symptoms of HF. PPCM can be difficult to diagnose because symptoms of HF can mimic those of pregnancy. PPCM can be a major cause of maternal morbidity and mortality, especially in some minority groups such as Africans and African Americans (Givertz, 2013). Most affected women recover normal heart function; however, some will progress to severe HF requiring mechanical support or heart transplantation. Even when the heart recovers, another pregnancy may be associated with a risk of recurrent HF (Givertz, 2013). Additionally, women with significant left ventricular dysfunction are at increased risk for future cardiovascular events (McNamara et al., 2015).

DIFFERENTIAL DIAGNOSES

Stroke

Definition, Scope, and Etiology. According to the 2015 AHA statistics, cardiovascular health encompasses several clinical conditions, including cerebrovascular disease and stroke. Stroke is currently the fifth leading cause of death and the leading cause of disability in adults in the United States; it is the third leading cause of death among women. Because of several important treatment modalities for acute stroke and because there has been a nationwide surge in establishing certified stroke centers, more patients are surviving their first stroke; there are currently 7 million stroke survivors, a majority of which are women. An additional 3.6 million people are projected to survive a stroke within the next 2 decades, and more than half of those individuals will be women. With a projected larger aging population, older women are expected to make up a majority of the stroke survivor population (Mozaffarian et al., 2015). The reasons for these statistics are multifold and include some of the following stark facts:

- Women live longer than men and therefore have a higher lifetime stroke risk than men.
- Women tend to have gaps in knowledge about stroke symptoms and stroke treatment options and therefore do not seek acute stroke care.
- Older women have a poorer functional recovery from stroke than men, as they frequently lack a support system to assist with rehabilitation and lifestyle and stroke-prevention strategies.
- Women have a higher rate of recurrent stroke compared with men.
- Stroke mortality is higher among women and is likely related to longer life expectancy.
- Women have been underrepresented in clinical trials related to stroke treatment and prevention and, as a result, may not be afforded gender-specific, evidence-based treatment.
- Women have sex-specific stroke risk factors, including pregnancy, gestational HTN, OCP use, menopause, and higher rates of other cardiovascular conditions.

In 2014, the AHA Stroke Association in collaboration with the Council on Cardiovascular and Stroke Nursing, the Council on Clinical Cardiology, the Council on Epidemiology and Prevention, and the Council for High Blood Pressure Research endorsed the first guideline dedicated to stroke risk and prevention in women. The AHA Science Advisory and Coordinating Committee approved a Healthcare Statement that summarized data on stroke risk factors unique to women and proposed a female-specific risk score to better capture adult women's stroke risk (Bushnell et al., 2014). Given that the majority of the population will be older women with multiple cardiovascular and cerebrovascular risk factors, this guideline provides an excellent reference for clinicians that prescribe both primary and secondary stroke-prevention strategies,

Stroke has been defined as a sudden death of brain cells due to the lack of oxygen caused by a blockage of blood flow (resulting in an ischemic stroke) or rupture of an artery in the brain (resulting in a hemorrhagic stroke). Approximately 87% of strokes are ischemic in nature, and 13% are hemorrhagic. Hemorrhagic stroke is further divided into ICH (10%) and subarachnoid hemorrhage (SAH) (3%) (Sacco et al., 2013).

Although women have an overall lower incidence of ischemic stroke than men, elderly women (older than 85 years) have a similar or higher incidence of ischemic stroke. Longevity and survival after their index stroke give women both a higher lifetime stroke risk and a higher stroke mortality rate.

Risk Factors. Table 43.4, taken from the 2014 AHA Guidelines, highlights stroke risk factors and the unique gender-specific factors, as well as those that are more prevalent in women than in men.

Symptoms. Strokes usually present as a syndrome in which patients experience the sudden onset of neurological deficits; the constellation of symptoms help localize the region in the central nervous system that has been injured. Public awareness campaigns have highlighted the most common symptoms by using the acronym F.A.S.T., which stands for *F*acial weakness or drooping, weakness in the *A*rm, *S*peech problems, and *T*ime, emphasizing the importance of calling 911 and seeking medical help immediately. Clinicians are familiar with the five "suddens": unilateral numbness/weakness in face/arm/leg, confusion, trouble speaking, severe headache, trouble seeing in one or both eyes, and trouble walking/lack of coordination. These "suddens"

TABLE 43.4	Stroke Risk Factors, Categorized by Those That Are Sex-Specific, Stronger, or More Prevalent in Woman or Are Similar Between Women and Men		
RISK FACTOR	**SEX-SPECIFIC RISK FACTORS**	**RISK FACTORS THAT ARE STRONGER OR MORE PREVALENT IN WOMEN**	**RISK FACTORS WITH SIMILAR PREVALENCE IN MEN AND WOMEN BUT UNKNOWN DIFFERENCE IN IMPACT**
Pregnancy	X		
Pre-eclarnpsia	X		
Gestational diabetes	X		
Oral contraceptive use	X		
Postmenopausal hormone use	X		
Changes in hormonal status	X		
Migraine with aura		X	
Atrial fibrillation		X	
Diabetes mellitus		X	
Hypertension		X	
Physical inactivity			X
Age			X
Prior cardiovascular disease			X
Obesity			X
Diet			X
Smoking			X
Metabolic syndrome			X
Depression		X	
Psychosocial stress		X	

highlight symptoms that indicate further evaluation is needed.

Patients may also present with symptoms of sudden onset of vertigo with vomiting, unexplained syncope, or altered mental status that precedes the symptoms already discussed and heightens suspicion for a cerebrovascular event.

Evaluation/Assessment. Although there are some common features to symptom presentation that may be indicative of stroke type, the diagnosis requires a detailed history, rapid imaging, and comprehensive neurologic exam.

Differential Diagnoses
ISCHEMIC STROKE

Definition, Scope, and Etiology. The classifications of ischemic stroke are generally divided into five subtypes. These classifications reflect a proposed etiology of ischemic stroke and serve as a guide for the appropriate treatments for secondary stroke prevention. Approximately 30% of patients who present with an ischemic stroke are diagnosed with large vessel disease, referring to atherosclerosis leading to stenosis or occlusion of a major artery in the brain or artery leading to the brain (including the carotid or vertebral arteries). An additional 20% of ischemic strokes are thought to be cardio embolic in nature, in which patients with vessel occlusions may have had an embolus travel from the heart (such as in AF). Approximately 15% of patients are diagnosed with small vessel disease, which refers to stenoses of the smaller vessels (deeper in the brain) typically related to long-standing diabetes or hyperlipidemia. Stroke patients who fall into the category of "other" are patients for whom their stroke may result from vasculopathies or hypercoagulable states. Nearly 30% of patients have a final diagnosis of "cryptogenic" stroke such that despite a comprehensive diagnostic work-up, there is no identified cause for their stroke.

Evaluation/Assessment and Diagnostic Studies. In addition to a careful medical history, diagnostic imaging (such as an MRI) and other studies (such as an echocardiogram) help to identify a suspected stroke etiology and guide secondary stroke prevention therapies.

TRANSIENT ISCHEMIC ATTACK
Definition. The term *transient ischemic attack (TIA)* is frequently used to describe stroke symptoms that are transient in nature, and have been too often and mistakenly considered a less urgent medical issue. Traditionally, TIAs have been defined as events in which focal neurological symptoms last less than 24 hours; however, the more routine use of neuroimaging studies such as a head CT scan or MRI have demonstrated that even patients with stroke symptoms lasting just several hours have evidence of infarction on CT or MRI. This has led to a more current definition of TIA, which is "a brief episode of neurological dysfunction caused by focal brain or retinal ischemia, with clinical symptoms typically lasting less than one hour, and without evidence of acute infarction" (Easton et al., 2009, p. 2277).

Evaluation/Assessment. A valuable risk-assessment tool called the $ABCD^2$ score used to predict short-term stroke risk after a TIA was developed by Johnston et al. (2007) and considered five items that were assigned points to determine the 2-, 7-, 30-, and 90-day stroke risk. The seven-point scoring scale is based on age, blood pressure, clinical features, duration of symptoms, and history of diabetes. Based on the patient's score, practitioners can make clinical decisions regarding the benefit of recommending hospital admission for urgent work-up and treatment (see Figure 43.3).

INTRACEREBRAL HEMORRHAGE. Spontaneous, nontraumatic intracerebral hemorrhage (ICH) is the most common of the hemorrhages in which blood vessel rupture causes bleeding into the brain parenchyma. Uncontrolled HTN is the principal cause; other secondary causes include cerebral amyloid angiopathy (CAA), intracranial aneurysm rupture, vasculitis, and hemorrhagic transformation after an ischemic stroke. The incidence of ICH and mortality resulting from ICH in women is reportedly lower than in men, but after the age of 65 years, there were similar mortality risks.

SUBARACHNOID HEMORRHAGE. SAH occurs when an intracranial aneurysm ruptures and blood enters the spaces around the brain tissue. The incidence of SAH is higher in women and is noted after the age of 55 years. Women have a higher risk of SAH resulting primarily from the prevalence and location of cerebral aneurysms (Algra, Klijn, Helmerhorst, Algra, & Rinkel, 2012). These statistics underscore the fact that women in all age groups can be at risk for any one or more of these ischemic stroke subtypes, so a thorough health history and gender-specific risk factor profile help direct therapies for both primary and secondary ischemic stroke prevention.

Treatment/Management. In the primary care setting, it is critical to recognize the symptoms of stroke and quickly have the patient transported to an emergency care facility. In the emergency facility, the goal is to stabilize, assess, and image the patient within 60 minutes of presentation (Adams et al., 2007). Rapid identification, diagnosis, and initiation of treatment are the key to minimizing the residual effects of stroke.

After patient discharge from the acute care setting, management focuses on rehabilitation. Rehabilitation programs are interdisciplinary with physical therapy, speech therapy, and a number of others as needed to minimize an individual residual effects.

Secondary Prevention. After a stroke that is not cardioembolic, the AHA and American Stroke Association recommend antiplatelet agents to decrease the risk for a second stroke or other cardiac events. Specifically, aspirin (50–325 mg/day) alone or in combination with dipyridamole extended release or clopidogrel alone (Adams et al., 2008). Consistent evaluation for adherence and encouragement to continue with therapy are important, as approximately 25% of patients stop taking their medications within 3 months after their stroke (Bushnell et al., 2010).

ABCD² Score

The ABCD² score is a risk-assessment tool designed to improve the prediction of short-term stroke risk after a TIA. The score is optimized to predict the risk of stroke within 2 days after a TIA but also predicts stroke risk within 90 days. The ABCD² score is calculated by summing uppoints for five independent factors.

RISK FACTOR	POINTS	SCORE
Age ≥60 years	1	
Blood pressure Systolic BP ≥ 140 mmHg *OR* Diastolic BP ≥ 90 mmHg	1	

Clinical features of TIA (*choose one*)
  Unilateral weakness with or without speech impairment *OR*
  Speech impairment without unilateral weakness
	2
	1	

Duration
  TIA duration ≥ 60 minutes
  TIA duration 10–59 minutes
	2
	1	

Diabetes	1	
Total ABCD² score	0–7	

Using the ABCD² Score

Higher ABCD² scores are associated with a greater risk of stroke during the 2, 7, 30, and 90 days after a TIA (Figure). The authors of the ABCD² score made the following recommendations for hospital observation

ABCD² Score	2-Day Stroke Risk	Comment
0–3	1.0%	Hospital observation may be unnecessary without another indication (e.g., new atrial fibrillation)
4–5	4.1%	Hospital observation justified in most situations
6–7	8.1%	Hospital observation worthwhile

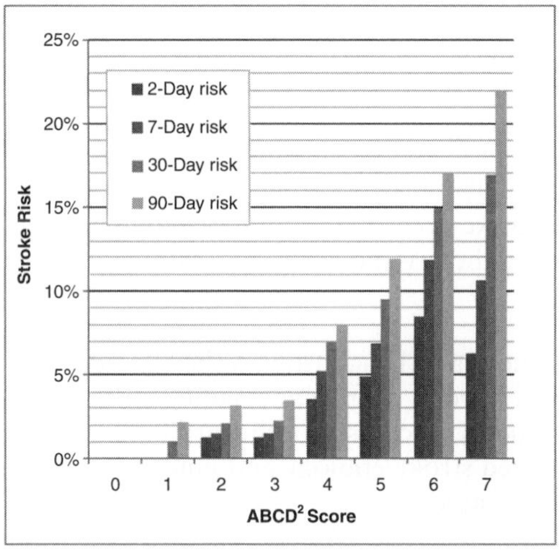

FIGURE 43.3

Transient ischemic attack (TIA): Prognosis and key management considerations.

Reprinted from Johnston et al. (2007). Copyright © 2007, with permission from Elsevier.

■ FUTURE DIRECTIONS

Much has been learned about women and heart disease during the past several years, and there is now clear evidence that CVD in women is indeed different from CVD in men. Clinicians need to continue to advocate for women who are at risk for heart disease and strive to provide best practices for preventing, identifying, and treating heart disease in women.

Future research will provide more data regarding unique symptoms and presentations among women, as well as treatment modalities that have superior outcomes for women. In the interim, aggressive preventative measures, early recognition, and aggressive management are critical.

■ REFERENCES

Abizaid, A., & Costa, J. R. (2010). New drug-eluting stents: An overview on biodegradable and polymer-free next-generation stent systems. *Circulation. Cardiovascular Interventions, 3*(4), 384–393.

Adams, H. P., del Zoppo, G., Alberts, M. J., Bhatt, D. L., Brass, L., Furlan, A., . . . Wijdicks, E. F.; American Heart Association; American Stroke Association Stroke Council; Clinical Cardiology Council; Cardiovascular Radiology and Intervention Council; Atherosclerotic Peripheral Vascular Disease and Quality of Care Outcomes in Research Interdisciplinary Working Groups. (2007). Guidelines for the early management of adults with ischemic stroke: A guideline from the American Heart Association/American Stroke Association Stroke Council, Clinical Cardiology Council, Cardiovascular Radiology and Intervention Council, and the Atherosclerotic Peripheral Vascular Disease and Quality of Care Outcomes in Research Interdisciplinary Working Groups: The American Academy of Neurology affirms the value of this guideline as an educational tool for neurologists. *Stroke, 38*(5), 1655–1711.

Adams, R. J., Albers, G., Alberts, M. J., Benavente, O., Furie, K., Goldstein, L. B., . . . Schwamm, L. H.; American Heart Association; American Stroke Association. (2008). Update to the AHA/ASA recommendations for the prevention of stroke in patients with stroke and transient ischemic attack. *Stroke, 39*(5), 1647–1652.

Agabiti-Rosei, E., & Muiesan, M. L. (2002). Left ventricular hypertrophy and heart failure in women. *Journal of Hypertension. Supplement, 20*(2), S34–S38.

Agarwal, S. K., Shawl, F., Raman, V. K., & Binbrek, A. S. (2008). Very late thrombosis of drug-eluting stents: A brief literature review and case example. *Journal of Invasive Cardiology, 20*(12), 655–658.

Akashi, Y. J., Goldstein, D. S., Barbaro, G., & Ueyama, T. (2008). Takotsubo cardiomyopathy: a new form of acute, reversible heart failure. *Circulation, 118*(25), 2754–2762.

Al-Aqeedi, R. F., Al Suwaidi, J., Singh, R., & Al Binali, H. A. (2012). Does prior coronary artery bypass surgery alter the gender gap in patients presenting with acute coronary syndrome? A 20-year retrospective cohort study. *BMJ Open, 2*(6).

Alberti, K. G., & Zimmet, P. Z. (1998). Definition, diagnosis and classification of diabetes mellitus and its complications. Part 1: Diagnosis and classification of diabetes mellitus provisional report of a WHO consultation. *Diabetic Medicine, 15*(7), 539–553.

Algra, A. M., Klijn, C. J., Helmerhorst, F. M., Algra, A., Rinkel, G. J. (2012). Female risk factors for subarachnoid hemorrhage: A systematic review. *Neurology, 79*(12), 1230–1236.

American College of Obstetricians and Gynecologists. (1996). *Hypertension in pregnancy*. ACOG Technical Bulletin No. 219. Washington, DC: Author.

American Diabetes Association. (2015). Standards of diabetes care. *Diabetes, 38*(Suppl. 1), S1–S93.

Amsterdam, E. A., Wenger, N. K., Brindis, R. G., Casey, D. E., Ganiats, T. G., Holmes, D. R, . . . Zieman, S. J. (2014). ACC/AHA guideline for the management of patients with non–ST-elevation acute coronary syndromes: A report of the American College of Cardiology/American Heart Association Task Force on Practice Guidelines [published online ahead of print September 23, 2014]. *Circulation, 64*(24), 2645–2687. doi:10.1161/CIR.0000000000000134

Anderson, J. L., Horne, B. D., Stevens, S. M., Grove, A. S., Barton, S., Nicholas, Z. P., . . . Carlquist, J. F.; Couma-Gen Investigators. (2007). Randomized trial of genotype-guided versus standard warfarin dosing in patients initiating oral anticoagulation. *Circulation, 116*(22), 2563–2570.

Anderson, M., Peterson, E. D., Brennan, J. M., Raol, S. V., Dail, D., Anstrom, K. J., . . . Douglas, P. S. (2012). Acute and long-term outcomes of coronary stenting in women vs. men: Results from the National Cardiovascular Data Registry® Centers for Medicare & Medicaid Services® Cohort. *Circulation, 112*, 2190–2199. doi:10.1161/CIRCULATIONAHA.112.111369

Anter, E., Jessup, M., & Callans, D. J. (2009). Atrial fibrillation and heart failure: Treatment considerations for a dual epidemic. *Circulation, 119*(18), 2516–2525.

Antithrombotic Trialists Collaboration. (2002). Collaborative meta-analysis of randomized trials of antiplatelet therapy for prevention of death, myocardial infarction, and stroke in high risk patients. *BMJ, 324*, 71–86.

Ashley, E. A., Raxwal, V., & Froelicher, V. (2001). An evidence-based review of the resting electrocardiogram as a screening technique for heart disease. *Progress in Cardiovascular Diseases, 44*(1), 55–67.

August, P., & Oparil, S. (1999). Hypertension in women. *Journal of Clinical Endocrinology and Metabolism, 84*(6), 1862–1866.

Ayas, N. T., White, D. P., Manson, J. E., Stampfer, M. J., Speizer, F. E., Malhotra, A., & Hu, F. B. (2003). A prospective study of sleep duration and coronary heart disease in women. *Archives of Internal Medicine, 163*(2), 205–209.

Bach, D. (2014). 2014 AHA/ACC guideline for the management of patients with valvular heart disease: A report of the American College of Cardiology/American Heart Association Task Force on Practice Guidelines. Summary. Retrieved from http://www.acc.org/latest-in-cardiology/journal-scans/2014/03/17/13/59/2014-aha-acc-guideline-for-the-management-of-patients-with-vhd

Bairey Merz, C. N., Shaw, L. J., Reis, S. E., Bittner, V., Kelsey, S. F., Olson, M., . . . Sopko, G.; WISE Investigators. (2006). Insights from the NHLBI-Sponsored Women's Ischemia Syndrome Evaluation (WISE) Study. Part II: Gender differences in presentation, diagnosis, and outcome with regard to gender-based pathophysiology of atherosclerosis and macrovascular and microvascular coronary disease. *Journal of the American College of Cardiology, 47*(Suppl. 3), S21–S29.

Balady, G. J., Williams, M. A., Ades, P. A., Bittner, V., Comoss, P., Foody, J. M., . . . Southard, D.; American Heart Association Exercise, Cardiac Rehabilitation, and Prevention Committee, the Council on Clinical Cardiology; American Heart Association Council on Cardiovascular Nursing; American Heart Association Council on Epidemiology and Prevention; American Heart Association Council on Nutrition, Physical Activity, and Metabolism; American Association of Cardiovascular and Pulmonary Rehabilitation. (2007). Core components of cardiac rehabilitation/secondary prevention programs—2007 update: A scientific statement from the American Heart Association Exercise, Cardiac Rehabilitation, and Prevention Committee, the Council on Clinical Cardiology; the Councils on Cardiovascular Nursing, Epidemiology and Prevention, and Nutrition, Physical Activity, and Metabolism; and the American Association of Cardiovascular and Pulmonary Rehabilitation. *Circulation, 115*(20), 2675–2682.

Ballantyne, C. M., O'Keefe, J. H., & Gotto, A.M. (2005). *Dyslipidemia essentials*. Royal Oak, MI: Physicians Press.

Barnard, D. D. (2005). Heart failure in women. *Current Cardiology Reports, 7*(3), 159–165.

Baroletti, S., & Dell'Orfano, H. (2010). Medication adherence in cardiovascular disease. *Circulation, 121*(12), 1455–1458.

Bell, D. S. (1995). Diabetic cardiomyopathy: A unique entity or a complication of coronary artery disease? *Diabetes Care, 18*(5), 708–714.

Bhardwaj, S., Selvarajah, S., & Schneider, E. B. (2013). Muscular effects of statins in the elderly female: A review. *Clinical Interventions in Aging, 8*, 47–59.

Bjarnason-Wehrens, B., Grande, G., Loewel, H., Völler, H., & Mittag, O. (2007). Gender-specific issues in cardiac rehabilitation: Do women with ischaemic heart disease need specially tailored programmes? *European Journal of Cardiovascular Prevention and Rehabilitation, 14*(2), 163–171.

Blanc, J. J., Etienne, Y., Gilard, M., Mansourati, J., Munier, S., Boschat, J., . . . Lurie, K. G. (1997). Evaluation of different ventricular pacing sites in patients with severe heart failure: Results of an acute hemodynamic study. *Circulation, 96*(10), 3273–3277.

Blecker, S., Paul, M., Taksler, G., Ogedegbe, G., & Katz, S. (2013). Heart failure–associated hospitalizations in the United States. *Journal of the American College of Cardiology, 61*(12), 1259–1267.

Blomström-Lundqvist, C., Scheinman, M. M., Aliot, E. M., Alpert, J. S., Calkins, H., Camm, A. J., . . . Trappe, H. J.; European Society of Cardiology Committee, NASPE-Heart Rhythm Society. (2003). ACC/AHA/ESC guidelines for the management of patients with supraventricular arrhythmias—Executive summary: A report of the American College of Cardiology/American Heart Association Task

Force on Practice Guidelines and the European Society of Cardiology Committee for Practice Guidelines (Writing Committee to Develop Guidelines for the Management of Patients with Supraventricular Arrhythmias) developed in collaboration with NASPE-Heart Rhythm Society. *Journal of the American College of Cardiology, 42*(8), 1493–1531.

Bonow, R. O., Carabello, B. A., Chatterjee, K., de Leon, A. C., Faxon, D. P., Freed, M. D., . . . Riegel, B. (2006). ACC/AHA 2006 guidelines for the management of patients with valvular disease: A report of the American College of Cardiology/American Heart Association Task Force on Practice Guidelines (Writing Committee to Develop Guidelines for the Management of Patients with Valvular Heart Disease). *Journal of the American College of Cardiology, 48*, e1–e148.

Bristow, M. R., & Lowes, B. D. (2005). Management of heart failure. In D. P. Zipes, P. Libby, R. O. Bonow, & E. Braunwald (Eds.), *Braunwald's heart disease* (7th ed.). Philadelphia, PA: Elsevier Saunders.

Bristow, M. R., Saxon, L. A., Boehmer, J., Krueger, S., Kass, D. A., De Marco, T., . . . Feldman, A. M.; Comparison of Medical Therapy, Pacing, and Defibrillation in Heart Failure (COMPANION) Investigators. (2004). Cardiac-resynchronization therapy with or without an implantable defibrillator in advanced chronic heart failure. *New England Journal of Medicine, 350*(21), 2140–2150.

Brown, B. G., Zhao, X. Q., Chait, A., Fisher, L. D., Cheung, M. C., Morse, J. S., . . . Albers, J. J. (2001). Simvastatin and niacin, antioxidant vitamins, or the combination for the prevention of coronary disease. *New England Journal of Medicine, 345*(22), 1583–1592.

Bugiardini, R., & Bairey Merz, C. N. (2005). Angina with "normal" coronary arteries: A changing philosophy. *Journal of the American Medical Association, 293*(4), 477–484.

Burke, A. P., Kolodgi, F., Farb, A., & Virmani, R. (2003). Gender differences in coronary plaque morphology in sudden coronary death [abstract], *Circulation, 108*, IV165.

Burke, J. G., Ehler, F. A., Kruse, J. T., Parker, M. A., Goldberger, J. J., & Kadish, A. H. (1997). Gender-specific differences in the QT interval and the effect of autonomic tone and menstrual cycle in healthy adults. *American Journal of Cardiology, 79*, 178–181.

Burt, V. L., Cutler, J. A., Higgins, M., Horan, M. J., Labarthe, D., Whelton, P., . . . Roccella, E. J. (1995). Trends in the prevalence, awareness, treatment, and control of hypertension in the adult U.S. population: Data from the health examination surveys, 1960 to 1991. *Hypertension, 26*(1), 60–69.

Bushnell, C., McCullough, L. D., Awad, I. A., Chireau, M. V., Fedder, W. N., Furie, K. L., . . . Walters, M. R.; American Heart Association Stroke Council; Council on Cardiovascular and Stroke Nursing; Council on Clinical Cardiology; Council on Epidemiology and Prevention; Council for High Blood Pressure Research. (2014). Guidelines for the prevention of stroke in women: a statement for healthcare professionals from the American Heart Association/American Stroke Association. *Stroke, 45*(5), 1545–1588.

Bushnell, C. D., Zimmer, L. O., Pan, W., Olson, D. M., Zhao, X., Meteleva, T., . . . Peterson, E. D.; Adherence Evaluation After Ischemic Stroke–Longitudinal Investigators. (2010). Persistence with stroke prevention medications 3 months after hospitalization. *Archives of Neurology, 67*(12), 1456–1463.

Cabin, H. S., Clubb, K. S., Hall, C., Perlmutter, R. A., & Feinstein, A. R. (1990). Risk for systemic embolization of atrial fibrillation without mitral stenosis. *American Journal of Cardiology, 65*(16), 1112–1116.

Calles-Escandon, J., Garcia-Rubi, E., Mirza, S., & Mortensen, A. (1999). Type 2 diabetes: one disease, multiple cardiovascular risk factors. *Coronary Artery Disease, 10*(1), 23–30.

Cannon, R. O., Quyyumi, A. A., Mincemoyer, R., Stine, A. M., Gracely, R. H., Smith, W. B., . . . Waclawiw, M. A. (1994). Imipramine in patients with chest pain despite normal coronary angiograms. *New England Journal of Medicine, 330*(20), 1411–1417.

Carabello, B. A., & Crawford, F. A. (1997). Valvular heart disease. *New England Journal of Medicine, 337*(1), 32–41.

Casella, I. B., Presti, C., Porta, R. M., Sabbag, C. R., Bosch, M. A., & Yamazaki, Y. (2008). A practical protocol to measure common carotid artery intima-media thickness. *Clinics (São Paulo, Brazil), 63*(4), 515–520.

Chan, D. C., Heidenreich, P. A., Weinstein, M. C., & Fonarow, G. C. (2008). Heart failure disease management programs: A cost-effectiveness analysis. *American Heart Journal, 155*(2), 332–338.

Chen, W., Woods, S. L., & Puntillo, K. A. (2005). Gender differences in symptoms associated with acute myocardial infarction: A review of the research. *Heart & Lung: The Journal of Critical Care, 34*(4), 240–247.

Chien, C. L., Lee, C. M., Wu, Y. W., Chen, T. A., & Wu, Y. T. (2008). Home-based exercise increases exercise capacity but not quality of life in people with chronic heart failure: A systematic review. *The Australian Journal of Physiotherapy, 54*(2), 87–93.

Chirillo, F., Salvador, L., & Cavallini, C. (2006). Medical and surgical treatment of chronic mitral regurgitation. *Journal of Cardiovascular Medicine, 7*(2), 96–107.

Chobanian, A. V., Bakris, G. L., Black, H. R., Cushman, W. C., Green, L. A., Izzo, J. L., . . . Roccella, E. J.; Joint National Committee on Prevention, Detection, Evaluation, and Treatment of High Blood Pressure. National Heart, Lung, and Blood Institute; National High Blood Pressure Education Program Coordinating Committee. (2003). Seventh report of the Joint National Committee on Prevention, Detection, Evaluation, and Treatment of High Blood Pressure. *Hypertension, 42*(6), 1206–1252.

Chow, G. V., Marine, J. E., & Fleg, J. L. (2012). Epidemiology of arrhythmias and conduction disorders in older adults. *Clinics in Geriatric Medicine, 28*(4), 539–553.

CIBIS-II Investigators and Committees. (1999). The Cardiac Insufficiency Bisoprolol Study II (CIBIS-II). *Lancet, 353*, 9–13.

Cohen, A., Pieper, C. F., Brown, A. J., & Bastian, L. A. (2006). Number of children and risk of metabolic syndrome in women. *Journal of Women's Health (2002), 15*(6), 763–773.

Colilla, S., Crow, A., Petkun, W., Singer, D. E., Simon, T., & Liu, X. (2013). Estimates of current and future incidence and prevalence of atrial fibrillation in the U.S. adult population. *American Journal of Cardiology, 112*(8), 1142–1147.

Concannon, T. W., Griffith, J. L., Kent, D. M., Normand, S. L., Newhouse, J. P., Atkins, J., . . . Selker, H. P. (2009). Elapsed time in emergency medical services for patients with cardiac complaints: Are some patients at greater risk for delay? *Circulation. Cardiovascular Quality and Outcomes, 2*(1), 9–15.

Connolly, S. J., Ezekowitz, M. D., Yusuf, S., Eikelboom, J., Oldgren, J., Parekh, A., . . . Wallentin, L.; RE-LY Steering Committee and Investigators. (2009). Dabigatran versus warfarin in patients with atrial fibrillation. *New England Journal of Medicine, 361*(12), 1139–1151.

Cortés, O., & Arthur, H. M. (2006). Determinants of referral to cardiac rehabilitation programs in patients with coronary artery disease: a systematic review. *American Heart Journal, 151*(2), 249–256.

Cox, J. L., & Gardner, M. J. (1993). Treatment of cardiac arrhythmias during pregnancy. *Progress in Cardiovascular Diseases, 36*(2), 137–178.

Curry, J. J., & Quintana, F. J. (1970). Myocardial infarction with ventricular fibrillation during pregnancy treated by direct current defibrillation with fetal survival. *Chest, 58*(1), 82–84.

Diabetes Atherosclerosis Intervention Study Investigators. (2001). Effect of fenofibrate on progression of coronary artery disease in Type 2 diabetes: The Diabetes Atherosclerosis Intervention Study, a randomised trial. *Lancet, 357*, 905–910.

DiMatteo, M. R. (2004). Variations in patients' adherence to medical recommendations: A quantitative review of 50 years of research. *Medical Care, 42*(3), 200–209.

Ditewig, J. B., Blok, H., Havers, J., & van Veenendaal, H. (2010). Effectiveness of self-management interventions on mortality, hospital readmissions, chronic heart failure hospitalization rate and quality of life in patients with chronic heart failure: a systematic review. *Patient Education and Counseling, 78*(3), 297–315.

Dolor, R. J., Melloni, C., Chatterjee, R., Allen, N.M., LaPointe, A., Williams, J.B., . . . Patel, M. R. (2012). *Treatment strategies for women with coronary artery disease*. Rockville, MD: Agency for Healthcare Research and Quality (US). Retrieved from https://effectivehealthcare .ahrq.gov/ehc/products/218/1226/CER66_Treatment-of-Women-with-CAD_ExecutiveSummary_20120816.pdf

Douglas, P. S., & Ginsburg, G. S. (1996). The evaluation of chest pain in women. *New England Journal of Medicine, 334*, 1311–1315.

Drazen, J. M., Jarcho, J. A., Morrissey, S., & Curfman, G. D. (2008). Cholesterol lowering and ezetimibe. *New England Journal of Medicine, 358*, 1507–1508.

Dukes, J. W., Dewland, T. A., Vittinghoff, E., Mandyam, M. C., Heckbert, S. R., Siscovick, D. S., . . . Marcus, G. M. (2015). Ventricular ectopy as a predictor of heart failure and death. *Journal of the American College of Cardiology, 66*(2), 101–109. doi:10.1016/j.jacc.2015.04.062

Duvall, W. L. (2003). Cardiovascular disease in women. *Mount Sinai Journal of Medicine, 70*(5), 293–305.

Easton, J. D., Saver, J. L., Albers, G. W., Alberts, M. J., Chaturvedi, S., Feldmann, E.,...Sacco, R. L.; American Heart Association; American Stroke Association Stroke Council; Council on Cardiovascular Surgery and Anesthesia; Council on Cardiovascular Radiology and Intervention; Council on Cardiovascular Nursing; Interdisciplinary Council on Peripheral Vascular Disease. (2009). Definition and evaluation of transient ischemic attack: A scientific statement for healthcare professionals from the American Heart Association/American Stroke Association Stroke Council; Council on Cardiovascular Surgery and Anesthesia; Council on Cardiovascular Radiology and Intervention; Council on Cardiovascular Nursing; and the Interdisciplinary Council on Peripheral Vascular Disease. The American Academy of Neurology affirms the value of this statement as an educational tool for neurologists. *Stroke, 40*(6), 2276–2293.

Eckel, R. H., Jakicic, J. M., Ard, J. D., de Jesus, J. M., Houston Miller, N., Hubbard, V. S.,...Yanovski, S. Z. (2014). 2013 AHA/ACC guideline on lifestyle management to reduce cardiovascular risk. *Circulation, 63,* 2960–2984.

Elkayam, U., & Bitar, F. (2005). Valvular heart disease and pregnancy. *Journal of the American College of Cardiology, 46*(2), 223–230.

Elkayam, U., & Goodwin, T. M. (1994). Safety and efficacy of intravenous adenosine therapy for supraventricular tachycardia during pregnancy: Results of a national survey [Abstract]. *Journal of the American College of Cardiology, 23,* 91A.

Fairweather, D., & Rose, N. R. (2004). Women and autoimmune diseases. *Emerging Infectious Diseases, 10*(11), 2005–2011.

Farley, T. M., Meirik, O., Chang, L., & Poulter, N. R. (1999). Combined oral contraceptives, smoking, and cardiovascular risk. *Journal of Epidemiology and Community Health, 52,* 775–785.

Fihn, S. D., Gardin, J. M., Abrams, J., Berra, K., Blankenship, J. C., Dallas, A. P.,...Williams, S. V. (2012). 2012 ACCF/AHA/ACP/AATS/PCNA/SCAI/STS guideline for the diagnosis and management of patients with stable ischemic heart disease: A report of the American College of Cardiology Foundation/American Heart Association Task Force on practice guidelines, and the American Association for Thoracic Surgery, Preventive Cardiovascular Nurses Association, Society for Cardiovascular Angiography and Interventions, and Society of Thoracic Surgeons. *Journal of the American College of Cardiology, 60,* e44–e164.

Finn, A. V., Nakano, M., Narula, J., Kolodgie, F. D., & Virmani, R. (2010). Concept of vulnerable/unstable plaque. *Arteriosclerosis, Thrombosis, and Vascular Biology, 30,* 1282–1292.

Ford, E. E., Ajani, U.A., Croft, J. B., Critchley, J.A., Labarthe, D. R., Kottke, T. E.,...Capewell, S. (2007). Explaining the decrease in U.S. deaths from coronary disease, 1980–2000. *New New England Journal of Medicine, 356,* 2388–2398.

Ford, E. S., Giles, W. H., & Dietz, W. H. (2002). Prevalence of the metabolic syndrome among US adults: Findings from the third National Health and Nutrition Examination Survey. *Journal of the American Medical Association, 287,* 356–359.

Fraker, T. D., Jr., & Fihn, S. D., writing on behalf of the 2002 Chronic Stable Angina Writing Committee. (2007). Chronic Angina Focused Update of the ACC/AHA 2002 Guidelines for the Management of Patients With Chronic Stable Angina: A report of the American College of Cardiology/American Heart Association Task Force on Practice Guidelines (Writing Group to Develop the Focused Update of the 2002 Guidelines for the Management of Patients With Chronic Stable Angina). *Journal of the American College of Cardiology, 50*(23), 2264–2274. doi:10.1016/j.jacc.2007.08.002

Friberg, L., Benson, L., Rosenqvist, M., & Lip, G.Y. (2012). Assessment of female sex as a risk factor in atrial fibrillation in Sweden: Nationwide retrospective cohort study. *BMJ, 344,* e3522.

Fuster, V., Ryden, L. E., Cannom, D. S., Crijns, H. J., Curtis, A. B., Ellenbogen, K. A., ... Le Heuzey, J. Y. (2006). ACC/AHA/ESC 2006 guidelines for the management of patients with atrial fibrillation: A report of the American College of Cardiology/American Heart Association Task Force on Practice Guidelines and the European Society of Cardiology Committee for Practice Guidelines (Writing Committee to Revise the 2001 Guidelines for the Management of

Patients with Atrial Fibrillation). *Journal of the American College of Cardiology, 48,* e149–e246.

Gandhi, P. U., & Pinney, S. (2014). Management of chronic heart failure: Biomarkers, monitors, and disease management programs. *Annals of Global Health, 80,* 46–54.

Ghali, J. K., Pina, I. L., Gottlieb, S. S., Deedwania, P. C., & Wikstrand, J. C. (2002). Metoprolol CR/XL in female patients with heart failure: Analysis of the experience in Metoprolol Extended Release Randomized Intervention Trial in Heart Failure (MERIT-HF). *Circulation, 105,* 1585–1591.

Gialdini, G., Nearing, K., Bhave, P. D., Bonuccelli, U., Iadecola, C., Healey, J. S., & Kamel, K. (2014). Perioperative atrial fibrillation and the long-term risk of ischemic stroke. *Journal of the American Medical Association, 312*(6), 616–622. doi:10.1001/jama.2014.9143

Giamouzis, G., Kalogeropoulos, A., Georgiopoulou, V., Laskar, S., Smith, A. L., Dunbar, S.,...Buter, J. (2011). Hospitalization epidemic in patients with heart failure: Risk factors, risk prediction, knowledge gaps, and future directions. *Journal of Cardiac Failure, 17,* 54–75.

Giardina, E. V., Sciacca, R. R., Foody, J. M., D'Onofrio, G., Villablanca, A. C., Leatherwood, S.,...Haynes, S. G. (2011). The DHHS office on women's health initiative to improve women's heart health: Focus on knowledge and awareness among women with cardiometabolic risk factors. *Journal of Women's Health, 20,* 6, 893–890. doi:10.1089/jwh,2010.2448

Giugliano, R. P., Ruff, C. T., Braunwald, E., Murphy, S. A., Wiviott, S. D., Halperin, J. L.,...Antman, E. M. (2013). Exoxaban versus warfarin in patients with atrial fibrillation. *New England Journal of Medicine, 369,* 2093–2104. doi:10.1056/NEJMoa1310907

Givertz, M. M. (2013). Peripartum cardiomyopathy. *Circulation, 127,* e622–e626. doi:10.1161/CIRCULATIONAHA.113.001851

Givertz, M. M., Colucci, W. S., & Braunwald, E. (2005). Clinical aspects of heart failure: Pulmonary edema, high-output failure. In D. P. Zipes, P. Libby, R. O. Bonow & E. Braunwald (Eds.), *Braunwald's heart disease* (7th ed., pp. 539–568). Philadelphia, PA: Elsevier Saunders.

Goldberg, A. C. (1998). Clinical trial experience with extended-release niacin (Niaspan): Dose related escalation study. *American Journal of Cardiology, 82,* 35U–38U.

Golden, K. E., Chang, A. M., & Hollander, J. E. (2013). Sex preferences in cardiovascular testing: The contribution of the patient-physician discussion. *Academic Emergency Medicine, 20*(7), 1–14. doi:10.1111/acem.12169

Gopalakrishnan, P., Ragland, M. M., & Tak, T. (2009). Gender differences in coronary artery disease: Review of diagnostic challenges and current treatment. *Postgraduate Medicine, 2,* 60–68. doi:10.3810/pgm.2009.03.1977

Gotto, A., & Pownall, H. (1999). *Manual of lipid disorders* (2nd ed.). Baltimore, MD: Lippincott Williams & Wilkins.

Grana, R., Benowitz, N., & Glantz, S. A. (2014). Contemporary reviews in cardiovascular medicine, e-cigarettes: A scientific review. *Circulation, 129,* 1972–1986. doi:10.1161/CIRCULATIONAHA.114.007667

Granger, C. B., Alexander, J. H., McMurphy, J. J., Lopes, R. D., Hylak, E. M., Hanna, M.,...Wallentin, L. (2011). Apixaban versus warfarin in patients with atrial fibrillation. *New England Journal of Medicine, 365,* 981–992.

Greenland, P., Smith, S. C., & Grundy, S. M. (2001). Improving coronary heart disease risk assessment in asymptomatic people: Role of traditional risk factors and noninvasive cardiovascular tests. *Circulation, 104,* 863–1867.

Gu, Q., Burt V. L., Paulose-Ram, R., & Dillon, C. F. (2008). Gender differences in hypertension treatment, drug utilization patterns, and blood pressure control among U.S. adults with hypertension: Data from the National Health and Nutrition Examination Survey 1999–2004. *American Journal of Hypertension, 21,* 789–798.

Gulati, M., Pandey, D. K., Arnsdorf, M. F., Lauderdale, D. S., Thisted, R. A., Wicklund, R. H.,...Black, H. R. (2003). Exercise capacity and the risk of death in women: The St James Women Take Heart Project. *Circulation, 108,* 1554–1559. doi:10.1161/01.CIR.0000091080.57509.E9

Gulati, M., Shaw, L. J., & Bairey Merz, C. N. (2012). Myocardial ischemia in women—lessons from the NHLBI WISE Study. *Clinical Cardiology, 35*(3), 141–148. doi:10.1002/clc.21966

Gunderson, E. P., Lewis, C. E., Wei, G. S., Whitmer, R. A., Quesenberry, C. P., & Sidney, S. (2007). Lactation and changes in maternal metabolic risk factors. *Obstetrics & Gynecology, 109*(3), 729–738.

Guru, V., Fremes, S. E., Austin, P. A., Blackstone, E. H., & Tu, J. V. (2006). Gender differences in outcomes after hospital discharge from coronary artery bypass grafting. *Circulation, 113*, 507–516.

Guyton, A. C., & Hall, J. E. (2006). *Textbook of medical physiology.* Philadelphia, PA: WB Saunders.

Gylling, H., Radhakrishnan, R., & Miettinen, T. (1997). Reduction of serum cholesterol in postmenopausal women with previous myocardial infarction and cholesterol malabsorption induced by dietary sitostanol ester margarine. *Circulation, 96*, 4226–4231.

Hajjar, I., & Kotchen, T. A. (2003). Trends in the prevalence, awareness, treatment and control of hypertension in the United States, 1998–2000. *Journal of the American Medical Association, 290*, 199–206.

Hall, J. M., Levant, S., & DeFrances, C. J. (2012). *Hospitalization for congestive heart failure: United States, 2000–2010.* U.S. Department of Health and Human Services, Centers for Disease Control and Prevention, National Center for Health Statistics.

Harjari, K. J. (1999). Potential new cardiovascular risk factors: Left ventricular hypertrophy, homocysteine, lipoprotein(a), triglycerides, oxidative stress, and fibrinogen. *Annals of Internal Medicine, 131*, 376–386.

Harrison, M. B., Browne, G. B., Roberts, J., Tugwell, P., Gafni, A., & Graham, I. (2002). Quality of life of individuals with heart failure: A randomized trial of the effectiveness of two models of hospital-to-home transition. *Medical Care, 40*, 271–282.

Heart Protection Study Collaborative Group. (2002). MRC/BRF Heart Protection Study of cholesterol lowering with simvastatin in 20,536 high-risk individuals: A randomised placebo-controlled trial. *Lancet, 36*, 7–22.

Hector, I., Michelena, B. D., Powell, P. A, Brady, P. A., Friedman, M. D., & Ezekowitz, M. D. (2010). Gender in atrial fibrillation: Ten years later. *Gender Medicine, 7*(3), 206–217.

Heer, T., Schiele, R., Schneider S., Git, A. K., Wienbergen, H., Gottwik, M.,…Senges, J. (2002). Gender differences in acute myocardial infarction in the era of thrombolytic reperfusion (the MITRA registry). *American Journal of Cardiology, 89*, 511–517.

Heo, S., Moser, D. K., & Widener, J. (2007). Gender differences in the effects of physical and motional symptoms on health-related quality of life in patients with heart failure. *European Journal of Cardiovascular Nursing, 6*, 146–152.

Hernesniemi, J. A., Seppälä, I., Lyytikäinen, L. P., Mononen, N., Oksala, N., Hutri-Kähönen, N.,…Lehtimäki, T. (2012). Genetic profiling using genome-wide significant coronary artery disease risk variants does not improve the prediction of subclinical atherosclerosis: The Cardiovascular Risk in Young Finns Study, the Bogalusa Heart Study and the Health 2000 Survey: A meta-analysis of three independent studies. *PLoS One, 7*, e28931.

Hillis, L. D., Smith, P. K., Anderson, J. L., Bittl, J. A., Bridges, C. R., Byrne, J. G.,…Winniford, M. D. (2011). 2011 ACCF/AHA guideline for coronary artery bypass graft surgery: A report of the American College of Cardiology Foundation/American Heart Association Task Force on Practice Guidelines. *Circulation, 124*, e652–e735.

Hohnloser, S. H. (2011). Stroke prevention versus bleeding risk in atrial fibrillation: A clinical dilemma. *Journal of the American College of Cardiology, 57*, 181–183.

Holmes, M. V., Harrison, S., Talmud, P. J., Hingorani, A. D., & Humphries, S. E. (2011). Utility of genetic determinants of lipids and cardiovascular events in assessing risk. *Nature Reviews Cardiology, 8*, 207–221.

Hongo, R. H., & Scheinman, M. M. (2005). Arrhythmia and arrhythmia management. In N. K. Wenger & P. Collins (Eds.), *Women and heart disease* (2nd ed., pp. 523–536). London, UK: Taylor & Francis Group.

Humphries, K. H., Kerr, C. R., Connolly, S. J., Klein, G., Boone, J. A., Green, M.,…Newman, D. (2001). New-onset atrial fibrillation: Sex differences in presentation, treatment and outcome. *Circulation, 103*, 2365–2370.

Hunt, S. A. et al. (2005). ACC/AHA 2005 guideline update for the diagnosis and management of chronic heart failure in the adult: A report of the American College of Cardiology/American Heart Association Task Force on Practice Guidelines (Writing Committee to Update the 2001 Guidelines for the Evaluation and Management of Heart Failure). Retrieved from http://circ.ahajournals.org/content/112/12/e154.full .pdf+html

Huxley, R. R., & Woodward, M. (2011). Cigarette smoking as a risk factor for coronary heart disease in women compared with men: A systematic review and meta-analysis of prospective cohort studies. *Lancet, 378*, 1297–1305.

Inglis, S. C., Clark, R. A., McAlister, F. A., Ball, J., Lewinter, C., Cullington, D., & Cleland, J. G. F. (2010). Structured telephone support or tele-monitoring programmes for patients with chronic heart failure. *The Cochrane Database of Systematic Reviews, 8*, CD007228.

Iung, B., & Vahanian, A. (2014). Epidemiology of acquired valvular heart disease. *Canadian Journal of Cardiology, 9*, 962–970. doi:10.1016/j .cjca.2014.03.022

Jackevicius, C. A., Ping, L., & Tu, J. V. (2008). Prevalence, predictors, and outcomes of primary nonadherence after acute myocardial infarction. *Circulation, 117*, 1028–1036. doi:10.1161/ CIRCULATIONAHA.107.706820

Jackevicius, C. A., Tu, J. V., Ko, D. T., Krumholtz, H. M. (2008). Use of ezetimibe in the United States and Canada. *New England Journal of Medicine, 358*, 1819–1828.

Jackson, G. (2005). Stable angina pectoris (recognition and management). In N. K. Wenger & P. Collins (Eds.), *Women and heart disease* (2nd ed., pp. 195–204). London, UK: Taylor & Francis Group.

Jacobs, A. K. (2003). Coronary revascularization in women in 2003: Sex revisited. *Circulation, 107*, 375–377.

Jacobs, A. K. (2009). The efficacy of drug-eluting stents in women. A window of opportunity. *JACC: Cardiovascular Interventions, 2*, 611–613. Retrieved from http://interventions.onlinejacc.org

James, P. A., Oparil, A., Carter, B. L., Cushman, W. C., Dennison-Himmelfarb, C., Handler, J.,…Ortiz, E. (2013). 2014 Evidence-based guideline for the management of high blood pressure in adults: Report from the panel members appointed to the Eighth Joint National Committee (JNC 8). *Journal of the American Medical Association, 311*(5), 507–520. doi:10.1.1001/jama.2013.28442

January, C., Wann, S. L., Alpert, J. S., Calkins, H., Cigarroa, J. E., Cleveland, J.C. Jr.,…Yancy, C. W. (2014). 2014 AHA/ACC/HRS guideline for the management of patients with atrial fibrillation: Executive summary. *Journal of the American College of Cardiology, 64*, 2246–2280.

Jessup, M., Abraham, W. T., Casey, D. E., Feldman, A. M., Francis, G. S., Ganiats, T. G.,…Yancy, C. W., writing on behalf of the 2005 Guideline Update for the Diagnosis and Management of Chronic Heart Failure in the Adult Writing Committee. (2009). Focused update ACCF/AHA guidelines for the diagnosis and management of heart failure in adults. *Journal of the American College of Cardiology, 53*, 1343–1382.

Jneid, H., Anderson, J. L., Wright, R. S., Adams, C. D., Bridges, C. R., Casey, D. E.,…Zidar, J. P. (2012). ACCF/AHA focused update of the guideline for the management of patients with unstable angina/non–ST-elevation myocardial infarction (updating the 2007 guideline and replacing the 2011 focused update): A report of the American College of Cardiology Foundation/American Heart Association Task Force on Practice Guidelines. *Journal of the American College of Cardiology, 60*, 645–681.

Johansson, P., Dahlstrom, U., & Brostrom, A. (2006). Factors and interventions influencing health-related quality of life in patients with heart failure: A review of the literature. *European Journal of Cardiovascular Nursing, 1*, 5–15.

Johnson, B. D., Shaw, L. J., Buchthal, S. D., Bairey Merz, C. N., Kim, H. W., Scott, K. N.,…Pohost, G. M. (2004). Prognosis in women with myocardial ischemia in the absence of obstructive coronary disease: Results from the National Institutes of Health—National Heart, Lung, and Blood Institute–Sponsored Women's Ischemia Syndrome Evaluation (WISE). *Circulation, 109*, 2993–2999.

Johnston, S. C., Rothwell, P. M., Huynh-Huynh, M. N., Giles, M. F., Elkins, J. S., & Sidney, S. (2007). Validation and refinement of scores to predict very early stroke risk after transient ischemic attack. *Lancet, 369*, 283–292.

Jones, L. W., Haykowsky, M. J., Swartz, J. J., Douglas, P. S., & Mackey, J. R. (2007). Early breast cancer therapy and cardiovascular injury. *Journal of the American College of Cardiology, 50*, 1435–41.

Kannel, W. B., & Abbott, R. D. (1986). A prognostic comparison of asymptomatic left ventricular hypertrophy and unrecognized myocardial infarction: The Framingham Study. *American Heart Journal, 111*, 391–397.

Karapolat, H., Demir, E., Bozkaya, Y. T., Eyigor, S., Nalbantgil, S., Durmaz, B., & Zoghi, M. (2009). Comparison of hospital-based versus home-based exercise training in patients with heart failure: Effects on functional capacity, quality of life, psychological symptoms, and hemodynamic parameters. *Clinical Research in Cardiology, 98*, 635–642.

Kaski, J. C. (2006). Cardiac syndrome X in women: The role of oestrogen deficiency. *Heart, 92*(3), iii5–iii9.

Kastelein, J. J., Akdim, F., Stroes, E. S., Zwinderman, A. H., Bots, M. L., Stalenhoef, A. F., & Visseren, F. L. (2008). Simvastatin with or without ezetimibe in familial hypercholesterolemia. *New England Journal of Medicine, 358,* 1431–1443.

Kern, M. J. (2005). Coronary blood flow and myocardial ischemia. In D. P. Zipes, P. Libby, R. O. Bonow, & E. Braunwald (Eds.), *Braunwald's heart disease* (7th ed., pp. 1103–1128). Philadelphia, PA: Elsevier Saunders.

Khot, U. N., Khot, M. B., Bajzer, C. T., Sapp, S. K., Ohman, E. M., Ellis, S. G.,…Topol, E. J. (2003). Prevalence of conventional risk factors in patients with coronary heart disease. *Journal of the American Medical Association, 290,* 898–904.

Kim, E., & Menon, V. (2009). Status of women in cardiovascular clinical trials. *Arteriosclerosis, Thrombosis and Vascular Biology, 29,* 279–283. doi:10.1161/ATVBAHA.108.179796

Kim M. H., Johnston, S. S., Chu, B. C., Dalal, M. R., & Shulman, K. L. (2011). Estimation of total incremental health care costs in patients with atrial fibrillation in the United States. *Circulation: Cardiovascular Quality and Outcomes, 4,* 313–320.

Klocke, F. J., Baird, M. G., Lorell, B. H., Bateman, T. M., Messer, J. V., Berman, D. S.,…Russell, R. O. (2003). ACC/AHA/ASNC guidelines for the clinical use of cardiac radionuclide imaging—executive summary. A report of the American College of Cardiology/American Heart Association Task Force on Practice Guidelines (ACC/AHA/ASNC Committee to Revise the 1995 Guidelines for the clinical use of cardiac radionuclide imaging. *Circulation, 108,* 1404–1418.

Kociol, R.D., Hammill, B.G., Fonarow, G. C., Klaskala, W., Mills, R. M., Hernandez, A. F., & Curtis, L. H. (2010). Generalizability and longitudinal outcomes of a national heart failure clinical registry: Comparison of Acute Decompensated Heart Failure National Registry (ADHERE) and non-ADHERE Medicare beneficiaries. *American Heart Journal, 160,* 885–892.

Koelling, T. M., Chen, R. S., Lubwama, R. N., L'Italien, G. J., & Eagle, K. A. (2004). The expanding national burden of heart failure in the United States: The influence of heart failure in women. *American Heart Journal, 147,* 74–78.

Kohli, P., & Gulati, M. (2010). Exercise stress testing in women; Going back to the basics. *Circulation, 122,* 2570–2580. doi:10.1161/CIRCULATIONAHA.109.914754

Konstam, M. A. (2012). Does home monitoring heart failure care improve patient outcomes? *Circulation, 125,* 820–827.

Kothawade, K., & Bairey Merz, C. N. (2011). Microvascular coronary dysfunction in women: Pathophysiology, diagnosis, and management. *Current Problems in Cardiology, 36*(8), 291–318. doi:10.1016/j.cpcardiol.2011.05.002

Krahn, A. D., Yee, R., Klein, G. J., & Morillo, C. (1995). Inappropriate sinus tachycardia: Evaluation and therapy. *Journal of Cardiovascular Electrophysiology, 6,* 1124–1128.

Kravitz, R. L., Hays, R. D., Sherbourne, C. D., DiMatteo, M. R., Rogers, W. H., Ordway, L., & Greenfield, S. (1993). Recall of recommendations and adherence to advice among patients with chronic medical conditions. *Archives of Internal Medicine, 153,* 1869–1878.

Krumholz, H. M., Anderson, J. L., Bachelder, B. L., Fesmire, F. M., Fihn, S. D., Foody, J. M.,…Nallamothu, B. K. (2008). ACC/AHA 2008 performance measures for adults with ST-elevation and non–ST-elevation myocardial infarction: A report of the American College of Cardiology/American Heart Association Task Force on Performance Measures (Writing Committee to Develop Performance Measures for ST-Elevation and Non–ST-Elevation Myocardial Infarction). *Circulation, 118,* 2598–2648.

Krumholz, H. M., Merrill, A. R., Schone, E. M., Schreiner, G. C., Chen, J., Bradley, E. H.,…Drye, E. E. (2009). Patterns of hospital performance in acute myocardial infarction and heart failure 30-day mortality and readmission. *Circulation: Cardiovascular Quality and Outcomes, 2,* 407–413.

Lakowski, S. G., Greenland, R. A., Wong, N. D., Schreiner, P. J., Herrington, D. M., Kronmal, R. A.,…Blumenthal, R. S. (2007). Coronary artery calcium scores and risk for cardiovascular events in women classified as "low risk" based on Framingham Risk Score: The Multi-Ethnic Study of Atherosclerosis (MESA). *Archives of Internal Medicine, 167*(22), 2437–2442.

Lane, D. A., & Lip, G. Y. (2012). Use of the CHA(2)DS(2)VASc and HAS-BLED scores to aid decision making for thromboprophylaxis in non-valvular atrial fibrillation. *Circulation, 126,* 860–865.

Lansky, A. J., Hochman, J. S., Ward, P. A, Montz, G. S., Fabunmi, R., Berger, P. B.,…Jacobs, A. K. (2005). Percutaneous coronary intervention and adjunctive pharmacotherapy in women: A statement for healthcare professionals from the American Heart Association. *Circulation, 111,* 940–953.

Leffler, S., & Johnson, D. R. (1992). Adenosine use in pregnancy: Lack of effect on the fetal heart rate. *American Journal of Emergency Medicine, 10,* 548–549.

Leon, A. S., Franklin, B. A., Costa, F., Balady, G. J., Berra, K. A., Stewart, K. J.,…Lauer, M. S. (2005). Cardiac rehabilitation and secondary prevention of coronary heart disease: An American Heart Association scientific statement from the Council on Clinical Cardiology (Subcommittee on Exercise, Cardiac Rehabilitation, and Prevention) and the Council on Nutrition, Physical Activity, and Metabolism (Subcommittee on Physical Activity), in collaboration with the American Association of Cardiovascular and Pulmonary Rehabilitation). *Circulation, 111,* 369–376.

Lerner, D. J., & Kannel, W. B. (1986). Patterns of coronary heart disease morbidity and mortality in the sexes: A 26-year follow-up of the Framingham population. *American Heart Journal, 111,* 383–390.

Lesman-Leegte, I., Jaarsma, T., Coyne, J. C., Hilege, H. L., Van Veldhuisen, D. J., & Sanderman, R. (2009). Quality of life and depressive symptoms in the elderly: A comparison between patients with heart failure and age- and gender-matched community controls. *Journal of Cardiac Failure, 15,* 17–23.

Levy, D., Kenchaia, S., Larson, M. G., Benjamin, E. J., Kupta, M. J., Ho, K. K.,…Vasen, R. S. (2002). Long term trends in the incidence of and survival with heart failure. *New England Journal of Medicine, 347,* 1397–1402.

Lewandowski, R., & Gracey, C. (2014). *Management of cardiovascular disease in women.* London, UK: Springer Publishing.

Libby, P. (2008). The pathogenesis, prevention, and treatment, of atherosclerosis. In D. L. Longo, A. S. Fauci, D. Kasper, S. L. Hauser, J. L. Jameson, & J. Loscalzo (Eds.), *Harrison's principles of internal medicine.* New York, NY: Blackwell Publishing.

Libby, P., & Therous, P. (2005). Basic science for clinicians: Pathophysiology of coronary artery disease. *Circulation, 111,* 481–3488.

Lindenfeld J., Albert N. M., Boehmer J. P., Collins S., Ezekowitz, J. A., Givertz, M. M.,…Walsh, M. N. (2010). Executive summary: HFSA 2010 comprehensive heart failure practice guideline. *Journal of Cardiac Failure, 16,* 475–539.

Lindenfeld, J., Albert, N. M., Boehmer, J. P., Collins, S. P., Ezekowitz, J. A., Givertz, M. M.,…Walsh, M. N. (2010). HFSA 2010 Comprehensive Heart Failure Practice Guideline. *Journal of Cardiac Failure, 16*(6), e1–194. doi: 10.1016/j.cardfail.2010.04.004

Lip, G. Y., Beevers, M., Churchill, D., Shaffer, L. M., & Beevers, D., G. (1997). Effect of atenolol on birth weight. *American Journal of Cardiology, 79,* 1436–1438.

Lip, G. Y., Nieuwlaat, R., Pisters, R., Lane, D. A., & Crijns, H. J. (2010). Refining clinical risk stratification for predicting stroke and thromboembolism in atrial fibrillation using a novel risk factor-based approach: The Euro Heart Survey on Atrial Fibrillation. *Chest, 137,* 263–272.

Lipton, R. B., & Bigal, M. E. (2005). The epidemiology of migraine. *American Journal of Medicine, 118,* S3–S19.

Lloyd-Jones, D. M., Hong, Y., Labarthe, D., Mozaffarian, D., Appel, L. J., Van Horn, L.,…Rosamond, W. D.; on behalf of the American Heart Association Strategic Planning Task Force and Statistics Committee. (2010). Defining and setting national goals for cardiovascular health promotion and disease reduction: The American Heart Association's Strategic Impact Goal through 2020 and beyond. *Circulation, 121,* 586–613.

Lloyd-Jones, D. M., Leip, E. P., Larson, M. G., D'Agostino, R. B., Beiser, A., Wilson, P. W., & Levy, D. (2006). Prediction of lifetime risk for cardiovascular disease by risk factor burden at 50 years of age. *Circulation, 113,* 791–798.

Lloyd-Jones, D. M., Nam, B. H., D'Agostino, R. B., Sr., Levy, D., Murabito, J. M., Wang, T. J.,…O'Donnell, C. J. (2004). Parental cardiovascular disease as a risk factor for cardiovascular disease in middle-aged adults: A prospective study of parents and offspring. *Journal of the American Medical Association, 291,* 2204–2211.

López-Pedrera, C., Pérez-Sánchez, C., Ramos-Casals, M., Santos-Gonzalez, M., Rodriguez-Ariza, A., & Cuadrado, M. J. (2011).

Cardiovascular risk in systemic autoimmune diseases: Epigenetic mechanisms of immune regulatory functions. *Clinical and Developmental Immunology, 2012,* 1–10. doi:10.1155/2012/974648

Loscalzo, J., Weinfeld, M., Fless, G. M., & Scanu, A. M. (1990). Lipoprotein(a), fibrin binding, and plasminogen activation. *Arteriosclerosis, 10,* 240–245.

Lowery, J., Hopp, F., Subramanian, U., Wiitala, W., Welsh, D. E., Larkin, A., ... Vaitkevicius, P. (2012). Evaluation of a nurse practitioner disease management model for chronic heart failure: A multi-site implementation study. *Congestive Heart Failure, 18,* 4–71.

Lui, K., Ballew, C., Jacobs, D. R., Sidney, S., Savage, P. J., Dyer, A., ... Blanton. M. M. (1989). Ethnic differences in blood pressure, pulse rate, and related characteristics in young adults: The CARDIA study. *Hypertension, 14,* 218–226.

Lundberg, G., & King, M. D. S. (2012). Coronary revascularization in women. *Clinical Cardiology, 35*(3), 156–159.

Macedo, A. F., Bell, J, McCarron, C., Conroy, R., Richardson, J., Scowcroft, A., ... Rotheram, N. (2015). Determinants of oral anticoagulation control in new warfarin patients: An analysis using data from clinical practice research datalink. *Thrombosis Research, 136,* 250–260. doi:10.1016/j/thromborese.2015.060007

Madias, J. E. (2006). ECG changes and voltage attenuation in congestive heart failure. *Hospital Chronicles, Supplement,* 27–30.

Manzi, S., Meilahn, E. N., Rairie, J. E., Conti, C. G., Medsgar, T. A., Jansen-McWilliams, L., ... Kuller, L. H. (1997). Age-specific incidence rates of myocardial infarction and angina in women with systemic lupus erythematosus: Comparison with the Framingham study. *American Journal of Epidemiology, 145,* 408–415.

Maron, B. J., Towbi, J. A., Thiene, G., Antelevitich, C., Corrado, D., Moss, A. J., ... Young, J. B. (2006). Contemporary definitions and classification of the cardiomyopathies: An American Heart Association Scientific Statement from the Council on Clinical Cardiology, Heart Failure and Transplantation Committee; Quality of Care and Outcomes Research and Functional Genomics and Translational Biology Interdisciplinary Working Groups; and Council on Epidemiology and Prevention. *Circulation, 113*(14), 1807–1816.

Marzolini, S., Brooks, D., & Oh, P. I. (2008). Sex differences in completion of a 12-month cardiac rehabilitation programme: An analysis of 5922 women and men. *European Journal of Cardiovascular Prevention and Rehabilitation,* (6), 1–6. doi:10.1097/HJR.0b013e32830c1ce3

McAlister F. A., Stewart, S., Ferrua, S., & McMurray, J. J. (2004). Multidisciplinary strategies for the management of heart failure patients at high risk for admission: A systematic review of randomized trials. *Journal of the American College of Cardiology, 44,* 810–819.

McMurray, J. J., with the Task Force for the Diagnosis and Treatment of Acute and Chronic Heart Failure 2012 of the European Society of Cardiology. Developed in collaboration with the Heart Failure Association (HFA) of the ESC. (2012). ESC guidelines for the diagnosis and treatment of acute and chronic heart failure 2012. *European Heart Journal, 33,* 1787–1847. doi:10.1093/eurheartj/ehs104

McNamara, D. M., Elkayam, U, Alharethi, R., Damp, R., Hsich, E., Ewald, G., ... Fett, J. D. (2015). Clinical outcomes for peripartum cardiomyopathy in North America. Results of the IPAC Study (Investigations of Pregnancy-Associated Cardiomyopathy). *Journal of the American College of Cardiology, 66*(8), 905–914. doi:10.1016/j .jacc.2015.06.1309

McSweeney, J. C., Cleves, M. A., Zhaom W., Lefler, L. L., & Yang, S. (2010). Cluster analysis of women's prodromal and acute myocardial infarction symptoms by race and other characteristics. *Journal of Cardiovascular Nursing, 25*(4), 311–322. doi:10.1097/ JCN.0b013e3181cfba15

McSweeney, J. C., Cody, M., O'Sullivan, P., Elberson, K., Moser, D. K., & Garvin, B. J. (2003). Women's early warning symptoms of acute myocardial infarction. *Circulation, 108,* 2619–2623.

Meagher, E. A. (2004). Addressing cardiovascular disease in women: Focus on dyslipidemia. *Journal of American Board of Family Practice, 17,* 424–437.

Mehta, S. R., Yusuf, S., Peters, R. J., Bertran, M. E., Lewis, B. S., Natarajan, M. K., ... Fox, A. A. (2001). Clopidogrel in Unstable angina to prevent Recurrent Events trial (CURE) Investigators. Effects of pretreatment with clopidogrel and aspirin followed by long-term therapy in patients undergoing percutaneous coronary intervention: The PCI:CURE study. *Lancet, 358,* 527–533.

Melloni, C., Berger, J. S., Wang, T., Gunes, F., Stebbins, A., Pieper, K. S., ... Newby, K. (2010). Representation of women in randomized clinical trials of cardiovascular disease prevention. *Circulation. Cardiovascular Quality and Outcomes, 3,* 1–8.

Meyer, J. S., Mehdirad, A., Salem, B. I., Kulikowska, A., & Kulikowski, P. (2003). Sudden arrhythmia death syndrome: Importance of the long QT syndrome. *American Family Physician, 68*(3), 483–488.

Michelena, H. I., Powell, B. D., Brady, P. A., Friedman, P. A., & Ezekowitz, M. D. (2010). Gender in atrial fibrillation: Ten years later. *Gender Medicine, 3*(7), 206–217.

Michowitz, Y., Rahkovich, M., Oral, H., Zado, E. S., Tilz, R., John, S., ... Belhassen, B. (2014). Effects of sex on the incidence of cardiac tamponade after catheter ablation of atrial fibrillation: Results from a worldwide survey in 34,943 atrial fibrillation ablation procedures. *Circulation: Arrhythmia and Electrophysiology, 7,* 274–280.

Mieres, J. H., Shaw, L. J., Arai, A., Budoff, M. J., Flamm, S. D., Hundley, W. G., ... Wenger, N. K. (2005). Role of noninvasive testing in the clinical evaluation of women with suspected coronary artery disease: Consensus statement from the Cardiac Imaging Committee, Council on Clinical Cardiology, and the Cardiovascular Imaging and Intervention Committee, Council on Cardiovascular Radiology and Intervention, American Heart Association. *Circulation, 111,* 682–696.

Mieres, J. H., Shaw, L. J., Hendel, R. C., Miller, D. D., Bonow, R. O., Berman, D. S., Heller, G. V., ... Walsh, M. N. (2003). A report of the American Society of Nuclear Cardiology Task Force on women and heart disease (writing group on perfusion imaging in women). *Journal of Nuclear Cardiology, 10,* 95–101.

Miettinen, T. A., Puska, P. P., Gylling, H., Vanhanen, H., & Vartianen, E. (1995). Reduction of serum cholesterol with sitostanol-ester margarine in a mildly hypercholesterolemic population. *New England Journal of Medicine, 333,* 1308–1312.

Miller, J. M., & Zipes, D. P. (2005). Therapy for cardiac arrhythmias. In D. P. Zipes, P. Libby, R. O. Bonow, & E. Braunwald (Eds.), *Braunwald's heart disease* (7th ed., pp. 713–766). Philadelphia, PA: Elsevier Saunders.

Milner, K. A., Funk, M., Arnold, A., & Vaccarino, V. (2002). Typical symptoms are predictive of acute coronary syndromes in women. *American Heart Journal, 143,* 283–288.

Mookadam, M., Shamoun, F. E., & Mookadam, F. (2015). Novel anticoagulants in atrial fibrillation: A primer for the primary physician. *The Journal of the American Board of Family Medicine, 28,* 510–522.

Mora, S., Glynn, R. J., Hsia, J., MacFadyen, J. G., Genest, J., & Ridker, P. M. (2010). Statins for the primary prevention of cardiovascular events in women with elevated high-sensitivity C-reactive protein or dyslipidemia: Results from the Justification for the Use of statins in Prevention: an Intervention Trial Evaluating Rosuvastatin (JUPITER) and meta-analysis of women from primary prevention trials. *Circulation, 121,* 1069–1077.

Morris, D. C. (2005). Acute coronary syndromes. In N. K. Wenger & P. Collins (Eds.), *Women and heart disease* (2nd ed., pp. 237–249). London, UK: Taylor & Francis Group.

Mosca, L. (2005). Management of dyslipidemia in women in the post-hormone therapy era. *Journal of General Internal Medicine, 20,* 297–305.

Mosca, L., Banka, C. L., Benjamin, E. J., Berra K., Bushnell, C., Dolor, R. J., ... Wenger, N. K. (2007). Evidence-based guidelines for cardiovascular disease prevention in women: 2007 update. *Circulation, 115,* 1–21.

Mosca, L., Benin, E. J., Berra, K., Benzanon, J. L., Dolor, R. J., Lloyd-Jones, D. M., ... Wenger, N. K. (2011). Effectiveness-based guidelines for the prevention of cardiovascular disease in women—2011 update. *Circulation, 123,* 1243–1262.

Mosca, L., Hammond, G., Mochari-Greenberger, H., Towfighi, A., & Albert, M. A.; on behalf of the American Heart Association Cardiovascular Disease and Stroke in Women and Special Populations Committee of the Council on Clinical Cardiology, Council on Epidemiology and Prevention, Council on Cardiovascular Nursing, Council on High Blood Pressure Research, and Council on Nutrition, Physical Activity and Metabolism. (2013). Fifteen-year trends in awareness of heart disease in women: Results of a 2012 American Heart Association National Survey. *Circulation, 11,* 1254–1263. doi:10.1161/CIR.0b013e318287cf2f

Mosca, L., Linfante, A. H., Benjamin, E. J., Berra, K., Hayes, S. N., Walsh, B. W.,...Simpson, S. L. (2005). National Study of Physician Awareness and Adherence to Cardiovascular Disease Prevention Guidelines. *Circulation, 111*, 499–510. doi:10.1161/01.CIR.0000154568.43333.82

Mozaffarian, D., Benjamin, E. J., Go, A. S., Arnett, D. K., Blaha, M. J., Cushman, M.,...Turner, M. B.; on behalf of the American Heart Association Statistics Committee and Stroke Statistics Subcommittee. (2015). Heart disease and stroke statistics—2015 update: A report from the American Heart Association. *Circulation, 131*, e29–e322. doi:10.1161/CIR.0000000000000152

Mukamal, K. J., Maclure, M., Muller, J. E., & Mittleman, M. A. (2008). An exploratory prospective study of marijuana use and mortality following acute myocardial infarction. *American Heart Journal, 155*(3), 465–470. doi:10.1016/j.ahj.2007.10.049

Mulders, T. A., Meyer, Z., van der Donk, C., Kroon, A. A., Ferreira, I., Stehouwer, C. D., & Pinto-Sietsma, S. J. (2011). Patients with premature cardiovascular disease and a positive family history for cardiovascular disease are prone to recurrent events. *International Journal of Cardiology, 153*(1), 64–67.

National Center for Health Statistics. National Health Interview Survey. (2013). *Public-use data file and documentation.* Retrieved from http://www.cdc.gov/nchs/nhis/quest_data_related_1997_forward.htm

National Cholesterol Education Program (NCEP) Expert Panel on Detection, Evaluation, and Treatment of High Blood Cholesterol in Adults (Adult Treatment Panel III). (2002). Third Report of the National Cholesterol Education Program (NCEP) Expert Panel on Detection, Evaluation, and Treatment of High Blood Cholesterol in Adults (Adult Treatment Panel III) final report. *Circulation, 106*, 3143–3421.

National Heart, Lung, and Blood Institute (NHLBI). (2001). Third report of the National Cholesterol Education Program (NCEP) expert panel on detection, evaluation, and treatment of high blood cholesterol in adults (Adult Treatment Panel III). *Circulation, 306*, 3143–3407. Retrieved from http://circ.ahajournals.org

National Heart, Lung, and Blood Institute, National Cholesterol Education Program. (2002). Third report of the expert panel on detection, evaluation and treatment of high blood cholesterol in adults (ATP III), full report, May 2001. *Circulation, 106*, 31–43.

Neimann, L., Shin, D. B., Wang, X., Margolis, D. J., Troxel, A. B., & Gelfand, J. M. (2006). Prevalence of cardiovascular risk factors in patients with psoriasis. *Journal of the American Academy of Dermatology, 55*(5), 829–883. doi:10.1016/j.jaad.2006.08.040

Newby L. K., LaPointe, N. M., Chen, A. Y., Kramer, J. M., Hammill, B. G., DeLong, E. R.,...Califf, R. M. (2006). Long-term adherence to evidence-based secondary prevention therapies in coronary artery disease. *Circulation, 113*, 203–212.

Nishimura, R. A., Otto, C. M., Bonow, R. O., Carabello, B. A., Erwin, J. P., Guyton, R. A.,...Thomas, J. D. (2014). AHA/ACC guideline for the management of patients with valvular heart disease: Executive summary: A report of the American College of Cardiology/American Heart Association Task Force on Practice Guidelines. *Circulation, 129*, 1–96.

Novella, S., Dantas, A. P., Segarra, G., Medina, P., & Hermenegildo, C. (2012). Vascular aging in women: Is estrogen the fountain of youth? *Frontiers in Physiology, 3*, 1–8. doi:10.3389/fphys.2012.00165

O'Gara, P. T., Kushner, F. G., Ascheim, D. D., Casey, D. E., Chung, M. K., de Lemos J. A.,...Zhao, D. X. (2013). 2013 ACCF/AHA guideline for the management of ST-elevation myocardial infarction: A report of the American College of Cardiology Foundation/American Heart Association Task Force on Practice Guidelines. *Circulation, 127*, 529–555.

O'Leary, D. H., Polak, J. F., Kronmal, R. A., Monolia, T., Burke, M. S., & Wolfson, S. K. (1999). Carotid intima-media thickness as a risk factor for myocardial infarction and stroke in older adults. Cardiovascular Health Study Collaborative Research Group. *New England Journal of Medicine, 340*, 14–22.

Oakley, C., Child, A., Jung, B., Prespitaro, P., Tornos, P., Klein, W.,...Poumeyrol-Jumeau, D. (2003). Expert consensus document of management of cardiovascular diseases during pregnancy. The Task Force on the Management of Cardiovascular Diseases During Pregnancy of the European Society of Cardiology. *European Heart Journal, 24*, 761–781.

Ogburn, P. L., Schmidt, G., Linman, J., & Cefalo, R. C. (1992). Paroxsymal tachycardia and cardioversion during pregnancy. *Journal of Reproductive Medicine, 27*, 359–366.

Oldridge, N. B., Guyatt, G., Jones, N., Crowe, J., Singer, J., Feeny, D.,...Torance, G. (1991). Effects of quality of life with comprehensive rehabilitation after acute myocardial infarction. *American Journal of Cardiology, 67*, 1084–1089.

Oparil, S. (2006). Women and hypertension: What did we learn from the Women's Health Initiative? *Cardiology Review, 14*, 267–275.

Orshal, J. M., & Khalil, R. A. (2004). Gender, sex hormones, and vascular tone. *American Journal of Physiology. Regular, Integrative Comparative Physiology, 286*, R233–R249.

Os, I., Bratland, B., Dahlof, B., Gisholt, K., Syvertsen, J. O., & Tretli, S. (1994). Female preponderance for lisinopril-induced cough in hypertension. *American Journal of Hypertension, 7*, 1012–1015.

Osnabrugge, R. L. J., Mylotte, D., Head, S. J., Van Mieghem, N. M., Nkomo, V. T., LeReun, C. M.,...Kappetein, A. P. (2013). Aortic stenosis in the elderly: Disease prevalence and number of candidates for transcatheter aortic valve replacement: A meta-analysis and modeling study. *Clinical Research: Heart Valve Disease, 62*(11), 1002–1012. doi:10.1016/j.jacc.2013.05.015

Packer, M., Coats, A. J. S., Fowler, M. B., Katus, H. A., Krum, H., Mohacsi, P., ... DeMets, D. L. (2001). Carvedilol Prospective Randomized Cumulative Survival Study Group (COPERNICUS): Effect of carvedilol on survival in severe chronic heart failure. *New England Journal of Medicine, 344*(22), 1651–1658.

Pandya, A., Sy, S., Cho, S., Weinstein, M. C., & Gaziano, T. A. (2015). Cost-effectiveness of 10-year risk thresholds for initiation of statin therapy for primary prevention of cardiovascular disease. *Journal of the American Medical Association, 314*, 142–150. doi:10.1001/jama.2015.6822

Pasternak, R. C., Smith, S. C, Bairey Merz, C. N., Grundy, S. M., Cleeman, J. J., & Lenfant, L. (2002). ACC/AHA/NHLBI clinical advisory on the use and safety of statins. *Circulation, 106*, 1024–1028.

Pate, R. R., Blair, S. N., Durstine, J. L., Eddy, D. L., Hanson, P., Painter, P., ... Wolfe, L. A. (1991). *Guidelines for exercise testing and prescription* (4th ed.). Philadelphia, PA: Lea and Febiger.

Patel, H., Rosengren, A., & Ekman I. (2004). Symptoms in acute coronary syndromes: Does sex make a difference? *American Heart Journal, 148*, 27–33.

Patel, M. R., Mahaffey, K. W., Garg, J., Pan, G., Singer, D. E., Hacke, W.,...Califf, R. M. (2011). Rivaroxaban versus warfarin in nonvalvular atrial fibrillation. *New England Journal of Medicine, 365*, 883–891.

Pearson, T. A., Mensah, G. A., Alexander, R. W., Anderson, J. L., Cannon, R. O., Criqui, M.,...Vinicor, F. (2003). Markers of inflammation and cardiovascular disease: Application to clinical and public health practice: A statement for healthcare professionals from the Centers for Disease Control and Prevention and the American Heart Association. *Circulation, 107*(3), 499–511.

Pemu, P. I., & Ofili, E. (2008). Hypertension in women. Part I. *The Journal of Clinical Hypertension, 10*, 406–410.

Perez-Silva, A., & Merino, J. L. (2011). Tachyarrhythmias and pregnancy. *European Society of Cardiology, E-Journal Cardiology Practice, 9*(3). Retrieved from http://www.escardio.org/communities/councils/ccp/e-journal/volume9/Pages/Tachyarrhythmias-Pregnancy-Perez-Silva-A-Merino-JL.aspx#.UdO5JYN-_yo

Pignone, M., Fowler-Brown, A., Pletcher, M., & Tice, J. A. (2003). *Screening for asymptomatic coronary artery disease: A systematic review for the U.S. Preventative Services Task Force.* Systematic Evidence Reviews, Number 22. Prepared by the Research Triangle Institute—University of North Carolina Evidence-based Practice Center under Contract No. 290–97-0011. Rockville, MD: Agency for Healthcare Research and Quality. Retrieved from http://www.ahrq.gov/downloads/pub/prevent/pdfser/chdser.pdf

Pina, I. L., & Daoud, S. (2005). Heart failure in women. In N. K. Wenger & P. Collins (Eds.), *Women and heart disease* (2nd ed., pp. 419–431). London, UK: Taylor & Francis Group.

Pollack, C. V., Reilly, P. A., Eikelboom, J., Glund, S., Verhamme, P., Bernstein, R. A.,...Weitz, J. I. (2015). Idarucizumab for dabigatran reversal. *New England Journal of Medicine, 373*, 511–520. doi:10.1056/NEJMoa1502000

Preis, S. R., Hwang, S. J., Coady, S., Pencina, M. J., D'Agostino, R. B., Savage, P. J.,...Fox, C. S. (2009). Trends in all-cause and cardiovascular disease mortality among women and men with diabetes mellitus in the Framingham Heart Study, 1950–2005. *Circulation, 119*, 1728–1735.

Pursnani, A., Massaro, J. M., D'Agostino, R. B., O'Donnell, C. J., & Hoffmann, U. (2015). Guideline-based statin eligibility, coronary artery calcification, and cardiovascular events. *Journal of the American Medical Association, 314*, 134–141. doi:10.1001/jama.2015.7515

Redberg, R. F., & Shaw, L. J. (2003). Diagnosis of coronary artery disease in women. *Progress in Cardiovascular Diseases, 46*, 39–258.

Reis, S. E., Holubkov, R., Conrad Smith A. J., Kelsey, S. F., Sharaf, B. L., Reichek, N.,...Pepine, C. J.; WISE Investigators. (2001). Coronary microvascular dysfunction is highly prevalent in women with chest pain in the absence of coronary artery disease: Results from the NHBLI WISE study. *American Heart Journal, 141*, 735–741.

Ridker, P. M., Cook, N. R., Lee, I. M., Gordon, D., Gaziano, M., Manson, J. E.,...Buring, J. (2005). A randomized trial of low-dose aspirin in the primary prevention of cardiovascular disease in women. *New England Journal of Medicine, 352*, 1293–1304.

Ridker, P. M., Hennekens, C. H., Buring, J. E., & Rifai, N. (2000). C-reactive protein and other markers of inflammation in the prediction of cardiovascular disease in women. *New England Journal of Medicine, 342*, 836–843.

Ridker, P. M., Rifai, N., Rose, L., Buring, J. E., & Cook, N. R. (2002). Comparison of C-reactive protein and low-density lipoprotein cholesterol levels in the prediction of first cardiovascular events. *New England Journal of Medicine, 327*, 1557–1565.

Rifai, N., & Ridker, P. M. (2001). High-sensitivity C-reactive protein: A novel and promising marker of coronary heart disease. *Clinical Chemistry, 3*, 403–411.

Rosengren, A., & Hasdai, D. (2005). Acute coronary syndromes—thrombolysis, angioplasty. In N. K. Wenger & P. Collins (Eds.), *Women and heart disease* (2nd ed., pp. 237–247). London, UK: Taylor & Francis Group.

Rossouw, J. E., Anderson, G. L, Prentice, R. L., LaCroix, A. Z., Kooperberg, C., Stefanick, M. L.,...Ockene, J.; Writing Group for Women's Health Initiative Investigators. (2002). Risks and benefits of estrogen plus progestin in healthy postmenopausal women: Principal results from the Women's Health Initiative randomized controlled trial. *Journal of the American Medical Association, 288*, 321–333.

Sacco, R. L., Kasner, S. E., Broderick, J. P., Caplan, L. R., Connors, J. J., Culebras, A.,...Vinters, H. V.; American Heart Association Stroke Council, Council on Cardiovascular Surgery and Anesthesia; Council on Cardiovascular Radiology and Intervention; Council on Cardiovascular and Stroke Nursing; Council on Epidemiology and Prevention; Council on Peripheral Vascular Disease; Council on Nutrition, Physical Activity and Metabolism. (2013). An updated definition of stroke for the 21st century: A statement for healthcare professionals from the American Heart Association/American Stroke Association. *Stroke, 44*(7), 2064–2089.

Salisbury, A. C., Reid, K. J., Marso, S. P., Amin, A. P., Alexander, K. P., Wang, T. Y.,...Kosiborod, M. (2014). Blood transfusion during acute myocardial infarction: Association with mortality and variability across hospitals. *Journal of the American College of Cardiology, 64*, 811–819.

Salmon, J. F., & Roman, M. J. (2008). Subclinical atherosclerosis in rheumatoid arthritis and systemic erythematosus. *American Journal of Medicine, 121*(1), S3–S8.

Sanghavi, D., George, M., Bencic, S., Bleiberg, S., Alawa, N., Shaljian, M., & McClellan, M. B. (2014). Treating congestive heart failure and the role of payment reform. ERIES, The Merkin Series on Innovation in Care Delivery. Retrieved from http://www.brookings.edu/research/papers/2014/05/21-congestive-heart-failure-hospital-aco-case-study#recent_rr

Scanu, A. M., Lawn, R. M., & Berg, K. (1991). Lipoprotein(a) and atherosclerosis. *Annals of Internal Medicine, 111*, 209–218.

Scheinman, M. M., & Huang, S. (2003). The 1998 NASPE prospective catheter ablation registry. *Pacing and Clinical Electrophysiology, 23*, 1020–1028.

Schnohr, P., Lange, P., Scharling, H., & Jensen, J. S. (2006). Long-term physical activity in leisure time and mortality from coronary heart disease, stroke, respiratory diseases, and cancer: The Copenhagen City Heart Study. *European Journal of Cardiovascular Prevention and Rehabilitation, 13*(2), 173–179.

Schürks, M., Rist, P. M., Bigal, M. E., Buring, J. E., Lipton, R. B., & Kurth, T. (2009). Migraine and cardiovascular disease: Systematic review and meta-analysis. *BMJ, 339*, 1–11. doi:10.1136/bmj.b3914

Sesso, H. D., Lee, I. M., Gaziano, J. M., Rexrode, K. M., Glynn, R. J., & Buring, J. E. (2001). Maternal and paternal history of myocardial infarction and risk of cardiovascular disease in men and women. *Circulation, 104*, 393–398.

Shah, A. J., Ghasemzadeh, N., Zaragoza-Macias, E., Patel, R., Eapen, D. J., Neeland, I. J.,...Vaccarino, V. (2014). Sex and age differences in the association of depression with obstructive coronary artery disease and adverse cardiovascular events. *Journal of the American Heart Association, 3*, e000741. doi:10.1161/JAHA.113.000741

Shai, I., Rimm, E. B., Hankinson, S. E., Cannuscio, C., Curhan, G., Manson, J. E.,...Ma, J. (2005). Lipoprotein(a) and coronary heart disease among women: Beyond a cholesterol carrier? *European Heart Journal, 26*, 1633–1639.

Shaw, L. J., Bairey Merz, C. N., Pepine, C. J., Reis, S. E., Bittner, V., Kelsey, S. F.,...Sopko, G. (2006). Insights from the NHLBI-sponsored Women's Ischemia Syndrome Evaluation (WISE) study. Part I: Gender differences in traditional and novel risk factors, symptom evaluation, and gender-optimized diagnostic strategies. *Journal of the American College of Cardiology, 47*, S4–S20.

Shekelle, P. G., Rich, M. W., Morton, S. C., Atkinson, S. W., Tu, W., Maglione, M.,...Stevenson, L. W. (2003). Efficacy of angiotensin-converting enzyme inhibitors and beta-blockers in the management of left ventricular systolic dysfunction according to race, gender, and diabetic status: A meta-analysis of major clinical trials. *Journal of the American College of Cardiology, 41*, 1529–1538.

Shipton, B., & Wahba, H. (2001). Valvular heart disease: Review and update. *American Family Physician, 63*, 2201–2208.

Shoob, H., Croft, J., Ayala, C., & Mensah, G. (2006). Valvular heart disease surveillance in the United States, 1980–2000 (Abstract). *Journal of the American College of Cardiology, 47*(Suppl. A), 276.

Shotan, A., Ostrzega, E., Mehra, A., Johnson, J. V., & Elkayam, U. (1997). Incidence of arrhythmias in normal pregnancy and relation to palpitations, dizziness, and syncope. *American Journal of Cardiology, 79*(8), 1061–1064.

Shufelt, C. L., & Bairey Merz, C. N. (2009). Contraceptive hormone use and cardiovascular disease. *Journal of the American College of Cardiology, 53*(3), 221–231. doi:10.1016/j.jacc.2008.09.042

Shufelt, C. L., Thomson, L. E. J., Goykham, P., Agarwal, M., Mehta, P. K., Sedlak, T.,...Bairey Merz, C. N. (2013). Cardiac magnetic resonance imaging myocardial perfusion reserve index assessment in women with microvascular coronary dysfunction and reference controls. *Cardiovascular Diagnosis and Therapy, 3*(3), 153–160. doi:10.3978/j.issn.2223-3652.2013.08.02

Stauffer, B. D., Fullerton, C., Fleming, N., Ogola, G., Herrin, J., Stafford, P. M., & Ballard, D. J. (2014). Effectiveness and cost of a transitional care program for heart failure: A prospective study with concurrent controls. *Archives of Internal Medicine, 171*(14), 1238–1242. doi:10.1001/archinternmed.2011.274

Stewart, S., Ekman, I., Ekman, T., Odén, A., & Rosengren, A. (2010). Population impact of heart failure and the most common forms of cancer: A study of 1 162 309 hospital cases in Sweden (1988 to 2004). *Circulation. Cardiovascular Quality and Outcomes, 3*, 573–580.

Stewart, S., Hart, C. L., Hole, D. J., & McMurray, J. J. (2002). A population-based study of the long-term risks associated with atrial fibrillation: A 20-year follow-up of the Renfrew-Paisley study. *American Journal of Medicine, 113*, 359–364.

Stone, N., Robinson, J. G., Lichenstein, A. H., Bairey Merz, C. N., Blum, C. B., Eckel, R. H., & Goldberg, A. C. (2014). 2013 ACC/AHA Guideline on the treatment of blood cholesterol to reduce atherosclerotic cardiovascular risk in adults: A report of the American College of Cardiology/American Heart Association Task Force on Practice Guidelines. *Circulation, 129*, S1–S45. doi:10.1161/01.cir.0000437738.63853.7a

Suaya, J. A., Shepard, D. S., Normand, S. L., Ades, P. A., Prottas, J., & Stason WB. (2007). Use of cardiac rehabilitation by Medicare beneficiaries after myocardial infarction or coronary bypass surgery. *Circulation, 116*, 1653–1662.

Suk Danik, J., Rifai, N., Buring, J. E., & Ridker, P. M. (2006). Lipoprotein(a), measured with an assay independent of apolipoprotein(a) isoform size, and risk of future cardiovascular events among initially healthy women. *Journal of the American Medical Association, 296*(11), 1363–1370.

Taneja, T., Mahnert, B. W., Passman, R., Goldberger, J., & Kadish, A. (2001). Effects of sex an age on electrocardiographic and cardiac electrophysiological properties in adults. *Pacing and Clinical Electrophysiology, 24,* 16–21.

Thanassoulis, G., Peloso, G. M., Pencina, M. J., Hoffmann, U., Fox, C. S., Cupples, L. A.,…O'Donnell, C. J. (2012). A genetic risk score is associated with incident cardiovascular disease and coronary artery calcium: The Framingham Heart Study. *Circulation. Cardiovascular Genetics, 5,* 113–121.

Theal, M., Sleik, K., Anand, S., Yi, Q., Yusuf, S., & Lonn, E. (2004). Prevalence of mitral valve prolapse in ethnic groups. *Canadian Journal of Cardiology, 20*(5), 511–515.

Thompson, P., Buchner, D., Pina, I. L., Balady, G. J., Williams, M. A., Marcus, B. H.,…Wenger, N. K. (2003). Exercise and physical activity in the prevention and treatment of atherosclerotic cardiovascular disease: A statement from the Council on Clinical Cardiology (Subcommittee on Exercise, Rehabilitation, and Prevention) and the Council on Nutrition, Physical Activity, and Metabolism (Subcommittee on Physical Activity). *Circulation, 107,* 3109–3116.

Tietjen, G. E. (2007). Migraine as a systemic disorder. *Neurology, 68,* 1555–1556.

Tracy, C. M., Epstein, A. E., Darbar, D., DiMarco, J. P., Dunbar, S. B, Estes N.,…Varosy, P. D. (2012). 2012 ACCF/AHA/HRS focused update of the 2008 guidelines for device-based therapy of cardiac rhythm abnormalities: A report of the American College of Cardiology Foundation/American Heart Association Task Force on Practice Guidelines. *Journal of the American College of Cardiology, 60,* 1297–1313.

U.S. Department of Agriculture (USDA) and U.S. Department of Health and Human Services (USDHHS). (2010). *Dietary guidelines for Americans* (7th ed.). Washington, DC: U.S. Government Printing Office.

U.S. Department of Health and Human Services (USDHHS). (2014). *The health consequences of smoking—50 years of progress: A report of the surgeon general.* Atlanta, GA: U.S. Department of Health and Human Services, Centers for Disease Control and Prevention, National Center for Chronic Disease Prevention and Health Promotion, Office on Smoking and Health.

Vaccarino, V., Shah, A. J., Rooks, C., Ibeanu, I., Nye, J. A., Pimple, P.,…Raggi, P. (2014). Sex differences in mental stress-induced myocardial ischemia in young survivors of an acute myocardial infarction. *Psychosomatic Medicine, 76*(3), 71–80. doi:10.1097/PSY.0000000000000045

Vasan, R. S., Bieser, A., Seshadri, S., Larson, M. G., Kannel, W. B., D'Agostino, R. B., & Levy, D. (2002). Residual lifetime risk for developing hypertension in middle aged women and men: The Framingham Study. *Journal of the American Medical Association, 287*(8), 1003–1010.

Vasan, R. S., & Levy, D. (2000). Defining diastolic heart failure: A call for standardized diagnostic criteria. *Circulation, 101,* 2118–2121.

Volgman, A. S., Manankil, M. F., Mookherjee, D., & Trohman, R. G. (2009). Women with atrial fibrillation: Greater risk, less attention. *Gender Medicine, 6*(3), 419–432.

Wang, T. J., Pencina, M. J., Booth, S. L., Jacques, P. F., Ingelsson, E., Lanier, K.,…Vasan, R. S. (2010). Vitamin D deficiency and risk of cardiovascular disease. *Circulation, 117,* 503–511. doi:10.1161/CIRCULATIONAHA.107.706127

Wenger, N. (1999). Should women have a different risk assessment than men for the primary prevention of coronary heart disease? *Journal of Women's Health Gender Based Medicine, 8,* 465–467.

Wenger, N. (2012). Women and coronary heart disease: A century after Herrick: Understudied, underdiagnosed, and undertreated. *Circulation, 126,* 604–611.

Wenger, N. K. (2002). Women, heart failure, and heart failure therapies. *Circulation, 105,* 1526–1528.

Wexler, R., Elton, T., Pleister, A., & Feldman, D. (2009). Cardiomyopathy: An overview. *American Family Physician, 79*(9), 778–784.

Wilcox, J. E., Fonarow, G. C., Zhang, Y., Albert, N. M., Curtis, A. B., Gheorghiade, M.,…Yancy, C. W. (2014). Clinical effectiveness of cardiac resynchronization and implantable cardioverter-defibrillator therapy in men and women with heart failure: Findings from IMPROVE HF. *Circulation: Heart Failure, 7*(1), 146–153.

Wilson, W., Taubert, K. A., Gewitz, M., Lockhart, P. B., Baddour, L. M., Levison, M., . . . Durack, D. T. (2007). Prevention of infective endocarditis: Guidelines from the American Heart Association Rheumatic Fever, Endocarditis, and Kawasaki Disease Committee, Council on Cardiovascular Disease in the Young, and the Council on Clinical Cardiology, Council on Cardiovascular Surgery and Anesthesia, and the Quality of Care and Outcomes Research Interdisciplinary Working Group. *Circulation, 116*(15), 1736–1754.

Wolf, P. A., Abbott R. D., & Kannel, W. B. (1991). Atrial fibrillation as an independent risk factor for stroke: The Framingham Study. *Stroke, 22,* 983–988.

Yancy, C. W., Jessup, M., Bozkurt, B., Butler, J., Casey, D. E., Jr., Drazner, M. H.,…Wilkoff, B. L. (2013). 2013 ACCF/AHA guideline for the management of heart failure: A report of the American College of Cardiology Foundation/American Heart Association Task Force on Practice Guidelines. *Circulation, 128,* e240–e327.

Young, J. B., & Mills, R. M. (2001). *Clinical management of heart failure.* New York, NY: Professional Communications.

Young, W., Gofman, J. W., Tandy, R., & Waters, E. S. G. (1960). The quantitation of atherosclerosis III: The extent of correlation of degrees of atherosclerosis within and between the coronary and cerebral vascular beds. *American Journal of Cardiology, 6*(2), 300–308. doi:10.1016/0002–9149(60)90319–2

Yusef, P. F., Hawken, S., Ôunpuu, S., Dans, T., Avezum, A., Lanas, F.,…Lisheng, L. on behalf of the INTERHEART Study Investigators. (2004). Effect of potentially modifiable risk factors associated with myocardial infarction in 52 countries (the INTERHEART study): Case-control study. *Lancet, 364*(9438), 937–952. doi:http://dx.doi.org/10.1016/S0140–6736(04)17018–9. Retrieved from http://www.sciencedirect.com/science/article/pii/S0140673604170189

Zipes, D. P., Camm, A. J., Borggrefe, M., Buxton, A., Chaitman, B., Fromer, A.,…Tracy, C. (2006). ACC/AHA/ESC guidelines for management of patients with ventricular arrhythmias and the prevention of sudden cardiac death—Executive summary. A report of the American College of Cardiology/American Heart Association Task Force on Practice Guidelines and the European Society of Cardiology Committee for Practice Guidelines (Writing Committee to Develop Guidelines for the Management of Patients with Ventricular Arrhythmia and the Prevention of Sudden Cardiac Death). *Journal of the American College of Cardiology, 48,* 1064–1108.

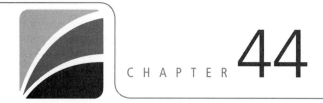

CHAPTER 44

Endocrine-Related Problems

Adrienne Berarducci

The endocrine system and nervous system control all physiologic processes in the body. The endocrine system acts as a chemical communication network that coordinates physiologic function through hormones that are released into the bloodstream from specific cells within ductless glands. Similar to other communication systems, the endocrine system is composed of transmitters (hormone-producing cells), signals (hormones), and receptors. Once in the circulation and extracellular fluid, hormones affect the function of target tissues. Hormonal mechanism of action is generally described by the particular effects they have on target cells. Table 44.1 depicts the effects of common endocrine disorders on target organs. Endocrine hormones are secreted into the bloodstream and bind to distant target cells. Paracrine hormones are those that exert an effect on cells of the organ from which they are released. Autocrine hormones affect the same cells from which they are produced. Hormones can be peptides or proteins (e.g., prolactin, adrenocorticotropic hormone [ACTH], insulin); steroids that are derived from cholesterol (e.g., sex hormones, adrenal steroids); amino acid derivatives (epinephrine, norepinephrine, thyroid hormones); or fatty acid derivatives (e.g., prostaglandins, leukotrienes).

All hormones bind selectively to receptors either in or on the surface of target cells. Intracellular receptors interact with hormones that modulate genetic function (e.g., corticosteroids, thyroid hormone). Hormones that bind with receptors on the target cell surface control enzyme activity or regulate ion channels (e.g., growth hormone, thyrotropin-releasing hormone).

HYPOTHALAMIC–PITUITARY RELATIONSHIPS

Endocrine organ functions within the body are modulated by pituitary hormones. An exception is secretion of insulin by the pancreas, which is primarily controlled by blood glucose level. Pituitary hormone secretion is controlled by the hypothalamus.

The hypothalamic–pituitary axis is the feedback system that controls interaction between the hypothalamus and pituitary gland. Input from all areas of the central nervous system is received by the hypothalamus to feed back information to the pituitary, which then releases specific hormones that stimulate endocrine glands throughout the body. The hypothalamus detects changes in circulating levels of hormones produced by these endocrine glands and either increases or decreases its stimulation of the pituitary to maintain homeostasis.

THYROID DISORDERS

The thyroid gland is one of the largest endocrine glands. It secretes thyroid hormone in response to signals received from the hypothalamus through the pituitary and functions through a negative feedback mechanism (Figure 44.1). Patients may present with signs of either thyroid excess or deficiency.

Hypothyroidism

DEFINITION AND SCOPE

Hypothyroidism results when the thyroid gland is unable to produce sufficient levels of thyroid hormone (T_3 and T_4). Primary hypothyroidism is relatively common, with incidence increasing with age. About 4.6% of the U.S. population 12 years of age and older have hypothyroidism (Lee, 2015). The exact prevalence varies by causative factors and is influenced by both geographic location and environmental factors. The incidence of Hashimoto's thyroiditis ranges from 0.3 to five per 1,000 and is 10 to 20 times more common in women than in men (Gardner & Shoback, 2011). Subclinical hypothyroidism is present in about 2% of the adult population and progresses to overt hypothyroidism in about 5% to 18% of patients (American Association of Clinical Endocrinologists [AACE] Thyroid Task Force, 2006).

ETIOLOGY

Hypothyroidism is a common endocrine disorder resulting from thyroid hormone deficiency. Most commonly, this is

TABLE 44.1	Clinical Manifestations of Endocrine Disorders
SIGNS AND SYMPTOMS	**POSSIBLE DISORDER**
Anemia	Adrenal problems, thyroid problems
Anorexia/nausea	Adrenal problems, diabetes (DKA and HHS), thyroid disorders
Menstrual changes	Adrenal problems, PCOS, thyroid conditions, menopause, hyperprolactinemia
Nervousness	Adrenal and thyroid problems
Weakness/fatigue	All endocrine problems
Bowel Changes	
Constipation	Diabetic neuropathy, hypothyroidism
Diarrhea	Hyperthyroidism
Hair Changes	
Hirsutism	PCOS, Cushing's syndrome
Hair loss	Hypothyroidism
Thermal Changes	
Fever	Adrenal and thyroid problems
Decreased temperature	Diabetes, thyroid
Weight Changes	
Loss	Adrenal (AI), thyroid (hyper), diabetes
Gain	Cushing's syndrome, thyroid (hypo)

AI, adrenal insufficiency; DKA, diabetic ketoacidosis; HHS, hyperosmolar hyperglycemia; PCOS, polycystic ovary syndrome.
Data from Gardner and Shoback (2011).

due to loss of functional thyroid tissue or a defect in hormone synthesis. It may also occur in response to pathology of the pituitary gland or hypothalamus.

Autoimmune thyroid disease (Hashimoto's thyroiditis) is the most common cause of hypothyroidism in the United States and other geographic areas where iodine intake is adequate. Worldwide, however, iodine deficiency remains the leading cause. Iatrogenic hypothyroidism can occur postpartum, following partial or complete surgical removal of the thyroid gland, from radioactive iodine (RAI) ablation, or may be drug-induced (e.g., lithium, alpha interferon, amiodarone, iodine). Secondary hypothyroidism is rare and occurs with disorders of the pituitary and hypothalamus that cause alterations in thyroid-stimulating hormone (TSH) production (e.g., pituitary adenoma). Congenital hypothyroidism occurs in infants born with a thyroid that is not

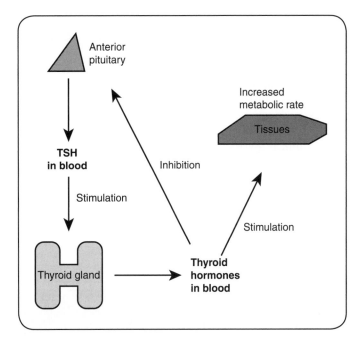

FIGURE 44.1
Thyroid negative feedback system.
TSH, thyroid-stimulating hormone.

fully developed or does not function properly. If untreated, congenital hypothyroidism can lead to mental dysfunction and growth failure. Newborns in the United States are generally screened for hypothyroidism as early detection and treatment can prevent these sequelae (Park & Chatterjee, 2005). Other causes are presented in Box 44.1.

RISK FACTORS

Numerous risk factors are associated with hypothyroidism (Table 44.2). They include: previous history of a thyroid disorder (e.g., goiter); partial or total thyroidectomy; radiation to the thyroid, neck, or chest; family history of thyroid disease; history of other autoimmune diseases (e.g., Sjogren's syndrome, rheumatoid arthritis, lupus); pernicious anemia; type 1 diabetes; Turner's syndrome; age greater than 60 years; or having been pregnant or delivered a baby within the past 6 months (Golden, Robinson, Saldanha, Anton, & Ladenson, 2009).

SYMPTOMS

Clinical manifestations of hypothyroidism result from reduced metabolic activity and metabolic rate (Zbhuvana, Krishnaswamy, & Periris, 2002). Thyroid hormone deficiency can cause multiple symptoms affecting a number of systems: central nervous, cardiovascular, musculoskeletal, and reproductive. Hypothyroidism has multiple symptoms that can vary greatly from person to person. Common symptoms include: fatigue; weight gain; a puffy face and/ or eyelids; dull facial expression; cold intolerance; joint and muscle pain; constipation; dry skin; dry, thinning hair; decreased sweating; heavy or irregular menstrual periods and impaired fertility; hoarseness; slow speech; blurred

BOX 44.1   CAUSES OF HYPOTHYROIDISM

Graves' disease (diffuse toxic goiter)
Plummer's disease (toxic multinodular goiter)
Toxic adenoma
Subacute thyroiditis
Subclinical thyroiditis
Iodine induced
Excessive pituitary production of thyroid-stimulating
    hormone

Data from Gardner and Shoback (2011); Bauer and McPhee (2006).

BOX 44.2   COMMON SYMPTOMS ASSOCIATED WITH HYPOTHYROIDISM

Fatigue
Weight gain
Puffy face and/or eyelids
Dull facial expression
Cold intolerance
Joint and muscle pain
Constipation
Dry skin and hair
Decreased sweating
Heavy or irregular menstrual periods
Impaired fertility
Hoarseness and/or slow speech
Blurred vision
Decreased hearing
Carpal tunnel syndrome
Depression
Confusion
Bradycardia

TABLE 44.2	Risk Factors for Primary and Secondary Hypothyroidism
TYPE OF HYPOTHYROIDISM	**SELECT CAUSES AND RISK FACTORS**
Primary	Older than 60 years Female History of hyperthyroidism or goiter Family history of hypothyroidism History of radiation therapy to neck Surgical removal of partial/complete thyroid Radioactive iodine ablation
Iatrogenic	Use of lithium Use of amiodarone Use of exogenous iodine Use of alpha interferon
Secondary	Pituitary adenoma Pituitary ablative therapy Peripheral thyroid hormone resistance
Congenital	Immature/underdeveloped thyroid gland

Data from Gardner and Shoback (2011); Park and Chatterjee (2005).

vision; decreased hearing; carpal tunnel syndrome; depression; confusion; and bradycardia (Box 44.2). However, hypothyroidism develops slowly and many patients do not notice symptoms.

Symptoms more specific to Hashimoto's disease are painless thyroid enlargement, subjective fullness in the throat, and exhaustion and transient neck pain with or without sore throat. Hypothyroidism is a contributor to hypercholesterolemia; therefore, individuals with hypercholesterolemia should be screened for hypothyroidism. In rare instances, severe, untreated hypothyroidism may lead to myxedema, an extreme form of hypothyroidism that results in an altered mental status, hypothermia, bradycardia, hypercarbia, and hyponatremia. Ascites, pericardial effusion, and cardiomegaly may be present and can lead to cardiogenic shock. This life-threatening condition occurs most commonly in individuals with hypothyroidism in whom the condition has not been diagnosed and who are exposed to physical stress, such as hypothermia, infection, myocardial infarction, stroke, or medical intervention (e.g., surgery or hypnotic drugs). Myxedema requires immediate hospitalization and intensive treatment.

EVALUATION/ASSESSMENT

History • Symptoms of hypothyroidism are generally very subtle and gradual and may be mistaken for symptoms of depression and other illnesses. With suspected hypothyroidism and health maintenance encounters, providers need to take a detailed, deliberate approach in evaluating risk factors and symptoms as the obscure presentation may make them unnoticeable in some patients.

Physical Examination • Evaluation of the woman with hypothyroidism may reveal subtle changes, and detection requires careful physical assessment. Physical signs may include: weight gain, slow speech and movements, xerosis, pallor, coarse and brittle hair, alopecia of varying degrees and patterns, dull and/or coarse facial expression, periorbital puffiness, macroglossia, simple or nodular goiter, bradycardia, hoarseness, edema, decreased systolic and increased diastolic blood pressure, and hyporeflexia with delayed relaxation phase. Other clinical manifestations can occur related to different causes of hypothyroidism such as pituitary enlargement or adenoma and with diffuse or multinodular goiter (Garber et al., 2012).

DIFFERENTIAL DIAGNOSES

Differential diagnoses can be extensive as many of the symptoms of hypothyroidism are nonspecific. Special consideration should be given to the possible presence of ischemic heart disease, liver abnormalities, and depression. Women presenting with menstrual irregularity and/or infertility may also have underlying metabolic disease. Other possible causes of the symptoms include eating disorders, HIV infections, sepsis, diabetes, and renal failure (Gardner & Shoback, 2011).

DIAGNOSTIC STUDIES

Third-generation TSH serum assays are considered the most sensitive screening tool for primary hypothyroidism. In the presence of TSH levels elevated above the reference range, measurement of serum-free thyroxine (T_4) or the free thyroxine index (FTI), which serves as a surrogate of the free hormone level, should be obtained. Measurement of triiodothyronine (T_3) is not recommended.

Elevated TSH with decreased T_4 or FTI indicates hypothyroidism. Elevated TSH (usually 4.5–10.0 mIU/L) with normal free T_4 or FTI is considered mild disease or subclinical hypothyroidism (Garber et al., 2012).

The complete blood count and metabolic profile may also exhibit abnormalities in patients with hypothyroidism and may include: anemia, dilutional hyponatremia, hyperlipidemia, reversible increased creatinine, and elevated transaminases and creatinine kinase (Kreisman & Hennessey, 1999).

Although no universal screening guidelines exist for thyroid disease in adults, the American Thyroid Association (ATA) recommends screening at age 35 years and every 5 years thereafter, with closer attention to high-risk individuals, such as pregnant women, women older than 60 years, individuals with type 1 diabetes or other autoimmune disorders, and those with a history of neck irradiation (Ladenson et al., 2000).

TREATMENT/MANAGEMENT OF PRIMARY HYPOTHYROIDISM

The goal of hypothyroidism treatment is to restore a state of euthyroidism, accomplished with thyroid replacement therapy. As with all treatment, it should be tailored to the individual. Education should provide an understanding of the disease and its treatment. Referral to an endocrinologist is appropriate for those in whom euthyroidism is difficult to achieve (Box 44.3).

Self-Management Measures • Self-management measures are most often geared toward managing the many symptoms that patients can experience with hypothyroidism (Table 44.3). Women who experience significant fatigue need to be cautioned to pace their activities and achieve adequate rest, especially until a euthyroid state is achieved. Measures for managing constipation may include increasing fluids, increasing dietary fiber, and using stool softeners.

Complementary and Alternative Medicine • The extant scientific literature does not recommend complementary

---

BOX 44.3   PATIENTS WITH HYPOTHYROIDISM WHO MAY REQUIRE REFERRAL TO ENDOCRINOLOGY

Patients younger than 18 years
Patients who are unresponsive to therapy
Patients who are pregnant
Patients with cardiovascular disease
Patients with other endocrine disorders
Patients with thyroid nodules

---

and alternative medicine (CAM) modalities specifically for hypothyroidism. Some women use CAM therapies to manage symptoms of the disorder such as fatigue, weight changes, and hair and skin changes; however, their use should be discussed with their clinician.

Pharmacotherapeutics • Updated guidelines from Jonklaas et al. (2014) indicate that levothyroxine (LT_4) as monotherapy remains the treatment of choice for hypothyroidism. Levothyroxine produces stable levels of both T_3 and T_4. The dosage is approximately 1.6 mcg/kg/d, taken every morning on an empty stomach. When initiating levothyroxine, the patient's weight, lean body mass, pregnancy status, etiology of thyroid disorder, degree of TSH elevation, age, and comorbidities, including the presence of cardiac disease, are considered.

Clinical benefits of LT_4 replacement can begin to be appreciated in as little as 3 to 5 days and generally plateau at 6 weeks. Until TSH levels are within target range, 1.0 to 2.0 U/mL, LT_4 dosing changes are made every 6 to 8 weeks. Serum TSH levels within the normal reference range commonly require several months of monitoring and dose titration. Dosing aspects of LT_4 treatment are depicted in Table 44.4.

Once the LT_4 dose is stabilized, annual monitoring of serum TSH and clinical evaluation is maintained. Overtreatment must be monitored and dose reductions initiated promptly. Women need to be aware of symptoms of overtreatment to avoid potential health threats, such as tachycardia, palpitations, angina, increased sweating, nervousness, atrial fibrillation, increased nervousness, fatigue, headache irritability, insomnia, and tremors. Excessive LT_4 can also cause bone loss over time.

Consideration should be given to causes other than hypothyroidism in patients who remain symptomatic despite normalization of their TSH level. This may indicate dysfunctional conversion of T_4 to T_3 in the brain. Combination LT_4/liothyronine (LT_3) therapy may benefit these individuals; however, this is rarely observed.

Considerations for Special Populations • The bioequivalence of various brands of levothyroxine can also be problematic. Because bioequivalence has been based on total T_4 measurements instead of TSH levels, bioequivalence does not equal therapeutic equivalence. The woman should be

TABLE 44.3	Clinical Findings in Hypothyroidism	
SYSTEM	**SYMPTOMS**	**SIGNS**
General	Fatigue/lethargy	Periorbital edema
	Weakness	Pallor
Endocrine	Swelling of thyroid	Goiter
	Menorrhagia	Galactorrhea
Metabolic	Cold intolerance	Hypothermia
	Weight gain	Obesity
Psychiatric	Depression	Depression
Musculoskeletal	Arthralgia, myalgia	
Skin	Decreased perspiration	Brittle nails
	Hair loss	Reduced skin turgor, alopecia/coarse hair, carotenemia
Gastrointestinal	Constipation	Megacolon
	Decreased appetite	
Respiratory	Snoring	Hypoventilation, sleep apnea
Cardiovascular bradycardia	Dyspnea	Hypertension,[a] pericardial effusion, cardiomegaly/CHF
Nervous system	Paresthesia	Bradykinesia
	Numbness	Distal sensory loss
	Unsteadiness	Ataxia
	Reduced mentation	Dementia, hyporeflexia, pseudomyotonia, visual disturbances[b]

[a]Diastolic hypertension.
[b]Findings in secondary hypothyroidism.
CHF, congestive heart failure.
Reprinted with permission from Guha, Krishnaswamy, and Peiris (2002).

TABLE 44.4	Dosing Aspects of LT$_4$ Treatment
POPULATION	**DOSING OF LT$_4$**
Young, healthy patients	Start at anticipated full replacement dose
Elderly patients	One fourth to one half of the anticipated full replacement dose and titrate slowly after no less than 4 to 6 weeks
Known ischemic heart disease	One fourth to one half of the anticipated full replacement dose and titrate slowly after no less than 4 to 6 weeks
Mild to moderate hypothyroidism	Start LT$_4$ at 50 to 75 mcg daily

LT$_4$, levothyroxine.
Data from Jonklaas et al. (2014).

maintained on a consistent brand of levothyroxine. If the brand is changed for any reason, then TSH levels should be repeated in 4 to 6 weeks and the dose adjusted as needed to maintain euthyroidism (Jonklaas et al., 2014).

Several conditions may require special dosing and monitoring of therapy for hypothyroidism. If dosage of levothyroxine is much higher than anticipated to maintain normal range TSH, consider evaluation for gastrointestinal disorders that may interfere with absorption. These include disorders such as *Helicobacter pylori*–related peptic ulcer disease and gastritis, gastroparesis, and celiac disease. Significant weight changes should also prompt closer patient monitoring.

TSH and LT$_4$ monitoring requirements may increase when initiating or discontinuing estrogen because exogenous estrogen may affect levothyroxine requirements. Numerous other pharmacotherapeutics can interfere with thyroxine metabolism and require closer monitoring of symptoms and TSH levels upon initiation, maintenance, and discontinuation. They include: calcium supplements, phenytoin, phenobarbital, sertraline, carbenzamine, rifampin, proton pump inhibitors, tyrosine kinase inhibitors, bile acid sequestrants, selective estrogen receptor dulators, and cytoprotective agents.

Untreated hypothyroidism in pregnancy increases maternal and fetal risks, such as hypertension, preeclampsia, anemia, cardiac dysfunction, spontaneous abortion, low birth weight, and fetal death (see Chapter 38). Even mild, untreated maternal hypothyroidism has been associated with cognitive dysfunction in the child. Thyroid hormone demand increases by 30% to 50% during pregnancy and will likely require an increased dose of levothyroxine. Levothyroxine has been assigned to pregnancy category A by the FDA and replacement when warranted should be maintained during pregnancy. A naturally occurring hormone, it is normally found in both maternal and fetal circulation. Levothyroxine is excreted into human milk in small amounts. In replacement doses, it is not expected to cause adverse effects in the nursing infant. The manufacturer recommends that caution be used when administering levothyroxine to nursing women. However, adequate replacement doses of levothyroxine are needed to maintain normal lactation.

Current recommendations indicate that pregnant women should receive levothyroxine replacement therapy with the dose titrated to achieve a TSH concentration within the trimester-specific reference range. During the first half of pregnancy, serum TSH should be monitored every 4 months with levothyroxine dosing adjustments to maintain the trimester-specific TSH range. TSH should be reevaluated during the second half of pregnancy. For women already taking levothyroxine for hypothyroidism, two additional doses of their current levothyroxine dose per week with several days' separation may be started as soon as pregnancy is confirmed (Stagnaro-Green et al., 2011).

Elderly women with new onset hypothyroidism should be started at a dose of 25 to 50 mcg daily and increased slowly by 12.5 to 25 mcg every 6 to 8 weeks. Reference ranges of serum TSH levels are higher in older populations (e.g., above 65 years), and so higher serum TSH targets may be appropriate for elderly women (Jonklass et al., 2014).

TREATMENT/MANAGEMENT OF SUBCLINICAL HYPOTHYROIDISM

Significant controversy persists regarding the treatment of subclinical hypothyroidism (Cooper & Biondi, 2012). Studies have suggested that treatment of these patients improves symptoms, prevents progression to overt hypothyroidism, and may be cardioprotective. However, an evidence-based consensus statement issued by the AACE, American Thyroid Association (ATA), and the Endocrine Society (TES) (2004) recommends against routine treatment if the TSH is between 4.5 and 10 m/U/L. In a separate statement, they recommended measuring thyroid antibodies in the presence of elevated TSH without symptoms. If antibodies are present and the TSH is above 5 m/U/L, treatment should be considered. Although patients are usually asymptomatic, there are potential associated risks. Thus, these patients should be followed every 3 months until they are stable, as evidenced by both clinical and laboratory evaluation. Individualized care was recommended in both statements (Gharib et al., 2004).

Hyperthyroidism

DEFINITION AND SCOPE

Hyperthyroidism is characterized by overproduction of triiodothyronine (T_3) and/or thyroxine (T_4). Symptoms develop in response to the effects of the excessive circulating thyroid hormone levels. The prevalence in the general population is low with peak incidence between the ages of 20 to 40 years (AACE Thyroid Task Force, 2006; Gardner & Shoback, 2011). Subclinical hyperthyroidism affects about 2% of the adult population and is thought to be related to oversensitivity of the pituitary gland in responding to minor elevations in T_3 and T_4. The clinical significance relates to progression to overt hyperthyroidism and possible effects on the cardiac and skeletal systems. In the older patient with subclinical hyperthyroidism, the risk of atrial fibrillation is increased threefold (AACE Thyroid Task Force, 2006; Gardner & Shoback, 2011).

ETIOLOGY

The most common causes include Graves' disease (an autoimmune disorder), toxic multinodular goiter, and toxic adenoma. A variety of disorders cause hyperthyroidism (Box 44.4), with the most common being Graves' disease,

---

BOX 44.4   CAUSES OF HYPERTHYROIDISM

Graves' disease (diffuse toxic goiter)
Plummer's disease (toxic multinodular goiter)
Toxic adenoma
Subacute thyroiditis
Subclinical thyroiditis
Excessive pituitary production of thyroid-stimulating hormone
Taking large amounts of tetraiodothyronine (through dietary supplements or medication)
Tumors of the ovaries
Tumors of the thyroid or pituitary gland

Source: Data from Gardner and Shoback (2011).

---

which accounts for 70% to 80% of the cases. More common in women than men, hyperthyroidism tends to run in families.

SYMPTOMS

Many of the presenting symptoms of hyperthyroidism are nonspecific: fatigue, nervousness, irritability, and heat intolerance with increased sweating are found in 80% to 96% of patients. Other symptoms may include weakness, weight loss, dyspnea, depression, alteration in appetite, menstrual irregularities, infertility, and increasing frequency of and changes in stool.

EVALUATION/ASSESSMENT

Physical examination includes a thorough assessment of the neck and thyroid gland. About 90% of patients with Graves' disease who are younger than 50 years will have a firm, diffuse goiter. Any thyroid nodule should be evaluated (see section "Thyroid Nodule"). Thyroid tenderness may indicate the presence of thyroiditis and is not usually seen in uncomplicated Graves' disease. About 75% of patients with Graves' disease will have a thyroid bruit (Gharib et al., 2010; Gardner & Shoback, 2011).

On general inspection, the hair may be fine and silky. Nails may develop ridges and plates may have an irregular separation from the bed (onycholysis). Skin may be hyperpigmented, especially over the extensor surfaces of the elbows, knees, and small joints. Tachycardia (resting heart rate over 90 beats per minute) is found in about 96% of patients with hyperthyroidism and about 20% have atrial fibrillation, either of which may be experienced subjectively as palpitations. Increased cardiac output may be reflected by wide pulse pressure when measuring the blood pressure, and murmurs are common as well. A neurological exam may reveal hand tremors or hyperactive reflexes. If tremor is not readily seen, a piece of paper is placed on the outstretched hand; the tremors can then be seen easily (Bahn et al, 2011; Hueston, 2011; Ladenson, 2010; Mandel, Larson, & Davies, 2011)

A detailed eye examination is needed as hyperthyroidism is associated with several ocular abnormalities. The patient should be evaluated for lid lag, stare, periorbital edema, and proptosis. Ophthalmic involvement in hyperthyroidism is due to lymphocyte and fluid infiltration into the periorbital tissues, causing an inflammatory response. This compresses the optic nerve and may lead to loss of vision (Hueston, 2011; Ladenson, 2010).

DIFFERENTIAL DIAGNOSES

The main differential diagnoses to consider include: TSH-induced hyperthyroidism, which can be caused by a pituitary adenoma secreting TSH or a problem in the feedback mechanism; euthyroid hyperthyroxinemia, caused by serum thyroid hormone-binding protein abnormalities; and low serum levels of TSH without hyperthyroidism, which may be seen in patients recovering from hyperthyroidism, with nonthyroid illnesses (e.g., requiring high dose glucocorticoid therapy), and with central hypothyroidism.

DIAGNOSTIC STUDIES

As with hypothyroidism, laboratory evaluation of hyperthyroidism begins with TSH levels. Hyperthyroidism is suggested when TSH levels are lower than normal; total T_3 (TT_3) and FT_4 levels should then be measured to aid in diagnosis. While not usually measured, thyroid-stimulating immunoglobulin (TSI) may be helpful, especially during pregnancy. Immunoglobulins are present in both Graves' disease and thyroiditis. Ultrasound is sometimes performed to measure the size of the entire thyroid gland, as well as any masses within it. It may also distinguish if the mass is solid or cystic. CT or MRI of the head is done if a pituitary tumor is suspected. Thyroid radioiodine uptake and scan can help determine the cause. Subclinical hyperthyroidism is identified in the instance of low TSH with normal T_3 and T_4 levels in asymptomatic women (Bahn et al., 2011).

TREATMENT/MANAGEMENT OF OVERT CLINICAL HYPERTHYROIDISM

Once diagnosed, three treatment options are available: surgery, antithyroid medications, and RAI. Treatment is determined based on the etiology and the woman's preference. Each option carries its own set of benefits and risks (Gardner & Shoback, 2011).

Several presentations require referral. Women with ocular involvement in Graves' disease require referral to an ophthalmologist for evaluation and long-term follow-up. Urgent referral is needed for those with eye pain, injected sclerae, or a change in vision. Radioactive sodium iodine (I_{131}) may exacerbate Graves' ophthalmopathy; these women should be referred to an endocrinologist. If surgery is the best treatment option, referral to a surgeon is warranted. Thyroid storm (Box 44.5) is a medical emergency and requires immediate referral (Bahn et al., 2011; Gardner & Shoback, 2011).

Self-Management Measures • Self-management measures are designed to reduce symptoms. Women should avoid caffeine and other stimulants as these may make palpitations

---

BOX 44.5   SIGNS OF THYROID STORM

Increased temperature up to 104°F
Unexplained jaundice
Tachycardia
CHF
Atrial fibrillation

CNS Symptoms

Agitation
Delirium
Seizure/coma

GI Symptoms

Nausea
Vomiting
Diarrhea

CHF, congestive heart failure; CNS, central nervous system; GI, gastrointestinal.
Data from Gardner and Shoback (2011).

---

and tremors worse. Once therapy has been initiated, careful balancing of diet and exercise is needed as weight gain is common.

Complementary and Alternative Medicine • Chinese herbal medicines are sometimes used instead of or in combination with antithyroid medications. These medicines generally include a combination of multiple plant and root products. The herbs are intended to weaken thyroxine's biological effects, reduce transformation of T_4 to T_3, and modulate the immune system or sympathetic nerve function (Chen, 2008). Although demonstrated to improve symptoms and reduce relapse rates and adverse effects (i.e., agranulocytosis) in one meta-analysis, strong evidence supporting the use of Chinese herbs for hyperthyroidism is lacking (Zeng, Yuan, Wu, Yan, & Su, 2007).

Surgery • Surgical management may be the treatment of choice for women with a very enlarged gland or multinodular goiter, especially in the presence of dysphagia. Surgery is the treatment of choice for those with Graves' opthalmopathy as I_{131} often worsens the ophthalmopathy. Patients are treated first with antithyroid hormones to reach a euthyroid state. Potential complications include hypoparathyroidism and vocal cord injury and occur in about 1% of patients. Near total thyroidectomy is usually done and will induce hypothyroidism, requiring lifetime thyroid replacement. If too much of the thyroid gland is left behind, Graves' disease can recur (Bahn et al., 2011).

Pharmacotherapeutics

Antithyroid Medications. Antithyroid medications are given in an attempt to lower the overall thyroid level by suppressing production of thyroid hormone. The most common medications used in managing hyperthyroidism are methimazole (MMI) and propylthiouracil (PTU). The starting dose depends on the severity of the hyperthyroidism. Prior to initiating antithyroid drug therapy, a baseline complete blood count, including white count with differential, and a liver profile including bilirubin and transaminases should be evaluated.

Currently, it is recommended that MMI be used for the treatment of Graves' disease in most patients. PTU is not recommended for initial use except during the first trimester of pregnancy when it is preferred; in the presence of thyroid storm; and in patients with minor reactions to MMI who refuse RAI therapy or surgery. At the initiation of MMI therapy, 10 to 20 mg daily will generally restore euthyroidism, following which the dose can be titrated to a maintenance level of 5 to 10 mg daily. Risks of major side effects are lower with MMI as compared with PTU, and MMI can be given as a single daily dose. Due to a shorter duration of action, PTU is generally administered two or three times daily. Depending on the severity of hyperthyroidism, starting doses generally range between 50 and 150 mg three times daily. Once clinical findings and thyroid function tests indicate euthyroid state, reduction of PTU dose to 50 mg two to three times daily is usually sufficient (Bahn et al., 2011).

Patients need to be monitored for adverse reactions. The most common side effect is a transient skin rash that can be managed with antihistamines. Although rare, agranulocytosis is a serious side effect requiring discontinuation of the medication. Symptoms of agranulocytosis include sore throat, fever, painful mouth ulcers, anal ulcerations, depressed immune response, and increased bacterial infections, and should be evaluated with complete blood count and red blood cell indices. The woman should stop her medication and call her clinician if these symptoms develop (Bahn et al., 2011).

RAI Therapy. The goal of RAI (I_{131}) treatment is to ablate the thyroid tissue. Because it works quickly, RAI tends to minimize the morbidity associated with hyperthyroidism. As with surgery, pretreatment with antithyroid medications is frequently used to achieve a euthyroid state, especially in older patients. Because most patients (80%) become hypothyroid following I_{131} treatment, thyroid replacement for life is generally needed. A pregnancy test should be obtained within 48 hours prior to treatment in any female of childbearing age who is to be treated with RAI. Verification of a negative pregnancy test prior to RAI is mandatory. Patients choosing I_{131} must be counseled to avoid close contact with children less than 8 years of age and with pregnant women. Breastfeeding is contraindicated for at least 2 weeks after receiving treatment (Bahn et al., 2011; Gardner & Shoback, 2011).

Beta-blockers may be used with I_{131} as adjunctive therapy to provide symptomatic relief and help stabilize the woman. Nondihydropyridine calcium-channel blockers are helpful if she cannot tolerate beta-blockers due to side effects such as light-headedness or drowsiness. These medications are discontinued as soon as she is euthyroid.

Considerations for Special Populations • Pregnancy presents some special concerns. I_{131} is contraindicated in both pregnancy and breastfeeding. Antithyroid medications may cross the placenta and oversuppression can adversely affect the fetus. PTU is the medication of choice and is given in the lowest possible dose to maintain euthyroidism, which is important to both maternal and fetal well-being. The need for antithyroid medications usually decreases during pregnancy and so close monitoring of TSH, T_3, and T_4 is advised. Hyperthyroidism in pregnant women is usually managed in collaboration with an endocrinologist.

TREATMENT/MANAGEMENT OF SUBCLINICAL HYPOTHYROIDISM

Management of subclinical hyperthyroidism is a widely debated subject as there is a paucity of long-term studies of subclinical hyperthyroidism treatment. Subclinical hyperthyroidism is defined by a low serum TSH level in the presence of normal range thyroid hormone levels. Management requires careful monitoring of thyroid function through clinical and laboratory evaluation. Treatment is currently recommended for patients 65 years of age and older, and in the presence of osteoporosis and atrial fibrillation. If treated, antithyroid drugs are usually used; however I_{131} is also an option (Palacios, Pascual-Corrales, & Galofre, 2012).

Thyroid Nodule

DEFINITION AND SCOPE

Thyroid nodules are a fairly common clinical finding in the United States. Based on palpation alone, current estimates suggest that prevalence is approximately 3% to 7% of adults. Approximately 300,000 new thyroid nodules are diagnosed annually in the United States. It is usually found during routine physical examination or as an incidental finding during color doppler studies of the carotid artery or other imaging studies performed for unrelated reasons.

ETIOLOGY

Thyroid nodules can be either benign or malignant, and hence, the major reason for evaluation is to exclude a malignant nodule. Causes of thyroid nodules include benign nodular goiter, chronic lymphocytic thyroiditis, simple or hemorrhagic cysts, follicular adenomas, subacute thyroiditis, and various histological primary and metastatic carcinomas (Gharib et al., 2010).

RISK FACTORS

A history of previous diseases or treatments involving the head and neck, recent pregnancy, and rapidity of onset and rate of growth of the neck mass should be documented. The malignancy rate is three- to fourfold higher for thyroid nodules found during childhood and adolescence as compared with adults. Thyroid cancer risk is also higher in males and in the elderly.

SYMPTOMS

Although clinical signs help with risk assessment, most women with thyroid nodules experience little or no symptoms.

EVALUATION/ASSESSMENT

A family history is important for the diagnosis as both benign and malignant nodules can be familial. It is critical to ascertain family history of thyroid cancer, familial adenomatous polyposis, and multiple endocrine neoplasia syndrome as these disorders are associated with a very high risk of development of thyroid cancer.

DIAGNOSTIC STUDIES

High-resolution ultrasound imaging, third-generation serum thyrotropin (TSH) assay, and fine-needle aspiration (FNA) biopsy are the basis for evaluation and management of thyroid nodules.

TREATMENT/MANAGEMENT

All patients with new and/or changing nodules should be referred to an endocrinologist for further evaluation and FNA (Gharib et al., 2010).

■ PARATHYROID DISEASE

Parathyroid hormone (PTH) is secreted from four small glands adjacent to the thyroid gland. Secretion is based on a feedback loop. PTH aids in regulating serum calcium levels. Any disruption in PTH secretion can cause serum calcium concentrations to fluctuate outside of the narrow normal range of 8.5 to 10.5 mg/dL (normal range may vary by laboratory) (Shoback, Sellmeyer, & Bikle, 2011).

Maintaining this concentration requires the coordinated effects of multiple systems and organs such as the kidneys, intestines, and skeleton (Shoback, Sellmeyer, & Bikle, 2011). When plasma calcium levels fall, PTH secretion increases. PTH stimulates more efficient renal calcium reabsorption and intestinal calcium absorption. Excessive amounts of PTH activate bone remodeling to support extracellular fluid calcium at the expense of skeletal integrity (Moe, 2008).

Hyperparathyroidism

DEFINITION, SCOPE, AND ETIOLOGY

Hyperparathyroidism (HPT), overactivity of the parathyroid glands, is the most common cause of hypercalcemia and is present in about 1% of the adult population, but is more common in older postmenopausal women. Women have a two- to fourfold increased likelihood of developing HPT over men. The most common cause is a single adenoma of the parathyroid gland. Other causes of HPT include vitamin D deficiency, chronic kidney disease, hyperplasia of one or more of the parathyroid glands, and parathyroid cancer, although this is rare and accounts for less than 1% of all cases.

SYMPTOMS

The clinical manifestations of HPT involve multiple systems. The most common features are nephrolithiasis, bone fracture, constipation, abnormal cognitive function, depression, and hypertension (El-Hajj Fuleihan, 2014). Hence, the mnemonic "moans, groans, stones, bones and thrones with psychic overtones."

EVALUATION/ASSESSMENT AND DIAGNOSTIC STUDIES

About 90% of those with HPT have an elevated PTH. Serum calcium levels are also abnormally high. Because low vitamin D levels are also associated with HPT, evaluating serum 25-OH vitamin D is appropriate (Marcocci & Cetani, 2011).

TREATMENT/MANAGEMENT

The treatment of choice is surgical removal of the abnormal gland, which is curative 95% to 98% of the time. Surgical complications can include laryngeal nerve damage, recurrent HPT, or permanent hypoparathyroidism. Surgery is suggested if serum calcium levels are greater than 12 mg/dL on multiple occasions or if there is a 20% rise from baseline. Serum calcium and bone mineral density are evaluated annually after surgery. Medications are not used to treat HPT (Bilezikian, Khan, & Potts, 2009; El-Hajj Fuleihan, 2014).

Hypoparathyroidism

DEFINITION AND ETIOLOGY

The most common cause of hypoparathyroidism, reduced function of the parathyroid glands, is neck surgery, such as surgery on the thyroid gland or neck neoplasms. Within hours of parathyroid gland removal, calcium concentration decreases while inorganic phosphorus increases. Urinary calcium excretion also increases. Although idiopathic disease is rare, if present, it is associated with autoimmune problems in multiple endocrine glands (Bilezikian, Khan, Potts, Brandi, et al., 2011; Gardner & Shoback, 2011).

SYMPTOMS, EVALUATION/ASSESSMENT, AND DIAGNOSTIC STUDIES

The history seeks information about risk factors and symptoms such as muscle cramps, dermatological problems (dry skin, brittle nails, dermatitis), and cataract development. Clinical signs of hypoparathyroidism include neuromuscular irritability such as a positive Chvostek's or Trousseau's sign. Diagnosis is made with a low or low-normal serum PTH (Gardner & Shoback, 2011).

TREATMENT/MANAGEMENT

Hypoparathyroidism is treated with calcium and vitamin D supplementation. If acute, 10% calcium gluconate can be given intravenously (Gardner & Shoback, 2011; Moe, 2008).

Long-term daily therapy is 1.5 to 3 g of oral elemental calcium with vitamin D (up to 1,000 IU). The goal is a serum calcium level between 8 and 9 mg/dL.

■ METABOLIC SYNDROME

Definition and Scope

Metabolic syndrome is a clustering of several cardiometabolic risk factors that greatly increase the risk of cardiovascular disease (CVD) and type 2 diabetes. The syndrome, as described by both the WHO and National Cholesterol Education Program (NCEP), includes a group of disorders: hyperinsulinemia/abnormal glucose tolerance, obesity, dyslipidemia, hypertension, and proinflammatory, prothrombotic state.

There are an estimated 47 million individuals (approximately 24%) with metabolic syndrome in the United States. The overall prevalence of 23.7% changes with age, affecting 6.7% of young adults (20–29 years), 43.5% of adults aged 60 to 69 years, and 42% of those older than 70 years. Ethnicity is also a factor: more Hispanic Americans are affected (31.9%) than non-Hispanic Whites (23.8%) and African Americans (21.6%). Gender differences place African American and Hispanic women at highest risk (Ford, Giles, & Dietz, 2002; Meigs, 2015).

Etiology

Several explanations have been suggested that describe the etiology of the metabolic syndrome. The American Association of Endocrinology (AAE) stresses the importance of insulin resistance; however, the AAE does not recognize obesity as a component of metabolic syndrome (Einhorn, Reaven, & Cobin, 2009). Initial definition by the WHO considered insulin resistance a major component of the metabolic syndrome (Alberti & Zimmet, 1998). NCEP: ATP III (2001), which developed a widely accepted definition, suggests equal weight to any of the components of the syndrome: fasting blood glucose, glucose intolerance, obesity (measured as waist circumference), hypertension, and dyslipidemia. The International Diabetic Federation (IDF) considers central obesity, insulin resistance, and a proinflammatory/prothombotic state as important causative factors in the metabolic syndrome (Nesto, 2003).

The underlying pathophysiology of metabolic syndrome is insulin resistance accompanying abnormal adipose deposition and function. Defined as a state in which the concentration of insulin is associated with an abnormal glucose response, this can lead to several pathogenic conditions (Freeman, 2006). Clinically, there is an imbalance of the amount of insulin required to maintain normal glucose levels, and the body is unable to control both hepatic glucose output and muscle glucose utilization (Masharani & German, 2011). Insulin regulation of protein and fat metabolism are disrupted.

Obesity and disorders of the adipose tissue play an important role in metabolic syndrome. Fat distribution and overall total body weight may be critical factors in pathogenesis. Obesity contributes to insulin resistance and to both hypertension and dyslipidemia. Excessive visceral adipose tissue releases several protein substances. Obesity also plays a role in endothelial dysfunction. The proinflammatory state is related to elevated C-reactive protein (CRP), fibrinogen, and other cytokines (Bentley-Lewis, Koruda, & Seely, 2007).

Hypertension is also related to insulin resistance, likely through sodium reabsorption pathways. The increase in sympathetic outflow and sodium reabsorption is thought to counter the vasodilatory effect, causing elevated blood pressure (Meigs, 2015). Insulin resistance causes an abnormality in the regulation of free fatty acids (FFA). This can lead to an increase in plasma lipid levels that may be diverted to the liver, promoting fatty liver disease or nonalcoholic steatohepatitis (NASH). Lipid levels increase, especially triglycerides (TG) and very low-density lipoprotein cholesterol (VLDL-C), while high-density lipoprotein cholesterol (HDL-C) levels remain low, promoting atherogenic dyslipidemia.

Several independent factors also play a role in the pathogenesis of metabolic syndrome, including age and ovarian failure in women. As estrogen levels decline in postmenopausal women, intra-abdominal fat increases, the lipid profile shifts in an atherogenic direction, and insulin resistance increases as observed by a rise in both glucose and insulin levels (Bentley-Lewis, Koruda, & Seely, 2007).

Risk Factors

Risk factors for metabolic syndrome are related to each of the components and to the syndrome overall. It remains unclear whether metabolic syndrome has a single cause, although it appears that multiple risk factors precipitate the syndrome. Insulin resistance and central obesity appear to be the most important precipitating factors. In most individuals, metabolic syndrome is lifestyle mediated, with those following a high fat, high concentrated sugar diet and having a sedentary lifestyle at greatest risk. Other risk factors include genetic predisposition, increased age, ethnicity, increased weight, postmenopausal status, low household income, smoking, and soft drink consumption (Alberti et al., 2009). Conflicting evidence exists regarding alcohol consumption and metabolic syndrome. Excessive alcohol intake is associated with numerous illnesses, although studies indicate that light to moderate drinking has a cardioprotective effect. There is a need for more prospective studies to determine the relationship between alcohol consumption and metabolic syndrome (Fujita & Takei, 2011).

Evaluation/Assessment and Diagnostic Studies

Several criteria have been proposed over the past decade to establish the diagnosis of metabolic syndrome. Diagnostic criteria developed by the NCEP Adult Treatment Panel III (ATP III; 2001) based on common clinical measures, including waist circumference, TG, HDL-C, blood pressure, and fasting glucose level, continue to be used with minor modifications. Modifications to the original diagnostic criteria include waist circumference adjustment to lower thresholds for individuals or ethnic groups predisposed to insulin resistance; designation of abnormal for the measures of TG, HDL-C, and blood pressure if an individual is taking

TABLE 44.5	Metabolic Syndrome Diagnostic Criteria
PARAMETER	**DIAGNOSTIC THRESHOLD**
Fasting blood sugar	≥ 100 mg/dL (or receiving medication for hyperglycemia)
Blood pressure	≥ 130/85 mmHg (or receiving medication for hypertension)
Triglycerides	≥ 150 mg/dL (or receiving medication for hypertriglyceridemia)
HDL-C	< 40 mg/dL in men or < 50 mg/dL in women (or receiving medication for reduced HDL-C)
Waist circumference	≥ 102 cm (40 in.) in men or ≥ 88 cm (35 in.) in women; if Asian American, ≥ 90 cm (35 in.) in men or ≥ 80 cm (32 in.) in women

Three of the five diagnostic criteria must be met to establish a diagnosis of metabolic syndrome.
HDL-C, high-density lipoprotein cholesterol.
Source: Data from Grundy et al. (2005).

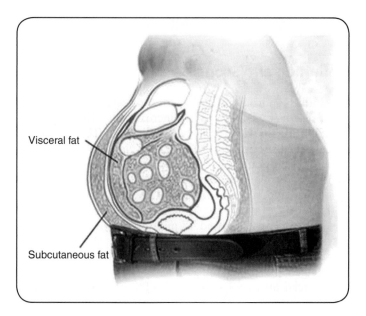

FIGURE 44.2
Subcutaneous versus visceral fat.

pharmacotherapeutics to treat these factors; delineating a threshold for both systolic and diastolic hypertension; and, in accordance with the American Diabetes Association (ADA), lowering the threshold for impaired fasting glucose level to 100 mg/dL. Metabolic syndrome is diagnosed when any three of the five diagnostic criteria exist, suggesting a multicausal etiology (Grundy et al., 2005). Diagnostic criteria for metabolic syndrome are depicted in Table 44.5.

Components of Metabolic Syndrome

OBESITY

Definition and Scope • Obesity, defined as a body mass index (BMI) of 30 kg/m² or greater, contributes to several conditions associated with metabolic syndrome. It is a common, serious, and costly disorder affecting more than one third of American adults (Bray, 2014). The presence of excessive weight is important, and the distribution of fat is critical to the metabolic syndrome diagnosis.

Etiology • Obesity is the accumulation of subcutaneous and visceral fat; it is the visceral fat (central obesity) (Figure 44.2) that is problematic. Visceral fat is thought to be more predictive of metabolic syndrome than total body weight.

Evaluation/Assessment • Because the main concern is central obesity, measurement of waist circumference or calculation of the waist-to-hip ratio should be done. Central obesity is identified when waist circumference is greater than 35 inches in women or when the waist-to-hip ratio is greater than 0.85 in women. To accurately measure the waist, the tape measure should be placed on the upper border of the iliac crest. Have the patient exhale and then

measure without compressing the skin. The hips are measured at the widest point, again without compressing the skin. Data suggest that waist circumference is more reflective of cardiovascular disease (CVD) in women than is BMI and is also associated with higher risk for development of type 2 diabetes and all-cause mortality (Expert Panel Report, 2014; Meigs, 2015).

BMI and waist circumference are screening tools to be included in all women's health encounters. Decisions to treat obesity are determined by BMI, comorbidities, and waist circumference.

Treatment/Management • Weight loss should be encouraged at a BMI of 25 or greater with just one comorbidity, and elevated waist circumference is considered a comorbidity. Counseling regarding dietary factors, exercise requirements, and weight management programs should be incorporated into treatment plans for all women who are overweight or obese or at high risk for obesity. It is critical that weight management programs include individual and/or group-based psychological/behavioral interventions.

Pharmacotherapy. Pharmacologic treatment (Orlistat) should be considered in adults as an adjunct to lifestyle interventions in the management of obesity. Current recommendations suggest that women with a BMI of 28 kg/m² or more (with comorbidities) or BMI 30 kg/m² or more should be considered on an individual case basis following careful assessment of risk/benefit and patient willingness to accept pharmacologic intervention.

Surgery. Bariatric surgery is an option for those women in whom previous attempts at weight loss have failed or are physically unattainable when the following criteria are met: BMI 35 kg/m² or more and/or presence of one or more severe comorbidities that are expected to improve significantly with weight reduction (e.g., immobility, arthritis, type 2 diabetes) (Expert Panel Report, 2014).

ACANTHOSIS NIGRICANS

Definition and Scope • Acanthosis nigricans, which is caused by an increase in melanocytes and epidermal papillomatosis, is a common finding with metabolic syndrome. This skin change is characterized by hyperpigmented, hyperkeratotic plaque-like lesions found especially in intertrigenous areas such as the axillae, neck, groin, under the breast, and the vulva. The skin is also hyperplastic and has a velvety or mossy appearance. It can occur in healthy individuals as well as in numerous health disorders and with exogenous hormone therapy including growth hormone and birth control pills. It is most commonly seen in individuals of African descent, partly because it is easier to visualize on darker skin.

Etiology and Risk Factors • When acanthosis nigricans develops in women who are not obese, a diagnostic work-up should be done. In rare instances, it is associated with lymphoma or malignancies of the gastrointestinal or genitourinary tract. In these cases, acanthosis nigricans may also appear on the lips, palms, and soles of feet and is generally severe. Occasionally acanthosis nigricans is congenital or due to an endocrine disorder such as diabetes, gonadal disorders, and thyroid disease (Habif, 2009).

Evaluation/Assessment and Diagnostic Studies • Acanthosis nigricans is usually diagnosed by inspection of affected areas. Skin biopsies are occasionally required for atypical cases.

Treatment/Management • Treatment is cosmetic only and includes topical tretinoin, 20% urea, alpha hydroxyacids, lactic or salicylic acid prescriptions, and laser resurfacing.

HYPERTENSION

Hypertension is a critical factor in the constellation of disorders that define the metabolic syndrome. Approximately 70 million (29%) American adults have hypertension. Of these individuals, slightly more than half (52%) have their blood pressure under control. Additionally, it is estimated that one in three adults in the United States are prehypertensive (Nwankwo, Yoon, Burt, & Gu, 2013). For a comprehensive overview of hypertension in women, see Chapter 43.

IMPAIRED GLUCOSE TOLERANCE

While glucose levels may range from normal to elevated, hyperinsulinemia is always manifested. The ADA and AACE recognize the connection of diabetes to insulin resistance and the metabolic syndrome. An important part of metabolic syndrome treatment is prevention of diabetes and CVD. The WHO criteria require glucose abnormalities to make a diagnosis of the metabolic syndrome, while the NCEP does not. In an 8-year Japanese study comparing these two definitions of metabolic syndrome, only the WHO criteria with its emphasis on abnormal glucose tolerance was predictive

of the development of CVD in women. These data support a link between diabetes and the metabolic syndrome; both are related to the development of CVD.

DYSLIPIDEMIA

Patients with metabolic syndrome have an abnormal, atherogenic lipid profile (see Chapter 43). TG levels are typically elevated and serum HDL-C levels are low. Serum low-density lipoprotein cholesterol (LDL-C) levels are increased, and the size and density of the LDL particles are reduced. The reduced particle size can lead to further development of atherosclerosis; thus, treatment is aimed at restoring the lipid profile to normal.

PROINFLAMMATORY, PROTHROMBOTIC STATE

Proinflammatory, prothrombotic state abnormalities are derived largely from the secretory activity of adipose tissue, particularly visceral fat. Adipocytes release adipokines such as leptin, interleukin (IL) 6, and plasminogen activator inhibitor-1 (PAI-1), all markers for CVD risk. The clinical value of measuring these markers and CRP is unknown and should be considered for use in clinical practice only in settings that are assessing CVD risk. Both the American Heart Association (AHA) and Centers for Disease Control and Prevention (CDC) list CRP testing as optional; the decision to test is based on clinical judgment (Bray, 2015).

Differential Diagnoses

The differential diagnosis involves looking at the entire constellation of problems that make up metabolic syndrome. The clinician must consider whether other causes explain the presence of hypertension, glucose abnormalities, or dyslipidemia. Other potential causes must be identified and managed. For example, in hypertensive women, secondary causes such as renovascular disease, obstructive sleep apnea, and disorders of renin and aldosterone metabolism may need exploration (Tasali & Ip, 2008). In the presence of a strong family history of dyslipidemia, hereditary dyslipidemia may need to be excluded. Hyperglycemia can present with thyroid disorders and rare endocrinopathies including pheochromocytomas and glucagonomas, and if the situation warrants, may need extensive work-up. If no other causes are present, then metabolic syndrome is identified as the primary diagnosis.

Diagnostic Studies

Preliminary laboratory studies in women suspected of having metabolic syndrome should include complete metabolic (chemistry) panels to evaluate serum glucose, renal function (creatinine, blood urea nitrogen [BUN], and estimated glomerular filtration rate [eGFR]), and lipid profile (TG, HDL-C, and LDL-C). In women with a family history of heart disease or other atherosclerotic disorder, consideration should be given for studies of lipoprotein(a), apolipoprotein-B100, high-sensitivity CRP, homocysteine, and fractionated LDL-C (Bray, 2015; Yaffe, 2007).

As previously discussed, factors associated with metabolic syndrome are found in other disorders and, as such, warrant assessment. These include thyroid function tests, liver function tests, hemoglobin A$_1$C, and uric acid. Extant data indicate that elevated TSH is associated with a higher prevalence of metabolic syndrome (Heima et al., 2012). Women with metabolic syndrome are more likely than the general population to have hyperuricemia, and this has been attributed to the proinflammatory nature of the syndrome (Puig & Martínez, 2008).

Imaging studies may be indicated for women with symptoms or signs of the many complications of the syndrome, including cardiovascular disease. Complaints of chest pain, shortness of breath, significant fatigue, dyspnea, or claudication may necessitate additional diagnostic testing with electrocardiography (rest/stress ECG), ultrasonography (vascular or rest/stress echocardiography), stress single-photon emission computed tomography (SPECT), cardiac positron emission tomography (PET), or other imaging studies.

Exacerbating factors such as obstructive sleep apnea should also be investigated. Polysomnography (sleep study) should be considered in women reporting snoring, periods of pauses in breathing, and/or daytime drowsiness. This is critical in the obese woman (Lam & Ip, 2007; Tasali & Ip, 2008).

Cardiovascular risk should be assessed using the American Heart Association/American College of Cardiology (Goff et al., 2014) calculator (available at http://tools.cardiosource.org/ASCVD-Risk-Estimator) to determine the risk of developing a first atherosclerotic cardiovascular disease (ASCVD) event. Risk factors that assess the 10-year and lifetime risk of an ASCVD event are: gender, age, race, total cholesterol level, HDL-C level, systolic blood pressure, treatment for hypertension, diabetes, and smoking status (see Chapter 43).

Treatment/Management

Metabolic syndrome is managed through focused treatment of each component. The primary goal is prevention of ASCVD and type 2 diabetes, achieved through risk reduction. The goals overlap as prevention of type 2 diabetes and treatment of other conditions are important factors in the prevention of ASCVD (Bray, 2015).

SELF-MANAGEMENT MEASURES

Lifestyle changes and management of obesity are the most important initial steps in treating metabolic syndrome. The major goal is lifestyle change to treat the underlying causes of obesity and physical inactivity and is essential for successful management of each metabolic syndrome component. For both long- and short-term risk reduction, therapeutic lifestyle changes (TLC) are first-line therapy for all women with metabolic syndrome. TLC include both dietary and exercise modification and have been demonstrated to effectively reduce progression to diabetes and development of CVD. Reduction of some of the major risk factors such as smoking, stress, and sedentary lifestyle are important components of management goals and referral for appropriate intervention is indicated to support women attempting TLC (Bray, 2015).

As with obesity, reduction in caloric intake and avoidance of high glycemic index foods and saturated fats are indicated. Not surprisingly, research indicates that the typical American diet is associated with a higher risk for developing metabolic syndrome; the opposite has been demonstrated in populations adhering to a typical Mediterranean diet (Yoneda et al., 2008). It is essential for diet modification programs to include a behavioral component as discussed in the obesity section, and referral for structured dietary modifications and weight loss may be warranted.

Exercise is an essential intervention in preventing and treating metabolic syndrome and obesity. Aerobic exercise, as opposed to resistance training, is recommended at least 5 days per week (Bateman et al., 2011; Roberts, Hevener, & Barnard, 2013). Exercise programs should be tailored to the individual woman to achieve the best outcomes. (See Chapters 13 and 14 for details about diet and exercise modifications used for women with metabolic syndrome, as well as information on supporting behavior change.)

PHARMACOTHERAPEUTICS

Medication therapies are used according to current authoritative guidelines for each component of the metabolic syndrome.

Dyslipidemia • Many patients will require lipid-modifying medications to control dyslipidemia, even those patients who achieve success in instituting and maintaining TLC. The goal for lipid management is threefold: to lower LDL-C, raise HDL-C, and lower TG, all of which help reduce CVD risk (Stone et al., 2014). As the goal is threefold, multiple medications may be needed. The use of multiple medications has been shown to achieve better lipid control. It is widely accepted to initiate statins (3-hydroxy-3-methylglutaryl coenzyme A [HMG-CoA] reductase inhibitors) in the presence of elevated LDL-C levels (Stone et al., 2013; Towne & Thara, 2008). Treatment of decreased HDL-C remains controversial, but may include niacin; however, careful monitoring is required as high doses may exacerbate hyperglycemia (Ito, 2004). Women with atherogenic dyslipidemia (elevated TG with low HDL-C), especially if overweight or obese, may benefit from fibrate medications; however, current recommendations for the treatment of cholesterol disorders emphasize statins over nonstatin medications (Stone et al., 2013).

Hypertriglyceridemia is amenable to both fibrates and niacin. Caution should be employed when prescribing fibrates due to well-documented drug interactions, especially when used in combination with statins. Omega-3 fatty acids may also help in lowering TG levels (see Chapter 43).

Hypertension • The goal of antihypertensive therapy in patients with metabolic syndrome is a blood pressure of less than 140/90 mmHg for most populations and 150/90 mmHg for patients aged 60 years or older. Treatment guidelines follow the Eighth Joint National Committee on Prevention, Detection, Evaluation, and Treatment of High Blood Pressure (JNC 8) (James et al., 2014) (see Chapter 43).

Insulin Resistance • Insulin resistance is first managed with TLC. There is no set limit for how long TLC alone are tried to manage insulin resistance. The woman should be evaluated with fasting glucose every 3 months; TLC have been shown to more effectively prevent metabolic syndrome as compared with metformin and placebo (cumulative incidence of metabolic syndrome at year 3 was 51% for placebo, 45% with metformin, and 34% for TLC). TLC should be the focus of initial and ongoing education about treatment for insulin resistance and should be maintained when pharmacotherapy is initiated.

The AACE recommends that clinicians use their judgment in making the decision to initiate pharmacotherapy and that pharmacotherapy should be considered when fasting blood glucose or A_1C levels begin to rise. The goal of pharmacotherapy is to reduce insulin resistance, and this includes the use of metformin and/or thazolidinediones (TZDs). Due to its extensive use and proven safety record, metformin is used most commonly. Titrating metformin from 500 mg once daily to 1000 mg twice daily in increments of 500 mg every 3 to 5 days will help to avoid common gastrointestinal side effects such as abdominal discomfort, diarrhea, gas, and bloating. Liver and renal function are evaluated prior to initiating metformin and monitored at least yearly. Renal dysfunction, heart failure, current liver disease, metabolic acidosis, and current alcohol abuse are contraindications to the use of metformin (Bray, 2015).

TZDs, including rosiglitazone and pioglitazone, have also been investigated for controlling insulin resistance and preventing diabetes in patients with the metabolic syndrome; however, no outcome data for CVD prevention in those with either the metabolic syndrome or diabetes exist as yet. As with any medication therapy, balancing the risks and side effects with the potential benefits must be considered (Grundy et al., 2005).

Proinflammatory, Prothrombotic State • No currently available pharmacotherapeutics are recommended for treatment of the proinflammatory/prothrombotic state.

Preventive Cardiovascular Treatment • Along with diet, exercise, and lifestyle behavior modifications, women may benefit from aspirin therapy (81 mg/d). Aspirin therapy is indicated if they have at least one significant risk for a cardiovascular event, if not contraindicated due to other comorbidities or current pharmacotherapeutic therapy (Blaha et al., 2008).

Surgical Considerations • Although surgical interventions for metabolic syndrome are not currently recommended, bariatric surgery referral may be considered for morbidly obese women when weight loss is not or cannot be achieved via diet and exercise.

■ DIABETES

Definition and Scope

The ADA defines type 1 diabetes as an absolute insulin deficiency related to beta-cell dysfunction. Type 2 diabetes mellitus is defined as a progressive insulin secretory defect related to insulin resistance. Prediabetes exists when blood glucose levels are higher than normal but not high enough to be diagnosed as diabetes. The ADA defines "gestational diabetes" as the development of diabetes during pregnancy (ADA, 2014) (see Chapter 38).

In the United States, it is estimated that nearly 26 million Americans have diabetes and an additional 79 million are prediabetic. Diabetes affects over 8% of the U.S. population across their life span. The Centers for Disease Control and Prevention (2011) reports that 11.3% of Americans 20 years of age and older are diabetic. In American adults 65 years of age and older, nearly 25% are affected. Alarmingly, approximately 27%, or 7 million Americans, are not aware that they have diabetes. In 2010, over 200,000 Americans 20 years of age or younger had either type 1 or type 2 diabetes. Diabetes was the seventh leading cause of death in the United States in 2013 and the leading cause of disabilities. The risk of death in people with diabetes is two times as great as in those who do not have the disease (CDC, 2015).

Type 2 diabetes accounts for approximately 90% to 95% of all diagnosed cases of diabetes. Current estimates suggest that approximately 40% of American adults will develop diabetes, primarily type 2. Recent data suggest that more than 50% of ethnic minorities will develop diabetes in their lifetime. The primary reason for the increased incidence of diabetes is the obesity epidemic in the United States (Gregg et al., 2014; Hackethal, 2014). Estimates suggest that 79 million or 35% of American adults aged 20 years and older have prediabetes and will subsequently develop diabetes in their lifetime (CDC, 2011).

The most common metabolic disease of childhood, type 1 diabetes affects approximately 1 in every 400 to 600 children and adolescents and accounts for 5% of all diagnosed cases of diabetes in adults. According to the CDC, the total incidence of type 1 diabetes is approximately 1 million Americans. CDC estimates indicate that 15,600 new cases of type 1 diabetes were diagnosed for each year from 2002 to 2005 in young people. In individuals less than 10 years of age, the annual rate of new cases was 19.7 per 100,000 population. In those older than 10 years, the annual rate of newly diagnosed cases was 18.6 per 100,000 population (CDC, 2011).

In children, type 1 diabetes mellitus generally starts around age 4 years or older, with an abrupt onset. Peak incidence of onset in children is age 11 to 13 years. In adults, generally in their late 30s and early 40s, type 1 diabetes tends to present less aggressively. The slower onset form of type 1 diabetes seen in adults is referred to as latent autoimmune diabetes of the adult or LADA (CDC, 2011).

Etiology

TYPE 1 DIABETES

Type 1 diabetes mellitus occurs due to lymphocytic infiltration and destruction of insulin-secreting beta cells in the islets of Langerhans in the pancreas. The resulting decline in beta-cell mass leads to reduced insulin secretion; over time, there is insufficient available insulin to maintain normal blood glucose levels. Generally, hyperglycemia develops after destruction of 80% to 90% of the beta cells and diabetes may then be diagnosed. Exogenous insulin is required to reverse this catabolic condition, prevent diabetic ketosis, decrease hyperglucagonemia, normalize the metabolism of lipids and proteins, and to sustain life.

Autoimmunity is currently considered the major factor in developing type 1 diabetes mellitus and may also be associated with other autoimmune diseases such as Addison's disease, Hashimoto's thyroiditis, and Graves' disease (Borchers, Uibo, & Gershwin, 2010). Less common causes of type 1 diabetes mellitus include pancreatitis, pancreatic cancer, or pancreatic surgery.

TYPE 2 DIABETES

The pathophysiology of type 2 diabetes is a spectrum of metabolic process abnormalities affecting glucose metabolism; insulin resistance is central. As discussed previously (see "Metabolic Syndrome"), insulin resistance leads to higher levels of circulating insulin as well as hyperglycemia due to the inability of the body to use insulin in both muscle and adipose tissue. Over time, the pancreas cannot produce enough insulin to keep up with the demand, and a relative insufficiency of insulin is created, resulting in hyperglycemia. Just as with the metabolic syndrome, type 2 diabetes is usually associated with multiple metabolic comorbidities.

The etiology of type 2 diabetes is multifactorial and involves both environmental and genetic factors. Extant data suggests that type 2 diabetes develops in response to excessive calorie intake without sufficient caloric expenditure and/or obesity in individuals with a susceptible genetic type. Nearly 90% of type 2 diabetics are obese; however, racial and ethnic factors influence the development of type 2 diabetes. Excess weight is a recognized risk factor for developing type 2 diabetes; however, individuals of Asian ancestry are at an increased risk for diabetes at lower weight levels when compared with persons of European ancestry. A greater risk for developing type 2 diabetes is also present in White individuals in the presence of hypertension and prehypertension as compared with African Americans (WHO Expert Consultation, 2004). Genetic variants can be attributed to only about 10% of the inheritable component in type 2 diabetes (Billings & Florez, 2010). Secondary diabetes can develop in individuals due to glucocorticoid therapy and in insulin-antagonistic disorders such as Cushing's syndrome, pheochromocytoma, and acromegaly.

Risk Factors

Risk factor assessment is an essential component of screening for diabetes and prediabetes. Women with any of the following risk factors should be screened at least every 3 years. In the presence of two or more risk factors, screening should occur annually (AACE, 2015).

- Family history of type 2 diabetes in a first-degree relative (such as parent or sibling)
- Age greater than 45 years, although type 2 diabetes is occurring with greater frequency in younger individuals.
- Sedentary lifestyle
- BMI greater than or equal to 30 kg/m²
- BMI 25 to 29.9 kg/m² in the presence of other risk factors such as ethnicity
- High-risk ethnicity including Hispanic, Native American, African American, Asian American, or Pacific Islander ancestry
- Prior history of impaired glucose tolerance (IGT) or impaired fasting glucose (IFG) or metabolic syndrome
- Hypertension (greater than 140/90 mmHg) or on antihypertensive therapy
- Dyslipidemia (HDL cholesterol level less than 35 mg/dL or TG level greater than 250 mg/dL)
- History of gestational diabetes or delivering a baby with a birth weight over 9 lbs
- Polycystic ovarian syndrome
- Nonalcoholic fatty liver disease
- Chronic or prolonged glucocorticoid therapy
- Antipsychotic drug therapy for schizophrenia or severe bipolar disorder
- Sleep disorders such as obstructive sleep apnea, chronic sleep deprivation, and night shift workers with glucose intolerance

Evaluation/Assessment

There are many differences between type 1 diabetes and type 2 diabetes (Table 44.6), and proper diagnosis is essential for management.

HISTORY

Many of the signs and symptoms of type 1 diabetes and type 2 diabetes are the same; however, their presentation is usually different (Table 44.6). Symptoms of type 1 diabetes have a rapid onset, while type 2 diabetes onset may be much slower, even insidious. In type 1 diabetes, polyuria and polydipsia are considered classic presenting signs; polyphagia with weight loss, blurred vision, and fatigue can also present. Type 2 diabetes can be largely asymptomatic; however, common presenting symptoms include fatigue, blurred vision, and candidal infections, as well as the classic symptoms of polydipsia, polyuria, polyphagia, weakness, and unexplained weight loss. Symptoms of autonomic neuropathy (dysphagia, bloating, change in bowel habits, and urinary and sexual dysfunction) as well as peripheral neuropathy (paresthesias of extremities) may be the first sign of type 2 diabetes. Chronic anovulation leading to oligomenorrhea or amenorrhea suggests an increase in the risk of type 2 diabetes, especially if accompanied by signs of hyperandrogenism. Women with a history of gestational diabetes or a history of large babies (over 9 lbs) are known to be at increased risk of developing type 2 diabetes (Wass, Stewart, Amiel, & Davies, 2011).

TABLE 44.6	Comparison of Type 1 and Type 2 Diabetes	
	TYPE 1	**TYPE 2**
Indicator % of occurrence of each	5%–10%	90%–95%
Age of diagnosis	Young, usually younger than 40 years	Older than 40 years usually
Condition in discovery	Mild to severe	Not ill, usually have mild symptoms
Cause	Absent or severely decreased insulin production	Insulin resistance or insulin secretory deficiency
Insulin levels	None to small amount	Markedly elevated early; later may see decrease

Adapted from Beasler (2014).

TABLE 44.7	Physical Findings in Diabetes	
EXAMINATION	**FINDING**	**INTERPRETATION**
General appearance	Altered level of consciousness	Suggest DKA
	Fruity breath	
	Loss of subcutaneous fat and muscle wasting	Suggest insulin deficiency
Height/weight BMI	BMI > 25	Present in 80% of type 2 diabetes
Fundoscopic examination (dilated)	Retinopathy	Suggest microvascular disease
	Microaneurysm	
	Exudate, hemorrhage, macular edema	
	Small, poorly responsive pupils	Suggest autonomic neuropathy
Oral examination	Gum disease	Suggest poor glycemic control
Thyroid examination	Wide range of findings from normal to abnormal	If abnormal, can suggest thyroid-caused symptoms or type 1 diabetes as it is associated with increased autoimmune disease
Skin	Acanthosis nigricans	Suggest type 2 diabetes
Cardiac examination	Cardiomegaly or gallop rhythm, little variation in rhythm with deep inspiration	CHF Autonomic neuropathy
Abdominal	Hepatomegaly	CHF
Pulses	Bruit (carotid/femoral) decrease/absent peripheral pulse	PVD
	Atrophy of subcutaneous skin and hair loss—legs and ankle brachial blood pressure index ↓0.9	
Feet	Foot ulcer, unrecognized trauma, infection, neuropathic arthropathy	PVD Sensory neuropathy Neuropathy disorders
CNS	Abnormalities suggest neuropathic disease	Place and type can suggest sensory peripheral or autonomic neuropathy

BMI, body mass index; CHF, congestive heart failure; CNS, central nervous system; DKA, diabetic ketoacidosis; PVD, peripheral vascular disease.
Data from American Diabetes Association: Clinical Practice Recommendations (2015).

PHYSICAL EXAMINATION

A thorough physical examination (Table 44.7) is performed to identify presenting signs of diabetes, rule out secondary diabetes, and evaluate other problems associated with the presenting signs and symptoms. Evaluation for signs of complications and target organ damage (Table 44.8), such as peripheral neuropathy and visual changes, are done at each visit.

Differential Diagnoses

The major diagnostic challenge is to differentiate between the possible causes of the patient's presenting symptoms. Fatigue and weakness can be presenting symptoms of thyroid disorders, anemia, chronic fatigue syndrome, diabetes, depression, and other conditions. Skin problems such as pruritus and dry skin also can present with several conditions. The urinary symptoms of diabetes can mimic the presence of a urinary tract infection (UTI).

Diagnostic Studies

Updated 2015 guidelines suggest differences in the diagnostic criteria for type 1 and type 2 diabetes. The criteria for diagnosing type 2 diabetes are summarized in Table 44.8.

The final differential between the two depends on the history, presentation of symptoms, physical examination, and plasma glucose studies. Routine screening for type 2 diabetes in adults older than 45 years is recommended because of the general lack of clinical symptoms in early hyperglycemia. While past experts recommended fasting plasma glucose as the initial screen, the 2-hour oral glucose tolerance test (OGTT) is a better predictor among patients with impaired fasting glucose. Patients who have a higher-than-normal glucose level that does not meet criteria for the diagnosis of diabetes are considered to be at particularly high risk for the development of diabetes and are frequently referred to as having prediabetes.

Once the diagnosis of type 2 diabetes is confirmed, a number of tests are done to guide management. Along with self-monitoring (see management), a glycosylated hemoglobin A_1C is assessed quarterly. The A_1C measures the level of control during the previous 2- to 3-month period. The higher the A_1C value, the poorer the glucose control. Maintaining an A_1C of less than 6.5% is recommended; however, the closer to normal (5.5% or lesser) the levels are, the less likely individuals are to develop long-term sequelae. A_1C results should be interpreted with caution in African Americans and in women with various anemias, hemoglobinopathies, and severe renal or hepatic disease (AACE, 2015).

Microalbumin is generally assessed at the time of diagnosis to identify microalbuminuria, which is present with early renal disease and may require treatment. Serum creatinine is also done yearly, and the estimated glomerular filtration rate (eGFR) is calculated in all adults. An EKG should be performed on all adults as a baseline. Diabetes is one of the greatest risk factors for CVD and congestive heart failure (CHF), and routine screening is needed. Dyslipidemia is also frequently seen with diabetes and should be screened for annually. Aggressive management of dyslipidemia is recommended by both the ADA and the AACE. An exercise stress test is considered in women older than 35 years, or older than 25 years if she has had diabetes for 15 years or more. Liver function studies are often needed as a baseline before starting medication (AACE, 2015).

Screening for gestational diabetes should occur between 24 and 28 weeks of gestation via 2-hour OGTT. Gestational diabetes is diagnosed if any of the three criteria are met with 2-hour OGTT: FPG greater than 92 mg/dL and/or 1-hour PG 180 mg/dL or more and/or 2-hour PG 153 mg/dL or more (AACE, 2015).

Type 1 diabetes may be present in both lean and overweight or obese girls and women. As it is generally characterized by insufficient endogenous insulin and exogenous insulin dependence, diagnosis requires documentation of C-peptide and insulin levels in addition to assessment of autoantibodies.

Treatment/Management

The goals for management are threefold: restore and maintain normal blood glucose levels, prevent target organ damage, and control and/or prevent comorbidities. Meeting these goals requires a partnership between the clinician and patient. Diabetes cannot be adequately controlled without systematic intensive therapy that is monitored by the woman. The best approach to management is a multidisciplinary team that includes the patient, an endocrinologist, primary care provider, diabetes educator, and nutritionist. For any treatment to succeed, the patient must understand the disease, treatment, and her role in management.

TABLE 44.8	Prediabetes and Diabetes Diagnostic Criteria for Nonpregnant Adults	
NORMAL	**PREDIABETES**	**DIABETES[a]**
FPG < 100 mg/dL	Impaired fasting glucose FPG ≥ 100–125 mg/dL	FPG > 126 mg/dL
2-hour PG < 140 mg/dL	Impaired glucose tolerance 2-hour PG ≥ 140 to 199 mg/dL	2-hour PG ≥ 200 mg/dL Random PG ≥ 200 mg/dL in the presence of clinical symptoms
A_1C < 5.5%	A_1C 5.5%–6.4%	A_1C ≥ 6.5%

[a]Diagnosis of diabetes is confirmed when a repeated serum test again demonstrates elevated levels.
2-hour PG, plasma glucose performed 2 hours after 75-g oral glucose load;
FPG, fasting plasma glucose; PG, plasma glucose.
Adapted from American Association of Clinical Endocrinologists and American College of Endocrinology (2015).

Along with diet, exercise, and glycemic control, it is important to address other lifestyle behaviors and comorbidities. In order to obtain optimal outcomes, aggressive treatment is needed. It is important to address the issues of smoking, dyslipidemia, and hypertension. Patients should be encouraged to stop smoking and referral for smoking cessation assistance may be warranted. Intensive hypertension management to reduce blood pressure to less than 140/90 mmHg should be started (ADA, 2016). LDL should be treated to reach the target of less than 100 mg/dL. If CVD diagnosis is already established, the goal for blood pressure is less than 120/80 mmHg if this can be safely achieved, and the LDL target is less than 70 mg/dL. These therapies, along with good glycemic control (A_1C less than 6.5%), help to prevent the long-term problems associated with diabetes (AACE, 2015).

Referral to specialty clinicians may be needed when caring for women with diabetes. Consider referral to nephrology if the eGFR is abnormal. Referral to cardiology is warranted if evidence of CVD is identified. Annual ophthalmologic evaluation is recommended. Most women are referred to podiatry for foot care, and referral to neurology may be needed if peripheral neuropathy develops. Other referrals are initiated as needed for management of sequelae.

SELF-MANAGEMENT MEASURES

Self-Monitoring of Blood Glucose • A large part of patient education focuses on self-management. One of the most critical techniques is self-monitoring of blood glucose (SMBG). SMBG provides immediate feedback on current glucose levels, and can help determine any actions needed. SMBG together with the periodic A_1C directs the glycemia treatment modalities: diet, exercise, and medication. SMBG should be done before and after each meal and at bedtime until good control is accomplished; then the timing and frequency of SMBG is determined by the patient's needs. Pre- and postprandial goals recommended for capillary blood by the ADA are 90 to 130 mg/dL preprandial and less than 180 mg/dL at peak postprandial (ADA, 2015).

Hyperglycemia and Hypoglycemia • Once SMBG is established, women need to know how to manage the results.

Education includes managing hyper- and hypoglycemia, medication use, changes in response to illness, and when to contact her clinician. Hypoglycemia can develop with treatment, and is more common in those with very tight control. Patients are taught to recognize and manage hypoglycemia (glucose less than 60 mg/dL). The symptoms of hypoglycemia vary and are additive (Table 44.9). If she is conscious and able to follow commands, hypoglycemia is treated by administering oral carbohydrates (e.g., glucose tablets, two tablespoons of raisins, half cup of a full sugar soda beverage, or one cup of milk). Blood glucose levels are rechecked within 30 to 60 minutes; if she is still hypoglycemic, further intake of carbohydrates is needed. Once stabilized, the woman should consume a snack or meal to avoid recurrence. Severe hypoglycemia can be an emergency requiring emergency room treatment with parenteral glucagon. Severe hyperglycemia can be managed with insulin; the woman should call her clinician or go to the emergency room if she is experiencing symptoms of diabetic ketoacidosis. Illness can precipitate elevations in blood glucose; however, the only medication that can be altered to meet these needs is insulin. The woman should contact her clinician if she is experiencing persistent hyperglycemia of more than 250 mg/dL (AACE, 2015; ADA, 2015).

Exercise • Another vital part of diabetes management is physical activity. Exercise has been shown to lower blood glucose, reduce A_1C, increase insulin sensitivity, decrease the need for insulin, and increase the number of insulin receptors. Physical activity, including moderate intensity aerobic exercise (59%–70% of maximum heart rate), flexibility, and resistance training, should be done for a minimum of 150 minutes/week. Careful balance between insulin and glucose needs to be maintained for safe exercise in patients with type 1 diabetes. Patients with type 1 diabetes should have a readily available source of carbohydrate when exercising in case of hypoglycemia. With repeated exercise, patients can determine their individual reaction and learn to adjust food and insulin to meet their needs. Exercise helps to reduce insulin resistance and can help with weight management, especially when combined with dietary modifications. Exercise for women with diabetes should include three components: aerobic exercise, flexibility training and resistance training. One

TABLE 44.9	Symptoms of Hypoglycemia		
LEVEL OF HYPOGLYCEMIA	**MILD**	**MODERATE**	**SEVERE**
Common symptoms	■ Pallor ■ Diaphoresis ■ Tachycardia ■ Palpitations ■ Hunger ■ Paresthesias ■ Shakiness/tremor	Symptoms of mild plus: ■ Inability to concentrate ■ Confusion ■ Slurred speech ■ Irrational or uncontrolled behavior ■ Slowed reaction time ■ Blurred vision ■ Somnolence ■ Extreme fatigue	Symptoms of mild and moderate plus: ■ Disoriented behavior ■ Loss of consciousness ■ Inability to wake up ■ Seizures ■ Impaired neurological function

Adapted from American Diabetes Association: Clinical Practice Recommendations (2015); AACE (2015).

hour of moderate intensity aerobic exercise provides the same benefit as a 700-calorie reduction in food intake. While many patients cannot exercise for 150 min/wk, any exercise helps to improve glycemic control. Resistance training improves insulin sensitivity at about the same rate as aerobic exercise and increases both metabolic rate and muscle mass. High intensity resistance training (three sets, three times per week) can reduce A$_1$C by 1.1% to 1.2% (AACE, 2015).

MEDICAL NUTRITION THERAPY

Medical nutrition therapy (MNT) is an integral part of diabetes management and plays a critical role in controlling the metabolic parameters of the disease. The same types of dietary changes used with TLC apply to MNT for women with diabetes. Weight loss of 5% to 10% should be encouraged in all overweight and obese patients. In type 2 diabetes, weight management to reduce insulin resistance is recommended. A moderate decrease in caloric intake (250–500 k/cal/d) can result in a slow and consistent weight loss. Fasting should be avoided as a method to reduce weight and meals and snacks should be eaten on a regular schedule. Current recommendations suggest a plant-based diet consisting of fresh fruits and vegetables, low-glycemic index carbohydrates, and low saturated fats. Meats should be lean, and processed meats should be avoided. Making healthier choices can help reduce caloric intake and provide a starting point for quantity reduction. For example, fruit or raw vegetables for a snack instead of crackers and cheese may reduce caloric intake by 150 calories per day. Micronutrient and vitamin supplementation is not recommended in the absence of insufficiency or deficiency (AACE, 2015).

COMPLEMENTARY AND ALTERNATIVE MEDICINE

Cinnamon may aid in reducing blood sugar levels; however, research is limited and it should be avoided in women with liver disorders.

PHARMACOTHERAPEUTICS

Medication Therapy for Type 2 Diabetes • As the pathophysiology of type 2 diabetes is multifactorial, treatment is likely to require multiple therapies. The choice for oral therapy can be complex. If glycemic control is not achieved after 3 to 6 months of lifestyle management, a program of medication therapy should be initiated. This clinical decision is usually based on glucose level as well as evidence of target organ damage. Many noninsulin and insulin medications, which provide an opportunity to truly tailor a regimen and individualize care, are available.

There are a number of considerations in selecting a treatment regimen. First, the underlying pathology must be considered. How severe is the hyperglycemia? Are both insulin resistance and insulin deficiency present? Is glucose toxicity (glucose more than 600 mg/dL) present? The age and weight of the woman and comorbidities also need to be considered. Each class of medication carries its own set of side effects and precautions that must be weighed.

Medication therapy usually involves multiple medications from different classes and both noninsulin medications and insulin are considered first-line therapy. Clinicians should refer to full prescribing information when selecting and initiating diabetes medication for dosing, precautions, contraindications, and interactions. Agents used in diabetic therapy include insulin and the following noninsulin medications: biguanides (Metformin), sulfonylureas (SU), meglitinide derivatives, alpha-glucosidase inhibitors (AGi), thiazolidinediones (TZDs), glucagon-like peptide-1 (GLP-1) agonists, dipeptidyl peptidase IV (DPP-4) inhibitors, selective sodium-glucose transporter-2 (SGLT-2) inhibitors, amylinomimetics, bile acid sequestrants, and dopamine agonists. Table 44.10 summarizes critical factors to be considered when prescribing noninsulin diabetes agents.

Weight loss in the presence of poorly controlled blood glucose suggests insulin deficiency. The pattern of SMBG levels throughout the day is most helpful in determining which medication to use because medications are used to target hyperglycemia occurring at different times. Additionally, the A$_1$C level at the time of initiation of a medication regime guides the selection of pharmacological agents. In women who begin pharmacological treatment for type 2 diabetes with a baseline A$_1$C level less than 7.5%, monotherapy is recommended. If the glycemic goal is not met after 3 months, a second agent should be added. With a baseline A$_1$C level greater than or equal to 7.5%, metformin or another first-line agent should be augmented with a second noninsulin or insulin agent. If glycemic control is not achieved in 3 months, a third agent should be added. For women with a baseline A$_1$C level greater than or equal to 9.0%, in the absence of overt symptoms, dual or triple therapy should be employed. If overt symptoms are present, insulin and possibly noninsulin therapy should be used. Lifestyle modifications along with medically assisted weight loss should be incorporated in all therapeutic plans to achieve and maintain glycemic control. Table 44.11 summarizes pharmacological agent choices for glycemic control based on baseline A$_1$C level.

Noninsulin Agents • When lifestyle changes are not sufficient to achieve glycemic control, typically patients are started on noninsulin agents. For women who are overweight, metformin is usually the first agent prescribed. If single therapy does not work, or if the woman's A$_1$C is 7.5% or greater, additional agents are added. Many women require treatment with two, three, or more different medicines. If oral-agent combinations are ineffective, an injected medicine such as an incretin-based medicine, amylin analog, or insulin may be prescribed. Combinations of noninsulin and insulin agents are used because different drugs target different parts of the glycemic regulation system. Table 44.10 summarizes critical factors to be considered when prescribing noninsulin diabetes agents.

Insulin Therapy

Type 1 Diabetes Mellitus. With type 1 diabetes, insulin therapy is required for survival and must be started at diagnosis. As intensive therapy is recommended, the clinician may choose to refer these patients for management

TABLE 44.10 Noninsulin Agents

CLASS	ACTION	FASTING GLUCOSE LOWERING	POSTPRANDIAL GLUCOSE LOWERING	NAFLD BENEFIT	HYPOGLYCEMIA	WEIGHT	RENAL/GU EFFECTS	GI ADVERSE EFFECTS
Alpha-glucosidase inhibitors	Delay carbohydrate absorption from intestine	Neutral	Moderate	Neutral	Neutral	Neutral	Neutral	Moderate
Amylin analog	Decrease glucagon secretion Slow gastric emptying Increase satiety	Mild	Moderate-marked	Neutral	Neutral	Loss	Neutral	Moderate
Biguanide	Decrease hepatic glucose production Increase muscle uptake of glucose	Moderate	Mild	Mild	Neutral	Slight loss	Contraindicated in moderate to severe chronic kidney disease	Moderate
Bile acid sequestrant	Possibly decrease hepatic glucose production and increase incretin levels	Mild	Mild	Neutral	Neutral	Neutral	Neutral	Moderate
DPP-4 inhibitors	Increase glucose-dependent insulin secretion Decrease secretion of glucagon	Mild	Moderate	Neutral	Neutral	Neutral	Dose adjustment necessary if renal impairment present (except linagliptin)	Neutral

(continued)

TABLE 44.10   Noninsulin Agents (continued)

CLASS	ACTION	FASTING GLUCOSE LOWERING	POSTPRANDIAL GLUCOSE LOWERING	NAFLD BENEFIT	HYPOGLYCEMIA	WEIGHT	RENAL/GU EFFECTS	GI ADVERSE EFFECTS
Dopamine-2 agonist	Activates dopaminergic receptors	Neutral	Mild	Neutral	Neutral	Neutral	Neutral	Moderate
Glinides	Increase insulin secretion	Mild	Moderate	Neutral	Mild-moderate	Gain	Increased risk of hypoglycemia	Neutral
GLP-1 receptor agonists	Increase glucose-dependent insulin secretion Decrease glucagon secretion Slow gastric emptying Increase satiety	Mild-moderate	Moderate marked	Mild	Neutral	Loss	Contraindicated if creatinine clearance <30 mg/mL	Moderate
SGLT-2 inhibitors	Increase urinary excretion of glucose	Moderate	Mild	Neutral	Neutral	Loss	GU infection risk	Neutral
Sulfonylureas	Increase insulin secretion	Moderate	Moderate	Neutral	Moderate to severe	Gain	Increased risk of hypoglycemia	Neutral
Thiazolidinediones	Increase glucose uptake in muscle and fat Decrease hepatic glucose production	Moderate	Mild	Moderate	Neutral	Gain	Potential to worsen fluid retention	Neutral

DPP-4, dipeptidyl peptidase IV; GLP-1, glucagon-like peptide-1; GU, genitourinary; NAFLD, Non-alcoholic fatty liver disease; SGLT-2, sodium-glucose transporter-2.
Adapted from American Association of Clinical Endocrinologists and American College of Endocrinology (2015).

TABLE 44.11	Pharmacological Interventions for Glycemic Control			
A₁C LEVEL < 7.5%	**A₁C LEVEL ≥ 7.5%**		**A₁C LEVEL ≥ 9.0%**	
Monotherapy	**Dual Therapy**	**Triple Therapy**	**Asymptomatic**	**Symptomatic**
Metformin GLP-1RA SGLT-2i DPP-4i AGi TZD SU/GLN	Metformin or other first-line agent plus one of the following: GLP-1RA SGLT-2i DPP-4i AGi TZD SU/GLN Basal insulin Colesevelam BromocriptineQR	Metformin or other first-line agent and second-line agent plus one of the following: GLP-1RA SGLT-2i DPP-4i AGi TZD SU/GLN Basal insulin Colesevelam BromocriptineQR	Dual or triple therapy	Insulin and possibly noninsulin agents
If glycemic control not achieved in 3 months, advance to dual therapy	If glycemic control not achieved in 3 months, advance to triple therapy	If glycemic control not achieved in 3 months, add or intensify insulin therapy	If glycemic control not achieved in 3 months, add or intensify insulin therapy	If glycemic control not achieved in 3 months, intensify insulin therapy

AGi, alpha-glucosidase inhibitors; DPP-4i, dipeptidyl peptidase IV inhibitors; GLP-1RA, glucagon-like peptide-1; SGLT-2i, selective sodium-glucose transporter-2; SU/GLN, sulfonylureas/ glucagon-like peptide; TZD, thiazolidinedione.
Adapted from American Association of Clinical Endocrinologists and American College of Endocrinology (2015).

by a clinical endocrinologist. For most patients with type 1 diabetes, physiological regimens using insulin analogs should be prescribed. Patients should be started on multiple daily injections of one to two doses of basal insulin to most closely approximate normal pancreatic function. Basal insulin is used in combination with rapid-acting prandial insulin before each meal. The insulin dose is determined by the woman's weight, blood glucose level, activity, and food intake, and thus requires intensive self-monitoring. Alternatively, insulin may be administered via continuous subcutaneous infusion (insulin pump) using rapid-acting insulin analog. A clear understanding by the patient of the treatment and how it works is critical to success. Insulins differ in their onset, peak, and duration, and they are selected to meet individual metabolic needs.

The initial insulin dose for type 1 diabetes is based on body weight with a recommended starting dosage of 0.4 to 0.5 units per kilogram daily. Daily basal dosing should represent 40% to 50% of the daily insulin dose administered as either a daily injection of a basal analogue or to doses of NPH insulin. Prandial insulin dosage should represent 50% to 60% of total daily insulin dose and should be administered in divided doses 15 minutes prior to each meal based on estimating the carbohydrate content of each meal.

Type 2 Diabetes Mellitus. In some patients with type 2 diabetes, the beta cells cannot meet the demand for insulin. When glycemic control cannot be achieved with TLC and noninsulin agents, insulin is started. Because insulin resistance is a major factor in type 2 diabetes, treatment with an agent that lowers insulin resistance (Table 44.10) may be needed in addition to insulin. Insulin may be needed

initially to help control hyperglycemia; if the patient is able to modify other factors, such as obesity, she may be able to discontinue the insulin in the future.

Complications

Complications related to diabetes are of special concern for women (Table 44.12). Two factors increase the risks associated with heart disease in women with diabetes. First, she loses the natural protection to CVD that is seen in other premenopausal women. Second, among people with diabetes who have a cardiac event, women have a lower survival rate. Of the women who do survive, the quality of life is poorer than that of men. Mortality rates are higher in women with diabetes. While diabetic retinopathy is a problem for all patients with diabetes, women are more likely to develop the proliferative form of the disease and more likely to lose their sight. Aggressive management is important to prevent these complications.

Considerations for Special Populations

WOMEN OF CHILDBEARING AGE

Women have a unique burden with diabetes because of the progression of the disease as well as its effect on pregnancy. Diabetes can cause difficulties in pregnancy such as increased risk of pregnancy loss at all stages and increased birth defects (see Chapter 38). Gestational diabetes (see Chapter 38), which increases the mother's risk of developing diabetes later in life, complicates 2% to 5% of all pregnancies (CDC, 2010).

TABLE 44.12	Complications of Diabetes
COMPLICATION	**STATISTICS**
CVD/stroke	
Death	68% of the deaths in diabetics are related to CVD 16% of the deaths in diabetics are related to stroke
CVD	Risk two to four times higher
Stroke	Risk two to four times higher
Hypertension	67% of diabetics have BP 140/90 or greater
Eyes (blindness)	Leading cause of blindness in adults, 28.5% of adults older than 40 years have diabetic retinopathy
Kidney disease	Leading cause of end-stage renal disease
Nervous system disease	60%–70% of diabetics have CNS damage (peripheral neuropathy, sexual dysfunction, gastroparesis, carpal tunnel syndrome)
Amputation	Leading cause of lower limb amputations (nontraumatic)
Dental disease	One third of diabetics have severe periodontal disease with tooth loss
Complications of pregnancy	Increased incidence of birth defects Spontaneous abortion in up to 20% of pregnancies Large babies

BP, blood pressure; CNS, central nervous system; CVD, cardiovascular disease. Data from Centers for Disease Control and Prevention (2011).

OLDER WOMEN

Close monitoring is especially important for older women. As older women are more likely to have other existing health conditions, the likelihood of medication interactions is increased. Concerns with hyper- and hypoglycemia are higher in older women who may have increased risks for falls or other medical conditions that can cause similar symptoms. Furthermore, poor glucose control can act synergistically with other health problems to accelerate complications (CDC, 2010).

WOMEN IN PRISON

In 2010, there were 113,000 women offenders incarcerated in state and federal facilities in the United States compared with 1,500,000 male inmates (Bureau of Justice, 2012). An estimated 4.8% of the incarcerated population, or around 80,000, have diabetes. Patient advocacy and diligence are required to assure that the same standard of care for diabetes is applied and met for incarcerated women as has been proven effective for all people with diabetes (ADA, 2014).

■ HYPOTHALAMUS AND PITUITARY GLAND DISORDERS

Many consider the pituitary the "master gland." The hypothalamus and pituitary gland form a unit that controls many endocrine system functions. Thyroid, adrenal, and gonadal functions are controlled by this unit as well as a wide range of physiologic activities. Additionally, neuroendocrinologic function, which includes regulation of the endocrine system and modulation of nervous system activity, are dependent on this unit (Carroll, Aron, Finding, & Tyrell, 2011).

Hyperprolactinemia

DEFINITION AND SCOPE

Hyperprolactinemia is a condition of elevated serum prolactin, an amino acid protein produced in the lactotroph cells of the anterior pituitary gland. Dopamine has the predominant inhibitory influence in the regulation of prolactin secretion. Prolactinemia may occur as a physiologic, pharmacologic or pathologic response.

In the United States, hyperprolactinemia occurs in less than 1% of the general population and in 5% to 14% of women with secondary amenorrhea. Nearly 75% of women who present with galactorrhea and amenorrhea are found to have hyperprolactinemia. Prolactin-secreting tumors are found in nearly one third of these women (Lee, Oh, Yoon, & Choi, 2012).

ETIOLOGY

Physiologic hyperprolactinemia generally produces mild to moderate symptoms and most commonly occurs due to nipple stimulation and lactation in the first 4 to 6 weeks postpartum. With pregnancy, there is a steady increase in prolactin that peaks at the time of delivery. Nipple stimulation further increases the levels of prolactin, allowing for breastfeeding. Without nipple stimulation, levels return to normal in 4 to 6 weeks. Physiologic hyperprolactinemia can also be mediated by stress, such as myocardial infarction, hypoglycemia, or surgery. Other causes include sleep, food ingestion, and physical exercise. Pharmacologic agents that affect the hypothalamic dopamine system and/or pituitary dopamine receptors can also stimulate prolactin release, resulting in hyperprolactinemia. Serum levels of prolactin increase within hours of medication dosing and will return to normal within 4 days of discontinuation. Several classes of medications (Table 44.13) can lead to this disorder. Withdrawal from the medication is curative. Not all medications in any one class cause hypersecretion, so changing agents may resolve the problem (Melmed et al., 2011; Serri et al., 2006; Snyder, 2014).

The major pathological causes of hyperprolactinemia are pituitary tumor, decreased dopamine inhibition of prolactin, hypothyroidism, chronic renal disease, or hypothalamic or pituitary disorders (e.g., head trauma, pituitary adenoma, or sarcoidosis). Hyperprolactinemia is also associated with insulin resistance and may be seen with the metabolic syndrome, polycystic ovarian syndrome (PCOS), or

TABLE 44.13	Selected Drugs Known to Cause Hyperprolactinemia and/or Galactorrhea[a]
DRUG CLASS	**DRUG**
Antipsychotic	Haldol
	Orap
	Zyprexa
	Risperdal
Antidepressant	Anafranil
	Norpramin
Gastrointestinal	Tagamet (IV)
	Reglan
Antihypertensives	Aldomet
	Reserpine
	Verapamil
Opiates	Codeine
	Morphine

[a]A selected sample of drugs. List not comprehensive.
Data from Snyder (2015).

diabetes. This may be related to the proinflammatory state thought to be present in these conditions, which seems to be independent of BMI (Melmed et al., 2011; Snyder, 2014).

SYMPTOMS AND EVALUATION/ASSESSMENT

Galactorrhea, defined as milk or milk-like secretion from the breast, is the most common presenting symptom. Eighty percent of nonpregnant or lactating women with galactorrhea have hyperprolactinemia. Oligomenorrhea or amenorrhea leading to suboptimal fertility is another common symptom. The suboptimal fertility can be in the form of either difficulty getting pregnant or recurrent spontaneous abortion. Symptoms such as headache, visual changes, and cranial neuropathies may indicate a mass and need to be evaluated accordingly. In patients experiencing increased intracranial pressure due to a mass, the presenting symptom may be seizures. A complete breast and pelvic exam should be completed (Snyder, 2015).

DIFFERENTIAL DIAGNOSES

All causes of oligomenorrhea, amenorrhea, and infertility, including PCOS, are part of the differential. Acute inflammatory diseases (e.g., sarcoidosis, histiocytosis) can also be the cause. Medications, benign and malignant tumors, hypothyroidism, chronic liver and renal disease, and normal physiological changes (e.g., pregnancy and increased breast stimulation) must be considered as well (Melmed et al., 2011).

DIAGNOSTIC STUDIES

The primary diagnostic test is serum prolactin. The diagnosis of hyperprolactinemia is made when serum prolactin levels are found on two separate occasions to be above the norm established for the laboratory used. Prolactin secretion is pulsatile; it increases with sleep, stress, pregnancy, and chest wall stimulation or trauma, and therefore must be drawn after fasting. Serum prolactin levels between 20 and 200 µg/L can be found in women with hyperprolactinemia due to any cause. Serum prolactin levels above 200 µg/L generally indicate the presence of a pituitary (lactotroph) adenoma. Dedicated pituitary MRI should be obtained if pituitary adenoma is suspected. Mammogram should be considered.

TREATMENT/MANAGEMENT

Management of drug-induced hyperprolactinemia includes discontinuation of the medication or substitution of an alternative medication and estrogen replacement in women with long-term hypogonadism. Dopamine agonists are often used for treatment of prolactinomas and require endocrinology referral. Oral contraceptives are used for women with amenorrhea due to prolactinomas. Resistant and malignant prolactinomas generally require increasing doses of dopamine agonists and/or transphenoid surgery, radiation therapy, as well as other chemotherapeutics (Melmed et al., 2011).

Self-Management Measures • For women with physiologic causes of hyperprolactinemia, the condition will remit once the cause is removed. In the case of increased nipple stimulation, if it is self- or partner-induced, counseling or referral for evaluation of the behavior may be warranted. Referral may also be warranted in women with excess stress and limited coping skills.

Pharmacotherapeutics • When possible, the treatment of choice is medical management with a dopamine agonist. The two most common medications are bromocriptine (Parlodel) and cabergoline (Dostinex). Treatment may not need to be continued indefinitely. If medications are withdrawn, monitoring for recurrence is warranted.

CONSIDERATIONS FOR SPECIAL POPULATIONS

The issues for pregnant women are mainly related to the effect of dopamine agonists in pregnancy. Bromocriptine has been studied and does not seem to cause fetal damage. Less data are available on the other medications currently used. Patients should be monitored for worsening symptoms. There is approximately a 25% chance that a tumor will increase in size. Periodic checks of prolactin levels are not useful as levels normally increase during pregnancy. The signs and symptoms the woman is experiencing at each prenatal visit can be used to follow the disease course. As abnormalities of the visual field and/or severe headaches can signify an increase in tumor size, assessment for both is critical. If present, neuroimaging (MRI) without gadolinium is indicated (Melmed et al., 2011).

Polycystic Ovarian Syndrome

DEFINITION AND SCOPE

PCOS is one of the most common endocrine disorders of reproductive-age women in the United States, presenting as menstrual irregularity and evidence of androgen excess. With a prevalence of 4% to 12% of premenopausal women, it is responsible for 75% of anovulatory infertility. Incidence is higher in Native American and Hispanic women when compared with Caucasians and African Americans (Ehrmann, 2005). While PCOS has always been associated with infertility and increased risk of endometrial and ovarian cancer, it is also recognized as a significant risk factor for metabolic diseases, such as diabetes, dyslipidemia, and cardiovascular disease (Azziz et al., 2004; Ovalle & Azziz, 2002). Although some studies have suggested an increased risk for breast cancer in women with PCOS, findings from a recent meta-analysis refute this (Barry, Azizia, & Hardiman, 2014).

ETIOLOGY

PCOS develops in the context of abnormalities of the hypothalamic–pituitary–ovarian axis, insulin resistance, and altered adipocyte function (Sachdeva, 2010). Together these factors and perhaps genetic abnormalities cause increased androgen levels, decreased ovulatory function, and increased metabolic risk.

PCOS is associated with abnormal androgen and estrogen metabolism and in the control of androgen production. Women with PCOS may have high serum male sex steroid levels including testosterone, androstenedione, and dehydroepiandrosterone sulfate (DHEA-S). However, normal levels of the aforementioned hormones may be encountered in these patients.

Women with PCOS often have insulin resistance and hyperinsulinemia, both of which are markedly increased in the presence of obesity. Defects in insulin receptor signaling pathways are thought to promote insulin resistance in PCOS patients, and elevated insulin levels may have gonadotropin-augmenting effects on ovarian function. Increased androgenicity is thought to occur from suppression of hormone-binding globulins in the liver due to hyperinsulinemia (Barber, McCarthy, Wass, & Franks, 2006).

Insulin resistance in PCOS has been associated with low levels of adiponectin, a hormone secreted by adipocytes that help regulate glucose levels and metabolism of lipids. Interestingly, both obese and nonobese women with PCOS have lower levels of adiponectin than women who do not have PCOS (Toulis et al., 2009).

Although controversial, as not all experts agree, one proposed mechanism for anovulation and elevated androgen levels suggests that oversecretion of leutenizing hormone (LH) may lead to changes in the LH to follicle-stimulating hormone (FSH) ratio (LH:FSH). This, in turn, causes abnormal gonadotropic releasing hormone (GnRH) levels. As a result, the ovaries cannot aromatize androgens to estrogens, which leads to decreased estrogen levels and consequent anovulation. Anovulation results in a lack of progesterone needed to protect the endometrium. With high LH levels and steady-state FSH, follicles may start to develop but do not reach maturity. This can account for the typical polycystic ovary seen on ultrasound imaging (Barbieri & Ehrmann, 2015; Freeman, 2006).

RISK FACTORS

PCOS is a genetically heterogeneous syndrome in which the genetic contributions remain incompletely described; however, studies of family members with PCOS indicate that an autosomal dominant mode of inheritance occurs. Fathers of PCOS patients may be abnormally hairy. Mothers may have oligomenorrhea and siblings may have oligomenorrhea and hirsutism. Family history of type 2 diabetes in a first-degree relative has also been indicated as a risk factor for PCOS, impaired glucose tolerance, type 2 diabetes, and metabolic abnormalities (Ehrmann, 2005).

SYMPTOMS AND EVALUATION/ASSESSMENT

Women with PCOS usually present with multiple symptoms, although not all are present in any one person.

History • Thorough investigation of a woman's personal and family health history are warranted to determine significant risk factors for PCOS. Family history may include menstrual disorders, adrenal enzyme deficiencies, infertility, hirsutism, obesity, metabolic syndrome, and diabetes. A comprehensive menstrual history is needed to identify the most common presenting symptom: menstrual irregularities. These abnormalities typically begin at menarche. Oligomenorrhea and secondary amenorrhea are the most common. Some women also experience dysfunctional uterine bleeding. Infertility is common with PCOS; thus, asking about attempts at conception is important. Other symptoms to discuss are hirsutism, acne, and alopecia (American College of ACOG, 2009).

Physical Examination • The goal of the physical exam is twofold: to exclude other causes of the symptoms and to identify risk factors for chronic disease. AACE advocates using the Rotterdam criteria to establish the diagnosis of PCOS in the presence of two of the following criteria: androgen excess, ovulatory dysfunction, or polycystic ovaries. Note that the presence of polycystic ovary is not needed for diagnosis (Legro et al., 2013).

Women suspected of having PCOS should be evaluated for hypertension, obesity, dermatological changes, virilization, and pelvic masses. Obesity (BMI of 30 or greater) with central adiposity is present in approximately 50% of women with PCOS. A waist-to-hip ratio of greater than 0.85 is diagnostic of central obesity. The obesity is thought to be related to both androgen excess and insulin resistance (Moran, Hutchinson, Norman, & Teede, 2011).

Enlarged ovaries are present in 50% to 75% of women with PCOS. This enlargement is due to the formation of cysts that give the syndrome its name as well as an increase in the ovarian stroma. The ovarian changes are a result of the disease and are not a cause of the syndrome. While polycystic ovaries are present in a large number of women, irregular menstrual patterns and signs of androgen excess are more common and better predictors of the disorder (Legro et al., 2013).

Skin and hair changes are also common. Alopecia or male pattern balding occurs in up to 25% of women and can be distressing. This symptom is related to the excessive level of androgens. Insulin resistance can lead to the development of acanthosis nigricans, as is seen with metabolic syndrome (Moran, Hutchinson, Norman, & Teede, 2011; Norman, Dewailly, Legro, & Hickey, 2007).

Differential Diagnoses • The differential diagnoses to be considered depend on the presenting symptoms. PCOS should be assessed in any woman with an abnormal menstrual pattern that is coupled with signs and symptoms of excessive androgens. In women of all ages, other causes of hyperandrogenism need to be ruled out, such as medication-induced issues, hyperprolactinemia, adrenal hyperplasia (Cushing's syndrome), and androgen-producing tumors. Virilization is not usually seen with PCOS; if present, may suggest adrenal hyperplasia or androgen-secreting tumor. Thyroid dysfunction can mimic some of the symptoms and should be ruled out (ACOG, 2009).

Diagnostic Studies • Current AACE guidelines do not recommend routine hormonal laboratory studies or ultrasonography to establish the diagnosis of PCOS in adult women if frank symptoms are present. The guidelines advise that an adult woman can be diagnosed with PCOS if she has at least two of the following symptoms: excess androgen, ovulatory dysfunction, or polycystic ovaries. During the perimenopausal transition and postmenopause, diagnosis should be based on documented, chronic oligomenorrhea, as well as hyperandrogenism during the reproductive years. Polycystic ovaries visualized on ultrasonography may provide supportive evidence although this is not likely in the postmenopausal woman. In addition, any diagnosis of PCOS must rule out other androgen-excess disorders. Clinicians should screen patients for endometrial cancer, mood disorders, obstructive sleep apnea if obese, diabetes, and cardiovascular disease. In adolescents with persistent oligomenorrhea, diagnosis of PCOS should be based on clinical presentation and hormonal analysis once other possible etiologies have been excluded (Legro et al., 2013).

When indicated, laboratory tests are used to rule out other causes of the symptoms and to document PCOS abnormalities. Measurement of serum 17-hydroxyprogesterone levels after a cosyntropin stimulation test can be used to exclude late-onset adrenal hyperplasia. If Cushing's syndrome is suspected, 24-hour urine for free cortisol and creatinine should be obtained. A dexamethasone suppression test is also useful in assessing for Cushing's syndrome. Serum insulin-like growth factor (IGF)-1 is a highly sensitive and specific biomarker of growth hormone excess and is used to rule-out acromegaly only if there is a clinical suspicion of this disorder. Hyperprolactinemia can be excluded by obtaining a fasting serum prolactin level. OGTT (2-hour GTT) is recommended to evaluate for type 2 diabetes. Thyroid function tests, specifically third-generation TSH and free T_4, should be obtained to exclude hypothyroidism (Barbieri & Ehrmann, 2015; Legro et al., 2013).

Elevated levels of total or free testosterone can confirm the androgen excess; however, they do not diagnose the cause. The typical range for elevated testosterone levels with PCOS is more than 50 ng/dL of total or more than 0.9 ng/dL of free testosterone. Levels are much higher in the presence of an androgen-secreting ovarian tumor (Legro et al., 2013). Depending on the androgen measured, up to 90% of women with PCOS will have elevated blood levels. LH and FSH levels may also be useful. An LH-to-FSH ratio of greater than 3 is often present in PCOS. Serum estradiol levels are usually normal, while serum estrone is elevated due to the conversion of androgen to estrone in the adipose tissue. Sex hormone-binding globulin (SHBG) is usually decreased. Currently, the SHBG test is performed as a baseline study to determine the free androgen index (FAI), especially when ovarian mass or tumor is suspected. Several tests are available to determine insulin levels; however, the results of these tests are not well defined and as such not recommended (Legro et al., 2013; Royal College of Obstetricians and Gynaecologists, 2007). Current, accepted guidelines should be used to screen for hyperlipidemia and hypertension. In obese women, the same screening measures used in metabolic syndrome should be employed. Frequency of rescreening depends on the initial results. If the results are abnormal, then rescreening may be indicated in 3 to 6 months, as opposed to 1 to 5 years or at the usual age for general screening.

Imaging studies such as transvaginal pelvic/ovarian ultrasonography are performed when the manual pelvic examination is inadequate, in the presence of abdominal and/or pelvic pain, when testosterone levels are excessively elevated (greater than 200 ng/dL), and to assess for endometrial thickness or anatomical etiology in the presence of amenorrhea. If a solid mass or tumor is suspected, CT or MRI should be obtained to assess the adrenal glands and ovaries. MRI is preferred for imaging the ovaries in very obese women as the ovaries may not always be visualized with transvaginal ultrasonography and in adolescents and women in whom transvaginal ultrasonography may be inappropriate (Lalwani et al., 2012; Trivax & Azziz, 2007).

Treatment/Management • Goals for the management of PCOS are to decrease androgen levels; control symptoms; prevent long-term problems; reduce BMI; decrease cardiovascular risk, including dyslipidemia; protect the endometrium; delay or prevent diabetes; decrease blood pressure; and induce ovulation if pregnancy is desired.

Self-Management Measures. First-line treatment modalities include TLC. Although the role of exercise, healthy diet, and weight reduction in improving PCOS is unclear, it is recommended for overweight and obese women for other health benefits, primarily reduction of cardiovascular and diabetes risk (Legro et al., 2013). Setting realistic goals that are acceptable to the patient are important to the success of TLC.

Pharmacotherapeutics. An Endocrine Society task force developed new evidence-based guidelines for the treatment of PCOS in 2013 using the Grading of Recommendations,

Assessment, Development, and Evaluation (GRADE) system to rate the strength and quality of recommendations. These guidelines are summarized in the following text (Legro et al., 2013).

HORMONAL CONTRACEPTIVES. Current guidelines recommend hormonal contraceptives (including pill, patch, vaginal ring) as first-line therapy for women with menstrual abnormalities and PCOS-related hirsutism and/or acne. As with use of hormonal contraceptives for prevention of pregnancy, screening for contraindications using established guidelines (U.S. Medical Eligibility Criteria for Contraceptive Use, 2010) is imperative.

METFORMIN. Use of metformin is indicated for women with PCOS with an established diagnosis of type 2 diabetes or impaired glucose tolerance who have been unsuccessful with lifestyle modifications. It is also recommended as second-line therapy for women with PCOS who have menstrual irregularities and cannot tolerate hormonal contraceptives or in whom hormonal contraceptives are contraindicated. Current guidelines do not recommend metformin as first-line therapy for women with PCOS for treatment of hirsutism and/or acne, for prevention of pregnancy complications, or for treatment of obesity.

TREATMENT OF INFERTILITY. Clomiphene citrate or comparable estrogen modulators (e.g., letrozole) is the recommended first-line therapy for anovulatory infertility. Women with PCOS having in vitro fertilization should be prescribed metformin as adjuvant therapy for infertility to prevent ovarian hyperstimulation syndrome.

OTHER PHARMACOTHERAPEUTICS. Treatment of PCOS should not include insulin sensitizers such as inositols due to lack of documented benefit or thiazolidinediones owing to safety concerns. Current expert opinion does not recommend the use of statin therapy for hyperandrogenism and anovulation in women with PCOS as sufficient risk–benefit data are lacking. Statins are recommended for women with PCOS who meet indications of current expert recommendations for statin therapy (Stone, Robinson, Lichtenstein, et al., 2014).

Treatment/Management of Adolescents • When the goal of treatment is to relieve anovulatory symptoms, treat hirsutism and/or acne, or prevent pregnancy in adolescents with suspected PCOS, hormonal contraceptives are considered first-line therapy. However, optimal duration of contraceptive use has not been established for this population.

If the adolescent has impaired glucose tolerance and/or metabolic syndrome, metformin may be considered, although optimal duration of this therapy has not been established.

Treatment/Management of Premenarchal Girls • For girls with advanced pubertal development (Tanner stage IV or above of breast development) accompanied by clinical and biochemical indicators of hyperandrogenism, initiation of hormonal contraceptives is suggested.

■ ADRENAL DISORDERS

The major function of the adrenal gland is the biosynthesis of steroids. As with the reproductive system, the regulation of these steroids is by a feedback mechanism. Aldosterone, the major mineralocorticoid, influences ion transport and plays a role in controlling blood pressure. Cortisol, the major glucocorticoid, is important in the regulation of many body systems including fetal lung maturity, bone remodeling, and calcium absorption. The third major group of steroids released from the adrenal gland is androgens. Dehydroepiandrosterone (DHEA), androsteredione, and testosterone are all released into circulation. Excess androgen can originate from either ovarian (PCOS) or adrenal sources.

Addison's Disease

DEFINITION

The most common cause of primary adrenal insufficiency is Addison's disease.

SYMPTOMS

The signs and symptoms related to the underproduction of cortisol are outlined in Table 44.14. Of these, the most common presenting symptoms are fatigue, weakness, and skin hyperpigmentation.

DIAGNOSTIC STUDIES

Initial testing for adrenal insufficiency is a fasting early morning serum cortisol.

TREATMENT/MANAGEMENT

All forms of adrenal insufficiency are treated with glucocorticoid replacement with prednisone, hydrocortisone, or dexamethasone. In addition, fludrocortisones are used to replace mineralocorticoid deficiency (Nieman, 2013).

Cushing's Syndrome

DEFINITION, SCOPE, AND ETIOLOGY

Oversecretion of glucocorticoids is known as Cushing's syndrome. The most common presentation (65%–70%) is due to oversecretion of ACTH by a pituitary adenoma and is eight times more likely to occur in women. The increased amplitude and duration of ACTH secretion usually results in bilateral hyperplasia of the adrenal gland, leading to increased secretion of adrenocortical hormones and androgens.

SYMPTOMS

As with Addison's disease, the effects of Cushing's syndrome are manifest throughout the body (Table 44.14). The clinical signs and symptoms depend on the degree and duration of excess of all three steroids secreted in the

TABLE 44.14	Comparison of Addison's Disease and Cushing's Syndrome	
TARGET	**ADDISON'S**	**CUSHING'S**
Liver	↓ Hepatic glucose output and glycogen storage	↑ Hepatic glucose output ↑ Hepatic glycogen stores
Adipose tissue	↓ Adipose tissue ↓ Lipolysis	Central obesity Mood faces, buffalo hump
Muscle	Weakness ↓ Muscle glycogen ↓ Urinary nitrogen excretion	Weakness and wasting ↑ Urinary nitrogen excretion
Plasma glucose	Hypoglycemia ↑ Insulin sensitivity	↓ Insulin sensitivity → diabetes IGT
Hypothalamus pituitary	Oligomenorrhea	Oligomenorrhea
Kidney Calcium homeostasis Sodium, potassium, ECF	Retardation of bone growth ↓ Growth hormone, ↓ ECF volume Hyponatremia Hyperkalemia	Hypercalciuria, hypokalemic acidosis, secondary hyperthyroidism, retardation of bone growth
Pancreas	Hypoinsulinemia	Hyperinsulinemia
Carrier protein		↓ in total T$_4$
Skin	Hyperpigmentation	Easy bruising, dermal atrophy
Breast		Galatorrhea
Heart	↓ Peripheral resistance Orthostatic hypotension	Hypertension
CNS	Depression ↓ Appetite ↓ Intraocular pressure	Euphoria → Depression ↑ Appetite Sleep disturbance Impaired memory Cataracts, ↑ ocular pressure

↓ = decreased; ↑ = increased; CNS, central nervous system; ECF, extracellular fluid; IGT, impaired glucose tolerance.
Data from Nieman (2013, 2015).

adrenal gland and vary according to the increases in the different hormones. Presenting symptoms vary depending on the system involved. Most women experience fatigue. Changes in their menstrual patterns (oligomenorrhea, amenorrhea) often prompt them to seek evaluation. Over time, problems such as osteoporosis, diabetes, hypertension, and CVD develop.

DIAGNOSTIC STUDIES

The two tests most commonly used to diagnose Cushing's syndrome are 24-hour urine for free cortisol and the overnight dexamethasone suppression test (Nieman, 2013).

TREATMENT/MANAGEMENT

Treatment of Cushing's syndrome is aimed at the primary cause of the disease and can involve medication, surgery, or irradiation. Treatment goals are threefold: reversal of clinical signs and symptoms, removal of tumors, and avoidance of dependence on medication. While all three goals are important, the first goal takes priority (Nieman, 2013). Untreated Cushing's syndrome is fatal, caused by the hypercortisol state and its complications. Any patient with symptoms suggestive of adrenal disorders requires referral to an endocrine specialist.

■ HIRSUTISM

Definition, Scope, Etiology, and Risk Factors

Hirsutism, the development of excess body hair in women, can be associated with several disease processes and is present in 5% to 10% of women (Sachdeva, 2010). Of particular interest in women's health is its association with PCOS, hyperprolactinemia, and insulin resistance; with PCOS accounting for 80% to 90% of all cases (Talaei, Adgi, & Mohamadi Kelishadi, 2013). It is most often caused by an increase in secreted or converted free androgens in circulation. It may also be related to certain medications including testosterone, progestin, phenobarbital, phenytoin, and minoxidil. Between 5% and 10% of hirsutism may be due to racial/ethnic differences and is considered normal. Women of Mediterranean descent tend to have more body hair than other ethnic groups.

Symptoms and Evaluation/Assessment

The hair appears in androgen-dependent areas such as the upper lip, chin, chest, lower abdomen, back, and thighs. Assessment is aimed at identifying the reason for the androgen excess. The basic approach is to document the degree of androgen excess as well as exclude any rare yet serious causes such as an androgen-secreting tumor. Abrupt, rapid onset usually over less than 1 year as well as onset later in life may be signs of an androgen-secreting tumor. Signs of virilization can signal not only an ovarian tumor but also developing Cushing's syndrome. A complete menstrual history that includes age of menarche, regularity of cycle, symptoms of ovulation, and pregnancy history can indicate underlying causes. A complete medication history, including current and past use of medications known to cause hirsutism, is also important.

The physical exam includes evaluation for other signs of hyperandrogenism such as seborrhea, alopecia, and acne. Any signs of virilization are noted and described (Bode, Seehusen, & Baird, 2012; Sachdeva, 2010).

TABLE 44.15	Laboratory Findings With Hyperandrogenism
CAUSE	FINDING
Cushing's syndrome	↑ Cortisol level Dexamethasone suppression: negative
Adrenal tumor	↑ Testosterone and DHEA level
Ovarian tumor	↑ Testosterone level DHEA level low
Hyperprolactinemia	↑ Prolactin level
Insulin resistance	↑ Glucose ↑ Lipids ↑ Insulin
PCOS	LH/FSH ratio ↑ 3 ↑ Insulin
Idiopathic	Normal laboratory findings

↓ = decreased; ↑ = increased; DHEA, dehydroepiandrosterone; FSH, follicle-stimulating hormone; LH, luteinizing hormone; PCOS, polycystic ovarian syndrome.
Data from Sachdeva (2010) and Talaei, Adgi, and Mohamadi Kelishadi (2013).

Diagnostic Studies

Several laboratory tests are ordered to help establish the cause and rule out various syndromes associated with hyperandrogenism (Table 44.15). Total and bioavailable testosterone are usually elevated and provide a diagnosis of androgen excess. Serum 17-hydroxyprogesterone should be evaluated if congenital adrenal hyperplasia is suspected. If the woman presents with signs of Cushing's syndrome, 24-hour urine-free cortisol should be measured. An elevated DHEA-S level suggests an adrenal source and can signal an adrenal tumor; if present, evaluation for a tumor is done using CT, MRI, and/or ultrasound. Pelvic ultrasonography should be performed if ovarian mass or PCOS is suspected. Serum TSH should be measured and will be elevated in hirsutism (Bode, Seehusen, & Baird, 2012; Sachdeva, 2010).

Treatment/Management

Management of the disorders that cause hirsutism is discussed in the pertaining chapter sections. The focus of management is cosmetic and encompasses two approaches: hair removal and suppression of hair growth. Shaving, topical depilatories, waxing, laser treatment, and electrolysis are options for reducing hair growth. Medications, including eflornithine hydrochloride cream 13.9% (Vaniqa cream) and spironolactone, can also be used. There is some evidence that hormonal contraception can suppress adrenal production of androgens

FUTURE DIRECTIONS

The endocrine system is complex and affects multiple other body systems. Problems can affect women in multiple

ways, and often the presentation for a single problem varies from one patient to another. A careful history and physical exam coupled with appropriate diagnostic studies assists with identifying the most likely diagnosis and developing an appropriate evidence-based management plan. Future research will provide additional information for identification and treatment of these problems in women.

■ REFERENCES

American Association of Clinical Endocrinologists (AACE), American Thyroid Association (ATA), Endocrine Society (TES). (2004). Joint statement RE: FDA approval of generic levothyroxine preparations as equivalent to brand preparations. Retrieved from http://www.aace.com/files/position-statements/levothyroxine.php

Alberti, K. G., Eckel, R. H., Grundy, S. M., Zimmet, P. Z., Cleeman, J. I., Donato, K. A.,...Smith, S. C., Jr. (2009). International Diabetes Federation Task Force on Epidemiology and Prevention; National Heart, Lung, and Blood Institute; American Heart Association; World Heart Federation; International Atherosclerosis Society; International Association for the Study of Obesity. *Circulation, 120*(16), 1640–1645.

Alberti, K. G., & Zimmet, P. Z. (1998). Definition, diagnosis and classification of diabetes mellitus and its complications. Part 1: diagnosis and classification of diabetes mellitus provisional report of a WHO consultation. *Diabetic Medicine, 15*, 539–553.

American Association of Clinical Endocrinologists and American College of Endocrinology. (2015). Clinical practice guidelines for developing a diabetes mellitus comprehensive care plan. *Endocrine Practice, 21*(4, Suppl. 1), 1–87.

American Association of Clinical Endocrinologists/American Thyroid Association/Endocrine Society; Gharib, H., Tuttle, R. M., Baskin, H. J., Fish, L. H., Singer, P. A., & McDermott, M. T. (2004). Subclinical thyroid dysfunction: A joint statement on management from the American Association of Clinical Endocrinologists, the American Thyroid Association, and The Endocrine Society. *Endocrinology Practice, 10*(6), 497–501.

American Association of Clinical Endocrinologists (AACE) Thyroid Task Force. (2006). Medical guidelines for clinical practice for the evaluation and treatment of hyperthyroidism and hypothyroidism. Amended version. *Endocrine Practice, 8*(6), 457–467.

American College of Cardiology, American Heart Association. ASCVD Risk Estimator. (2014). Retrieved from http://tools.cardiosource.org/ASCVD-Risk-Estimator

American College of Obstetricians and Gynecologists. (2009). *Polycystic ovary syndrome.* Washington, DC: American College of Obstetricians and Gynecologists. ACOG practice bulletin No. 108. Retrieved from www.guideline.gov

American Diabetes Association (ADA). (2014). Diabetes management in correctional institutions. *Diabetes Care, 37*(Suppl. 1), S104–S111.

American Diabetes Association: Clinical Practice Recommendations (2015). Retrieved from http://professional.diabetes.org/ResourcesForProfessionals.aspx?cid=84160

American Diabetes Association (ADA). (2016). Standards of medical care in diabetes—2016 Summary of revisions. *Diabetes Care, 39*(S1), S4–S5. Retrieved from http://care.diabetesjournals.org/content/39/Supplement_1/S4

Azziz, R., Woods, K. S., Reyna, R., Key, T. J., Knochenhauer, E. S., & Yildiz, B. O. (2004). The prevalence and features of the polycystic ovary syndrome in an unselected population. *Journal of Clinical Endocrinology and Metabolism, 89*(6), 2745–2749.

Bahn, R. S., Burch, H. B., Cooper, D. S., Garber, J. R., Greenlee, M. C., Klein, I.,...Stan, M. N.; American Thyroid Association, American Association of Clinical Endocrinologists. (2011). Hyperthyroidism and other causes of thyrotoxicosis: Management guidelines of the American Thyroid Association and American Association of Clinical Endocrinologists. *Thyroid, 21*(6), 593–646.

Barber, T. M., McCarthy. M. I., Wass, J. A., & Franks, S. (2006). Obesity and polycystic ovary syndrome. *Clinical Endocrinology, 65*(2), 137–145.

Barbieri, R. L. (2014). The endocrinology of the menstrual cycle. *Methods in Molecular Biology, 1154*, 145–169.

Barbieri, R. L., & Ehrmann, D. A. (2015). Diagnosis of polycystic ovary syndrome. *UpToDate*. Retrieved from http://www.uptodate.com/contents/diagnosis-of-polycystic-ovary-syndrome-in-adults

Barry, J. A., Azizia, M. M., & Hardiman, P. J. (2014). Risk of endometrial, ovarian and breast cancer in women with polycystic ovary syndrome: A systematic review and meta-analysis. *Human Reproduction Update, 20*(5), 748–758.

Bateman, L. A., Slentz, C. A., Willis L. H., Shields, A. T., Piner, L. W., Bales, C. W.,...Kraus, W. E. (2011). Comparison of aerobic versus resistance exercise training effects on metabolic syndrome (from the Studies of a Targeted Risk Reduction Intervention Through Defined Exercise—STRRIDE-AT/RT). *American Journal of Cardiology, 108*(6), 838–844. Retrieved from http://reference.medscape.com/medline/abstract/21741606

Bauer, D. C., & McPhee, S. J. (2006). Thyroid disease. In S. J. McPhee & W. F. Ganong (Eds.), *Pathophysiology of disease: An introduction to clinical medicine* (5th ed.). New York, NY: Lange Medical Books/McGraw-Hill.

Beasler, R. S. (2014). *Joslin's diabetes deskbook: A guide for primary care providers,* Boston, MA: Joslin Diabetes Center.

Bentley-Lewis, R., Koruda, K., & Seely, E. W. (2007). The metabolic syndrome in women. *Nature Clinical Practice Endocrinology and Metabolism,* (10), 696–704.

Bilezikian, J. P., Khan, A. A., & Potts, J. T. (2009). Guidelines for the management of asymptomatic primary hyperparathyroidism: Summary statement from the Third International Workshop. *Journal of Clinical Endocrinology & Metabolism, 94*(2), 335–339.

Bilezikian, J. P., Khan, A., Potts, J. T., Brandi, M. L., Clarke, B. L., Shoback, D.,...Sanders, J. (2011). Hypoparathyroidism in the adult: Epidemiology, diagnosis, pathophysiology, target-organ involvement, treatment, and challenges for future research. *Journal of Bone and Mineral Research, 26,* 2317–2337.

Billings, L. K., & Florez, J. C. (2010). The genetics of type 2 diabetes: What have we learned from GWAS? *Annals of the New York Academy of Sciences, 1212,* 59–77.

Blaha, M. J., Bansal, S., Rouf, R., Golden, S. H., Blumenthal, R. S., & Defilippis, A. P. (2008). A practical "ABCDE" approach to the metabolic syndrome. *Mayo Clinic Proceedings, 83*(8), 932–941.

Bode, D., Seehusen, D. A., & Baird, D. (2012). Hirsutism in women. *American Family Physician, 85*(4), 373–380.

Borchers, A. T., Uibo, R., Gershwin, M. E. (2010). The geoepidemiology of type 1 diabetes. *Autoimmunity Reviews, 9,* A355–A365.

Bray, G. A. (2014). *Obesity in adults: Prevalence, screening and evaluation.* UpToDate. Retrieved from http://uptodateonline.com

Bray, G. A. (2015). *Obesity in adults: Overview of management.* UpToDate. Retrieved from http://uptodateonline.com

Bureau of Justice. (2012). *Bureau of Justice Statistics.* Retrieved from http://www.ojp.usdoj.gov/bjs

Carroll, T. B., Aron, D. C., Finding, J. W., & Tyrell, J. B. (2011). Glucocorticoids and adrenal androgens. In D. Gardner & D. Shoback (Eds.), *Greenspan's basic and clinical endocrinology* (9th ed.). New York, NY: Lange Medical Books/McGraw Hill.

Centers for Disease Control and Prevention (CDC). (2010). Diabetes and women's health across the life stages: A public health perspective. Retrieved from http://www.cdc.gov/diabetes/pubs/pdf/women.pdf

Centers for Disease Control and Prevention (CDC). (2011). National diabetes fact sheet: National estimates and general information on diabetes and prediabetes in the United States. Retrieved from http://www.cdc.gov/diabetes/pubs/pdf/ndfs_2011.pdf

Centers for Disease Control and Prevention. (2015). Top 10 leading causes of death: United States, 2013. Retrieved from http://blogs.cdc.gov/nchs-data-visualization/2015/06/01/leading-causes-of-death

Chen, J. (2008). *Chinese herbal formulas and applications.* City of Industry, CA: AOM Press.

Cooper, D. S., & Biondi, B. (2012). Subclinical thyroid disease. *Lancet, 379*(9821), 1142–1154.

Ehrmann, D. A. (2005). Polycystic ovary syndrome. *New England Journal of Medicine, 352,* 1223–1236.

Einhorn, D., Reaven, G. M., & Cobin, R. H. (2009). American College of Endocrinology position statement on the insulin resistance syndrome. *Endocrine Practice, 9,* 236–252.

El-Hajj Fuleihan, G. (2014). *Primary hyperthyroidism: Beyond the basics.* UpToDate. Retrieved from http://updateonline.com

Expert Panel Report. (2014). Guidelines for the management of overweight and obesity in adults. *Obesity, 22,* S41–S68.

Ford, E. S., Giles, W. H., & Dietz, W. H. (2002). Prevalence of the metabolic syndrome among US adults: Findings from the Third National Health and Nutrition Examination Survey. *Journal of the American Medical Association, 287,* 356–359.

Freeman, S. B. (2006). The metabolic syndrome revisited. *Women's Healthcare: A Practical Journal for Nurse Practitioners, 5*(4), 52–72.

Fujita, N., & Takei, Y. (2011). Alcohol consumption and metabolic syndrome. *Hepatology Research, 41*(4), 287–295.

Gardner, D., & Shoback, D. (2011). *Greenspan's basic and clinical endocrinology* (9th ed.). New York, NY: Lange Medical Books/McGraw Hill.

Gharib, H., Papini, E., Paschke, R., Duick, D. S., Valcavi, R., Hegedüs, L., & Vitti, P. (2010). AACE/AME/ETA Task Force on Thyroid Nodules. American Association of Clinical Endocrinologists, Associazione Medici Endocrinologi, and European Thyroid Association medical guidelines for clinical practice for the diagnosis and management of thyroid nodules: Executive summary of recommendations. *Journal of Endocrinolical Investment, 33*(Suppl. 5), 51–56.

Gharib, H., Tuttle, R. M., Baskin, H. J., Fish, L. H., Singer, P. A., & McDermott, M. T. (2004). Subclinical thyroid dysfunction: A joint statement on management from the American Association of Clinical Endocrinologists, the American Thyroid Association, and the Endocrine Society. *Journal of Clinical Endocrinology & Metabolism, 90*(1), 586–587.

Goff, D. C., Jr., Lloyd-Jones, D. M., Bennett, G., Coady, S., D'Agostino, R. B., Sr., Gibbons, R.,...Tomaselli, G. F. (2014). ACC/AHA guideline on the assessment of cardiovascular risk: A report of the American College of Cardiology/American Heart Association Task Force on Practice Guidelines. *Circulation, 129*(25, Suppl. 2), S49–S73.

Golden, S. H., Robinson, K. A., Saldanha, I., Anton, B., & Ladenson, P. W. (2009). Prevalence and incidence of endocrine and metabolic disorders in the United States: A comprehensive review. *Journal of Clinical Endocrinology & Metabolism, 94*(6), 1853–1878.

Goodman, N. F., Cobin, R. H., Futterweit, W., Glueck, J. S., Legro, R. S., & Carmina, E. (2015). American Association of Clinical Endocrinologists, American College of Endocrinology, and Androgen Excess and PCOS Society Disease State Clinical Review: Guide to the best practices in the evaluation and treatment of polycystic ovary syndrome—Part 1. *Endocrine Practice, 21*(11), 1291–1230.

Grundy, S. M., Cleeman, J. I., Daniels, S. R., Donato, K. A., Eckel, R. H., Franklin, B. A.,...Costa, F. (2005). AHA scientific statement: Diagnosis and management of the metabolic syndrome. An American Heart Association/National Heart, Lung, and Blood Institute Scientific Statement: Executive Summary. *Circulation, 112,* 285–290.

Guha, B., Krishnaswamy, G., & Peiris, A. (2002). The diagnosis and management of hypothyroidism. *Southern Medical Journal, 95*(5), 475–480.

Habif, T. P. (2009). Cutaneous manifestations of internal disease. In T. P. Habif (Ed.), *Clinical dermatology* (5th ed., Chapter 26, pp. 975-995). Philadelphia, PA: Mosby Elsevier.

Hackethal, V. (2014). 2 in 5 American adults will develop diabetes. *Medscape Medical News.* Retrieved from http://www.medscape.com/viewarticle/829833

Heima, N. E., Eekhoff, E. M., Oosterwerff, M., Lips, P., van Schoor, N., & Simsek, S. (2012). Thyroid function and the metabolic syndrome in older persons: A population-based study. *European Journal of Endocrinology.* Retrieved from http://reference.medscape.com/medline/abstract/23093697

Hueston, W. J. (2011). Hyperthyroidism. In E. T. Bope, R. Kellerman, & R. E. Rakel (Eds.), *Conn's current therapy* (pp. 681–683). Philadelphia, PA: Saunders.

Ito, M. K. (2004). The metabolic syndrome: Pathophysiology, clinical relevance, and use of niacin. *Annals of Pharmacotherapy, 38*(2), 277–285.

James, P. A., Oparil, S., Carter, B. L., Cushman, W. C., Dennison-Himmelfarb, C., Handler J.,...Ortiz, E. (2014). Evidence-based guideline for the management of high blood pressure in adults: Report by the panel appointed to the Eighth Joint National Committee (JNC 8). *Journal of the American Medical Association, 311*(5), 507–520. doi:10.1001/JAMA.2013.284427

Jonklaas, J., Bianco, A. C., Bauer, A. J., Burman K. D., Cappola, A. R., Celi, F.,...Sawka, A. M.; American Thyroid Association Task Force on Thyroid Hormone Replacement. (2014). Guidelines for the treatment of hypothyroidism: Prepared by the American Thyroid Association task force on thyroid hormone replacement. *Thyroid, 24*(12), 1670–1751.

Kreisman, S. H., & Hennessey, J. V. (1999). Consistent reversible elevations of serum creatinine levels in severe hypothyroidism. *Archives of Internal Medicine, 159*(1), 79–82.

Ladenson, P. W. (2010). Thyroid. In E. G. Nabel (Ed.), *ACP medicine* (Section 3, Chapter 1). Hamilton, ON: BC Decker.

Ladenson, P. W., Singer, P. A., Ain, K. B., Bagchi, N., Bigos, S. T., Levy, E. G.,...Cohen, H. D. (2000). American Thyroid Association guidelines for detection of thyroid dysfunction. *Archives of Internal Medicine, 160*(11), 1573–1575.

Lalwani, N., Patel, S., Ha, K. Y., Shanbhogue, A. K., Nagar, A. M., Chintapalli, K. N., & Prasad, S. R. (2012). Miscellaneous tumour-like lesions of the ovary: Cross-sectional imaging review. *British Journal of Radiology, 85*(1013), 477–486.

Lam, J. C., & Ip, M. S. (2007). An update on obstructive sleep apnea and the metabolic syndrome. *Current Opinion in Pulmonary Medicine, 13*(6), 484–489.

Lee, S. L. (2015). Hyperthyroidism. *Medscape emedicine.* Retrieved from http://emedicine.medscape.com/article/121865-overview

Lee, D.-Y., Oh, Y.-K., Yoon, B.-K., & Choi, D. (2012). Prevalence of hyperprolactinemia in adolescents and young women with menstruation-related problems. *American Journal of Obstetrics & Gynecology, 206*, 213e1–213e5.

Legro, R. S., Arslanian, S. A., Ehrmann, D. A., Hoeger, K. M., Hassan Murad, M., Renato Pasquali, R., & Welt, C. K. (2013). Diagnosis and treatment of polycystic ovary syndrome: An Endocrine Society Clinical Practice Guideline. *Journal of Clinical Endocrinology & Metabolism, 98*(12), 4565–4592.

Mandel, S. J., Larson, P. R., & Davies, T. F. (2011). Thyrotoxicosis. In S. Melmed, K. S. Polansky, P. R. Larsen, & H. R. Kronenberg (Eds.), *Williams textbook of endocrinology* (12th ed., pp. 362–405). Philadelphia, PA: Saunders.

Marcocci, C., & Cetani, F. (2011). Primary hyperparathyroidism. *New England Journal of Medicine, 365*, 2389–2397.

Masharani, U., & German, M. S. (2011). Pancreatic hormones and diabetes mellitus. In D. Gardner & D. Shoback (Eds.), *Greenspan's basic and clinical endocrinology* (9th ed.). New York, NY: Lange Medical Books/McGraw Hill.

Meigs, J. B. (2015). *The metabolic syndrome (insulin resistance or Syndrome X).* UpToDate. Retrieved from http://uptodateonline.com

Melmed, S., Casanueva, F. F., Hoffman. A. R., Kleinberg, D. L., Montori, V. M., Schlechte, J. A., & Wass, J. A.; Endocrine Society. (2011). Diagnosis and treatment of hyperprolactinemia: An Endocrine Society clinical practice guideline. *Journal of Clinical Endocrinology & Metabolism, 96*(2), 273–288.

Moe, S. M. (2008). Disorders involving calcium, phosphorus and magnesium. *Primary Care, 35*(2), 215–vi.

Moran, L. J., Hutchison, S. K., Norman, R. J., & Teede, H. J. (2011). Lifestyle changes in women with polycystic ovary syndrome. *The Cochrane Database of Systematic Reviews, 16*(2), CD007506. Retrieved from http://www.ncbi.nlm.nih.gov/pubmed/21328294

NCEP/ATP III. (2001). Executive summary of the third report of the National Cholesterol Education Program (NCEP) expert panel on detection, evaluation, and treatment of high blood cholesterol in adults (adult treatment panel III). *Journal of the American Medical Association, 285*, 2486–2497.

Nesto, R. W. (2003). The relation of insulin resistance syndromes to risk of cardiovascular disease. *Review of Cardiovascular Medicine, 4*(6), S11–S18. Retrieved from http://www.ncbi.nlm.nih.gov/pubmed/14668699

Nieman, L. K. (2013). *Epidemiology and clinical manifestations of Cushing's syndrome.* UpToDate. Retrieved from http://www.uptodate.com/contents/epidemiology-and-clinical-manifestations-of-cushings-syndrome

Nieman, L. K. (2015). *Treatment of adrenal insufficiency.* UpToDate. Retrieved from http://uptodateonline.com

Norman, R. J., Dewailly, D., Legro, R. S., & Hickey, T. E. (2007). Polycystic ovary syndrome. *Lancet, 370*, 685–697.

Nwankwo, T., Yoon, S. S., Burt, V., & Gu, Q. (2013). Hypertension among adults in the US: National Health and Nutrition Examination Survey, 2011–2012. NCHS Data Brief, No. 133. Hyattsville, MD: National Center for Health Statistics, Centers for Disease Control and Prevention, U.S. Department of Health and Human Services.

Ovalle, F., & Azziz, R. (2002). Insulin resistance, polycystic ovary syndrome, and type 2 diabetes mellitus. *Fertility and Sterility, 77*, 1095–1105.

Palacios, S. S., Pascual-Corrales, E., & Galofre, J. C. (2012). Management of subclinical hyperthyroidism. *International Journal of Endocrinology and Metabolism, 10*(2), 490–496.

Park, S. M., & Chatterjee, V. K. (2005). Genetics of congenital hypothyroidism. *Journal of Medical Genetics, 42*(5), 379–389.

Puig, J. G., & Martínez, M. A. (2008). Hyperuricemia, gout and the metabolic syndrome. *Current Opinion in Rheumatology, 20*(2), 187–191.

Roberts, C. K., Hevener, A. L., & Barnard, R. J. (2013). Metabolic syndrome and insulin resistance: Underlying causes and modification by exercise training. *Comprehensive Physiology, 3*(1), 1–58. Retrieved from http://reference.medscape.com/medline/abstract/21741606

Royal College of Obstetricians and Gynaecologists. (2007). *Long-term consequences of polycystic ovary syndrome.* London, UK: Royal College of Obstetricians and Gynaecologists; Green-top guideline; No. 33. Retrieved from www.guideline.gov

Sachdeva, S. (2010). Hirsutism evaluation and treatment. *Indian Journal of Dermatology, 55*(1), 3–7. Retrieved from http://www.ncbi.nlm.nih.gov/pmc/articles/PMC2856356

Serri, O., Li, L., Mamputu, J. C., Beauchamp, M. C., Maingrette, F., & Renier, M. F. (2006). The influences of hyperprolactinemia and obesity on cardiovascular risk markers: Effects of cabergoline therapy. *Clinical Endocrinology, 64*(4), 366–370.

Shoback, D., Sellmeyer, D., & Bikle, D. D. (2011). Metabolic bone disease. In D. Gardner & D. Shoback (Eds.), *Greenspan's basic and clinical endocrinology* (9th ed., pp. 227–284). New York, NY: Lange Medical Books/McGraw Hill.

Snyder, P. J. (2014). Clinical manifestations and evaluation of hyperprolactinemia. UpToDate. Retrived from http://uptodateonline.com

Stagnaro-Green, A., Abalovich, M., Alexander, E., Azizi, F., Mestman, J., Negro, R.,... Wiersinga, W.; American Thyroid Association Taskforce on Thyroid Disease During Pregnancy and Postpartum. (2011). Guidelines of the American Thyroid Association for the diagnosis and management of thyroid disease during pregnancy and postpartum. *Thyroid, 21*(10), 1081–1125. doi:10.1089/thy.2011.0087

Stone, N. J., Robinson, J. G., Lichtenstein, A. H., Bairey-Merz, C. N., Blum, C. B., Eckel, R. H.,...Wilson, P. W. (2014). 2013 ACC/AHA guideline on the treatment of blood cholesterol to reduce atherosclerotic cardiovascular risk in adults: A report of the American College of Cardiology/American Heart Association Task Force on Practice Guidelines. *Journal of the American College of Cardiology, 63*(25, Pt. B), 2889–2934.

Talaei, A., Adgi, Z., & Mohamadi Kelishadi, M. (2013). Idiopathic hirsutism and insulin resistance. *International Journal of Endocrinology,* vol. 2013, Article ID 593197, 5 pages, doi:10.1155/2013/593197. Retrieved from http://www.hindawi.com/journals/ije/2013/593197/cta

Tasali, E., & Ip, M. S. (2008). Obstructive sleep apnea and metabolic syndrome: Alterations in glucose metabolism and inflammation. *Proceedings of the American Thoracic Society, 5*(2), 207–217.

Toulis, K. A., Goulis, D. G., Farmakiotis, D., Georgopoulos, N. A., Katsikis, I., Tarlatzis, B. C., ... Panidis, D. (2009). Adiponectin levels in women with polycystic ovary syndrome: A systematic review and a meta-analysis. *Human Reproduction Update, 15*(3), 297–307.

Towne, S. P., & Thara, E. (2008). Do statins reduce events in patients with metabolic syndrome? *Current Atherosclerosis Report, 10*(1), 39–44.

Trivax, B., & Azziz, R. (2007). Diagnosis of polycystic ovary syndrome. *Clinical Obstetrics and Gynecology, 50*, 168–177.

U.S. Medical Eligibility Criteria for Contraceptive Use. (2010). *MMWR Recommendations and Reports, 59*, 1–86. Retrieved from http://www.cdc.gov/mmwr/pdf/rr/rr59e0528.pdf

Wass, J. A. H., Stewart, P. M., Amiel, S. A., & Davies, M. C. (2011). In J. A. H. Wass, P. M. Stewart, S. A. Amiel, M. J. Davies (Eds.), *Oxford textbook of endocrinology and diabetes* (2nd ed.). Oxford, UK: Oxford University Press.

WHO Expert Consultation. (2004). Appropriate body-mass index for Asian populations and its implications for policy and intervention strategies. *Lancet, 363*, 157–163.

Yaffe, K. (2007). Metabolic syndrome and cognitive decline. *Current Alzheimer Research, 4*(2), 123–126.

Yoneda, M., Yamane, K., Jitsuiki, K., Nakanishi, S., Kamei, N., Watanabe, H., & Kohno, N. (2008). Prevalence of metabolic syndrome compared between native Japanese and Japanese-Americans. *Diabetes Research and Clinical Practice, 79*(3), 518–522.

Zbhuvana, G., Krishnaswamy, G., & Periris, A. (2002). The diagnosis and management of hypothyroidism. *Southern Medical Journal, 95*(5), 475–408.

Zeng, X, Yuan, Y., Wu, T., Yan, L., & Su, H. (2007). Chinese herbal medicines for hyperthyroidism. *The Cochrane Database of Systematic Reviews, 2007*(2), CD005450. doi:10.1002/14651858.CD005450.pub2

CHAPTER 45

Chronic Illness and Women

Tara F. Bertulfo • Theresa G. Rashdan

As a nation, we spend 86% of our health care dollars on the treatment of chronic diseases. These persistent conditions—the nation's leading causes of death and disability—leave in their wake deaths that could have been prevented, lifelong disability, compromised quality of life, and burgeoning health care costs.
—Centers for Disease Control and Prevention (CDC, 2015)

Several chronic diseases disproportionately affect women. It is important to monitor for these health concerns and follow current best practices for managing them. With careful management, the negative effects of chronic conditions can be reduced. Assisting women to attend to their health and maximize their wellness requires skill as many women put their own health needs after those of their family members (see Chapter 9).

■ DEFINITION AND SCOPE

"Chronic disease" is defined as a disease that can be controlled, but not cured, typically lasting 6 months or longer (Center for Managing Chronic Disease, 2011). These conditions usually develop slowly, often over a period of months or years.

Chronic diseases are prevalent in the United States and are a significant cause of death and disability. This trend is a dramatic break from the past, when infectious disease and trauma were the primary causes of death and disease. The CDC estimates that as of 2012, about half of all adults—117 million people—have one or more chronic health conditions. Seven of the top ten causes of death in 2010 were chronic diseases (CDC, 2012). Two of these chronic diseases—heart disease and cancer—together accounted for nearly 48% of all deaths (CDC, 2014).

The risk of chronic disease increases in women of child-bearing age who have certain pregnancy complications. Up to 50% of women with a history of gestational diabetes will develop type 2 diabetes within 5 years of pregnancy. Women with hypertension during pregnancy are about three times as likely to develop chronic hypertension and two times

as likely to develop heart disease later in life. Women with severe preeclampsia are about six times as likely to develop chronic hypertension (Division of Reproductive Health, 2011). The risk of developing a chronic disease also increases with age. Thus, increased longevity has resulted in the increased prevalence of many chronic diseases. Chronic conditions such as diabetes, obesity, osteoporosis, and HIV/AIDS can affect all aspects of a woman's life (Agency for Healthcare Research and Quality [AHRQ], 2012).

According to data from the 2008 National Health Interview Survey (NHIS), women in all age groups are more likely than men to have one, two, three, or more chronic conditions. These data (shown in Table 45.1) are categorized by sex and are broken down into three age categories: 55 years and older, 55 to 64 years, and 65 years and older. The six possible chronic conditions are arthritis, current asthma, cancer, cardiovascular disease, chronic obstructive pulmonary disease (COPD), and diabetes.

The National Center for Health Statistics (NCHS) tracks the prevalence of selected chronic conditions; the 2012 data regarding women 18 years of age and older are presented in Table 45.2. Among the most common conditions are arthritis, joint and back problems, hypertension, sinusitis, heart disease, and asthma (NCHS, 2014).

The NHIS is the principal source of information on the health of the civilian noninstitutionalized population of the United States and is one of the major data collection programs of the NCHS, CDC. A wide range of questions about health and health practices are asked. This survey demonstrates that when faced with chronic disease, a significant number of adult women experience substantial activity limitations, such as the inability to walk a quarter of a mile or climb 10 steps without resting. These data are given in Table 45.3.

■ ETIOLOGY

The cause or etiology of a chronic disease is typically multifactorial. These factors might be the physical, social, and psychological environment; biology and genetics, including sex; lifestyle and associated risks; or a combination of the factors

TABLE 45.1	Percentage of Adults Age 55 Years and Older (Total, Male and Female), With One or More, Two or More, or Three or More of a Possible Six Chronic Conditions: United States, 2008					
	TOTAL		**MALE**		**FEMALE**	
	%	SE	%	SE	%	SE
AGE 55 YEARS AND OVER	(*n* = 70,688,633)		(*n* = 32,130,140)		(*n* = 38,558,493)	
1+ chronic conditions	78.0	0.6	75.3	0.9	80.1	0.7
2+ chronic conditions	47.0	0.7	41.8	1.0	51.3	0.9
3+ chronic conditions	19.0	0.5	16.1	0.7	21.4	0.7

Source: CDC/National Center for Health Statistics: National Health Interview Survey.

TABLE 45.2	Age-Adjusted Percentages of Selected Diseases and Conditions Among Adults Aged 18 Years and Older, by Selected Characteristics: United States, 2012
CONDITION	**AGE-ADJUSTED PERCENTAGE**
Heart disease	9.7
Hypertension	23.2
Stroke	2.6
Emphysema	1.3
Asthma	9.8
Sinusitis	14.5
Chronic bronchitis	4.3
Cancer	8.6
Breast cancer	2.4
Cervical cancer	1.1
Diabetes	8.3
Ulcers	6.7
Kidney disease	1.5
Liver disease	1.3
Arthritis	23.2
Chronic joint symptoms	27.0
Back pain	29.6
Migraines/severe headaches	18.9
Feelings of sadness all or most of the time	3.2

Source: National Center for Health Statistics (NCHS) and Centers for Disease Control and Prevention (CDC), 2014.

TABLE 45.3	Physical Activities That Are Very Difficult or Cannot Be Done at all
PHYSICAL ACTIVITY	**PERCENTAGE OF WOMEN REPORTING DIFFICULTY**
Any physical difficulty	16.4
Walk a quarter of a mile	6.1
Climb 10 steps without resting	9.8
Stand for 2 hours	3.3

Source: National Center for Health Statistics (NCHS), Centers for Disease Control and Prevention (CDC), 2014.

(Fish, 2008; Pennell, Galligan, & Fish, 2012). There may also be a long stage of subclinical disease during which the disease process has begun yet symptoms have not yet appeared.

Multiple factors may interact and combine in specific ways to place the individual at higher risk for developing disease than if a single factor were present alone. For example, an obese woman who smokes is at greater risk for developing cardiovascular disease than an obese woman who is not a smoker. The cumulative effect of these factors increases the individual's risk for developing a chronic disease. Therefore, a multiple causation approach is often used to guide investigations of chronic diseases (Dever, 1991).

Chronic illness trajectory refers to the overall course of a person's experience as a result of the illness over time. This trajectory can describe not only pathological changes but also other aspects of the disease such as symptom experience, physical functioning, quality of life, social or role performance, and other variables (Corbin & Strauss, 1988). Each aspect of the disease progression is considered an outcome; its trajectory can be monitored.

Unlike acute conditions, which are often self-limiting, chronic conditions are generally not easily curable or self-limiting. A chronic disease can vary over time, sometimes transiently improving, often worsening. Chronic diseases can be ongoing such as diabetes, or they can be reoccurring, such as with depression. The course of a specific illness depends on the characteristics of the condition (e.g., relapsing, episodic), characteristics of the individual (e.g., age, gender), and psychological, family, and sociocultural factors.

Health care providers can use the concept of illness trajectory to identify and understand the specific needs of patients and families as the patient moves along the continuum of chronic illness. It is useful for providers to have a general understanding of the usual course of a disease. The patient and provider can then compare the patient's course of the disease with the usual progression. If the disease is characterized by general deterioration, then slowing the progression of the disease represents a major therapeutic success. On the other hand, if the patient's disease is progressing faster than is typical, this could invoke analysis and redesign of the treatment plan. More data are needed regarding the typical progression of the multiple outcomes of common chronic diseases so that providers and patients can evaluate the success of the treatment regimen.

■ TREATMENT/MANAGEMENT OF CHRONIC ILLNESS

Unlike acute care, in which the goal of treatment is typically to cure, in chronic care, the goal is to manage the disease and help the patient cope with its effects. In chronic care, an ideal outcome might be that the disease stabilizes and the patient achieves a "new normal." Often this is a state of being in which the patient learns to function at a new normal and to accept the illness as a part of his or her life.

The effects of chronic disease on the individual are often substantial, affecting physical health, physical functioning, symptom experience, quality of life, and social and role performance. Chronic diseases such as diabetes, heart failure, hypertension, arthritis, and lung disease are associated with significant underlying pathology. Factors related to the disease itself, such as the type of organ damage, disease severity, treatment regime, personal factors (such as individual coping ability), and social support, can influence whether the chronic disease is associated with altered physical functioning or disability. Chronic conditions frequently cause disabling symptoms such as pain and fatigue and may have a profound influence on the individual and her family. All of these factors are considered in managing the patient.

The term "chronic disease" invokes the pathological manifestations of the disease. However, because the effects of the disease are generally much broader, the term "chronic illness" is used to refer to the individual's experience with the disease. Clinicians and researchers are increasingly aware of the influence of the individual's experience with the disease on its course and outcomes. Therefore, in this chapter, aspects of both the chronic disease and the experience of having this disease are addressed. For similar reasons, treatment is referred to as chronic care, not chronic disease care.

Goals of chronic care include slowing the rate of decline due to the disease, reducing the frequency of disease exacerbations or complications, mitigating the functional impairment, maximizing the quality of life, reducing hospitalizations, and maintaining a sense of normalcy. Chronic care services also address the woman's experience of the disease, the impact of the disease on her daily life and functioning, and the suffering caused by the disease. Chronic care requires significant emphasis on health promotion, to slow or reverse the progression of the disease.

The care paradigm for chronic disease is very different from that for an acute medical problem. When a patient presents with an acute problem such as a fractured bone, the clinician, the expert, provides direct and immediate interventions to correct or cure the underlying problem and treat the related symptoms. The patient receives the care, often somewhat passively. With chronic care, the ideal circumstance involves the patient partnering with her clinician to design and implement a plan of care. This plan incorporates biological disease management with health promotion to slow disease progression. The plan of care includes supportive services such as counseling related to diet, exercise, lifestyle, and self-care. Psychological care services may be required to assist in the adjustment to the condition. In addition, women frequently use complementary and alternative approaches to health care, and these approaches should be integrated into the plan of care.

In individuals who are well, self-care focuses on self-improvement. In the face of a chronic illness, it is critical that the patient partner with the clinician to plan her chronic care (Jaarsma, Riegel, & Strömberg, 2012). The patient lives with her illness and sees the clinician only occasionally and then typically for brief visits. The patient must monitor her condition on a day-to-day basis and recognize deterioration or improvement. It is important to educate patients on how to prepare for the clinician encounter, so that they are able to take an active role in monitoring, managing, and decision making. Patient-centered care mandates that the patient be the primary decision maker in managing the disease and its effects. Therefore, chronic care requires developing skills in decision counseling and decision support. The clinician can make recommendations based on science and experience regarding surgical or medical and pharmaceutical treatments; the well-informed patient will be able to choose among the options based on her own analysis.

Women with chronic illness live with symptoms and disabilities that they often must manage for their lifetime and that require collaborative partnerships with clinicians to assist them in integrating self-care into their daily activities. This requires that clinicians are not only knowledgeable about managing medical treatment regimens but also able to provide emotional and intangible support, including ongoing patient and family education and counseling.

Caring for a woman with a chronic illness necessitates caring for her family as well. Chronic illness changes family members' roles, responsibilities, and boundaries, especially when the traditional caregiver, the woman, is the one who is ill. It can disrupt her self-image and self-esteem. It can result in uncertain and unpredictable futures. Moreover, it can trigger distressing emotions—anxiety, depression, resentment, feelings of helplessness, as well as illness-related factors such as permanent changes in physical appearance or bodily functioning.

A woman who is chronically ill may feel guilty about the demands that her illness makes on the family. She may resent the change in roles and responsibilities caused by the limitations imposed by the illness, and she must deal with the threat to her role autonomy (Lawrence, 2012).

Often the focus of care of the chronically ill is the individual with the disease, the management of symptoms, and prognosis (Eggenberger, Meiers, Krumwiede, Bliesmer, & Earle, 2011). However, supporting families with chronic illness is a critical concern for all health care providers. While the care of the individual with the illness is essential, the care of the family must be simultaneously addressed. To support the struggling that families experience, simply recognizing the issues openly may be what is needed. In this manner, the woman's family can use their own interactions to situate the illness within the evolving family and best identify their own strategies for accomplishing family goals (Eggenberger et al., 2011). Including care directed at family processes may have profound effects on individual and family outcomes because individual health and family health are interdependent (Eggenberger et al., 2011). To facilitate women's coping with chronic illness, clinicians need to consider the various types, sources, and benefits of support available.

■ SELECTED CHRONIC ILLNESSES

Chronic Obstructive Pulmonary Disease

DEFINITION AND SCOPE

COPD is the third leading cause of death in the United States (Hoyert & Xu, 2011). The number of women who die from COPD exceeds that of men (CDC, 2012).

ETIOLOGY, RISK FACTORS

COPD is a common, preventable, and treatable disease characterized by persistent airflow limitation that is usually progressive and associated with an enhanced chronic inflammatory response in the airways and the lungs to noxious particles or gases (Global Initiative for Chronic Obstructive Lung Disease [GOLD], 2015, p. 5). Risk factors associated with COPD include tobacco smoke, indoor and outdoor pollution, and occupational dusts and chemicals.

SYMPTOMS

Symptoms of COPD include dyspnea, chronic cough, and chronic sputum production.

EVALUATION/ASSESSMENT

Clinical physical findings in COPD may include the following: prolonged forced expiratory time, tachypnea, cyanosis, tachycardia, end-expiratory wheezes on forced expiration, decreased breath sounds, and/or inspiratory crackles, hyperresonance on percussion, and signs of cor pulmonale.

DIAGNOSTIC TESTING

In order to make a clinical diagnosis of COPD, spirometry is required. To diagnose COPD, the $FEV_1/FVC < 0.70$ confirms the presence of persistent airflow limitation.

TREATMENT/MANAGEMENT

With the growing burden of COPD among women, understanding the clinical presentation and providing access to care is important (Martinez et al., 2012). Smoking cessation is one of the most important interventions that can potentially slow COPD disease progression. FEV_1 decreases by approximately 25 to 30 mL/year starting at age 35 years; however, the rate of decline is faster (threefold to fourfold) in smokers.

Pharmacologic treatment is used to reduce symptoms and the frequency and severity of exacerbations. Medications include bronchodilators, inhaled corticosteroids, or combination inhaled corticosteroid/bronchodilator therapy and preventive vaccines. Nonpharmacologic treatments include oxygen therapy and pulmonary rehabilitation. Oxygen therapy has been shown to improve survival and quality of life in patients with COPD and chronic hypoxemia. Pulmonary rehabilitation improves functional status and quality of life.

Asthma

DEFINITION AND SCOPE, ETIOLOGY

Asthma refers to a disorder of variable expiratory airflow obstruction that arises in association with symptoms of wheezing, cough, and dyspnea. Inflammation of the airways may increase airway responsiveness that allows triggers to initiate bronchoconstriction. Asthma causes increased mucous secretions that can occlude the airway.

Asthma is one of the leading chronic conditions in the United States. It has marked health disparities, especially in older women where the highest mortality rate is seen (Baptist, Hamad, & Patel, 2014). In women above 65 years of age, the death rate is approximately four times higher than the overall mean rate (Akinbami et al., 2012).

RISK FACTORS

Hormones may explain the increased risk for asthma among women. Estrogen and progesterone affect airway caliber and asthma exacerbations. Postmenopausal women taking hormone therapy (HT) have a 2.24-fold increase in asthma diagnosis as compared with women not taking HT (Barr et al., 2004).

EVALUATION/ASSESSMENT

Patients presenting with asthma may have the following clinical findings: tachypnea, nasal flaring, tachycardia, hyperresonance, prolonged expiration, wheezing, diminished lung sounds, sputum production, and nocturnal cough and wheezing. The lung exam often reveals diminished airflow with wheezing as a major characteristic. Diagnosis is made based on recurrence of symptoms and the severity of disease is determined based on symptoms.

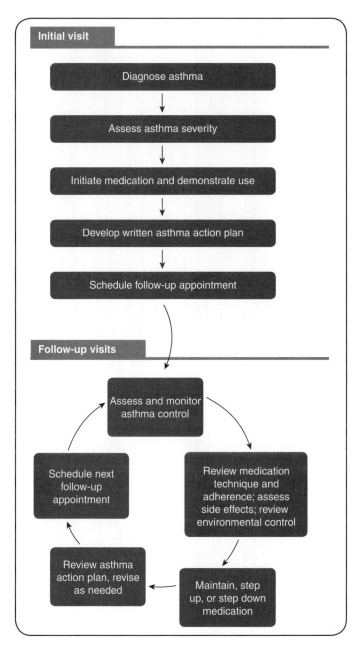

FIGURE 45.1
Asthma management.
Source: https://www.nhlbi.nih.gov/files/docs/guidelines/asthma_qrg.pdf

DIFFERENTIAL DIAGNOSES

Asthma is differentiated from other chronic restrictive airway diseases such as reactive airway, COPD, and chronic bronchitis.

DIAGNOSTIC TESTING

Pulmonary function studies, pre- and postbronchodilator, are the main diagnostic tests used to identify asthma. Women also use peak flow meters to monitor their respiratory function and guide self-care (see Treatment/Management section).

TREATMENT/MANAGEMENT

During the initial visit for asthma, severity is determined and a treatment plan is established. Follow-up visits include

reassessment of symptoms and adjustment of the management plan as needed (Figure 45.1). Medications used to manage asthma include bronchodilators and inhaled steroids. Identification and avoidance of triggers that cause exacerbations is important. Medications are prescribed in a stepwise manner based on symptom severity (see Figure 45.2). When symptoms are increasing, the woman uses a peak flow meter to determine how limited her airflow has become (Willems, Joore, Hendriks, Wouters, & Severens, 2006). Short-acting bronchodilators are used, preferably with a spacer, to relieve symptoms and to reopen her airways. If home care is unsuccessful, she is educated to seek clinical care.

Celiac Disease

DEFINITION, ETIOLOGY, AND SYMPTOMS

Celiac disease (CD) is a common chronic condition caused by an inflammatory response to ingestion of gluten proteins. The effect of gluten causes atrophy of the villous of the small intestine in CD, which may lead to nutrient malabsorption (Hopman et al., 2008). The presenting symptoms are a wide array of gastrointestinal (GI) manifestations including diarrhea, weight loss, and malabsorption.

CD occurs at the same frequency in both sexes; however, women are diagnosed more frequently than men (2:1). Unfortunately, women report a lower quality of life (Hallert, Grännö, et al., 1998; Hallert, Sandlund, & Broqvist, 2003; Zarkadas et al., 2006). The prevalence of CD was as high in first- and second-degree relatives without symptoms as in relatives with symptoms, highlighting the importance of genetic predisposition as a risk factor for CD (Fasano et al., 2003). African American patients are less frequently diagnosed.

DIFFERENTIAL DIAGNOSES

Differential diagnoses for CD include: Crohn's disease, ulcerative colitis (UC), tropical sprue, Zollinger–Ellison syndrome, autoimmune enteropathy, T-cell lymphoma, and combined immunodeficiency states.

DIAGNOSTIC STUDIES

Initial diagnostic testing for CD includes serological studies while the woman is on a gluten-containing diet. The two initial tests are immunoglobulin A (IgA) and anti-tissue transglutaminase (tTG). If CD is the primary working diagnosis, an endoscopy with intestinal biopsy should be performed regardless of the serological tests. Although genetic testing may be performed, it should be saved for patients with atypical presentation of the disease (Rubio-Tapia, Hill, Kelly, Calderwood, & Murray, 2013).

TREATMENT/MANAGEMENT

The gold standard of treatment for CD is complete elimination of gluten from the diet. Glutens are the components found in rye, wheat, and barley grains. Patients are taught how to read food labels and to request gluten-free options when dining out. See Table 45.4.

Level of severity (Columns 2–5) is determined by events listed in Column 1 for both impairment (frequency and intensity of symptoms and functional limitations) and risk (of exacerbations). Assess impairment by patient's or caregiver's recall of events during the previous 2 and 4 weeks; assess risk over the last year. Recommendations for initiating therapy based on level of severity are presented in the last row.

Components of Severity		Intermittent			Persistent								
					Mild			Moderate			Severe		
		Ages 0 to 4 years	Ages 5 to 11 years	Ages ≥ 12 years	Ages 0 to 4 years	Ages 5 to 11 years	Ages ≥ 12 years	Ages 0 to 4 years	Ages 5 to 11 years	Ages ≥ 12 years	Ages 0 to 4 years	Ages 5 to 11 years	Ages ≥ 12 years
Impairment	Symptoms	≤ 2 days/week			> 2 days/week but not daily			Daily			Throughout the day		
	Nighttime awakenings	0	≤2x/month	≤2x/month	1–2x/month	3–4x/month	3–4x/month	3–4x/month	>1x/week but not nightly	>1x/week but not nightly	>1x/week	Often 7x/week	Often 7x/week
	SABA use for symptom control (not to prevent EIB)	≤ 2 days/week			> 2 days/week but not daily	> 2 days/week but not more than once on any day	> 2 days/week and not more than once on any day	Daily	Daily	Daily	Several times per day	Several times per day	Several times per day
	Interference with normal activity	None			Minor limitation			Some limitation			Extremely limited		
	Lung function ↑ FEV₁ (% predicted)	Not applicable	Normal FEV₁ between exacerbations > 80%	Normal FEV₁ between exacerbations > 80%	Not applicable	> 80%	> 80%	Not applicable	60%–80%	60%–80%	Not applicable	< 60%	< 60%
	↑ FEV₁/FVC		> 85%	Normal		> 80%	Normal		75%–80%	Reduced 5%		< 75%	Reduced > 5%
Risk	Asthma exacerbations requiring oral systemic corticosteroids	0–1/year			≥ 2 exacerb. in 6 months, or wheezing ≥ 4x per year lasting >1 day AND risk factors for persistent asthma	≥ 2/year	≥ 2/year						

Generally, more frequent and intense events indicate greater severity.

Consider severity and interval since last asthma exacerbation. Frequency and severity may fluctuate over time for patients in any severity category. Relative annual risk of exacerbations may be related to FEV₁.

Recommended Step for Initiating Therapy (See "Stepwise Approach for Managing Asthma Long Term," page 7)	Step 1			Step 2			Step 3	Step 3 medium-dose ICS option	Step 3	Step 3	Step 3 medium-dose ICS option or Step 4	Step 4 or 5

In 2–6 weeks, depending on severity, assess level of asthma control achieved and adjust therapy as needed.
Consider short course of oral systemic corticosteroids.
For children 0–4 years old, if no clear benefit is observed in 4–6 weeks, consider adjusting therapy or alternate diagnoses.

The stepwise approach is meant to help, not replace, the clinical decision making needed to meet individual patient needs.

FIGURE 45.2
Classification of asthma severity.

Source: U.S. Department of Health and Human Services.

TABLE 45.4	Gluten-Containing and Gluten-Free Foods			
GLUTEN-FREE FOODS		**FOODS-CONTAINING GLUTEN**		**CHECK THE LABEL**
Amaranth	Glucose syrup	Barley	Malt	Dextrin made from wheat
Arrowroot	Herbs	Some flavorings added to foods	Seitan	Tofu
Buckwheat	Lecithin	Gluten	Teriyaki Sauce	
Citric acid	Maltodextrin	Guar Gum	Triticale	
Corn	Millet Montina Quinoa Yeast	Hydrolyzed vegetable protein	Wheat—bulgur, durum, einkorn, farina, graham, kamut, semolina, and spelt	

Source: Gluten Free Living (2013).

Inflammatory Bowel Disease

DEFINITION AND SCOPE

Inflammatory bowel disease (IBD) describes chronic autoimmune diseases that cause inflammation of the GI tract. The two chronic diseases in this category are UC and Crohn's disease.

IBD is commonly diagnosed during women's reproductive years, with the highest incidence of disease onset occurring between 20 and 29 years of age (Molodecky et al., 2012).

ETIOLOGY

UC and Crohn's disease share certain clinical findings; however, they have important differences that influence their management (Greenberger, Blumberg, & Burakoff, 2012). UC is a chronic, recurrent disease characterized by diffuse mucosal inflammation of the colon. Crohn's disease is a chronic, recurrent disease characterized by patchy, transmural inflammation of any part of the GI mucosa from the mouth to the anus. IBD is a lifelong illness with profound psychosocial, emotional, and economic impacts.

RISK FACTORS

Use of hormonal contraceptives by women with IBD may increase disease relapse and risk of other adverse health outcomes, including thrombosis. Additionally, IBD-related malabsorption might interfere with the effectiveness of oral contraceptives (Molodecky et al., 2012).

SYMPTOMS, EVALUATION/ASSESSMENT

Patients with IBD can present with a variety of symptoms that need to be differentiated from other GI diseases as well as differentiated between UC and Crohn's disease. Patients with mild UC present with frequent loose bowel movements associated with cramping; often there is blood and mucus in the stool. With more severe UC, the patient experiences more frequent stools (more than 10 per day and often at night) and more blood and mucus in the stool. The patient could have tachycardia, fever, weight loss, and signs of undernutrition such as hypoproteinemia and peripheral edema.

The patient with Crohn's disease commonly presents with abdominal cramping and tenderness, fever, anorexia, weight loss, and pain. There may be intermittent blood loss in the stool. The loss of mucosa could be sufficient to interfere with bile salt absorption, producing steatorrhea. If the bowel perforates, peritonitis will occur.

TREATMENT/MANAGEMENT

Treatment for IBD is multifaceted and includes the use of medication, alterations in diet and nutrition, and sometimes surgical procedures to repair or remove affected portions of the GI tract. Aminosalicylates (5-ASA) and corticosteroids are usually the first line of treatment for IBD. If these treatments are unsuccessful, an immunomodulator or biological treatment such as a tumor necrosis factor (TNF) blocker may be indicated as an ongoing treatment to decrease the inflammatory response and ideally achieve remission. In addition, because stress is often associated with IBD "flares," methods of stress reduction and relaxation such as meditation or yoga are often prescribed.

■ RHEUMATIC DISORDERS

Osteoarthritis

DEFINITION AND SCOPE

Osteoarthritis (OA) is the most common form of arthritis and common cause of disability among older people. Women have higher rates of OA, and it is more prominent after age 50 years.

ETIOLOGY, RISK FACTORS, AND SYMPTOMS

OA of the knee is characterized by degeneration of the articular cartilage, morphological changes to the subchondral bone, and damage to the surrounding soft tissue (Felson et al., 2000). These structural changes lead to joint pain, quadriceps muscle weakness, reduced range of motion, and joint instability (Fitzgerald, Piva, & Irrgang, 2004; Messier, Loeser, Hoover, Semble, & Wise, 1992). As a result, most individuals with symptomatic knee OA report difficulty with walking, stair climbing, rising from a car, or carrying heavy loads. Early in the disease, patients may experience stiffness upon arising, which recedes with activity. As the disease progresses, stiffness and joint pain with movement becomes more constant. Incidence of OA increases with aging and is more common in those who have family members with the disease.

EVALUATION/ASSESSMENT

The physical exam may reveal joint erythema, warmth, and edema as well as limited range of motion and crepitus. Heberden's nodes may be present at the distal interphalangeal joints. Bouchard's nodes may be present at the middle interphalangeal joints.

DIFFERENTIAL DIAGNOSES

The differential diagnoses for joint pain, joint edema, and fatigue include:

- Infection
- Other connective tissue disorders (e.g., lupus, scleroderma)
- Fibromyalgia
- Rheumatoid arthritis (RA)
- Gout

DIAGNOSTIC TESTING

OA is usually diagnosed with an x-ray. The x-ray will typically reveal:

- Cartilage loss, joint space narrowing
- Increased bone density at narrowed joint spaces (in response to increased friction with cartilage loss)
- Osteophytes
- Bone erosion

TREATMENT/MANAGEMENT

Chronic pain and disability are often associated with OA. Treatment encompasses both nonpharmacological and pharmacological approaches. Nonpharmacological treatment may include weight loss, rest, physical therapy and structured exercise programs, assistive devices (canes, raised toilet seats, and walkers), heat and cold therapy, supportive orthotic shoes, and use of transcutaneous electrical stimulation. Other nonpharmacological treatments may include participation in tai chi programs and treatment with traditional Chinese acupuncture. Pharmacological recommendations may include the following: topical capsaicin, topical nonsteroidal anti-inflammatory drugs (NSAIDs), and oral NSAIDs, including cyclooxygenase-2 (COX-2) selective inhibitors.

Rheumatoid Arthritis

DEFINITION AND SCOPE

RA is a chronic, inflammatory autoimmune disease. It is a systemic illness and may involve other organ systems of the body. RA is three times more common in women than in men (Forslind, Hafström, Ahlmén, & Svensson, 2007).

ETIOLOGY

The exact cause of RA is unknown. It is thought to be an autoimmune process; however, the cause that initiates the autoimmune response is also unknown. There may be a genetic factor as RA has a hereditary component.

RISK FACTORS

Risk factors for RA include female gender, middle age (onset usually occurs between 40 and 60 years of age), family history of RA, smoking, environmental exposures, and obesity.

SYMPTOMS

The most common symptoms of arthritis include pain, fatigue, joint deformity, stiffness, and swelling. Symptoms of pain, joint swelling, and fatigue are intermittent and can be severe, debilitating, and unpredictable, and often curb function and limit daily life (De Cock et al., 2013).

Women with arthritis must deal with an uncertain prognosis, medical regimen, and multiple losses—a loss in mobility, the inability to work, and an altered self-identity due in part to a changed bodily appearance and changes in leisure activities frequently accompany RA.

DIAGNOSIS OF RA: CLASSIFICATION CRITERIA

The American College of Rheumatology (ACR) and the European League Against Rheumatism (EULAR) worked together to develop the 2010 Rheumatoid Arthritis Classification Criteria for RA (Aletaha et al., 2010) (Table 45.5).

- Add score of categories A–D; a score of $\geq$ 6/10 is needed for classification of a patient as having definite RA.

TREATMENT/MANAGEMENT

RA treatment is focused on arresting disease progression and reducing disability. As with OA, both nonpharmacologic and pharmacologic approaches are important. Nonpharmacologic approaches may include occupational therapy, physical therapy, modifying the home environment, and so forth. Pharmacologic management includes disease-modifying antirheumatic drugs (DMARDs) and medications to manage pain.

Lupus

DEFINITION AND SCOPE

Systemic lupus erythematosus (SLE) is an autoimmune disease affecting multiple organs with immunological and clinical manifestations. The disease affects the skin, joints, kidneys, blood cells, and nervous system (Cervera, Khamashta, & Hughes, 2009). Once thought to be a disease striking reproductive age women, the onset has been noted to be diagnosed in women older than the age of 50 years. The later age of onset affects the clinical presentation, disease course, response to treatment. and prognosis of SLE. Newly diagnosed patients have increased anxieties about fatal chronic illness with unpredictable flares and potential disability.

TABLE 45.5	Classification Criteria for Rheumatoid Arthritis (RA)

Target population to be tested should have at least one joint with definite clinical swelling[a] and with the synovitis not better explained by another disease.

CRITERIA	SCORE
A. The number and size of joints that are swollen	
1 Large joint	0
2–10 Large joints	1
1–3 Small joints (with or without involvement of large joints)	2
4–10 Small joints (with or without involvement of large joints)	3
> 10 Joints (at least 1 small joint)	5
B. Serology	
Negative RF and negative ACPA	0
Low-positive RF or low-positive ACPA	2
High-positive RF or high-positive ACPA	3
C. Acute phase reactants	
Normal CRP and normal ESR	0
Abnormal CRP or abnormal ESR	1
D. Duration of symptoms	
< 6 weeks	0
< 6 weeks	1

Add score of categories A–D; a score of ≥ 6/10 is needed for classification of a patient as having definite RA.

[a]The criteria are aimed at classification of newly presenting patients. In addition, patients with erosive disease typical of RA with a history compatible with prior fulfillment of the 2010 criteria should be classified as having RA. Patients with long-standing disease, including those whose disease is inactive (with or without treatment) and who, based on retrospectively available data, have previously fulfilled the 2010 criteria should be classified as having RA.
ACPA, antibodies to citrullinated protein antigens; CRP, c-reactive protein; ESR, erythrocyte sedimentation rate; RF, rheumatoid factor.
Source: Republished with permission from John Wiley & Sons, Inc., from Arthritis & rheumatism by American College of Rheumatology; American Rheumatism Association; Arthritis Foundation; permission conveyed through Copyright Clearance Center, Inc.

SYMPTOMS AND EVALUATION/ASSESSMENT

SLE often presents with a butterfly-shaped rash on the face. Other presentations can be nonspecific (e.g., hematuria), and the diagnosis of SLE requires the health care provider to take a thorough history, a complete physical examination, and interpretation of diagnostic tests.

The guidelines for diagnosis include both a clinical and an immunological group. Criteria need not be present simultaneously. The clinical criteria include acute cutaneous lupus, chronic cutaneous lupus, oral ulcers, nonscarring

alopecia (hair loss), synovitis, serositis, renal involvement, neurological involvement, hemolytic anemia, leukopenia, and thrombocytopenia. The immunological criteria include elevated antinuclear antibodies (ANA), elevated anti-ds-DNA, anti-Smith antibodies, antiphospholipid antibodies, low complement, and direct Coombs test in the absence of hemolytic anemia (1997 update of the 1982 American College of Rheumatology classification criteria for systemic lupus erythe-matosus [Hochberg, 1997]).

A classification of SLE is made if: (a) a patient satisfies four of the SLICC criteria (including at least one immunological criterion and at least one clinical criteria); or (b) if a patient has biopsy-proven nephritis (inflammation of the kidney) compatible with SLE in the presence of either ANA or anti-ds-DNA (1997 update of the 1982 American College of Rheumatology classification criteria for systemic lupus erythe-matosus [Hochberg, 1997]).

TREATMENT/MANAGEMENT

Treatment for SLE includes NSAIDs for less severe symptoms, local or systemic corticosteroids for acute exacerbations, and systemic corticosteroids for severe manifestations. It is usually managed primarily by a clinician with rheumatology expertise.

Headaches/Migraines

DEFINITION AND SCOPE

Migraine and other recurrent headache disorders cause personal suffering and decreased economic productivity (Burch, Loder, Loder, & Smitherman, 2015). The frequency of occurrence of headache is two to three times more common in women than in men (Burch et al., 2015), and migraines and other severe or frequent headaches are more prevalent in women than in men, especially during the reproductive years (Loder, Sheikh, & Loder, 2015). The prevalence ratio is consistent across all racial and ethnic groups (Smitherman, Burch, Sheikh, & Loder, 2013). Interestingly, U.S. military personnel have lower headache rates than the general population.

ETIOLOGY

Although the cause of headaches is multifactorial, there is strong evidence that sex hormones, estrogen in particular, play an important role (Chai, Peterlin, & Calhoun, 2014).

RISK FACTORS

Multiple triggers exist for migraine headaches; some common ones are wine (red or white), strong cheeses, caffeine, and noxious gases. Health disparities exist related to diagnosis and treatment of headaches among Black and Hispanic individuals (Loder et al., 2015).

SYMPTOMS

Common presenting symptoms include severe headache, bilateral or unilateral; photophobia; photophonia; and nausea. The following symptoms increase the odds of finding a pathological abnormality on neuroimaging: worst headache of her life, rapidly increasing headache frequency, history of lack of coordination, history of localized neurological signs or a history of subjective numbness or tingling, and history of headache causing awakening from sleep (Silberstein, 2000).

EVALUATION/ASSESSMENT

A careful history is needed to identify possible triggers, patterns, and associated symptoms. The physical examination focuses on identifying any neurological deficits.

DIFFERENTIAL DIAGNOSES

When a woman first presents with a headache, it is classified (e.g., migraine, tension, etc.). Differential diagnoses that need to be ruled out include central lesions, cerebral mass, and increased intracranial pressure.

DIAGNOSTIC STUDIES

A diagnosis of migraine headache is usually made based on clinical history and physical exam. For women with worrisome symptoms (see the preceding Symptoms section) or findings of neurological abnormalities, head CT or MRI/MRA is warranted.

TREATMENT/MANAGEMENT

Treatment for acute headaches includes migraine aborting agents such as triptans (sumatriptan and zolmitriptan), frovatriptan for short-term menstrually associated migraine (MAM) prevention, and pain medications. Antiemetics are frequently also used due to the concomitant presentation of nausea with migraine. Preventive strategies include avoiding triggers, which can effectively be identified through documenting a headache diary. Preventive medications are useful for women who experience moderate to severe migraines frequently and include beta-blockers, for example, metoprolol, proprandolol; and antiepileptic drugs (AEDs), for example, sodium valproate and topiramate (Silberstein et al., 2012). Lamotrigine has been found ineffective for migraine prevention (Silberstein et al., 2012).

■ FUTURE DIRECTIONS

Chronic diseases are very common among women, affecting not only physical health but also physical functioning, symptom experience, quality of life, and role performance. The U.S. health care system is designed to respond promptly and effectively to cure and manage acute problems. However, in chronic disease, a different paradigm is needed. The goals of chronic treatment are to mitigate the disease progression and limit the effects of the disease on the woman's day-to-day life. These goals are best accomplished when the woman partners with her clinician to make treatment decisions and to monitor disease and symptom progression. Clinicians

need to be sensitive to the long-term implications of chronic disease, and to approach each individual's situation from a holistic standpoint.

As research on the Human Genome Project continues, some chronic diseases may be identifiable earlier, thus reducing overall disability. However, patient responses to knowing they carry a genetic risk for developing a disease, or that they have a disease that is subclinical, will need to be carefully monitored. The stress related to knowing a disease is coming may have negative consequences on physical and mental health.

■ REFERENCES

Agency for Healthcare Research and Quality (AHRQ). (2012). *Cardiovascular disease and other chronic conditions in women: Recent findings (program brief)*. Retrieved from http://www.ahrq.gov/research/findings/factsheets/women/womheart/index.html

Akinbami, L. J., Moorman, J. E., Bailey, C., Zahran, H. S., King, M., Johnson, C. A., & Liu, X. (2012). Trends in asthma prevalence, health care use, and mortality in the United States, 2001–2010. *NCHS Data Brief, 94*, 1–8.

Aletaha, D., Neogi, T., Silman, A. J., Funovits, J., Felson, D. T., Bingham, C. O.,…Hawker, G. (2010). 2010 Rheumatoid arthritis classification criteria: An American College of Rheumatology/European League Against Rheumatism collaborative initiative. *Arthritis and Rheumatism, 62*(9), 2569–2581.

American College of Rheumatology. (2010). *Criteria*. Retrieved from http://www.rheumatology.org/practice/clinical/classification/ra/ra_2010.asp

Baptist, A. P., Hamad, A., & Patel, M. R. (2014). Special challenges in treatment and self-management of older women with asthma. *Annals of Allergy, Asthma & Immunology, 113*(2), 125–130.

Barr, R. G., Wentowski, C. C., Grodstein, F., Somers, S. C., Stampfer, M. J., Schwartz, J.,…Camargo, C. A. (2004). Prospective study of postmenopausal hormone use and newly diagnosed asthma and chronic obstructive pulmonary disease. *Archives of Internal Medicine, 164*(4), 379–386.

Burch, R. C., Loder, S., Loder, E., & Smitherman, T. A. (2015). The prevalence and burden of migraine and severe headache in the United States: Updated statistics from government health surveillance studies. *Headache, 55*(1), 21–34.

Center for Managing Chronic Disease. (2011). *What is chronic disease?* Retrieved from http://cmcd.sph.umich.edu/what-is-chronic-disease.html

Centers for Disease Control and Prevention (CDC). (2012). Chronic obstructive pulmonary disease among adults—United States 2011. *MMWR. Morbidity and Mortality Weekly Report, 61*(46), 938–943.

Centers for Disease Control and Prevention (CDC). (2014). *Chronic diseases: The leading causes of death and disability in the United States*. Retrieved from http://www.cdc.gov/chronicdisease/overview/index.htm

Centers for Disease Control and Prevention (CDC). (2015). *Chronic disease prevention and health promotion*. Retrieved from http://www.cdc.gov/chronicdisease/

Cervera, R., Khamashta, M. A., & Hughes, G. R. (2009). The Euro-lupus project: Epidemiology of systemic lupus erythematosus in Europe. *Lupus, 18*(10), 869–874. doi:10.1177/0961203309106831

Chai, N. C., Peterlin, B. L., & Calhoun, A. H. (2014). Migraine and estrogen. *Current Opinion in Neurology, 27*(3), 315–324.

Corbin, J., & Strauss, A. (1988). *Unending work and care: Managing chronic illness at home*. San Francisco, CA: Jossey-Bass.

De Cock, D., Meyfroidt, S., Joly, J., Van der Elst, K., Westhovens, R., Verschueren, P.; CareRA Study Group*. (2013). A detailed analysis of treatment delay from the onset of symptoms in early rheumatoid arthritis patients. *Scandinavian Journal of Rheumatology, 43*(1), 1–8.

Dever, G. E. A. (1991). *Community health analysis: Global awareness at the local level* (2nd ed.). Gaithersburg, MD: Aspen.

Division of Reproductive Health, National Center for Chronic Disease Prevention and Health Promotion, Centers for Disease Control and

Prevention (CDC). (2011). *Preventing and managing chronic disease to improve the health of women and infants.* Retrieved from https://idph.iowa.gov/Portals/1/Files/FamilyHealth/2012_cdc_factsheet.pdf

Eggenberger, S. K., Meiers, S. J., Krumwiede, N., Bliesmer, M., & Earle, P. (2011). Reintegration within families in the context of chronic illness: A family health promoting process. *Journal of Nursing and Healthcare of Chronic Illness, 3,* 283–292. doi:10.1111/j.1752–9824.2011.01101.x

Fasano, A., Berti, I., Geraduzzi, T., Tarcisio, N., Colletti, R. B., Drago, S., ...Horvath, K. (2003). Prevalence of celiac disease in at-risk and not-at-risk groups in the United States. *Archives of Internal Medicine, 163,* 286–292.

Felson, D. T., Lawrence, R. C., Dieppe, P. A., Hirsch, R., Helmick, C. G., Jordan, J. M.,...Fries, J. F. (2000). Osteoarthritis: New insights. Part 1: The disease and its risk factors. *Annals of Internal Medicine, 133*(8), 635–646.

Fish, E. N. (2008). The X-files in immunity: Sex-based differences predispose immune responses. *Nature Reviews Immunology, 8,* 737–744.

Fitzgerald, G. K., Piva, S. R., & Irrgang, J. J. (2004). Reports of joint instability in knee osteoarthritis: Its prevalence and relationship to physical function. *Arthritis Rheumatology, 51*(6), 941–946

Forslind, K., Hafström, I., Ahlmén, M., & Svensson, B; BARFOT Study Group. (2007). Sex: A major predictor of remission in early rheumatoid arthritis? *Annals of Rheumatological Disease, 66,* 46–52.

Global Initiative for Chronic Obstructive Lung Disease (GOLD). (2015). *Pocket guide to COPD diagnosis, management, and prevention: A guide for health care professionals* (Updated 2015). Retrieved from http://www.goldcopd.it/materiale/2015/GOLD_Pocket_2015.pdf

Gluten Free Living. (2013). *Ingredients index.* Retrieved from www.glutenfreeliving.com/ingredient.php

Greenberger, N., Blumberg, R., & Burakoff, R. (2012). *Current diagnosis and treatment: Gastroenterology, hepatology, & endoscopy* (2nd ed.). New York, NY: McGraw-Hill.

Hallert, C., Grännö, C., Grant, C., Hultén, S., Midhagen, M., Ström, H., ...Wickström, T. (1998). Quality of life of adult celiac patients treated for 10 years. *Scandinavian Journal of Gastroenterology, 33,* 933–938.

Hallert, C., Sandlund, O., & Broqvist, M. (2003). Perceptions of health-related quality of life of men and women living with celiac disease. *Scandinavian Journal of Caring Sciences, 17*(3), 301–307.

Hopman, E. G., von Blomberg, M. E., Batstra, M. R., Morreau, H., Dekker, F. W., Koning, F.,...Mearin, M. L. (2008). Gluten tolerance in adult patients with celiac disease 20 years after diagnosis? *European Journal of Gastroenterology & Hepatology, 20*(5), 423–429.

Hoyert, D. L., & Xu, J. (2011). *Deaths: Preliminary data for 2011.* National Vital Statistics Reports. Hyattsville, MD: National Center for Health Statistics. Retrieved from http://www.cdc.gov/nchs/data/nvsr/nvsr61/nvsr61_06.pdf

Jaarsma, T., Riegel, B., & Strömberg, A. (2012). A middle-range theory of self-care of chronic illness. *Advances in Nursing Science, 35*(3), 194–204.

Lawrence, E. (2012). *The impact of chronic illness on the family. IG Living.* Retrieved from http://www.igliving.com/magazine/articles/IGL_2012-06_AR_The-Impact-of-Chronic-Illness-on-the-Family.pdf

Loder, S., Sheikh, H. U., & Loder, E. (2015). The prevalence, burden, and treatment of severe, frequent, and migraine headaches in US minority populations: Statistics from National Survey studies. *Headache, 55*(2), 214–228.

Martinez, C. H., Raparla, S., Plauschinat, C. A., Giardino, N. D., Rogers, B., Beresford, J.,...Han, M. K. (2012). Gender differences in symptoms and care delivery for chronic obstructive pulmonary disease. *Journal of Women's Health (2002), 21*(12), 1267–1274.

Messier, S. P., Loeser, R. F., Hoover, J. L., Semble, E. L., & WIse, C. M. (1992). Osteoarthritis of the knee: Effects on gait, strength, and flexibility. *Archives of Physical Medicine and Rehabilitation, 73*(1), 29–36.

Molodecky, N. A., Soon, I. S., Rabi, D. M., Ghali, W. A., Ferris, M., Chernoff, G.,...Kaplan, G. G. (2012). Increasing incidence and prevalence of the inflammatory bowel diseases with time, based on systematic review. *Gastroenterology, 142*(1), 46–54.e42; quiz e30.

National Center for Health Statistics (NCHS), Centers for Disease Control and Prevention (CDC). (2009). *Percent of U.S. adults 55 and over with chronic conditions.* Retrieved from http://www.cdc.gov/nchs/health_policy/adult_chronic_conditions.htm

National Center for Health Statistics (NCHS), Centers for Disease Control and Prevention (CDC). (2014). *Summary health statistics for U.S. adults: National Health Interview Survey, 2012.* DHHS Publication No. 2014–1588. Hyattsville, MD: U.S. Department of Health and Human Services.

Pennell, L. M., Galligan, C. L., & Fish, E. N. (2012). Sex affects immunity. *Journal of Autoimmunity, 38*(2–3), J282–J291.

Rubio-Tapia, A., Hill, I. D., Kelly, C. P., Calderwood, A. H., & Murray, J. A.; American College of Gastroenterology. (2013). ACG clinical guidelines: Diagnosis and management of celiac disease. *American Journal of Gastroenterology, 108*(5), 656–676; quiz 677.

Silberstein, S. D. (2000). Practice parameter: Evidence-based guidelines for migraine headache (an evidence-based review): Report of the Quality Standards Subcommittee of the American Academy of Neurology. *Neurology, 55*(6), 754–762.

Silberstein, S. D., Holland, S., Freitag, F., Dodick, D. W., Argoff, C., & Ashman, E.; Quality Standards Subcommittee of the American Academy of Neurology and the American Headache Society. (2012). Evidence-based guideline update: Pharmacologic treatment for episodic migraine prevention in adults: Report of the Quality Standards Subcommittee of the American Academy of Neurology and the American Headache Society. *Neurology, 78*(17), 1337–1345.

Smitherman, T. A., Burch, R., Sheikh, H., & Loder, E. (2013). The prevalence, impact, and treatment of migraine and severe headaches in the United States: A review of statistics from national surveillance studies. *Headache, 53*(3), 427–436.

U.S. Department of Health and Human Services. (2011). *Asthma care quick reference: Diagnosing and managing asthma.* Retrieved from http://www.nhlbi.nih.gov/files/docs/guidelines/asthma_qrg.pdf

Willems, D. C., Joore, M. A., Hendriks, J. J., Wouters, E. F., & Severens, J. L. (2006). Cost-effectiveness of self-management in asthma: A systematic review of peak flow monitoring interventions. *International journal of Technology Assessment in Health Care, 22*(4), 436–442.

Zarkadas, M., Cranney, A., Case, S., Molloy, M., Switzer, C., Graham, I. D.,...Burrows, V. (2006). The impact of a gluten-free diet on adults with coeliac disease: Results of a national survey. *Journal of Human Nutrition and Dietetics, 19*(1), 41–49.

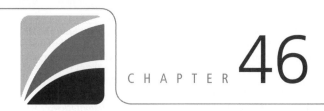

CHAPTER 46

Care of Women With Disabilities

Tracie Harrison

By midlife, few women can say that disability has not profoundly affected their lives. Women have some of the highest rates of disabling conditions when compared with men, which are 20.3% and 17.3%, respectively (U.S. Census, 2010). Moreover, 6 out of 10 people who provide support to people with disabilities are female (Family Caregiver Alliance, 2016; National Alliance for Caregiving [NAC], 2015).

It is now time for women's health advanced practice nurses (APNs) to be well prepared in providing care to women aging with and into disability; aspects of care once reserved for specialists in rehabilitation therapies are now in the domain of the APN in primary care. Along with the increased expectations for providing more expansive primary care to women with disabilities, primary care visits now require APNs to be judicious with their time. They need to be knowledgeable, focused, pragmatic, and organized with a bountiful set of resources for the health benefit of women with a growing number of disabling conditions, circumstances, and environments. APNs are called upon to provide not only primary care, but disability health care for women, incorporating anticipatory guidance regarding the health-related concerns and needs of women with varying degrees of functional limitations (FLs).

This chapter begins with definitions that facilitate understanding of the problems facing women aging with/or into disability, including the process of disablement. Next, several social and economic conditions confronting women with disabilities are discussed. Finally, the evidential basis for an assessment to guide preemptive primary care for women living with disability is proposed.

■ BACKGROUND

Several standpoints on aging and disability form an essential foundation for APNs providing care for women with disabilities. The first is related to how disability may progress over time, often called the disablement process (Verbrugge & Jette, 1994). Disablement is the progression from pathological change in cellular function to impaired organ function, to experiencing limitations in physical function, and finally to losing valuable social roles. Impairments, such

as diabetes and congestive heart failure, and FL, such as paralysis and shortness of breath, have a way of weaving their way through all domains of women's health, leaving a profound effect on the female body. Disability, which is the inability to carry out relevant roles due to the social impact of either a physical impairment or an FL, may be the result of quickly advancing or even mismanaged impairment and FL. The progression from a state of poor cellular or organ function to the point at which the body is no longer able to walk or stand is considered an organ system impairment; this condition has often been the focus of medical providers concerned with providing billable services over the years. The movement from disease to disability has not traditionally been a primary concern of medicine; for example, a woman's loss of employment due to her inability to lift boxes at work, manage bills at home, or go to the park with her dog are each examples of how disease may become a disability but may not be under the purview of the practicing physician. Yet, within this view of the disablement process, these physical, mental, and social states of being are all intertwined, and treatment is incomplete if all areas are not addressed.

In providing care to women with disabilities, it may be helpful to understand the differences that occur between women who were born with or who acquired an FL early in life, and those who acquired an FL later in life, such as after age 65. This distinction can be helpful in understanding women's physiology, psychology, and social responses/needs. This distinction extends beyond the fact that both groups of women live with disabilities for a considerable amount of time, sometimes referred to by many in medicine and nursing as disease or "abnormal." Another distinction that may be helpful is between those who have a condition that is "age-related" and those with a condition that is "ageing-related" (Ritchie & Kildea, 1995; Turner, Barnwell, Al-Chalabi, & Eisen, 2012). This categorization reflects how pathology and impairment conditions accumulate and evolve with age. The mean age of onset may show that the disease is one that is *aged* into; for instance, men and women may develop a cardiomyopathy on average by age 65 years. There is beginning evidence that women's physiology as compared with men's physiology may put them at increased risk with ageing (Mellor et al., 2014). A condition is age related when it occurs within a comparatively older age range and is ageing related when it is due to the changes that occur with age.

The comparison between women with early onset disability, such as cerebral palsy and spinal muscle atrophy, and those with later onset disability, such as stroke and osteoarthritis, may or may not create a substantial difference in the types of services they need. Comparison of the two groups of women may, however, create an understanding of how they respond to the type and timing of services offered. For instance, in a grounded theory study of 45 women with an FL, timing, resources, and meaning of impairment, along with exposure to an accessible environment post-FL, made a difference in how women with a disability promoted health over time (Harrison, Umberson, Lin, & Cheng, 2010). Timing of onset made a difference in which skills were developed for adapting to an environment. Timing of impairment, which may not only predefine a woman's identity and status in society as being disabled but also give her the time and confirm the absolute necessity of crafting unique skills for performing her roles, makes a difference in women's health. Although researchers often define aging as a slow process (Bauer, Wieck, Petersen, & Baptista, 2015), women with early onset disabilities frequently describe the aging process as short and unpredictable (Harrison, 2006). These include women with spinal cord injury, multiple sclerosis, paralytic polio with or without post-polio syndrome, and spinal muscle atrophy. Differences between women who are aging with a disability and women who age into them later in life are critical considerations for APNs working collaboratively to plan the best course of action, which is often a challenge due to limited resources.

Due to the high prevalence of disability among women, this group, in general, is often faced with disability-associated poverty and inequity. Once a limitation occurs, women have historically been without economic support that could help them transition into a new role, gain needed disability resources, or carry them through to old age with housing and food. In part, this occurs because once FL is part of women's lives, they tend to have very low employment rates. For instance, overall labor participation rates are lower for people with FL than for people without; the percent of women older than 16 years not in the labor force is 53.5%, as compared with women with FL, which is 14.5% (Bureau of Labor Statistics [BLS], 2015). When women with FL are compared with men with FL, 14.5% of women with FL are employed as compared with 20.0% of men with FL (BLS, 2015). To demonstrate that women are not to be blamed for this inequity, but instead considered survivors of it, the system-level inequities that lead to the aforementioned employment distribution are discussed. Awareness of the social determinants of disablement is essential to ensure that women receive needed support.

■ WOMEN AGING WITH DISABILITIES, POLICIES, AND SOCIOECONOMIC HARDSHIP

According to Hirschman (2013), the "able-bodied man" was the center of political thought when the foundation of political freedom was established in this country; equality

and justice were defined for our nation by our forefathers on the basis of equality of right, thereby leaving women with disabilities out of the discourse among human beings who are "in a state of perfect freedom to order their actions, and dispose of their possessions, and persons as they think fit" (p. 167). Understanding that women living with disability have the right to services that enable their freedom within our society requires consideration in order to ensure social justice in health and health care (Hirschman, 2012).

Hirschman (2013) argues that women with disabilities were without an equality of right as originally conceived; instead, they had the equality of right to envision a life and to achieve that through the combined rights of a community of people functioning with them and on their behalf. In other words, women with disabilities may suffer from our societies' view that individuals bears sole responsibility for their independent ability to maintain a job, working for their own long-term benefit in this country. However, the community may benefit from the unique knowledge and standpoint of a woman with a disability. If we act on each other's behalf, we might come to create a more sustainable environment for all workers in the community, enhancing the well-being of all. Policies related to illness and injury in the United States relegate the individual woman to a state of poverty. APNs must negotiate on behalf of women living with disability or risk being of little benefit to them. Policies related to work are discussed here due to their high significance in the lives of women/women with disabilities.

Injuries and illnesses that occur early in women's lives may lead to lasting FL and result in disability, which is of considerable concern to gerontologists, epidemiologists, political and administrative leaders, economists, and demographers, as well as the APN. Early onset injuries and illnesses increase the risk for loss of benefits, income, and health over the life course through two major mechanisms: injuries may result in the loss of work incentive and/or ability, and injuries may exacerbate a preexisting condition. Both mechanisms push people out of the job market earlier than needed (Harrison et al., 2013).

APNs are often needed to assist with the paperwork that can make a difference in the lives of women with severe FL, whether that was gained on the job or not. Most important to realize is that policies that support the injured workers on the state or federal level in the event they are unable to work are in the domain of the APN. First, worker compensation benefits cover only injuries arising out of and during employment that are approved as work related by the employer, depending on the state's unique set of laws. Quite the reverse, Social Security Disability Insurance (SSDI) benefits are federally managed and paid to workers with permanent impairments rendering them unable to maintain gainful employment; it does not matter if the employee can prove the injury occurred on the job or not (O'Leary, Boden, Seabury, Ozonoff, & Scherer, 2012). Both workers' compensation and SSDI programs are designed to ensure that workers do not accrue more than 80% of a capped wage so that people do not profit or benefit from FL and unemployment.

Work-related injury is a major cause of FL and permanent job loss in the United States for those without early onset FL (see Chapter 17 on occupational health). A significant portion of the U.S. population experiences permanent economic loss, as well as pain and suffering, due to occupational injuries (O'Leary et al., 2012). In 2009, 1.2 million nonfatal job-related accidents led to time away from work; this rate of injury did not significantly change for 2010 (BLS, 2011) and changed relatively little in 2014 (BLS, 2015). In fact, three million workplace injuries occurred in 2010 (BLS, 2011). Of those, there were 118 of 10,000 severely injured workers who required time off from work due to their injuries. The average number of days off work was 8. Although the highest percentage of work-related injuries occurred in people younger than 45 years, injuries continued to occur in people older than 65 years (BLS, 2011, 2015). Indeed, more than 17% of all workplace accidents were reported in people aged 55 years and older. Injuries among those older than 55 years resulted in the highest number of days off work due to injury among all adult workers. Further, women and Hispanics were at an especially high risk for job-related injuries, due to their high participation in industries such as nursing homes that have a higher-than-average injury rate (BLS, 2011). These injuries are only those reported as meeting the definition for work-related injuries by employees *and* employers. They do not cover those injuries that may occur and result in an exacerbation of mental or physical illness causing worsened FL.

In our nation's social safety net in place for the injured worker, the SSDI is to be the last rung available to prevent the suffering of our disabled workforce, which is tied to their payments into the system over their lifetime of working. It is provided under the Old-Age, Survivors, and Disability Insurance program and administered through the Social Security Administration. Kaye (2010) asserted that people with FLs exit the job market during these times of economic stress due to a push from work conditions and life circumstance that generate internal and physical surroundings that exacerbate a preexisting condition. Kaye noted that job losses between 2008 and 2010 (time of recession) were greater among workers with FL than among those without, which caused the portion of U.S. workers with FL to decrease significantly. Kaye suggested that despite the Americans with Disabilities Act, FL does not provide protection from unemployment; in fact, it is a risk factor for job loss. Long-term joblessness, defined as being without employment for more than one year, can have a negative impact on health (Couch, Reznik, Tamorini, & Iams, 2013).

Looking further into these reasons for exiting the job market and the variations in outcomes once people do exit, Meseguer (2013) reported that despite the federal guidelines for SSDI being the same across the states, the outcomes vary by state. In his analysis, the primary provider's recording of diagnosis code was the largest contributor on the basis of which an individual was selected initially for benefits. The persons' requests for reevaluation of paper work applications were seldom overturned, but their requests for a hearing quite often resulted in SSDI acceptance. This indicates the need for careful documentation that accurately reflects the ongoing condition of the person with the FL. It is costly to society for the state to hold judicial hearings to truly understand the state of FL the person is living with at the time.

In order to investigate the current status of the literature, a review was performed in PubMed, Web of Science, CINAHL, and PsychInfo using the following search terms: "Workers' compensation & Women"; "Workers' compensation & Women & Disability & Return to work"; and "Workers' compensation & Gender & Disability & Return to work". After titles and abstracts were reviewed for applicability to the project, a total of 112 articles were included in the review from the initial 673 identified. Policy and research that specifically addressed the woman's experience were also integrated. Based on the literature, a total of eight factors were identified that influence the employment experience of women with FL.

First, the literature suggests that women who perform physically demanding jobs for low wages are more likely to be injured with resulting FL than those who perform higher paying, white collar jobs (Guthrie & Jansz, 2006; Stover, Wickizer, Zimmerman, Fulton-Kehoe, & Franklin, 2007). This is the "expendable worker" phenomenon. Expendable workers are paid to do high-risk jobs for low compensation. When they are injured, their injury benefit is based upon their preinjury wages. If they cannot return to work, their positions are filled by choosing from a pool of nonskilled workers. The women who perform these high-risk/low-wage jobs are less likely to move out of poverty if they remain in these jobs over time. Injury may be perceived by women as one mechanism to exit their high-risk, low-wage jobs.

Second, women often take jobs that have gender-related risks and associated low benefits. These jobs may have a different pattern of injury and pain than what men experience in their jobs (Stover et al., 2007). Treaster and Burr (2004) conducted a review of the literature on gender differences in upper extremity musculoskeletal disorders (UEMSDs), finding that women were significantly more likely than men to suffer from diverse kinds of UEMSDs. Stover et al. (2007) examined 81,077 compensation claims from workers who had experienced 4 or more days of work leave due to occupational injuries in Washington state. The 10 predictors for a long-term disability came from demographic and situational factors such as age, gender, delay of the first medical treatment after injury, specific industry, or types of occupation. Gender (female) was a strong factor with a moderate effect size (odds ratio of long-term disability was 1.56 to that of male workers). Stover et al. pointed out that 30% of workers' compensation was claimed by women, but women represented 40% of upper extremity nontraumatic musculoskeletal disorders. According to Harrold, Savageau, Pransky, and Benjamin (2008), women's injuries were more often a result of routine job tasks and of gradual onset than were men's injuries. Women had worse long-term outcomes than men, including lower job stability and postinjury income. Being female was independently associated with a negative employer response to the injured worker.

The third factor is women's low level of political influence in the job bargaining arena. Not only do women have gender-specific jobs and experience injuries with low benefits, they also have an associated low level of bargaining power to improve this situation. The jobs that women perform have associated low benefits that place them at risk for aging into poverty because society has provided a low level of importance and reimbursement for the services they provide, and they are less likely to be in positions to bargain for the needs of other women. In fact, according to Guthrie and Jansz (2006), the issues of gender inequality in the workers' compensation system come directly out of the industrial environment. Women tend to work within different industries or "in gender-segregated circumstances," which provide them with smaller paychecks and do not allow equal bargaining power.

Fourth are the effects of gender and age on a worker's capacity to endure workplace injuries. For instance, women have a particularly high risk for injury (Cheadle, Franklin, & Wolfhagen, 1994). According to Saleh, Fuortes, Vaughn, and Bauer (2001), the rates of being injured from lifting, falling, noxious exposures, repetitive motions, and carpal tunnel syndrome for women were significantly higher than those for men. Likewise, the rates of claims of pain, sprains, bruises, burns, concussion, and inhalation injury were higher for women than for men. Although women in Saleh et al.'s (2001) study were not at higher risk from every single cause or claim of injuries than men, the overall rate for women to be injured or involved in a claim was 1.36-fold higher in terms of relative risk ($p < .05$) than for men.

Age, however, often potentiates the effect of gender, making older women at higher risk than younger women in work settings. This was evident when age and gender were reported as predictors of longer duration of sick leave after an occupational injury (Steenstra, Verbeek, Heymans, & Bongers, 2005; Stover et al., 2007). Based on their systematic review of work-related lower back pain (LBP), Steenstra et al. (2005) stated that radiating pain, higher levels of disability at inception, and social dysfunction, social isolation, and older age (particularly 51 years or older) had a stronger effect on a prolonged sick leave than did any of the other factors. Based on data from a population-based research study with more than 8,500 Michigan workers with compensable injury, gender was one factor, along with others such as older age, greater number of dependents, type of industry (construction), and occupation (white collar job), which explained prolonged duration of missed work time (Oleinick, Gluck, & Guire, 1996).

The fifth contributor is the workers' compensation process. Injured workers report a lack of respect and voice in the compensation and rehabilitation processes (Beardwood, Kirsh, & Clark, 2005; Kirsh & McKee, 2003; Sager & James, 2005). Studies have reported that workers perceive an unrealistically short recovery time for any medical and/or rehabilitating treatment, with little or no help for their symptoms (Kirsh & McKee, 2003). Furthermore, they also report very limited opportunities to be included in the decision-making process regarding their medical or rehabilitation choices (Beardwood, Kirsh, & Clark, 2005; Sager & James, 2005). Men and women share this risk of poor treatment in the return to work (RTW) process.

The sixth factor is the lower levels of treatment efficacy for pain and injury among women when compared with men. Women have had more difficulties managing their pain after an injury than have men, which has resulted in higher levels of disability for women than for men (Adams et al., 2008; Tait & Chibnall, 2005). Tait and Chibnall (2005) reported that women with lower back injury were more sensitive to certain types of pain-related activities when compared with men. In their study of psychometric characteristics using the Pain Disability Index (PDI), researchers found that women had

more pain-related disability than men. Furthermore, women's pain management has been reportedly worse when other factors impacting on their pain were taken into account. For instance, women experience the "pain-augmenting" effects of depression more often than men (Adams et al., 2008).

Seventh, once an FL occurs, employer attitudes may make it difficult for people with disabilities to qualify for jobs with high salaries and benefits despite their qualifications. This is the "low-return phenomenon," reflecting perceptions of workers with disabilities that they have a low economic return for their employer (Pentland, Tremblay, Spring, & Rosenthal, 1999). People with disabilities may require accommodations in the employment setting, creating a perceived risk or cost to the employer or a tension between themselves and their coworkers. On the contrary, employers may believe that hiring an employee with a disability is a noble service, if they consider the issue at all. However, taking the steps to recruit and reward workers with functional impairments for high pay positions may be less common, as evidenced by the fact that rates of disability are highly correlated to income, with the highest rates of work limitations being reported in "workers at the bottom of the income distribution" (Munnell & Sass, 2008, p. 31).

Finally, women are vulnerable to the poverty effects of age and disability due to a lifetime of differences in financial gains, incentives, and obligations as compared with men (Munnell & Sass, 2008). Women are understood to move in and out of the job market due to family obligations that require attention while adding financial obligations without compensation. This also causes a lack of access to social capital that may have an effect on the ability to negotiate and gain compensation once their family obligations stabilize. Moving in and out of the job market without accumulation of substantial benefits and social capital puts women workers at a disadvantage in the event of an injury. Any initial loss of benefits and resources due to a job hiatus may never be regained over time (Munnell & Sass, 2008). Not having the connections and/or benefits to manage a workplace injury exacerbates the physical problems and pushes women out of the job market and into poverty.

In summary, the previous literature provides a litany of reasons for the socioeconomic issues faced by women aging with disabilities during adulthood, which may fall in the domain of APN intervention.

■ RISK FOR HEALTH DECLINE AMONG WOMEN WITH DISABILITIES

Published tools validated for the classification of disability for work-eligibility-related purposes include those developed by McDonough et al. (2013). The purpose of the assessment guide (Table 46.1) is to focus understanding of the needs for ongoing care and assessment of women living with disabilities. The factors included in this guide are grounded in the assumption that women with disabilities should receive preemptive primary care that works to eliminate modifiable factors that worsen health with age.

TABLE 46.1	Assessment Guide for Women Aging With Disabilities: Risk Factors for Health Decline

Age

- 60 plus with later onset disability
- 40 plus with early onset disability
- Age since onset of functional limitation changes the risk for mortality; alter health promotion activities in response

Age of Menopause

- Postmenopausal musculosketal changes
- Time since ovulation
- Oophorectomy early in life

Oral Health

- Yearly oral evaluations by dentist
- Goal: no ongoing periodontal disease
- Risk factor: loss of teeth
- Risk factor: fewer than nine teeth left

Physical Activity

- Planned physical activity at least 3 d/wk
- The ability to maintain support in this goal diminishes during exacerbations

Cognitive Decline

- Mild cognitive impairment with age
- Dementia onset
- Might look into interventions to address

Long-Term Use of Accommodations

- Manual wheelchair use is a risk factor
- History of painful injuries in arms and shoulders
- Lack of mobility
- Never dismiss musculoskeletal complaints
- May need to address pain management routine as age and wear/tear continues

Musculoskeletal Health

- Notable decline in strength
- May need to change accommodations to something less risky for injury or decline

Mental Health

- History of depression
- History of posttraumatic stress disorder
- History of multiple mood disorders

Sensory Ability

- Notable loss of vision with accommodation
- Notable loss of hearing with accommodation
- Refer for evaluations and provide well-written notes

Risk factors for a decline in health among women with disabilities have been identified in published literature. There is, however, an exception for women with disabilities and women without disabilities who report current pregnancy; they tend to have better health risk profiles, such as less tobacco use and fewer mental health issues (Iezzoni, Yu, Wint, Smeltzer, & Ecker, 2015). The tool presented here is intended to begin a conversation about women living with disability and how we can assist them with risk factors specific to them. Nine risk factors defined at this time are: age,

menopausal status, muscular fitness, oral health, physical activity, long-term use of accommodations, menopause, cognitive decline, and mental health. These are discussed in the following sections of this chapter.

Age

Age is the springboard for the risk assessment of health outcomes in all women, including women with disabilities. As women at any age may have disabilities and this discussion is focused on women with an already notable disability, age is an important consideration due to both age-related and aging-dependent changes in the body that occur over time.

Some authors define "aging" using a series of notable demarcations of damage in cells, organs, tissues, and so on (Huang et al., 2015). Others view aging as growth in personality, wit, and wisdom. Within this model of risk factors, age will be described as a complex process of variable rates of change in numerous domains of life, each leading to positive and/or negative consequences for the function and performance of the woman. This definition allows for multiple interpretations of the impact of age on the health of women with a disability.

First, within any developmental age group, an APN should attend to both the psychosocial risk factors for the loss of social roles and the biological risk factors for physical loss. Allowing these possible developmental roles to guide the conversation, an ANP can assess whether a woman is able to meet the role expectations she finds important to her at that age or during that time period, which serves as an approach to assessing levels of disability. Because a woman's roles shift over time, her perspective on her ability to meet valued role expectations should be reassessed periodically.

Age may also potentiate the effect of gender, placing older women at higher risk than younger women for illnesses or impairments, such as cancer. For instance, in the case of cancer, there are six common hallmarks of aging along with the disease: genomic instability, epigenetic alteration, aberrant telomeres, reprogrammed metabolism, impaired degradation, and impaired immune-inflammatory response (Huang et al., 2015). Without going into each of these processes, suffice it to say that aging women are at higher risk for aging-related diseases such as those cancers unique to women. These include breast, vaginal, and cervical cancers. Women with disabilities bear the same risk. Maintaining an attitude of awareness of risk for women with disabilities is essential in primary disability health care.

Women with early onset disabilities have reported being told by physicians that their life expectancy would be shorter than those without disabilities, and that they should plan their lives accordingly (McBryde Johnson, 2005). This experience is commonly reported by women with early onset disabilities, who on average live shorter periods of time, such as those with spinal muscle atrophy or spinal cord injuries. The need for them to plan for the changes occurring with aging were not part of their life plan, due to the fact that they did not anticipate a long life span. Nonetheless, many women who experience disability early in life do age into their later years. Consequently, a part of the APN primary care visit is assessment of women's readiness for retirement, shift in accommodations, and the loss of family members, providers, and attendants over time.

In an important review article by Karvonen-Gutierrez (2015), the author reported that midlife women may be at the most high-risk period of their lives. This is the time when women accumulate mobility disability at a higher rate than in previous years and that rate of mobility disability affects their ability to perform necessary and socially important roles. Another critical thing to mention about midlife is that this is the time when we lose many women who are aging with early onset disability. Hence, it is important for the practitioner to look at those women who are middle aged as being at a critical period for intervention; this refers to women who are both aging into and aging with a disability.

Awareness that life may be shortened or at heightened risk given the differences in the women's bodies at a common social and developmental period, midlife, is not without merit. Women with early onset disabilities may not have the same life span as someone without a disability. Women without disabilities may be at higher risk during periods of high developmental role performance. Campbell et al. (1999) express concern that those with early onset conditions may have accelerated aging. This is because they may have been exposed to excessive (a) environmental barriers (e.g., slick floors and no elevators), (b) pathological conditions (e.g., tuberculosis), (c) medical-exposure risk (e.g., excessive x-rays), (d) general wear and tear of the body (e.g., straining with pain to carry heavy objects), and (e) high levels of endogenous stressors for a long period of time due to the aforementioned, all of which contribute to shortening their life expectancy. These excessive exposures may wear all women down with heightened effects at midlife.

Age of Menopause

As women complete the transition to menopause, previous function may worsen due to problems such as arthritic pain and swelling (Szoeke, Cicuttini, Guthrie, & Dennerstein, 2005), skin fragility, diminished strength, decreased pulmonary function, and incontinence (Kapoor, Thakar, & Sultan, 2005). After menopause, women may have a decrease in overall muscle mass and an increase in adipose tissue. For women with long-standing FLs, such as those with spinal cord injuries, an increase in adipose tissue with decreasing muscle can alter the ability to remain agile and to transfer without assistance. Loss of muscle mass may decrease women's activity level, contributing to weight gain and diminishing socialization. It may also place them at risk for injury as transfers, with or without assistance, become more difficult. The period after menopause is a good time to reassess women's use of appropriate accommodations for their ambulatory and other needs.

The actual experience of menopause is similar for women with and without disabilities (Vanderakke & Glass, 2001). There is, however, concern that treatments for problems experienced during or around that period might cause women with disabilities to forgo needed care. For instance, McColl (2002) points out that access to hysterectomy or bladder repair surgeries might be a challenge, depending on the nature of the woman's disabling physical condition, her financial resources, and her access to support after a surgery.

Oral Health

Oral health reflects a complex attitude toward teeth, appearance, oral hygiene, dental practices, and availability, as well as socioeconomic access to dental care. First, periodontal disease has been associated with coronary disease, diabetes, stroke, and rheumatoid arthritis (Hoyuela, Furtado, Chiari, & Natour, 2015). Studies linking worsening of multiple sclerosis and dental pathology have been mixed (Dulamea, Boscaiu, & Sava, 2015). The risk for the spread of infection from the mouth to other areas in the body is a concern, especially during operative procedures. Lampley, Huang, Arnold, and Parvizi (2014) indicated that periodontal disease has been considered a possible link to infection in people who have artificial joint replacement, culminating in lengthy operative and convalescent periods. The need for dental clearance preoperatively is often a matter of provider preference and is currently being debated (Lampley et al., 2014).

Periodontal disease can be painful, disabling, and life threatening, thus increasing risk for poor health among women living with disability. Finally, Holm-Pedersen, Schultz-Larsen, Christiansen, and Avulund (2008) found that disability was significantly associated with tooth loss. These researchers set out to follow 573 nondisabled people for 20 years, which dwindled down to a total of 78 people by the end. They found that having one to nine teeth (e.g., edentulous) was associated with disability onset at age 75 and 80 years. They also found that being edentulous at 70 years was predictive of a higher risk for mortality than for women who were not edentulous. Ensuring that women take care of their teeth as part of their health promotion is essential, and it may provide lasting health protection.

Physical Activity

Physical activity is an important dimension in the lives of women with disabilities. It affects how women view their potential for action and their views regarding their body. Rolfe, Yoshida, Renwick, and Bailey (2009) conducted a qualitative study on exercise in women with disabilities. They reported that "women described how exercise improves their psychosocial health and well-being, fosters a sense of independence and accomplishment, and increases their awareness of their body's abilities and limitations" (p. 748). It is clear from this group's opinion that exercise has the potential to improve perceptions of self.

Cognitive Decline

There are studies that demonstrate a relationship between FLs and cognitive ability. As suggested by Gothe et al. (2014), despite the reports that cognitive and physical function tend to decline together with age, there are new reports that cognitive decline may be a precursor to functional decline. The positive aspect of this work is the focus on strategies to improve cognitive function, which might possibly stave off functional decline as well. Monitoring for cognitive decline and its root cause may help with understanding a woman's risk for problems and her ability to adapt. Women with disabilities have routinely reported that their ability to maintain activity in their communities has been dependent on their ability to solve problems, to identify threats to their current functional routine, and to think of new ways to overcome structural, emotional, and interpersonal barriers (Harrison et al., 2010; Harrison et al., 2013).

Long-Term Use of Accommodations

As women use accommodations in their daily mobility routine, injury, strain, and/or chronic pain often happen (Nawoczenski, Riek, Greco, Staiti, & Ludewig, 2012). This is especially true of women who use a manual wheelchair for mobility: the regular push and pull of the wheel can lead to painful strain. The most commonly reported problem among those using manual wheelchairs is shoulder impingement syndrome, which might be further differentiated as either subacromial or internal impingement (Nawoczenski et al., 2012). Furthermore, transfers from seat to seat with arms instead of the lower body can lead to wear and tear on the upper arm joints and soft tissues. This is often seen in women with spinal cord injury for various reasons, which include (a) vascular occlusion, progressive resorption of the clavicle at the end region, (b) clavicle malalignment during movement of the wheelchair, (c) a bent posture while sitting in the wheelchair, and (d) finally, altered muscle growth, due to variations in muscle development related to how the muscles are used (Giner-Pascual et al., 2011). Giner-Pascual et al. (2011) reported that if men and women used a wheelchair seat positioned parallel to the ground, as compared with a seat tilted at an angle, they were at an increased risk for structural injury in their shoulders and subsequent pain.

The use of accommodations, such as canes and wheelchairs, can have a positive effect on the body. For instance, in a study of older adults with hemiparesis, one-sided paralysis, adults were significantly faster with a stronger gait if they used a cane for sit-to-stand transfers than if they did not (Hu et al., 2013). The person with hemiparesis was able to extend his or her paralyzed knee more and balance the load in movement. It is suggested that the strategy of using a cane during sit-to-stand transfer from seat to wheelchair and afterward during movement can help prevent falls as well. This is because the cane keeps the body from swaying, for example, it keeps the load balanced. It is important that the provider balance his or her understanding of negative outcomes with accommodations with that of good outcomes, and make the most appropriate person-centered recommendations he or she can over time.

Musculoskeletal Health

Changes in the musculoskeletal system can evolve into disease pathology, such as osteoarthritis or osteoporosis. These aging-related disease shifts are most notable in the movement from osteopenia to osteoporosis (Freemont & Hoyland, 2007). The age-related changes we all face include: (a) losses in bone tissues with subsequent weakness; (b) lack of cushioning effects of water between the joints, which results in osteoarthritis; (c) loss of elasticity in the ligaments that stretch and return to prior shape; (d) losses of muscle mass and power, often partly due to denervation; (e) redistribution of fat; (f) stiffening of collagen and elastin; as well as (g) change in humoral factors that mediate growth, development, and life span (Freemont & Hoyland, 2007).

For women with disabilities, the loss of strength can make a difference in their being independent. For instance, losses of muscle strength may prevent a woman from transferring from her wheelchair to her car seat. Further, sarcopenia with loss in muscle strength tends to be more common in postmenopausal women (Anagnostis, Dimopoulou, Karras, Lambrinoudaki, & Goulis, 2015). This is consistent with a study by Andrews et al. (2014), who wrote that muscle strength was strongly associated with physical disability in women with lupus, even after adjustment for covariates. The recommendation that vitamin D may be helpful in the prevention of sarcopenia in this population might be worthy of consideration by women with disabilities (Anagnostis et al., 2015).

Women with a disability enter into postmenopausal, musculoskeletal changes with varying degrees of muscle strength due to earlier onset FLs. There is a need to prepare the woman and her family for changes in her ability that come with age, as well as the changes that occur in people who are aging alongside her. The type of accommodation that worked at age 35 years to lift a woman from her wheelchair to her bed might not work at age 60 years. A thorough musculoskeletal assessment at baseline and a periodical assessment over time are warranted. A change of equipment might be needed through occupational or physical therapy. This is important given the evidence that overall happiness among people with polio-related disability was significantly related to their assistive technology (Spiliotopoulou, Fowkes, & Atwal, 2012).

Mental Health

In a study of predictive factors of increasing functional decline among 1,187 men and women (63% women) age 60 years or older with multiple disabling conditions, investigators found that among older women mental health was the main outcome predictor of activities of daily living (Laan et al., 2013). For men, the predictors were transient ischemic attacks and myocardial infarction. Women tended to respond physically to their mental state. In a study of early aging among people with posttraumatic stress disorder (PTSD), Lohr et al. (2015) reported that 7 of 10 studies reported higher mortality for those with PTSD. They also found higher proinflammatory markers in those with PTSD. Although this finding was not specific to women, the relationship of mental health to physical disability in aging women is noteworthy. Therefore, assessment for mental health issues such as depression and PTSD is important as a basis for mental health treatment when warranted.

Sensory Ability

In the aforementioned study by Laan et al. (2013), vision was also an independent predictor of decline among older women. The risk for losses when the woman with a disability loses her hearing or vision can result in institutionalization if accommodations are not planned for and made.

Health Promotion

There are studies that address our clinical need for an overall healthy lifestyle guide/program for women with disabilities. For instance, Stuifbergen, Becker, Blozis, Timmerman, and Kulberg (2003) tested in a randomized control trial the wellness intervention they created for women with multiple sclerosis. They integrated an educational and skill-building lifestyle change program, along with a supportive telephone follow-up. The lifestyle change program consisted of eight sessions over an 8-week period; it guided participants in self-assessment of behaviors, resources, and barriers and supported specific strategies aimed at building self-efficacy for health behaviors. This program has also been tested in low-income cancer survivors (Meraviglia, Stuifbergen, Morgan, & Parsons, 2015). It might supplement the care that is provided in the clinical setting to ensure that the provider and the woman with the disability are working together in the best direction. Looking at the trajectory of disability (Harrison & Stuifbergen, 2005), engaging a midlife group of women in health promotion activities might be an excellent way to prepare them for the future. However, starting earlier with women who have early onset disabilities, for example, young adulthood, might be best for this group. In this way, the possibility of midlife mortality might be diminished.

◼ SUMMARY

This chapter began with consideration of definitions that facilitate understanding of the problems faced by women who are aging with/or into disability. Socioeconomic conditions confronting women with disabilities were discussed. The impact the provider has on the outcomes of the woman with the disability cannot be understated. The provider can write a referral that helps to support her work role or prevent her continuation without services.

Finally, the evidential basis for an assessment tool to guide preemptive care for women living with disability was proposed. To support APNs providing primary health care to women with disabilities, an assessment tool incorporating nine risk factors salient for decline among women with physical disabilities was provided. The tool is intended as a guide for assessment, not as a predictive measure, and is designed to support APNs as they venture beyond the disease-central focus they have been prepared to address and assist women with managing aging, disability, and any relevant barriers set before them. Despite knowing that few providers currently have

the requisite knowledge of disability-related health care (Iezzoni, 2006), APNs are being called upon to provide disability-related health care focusing on health promotion in the context of FL for the prevention of exacerbations and comorbidities. In addition, APNs can provide access to the appropriate consultations and services and provide for the elimination of social and cultural barriers to health over the life course (Menter et al., 1991). Again, it is expected that women with disabilities have issues related to bowel movements and pain care on an ongoing basis. The need to treat the pain reported with a supportive, essentially stable approach to their pain management regime must go without saying.

◼ REFERENCES

Adams, H., Thibault, P., Davidson, N., Simmonds, M., Velly, A., & Sullivan, M. J. (2008). Depression augments activity-related pain in women but not in men with chronic musculoskeletal conditions. *Pain Research & Management, 13*(3), 236–242.

Anagnostis, P., Dimopoulou, C., Karras, S., Lambrinoudaki, I., & Goulis, D. (2015). Sarcopenia in post-menopausal women: Is there any role for vitamin D? *Maturitas, 82*(1), 56–64.

Andrews, J. S., Trupin, L., Schmajuk, G., Barton, J., Margaretten, M., Yazdany, J.,…Katz, P. P. (2014). Muscle strength, muscle mass, and physical disability in women with systemic lupus erythematosus. *Arthritis Care & Research, 67*(1), 120–127.

Bauer, M. E., Wieck, A., Petersen, L. E., & Baptista, T. A. A. (2015). Neuroendocrine and viral correlates of premature immunosenescence. *Annals of the New York Academy of Sciences, 1351*, 11–21.

Beardwood, B. A., Kirsh, B., & Clark, N. J. (2005). Victims twice over: Perceptions and experiences of injured workers. *Qualitative Health Research, 15*(1), 30–48.

Bureau of Labor Statistics (BLS). (2011). *Women at work*. Retrieved from http://www.bls.gov/spotlight/2011/women

Bureau of Labor Statistics (BLS). (2012). *Union members summary*. Retrieved from http://www.bls.gov/news.release/union2.nr0.htm

Bureau of Labor Statistics (BLS). (2015). Persons with a disability: Labor force characteristics—2014. Retrieved from http://www.bls.gov/news.release/pdf/disabl.pdf

Campbell, M. L., Sheets, D., & Strong, P. (1999). Secondary health conditions among middle-aged individuals with chronic physical disabilities: Implications for unmet needs for services. *Assistive Technology Journal, 11*, 205–213.

Cheadle, A., Franklin, G., & Wolfhagen, C. (1994). Factors influencing the duration of work related disability: A population-based study of Washington State Workers' Compensation. *American Journal of Public Health, 84*, 190–196.

Couch, K., Reznik, G., Tamorini, C., & Iams, H. M. (2013). Economic and health implications of long-term unemployment: Earnings, disability benefits, and mortality. *Research in Labor Economics, 100*(1), 572–589.

Dulamea, A. O., Boscaiu, V., & Sava, M. M. (2015). Disability status and dental pathology in multiple sclerosis patients. *Multiple Sclerosis and Related Disorders, 4*(6), 567–571.

Family Caregiver Alliance. (2016). Selected caregiver statistics. Retrieved from https://www.caregiver.org/women-and-caregiving-facts-and-figures

Freemont, A. J., & Hoyland, J. A. (2007). Morphology, mechanism, and pathology of musculoskeletal ageing. *Journal of Pathology, 211*(2), 252–259.

Giner-Pascual, M., Alcanyis-Alberola, M., Gonalez, M., Rodriquez, M., & Querol, F. (2011). Shoulder pain in cases of spinal injury: Influence of the position of the wheelchair seat. *International Journal of Rehabilitation Research, 34*(4), 282–289.

Gothe, N. P., Fanning, J., Awick, E., Chung, D., Wojcicki, T. R., Olson, E. A.,…McAuley, E. (2014). Executive function processes predict mobility outcomes in older adults. *Journal of the American Geriatrics Society, 62*, 285–290.

Guthrie, R., & Jansz, J. (2006). Women's experience in the workers' compensation system. *Journal of Occupational Rehabilitation, 16*, 485–499.

Harrison, T. (2006). A qualitative analysis of the meaning of aging for women with disabilities with implications for health policy. *Advances in Nursing Science, 29*(2), E1–E18.

Harrison, T., LeGarde, B., Kim, S. H., Blozis, S., Walker, J., & Umberson, D. (2013). Women's experience with workplace injury. *Policy, Politics & Nursing Practice, 14*(1), 16–25.

Harrison, T., & Stuifbergen, A. (2005). A hermeneutic phenomenological analysis of aging with a childhood onset disability. *Health Care for Women International, 26*, 731–747.

Harrison, T., Umberson, D., Lin, L. C., & Cheng, H. R. (2010). Timing of impairment and health-promoting lifestyles in women with disabilities. *Qualitative Health Research, 20*, 816–829.

Harrold, L. R., Savageau, J. A., Pransky, G., & Benjamin, K. (2008). Understanding the role of sex differences in work injuries: Implications for primary care practice. *Disability and Rehabilitation, 30*(1), 36–43.

Hirschman, N. J. (2012). Disability as a new frontier for feminist intersectionality research, *Politics & Gender, 8*(3), 396–405.

Hirschman, N. J. (2013). Freedom and (dis) ability in early modern political thought. In A. P. Hobgood and D. H. Wood (Eds.), *Recovering disability in early modern England* (pp. 167–186). Columbus, OH: Ohio State University Press.

Holm-Pedersen, P., Schultz-Larsen, K., Christiansen, N., & Avulund, K. (2008). Tooth loss and subsequent disability and mortality in old age. *Journal of the American Geriatrics Society, 56*, 429–435.

Hoyuela, C. P. S., Furtado, R. N. V., Chiari, A., & Natour, J. (2015). Orofacial evaluation of women with rheumatoid arthritis. *Journal of Oral Rehabilitation, 42*, 370–377.

Hu, P. T., Lin, K. H., Lu, T.-W., Tang, P.-F., Hu, M.-H., & Lai, J. S. (2013). Effect of a cane on sit-to-stand transfer in subjects with hemiparesis. *American Journal of Physical Medicine & Rehabilitation, 92*(3), 191–202.

Huang, J., Xie, Y., Sun, X., Zeh, H. G., Kang, R., Lotze, M., & Tang, D. (2015). DAMPs ageing and cancer: The "DAMP Hypothesis." *Ageing Research Reviews, 24*, 3–16.

Iezzoni, L. I. (2006). Going beyond disease to address disability. *New England Journal of Medicine, 355*, 976–979.

Iezzoni, L. I., Yu, J., Wint, A. J., Smeltzer, S. C., & Ecker, J. L. (2015). Health risk factors and mental health among U.S. women with and without chronic physical disabilities by whether women are currently pregnant. *Maternal Child Health Journal, 19*, 1364–1375.

Kapoor, D. S., Thakar, R., & Sultan, A. H. (2005). Combined urinary and faecal incontinence. *International Urogynecology Journal, 16*, 321–328.

Karvonen-Gutierrez, C. A. (2015). The importance of disability as a health issue for mid-life women. *Women's Midlife Health, 1*(10). doi: 10.1186/s40695-015-0011-x

Kaye, H. S. (2010). The impact of the 2007–09 recession on workers with disabilities. *Monthly Labor Review, 133*(10), 1–15.

Kirsh, B., & McKee, P. (2003). The needs and experiences of injured workers: a participatory research study. *Work, 21*(3), 221–231.

Laan, W., Bleijenberg, N., Drubbel, I., Numans, M. E., de Wit, N. J., & Schuurmans, M. J. (2013). Factors associated with increasing functional decline in multi-morbid independently living older people. *Maturitas, 75*, 276–281.

Lampley, A., Huang, R. C., Arnold, W., & Parvizi, J. (2014). Total joint arthroplasty: Should patients have preoperative dental clearance? *Journal of Arthroplasty, 29*, 1087–1090.

Lohr, J. B., Palmer, B. W., Eidt, C. A., Aailaboyina, S., Mausbach, B. T., Wolkowitz, O. M.,...Jeste, D. V. (2015). Is post-traumatic stress disorder associated with premature senescence? A review of the literature. *American Journal of Geriatric Psychiatry, 23*(7), 709–725.

McBryde Johnson, H. (2005). *Too late to die young.* New York, NY: Henry Holt and Company.

McColl, M. A. (2002). A house of cards: Women, aging and spinal cord injury. *Spinal Cord, 40*, 371–373.

McDonough, C. M, Jette, A. M., Pengsheng, M., Bogusz, K., Marfeo, E. E., Brandt, D. E.,...Rasch, E. (2013). Development of a self-report physical function instrument for disability assessment: Item pool construction and factor analysis. *Archives of Physical Medicine and Rehabilitation, 94*(9), 1653–1660.

Mellor, K. M., Curl, C. L., Chandramouli, C., Pedrazzini, T., Wendt, I., & Delbridge, L. (2014). Ageing-related cardiomyocyte functional decline is sex and angiotensin II dependent. *Age, 36*, 1155–1167.

Menter, R. R., Whiteneck, G. G., Charlifue, S. W., Gerhart, K., Solnick, S., Brooks, C., & Huges, L. (1991). Impairment, disability, handicap, and medical expenses of persons aging with spinal cord injury. *Paraplegia, 29*, 613–619.

Meraviglia, M., Stuifbergen, A., Morgan, S., & Parsons, D. (2015). Low-income cancer survivors use of health-promoting behaviors. *MedSurg Nursing, 24*(2), 101–106.

Meseguer, J. (2013). Outcome variation in the Social Security disability administration: The role of primary diagnoses. *Social Security Bulletin, 73*(2), 39–75.

Munnell, A. H., & Rutledge, M. (2013). The effects of the Great Recession on the retirement security of older workers. *Annals of the American Academy of Political and Social Science, 650*(1), 124–142.

Munnell, A., & Sass, S. (2008). *Working longer: The solution to the retirement income challenge.* Washington, DC: Brookings Institution Press.

National Alliance for Caregiving (NAC). (2015). *Caregiving in the USA 2015.* Retrieved from http://www.caregiving.org/wp-content/uploads/2015/05/2015_CaregivingintheUS_Executive-Summary-June-4_WEB.pdf

Nawoczenski, D. A., Riek, L. M., Greco, L., Staiti, K., & Ludewig, P. M. (2012). Effects of shoulder pain on shoulder kinematics during weight-bearing tasks in persons with spinal cord injury. *Archives of Physical Medicine and Rehabilitation, 93*(8), 1421–1430.

O'Leary, P., Boden, L. I., Seabury, S. A., Ozonoff, A., & Scherer, E. (2012). Workplace injuries and the take-up of Social Security disability benefits. *Social Security Bulletin, 72*(3), 1–18.

Oleinick, A., Gluck, J. V., & Cuire, K. (1996). Concordance between ANSI occupational back injury codes and claim form diagnoses and a lower bound estimate of the fraction associated with disc displacement/herniation. *American Journal of Industrial Medicine, 30*, 556–568.

Orrenius, P. M., & Zavodny, M. (2009). Do immigrants work in riskier jobs? *Demography, 46*(3), 535–551. doi:10.1353/dem.0.0064

Pentland, W., Tremblay, M., Spring, K., & Rosenthal, C. (1999). Women with physical disabilities: Occupational impacts of ageing. *Journal of Occupational Science, 6*(3), 111–123.

Reno, V., Williams, C. T., & Sengupta, I. (2003/2004). Workers' compensation, Social Security disability insurance, and the offset: A fact sheet. *Social Security Bulletin, 65*(4), 3–6.

Ritchie, K., & Kildea, D. (1995). Is senile dementia "age-related"?— Evidence from meta-analysis of dementia prevalence in the oldest old. *Lancet, 346*(8980), 931.

Rolfe, D. E., Yoshida, K., Renwick, R., & Bailey, C. (2009). Negotiating participation: How women living with disabilities address barriers to exercise. *Health Care for Women International, 30*, 743–766.

Sager, L., & James, C. (2005). Injured workers' perspectives of their rehabilitation process under the New South Wales Workers Compensation System. *Australian Occupational Therapy Journal, 52*(2), 127–135.

Saleh, A., Fuortes, L., Vaughn, T., & Bauer, E. P. (2001). Epidemiology of occupational injuries and illnesses in a university population: A focus on age and gender differences, 39. *American Journal of Industrial Medicine, 39*(6), 581–586.

Spiliotopoulou, G., Fowkes, C., & Atwal, A. (2012). Assistive technology and prediction of happiness in people with post-polio syndrome. *Disability & Rehabilitation: Assistive Technology, 7*(3), 199–204.

Steenstra, I. A., Verbeek, J. H., Heymans, M. W., & Bongers, P. M. (2005). Occupational and environmental medicine. *British Medical Journal, 62*(12), 851–860.

Stover, B., Wickizer, T., Zimmerman, F., Fulton-Kehoe, D., & Franklin, G. (2007). Prognostic factors of long-term disability in a workers' compensation system. *Journal of Occupational and Environmental Medicine, 49*, 31–40.

Stuifbergen, A., Becker, H., Blozis, S., Timmerman, G., & Kulberg, V. (2003). A randomized clinical trial of a wellness intervention for women with multiple sclerosis. *Archives of Physical Medicine & Rehabilitation, 84*, 467–476.

Stuifbergen, A., Becker, H., Perez, F., Morison, J., Kulberg, V., & Todd, A. (2012). A randomized controlled trial of a cognitive rehabilitation intervention for persons with multiple sclerosis. *Clinical Rehabilitation, 26*(10), 882–893.

Szoeke, C. E. I., Cicuttini, F. M., Guthrie, J. R., & Dennerstein, L. (2005). Factors affecting the prevalence of osteoarthritis in healthy middle-aged women: Data from the longitudinal Melbourne women's midlife health project. *Bone, 39,* 1149–1155.

Tait, R. C., & Chibnall, J. T. (2005). Factor structure of the pain disability index in workers' compensation claimants with low back injuries. *Archives of Physical Medicine and Rehabilitation, 86*(6), 1141–1146.

Timmerman, G. M., Calfa, N. A., & Stuifbergen, A. (2013). Correlates of body mass index in women with fibromyalgia. *Orthopaedic Nursing, 32,* 113–119.

Treaster, R., & Burr, D. (2004). Gender differences in prevalence of upper extremity musculoskeletal disorders. *Ergonomics, 47*(5), 495–526.

Turner, M. R., Barnwell, J., Al-Chalabi, A., & Eisen, A. (2012). Young-onset amyotrophic lateral sclerosis: Historical and other observations. *Brain, 135,* 2883–2891.

U.S. Census (2010). *Disability.* Retrieved from https://www.census.gov/people/disability/publications/disab10/table_2.pdf

Vanderakke, C. V., & Glass, D. D. (2001). Menopause and aging with disability. *Physical Medicine & Rehabilitation Clinics of North America, 12,* 133–151.

Verbrugge, L. M., & Jette, A. M. (1994). The disablement process. *Social Science & Medicine, 38,* 1–14.

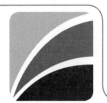

Index